A LETTER FROM THE AUTHORS

Dear Nursing Student,

Welcome to your pediatric nursing course and to the challenge of becoming a successful nurse! You know the importance of your classroom education and clinical experience, but you may not realize the importance of the educational materials that you use in preparation for your career. We believe that this textbook and its many resources will help you become successful in reaching your goals. In fact, that's why we wrote this book and why we've revised it with the feedback from professors, students, and practicing pediatric nurses in mind.

Success for your classroom, clinical, and NCLEX-RN® experiences are ensured through the features that we have included in this book. They will help you to focus your studying on the most important information. Read your text before you attend class to get the maximum from your instructor's lecture and direction. Study and apply the concepts you've learned by engaging in the activities and features on the Prentice Hall Nursing MediaLink DVD-ROM and Companion Website. Practice for the NCLEX-RN® exam by taking advantage of the review questions found on both resources. Finally, give yourself the added benefit of getting enough sleep, exercise, and good nutrition so you will enjoy good health and consequently perform better in all your educational experiences.

We wish you success in your course and in all your future endeavors!

Sincerely,

Jane W. Ball and Ruth C. Bindler

FOCUS FOR SUCCESS...*on the NCLEX-RN® REXAM*

Feature	Description	Benefit
Your Prentice Hall Nursing MediaLink DVD-ROM contains...		
Approximately 300 NCLEX-RN®-style questions	Each question contains rationales and identifies the step of the nursing process, client care level, and a test-taking strategy.	Practicing with these questions will improve your chances of passing the NCLEX-RN® exam.
The Companion Website (www.prenhall.com/ball) contains...		
Approximately 300 additional NCLEX-RN®-style questions	These questions are in addition to those on the DVD-ROM and contain the same components.	Practicing with these questions will improve your chances of passing the NCLEX-RN® exam.

Also available:

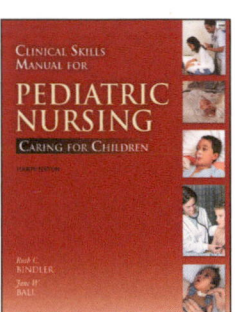

Clinical Skills Manual for Pediatric Nursing, Fourth Edition by Ruth Bindler and Jane Ball (ISBN 0-13-613554-4)

Provides procedures with step-by-step instructions, rationales, and photographs to help you perform pediatric skills successfully.

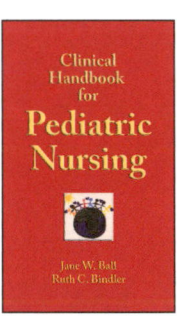

Clinical Handbook for Pediatric Nursing by Jane Ball and Ruth Bindler (ISBN 0-13-113316-0)

Critical information for quick reference in the clinical setting.

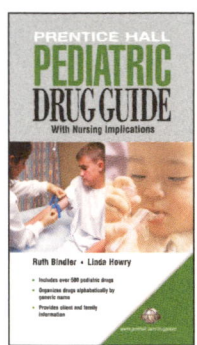

Prentice Hall Pediatric Drug Guide by Bindler, Howry, Wilson, Shannon and Stang (ISBN 0-13-119615-4)

Provides easy access to information and nursing care related to medications administered to children of all ages.

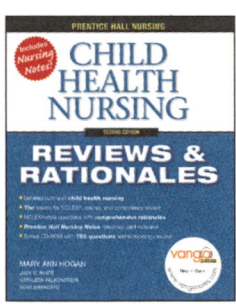

Child Health Nursing: Reviews & Rationales by Mary Ann Hogan (ISBN 0-13-243711-2)

Provides both course and NCLEX-RN® review featuring 750 practice questions, NCLEX® Alerts, and more.

Student Assessment .... Real Nursing Skills .... Customized Study Plans ...
The path to student success and nursing excellence!

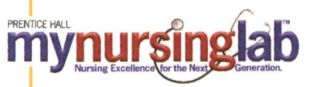

MyNursingLab is a user-friendly site that gives students the opportunity to test themselves on key concepts and skills. By using *MyNursingLab*, students can track their own progress through the course and use customized, media-rich study plan activities to help them achieve success in the classroom, in clinical, and ultimately on the NCLEX-RN®. *MyNursingLab* can also help you, the instructor, to monitor class progress as students move through the curriculum.

To take a tour and see the power of **mynursinglab** go to **www.prenhall.com/nursing**.

Feature	Description	Benefit	Page
Your textbook contains...			
Nursing Management	These sections highlight the nursing process in relation to the chapter topic.	Learning the application of the nursing process will improve your client care in your clinical experiences.	**684**
Collaborative Care	Parts of the chapter discuss other healthcare providers with whom you will partner.	Understanding all aspects of your clients' care will allow you to provide informed nursing care.	**684**
Nursing Care Plan	These charts use NIC and NOC criteria to provide the goal, intervention, rationale, and outcome for specific conditions.	These familiarize you with developing plans of care and to think about the reason for actions and intended results.	**703**
Evidence-Based Practice	Boxes with recent nursing research present implications for nursing action.	These boxes challenge you to consider evidence and incorporate it into your nursing practice.	**693**
Complementary Therapy	These boxes tell you about therapies that may be connected with cultural groups, beliefs, or practices.	You will increase your awareness of practices or beliefs that may influence health care.	**688**
Clinical Tip	These are tips about practical actions related to the topic.	Your transition from classroom to clinical will be smoother by using these helpful practices.	**683**
Nursing Alert	These boxes contain warnings about the topic.	Knowing the hazards will help you be better prepared for clinical success.	**683**
Families Want to Know	These offer information about specific topics that families need to know when caring for their child.	You can use these as guides for educating patients and families.	**690**
Medications Used to Treat	Drug information contains indication or action, side effects, and implications for nursing care.	Knowing the implications for nursing care equips you for your clinical experience.	**697**
Culture	These offer diverse perspectives and cultural variations and indicate their impact on health care.	Understanding cultural differences will help you know what to ask your patients and their families.	**722**
Clinical Manifestations	These features present the etiology, clinical presentation, and clinical therapy for selected conditions.	You will recognize these signs when seen in clinical and know what action to take.	**687**
Community Care	Boxes contain information about how a condition can impact a child's life in the community.	You will be better equipped to teach families what to expect and what action to take on behalf of their children.	**730**
Your Prentice Hall MediaLink DVD-ROM contains...			
Videos	Videos show procedures, skills, and information you need to know.	These videos present information you will need to know for clinical. For instance, the Developmental Milestones video presents children of various ages to help you prepare for assessments.	
The Companion Website (www.prenhall.com/ball) contains...			
Case Studies, Care Plans, Critical Thinking Exercises	These chapter-related exercises challenge you to apply the material you have read.	Completing these exercises helps you rehearse appropriate nursing care responses to real-life scenarios.	

Instructor's Resource Manual	• Concepts for Lecture • Learning Outcomes with PowerPoint lecture slides that support them • Suggestions for Classroom Activities • Suggestions for Clinical Activities • Resource Library—including Media Gallery and Image Gallery • Testbank with more than 450 NCLEX-RN®-style test questions from the Instructor's Resource DVD-ROM • List of videos and animations from Prentice Hall Nursing MediaLink DVD-ROM
Instructor's Resource DVD-ROM	• Comprehensive PowerPoint lecture slides for every chapter, fully customizable • Classroom Response System questions set in PowerPoint slides (ask your Prentice Hall representative for more information about hardware to enhance your presentation) • First Day of Class presentation to show students how to use this textbook • Complete Image Gallery in PowerPoint • TestGen Test Item File with questions in all NCLEX-RN® formats, including questions mapped to the chapter learning outcomes and the clinical competencies • Link to the Prentice Hall Instructor's Resource Center for additional resources *Ask your Prentice Hall Representative if you require a CD-ROM version of this resource.*
Online Course Management	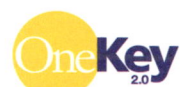 Prentice Hall OneKey is an open-access, integrated online course management system for schools using BlackBoard and WebCT platforms that provides the following: **For Students** NCLEX-RN®-style Review Questions Case Studies Care Plan Activities WebLinks E-mail Communication **For Instructors** Test Item Files PowerPoint Presentations Media Gallery Resources Discussion Board Class Announcements **For a preview go to:** http://cms.prenhall.com/blackboard/index.html 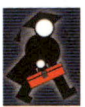 http://cms.prenhall.com/webct/index.html *Ask your Prentice Hall Representative for more information and packaging options for including* **MyNursingLab** *and* **Prentice Hall OneKey** *in your curriculum.*

Jane W.
BALL

Ruth C.
BINDLER

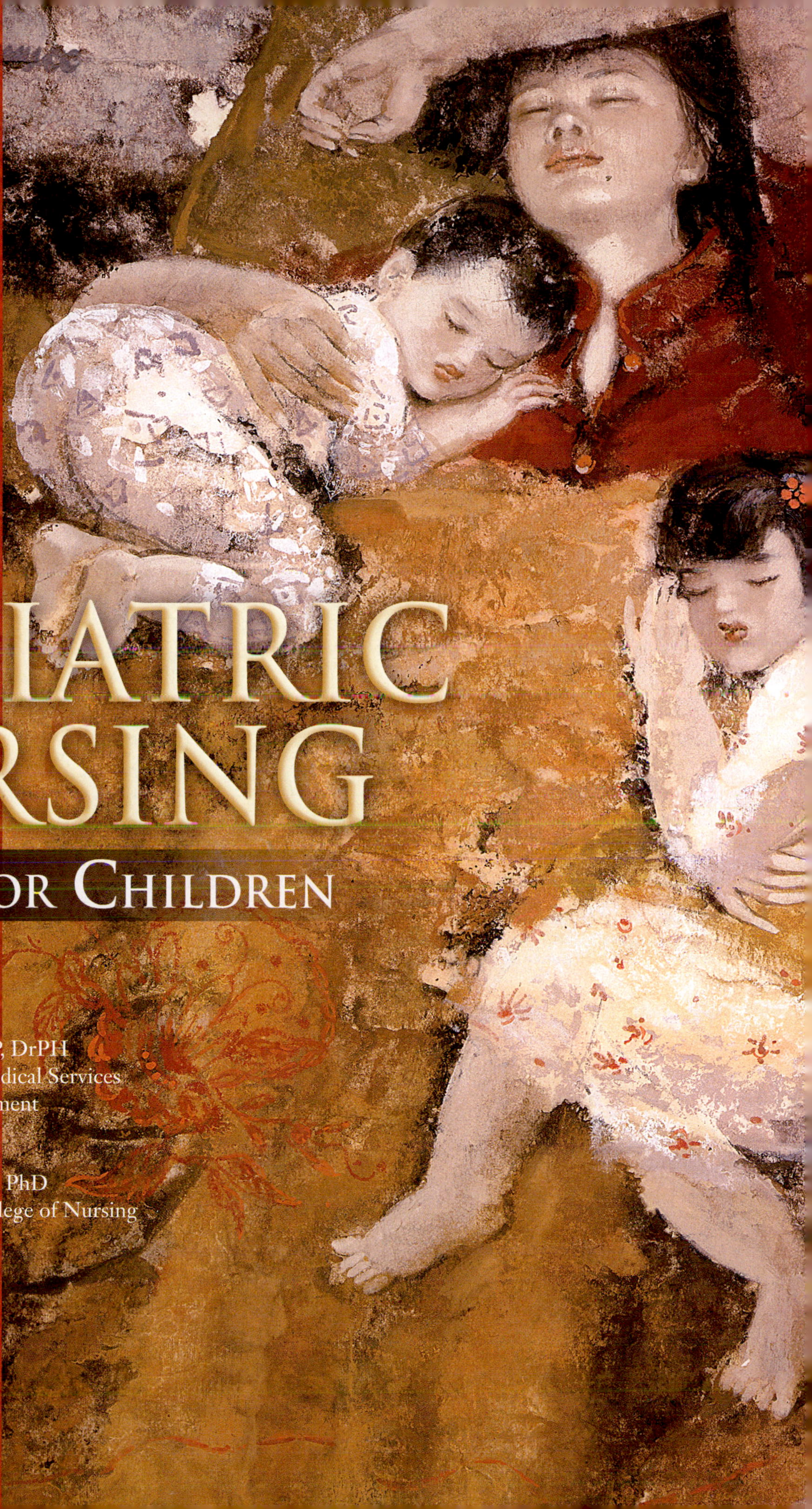

PEDIATRIC NURSING

CARING FOR CHILDREN

FOURTH EDITION

Jane W. Ball, RN, CPNP, DrPH
Consultant in Emergency Medical Services
and Trauma System Development
Gaithersburg, Maryland

Ruth C. Bindler, RNC, PhD
Professor, Intercollegiate College of Nursing
Washington State University
Spokane, Washington

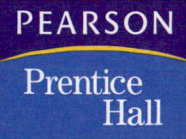
PEARSON

Prentice
Hall

Library of Congress Cataloging-in-Publication Data

Pediatric nursing: caring for children/ [edited by] Jane W. Ball, Ruth C. Bindler. —
4th ed.
    p. ; cm.
    Includes bibliographical references and index.
    ISBN 0-13-220871-7
    I. Ball, Jane. II. Binder, Ruth McGillis.
    [DNLM: 1. Pediatric Nursing—methods. 2. Child. 3. Infant. 4. Nursing
Assessment—methods. WY 159 P3733 2008]
    RJ245. P4414 2008
    618. 92'00231—dc22

2006035667

Publisher: Julie Levin Alexander
Assistant to Publisher: Regina Bruno
Editor-in-Chief: Maura Connor
Executive Acquisitions Editor: Pamela Lappies
Associate Editor: Michael Giacobbe
Development Editor: Kim Wyatt
Managing Editor, Development: Marilyn Meserve
Editorial Art Manager: Patrick Watson
Media Product Manager: John J. Jordan
Director of Marketing: Karen Allman
Senior Marketing Manager: Francisco del Castillo
Marketing Coordinator: Michael Sirinides
Managing Editor, Production: Patrick Walsh
Production Editor: Amy Gehl, Carlisle Editorial Services
Production Liaison: Anne Garcia
Media Project Manager: Stephen Hartner
Manufacturing Manager: Ilene Sanford
Manufacturing Buyer: Pat Brown
Senior Design Coordinator: Maria Guglielmo
Printer/Binder: RR Donnelley, Willard
Composition: Carlisle Publishing Services
Interior Design: Christine Cantera
Cover Design: Christine Cantera
Cover Illustration: "Dreaming" by Yihang Pan. Used by permission of Chinese Art Net.
Cover Printer: Phoenix Color
Director, Image Resource Center: Melinda Patelli
Manager, Rights and Permissions: Zina Arabia
Manager, Visual Research: Beth Brenzel
Manager, Cover Visual Research and Permissions: Karen Sanatar
Image Permission Coordinator: Kathy Gavilanes

DEDICATION

To our mentors—those who matched
our passion for child health care.

Notice: Care has been taken to confirm the accuracy of information presented in this book. The authors, editors, and the publisher, however, cannot accept any responsibility for errors or omissions or for consequences from application of the information in this book and make no warranty, express or implied, with respect to its contents.

The authors and publisher have exerted every effort to ensure that drug selections and dosages set forth in this text are in accord with current recommendations and practice at time of publication. However, in view of ongoing research, changes in government regulations, and the constant flow of information relating to drug therapy and drug reactions, the reader is urged to check the package inserts of all drugs for any change in indications of dosage and for added warnings and precautions. This is particularly important when the recommended agent is a new and/or infrequently employed drug.

Pearson Education Ltd.
Pearson Education Singapore, Pte. Ltd.
Pearson Education Canada, Ltd.
Pearson Education—Japan
Pearson Education Australia PTY, Limited

Pearson Education North Asia Ltd.
Pearson Educación de Mexico, S.A. de C.V.
Pearson Education Malaysia, Pte. Ltd.
Pearson Education, Upper Saddle River, New Jersey

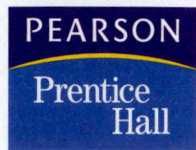

10 9 8 7 6 5 4 3 2 1
ISBN-13: 978-0-13-220871-0
ISBN-10: 0-13-220871-7

BRIEF TABLE OF CONTENTS

JANE W. BALL graduated from the Johns Hopkins Hospital School of Nursing, and subsequently received a BS from the Johns Hopkins University. She worked in the surgical, emergency, and outpatient units of the Johns Hopkins Children's Medical and Surgical Center, first as a staff nurse and then as a pediatric nurse practitioner. Thus began her career as a pediatric nurse and advocate for children's health needs. Jane obtained both a master of public health and doctor of public health degree from the Johns Hopkins University Bloomberg School of Public Health with a focus on maternal and child health. After graduation she became the chief of child health services for the Commonwealth of Pennsylvania Department of Health. In this capacity she oversaw the state-funded well-child clinics and explored ways to improve education for the state's community health nurses. After relocating to Texas, she joined the faculty at the University of Texas at Arlington School of Nursing to teach community pediatrics to registered nurses returning to school for a BSN. During this time she became involved in writing her first textbook, *Mosby's Guide to Physical Examination*, which is currently in its sixth edition. After relocating to the Washington, DC, area, she joined Children's National Medical Center to manage a federal project to teach instructors of emergency medical technicians from all states about the special care children need during an emergency. Exposure to the shortcomings of the emergency medical services system in the late 1980s with regard to pediatric care was a career-changing event. With federal funding, she developed educational curricula for emergency medical technicians and emergency nurses to help them provide improved care for children. A textbook entitled *Pediatric Emergencies, A Manual for Prehospital Providers* was developed from these educational ventures. For 15 years she has managed the federally funded Emergency Medical Services for Children's National Resource Center. As executive director, Dr. Ball directed the provision of consultation and resource development for state health agencies, health professionals, families, and advocates about successful methods to improve the healthcare system so that children get optimal emergency care in all healthcare settings. She recently left this position to devote more time to writing and to become a consultant on emergency medical services and state trauma system development.

RUTH C. MCGILLIS BINDLER received her BSN from Cornell University—New York Hospital School of Nursing in New York. She worked in oncology nursing at Memorial-Sloan Kettering Cancer Center in New York, and then moved to Wisconsin and became a public health nurse in Dane County, Wisconsin. Thus began her commitment to work with children as she visited children and their families at home, and served as a school nurse for several elementary, middle, and high schools. Due to this interest in child healthcare needs, she earned her MS in child development from the University of Wisconsin. A move to Washington State was accompanied by a new job as a faculty member at the Intercollegiate Center for Nursing Education in Spokane, Washington. Dr. Bindler has been fortunate to be involved for over 30 years in the growth of this nursing education consortium, which is a combination of public and private universities and colleges and is now the Washington State University/Intercollegiate College of Nursing. She has taught theory and clinical courses in child health nursing, cultural diversity and health, graduate research, pharmacology, and assessment, as well as serving as lead faculty for child health nursing. She is presently interim associate dean for the college's graduate programs. Her first professional book, *Pediatric Medications*, was published in 1981, and she has continued to publish articles and books in the areas of pediatric medications and pediatric health. Research efforts are focused in the area of childhood obesity, type 2 diabetes, metabolic syndrome, and cardiovascular risk factors in children. Ethnic diversity has been another theme in her work. She facilitates international and other diversity experiences for students and performs research with culturally diverse children. Dr. Bindler believes that her role as a faculty member has enabled her to learn continually, to foster the development of students in nursing, and to participate fully in the profession of nursing. In addition to teaching, research, publication, and leadership, she enhances her life by service in several professional and community activities, and by activities with her family.

We are grateful to all the nurses, both clinicians and educators, who reviewed the manuscript of this text. Their insights, suggestions, and eye for detail helped us prepare a more relevant, useful, and current book, reflective of the present time and of the essential components of learning in the field of child health nursing.

Patricia T. Alpert, University of Nevada

Joan Becker, El Centro Community College

Laura Bowers, Columbus Children's Hospital

Sharen Brady, Weber State University

Nancy Brauhn, Mount Mercy College

Gwendolyn Brown, Hampton University

Jane Brown, Walters State Community College

Linda Burkett, Children's Hospital Los Angeles Center for Endocrinology, Diabetes and Metabolism

Eva Caldwell, Armstrong Atlantic State University

Susan Caulkins, Central Carolina Technical College

Ellen Christian, University of Massachusetts–Dartmouth College of Nursing

Joyce Clay, Richland Community College

Donna Eberly, Western Iowa Tech Community College

Alison Fisher, Del Mar College

Rachel Francols, Mount Mercy College

Laura Hammond, Seattle Central Community College

Erin Hart, Massachusetts General Hospital for Children

Laurie Hartjes, University of Wisconsin–Madison

Debra Hearington, Virginia Commonwealth University

Leslie Hoover, Lansing Community College

Susan Hudson, Kishwaukee College

Dawn Hughes, Mount Carmel College of Nursing

Linda R. Hunter, Florida Community College at Jacksonville

Karrie S. Ingalsbe, Mennonite College of Nursing at Illinois State University

Nancy Jackson, New York University

Amy Johnson, University of Delaware, School of Nursing

Sharon Donohue Kappel, Louisiana State University Health Sciences Center School of Nursing

Sheila Kenning, Skagit Valley College

Kathryn Kushto-Reese, The Johns Hopkins University School of Nursing

Anita Kyle, Texas Women's College of Nursing

Joanne M. McBroome, Texarkana College

Denise Ogletree McGuinn, McGuinn & Associates

Mikki Meadows-Oliver, Yale University School of Nursing

Marcl Mechtel, Johns Hopkins University

Sara H. Mitchell, Georgia Baptist College of Nursing of Mercer University

Alison Moriarty Daley, Yale University School of Nursing

Louise Niemer, Northern Kentucky University

Casey Norris, East Tennessee Children's Hospital

Gen M. Owens, Children's Medical Center–Dallas

Pamela Penney, Renton Technical College

Dawn M. Pope, University of Wisconsin–Oshkosh

Marisue Rayno, Luzeme County Community College

Katherine Roberts, Lamar University, Department of Nursing

Sarah Roland, Central Carolina Technical College

Eileen Rosen, Jackson Health System

Marty Rucker, Walters State Community College

Margaret P. Rudd-Arleta, University of Massachusetts–Dartmouth

Cynthia Schmus, Children's Hospital of Philadelphia

Judy Scott, Community College of Southern Nevada

Lisa South, University of Alabama School of Nursing at University of Alabama at Birmingham

Joanna Spahis, Children's Medical Center of Dallas

Dr. Diana Tattoni, Children's Regional Medical Center in Seattle, Renton Technical College

Theresa Turick-Gibson, Hartwick College

Diane Van Os, Westminster College

Jo Wade, University of Tennessee–Knoxville

Jane K. Walker, Walters State Community College

Terri L. Walker, Oklahoma City Community College

Donna Wilsker, Lamar University

Ronda M. Wood, Long Beach City College

Kelly K. Zinn, Clarkson College

PREFACE

Pediatric nursing, like all of health care, is constantly changing. Student nurses must learn what helps them to provide safe, effective, and excellent care today, while integrating new knowledge and skills needed for nursing practice in the next generation. Faculty have the responsibility of teaching students to provide pediatric nursing care today, while equipping them to meet tomorrow's unknown healthcare challenges.

Preparation for Nursing Excellence

The goal of the fourth edition of this textbook is to provide core pediatric nursing knowledge that prepares students for excellence in nursing, and to offer the tools of critical thinking needed to apply this learning to future challenges. Students must learn to question, to evaluate the research and experiences of others, to apply information in many settings, and to constantly adapt to changes while providing high-quality nursing care.

This textbook reflects a multitude of approaches to learning that can be helpful to all students. We acknowledge that many students learn pediatric nursing in a very short time period. Therefore, the approaches in this textbook are designed to help all students assess the child's needs and to make care decisions based on the standards of pediatric nursing practice.

Realities of Pediatric Nursing

The first edition of this textbook focused on the nursing care of children and their families in acute care environments. In the subsequent editions, the focus was broadened to reflect the increasing delivery of pediatric health care in community settings, such as home, school, and health centers. Many procedures are performed in short-stay units, and long-term care is often provided at home for children with complex health conditions. Families are often the providers of care and case managers for children with complex healthcare conditions. Technological advances are resulting in earlier diagnoses and new therapies; this content is integrated throughout the textbook

Pediatric nursing care is provided within the context of a rapidly changing society. An examination of the major morbidities and mortalities of childhood guided the addition of new material and topics throughout the text. Chapters have been added on the family, care in chronic conditions, and health promotion across the life span. Current challenges for children have guided the further development of chapters on childhood nutrition, and on societal and environmental influences on child health.

Many graduating nurses practice in acute care facilities, and this textbook continues to emphasize the information necessary to prepare students for working in hospitals. In addition, the information provided in this textbook will enable graduates to assume positions in ambulatory care facilities, home health nursing, schools, and a variety of other settings. Effective communication methods, principles of working with families, and knowledge of pathophysiologic, psychologic, and environmental factors found in this book can all be applied to a wide variety of settings.

Another major change in our society involves access to information and reliance on the Internet. Nurses must learn to obtain information and then analyze and judge the quality of information they find. In this edition, MediaLink icons send the student online to obtain the latest information available on many topics. Nurses must also assist children and family members to use the Internet wisely to help them in making healthcare decisions.

Organization and Integrated Themes

We have organized *Pediatric Nursing: Caring for Children*, Fourth Edition, first to present important information—on growth and development, family-centered care, physical assessment, nutrition, health promotion, health issues in today's world, and children's responses to illness and injury—needed to care for all children in different healthcare settings. Following the introductory chapters, this book is organized by body systems to facilitate the student's ability to locate information, focus studying, and prepare for clinical experiences with children and families. The organizational framework also eliminates redundancy, so that the student uses time efficiently.

In addition to the significant revisions made to all chapters to update clinical information and resources, we added six new chapters to reflect the emphasis on health promotion and family-centered care:

Chapter 2: Family-Centered Care: Theory and Application

Chapter 7: Introduction to Health Promotion and Health Maintenance

Chapter 8: Health Promotion and Health Maintenance for the Newborn and Infant

Chapter 9: Health Promotion and Health Maintenance for the Young and School-Age Child

Chapter 10: Health Promotion and Health Maintenance for the Adolescent

Chapter 12: Nursing Considerations for the Child with a Chronic Condition

The recently developed **Bindler-Ball Child Healthcare Model** illustrates the important core value: that all children need health promotion and health maintenance interventions, no matter where they seek health care or what health conditions they may be experiencing.

The nursing process is used as the framework for nursing care. **Nursing Management** is the major heading, with subheadings of **Nursing Assessment and Diagnosis, Planning and Implementation,** and **Evaluation**. When it is appropriate to focus on care in a specific setting, Hospital-Based Care, Discharge Planning, and Community Care are separated into sections. We feature nursing care plans throughout the text to help students approach care from the nursing process perspective. **Nursing Care Plans** include nursing intervention classifications (NIC) and nursing outcome classifications (NOC).

Several major concepts are integrated throughout the textbook to encourage the student to think creatively and critically about nursing care. These major themes are interwoven throughout the text through the features and supplements.

■ **Nursing care** is the critical and central core of this textbook. Nursing assessment and management are emphasized in all sections of the book, with nurses shown providing care in a variety of settings.

■ **Critical thinking and problem-solving principles** are integrated in the organization, pedagogy, writing style, evidence-based practice features, research boxes, DVD-ROM exercises, and art captions. Students practice critical thinking in their everyday lives, but need help to apply these concepts to the practice of nursing. This book and the accompanying learning materials help students understand how their normal curiosity and problem-solving ability can be applied to pediatric nursing.

■ **Communication** is one of the most important skills that students need to learn. Effective communication with children is challenging because they communicate differently according to their developmental levels. Family members have communication needs in addition to those of their children. This book integrates communication skills by applied examples that help the student to communicate effectively with children and their families.

■ **Teaching** about health care is an integral part of the pediatric nurse's responsibilities. Since hospitalizations are short and families increasingly care for children at home, information about healthcare needs and procedures have become even more important.

■ **Developing cultural competence** is critical for all nurses in the increasingly diverse community of today's world. Students have all met people from different ethnic and cultural groups but they need help to understand, respect, and integrate differing beliefs, practices, and healthcare needs when providing care.

■ **Growth and development considerations** and **physical assessment** are central to the effective practice of pediatric nursing. A separate chapter is devoted to each area, Chapters 3 and Chapter 5, respectively. In addition, both topics are integrated where appropriate in narrative, figures, captions, and on the Prentice Hall Nursing MediaLink DVD-ROM.

■ **Community care** is an increasing part of nursing responsibilities. To assist students in transferring knowledge to caring for children in community settings, both narrative and boxes address this information in nursing management sections of chapters. In addition, an entire chapter is devoted to nursing care in the community and directly addresses the nurse's roles in these settings.

In addition to being interwoven in the narrative and reflected in the art that accompanies it, these themes and others are highlighted in the many chapter features in the text and in the supplements that students can use to augment their learning.

HOW TO USE THIS TEXTBOOK

➤ This textbook will help you focus your attention on the information you need to know for success in your class, in clinical, and on the NCLEX-RN® exam. The many boxes, tables, and charts highlight the important material to learn, and the drawings and photographs offer visual descriptions to help you understand key concepts. To assist you to take full advantage of all it has to offer, read through the information that follows and refer to the boxes and sections described as you study.

The **case study** at the start of each chapter focuses on a child with a specific nursing care need that relates to the chapter topic. The scenario provides you with a context for the information that follows.

Also at the start of each chapter is a list of **Learning Outcomes** to point out what you should learn after reading and studying the information in the chapter.

A list of the words that are essential to understanding the material appears under the **Key Terms** heading. Following each term in boldface is the page number on which you can find the word defined in the text.

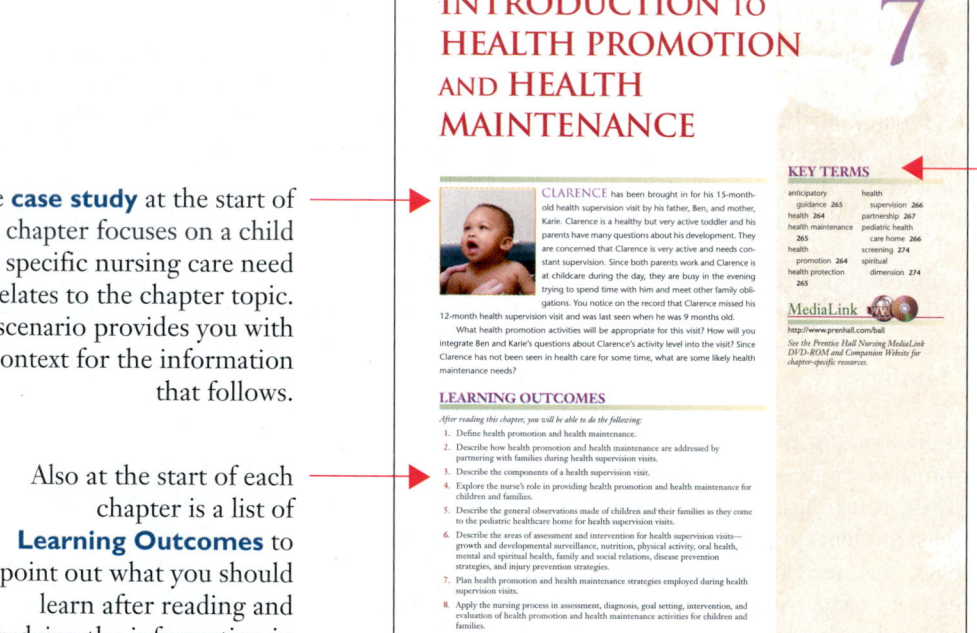

Pathophysiology Illustrated boxes contain illustrations that visually explain the pathophysiology of certain conditions to increase your understanding of the condition and its treatment.

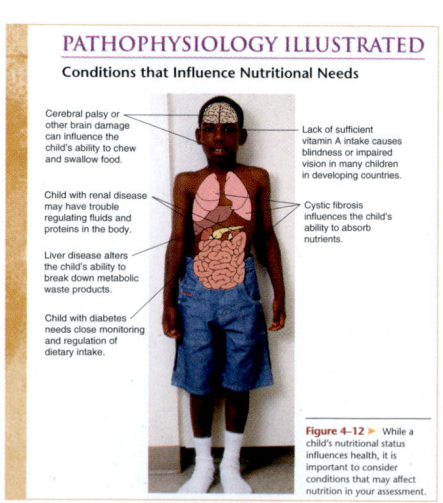

Figure 4–12 ▶ While a child's nutritional status influences health, it is important to consider conditions that may affect nutrition in your assessment.

FOCUS ON

The **Focus on** . . . section appears at the start of each body system chapter. It gives you key information to review and an easy reference to use as you read the chapter.

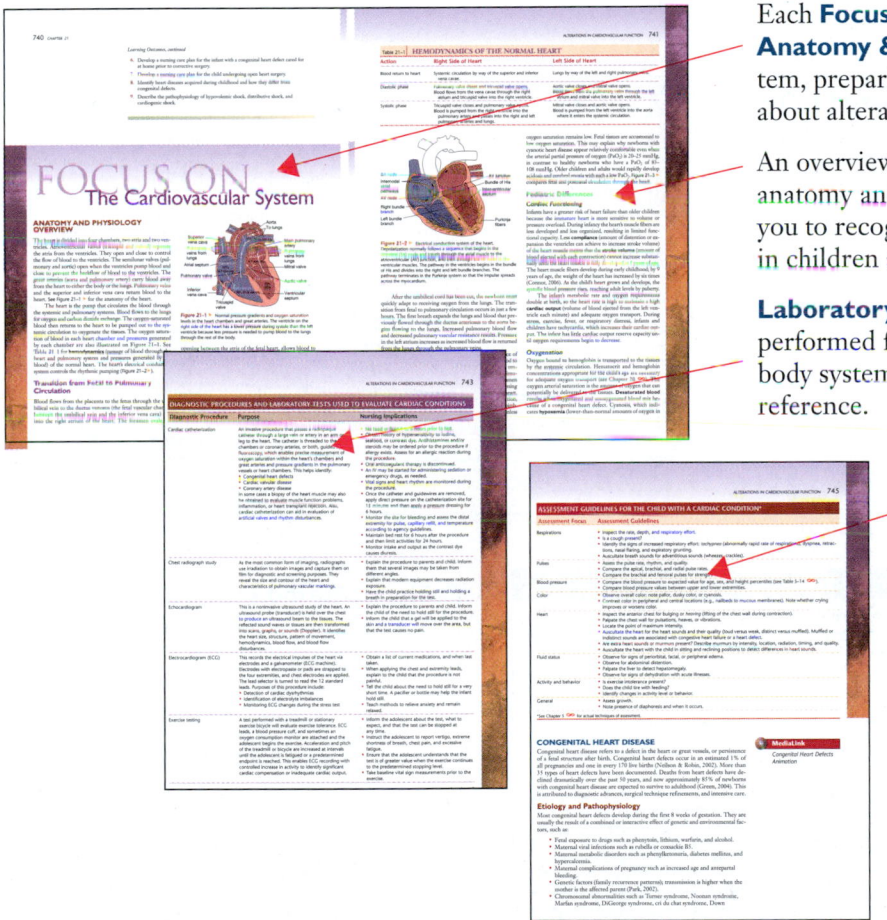

Each **Focus on** . . . section starts with a quick **Anatomy & Physiology Review** of the body system, preparing you for the material in the chapter about alterations to that system in children.

An overview of **Pediatric Differences** in the anatomy and physiology of the body system helps you to recognize physical and mental differences in children at various ages.

Laboratory and Diagnostic Tests commonly performed for health conditions related to the body system are described in chart format for easy reference.

The **Guidelines for Assessment** chart includes tips or instructions for performing a focused assessment for health conditions related to the body system.

AS CHILDREN GROW

Sinus Development

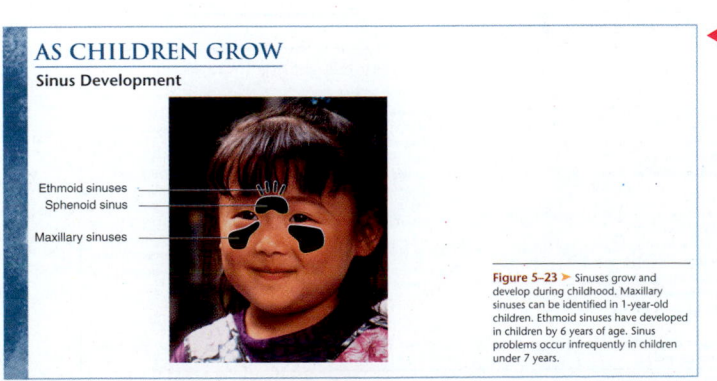

Ethmoid sinuses
Sphenoid sinus
Maxillary sinuses

Figure 5–23 ▶ Sinuses grow and develop during childhood. Maxillary sinuses can be identified in 1-year-old children. Ethmoid sinuses have developed in children by 6 years of age. Sinus problems occur infrequently in children under 7 years.

As Children Grow boxes illustrate the anatomic and physiologic differences between children and adults. This visual feature will help you to consider developmental differences when working with children of different age groups.

Clinical Manifestations charts present the etiology, clinical presentation, and often the clinical therapy for selected conditions to help you recognize these signs in clinical settings.

CLINICAL MANIFESTATIONS OF DIETARY DEFICIENCIES/EXCESSES

Nutrient	Deficiency Manifestation	Excess Manifestation
Vitamin A	Night blindness Skin dryness and scaling	Headache Drowsiness Hepatomegaly
Vitamin C	Abnormal hair (coiled shape) Skin abnormalities (dermatitis and lesions) Purpura Bleeding gums Joint tenderness Sudden heart failure	Usually none—excess is excreted in urine
Vitamin D	Rib abnormalities Bowed legs	Drowsiness
B vitamins	Weakness Decreased deep tendon reflexes Dermatitis	Usually none—excess is excreted in urine
Protein	Hepatomegaly Edema Scant, depigmented hair	Kidney failure
Carbohydrate	Emaciation Decreased energy Retarded growth and development	Overweight

Medications Used to Treat boxes prepare you for administering medications for specific conditions during your clinical experience.

MEDICATIONS USED TO TREAT
Symptomatic Laryngotracheobronchitis

Medication	Action/Indication	Nursing Implications
Beta-agonists and beta-adrenergics (e.g., albuterol, racemic epinephrine): aerosolized through face mask	Rapid-acting bronchodilator, decreases bronchial and tracheal secretions and mucosal edema, used to decrease symptoms of moderate to severe respiratory distress; and constriction of subglottic mucosa and submucosal capillaries. Used until dexamethasone begins working.	Provides only temporary relief; improvement in 30 minutes that lasts about 2 hours, it gives time for the steroid to work; the child may experience tachycardia (160–200 beats/min) and hypertension; dizziness, headache, and nausea; may necessitate stopping medication; reduces the need for artificial airway.
Corticosteroids (e.g., dexamethasone): IM, PO, nebulized budesonide	Anti-inflammatory, used to decrease edema; has a long half-life of 36–54 hours.	The child may experience cardiovascular symptoms (hypertension): requires close observation for individual response; children less frequently need emergency airways; stridor resolves faster.

Evidence-Based Practice boxes present recent nursing research, discuss implications, and challenge you to incorporate this information into your nursing practice through activities.

EVIDENCE-BASED PRACTICE

Reducing Injuries in Childcare Centers

Clinical Question

What are the most common injuries that occur in childcare settings and how do the types of injuries vary by the age of the child?

Evidence

Injury data was collected for a full year from incident reports about the types of injuries occurring to children in two urban childcare centers. A total of 131 children between 6 weeks and 7 years of age (mean age of 24 months) were enrolled full- or part-time in the centers. During the year, a total of 897 incident reports identified 1023 injuries. The distribution of injuries was as follows: bites (39%), falls (23%), bumps and bruises (22%), and scratches, cuts, blisters, and fracture (16%). Only 2 children required medical attention, while the remainder received first aid on site. Infants and toddlers (0 to 36 months of age) had the highest frequency of injury, reflecting in large part the high frequency of biting reported in this age group. Approximately 60% of all injuries occurred in the morning hours (Waibel & Misra, 2003).

Implications

Understanding the type of injuries that happen in childcare centers, the age group most affected, and other information, such as time of day, provides the nurse with important information to help the childcare center to promote the health of enrolled children and make efforts to reduce injuries. Injury prevention strategies can potentially be developed based upon collected data. The number of minor injuries in childcare centers also illustrates the importance of having childcare center staff trained in first aid. It is also important to have guidelines for management of injuries and notification of parents when injuries happen.

Critical Thinking

Consider the distribution of injuries and identify potential strategies that could be used to reduce the number of biting and falling incidents. What actions could the childcare center workers take to reduce the number of incidents that occur during morning hours? Outline the first aid guidelines that a childcare center should have in place to manage each of the most common injuries reported. What guidelines should exist for notifying parents about injuries that occur?

Families Want to Know boxes offer specific information for you to use in educating the families of the children in your care.

FAMILIES WANT TO KNOW

Using the Internet to Evaluate Complementary and Alternative Therapies

There are millions of web sites promoting complementary and alternative therapies that are often dangerously misleading. Provide families with guidelines for evaluating complementary and alternative therapies and other medical information on the Internet. Encourage families to use the following questions when looking for health information online to help evaluate the information found.

- Who runs this site?
- Who pays for the site? The source of funding can affect what content is presented and how.
- What is the purpose of the site? The purpose should be clearly stated to help you evaluate how much to trust the information.
- Where does the information come from? The original source of the information should be clearly stated if the organization in charge of the site did not create the information.

- How is the information selected? Determine if evidence is provided about the information rather than just opinions and advice.
- How current is the information? Look for the latest update of information.
- How does the site choose links to other sites? Determine if any criteria are used for decisions about who can link to the site.
- What information about you does the site collect, and why? Does the site ask you to subscribe or become a member? If so, personal information will be collected. Review any privacy policy or similar language before signing up for the site.
- How does the site manage interactions with visitors? Is there a chat room or other online discussion? Review the discussion carefully before joining in.

Data from: NCCAM (2002a). 10 things to know about evaluating medical resources on the Web. NCCAM Publication No. D142. Retrieved March 17, 2006, from www.nccam.nih.gov/health/webresources/.

ADDITIONAL TOOLS FOR CLINICAL SUCCESS

➤ The boxes that appear in the margins of this textbook equip you with practical knowledge that will benefit you in your clinical experience and throughout your nursing career.

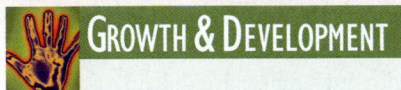

Growth and Development boxes highlight nursing care for various stages of development.

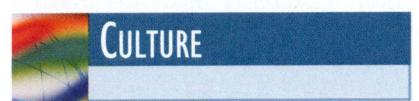

Culture boxes heighten your awareness of diverse perspectives and cultural variations and alert you to their impact on the health care of children.

COMPLEMENTARY THERAPY

Complementary Therapy boxes point out common alternative and complementary therapy practices, alert you to when you might encounter them, and explain how health care can be influenced by them.

Community Care boxes prepare you for the issues that nurses often face outside of the hospital environment.

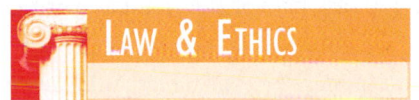

Law and Ethics boxes highlight the many issues challenging nurses today to help you be ready for your clinical experiences.

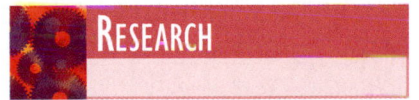

Research boxes provide quick summaries of recent nursing research, followed by an application question to hone your critical thinking skills.

Other Tools to Help You Use This Book Successfully:

- **Highlighted critical-thinking questions** draw attention to questions that ask you to think about the scenarios, images, or material you have just seen.

- **Nursing Care Plans** include NIC and NOC criteria and help you apply nursing care to specific conditions.

- **Cross-reference links** ∞ call your attention to page references for related material in other chapters.

- **MediaLink margin icons** **MediaLink** point out supplemental animations, videos, or media activities from your DVD-ROM or the Companion Website.

- **Skills Manual links** reference the appropriate skills in the Clinical Skills Manual for Pediatric Nursing.

- **Critical Thinking in Action** boxes at the end of each chapter provide a continuation of the opening scenario and challenge you to apply what you have learned. Answers to the questions are on the DVD-ROM.

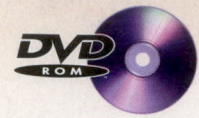

The Prentice Hall Nursing MediaLink DVD-ROM accompanying your textbook has many tools to help you study, including NCLEX-RN®-style questions, videos and animation, health promotion boxes, case studies, nursing tools, and a comprehensive audio glossary of key terms.

The **Clinical Skills Manual for Pediatric Nursing,** Fourth Edition, is a full-color, highly visual book that gives step-by-step instructions with color photographs on how to perform each skill. The material focuses on techniques specific to pediatric patients.

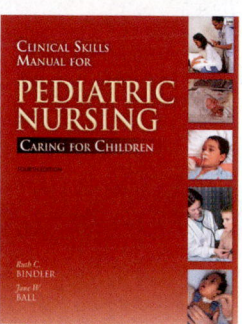

CLINICAL SKILLS MANUAL FOR
PEDIATRIC NURSING
CARING FOR CHILDREN

Ruth C.
BINDLER

Jane W.
BALL

The **Companion Website** at www.prenhall.com/ball is a text-specific, interactive online workbook that includes learning outcomes, chapter outlines, audio glossary of key terms, Thinking Critically exercises with essay responses, case studies, and additional NCLEX-RN®-style review questions with rationales. MediaLink Applications are research exercises linked to web sites. Also provided are links to web sites with related content.

RESOURCES FOR FACULTY SUCCESS

The **Instructor's Resource Manual** provides chapter-specific concepts for lectures, including PowerPoint Lecture Slides linked to learning outcomes. A complete testbank of approximately 450 NCLEX-RN®-style questions with rationales comprises the last half of the manual, with questions linked to learning outcomes for each chapter.

The **Instructor's Resource DVD-ROM** includes a test generator with testbank, customizable PowerPoint lecture slides, and a comprehensive collection of images from the textbook. It also provides access to all animations and videos on the Prentice Hall Nursing MediaLink DVD-ROM.

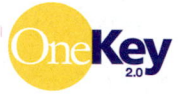

Prentice Hall OneKey Online Course Management is an open-access, integrated online course management system for schools using BlackBoard and WebCT platforms and provides you with the following:

For Students
NCLEX-RN® Review Questions
Case Studies
Care Plan Activities
WebLinks
E-mail Communication

For Instructors
Test Item Files
PowerPoint Presentations
Media Gallery Resources
Discussion Board
Class Announcements

For a Preview, go to:

cms.prenhall.com/webct/index.html

cms.prenhall.com/blackboard/index.html

Student Assessment .... Real Nursing Skills .... Customized Study Plans ... The path to student success and nursing excellence!

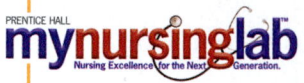

MyNursingLab is a user-friendly site that gives students the opportunity to test themselves on key concepts and skills in pediatric nursing. By using *MyNursingLab*, students can track their own progress through the course and use customized, media-rich, study plan activities to help them achieve success in the classroom, in clinical, and ultimately on the NCLEX-RN®. *MyNursingLab* can also help you, the instructor, to monitor class progress as students move through the curriculum.

To take a tour and see the power of **mynursinglab**, go to www.prenhall.com/nursing.

Ask your Prentice Hall Representative for more information and packaging options for including *MyNursingLab* and *Prentice Hall OneKey* in your curriculum.

ACKNOWLEDGMENTS

It is both exciting and challenging to have the opportunity to write a textbook. It is inspiring to observe the evolution of pediatric nursing practice, and to encourage nursing students to share our excitement and enthusiasm for working with children and their families. Although each edition carries its own unique set of challenges and circumstances, it continues to be a privilege to contribute to the education of the new generation of student nurses.

This edition has undergone significant changes and integrates some new features developed in collaboration with Prentice Hall Health. Our third edition editor, Maura Connor, had a dream and vision of the potential for development of this textbook that matched our own. Our present editor, Pamela Lappies, continues to work closely with us so that our views of pediatric nursing can best be conveyed to students and faculty. The vice president and publisher, Julie Alexander, enthusiastically supported this venture, and has supported us in decisions regarding changes, updates, and features for the text.

Our developmental editor, Kim Wyatt, has worked with us on several publications and is a tireless proponent for the approach, philosophy, and conceptual framework underlying the text. She explained our goals to others, and worked endlessly to enhance and organize the materials we provided. This effort could not have succeeded without her.

Kay J. Cowen contributed two chapters to this textbook, and we value her fresh approach to the information. We'd also like to acknowledge the contributions of Nancy Bowers and Jeanette Zaichken, nurse leaders who have contributed genetics and newborn expertise, respectively. The Prentice Hall Health executive development editor, Marilyn Meserve, was an important liaison for editorial consultation with Prentice Hall Health. We thank Anne Garcia, production editor; Patrick Walsh, production managing editor; and Frank del Castillo, senior marketing manager for their expertise and valuable contributions. Our thanks also go to Maria Guglielmo, design coordinator, for creating the fresh textbook design. Media editor John J. Jordan helped bring our media ideas to fruition, with the help of Stephen Hartner and Dorothy Cook. At Carlisle Publishing Services, we thank Amy Gehl for coordinating production, and Chris Feldman for his copyediting skills. Pat Gillivan of Triple SSS Press helped assemble content for the supplements.

The authors and Prentice Hall Health would also like to thank those who have enhanced the learning and teaching package for this text by contributing to the resources that accompany it. Diane Anderson, Texas Women's University; Stephanie Butkus, Kettering College of Medical Arts; and Wendy Bowles, Kettering College of Medical Arts, contributed to the DVD-ROM. Brent Thompson, West Chester University; and Rebecca Gesler, Spalding University, wrote content for the *Instructor's Resource Manual* and NCLEX-RN® review questions. We appreciate the effort they put into supporting the book to help students use it more effectively. We also appreciate Jack Yensen's work on the Instructor Resource DVD and Patrick Watson's management of the art program.

Finally, our families once again have supported us tirelessly through the revision process. They sacrificed by allowing us to work on the book when we could have been with them. Yet, they show others the book with pride. We could not have accomplished this without their love and patience.

Jane W. Ball
Ruth C. Bindler

SPECIAL FEATURES

MEDICATIONS USED TO TREAT

EVIDENCE-BASED PRACTICE

COMPLEMENTARY THERAPY

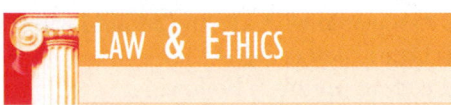

LAW & ETHICS

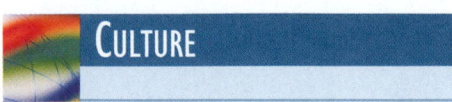

CULTURE

PATHOPHYSIOLOGY ILLUSTRATED

COMMUNITY CARE

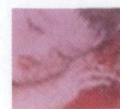

FAMILIES WANT TO KNOW

GROWTH & DEVELOPMENT

NURSING CARE PLAN

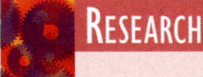

RESEARCH

CONTENTS

NURSE'S ROLE IN CARE OF THE CHILD:
Hospital, Community, and Home

1

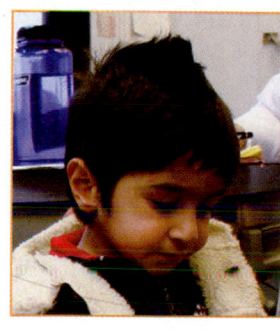

MANNY is a 3-year-old boy who has a seizure disorder that until a week ago was fairly well controlled by medication. He and his family receive their health care from the mobile care van that visits their neighborhood each week. A pediatric nurse and pediatrician collaborate in providing Manny's health care and monitoring his developmental progress.

Manny had a seizure in the last week. His phenytoin blood level, taken the day of the seizure, was slightly lower than the therapeutic range, but his parents report they have given his medication daily as prescribed. He might require a higher dosage of the same medication because he has grown, or maybe he needs a different medication. Because of the recent seizure, an electroencephalogram is ordered to identify any change in the electrical pattern of his brain. Other laboratory tests are also ordered, following the guidelines of the health center's clinical pathway for children with seizure disorders.

Over the past 2 years, Manny's family and the pediatric nurse have worked together to assure that Manny is treated as a healthy child with a chronic condition. The nurse has helped his parents to obtain information about his condition, to understand the action of his medication, and to take appropriate action when he has a seizure.

LEARNING OUTCOMES

After reading this chapter, you will be able to do the following:

1. Describe the continuum of pediatric health care.
2. Describe the roles for nurses in child health care.
3. Identify current societal influences on pediatric health care and nursing practice.
4. List the most common causes of child mortality and reasons for hospitalization by age group.
5. Contrast the policies for obtaining informed consent of minors with policies for adults.
6. Identify three unique pediatric legal and ethical issues in pediatric nursing practice.

KEY TERMS

advance
   directives **19**
advocacy **4**
assent **18**
autonomy **21**
beneficence **21**
case
   management **4**
clinical practice
   guidelines **6**
competence **18**
confidentiality **19**
continuity of
   care **4**
critical thinking **5**
emancipated
   minors **18**
ethics **20**

evidence-based
   practice **6**
family-centered
   care **8**
infant mortality **9**
informed
   consent **17**
justice **21**
mature minors **18**
moral dilemma **20**
morbidity **10**
nonmaleficence **21**
quality
   improvement **15**
risk
   management **15**

MediaLink

http://www.prenhall.com/ball

See the Prentice Hall Nursing MediaLink DVD-ROM and Companion Website for chapter-specific resources.

PEDIATRIC HEALTHCARE OVERVIEW

Nurses provide care to healthy children, as well as to those with illnesses, injuries, and chronic conditions such as seizures, in a wide variety of settings. Watching children grow, achieving milestones in development, and adapting to and managing their health conditions is rewarding to nurses, as they know that they made a contribution to their health and welfare. Fortunately, most children are healthy, experiencing only occasional short-term health problems, and nurses have the opportunity to help children and families to prevent disease and promote a healthy lifestyle. However, children with special healthcare needs require frequent contact with the healthcare system to achieve and maintain their optimal level of health.

Pediatric health care occurs along a continuum that reflects not only the various settings of care, but also the complexity and range of care needed by individual children and their families. For example, all children need health promotion and health maintenance services, but some children will need care for chronic conditions, acute illnesses and injuries, and even end-of-life care. See Figure 1–1 ➤ for the model of pediatric healthcare upon which this text is based.

The range of healthcare settings where pediatric nurses work includes the following:

- Different hospital locations, such as pediatric wards, intensive care units, newborn nursery, emergency department, radiology, and specialty clinics;
- Physician offices, clinics, and healthcare centers;
- The home of the child;
- Rehabilitation centers and residential treatment centers;
- Schools, childcare centers, and camps; and
- The community.

MediaLink

The Role of the Pediatric Nurse Video

Figure 1–1 ➤ The Bindler-Ball Continuum of Pediatric Health Care for Children and Their Families.
The outer bars represent the family, cultural, and community influence on the care that the child receives, either through the services sought by the family or the services provided in the community. Cultural influences include the family's decision to seek health care and follow recommendations, as well as the healthcare provider's cultural competence in caring for a child and family.

The inner categories represent the different types of health care needed by children. All children need health promotion and health maintenance services, represented by the base of the triangle. Notice the wave and arrows representing the upward and downward movement between the levels of care as the child's condition changes.

Children may be healthy with episodic acute illnesses and injuries. Some children develop a chronic condition for which specialized health care is needed. A child's chronic condition may be well controlled, but acute episodes (such as with asthma) or other illnesses and injuries may occur, but the child also needs health promotion and health maintenance services. A few children develop a life-threatening illness and ultimately need end-of-life care. A healthy child can also experience a catastrophic injury that causes death. The family then needs supportive end-of-life care.

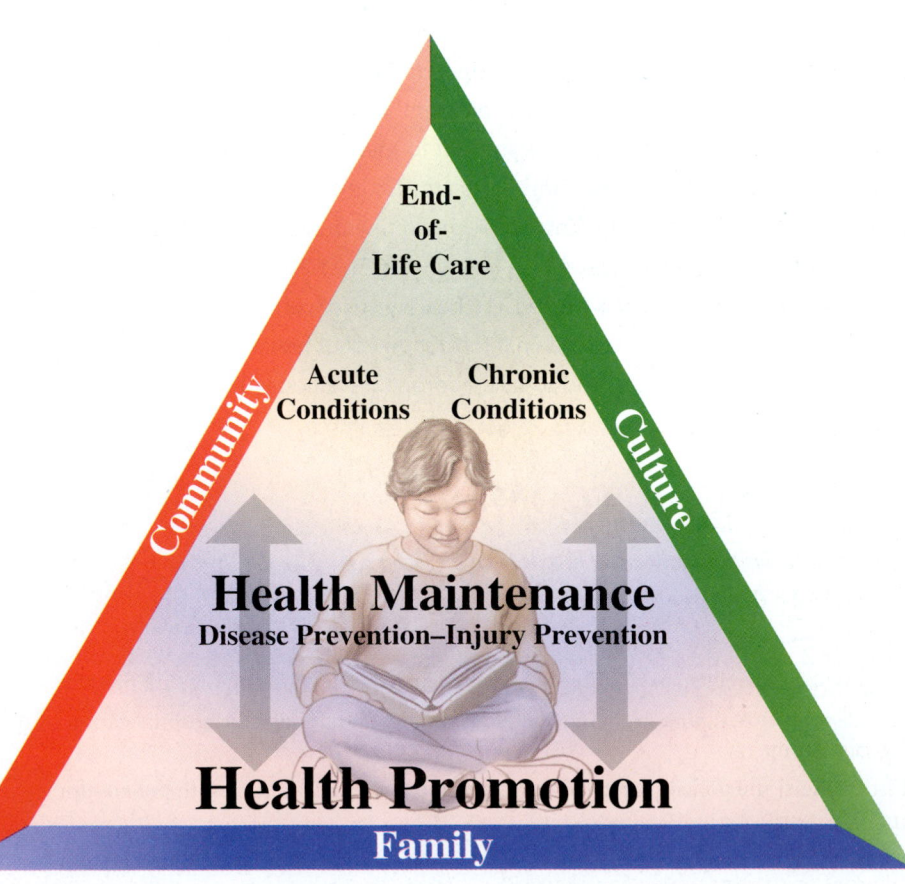

Nurses play a very significant role in the provision of health care for children. Nurses have varied responsibilities in the different settings in collaboration with many different healthcare providers, such as physicians, social workers, pharmacists, optometrists, psychologists, dentists, nutritionists, speech therapists, and physical and occupational therapists.

Think about the role of the nurse in working with children who have seizures. In how many different settings could you find nurses providing care to children with seizures? Does the type of nursing care provided to children by nurses differ among these settings? Regardless of the setting in which nurses work, assessment, nursing care interventions, and patient education are universal roles for nurses. This chapter defines the various roles for the nursing care of children and reviews concepts important to pediatric nursing.

ROLE OF THE NURSE IN PEDIATRICS

Pediatric nursing focuses on protecting children from illness and injury; assisting them to attain optimal levels of health, regardless of health problems; and rehabilitation. This focus is consistent with the American Nurses Association (2004, p. 7) definition of the scope of nursing practice: "the protection, promotion, and optimization of health and abilities, prevention of illness and injury, alleviation of suffering through the diagnosis and treatment of human response, and advocacy in the care of individuals, families, communities, and populations." The nursing roles in caring for children and their families include direct care, patient education, advocacy, and case management.

Nurses who specialize in pediatrics apply foundational knowledge provided during nursing education such as the nursing process, anatomy and physiology, physical assessment, healthcare condition recognition and management, and the full range of nursing skills. Pediatric nurses then add additional competencies related to the care of children and their families. The special knowledge and skills that nurses caring for children must acquire and apply are listed in Box 1–1.

Direct Nursing Care

The primary role of pediatric nurses is to provide direct nursing care to children and their families. The nursing process provides the framework for delivery of direct pediatric nursing care. The nurse assesses the child, identifies the nursing diagnoses that describe the responses of the child and family to the health promotion and health maintenance plan, and identifies any illness or injury experienced. The nurse then implements and evaluates nursing care. This care is designed to meet the child's physical and emotional needs. It is tailored to the child's developmental stage, giving the child additional responsibility for self-care with increasing age. Planned care is offered in a sensitive manner, compatible with the child's and family's cultural beliefs. The care is also provided in collaboration with the family, using family-centered care principles (see Chapter 2 ∞).

Nurses play an important role in minimizing the psychologic and physical distress experienced by children and their families. Providing support to children and their families is one component of direct nursing care. This often involves listening to the concerns of children and parents, being present during stressful or emotional experiences, and implementing strategies to help children and family members cope (see Chapter 2 ∞). Nurses can help families by suggesting ways to support their children in the hospital, in out-of-hospital settings, and in the home.

Patient Education

The education of children and their families improves treatment results. In pediatric nursing, patient education is especially challenging, because nurses must be prepared to work with children at various levels of understanding. Rather than give simple facts, the goal of patient education is to help the child and family to make informed choices about health and healthy behaviors.

As patient educators, nurses help children adapt to the hospital setting and prepare them for procedures (Figure 1–2 ➤). Most hospitals encourage a parent to stay with

BOX 1–1

EXPECTED COMPETENCIES OF THE PEDIATRIC NURSE

The Society of Pediatric Nursing has identified these standards for the generalist pediatric nurse:

- An understanding of the unique anatomical, physiological, and developmental differences among neonates, infants, children, and adolescents, as well as the needs unique to the growth and development of children who have chronic conditions and their families;
- The ability to care for children and promote their health in the context of their families;
- The ability to communicate effectively with children, families, and other healthcare providers, demonstrating sensitivity to cultural issues, especially those related to how the family and healthcare providers meet the children's healthcare needs;
- The provision of safety assurance and injury prevention to children and their families;
- The ability to provide for the exceptional needs of children with episodic injuries or illnesses;
- An understanding of the economic, social, and political influences outside the family that have an impact on children's health and development and family functioning; and
- An understanding of the ethical, moral, and legal dilemmas involving children, families, and healthcare professionals.

Reprinted with permission from Society of Pediatric Nurses and American Nurses Association. (2003). *Scope and standards of pediatric nursing practice.* Washington, DC: Nursesbooks.org, pp. 7–8.

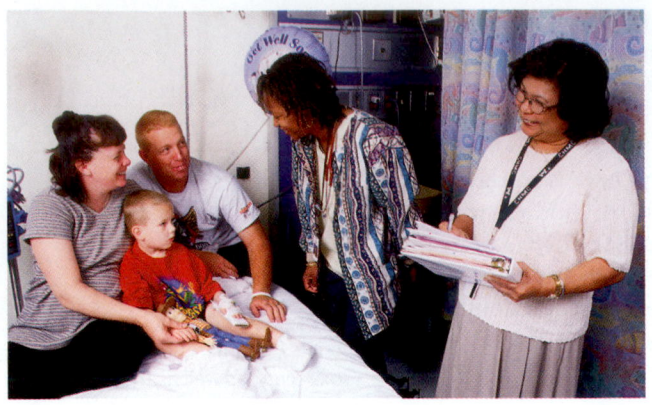

Figure 1–2 ▶ Explaining procedures can reduce the patient's and family's fears and anxieties about what to expect as well as teach procedures and proper home care.

the child and to provide much of the direct and supportive care. Nurses teach parents to watch for important signs and responses to therapies, to increase the child's comfort, and even to provide advanced care. Taking an active role prepares the parent to assume total responsibility for care after the child leaves the hospital.

Planning and preparation, as well as an understanding of the child's developmental level, are needed to effectively educate children and parents. An assessment of the child's and family's knowledge about the condition or health practices, past experiences, and their attitudes and beliefs is a starting point for education. The nurse needs to think about strategies and resources available to help the child and family learn about the health condition. Outcomes of education can be evaluated during future visits, particularly for children receiving ongoing health promotion and health maintenance care and for those with a chronic condition that requires home management.

Patient Advocacy

Advocacy—acting to safeguard and advance the interests of another—is directed at enabling the child and family to adjust to the changes in the child's health in their own way. To be an effective advocate, the nurse must be aware of the child's and the family's needs, the family's resources, and the healthcare services available in the hospital and the community. The nurse can then assist the family and the child to make informed choices about these services and to act in the child's best interests.

As advocates, nurses often serve on committees to ensure that the policies and resources of healthcare agencies meet the psychosocial needs of children and their families. The nurse must also protect the child and family by taking appropriate actions related to any incidents of incompetent, unethical, or illegal practices by any member of the healthcare team.

Case Management

What happens when a child has significant health problems? Can you handle it all? When a child has a significant health problem or handicapping condition, healthcare professionals (physicians, nurses, social workers, physical and occupational therapists, and other specialists) create an interdisciplinary plan to meet the child's medical, nursing, developmental, educational, and psychosocial needs. Because nurses spend time with the child and family while providing nursing care for the child and family, they often know more than other healthcare professionals about the family's wishes and resources. As a member of the interdisciplinary care plan team, one important role for the nurse is to serve as the family's advocate to ensure that the care plan considers the family's wishes and contains appropriate services. The nurse often becomes the child's case manager, coordinating the implementation of the interdisciplinary care plan. Sometimes the parent or a social worker becomes the case manager.

Case management is a process of coordinating the delivery of healthcare services in a manner that focuses on both quality and cost outcomes. This is often a collaborative practice with other healthcare providers that promotes **continuity of care**, an interdisciplinary process of facilitating a patient's transition between and among settings based on changing needs and available resources. The nurse case manager has control over the use of healthcare resources that are considered appropriate for the patient's condition and links the child and family to these services. The goal is to help the child and family have the best healthcare outcome and decrease fragmentation of care, while controlling the cost of healthcare services. Case management may be used for care of the patient when hospitalized as well as for long-term care of chronic conditions.

Discharge planning is a form of case management. Good discharge planning promotes a smooth, rapid, and safe transition into the community and improves the results of treatment begun in the hospital. To be a discharge planner, the nurse needs to know about community medical resources, home care agencies qualified to care for

---

CULTURE

Literacy and Communication

Many parents cannot read above a fifth-grade level. Some tips for developing patient education materials at an appropriate reading level include the following:

- Use short familiar words with one or two syllables
- Substitute simple language that defines a medical term rather than using the term
- Use short sentences
- Use active voice (subject–verb–object) rather than passive voice (e.g., a side effect is loss of appetite.)
- Use numerals rather than spelling out the number
- Use a computer program to check reading level

children, educational interventions, and services reimbursed by the child's health plan or other financial resources.

Research

Research is conducted to determine effective methods for treating a child's health condition or providing care. Innovations in care are evaluated to determine if practice is improved. Research provides a scientific basis for nursing practice. Pediatric nurses are responsible for keeping current with new pediatric research findings and identifying when changes in practice are needed. This research is also used in developing healthcare facility-specific evidence-based practice guidelines. In collaboration with advanced practice nurse researchers or other health professionals, pediatric nurses can help identify research questions, assist with the design of research studies, and collect data.

NURSING PROCESS IN PEDIATRIC CARE

Pediatric nurses use the nursing process to identify and solve problems and to plan patient care, the same process used for other patients. Consider how the five steps of the nursing process relate to children.

- *Assessment* involves collecting patient and family data and performing physical examinations during community-based health services, at admission, periodically during the child's hospitalization, and when home care services are provided. The nurse analyzes and synthesizes data to make a judgment about the patient's problems.
- *Nursing diagnoses* describe the health promotion and health patterns that nurses can manage. Once health patterns have been identified, specific nursing actions can be planned. The North American Nursing Diagnosis Association (NANDA) has responsibility for endorsing the standard language for these nursing diagnoses to describe the health promotion and health patterns that nurses can independently manage. Each nursing diagnosis has defining characteristics and related factors or risk factors.
- *Nursing care plans* are based on goals that will improve the child's or family's dysfunctional health patterns. Specific expected outcomes should be realistic. Nursing care plans have nursing intervention classifications (NIC) and nursing outcome classifications (NOC). NIC provides a standard language for general nursing actions that are specific for a nursing diagnosis. NOC provides a standard language for patient states or behaviors that should be monitored in children and families with a specific nursing diagnosis.

Standard care plans for specific diagnoses are often used in the pediatric unit of the hospital and by home health agencies. The nurse is responsible for individualizing standard care plans based on data collected from the child's assessment and from evaluation of the child's response to care. The family and the nurse (and the child, when old enough) should agree with the care plan goals. Individualized nursing action plans provide directions for nursing care.

- *Implementation* is the carrying out of interventions outlined in the nursing care plan. Interventions may be modified if the child's responses are undesirable.
- *Evaluation* is the use of specific objective and subjective measures (often called outcome measures or criteria) to assess the child's and family's progress in reaching the goals defined in the nursing care plan. Following the evaluation of their progress toward the goals, the nursing care plan may be modified. For example, as the child's condition improves and goals are attained, new goals and nursing action plans must be defined. Data from ongoing assessments are collected to guide the revision of the care plan.

Critical Thinking

Critical thinking, an individualized, creative thinking or reasoning process that the nurse uses to solve problems, plays an important role in the nursing process. The process of critical thinking involves identifying the specific problem or issue that needs to be addressed or the goal to be achieved. Information is collected from multiple sources, including the child, family, health facility, and community, in addition to research, experts, and published literature. The nurse then creatively analyzes all the information to make judgments about clinical actions. Additional considerations such as professional standards, ethics, and cultural values of the child and family are integrated into the problem-solving process. Once a solution or action is identified, the nurse then must evaluate the impact or outcome of that action to improve the strategy or care provided (Alfaro-LeFevre, 2004).

Clinical Practice Guidelines and Clinical Pathways

Clinical practice guidelines are comprehensive interdisciplinary care plans for a specific condition, which describe the sequence and timing of interventions that should result in expected patient outcomes. The care plans are increasingly evidence based, using research findings, judgments of healthcare experts, and group consensus to identify the most effective practices for a specific health condition. Often a national organization will develop a clinical practice guideline for a specific health condition, such as the asthma guidelines developed by the National Asthma Education Program of the National Institutes of Health (see Chapter 20 ∞).

Clinical pathways (critical pathways) are structured care plans for a specific patient problem that outline key events and timing in a step-wise manner for the management of a child by multiple healthcare professionals. They often describe the specific application of clinical practice guidelines developed by national organizations to the local hospital setting, establishing criteria for short-term and long-term patient outcomes (Napolitano, 2005). The goal is to improve the continuity and coordination of care among the different healthcare professionals and efficiency in care provided.

Evidence-Based Practice

Evidence-based practice is a problem-solving approach that integrates the best research evidence with a nurse's clinical expertise and the patient's values or preferences (Melnyk, 2004). To integrate the best research evidence, the nurse or other health professional must analyze and evaluate all clinical studies related to a specific health condition or clinical problem. It is a method to ensure that the latest information known about providing care (nursing care as well as what is known by other healthcare disciplines) to children with a particular health problem is included in the nursing care plan. However, clinical judgment is needed to determine if the research findings fit the population being served in the healthcare setting. The preferences of the child and family must also be considered. New evidence may alter the way care is provided because it has been revealed that the children have a better outcome or perhaps the cost of care is reduced with the new procedure or treatment. Once the nursing care plan, clinical practice guideline, or clinical pathway is modified based upon the new evidence, data need to be collected to determine if the expected outcomes are seen in the population served by the healthcare setting.

SETTINGS FOR PEDIATRIC NURSING CARE

Pediatric nurses function in a variety of settings within the hospital. Acute care may be provided in the emergency department, observation or short-stay unit, postanesthesia unit, intensive care unit, general pediatric inpatient unit, and various outpatient clinics. In rehabilitation centers, nurses provide inpatient and ambulatory care to help restore children to an optimal state and plan for discharge management of chronic conditions. Pediatric nurses working with children and families on a general pediatric hospital unit promote health improvement in the following ways:

- By gathering data and assessing the health of children and their families
- By providing ordered medical therapies
- By providing nursing care in a manner that preserves as many of the child's and family's normal routines as possible while maintaining the family unit

- By working with the family and healthcare team to develop an individualized healthcare plan and a discharge plan, or to implement a clinical practice guideline

The hospital stay is now integrated into a continuum that allows children to complete therapy at home, at school, or in other community settings. Pediatric nurses assist families in making the transition from the acute hospital setting to the home, rehabilitation center, or long-term care facility. Managing the child's transition from acute care to another setting involves planning the discharge, implementing interdisciplinary plans, helping the family to develop an emergency care plan in the event the child has an unexpected healthcare crisis, and collaborating with a broad range of healthcare professionals.

Pediatric nurses also work in several community healthcare settings (see Chapter 11 ∞):

- In pediatricians' offices and healthcare centers, nurses assess children, provide telephone counseling, and support and counsel families about growth, development, and nutrition.
- In clinic settings, nurses assess children, assist with medical procedures, and educate families to ensure the continuous management of the children's healthcare problems.
- In home health agencies, nurses provide home care to children who require their services. Children need medical treatment and nursing care for acute, self-limited, chronic, and terminal conditions. This may involve visits for specific interventions such as medication administration or "private duty" (one-to-one) nursing care.
- In schools, nurses assess children, monitor their health status, and provide health education to teachers and children. Many children who are assisted by technology or have chronic conditions attend school.

CONTEMPORARY CLIMATE FOR PEDIATRIC NURSING CARE

In 2000 more than 81 million children under the age of 20 years lived in the United States. They accounted for 28.1% of the population (Anderson & Smith, 2005). (See Figure 1–3 ➤ for a distribution of the population by age group.) The racial and ethnic diversity of children in the United States has increased and is currently estimated as follows (Federal Interagency Forum on Child and Family Statistics, 2005):

- White, non-Hispanic—60%
- Black, non-Hispanic—16%
- Hispanic—19%
- Asian—4%
- Native American or Alaskan Native—1%

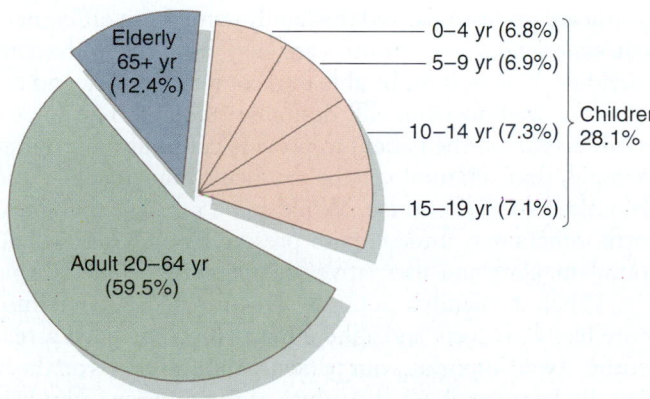

Figure 1–3 ➤ At the time of the U.S. Census 2000, children under 20 years of age accounted for 28.1% of the population in the United States. Data from: Anderson, R. N., & Smith, B. L. (2005). Deaths: Leading causes for 2002. *National Vital Statistics Reports, 53*(17). Hyattsville, MD: National Center for Health Statistics.

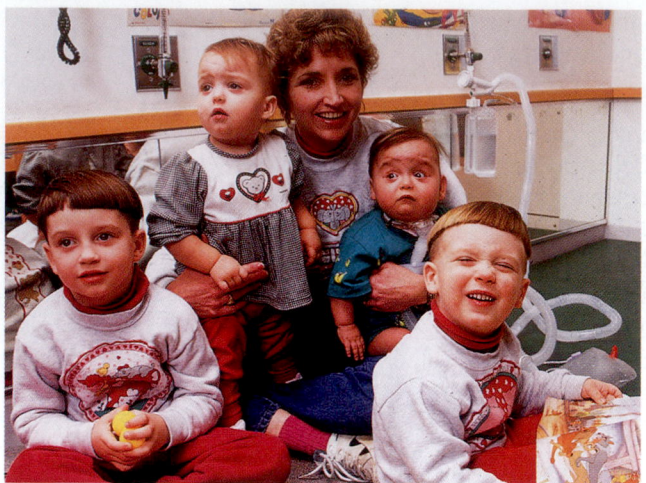

Figure 1–4 ➤ Many facilities now encourage family visitation for children with health problems that require long-term hospitalization. Extended family visits enable parents to learn about the child's care, and provide siblings with opportunities to interact with the hospitalized child.

Family-Centered Care

Recognizing the family as the constant influence and support in a child's life is the foundation for developing a trusting relationship with families. The family is the principal caregiver and support for the child, and the family is important in helping the child recover from an illness or injury (Figure 1–4 ➤). Efforts to address and meet the emotional, social, and developmental needs of children and families seeking health care in all settings is a concept known as **family-centered care**. Families are often considered partners in care, learning about children's conditions and participating in decisions regarding their care. Thus, families gain greater confidence and competence in caring for their children, which has become even more important as families play an ever increasing role in providing care for children's healthcare problems. The key elements of family-centered care are described in Chapter 2 ∞.

Culturally Sensitive Care

The U.S. population has a varied mix of cultural groups, with ever increasing diversity. More than 33% of all children less than 20 years of age are from families of minority populations (U.S. Census, 2001). By the year 2020, it is expected that the proportion of children who are of Hispanic origin will increase to one child in every five (Federal Interagency Forum on Child and Family Statistics, 2005). It is also important to recognize the diversity among the non-Hispanic White population as they represent many cultural groups, such as immigrants from former Soviet bloc countries.

Culture develops from socially learned beliefs, lifestyles, values, and integrated patterns of behavior that are characteristic of the family, cultural group, and community. The cultural background and values of children and their parents are often quite different from those of the nurse. Specific elements that contribute to a family's value system include the following:

- Religion and social beliefs
- Presence and influence of the extended family, as well as socialization within the ethnic group
- Communication patterns
- Beliefs and understanding about the concepts of health and illness
- Permissible physical contact with strangers
- Education

Specific differences in beliefs between families and healthcare providers are common in the following areas: help-seeking behaviors, causes of diseases or illnesses, death and dying, caretaking and caregiving, and childrearing practices.

These elements in differing degrees influence the cultural beliefs and values of an ethnic group, making the group unique. Misunderstandings may occur when the healthcare professional and the family come from different cultural groups. In addition, past experiences with health care may have made the family angry or suspicious of providers. Nurses must be able to recognize, respect, and respond to ethnic diversity in a way that leads to a mutually desirable outcome. The nurse must identify culturally relevant facts about the patient to provide culturally appropriate and competent care. For example, some cultural groups practice complementary and alternative therapies that are unknown to the nurse. While some of these therapies are beneficial or cause no harm, others may interact with prescribed medications and cause harm. Examples of complementary and alternative therapies are included throughout the textbook.

When the family's cultural values are incorporated into the care plan, the family is more likely to accept and adhere to the recommended care, especially in the home care setting. Avoid imposing your personal cultural values on the children and families in your care. By learning about the values of the different ethnic groups in the community—

religious beliefs that have an impact on healthcare practices, beliefs about common illnesses, and specific healing practices—you can develop an individualized nursing care plan for each child and family.

PEDIATRIC HEALTH STATISTICS

Mortality

Children have different healthcare problems than adults, and the problems may depend on age and development. For example, the leading causes of **infant mortality** (death occurring during the first year of life) vary according to the age of the infant (Figure 1–5 ➤).

The leading causes of death in neonates (birth to 28 days of age) are congenital anomalies, low birth weight, respiratory distress syndrome, and maternal complications of pregnancy. Sudden infant death syndrome accounts for nearly 28% of deaths to infants in the postneonatal period (between 1 and 12 months of age). Figure 1–5 shows the relative frequency of other major causes of death in the postneonatal period. The mortality rate for Black infants is at least 2 times that of Whites (Hoyert, Kung, & Smith, 2005).

The most common cause of death for children between 1 and 19 years of age is unintentional injury. The major causes of death from unintentional injury in childhood include motor vehicle crashes (passengers and pedestrians), drowning, fires and burns, firearms, and suffocation. Congenital malformations, cancer, and diseases of the heart are the most common medical causes of death. Figure 1–6 ➤ shows the distribution of the leading causes of death by age group.

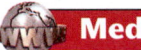

> **CULTURE**
>
> **Integration of Traditional Practice**
>
> Conflicts can occur within a family when traditional rituals and practices of the family's elders do not conform to current healthcare practices. When cultural values are not part of the nursing care plan, parents may be forced to decide whether the family's beliefs should take priority over the healthcare professional's guidance when caring for the child at home. Make an effort to understand the family's traditional health practices and to integrate them into the care plan.

> **MediaLink**
>
> *Child Health Statistics*

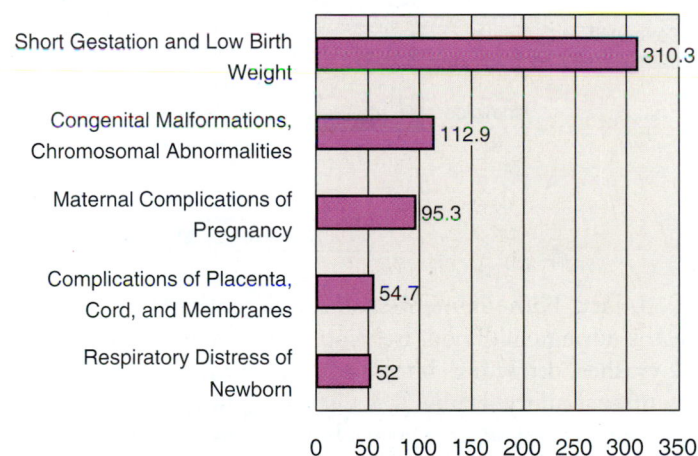

A. Leading Causes of Neonatal Mortality

- Short Gestation and Low Birth Weight — 310.3
- Congenital Malformations, Chromosomal Abnormalities — 112.9
- Maternal Complications of Pregnancy — 95.3
- Complications of Placenta, Cord, and Membranes — 54.7
- Respiratory Distress of Newborn — 52

(0, 50, 100, 150, 200, 250, 300, 350)

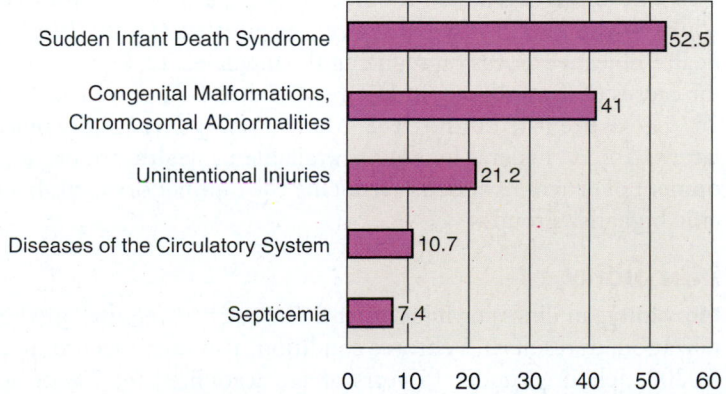

B. Leading Causes of Postneonatal Mortality

- Sudden Infant Death Syndrome — 52.5
- Congenital Malformations, Chromosomal Abnormalities — 41
- Unintentional Injuries — 21.2
- Diseases of the Circulatory System — 10.7
- Septicemia — 7.4

(0, 10, 20, 30, 40, 50, 60)

Figure 1–5 ➤ Age-specific death rate per 1000 live births in the United States for infants in 2002. A, Neonatal mortality (in infants up to 28 days old) and B, Postneonatal mortality (in infants between 28 days and 1 year old). In 1993 the mortality rate for Sudden Infant Death Syndrome was 109.5 per 100,000 live births. What could account for this dramatic rate reduction? (See Chapter 20 ∞ to find the answer.) Data from: Anderson, R. N., & Smith, B. L. (2005). Deaths: Leading causes for 2002. *National Vital Statistics Reports, 53*(17). Hyattsville, MD: National Center for Health Statistics.

A. Leading Causes of Death to Children 1-9 Years

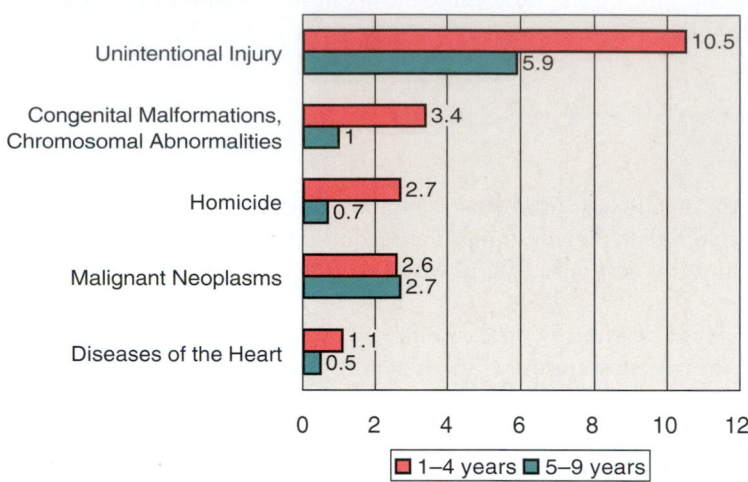

B. Leading Causes of Death for Children 10-19 Years

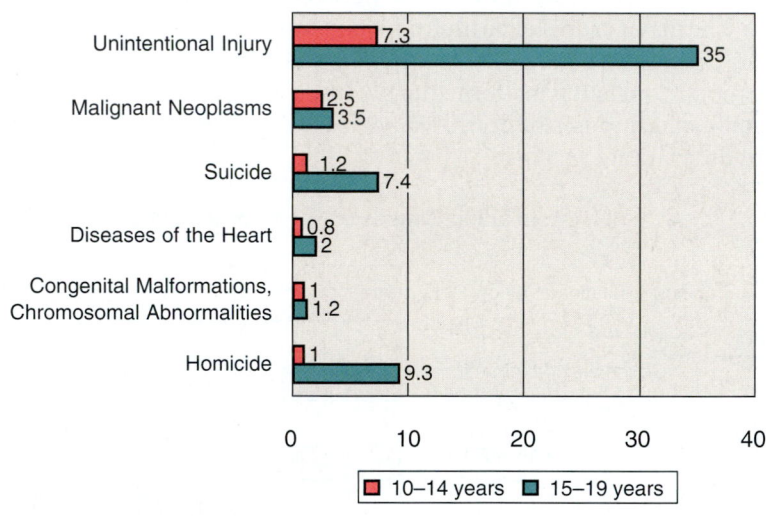

Figure 1–6 ▶ Age-specific death rate per 100,000 children in the United States in 2002. A, Death rates for children between 1 and 9 years of age and B, Death rates for children between 10 and 19 years of age. The leading cause of death in children in all age groups was unintentional injury. Why do you think that is? Which type of injury has the highest rate of death? Drowning? Fires and burns? Motor vehicle crashes? See Table 1-1 for the answer. Data from: Anderson, R. N., & Smith, B. L. (2005). Deaths: Leading causes for 2002. *National Vital Statistics Reports, 53*(17). Hyattsville, MD: National Center for Health Statistics.

BOX 1–2
HEALTHY PEOPLE 2010 GOALS

Goal 1: Help individuals of all ages increase life expectancy and improve their quality of life.
Goal 2: Eliminate health disparities among segments of the population, including differences that occur by gender, race or ethnicity, education or income, disability, geographic location, or sexual orientation.

From: U.S. Department of Health and Human Services. *Healthy People 2010.* (2nd ed.). With *Understanding and Improving Health and Objectives for Improving Health,* 2 vols. Washington, DC: U.S. Government Printing Office, November 2000.

Injury, both unintentional and intentional, contributes to many preventable deaths during childhood. Leading causes of unintentional injury include motor vehicle crashes, drowning, burns, and suffocation. Firearms are a major contributor to intentional injury deaths. It is disturbing to note that violence-related deaths (homicide and suicide) occur at such a high rate in children. Table 1–1 illustrates the leading causes of injury deaths by age group. Many injury prevention programs have been implemented by state health departments, healthcare facilities, and national organizations to reduce the number of children who die unnecessarily.

The U.S. government set objectives to improve the health of children and young adults in the 21st century in the report entitled *Healthy People 2010*. These national health objectives focus on reducing the incidence of death and disability from the major causes of death shown in Figures 1–5 and 1–6, as well as Table 1–1. *Healthy People 2010* goals are listed in Box 1–2. Many *Healthy People 2010* objectives are included in later chapters. Federal funding is available to healthcare organizations for the development of programs aimed at reducing the number of deaths from these factors in specific high-risk groups.

Morbidity

Morbidity, an illness or injury that limits activity, requires medical attention or hospitalization, or results in a chronic condition, also varies according to the age of the child. In 2003, children under 15 years of age accounted for 7% of hospital discharges and

Table 1–1	FIVE LEADING CAUSES OF INJURY DEATH BY AGE GROUP, 2000–2002*				
	Ranking				
Age Group	First	Second	Third	Fourth	Fifth
Under 1 year	Suffocation	Motor vehicle	Homicide, unspecified cause	Homicide, specified cause	Drowning
1 to 4 years	Motor vehicle	Drowning	Fire, burns	Suffocation	Homicide
5 to 9 years	Motor vehicle	Drowning	Fire, burn	Homicide, firearm	Suffocation
10 to 14 years	Motor vehicle	Drowning	Suicide, suffocation	Homicide, firearm	Suicide, firearm
15 to 19 years	Motor vehicle	Homicide, firearm	Suicide, firearm	Suicide, suffocation	Poisoning

*Shaded boxes indicate unintentional injuries.

Data from: National Center for Injury Prevention and Control. (2004). 10 leading causes of injury deaths, United States 2000–2002, all races, both sexes, accessed August 24, 2005, from http://webapp.cdc.gov/cgi-bin/broker.exe

their average length of stay was 4.5 days (DeFrances, Hall, & Podgornik, 2005). Figure 1–7 ➤ compares the leading causes of hospitalization of children by age group in 1993 and 2003. Respiratory diseases are the leading cause of hospitalization in children between 1 and 9 years of age, while mental disorders are a leading cause of hospitalization in children and adolescents between 10 and 21 years. Childbirth is among the leading causes of hospitalization in adolescents between 15 and 21 years of age (Fingerhut, 2005). What do you think could account for the increase in hospital discharges for mental disorders in children and adolescents from 10 to 21 years? See Chapter 6 ∞.

HEALTHCARE ISSUES
Healthcare Financing

Not all children in the United States have access to healthcare. In 2004, 8.5 million children, or 11.7% of those below 18 years of age, had no health insurance, and 29.4% were covered by public insurance programs such as Medicaid and the State Child Health Insurance Program (SCHIP). Private insurance covered 58.9% of children under 18 years of age (Rhoades, 2005) (Figure 1–8 ➤).

Family members pay approximately 21% of their children's healthcare expenditures out-of-pocket. Families who live in poverty still pay a considerably greater proportion of their income for out-of-pocket medical expenses than families who are not living in poverty, even with greater access to public insurance for children (Wong, Galbraith, Kim, et al., 2005). Children living in poverty are also more likely to have breaks in health insurance coverage that seriously jeopardize consistent care for chronic conditions and preventive health services (Satchell & Pati, 2005). Efforts to provide universal access to health care for children continue. States are allocated federal funds to encourage enrollment of children up to 200% of the federal poverty level (Kenney & Chang, 2004). As of June 2003, 3.9 million children were enrolled (Kenney & Chang, 2004).

Despite the availability of SCHIP, many eligible children are not enrolled. Reasons why families have not enrolled their eligible children may include:

- Believe their income is too high to qualify,
- Have obtained other insurance like Medicaid,
- Have difficulty with application procedure and required documentation,
- Lack of skills in negotiating the system to get coverage.

Nurses can play an important role in encouraging families to investigate their eligibility for the program. Obtain current guidelines in your state about eligibility

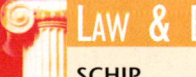

LAW & ETHICS

SCHIP
Congress created the State Child Health Insurance Program in 1997 to provide health insurance for children when their family's income was too high to qualify for Medicaid but not high enough to pay for private insurance coverage (Kenney & Chang, 2004). Each state decides eligibility requirements for children and families.

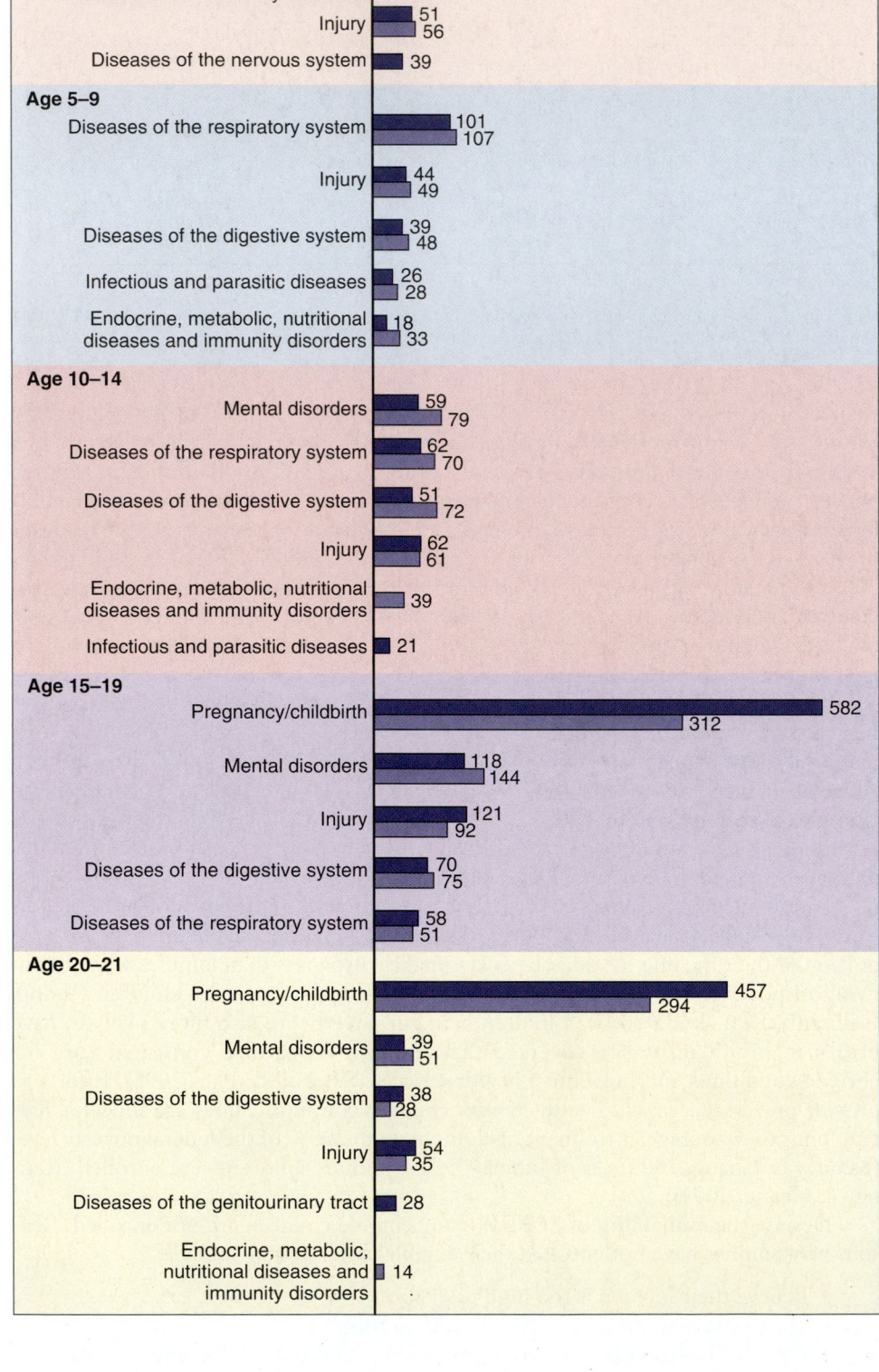

Figure 1-7 ➤ The leading causes of hospitalization in the United States in 2003 are much the same as those in 1993 in those 21 years of age and younger, but the number of hospital discharges [in 1000s] have changed for some causes. What do you think might account for the rise in hospital discharges for mental disorders? What do you think the current hospital discharge numbers are today?

Data from: Fingerhut, L. A. (2005). National hospital discharge survey. Unpublished data; and National Center for Health Statistics. (1999). National Hospital Discharge Survey. Unpublished Data.

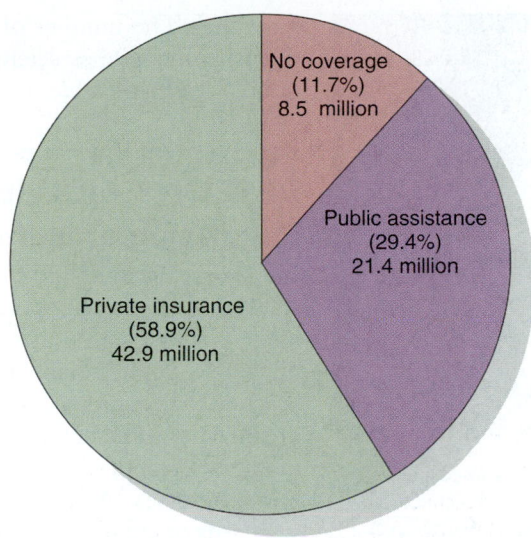

No coverage
(11.7%)
8.5 million

Public assistance
(29.4%)
21.4 million

Private insurance
(58.9%)
42.9 million

Figure 1–8 ➤ In the United States, how is health care of children paid for? These data from 2004 show that our taxes support 41% of the costs. What can you do to help? Something as simple as counseling parents about injury prevention and providing immunizations while a child is under care for other problems can prevent potential health problems. Part of good nursing care is supporting the well-being of the child in addition to caring for the presenting problem.
Data from: Rhoades, J. A. (2005). Health insurance status of children in America, 1996–2004: Estimates for the U.S. civilian noninstitutionalized population under age 18, Statistical Brief #85, Rockville, MD: Agency for Healthcare Research and Quality, accessed October 28, 2005, from http://www.meps. ahrq.gov/papers/st85/stat85.pdf

requirements and coverage benefits. For example, some states require a monthly premium or co-pay for healthcare visits.

Medicaid provides coverage to children and individuals with disabilities who meet income level qualifications set by the state. Children covered under the Temporary Assistance to Needy Families (TANF) are usually eligible. For covered health services see Box 1–3. This is a comprehensive and preventive child health program for individuals under 21 years.

Healthcare Technology

Research and technology have enabled many children with congenital anomalies and low birth weights to survive, with and without chronic conditions. Lifesaving technology has also created such burdens as high costs of health care and stresses on the functioning of the child's family. Technologic advances have resulted in the design of portable medical and infusion therapy equipment for home care. Many children are dependent upon or assisted by technology for physiologic functions. Some families have regained control over their lives by creating intensive care units in their homes (Figure 1–9 ➤). Examples of technology children may require in the home setting include ventilators, feeding tubes and intravenous or central lines along with their associated pumps, cardiorespiratory monitors, peritoneal dialysis, and pacemakers. Generators are often used in case of power outages, and emergency transport and helicopter landing sites may be

---

BOX 1–3

PREVENTIVE HEALTH SERVICES COVERED UNDER THE EARLY PERIODIC SCREENING, DIAGNOSTIC, AND TREATMENT (EPSDT) SERVICE OF MEDICAID

- Comprehensive health and developmental history
- Comprehensive unclothed physical examination
- Appropriate immunizations
- Laboratory tests (statewide screening requirements and lead toxicity screening)
- Health education
- Vision services—screening, treatment for defects in vision, including eyeglasses
- Dental services—dental screening, relief of pain and infection, restoration of teeth, and maintenance of dental health
- Hearing services—diagnosis and treatment of hearing defects, including hearing aids
- Other necessary health care—to correct or ameliorate defects, physical and mental illnesses, and conditions discovered by the screening process

Note: Data from: Centers for Medicare and Medicaid Services. (2003). Medicaid and EPSDT, accessed January 3, 2006, http://www.cms.gov/medicaid/ epsdt/

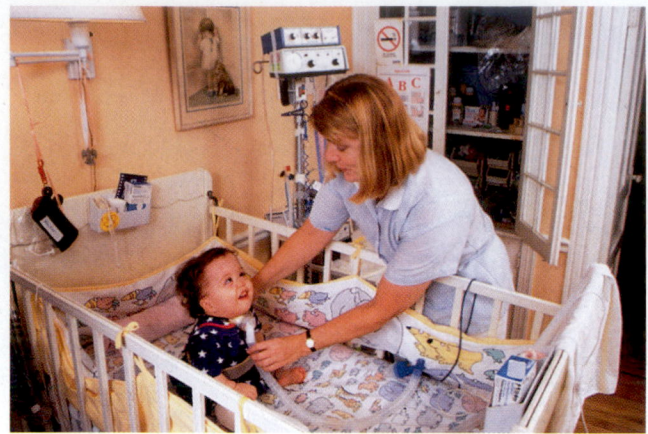

Figure 1–9 ▶ It is often desirable from a family and cost perspective to provide health care in the home, and technologic advances have made this possible. But is it really less costly to provide care in the home for a child with technology assistance? How does one factor in parents' out-of-pocket expenses for medical supplies that are not reimbursed? Lost time from work or the need for a parent to discontinue employment to care for the child? What is the emotional strain on families who care for their child 24 hours a day, 7 days a week? What support is needed by these families to continue providing this level of care at home? See Chapters 11 and 12 ∞ for answers.

identified. The number of children assisted by technology continues to increase as scientific and technological advances continue. See Chapter 12 ∞.

LEGAL CONCEPTS AND RESPONSIBILITIES

Regulation of Nursing Practice

Nurses are accountable for their professional actions, and each state regulates nursing practice with a nurse practice act. A state's nurse practice act defines the legal roles and responsibilities of nurses. As professionals, nurses set standards for education and practice that conform to state regulations. Professional nursing organizations and state agencies that accredit nursing programs modify the standards for nursing education as the science of nursing progresses. Nurses in professional organizations develop standards of nursing practice. These standards describe the public and patient responsibilities for which nurses are accountable.

Standards of clinical nursing practice developed by the American Nurses Association in 2004 define standards for both nursing care and performance. Standards of care describe the competent level of nursing care using the nursing process and form the foundation of clinical decision making. Standards of performance describe the nurse's behavior in the professional role and include such criteria as quality of care, performance appraisal, collegiality, resource utilization, ethics, research, education, and collaboration. The Society of Pediatric Nurses in collaboration with the American Nurses Association has also developed specific standards of pediatric clinical nursing practice. See Box 1–4.

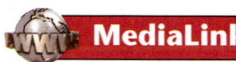

MediaLink

Professional Nursing Organizations

BOX 1–4

PROFESSIONAL PRACTICE STANDARDS FOR PEDIATRIC NURSING PRACTICE

Standards of Care for the Pediatric Nurse Include:

- Collecting health data
- Analyzing the assessment data in determining diagnoses
- Identifying expected outcomes individualized to the child and family
- Developing a plan of care that prescribes interventions to attain expected outcomes
- Implementing the interventions identified in the plan of care

Standards of Performance for the Pediatric Nurse Include:

- Systematically evaluating the quality and effectiveness of pediatric nursing practice
- Evaluating own nursing practice in relation to professional practice standards and relevant statutes and regulations
- Acquiring and maintaining current knowledge and competence in pediatric nursing practice
- Interacting with and contributing to the professional development of peers, colleagues, and other healthcare providers
- Making assessments and recommendations and taking action on behalf of children and their families in an ethical manner
- Collaborating with the child, family, and other healthcare providers in providing patient care
- Contributing to nursing and pediatric health care through the use of research methods and findings
- Considering factors related to safety, effectiveness, and cost in planning and delivering care

Reprinted with permission from American Nurses Association & the Society of Pediatric Nurses. (2003). *Scope and standards of pediatric nursing practice.* Washington, DC: nursebooks.org, American Nurses Association, 600 Maryland Ave SW, Suite 100W, Washington, DC 20024-2571.

Accountability and Risk Management

Accountability

The family entrusts the child's care to the healthcare team. Family members expect this team to provide good medical and nursing care and to avoid mistakes that cause harm. Nurses are personally accountable for expanding their knowledge base, staying current regarding changes in medical and nursing care for specific conditions, recognizing important changes in the child's condition that require intervention, and taking action as necessary to protect the child.

Patient Safety

Children are at a higher risk for medical error than other patients and also may be more vulnerable to harm when errors are made because of their immature physiology (Hughes & Edgerton, 2005). Most errors in medical care within hospitals are "systems errors," such as incorrect transcription of physician orders, malfunctioning equipment used for administering medications, and delayed medication delivery by the pharmacy, rather than being the error of a single individual. (See Evidence-Based Practice: Medication Errors, on page 16). The Joint Commission on Accreditation of Healthcare Organizations has identified patient safety as an important responsibility with requirements that must be met for accreditation (Burke, 2005).

Reasons for the increase in medical error among children include the following (Hughes & Edgerton, 2005):

- Medication dosage calculations are more complex. Many medications are produced in adult concentrations requiring dilution, or dosages must be calculated based upon weight. This means the optimal dose is based on mg/kg and divided by number of doses to be given each day. An additional problem is that children often need suspensions or liquid preparations, adding to the dosage calculation complexity. Not only is the correct dose calculated, but also the amount of liquid preparation with that dose must be calculated. Errors in these mathematical calculations are common.
- The misplacement of a decimal in the medication dosage calculation can result in an overdose that can cause harm to the child or even death. Critically ill and injured children do not have the reserves to deal with an overdose of medication like a healthy older child or adult.
- Many drug preparations require dilution to achieve the small dosage required by infants.
- Medications are sometimes prescribed that are not yet approved by the Food and Drug Administration for use in children.
- Young children cannot communicate well if they are having a reaction to the medication.

Families with limited English proficiency are potentially at risk for medical errors even when using a hospital interpreter. Errors such as omitting instructions on dose, frequency, and duration of medications can be made by interpreters and have potential clinical consequences (Flores, Laws, Mayo, et al., 2003). Healthcare facilities are challenged to implement strategies that will reduce medical errors in all child patients.

Risk Management

Healthcare institutions make every effort to promote optimal patient care and reduce liability by various activities. **Risk management** is a process established by a healthcare institution to identify, evaluate, and reduce the risk of injury to patients, staff, and visitors, and thus reduce the institution's liability. This involves the study of causes of medical errors within a healthcare institution and implementing system changes to prevent future errors similar to those studied. Several strategies developed to reduce medication errors in children are listed in Box 1–5.

Quality improvement is the continuous study and improvement of the processes and outcomes of providing healthcare services to meet the needs of patients, by examining the systems and processes of how care and services are delivered.

CLINICAL TIP

Policy and procedure manuals should be current and provide guidance on patient care and the use of technology specifically related to potentially serious situations. Nurses often participate as committee members in the development and revision of these policy and procedure manuals.

EVIDENCE-BASED PRACTICE

Medication Errors

Clinical Question

Adverse drug events occur in children and can have serious consequences because of the child's immature physiology. For children cared for in the hospital, is there a better method of reducing medication errors than a weight-based dosing reference for commonly used medications?

Evidence

An epidemiologic study was conducted at two urban teaching hospitals to determine the rates of medication errors and adverse drug events with the potential to injure the patient among hospitalized children. Medication errors were defined as errors in drug ordering, transcribing, dispensing, administering, and monitoring. Errors were found in 5.7% of all medication orders (often at the stage of drug ordering), and medication error rates were similar across different types of pediatric units. The majority of errors were related to doses, followed by administration errors. Errors with the greatest potential for harm occurred in infants cared for in the neonatal intensive care unit (Kaushal, Bates, Landrigan, et al., 2001). Medication errors occur more frequently in seriously ill children who are hospitalized longer and undergo more medical procedures. Both of these factors increase the child's likelihood of being affected by a medication error (Slonim, LaFleur, Ahmed, et al., 2003). A study examining the role of nurses and pharmacists in identifying pre-scribing errors prior to drug administration was conducted at a British hospital over two 2-week periods. Two life-threatening drug errors were detected, one by the nurses and one by the pharmacists. Nurses identified almost 50% of the errors in each study period. In 50% of cases of nurse intervention, the prescription was amended, versus 80% of the cases of pharmacist intervention. This study illustrates the importance of nurses and pharmacists in identifying errors in prescribed medications (Guy, Persaud, Davies, et al., 2003).

Implications

Medication errors are a serious problem in pediatrics because dosages are calculated by the weight of the child, and an error in the placement of a decimal results in a potential overdose or underdose. Confusion about the medication ordered can occur because of similarity in medication names or because of the difficulty reading a physican's handwriting. Nurses play an important role in reducing errors by verifying medications ordered and administering the correct dosage on time and in the correct manner (e.g., rate of IV infusion).

Critical Thinking Application

Identify the medication error reduction policies and strategies that exist in each health setting used for clinical practice. What other medication safety practices do nurses use routinely in these settings? Identify any potential areas of improvement in medication safety practice in these settings.

Nurses participate in the development of institutional policies and standards of nursing practice. Hospitals and home health agencies encourage the development of diagnosis-specific nursing care plans, interdisciplinary clinical practice guidelines, or clinical pathways that serve as minimal institutional standards of care.

During the development of institutional standards of care, indicators of effective care by pediatric nurses and other providers are identified. These indicators may measure either the process of care, the institution's systems, or the expected outcome of care for a specific patient condition. Patient records are regularly reviewed to identify

---

BOX 1–5
STRATEGIES TO REDUCE PEDIATRIC MEDICATION ERRORS

- Do not rely on memory; verify medication dosages and medication dosage calculations.
- Every prescription should include the child's weight and age, as well as the calculated dose and mg/kg dose. The dosage form (vial, tablet, or ampule) should not be used on the prescription, as medication preparations and concentrations may vary by pharmaceutical company.
- Prescription information should be written in legible printed letters to prevent confusion with other drugs having similar names.
- Abbreviations for medications and frequency of administration should not be used.
- The administration rate for all IV medications should be specified. Computerized IV pumps are becoming more available to increase safety.
- A zero should not be used after a whole number (e.g., 5.0 could be misread as 50) and this can potentially result in a 10-fold dosage increase.
- Drug interactions and patient allergies cause adverse drug events when the inappropriate medication is ordered. A computerized physician order system with clinical decision support can improve the system, reducing errors from poor handwriting and checking for drug interactions and allergies.
- Bar coding for medications as well as timers and alarms to remind nurses to administer medications are other strategies in development.
- Unit dose dispensing systems should be used.

Note: Data from: Levine, S. R., Cohen, M. R., Blanchard, N. R., Frederico, F., Magelli, M., Lomax, C., et al. (2001). Guidelines for preventing medication errors in pediatrics. *Journal of Pediatric Pharmacology and Therapeutics, 6,* 426–442.

deviations from the institutional standards or clinical practice guidelines/clinical pathways. When deviations from expected processes and outcomes are identified, opportunities to improve the system or processes of care provision are explored with all care providers. Recommendations for the revision of institutional standards to further improve care by nurses and other health providers in the institution often result.

Documentation of nursing care is an essential part of risk management and quality improvement. If a patient record is subpoenaed, documented care is considered the only care provided, regardless of the quality of undocumented care. The patient assessment, the nursing care plan, and the child's responses to medical therapies and nursing care, including the regularly scheduled evaluation of the patient's progress toward nursing goals, must all be documented accurately and sequentially. Nurses must also report any untoward incidents that could inhibit the patient's recovery.

LEGAL AND ETHICAL ISSUES IN PEDIATRIC CARE

Marvin, a 15-year-old boy with acute nonlymphocytic leukemia, has come out of remission with an acute onset of fever, joint pain, and petechiae (Figure 1–10 ➤). A hematopoietic stem cell (bone marrow) transplant is one of his therapeutic options. Although Marvin has agreed to a transplant if a suitable donor is found, he does not want to be resuscitated and placed on life support equipment should he have a cardiac arrest. He has talked extensively with the hospital chaplain and social worker and feels comfortable with his decision. His parents want an all-out effort to sustain his life until a donor is located.

Marvin's case illustrates the legal and ethical dilemmas in caring for children. At what age can children make an informed decision about whether to accept or refuse treatment? What happens when the parents and child have conflicting opinions about treatment? How are ethical decisions resolved?

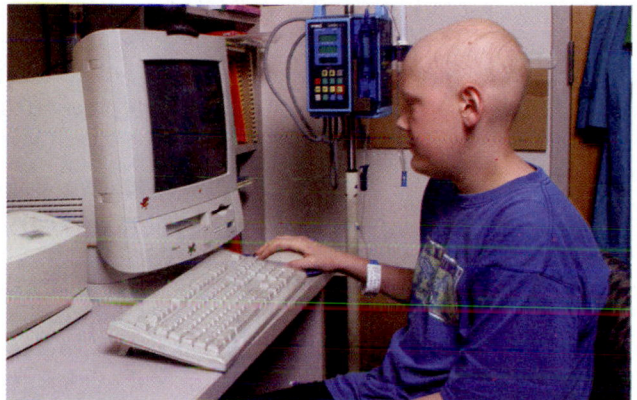

Figure 1–10 ➤ Marvin, a 15-year-old boy with acute nonlymphocytic leukemia, has definite opinions about his treatment, but his parents disagree. At what age can children make an informed decision about whether to accept or refuse treatment?

Informed Consent

Informed consent is a formal authorization by the child's parent or guardian allowing an invasive procedure to be performed or for participation in research. The physician is legally responsible for obtaining informed consent. In the case of research, the investigative researcher may formally designate a person to obtain informed consent. The nurse's role in obtaining informed consent includes the following: verifying that informed consent has been obtained prior to any procedure or research participation, alerting physicians to the need for informed consent, serving as a witness for informed consent, and responding to questions asked by parents and children.

Consent must be given voluntarily and prior to the procedure or research. Parents, as the legal custodians of minor children, are customarily requested to give informed consent on behalf of a child. Both children and parents must understand that they have the right to refuse treatment at any time. In an emergency, consent for treatment to preserve life or limb is not required.

When parents are divorced and have joint custody, in most cases either may give informed consent. When parents are divorced, some states limit the parental rights to give informed consent to the parent with custody. Obtain information about your state law regarding custody and who can provide informed consent for healthcare procedures and treatments. Obtain legal advice for complex family issues related to guardianship, divorced parents disagreeing over care, or a caregiver who is not the legal guardian.

Many children live in homes with a parent and other adult (stepparent, cohabiting unmarried adults, or grandparent) who does not have legal authority to sign consent. Proxy consent can be granted in writing by the parent to another adult so that children can obtain health care when needed (Berger, and Committee on Medical Liability, 2003).

Child Participation in Healthcare Decisions

A child is considered to have the cognitive capacity for **competence**, an ability to be involved in healthcare decisions requiring a certain degree of intellect, an ability to communicate, and an ability to remember. A child displays competence when he or she is able to use abstract reasoning, which occurs sometime during adolescence when abstract thinking skills have developed (Beidler & Dickey, 2001). Children under 18 or 21 years of age (the age of majority), depending on state law, are considered minor children, but they can legally give informed consent in the following circumstances:

- When they are minor parents of the child patient.
- When they are **emancipated minors** (economically self-supporting adolescents under 18 years of age, no longer living at home and not subject to parental control).
- When they are adolescents between 16 and 18 years of age seeking birth control, prenatal care, sexually transmitted infection care, mental health counseling, or substance abuse treatment (Anderson, Schaechter, & Brosco, 2005).
- Oregon permits minors of 15 years of age or older to give consent to hospital care, medical or surgical diagnosis, or treatment without the consent of the parent or guardian, and Alabama has a similar law for minors 14 years or older (Maradiegue, 2003).

Mature minors (14- and 15-year-old adolescents who are able to understand treatment risks) can give consent for treatment or refuse treatment in some states. In some cases the minor must convince a judge that he or she is mature enough to make an independent judgment about consent for treatment.

Children should become more actively involved in decision making about treatment procedures as their reasoning skills develop. **Assent**, the voluntary agreement to accept treatment or to participate in a research project, is the ability to have a basic understanding of what will be done, what is required for participation, and then agree or disagree with the proposed treatment or research. Children too young to give informed consent can be given age-appropriate information about their condition and asked about their care preferences. Their parents, however, make ultimate decisions regarding their care.

With regard to participation in research, federal guidelines state that children 7 years of age and older must receive developmentally appropriate information about a research project, their condition, and what they can expect with the tests and treatments before they give assent for enrollment in the study. If children disagree with participation, they dissent to the proposed treatment or research. Children should be given adequate time to ask questions and be told that they have the right to refuse to participate in the study. The child's refusal to participate should be respected (Hoehn & Nelson, 2004).

Child's Rights versus Parents' Rights

Parents or guardians have absolute authority to make choices about their child's health care except in the following cases:

- When the child and parents do not agree on major treatment options
- When the parents' choice of treatment does not permit lifesaving treatment for the child
- When there is a potential conflict of interest between the child and parents, such as with suspected child abuse or neglect

In cases when the child and parents do not agree on major treatment options, negotiation and compromise may be tried as a first step to avoid destruction of the family relationships. Medical consultation may be sought to identify other treatment options that might be acceptable to both the child and parents. An ethics committee usually becomes involved to help resolve the issue. In some cases, the court may be requested to appoint a proxy decision maker for the child or to determine that the child is capable of making a major treatment decision.

GROWTH & DEVELOPMENT

Consent Considerations

By 7 or 8 years of age, a child is able to understand concrete explanations about informed consent for research participation. By age 11 years, a child's abstract reasoning and logic are advanced. By age 14 years, an adolescent can weigh options and make decisions regarding consent as capably as an adult.

Confidentiality

The Health Insurance Portability and Accountability Act (HIPAA), P.L. 104-191, enacted by Congress in 1996, requires the confidential management of patient medical record data. The goal of the law is to protect the privacy of citizens by establishing standards for the management of confidential medical information. The rules developed for implementation of this law affect all persons who use medical and financial information in the healthcare system (Maradiegue, 2002). Each healthcare provider or organization has been required to develop policies to prevent the disclosure of protected health information. Patients have the right to control access to their health information (Maliszewski, 2003). Breaching confidentiality puts the nurse at risk for liability and legal action.

Confidentiality is an agreement between a patient and a provider that information discussed during the healthcare encounter will not be shared without the patient's permission. Concerns about privacy and the fear of disclosure of sensitive information to parents are a major reason why adolescents do not seek health care (Anderson, Schaechter, & Brosco, 2005). When the child is an emancipated or mature minor, most states permit healthcare providers to provide birth control, treatment for sexually transmitted infections including HIV, pregnancy and prenatal care, as well as mental health and substance abuse care without informing the child's parents (Anderson, Schaechter, & Brosco, 2005). However, state laws vary, and the nurse should know the state's law regarding confidentiality for emancipated minors. If the state law does not require the consent of the parent for the previous conditions, the consenting minor controls the healthcare decisions as well as the parent's access to the health information related to that care. However, the issue of minors giving consent is complicated by the healthcare system that holds the parents responsible for the financial costs of the healthcare services sought in confidence, and in some cases parents may get indirect information from health insurance bills. See Families Want to Know on page 20.

Patient Self-Determination Act

The federal Patient Self-Determination Act directs healthcare institutions to inform hospitalized patients about their rights, which include expressing a preference for treatment options and making **advance directives** (writing a living will or authorizing a durable power of attorney for healthcare decisions on the patient's behalf). Nurses often discuss these issues with patients and their families. Minor children and their parents should also be informed of their rights. Adolescents with serious acute or chronic conditions with a higher risk of death have a strong and legitimate interest in having a direct role in their healthcare decisions. They should be encouraged to talk with their parents about their healthcare wishes and to jointly prepare advance directives (Fletcher, 2004). Most state laws do not address the rights of minors to refuse treatment when treatment refusal will end in death (Zawistowski & Frader, 2003).

CLINICAL TIP

Breaching confidentiality is a potential problem for adolescents, who are just learning whom they can trust in the healthcare system. Make sure you openly discuss the limits of confidentiality for such things as mandatory reporting requirements with the patient and family. Inadvertent disclosure of personal information may lead to psychologic, social, or physical harm in some patients. If the child has a reportable disease, confidentiality may create a public health hazard. In such cases, the healthcare professional is obligated to report the presence of the disease to the appropriate state or county agency. Suspected cases of child abuse must be reported to the appropriate agency specified by state law.

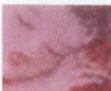

FAMILIES WANT TO KNOW

Providing Adolescents Confidentiality

Adolescents need a safe and confidential environment in which to discuss healthcare issues so that they seek health care when needed. Ways to promote confidentiality include the following actions:

- Assure that adolescents and parents talk separately to the healthcare provider about their concerns.
- Display and offer educational materials on confidentiality to adolescents and parents.
- Make sure all the doors are closed when collecting an adolescent's medical history or discussing sensitive issues.
- Ask if the adolescent is comfortable receiving messages and mail from the health professional using the contact information provided. If not, ask for alternate contact information for mail or phone messages.

- Create a comfortable atmosphere and environment for adolescents to discuss private concerns regarding their health.
- Make sure clinic literature distributed is small enough to fit into a purse or wallet.
- Make sure you and your health professional colleagues are fully informed about the laws in your state about the rights of adolescents to receive care without their parent's consent.
- Explain the parameters of confidentiality between you and the adolescent and his or her parents at the beginning of the healthcare visit.
- Discuss situations in which you need to breach confidentiality.

Adapted From: Simmons, M., Shalwitz, J., & Pollack, S. (2002). *Understanding confidentiality and minor consent in California: An adolescent provider toolkit.* San Francisco, CA: Adolescent Health Working Group, San Francisco Health Plan.

Do-Not-Resuscitate orders have become more common for children with terminal illnesses in which no further aggressive treatments are desired, but usual palliative and comfort care are provided. In many cases, these children are cared for at home or in a hospice program, but some still attend school. Implementation of Do-Not-Resuscitate orders for such children then becomes a community issue, to ensure that no resuscitation measures are initiated by any emergency care provider when the child has a life-threatening event. State health policies must be developed so children with these signed orders are easily identified and appropriate documentation of the orders is on file. See Chapter 14 ∞ for issues related to palliative and end-of-life care.

Ethical Issues

Ethics involves a rational process for considering all issues and determining the best course of action when there are conflicting choices (e.g., a **moral dilemma** or social value conflict) in the care of a patient. Ethics has become a prominent discipline because of significant developments (Mappes & DeGrazia, 2001):

- Because of major advances in medical research and resulting development of medical technology; for example, the ability to save the lives of severely impaired newborns, genetic testing, and gene therapy have resulted in challenges in making the best decision for the child and family.
- Health care is provided in an increasingly complex environment with multiple disciplines involved in patient care, consumer rights, managed care and the economic constraints associated with healthcare costs, and legal liability.

While decisions about care should be centered on what is best for the child, parents and healthcare providers collaborate in difficult decisions, and respect the family's and child's autonomy in decision making (Fleischman & Collogan, 2004). Ethical decision making is based on respect for persons and their ability to make decisions independently. Problems may develop because physicians, nurses, and parents have differing opinions about treatments for an infant or child with a serious or fatal condition.

Nurses often face ethical dilemmas when providing care to such a child. They witness parents struggling to decide among treatment options. Pediatric nurses have a responsibility to become knowledgeable about the moral and legal rights of their patients and families and to protect and support those rights. Nurses often initiate and partici-

CLINICAL TIP

No matter what decision parents make about their child's care they need to be reassured that they are trying to do what they think is the best thing for their child.

pate in discussions about the ethical issues involving their patients to effectively serve as the advocate for the child or family.

Approaches to ethical decision making take into account social-political philosophy, philosophy of law, moral philosophy, and moral theology as well as the concrete realities that medicine and biology contribute. An ethical framework for decision making is often used in healthcare institutions to guide individuals to determine an appropriate action. The four general ethical principles used in the development of a decision-making framework include (Silber & Batshaw, 2004):

- **Beneficence**—an obligation to act or to make a decision to benefit the patient, promoting the child's well-being in addition to working with parents and other family members
- Respect for patient's **autonomy**—right for self-determination or decision making, to protect the informed choices (consent and refusal) of patients capable of decision making
- **Nonmaleficence**—to prevent harm
- **Justice**—fairness in the use of scarce resources

A healthcare institution's ethics committee often serves the role of resolving conflicts about treatment decisions in one of the following ways:

- Performing individual case consultations
- Resolving a dispute between health professionals about the care to provide to a child
- Serving as a forum to discuss policies about institutional ethics
- Educating health professionals and the community about ethical concepts

An ethical consultation may be requested by healthcare providers as well as by the family. The committees often make treatment decisions using the process of data collection and evaluation outlined in Box 1–6. Courts should make ethical decisions only when healthcare professionals and parents are unable to agree about providing or withholding treatment.

> **BOX 1–6**
> ## STEPS IN ETHICAL PROBLEM SOLVING
>
> - Recognize that a potential or actual ethical dilemma exists
> - Collect as much information as possible:
>   - About the medical facts and the physician's goals
>   - About the child's and family's wishes or preferences
>   - About your values and beliefs
> - Identify if surrogate decision makers exist (i.e., court-appointed guardian)
> - State the dilemma as clearly as possible
> - Seek consultation on all possible courses of action or inaction
> - Identify the strengths and weaknesses of each therapeutic action
> - Identify the realistic expectations and benefits of each potential therapeutic action or inaction
> - Set goals and establish a decision-making process, and implement a plan of action
> - Evaluate the results

Withholding or Withdrawing Medical Treatment

Infant John, at 5 days of age, has a birth weight of 1200 grams, acute respiratory distress, and a severe intraventricular hemorrhage. See Figure 1–11 ➤. His physicians are seeking his parents' consent for surgical placement of a ventriculo-peritoneal shunt. Regardless of intensive medical care and planned surgical intervention, the infant is expected to have a severe handicap. The infant's condition is critical, and it is not certain how well the infant will respond to surgery. The parents, after much consideration and discussions with their family and pastor, have requested that comfort measures only be provided. They want life-sustaining treatment to be withheld, because they believe the additional procedures will cause excessive suffering for the infant, especially when the outcome is uncertain.

Parents are the recognized decision makers for infants, and they are entitled to full information about the risks and benefits of a procedure as well as the child's long-term prognosis. Factors important to parents in making their decision include the child's quality of life, degree of pain and suffering, likelihood of improvement, and physician recommendations (Sharman, Meert, & Sarnaik, 2005). Conflict may arise when parents choose to withhold therapy or request aggressive therapy on behalf of their child that differs from the healthcare providers' recommendations. The ethical principle of autonomy in making an informed decision is especially challenging when parents' rights to make such a decision is challenged by the healthcare system.

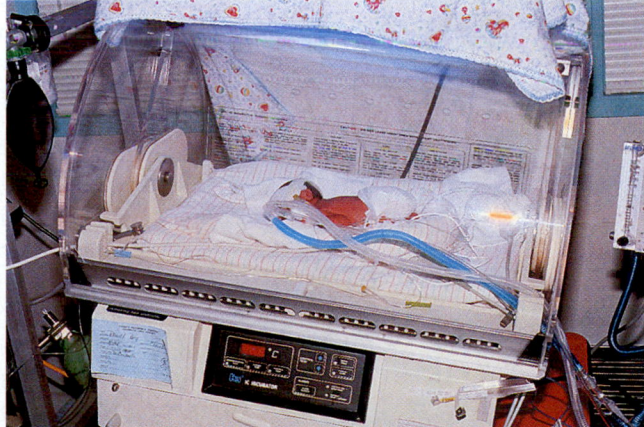

Figure 1–11 ➤ Due to technological advances that sustain life, parents must sometimes face difficult decisions. If an infant is certain to have severe handicaps, at what point should they decide to withhold or withdraw treatment?
Courtesy of Carol Harrigan, RNC, MSN, NNP.

Federal "Baby Doe" regulations were developed to protect the rights of infants with severe defects. When treatment has a reasonable chance of success and the infant will likely survive and be able to interact with the environment, even if burdened by a serious disability, the best interest of the infant is treatment (Silber & Batshaw, 2004). Physicians are not obligated to offer interventions that cause extreme pain and suffering when there is no or limited potential benefit. Treatments that only prolong life without improving quality of life are often considered to represent a misuse of expensive healthcare resources.

Genetic Testing of Children

With advances in genetics research, it is now possible to conduct genetic testing of infants for the presence of carrier status or the presymptomatic testing for a specific condition, such as Huntington disease or Duchenne muscular dystrophy. In some cases genetic testing can be performed to determine a child's predisposition to develop a condition, such as breast cancer (Ross, 2004). Often testing is possible for some conditions even when no definitive treatment for or prevention of the condition exists.

Important ethical issues are associated with genetic testing (Ross, 2004; Twomey, 2002). The benefits of screening when no therapy can be offered may include providing parents with information for future planning or reproductive decisions, or reducing anxiety.

- What is the potential risk (psychological harm, social stigma, discrimination in employment or insurance benefits) if an individual knows of the risk of developing a significant health condition or being a carrier of a health condition?
- Will parents seek unproven interventions for the child?
- Should newborn screening programs be mandatory or voluntary with informed consent required?

Genetic testing of children is a complex issue because of the different reasons for testing and the fact that decisions are made for children by parents. The strongest support for genetic testing occurs when the identification of a genetic condition will have a clear benefit to the child, such as initiation of early treatment. When children are old enough to understand, assent for genetic testing should be obtained and the child's decision should be honored.

Organ Transplantation Issues

The death of a child can benefit several other children through organ transplantation, and organ transplantation has become an accepted therapeutic option for some life-threatening conditions. The limited supply of organs has created numerous ethical issues. Which patients on the waiting list should receive the organs available? Should a patient with multiple congenital anomalies, disabilities, or abnormal chromosomes be eligible for a transplant? Should families be permitted to pay donor families for organs? Should the family's ability to pay for an organ transplant give a child higher priority for an organ? Should a patient receive a second organ transplant, replacing an organ deteriorating because of rejection? Should parents conceive another child hoping that the new baby is a potential stem cell donor for a child with an illness? If so, what pressures does this place on both children as they grow older? Each institution performing organ transplants develops guidelines for ethical decision making regarding these questions.

Research Issues

While legal issues regarding informed consent and assent for research have been discussed, there are additional ethical questions related to conducting research with children as subjects. Because of the ethical principles of beneficence and nonmaleficence, it is imperative that there be a risk-benefit ratio that is favorable to the individual child or to children in general. Harm must be considered from the perspective of the child and be sensitive to the child's reduced capacity to understand what is happening, and the effects of disruption, inconvenience, and novel situations on the child and family (Shevell, 2002). The potential for the treatment to influence the child differently than an adult due to developmental variation also must be considered.

SUMMARY

Many topics discussed in this chapter reflect the current challenges children and their families face in the healthcare system—access to health care, specific disease and injury risks, and ethical and legal concerns. Collaboration with parents and children is essential every step of the way:

- Obtaining informed consent and assent,
- Respecting that the parent is the expert with regard to the child's care,
- Acknowledging and supporting cultural values in the provision of care, and
- Preparing parents to assume ongoing complex healthcare responsibilities for their child.

Developing relationships with children and families is challenging, exciting, and ultimately gratifying for nurses who choose to specialize in pediatrics.

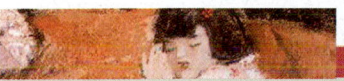

CRITICAL THINKING IN ACTION

EXAMINING THE SCOPE OF PEDIATRIC NURSING

Recall 3-year-old Manny, at the beginning of the chapter, who has a seizure disorder. He receives his care in a mobile van sent to his community by the local children's hospital. Manny has a regular source of care because his family income qualifies him for the State Child Health Insurance Program (SCHIP).

1. What health promotion and health maintenance services is Manny eligible for since the SCHIP in his state offers the same benefits as Medicaid?

2. Describe the different settings in which a child with a seizure disorder could receive health care.

3. List three specific injury prevention messages specific to Manny's age that should be provided to Manny's parents to reduce his risk for morbidity and mortality.

4. List specific steps that should be used in the healthcare setting to ensure that an error is avoided when prescribing Manny's seizure medication.

 Refer to your Prentice Hall Nursing MediaLink DVD-ROM for answers.

EXPLORE MediaLink 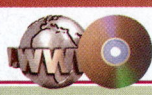 http://www.prenhall.com/ball

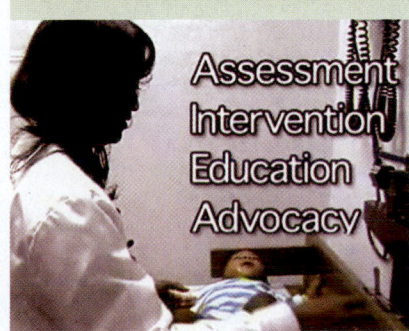

Resources for this chapter can be found on the Prentice Hall Nursing MediaLink DVD-ROM accompanying this textbook, and on the Companion Website at http://www.prenhall.com/ball.

DVD-ROM
Audio Glossary
NCLEX-RN® Review
Video
   The Role of the Pediatric Nurse

COMPANION WEBSITE
Audio Glossary
NCLEX-RN® Review
Case Study: Sickle Cell Crisis
Critical Thinking: Healthcare Settings
MediaLink Applications
   SCHIP
   Medicaid and SCHIP
WebLinks

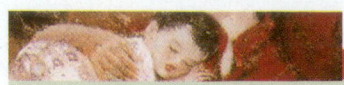

REFERENCES

Alfaro-LeFevre, R. (2004). *Critical thinking and clinical judgment*, (3rd ed). Philadelphia: W.B. Saunders, pp. 4–8.

American Nurses Association. (2004). *Scope and standards of practice*. Washington, DC: nursesbooks.org.

Anderson, R. N., & Smith, B. L. (2005). Deaths: Leading causes for 2002. *National Vital Statistics Reports*, 53(17). Hyattsville, MD: National Center for Health Statistics.

Anderson, S. L., Schaechter, J., & Brosco, J. P. (2005). Adolescent patients and their confidentiality: Staying within legal bounds. *Contemporary Pediatrics*, 22(7), 54–64.

Beidler, S. M., & Dickey, S. B. (2001). Children's competence to participate in healthcare decisions. *JONA's Healthcare Law, Ethics, and Regulation*, 3(3), 80–87.

Berger, J. E., and Committee on Medical Liability. (2003). Consent by proxy for nonurgent pediatric care. *Pediatrics*, 112(5), 1186–1195.

Burke, K. G. (2005). Executive summary: The state of the science on safe medication administration symposium. *American Journal of Nursing*, 105(3), 73–79.

DeFrances, C. J., Hall, M. J., & Podgornik, M. N. (2005, July 8). 2003 national hospital discharge survey, *Advance Data From Vital and Health Statistics, No. 359*. Hyattsville, MD: National Center for Health Statistics.

Federal Interagency Forum on Child and Family Statistics. (2005). America's children: Key national indicators of well-being 2005. Accessed August 10, 2005, from http://www.childstats.gov/americaschildren/index.asp

Fingerhut, L. (2005). Hospital discharges, ages 1 to 21 years, 2003. National Hospital Discharge Survey, unpublished data.

Fleischman, A. R., & Collogan, L. K. (2004). Addressing ethical issues in everyday practice. *Pediatric Annals*, 33(11), 740–745.

Fletcher, J. (2004). Adolescents and the Patient Self-Determination Act. *Pediatric Ethiscope*, 15(1). Washington, DC: Children's National Medical Center.

Flores, G., Laws, M. B., Mayo, S. J., Zuckerman, B., Abreu, M., Medina, L., & Hardt, E. J. (2003). Errors in medical interpretation and their potential clinical consequences in pediatric encounters. *Pediatrics*, 111(1), 6–14.

Guy, J., Persaud, J., Davies, E., & Harvey, D. (2003). Drug errors: What roles do nurses and pharmacists have in minimizing risk? *Journal of Child Health Care*, 7(4), 277–290.

Hoehn, K. S., & Nelson, R. M. (2004). Advising parents about children's participation in clinical research. *Pediatric Annals*, 33(11), 779–781.

Hoyert, D. L., Kung, H., & Smith, B. L. (2005). Deaths: Preliminary data for 2003. *National Vital Statistics Reports*, 53(15). Hyattsville, MD: National Center for Health Statistics.

Hughes, R. G., & Edgerton, E. A. (2005). First, do no harm: Reducing pediatric medication errors. *American Journal of Nursing*, 105(5), 79–92.

Kaushal, R., Bates, D. W., Landrigan, C., McKenna, K. J., Clapp. M. D., et al. (2001). Medication error and adverse drug events in pediatric patients. *Journal of the American Medical Association*, 285(16), 2114–2120.

Kenney, G., & Chang, D. I. (2004). The state children's health insurance program: Successes, shortcomings, and challenges. *Health Affairs*, 23(5), 51–62.

Levine, S. R., Cohen, M. R., Blanchard, N. R., Frederico, F., Magelli, M., Lomax, C., et al. (2001). Guidelines for preventing medication errors in pediatrics. *Journal of Pediatric Pharmacology and Therapeutics*, 6, 426–442.

Linnard-Palmer, L., & Kools, S. (2004). Parents' refusal of medical treatment based on religious and/or cultural beliefs: The law, ethical principles, and clinical implications. *Journal of Pediatric Nursing*, 19(5), 351–356.

Maliszewski, S. C. (2003). HIPAA privacy regulations. *Advance for Nurse Practitioners*, 11(1), 16.

Mappes, T. A., & DeGrazia, D. (2001). *Biomedical ethics* (5th ed.). Boston: McGraw Hill.

Maradiegue, A. (2002). The Health Insurance Portability and Accountability Act and adolescents. *Pediatric Nursing*, 28(4), 417–420.

Maradiegue, A. (2003). Minor's rights versus parental rights: Review of legal issues in adolescent healthcare. *Journal of Midwifery Womens Health*, 48(3), 170–177.

Melnyk, B. M. (2004). Integrating levels of evidence into clinical decision making. *Pediatric Nursing*, 30(4), 323–325.

Napolitano, L. M. (2005). Standardization of perioperative management: Clinical pathways. *Surgical Clinics of North America*, 85, 1321–1327.

National Center for Injury Prevention and Control. (2004). 10 leading causes of injury deaths, United States 2000–2002, all races, both sexes, accessed August 24, 2005, from http://webapp.cdc.gov/cgi-bin/broker.exe

Rhoades, J. A. (2005). Health insurance status of children in America, 1996–2004: Estimates for the U.S. civilian noninstitutionalized population under age 18, Statistical Brief #85, Rockville, MD: Agency for Healthcare Research and Quality, accessed October 28, 2005, from http://www.meps.ahrq.gov/papers/st85/stat85.pdf

Ross, L. F. (2004). Should children and adolescents undergo genetic testing? *Pediatric Annals*, 33(11), 762–769.

Satchell, M., & Pati, S. (2005). Insurance gaps among vulnerable children in the United States, 1999–2001. *Pediatrics*, 116(5), 1155–1161.

Sharman, M., Meert, K. L., & Sarnaik, A. P. (2005). What influences parents' decisions to limit or withdraw life support? *Pediatric Critical Care Medicine*, 6(5), 513–518.

Shevell, M. I. (2002). Ethics of clinical research in children. *Seminars in Pediatric Neurology*, 9(1), 46–52.

Silber, T., & Batshaw, M. L. (2004). Ethical dilemmas in the treatment of children with disabilities. *Pediatric Annals*, 33(11), 752–761.

Simmons, M., Shalwitz, J., & Pollack, S. (2002). *Understanding confidentiality and minor consent in California: An adolescent provider toolkit*. San Francisco, CA: Adolescent Health Working Group, San Francisco Health Plan.

Slonim, A., LaFleur, B. J., Ahmed, B. S., & Joseph, J. G. (2003). Hospital-reported medical errors in children. *Pediatrics*, 111(3), 617–621.

Twomey, J. G. (2002). Genetic testing of children: Confluence or collision between parents and professionals? *AACN Clinical Issues*, 13(4), 557–566.

U.S. Census. (2001). Population estimates for children by age and race. www.wonder.cdc/census

U.S. Department of Health and Human Services. (2000). *Healthy People 2010* (2nd ed.). Washington, DC: U.S. Government Printing Office.

Wong, S. T., Galbraith, A., Kim, S., & Newacheck, P. W. (2005, November). Disparities in the financial burden of children's healthcare expenditures. *Archives of Pediatric and Adolescent Medicine*, 159, 1008–1013.

Zawistowski, C. A., & Frader, J. E. (2003). Ethical problems in pediatric critical care: Consent. *Critical Care Medicine*, 31(5, suppl), S407–S410.

FAMILY-CENTERED CARE:
Theory and Application

2

KEY TERMS

adoption **42**
coping **47**
discipline **37**
ecomap **50**
family **26**
family
  adaptability **46**
family-centered
  care **27**
family cohesion **47**
family
  strengths **47**

foster care **40**
joint custody **31**
legal
  guardianship **42**
limit setting **34**
normalization **49**
parenting **34**
punishment **37**
resilience **48**

MediaLink

http://www.prenhall.com/ball

See the Prentice Hall Nursing MediaLink DVD-ROM and Companion Website for chapter-specific resources.

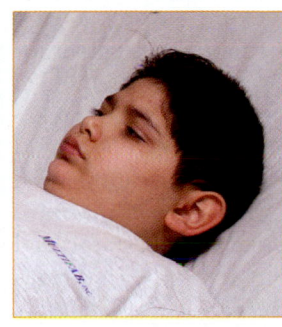

CASEY, a 16-year-old, is recuperating from injuries sustained in a motor vehicle crash in which he was the passenger. He was not wearing a seatbelt and experienced a brain injury after striking the windshield. His cognitive and motor functions are impaired. Following a 7-day acute care hospital stay, he was moved to an inpatient rehabilitation hospital where he has been for the past 5 days. He is much more responsive to stimuli and to family members 12 days after his injury. Physical therapy is provided twice a day to promote range of motion and muscle tone and to prevent contractures. Plans are being made to discharge him home with outpatient rehabilitation care within the next 5 days. A case manager will be assigned to coordinate his healthcare services.

Casey lives with his mother, two half-brothers (10 and 6 years old), and stepfather. Both his mother and stepfather are employed full time and are trying to determine how to manage care for Casey once he returns home. Casey's father has not been actively involved in his life since the divorce 12 years ago. Casey's grandparents reside in the same town and may provide some support to the family.

What family supports will Casey need as he continues his rehabilitation from the brain injury? What family assessment information is needed to effectively plan nursing care for this adolescent and his family? Does this family have strengths and coping strategies that will help them adapt to Casey's disability?

LEARNING OUTCOMES

After reading this chapter, you will be able to do the following:

1. Describe family-centered care and develop a nursing care plan for the child and family that integrates key concepts.

2. Describe characteristics of different types of families.

3. Identify four different parenting styles and analyze their impact on child personality development.

4. Describe the effect of major family changes on children, including divorce, gaining a stepparent, being placed in foster care, and adoption.

5. List the categories of family strengths that help families develop and cope with stressors.

6. Identify a variety of family support services that might be available in a community.

7. Delineate the advantages of using a family assessment tool.

8. Discuss nursing interventions for providing culturally sensitive and competent care to the child and family.

MediaLink

Defining Family Video

FAMILY AND FAMILY ROLES

The U.S. Census Bureau defines a **family** as individuals who are joined together by marriage, blood, adoption, or residence in the same household (Friedman, Bowden, & Jones, 2003). More broadly, however, a family may be a self-identified group of two or more persons joined together by sharing resources and emotional closeness. Family members can also include "honorary relatives" of the family, whether or not they are related by blood, marriage, or adoption, or even living in the same household. The family as defined by its members is likely to be dynamic, because membership often changes over time. For example, second marriages often integrate children into a newly formed family; and spouses of married children are integrated into an existing family while the newly married couple begins a new family. In today's world it is even more likely that families will live in different cities, states, or even countries than their extended families. So, there is no *typical* family (Figure 2–1 ➤).

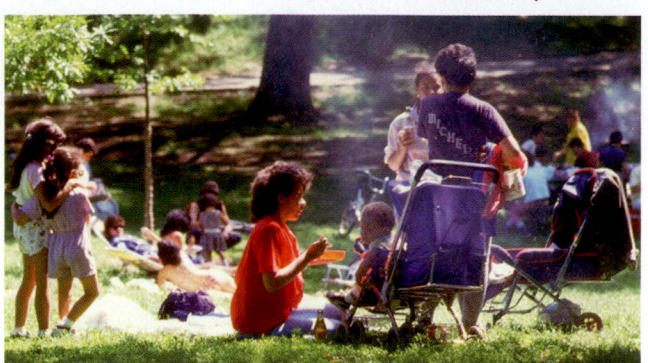

Figure 2–1 ➤ Families are diverse in their composition. In this case the extended family has gathered for a traditional holiday celebration.

Generally, family members depend upon each other for emotional, physical, and economic support. Families are guided by a common set of values or beliefs about the worth and importance of certain ideas and traditions. These values often bind family members together, and these values are greatly influenced by external factors including cultural background, social norms, education, environmental influences, socioeconomic status, and beliefs held by peers, coworkers, political and community leaders, and other individuals outside the family unit. Because of the influence of these external factors, a family's values may change considerably over the years, or members within a family may hold values that conflict with those of other family members.

A family is generally understood to be a safe haven for its members as they learn group values, norms, and acceptable behaviors. However, keep in mind that child abuse and neglect is a significant problem and can occur within any family configuration (see Chapter 6 ∞). Roles of the family include the following:

- Caring, nurturing, and educating children; teaching children how to get along in the world
- Maintaining the continuity of society by transmitting the family's knowledge, customs, values, and beliefs to children
- Receiving and giving love
- Preparing children to become productive members of society
- Meeting the needs of its members, including protection and economic support
- Serving as a buffer between its members and environmental and societal demands while advocating or addressing the interests and needs of the individual family members

Individual family members take on certain social and gender roles and hold a designated status within the family based on the values and beliefs that bind extended families together. These values and beliefs may evolve from the family's cultural values and practices, social norms, education, and other influences to which parents were exposed during childhood, adolescence, and early adult years. Parental roles, including childrearing practices and beliefs, are usually learned through a socialization process during childhood and adolescence.

Parents have important roles that involve childrearing and the long-term care of children until they reach adulthood. Depending upon their other roles in society, parents work to successfully nurture and rear children, helping them to meet role expectations. Parents must also meet the needs of the family unit and provide economic support for the family. Children also learn specific roles through a socialization process. Parents set expectations of behavior with discipline and modeling of appropriate behavior.

Ideally the family is a child's source of strength and support, the major constant in the child's life. Families are intimately involved in their children's physical and psychological well-being, and they play a vital role in the health promotion and health maintenance of their children. By respecting the family's role, strengths, and experiences with the healthcare system, nurses have an opportunity to develop an effective partnership with the child and family as they make healthcare decisions that promote the child's health. This partnership between nurses and families is known as family-centered care.

FAMILY-CENTERED CARE

Family-centered care is a philosophy of health care in which a mutually beneficial partnership develops between families and the nurse, and also other health professionals. In this way the priorities and needs of the family are addressed when the family seeks health care for the child. Each party respects the knowledge, skills, and experience that the other brings to the healthcare encounter. This is in contrast to family-focused care, in which health professionals provide care from the position of being the expert. In family-focused care the expert health professional directs care, tells the family what to do, and intervenes for the child and family as a unit.

History of Family-Centered Care

Family-centered care became integral to the nursing care of children when it was recognized that families had a significant role in promoting the psychosocial and developmental needs of children in the hospital. When parents were initially allowed to stay with hospitalized children, nurses and other health professionals noticed that children were quieter, happier, and recovering sooner. Research confirmed that children had decreased anxiety during procedures, needed less pain medication following surgery, and coped better during hospitalization (American Academy of Pediatrics, 2003). Eventually "rooming in" became a standard for hospital credentialing.

Gradually it became recognized that parental presence during certain medical procedures, and sometimes resuscitation, was also beneficial to children and their families (Lewandowski & Tesler, 2003, pp. 28–32). Parents are now invited to participate in patient conferences, serve on hospital advisory committees, and help educate health professionals about how to improve family-centered care (Figure 2–2 ➤).

Nurses have long embraced the family-centered care philosophy, and it is becoming more widely accepted by other health professionals, including pediatricians (American Academy of Pediatrics, 2003). The Society of Pediatric Nurses and the American Nurses Association have developed nursing practice guidelines for family-centered care. See Table 2–1.

Promoting Family-Centered Care

Collaborating with families in the provision of health care is essential to promote the best outcome when caring for children. Families have important knowledge to share about their child, their child's health condition, and how their child responds to various actions and events. They also need access to information that will make it possible for them to fully participate in planning and decision making.

Parents often need to assess their strengths in managing their ongoing family and caregiving responsibilities before planning how to add more caregiving responsibilities

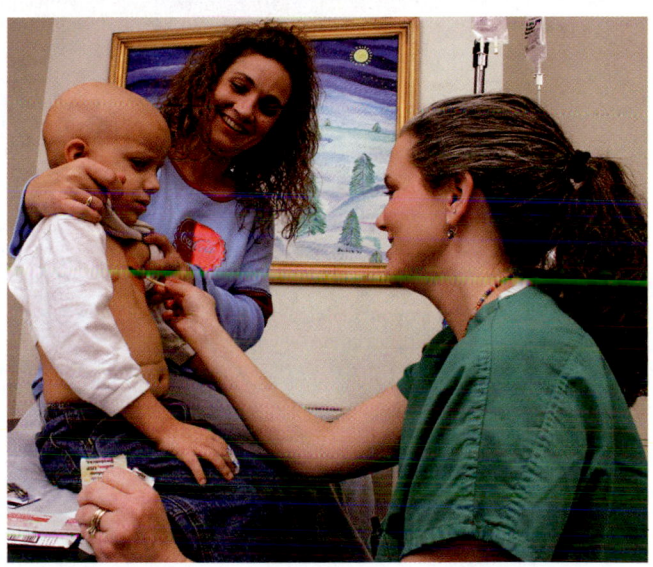

Figure 2–2 ➤ Health facility policies that permit a parent to be present during a procedure performed on a child are an example of a family-centered care policy. The parent plays an important role in providing security and comfort to this child who is having his port accessed for an IV infusion treatment.

CLINICAL TIP

Some healthcare facilities are developing family resource centers to provide consumer information and support. In most cases, the resource center is a consumer-oriented health library with staffing, but peer support services may also be coordinated through the center as well (Institute for Family Centered Care, 2004). Families can be supported to access useful information that helps them to become informed participants in decision making about their child's care. Resources can often be provided in the preferred language and appropriate reading level.

Table 2–1	ELEMENTS OF FAMILY-CENTERED CARE AND RECOMMENDATIONS FOR NURSING PRACTICE

Elements	Nursing Practice Recommendations
The Family at the Center: Incorporate into policy and practice the recognition that the family is the constant in a child's life, while the service systems and support personnel within those systems fluctuates, and that the illness or injury of a child affects all members of the family system.	• Establish a therapeutic relationship with the family. • Perform a comprehensive family assessment in collaboration with the family, identifying both strengths and needs. • Use the family assessment when working with the family to plan, implement, and evaluate care, considering the impact of the child's illness or injury on the entire family, with special attention to the siblings. • Provide siblings with information about their sibling's illness/injury at an appropriate developmental level and answer questions honestly. • Promote sibling visitation in hospital settings and participation in home care activities. • Identify extended family members who should receive information and be included in the educational process.
Family-Professional Collaboration: Facilitate family professional collaboration at all levels of hospital, home, and community care for: • Care of an individual child • Program development, implementation, evaluation, and evolution • Policy formation	• Develop provider-family relationships that are guided by goals and expectations of both the family and the provider. • Assure that parents are integral and critical collaborators in the decision-making process about their child's care. Involve children and adolescents in the decision-making process as appropriate for their cognitive and emotional development. • Assure parents 24-hour access to their children and facilitate their participation in the child's care. • Provide parents with the option to stay with their child during procedures and tests, and provide ways for the parent to support the child during the procedure. • Provide comfort and hygiene facilities for families who spend long hours at the facility or travel great distances. • Promote the family's development of expertise in the special care of their child, fostering family independence and empowerment. • Incorporate parents and children into the quality assessment/improvement process. • Integrate family members into institutional and community advisory groups and in policy development.
Family-Professional Communication: Exchange complete and unbiased information between families and professionals in a supportive manner at all times.	• Provide information about the child's problem, prognosis, and needs in a manner that respects the child and family as individuals and promotes two-way dialogue. • Encourage the family to share information about the child and the illness/injury so that care planning and decisions are made in the most informed and collaborative manner.
Cultural Diversity of Families: Incorporate into policy and practice the recognition and honoring of cultural diversity, strengths, and individuality within and across all families, including ethnic, racial, spiritual, social, economic, educational, and geographic diversity.	• Practice family-centered care in a culturally competent manner with respect and sensitivity for the wide range of families with diverse values and beliefs. • Seek to understand the family's beliefs and practices related to race, culture, and ethnicity when developing relationships and collaborating in the child's health care. • Seek to understand and respect the family's religious/spiritual beliefs and practices and integrate these into the child's care, as the family desires. • Assist the family to address care issues related to socioeconomic status, insurance status, geography, and access to health care. • Integrate training programs on diversity, cultural understanding, and culturally competent care into staff development programs.
Coping Differences and Support: Recognize and respect different methods of coping. Implement comprehensive policies and programs that provide families with the developmental, educational, emotional, spiritual, environmental, and financial supports needed to meet their diverse needs.	• Assess the strengths and weaknesses of the family's coping strategies and their resiliency factors and characteristics. Identify maladaptive coping mechanisms and assist the family to augment their coping efforts. • Assess and support the family's needs and desires for support and assist the family in accessing and accepting assistance from support networks as needed or desired.
Family-Centered Peer Support: Encourage and facilitate family-to-family support and networking.	• Educate parents about parent-to-parent and family support resources and assist them to access such resources in the institution and community. • Provide access to psychoeducational groups that might be useful to parents, siblings, or ill/injured children.
Specialized Service and Support Systems: Ensure that hospital, home, and community service and support systems for children needing specialized health and developmental care and their families are flexible, accessible, and comprehensive in responding to diverse family-identified needs.	• Provide collaborative, flexible, accessible, comprehensive, and coordinated services to children and their families. • Provide comprehensive case management/care coordination for children and families with on-going care needs. • Along with families, take an active role in advocating for the needs of ill and injured children.
Holistic Perspective of Family-Centered Care: Appreciate families as families and children as as children, recognizing that they possess a wider range of strengths, concerns, emotions, and aspirations beyond their need for specialized health and developmental services and support.	• Encourage attention to the normal developmental needs and developmental tasks of the entire family unit and individual family members. • Encourage and facilitate the development of individual and family identities beyond a focus on illness or injury. • Facilitate "normalization" as valued and desired by the family.

Reprinted with permission from the American Nurses Association and Society of Pediatric Nurses, *Family-centered care: Putting it into action.* © 2003. Nursesbooks.org, Silver Spring, MD.

to their routine. Strategies that the nurse and parents collaboratively develop for the child's care must mesh with the family's cultural and ethnic illness-related behaviors, experiences, and beliefs (Sullivan-Bolyai, Sadler, Knafl et al., 2004). The child's opinions should also be integrated in the strategies for care. In almost all cases, the child leaves the healthcare setting and the family assumes responsibility for provision of needed care in the home. The family caregivers must not feel alienated from a healthcare system they need for continuing assistance. See Families Want to Know: Guidelines for Effective Collaboration below.

Family involvement is also valuable in the development of policies and guidelines for family-centered care in all types of healthcare settings. Their experiences while receiving care in the healthcare setting may reveal valuable insights, perspectives, and realities that could lead to improved quality of care and satisfaction with care. Examples of feedback that could be provided include the following: how comfortable they felt in the setting, if provided information was understood, and what attitudes they sensed from health professionals (Hanson & Randall, 1999). Parents who have been supported to develop leadership skills can be empowered to serve on advisory boards or councils and represent the family and community perspective. Guidelines for working with families as advisors and tools for assessing the family-centered policies in various healthcare settings are available from the Institute of Family-Centered Care.

Parents can also serve a valuable role in family-to-family support networks by serving as mentors to new families entering the healthcare system for a new chronic condition. Parents may also help raise awareness about specific healthcare issues, serve as advocates for public policy issues, and assist with fundraising activities.

FAMILY COMPOSITION

Families are diverse in structure, roles, and relationships. Various types of families—both those considered traditional and nontraditional—exist in contemporary American society. The following list identifies common types of family structure.

Nuclear Family

In the nuclear family, children live with both biological parents, and no other relatives or persons live in the household. One parent may stay home to rear the children while the other parent works, but more commonly, both parents are employed by choice or necessity. Two-income families must address important issues such as childcare

---

CULTURE

Family-Centered Care

When working to establish a family-centered relationship with families of various ethnic groups, consider the possibility that an extended family may need to be consulted. For example, Native Americans may consult tribal elders (considered part of the extended family) before agreeing to health care for their child. In some Hispanic cultures, major decisions for the child's health care include input from grandparents and other extended family members. It is important for the nurse to learn more about the strengths of the family network to better assist the family in planning the child's care at home (Ochieng, 2003).

CLINICAL TIP

When providing care to children, recall that the family is central to all healthcare interventions with parents and child as the partners in care. It is important to consider how a healthcare setting's written policies, procedures, and literature for families refer to families and what attitudes these materials convey. Words like *policies, allowed,* and *not permitted* imply that hospital personnel have authority over families in matters concerning their children. Words like *guidelines, working together,* and *welcome* communicate an openness and appreciation for families in the care of their children.

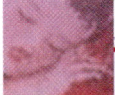

FAMILIES WANT TO KNOW

Guidelines for Effective Collaboration

Parents have a role in developing an effective collaborative relationship with nurses and other health professionals. Parents often become experts in their child's health condition, and learn to advocate for their child. They also must learn to communicate effectively with the health professionals caring for their child, and in the process develop a trusting relationship.

Tips for improved communication include the following (Allshouse & Goldberg, 2003):

- Keep a journal that includes your observations about your child's behavior, eating habits, illness, temperature, or anything else that might be helpful to the healthcare providers caring for your child.
- Keep a copy of your child's medical records, including test and procedure results.
- Write out questions and do not hesitate to ask for clarification if you don't understand an answer provided.

- Be realistic about what you can expect from your child's nurses and doctors. They cannot solve all your problems or answer all your questions. They also can become frustrated at times by the child's condition or lack of answers to questions. Try to let your healthcare providers know you appreciate their time and efforts on behalf of your child.

Communication tips for nurses include:

- Provide information and honestly discuss issues of concern to both the family and healthcare providers.
- Creatively problem solve and identify options for needed care that conform to the family's values and functioning.
- Demonstrate respect for the family's choices and methods for providing needed care.
- Continue to collaborate with the child and family and be willing to continue problem solving as new issues arise.

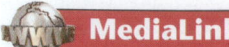
MediaLink

Institute of Family-Centered Care

arrangements, household chores, and how to assure quality family time. Important nursing considerations include:

- Respecting a parent who stays home to rear the children while appreciating the value of childrearing.
- Helping parents to develop strategies to assure that the child's health promotion needs are met, such as a nutritious diet with appropriate calories and adequate physical exercise.

Blended or Reconstituted Family

This type of nuclear family includes two parents with biological children from a previous marriage or relationship who marry or cohabitate. This family structure has become increasingly common because of high rates of divorce and remarriage. Potential advantages to the children may include better financial support and a new supportive role model. Stressors that can cause challenges in forming a cohesive family unit may include lack of a clear role for or acceptance of the stepparent, financial stresses when two families must be supported by stepparents, and communication problems. Parents in the blended family also may have difficulties overcoming differences in parenting styles, discipline strategies, and values. Important nursing considerations include directing families to resources that may help reduce the potential conflicts associated with different parenting styles, discipline, and manipulative behaviors by children that can develop with the blended family. See the discussion on page 44 regarding stepparenting.

Another type of blended family is two parents with adoptive or foster children, sometimes including biological children. Many parents choose adoption because of infertility. In other cases, a couple or single adult chooses to adopt a child or take in foster children for personal, religious, or family reasons. The adoptive or foster parent is often a relative of the child. See the discussion beginning page 45 regarding foster care and adoption.

Extended Family

Extended families exist when one parent or a couple shares expenses as well as household and childrearing responsibilities with grandparents, the sibling of a parent, or other relatives. According to the U.S. Bureau of the Census, 4.1 million children live in an extended family with at least one parent and usually a grandparent (U.S. Census Bureau, 2002). This type of family is common in recent immigrant families as well as working class families. For example, in a multigenerational (three generations in the same household) family living arrangement, the grandparents may be invited to live in the family home, or the family moves into the grandparents' home on a temporary basis. Families may reside together to share housing expenses and childcare. However, in many cases, the child may be residing with the grandparent and one parent because of issues associated with unemployment, parental separation, parental death, or parental substance abuse. Grandparents may raise children due to the inability of parents to care for children. Grandparents endure emotional, physical, and financial stresses when taking on the childrearing role of one or more grandchildren (Figure 2–3 ➤).

Another example of an extended family is the extended relative network family in which two nuclear families of primary relatives or unmarried relatives live in close proximity to each other. The family shares a social support network in which chores, goods, and services are exchanged. This type of family model is common in the Latino community.

Single-Parent Family

The family of a single parent is formed when the mother or father is widowed, divorced, abandoned, or separated. According to the 2000 Census, of the 11.3 million single-parent families with children under 18 years in the United States, approximately 30% are single-father families (Annie E. Casey Foundation, 2004). Single-mother households make up 7% of all U.S. households (Council on Contemporary Families, 2003). In 2000, 26.7% of children less than 18 years lived with a single parent, and almost one in ten children lived with a never-married parent (Lugaila & Overturf, 2004; U.S. Department of

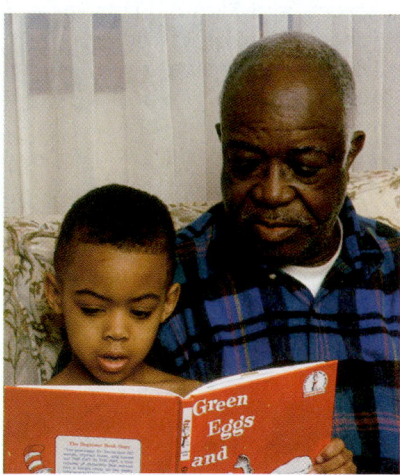

Figure 2–3 ➤ This child lives with his mother and grandparents following the divorce of his parents. The special attention provided by his grandfather is helping him to adapt to the change in his family, and it enables the mother to work, feeling confident that her son is safely cared for before and after school.

Health and Human Services, 2001). Reasons for the increasing rate of single-parent families include the following (Friedman, Bowden, & Jones, 2003):

- High rates of divorce
- The large amount of financial aid to one-parent families with dependent children
- The loss of stigma associated with unwed motherhood
- The growth in number of births to never-married mothers

Single-parent families often face difficulties because the sole parent may lack social and emotional support, need assistance with childrearing issues, and face financial strain. Single-parent families experience higher rates of poverty, which has important implications for the children (Denham, 2005). Depending upon social support and family resources, the single parent may be stressed from working to support the family, household responsibilities, serving as both mother and father, and attempting to have a personal life. Single mothers are often impoverished due to lack of child support, inequitable pay for work performed, work skill deficiencies, and cutbacks in social welfare programs. Important nursing considerations for working with single parents is to assess their strengths and needs in providing care to the child, such as afterschool and back-up childcare arrangements that enable the parent to fulfill work commitments (Figure 2–4 ➤). Determine if the child has access to all resources available to support growth and development, such as school breakfast and lunch programs that provide nutritional support.

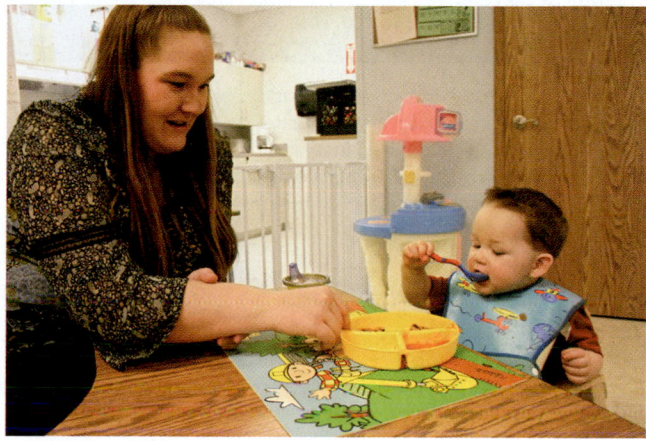

Figure 2–4 ➤ Adolescents often become single parents and face challenges balancing school, personal time, and care of the infant.

Binuclear Family

In a post-divorce family the biological children can be members of two nuclear households, with co-parenting by the father and the mother. The children alternate between the two homes, spending varying amounts of time with both parents in a situation called co-parenting, usually involving joint custody. **Joint custody** is a legal situation in which both parents have equal responsibility and legal rights, regardless of where the children live. The binuclear family is a model for effective communication. It enables both biological parents to be involved in a child's upbringing and provides additional support and role models from extended family members. Special nursing considerations in this family type involve assuring that health promotion guidance and education for care of the child with an acute or chronic condition are communicated effectively to both biological parents.

Heterosexual Cohabitating Family

In this family type, a heterosexual couple that may or may not have children lives together outside of marriage. This may include never-married individuals as well as divorced or widowed persons. According to the 2000 U.S. Census, approximately 2.9 million children under 18 years of age live with a parent and unmarried partner (Peterson, 2003). Biological children may result from the relationship, or in some cases children of one parent are present and help form a blended type of cohabitating family. Special concerns exist regarding the increased likelihood of the couple separating— approximately 50% in 5 years versus 20% for married couples (Peterson, 2003). These families are more unstable for the children because of the disruption associated with separation (American Academy of Pediatrics Task Force on the Family, 2003). An important nursing consideration for children who live in informal stepfamilies is that the nonbiological parent has no legal authority to seek emergency medical care for the child. However, in the case of a true emergency that could result in loss of life or diminished functioning, health professionals are obligated to provide care and obtain consent as soon as possible afterwards. The nonbiological parent also may not have any knowledge of the child's medical history.

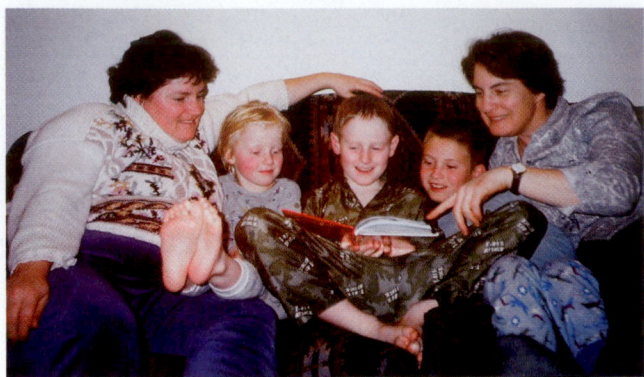

Figure 2–5 ➤ No evidence exists to indicate that children raised in a homosexual family are at any greater developmental risk or dysfunction than a child raised in a heterosexual family (Ariel & McPherson, 2000). These parents are as firmly dedicated as heterosexual families to promoting the growth and development of their children.

Gay and Lesbian Family

A gay or lesbian family involves two adults of the same sex who live together as domestic partners with or without children, or a gay or lesbian single parent rearing a child. Children in these families may be from a previous heterosexual union, or be born to or adopted by one or both member(s) of the same-sex couple. For example, a biological child may be born to one of the partners through artificial insemination or through a surrogate mother. According to the 2000 U.S. Census, 96% of all U.S. counties have at least one gay or lesbian couple with children under 18 years in the household (Urban Institute, 2003a).

Lesbian and gay couples function much like heterosexual couples, and children who are adopted or born into the family are highly valued (Figure 2–5 ➤). Small studies that have evaluated children reared by same-sex couples found no significant differences in childrearing or in the children's adjustment from children reared in other types of families. These children have been found to have the same advantages and expectations for health, adjustment, and development as children born into heterosexual families (American Academy of Pediatrics, 2002a). Lesbian and gay parents are believed to be as effective as heterosexual couples in providing a supportive and healthy environment for their children (American Psychological Association, 2004).

Children in these families sometimes have only one biological or adoptive legal parent. The other partner is the co-parent and has no legal parental status in the majority of states. Only seven states (California, Connecticut, Massachusetts, New Jersey, New York, Pennsylvania, Vermont) and the District of Columbia have considered legislative actions to ensure the security of children whose parents are gay or lesbian by guaranteeing access to the second-parent of joint adoption rights (Urban Institute, 2003a). Co-parent adoption would help maintain the child's rights to a continuing relationship if the legal parent dies or becomes incapacitated, or if the parents separate. Either parent could then provide consent for health care and make other important decisions on behalf of the child. Financial support of the child is more assured if one parent dies or parents separate. Nursing considerations in this type of family involve respect for the relationship between partners and recognition of the nurturing capacity in these families.

> ### NURSING ALERT
>
> It is important to identify the biological or adoptive parent, or a caregiver's legal documentation proving the right to medical decision making, when obtaining consent for the child's health care.

> ### LAW & ETHICS
>
> **Medical and Family Leave Act**
> Eligible parents of newborns and adopted children are entitled to 12 weeks of unpaid leave during any 12-month period initially authorized under the federal Medical and Family Leave Act of 1993. Vacation or sick leave may often be used to pay for time away from work. This act also applies if a child, spouse, or parent of the employee develops a serious health condition. The employee is entitled to return to the previous position or an equivalent position with all the same pay, benefits, and other conditions (Family and Medical Leave, 1999).

FAMILY FUNCTIONING
Transition to Parenthood

Choosing to become a parent is a major life change for adults. Couples experience significant family and cultural pressure to have a child. Mothers may be eager to have a child, but be concerned about fulfilling all of the expectations of others (father, the baby, other children, her parents, close friends, and employer). Fathers anticipate increased responsibility and are concerned about their ability to provide adequate support for the family.

At the time of birth the parents experience stresses and challenges along with feelings of pride and excitement. Mothers and fathers both make adjustments to their lifestyles to give priority to parenting. The baby is dependent for total care 24 hours a day and this often results in sleep deprivation, irritability, less personal time, and less time for the couple's relationship. In addition, the family often experiences a change in financial status.

Several factors influence how well the parents adjust to their new role. Social support provided to the mother, especially by the father, is important for the mother's adjustment. Marital happiness during pregnancy is an important adjustment factor for both parents. Infants with significant health conditions or those with difficult temperaments can cause extra stress for the parents and affect their adjustment to the parenting role.

With the birth of the first child, mothers and fathers both have challenges related to renegotiating their employment to accommodate family and childcare time. Fathers are sometimes additionally challenged to develop closeness with the infant and to learn how to care for the infant, especially when they may not have had role models or any childcare experience. Most parents find that caring for infants and children takes more time than anticipated.

Nurses can help parents through this important transition by listening to the challenges described by the parents during the infant's first health visits. Encourage fathers as well as mothers to attend and participate in health promotion visits with the healthcare provider so that positive parenting can be supported. Answer questions and offer ideas to address described problems that the parents may be too tired to solve on their own. Help them recognize that frustrations and feelings they have regarding the challenges of infant care are normal. Encourage both parents to become active in caring for the infant and to gain comfort in that care. Help each parent find activities that they enjoy with regard to infant care to encourage interaction and bonding with the infant.

Parental Influences on the Child

The qualities of family relationships and of family behaviors are important aspects of family strengths and family functioning. Positive family relationships are characterized by parent-child warmth and supportiveness. Warm parent-child relationships can buffer children from stress and promote positive cognitive and social outcomes. Parents who are warm and place high demands on their children for appropriate behavior have children who tend to be content, self-reliant, self-controlled, and open to learning in school.

Mothers and fathers each contribute to the psychological, emotional, and social health and development of their children. Both parents provide affection, nurturing, and comfort. They teach children life skills and healthy lifestyles. Fathers play an important role in the sexual identity and gender role development of their children. They promote the social competence, academic achievement, and problem-solving abilities of their children (American Academy of Pediatrics, 2004).

Family Size

The size of the family influences the amount of attention given to children. In small families parents often have more time to give attention to the children, to encourage achievement, to meet family expectations, and to support involvement in community activities. Children in larger families are encouraged to be cooperative to support family functioning. The child usually receives less personal attention from the parents and often turns to others in the family to get needed support. Family finances may be more limited. Children may adopt a specialized family role to gain recognition, such as the "responsible one," "the clown," or "the black sheep."

Sibling Relationships

Siblings are the first peers of a child and often have a life-long relationship lasting up to 70 or more years. Siblings, especially those of the same gender, who are closer in age tend to have a closer relationship because they often share many common experiences through childhood and adolescence. In general, the parents have greater influence than siblings on children who are more widely spaced in age. However, the older sibling may be a very strong role model for younger siblings.

Sibling rivalry exists between children at times in all families. Within the family children learn to share, compete, and compromise with siblings. Some siblings take on roles such as protector, problem solver, friend, and supporter for dealing with issues in the family and in the environment. Some siblings learn to work well together to maintain privacy or to form a coalition for negotiating with the parents. An older sibling helps reinforce rules and roles in the family by prompting and inhibiting certain patterns of behavior in the younger siblings. However, one sibling may test the waters by breaking a previously implicit rule to determine what rule flexibility is allowed in the family (Figure 2–6 ▶).

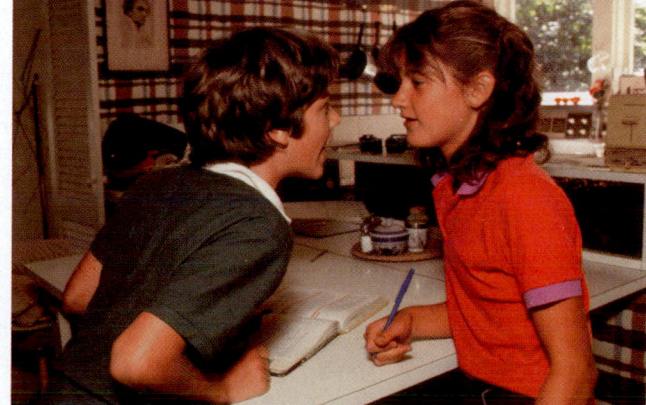

Figure 2–6 ▶ Siblings often argue with each other over possessions or perceived slights.

Children develop different personalities because of a need to establish distinct identities for themselves and be seen as unique in the family. It has not been possible to reproduce earlier research findings that birth order was associated with specific personality traits of individual children in a family (Craig & Baucum, 2002). Siblings may share some experiences, but they are often exposed to different environmental experiences that help shape their personalities (Craig & Baucum, 2002). First-born children do have some advantages, such as more favorable treatment in the family. First-born children do have slightly higher IQs and greater achievement in school and in their careers (Craig & Baucum, 2002). Their intellectual development may be enhanced through experiences of teaching their younger siblings.

CULTURE

Family Structure and Roles

A family's structure and roles are largely dependent upon cultural influence. For example, culture may determine who has authority (head of household) and is the primary decision maker for other members of the family. Sometimes the decision-maker role varies by the type of decisions to be made. For example, in some cultures such as Hispanic, decisions regarding the health care of children are primarily the responsibility of the female, while other decisions are male dominated. Family dominance patterns may be *patriarchal*, as may be seen in Appalachian cultures; *matriarchal*, as may be seen in African American cultures; or more *egalitarian*, as may be seen in European-American cultures.

PARENTING

The family is an important component in the lives of all children, and it plays an essential role in fostering the development of infants, children, and youth. A significant concept in families is that of parenting. **Parenting** is a leadership role in the family in which children are guided to learn acceptable behaviors, beliefs, morals, and rituals of the family and to become socially responsible contributing members of society. The manner in which children are parented, in combination with their individual personality traits and characteristics, influences their developmental outcomes.

Parents have responsibility for providing stability to children with nurturance, safety, and structure in a family that undergoes frequent changes over time. The child needs to have physical and emotional space to grow and develop. This space enables the child to personally find the relationship balance between closeness and distance, as well as safety and risk. Parents also provide their children with the values, beliefs, rituals, and behaviors learned and transmitted across family generations. To be successful in parenting, parents must have a certain flexibility that enables the family to adapt and adjust to family changes with time and other significant stressors and challenges.

To be successful, parents should implement reasonable **limit setting** (established rules or guidelines for behavior) on children's autonomy, while they learn values and self-control. Yet at the same time, parents need to foster the child's curiosity, initiative, and sense of competence. Parents use different styles to parent their children. Parental warmth and control are two major factors that are important in the development of children. Parental warmth refers to the amount of affection and approval displayed. Parental control refers to how restrictive the parents are regarding rules. See Table 2–2 for the characteristics associated with parental warmth and control.

Table 2–2	CHARACTERISTICS OF SIGNIFICANT PARENTING ATTRIBUTES	
Parenting Attribute	**Parental Warmth**	**Parental Control**
High level	Warm, nurturing	Restrictive control of behavior
	Express affection and smile at children frequently	Survey and enforce compliance with rules
	Limit criticism, punishment	Encourage children to fulfill their responsibilities
	Express approval of child	May limit freedom of expression
Low level	Cool, hostile	Permissive, minimally controlling
	Quick to criticize or punish	Make fewer demands
	Ignore children	Fewer restrictions on behavior or expression of emotion
	Rarely express affection or approval	Permit freedom in exploring environment
	Rejection may be seen	

Diana Baumrind (1971), an important contemporary child developmentalist, proposed classifications of parenting styles that are still well accepted today. She identified three main types of parenting styles (*authoritarian*, *authoritative*, and *permissive*) and described the influences each style has on children. One additional parenting style, called *indifferent*, exists in some families. While families will generally tend to use one style, they may vary their style for certain situations. See Table 2–3 for characteristics or parenting styles by warmth and control and associated child outcomes.

Authoritarian Parents

Authoritarian parents tend to be punitive and adhere to rigid rules, or be more dictatorial. Parents who use this style might say, "Because I'm your parent, that's why," "A rule is a rule," or "Just do what I say." While this style sets firm limits, those limits or rules are not negotiable or open to any discussion. Parents expect family beliefs and principles to be accepted without question. Children have no opportunity to participate in the family decision-making process. Children with authoritarian parents do not develop the skills to examine why a certain behavior is desirable or how their actions might influence others.

Authoritative Parents

Authoritative parents use firm control to set limits, but they establish an atmosphere with open discussion, or are more democratic. Limits for behavior are clear and reasonable, but the child is encouraged to talk about why certain behaviors occurred and how the situations might be handled differently another time. Parents provide explanations about inappropriate behaviors at the child's level of understanding. Children are allowed to express their opinions and objections, and some flexibility is permitted when appropriate. However, parents make it clear that they are the ultimate authority for decisions. Children with authoritative parents develop a sense of social responsibility since they converse about their responsibilities and approaches.

Table 2–3	PARENTING STYLES BY LEVEL OF WARMTH AND CONTROL		
Parenting Style	**Warmth/Control**	**Behavior of Parents**	**Child Outcomes**
Authoritarian	High control Low warmth	Highly controlling, issues commands and expects them to be obeyed Little communication with children, avoids lengthy verbal discussions with children Inflexible rules Permits little independence	No negotiation skills No ability to direct and initiate own activities Frustrated in efforts to achieve autonomy May become fearful, withdrawn, and unassertive Girls often passive and dependent during adolescence Boys often rebellious and aggressive
Authoritative	Moderately high control High warmth	Sets reasonable limits on behavior Accepts and encourages growing autonomy of children Open communication with children Flexible rules	More willingly accept restrictions Tend to be more self-reliant, self-controlled, and socially competent Higher self-esteem Better school performance
Permissive	Low control High warmth	Few or no restraints Unconditional love Communication flows from child to parent Much freedom and little guidance No limit setting	Often unable to cooperate and negotiate with others May become rebellious, aggressive, or socially inept, self-indulgent, or impulsive May have difficulty being accepted by peers or being accepted and effective in a work setting May be creative, active, and outgoing
Indifferent	Low control Low warmth	No limit setting Lack affection for children Parents focused on stress in own life Parents may show hostility or neglect	Often have the worst outcomes such as destructive impulses and delinquent behavior

Adapted From: Craig, G. J., & Baucum, D. (2002). *Human development* (9th ed.). Upper Saddle River, NJ: Prentice Hall, pp. 303–304.

Permissive Parents

Permissive parents show a great deal of warmth, but set few controls or restraints on the child's behavior. Parents are so intent on showing unconditional love that they fail in performing some important parenting functions. Children are allowed to regulate their own behavior. Discipline is inconsistent and parents may threaten punishment but not follow through. Both extremes result in excessive permissiveness, and the child does not learn socially acceptable limits of behavior. As the parent does not impose any controls on the child, the child ends up controlling the parents.

Indifferent Parents

Indifferent parents do not display much interest in their children or in their roles as parents. They do not demonstrate affection or approval of the children, and they do not set limits or controls on the children. This may occur because they don't care, or because their lives are so stressed that there is no time or energy left for the children (Craig & Baucum, 2002).

Parent Adaptability

Parents who are able to adapt their behavior to meet the needs of children at different developmental stages are also more effective. Eleanor Maccoby (1980) expanded upon Diana Baumrind's perspectives on parenting style by examining how parents and children interact during the parenting process. Parenting styles may change as the child grows older. For example, parents may use negotiation to help the child develop problem-solving skills and to learn how to compromise and get along with others. This enables the child to have more self-control and self-responsibility over time. Parents and some children can develop shared goals and jointly participate in decision making while other children require constant negotiation for decision making. See Families Want to Know: Guidelines for Promoting Acceptable Behavior in Children.

Assessing Parenting Styles

Nurses assess parenting styles by asking families how they handle situations that require limit setting. As previously described, an authoritative style is preferred because of its positive outcomes for child behavior and learning. The nurse in all settings is often in a position to discuss parenting styles and to offer suggestions for managing certain types of child behaviors that are frustrating to the family. Keep in mind that children are all different and parents often must vary their parenting styles for different children in the family. For example, the child's temperament is often tied to their

CULTURE

Influences on Parenting

Some cultural influences on parenting are associated with chosen lifestyle. For example, living in a predominantly ethnic neighborhood makes it possible to participate in special ethnic events that help teach the child about the culture. Parents use the community for social contacts that help to reinforce patterns of parenting and to establish behavioral expectations of their children. Frequent contact or living with the extended family helps the child learn family and ethnic traditions, behaviors, and values. Children may be sent to religious or parochial schools that foster values important to the family.

FAMILIES WANT TO KNOW

Guidelines for Promoting Acceptable Behavior in Children

- Set realistic expectations and directions for behavior based upon the child's age and understanding; consistently enforce the expected directions and behaviors.
- Focus on promoting appropriate and desirable behaviors in the child:
  - Model or suggest appropriate behavior
  - Review expected behavior for special situations, such as a family party, going to the movies, or other social event
  - Help the child distinguish between inside and outside voice and behaviors, and
  - Praise or reward the child using appropriate behaviors.
- Tell the child about his or her inappropriate behavior as soon as it begins and offer guidelines for behavior change or provide a distraction.
- When reprimanding the child, focus on the behavior rather than stating that the child is bad. Explain how the behavior is

inappropriate; how it makes you, as the parent, and any other person involved feel. Avoid ridicule or accusation that can take the form of shame or criticism. These actions can have an impact on the child's self-esteem if repeated often enough.
- Be alert for situations when the child could potentially misbehave, such as when tired or overexcited. Use a distraction to control or calm the child.
- Help children gain self-control with friendly reminders (e.g., count to three, as soon as the clothes are on the doll, as soon as you finish the game) regarding the timing for transition to the next event of the day, such as bedtime, putting the toys away, or washing hands before dinner.
- Discuss reasons and social rules for expected behaviors when the child is old enough to understand.

behavioral style. (See Chapter 3 ∞ for more information on child temperament.) One child may need very clear limits set with discussion and reinforcement needed, while a sibling may immediately respond to the parents' limit setting without a need for discussion of the situation.

Discipline and Limit Setting

Discipline is a method for teaching children the rules for how to behave in society and what is expected in different circumstances. **Punishment** is the action taken to enforce the rules when the child misbehaves. Parenting styles play an important role in the type of discipline and punishment used with children. When clear limits are set and consistently maintained, as with authoritative parenting, punishment may be needed less often. Limit setting and firm control of those limits are important discipline methods used so children learn to what extent they can safely and independently operate within the environment. Firm limits also help children to feel secure because they are reassured by consistency and the sense of protection perceived by the limits. Punishment helps children learn that there are consequences for misbehavior, and that other individuals may be affected by that behavior. This helps children develop a sense of responsibility for their behavior.

Various strategies are used for discipline and punishment by children. Strategies selected by parents are often associated with the parents' ethnicity, emotions, and mental health. A recent strategy revealed the following common strategies were used among children between 19 and 35 months of age (Regalado, Sareen, Inkelas et al., 2004):

- Reasoning—a discipline method explaining why a behavior or action is inappropriate.
- Time-out—a punishment method of placing the child in a location away from toys and attention as a consequence of misbehavior (Figure 2–7 ➤).
- Experiencing a consequence—allowing the child to learn important lessons associated with misbehavior, such as taking away a toy by using a time-out, withdrawing privileges, and providing no dessert if the child misses dinner or does not eat nutritious foods.
- Corporal punishment—spanking or inflicting pain with a paddle, whip, or other object is one of the most widely used techniques for punishing children (Slade & Wissow, 2004). This form of punishment is not recommended as it teaches children that violence is acceptable. If parents are out of control or in a rage, the child may be seriously injured.
- Scolding or yelling—use of harsh language directed at the child.
- Behavior modification—giving positive rewards or reinforcement for good behavior or consistently ignoring inappropriate behavior to minimize the behavior. This encourages children to behave in specified ways; see Chapters 9 and 10 ∞ for age-specific discipline and punishment strategies.

Discussion of inappropriate behaviors and the reason for limit setting (methods of discipline) will help the child to understand why certain behaviors are wrong. Personal stories and fables can also be used to help children understand social and moral values or to better understand acceptable behavior.

SPECIAL FAMILY CONSIDERATIONS

Divorce and Its Effects on Children

The average age of children at the time of their parents' divorce in the United States is 7 years (Sammons, 2003). Approximately 1 million children per year are involved in divorce (American Academy of Pediatrics Task Force on the Family, 2003). Children are affected in many ways when the family breaks apart due to divorce, even though there have often been many periods of stress and tension in the home before the actual separation and divorce occur. Many children believe they are at fault for the separation and divorce, having said or done something to make the parent leave. When one parent leaves, the children may feel abandoned and divorced by that parent. They may also fear being abandoned by the remaining parent (Table 2–4).

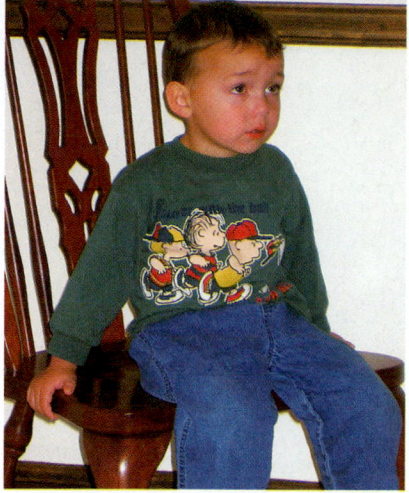

Figure 2–7 ➤ One effective discipline method is to remove the child to an isolated area where no interaction with children and adults can occur and no toys are present. This is used to demonstrate that there is a consequence to misbehavior. For older children, consider the loss of phone, computer, or other privileges.

CLINICAL TIP

Nurses have an important educational role in helping parents identify an appropriate discipline method and to take an authoritative role with their children. Encourage and educate parents about the need to be in charge, to set the rules, and to stand by them so that children learn how to behave.

Table 2–4	POTENTIAL EFFECTS OF DIVORCE ON CHILDREN OF DIFFERENT AGES
Age (years)	**Behavior**
3–5	Fear, anxiety, and dread in daily life events Regression Searching and questioning Self-blame Increased aggression
6–8	Extreme sadness Fantasies and panic Worries about lack of food, money, caretaking
9–12	Intense anger Somatic complaints Confused self-identity
13–18	Withdrawal from family Concern about sex and marriage Sense of loss Anger

Note: Adapted from Wallerstein, J. & Kelly, J. (2000). *Surviving the breakup*. New York: Harper Collins.

Children may become engaged in the disputes of parents, and experience conflicts of loyalty when parents fight for their affection. Sometimes parents are so stressed their customary parenting styles become inconsistent. They may be unable to provide the warmth, affection, and support that the children need during this time. When the divorce involves a lot of conflict and hostility, the children may have increased problems with adjustment. Battles over custody, child support, property division, and visitation rights all cause more distress for the children. When children must make a lot of changes in their lives, in addition to the parents' separation (new home, different school), their adjustment is made more difficult as their sense of order is upset. Predictable routines change and children may test limits to see if they still apply. The more changes they must make in the period immediately after the divorce, the more challenging is their adjustment.

The disruption associated with divorce is linked to academic and behavior problems among children, including depression, antisocial behavior, impulsive/hyperactive behavior, and school behavior problems (Amato, 2000).

- Infants and toddlers sense the tensions in the home and respond with increased irritability or tantrums, disturbance in eating and sleeping patterns, and regression in toilet training.
- Preschoolers and school-age children exhibit their anxiety and distress about the separation and divorce by "acting out," pestering siblings more, becoming overly demanding of either parent, being clingy or regressive, or being defiant or argumentative. They may also develop nervous habits, and begin bed-wetting.
- Older school-age children and adolescents may become angry, take risks with drugs or sex, develop school problems, disengage or withdraw from family and friends, or have other signs of depression or distress. Some children develop extremely destructive behavior such as suicide, drug abuse, and violence.

Nurses can assist families experiencing divorce by inquiring about the circumstances and changes that the child is experiencing. When parents are well-adjusted, adapt well following the divorce, and the quality of parenting is good, children adapt better following the divorce (American Academy of Pediatrics Task Force on the Family, 2003). Talk with parents about the child's fears of abandonment and concerns, reminding parents that even infants and toddlers can sense tensions in the home. Remind parents about the need to keep children out of the middle of confrontations, and to maintain limits of acceptable behavior. Encourage parents to avoid saying negative statements about the other parent and encourage parents to make every effort to maintain the relationship with the children. And most important, help parents recognize their children's needs for love and security during this difficult period.

The quality of the relationship between the divorced parents has an important impact on the future relationships their children have with them as adults. When divorced parents are able to minimize the conflict and continue sharing parenting (even in a minimal way), better maintenance of family and kinship ties (e.g., grandparents, stepparents, and half-siblings) results (Ahrons, 2003).

Fathers who do not live with their children but live nearby are more likely to have involvement with their children if they have a good relationship with the child's mother, financial resources, and work experience. The relationship between father and child may be improved when the father can interact with the child in a conflict-free environment. Factors that negatively affect ongoing involvement with the child include conflicts with the mother, lack of financial resources, geographic distance, and a new spouse or partner (Halle & Le Menestrel, 2002). See Families Want to Know: Promoting Relationships with Parents Following Separation and Divorce below.

Stepparenting

When divorced or widowed parents remarry, the child may respond with ambivalence, divided loyalty, anger, or uncertainty. Many changes in lifestyles, routines, and interaction patterns for the child and entire family should be anticipated and addressed early in the formation of the new family relationship. When a stepparent joins a ready-made family, opportunities for improved emotional and financial support of the child can result, but the development of a new cohesive family requires many adjustments by all family members.

Blending two families often results in the need to identify or negotiate new customs, traditions, rituals, and routines for the family. Children may fear or experience losses such as a close relationship with the noncustodial parent, neighborhood friends if a move was required, contact with grandparents, and family traditions. Discussions with children about their feelings may help the new family develop plans that ease the transition.

Stepparents must adjust to the habits and personality of the child and then work to gain trust and acceptance. If the child has not accepted the divorce or loss of a biological parent, developing a trusting, affectionate, and respectful relationship with the stepparent is more challenging. Sharing in childrearing decisions and responsibilities is an important task for stepparents. Determining acceptable stepparent roles and the role of the joint or noncustodial parent needs to be discussed and negotiated. Discipline is a challenge in most stepparent families. Standards of behavior, as well as who, when, and how discipline is used, need to be agreed upon within the family, and those guidelines need to be consistently maintained. Discipline by a stepparent is challenging until a bond develops between the stepparent and stepchild. Feelings and development of this bond cannot be forced. Time and honest communication are needed to make a successful transition to stepparenting and to gain the child's trust.

Stepparents are additional parents, not replacement parents. Adjustment of the child to the stepparent and the stepparent to the child are needed. The stepparent should

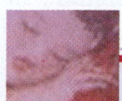

FAMILIES WANT TO KNOW

Promoting Relationships with Parents Following Separation and Divorce

Guidelines that may help to reduce conflict and to foster maintenance of a close relationship between the child and each parent include the following:

- Develop a way to stay in touch with the child even when apart, such as phone calls, faxes, or e-mail.

- Encourage a liberal visitation schedule so that each parent has time to be a normal parent. Overnight stays rather than a few hours at a time allow for more normal interactions.
- When parents have difficulty minimizing conflict in front of the child, transition the child to the other parent after school or childcare, or from a friend's home. This keeps the child from feeling responsible for the conflict.

CLINICAL TIP

Identify the parent who can legally provide consent for medical treatment when there has been a divorce and potentially a remarriage. In some states the noncustodial parent cannot give consent. The stepparent cannot give consent unless the custodial parent grants written permission. Stepparents or other family members may also not know the child's medical history. Identify the legal framework for informed consent with regards to these children so that care is provided in an appropriate and responsible manner.

COMMUNITY CARE

Grandparent-headed Households

Approximately 2.3 million grandparent-headed households are raising 3.9 million children under 18 years, sometimes in association with the parents. Of these children, 1.5 million are being raised completely by the grandparents, in an effort to keep these children out of the foster care system (Dowdell, 2004). Challenges faced by these grandparents include the following: poverty, no health insurance for the children, personal stress related to caring for an infant or young child, strained relationships with parents due to custody issues, challenges in enrolling the children in school, difficulty in providing needed transportation, and lack of affordable and appropriate housing (FRIENDS National Resource Center for Community-Based Family Resource and Support Programs, 2001).

try to establish a position in the child's life that is different from that of the missing biological parent, rather than competing with the biological parent. Men who live with their biological children and stepchildren, and those men who become stepparents when the children are young, tend to be more involved in parenting their stepchildren (Halle & Le Menestrel, 2002). Stepmothers often have more challenges than stepfathers adjusting to their new role. This may be because they spend more time with the children.

Contact with the biological parent often continues through custody arrangements, financial support, and visitation. Children may actually move between two households, adding to the complexity and stressors in their lives. Children may have divided loyalties between the two sets of parents. Power conflicts may emerge if the biological parents do not make efforts to cooperate in parenting decisions. A parenting coalition between all parents in the two families can reduce the conflicts and tensions that can emerge when parents agree to work together for the child's benefit.

FOSTER CARE

Foster care is the provision of protection and shelter for a child in an approved living situation away from the family of origin. It is legally coordinated by the state's child welfare system. The goal of foster care is to ensure the safety and well-being of vulnerable children. Approximately 542,000 children were in foster care at the end of 2001, a substantial increase over the 302,000 children in foster care in 1980 (Chipungu & Bent-Goodley, 2004). Of the approximate 1.4 million children who do not live with either a parent or a grandparent, 40% are in foster care (U.S. Department of Health and Human Services, 2002).

The average length of stay in foster care is approximately 33 months; however, some children stay for shorter or longer times (U.S. Department of Health and Human Services, 2003). Children enter the foster care system for many reasons. Neglect, often as a consequence of poverty, is a major reason children are placed in foster care (Gottesman, 2001). An estimated 275,000 children were placed in foster care as a result of child abuse investigations or assessments (Chipungu & Bent-Goodley, 2004). Racial distribution of children in foster care is 38% African American, 37% Caucasian, 17% Latino, 2% Native American, 1% Pacific Islander, and 5% of unknown race (Chipungu & Bent-Goodley, 2004).

Each state has guidelines regarding qualifications and standards for foster care parents and the process for becoming a foster parent. In an effort to ensure that the child is placed in a safe and nurturing environment, state guidelines used to investigate the home often include an interview with the interested adults to check for readiness to be a foster parent, health of all family members, legal background checks, and safety of the residence. Foster parents are also required to have initial training and annual continuing education.

Foster parents may be relatives (kinship care) or unrelated families with whom the child has a strong emotional bond. However, many children needing foster care are placed in extended families, as there are fewer suitable nonkinship family foster homes. While there are psychological benefits in keeping the child within the extended family, especially for helping the child learn and understand cultural and family values, the kinship foster parents have more challenges than other foster parents. They may be older, in poorer health, have less income, and have less education. In many states, kinship foster parents receive less funding than licensed foster care parents, even though their costs are identical (Bass, Shields, & Behrman, 2004). In addition, they tend to receive less supervision and family service support than in nonkinship foster care (Green, 2004).

Foster Parenting

Foster parenting is very demanding. Children placed in foster care often have more problems than other children from the same socioeconomic background, such as chronic medical conditions, birth defects, emotional or mental health disorders, and school-related problems (Schneiderman, 2004; Sobel & Healy, 2001). Foster parents must provide for the daily needs of children, support them emotionally, and provide appropriate responses to their behaviors. They provide transportation to medical appointments, mental health counseling, and court hearings. They coordinate visits with birth parents and caseworkers, and they also advocate for the child in school settings. When the child has complex problems or needs, the challenge of caring for the foster child is even greater. Foster parents receive some funding to care for children, but it is often inadequate for the child's needs, and the family often subsidizes the child's care from their own funds.

Many parents become frustrated with the challenges and stop serving as foster parents after 1 year (Chipungu & Bent-Goodley, 2004). Some of these challenges include the following: complicated and time-consuming paperwork for health and other financial resources, negative perceptions about foster parents who use food stamps, and being required to open the home to social services and court services personnel (Sobel & Healy, 2001). When the child must be moved to a different foster family, this may further exacerbate the ongoing stress that the individual child has in the foster care system.

Much of the child's adjustment rests with the stability of the family and available resources. Even though foster care is intended to be a temporary short placement—until the child can be returned home or an adoptive home is found—placed children may actually reside with the foster family for a lengthy time. For children who have come from an environment that has been unstable, abusive, or neglectful, the foster care home can be supportive to the child's health status, development, and academic achievement.

Children who have experience with the foster care system are more likely to have compromised development (behavioral problems, emotional problems, poor school adjustment) and higher levels of risky sexual behavior (Wertheimer, 2002). Many of the problems are thought to be tied to the reason foster care was sought, such as physical or sexual abuse, neglect, or abandonment. For the optimal psychological outcome of children placed in foster care, efforts should be made for permanent placement of the child as rapidly as possible so the child perceives a sense of belonging and develops psychological ties.

Foster parents caring for children need to provide continuity, consistency, and predictability. Foster parents should be encouraged to do the following (American Academy of Pediatrics, 2000):

- Give the child lots of love and attention;
- Be consistent with love, stimulation, and discipline;
- Use developmentally appropriate methods to stimulate the child such as holding, conversation, reading, music, and toys; and
- Help the child develop language.

Health Status of Foster Children

Children in foster care have a high prevalence of chronic and complex health conditions and may be in poor health if prior healthcare needs have not been addressed. Efforts to assure that children receive appropriate health care while in foster care are challenged by various barriers, such as an incomplete health history obtained from the parents, insufficient funding for needed health services, prolonged waits for community-based medical and mental health services, poor coordination of services with lack of communication between health professionals, and poor communication between health and community welfare professionals (American Academy of Pediatrics, 2002b).

Every child entering foster care should receive an initial health screening, followed by a more comprehensive health assessment within a month. Findings and recommendations from the health assessment and additional health evaluations should be incorporated into the child's social service case plan. Nurses can play an important role in partnering with foster parents to arrange for and obtain the services needed by the child. Foster parents need to be supported in their efforts to be the caring adult for these children, helping them to develop self-esteem and resilience.

Transition to Permanent Placement

While many children are reunited with birthparents, it is not possible for many other children. Foster care is not intended to be a long-term solution for a safe and secure home for the child. The Adoption and Safe Families Act of 1997 (P.L. 105-89) led to significant changes in child welfare. Timelines were shortened for decision making about permanent placement of children, and incentives were established for states to encourage adoption. States were given guidelines regarding when reasonable efforts to reunite children with birthparents were no longer necessary, and action is required in certain circumstances to terminate parental rights. Kinship foster care was formally recognized. **Legal guardianship** (a permanent placement option for the child, often with relatives, in which parental rights are not terminated) was established as an alternative to **adoption** (a legal relationship between the child and parents not related by birth in which the adoptive parents assume all legal and financial responsibility for the child). Long-term foster care was eliminated as a permanent placement option in nonkinship care, but it could continue for kinship foster care to promote stability for the involved children (Bass, Shields, & Behrman, 2004).

For those children with kinship foster care, adoption is often not perceived as the best option. Legal guardianship enables the child to retain legal connections with the birth family and relationship with the extended family. The guardian assumes limited financial liability for the child's care. Legal guardianship can be reversed at a future point in time if the birth parents petition the court.

Many children stay in foster care until they reach 18 years and are no longer eligible for services. States are required to track outcomes for the youth served (Barbell & Freundlich, 2001).

ADOPTION

Adoption is a legal relationship between the child and parents not related by birth in which the adoptive parents assume all legal and financial responsibility for the child. Motivations for adoption of a child vary with the families seeking adoption. In some cases couples have infertility problems and are unable to have a biological child. In other cases when the family already has one or two biological children, the reasons could include the following:

- Providing a home to a child who needs one or a desire for a larger family without additional biological children.
- Fertility issues requiring invasive medical procedures are too extensive, expensive, or psychologically overwhelming for a subsequent pregnancy.
- Adoption of a foster child with whom the family has established strong bonds.
- Adoption by a family relative or stepparent.

The supply of healthy infants available for adoption is much smaller than the number of families who want to adopt. Most children in the United States available for adoption are older children, often of minority populations or of mixed races, and those with special healthcare needs. As of September 2001, 126,000 children under 16 years of age were awaiting adoption from the foster care system (U.S. Department of Health and Human Services, 2003). Because most families choosing to adopt children prefer to have an infant, many children have been adopted from foreign nations. Since 1995, the nations that have provided the largest number of orphans for adoption in the United States include mainland China, Russia, Guatemala, and South Korea (U.S. Department of State, 2004). Adopted children account for approximately 2.5% of all children under 18 years in the United States (Kreider, 2003).

Legal Aspects of Adoption

Adoption is controlled by individual state law. Adoption may be arranged through an authorized agency, such as a licensed social service agency. Any family who wants to adopt a child is required by state law to undergo a home study. This is a process in which parents are interviewed about a large number of topics and issues, as well as being provided education and guidelines to prepare for the adoption. Some adoptions are arranged through independent agencies in collaboration with physicians, lawyers, nurses, and members of the clergy. Family home studies are not always conducted in the case of independent adoptions. The National Adoption Information Clearing-house provides information about state adoption laws.

Birth mothers and birth fathers are each required to relinquish legal rights to a child before an adoption can occur. The legal period between the child's birth and when the birth mother relinquishes legal rights varies by state. Efforts are made to assure that the birth mother is not coerced into relinquishing legal rights to the child immediately after birth. In an open adoption, the birth mother and adoptive parents often have contact with each other prior to the birth and have jointly planned potential future contacts between the child and biological mother. In some adoptions, birth mothers write a letter to the child that is given to the child at an appropriate age.

Preparation for Adoption

Parents often benefit from preadoption counseling. Such counseling may help provide the support and reassurance needed about parenting, the adoptive process, and a connection to support groups or other families with adopted children. Parents may wonder about their ability to love and parent the child, and have concerns about the responses of relatives, other children, and friends, especially if the child is from a different ethnic or racial group. Children already present in the family need to be reassured that they will not be displaced by the new child. Families need information about the child's understanding of what adoption means and guidance to help inform the child about being adopted.

Responses by Adopted Children

Children vary in their understanding and response to adoption by age (Borchers & Committee on Early Childhood, Adoption, and Dependent Care, American Academy of Pediatrics, 2003):

- Children under 3 years of age do not recognize a difference between being adopted into a family versus being a biological child in the family.
- Starting at about 3 years of age children like to hear about their adoption story and they begin to ask what adoption means. Children adopted at this age may experience the separation from their other family and relatives. They are aware of physical differences between themselves and the adoptive family when they are of a different race or ethnic group. They may be fearful of abandonment by the adoptive family.
- By 5 years of age adopted children begin to recognize they are different from most of their peers who were not adopted. Some children develop a feeling of responsibility for their biological parent's decision not to keep them.
- School-age children may fantasize about their biological family and what their life might have been like if they were not adopted. Their self-esteem may be affected as they think there was a flaw in them that was the reason biological parents gave them up for adoption.
- Adolescents may continue to fantasize about the "ideal" biological family and try out identities similar to what they know or imagine about their biological parents. They may also become angry that their own life experience is different from societal norms. Adoption issues continue into young adulthood as the individual deals with aspects of loss or rejection by the birth family and attempts to determine an identity (Cox & Lieberthal, 2005). They may choose to seek information about their biological family through a reunion registry. See Families Want to Know: Informing the Child About Adoption on the next page.

Children who are older when adopted must also make the commitment to the family relationship. They often have a memory of parents and other caregivers, so developing a close relationship with the adoptive parents takes more time. It may also be more challenging for the adoptive parents to develop as strong an emotional bond to

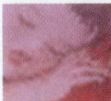

FAMILIES WANT TO KNOW

Informing the Child About Adoption

Most parents have anxiety about when and how to tell the child that he or she was adopted. There is no perfect age to tell the child about the adoption, so look for when the child is potentially ready to hear the information.

- Some authorities believe the child should be told at such a young age that the child will always know that he or she is adopted. This may be especially important when the child is of a different ethnic or racial group.
- The terms *adoption, adopted, birth family,* or *biologic family* should be part of the family's natural conversation (Borchers et al., 2003).
- Avoid waiting for "just the right moment" to tell the child. Make sure the child is told before a third party is likely to say something. If this happens the child may wonder what other information has not yet been shared.
- Tell the child in a matter-of-fact manner about the adoption. Let the child know how much he or she was wanted and specifically chosen because of some special characteristics. Make sure the child understands that his or her place in the family is permanent.

The adoptive family's commitment to the child should be repeated frequently.

- Be willing to honestly discuss the child's biological family and the adoption process so the child feels comfortable asking questions. More discussion about adoption will be needed as the child grows older, especially when the child begins to ask at about 5 to 6 years of age why he or she was not wanted by the biological parents. Anticipate that the child will grieve about the loss of the birth parents.
- As the child grows older and asks for more information about the birth parents, provide what information is known and try to help the child deal with difficult to hear information. Help the child decide what information to share with strangers, friends, and extended family members.
- Recognize that the adolescent may fantasize about the birth parents and want to find them. Listening to their concerns and providing support during this challenging time of development is important.

the older child as occurs when an infant is adopted. Even when a serious commitment has been made to adopt an older child, adjustment of the family and child may be difficult for everyone. Counseling may be helpful to some families during the transition process. See Box 2–1 for family resources related to adoption.

International Adoptions

Internationally adopted children often need special healthcare services. These children may be at risk for medical, developmental, and emotional problems that are uncommon in children born in the United States. Nurses that work with families that have adopted children from other countries provide a comprehensive evaluation of the child to detect potential developmental problems and health conditions as soon as the child is brought into the country. Examples of health problems that could potentially exist include infectious diseases (tuberculosis, hepatitis B and C) and parasites; various medical conditions such as fetal alcohol syndrome, mental retardation, lead poisoning; and incomplete immunizations (Narad & Mason, 2004).

BOX 2–1
ADOPTION RESOURCES FOR FAMILIES

Adamec, C. (1993). *Explaining adoption to your child.* Rockville, MD: National Adoption Information Clearinghouse.

Keck, G. C., & Kupecky, R. M. (1995). *Adopting the hurt child: Hope for families with special needs kids. A guide for parents and professionals.* Colorado Springs, CO: Pinon Press.

Keefer, B., & Schooler, J. E. (2000). *Telling the truth to your adopted or foster child: Making sense of the past.* Westport, CT: Bergin & Garvey.

Matthew, T. (1999). *Our own: Adopting and parenting the older child.* Longmont, CO: Snowcap Press.

Melina, L. R. (1998). *Raising adopted children: Practical reassuring advice for every adoptive parent.* New York: Harper Perennial.

Root, M. P. P., & Kelley, M. (Eds.). (2003). *Multiracial child resource book: Living complex identities.* Seattle: Mavin Foundation. http://www.mavinfoundation.org

Steinberg, G., & Hall, B. (2000). *Inside transracial adoption.* Indianapolis, IN: Perspectives Press.

Watkins, M., & Fisher, S. (1993). *Talking with young children about adoption.* New Haven, CT: Yale University Press.

Emotional and psychological problems may be the result of long-term institutionalization in an orphanage, such as inconsistency in interpersonal development and delayed developmental milestones. The child and family may need counseling and support to help the child adjust to being part of a family. The initial response of the child who has been in an orphanage to the new parents may be crying or turning away. Children need a transition period of several months to adjust to a different daily routine and to bond with the parents. Exposing the child to large numbers of family members or to busy environments may be stressful to the child. The nurse may become involved in providing counseling to the family trying to integrate the adoptive child into the family's life and routine (Figure 2–8 ➤). As the child grows, efforts to help the child understand the cultural birth heritage are also important.

FAMILY THEORIES

Families must be understood in their own context. It is important to understand each family's strengths and uniqueness and how the family and its members respond to the complex and often conflicting demands for time and attention. Many families live in a stressed state due to inadequate finances, healthcare concerns, relationship challenges, and other pressures. Nurses need to be able to assess family strengths and support mechanisms, to identify coping strategies, and to determine when families have overextended their resources and need additional support. In some cases nurses can provide the additional support needed, and at other times referral to other health professionals is appropriate to address the family's needs.

Family social system theories are helpful in understanding family functioning, environment-family interchange, family changes over time, and family response to health and illness. A brief review of family theories provides a context about family functioning that can assist with planning nursing care and developing future partnerships with families and their children.

Each family has structure and functions to help it maintain stability while responding continuously to various stresses and strains within the family and in the family's interactions and functioning within the community. Families develop and modify

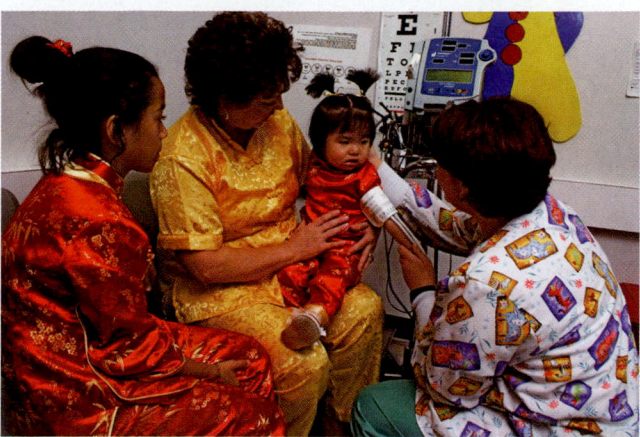

Figure 2–8 ➤ Adopted children who are of mixed race or a different ethnic group than the parents may cause a few additional challenges for the adoptive parents. Family members may be less supportive of the adoption initially. Because the children may have different physical characteristics, the family may capture more attention than it wishes. The family needs to learn to appreciate the different cultures represented in the newly formed family.

their responses and functioning over time to adapt or be tolerant of family, community, and environmental changes. Family processes include the behaviors and strategies that help to regulate space, time, energy, and other aspects of family functioning to promote family stability, growth, and control.

Family Development Theory

Family development refers to the dynamic changes that a family experiences over time, including changes within the family and in response to societal pressures. Family development includes relationships, communication patterns, roles, and changes in interactions. Over the years many models and frameworks of family development have been proposed. These developmental frameworks observe a family's progression over time by identifying specific developmental tasks or typical stages in family life. There are predictable stages in the life cycle of every family, but they follow no rigid pattern. Duvall's eight stages in the family life cycle of a traditional nuclear family have been used as the foundation for contemporary models of the family life cycle. The following stages describe the developmental processes and role expectations for different family types (Duvall & Miller, 1985):

- Beginning family, newly married couples (While this was the norm when the model was developed, today's families form by many different types of relationships.)
- Childbearing family (oldest child is an infant through 30 months of age)
- Families with preschool children (oldest child is between 2.5 and 6 years of age)
- Families with school children (oldest child is between 6 and 13 years of age)
- Families with teenagers (oldest child is between 13 and 20 years of age)
- Families launching young adults (all children leave home)
- Middle-age parents (empty nest through retirement)
- Family in retirement and old age (retirement to death of both spouses)

The stages provide a method for anticipating transitions and potential stressors with family role changes that occur at different points along the developmental continuum for different family types. However, life cycle stages have been developed for the more contemporary blended families, dual career families, and others (Friedman, Bowden, & Jones, 2003).

It is helpful to understand the family's developmental stage because it enables the nurse to analyze the family growth and health promotion needs. Understanding developmental transitions and potential stressors can then help the nurse identify the types of teaching and anticipatory guidance that might be needed.

Family Systems Theory

Family systems theory evolved from "general systems theory" in which there is interaction between the components (family members) of the system (family) and between the system and the environment. A family is a living social system, consisting of a small group of individuals who are closely interrelated and interdependent while collaborating to attain family functions and goals; therefore, the family is more than the sum of its members. In family systems theory, due to the amount of interrelationship and interdependence in the family, it is recognized that any change or stressor experienced by one or more family members has an impact on the entire family and causes disruption. Families are adaptable, and can change interactions and behaviors associated with the disruption in response to positive feedback. The family is a system that may or may not exchange materials, energy, and information with its physical, social, and cultural environments. An *open family* seeks information and resources, and actively interacts with the community to solve problems. A *closed family* views change and offered support as a threat. Resistance to outside influences is a strategy the family uses to maintain control. These characteristics have an effect on **family adaptability**—the capacity to modify behavior and change as the situation demands.

This theory encourages nurses to see the child and parents as participating members of a whole family. It encourages looking at the processes within the family and the relationships between subsystems (spouse, parent-child, and siblings) and suprasystems (the community within which it is embedded). Stress and crises motivate the family to mobilize its resources and to begin problem solving.

Using this information, the nurse can assess the effects of illness or injury on the entire family system and the reciprocal effects of the family on the illness or injury. Assessing how open or closed the family is to information and resources is important in planning nursing care. Open families will be more receptive to referrals and interventions from health professionals. The nurse will need to work with the closed family to establish trust and acceptance before the family is receptive to ideas and interventions proposed.

Family Stress Theory

Families experience many stressors as an inevitable part of life. Some stressors are positive, such as the birth of a child that leads to transitions within the family. Other stressors are unexpected and not considered positive, such as learning that a child has a serious health condition. All stressors demand a response from the family members that can lead to change within the family's interactions among its members and with the environment. Stressors are also cumulative and can come from many sources (work demands, school issues, extended family demands, achieving quality family time, and community roles). Most families have developed coping strategies to deal with daily routine stressors. Unexpected events are often more stressful as the family has not had time to review resources and prepare a response.

No one theory is sufficient for viewing the needs and behaviors of all families. The theories previously described continue to evolve as new researchers identify new or broadened explanations for behaviors, so it is difficult to attach one specific theorist to each family theory. When assessing families, you may also find it useful to consider more than one of these theories with the particular families to help you understand the full set of behaviors associated with individual families and to plan effective nursing interventions.

FAMILY ASSESSMENT

Families must be understood in their own context. It is important to understand each family's strengths and uniqueness and how the family and its members respond to the complex and often conflicting demands for time and attention. Nurses need to be able to assess family strengths and support mechanisms; to identify strategies for **coping**, the use of learned behavioral and cognitive strategies to manage or relieve perceived stress; and to determine when families have overextended their resources and need additional support. In some cases nurses can provide the additional support needed, and at other times referral to other health professionals is appropriate to address the family's needs.

Children and families live their lives within a variety of settings and interact with those settings in ways that directly or indirectly influence behaviors and learning. Because of these environmental influences on the family, it is important to consider the relationship of the family with the social networks within the community.

Family Stressors

A child's illness or injury impacts the entire family. Such a stressor demands a response from the family members that can lead to change within the family's interactions among its members and with the environment. Identifying how families respond to the stress of illness or injury of a child or other family member is important because of the potential hardships it causes the entire family.

Many families live in a stressed state due to inadequate finances, healthcare concerns, relationship challenges, and other pressures.

Family Strengths

Family strengths are the relationships and processes that support and protect families and family members during times of adversity and change. These strengths help maintain **family cohesion** (the amount of attachment and emotional bonding between family members) while supporting the development and well-being of individual

CLINICAL TIP

Family strengths helpful in managing stressors include the following:

- The ability of family members to listen and to discuss their concerns
- Shared family values and beliefs with common perceptions of reality, willingness to have hope, and know that change is possible
- Support and reinforcement by extended family members, and a feeling of belonging
- Self-care abilities for health problems
- Problem-solving skills using negotiation and everyday experiences as resources
- Focus on the present rather than past events or disappointments

family members (Moore, Chalk, Scarpa et al., 2002). There are four types of strengths that enable families to develop, adapt to change, and cope with challenges (Feeley & Gottlieb, 2000):

- Individual or family traits, such as optimism or resilience
- Individual or family assets, such as finances
- Individual or family capabilities, skills, and competencies, such as problem solving
- Another quality less permanent than a trait or asset, such as motivation

Identifying the family's **resilience**, their capacity to develop their strengths and abilities, to "bounce back" from the stresses and challenges faced, and to eliminate or minimize negative outcomes, is an important focus for family assessment prior to planning nursing interventions. Resilience of children is discussed in Chapter 6 ∞ .

When a family can control and deal with events satisfactorily, they gain a sense of competence, making them more resilient, in contrast to families who are overwhelmed by traumatic experiences. Characteristics of a resilient family include the following (Benard, 2004):

- Social competence, involving cultural flexibility, empathy, and caring
- Developing competence in communication skills
- Problem solving that involves planning, help-seeking, and critical and creative thinking that enables them to make decisions
- Maintaining family flexibility and adapting to changing circumstances, while maintaining a commitment to the family as a unit
- Having a sense of purpose and belief in a positive outcome (can set goals, have optimism and faith)
- Connectedness and maintenance of supportive relationships outside the family

Most families have the capacity for resilience. Often nursing support is needed to help family members learn new skills, make adaptations, and gain confidence in their abilities to manage the challenges they face. Potential resources include religious faith, finances, social support, physical health, family flexibility, and family coping mechanisms. If resources are diminished and the family defines the stressor as significant enough to cause a crisis, then the family will be susceptible to more serious disruption by the event. Nurses need to help families identify their strengths and areas for improvement that will lead to increased resiliency.

Functional families use a variety of coping strategies for stress management and they successfully reduce stress. Coping strategies of dysfunctional families are defensive and do not effectively manage the stress. See Table 2–5 for coping strategies used by functional and dysfunctional families.

Recognition of family strengths can be used to develop a rapport and relationship with the family. You should focus on family competence, and acknowledge and validate family members' emotions. Once the family recognizes the strengths it brings to the management of their child's healthcare problem, the family will more likely become an effective partner in the process. The nurse can often help families recognize that the strengths used in prior life experiences may transfer to the current healthcare experience.

Collecting Data for Family Assessment

To obtain an accurate and concise family assessment, the nurse needs to establish a trusting relationship with the child and family. Identify the parent's and the child's greatest concern, and expect these concerns to be different. It is important to acknowledge these multiple concerns and demonstrate respect for the diversity of the family. The goal is to obtain family information that will be helpful in planning nursing interventions that will help the family care for the child and improve the child's outcomes while valuing each person within the family.

Information about the family is collected continuously during the healthcare process, through interviews, observations of the family interactions, reports from other

Table 2–5	COPING STRATEGIES USED BY FUNCTIONAL FAMILIES AND DYSFUNCTIONAL FAMILIES

Functional Family Coping Strategies	Dysfunctional Family Coping Strategies
• Family relationships—increased structure and organization within the home and family, strengthening family cohesion, and increased role flexibility of family members. • Gathering information and knowledge, family joint problem solving. • **Normalization**—the process of family management that involves acknowledging a life-changing situation, such as the child has a chronic health problem, but family makes an effort to lead a normal life. Family life is normal because the impact of the condition on the family functioning is minimized as demonstrated by behaviors, rituals, and routines that show others that the family is normal. • Passive acceptance about an event or situation about which little or nothing can be done and determining that it is something that will take care of itself over time. • Direct, open, honest, and clear communication. • Use of humor and laughter. • Maintaining active linkages with the community and using social support networks. • Spiritual supports.	• Denial of family problems. • Exploitation of family members such as by scapegoating (negatively labeling and stigmatizing a family member, often a child) to avoid examining the real problem in the family. • Use of threat or withdrawal of affection and support to keep family members together at the expense of the emotional health of its members. • Myths or images the family has of itself that obscure reality and enable the family to deny some of its problems. • Extreme dominance and submission patterns. • Family addictions (drug or alcohol). • Domestic violence (partner, child, sibling to sibling, and elder abuse).

Data from: Friedman, M. M., Bowden, V. R., & Jones, E. G. (2003). *Family nursing: Research, theory, and practice* (5th ed., pp. 476–494). Upper Saddle River, NJ: Prentice Hall.

healthcare providers or agencies working with the family, and with a family assessment tool. Family assessment data that are important to collect include the following:

- Name, age, sex, and family relationship of all people residing in the household
- Family type, structure, roles, and values
- Cultural associations, including cultural norms and customs related to childrearing and infant feeding
- Faith-based affiliations
- Support systems network, including extended family, friends, and faith-based and community associations
- Communication patterns, including language barriers
- Environmental data—place of residence, condition of housing, number of persons living in the residence, sleeping arrangements, play areas, and neighborhood characteristics

See Chapter 5 ∞ for suggested data to collect about the psychosocial history and daily living patterns. Observation of the home and family members is recommended in some cases to obtain valuable information about family functioning.

Family Assessment Tools

Family assessment tools can be used to gather additional information about the family's functioning and can place particular focus on family stresses, coping strategies, and family strengths. Information about the way the family functions in nurturing its members, problem solving, and communicating may help identify strategies that are potentially more effective for management of the child's health care. They enable the nurse to work more effectively with the family, such as collaborating with the family in planning for health maintenance and health promotion strategies.

Family Ecomap

An **ecomap** illustrates the family's relationships and interactions with the social networks in the community, enabling the nurse and other healthcare providers to visualize the family's social network. By having the family participate in the preparation of the ecomap, it is possible to have some information about how the family perceives or receives social support, as well as the strength of family relationships with significant other persons and organizations. The ecomap provides an opportunity to identify the community resources being used by the family and to highlight any potential community resources that may help promote the family's health. See Figure 2–9 ➤ for a sample ecomap for Casey's family from the chapter opener.

Family APGAR

The Family APGAR is a quick five-item questionnaire that may be used as an initial screening tool for family assessment. The five family concepts measured include family adaptability, partnership, growth, affection, and resolve. See Table 2–6. The five-item questionnaire can be administered quickly to family members over 10 years of age. Ask all family members to complete a separate copy of the questionnaire to gain a picture of the family's perspective on family functioning. Be more concerned if the majority of responses fall in the "hardly ever" category or responses vary a lot among family members. This may indicate a family that needs much more support to cope with the demands of daily life and management of the child's condition.

MediaLink

HOME Inventory

Home Observation for Measurement of the Environment (HOME)

The HOME Inventory is an assessment tool developed to measure the quality and quantity of stimulation and support available to the child in the home environment (Caldwell & Bradley, 1984). Four age-specific scales are available (birth to 3 years, 3–6 years, 6–10 years, and 10–15 years). Examples of subscales within each age-specific scale include parental responsivity, acceptance of child, the physical environment, learning materials, variety in experience, and parental involvement. Data are collected during an informal,

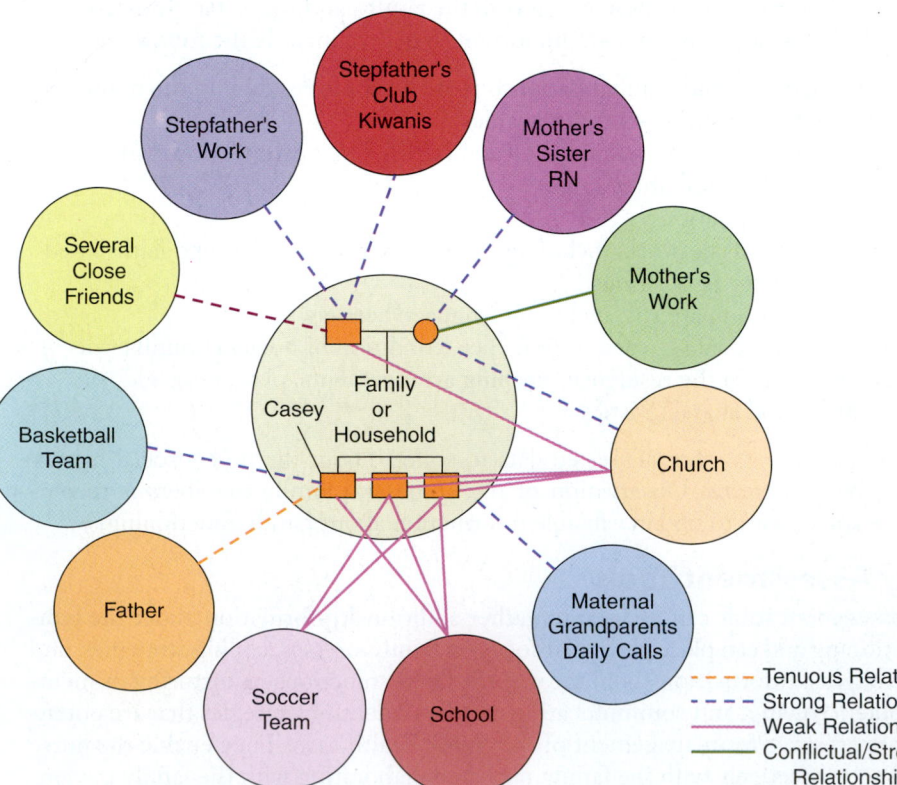

Ecomap of Casey's Family

Figure 2–9 ➤ An ecomap illustrates the family's relationships and interactions with groups and individuals in the immediate external environment.

Table 2–6	THE FAMILY APGAR QUESTIONNAIRE

Directions:

The following questions have been designed to help us better understand you and your family. You should feel free to ask questions about any item in the questionnaire.

The space for comments should be used when you wish to give additional information or if you wish to discuss the way the question is applied to your family. Please try to answer all questions.

Family is defined as the individual(s) with whom you usually live. If you live alone, your "family" consists of persons with whom you now have the strongest emotional ties.*

For each question, check only one box.

	Almost Always 2	Some of the Time 1	Hardly Ever 0
I am satisfied that I can turn to my family for help when something is troubling me. Comments:_____ _____			
I am satisfied with the way my family talks over things with me and shares problems with me. Comments:_____ _____			
I am satisfied that my family accepts and supports my wishes to take on new activities or directions. Comments:_____ _____			
I am satisfied with the way my family expresses affection and responds to my emotions, such as anger, sorrow, and love. Comments:_____ _____			
I am satisfied with the way my family and I share time together. Comments:_____ _____			

*According to which member of the family is being interviewed, the interviewer may substitute for the word *family* either *spouse*, *significant other*, *parents*, or *children*.
Responses are scored either (2, 1, 0) and summed. The total score ranges from 0 to 10. The larger the score, the greater amount of satisfaction with family functioning.
Note: From Smilkstein, G. (1978). The family APGAR: A proposal for a family function test and its use by physicians. *Journal of Family Practice, 6*(6), 1231–1239.

low-stress interview and observation over 45 to 90 minutes in the home setting. The child's primary caregiver and child must be present and awake during the interview. Observation of the parent–child interaction is an essential part of the assessment. The intent is to allow family members to act normally. Assessment of the home environment will help to identify factors that promote the child's growth and development. Examples of nursing interventions that could result from the HOME assessment include items that can be used in the home for toys and strategies for interacting with the child to promote learning.

Friedman Family Assessment Tool

The Friedman Family Assessment Tool (FFAM), developed by Marilyn Friedman, has been developed to assist nurses with family assessment. This tool provides a method to examine the whole family in the context of the larger community where the family resides. Information is collected in an interview process about a family's relationships, functioning, strengths, and problems. The short form for this assessment tool is provided in Box 2–2.

BOX 2–2
FRIEDMAN FAMILY ASSESSMENT TOOL

The following form is shortened for ease in assessing a family. If you are not sure what data should be covered in each of the assessment areas below, please refer to the original reference where more detailed questions/areas are presented.

Before using the following guidelines in completing family assessments, note that not all areas included below will be germane for each of the families visited. The guidelines are comprehensive and allow depth when probing is necessary. Do not feel that every subarea needs to be covered when the broad area of inquiry poses no problems to the family or concern to the health worker. Second, by virtue of the interdependence of the family system, one will find unavoidable redundancy. The assessor should try not to repeat data, but to refer the reader back to sections where this information has already been described.

Identifying Data

1. Family Name
2. Address and Phone
3. Family Composition: The Family Genogram
4. Type of Family Form
5. Cultural (Ethnic) Background
6. Religious Identification
7. Social Class Status
8. Social Class Mobility

Developmental Stage and History of Family

9. Family's Present Developmental Stage
10. Extent of Family Developmental Tasks Fulfillment
11. Nuclear Family History
12. History of Family of Origin of Both Parents

Environmental Data

13. Characteristics of Home
14. Characteristics of Neighborhood and Larger Community
15. Family's Geographical Mobility
16. Family's Associations and Transactions with Community

Family Structure

17. Communication Patterns
    Extent of Functional and Dysfunctional Communication (types of recurring patterns)
    Extent of Emotional (Affective) Messages and How Expressed
    Characteristics of Communication Within Family Subsystems
    Extent of Congruent and Incongruent Messages
    Types of Dysfunctional Communication Processes Seen in Family
    Areas of Closed Communication
    Familial and Contextual Variables Affecting Communication
18. Power Structure
    Power Outcomes
    Decision-making Process
    Power Bases
    Variables Affecting Family Power
    Overall Family System and Subsystem Power (Family Power Continuum Placement)
19. Role Structure
    Formal Role Structure
    Informal Role Structure
    Analysis of Role Models (optional)
    Variables Affecting Role Structure
20. Family Values
    Compare the family to American core values or family's reference group values and/or identify important family values and their importance (priority) in family.
    Congruence Between the Family's Values and the Family's Reference Group or Wider Community
    Disparity in Value Systems
    Presence of Value Conflicts in Family
    Effect of the Above Values and Value Conflicts on Health Status of Family

Family Functions

21. Affective Function
    Mutual Nurturance, Closeness, and Identification
    Separateness and Connectedness
    Family's Need–Response Patterns
22. Socialization Function
    Family Child-rearing Practices
    Adaptability of Child-rearing Practices for Family Form and Family's Situation
    Who Is (Are) Socializing Agent(s) for Child(ren)?
    Value of Children in Family
    Cultural Beliefs That Influence Family's Child-rearing Patterns
    Social Class Influence on Child-rearing Patterns
    Estimation About Whether Family Is at Risk for Child-rearing Problems and if So, Indication of High-risk Factors
    Adequacy of Home Environment for Children's Needs to Play
23. Health Care Function
    Family's Health Beliefs, Values, and Behavior
    Family's Definitions of Health–Illness and Its Level of Knowledge
    Family's Perceived Health Status and Illness Susceptibility
    Family's Dietary Practices
    Adequacy of Family Diet (recommended 3-day food history record)
    Function of Mealtimes and Attitudes Toward Food and Mealtimes.
    Shopping (and its planning) practices.
    Person(s) Responsible for Planning, Shopping, and Preparation of Meals.
    Sleep and Rest Habits
    Physical Activity and Recreation Practices
    Family's Therapeutic and Recreational Drug, Alcohol, and Tobacco Practices
    Family's Role in Self-care Practices
    Medically Based Preventive Measures (physicals, eye and hearing tests, immunizations, dental care)
    Complementary and Alternative Therapies
    Family Health History (both general and specific diseases— environmentally and genetically related)
    Health Care Services Received
    Feelings and Perceptions Regarding Health Services
    Emergency Health Services
    Source of Payments for Health and Other Services
    Logistics of Receiving Care

Family Stress, Coping, and Adaptation

24. Family Stressors, Strengths, and Perceptions
    Stressors Family Is Experiencing
    Strengths That Counterbalance Stressors
    Family's Definition of the Situation
25. Family Coping Strategies
    How the Family Is Reacting to the Stressors
    Extent of Family's Use of Internal Coping Strategies (past/present)
    Extent of Family's Use of External Coping Strategies (past/present)
    Dysfunctional Coping Strategies Utilized (past/present; extent of use)
26. Family Adaptation
    Overall Family Adaptation
    Estimation of Whether Family Is in Crisis
27. Tracking Stressors, Coping, and Adaptation Over Time

From Friedman, M. M., Bowden, V. R., & Jones, E. G. (2003). *Family nursing: Research, theory, and practice* (5th ed., pp. 593–594). Upper Saddle River, NJ: Prentice Hall.

FAMILY SUPPORT SERVICES

Family support services exist in all communities with a purpose of supporting families in the rearing of healthy children. Social support is information that can result in one of the following outcomes: feeling cared for, belief that one is valued or loved, or sense of belonging to a reciprocal network (American Academy of Pediatrics Task Force on the Family, 2003). Contemporary lifestyles (divorced parents, single parents, mothers in the labor force, more time away from children, and parents separated from extended families and natural support systems) stress families trying to provide for their children's needs. In other cases families are stressed because of economics, living in or near poverty, or even being homeless. See Chapter 6 ∞. Many communities have worked to develop social support programs to support the health and development of children and to promote family positive relationships. Examples of these family support services include the following:

- Head Start and Early Head Start
- Before- and afterschool programs for children of working parents
- School-based health and counseling services
- Play groups for preschool children
- Peer support groups
- Social service programs offered by the faith community
- Home visiting programs for high-risk children and parents
- Job skills training, adult education, and literacy programs
- Crisis care and respite care programs

Many of these family support services work to promote positive family relationships, parental competencies, and behaviors that contribute to the health and development of the children and family. Most programs are designed with the premise that no family is entirely self-sufficient and most can benefit from some external support.

Think about the formal and informal family support services in your community. Nurses play an important role in helping to link families to the types of community support services they need after performing a family assessment and collaborating with families to identify and seek assistance most beneficial to their needs.

■ NURSING MANAGEMENT

The goal of family-centered nursing management is to assess and help families recognize their strengths and resiliency. This information can then be used in collaboratively planning the nursing care with the child and families.

Nursing Assessment and Diagnoses

The presence of a newly acquired disability, such as has occurred in Casey's family, adds a dimension of developmental risk. The child and family members may respond with either psychological or behavioral problems, or they may respond in a more positive manner.

Collect the psychosocial history and daily living patterns data from the family and child. Assessment of the culturally diverse child and family additionally includes determining the family's healthcare practices such as health traditions, health beliefs, health-seeking behaviors, healthcare practitioner, and religion or spirituality.

Select the appropriate family assessment tool to collect information that can help evaluate the family's strengths and resources. Analyze the information collected and focus on key information that will help develop a plan of care for the child and family. Determine how this condition influences family functioning.

- Identify how all of the family members have responded to the child's acute condition and disability.
- Obtain information about how the family is considering management of the child's care at home.

- Determine if other family issues or stressors must be integrated into the plan of care.
- Identify the family's expectations of different health professionals and facilities to help manage the child's care.
- Prepare an ecomap and genogram.

Examples of nursing diagnoses that may result from the family and home assessment include:

- Compromised Family Coping related to multiple simultaneous stressors
- Interrupted Family Processes related to child with a significant disability requiring alteration in family functioning
- Risk for Caregiver Role Strain related to child with a newly acquired disability and the associated financial burden
- Impaired Social Interaction (Parents and Child) related to lack of family or respite support

Planning and Implementation

Families need support to increase their resources and coping behaviors so they can successfully manage the multiple stressors, strains, and problems of daily living along with the child's chronic condition.

Establishing a therapeutic relationship with the family is an important intervention. This relationship should be characterized by empathy and trust, as well as the development of mutually identified goals for the child's care. To help families develop resiliency, focus on family competence and strengths. Acknowledge and validate their emotions. Provide information in a clear, timely, and sensitive manner. Ask questions that help direct the family's thinking rather than providing them with all of the answers. Work with families by teaching them to identify solutions until they are able to independently problem solve. Linkage with other families who have faced similar situations may be helpful.

Assist the family to begin planning for ongoing care using family-centered principles:

- Identify the primary decision maker for the child's health care.
- Discuss the family's goals for managing the child's care in the home setting.
- Consider how the family's strengths and previous family problem-solving experiences can be integrated into the intervention.
- Consider the family's ethnic and religious background in developing intervention recommendations. Partner with the child and family to assist them in determining how they can incorporate prescribed therapies with their healthcare practices. Ensure that the child and family understand the child's illness, treatment, or health promotion. Apply culturally sensitive techniques when dispelling any cultural myths.
- Offer the family one or more potential interventions rather than trying to force one intervention. Be open to modifying the intervention or devising an alternate intervention to better match the family's lifestyle preferences.
- Identify the type of support or assistance the family would like to have.

Identify potential resources in the community that match the child's and the family's needs for support. Collaborate with the family to discuss those resources and to select those that are acceptable to the family. Collaborate with a multidisciplinary team including social workers to assist the family in receiving assistance for barriers such as transportation, financial issues, geographic barriers, and any other barriers to the child's health care. Make sure the family has a coordinator of care, especially when a family member initially seems to be unable to assume the case management role. Assist families in obtaining resources by such actions as role rehearsal, providing instructions and support when making an initial call, or connecting with another family support person who can help with resource linkage. Refer families with moderate or severe dysfunction to community resources for social support and counseling as appropriate.

CULTURE

Traditional Healthcare Providers

When appropriate, collaborate with the family to determine the role traditional healthcare providers and other practitioners, such as folk healers, curandero or curandera, and spiritualists, will have in the care of the child. Encourage collaboration and communication between practitioners to ensure continuity of care.

Evaluation

Expected outcomes of nursing care include:

- The family assumes the role of case manager or works effectively with an assigned case manager to implement the interventions recommended by the nurse and healthcare team.
- The care needed by the child with an acquired disability is provided by the family according to recommended guidelines.

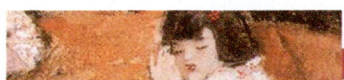

CRITICAL THINKING IN ACTION

FAMILY-CENTERED CARE

Think about Casey and his family from the beginning of the chapter. Casey's family is coping with his initial survival of a serious brain injury, and facing a long rehabilitation process. The family is just now recognizing that life as they have known it is changing.

Casey is totally dependent for care including bathing, toileting, feeding, and mobilizing. While he is expected to regain self-care abilities, the impact of the injury on his cognitive ability and future functioning is unknown.

Casey's extended family has provided support to the family during the past 12 days, but the level of support in the future weeks will decrease because of other family obligations. Casey's mother has already initiated a leave of absence from work so she can care for him when he returns home; however, this will mean the family has reduced income during that time period. Casey's younger brothers have been able to visit him, and they are very anxious because Casey cannot talk with them. They have been trying to avoid bothering their mother and father during this time, but they are wondering when life will be more normal and they can again participate in their usual afterschool activities.

1. What information about the family strengths, needs, and resilience can be identified from the chapter opening scenario, the ecomap on page 50, and the previous information?

2. What additional information would be helpful to know about family strengths and needs prior to developing a nursing care plan?

3. Based on your assessment of the family and challenges facing them, list at least one nursing diagnosis (additional to those listed on page 54) that addresses issues important for planning nursing care for Casey and his family.

4. Describe the use of family-centered care principles in planning Casey's nursing care in collaboration with the family.

5. What potential parenting issues could this family anticipate for Casey and his brothers?

 Refer to your Prentice Hall Nursing MediaLink DVD-ROM for answers.

EXPLORE MediaLink 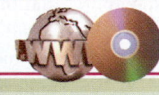 http://www.prenhall.com/ball

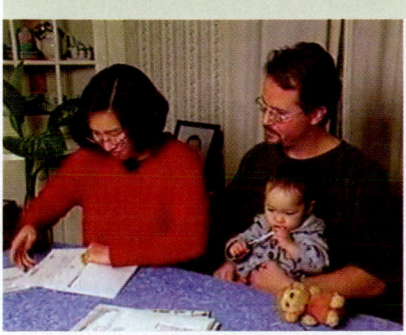

Resources for this chapter can be found on the Prentice Hall Nursing MediaLink DVD-ROM accompanying this textbook, and on the Companion Website at http://www.prenhall.com/ball.

DVD-ROM
Audio Glossary
NCLEX-RN® Review
Video
   Defining Family

COMPANION WEBSITE
Audio Glossary
NCLEX-RN® Review
Case Study: Family-Centered Care
Critical Thinking
   Family Support Services
   The Nursing Process and Family-Centered Care
MediaLink Application: Assessment of Healthcare
   Settings for Family-Centered Care
WebLinks

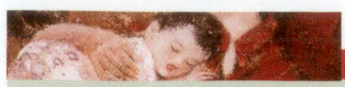

REFERENCES

Ahrons, C. R. (2003). The facts about divorce. Council on Contemporary Families. Accessed March 24, 2004, from http://www.contemporaryfamilies.org/public/fact2.php

Allshouse, C., & Goldberg, P. F. (2003). *Working with doctors: A parent's guide to navigating the health system.* Minneapolis, MN: Pacer Center, Inc.

Amato, P. R. (2000). The consequences of divorce for adults and children. *Journal of Marriage and the Family, 62*(4), 1269–1287.

American Academy of Pediatrics. (2004). Fathers and pediatricians: Enhancing men's roles in the care and development of their children. *Pediatrics, 113*(5), 1406–1411.

American Academy of Pediatrics Committee on Early Childhood, Adoption, and Dependent Care. (2000). Developmental issues for young children in foster care. *Pediatrics, 106*(5), 1145–1150.

American Academy of Pediatrics Committee on Early Childhood, Adoption, and Dependent Care. (2002b). Health care of young children in foster care. *Pediatrics, 109*(3), 536–541.

American Academy of Pediatrics Committee on Hospital Care and the Institute of Family Centered Care. (2003). Family-centered care and the pediatrician's role. *Pediatrics, 112*(3), 691–696.

American Academy of Pediatrics Committee on Psychosocial Aspects of Child and Family Health. (2002a). Coparent or second parent adoption by same-sex parents. *Pediatrics, 109*(3), 339–340.

American Academy of Pediatrics Task Force on the Family. (2003). Family pediatrics: Report on the Task Force on the Family. *Pediatrics, 111*(6), 1541–1571.

American Psychological Association. (2004). Sexual orientation, parents, and children: APA Policy Statement, accessed May 6, 2006, from http://www.apa.org/pi/lgbc/policy/parents.html

Annie E. Casey Foundation. (2004). 2000 Census data—Living arrangements profile for United States. KIDS COUNT census data online. Accessed March 1, 2004, from http://www.aecf.org

Ariel, J., & McPherson, D. (2000). Therapy with lesbian and gay families and their children. *Journal of Marital and Family Therapy, 26*(4), 421–432.

Barbell, K., & Freundlich, M. (2001). Foster care today. Washington, DC: Casey Family Programs. Accessed February 11, 2004, from http://www.casey.org

Bass, S., Shields, M. K., & Behrman, R. E. (2004). Children, families, and foster care: Analysis and recommendations. *The Future of Children, 14*(1), 5–29.

Baumrind, D. (1971). Current patterns of parental authority. *Developmental Psychology, 4,* 1–103.

Benard, B. (2004). The foundations of the resiliency framework: From research to practice. Accessed October 7, 2005, from http://www.resiliency.com/htm/research.htm

Borchers and Committee on Early Childhood, Adoption, and Dependent Care, American Academy of Pediatrics. (2003). Families and adoption: The pediatrician's role in supporting communication. *Pediatrics, 112*(6), 1437–1441.

Caldwell, B. M., & Bradley, R. H. (1984). *The Home Observation for Measurement of the Environment.* Little Rock, AR: University of Arkansas.

Chipungu, S. S., & Bent-Goodley, T. B. (2004). Meeting the challenges of contemporary foster care, *The Future of Children, 14*(1), 75–93.

Council on Contemporary Families. (2003). America's changing families: The 2000 Census. Accessed March 24, 2004, from http://www.contemporaryfamilies.org/public/families.php

Cox, S. S., & Lieberthal, J. (2005). Intercountry adoption: Young adult issues and transition to adulthood. *Pediatric Clinics of North America, 52,* 1495–1506.

Craig, G. J., & Baucum, D. (2002). *Human development* (9th ed.). Upper Saddle River, NJ: Prentice Hall.

Denham, S. A. (2005). Family structure, function, and process. In S. M. H. Hanson, V. Gedaly-Duff, & J. R. Kaakinen, *Family health care nursing* (3rd ed., pp. 119–156). Philadelphia: F. A. Davis.

Dowdell, E. B. (2004). Grandmother caregivers and caregiver burden. *Maternal Child Nursing, 29*(5), 299–304.

Duvall, E. M., & Miller, B. L. (1985). *Marriage and family development* (6th ed.). New York: Harper & Row.

Family and Medical Leave, Public Law 103-3, February 5, 1999. 5 U.S.C. 6381–6387; 5 CFR part 630, subpart L. Accessed July 9, 2004, from http://www.opm.gov/pca/leave/HTMS/fmlafac2.asp

Feeley, N., & Gottlieb, L. N. (2000). Nursing approaches for working with family strengths and resources. *Journal of Family Nursing, 6*(1), 9–24.

Friedman, M. M., Bowden, V. R., & Jones, E. G. (2003). *Family nursing: Research, theory, and practice* (5th ed.). Upper Saddle River, NJ: Prentice Hall.

FRIENDS National Resource Center for Community-Based Family Resource and Support Programs. (2001). Family support and intergenerational programming (Fact sheet Number 5). Chapel Hill, NC: Author. Accessed February 11, 2004, from http://www.friendsnrc.org

Gottesman, M. M. (2001). Children in foster care: A nursing perspective on research, policy, and child health issues. *Journal of the Society of Pediatric Nurses, 6*(2), 55–64.

Green, R. (2004). The evolution of kinship care policy and practice. *The Future of Children, 14*(1), 131–149.

Halle, T., & Le Menestrel, S. (2002). How do social, economic, and cultural factors influence fathers' involvement with their children? Child Trends Research Brief. Accessed December 5, 2003, from http://www.childtrends.org

Hanson, J. L., & Randall, V. F. (1999). Evaluating and improving the practice of family-centered care. *Pediatric Nursing, 25*(4), 445–449.

Institute for Family Centered Care. (2004). Patient and family resource centers. Accessed on March 12, 2004, from http://www.familycenteredcare.org/special_topics/familyresource/main.html

Kreider, R. M. (2003). *Adopted children and stepchildren: 2000. CENSR-6RV.* Washington, DC: U.S. Census Bureau.

Lewandowski, L. A., & Tesler, M. D. (Eds.). (2003). *Family-centered care: Putting it into action. The SPN/ANA guide to family-centered care.* Washington, DC: American Nurses Association.

Lugaila, T., & Overturf, J. (2004). *Children and the households they live in: 2000. CENSR-14.* Washington, DC: U.S. Census Bureau.

Maccoby, E. E. (1980). *Social development: Psychological growth and the parent-child relationship.* New York: Harcourt Brace Jovanovich.

Meyers, T. A., Eichhorn, D. J., & Guzzetta, C. E. (1998). Do family members want to be present during CPR? A retrospective study. *Journal of Emergency Nursing, 24*(5), 400–405.

Moore, K. A., Chalk, R., Scarpa, J., & Vandivere, S. (2002). Family strengths: Often overlooked, but real. Child Trends Research Brief. Accessed December 5, 2003, from http://www.childtrends.org

Munro, H., & D'Errico, C. (2000). Parental involvement in perioperative anesthetic management. *Journal of PeriAnesthesia Nursing, 15*(6), 397–400.

Narad, C., & Mason, P. W. (2004). International adoptions: Myths and realities. *Pediatric Nursing, 30*(6), 483–487.

Ochieng, B. M. N. (2003). Minority ethnic families and family-centered care. *Journal of Child Health Care, 7*(2), 123–132.

Peterson, K. S. (2003). Unmarried with children: For better or worse? *USA Today,* September 18, 1A, 8A.

Powers, K. S., & Rubenstein, J. S. (1999). Family presence during invasive procedures in pediatric intensive care unit: A prospective study. *Archives of Pediatric and Adolescent Medicine, 153,* 955–958.

Regalado, M., Sareen, H., Inkelas, M., Wissow, L. S., & Halfon, N. (2004). Parents' discipline of young children: Results from the national survey of early childhood health. *Pediatrics, 113*(6), 1952–1958.

Sacchetti, A., Paston, C., & Carraccio, C. (2005). Family members do not disrupt care when present during invasive procedures. *Academic Emergency Medicine, 12*(5), 477–479.

Sammons, W. (2003). Divorce: How you can help the family. *Contemporary Pediatrics, 20*(9), 33–35.

Schneiderman, J. U. (2004). The health of children in foster care. *Journal of School Nursing, 20*(6), 343–351.

Slade, E. P., & Wissow, L. S. (2004). Spanking in early childhood and later behavior problems: A prospective study of infants and young toddlers. *Pediatrics, 113*(5), 1321–1330.

Sobel, A., & Healy, C. (2001). Fostering health in the foster care maze. *Pediatric Nursing, 27*(5), 493–497.

Sullivan-Bolyai, S., Sadler, L., Knafl, K. A., & Gillis, C. L. (2004). Great expectations: A position description for parents as caregivers: Part II. *Pediatric Nursing, 30*(1), 52–56.

Urban Institute. (2003a). *Gay and lesbian families in the Census: Couples with children.* Washington, DC: Author, Accessed January 28, 2004, from http://www.urban.org

Urban Institute. (2003b). *Who will adopt the foster care children left behind.* Washington, DC: Author. Accessed February 1, 2004, from http://www.urban.org

U.S. Bureau of Census. (2002). Living arrangements of children under 18 years of age: 1960 to present. Retrieved May 5, 2004, from http://www.census.gov/population/hh-fam/tabCH-1.xls

U.S. Department of Health and Human Services. (2001). Indicators of welfare reform. Annual Report to Congress 2001. Table Birth 4. Washington, DC.

U.S. Department of Health and Human Services. (2002). The AFCARS report, number 7: Interim FY 2000 estimates. Accessed December 28, 2003, from http://www.acf.hhs.gov/programs/cb

U.S. Department of Health and Human Services. (2003). National Adoption and Foster Care Statistics. Accessed February 11, 2004, from http://www.acf.hhs.gov/programs/cb/dis/afcars/publications/afcars.htm

U.S. Department of State. (2004). Immigrant visas issued to orphans coming to the U.S. Accessed February 11, 2004, from http://travel.state.gov/orphan_numbers.html

Wallerstein J. & Kelly, J. (2000). *Surviving the breakup.* New York: Harper Collins.

Wertheimer, R. (2002). Youth who "age out" of foster care: Troubled lives, troubling prospects. Child Trends Research Brief. Accessed December 5, 2003, from http://www.childtrends.org

3

GROWTH AND DEVELOPMENT

KEY TERMS

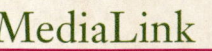 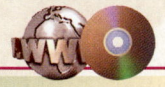

http://www.prenhall.com/ball

See the Prentice Hall Nursing MediaLink DVD-ROM and Companion Website for chapter-specific resources.

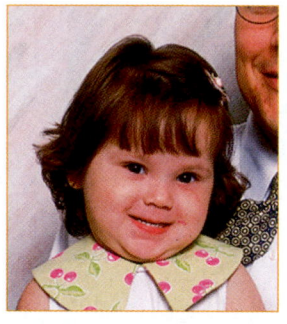

MICHAEL and Alyssa had tried for several years to have a biological child. After an unsuccessful in vitro fertilization, they decided to adopt a child. They explored opportunities with adoption agencies, and learned that international adoption was possible. They adopted 2-year-old Irena from Romania several months ago. Despite the adoption agency's thorough investigation of Michael and Alyssa, the couple received only scant information about Irena's history. She was surrendered to an orphanage by her mother when she was about 7 months old; the mother stated that the pregnancy and delivery were normal. She was giving up the child because she had two older children to care for and her husband had left home nearly a year before and had not been heard from since. Irena appears small for her age, but is thriving in her new environment. She is learning to say a few English words and is responding appropriately to care and interactions. How can the nurse work with Michael and Alyssa to ensure special attention to Irena's growth and healthcare needs? What will Irena's cultural needs be as she grows older?

LEARNING OUTCOMES

After reading this chapter, you will be able to do the following:

1. Describe major theories of development as formulated by Freud, Erikson, Piaget, Kohlberg, social learning theorists, and behaviorists.

2. Plan nursing interventions for children that are appropriate for the child's developmental state, based on theoretical frameworks.

3. Explain contemporary developmental approaches such as temperament theory, ecologic theory, and the resilience framework.

4. Recognize major developmental milestones for infants, toddlers, preschoolers, school-age children, and adolescents.

5. Synthesize information from several theoretical approaches to plan assessments of the child's growth and developmental milestones.

6. Describe the role of play in the growth and development of children.

7. Use data collected during developmental assessments to plan activities that promote development of children and adolescents.

INTRODUCTION

Children develop as they interact with their surroundings. They learn skills at different ages, but the order in which they learn them is universal. Development is affected by factors such as nutrition and cultural practices, as well as the social situation in the country or neighborhood. While Irena will develop in a unique manner influenced by her genetic makeup, life experiences, and the interaction between these factors, certain principles of development can assist her parents and the nurse in fostering positive adaptations for her.

In this chapter, you will learn general principles of growth and development and will explore several theories related to childhood development, as well as their nursing applications. Each age group, from infancy through adolescence, is described in detail. Developmental milestones, physical and cognitive characteristics, play patterns, and communication strategies are presented. This basic information will help you provide developmentally appropriate care for children in each age group. You can apply these concepts to all children, including special situations such as the one described in the opening scenario.

To highlight the important facets of development that are explored in this chapter, let us begin by examining some of Irena's characteristics (Figure 3–1 ➤).

> *Physical Growth and Development*—Although many international adoptees are small for their age, Irena appears well nourished. (See Chapter 4 ∞ for a discussion of nutritional needs during toddlerhood.) Her gross motor skills, including walking up steps, running, and kicking a ball, are well developed.

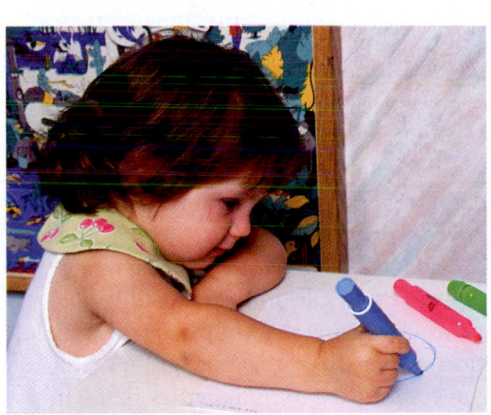

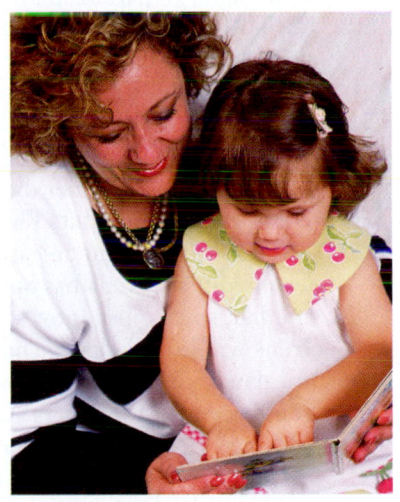

A

B

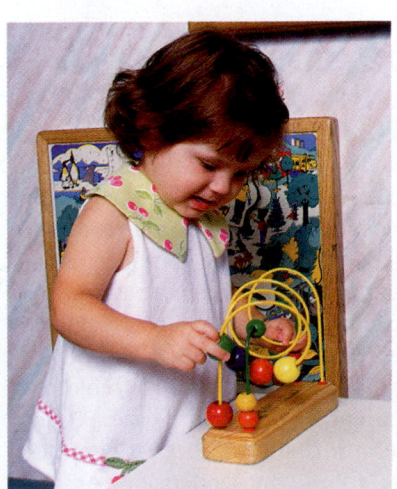

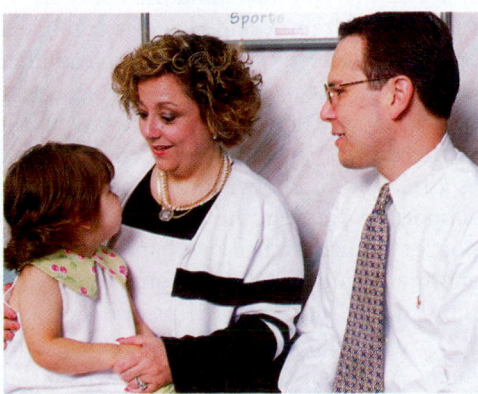

C

D

Figure 3–1 ➤ Observing the activities of a child provides information about developmental status. A, Irena shows fine motor skills as she begins to scribble and color in a circle provided by a parent. B, The parent provides positive reinforcement for activities. C, Cognitive development is enhanced as toddlers manipulate objects. D, Irena's parents provide comfort and a trusting environment.

Fine motor skills are evident in her ability to brush teeth and dress with help, scribble on paper, and build a tower of cubes.

Cognitive Development—Cognitive development relates to intellectual or thinking processes. It is hard to identify Irena's cognitive stage at this time, as she knows only a few English words and is shy during interactions with strangers. As she adapts to her new home, frequent assessments of her cognitive development will be necessary. Physical and cognitive developmental milestones determine injury prevention strategies. Injuries are a common cause of death and hospitalization during childhood. (See Chapter 1 ∞ for statistics about the relationship of injury to morbidity and mortality in childhood.) Nurses use **anticipatory guidance**, predicting the upcoming developmental tasks or needs of a child and performing appropriate teaching related to them, to discuss safety hazards and injury prevention for children of various ages with their parents. See Chapters 7–10 ∞ for specific anticipatory measures during health supervision visits at each age.

Psychosocial Development—There are several components of psychosocial development. For our purposes we will analyze the play and interactional patterns at each age, will apply information about temperament and personality, and then discuss communication skills.

Play—Irena is observed playing with toys and making sounds with her dolls. This is expected behavior, as toddlers often engage in solitary play. Toddlers also begin to enjoy the presence of other children, even though they do not yet play cooperatively with them. Irena's parents can encourage the emergence of parallel play with other toddlers by arranging to have Irena play with other children. The parents can be available at first so that Irena feels secure; once she shows comfort with other children, parents can gradually increase their absence during these playtimes.

Personality and Temperament—Irena has been demonstrating what experts term an "easy" temperament; that is, she has readily acquired a regular schedule for eating and sleeping, her mood is generally pleasant, and she is easily comforted when upset. These temperamental characteristics will form a critical link to communication with family, teachers, and friends.

Communication—Irena has only learned a few words. This is abnormal for a toddler, since most know several hundred words. However, it is expected that Irena will learn language quickly as she adapts. Michael and Alyssa should speak with Irena often, pointing out names of people and objects. Positive reinforcement for Irena's attempts at speech can involve smiles, phrases such as "that's right," and further elaboration such as "Yes, that is a bus; it's a big, yellow bus." What else can you suggest to her parents as activities that will enhance speech development?

PRINCIPLES OF GROWTH AND DEVELOPMENT

It is essential to understand the concepts of growth and development when learning to care for children. A skilled pediatric nurse integrates knowledge of physical growth and psychosocial development into each child healthcare encounter. **Growth** refers to an increase in physical size. Growth represents quantitative changes such as height, weight, blood pressure, and number of words in the child's vocabulary. **Development** refers to an increase in capability or function. Developmental skills unfold in a complex manner as a relationship between the child's innate, unfolding capabilities and the stimuli and support provided in the environment. Examples include the ability to sit without support or to throw a ball overhand. The quantitative and qualitative changes in body organ functioning, ability to communicate, and performance of motor skills unfold over time and are key components in the process of planning pediatric health care.

Each child displays a unique maturational pattern during the process of development. Although the exact age at which skills emerge differs, the sequence or order of skill performance is uniform among children. Skill development proceeds according to

GROWTH & DEVELOPMENT

Adoptees

While it is important for nurses to know usual developmental milestones, nurses must also be able to adapt information about development to specific circumstances. Some children will be slow to develop certain skills because they have a chronic illness or have had limited experiences with other children. An example chosen to demonstrate the application of development in special circumstances in this chapter is that of adoption. Many international adoptees are small in size, due to poor nutrition of the mother during pregnancy and of the infant after birth, and to growth delay related to emotional issues. The child should be examined closely at the time of adoption for length, weight, and head circumference. Within 6 months of arrival, most children show improvement in growth patterns. If growth does not improve by this time, the child is further assessed for problems such as intestinal parasites, chronic diseases, or other medical problems (Chen, Barnett, & Wilson, 2003; Miller, 2000; Barnett & Chen, 2005). The psychosocially based condition called eating disorder of infancy and childhood should also be considered (see Chapter 4 ∞ for a thorough description of this condition).

Although it is expected that international adoptees may have some developmental delays and often improve dramatically after adoption, testing of development, including verbal skills, upon arrival with their adoptive family is important. It provides a baseline upon which to measure future developmental test results and provides information needed to help parents encourage and stimulate the child appropriately (Miller, 2000). See Chapter 7 ∞ for a description of the Denver II Developmental Test.

The moment when the child meets an adoptive parent may be seen as joyous by the parent but can be traumatic for the young child who is separated from the adults who are familiar (Miller, 2005). Parents need preparation for establishing trust with the child. Institutionalization and multiple foster care placements in the child's past can result in emotional neglect, growth and developmental delays, and behavior problems among adoptees. In addition, attachment disorders and posttraumatic stress disorder may occur in some children in the adoptive home (Nickman, Rosenfeld, Fine et al., 2005). Parents need a thorough understanding of normal growth and development, as well as an understanding of the effects of the child's early life experience on the child's needs (Narad & Mason, 2004). Nurses perform careful developmental monitoring, assist adoptive parents in fostering normal growth and development, and provide referral to additional resources when needed. Integration into the school system for children of school age will necessitate special planning and the establishment of an individualized education plan or IEP (see Chapter 11 ∞ for further information about IEPs) (Dole, 2005).

---

two processes: from the head downward and from the center of the body out to the extremities. Development that proceeds from the head downward through the body and toward the feet is called **cephalocaudal development** (Figure 3–2 ➤). For example, at birth, an infant's head is much larger proportionately than the trunk or extremities. Similarly, infants learn to hold up their heads before sitting, and to sit before standing. Skills such as walking that involve the legs and feet develop last in infancy. Development that proceeds from the center of the body outward to the extremities is called **proximodistal development** (see Figure 3–2). For example, infants are first able to control the trunk, then the arms; only later are fine motor movements of the fingers possible. Pediatric nurses use these concepts of predictable and sequential developmental direction to analyze the infant's and child's present state and to assist parents to plan ways to encourage and support the next emerging developmental abilities.

During the childhood years, extraordinary changes occur in all aspects of development. Physical size, motor skills, cognitive ability, language, sensory ability, and psychosocial patterns all undergo major transformations. Nurses study normal patterns of development so they can perform thorough pediatric assessments and identify children who demonstrate slow or abnormal

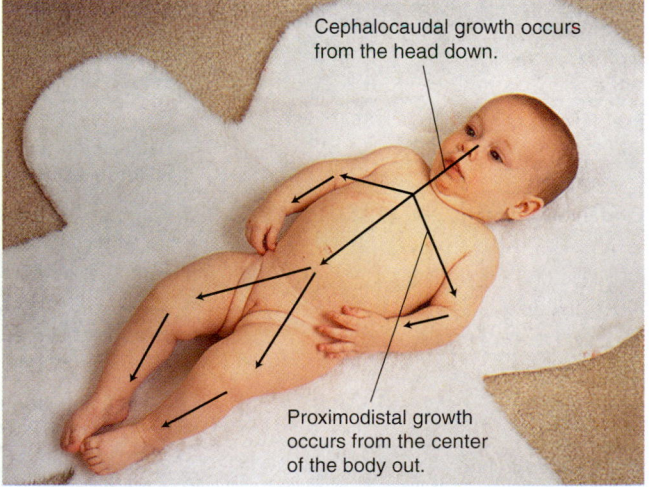

Cephalocaudal growth occurs from the head down.

Proximodistal growth occurs from the center of the body out.

Figure 3–2 ➤ In normal cephalocaudal growth, the child gains control of the head and neck before the trunk and limbs. In normal proximodistal growth, the child controls arm movements before hand movements. For example, the child reaches for objects before being able to grasp them. Children gain control of their hands before their fingers; that is, they can hold things with the entire hand before they can pick something up with just their fingers.

Infancy—Birth to 12 months. Includes infants or babies up to 1 year of age who require a high level of care in daily activities.

Toddlerhood—1–3 years. Characterized by increased motor ability and independent behavior.

Preschool—3–6 years. The preschooler refines gross and fine motor ability and language skills and often participates in a preschool learning program.

School age—6–12 years. Begins with entry into a school system and is characterized by growing intellectual skills, physical ability, and independence.

Adolescence—12–18 years. Begins with entry into the teen years. Mature cognitive thought, formation of identity, and influence of peers are important characteristics of adolescence.

development. These assessments can guide the nurse in planning interventions for the child and family, such as referring the child for a diagnostic evaluation or rehabilitation, or teaching the parents how to provide adequate stimulation for the child. When development is proceeding normally, the nurse uses the knowledge of usual patterns to plan teaching approaches based on the child's cognitive and language ability, to offer appropriate toys and activities during illness, and to respond therapeutically during interactions with the child.

MAJOR THEORIES OF DEVELOPMENT

Child development is a complex process. Many theorists have attempted to organize their observations of behavior into a description of principles or a set of stages. Each theory focuses on a particular facet of development. Most developmental theorists separate children into age groups by common characteristics. See Box 3–1 and Table 3–1.

Freud's Theory of Psychosexual Development
Theoretical Framework

The psychoanalytic techniques used by Freud led him to believe that early childhood experiences form the unconscious motivation for actions in later life. He developed a theory that sexual energy is centered in specific parts of the body at certain ages. Unresolved conflict and unmet needs at a certain stage lead to a fixation of development at that stage (Lerner, 2002).

Freud viewed the personality as a structure with three parts: the *id*, the basic sexual energy that is present at birth and drives the individual to seek pleasure; the *ego*, the realistic part of the person, which develops during infancy and searches for acceptable methods of meeting impulses; and the *superego*, the moral and ethical system, which develops in childhood and contains a set of values and conscience (Craig & Baucum, 2002). The ego diverts impulses and protects itself from excess anxiety by use of

Table 3–1	MAJOR DEVELOPMENTAL THEORISTS	
Theorist	**Years of Life**	**Background**
Sigmund Freud	1856–1939	Freud was a physician in Vienna, Austria. His work with adults who were experiencing a variety of nervous disorders led Freud to develop the approach called psychoanalysis, which explored the driving forces of the unconscious mind.
Erik Erikson	1902–1994	Erikson studied Freud's theory of psychoanalysis under Freud's daughter, Anna, but later established his own developmental theory emphasizing the psychosocial nature of individuals. Erikson's theory is one of the few that addresses development over the entire life span.
Jean Piaget	1896–1980	Piaget was a 20th-century Swiss scientist who watched his own three children carefully and wrote detailed journals of their behaviors and verbalizations. He studied the intellectual abilities of children, focusing on child psychology and its application to education.
Lawrence Kohlberg	1927–1987	Kohlberg used Piaget's cognitive stage theory as the basis for his theory of moral development. He worked with children in his native Germany and in many other countries, including Kenya, Taiwan, and Mexico.
Albert Bandura	b. 1925	Bandura is a Canadian who has conducted psychologic research at Stanford University for many years. He believes that children learn from their social environment, particularly by modeling the observed behaviors of others.
John Watson	1878–1958	Watson was an American scientist who applied the work of animal behaviorists, such as Ivan Pavlov and B. F. Skinner, to children.
Urie Bronfenbrenner	1917–2005	Bronfenbrenner established the ecologic theory of development and served as a professor at Cornell University. He viewed the child as interacting with the environment at different levels, or systems. This revolutionary approach emphasizes the series of mutual interactions between the child and the various systems.
Stella Chess and Alexander Thomas Chess (b.1914); Thomas (1914–2003)		Chess and Thomas are psychiatrists who began the New York Longitudinal Study in 1956 with 141 children, which they expanded in 1961 with 95 additional children. Most of these individuals are still being assessed periodically as adults. Their research identified characteristics of personality and provides a basis for the ongoing study of temperament (Chess & Thomas, 1995).

defense mechanisms, which are unconscious techniques that distort reality to protect the self from excessive anxiety (Table 3–2).

Stages

ORAL (BIRTH TO 1 YEAR)   The infant derives pleasure largely from the mouth, with sucking and eating as primary desires.

ANAL (1 TO 3 YEARS)   The young child's pleasure is centered in the anal area, with control over body secretions as a prime force in behavior.

PHALLIC (3 TO 6 YEARS)   Sexual energy becomes centered in the genitalia as the child works out relationships with parents of the same and opposite sexes.

LATENCY (6 TO 12 YEARS)   Sexual energy is at rest in the passage between earlier stages and adolescence.

GENITAL (12 YEARS TO ADULTHOOD)   Mature sexuality is achieved as physical growth is completed and relationships with others occur.

Nursing Application

Freud's theory has been criticized for several reasons—he developed a theory of childhood based on his work with adults, primarily women who sought help in dealing with emotional issues; he viewed males as dominant; and he ignored the effects of culture and other experiences. However, some parts of his theory can be applied in nursing. Freud emphasized the importance of meeting the needs of each stage in order to move successfully into future developmental stages. The crisis of illness can interfere with normal developmental processes and add challenges for the nurse who is striving to meet an ill child's needs. For example, the importance of sucking in infancy guides the nurse to provide a pacifier for the infant who cannot have oral fluids. The preschool child's concern about sexuality guides the nurse to provide privacy and clear explanations during any procedures involving the genital area. It may be necessary to teach parents that masturbation by the young child is normal and to help parents deal with it. The adolescent's focus on relationships suggests that the nurse should include questions about significant friends during history taking. Table 3–3 summarizes ways in which the nurse can apply these theoretical concepts to the care of children.

Erikson's Theory of Psychosocial Development
Theoretical Framework

Erikson's theory establishes psychosocial stages during eight periods of human life. For each stage, Erikson identifies a crisis, that is, a particular challenge that exists for healthy personality development to occur (Erikson, 1963, 1968). The word *crisis* in this context refers to normal maturational social needs rather than to a single critical event.

Table 3–2	COMMON DEFENSE MECHANISMS USED BY CHILDREN	
Defense Mechanism	**Definition**	**Example**
Regression	Return to an earlier behavior	A previously toilet-trained child becomes incontinent when separated from parents during a hospitalization.
Repression	Involuntary forgetting of uncomfortable situations	An abused child cannot consciously recall episodes of abuse.
Rationalization	An attempt to make unacceptable feelings acceptable	A child explains hitting another because "he took my toy."
Fantasy	A creation of the mind to help deal with unacceptable fear	A hospitalized child who is weak pretends to be Superman.

Table 3–3	**NURSING APPLICATIONS OF THEORIES OF FREUD, ERIKSON, AND PIAGET**

Age Group	Developmental Stages	Nursing Applications
Infant (birth to 1 year)	Oral stage (Freud): The baby obtains pleasure and comfort through the mouth.	When a baby is NPO, offer a pacifier if not contraindicated. After painful procedures, offer a baby a bottle or pacifier or have the mother breast-feed.
	Trust versus mistrust stage (Erikson): The baby establishes a sense of trust when basic needs are met.	Hold the hospitalized baby often. **(1)** Offer comfort after painful procedures. Meet the baby's needs for food and hygiene. Encourage parents to room in. Manage pain effectively with use of pain medications and other measures.
	Sensorimotor stage (Piaget): The baby learns from movement and sensory input.	Use crib mobiles, manipulative toys, wall murals, and bright colors to provide interesting stimuli and comfort. Use toys to distract the baby during procedures and assessments.
Toddler (1–3 years)	Anal stage (Freud): The child derives gratification from control over bodily excretions.	Ask about toilet training and the child's rituals and words for elimination during admission history. Continue the child's normal patterns of elimination in the hospital. Do not begin toilet training during illness or hospitalization. Accept regression in toileting during illness or hospitalization. Have potty chairs available in hospital and childcare centers. Allow self-feeding opportunities.
	Autonomy versus shame and doubt stage (Erikson): The child is increasingly independent in many spheres of life.	Encourage child to remove and put on own clothes, brush teeth, or assist with hygiene. **(2)** If restraint for a procedure is necessary, proceed quickly, providing explanations and comfort.
	Sensorimotor stage (end); preoperational stage (beginning) (Piaget): The child shows increasing curiosity and explorative behavior. Language skills improve.	Ensure safe surroundings to allow opportunities to manipulate objects. Name objects and give simple explanations.
Preschooler (3–6 years)	Phallic stage (Freud): The child initially identifies with the parent of the opposite sex but by the end of this stage has identified with the same-sex parent.	Be alert for children who appear more comfortable with male or female nurses, and attempt to accommodate them. Encourage parental involvement in care. Plan for playtime and offer a variety of materials from which to choose.
	Initiative versus guilt stage (Erikson): The child likes to initiate play activities.	Offer medical equipment for play to lessen anxiety about strange objects. **(3)** Assess children's concerns as expressed through their drawings. Accept the child's choices and expressions of feelings.
	Preoperational stage (Piaget): The child is increasingly verbal but has some limitations in thought processes. Causality is often confused, so the child may feel responsible for causing an illness.	Offer explanations about all procedures and treatments. Clearly explain that the child is not responsible for causing the illness.

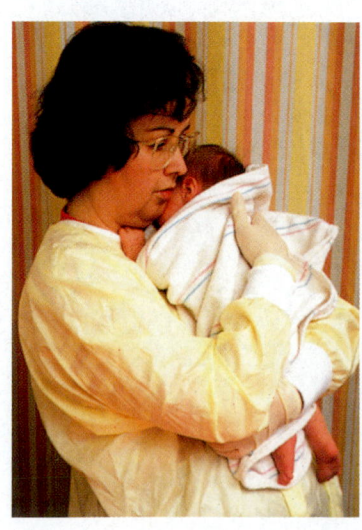

(1)

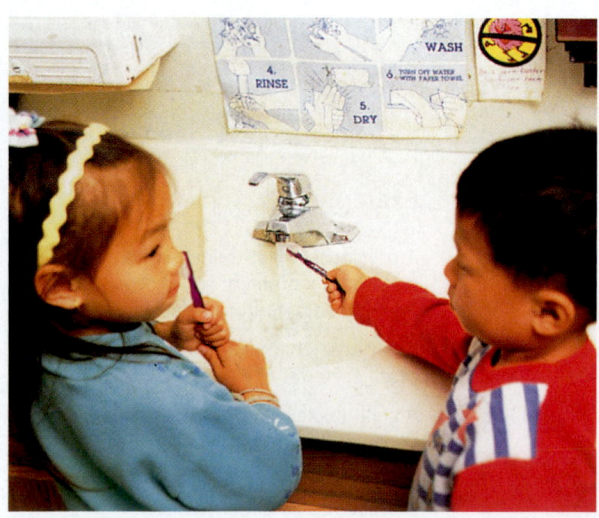

(2)

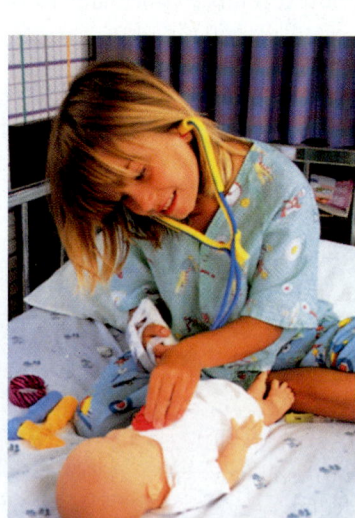

(3)

Table 3–3	**NURSING APPLICATIONS OF THEORIES OF FREUD, ERIKSON, AND PIAGET (continued)**	
Age Group	**Developmental Stages**	**Nursing Applications**
School age (6–12 years)	Latency stage (Freud): The child places importance on privacy and understanding the body.	Provide gowns, covers, and underwear. Knock on door before entering. Explain treatments and procedures.
	Industry versus inferiority stage (Erikson): The child gains a sense of self-worth from involvement in activities.	Encourage the child to continue school work while hospitalized. Encourage the child to bring favorite pastimes to the hospital. **(4)** Help child adjust to limitations on favorite activities.
	Concrete operational stage (Piaget): The child is capable of mature thought when allowed to manipulate and see objects.	Give clear instructions about details of treatment. Show the child equipment that will be used in treatment.
Adolescent (12–18 years)	Genital stage (Freud): The adolescent's focus is on genital function and relationships.	Ensure access to gynecologic care for adolescent girls. Provide information on sexuality. Ensure privacy during healthcare. Have brochures and videos available for teaching about sexuality.
	Identity versus role confusion stage (Erikson): The adolescent's search for self-identity leads to independence from parents and reliance on peers.	Provide a separate recreation room for teens who are hospitalized. **(5)** Take health history and perform examinations without parents present. Introduce adolescent to other teens with the same health condition.
	Formal operational stage (Piaget): The adolescent is capable of mature, abstract thought.	Give clear and complete information about health care and treatments. Offer both written and verbal instructions. Continue to provide education about the disease to the adolescent with a chronic illness, as mature thought now leads to greater understanding.

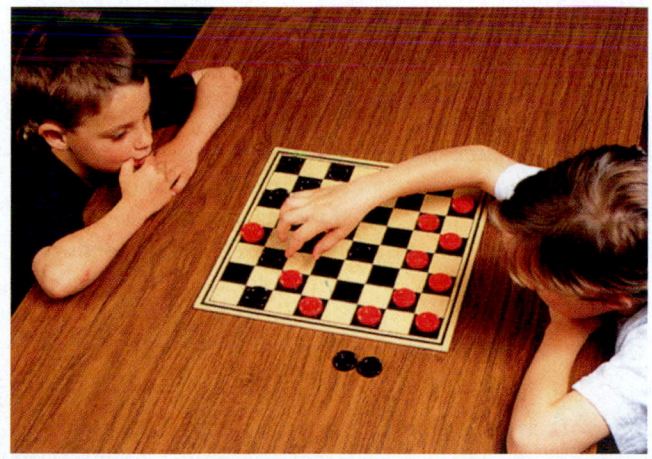

(4)

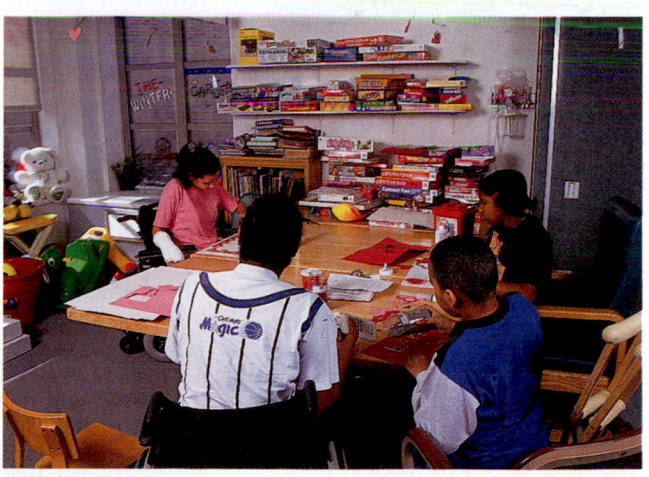

(5)

Each developmental crisis has two possible outcomes: When needs are met, the consequence is healthy and the individual moves on to future stages with particular strengths. When needs are not met, an unhealthy outcome occurs that will influence future social relationships.

Stages

TRUST VERSUS MISTRUST (BIRTH TO 1 YEAR)   The task of the first year of life is to establish trust in the people providing care. Trust is fostered by provision of food, clean clothing, touch, and comfort. If basic needs are not met, the infant will eventually learn to mistrust others.

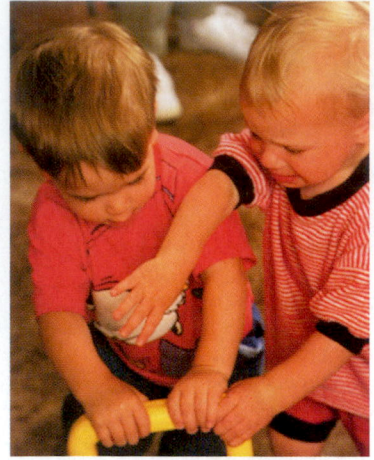

A

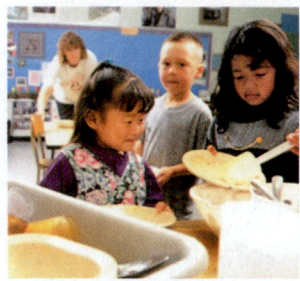

B

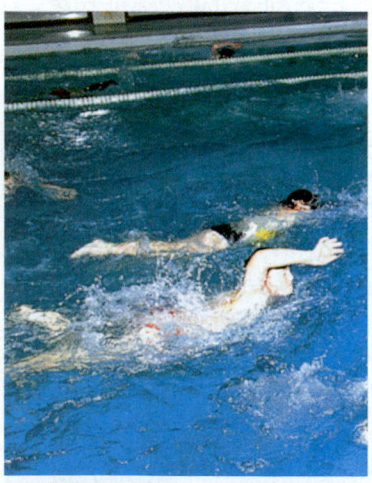

C

Figure 3–3 ▶ Erikson's Psychosocial Stages. A, The toddler shows *autonomy* by exerting control over toys and activities. B, Preschoolers demonstrate *initiative* by planning and carrying out activities. C, School-age children excel at *industry* when they take pride in accomplishments, such as those achieved in sporting activities.

AUTONOMY VERSUS SHAME AND DOUBT (1 TO 3 YEARS) The toddler's sense of autonomy or independence is shown by controlling body excretions, saying no when asked to do something, and directing motor activity. Children who are consistently criticized for expressions of autonomy or for lack of control—for example, during toilet training—will develop a sense of shame about themselves and doubt in their abilities (Figure 3–3 ▶).

INITIATIVE VERSUS GUILT (3 TO 6 YEARS) The young child initiates new activities and considers new ideas. This interest in exploring the world creates a child who is involved and busy. Constant criticism, however, leads to feelings of guilt and a lack of purpose.

INDUSTRY VERSUS INFERIORITY (6 TO 12 YEARS) The middle years of childhood are characterized by development of new interests and by involvement in activities. The child takes pride in accomplishments in sports, school, home, and community. If the child cannot accomplish what is expected, however, the result will be a sense of inferiority.

IDENTITY VERSUS ROLE CONFUSION (12 TO 18 YEARS) In adolescence, as the body matures and thought processes become more complex, a new sense of identity or self is established. The self, family, peer group, and community are all examined and redefined. The adolescent who is unable to establish a meaningful definition of self will experience confusion in one or more roles of life.

Nursing Application

Erikson's theory is directly applicable to the nursing care of children. Health promotion and health maintenance visits in the community provide opportunities for helping caregivers meet children's needs. Parents benefit from learning what the child's developmental tasks are at each stage and from discussing ideas about how to encourage healthy psychosocial development. Such discussions may also highlight parental concerns and provide a forum for reassurance about normal developmental characteristics.

The child's usual support from family, peers, and others is interrupted by hospitalization. The challenge of hospitalization also adds a situational crisis to the normal developmental crisis a child is experiencing. Although the nurse may meet many of the hospitalized child's needs, continued parental involvement is necessary both during and after hospitalization to ensure progression through expected developmental stages (see Table 3–3). Asking parents about the child's developmental progression offers clues to activities and provides information about the child's psychosocial needs during hospitalization.

Piaget's Theory of Cognitive Development
Theoretical Framework

Based on his observations and work with children, Piaget formulated a theory of cognitive (or intellectual) development. He believed that the child's view of the world is influenced largely by age and maturational ability. Given nurturing experiences, the child's ability to think matures naturally (Ginsberg & Opper, 1988; Piaget, 1972). The child incorporates new experiences via **assimilation** and changes to deal with these experiences by the process of **accommodation**. An example of assimilation occurs when the infant uses reflexes to suck on objects that touch the lips. With more experiences the infant accommodates by realizing that not all objects are pleasant to suck; cognitive structures change to integrate and learn from the experiences of sucking.

Stages

SENSORIMOTOR (BIRTH TO 2 YEARS) Infants learn about the world by input obtained through the senses and by their motor activity. Six substages are characteristic of this stage.

Use of Reflexes (Birth to 1 Month)   The infant begins life with a set of reflexes such as sucking, rooting, and grasping. By using these reflexes, the infant receives stimulation via touch, sound, smell, and vision. The reflexes thus pave the way for the first learning to occur.

Primary Circular Reactions (1 to 4 Months)   Once the infant responds reflexively, the pleasure gained from that response causes repetition of the behavior. For example, if a toy grasped reflexively makes noise and is interesting to watch, the infant will grasp it again (Figure 3–4a ➤).

Secondary Circular Reactions (4 to 8 Months)   Awareness of the environment grows as the infant begins to connect cause and effect. The sounds of bottle preparation will lead to excited behavior. If an object is partially hidden, the infant will attempt to uncover and retrieve it.

Coordination of Secondary Schemes (8 to 12 Months)   Intentional behavior is observed as the infant uses learned behavior to obtain objects, create sounds, or engage in other pleasurable activity. **Object permanence** (the knowledge that something continues to exist even when out of sight) begins when the infant remembers where a hidden object is likely to be found; it is no longer "out of sight, out of mind." However, the concept of object permanence is not fully developed. The infant knows the parent well, objects to new people, and seems very worried when the parent leaves. Other caretakers may be rejected as the infant does not understand that the parent will return. This phase of "stranger anxiety" is quite common and heralds the infant's growing recognition of and desire to be cared for by the parent.

Tertiary Circular Reactions (12 to 18 Months)   Curiosity, experimentation, and exploration predominate as the toddler tries out actions to learn results. Objects are turned in every direction, placed in the mouth, used for banging, and inserted in containers as their qualities and uses are explored (Figure 3–4b ➤).

Mental Combinations (18 to 24 Months)   Language provides a new tool for the toddler to use in understanding the world. Language enables the child to think about events and objects before or after they occur. Object permanence is now fully developed as the child actively searches for objects in various locations and out of view. The child who has had successful separations from the parents followed by return, such as hours spent in another's home or childcare center, begins to understand that the missing parent will return (Figure 3–4c ➤).

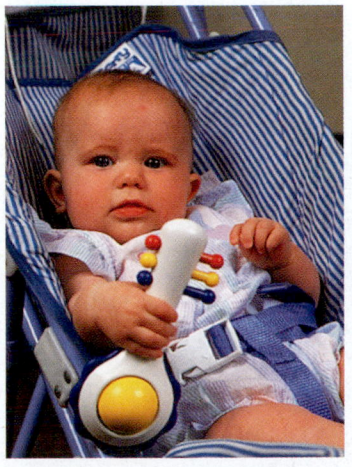   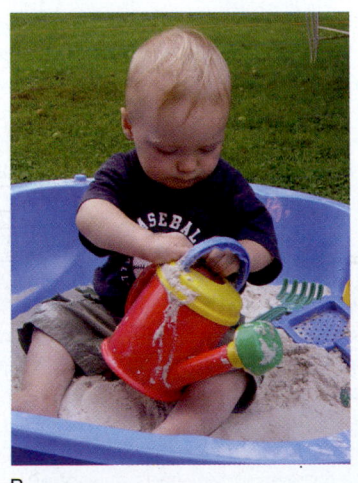   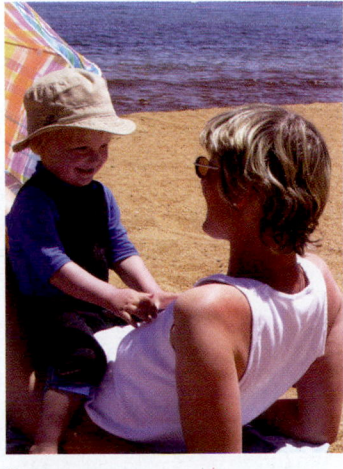

A   B   C

Figure 3–4 ➤ Piaget's Cognitive Stages. A, A young infant displays *primary circular reactions* when a reflexive response, such as shaking a rattle, results in pleasure and is repeated. B, As the infant becomes a toddler, *tertiary circular reactions* are demonstrated when the child experiments with objects by turning them, placing them in the mouth, and banging them. C, Toddlers and preschoolers demonstrate *mental combinations* as they increasingly use language to describe and understand their worlds.

PREOPERATIONAL (2 TO 7 YEARS)   The young child thinks by using words as symbols, but logic is not well developed. During the *preconceptual substage* (2 to 4 years), vocabulary and comprehension increase greatly, but the child shows **egocentrism** (that is, an inability to see things from the perspective of another). In the *intuitive substage* (4 to 7 years), the child relies on **transductive reasoning** (that is, drawing conclusions from one general fact to another). For example, if a child disobeys a parent and then falls and breaks an arm that day, the child may ascribe the broken arm to bad behavior. Cause-and-effect relationships are often unrealistic or a result of **magical thinking** (the belief that events occur because of thoughts or wishes). Additional characteristics noted in the thought of preschoolers include **centration**, or the ability to consider only one aspect of a situation at a time, and **animism**, or ascribing life to inanimate objects because they move, make noise, or have certain other qualities.

CONCRETE OPERATIONAL (7 TO 11 YEARS)   Transductive reasoning has given way to a more accurate understanding of cause and effect. The child can reason quite well if concrete objects are used in teaching or experimentation. The concept of **conservation** (that matter does not change when its form is altered) is learned at this age.

FORMAL OPERATIONAL (11 YEARS TO ADULTHOOD)   Fully mature intellectual thought has now been attained. The adolescent can think abstractly about objects or concepts and consider different alternatives or outcomes.

Nursing Application

Piaget's theory is essential to pediatric nursing. The nurse must understand a child's thought processes in order to design stimulating activities and meaningful, appropriate teaching plans. Health teaching is tailored to understanding of cognitive stages. For example, understanding a child's concept of time suggests to the nurse how far in advance to prepare that child for procedures. Similarly, the nurse's decision to offer manipulative toys, read stories, draw pictures, or give the child reading material to explain healthcare measures depends on the child's cognitive stage of development (see Table 3–3). Refer back to the opening scenario and 2-year-old Irena. What activities will you plan for Irena during a healthcare visit based on her expected cognitive level? How can you encourage her cognitive development? What activities will you suggest for her parents at home?

RESEARCH

Cognitive Theories

All developmental theories are simply that—theories. A theory is developed to explain a collection of observations or facts and to predict future occurrences. As such, no theory can explain all of reality and all have some strengths and some weaknesses. While Piaget's theory of cognitive development provides a useful framework to examine and understand the thought process of young children, like all theories, it is not perfect. He developed the theory mainly by observation of his own three children. It may lack some applicability in cross-cultural contexts, and it does not explain the importance of social contexts in learning. Two other important cognitive theories help to expand the work of Piaget and may provide assistance for nurses planning to teach young children:

1. Lev Vygotsky (1896–1934) agreed with Piaget's theory of the child's cognition. However, he believed that children are embedded in social contexts that influence learning. As parents and others guide and assist children they learn tasks that were impossible for them to master alone. He also viewed the social structure of language as essential to development of thought (Santrock, 2005; Vygotsky, 1962).
2. Information processing is another theory about cognitive development that views attention and memory as the most important parts of learning, rather than the structures described by Piaget. Infants tend to habituate or become bored with the same stimuli and therefore are more attentive to, and learn from, new stimuli that are introduced to them. Both long-term and short-term memory are important to learning. The older child actively engages in strategies to assist with memorization, thereby playing an active part in learning (Meltzoff & Gopnick, 1997; Santrock, 2005).

Kohlberg's Theory of Moral Development
Theoretical Framework

Lawrence Kohlberg's focus is on a particular type of cognitive development concerned with moral decisions. He presented stories involving moral dilemmas to children and adults and asked them to solve the dilemmas. Kohlberg then analyzed the motives people expressed when making decisions about the best course to take. Based on the explanations given, Kohlberg established three levels of moral reasoning. Although he provided age guidelines, he stated that they are approximate and that many people never reach the highest (postconventional) stage of development (Santrock, 2005).

Kohlberg's work has been criticized for insensitivity to cultural differences in moral reasoning, lack of consideration of the family in moral development, an emphasis on moral reasoning rather than actual actions, and for sexual bias. However, it remains a useful framework to help understand moral decision making.

Stages

PRECONVENTIONAL (4 TO 7 YEARS)   Decisions are based on the desire to please others and to avoid punishment.

CONVENTIONAL (7 TO 11 YEARS)   Conscience or an internal set of standards becomes important. Rules are important and must be followed to please other people and "be good."

POSTCONVENTIONAL (12 YEARS AND OLDER)   The individual has internalized ethical standards on which to base decisions. Social responsibility is recognized. The value in each of two differing moral approaches can be considered and a decision made.

Nursing Application

Decision making is required in many areas of health care. Children can be assisted to make decisions about health care and to consider alternatives when available. The nurse should keep in mind that young children may agree to participate in research simply because they want to comply with adults and appear cooperative. Guidelines for child participation in research are available (see Chapter 1 ∞).

Parents can be provided with information so that they can assist their children in moral judgments. Encourage talking with a child or adolescent about how a given decision was made. Parents can then add information and help the child learn to integrate more factors into decision making. Talking about the process is important in helping children progress to higher stages of moral development. Focusing on the feelings of others, using positive discipline techniques, and clearly identifying positive and negative behaviors are important.

Social Learning Theory
Theoretical Framework

Bandura, a contemporary psychologist, believes that children learn attitudes, beliefs, customs, and values through their social contacts with adults and other children. Children imitate (or model) the behavior they see; if the behavior is positively reinforced, they tend to repeat it. However, Bandura also believes that people can consciously choose how to act, such as deciding to handle problems by talking rather than using violence. The external environment (the behavior of others) and the child's internal processes are both key elements in the behaviors the child manifests (Bandura, 1986, 1997a).

Bandura believes that an important determinant of behavior is **self-efficacy**, or the expectation that someone can produce a desired outcome. For example, if adolescents believe they can avoid use of drugs or alcohol, they are more likely to do so. A child who has confidence in his or her ability to exercise regularly or lose weight has a greater chance of success with these behavior changes. Parents who have confidence in their ability to care adequately for their infants are more likely to do so (Bandura, 1997b). See Evidence-Based Practice: Self-Efficacy on the next page.

EVIDENCE-BASED PRACTICE

Self-Efficacy

Clinical Question

How can nurses use the concept of self-efficacy when planning interventions for children and families?

Evidence

Nurses often provide information for parents and children that will encourage them to adopt healthy lifestyles. Providing information may not be enough; many of us know about health behaviors but do not consistently apply them. The concept of self-efficacy helps to explain why some people take on healthy behaviors while others do not. People who are convinced they can make a positive change are more likely to do so. A number of research projects test and apply self-efficacy in teaching about health. Two examples follow.

- Few effective interventions have been found that prevent or lower obesity rates in early adolescents. Nurses tested a health promotion program designed to increase self-efficacy and provide information in a group of 60 middle school youth, matched with 57 youth who did not receive the teaching. Children who had low self-efficacy scores tended to have greater consumption of high-fat foods. The intervention was associated with significantly lowered fat in the diet. Approaches that address diet choices, consciousness, efficacy, and other behavioral factors are more likely to contribute to dietary change than simple presentation of facts about dietary intake (Frenn, Malin, & Bansal, 2003).

- Violence among youth is a complex problem that presents challenges to nurses in many settings. The authors examined factors that influence extent and likelihood of youth violence among 318 middle school students. Self-efficacy was identified as a key concept for testing, and was defined as the confidence of students to avoid engaging in physically violent behaviors. Lower self-efficacy was associated with, and a strong predictor of, more frequent violent behaviors. Interventions can be targeted at increasing students' self-efficacy so that violent behaviors will decrease (Riner & Saywell, 2002).

Implications

When planning interventions to encourage health behaviors in children and adolescents, assess the youth's belief that the new behaviors are important and that they can be adopted. Include interventions that demonstrate that others have adopted the health behaviors and plan approaches to enhance the child's belief in ability to change.

Critical Thinking

Plan a teaching project about the importance of physical activity for presentation to a group of 12-year-olds. What approaches will enhance the self-efficacy of the children? How would interventions to enhance self-efficacy differ for young elementary schoolchildren compared to those in middle or high school? What theoretical approaches discussed earlier in this chapter help you to understand the cognitive abilities of children at various ages and suggest ways to influence their self-efficacy?

References

Frenn, M., Malin, S., & Bansal, N. K. (2003). Stage-based interventions for low-fat diet with middle school students. *Journal of Pediatric Nursing, 18,* 36–45.

Riner, M. E., & Saywell, R. M. (2002). Development of the Social Ecology Model of Adolescent Interpersonal Violence Prevention (SEMAIVP). *Journal of School Health, 72,* 65–70.

Nursing Application

The importance of modeling behavior can readily be applied in health care. Children are more likely to cooperate if they see adults or other children performing a task willingly. A frightened child may watch another child perform vision screening or have blood drawn and then decide to allow the procedure to take place. Contact with positive role models is useful when teaching children and adolescents self-care for chronic diseases such as diabetes. Positive reinforcement should be given for desired performance.

Nurses can utilize the concept of self-efficacy to increase the chance of success with lifestyle behavior changes. For example, encouraging youth who are trying to quit smoking, providing them with role models, and pointing out parental successes with their children all demonstrate methods of fostering self-efficacy.

Behaviorism

Theoretical Framework

John Watson studied the research of Pavlov and Skinner, who demonstrated that actions are determined by responses from the environment. Pavlov and, later, Skinner worked with animals, presenting a stimulus such as food and pairing it with another stimulus such as a ringing bell. Eventually the animal being fed began to salivate when the bell rang. As Skinner and then Watson began to apply these concepts to children, they showed that behaviors can be elicited by positive reinforcement, such as a food treat, or extinguished by negative reinforcement, such as by scolding or withdrawal of attention. Watson believed that he could make a child into anyone he desired—from a professional to a thief or beggar—simply by reinforcing behavior in certain ways (Santrock, 2005).

Nursing Application

Behaviorism has been criticized for its simplicity and its denial of the inherent capability of persons to respond willfully to events in the environment. This theory does, however, have some use in health care. When particular behaviors are desired, positive reinforcement can be established to encourage these behaviors. Behavioral techniques are also used to alter the behavior of children who misbehave or to teach skills to children who are physically challenged. Parents often use reinforcement in toilet training and other skills learned in childhood. Indeed, combining behaviorism with social learning theory can be beneficial. For example, children might have desired activities, such as tooth brushing, modeled by an adult or older child (social learning theory), and be rewarded (behaviorism) for carrying out the activity on a regular basis.

Ecologic Theory

Theoretical Framework

You may have noticed that there is controversy among theorists concerning the relative importance of heredity versus environment—or nature versus nurture—in human development. **Nature** refers to the genetic or hereditary capability of an individual. **Nurture** refers to the effects of the environment on a person's performance (Box 3–2). Piaget believed in the importance of internal cognitive structures that unfold at their appointed times, given any environment that provides basic opportunities. He emphasized the strength of nature. The behaviorist John Watson, however, believed that behaviors are primarily shaped by environmental responses; he thus stressed the predominance of nurture. Contemporary developmental theories increasingly recognize the interaction of nature and nurture in determining the child's development.

The ecologic theory of development was formulated by Urie Bronfenbrenner to explain the child's unique relationship in all of life's settings, from close to remote (Bronfenbrenner, 1986, 2005; Bronfenbrenner, McClelland, Ceci, Moen, & Wethington, 1996). **Ecologic theory** emphasizes the presence of mutual interactions between the child and these various settings. Neither nature nor nurture is considered of more importance. Bronfenbrenner believes each child brings a unique set of genes—and specific attributes such as age, gender, health, and other characteristics—to his or her interactions with the environment. The child then interacts in many settings at different levels or systems (Figure 3–5 ➤).

Levels or Systems

MICROSYSTEM This level is defined as the daily, consistent, close relationships such as home, childcare, school, friends, and neighbors. For the child with a chronic illness requiring regular care, the healthcare providers may even be part of the microsystem. In the ecologic model, the child influences each of these settings in addition to being influenced by them, with reciprocal interactions. Consider how Irena's microsystems have changed. Initially her mother and siblings were the important persons in her daily life, then the orphanage staff and other children, and finally Michael and Alyssa and their families and friends. How might these changes have influenced Irena? What stability is needed now to foster her ability to form relationships?

MESOSYSTEM This level includes relationships of microsystems with one another. For example, two microsystems for most children are the home and the school. The relationships between these microsystems are shown by parents' involvement in their children's school. This involvement, in turn, influences the effects of the home and school settings on the children.

EXOSYSTEM This level is composed of those settings that influence the child even though the child is not in close daily contact with the system. Examples include the parents' jobs and the governing board of the local school district. Although the child may not go to the parents' workplaces, he or she can be influenced by policies related to health care, sick leave, inflexible work hours, overtime, travel, or even by the mood of the boss (through its impact on the parent). The child's needs may influence a

---

BOX 3–2
NATURE VERSUS NURTURE

Does nature or nurture have primary importance in the theories of Erikson, Kohlberg, Freud, and social learning? Think about whether each of the theories emphasizes the role of heredity (nature) or the role of the environment (nurture) in influencing the development of children.

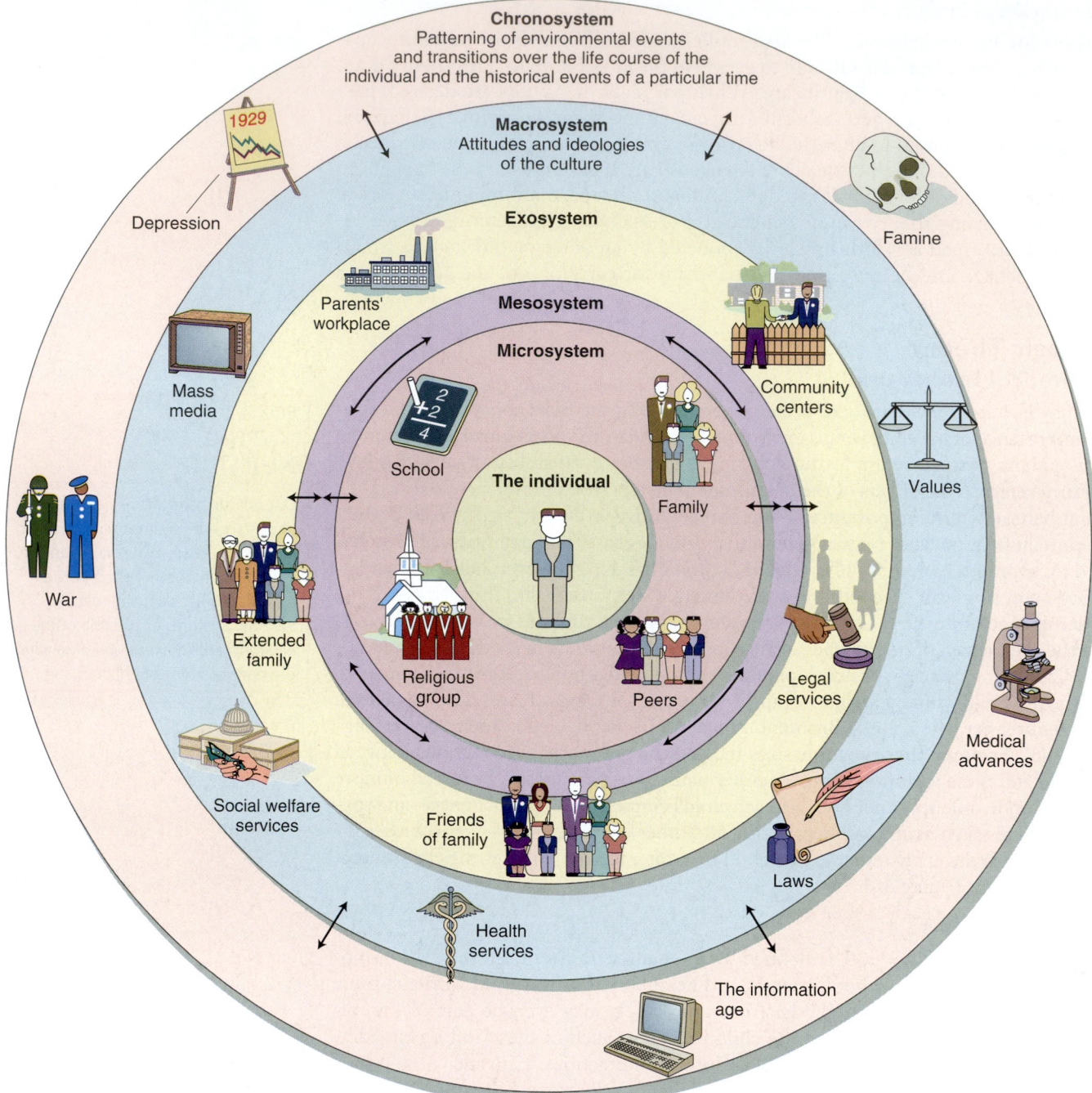

Figure 3–5 ➤ Bronfenbrenner's ecologic theory of development views the individual as interacting within five levels or systems.
Note: Redrawn from Santrock, J. W. (2005). *Life span development*. Madison, WI: Brown & Benchmark. Based on Brofenbrenner's (1979, 1986) works in Contexts of child rearing: Problems and prospects. *American Psychologist, 34,* 844–850; and Ecology of the family as a context for human development: Research perspectives. *Developmental Psychology, 22,* 723–742.

parent to give up a certain job or to work harder to obtain money for the child's education. Likewise, when a local school board votes to ban certain books or to finance a field trip, the child is influenced by these decisions; the child, in turn, can help establish an atmosphere that will guide future school board decisions.

MACROSYSTEM   This level includes the beliefs, values, and behaviors expressed in the child's environment. Culture is a powerful influence in the macrosystem, as is the political system. For instance, a democratic system creates different beliefs, values, and even eating practices than an anarchic system.

CHRONOSYSTEM   This final level brings the perspective of time to the previous settings. The time period during which the child grows up influences views of health and illness. For example, the experiences of children with influenza in the 19th versus 20th centuries were quite different.

Nursing Application

Nurses use ecologic theory when they assess the child's settings to identify influences on development. Table 3–4 provides an assessment tool based on this theory. Interventions are planned to enhance the strengths of the child's settings and to improve on areas that are not supportive. Ask yourself the following questions:

- How does the child influence each system?
- How is the child influenced by each system?
- What interventions should be planned for the child?

Temperament Theory

Theoretical Framework

In contrast to behaviorists such as Watson or maturational theorists such as Piaget, Chess and Thomas (1995, 1996) recognize the innate qualities of personality that each individual brings to the events of daily life. They, like Bronfenbrenner, viewed the child as an individual who both influences and is influenced by the environment. However, Chess and Thomas focused on one specific aspect of development—the wide spectrum of behaviors possible in children, identifying nine parameters of response to daily events (Box 3–3). Infants generally display clusters of responses, which Chess and Thomas have classified into three major personality types (Box 3–4). Although most children do not demonstrate all behaviors described for a particular type, they usually show a grouping indicative of one personality type (Chess & Thomas, 1995, 1996).

Longitudinal research has demonstrated that personality characteristics displayed during infancy are often consistent with those seen later in life. The ability to predict future characteristics is not possible, however, because of the complex and dynamic interaction of personality traits and environmental reactions.

Many other researchers have expanded the work of Chess and Thomas, developing assessment tools for temperament types. The concept of "goodness of fit" is an outgrowth of this theory. Goodness of fit refers to whether parents' expectations of their child's behavior are consistent with the child's temperament type. There is a "good fit" when the properties of the environment are in accord with the child's capabilities, characteristics, and style of behavior (Chess & Thomas, 1999; Turecki, 2003). As an example of lack of good fit, an active infant who reacts strongly to verbal stimuli may be unable to sleep when placed in a room with older siblings. A child who is slow to warm

Table 3–4	ASSESSMENT OF ECOLOGIC SYSTEMS IN CHILDHOOD—BRONFENBRENNER			
Microsystems	**Mesosystems**	**Exosystems**	**Macrosystems**	**Chronosystems**
Parents	Parents' involvement in childcare or school	Community centers	Cultural group membership	Child's age
Significant others in close contact	Parents' involvement in community	Local political influences	Beliefs and values of group	Parents' ages
Childcare arrangements	Parents' relationships with significant others (e.g., grandparents, care providers)	Parents' work	Political structure	
School		Parents' friends and activities		
Neighborhood contacts	Influences of religious community (e.g., church, synagogue mosque) or parents and school	Social services		
Clubs		Health care		
Friends, peers		Libraries		
Religious community, (e.g., churches, synagogues, mosques)				

BOX 3–3
NINE PARAMETERS OF PERSONALITY—CHESS AND THOMAS

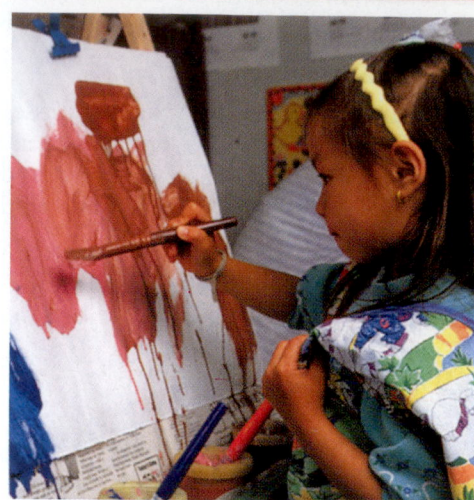

1. **Activity level.** The degree of motion during eating, playing, sleeping, or bathing. Scored as high, medium, or low.
2. **Rhythmicity.** The regularity of schedule maintained for sleep, hunger, or elimination. Scored as regular, variable, or irregular.
3. **Approach or withdrawal.** The response to a new stimulus such as a food, activity, or person. Scored as approachable, variable, or withdrawn.
4. **Adaptability.** The degree of adaptation to new situations. Scored as adaptive, variable, or nonadaptive.
5. **Threshold of responsiveness.** The intensity of stimulation needed to elicit a response to sensory input, objects in the environment, or people. Scored as high, medium, or low.
6. **Intensity of reaction.** The degree of response to situations. Scored as positive, variable, or negative.
7. **Quality of mood.** The predominant mood during daily activity and in response to stimuli. Scored as positive, variable, or negative.
8. **Distractibility.** The ability of environmental stimuli to interfere with the child's activity. Scored as distractible, variable, or nondistractible.
9. **Attention span and persistence.** The amount of time devoted to activities (compared with other children of the same age) and the degree of ability to stick with an activity in spite of obstacles. Scored as persistent, variable, or nonpersistent.

Note: Adapted from Chess, S., & Thomas, A. (1996). *Temperament: Theory and practice.* Philadelphia: Brunner/Mazel Publishers.

up may not perform well in the first few months at a new school, much to parents' disappointment. When parents understand a child's temperament characteristics, they are better able to shape the environment to meet the child's needs.

Nursing Application

The concept of personality type or temperament is a useful one for nurses (McClowry & Galehouse, 2002). Nurses can assess the temperament of young children and alter the environment to meet their needs. This may involve moving a hospitalized child to a single room to ensure adequate rest if the child is easily stimulated, or allowing a shy child time to become accustomed to new surroundings and equipment before beginning procedures or treatments.

Parents are often relieved to learn about temperament characteristics. They learn to appreciate their children's qualities and to adapt the environment to meet the children's needs. A burden of guilt can also be lifted from parents who feel that they are responsible for their child's actions. The nurse can teach parents ways of enhancing goodness of fit between the child's personality and the environment (Table 3–5). See further suggestions for helping parents understand temperament during health promotion and health maintenance visits in Chapters 8 through 10 ∞.

Resiliency Theory
Theoretical Framework

Why do some children coming from similar backgrounds have such different behavioral outcomes? A theory that examines both the individual's characteristics as well as the interaction of these characteristics with the environment is the resiliency model. **Resilience** is the ability to function with healthy responses, even with significant stress and adversity (Stewart, Reid, & Mangham, 1997). In this model, the individual or family members experience a crisis that provides a source of stress, and the family interprets

BOX 3–4
PATTERNS OF TEMPERAMENT—CHESS AND THOMAS

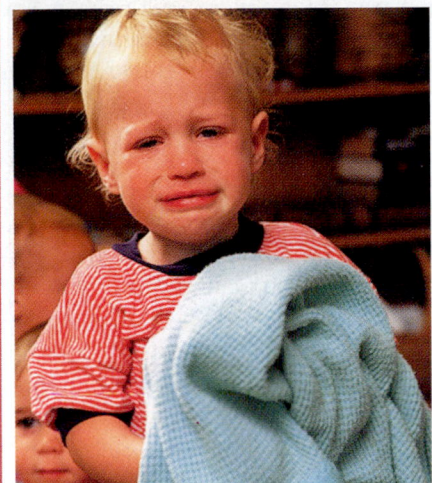

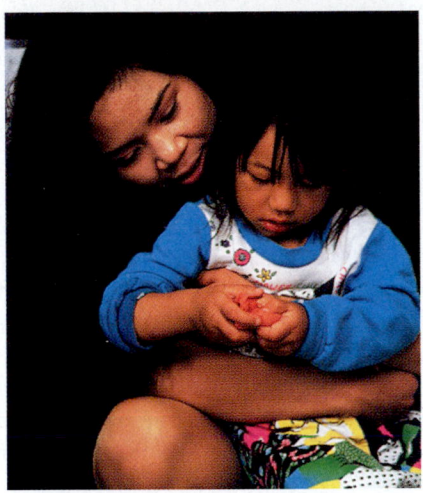

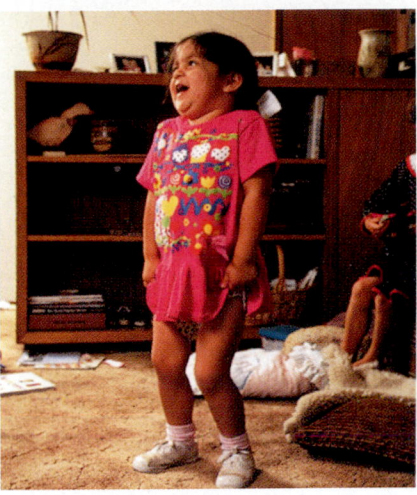

The "difficult" child displays irregular schedules for eating, sleeping, and elimination; adapts slowly to new situations and persons; and displays a predominantly negative mood. Intense reactions to the environment are common. About 10% of children in the New York Longitudinal Study displayed this personality type.

The "slow-to-warm-up" child has reactions of mild intensity and slow adaptability to new situations. The child displays initial withdrawal followed by gradual, quiet, and slow interaction with the environment. About 15% of children in the New York Longitudinal Study displayed this personality type.

The "easy" child is generally moderate in activity; shows regularity in patterns of eating, sleeping, and elimination; and is usually positive in mood and when subjected to new stimuli. The easy child adapts to new situations and is able to accept rules and work well with others. About 40% of children in the New York Longitudinal Study displayed this personality type.

*The remaining 35% of children studied showed some characteristics of each personality type.

or deals with the crisis based on resources available. Families and individuals have **protective factors** that provide strength and assistance in dealing with crises, and **risk factors** that promote or contribute to their challenges. Risk and protective factors can be identified in children, in their families, and in their communities (see Chapter 6 ∞ for further description of the interplay of social and environmental factors with individual characteristics). A crisis for a young child might be a transfer to a new childcare provider. Protective factors could involve past positive experiences with new people, an "easy" temperament, and awareness of the new childcare provider about adaptation needs of young children to new experiences. Risk factors for a similar child might be repeated moves to new care providers, limited close relationships with adults, and a "slow-to-warm-up" temperament.

Table 3–5	WAYS TO IMPROVE GOODNESS OF FIT BETWEEN PARENT AND CHILD
Child's Behavior	**Parent's Activity**
Extremely active	Plan periods of active play several times in a day. Have restful periods before bedtime to foster sleep.
Shy	Allow time to adapt at own pace to new people and situations.
Easily stimulated	Have quiet room for sleeping as an infant. Have quiet room for homework as a school-age child.
Short attention span	Provide projects that can be completed in a short period. Gradually encourage longer periods at activities.

BOX 3–5

ASSESSMENT QUESTIONS TO DETERMINE RESILIENCE CAPABILITY

Questions to Determine Risk Factors

- Describe the event that occurred and what it has been like for your family.
- What other stressors do you have in your family right now?
- Are there financial worries?
- Are there things you think and worry about late at night?
- Describe your job, your friends.
- Describe your typical day.
- Describe your neighborhood.
- Do you have friends, people to call in emergencies?

Questions to Determine Protective Factors

- What gives you strength?
- How do you deal with this stress?
- What do you think you do well in your family?
- Who do you call when you need help?
- Do you have a computer? Internet access?
- Are you religious? Spiritual?
- Do you exercise regularly?
- How do you spend free time?

Once confronted by a crisis, the child and family first experience the **adjustment phase**, characterized by disorganization and unsuccessful attempts at meeting the crisis. In the **adaptation phase**, the child and family meet the challenge and use resources to deal with the crisis (Malone, 1998). Adaptation may lead to increasing resilience as well when the child and family learn about new resources and inner strengths and develop the ability to deal more effectively with future crises. The model and examples are described in Table 3–6.

Nursing Application

Nurses gather information about the individual characteristics, prior life experiences, and environmental factors that act as protective and risk factors for children. Box 3–5 lists questions that can be helpful as the nurse gathers information from a child or family members. Nurses then use concepts of resiliency theory in planning interventions for children and families. Nursing strategies can target risk factors, such as encouraging family behaviors to ensure gun safety by teaching about use of gun trigger locks and locked gun cabinets in families with firearms. In addition, protective factors can be emphasized, such as encouraging holding and verbalization to parents of infants to provide an environment that meets needs for trust establishment and speech development.

INFLUENCES ON DEVELOPMENT

As we have seen, both nature and nurture are important in determining individual patterns of development. The interaction of these two forces can explain differences in time frames for acquisition of developmental skills, personality variations between identical twins, and other unique characteristics of individuals. The genetic and environmental factors that contribute to individual differences are explored in more detail next.

Genetics

Each child inherits 23 chromosomes from the mother's egg and 23 from the father's sperm, resulting in a unique individual with 46 chromosomes. Two of these are **sex chromosomes**, and determine the child's gender; the rest are called **autosomal chromosomes**, and govern all remaining characteristics. Every chromosome carries many genes that determine physical characteristics, intellectual potential, personality type, and other traits. Children are born with the potential for certain features; however, their interaction with the environment influences how and to what extent particular

Table 3–6	COMPONENTS OF RESILIENCY MODEL	
Component	**Meaning**	**Example**
A = Crisis event or health challenge	Nature of healthcare challenge	Parent leaving home
V = Vulnerability; risk factors	Stresses and risks related to dealing with the health challenge	Prior abandonment; financial instability; child's developmental understanding of abandonment
T = Typology	Family methods of functioning	Reliance on extended family; parent alcoholism
B = Protective factors	Strengths for dealing with challenge	Child's desire to succeed in school; positive role modeling of maternal grandparents
C = Appraisal	Family's interpretation of crisis event	Abandonment by loved one; inability to trust others
PS = Problem-solving or coping techniques	Skills that help family work toward solution	Use of community resources; acceptance of school and community counselors; child's involvement in classroom activities
X = Response	Positive or negative response to tension created by the health challenge	Remaining parent using counseling available; child identifying with a teacher in school; establishment of sense of mutual interdependence among remaining family members

Data from Malone, J. A. (1998). *The resiliency model of family stress, adjustment, and adaptation.* In B. Vaughan-Cole, M. A. Johnson, J. A. Malone, & B. L. Walker, *Family Nursing Practice.* Philadelphia: W.B. Saunders, pg 42. Adapted.

traits are manifested. For example, a child may have the potential for a high level of intellectual performance, but because he or she lives in an unstimulating environment, that potential is never reached.

Since chromosomes and genes carry messages that encode for certain characteristics, they also can carry diseases. Children can be affected by chromosomal disorders, which involve either altered numbers or structure of chromosomes. Whereas some of these mutations are incompatible with life and result in fetal death, others can lead to live births. Chromosomal disorders are caused by an array of factors such as radiation exposure, parental age, or parental disease states, but their causes are often unknown. Some chromosomal disorders are outlined in Table 3–7. A disorder known as fragile X results from a different abnormality when there is a fragile site on the X chromosome that is susceptible to chromosome breakage. See Chapter 27 ∞ for a discussion of the chromosomal disorders Down syndrome and fragile X that result in mental retardation.

Some children also inherit genes that lead to diseases such as cystic fibrosis or may have a mutation that manifests in the disease (see Box 3–6 for types of genetic disease transmission). A family history of these diseases is usually present, although they may appear without an identifiable history, because genes sometimes mutate, leading to an initial incidence of a genetic disorder.

In 1988, the U.S. Congress began funding research for mapping of all human genes, and many other nations set similar goals. The **Human Genome Project** was an international effort to determine the exact DNA sequences of every human gene. In 2000, a working draft of the human genome was achieved, several years ahead of schedule. This information about the human genetic code is freely provided to the scientific community and to the public. What does this mean for health care of children? First, it has already led to identifying the gene associated with certain abnormalities such as fragile X and cystic fibrosis (National Human Genome Research Institute, 2005; Williams, 2000). Once these genes are identified, it is possible to detect their presence in carriers, which will lead to better genetic counseling. New genetic material might be inserted into cells to provide important missing information, or medications can be specifically designed to target the disease on a molecular level. However, there have been concerns about ethical considerations with genetic research. What guidelines are needed to protect children and families so that genetic testing does not lead to discrimination in employment or health insurance? Who should be tested for genetic diseases, and who should have access to results? Since children cannot yet give informed

LAW & ETHICS

Genetic Considerations

The explosion in knowledge and clinical therapy related to genetics are offering challenges to those in healthcare professions. Just because a genetic test for a disease can be performed, should it be done on all newborns? What might be the potential harmful uses of information obtained about someone's genetic information? What forms of disadvantage and discrimination might occur if someone was known to carry a gene for breast cancer, a neurological disease, or Alzheimer's disease? What information do parents need about genetic screening tests available to their children? The rapidly advancing technology demands a focus on the ethical aspects of use of genetic tests and information. The Ethical, Legal, and Social Implications (ELSI) program of the National Human Genome Research Institute has been established to explore these issues (American Academy of Pediatrics, 2000, 2001; National Human Genome Research Institute [NHGRI], 2005).

While the Health Insurance Portability and Accountability Act (HIPAA) protects against some forms of genetic discrimination, there are gaps related to prohibiting use of genetic information for establishing health insurance fees, requiring genetic testing for insurance coverage, and limiting disclosure of genetic information to employers. While a Genetic Information Nondiscrimination Act has been composed, it has not yet passed both houses of the U.S. Congress (NHGRI, 2005). Check on the status of the bill and on state laws in your state to ensure genetic nondiscrimination. See Chapter 1 ∞ for more information about HIPAA and Chapter 29 for information about prenatal screening tests.

Table 3–7	EXAMPLES OF CHROMOSOMAL ALTERATIONS		
Syndrome Name	**Chromosomal Variation**	**Gender Affected**	**Clinical Manifestations**
Cri du Chat Incidence: 1 in 20,000–50,000	Autosomal deletion syndrome 5p (large deletion on the short arm of chromosome 5)	Male and female	Low birth weight (<2.5 kg) Microcephaly Hypertelorism High-pitched, catlike cry Low-set and poorly formed ears Single transverse palmar crease Severe mental retardation Slow growth (Jones, 2005)
Down Syndrome Incidence: 1 in 800 Variable with maternal age Etiology: Nondisjunction 94% Mosaicism 2.4% Translocation 3.3% (See Chapter 27 ∞)	Trisomy 21 Epicanthal folds	Male and female	Flat occiput Hypotonia Congenital heart defects Single transverse palmar crease Short limbs High-arched palate that may cause protruding tongue Small nose Brushfield spots (white speckles on edge of iris) Absent Moro reflex Variable degrees of mental retardation (Nussbaum et al., 2001; Lashley, 2005)
Edwards Syndrome Incidence: 1 in 7,500 births	Trisomy 18	Male and female	Low-set malformed ears Hands held in a clenched fist Rocker bottom feet Small nails (hypoplastic) Prominent forehead Weak cry Small jaw (micrognathia) Poor suck Failure to thrive (Klug & Cummings, 2003; Nussbaum et al.,2001; Lashley, 2005)
Patau Syndrome Incidence: 1 in 20,000–25,000 births	Trisomy 13	Male and female	Cleft lip and palate Hands held in a clenched fist Multiple fingers or toes (polydactyly) Small head (microcephaly) Small or absent eyes Rocker bottom feet Severe growth and mental retardation Multiple system anomalies (Klug & Cummings, 2003; Nussbaum et al., 2001; Lashley, 2005)
Klinefelter Syndrome Incidence: 1 in 500 males (See Chapter 29 ∞)	47, XXY Trisomy	Male	Small testes Long legs Slim, tall stature Infertility Gynecomastia in 1/3 of adolescents Fifth finger clinodactyly Appear physically normal until puberty, then show signs of hypogonadism (Jones, 2005)
Triple X Syndrome Incidence: 1 in 1,000 females	47, XXX (Trisomy)	Female	Usually physically normal May be above average in stature May have behavioral problems during development transition from adolescent to early adulthood Usually have learning difficulties Mild depression (Jones, 2005)

Table 3–7	EXAMPLES OF CHROMOSOMAL ALTERATIONS (continued)		
Syndrome Name	**Chromosomal Variation**	**Gender Affected**	**Clinical Manifestations**
Turner Syndrome Incidence: 1 in 2,000 females (See Chapter 29 ∞)	45, XO Monosomy	Female	Short, webbed neck Loose skin around neck in infancy Congenital lymphedema with residual edema over the dorsum of the fingers and toes that can be seen at any age Ovarian dysgenesis Infertility Short stature Broad chest with widely spaced nipples Low posterior hairline Low birth weight (2,900 g average) Delayed bone maturation Cardiovascular and renal abnormalities (Jones, 2005)

consent for genetic testing (see Chapter 1 ∞ for a discussion of informed consent), it is recommended that children and adolescents should have genetic testing for a disease only when medical treatment could help if the disease is identified, or when another family member might benefit from the knowledge for his or her own health and the child will not be harmed by the testing (American Academy of Pediatrics, Committee on Genetics, 2000). When genetic testing is performed, counseling about the results must be made available. Some nurses are choosing special educational programs to enable them to work in the growing field of genetics and health care.

Prenatal Influences

Some Asian cultures calculate age from the time of conception. This practice acknowledges the profound influence of the prenatal period. Nurses work closely with pregnant families to encourage safe health practices.

The mother's nutrition and general state of health play a part in pregnancy outcome. Poor nutrition can lead to low-birth-weight infants and infants with compromised neurologic performance, slow development, or impaired immune status with resultant high disease rates. Low maternal stores of iron can result in anemia in the infant (American Academy of Pediatrics, 2004). Maternal smoking is associated with low-birth-weight infants. Ingestion of alcoholic beverages, including beer and wine, during pregnancy may lead to fetal alcohol syndrome or fetal alcohol effects. See Chapter 27 ∞ for a detailed description and a photo of this condition. Substance abuse by the mother may result in neonatal addiction, convulsions, hyperirritability, poor social responsiveness, and other neurologic disturbances of the infant, as well as changes in neurobehavioral and cognitive function of children (Huizink & Mulder, 2006) (see Chapter 26 ∞ for a discussion of neonatal withdrawal syndrome).

Even prescription or nonprescription drugs may adversely affect the fetus. This was brought to general attention with the drug thalidomide, commonly used in Europe to treat nausea during the 1950s. This drug resulted in the birth of infants with limb abnormalities to women who used the drug during pregnancy. Differences in physiology related to gastric emptying, renal clearance, drug distribution, and other factors contribute to variations in pharmacokinetics during pregnancy. Drugs can cause teratogenesis (abnormal development of the fetus) or mutagenesis (permanent changes in the fetus' genetic material) (McCarter-Spaulding, 2005). Certain drugs can cause bleeding, stained teeth, impaired hearing, or other defects in the infant. The U.S. Food and Drug Administration (FDA) has established risk categories for drugs in pregnancy.

Some maternal illnesses are harmful to the developing fetus. An example is rubella (German measles), which is rarely a serious disease for adults but can cause deafness, vision defects, heart defects, and mental retardation in the fetus if it is acquired by a

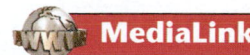
MediaLink

U.S. Food and Drug Administration

BOX 3–6
LAWS OF MENDELIAN INHERITANCE

Dominant inheritance: A gene that produces a trait whenever it is present. Achondroplasia dwarfism is one example.

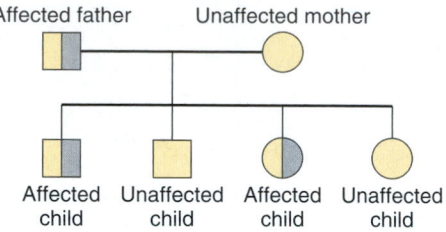

In each pregnancy there is a 50% chance that the child will have the characteristic.

Affected father   Unaffected mother

Affected child   Unaffected child   Affected child   Unaffected child

---

Recessive inheritance: A gene that produces a trait only when paired with another similar gene. Examples include cystic fibrosis, Tay-Sachs disease, and phenylketonuria.

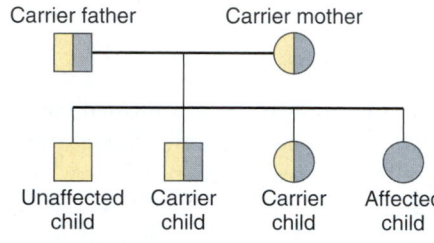

In each pregnancy, there is a 25% chance that the child will have the characteristic, a 25% chance that the child will be unaffected, and a 50% chance that the child will be a carrier of the characteristic.

Carrier father   Carrier mother

Unaffected child   Carrier child   Carrier child   Affected child

---

X-linked inheritance: A disease carried in either a dominant or recessive fashion on the X chromosome. Hemophilia is a common example of an X-linked disorder.

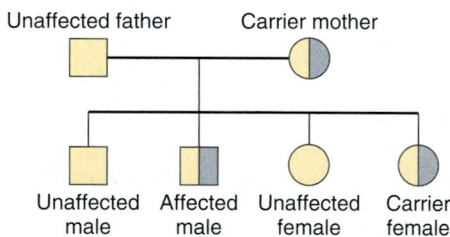

In each pregnancy with a male birth, there is a 50% chance that the child will have the characteristic and a 50% chance that the child will be unaffected. In each pregnancy with a female birth, there is a 50% chance that the child will be a carrier and a 50% chance that the child will be unaffected.

Unaffected father   Carrier mother

Unaffected male   Affected male   Unaffected female   Carrier female

---

Chromosome defect: Disorders caused by nondisjunction or translocation of chromosomes. Down syndrome is usually caused by a trisomy of chromosome 21.

---

pregnant woman. A fetus can also acquire diseases, such as acquired immunodeficiency syndrome (AIDS) and human immunodeficiency virus (HIV) infection or hepatitis B from the mother.

Radiation, chemicals, and other environmental hazards may adversely affect a fetus when the mother is exposed to these influences during her pregnancy. The best outcomes for infants occur when mothers eat well; exercise regularly; seek early prenatal care; refrain from use of drugs, alcohol, tobacco, and excessive caffeine; and follow general principles of good health.

Family and Parenting

An environmental factor that is extremely important in the development of children is the profile of family characteristics. The family is an important component in the lives of all children, and plays an essential role in fostering the development of youth. A significant concept in families is that of parenting. How children are parented interacts with their individual characteristics to influence risk and protective factors, personality characteristics, and developmental outcomes. Chapter 2 ∞ discusses types of families, frameworks used to understand families, the roles of families in fostering the development of children, and types of parenting styles.

The families into which children are born influence them profoundly. Children are supported in different ways and acquire different world views depending on such factors as whether they have one or two parents or stepparents, whether one or both parents work, how many siblings are present, and whether an extended family is close. Note should be made of variations in family structure such as single parent, homosexual parents, extended family, and stepparents. How might an adoptive home influence the child's development? Consider the 2-year-old Irena who was described in the opening scenario and was recently adopted from Romania. How have her birth and adoptive families influenced her development?

Cultural Influences

Another factor that influences child development is that of culture, through traditional practices and due to genetic variations among some ethnic groups. The traditional customs of the many cultural groups represented in North America influence the development of the children in these groups. Nutritional practices of various ethnic groups may influence the rate of growth for infants. In addition, development may be influenced by childrearing practices. For example, the Native American practice of carrying infants on boards often delays walking when it is measured against the norm for walking on some developmental tests. Children who are carried by straddling the mother's hips or back for extended periods have a low incidence of developmental dysplasia of the hip since this keeps their hips in an abducted position (Witt, 2003). It is important for nurses to take cultural practices into account when performing developmental screening; some tests may not be culturally sensitive and can inaccurately label a child as delayed when the pattern of development is simply different in the group, perhaps due to childrearing practices in the family. In these cases there is no lasting delay in any milestone but variation in acquiring skills may occur.

All cultural groups have rules regarding patterns of social interaction. Schedules of language acquisition are determined by the number of languages spoken and the amount of speech in the home. The particular social roles assumed by men and women in the culture affect school activities and ultimately career choices. Attitudes toward touching and other methods of encouraging developmental skills vary among cultures. Chapter 6 includes further description of other factors that influence child development such as school and childcare, community services, and additional community and family factors.

Genetic traits common in certain ethnic or cultural groups may predispose children for being at the upper or lower ranges of growth and influence other physical characteristics. Certain groups are more prone to develop certain diseases due to genetic variations (Table 3–8).

INFANT (BIRTH TO 1 YEAR)

Can you imagine tripling your present weight in a single year? Or becoming proficient in understanding fundamental words in a new language and even speaking a few? These and many more accomplishments take place in the first year of life. Starting as a mainly reflexive creature, the infant can walk and communicate by the year's end. Never again in life is development so swift (Figure 3–6 ➤).

Physical Growth and Development

The first year of life is one of rapid change for the infant. The birth weight usually doubles by about 5 months and triples by the end of the first year (Figure 3–7 ➤). Height increases by approximately 1 foot during this year. Teeth begin to erupt at about 6 months, and by the end of the first year the infant has six to eight deciduous teeth (see Chapter 5 ∞). Physical growth is closely associated with type and quality of feeding. See Chapter 4 ∞ for a discussion of nutrition in infancy.

Body organs and systems, although not fully mature at 1 year of age, function differently than they did at birth. Kidney and liver maturation helps the 1-year-old excrete drugs or other toxic substances more readily than in the first weeks of life. The changing body proportions mirror changes in developing internal organs. Maturation

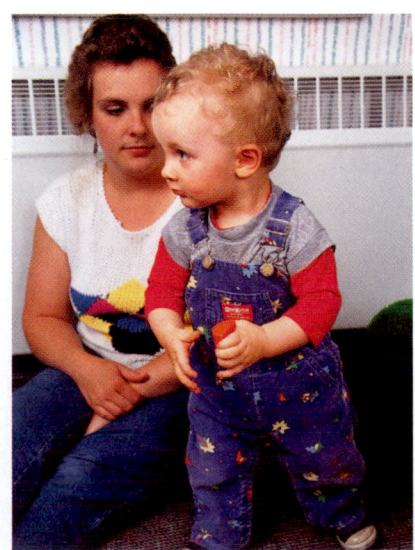

Figure 3–6 ➤ A 12-month-old child will have tripled his birth weight, learned to walk, and will begin to talk.

Table 3–8	DISEASES AND CONDITIONS MORE COMMON AMONG CULTURAL GROUPS	
Cultural Groups	**Disease/Condition**
African Americans	Sickle cell disease Hypertension Stomach and esophageal cancer Lactose intolerance
Asians/Pacific Islanders	Hypertension Stomach and liver cancer Lactose intolerance Thalassemia
American Indians/Aleuts/Eskimos	Diabetes Ear infections Accidents and suicides Cirrhosis of the liver Overweight
Hispanic Americans	Diabetes Overweight Lactose intolerance
Jews	Tay-Sachs disease Niemann-Pick disease Werdnig-Hoffman syndrome
Mediterraneans	G6PD deficiency β-Thalassemia Familial Mediterranean fever
United Kingdom	Cystic fibrosis Phenylketonuria Hereditary amyloidosis Hyperhomocysteinemia

Note: Adapted from Jarvis, C. (2004). *Physical examination and health assessment* (3rd ed.). Philadelphia: W.B. Saunders; and Spector, R. (2004). *Culture care: Guides to heritage assessment and health traditions.* Upper Saddle River, NJ: Prentice Hall Health.

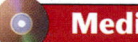

MediaLink

Developmental Milestones Child

of the nervous system is demonstrated by increased control over body movements, enabling the infant to sit, stand, and walk. Sensory function also increases as the infant begins to discriminate visual images, sounds, and tastes (Table 3–9). See Table 8–5 for a detailed list of the developmental milestones of the infant.

Cognitive Development

The brain continues to increase in complexity during the first year. Most of the growth involves maturation of cells, with only a small increase in cell number. This growth of

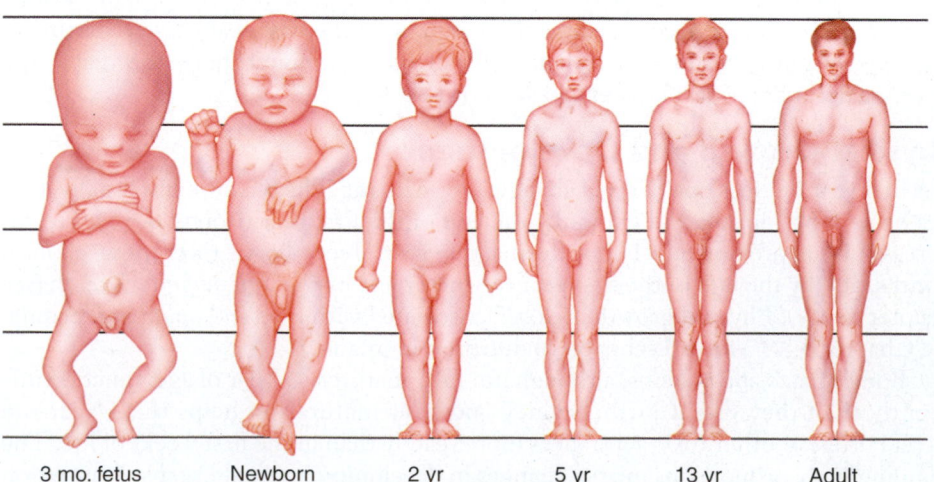

Figure 3–7 ➤ Body proportions at various ages.

| 3 mo. fetus | Newborn | 2 yr | 5 yr | 13 yr | Adult |

Table 3–9	GROWTH AND DEVELOPMENT MILESTONES DURING INFANCY			
AGE	**PHYSICAL GROWTH**	**FINE MOTOR ABILITY**	**GROSS MOTOR ABILITY**	**SENSORY ABILITY**
Birth to 1 month	Gains 5–7 oz (140–200 g)/week Grows 1.5 cm (1/2 in.) in first month Head circumference increases 1.5 cm (1/2 in.)/month	Holds hand in fist **(1)** Draws arms and legs to body when crying	Inborn reflexes such as startle and rooting are predominant activity May lift head briefly if prone **(2)** Alerts to high-pitched voices Comforts with touch **(3)**	Prefers to look at faces and black-and-white geometric designs Follows objects in line of vision **(4)**
2–4 months	Gains 5–7 oz (140–200 g)/week Grows 1.5 cm (1/2 in.)/month Head circumference increases 1.5 cm (1/2 in.)/month Posterior fontanel closes Eats 120 mL/kg/24 hr (2 oz/lb/24 hr)	Holds rattle when placed in hand **(5)** Looks at and plays with own fingers Brings hands to midline	Moro reflex fading in strength Can turn from side to back and then return **(6)** Decrease in head lag when pulled to sitting; sits with head held in midline with some bobbing When prone, holds head and supports weight on forearms **(7)**	Follows objects 180 degrees Turns head to look for voices and sounds

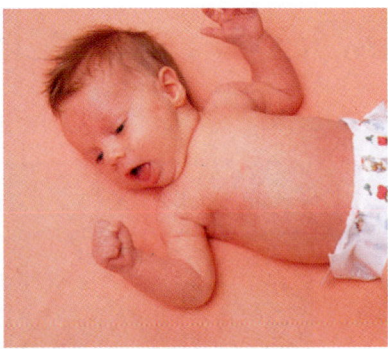

(1) Holds hand in fist

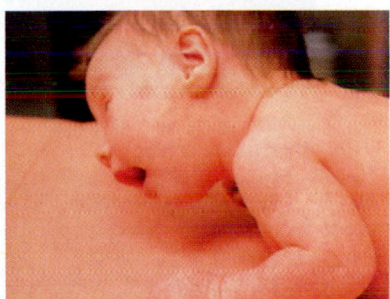

(2) May lift head

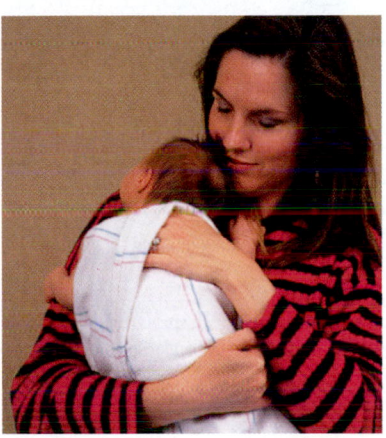

(3) Comforts with touch

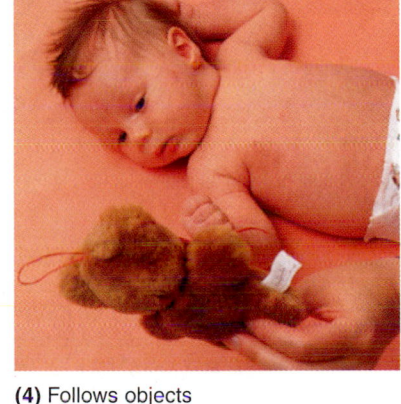

(4) Follows objects

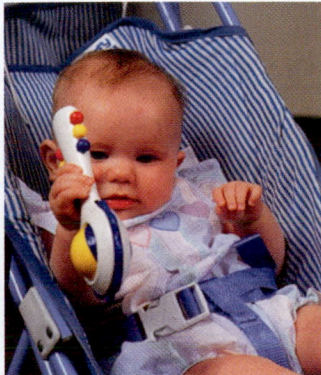

(5) Holds rattle

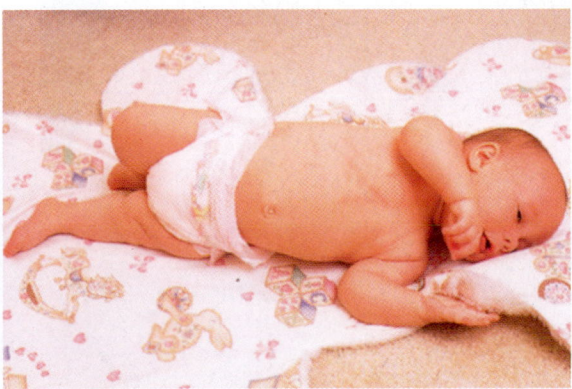

(6) Can turn from side to back

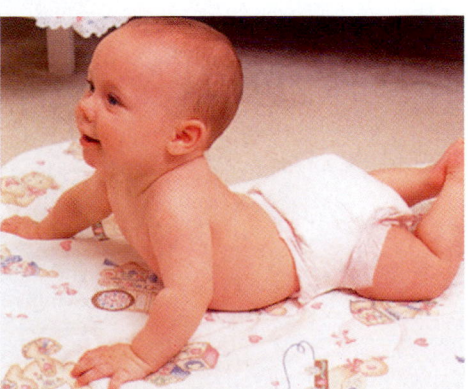

(7) Holds head up and supports weight with arms

(continues)

Table 3–9	**GROWTH AND DEVELOPMENT MILESTONES DURING INFANCY (continued)**			
AGE	**PHYSICAL GROWTH**	**FINE MOTOR ABILITY**	**GROSS MOTOR ABILITY**	**SENSORY ABILITY**
4–6 months	Gains 5–7 oz (140–200 g)/week Doubles birth weight 5–6 months Grows 1.5 cm (1/2 in.)/month Head circumference increases 1.5 cm (1/2 in.)/month Teeth may begin erupting by 6 months Eats 100 mL/kg/24 hr (1 1/2 oz/lb/24 hr)	Grasps rattles and other objects at will; drops them to pick up another offered object **(8)** Mouths objects Holds feet and pulls to mouth Holds bottle Grasps with whole hand (palmar grasp) Manipulates objects **(9)**	Head held steady when sitting No head lag when pulled to sitting Turns from abdomen to back by 4 months and then back to abdomen by 6 months When held standing supports much of own weight **(10)**	Examines complex visual images Watches the course of a falling object Responds readily to sounds

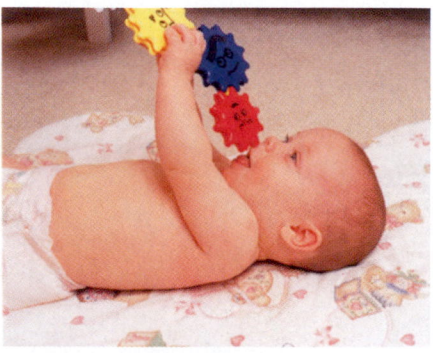

(8) Grasps objects at will

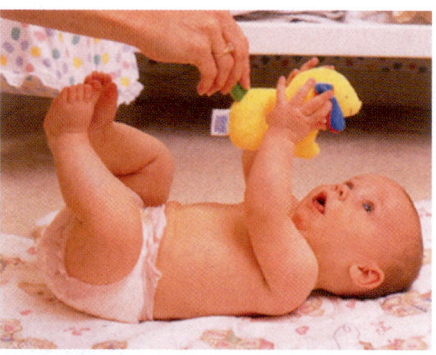

(9) Manipulates objects

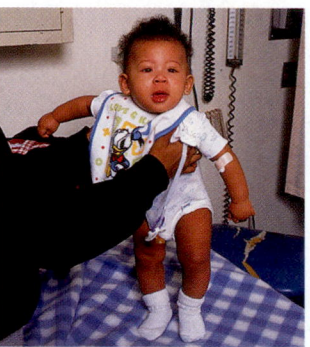

(10) Supports most of weight when held standing

6–8 months	Gains 3–5 oz (85–140 g)/week Grows 1 cm (3/8 in.)/month Growth rate slower than first 6 months	Bangs objects held in hands Transfers objects from one hand to the other Beginning pincer grasp at times	Most inborn reflexes extinguished Sits alone steadily without support by 8 months **(11)** Likes to bounce on legs when held in standing position	Recognizes own name and responds by looking and smiling Enjoys small and complex objects at play

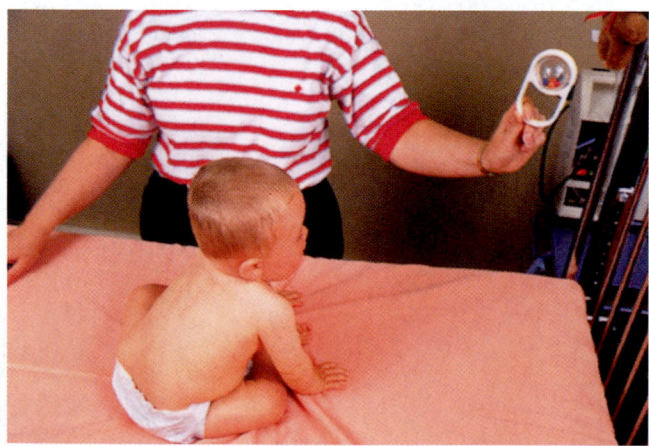

(11) Sits alone without support

Table 3–9	**GROWTH AND DEVELOPMENT MILESTONES DURING INFANCY (continued)**			
AGE	**PHYSICAL GROWTH**	**FINE MOTOR ABILITY**	**GROSS MOTOR ABILITY**	**SENSORY ABILITY**
8–10 months	Gains 3–5 oz (85–140 g)/week Grows 1 cm (3/8 in.)/month	Picks up small objects **(12)** Uses pincer grasp well **(14)**	Crawls or pulls whole body along floor by arms **(13)** Creeps by using hands and knees to keep trunk off floor Pulls self to standing and sitting by 10 months Recovers balance when sitting	Understands words such as "no" and "cracker" May say one word in addition to "mama" and "dada" Recognizes sound without difficulty

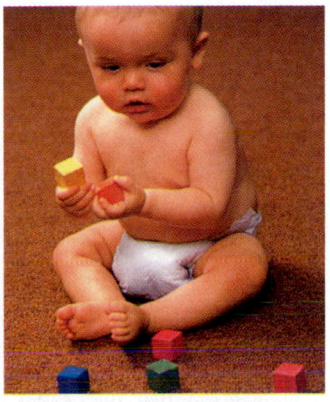

(12) Picks up small objects

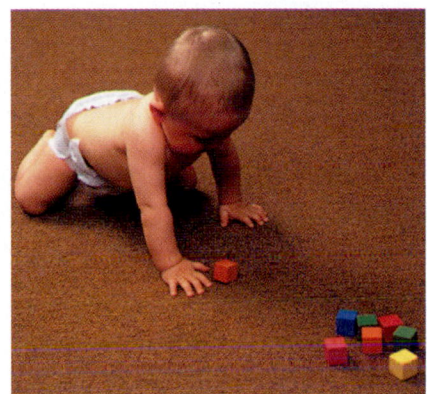

(13) Crawls or pulls body by arms

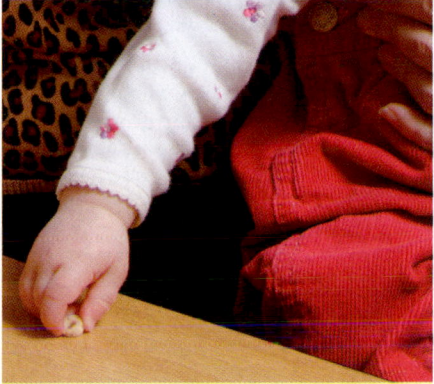

(14) Uses pincer grasp well

10–12 months	Gains 3–5 oz (85–140 g)/week Grows 1 cm (3/8 in.)/month Head circumference equals chest circumference Triples birth weight by 1 year	May hold crayon or pencil and make mark on paper Places objects into containers through holes **(15)**	Stands alone **(16)** Walks holding onto furniture Sits down from standing **(17)**	Plays peek-a-boo and patty cake

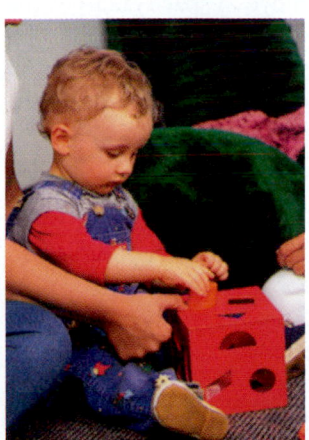

(15) Places objects in container through holes

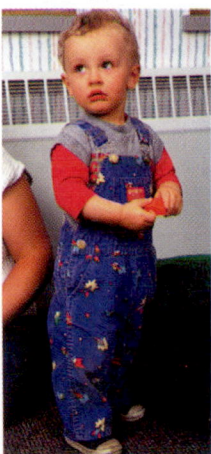

(16) Stands alone

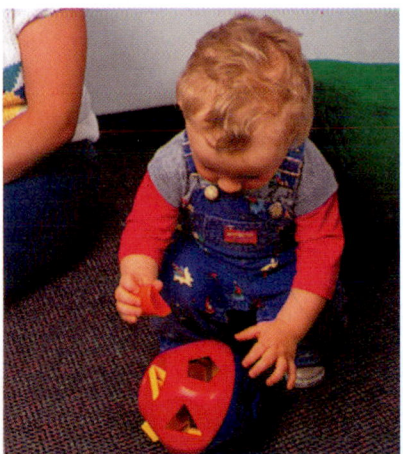

(17) Sits down from standing

the brain is accompanied by development of its functions. One has only to compare the behavior of an infant shortly after birth with that of a 1-year-old to understand the incredible maturation of brain function. The newborn's eyes widen in response to sound; the 1-year-old turns to the sound and recognizes its significance. The 2-month-old cries and coos; the 1-year-old says a few words and understands many more. The 6-week-old grasps a rattle for the first time; the 1-year-old reaches for toys and self-feeds.

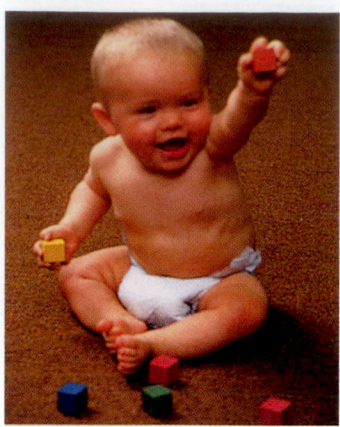

Figure 3–8 ➤ Garrett shows us that an 8-month-old child can play with blocks, demonstrating physical, cognitive, and social capabilities. Notice also his ability to sit well and engagement with his environment.

 MediaLink

Stages of Play Video

The infant's behaviors provide clues about thought processes. Piaget's work outlines the infant's actions in a set of rapidly progressing changes in the first year of life. The infant receives stimulation through sight, sound, and feeling, which the maturing brain interprets. This input from the environment interacts with internal cognitive abilities to enhance cognitive functioning.

Psychosocial Development

The infant relies on interactions with primary care providers to meet needs and then will establish a sense of trust in other adults and in children. As trust develops the infant becomes comfortable in interactions with a widening array of people.

Play

An 8-month-old infant is sitting on the floor, grasping blocks and banging them on the floor. When a parent walks by, the infant laughs and waves hands and feet wildly (Figure 3–8 ➤). The infant plays primarily alone with toys (**solitary play**) but enjoys the presence of adults or other children. Physical capabilities enable the infant to move toward and reach for objects of interest.

Cognitive ability is reflected in manipulation of the blocks to create different sounds. Social interaction enhances play. The presence of a parent or other person increases interest in surroundings and teaches the infant different ways to play.

The play of infants begins in a reflexive manner. When infants move extremities or grasp objects, they experience the foundations of play. They gain pleasure from the feel and sound of these activities, and gradually perform them purposefully. For example, when a parent places a rattle in the hand of a 6-week-old infant, the infant grasps it reflexively. As the hands move randomly, the rattle makes an enjoyable sound. The infant learns to move the rattle to create the sound and then finally to grasp the toy at will to play with it.

The next phase of infant play focuses on manipulative behavior. The infant examines toys closely, looking at them, touching them, and placing them in the mouth. The infant learns a great deal about texture, qualities of objects, and all aspects of the surroundings. At the same time, interaction with others becomes an important part of play. The social nature of play is obvious as the infant plays with other children and adults.

Toward the end of the first year, the infant's ability to move in space enlarges the sphere of play. Once infants crawl or walk, they can get to new places, find new toys, discover forgotten objects, or seek out other people for interaction. Play is a reflection of every aspect of development, as well as a method for enhancing learning and maturation (Table 3–10).

Personality and Temperament

Why does one infant frequently awaken at night crying while another sleeps for 8 to 10 hours undisturbed? Why does one infant smile much of the time and react positively to interactions while another is withdrawn around unfamiliar people and frequently frowns and cries? Such differences in responses to the environment are believed to be inborn characteristics of temperament. Infants are born with a tendency to react in certain ways to noise and to interact differently with people. They may display varying degrees of regularity in activities of eating and sleeping, and manifest a capacity for concentrating on tasks for different amounts of time (see Table 3–5).

Nursing assessment identifies personality characteristics of the infant that the nurse can share with the parents. With this information, the parents can appreciate more fully the uniqueness of their infant and design experiences to meet the infant's needs. Parents can learn to modify the environment to promote adaptation. For example, an infant who does not adapt easily to new situations may cry, withdraw, or develop another way of coping when adjusting to new people or places. Parents might be advised to use one or two baby-sitters rather than engaging new sitters frequently. If the infant is easily distracted when eating, parents can feed the infant in a quiet setting to encourage a focus on eating. Although the infant's temperament is unchanged, the ability to fit with the environment is enhanced.

Table 3–10	PSYCHOSOCIAL DEVELOPMENT DURING INFANCY	
Age	**Play and Toys**	**Communication**
Birth–3 months 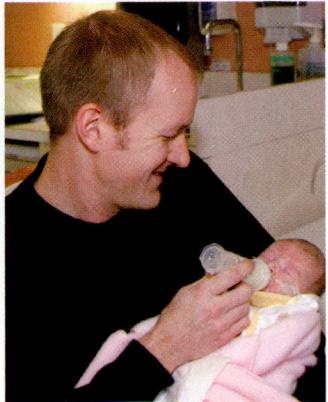	Prefers visual stimuli of mobiles, black-and-white patterns, mirrors Auditory stimuli are music boxes, tape players, soft voices Responds to rocking and cuddling Moves legs and arms while adult sings and talks Likes varying stimuli—different rooms, sounds, visual images	Coos Babbles Cries
3–6 months	Prefers noise-making objects that are easily grasped like rattles Enjoys stuffed animals and soft toys with contrasting colors	Vocalizes during play and with familiar people Laughs Cries less Squeals and makes pleasure sounds Babbles multisyllabically (mamamamama)
6–9 months	Likes teething toys Increasingly desires social interaction with adults and other children Soft toys that can be manipulated and mouthed are favorites	Increases vowel and consonant sounds Links syllables together Uses speechlike rhythm when vocalizing with others
9–12 months	Enjoys large blocks, toys that pop apart and go back together, nesting cups and other objects Laughs at surprise toys like jack-in-the-box Plays interactive games like peek-a-boo Uses push-and-pull toys	Understands "no" and other simple commands Says "dada" and "mama" to identify parents Learns one or two other words Receptive speech surpasses expressive speech

Communication

Even at a few weeks of age, infants communicate and engage in two-way interaction, and express comfort by soft sounds, cuddling, and eye contact. The infant displays discomfort by thrashing the extremities, arching the back, and crying vigorously. From these rudimentary skills, communication ability continues to develop until the infant speaks several words at the end of the first year of life (see Table 3–9). Nonverbal methods continue to be a primary method of communication between parent and child.

Nurses assess communication to identify possible abnormalities or developmental delays. Language ability may be assessed with the Denver II Developmental Test and other specialized language screening tools (see Chapter 7 ∞). Normal infants and toddlers understand (**receptive speech**) more words than they can speak (**expressive speech**). Abnormalities may be caused by a hearing deficit, developmental delay, or lack of verbal stimulation from caretakers. Further assessment may be required to pinpoint the cause of the abnormality.

Nursing interventions focus on providing a stimulating and comforting environment. Parents are encouraged to speak to infants and teach words. Hospital nurses should include the infant's known words when providing care, and provide nonverbal support by hugging and holding. Consider the family's cultural patterns for communications and development.

TODDLER (1 TO 3 YEARS)

Toddlerhood is sometimes called the first adolescence. An infant only months before, this child from 1 to 3 years is now displaying independence and negativism. Pride in newfound accomplishments emerges.

CULTURE

Reaching Developmental Milestones

In traditional Native American families, children are allowed to unfold and develop naturally at their own pace. Children thus wean and toilet-train themselves with little interference or pressure from parents. The nurse should be sensitive to the childrearing practices of the family and support them in these culturally accepted practices, rather than imposing a more structured approach to developmental milestones.

Physical Growth and Development

The rate of growth slows during the second year of life. Parents may become concerned because the child has a limited food intake and need reassurance that this is normal. See Chapter 4 ∞ for further discussion of nutrition in toddlerhood. By age 2 years, the birth weight has usually quadrupled and the child is about one-half of the adult height. Body proportions begin to change, with legs longer and head smaller in proportion to body size than during infancy (see Figure 3–7). The toddler has a pot-bellied appearance and stands with feet apart to provide a wide base of support. By approximately 33 months, eruption of deciduous teeth is complete, with 20 teeth present.

Gross motor activity develops rapidly (Table 3–11), as the toddler progresses from walking to running, kicking, and riding a tricycle (Figure 3–9 ➤). As physical maturation

Table 3–11	GROWTH AND DEVELOPMENT MILESTONES DURING TODDLERHOOD			
Age	**Physical Growth**	**Fine Motor Ability**	**Gross Motor Ability**	**Sensory Ability**
1–2 years	Gains 8 oz (227 g) or more per month Grows 3.5–5 in. (9–12 cm) during this year Anterior fontanel closes	By end of 2nd year, builds a tower of four blocks **(1)** Scribbles on paper **(2)** Can undress self **(3)** Throws a ball	Runs Walks up and down stairs **(5)** Likes push and pull toys	Visual acuity 20/50
2–3 years	Gains 1.4–2.3 kg (3–5 lb)/year Grows 5–6.5 cm (2–2.5 in.)/year	Draws a circle and other rudimentary forms Learns to pour Learning to dress self **(4)**	Jumps Kicks ball **(6)** Throws ball overhand	

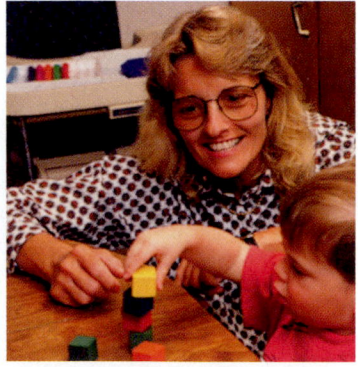

(1) Second year tower of four blocks

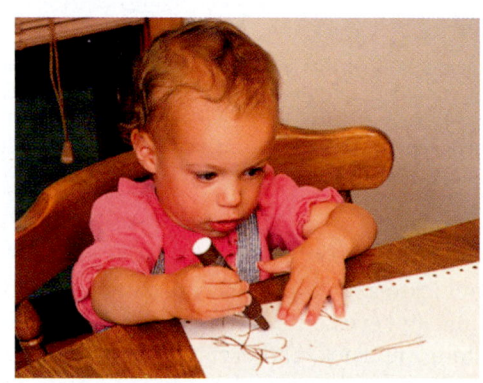

(2) Scribbles on paper

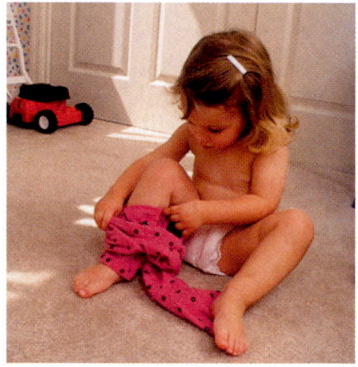

(3) Can undress self

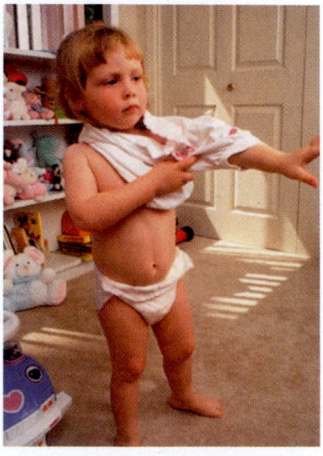

(4) Learning to dress self

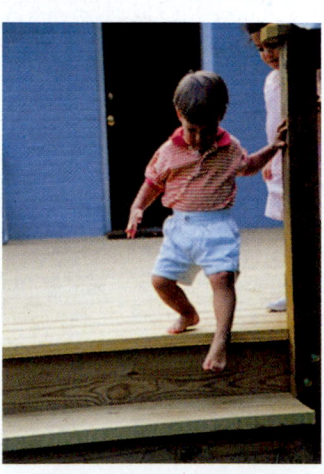

(5) Walks up and down stairs

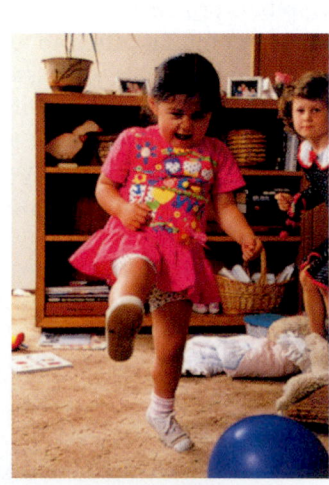

(6) Jumps and kicks ball

occurs, the toddler develops the ability to control elimination patterns. See Table 9–1 in Chapter 9 ∞ for a detailed list of the developmental milestones of toddlerhood.

Cognitive Development

During the toddler years, the child moves from the sensorimotor to the preoperational stage of development. The early use of language awakens in the 1-year-old the ability to think about objects or people when they are absent. Object permanence is well developed.

At about 2 years of age, the increasing use of words as symbols enables the toddler to use preoperational thought. Rudimentary problem solving, creative thought, and an understanding of cause-and-effect relationships are now possible.

Psychosocial Development

The toddler is soundly rooted in a trusting relationship and feels more comfortable in asserting autonomy and separating the self from primary care providers. It will be important to become an autonomous person while learning the patterns that promote interactions with adults and children.

Play

Many changes in play patterns occur between infancy and toddlerhood. The toddler's motor skills enable him or her to bang pegs into a pounding board with a hammer. The social nature of toddler play is also readily seen. Toddlers find the company of other children pleasurable, even though socially interactive play may not occur (Figure 3–10 ➤). Two toddlers tend to play with similar objects side-by-side, occasionally trading toys and words. This is called **parallel play**. This playtime with other children assists toddlers to develop social skills. Toddlers engage in play activities they have seen at home, such as pounding with a hammer and talking on the phone. This imitative behavior helps them to learn new actions and skills (Figure 3–11 ➤).

Physical skills are manifested in play as toddlers push and pull objects, climb in and out and up and down, run, ride a Big Wheel, turn the pages of books, and scribble with a pen. Both gross motor and fine motor abilities are enhanced during this age period.

Cognitive understanding enables the toddler to manipulate objects and learn about their qualities. Stacking blocks and placing rings on a building tower teach spatial relationships and other lessons that provide a foundation for future learning. Various kinds of play objects should be provided for the toddler to meet play needs. These play needs can easily be met whether the child is hospitalized or at home (Table 3–12).

Personality and Temperament

The toddler retains most of the temperamental characteristics identified during infancy, but may demonstrate some changes. The normal developmental progression of toddlerhood also plays a part in responses. For example, the infant who previously responded positively to stimuli, such as a new baby-sitter, may appear more negative in toddlerhood. The increasing independence characteristic of this age is shown by the toddler's use of the word *no*. The parent and child constantly adapt their responses to each other and learn anew how to communicate with each other.

Communication

Because of the phenomenal growth of language skills during the toddler period, adults should communicate frequently with children in this age group. Toddlers imitate words and speech intonations, as well as the social interactions they observe.

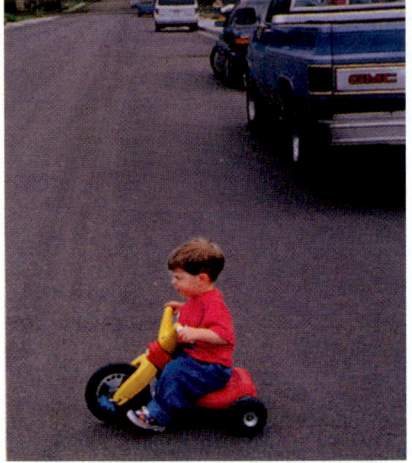

Figure 3–9 ➤ This toddler has learned to ride a Big Wheel, which he is doing right into the street. Toddlers must be closely watched to prevent injury. What other characteristics of toddlerhood can you identify? Notice the boy's short legs and arms.

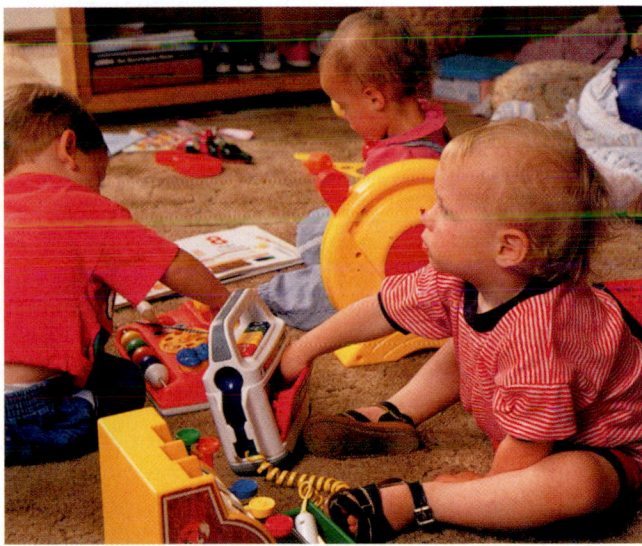

Figure 3–10 ➤ Mobility enlarges the sphere of play, allowing the child to seek new toys and spaces and to seek out people for interaction. Which psychosocial, cognitive, and motor skills do you see taking place in this photograph?

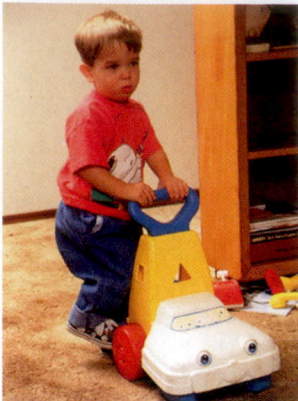

Figure 3–11 ➤ Imitative play such as pushing and pulling a vacuum allows the toddler to develop gross and fine motor skills. What are the benefits to the toddler from imitating behaviors of adults?

At the beginning of toddlerhood, the child may use four to six words in addition to "mama" and "dada." Receptive speech (the ability to understand words) far outpaces expressive speech. By the end of toddlerhood, however, the 3-year-old has a vocabulary of almost 1000 words and uses short sentences.

Communication occurs in many ways, some of which are nonverbal. Toddler communication includes pointing, pulling an adult over to a room or object, and speaking in **expressive jargon** (using unintelligible words with normal speech intonations as if truly communicating in words). Another communication method occurs when the toddler cries, pounds feet, displays a temper tantrum, or uses other means to illustrate dismay. These powerful communication methods can upset parents, who often need suggestions for handling them. It is best to verbalize the feelings shown by the toddler, for example, by saying, "You must be very upset that you cannot have that candy. When you stop crying you can come out of your room," and then to ignore further negative behavior. The toddler's search for autonomy and independence creates a need for such behavior. Sometimes an upset toddler responds well to holding, rocking, and stroking.

Parents and nurses can promote a toddler's communication by speaking frequently, naming objects, explaining procedures in simple terms, expressing feelings that the toddler seems to be displaying, and encouraging speech. The toddler from a bilingual home is at an optimal age to learn two languages. If the parents do not speak English, the toddler will benefit from a childcare experience because both languages can then be learned.

The nurse who understands the communication skills of toddlers is able to assess expressive and receptive language and communicate effectively, thereby promoting positive healthcare experiences for these children. Parents often need ideas of strategies for communication with the young child. See Families Want to Know: Communicating with a Toddler on page 91.

PRESCHOOL CHILD (3 TO 6 YEARS)

The preschool years are a time of new initiative and independence. Most children are in a childcare center or school for part of the day and learn a great deal from this social contact. Language skills are well developed, and the child is able to understand and speak clearly. Endless projects characterize the world of busy preschoolers. They may work with play dough to form animals, then cut out and paste paper, then draw and color (Figure 3–12 ➤).

Physical Growth and Development

Preschoolers grow slowly and steadily, with most growth taking place in long bones of the arms and legs. The short, chubby toddler gradually gives way to a slender, long-legged preschooler (Table 3–13).

Physical skills continue to develop. The preschooler runs with ease, holds a bat, and throws balls of various types. Writing ability increases, and the preschooler enjoys

Table 3–12	PSYCHOSOCIAL DEVELOPMENT DURING TODDLERHOOD	
Age	**Play and Toys**	**Communication**
1–3 years 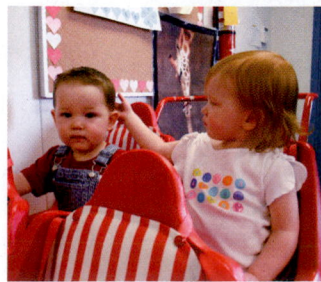	Refines fine motor skills by use of cloth books, large pencil and paper, wooden puzzles Facilitates imitative behavior by playing kitchen, grocery shopping, toy telephone Learns gross motor activities by riding Big Wheel tricycle, playing with soft ball and bat, molding water and sand, tossing ball or bean bag Cognitive skills develop by educational television shows, music, stories and books	Increasingly enjoys talking Exponential growth of vocabulary especially when spoken and read to Needs to release stress by pounding board, frequent gross motor activities, and occasional temper tantrums Likes contact with other children and learns interpersonal skills

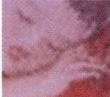

FAMILIES WANT TO KNOW

Communicating with a Toddler

Procedures such as drawing blood, getting immunizations, or even having ears checked can be frightening for a toddler. Parents and nurses can both apply effective communication that minimizes the trauma caused by such procedures. Share these tips with parents.

- Avoid telling toddlers about the procedure too far in advance. They do not have an understanding of time and can become quite anxious. Telling them just before the procedure begins is most appropriate.
- Use simple terminology. "We need to get a little blood from your arm. It will help us to find out if you are getting better." If the parent is willing, say, "Your Mom will hold your arm still so we can do it quickly." Approach positively and confidently.
- Give short, clear instructions. Do not give choices if none exist. Offer a choice of two alternatives when possible. "Would you like apple juice or grape juice after you drink this medicine?"
- Tell the toddler what you are doing; name objects.

- Allow the toddler to cry. Acknowledge that it must be frightening and that you understand. Encourge parents to allow the child to cry out during a procedure or other frightening event.
- If in a hospital, perform the procedure in a treatment room so that the toddler's bed and room are a safe haven.
- Be sure the toddler is restrained, with the joints above and below the procedure immobilized so the procedure can be quickly accomplished with the least trauma.
- Use a Band-Aid to cover up the site. This can reassure the toddler that the body is still intact.
- Allow the toddler to choose a reward such as a sticker after the procedure.
- Praise the toddler for cooperation and acknowledge that you know this was difficult.
- Comfort the toddler by rocking, offering a favorite drink, playing music, and holding. If parents are present, they can offer the comfort needed.

---

drawing and learning to write a few letters. See Table 9–1 in Chapter 9 ∞ for a detailed list of developmental milestones during the preschool period.

The preschool period is a good time to encourage good dental habits. Children can begin to brush their own teeth with parental supervision and help to reach all tooth surfaces. Parents should floss children's teeth, give fluoride as ordered if the water supply is not fluoridated (see Table 3–13), and schedule the first dental visit so the child can become accustomed to the routine of periodic dental care.

Cognitive Development

The preschooler exhibits characteristics of preoperational thought. Symbols or words are used to represent objects and people, enabling the young child to think about them. This is a milestone in intellectual development; however, the preschooler still has some limitations in thought (Table 3–14).

The preschooler's thought processes are important to understand in order to plan appropriate teaching for health care and development of health habits.

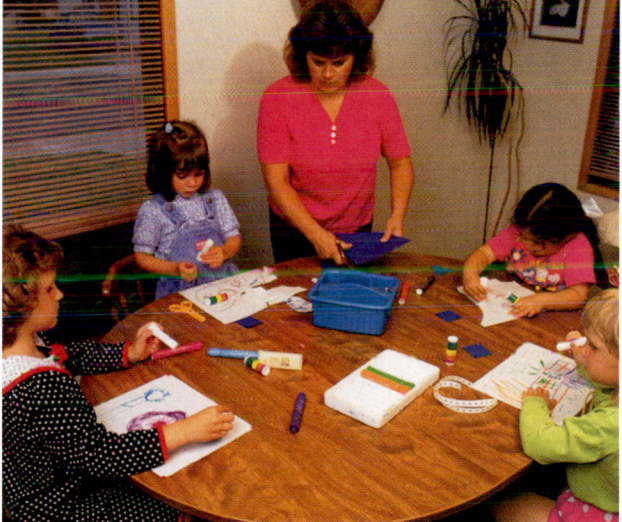

Figure 3–12 ➤ Preschoolers have well-developed language, motor, and social skills, and they can work creatively together on an art project, as this group is doing at an in-home childcare center.

Psychosocial Development

The preschooler is more independent in establishing relationships with others. The child interacts closely with children and adults as well as planning and carrying out activities.

Play

The preschooler has begun to play in a new way. Toddlers simply play side-by-side with friends, each engaging in his or her own activities; preschoolers interact with others during play. One child cuts out colored paper while her friend glues it on paper in a design. This new type of interaction is called **associative play** (Figure 3–13 ➤).

In addition to this social dimension of play, other aspects of play also differ. The preschooler enjoys large motor activities such as swinging, riding a tricycle, and throwing a ball. Increasing manual dexterity is demonstrated in greater complexity of drawings and manipulation of blocks and modeling. These changes necessitate planning of playtime to include appropriate activities. Preschool programs and child life departments in hospitals help meet this important need.

Table 3–13	**GROWTH AND DEVELOPMENT MILESTONES DURING THE PRESCHOOL YEARS**

Physical Growth

Gains 1.5–2/5 kg (3–5 lb)/year   Grows 4–6 cm (1 1/2–2 1/2 in.)/year

Fine Motor Ability

Uses scissors **(1)**
Draws circle, square, cross **(2)**
Draws at least a six-part person
Enjoys art projects such as pasting, stringing beads, using clay
Learns to tie shoes at end of preschool years **(3)**
Buttons clothes **(4)**
Brushes teeth **(5)**

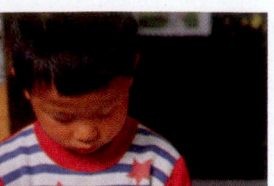
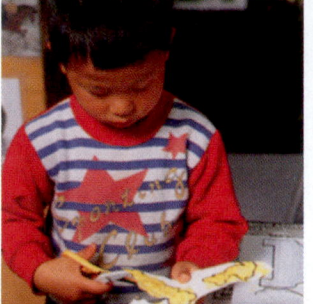

(1) Uses scissors

(2) Draws circle, square, cross

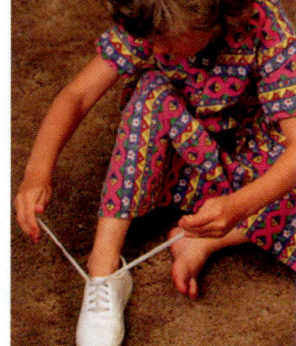
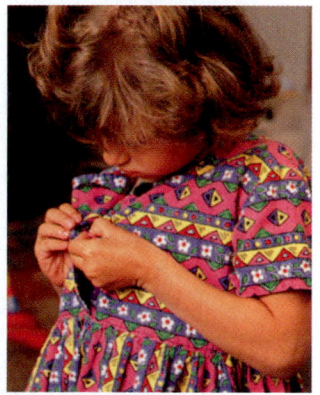
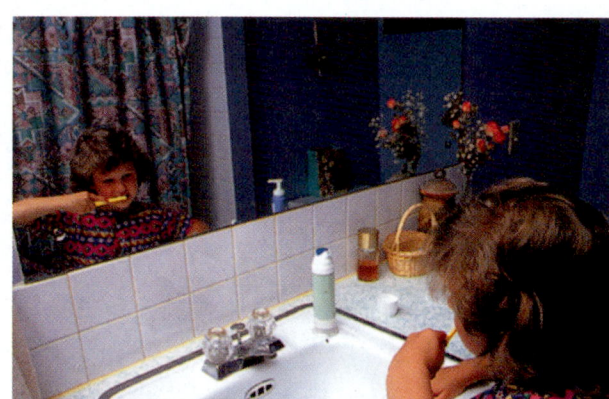

(3) Ties shoes

(4) Buttons clothes

(5) Brushes teeth

Gross Motor Ability

Throws a ball overhand
Climbs well **(6)**
Rides tricycle **(7)**

Sensory Ability

Visual acuity continues to improve
Can focus on and learn letters and numbers **(8)**

Fine Motor Ability

Eats three meals with snacks
Uses spoon, fork, and knife

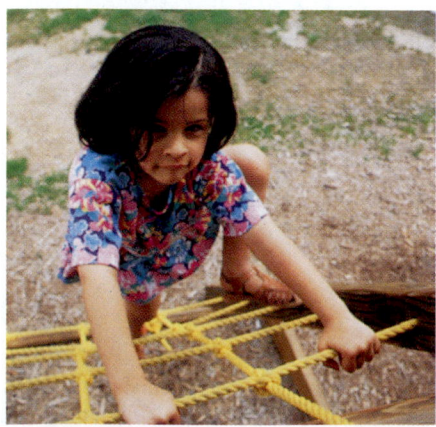
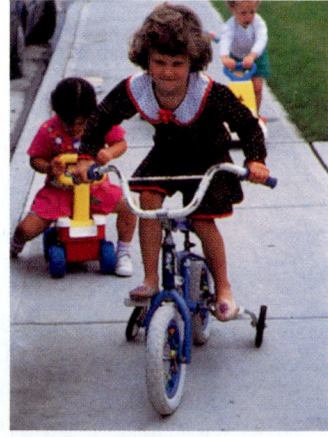
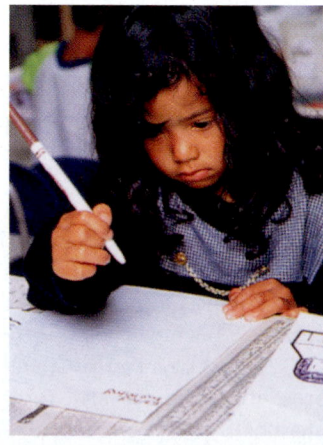

(6) Climbs well

(7) Rides tricycle or bicycle with training wheels

(8) Learns letters and numbers

Table 3–14	CHARACTERISTICS OF THOUGHT IDENTIFIED BY PIAGET		
Characteristic	**Definition**	**Development Stage**	**Nursing Implications**
Object permanence	Ability to understand that when something is out of sight it still exists	Sensorimotor period, especially in coordination of secondary schemes substage from 8–12 months	Before development of object permanence babies will not look for toys or other objects out of sight; as the concept is developing they are concerned when a parent leaves since they are not certain the parent will return.
Egocentrism	Ability to see things only from one's own point of view	Preoperational thought	Peers or others who have gone through an experience will not impress the preschooler; teaching should focus on what an experience will be like to the child.
Transductive reasoning	Connecting two events in a cause-effect relationship simply because they occur together in time	Preoperational thought	Ask the child what he or she thinks caused an occurrence; ask how the two events are connected; correct misconceptions to lessen child's guilt.
Centration	Focusing only on one particular aspect of a situation	Preoperational thought	Listen to the child's comments and deal with concerns in order to be able to present new concepts to the child.
Animism	Giving lifelike qualities to nonliving things	Preoperational thought	Ask preschool children to describe how a machine works, or how the trees move. Provide opportunities to learn about machines that may move and make noises (intravenous pumps, magnetic resonance imaging) to decrease fears.
Magical thinking	The belief that events occur because of one's thoughts or actions	Preoperational thought	Ask young children how they became ill, or what caused a parent or sibling's illness. Correct misconceptions when the child blames self for causing problems by wishing someone ill or having bad behavior.
Conservation	Knowledge that matter is not changed when its form is altered	Concrete operational thought	Before conservation of thought is reached, the child may think that gender can be changed when hair is cut; the leg under a cast is broken in separate pieces. Ask perceptions and clarify misconceptions.

Materials provided for play can be simple but should guide activities in which the child engages. Because fine motor activities are popular, paper, pens, scissors, glue, and a variety of other such objects should be available. The child can use them to create important images such as pictures of people, hospital beds, or friends. A collection of dolls, furniture, and clothing can be manipulated to represent parents and children, nurses and physicians, teachers, or other significant people. Because fantasy life is so powerful at this age, the preschooler readily uses props to engage in **dramatic play**, that is, the living out of the drama of human life (Figure 3–14 ➤).

The nurse can use playtime to assess the preschooler's developmental level, knowledge about health care, and emotions related to healthcare experiences. Observations about objects chosen for play, content of dramatic play, and pictures drawn can provide important assessment data. The nurse can also use play periods to teach the child about healthcare procedures and offer an outlet for expression of emotions (Table 3–15). Further information about play for hospitalized children is found in Chapter 13, while play therapy for children with psychological alterations is described in Chapter 27 ∞.

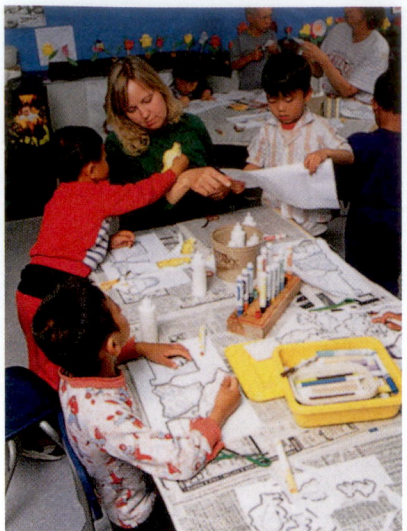

Figure 3–13 ➤ These preschoolers are participating in associative play, which means they can interact. One child is cutting out shapes, and the other is gluing them in place.

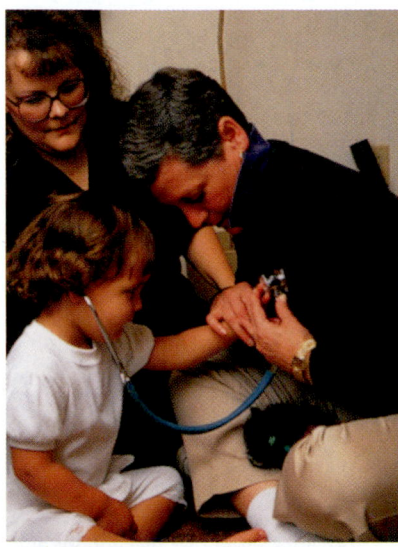

Figure 3–14 ➤ Jasmine is participating in dramatic play with a nurse while her mother looks on. In dramatic play, the child uses props to play out the drama of human life. It can be an excellent way for a nurse to assess the developmental level of children while talking to them. Notice that the child and the nurse are on the floor at the same level and the atmosphere is informal. Why is it important to be at the same level as the child?

Personality and Temperament

Characteristics of personality observed in infancy tend to persist over time. The preschooler may need assistance as these characteristics are expressed in the new situations of preschool or nursery school. An excessively active child, for example, will need gentle, consistent handling to adjust to the structure of a classroom. Encourage parents to visit preschool programs to choose the one that would best foster growth in their child. Some preschoolers enjoy the structured learning of a program that focuses on cognitive skills, whereas others are happier and more open to learning in a small group that provides much time for free play. Nurses can help parents to identify their child's personality or temperament characteristics and to find the best environment for growth.

Communication

Language skills blossom during the preschool years. The vocabulary grows to over 2000 words, and children speak in complete sentences of several words and use all parts of speech. They practice these newfound language skills by endlessly talking and asking questions.

The sophisticated speech of preschoolers mirrors the development occurring in their minds and helps them to learn about the world around them. However, this speech can be quite deceptive. Although preschoolers use many words, their grasp of meaning is usually literal and may not match that of adults. These literal interpretations have important implications for healthcare providers. For example, the preschooler who is told she will be "put to sleep" for surgery may think of a pet recently euthanized; the child who is told that a dye will be injected for a diagnostic test may think he is going to die; mention of "a little stick" in the arm can cause images of tree branches rather than of a simple immunization.

The child may also have difficulty focusing on the content of a conversation. The preschooler is egocentric and may be unable to move from individual thoughts to those the nurse is proposing, as the following conversation illustrates:

Nurse: I'd like to tell you about the operation that you will have tomorrow.
Sharisse: OK. Did you know my brother just got a new squirt gun?
Nurse: That's nice. Now, first thing in the morning you will wake up early and your foot will be scrubbed with a special soap.
Sharisse: The gun can spurt for about 40 feet—you have to pump it up.
Nurse: We'll talk about that later. Let me tell you about your operation now. After your foot is scrubbed, the nurse will measure your blood pressure and temperature and feel the pulse in your arm. Do you remember my doing those things today?
Sharisse: Yes. And I got a sticker when I came into the hospital today, too. Do you know that my Mom is going to stay here tonight?

During this interchange, Sharisse engages in **collective monologue**, in which separate conversations occur even though each person waits for the other to speak. Though waiting for the nurse to speak, Sharisse is not generally responding to the nurse's content but is instead focusing on content from her own mind. The nurse needs to respond to Sharisse's content and then reinsert more facts about the preparations for surgery.

Concrete visual aids such as pictures of a child undergoing the same procedure or a book to read together enhance teaching by meeting the child's developmental needs. Handling medical equipment such as intravenous bags and stethoscopes increases interest and helps the child to focus. Teaching may have to be done in several short sessions rather than one long session.

Some general approaches are:

- Allow time for the child to integrate explanations
- Verbalize frequently to the child
- Use drawings and stories to explain care
- Use accurate names for bodily functions
- Allow choices

Table 3–15	PSYCHOSOCIAL DEVELOPMENT DURING PRESCHOOL YEARS	
Age	**Play and Toys**	**Communication**
3–6 years 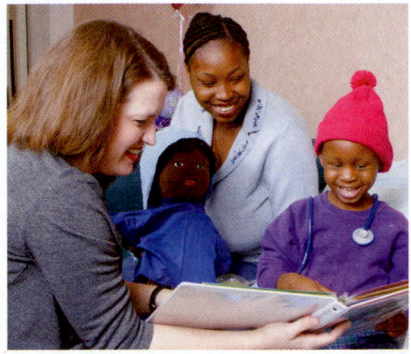	Associative play is facilitated by simple games, puzzles, nursery rhymes, songs Dramatic play is fostered by dolls and doll clothes, play houses and hospitals, dress-up clothes, puppets Stress is relieved by pens, paper, glue, scissors Cognitive growth is fostered by educational television shows, music, stories and books	All parts of speech are developed and used, occasionally incorrectly Communicates with a widening array of people Play with other children is a favorite activity Health professionals can • Verbalize and explain procedures to children • Use drawings and stories to explain care • Use accurate names for bodily functions • Allow the child to talk, ask questions, and make choices

SCHOOL-AGE CHILD (6 TO 12 YEARS)

Errol, 10 years old, arrives home from school shortly after 3 p.m. each day. He immediately calls his friends and goes to visit one of them. They are building models of cars and collecting baseball cards. Endless hours are spent on these projects and on discussions of events at school that day (Figure 3–15 ➤).

Nine-year-old Karen practices soccer two afternoons a week and plays in games each weekend. She also is learning to play the flute and spends her free time at home practicing. Although practice time is not her favorite part of music, Karen enjoys the performances and wants to play well in front of her friends and teacher. Her parents now allow her to ride her bike unaccompanied to the store or to a friend's house.

These two school-age children demonstrate common characteristics of their age group. They are in a stage of industry in which it is important to the child to perform useful work. Meaningful activities take on great importance and are usually carried out in the company of peers. A sense of achievement in these activities is important to develop self-esteem and to prevent a sense of inferiority or poor self-worth.

Physical Growth and Development

School age is the last period in which girls and boys are close in size and body proportions. As the long bones continue to grow, leg length increases (see Figure 3–7). Fat

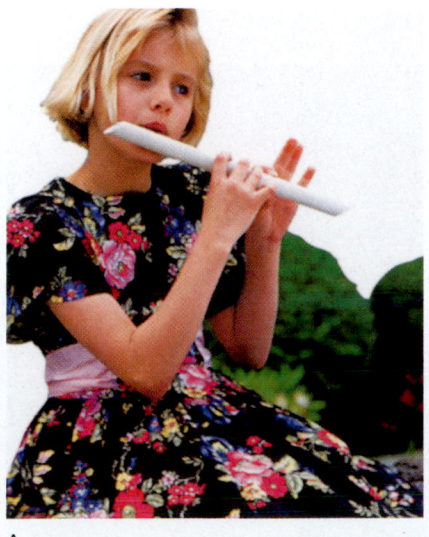

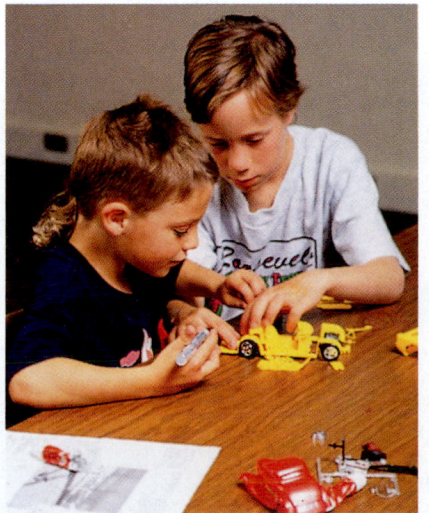

Figure 3–15 ➤ A, School-age children may take part in activities that require practice. This is a consideration when children are hospitalized and unable to practice or perform. Why? B, School-age children enjoy spending time with others the same age on projects and discussing the activities of the day. This is an important consideration when they are in an acute-care setting. When you are in the clinical setting, look for examples of this type of interaction taking place.

A

B

Table 3–16	GROWTH AND DEVELOPMENT MILESTONES DURING THE SCHOOL-AGE YEARS		
Physical Growth	**Fine Motor Ability**	**Gross Motor Ability**	**Sensory Ability**
Gains 1.4–2.2 kg (3–5 lb)/year Grows 4–6 cm (1 1/2–2 1/2 in.)/year	Enjoys craft projects Plays card and board games	Rides two-wheeler **(1)** Jumps rope **(2)** Roller skates or ice skates	Can read Able to concentrate for longer periods on activities by filtering out surrounding sounds **(3)**

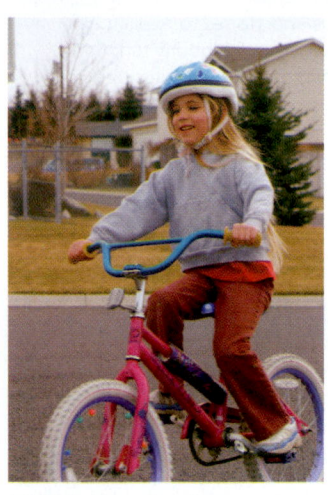

(1) Rides two-wheeler

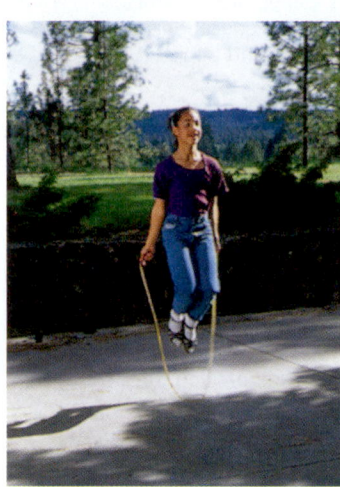

(2) Jumps rope

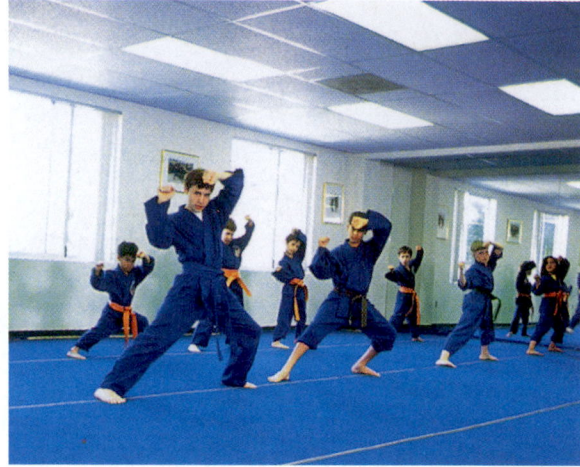

(3) Concentrates on activities for longer periods

gives way to muscle, and the child appears leaner. Jaw proportions change as the first deciduous tooth is lost at 6 years and permanent teeth begin to erupt. Body organs and the immune system mature, resulting in fewer illnesses among school-age children. Medications are less likely to cause serious side effects, because they can be metabolized more easily. The urinary system can adjust to changes in fluid status. Physical skills are also refined as children begin to play sports, and fine motor skills are well developed through school activities (Table 3–16 and Figure 3–16 ➤).

Although it is commonly believed that the start of adolescence (age 12 years) heralds a growth spurt, the rapid increases in size commonly occur during school age. Girls may begin a growth spurt as early as 9 or 10 years and boys a year or so later (Figure 3–17 ➤). Nutritional needs increase dramatically with this spurt.

The loss of the first deciduous teeth and the eruption of permanent teeth usually occur at about age 6 years, or at the beginning of the school-age period. Of the 32 perma-

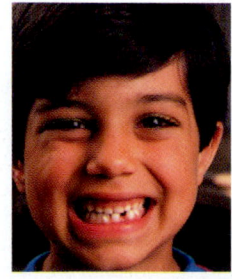

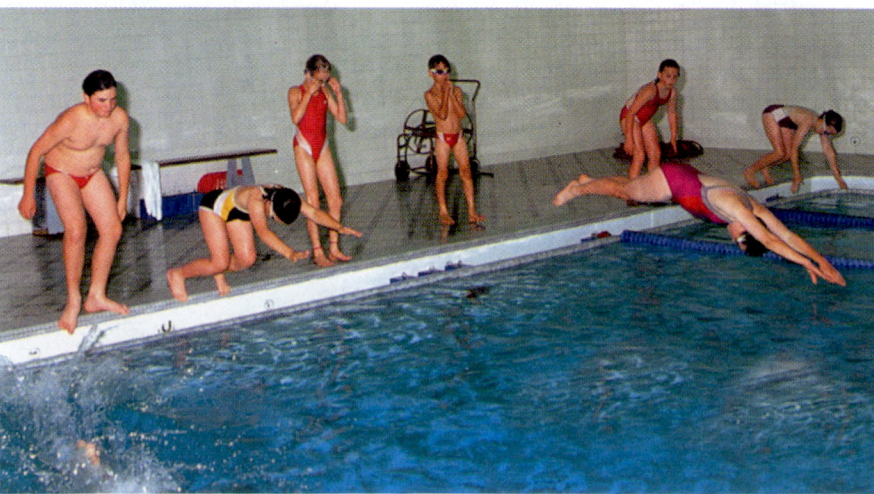

Figure 3–16 ➤ School-age girls and boys enjoy participating in sports. They begin to lose fat while developing their muscles, so they appear leaner than at earlier ages. Above photo, Front teeth are lost around age 6 years. The family may have rituals associated with the loss of teeth that could affect the child's behavior if he loses a tooth while in the hospital.

nent teeth, 22 to 26 erupt by age 12 years and the remaining molars follow during the teenage years (see Figure 3–16). The school-age child should be closely monitored to ensure that brushing and flossing are adequate, that fluoride is taken if the water supply is not fluoridated, that dental care is obtained to provide for examination of teeth and alignment, and that loose teeth are identified before surgery or other events that may lead to loss of a tooth.

Cognitive Development

The child enters the stage of concrete operational thought at about 7 years. This stage enables school-age children to consider alternative solutions and solve problems. However, school-age children continue to rely on concrete experiences and materials to form their thought content.

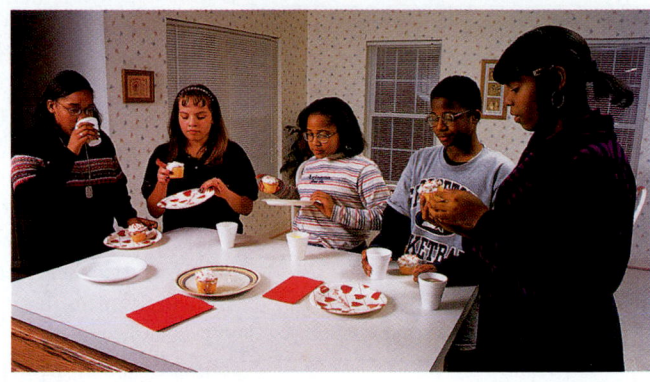

Figure 3–17 ➤ Because girls have a growth spurt earlier than boys, girls often are taller than boys of the same age. Remember what it was like at your first dance?

During the school-age years, the child learns the concept of conservation (that matter is not changed when its form is altered). At earlier ages, a child believes that when water is poured from a short, wide glass into a tall, thin glass, there is more water in the taller glass. The school-age child recognizes that although it may look like the taller glass holds more water, the quantity is the same. The concept of conservation is helpful when the nurse explains medical treatments. The school-age child understands that an incision will heal, that a cast will be removed, and that an arm will look the same as before once the intravenous infusion is removed.

Psychosocial Development

The school-age child has many friends and cooperatively interacts with others to accomplish tasks. The child develops a sense of accomplishment from activities and relationships.

Play

When the preschool teacher tries to organize a game of baseball, both the teacher and the children become frustrated. Not only are the children physically unable to hold a bat and hit a ball, but they seem to have no understanding of the rules of the game and do not want to wait for their turn at bat. By 6 years of age, however, children have acquired the physical ability to hold the bat properly and may occasionally hit the ball. School-age children also understand that everyone has a role—the pitcher, the catcher, the batter, the outfielders. They cooperate with one another to form a team, are eager to learn the rules of the game, and want to ensure that these rules are followed exactly (Table 3–17).

Table 3–17	PSYCHOSOCIAL DEVELOPMENT DURING THE SCHOOL-AGE YEARS	
Age	**Activities**	**Communication**
6–12 years 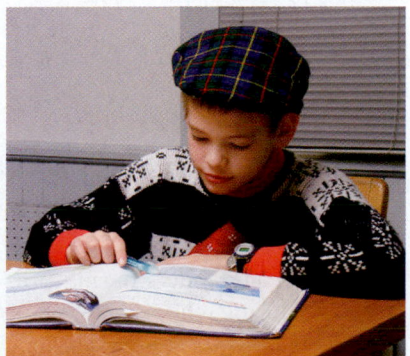	Gross motor development is fostered by ball sports, skating, dance lessons, water and snow skiing/boarding, biking A sense of industry is fostered by playing a musical instrument, gathering collections, starting hobbies, playing board and video games Cognitive growth is facilitated by reading, crafts, word puzzles, school work	Mature use of language Ability to converse and discuss topics for increasing lengths of time Spends many hours at school and with friends in sports or other activities Health professionals can: • Assess child's knowledge before teaching • Allow the child to select rewards following procedures • Teach techniques such as counting or visualization to manage difficult situations • Include both parent and child in healthcare decisions

The characteristics of play exhibited by the school-age child are cooperation with others and the ability to play a part in order to contribute to a unified whole. This type of play is called **cooperative play**. The concrete nature of cognitive thought leads to a reliance on rules to provide structure and security. Children have an increasing desire to spend much of their playtime with friends, which demonstrates the social component of play. Play is an extremely important method of learning and living for the school-age child. Active physical play has decreased in recent years as television viewing and playing of computer games have increased, leading to poor nutritional status and high rate of overweight among children. See Chapter 4 ∞ for further discussion of nutrition and physical activity in children.

When a child is hospitalized, the separation from playmates can lead to feelings of sadness and purposelessness. School-age children often feel better when placed in multibed units with other children. Games can be devised even when children are wheelchair bound (Figure 3–18 ➤). Normal, rewarding parts of play should be integrated into care. Many children enjoy music played through earphones or on CD players. Friends should be encouraged to visit or call a hospitalized child. Discharge planning for the child who has had a cast or brace applied should address the activities in which the child can participate and those the child must avoid. Reinforce the importance of playing games with friends.

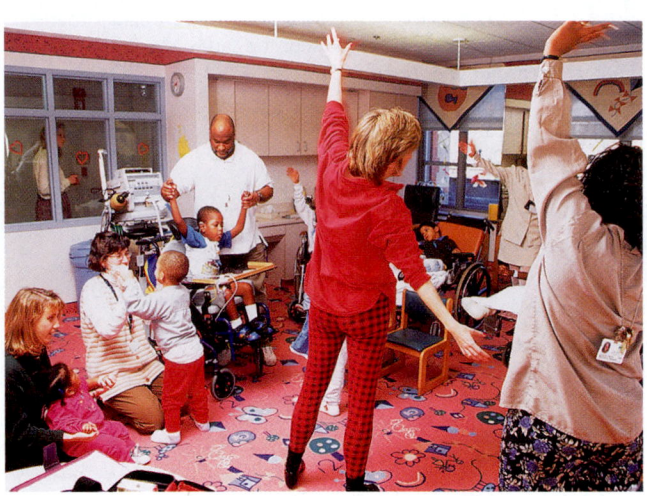

Figure 3–18 ➤ The nurse can help the child and family accept and adjust to new circumstances. Encouraging the child in a wheelchair to participate in group activities can help build confidence in physical skills. Positive self-esteem, goal attainment, personal satisfaction, and general health are the continued benefits.

Personality and Temperament

The enduring aspects of temperament continue to be manifested during the school years. The child classified as "difficult" at an earlier age may now have trouble in the classroom. Advise parents to provide a quiet setting for homework and to reward the child for concentration. For example, after homework is completed, the child may watch a television show. Creative efforts and alternative methods of learning should be valued. Encourage parents to see their children as individuals who may not all learn in the same way. The "slow-to-warm-up" child may need encouragement to try new activities and to share experiences with others, whereas the "easy" child will readily adapt to new schools, people, and experiences.

Communication

During the school-age years, the child should learn how to correct any lingering pronunciation or grammatical errors. Vocabulary increases, and the child learns about parts of speech in school. School-age children enjoy writing and can be encouraged to keep a journal of their experiences while in the hospital as a method of dealing with anxiety. The literal translation of words characteristic of preschoolers is uncommon among school-age children.

Some communication strategies helpful with the school-age child include:

- Provide concrete examples of pictures or materials to accompany verbal descriptions.
- Assess knowledge before planning the instruction.
- Allow child to select rewards following procedures.
- Teach techniques such as counting or visualization to manage difficult situations.
- Include child in discussions and history with parent.

Sexuality

Although children become aware of sexual differences between genders during preschool years, they deal much more consciously with sexuality during school age. As children mature physically, they need information about their bodily changes so that they can develop a healthy self-image and an understanding of the relationships between their bodies and sexuality. Children become interested in sexual issues and are often exposed to erroneous information on television shows, in magazines, or from friends and siblings. Schools and families need to use opportunities to teach school-age children factual information about sex and to foster healthy concepts of self and others. It is advisable to ask occasional questions about sexual issues to learn how much the child knows and to provide correct information when answers demonstrate confusion. Both friends and the media are common sources of erroneous ideas. Appropriate and inappropriate touch should be discussed, with lists of trusted people who can be approached (teachers, clergy, school counselors, family members, neighbors) to discuss any episodes with which the child feels uncomfortable. Recognize that even these trusted people can be implicated in inappropriate episodes, so encourage the child to go to more than one person, an important approach if the child is uncomfortable about a relationship with any individual.

ADOLESCENT (12 TO 18 YEARS)

Adolescence is a time of passage signaling the end of childhood and the beginning of adulthood. Although adolescents differ in behaviors and accomplishments, they are in a period of identity formation. If a healthy identity and sense of self-worth are not developed in this period, role confusion and purposeless struggling will ensue. The adolescents in your care will represent various degrees of identity formation, and each will offer unique challenges.

Physical Growth and Development

The physical changes ending in **puberty**, or sexual maturity, begin near the end of the school-age period. The prepubescent period is marked by a growth spurt at an average age of 10 years for girls and 13 years for boys, although there is considerable variation among children (see Figure 3–17). The increase in height and weight is generally remarkable and is completed in 2 to 3 years (Table 3–18). The growth spurt in girls is

Table 3–18	GROWTH AND DEVELOPMENT MILESTONES DURING ADOLESCENCE		
Physical Growth	**Fine Motor Ability**	**Gross Motor Ability**	**Sensory Ability**
Variation in age of growth spurt During growth spurt, girls gain 7–25 kg (15–55 lb) and grow 2.5–20 cm (2–8 in.); boys gain approximately 7–29.5 kg (15–65 lb) and grow 11–30 cm (41/2–12 in.)	Skills are well developed **(1)**	New sports activities attempted and muscle development continues **(2)** Some lack of coordination common during growth spurt	Fully developed

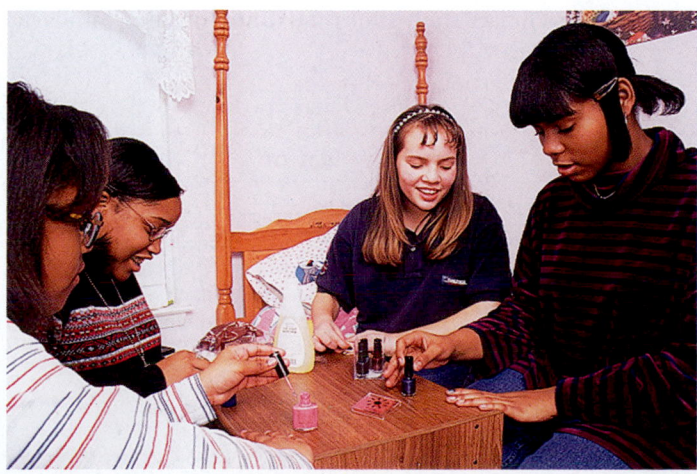

(1) Motor skills are well developed

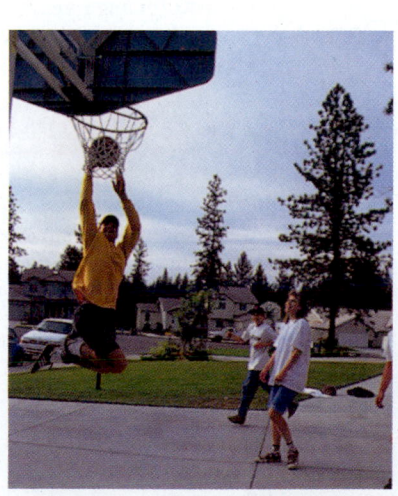

(2) New sports activities attempted

accompanied by an increase in breast size and growth of pubic hair. Menstruation occurs last and signals achievement of puberty. In boys, the growth spurt is accompanied by growth in size of the penis and testes and by growth of pubic hair. Deepening of the voice and growth of facial hair occur later, at the time of puberty. See Chapter 5 ∞ for a description of the pubertal stages.

During adolescence children grow stronger and more muscular and establish characteristic male and female patterns of fat distribution. The apocrine and eccrine glands mature, leading to increased sweating and a distinct odor to perspiration. All body organs are now fully mature, enabling the adolescent to take adult doses of medications.

The adolescent must adapt to a rapidly changing body for several years. These physical changes and hormonal variations offer challenges to identity formation.

Cognitive Development

Adolescence marks the beginning of Piaget's last stage of cognitive development, the stage of formal operational thought. The adolescent no longer depends on concrete experiences as the basis of thought but develops the ability to reason abstractly. Such concepts as justice, truth, beauty, and power can be understood. The adolescent revels in this newfound ability and spends a great deal of time thinking, reading, and talking about abstract concepts.

The ability to think and act independently leads many adolescents to rebel against parental authority. Through these actions, adolescents seek to establish their own identity and values.

Psychosocial Development

The adolescent is mature in relationships with others. The key aspect that the teen is working on during relationships and activities is to establish a meaningful identity.

Activities

Maturity leads to new activities. Adolescents may drive, ride buses, or bike independently (Research 3–2). They are less dependent on parents for transportation and spend more time with friends. Activities include participation in sports and extracurricular school activities, as well as "hanging out" and attending movies or concerts with friends (Table 3–19). The peer group becomes the focus of activities (Figure 3–19 ➤), regardless of the teen's interests. Peers are important in establishing identity and providing meaning. Although same-sex interactions predominate, boy-girl relationships are more common than at earlier stages. Adolescents thus participate in and learn from social interactions fundamental to adult relationships.

Personality and Temperament

Characteristics of temperament manifested during childhood usually remain stable in the teenage years. For instance, the adolescent who was a calm, scheduled infant and child often demonstrates initiative to regulate study times and other routines. Similarly,

RESEARCH

YRBS

The federal government administers questionnaires to a large cross-section of youth annually to monitor their behaviors related to risk behavior. The Youth Risk Behavior Surveillance (YRBS) system gathers data about six high-priority areas: unintentional and intentional injury, tobacco use, alcohol and other drug use, sexual behavior, dietary behavior, and physical inactivity. How can nurses use this information to plan appropriate interventions for populations of adolescents?

Table 3–19	PSYCHOSOCIAL DEVELOPMENT DURING ADOLESCENCE	
Age	**Activities**	**Communication**
12–18 years 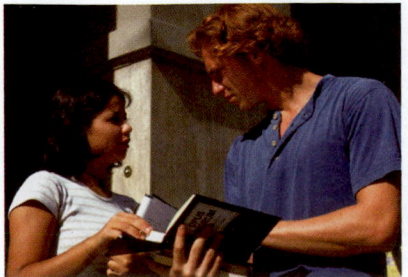	Sports—ball games, gymnastics, water and snow skiing/boarding, swimming, school sports School activities—drama, yearbook, class office, club participation Quiet activities—Reading, school work, television, computer, video games, music	Increasing communication and time with peer group—movies, dances, driving, eating out, attending sports events Applying abstract thought and analysis in conversations at home and school

the adolescent who was an easily stimulated infant may now have a messy room, a harried schedule with assignments always completed late, and an interest in many activities. It is also common for an adolescent who was an easy child to become more difficult because of the psychologic changes of adolescence and the need to assert independence.

Similar to the child's earlier ages, the nurse's role may be to inform parents of different personality types and to help them support the teen's uniqueness while providing necessary structure and feedback. Nurses can help parents to understand their teen's personality type and to work with the adolescent to meet expectations of teachers and others in authority.

Communication

All parts of speech are used and understood by the adolescent. Colloquialisms and slang are commonly used with the peer group. The adolescent often studies a foreign language in school, having the ability to understand and analyze grammar and sentence structure.

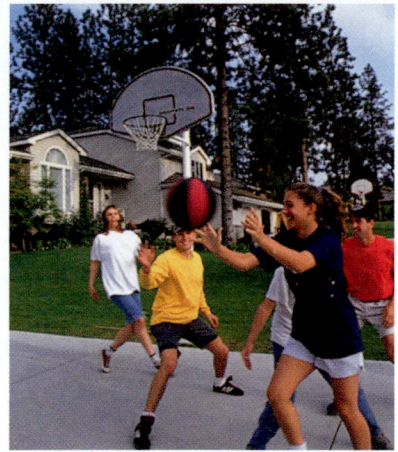

A

The adolescent increasingly leaves the home base and establishes close ties with peers. These relationships become the basis for identity formation. There is generally a period of stress or crisis before a strong identity can emerge. The adolescent may try out new roles by learning a new sport or other skills, experimenting with drugs or alcohol, wearing different styles of clothing, or trying other activities. It is important to provide positive role models and a variety of experiences to help the adolescent make wise choices.

The adolescent also has a need to leave the past, to be different, and to change from former patterns to establish a self-identity. Rules that are repeated constantly and dogmatically will probably be broken in the adolescent's quest for self-awareness. This poses difficulties when the adolescent has a health problem, such as diabetes or a heart problem, that requires ongoing care. Introducing the adolescent to other teens who manage the same problem appropriately is usually more successful than telling the adolescent what to do.

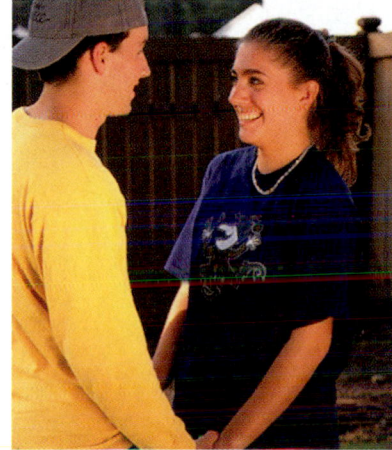

B

Privacy should be ensured during the taking of health histories or interventions with teens. Even if a parent is present for part of a history or examination, the adolescent should be given the opportunity to relay information or ask questions alone with the healthcare provider. The adolescent should be given a choice of whether to have a parent present during an examination or while care is provided. Most information shared by an adolescent is confidential. Some states mandate disclosure of certain information to parents such as an adolescent's desire for an abortion. In these cases, the adolescent should be informed of what will be disclosed to the parent. See Chapter 1 ∞ for further information about the legal implications of care for adolescents.

Figure 3–19 ➤ Social interaction between children of the same and opposite sex is as important inside the acute care setting as it is outside. *A*, Teenagers enjoy playing together. *B*, Emotional relationships form during adolescence.

Setting up teen rooms (recreation rooms for use only by adolescents) or separate adolescent units in hospitals can provide necessary peer support during hospitalization. Most adolescents are not pleased when placed on a unit or in a room with young children. Choices should be allowed when possible, and include preference for evening or morning bathing, the type of clothes to wear while hospitalized, timing of treatments, and visitation guidelines. Use of contracts with adolescents may increase adherence with healthcare recommendations. Firmness, gentleness, choices, and respect must be balanced during care of adolescent patients.

Some specific communication strategies that help with the adolescent include:

- Provide written and verbal explanations.
- Direct history and explanations to teen alone; then include parent.
- Allow for safe exploration of topics by suggesting that the teen is similar to other teens. ("Many teens with diabetes have questions about. . . . How about you?")
- Arrange meetings for discussions with other teens.

Sexuality

With maturation of the body and increased secretion of hormones, the adolescent achieves sexual maturity. This complex process involves growing interactions with members of the opposite sex, an interplay of the forces of society and family, and identity formation. The early adolescent progresses from dances and other social events with members of the opposite sex to the late adolescent who is mature sexually and may have regular sexual encounters. About 47% of all high school students in the United States have had intercourse and 34% are currently sexually active. Only 63% used a condom at their last sexual encounter, putting this age group at high risk of acquiring sexually transmitted infections (Grunbaum et al., 2004).

Teenagers need information about their bodies and emerging sexuality. They should understand the interests and forces they experience. Including sex education in school classes and healthcare encounters is important. Information on methods to prevent sexually transmitted diseases is given, with most school districts now providing some teaching on human immunodeficiency virus. Far more common risks to teens, however, are diseases such as gonorrhea, herpes, and hepatitis. Health histories should include questions on sexual activity, sexually transmitted diseases, and birth control use and understanding. Most hospitals routinely perform pregnancy screening on adolescent girls before elective procedures.

Adolescents will benefit from clear information about sexuality, an opportunity to develop relationships with adolescents in various settings, an open atmosphere at home and school where problems and issues can be discussed, and previous experience in problem solving and self-decision making. Sexual issues should be among topics that adolescents can discuss openly in a variety of settings. Alternatives and support for their decisions should be available.

Some adolescents identify with a sexual minority group such as lesbian, gay, bisexual, or transgendered. They are at particular risk of being stigmatized and harassed by other youth or adults. They are more likely to suffer a variety of problems such as isolation, rejection by significant others, violence, suicide, and taking sexual risks (Rew, Whittaker, Taylor-Seehafer, & Smith, 2005). Nurses are instrumental in helping these youths by providing information for them and their parents, integrating sexual minority content into sexual education curricula, and providing referrals for health and social care when needed. Nurses must examine their own beliefs and communication styles to provide culturally competent care. They can promote trust and acceptance among youth and in the general school community (Bakker & Cavender, 2003). See Chapter 6 ∞ for further information about the health issues related to homosexuality and other sexual minority practices.

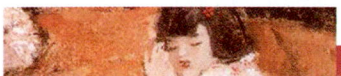

CRITICAL THINKING IN ACTION

GROWTH AND DEVELOPMENT

Consider Irena, who was introduced in the chapter opening scenario. She is 2 years of age and was recently adopted from Romania. Irena is adapting well but her parents have many questions. Since they have no other children and have limited experience with children, the parents, Michael and Alyssa, need information about toddler development as well as the unique needs of Irena.

1. Describe Irena's psychosocial needs. Consider the needs of all toddlers and, in addition, the particular support she needs to bond with her new parents.

2. What type of play most likely predominates in Irena's interactions with other children? What are the benefits of play with others?

3. Irena has been described as having an "easy" temperament by her parents. Describe the characteristics that Thomas and Chess identified for the child with an easy temperament.

4. Since Irena has only a few English words, develop a nursing care plan that involves several suggestions for her parents about how to assist her in learning new words. Can you integrate a plan to help Irena continue to speak the few Romanian words in her vocabulary?

Refer to your Prentice Hall Nursing MediaLink DVD-ROM for answers.

EXPLORE MediaLink

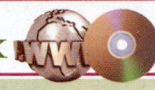

http://www.prenhall.com/ball

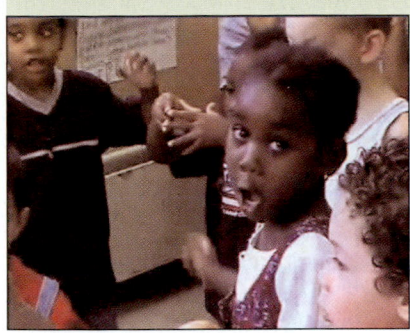

Resources for this chapter can be found on the Prentice Hall Nursing MediaLink DVD-ROM accompanying this textbook, and on the Companion Website at http://www.prenhall.com/ball.

DVD-ROM
Audio Glossary
NCLEX-RN® Review
Videos
  Child Developmental Milestones
  The Stages of Play

COMPANION WEBSITE
Audio Glossary
NCLEX-RN® Review
Care Plan Activity: Infant with Failure to Thrive
Case Study: Diabetic Risk Factors and the School-Age Child
Critical Thinking
  Preparing a Preschooler for a Procedure
  Theories of Development
MediaLink Application: Developmental Milestones
WebLinks

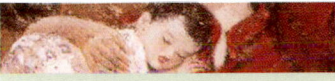

REFERENCES

American Academy of Pediatrics. (2004). *Pediatric nutrition handbook* (5th ed.). Elk Grove Village, IL: Author.

American Academy of Pediatrics, Committee on Bioethics. (2001). Ethical issues with genetic testing in pediatrics. *Pediatrics, 107,* 1451–1455.

American Academy of Pediatrics, Committee on Genetics. (2000). Molecular genetic testing in pediatric practice: A subject review. *Pediatrics, 106,* 1494–1497.

Bakker, L. J., & Cavender, A. (2003). Promoting culturally competent care for gay youth. *Journal of School Nursing, 19,* 65–72.

Bandura, A. (1986). *Social foundations of thought and actions: A social cognitive theory.* Englewood Cliffs, NJ: Prentice Hall.

Bandura, A. (1997a). *Self-efficacy: The exercise of control.* New York: W. H. Freeman.

Bandura, A. (1997b). *Self-efficacy in changing societies.* New York: Cambridge University Press.

Barnett, E. D., & Chen, L. H. (2005). Prevention of travel-related infectious diseases in families of internationally adopted children. *Pediatric Clinics of North America, 52,* 1271–1286.

Bronfenbrenner, U. (1986). Ecology of the family as a context for human development: Research perspectives. *Developmental Psychology, 22,* 723–742.

Bronfenbrenner, U. (Ed.). (2005). *Making human beings human: Bioecological perspectives on human development.* Thousand Oaks, CA: Sage Publications.

Bronfenbrenner, U., McClelland, P. D., Ceci, S. J., Moen, P., & Wethington, E. (1996). *The state of Americans.* New York: Free Press.

Chen, L. H., Barnett, E. D., & Wilson, J. E. (2003). Preventing infectious diseases during and after international adoption. *Annals of Internal Medicine, 139,* 371–378.

Chess, S., & Thomas, A. (1995). *Temperament in clinical practice.* New York: Guilford Press.

Chess, S., & Thomas, A. (1996). *Temperament: Theory and practice.* Philadelphia: Brunner/Mazel Publishers.

Chess, S., & Thomas, A. (1999). *Goodness of fit: Clinical applications from infancy through adult life.* Philadelphia: Brunner/Mazel Publishers.

Craig, G. J., & Baucum, C. (2002). *Human development* (9th ed.). Upper Saddle River, NJ: Pearson Education.

DeLoach Walworth, D. (2005). Procedural-support music therapy in the healthcare setting: A cost-effectiveness analysis. *Journal of Pediatric Nursing, 20,* 276–284.

Dole, K. N. (2005). Education and internationally adopted children: Working collaboratively with schools. *Pediatric Clinics of North America, 52,* 1445–1462.

Erikson, E. (1963). *Childhood and society.* New York: W.W. Norton.

Erikson, E. (1968). *Identity: Youth and crisis.* New York: W.W. Norton.

Field, T. (2002). Preterm infant massage therapy studies: An American approach. *Seminars in Neonatology, 7,* 487–494.

Frenn, M., Malin, S., & Bansal, N. K. (2003). Stage-based interventions for low-fat diet with middle school students. *Journal of Pediatric Nursing, 18,* 36–45.

Ginsberg, H., & Opper, S. (1988). *Piaget's theory of intellectual development* (3rd ed.). Paramus, NJ: Prentice Hall.

Grunbaum, J. A., Kann, L., Kinchen, S., Ross, J., Hawkins, J., Lowry, R., et al. (2004). Youth risk behavior surveillance—United States, 2003. *Morbidity and Mortality Weekly Report, 53* (SS02), 1–96.

Huizink, A. C., & Mulder, E. J. (2006). Maternal smoking, drinking, or cannabis use during pregnancy and neurobehavioral and cognitive functioning in human offspring. *Neuroscience and Biobehavior Review, 30,* 24–41.

Jarvis, C. (2004). *Physical examination and health assessment* (4th ed.). Philadelphia: W. B. Saunders.

Jones, K. L. (2005). Smith's recognizable patterns of human malformations (6th ed.). Philadelphia: Saunders.

Johnson, D. E. (2005). International adoption: What is fact, what is fiction, and what is the future? *Pediatric Clinics of North America, 52,* 1221–1246.

Klug, W. S. & Cummings, M. R. (2003). Concepts of genetics (7th ed.). Upper Saddle River, NJ: Prentice Hall.

Lashley, F. R. (2005). Clinical genetics in nursing practice (3rd ed.). New York: Springer.

Lerner, R. M. (2002). *Adolescence.* Upper Saddle River, NJ: Pearson Education.

Mainous, R. O. (2003). Infant massage as a component of developmental care: Past, present, and future. *Holistic Nursing Practice, 17,* 1–7.

Malone, J. A. (1998). The resiliency model of family stress, adjustment, and adaptation. In B. Vaughan-Cole, M. A. Johnson, J. A. Malone, & B. L. Walker. *Family nursing practice* (pp. 49–60). Philadelphia: W.B. Saunders.

McCarter-Spaulding, D. E. (2005). Medications in pregnancy and lactation. *MCN. American Journal of Maternal Child Nursing, 30,* 10–17.

McClowry, S., & Galehouse, P. (2002). Planning a temperament-based parenting program for inner-city families. *Journal of Child and Adolescent Psychiatry, 15,* 97–105.

Meltzoff, A., & Gopnick, A. (1997). *Words, thoughts, and theories.* Cambridge, MA: MIT Press.

Miller, L. C. (2000). Initial assessment of growth, development, and the effects of institutionalization in internationally adopted children. *Pediatric Annals, 29,* 224–233.

Miller, L. C. (2005). Immediate behavioral and developmental considerations for internationally adopted children transitioning to families. *Pediatric Clinics of North America, 52*, 1311–1330.

Narad, C., & Mason, P. W. (2004). International adoptions: Myths and realities. *Pediatric Nursing, 30*, 483–487.

National Human Genome Research Institute. (2005). Genetic discrimination. Retrieved January 30, 2006, from http://www.genome.gov/10002077

Nickman, S. L., Rosenfeld, A. A., Fine, P., MacIntyre, J. C., Pilowsky, D. J., Howe, R. A., Derdeyn, A., Gonzales, M. B., Forsythe, L., & Sveda, S. A. (2005). Children in adoptive families: Overview and update. *Journal of the American Academy of Child and Adolescent Psychiatry, 44*, 987–995.

Nussbaum, R. L., McInnes, R. R., Willard, H. G. & Boerkoel, C. F. (2001). Thompson & Thompson genetics in medicine (6th ed.). Philadelphia: Saunders.

Piaget, J. (1972). *The child's conception of the world.* Totowa, NJ: Littlefield, Adams Co.

Rew, L., Whittaker, T. A., Taylor-Seehafer, M. A., & Smith, L. R. (2005). Sexual health risks and protective resources in gay, lesbian, bisexual, and heterosexual homeless youth. *Journal for Specialists in Pediatric Nursing, 10*, 11–19.

Riner, M. E., & Saywell, R. M. (2002). Development of the social ecology model of adolescent interpersonal violence prevention (SEMAIVP). *Journal of School Health, 72*, 65–70.

Santrock, J. (2005). *Life-span development* (9th ed.). Boston: McGraw-Hill.

Spector, R. (2004). *Culture care: Guide to heritage assessment and health traditions* (3rd ed.). Upper Saddle River, NJ: Prentice Hall Health.

Stewart, M., Reid, G., & Mangham, C. (1997). Fostering children's resilience. *Journal of Pediatric Nursing, 12*, 21–31.

Turecki, S. (2003). The behavioral complaint: Symptom of a psychiatric disorder or a matter of temperament? *Contemporary Pediatrics, 20*, 111–119.

Vygotsky, L. (1962). *Thought and language.* Cambridge, MA: MIT Press.

Williams, J. K. (2000). Impact of genome research on children and their families. *Journal of Pediatric Nursing, 15*, 207–211.

Witt, C. (2003). Detecting developmental dysplasia of the hip. *Advances in Neonatal Care, 3*, 65–75.

INFANT, CHILD, AND ADOLESCENT NUTRITION

4

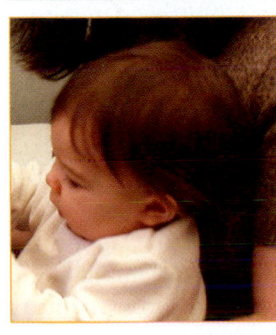

YVONNE is a 9-month-old infant who has been brought to the Women, Infant, and Child (WIC) clinic by her mother, Colleen. Her grandmother, Margarita, has also come since she will take Yvonne home by bus after the WIC appointment, and Colleen will return to work. Margarita cares for Yvonne during the day and likes to feed the baby her native Mexican dishes. Margarita speaks Spanish and demonstrates obvious pride in caring for Yvonne. The nurse weighs and measures Yvonne, takes a blood sample for hematocrit, and performs a 24-hour recall of Yvonne's intake. She finds that Yvonne breast-feeds in the morning and evening, takes an 8-ounce bottle of regular milk during the day, and eats soft table foods.

LEARNING OUTCOMES

After reading this chapter, you will be able to do the following:

1. Discuss major nutritional concepts pertaining to the growth and development of children.

2. Describe and plan nursing interventions to meet nutritional needs for all age groups from infancy through adolescence.

3. Integrate methods of nutritional assessment into nursing care of infants, children, and adolescents.

4. Discuss common nutritional problems of children in developed countries.

5. Apply the nursing process to care for children with disordered eating.

6. Discuss nursing implications for children with common nutritional disorders.

KEY TERMS

anemia **128**
anthropometric measurement **115**
atopy **138**
Body Mass Index (BMI) **116**
Dietary Reference Intakes (DRIs) **106**
early childhood caries **110**
ergogenic aids **140**
food allergy **137**
food insecurity **121**
food intolerance **137**

food jags **113**
food security **121**
lacto-ovovegetarians **142**
lacto-vegetarians **142**
macronutrients **106**
micronutrients **106**
physiologic anorexia **112**
pica **130**
Radioallergosorbent Test (RAST) **138**
vegans **142**
vegetarians **142**

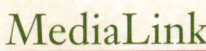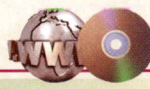

MediaLink

http://www.prenhall.com/ball

See the Prentice Hall Nursing MediaLink DVD-ROM and Companion Website for chapter-specific resources.

Adequate nutrition is an essential component of growth and development. The child's nutritional status begins before birth and is related to the mother's nutritional state. All children must be assessed for nutritional status, followed by teaching or other interventions to enhance health. Nurses are instrumental in giving parents information about normal nutritional needs of infants and young children. Common techniques to assess nutrition, such as measuring growth and monitoring hematocrit, provide needed information about whether the child's intake of nutrients is adequate. How can the nurse bridge the various settings in which children's nutritional needs are met, including the home, childcare settings, schools, and hospitals? The nurse caring for Yvonne must integrate information about Colleen's knowledge of infant nutrition and the grandmother's food patterns to plan culturally appropriate interventions.

While all children and parents can benefit from information about nutritional needs, some children have additional issues that must be considered. The nurse recognizes the special intake requirements of children with health conditions such as eating disorders, food allergies, cystic fibrosis, cerebral palsy, or diabetes. Nutrition monitoring is provided during childhood so that dietary counseling can be integrated with other teaching to promote development. The nurse plays an essential role in helping the family prepare for meeting the nutritional needs of a child who has special needs throughout childhood and in multiple settings. Some children have unique nutritional needs due to their social environments. However, parents may not be knowledgeable about their child's nutritional requirements. Perhaps the family is vegetarian and needs extra help to ensure intake of essential nutrients. If finances are limited, the family may need resources such as access to food stamps, food banks, or budget planning. The nurse considers the high rate of childhood obesity and common nutritional deficits when applying concepts of health promotion with families. Whatever the setting in which the nurse is employed, knowledge of nutrition must be integrated within nursing care.

GENERAL CONCEPTS IN NUTRITION

Nutrition refers to taking in food and assimilating it metabolically for use by the body. It is an essential component of life and therefore an important topic to consider in discussions of child growth and development. The body requires a wide array of intake products. **Macronutrients**, or the major building blocks of the body, are carbohydrates, proteins, and fats. Vitamins and minerals are **micronutrients**, or substances needed in small quantities for healthy body functioning. The need for nutrients is dependent on activity level, state of health and presence of disease or other stress, and age-related needs.

The **Dietary Reference Intakes (DRIs)** are a set of values established by the Food and Nutrition Board of the Institute of Medicine and the National Academy of Science that can be used to assess and plan intake for individuals of different ages. They commonly include four different values that can be considered by nursing, nutrition, and other health personnel (Table 4–1). While the DRI approach is used in the United States, other countries have developed their own approaches to dietary standards. For example, Canada uses Adequate Intake and Reference Nutrient Intake, and the United Kingdom uses Recommended Daily Nutrient Intakes. The aim of these standards is to provide a method of evaluating individual and population diets, and of planning nutrition programs and education. DRIs are generally specific to males and females in several age categories (Table 4–2). See Appendix B ∞ for a list of Dietary Reference Intakes for children and adolescents. For more detailed explanations of recommendations, consult the Dietary Guidelines for Americans (U.S. Department of Health and Human Services, 2005).

Although the DRIs provide useful information when evaluating diets, their use can be time consuming. What "quick check" can be performed to provide feedback about children's daily diets? Learn the Food Guide Pyramid and hang posters of it in schools, clinics, and hospitals. Posters and instructions about personalizing the pyra-

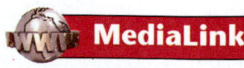

MediaLink

Dietary Guidelines

Table 4–1	DAILY REFERENCE INTAKES (DRIs)		
Term	**Definition**	**Use**	**Example**
Estimated Average Requirement (EAR)	Daily intake needed to meet the requirements of 50% of a certain age and gender group.	Evaluate intake of a group; plan for intake of a group.	Compare the daily intake of vitamin C of a class of children from 24-hour recalls to this number to learn how many do not meet average requirements; plan daily menu for a childcare center.
Recommended Dietary Allowance (RDA)	Daily intake needed to meet the requirements of most people (97–98%) of a certain age and gender group.	Set goal for daily intake.	Evaluate the dietary intake of an individual for a nutrient such as vitamin C; make recommendations to an individual for a daily menu.
Adequate Intake (AI)	Used when limited information on the needs for a vitamin is available and EAR is not available, usually because studies on its metabolism in the body are hard to carry out; rather than being based on metabolic studies, it is derived from the average intake of that nutrient by a healthy group of people.	Evaluate intake of a group; plan intake for a group.	See EAR.
Upper Intake (UI)	Upper tolerable intake level; maximum level unlikely to pose a health risk.	Limit fortification levels of foods and provide information to limit dietary supplements.	Consider intake of a fat-soluble vitamin such as vitamin A that is not readily excreted; include both food sources and supplements.

mid are available at the United States Department of Agriculture (USDA) web site. The Food Guide Pyramid provides a fast method of establishing children's nutritional needs; results are individualized according to the child's age, gender, and activity level. See Figure 4–1 ➤ for the Food Guide Pyramid. In addition, consult the appropriate web sites for alternative pyramids for vegetarians and those from various ethnic groups, such as Hispanic and Native American, as well as Canada's Food Guide to Healthy Eating.

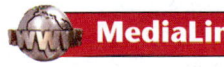
MediaLink

Alternative Food Pyramids

NUTRITIONAL NEEDS

Nutritional needs evolve during all of infancy and childhood. They support growth and development, and influence the child's progression along the developmental path. Nutritional intake helps to maintain the child's health and fosters a state of maximal potential or health promotion. Specific needs during each developmental stage are discussed in this section.

Infancy

From the first feeding of a few ounces of breast milk to a meal of soft table foods with the family at 1 year of age, the infant demonstrates an amazing growth in the ability to ingest and digest a wide variety of foods. Never again will the individual have such a high metabolic rate or high intake requirements in relation to size, or such a change in the types of foods eaten. Infants have an extremely fast rate of growth, since birth weight is usually doubled by about 5 months of age, and tripled by 12 months. Meeting nutritional needs is made difficult by the small size of the infant's stomach and the immaturity of the digestive system. The great physical activity also necessitates high caloric intake. Nutrient demands for protein and vitamins must be met for the cells of the nervous system and body organs to properly develop.

Table 4–2	DRI AGE GROUPS
Pregnancy and Lactation
Birth to 6 months
6–12 months
1–3 years
4–8 years
9–13 years
14–18 years
19–30 years
31–50 years
51–70 years
Over 70 years

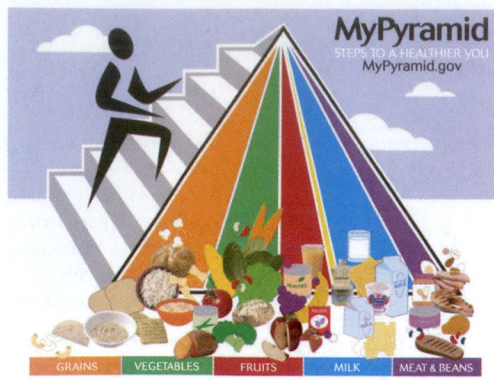

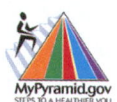

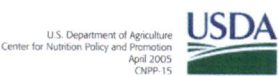

Figure 4–1 ➤ The Food Guide Pyramid is used to provide teaching about amounts of foods recommended for daily intake.
U.S. Department of Agriculture and U.S. Department of Health and Human Services. (2005). http://www.mypyramid.gov/downloads/miniposter.pdf

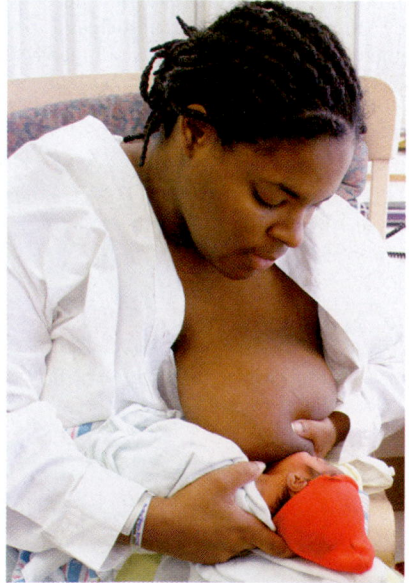

Figure 4–2 ➤ Breast-feeding offers many physical and emotional benefits for the infant. This new mother is learning to breast-feed her baby. How can nurses encourage mothers to have positive breast-feeding experiences?

Breast- and Bottle-Feeding

The natural first food, breast milk, should be encouraged for all infants (Figure 4–2 ➤). Many health groups have made clear statements about the benefits of breast-feeding. See Box 4-1. Breast milk can be the only food for the first 6 months, and should continue through 12 months of age, with addition of solid foods from 6 to 12 months. Many advantages to breast-feeding are recognized, including excellent nutritional balance, promotion of gastrointestinal function, fostering immune defense, psychological benefits, and economic advantage. Although breast milk is the best nutritional source for infants, there may be a need for some limited supplements.

BOX 4–1
BREAST-FEEDING RECOMMENDATIONS

A number of health-related groups strongly recommend breast-feeding and provide specific suggestions for healthcare professionals.

- The American Academy of Pediatrics believes that breast-feeding is the best source of nutrition for babies through the first birthday and should be encouraged by health professionals (AAP, Committee on Nutrition, 2004; and American Academy of Pediatrics, section on Breast-feeding, 2005). At each healthcare visit with an infant and mother, nurses can inquire about breast-feeding, encourage the mother to continue, or offer resources to assist with successful breast-feeding techniques.

- The American Diabetes Association and American Dietetic Association state that broad-based efforts are needed to break barriers to breast-feeding, citing that exclusive breast-feeding for 6 months, and breast-feeding with supplementary foods for at least 12 months, is the ideal feeding pattern for infants (American Diabetes Association, 2006; American Dietetic Association 2001). The nurse teaches about breast-feeding and supplementary foods at each healthcare encounter.

- The U.S. Preventive Services Task Force recommends breast-feeding education and behavioral counseling in 30- to 90-minute individual or group sessions with specially trained nurses or lactation specialists. The Canadian Task Force on Preventive Health Care also recommends counseling for women to encourage breast-feeding. The nurse recommends resources for counseling by lactation experts.

FAMILIES WANT TO KNOW

Supplements for Breast-Fed Babies

1. Each infant receives a vitamin K injection after birth to promote adequate blood clotting. After this time no further vitamin K is needed, as the baby manufactures this vitamin in the gut once he or she begins eating.

2. The need for vitamin D is not fully established, but 400 international units/day is recommended for infants who are breast-fed; live in northern climates and urban settings, especially in winter or if the baby is dark skinned; or is kept well covered when outside.

3. Iron is not needed unless the infant is not taking in other sources of food with iron by 4–6 months. The baby may need an iron source earlier if the mother was anemic during pregnancy or while breast-feeding.

4. Fluoride 0.25 mg is given after 6 months of age if water is not fluoridated to a level of 0.3 parts per million (ppm), or the baby is not drinking any water.

Providing breast-feeding information and instruction positively influences the number of women who decide to breast-feed and increases the number of months they choose to continue breast-feeding (Kramer, 2001). The most effective programs for encouraging breast-feeding are those that involve education and skill/problem-solving information given in at least one session by a health professional (U.S. Preventive Services Task Force, 2003). Some hospitals have lactation specialists who assist breast-feeding mothers; in others, nurses provide this service. Home visits, phone calls from hospital nursing staff, early visits after the birth to obstetric and pediatric offices, and resources such as LaLeche League can provide mothers with needed breast-feeding information and problem-solving suggestions.

The nurse encourages the mother to obtain adequate nutritional intake and sufficient rest, since both are needed for successful breast-feeding. Support programs are especially helpful to mothers who have difficulty breast-feeding, feel unsure how it will fit into their family and work life, are very young, or have an infant with problems related to feeding. Supplements may be needed for some infants. See Families Want to Know: Supplements for Breast-Fed Babies. The mother of a hospitalized infant will need special support to continue breast-feeding. The mother should be encouraged to come to the hospital to feed her baby on the same schedule as at home. If the infant cannot breast-feed, the hospital can provide an electric pump so the mother can maintain lactation. Often hospitals provide meals for the mother of a hospitalized baby so that she can maintain good nutrition and quality breast milk while she stays in the hospital with the baby.

Some women decide not to breast-feed or are unable to do so. After several months of breast-feeding, some mothers begin to use supplemental bottles when they are away from the infant. Nurses provide these mothers with information about formula preparation and feeding. Three types of formula are available—ready to feed, concentrate, and powder. All are nutritionally adequate for infants. The nurse can help parents decide which preparation of formula is best suited for their infant (Table 4–3)

NURSING ALERT

Safety Precautions

Formula can be mixed with tap water but must be refrigerated once mixed. Formula that the baby does not drink should be discarded after use and not kept for future feedings. This minimizes the chance for bacteria to multiply and to cause illness in the baby. When the family lives in older housing, caution them to run tap water for about 2 minutes before using it, and to use only cold water for formula preparation. These practices will minimize the chance that lead is leached from the older pipes in the house (see Chapter 6 ∞ for further discussion of lead poisoning). If the family has a well, the water should be tested for microorganisms before being used for the baby.

Table 4–3	ADVANTAGES AND DISADVANTAGES OF FORMULA PREPARATIONS		
Formula Preparation	**How Packaged**	**Advantages**	**Disadvantages**
Ready to feed	Bottles or cans	No preparation needed	Most expensive type of formula
Concentrate	Cans of concentrated liquid	Easy to add equal amounts of formula concentrate and water directly into bottle and shake	Can be incorrectly measured, leading to inadequate or unsafe nutrition for infant; requires access to clean water supply such as city tap water or bottled water; well water may have too high a mineral concentration
Powder	Cans	Least expensive type of formula	Can be incorrectly measured, leading to inadequate or unsafe nutrition for infant; requires shaking to mix thoroughly; requires access to clean water supply such as city tap water or bottled water; well water may have too high a mineral concentration

BOX 4–2
**COMMON BABY
FORMULAS**

Milk-Based Formulas

Enfamil
Similac
Good Start

Soy-Based Formulas

Isomil   Soyalac
Nursoy   Good Start Supreme Soy
Prosobee   RCF

Specialized Formulas

Lofenalac (low phenylketonuria)
Nutramigen (casein hydrolysate)
Pregestimil (casein hydrolysate)
Alimentum (casein hydrolysate)
MJ (casein hydrolysate)
Portagen (sodium caseinate)
Lactofree (lactose free)
Neocate (synthetic amino acids)
EleCare (amino acids)

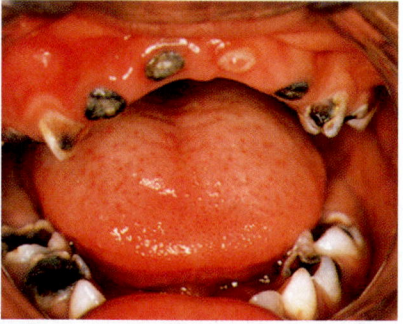

Figure 4–3 ➤ Early childhood caries. This child has had major tooth decay related to sleeping as an infant and toddler while sucking bottles of juice and milk. Courtesy of Dr. Lezley McIlveen, Department of Dentistry, Children's National Medical Center, Washington, DC.

> ## NURSING ALERT
>
> **Safety Precautions**
>
> Advise parents to use caution when providing finger foods to the infant. Hard foods and some soft and malleable ones slip easily into the throat and may cause choking. Avoid hot dogs, hard vegetables, candy, whole grapes, and chunks of peanut butter. Infants and other young children should always be supervised while eating. Be sure parents are familiar with techniques for airway obstruction removal and have emergency numbers clearly listed on their phones.

and teach methods of preparation. Some infants, such as those with phenylketonuria, or other metabolic disorders, or infants with cow milk allergy, require specialized formulas (Box 4–2). Breast- or bottle-feeding is discussed at each contact with health professionals to identify potential teaching needs.

During infancy and toddlerhood, nurses should carefully examine the patterns of breast- and bottle-feeding. **Early childhood caries** can occur when a young child is allowed to nurse or drink from a bottle for long periods, especially when sleeping (Figure 4–3 ➤). The milk, juice, or other fluid pools around the upper anterior teeth, salivary flow decreases, and acid buffering is decreased, resulting in tooth decay. Teach parents to avoid putting the child to bed with a bottle. Encourage pacifier use or a bottle of water instead. Mothers who breast-feed should also be cautioned to limit nursing to specific times so that milk will not pool in the infant's mouth during sleep.

Parents can be taught beginning dental care for the infant, which includes wiping the teeth off daily with a piece of moist gauze or a small infant toothbrush once the teeth erupt. Pediatric dentists advise the first dental visit within 6 months of the first tooth eruption, or no later than about 1 year of age (American Dental Association, n.d.). Have the parents select and establish contact with a dental provider during infancy.

Introduction of Supplemental Foods

When should other foods be added to the infant's diet? Although some parents add other foods when the infant is only days or weeks old, it is best to take cues from the infant's developmental milestones. The American Academy of Pediatrics recommends introducing semisolid foods at 4 to 6 months (AAP, Committee on Nutrition, 2004). Breast- or formula-feeding provides sufficient nutrients in most cases for the first 6 months, with complementary foods rich in iron needed at that age (American Academy of Pediatrics, 2005). Additionally, at about 6 months the extrusion reflex (or tongue thrust) decreases and the infant can sit well with support. The infant is also developing the ability to appreciate texture and to swallow nonliquid foods, and can indicate desire for food or turn away when full.

The first food added to the infant's diet is usually rice cereal. The advantages of introducing cereal first are that it provides iron at an age when the infant's prenatal iron stores begin to decrease, it seldom causes an allergic reaction, and it is easy to digest. One to 2 tablespoons are fed to the infant once or twice daily just before formula or breast-feeding. The infant may appear to spit out food at first because of normal back-and-forth tongue movement. Parents should not interpret this early feeding behavior as indicating dislike for the food. With a little practice, the infant will become adept at spoon-feeding.

Once the infant eats 1/4 cup of cereal twice daily, usually at 6 to 8 months of age, vegetables or fruits can be introduced (Table 4–4). By 8 to 10 months, most fruits and vegetables have been introduced and strained meats or other protein (e.g., tofu, cheese, mashed beans) can be added to the infant's diet. Finger foods are introduced during the second half of the first year as the infant's palmar and then finger grasps develop and as teeth begin to erupt (Figure 4–4 ➤). Infants enjoy toast, O-shaped cereal, finely sliced meats, cheese and tofu, and small pieces of cooked, softened vegetables. Avoid foods that may cause choking.

Certain foods are more commonly associated with the development of food allergies, and avoiding them in infancy may decrease allergy incidence. Recommendations for infants at risk due to a family history of allergy are to delay feeding of cow milk until 1 year; eggs until 2 years; and peanuts, nuts, fish, and shellfish until 3 years (AAP, Committee on Nutrition, 2004). See the discussion on food reactions later in this chapter for more information about food intolerance and allergy. As food and juice intake increase, formula or breast-feedings decrease in amount and frequency (Table 4–5). Nine-month-old Yvonne, introduced in the chapter opening scenario, is learning to eat supplemental foods and her mother needs help from the nurse to decide what foods fit into both the recommendations for her age and the ethnic patterns common in the family. She should remain on breast milk or formula until at least 1 year of age.

If breast-feeding is not chosen, or if supplemental feedings are given, only iron-fortified infant formula should be used during the first year of life. When breast-fed

Table 4–4	INTRODUCTION OF SOLID FOODS IN INFANCY	
Recommendation	**Rationale**	
Introduce rice cereal at 4–6 months.	Rice cereal is easy to digest, has low allergenic potential, and contains iron.	
Introduce fruits or vegetables at 6–8 months. Some healthcare providers recommend vegetable introduction before fruits.	Fruits and vegetables provide needed vitamins. Vegetables are not as sweet as fruits; introducing them first may enhance acceptability to the infant.	
Introduce meats at 8–10 months.	Meats are harder to digest, have high protein load, and should not be fed until close to 1 year of age when kidney function is mature.	
Use single-food prepared baby foods rather than combination meals.	Combination meals usually contain more sugar, salt, and fillers.	
Introduce one new food at a time, waiting at least 3 days to introduce another. Delay feeding eggs, strawberries, wheat, corn, fish, and nut products until close to 1 year of age.	If a food allergy or intolerance develops, it will be easy to identify. The foods listed are those most commonly associated with food allergy.	
Avoid carrots, beets, and spinach before 4 months of age. Have well water evaluated for nitrates (recommended level <10mg/L).	Nitrates in these foods and in water near agricultural runoff can be converted to nitrite by young infants, causing methemoglobinemia.	
Infants can be fed mashed portions of table foods such as carrots, rice, and potatoes.	This is a less expensive alternative to jars of commercially prepared baby food; it allows parents of various cultural groups to feed ethnic foods to infants.	
Avoid adding sugar, salt, spices when mixing own baby foods.	Infants need not become accustomed to these flavors; they may get too much sodium from salt or develop gastric distress from some spices.	
Avoid honey until at least 1 year of age.	Infants cannot detoxify *Clostridium botulinum* spores sometimes present in honey and can develop botulism.	

infants are not eating foods with iron by 4 to 6 months, supplemental iron may need to be added. Careful dietary assessment and discussion of intake by the nurse at health visits helps the practitioner decide if supplemental iron is needed.

Weaning is the term used when infants give up breast-feeding or a bottle and obtain most fluids by cup. At about 8–9 months the baby should be offered a cup with assistance provided so that learning about drinking from a cup can begin. By about 1 year of age, infants are usually able to drink most liquids from a cup with a lid. Bottles can then be slowly withdrawn and replaced by cups. Breast-feeding may continue if the parent and infant desire but introduction of other foods and a cup for drinking water or juice are still recommended. Infants should only be offered cups at meal and snack times so they become accustomed to drinking when thirsty rather than carrying a bottle or cup for much of the day, in order to decrease the chance for dental caries and increased calorie intake.

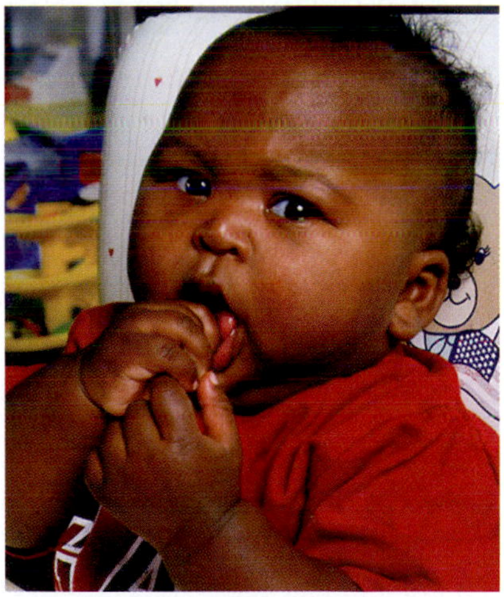

Table 4–5	INFANT NUTRITIONAL PATTERNS

Birth to 1 month
Eats every 2–3 hours, breast or bottle
Eats 2–3 ounces (60–90 mL) per feeding

2–4 months
Has coordinated suck–swallow
Eats every 3–4 hours
Eats 3–4 ounces (90–120 mL) per feeding

4–6 months
Begins baby food, usually rice cereal
Eats four or more times daily
Eats 4–5 ounces (100–150 mL) per feeding

6–8 months
Eats baby food such as rice cereal, fruits, and vegetables
Eats four times daily
Eats 6–8 ounces (160–225 mL) per feeding

8–10 months
Enjoys soft finger foods
Eats four times daily
Eats 6 ounces (160 mL) per feeding

10–12 months
Eats most soft table foods with family
Uses cup with lid
Attempts to feed self with spoon, though spills often
Eats four times daily
Eats 6–8 ounces (160–225 mL) per feeding

Figure 4–4 ▶ The infant who has developed the ability to grasp with thumb and forefinger should receive some foods that can be held in the hand.

CLINICAL TIP

Cow milk (including evaporated milk) can lead to bleeding and anemia, can interfere with absorption of nutrients, and has a high solute load (concentration) which the immature kidneys of the infant can have difficulty excreting. Cow milk should be avoided in the first year of life.

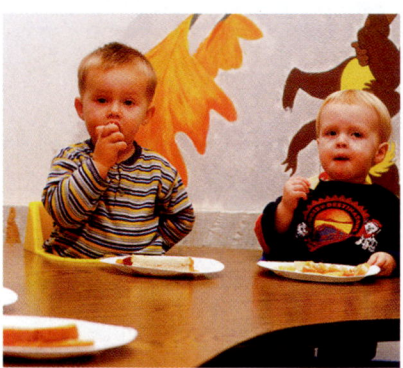

Figure 4–5 ➤ Toddlers should sit at a table or in a high chair to minimize the chance of choking and to foster positive eating patterns.

Parents who want to make infant foods at home can be encouraged and instructed about how to do so. Some commercially prepared foods have unnecessary additives such as salt, sugar, and food starch, and they may be costly for some families. Parents can easily blend fruits and vegetables the family is eating before adding salt, sugar, or seasoning. Prepared foods should be used promptly and stored in the refrigerator between feedings. Foods can also be placed into ice cube trays and frozen; a cube or two can be defrosted at mealtime. Caution parents not to use honey in foods for infants, as it can lead to infant botulism (Centers for Disease Control and Prevention, 2004a).

Toddlerhood

Why do parents of toddlers frequently become concerned about the small amount of food their children eat? Why do toddlers seem to survive and even thrive with minimal food intake? The toddler often displays the phenomenon of **physiologic anorexia**, caused when the extremely high metabolic demands of infancy slow to keep pace with the more moderate growth rate of toddlerhood. Although it can appear that the toddler eats nothing at times, intake over days or a week is generally sufficient and balanced enough to meet the body's demands for nutrients and energy.

Parents often need knowledge about types of foods that constitute a healthy diet. Some easy-to-prepare foods are high in salt and other additives, and can lead to exceeding the recommendation of *Healthy People 2010* (U.S. Department of Health and Human Services, 2000) for sodium intake. Provide alternatives to hot dogs, microwave meals, or fast foods with information about easy-to-prepare sliced meats, cheese, tofu, fruits, and vegetables. Healthy snacks for young children include yogurt, cheese, milk, slices of bread with peanut butter, thinly sliced fruits, and soft vegetables.

Advise parents to offer a variety of nutritious foods several times daily (three meals and two snacks) and let the toddler make choices from the foods offered. Offer foods only at mealtimes and have the child eat in a high chair or on a special seat at the table (Figure 4–5 ➤). Small portions are most appealing to the toddler. A general guideline for food quantity at a meal is 1 tablespoon of each food per year of age (see Table 4–6 for common serving sizes at various ages). The toddler should drink 16 to 24 ounces (1/2 to 3/4 L) of milk daily. Caution parents against giving the toddler more than 1 quart (1 L) of milk daily, since this interferes with the desire to eat other foods, leading to dietary deficiencies. Recall that the child should not be placed to bed with a bottle or allowed to carry a bottle of milk or juice around during the day, due to the risk of early childhood caries (see previous discussion in this chapter). In addition, parents should be cautioned to limit fruit juice to 4 to 6 ounces daily for children ages 1 to 6 years in order to decrease the opportunity for overweight, dental caries, and abdominal discomfort (American Academy of Pediatrics, Committee on Nutrition, 2001). Unpasteurized juice should never be used since it may contain pathogens, such as *E. coli*, *Salmonella*, and *Crytosporidium*, which are particularly harmful to young children (Centers for Disease Control and Prevention, 2005b). Using water to drink in combination with whole fruits, which provide fiber, is a healthier alternative. Avoid more than one meal weekly from a fast-food restaurant due to the generally high fat and low fiber content of such meals.

Learning how to eat with others is an important task of toddlerhood. The toddler displays characteristic autonomy or independence during mealtime. Advise parents to provide opportunities for self-feeding of food with fingers and utensils, and to allow some simple choices, such as type of liquid or cup to use. Young children should eat at a table with others, not be allowed to run and play while eating, and eat at specified meal and snack times. Because social skills are developing, the hospitalized toddler may develop positive eating habits if allowed to have meals with parents or other hospitalized children. See Chapter 13 ∞ for further suggestions about management of nutrition in hospitalized children.

Preschool

The preschooler's diet is similar to that of the toddler, but mealtime is now a more social event. Preschoolers like the company of others while they eat, and they enjoy help-

Table 4–6	**TYPICAL DAILY INTAKE AT VARIOUS AGES**					
	Breakfast	**Snack**	**Lunch**	**Snack**	**Dinner**	**Snack**
Infant 6 months	2 T rice cereal with 2 oz (60 mL) formula	4 oz (120 mL) formula or breast milk	6 oz (180 mL) formula or breast milk	6 oz (180 mL) formula or breast milk	2 T rice cereal with 2 oz (60 mL) formula, then 6 oz (180 mL) formula or breast milk	4 oz (120 mL) formula or breast milk
12 months	1/4 to 1/2 cup (60–120 mL) apple juice 4 T rice cereal with 4 oz (120 mL) milk	3 crackers 1/2 cup (120 mL) milk	1 thin slice (1/2 oz [14 g]) of turkey 1/2 cup soft cooked carrots 1 cup (240 mL) milk	1/2 slice of cheese 1/2 cup (120 mL) milk or water	1/4 cup plain pasta 1/4 cup thin-sliced apple chunks 1/2 cup (120 mL) milk	1/2 cup yogurt
Toddler	1/4 cup (60 mL) orange juice 1/4 cup cereal with 1/2 cup (120 mL) milk 1/4 banana	5 crackers 1/2 cup (120 mL) milk	2 thin slices (1 oz [28 g]) of turkey with 1/2 slice of bread 1/2 cup cooked carrots 1 cup (240 mL) milk	1 slice cheese 1/2 cup (120 mL) juice	1/4 cup plain pasta 1/4–1/2 cup thin-sliced apple chunks 1/2 cup (120 mL) milk	1/2 cup yogurt
Preschooler	1/2 cup (120 mL) orange juice 1/3 cup cereal with 3/4 cup (180 mL) milk 1/2 banana	5 crackers 1/2 orange 1/2 cup (120 mL) milk	3 thin slices (1 1/2 oz [42 g]) of turkey with 1/2 slice bread 1/4 cup cooked carrots 3/4 cup (180 mL) milk	1 slice cheese 1/2 cup (120 mL) juice	1/4–1/2 cup plain pasta with meat sauce 1/2 cup thin-sliced apple chunks 1/2 cup (120 mL) milk	1/2 cup yogurt
School-age child	1/2 cup (120 mL) orange juice 3/4 cup cereal with 1 cup (240 mL) milk 1/2 bagel with jam		4 thin slices (2 oz [56 g]) of turkey with 1 slice bread and condiments Apple 1 cup (240 mL) milk 1 oatmeal cookie	1 1/2 cups popcorn 1 cup (240 mL) lemonade	1/2 cup pasta with meat sauce Dinner salad 1 slice garlic bread 1 cup (240 mL) milk	1 cup pudding or yogurt
Adolescent	1/2 cup (120 mL) orange juice 1 cup cereal 1 cup (240 mL) milk 1 bagel with 1 T peanut butter and jam		3 oz (84 g) meat with 2 slices of bread plus condiments Apple 1 cup (240 mL) milk 1 oatmeal cookie	3 cups popcorn 1 cup (240 mL) lemonade	1 1/2 cup pasta with meat sauce 1 slice garlic bread Salad with dressing 1 cup (240 mL) milk	1 cup pudding Fruit

Note: The young infant should be fed as often as needed rather than on a strict schedule of meals and snacks. The amounts listed for the infant are averages based on a 24-hour recommended intake.

ing with food preparation and table setting (Figure 4–6 ➤). Involving them in these tasks can provide a forum for teaching about nutritious foods and principles of preparation such as the need for refrigeration, safety around stoves, and cleanliness. Limit visits to fast-food restaurants to about once weekly and use the opportunity to assist the child in making wise choices of nutritionally adequate foods in that setting.

Although the rate of growth is slow and steady during the preschool years, the child has periods of **food jags** (eating only a few foods for several days or weeks) and greater or lesser intake. Advise parents to assess food intake over a 1- or 2-week period rather than at each meal to obtain a more accurate impression of total intake. Food jags can be handled by providing the desired food along with other foods to foster choice. The child

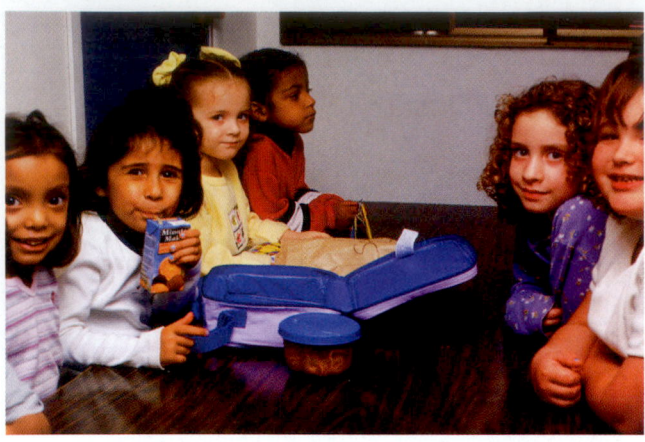
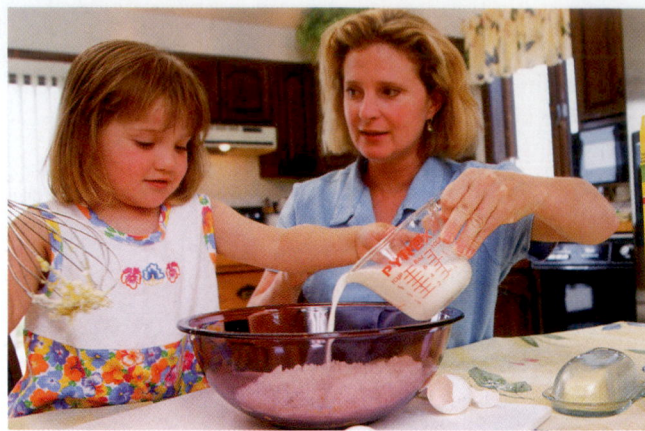

Figure 4–6 ➤ Preschoolers learn food habits by eating with others. Engaging them in food preparation enhances knowledge of food and promotes intake at meals.

who chooses not to eat at snack or mealtime should not be given other foods in between. Hunger will develop and the child will become accustomed to eating when food is provided. Three meals and two or three snacks daily are the norm (see Table 4–6). Limit fruit juice to 8 to 12 ounces daily.

The preschool period is a good time to continue encouraging good dental habits. Children can begin to brush their own teeth with parental supervision and help to reach all tooth surfaces. See Chapter 8 ∞ for recommended doses of fluoride when the water supply is not fluoridated. If the child has not yet visited a dentist, the first dental visit should be scheduled so the child can become accustomed to the routine of dental care.

School Age

The school-age years are a period of gradual growth when energy requirements remain at a steady level, although sometime during these years most children experience a preadolescent growth spurt. Girls may begin a growth spurt by 10 or 11 years, and boys a year or so later. Nutritional needs increase dramatically with this spurt, with large numbers of calories and increased amounts of other nutrients required (see Appendix B ∞ for Dietary Reference Intakes).

School-age children are increasingly responsible for preparing snacks, lunches, and even some other meals. These years are a good time to teach children how to choose nutritious foods and how to plan a well-balanced meal. Because school-age children operate at the concrete level of cognitive thought, nutrition teaching is best presented by using pictures, samples of foods, videotapes, handouts, and hands-on experience.

School-age children often prefer the types of foods eaten at home and may be resistant to new food items. A hospitalized child may refuse to eat, slowing the recuperative process. Encourage family members to bring favorite foods from home that meet nutritional requirements. This can be especially helpful when the hospital serves food only from the dominant cultural group. A child accustomed to a diet of rice, tofu, and vegetables may not enjoy a hospital meal of hamburger and fries. By school age, food has become strongly associated with social interaction, so it is beneficial to have children eat together or to invite family members to take the child off the unit to eat or to bring in food from home and eat with the child. Many hospitals allow children to plan a pizza night or sponsor other events to encourage eating in a social atmosphere.

Most children consume at least one meal daily in school. Although they may bring lunches to school, many children participate in the school lunch program, and perhaps the school breakfast program. Become familiar with the school district's policies in your area for providing foods, snacks, and reduced-price food to students in need. Over the past decade, many U.S. school systems have allowed vending machines for carbonated sweetened beverages and snacks to be installed. Part of the profits from these machines has enabled revenue-strapped school districts to enhance their incomes. However, schools are increasingly challenged about the presence of the machines, especially in light of the growing problem of overweight among youth. Some school districts have now limited the number of machines or the hours during which they can be used by students. Nurses are able to provide information for districts about the problems of obesity and the need for healthy foods for youth.

The loss of the first deciduous teeth and the eruption of permanent teeth usually occur at about 6 years, or at the beginning of the school-age period. Of the 32 permanent teeth, 22 to 26 teeth erupt by age 12 years, and the remaining molars follow in the teenage years. See Chapter 5 ∞ for the typical sequence of tooth eruption and Chapters 8, 9, and 10 ∞ for further information about dental needs during childhood. The school-age child should be closely monitored to ensure that brushing and flossing are adequate, that fluoride is taken if the water supply is not fluoridated, that dental care is obtained to provide for examination of teeth and alignment, and that loose teeth are identified before surgery or sports participation.

Adolescence

Most adolescents need well over 2000 calories daily to support the growth spurt, and some adolescent boys require nearly 3000 calories daily. When teenagers are active in a variety of sports, these requirements increase further. The pregnant or breast-feeding adolescent has even more challenging nutrient requirements, and maternity resources should be consulted to plan diets for these periods. Supplementary vitamins and minerals will be needed to enhance the pregnancy outcome. Because adolescents prepare much of their own food and often eat with friends, they need to be taught about good nutrition. Developing a diet that includes a large number of calories, meets vitamin and mineral requirements, and is acceptable to the teen may be a challenge. An adolescent who is hospitalized and does not like the hospital lunch sometimes has a soft drink and chips when a friend comes to visit; however, the teen may be receptive to offers of juice and pizza, a more nutritious meal. Small improvements should be viewed positively as they may lead to further changes.

Fast food represents a significant intake for many adolescents. It is commonly high in fat, calories, and sodium while being low in essential nutrients such as calcium, folic acid, riboflavin, vitamins A and C, and fiber. Many schools are redesigning cafeterias and food programs to entice more teens to eat at school rather than nearby fast-food restaurants. Adding fruits and salads and decreasing access to snack bars can enhance the quality of food intake (Cullen & Zakeri, 2004). School nurses play a vital role in helping to tailor a healthy school nutrition program. Remember that peer group influence is important, so group sessions in which adolescents eat lunch together can provide a forum for influencing food habits. (See Evidence-Based Practice: Adolescent Food Habits.) What other methods can you think of to encourage positive nutritional habits among teens?

NUTRITIONAL ASSESSMENT

What is the best indication that the child's nutrition is adequate? Which data collection methods provide the most accurate information about a child's dietary intake? The nurse plays an important role in assessing the diets of children and in seeking additional evaluation from dietitians and nutritionists in complex situations.

Physical and Behavioral Measurement

Growth Measurement

A common method used to evaluate the adequacy of diet is measurement of growth. **Anthropometric measurement** is the term used to refer to assessment of various parts of the body. Anthropometry of young children commonly includes weight, length, and head circumference. Standing height is substituted for length once the child can stand. Head circumference, also known as occipital-frontal circumference (OFC), is measured until the child is about 5 years. Additional measurements that may be included in special circumstances include chest circumference, mid-upper arm circumference, and

EVIDENCE-BASED PRACTICE

Adolescent Food Habits

Problem

Adolescents are largely independent in their food choices. They often eat "on the run" and are influenced by peers and the media. At the same time, rates of obesity are on an escalating trajectory upward. Nurses need to understand and apply evidence-based practice for influencing eating behaviors in adolescents.

Evidence

Two nurses conducted a literature review on adolescent nutrition publications in the last decade. Twenty-two articles on eating patterns, barriers, and nutrition interventions met their criteria for review and became the basis of their analysis. Important topics were family effects on adolescent eating, cultural and economic factors, school effects on diet, and community effects on adolescent eating behaviors. While the studies identified important influences on adolescent eating, the authors noted that there is a lack of information about ethnic minority group influences, socioeconomic factors, interventions that will assist adolescents to change unhealthy behaviors, and the role of parents in adolescent eating.

Implications

While adolescent nutritional intake is an important health concern, there is a limited body of knowledge to guide the health professional.

Findings of importance are that child and adolescent eating patterns set an important example for life and that the family eating patterns, school setting, and community influences must all be examined to identify risk and protective factors in the adolescent diet. Important barriers to adolescent healthy eating include availability of "junk food" snacks, lack of parental involvement in the lives of teens, and the media messages about food consumption.

Critical Thinking

1. What developmental stages of the adolescent provide both challenges to healthy eating and ability to make wise food choices?
2. Construct a list of questions about family food patterns that will help you identify risk and protective factors of the family.
3. Visit a local high school and then travel 1/2 mile in each direction from the school. Record the number of fast-food restaurants, billboards about foods, and any other food-related resources or media. Watch 2 hours of television at 3–5 p.m., when adolescents frequently arrive home. Record the number of food-related messages, what types of foods are advertised, and other observations.
4. How can you integrate knowledge about adolescent nutrition into your potential role as a school nurse at a high school?

Source: Jenkins, S., & Horner, S. D. (2005). Barriers that influence eating behaviors in adolescents. *Journal of Pediatric Nursing, 20,* 258–267.

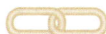

SKILLS 6–1 THROUGH 6–7:
Growth Measurements

CLINICAL TIP

To calculate body mass index (BMI), you must:

1. Be sure that weight is in kilograms. If it is in pounds, divide that number by 2.2 to get kilograms.
2. Change height measurement to meters. Because 1 meter = 39.37 inches (or 0.0254 meters = 1 inch), you must multiply the child's height in inches by 0.0254 to obtain height in meters.
3. Now square the number of meters.
4. You are ready to calculate BMI. Put kilograms of weight/height in meters squared and divide appropriately.

If a child weighs 26.5 pounds, convert to kilograms = 12 kg. The child's height is 34.5 inches = 0.8763 m. Because $m^2 = 0.7679$, BMI = 15.63.

Alternatively, visit the web site for the Centers for Disease Control and Prevention for calculation of BMI using metric or English units.

skinfold measurement at sites such as triceps, abdomen, and subscapular regions. The *Clinical Skills Manual* presents techniques for accurate measurement of weight, length, height, chest, and head circumference.

Once the measurements are collected, plot the readings on the appropriate standardized growth curves for weight, length to height, head circumference, and body mass index (Figure 4–7 ➤). **Body mass index (BMI)** is a calculation based on the child's weight and height, or length, and is calculated as kilograms of weight/m^2 of height. This is a useful calculation for determining if the child's height and weight are in proportion. Identify on the plots where the child falls in percentile for each measurement. Children normally fall between the 10th and 90th percentiles. A measurement below the 10th percentile, especially for BMI, may indicate undernutrition, whereas one over the 90th percentile can indicate overnutrition. It is important, however, to look at the differences between measurements. An infant in the 90th percentile for length, weight, and head circumference is proportional and may be a naturally large baby. However, a child who is consistently in the 10th percentile for all measurements, but is growing steadily and is at a normal development level, may simply be a small child. Much cultural and individual variation exists regarding size. See Appendix A ∞ for standardized growth curves by gender and age for infants, children, and adolescents. Visit our web site to find out more about the growth curves and a course in accurate assessment techniques.

Plot your measurements on the same growth curve with earlier percentiles for the child. When measurements follow the same percentile over time, growth is generally normal for the child and nutrition is likely adequate. However, a sudden or sustained change in percentile may indicate a chronic disorder, emotional difficulty, or a nutritional intake problem. Further assessment of physical status and dietary intake will be needed.

Additional Physical Measurements

Many observations from the physical assessment provide clues to nutritional status. Every body system can be affected by dietary intake, and a combination of certain symptoms may suggest specific nutritional problems. Some of the common Clinical Manifestations of dietary deficiencies and excesses are outlined on page 118.

Laboratory measurements can provide useful information when nutritional status is questionable. Some common studies include hematocrit and hemoglobin, serum

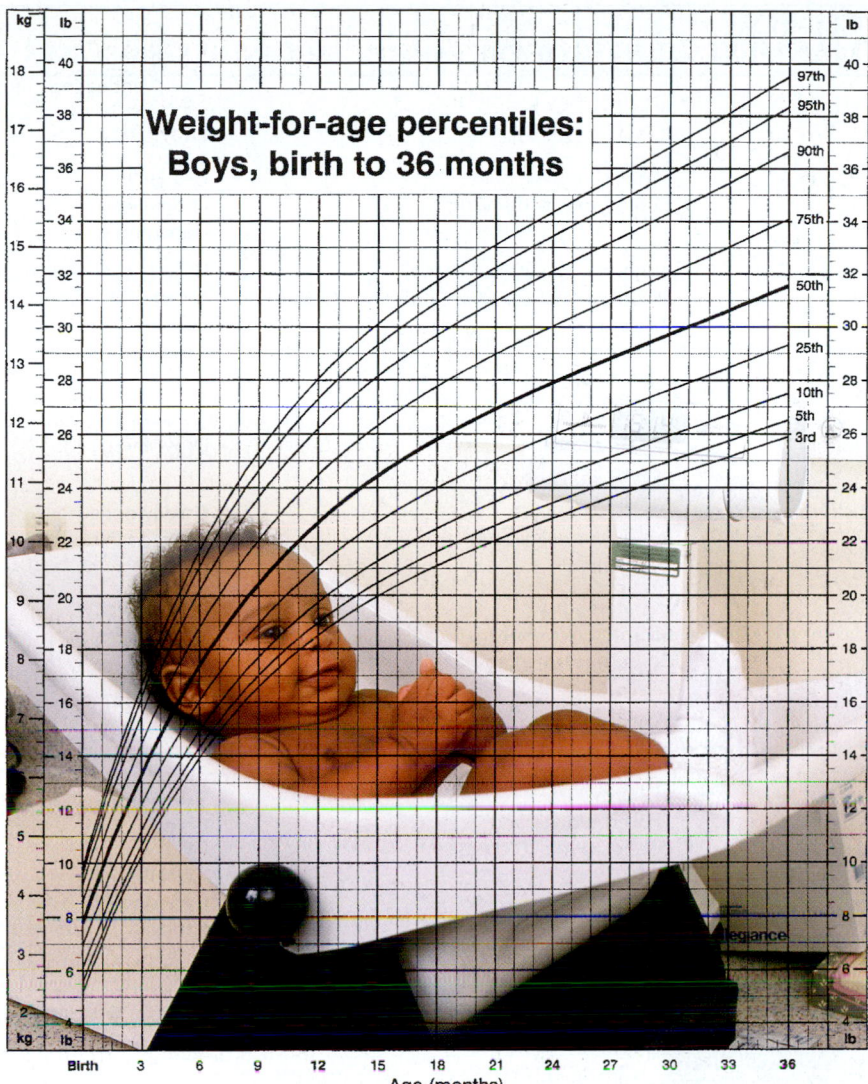

Weight-for-age percentiles:
Boys, birth to 36 months

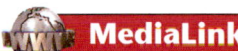

Figure 4–7 ➤ The nurse accurately
measures the child and then places height
and weight on appropriate growth grids
for the child's age and gender.

MediaLink

Growth Grids

CLINICAL TIP

If you measure a child and find
him or her to be either in very low or
high percentiles, try the following:

1. Measure again to check for
   accuracy.
2. Examine if length or height,
   weight, and head circumference
   are in similar percentiles. Is the
   child proportional?
3. Observe if the parents are very
   large or very small.
4. Look at the child's chart to see if
   the patterns have continued over
   time or if they represent a
   sudden change. Changes from
   one channel to another are of
   concern. For example, if the
   child has usually been in the 25th
   percentile for all measurements,
   and now suddenly is in the 90th
   percentile for head
   circumference or weight,
   additional assessments must be
   performed to identify the reason.

glucose and fasting insulin, lipids and lipoproteins, and liver and renal function studies. Adding some further measurements such as chest circumference and skinfolds
(measurement of fat at certain body sites such as triceps, scapular, and abdominal areas) may also be useful.

Dietary Intake

The mother's dietary intake during pregnancy may provide information about the
child's nutritional state and it can be assessed for pertinent information. Obtain detailed information about the child's dietary intake when there is a potential for nutritional deficiency due to disease, knowledge deficit, or socioeconomic status. After the
information is collected, compare the dietary intake with the recommended levels for
a child of that age and gender (see Figure 4–1 for Food Guide Pyramid recommendations, and Appendix B ∞ for Daily Reference Intakes). The 24-hour recall of intake,
food frequency questionnaire, and a dietary screening history provide a good overview
of the infant's or child's intake and eating patterns. A food diary provides information
about the child's precise food intake.

24-Hour Recall of Food Intake

The 24-hour diet recall is frequently used to assess the adequacy of the diet. People can
generally remember their intake in the past day, so results are fairly accurate; it is easy to
gather the data and analyze results; only a few minutes are needed. Ask the parent or child

CULTURE

Growth Grids

The revised growth grids now in use were standardized using a cross-section of the U.S. population and are generally reflective of most children. However, children from some other countries or cultures may fall outside of these curves. For example, new immigrants or adoptees may be in lower percentiles, and "catch up" over several months or years. Children of immigrants from developing countries tend to be larger than their parents. Even when small, children should follow normal growth patterns. For example, a child may remain at the 10th or 25th percentile for height, but continue to slowly grow and not fall to a lower percentile.

CLINICAL MANIFESTATIONS OF DIETARY DEFICIENCIES/EXCESSES

Nutrient	Deficiency Manifestation	Excess Manifestation
Vitamin A	Night blindness Skin dryness and scaling	Headache Drowsiness Hepatomegaly
Vitamin C	Abnormal hair (coiled shape) Skin abnormalities (dermatitis and lesions) Purpura Bleeding gums Joint tenderness Sudden heart failure	Usually none—excess is excreted in urine
Vitamin D	Rib abnormalities Bowed legs	Drowsiness
B vitamins	Weakness Decreased deep tendon reflexes Dermatitis	Usually none—excess is excreted in urine
Protein	Hepatomegaly Edema Scant, depigmented hair	Kidney failure
Carbohydrate	Emaciation Decreased energy Retarded growth and development	Overweight
Iron	Lethargy Slowed growth and developmental progression Pallor	Vomiting, diarrhea, abdominal pain Pallor Cyanosis Drowsiness Shock

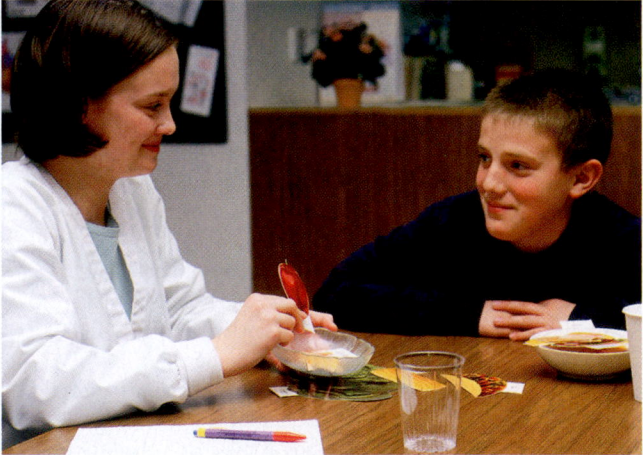

Figure 4–8 ➤ The nurse is interviewing a child about foods eaten in the last day. Note the models of food and dishes for accurate assessment of serving sizes.

to list all foods eaten during the past 24 hours (Figure 4–8 ➤). It is usually helpful to ask for a description of activities in the last day. Then start with the most recent event and move backwards, integrating food intake into the daily schedule. For example, you might begin by saying, "You mentioned you got up early to come to the clinic today. What did Sam eat at home before you left? Did he have a snack as you traveled here or after you arrived?" While asking about the foods eaten, inquire specifically about the following:

- All meals and snacks
- Amounts of each food item consumed (have various-size measuring cups, bowls, and plates so accurate amounts can be indicated)
- Types of specific foods used, such as whole milk versus nonfat or 2%, brand names of cereals, specific types of margarine or butter
- Additives used, such as condiments, table salt, spices, milk to mix formula
- Food preparation methods, including adding fats to cook, removal or retention of fats on meats
- Vitamins and supplements, types, and doses
- Whether the intake is representative of the typical diet (in situations such as illness or vacation, intake may be different than usual)

Once the 24-hour recall is obtained, intake analysis is next. First, a quick check can be done to compare servings of various food types with the Food Guide Pyramid, as described earlier. Next, a detailed analysis is done to compute calories, carbohydrate, protein, and fat intake and compare them with recommended amounts. All major vitamins and minerals are also computed and comparisons made to the DRIs. This computation may be done by hand, using a book of nutrients in common foods, or may be done on the computer. Several computer programs are available, and a federal government web site provides intake levels and comparisons to the RDAs—try computing your own 24-hour recall or that of a child in your clinical setting with the Healthy Eating Index.

Food Frequency Questionnaire

Food frequency questionnaires are available that can be easily administered to parents or children. Usually they ask about how often certain types of foods are eaten in a specified period such as a week. Questionnaires can be long and evaluate a total diet, or short to focus on specific items such as fruit and vegetable intake. A short questionnaire about milk intake or fruit and vegetable intake may be helpful before the start of a teaching project on nutrition to a class of school-age children. Knowing their usual intake of a food item can provide helpful information for the project. One example of the types of questions asked on a food frequency questionnaire is shown in Box 4-3.

BOX 4–3

SAMPLE QUESTIONS—YOUTH/ADOLESCENT QUESTIONNAIRE (YAQ)

1. Where do you usually eat breakfast?
   - Home
   - School
   - Don't eat breakfast
   - Other
2. Which cold breakfast cereal do you usually eat?
3. What type of milk do you usually drink?
   - Whole milk
   - 2% milk
   - 1% milk
   - Skim/nonfat milk
   - Don't know
   - Don't drink milk
4. How much milk (glass or with cereal) do you drink?
   - Never/less than one glass per month
   - One glass per week or less
   - Two to six glasses per week
   - One glass per day
   - Two to three glasses per day
   - Four or more glasses per day
5. How often do you eat pizza (two slices)?
   - Never/less than once per month
   - One to three times per month
   - Once per week
   - Two to four times per week
   - Five or more times per week
6. Do you eat peanut butter sandwiches (plain or with jelly, fluff, etc.)?
   - Never/less than one sandwich per month
   - One to three sandwiches per month
   - One sandwich per week
   - Two to four sandwiches per week
   - Five or more sandwiches per week

From Youth/Adolescent Questionnaire. (1995). Harvard Medical School. Channing Laboratory, 181 Longwood Avenue, Boston, MA 02115.

BOX 4–4
DIETARY SCREENING HISTORY FOR INFANTS

Overview Questions

What was the infant's birth weight?
At what age did the birth weight double and triple?
Was the infant preterm?
Does the infant have any feeding problems such as difficulty sucking and swallowing, spitting up, fatigue, or fussiness?

If Infant Is Breast-Fed

How long does the baby nurse at each breast?
What is the usual schedule for nursing?
Does the baby also take any milk or formula? Amount and frequency? What type?

If Infant Is Formula Fed

What formula is used? Is it iron fortified?
How is it prepared?
Do you hold or prop the bottle for feedings?
How much formula is taken at each feeding?
How many bottles are taken each day?
Does the baby take a bottle to bed for naps or nighttime?
    What is in the bottle?

If Infant Is Fed Other Foods

At what age did the baby start eating other foods?

Cereal	Finger foods
Fruit/juices	Meats
Vegetables	Other protein sources

Do you use commercial baby food or make your own?
Does the baby eat any table foods?
How often does the baby take solid foods?
How is the baby's appetite?
Do you have any concerns about the baby's feeding habits?
Does the baby take a vitamin supplement? Fluoride?
Have there been any allergic reactions to foods? Which ones?
Does the baby spit up frequently?
Have there been any rashes?
What types of stools does the baby have? Frequency? Consistency?

Dietary Screening History

Ask the parent about the infant's or child's eating habits using questions in Boxes 4–4 and 4–5. (Questions about adolescents eating patterns are in Box 4–6.) Responses provide information about the family's and individual youth's eating habits and food beliefs beyond that collected on a 24-hour dietary recall or food frequency questionnaire.

Food Diary

Parents are asked to keep a food diary when the child has a nutrition problem or disorder, such as malnutrition, obesity, or type 1 diabetes, that requires dietary management. All meals and snacks, with food preparation methods and quantities eaten over a 1- to 7-day period, are recorded. Eating patterns change significantly for holidays or family gatherings, so ask parents to select typical days for the food diary or to record specific events

---

BOX 4–5
DIETARY SCREENING HISTORY FOR CHILDREN

- What foods or beverages does the child dislike?
- What types of food or beverage does the child especially like?
- What is the child's typical eating schedule? Meals and snacks?
- Does the child eat with the family or at separate times?
- Where does the child eat each meal?
- Who prepares the food for the family?
- What method of cooking is used? Baking? Frying? Broiling?
- What ethnic foods are commonly eaten?
- Does the family eat in a restaurant frequently? What type?
- What type of food does the child usually order?
- Is the child on a special diet?
- Does the child need to be fed, feed himself or herself, need assistance eating, or need any adaptive devices for eating?
- What is the child's appetite like?
- Does the child take any vitamin supplements (iron, fluoride)?
- Does the child have any allergies? What types of symptoms?
- What types of regular exercise does the child get?
- Are there any concerns about the child's eating habits?

BOX 4–6

DIETARY SCREENING HISTORY FOR ADOLESCENTS

- How many times do you eat (meals and snacks) daily? What meals (breakfast, lunch, dinner) do you skip at least three times per week?
- How often do you eat food from fast-food restaurants? Which ones? What are your favorite meals from these restaurants?
- Do you have a special diet? Are there foods you avoid either because of dislike for the food or your own decision, such as vegetarianism?
- Which grains have you eaten in the last few days? Vegetables? Fruits? Milk and dairy products? Meat and meat alternatives? Fats and sweets?
- Are you concerned or satisfied about your weight? Have you tried to lose weight? If so, what methods have you used?
- Do you take vitamin pills? Herbal supplements? Protein powders? Other supplements?
- Do you drink alcohol? How much? Do you use street drugs or other drugs without prescription? If so, which ones?

Adapted from Story, M., Holt, K., & Sofka, D. (Eds.). (2002). *Bright futures in practice: Nutrition* (2nd ed.). Arlington, VA: National Center for Education in Maternal and Child Health, Nutrition Tools, Appendix.

---

affecting food intake. Including one weekday and one weekend day may provide the most accurate overview. Food diaries can provide a great deal of helpful information, but take the time and motivation to complete them well (Lee & Nieman, 2007). Be sure instructions are complete and that the form has a place to record amounts, preparation, events occurring, and where food was eaten. The nurse or parent may need to obtain the school lunch menu and talk with the school lunch personnel to add accurate school intake.

The nurse completes the nutritional assessment indicated for a child, and may consult with or refer the family to a dietitian or nutritionist for additional assessment and teaching.

COMMON NUTRITIONAL CONCERNS

Childhood Hunger

Although most Americans live in a "land of plenty," significant numbers of children periodically experience hunger. **Food security** is access at all times to enough nourishment for an active, healthy life. In contrast, **food insecurity** indicates an inability to acquire or consume adequate quality or quantity of foods in socially acceptable ways, or the uncertainty that one will be able to do so (Federal Interagency Forum on Child and Family Statistics, 2005). About 18% of U.S. children live in households that experience food insecurity at times. The proportion is much higher for certain groups in the population: 45% for those living in poverty, 38% for those where parents lack a high school diploma, 34% for those living with a single mother; and 31% for Blacks and Hispanics (Federal Interagency Forum, 2005).

A major cause of hunger in children is therefore poverty, and because one in five children is poor, many families may be unable to provide sustainable nutrition at all times (Children's Defense Fund, 2004). In some single-income families the head of household may be in the workforce, but with an income insufficient to provide for family food needs (see Chapter 1 ∞ for a description of Temporary Assistance for Needy Families [TANF]). Families may be ineligible for food assistance programs even though they are unable to purchase enough food for all their members. Children with special nutritional needs are at particular risk because it may be more costly to buy and prepare formula or foods for a child with allergies, diabetes, or an immune disorder.

Children who have insufficient dietary intake are at risk for a wide array of health problems. They may become anemic; experience a high rate of infectious disease due to lowered immune response; have slowed developmental maturation, delayed or stunted physical growth, and learning disorders; and be at greater risk of overweight, cardiovascular disease, and diabetes in adulthood (AAP, Committee on Nutrition, 2004). Subsequently, the national and individual cost of childhood hunger is great.

BOX 4–7
FOOD INSECURITY SCREENING

1. Does your household ever run out of money to buy food to make a meal?
2. Do you or members of your household ever eat less than you feel you should because there is not enough money for food?
3. Do you or members of your household ever cut the size of meals or skip meals because there is not enough money for food?
4. Do your children ever eat less than you feel they should because there is not enough money for food?
5. Do you ever cut the size of your children's meals or do they skip meals because there is not enough money for food?
6. Do your children ever say they are hungry because there is not enough food in the house?
7. Do you ever rely on a limited number of foods to feed your children because you are running out of money to buy food for a meal?
8. Do any of your children ever go to bed hungry because there is not enough money to buy food?

Scoring: 5–8 yes = hungry; 1–4 yes = risk of hunger

From the Washington State Department of Health.

Nurses are well positioned to evaluate families for food insecurity in a variety of hospital, clinic, school, and home settings. In addition to the assessment of the individual child's nutritional status, further questions can determine families with potential problems. Administer the screening tool to identify risk in families (Box 4–7). Most parents go without food themselves in order to feed their children, so food insecurity may not necessarily have directly impacted all children at risk. However, anxiety over providing food can be a very stressful event in families and diet quality deteriorates as insecurity increases. If families have experienced food insecurity or may be likely to at some time, be sure to provide them with access to community agencies and programs that can be of assistance. (See Families Want to Know: Community Resources for Food.) What resources are available in your community to help families with food insecurity?

Overweight and Obesity

After several decades of similar statistics regarding overweight in children, the numbers are now skyrocketing. The current incidence of overweight in the United States has been labeled as an epidemic and is associated with a wide array of health problems, such as the appearance of type 2 diabetes in youth (American Diabetes Association, Inc., 2003). See Chapter 29 ∞ for a discussion of diabetes. Additional problems such as stroke, gallbladder disease, arthritis, cardiovascular disease, sleep disturbances, hypertension, dyslipidemia, respiratory problems, certain cancers, interference with physical activity and

---

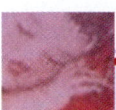

FAMILIES WANT TO KNOW

Community Resources for Food

Food Stamp Program—Eligibility based on household size and income; refer students and those with low incomes, especially when they have young children; education services often available

Child Nutrition Programs—School lunch, breakfast, and milk programs; free and lowered cost meals in schools; assist parents to apply

Special Child Programs—Summer programs, Head Start, childcare centers, and homeless children programs may provide nutritional support in some communities

Women, Infants, and Children (WIC)—Supplemental foods and nutrition education to pregnant, breast-feeding, and postpartum women and to their young children; assessment of child growth often included

Nutrition Education and Training Program—Nutrition education for teachers and school food service personnel

Community Services—May include food banks, field gleaning, and other programs

Find out what services are available to provide food and nutrition education in your community. Make a list for use in clinical settings with families.

activities of daily living, social stigma, discrimination, depression, and lower self-esteem have been related to obesity rates (Hagerty, Schmidt, Bernaix, & Clement, 2004; U.S. Centers for Disease Control and Prevention et al., 2004). Increasing obesity rates lead to earlier emergence of many of these health problems in youth and young adults. The Third National Health and Nutrition Examination Survey found that 11–15% of various child and adolescent groups are now overweight (U.S. Department of Health and Human Services, 2000). When using the 95th percentile of BMI as an indicator of overweight or obesity, 10% of 2- to 5-year-old children, and more than 15% of 6- to 19-year-olds, are affected (Institute of Medicine, 2005). Since overweight in childhood and adolescence frequently tracks into adulthood, the implications for health care are obvious.

Many reasons are cited for the increase in overweight children. The number of calories consumed by children is not generally increasing, but children tend to exercise less, particularly on a daily basis. They infrequently walk or ride bikes, either because of the convenience of driving or due to unsafe neighborhoods. Television viewing is very high among youth; television and other screen activities account for an average of 5.5 hours daily in the lives of children in the United States. Even the youngest children are affected; children under 6 years spend on average about 2 hours daily on screen activities, and 26% of those less than 2 years have television sets in their bedrooms (Rideout et al., 2003). These are alarming trends because children having > 2 hours of screen activities daily are 73% more likely to be at risk of obesity and related health problems such as type 2 diabetes mellitus (see Chapter 29) (Urrutia-Rojas & Menchaca, 2006). Inactive pursuits do not require high caloric energy, leading to an imbalance in intake and demand for calories. Additionally, sedentary pursuits such as television viewing are often accompanied by ingestion of high-calorie "junk" foods. Many of the sedentary behaviors of youth, such as television viewing and computer use, also subject them to the effects of the media which tends heavily toward advertisements of less healthy foods.

The percentage of calories from fat consumed in the United States is among the highest in the world. Although no more than 30% of calories should come from total dietary fat, and no more than 10% from saturated fat, about 32% of calories consumed by children in the United States are supplied by fat and 12% by saturated fat (Institute of Medicine, 2005). High levels of dietary fat are associated with higher cholesterol levels and decreased activity. The high rate of dietary fat is related to the large amount of fast food consumed, as fast-food restaurants are convenient and fit well into today's lifestyles. Another contributing factor to overweight is poor snacking habits, which have been on the increase in the last decade. Snacks of choice are often nutrient poor and calorie dense (Briefel & Johnson, 2004).

MediaLink

Children and Overweight Video

CULTURE

Overweight

Overweight is more common among some ethnic and socioeconomic groups. Lack of knowledge about foods and physical activity, limited access to fresh produce and safe places to exercise, easy access to increasing numbers of fast foods, and ethnic differences in metabolism may constitute risk factors. Lower income and Hispanic, African American, and Native American ethnic identities are associated with higher incidence of overweight, especially among women. National goals to eliminate health disparities in income and ethnic groups have been set (U.S. Department of Health and Human Services, 2000).

GROWTH & DEVELOPMENT

Diet and Physical Activity

The interaction between dietary intake and physical activity is complex. In an effort to examine the effects of decreased physical activity time and increased sedentary time, which are common in our cultures today, on increased obesity rates, researchers are designing studies to measure these interactions. One of the best ways to measure effects is to do so longitudinally, or over time. In one study, 106 preschoolers were followed from age 4 years to 11 years, with annual body measurements and parental information about children's television and video habits. Television viewing time was a predictor of body mass index (BMI) and skinfold measurement, and the effect was greater when children also had more total sedentary hours and higher fat diets (Proctor, Moore, Gao et al., 2003).

A group of 1970 British were measured at ages 5, 10, and 30 years and television viewing habits were assessed. Weekend television viewing time as a child was significantly related to BMI in adulthood (Viner & Cole, 2005). The implications for growth and development are clear: Television and other screen activities directly and indirectly influence rates of obesity. Nurses who are performing nutritional assessments should integrate questions about the amount of sedentary behaviors, such as television, videos, and computers, and the amount of physical activity. Recommend that no more than 2 hours daily be spent on "screen" activities and discourage all viewing by children less than 2 years. Provide ideas about alternative entertainment, particularly those that involve physical activity (Gentile, Oberg, Sherwood et al., 2004).

Nursing Management

Nurses can assist parents and children in building good nutritional and exercise habits throughout life, thus decreasing the incidence of overweight and its attendant health risks. Begin with an assessment of growth patterns starting early in life. Patterns of eating fast foods, meals on the run, and while watching television should be addressed in early health promotion and health maintenance visits. Caution parents that television viewing should be limited to a maximum of 2 hours daily, and that television and video games should not be placed in children's bedrooms. Daily exercise routines of at least 30 minutes can be included in most families. Also, teach about the Food Guide Pyramid and its integration into a healthy life. Healthy snacks include fruits, vegetables, grains, and nuts. "Super sizing" fast foods and eating out often should be avoided.

Risks for poor health often cluster in individuals and families because of both genetic factors and common lifestyles, so the nurse can be alert for situations in which parents are overweight, or children have elevated blood pressure, exercise infrequently, or are in upper percentiles for weight, BMI, or skinfold. Presence of risk factors necessitates further dietary and risk assessment so that a management plan can be implemented. See resources such as "Helping Your Overweight Child" and "Take Charge of Your Health: A Teenager's Guide to Better Health," and the accompanying Nursing Care Plan.

Food Safety

Every year in the United States, about 76 million people contract foodborne illnesses. Some are quite mild, whereas others can be severe. About 300,000 people are hospitalized and 5000 die from these illnesses (Morbidity and Mortality Weekly Report [MMWR], 2004). Children are at greater risk of severe illness and death from food and water than adults, due to their immature gastrointestinal and immune systems. Immuno-compromised children are at even greater risk. The most common pathogens are *Campylobacter*, *Salmonella*, *Shigella*, and *E. coli*; infants under 1 year are at extremely high risk of *Campylobacter*, *Rotavirus*, and *Salmonella* illness (Morbidity and Mortality Weekly Report [MMWR], 2004). A former common cause of food-related illness was hepatitis A. Although still prevalent in some parts of the country, effective management and prevention through immunization has decreased its incidence (see Chapter 24 ∞).

NURSING CARE PLAN   The Child Who Is Overweight

GOAL	INTERVENTION	RATIONALE	EXPECTED OUTCOME
1. Imbalanced Nutrition: More than Body Requirements related to excessive intake in comparison to metabolic needs			
	NIC Priority Intervention: **Weight Reduction Assistance:** *Facilitating loss of weight and body fat.*		*NOC Suggested Outcome:* **Weight Control:** *Personal actions resulting in achievement and maintenance of optimum body weight for health.*
Child will demonstrate adequate intake of all nutrients without excessive energy intake.			Child meets dietary requirements while achieving weight and body mass index goal.
	Perform thorough nutritional assessment of child.	Assessment assists in identification of dietary risks and strengths as well as health conditions related to nutrition.	
	Share results of the assessment with the child and family by showing weight, height, and body mass index grids.	Many families do not consider their child overweight. Concrete information about the child's size in comparison with recommendations assists in establishing the importance of weight management.	
	Identify with the child and family two to three target areas to begin weight management. Examples might include • Having fast food only once a week. • Switching to low-fat dairy products. • Keeping two more fresh fruits and vegetables in the house and two less snack foods.	Changing dietary patterns drastically is difficult and may lead to giving up the attempt at weight management. Partnering with the family to set goals enhances the chance of success.	
	Integrate nutrition information into each visit. Examples of topics include: • Dietary requirements for age group. • Effects of simple sugar and fat intake on weight. • Beneficial effects of fruits, vegetables, whole grains, and nonfat dairy. • Reading food labels. • Health choices in fast-food restaurants. • Calculation of fat content of foods.	Nutrition information is best learned in an ongoing program.	
	Use growth grids to help child and family establish a weight reduction or maintenance goal.	Goals motivate families to achieve desired health behaviors. The goal for a young child may be weight maintenance so that as the child grows in height, the correct proportion is reached, while weight reduction may be needed for older children or youth who are very obese.	

(continued)

NURSING CARE PLAN The Child Who Is Overweight (continued)

GOAL	INTERVENTION	RATIONALE	EXPECTED OUTCOME
2. Readiness for Enhanced Family Coping related to need to foster health of family member			
	NIC Priority Intervention: **Health System Guidance:** *Facilitating child's use of appropriate nutrition and health services to foster weight control.*		*NOC Priority Outcome:* **Health Promoting Behavior:** *Actions to promote, sustain, and increase wellness.*
Family will assist child to manage stressors and to develop new strategies to support weight control goals.			Child expresses satisfaction with family understanding and support of weight management goals.
	Include key family members in some of the counseling sessions with the overweight child.	Key family members are those who purchase food, provide support for the child, and participate in health decisions.	
	Encourage the family to eat together at least once daily if possible or to increase the number of meals eaten together each week.	The family is an important support system in weight loss programs. Eating as a family or in a social situation can provide a chance to promote healthy foods; intake is generally lower fat and calorie than when eating alone.	
	Seek a resource for the child to be monitored about twice monthly; this may be a healthcare provider office, nutritionist, school nurse, or other person.	Provides opportunity to monitor the child's progress and offer support, additional information, and problem-solving techniques.	
3. Activity Intolerance related to sedentary lifestyle			
	NIC Priority Intervention: **Exercise Promotion:** *Facilitating regular exercise to maintain and increase endurance and energy use.*		*NOC Priority Outcome:* **Endurance:** *Extent that energy enables the child to sustain activity.*
Demonstrated activity tolerance by adequate oxygenation, respiratory effort, and ability to speak during brisk walking, biking, or other activity.			Child demonstrates ability to engage in moderate activity for 60 minutes with minimal respiratory discomfort.
	Establish daily exercise routine beginning with 15–30 minutes of daily walking.	Starting with brief amounts of exercise makes the child feel comfortable and enhances the potential for success.	
	Gradually increase activity over 1–2 months until 60 minutes of daily exercise is maintained.	Gradual increase as the cardiovascular and respiratory systems adapt is generally comfortable for children; 60 minutes of moderate activity daily is recommended for children.	
	Use activities enjoyed by the child and suggest options as necessary; refer the family to community resources such as swimming pools, organized sports, and biking groups.	Activities the child enjoys will be more likely to remain in usual activity patterns; exercising with others in groups increases motivation.	

NURSING CARE PLAN   The Child Who Is Overweight (continued)

GOAL	INTERVENTION	RATIONALE	EXPECTED OUTCOME
3. Activity Intolerance related to sedentary lifestyle (continued)			
	Have families plan at least one to two activities they can do together each week.	This fosters family relationships and provides the child with support and motivation.	
	Limit screen activities to a maximum of 2 hours daily. Have child keep a log of hours of television, video games, computer, and other similar activities. Tell child never to snack while doing screen activities.	Increased use of screen activities is related to poor dietary habits and increased sedentary behaviors and excess weight.	
	Ask about use of tobacco in children in fifth grade or higher. Inquire about exposure to environmental tobacco smoke at all ages. Perform teaching to discourage tobacco use or offer cessation programs as needed.	Most adults who smoke began the habit in childhood; middle school years are the most common age for smoking initiation. Smoking by others in the household can be harmful to children. Smoking decreases respiratory reserves and worsens several cardiovascular disease risks.	
4. Chronic Low Self-Esteem related to weight			
	NIC Priority Intervention: **Self-Esteem Enhancement:** *Assisting the child to increase personal judgment of self-worth.*		*NOC Priority Outcome:* **Quality of Life and Self-Esteem:** *Expressed satisfaction with life circumstances and positive judgment of self-worth.*
Child expresses positive perception of self-worth and confidence in ability to deal with issues related to weight.			Child speaks positively about accomplishments in weight control management.
	Facilitate development of a positive outlook by exposing child to others who have been successful with weight loss.	Increases motivation and feelings of self-efficacy.	
	Praise child for weight loss, weight maintenance, increased physical activity, and other achievements. Help the child establish rewards for meeting goals, such as purchase of new clothing.	Enhances judgment of self-worth and pride in accomplishments.	
	Partner with parents so that they understand the value of praise and never label the child by derogatory words such as *fat*.	Family members are usually the most intimate support system for the child.	

Foodborne illness is transmitted by food preparation and storage practices, lack of adequate training of retail employees regarding foods and hygiene, and increasing amounts and types of foods being imported from various geographic areas. Some examples of contaminated foods in the last few years include undercooked hamburger meat and cross-contamination of salad bar items from meats, fish, unpasteurized apple cider, milk, raw or undercooked eggs, green onions, prepackaged salad and delicatessen meat, berries, and sprouts. While most infected persons experience acute gastroenteritis, some can develop complications such as hemolytic uremic syndrome or thrombocytic purpura. A wide array of other symptoms may include neurologic and respiratory problems, fever, jaundice, or arthritis. Health personnel should be alert to symptoms of foodborne illness and integrate teaching regularly so that families can decrease risks. See Families Want to Know: Foodborne Safety Guidelines.

Food may carry products other than microorganisms that can be harmful. An example is mercury, which may be concentrated in certain types of fish. This metal can cause harm to the developing nervous system of fetuses, infants, and young children when consumed regularly. The U.S. Food and Drug Administration (FDA) and Environmental Protection Agency (EPA) note that fish are an important part of a healthy diet, but that certain recommendations should be followed to lower the risk of mercury's detrimental effects. Women who may become pregnant, are pregnant or nursing, and young children should:

- Eliminate shark, swordfish, king mackerel, and tilefish from the diet.
- Eat up to 12 ounces (two average meals) a week of a variety of low-mercury fish and shellfish, such as shrimp, canned light tuna, salmon, pollock, and catfish. Albacore or white tuna has more mercury than light tuna so limit white tuna to one meal per week.
- Check for local advisories about safety of fish caught in local waters in your area. In the absence of advice, up to 6 ounces (one meal) per week may be eaten from local waters. Do not eat other fish during that week (FDA, 2004).

Common Dietary Deficiencies

Although there can be deficits in nearly all nutrients, certain deficiencies are more common in childhood. Either limitations in the food supply or patterns of dietary intake are the cause of most deficiencies, while children with certain disease processes, such as metabolic diseases, may have difficulty absorbing or using nutrients ingested (see Chapter 29 ∞ for a discussion of inborn errors of metabolism). The nutrient deficiencies present in a population are a result of genetic factors and characteristics of the food supply and intake patterns of particular groups.

Iron

Newborns have a store of iron obtained from their mothers in the uterus, if the maternal nutritional state was satisfactory and the baby is normal gestational age. Breast milk contains little iron, but the iron it does contain has high bioavailability. By 4 to 6 months of age, however, the baby's iron stores begin to decrease and a dietary source of iron must be added by about 6 months of age. Enriched rice cereal is commonly used to meet these initial iron needs. In babies who do not have adequate stores or do not take in enough iron, **anemia** (a reduction in the number of red blood cells) can result (Figure 4–9 ▶). Feeding cow milk during infancy can also cause anemia by irritating the gut and leading to small but consistent loss of blood from the gastrointestinal tract; cow milk should not be fed during the first year of life. When formulas are used, they should be iron fortified to help avoid iron deficiency anemia.

The other group most commonly deficient in iron is adolescent females, related to loss of blood in menses, metabolic need of the growth spurt, and poor dietary bal-

FAMILIES WANT TO KNOW

Foodborne Safety Guidelines

Four Key Food Safety Practices:
1. Clean: Wash hands and surfaces often.
2. Separate: Avoid cross-contamination.
3. Cook: Cook to proper temperatures.
4. Chill: Refrigerate promptly.

Source: U.S. Department of Health and Human Services. (2000). *Healthy People 2010*. Washington DC: U.S. Department of Health and Human Services. Retrieved April 13, 2001, from http://www.health.gov/healthypeople/document.html.

ance due to sporadic dieting. Further discussion of the symptoms and treatment of iron deficiency anemia can be found in Chapter 22 ∞. See Table 4–7 for food sources of iron.

Calcium

Calcium is an essential nutrient for bone development during childhood and adolescence. An increased intake of soda pop and fruit juices is related to a decrease in calcium intake, especially among adolescents. During the adolescent growth spurt, almost 40% of the adult bone mass is accumulated (AAP, Committee on Nutrition, 2004). Inadequate intake puts the person at risk for osteoporosis later in life, as there is minimal or no ability to make up for earlier deficits. Although genetic variables account for some of the influence on adult bone mass, increasing calcium intake has been shown to promote bone formation. While the recommended daily intake for adolescents is 1300 mg, the average intake for adolescent males is 1145 mg and for females is only 700 to 850 mg—only about half of the recommended level (Storey, Forshee, & Anderson, 2004). See Table 4–7 for common food sources of calcium.

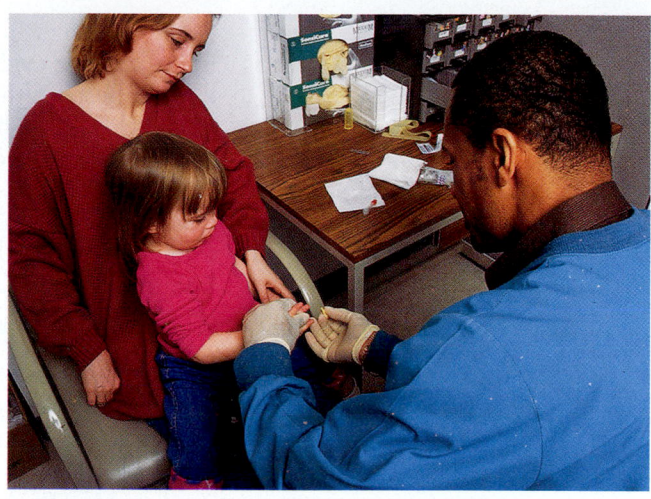

Figure 4–9 ► Head Start centers participate in screening programs to identify children at risk for anemia. This child sits on the mother's lap while the nurse performs a fingerstick to measure hematocrit. What is the expected hematocrit level in a young child?

Adolescents at highest risk for impaired bone development include female athletes and others who diet to a magnified degree to maintain slimness. These teens manifest the "female athlete triad" of disorder eating and excessive exercise leading to excessive thinness, amenorrhea, and osteopenia (Waldrop, 2005). A high rate of fractures and osteomalacia can result, in addition to an extreme risk of osteoporosis in adulthood. Asking about menstrual patterns, as well as exercise and diet, can be combined with physical measurements of height and weight to obtain pertinent information about the teen athlete. See the discussion of the other disordered eating patterns such as anorexia nervosa and bulimia nervosa later in this chapter.

Vitamin D

Vitamin D deficiencies are rare because the vitamin can be synthesized in the skin upon exposure to sunlight. However, an increased incidence in cases of vitamin D–deficient rickets has been observed in recent years. This vitamin is needed to enhance absorption of calcium so a lack of vitamin D can contribute to calcium deficiency as well. Human milk contains little vitamin D, and if infants are kept wrapped when outside, live in northern climates and rarely get outside in winter months, live in areas with high air pollution, have extensive sunscreens applied, or are dark in skin color, vitamin D deficiency can result. This has led to a recommendation by the American Academy of Pediatrics that all breast-fed infants receive a daily supplement of 200 international units of vitamin D (Gartner & Greer, 2003). Infant multivitamin preparations contain 400 international units and are recommended for breast-fed infants. Formula-fed infants and children ingesting regular milk receive adequate amounts as long as they drink 500 mL of fortified formula or milk daily. See Table 4–7 for common food sources of vitamin D.

GROWTH & DEVELOPMENT

Vitamin D Rickets

Vitamin D rickets virtually disappeared from the United States, but several cases have been identified in recent years. Suggested reasons for the resurgence include failure to provide vitamin D supplementation when breast-feeding is the sole source of intake for over 6 months, use of nonfortified products such as soy milk, and use of sunscreens or covers when infants are outside. Be alert for infants and toddlers with neurological conditions such as seizures, low height for age, slowness in learning to walk, and malformations (bowing) of spine, legs, and arms. Encourage sunscreen use, but be aware that children who are dark skinned or are kept covered due to religious beliefs may be at higher risk. Be certain that breast-fed babies receive vitamin D supplements until other vitamin D sources are added to the diet (Gartner & Greer, 2003).

Table 4–7	FOOD SOURCES OF CERTAIN NUTRIENTS		
Iron	**Calcium**	**Vitamin D**	**Folate**
• Meats	• Milk and milk products	• Milk and formulas fortified with the vitamin	• Bread and other products with flour
• Iron-fortified formula	• Egg yolks	• Eggs	• Yeast
• Iron-fortified baby cereal	• Grains	• Butter	• Spinach, avocado, green leafy vegetables
• Iron absorption is enhanced by vitamin C intake if taken together	• Legumes	• Margarine	• Beans and peas
• Iron is present in breast milk in a small amount, but is very well absorbed	• Nuts		• Liver
	• Soybeans		• Fruits

Folic Acid

Epidemiologic evidence has linked increasing maternal folic acid (the most common form of folate in the human body) intake with decreased incidence of neural tube defects such as spina bifida in offspring of mothers. More recently, cleft lip and palate incidence has also been found to decrease when folate intake increases. Folate levels are low among adolescents, putting them at particular risk of birth defects when they have infants. The Food and Drug Administration approved fortification of cereals and breads with folate to decrease the population risk of related congenital anomalies. All women from 15–45 years should consume 0.4 mg of folic acid daily and pregnant women should consume 0.6 mg daily. See Table 4–7 for common food sources of folate.

Protein-Energy Malnutrition

While the micronutrient deficiencies previously described are the most common problems in developed countries, macronutrient deficiencies are the most common nutritional problems worldwide. While kwashiorkor indicates protein deficiency, and marasmus is a lack of energy-producing calories, both deficiencies often occur together and are referred to as protein-energy malnutrition (PEM). Protein deficiency manifests with edema, leading to the large abdomens and rounded faces seen in severely malnourished children. Other symptoms include scant, depigmented hair; skin changes; and decreased serum proteins. It can occur following severe diarrhea or other infection in susceptible children. Caloric deficiency results in emaciation, decreased energy levels, and retarded development (see the Clinical Manifestations table on page 118). PEM may occur when a child is weaned in order for the mother to provide breast milk to a new baby. Adoptees and immigrants to developed countries sometimes manifest with at least mild PEM, so careful nutritional assessment is needed in order to provide adequate nutrition.

Disorders of Feeding and Eating

Deficiencies in food intake related to available nutrients and safety of the food supply were discussed in the previous section. In addition to these issues of availability, nutrient intake is affected by psychological issues of individuals as well. Disorders of food intake span the entire developmental spectrum, and can affect pregnant women, young children, and adolescents. They may be mild and occasional or severe among individuals (Kazis & Iglesias, 2003). Some of the most common disorders of feeding and eating are discussed in the following text.

Pica

Pica is an eating disorder characterized by ingestion of nonfood items or food items consumed in abnormal quantities or forms. Examples of ingested items include starch, peeling paint, paper, soil components, flour, and coffee grounds. Clinical manifestations include zinc and iron deficiencies as well as symptoms of lead or other poisoning (see Chapter 6 ∞) if these substances are contained in peeling paint or other ingested material. The disorder most commonly manifests in pregnancy when women have abnormal cravings for nonfood products and can seriously impair the developing fetus. Some children also manifest ingestion of abnormal amounts of nonfood items and fail to take in adequate nutrients from food. Treatment for children involves removing them from the substances, ensuring an adequate and nutritious diet, and treating any dietary deficiencies noted.

Feeding Disorder of Infancy and Early Childhood (Failure to Thrive)

Feeding disorder of infancy and early childhood, or failure to thrive (FTT), describes a syndrome in which infants or young children fail to eat enough food to be adequately nourished. This disorder accounts for 1–5% of pediatric hospitalizations in children under 1 year of age, and many more children are managed in community settings. From 5–10% of low-birth-weight infants are affected (Behrman, Kliegman, & Jenson, 2004).

ETIOLOGY AND PATHOPHYSIOLOGY The cause of FTT can be organic, as in congenital acquired immunodeficiency syndrome (AIDS) (see Chapter 17 ∞), inborn errors of metabolism (see Chapter 29 ∞), neurologic disease, and esophageal reflux (see Chapter 24 ∞). However, most cases of FTT are nonorganic in origin. FTT resulting from nonorganic causes is called feeding disorder of infancy or early childhood.

Infants and children whose parents or caretakers have depression, substance abuse, mental retardation, psychosis, or a history of abuse are at risk for this disorder. Parents may be socially and emotionally isolated, or may lack knowledge of infant nutritional and nurturing needs. A multifactorial and reciprocal interaction pattern may exist whereby the parent does not offer enough food or is not responsive to the infant's hunger cues, and the infant is irritable, not soothed, and does not give clear cues about hunger. Preterm and small-for-gestational-age babies more commonly have eating disorders (Block & Krebs, 2005).

CLINICAL MANIFESTATIONS   The characteristics of this feeding disorder are persistent failure to eat adequately with no weight gain or with weight loss in a child under 6 years of age, which is not associated with other medical conditions or mental disorders, and is not caused by lack of or unavailability of food (American Psychiatric Association Working Group on Eating Disorders, 2000). Infants with feeding disorders refuse food, may have erratic sleep patterns, are irritable and difficult to soothe, fall well under expected growth patterns, and are often developmentally delayed (Figure 4–10 ➤).

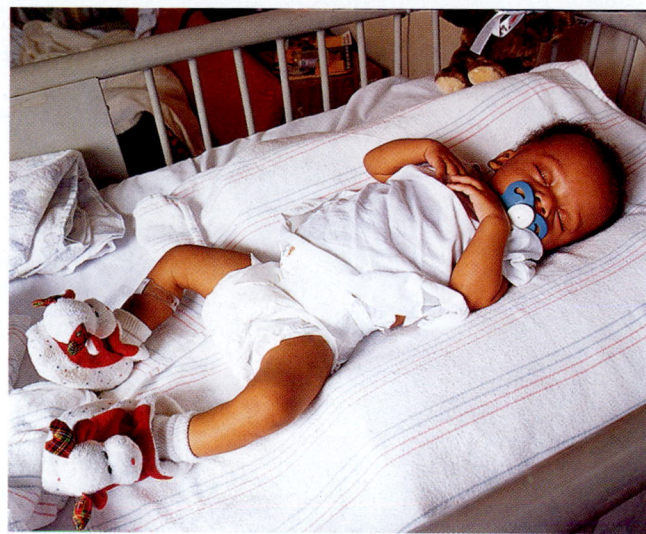

Figure 4–10 ➤ Infants with failure to thrive may not look severely malnourished, but they fall well below the expected weight and height norms for their age. This infant, who appears to be about 4 months old, is actually 8 months old. He has been hospitalized for examination of his failure to thrive and treatment of the eating disorder.

COLLABORATIVE CARE

A thorough history and physical examination are needed to rule out any chronic physical illness. The infant or child may be hospitalized so that healthcare providers can establish a routine for feeding and sleeping. The goals of treatment are to provide adequate caloric and nutritional intake, promote normal growth and development, and assist parents in developing feeding routines and responding to the infant's cues of physical and psychological hunger.

NURSING MANAGEMENT
Nursing Assessment and Diagnosis

Assessment of the child by the nurse is essential for establishing the best intervention plan. Accurate measurement of weight, height, BMI, and percentiles each time any child is seen for health care provides an important record of growth patterns over time. This helps in identification of the child with an eating disorder. The child's activity level, developmental milestones, and interaction patterns provide important information. When feeding the child, the nurse observes how the child indicates hunger or satiety, the ability of the child to be soothed, and general interaction patterns such as eye contact, touch, and cuddliness.

Parents are questioned about stresses in their lives; these may prevent appropriate interaction with the child. Asking about the pregnancy and delivery can elicit information about early disturbances in the child–parent relationship. Are there other children in the family and have eating problems occurred with them? Observe the child and parent behaviors while they feed the child; cues given by each person and interactional modes such as rocking, singing, talking, and body postures are important.

Following are nursing diagnoses pertinent for the young child with an eating disorder:

- Imbalanced Nutrition: Less than Body Requirements related to inability to ingest proper amounts of food

CULTURE

Growth Measurement

Each child should maintain a height and weight growth pattern similar to the population standard. Asian American children may normally be below the 5th percentile on growth charts and not have an eating disorder. Suspect an eating disorder when the infant or child falls one standard deviation below his or her own curve and either fails to gain weight or loses weight over several months.

- Delayed Growth and Development related to inadequate intake
- Risk for Impaired Parenting related to lack of knowledge about nutritional needs
- Fatigue related to malnutrition

Planning and Implementation

Nursing care centers on performing a thorough history and physical assessment, observing parent–child interactions during feeding times, and providing necessary teaching to enable parents to respond appropriately to their child's needs. The child is often hospitalized initially and evaluated for physical growth while staff members feed the child. Accurate weights, nutritional assessments, and developmental evaluation should be done to see if the child grows more normally. Additional diagnostic tests may be carried out at this time to rule out organic causes of the poor growth.

Once a diagnosis of nonorganic failure to thrive is confirmed, parents become involved in feeding the child. Observations of feeding and continued careful physical assessments are needed. The child's intake is carefully recorded at each meal or feeding. Parents are taught how to understand and respond to the child's cues of hunger and satiety. They are taught to hold, rock, and touch the infant during feedings, and to establish eye contact with infants and older children.

Upon discharge, referral to an agency that can continue monitoring the home situation is needed. This provides an opportunity to observe feeding during a home visit and evaluate stresses and behavior patterns among family members. Frequent growth measurement and development must be ensured so the child is adequately nourished. Parents may need referral to community resources to help them manage stressful situations in their lives and to enhance their parenting skills.

Evaluation

Expected outcomes of nursing care include the following:

- Adequate growth and normal development of the infant is achieved.
- An improved parent–child relationship is established.

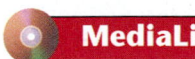

MediaLink

Anorexia Nervosa Video

Anorexia Nervosa

Anorexia nervosa is a potentially life-threatening type of disordered eating that occurs primarily in teenage girls and young women. An estimated 5% of young women and 1% of young men in the United States are affected by anorexia nervosa or a related eating disorder (American Dietetic Association, 2006). Incidence may be as high as 10% among college women, and 15–62% in female athletes (Kazis & Iglesias, 2003). Mortality rates are from 5–13% (Krassas, 2003). The typical patient is White and from a middle- to upper middle-class family. Age at onset varies, and incidence peaks at 12 to 13 years and again at 17 to 18 years.

ETIOLOGY AND PATHOPHYSIOLOGY Many causes are now thought to contribute to the onset of anorexia. Cultural overemphasis on thinness may contribute to the overconcern with dieting, body image, and fear of becoming fat experienced by many adolescents. Chemical changes have been found in the brain and blood of anorectic patients, leading to theories about a biological cause. Often a significant life stress, loss, or change precedes the onset of anorexia. Stress hormones are commonly elevated in anorectics and immune system function may be disturbed (Gluck, 2006).

Many authorities view family issues as contributory to anorexia. Intrafamilial conflicts and dysfunctional family patterns may occur when parents are overcontrolling and perfectionistic. The adolescent's eating behaviors may be an attempt to exercise independence and resolve internal psychologic conflicts.

The adolescent often engages in lengthy and vigorous exercise (up to 4 hours daily) to prevent weight gain. Laxatives or diuretics may be used to induce weight loss. As the disorder progresses, the adolescent perceives the ever-thinner body as becoming more beautiful. Youth may share weight loss techniques with anorectic friends and search out Internet sites that are positive about anorexia. The body responds to the abnormal eating behaviors as if starvation were occurring. Leukopenia, electrolyte imbalance, and hypoglycemia develop as a result of protein–energy malnutrition. Once the body mass decreases below a critical level, menstruation ceases.

CLINICAL MANIFESTATIONS Adolescents with anorexia are characterized by extreme weight loss accompanied by a preoccupation with weight and food, excessive compulsive exercising, peculiar patterns of eating and handling food, and distorted body image. They may prepare elaborate meals for others but eat only low-calorie foods. Characteristically, the fear of becoming fat does not decrease with continued weight loss. Accompanying signs and symptoms of depression, crying spells, feelings of isolation and loneliness, and suicidal thoughts and feelings are common. The disorder is often associated with mental illness such as obsessive-compulsive disorder, anxiety disorders (see Chapter 27 ∞), and history of abuse (American Dietetic Association, 2006).

Physical findings include cold intolerance, dizziness, constipation, abdominal discomfort, bloating, irregular menses, and malnutrition (Figure 4–11 ➤). Hypothalamic suppression can lead to disturbances of gynecologic function, osteoporosis, decreased bone density, and fractures (Krassas, 2003). Lanugo (fine, downy body hair) may be present. Fluid and electrolyte imbalances, especially potassium imbalances, are common. The child or adolescent is usually energetic despite significant weight loss. Extreme weight loss often leads to cardiac arrhythmias (bradycardia).

■ COLLABORATIVE CARE

Collaborative care focuses on early diagnosis of the disorder and referral for treatment, with follow-up to ensure continued interventions when needed.

Diagnostic Tests

Diagnosis is based on a comprehensive history, physical examination revealing characteristic clinical manifestations, and the *DSM-IV* criteria included in Box 4–8. Diagnostic tests commonly include hematocrit and hemoglobin, serum electrolytes, and serum vitamins and vitamin-precursors.

Clinical Therapy

The goal of treatment is to address the physiologic problems associated with malnutrition, as well as the behavioral and cognitive components of the disorder. The first phase of therapy involves management and stabilization of the abnormal serum electrolytes. Once that is accomplished, weight management is the major concern. A firm focus is placed on reaching a targeted weight with a gradual weight gain of 0.1 to 0.2 kg/day (0.25 to 0.5 lb/day). Enteral feedings or total parenteral nutrition (TPN) may be necessary to replace lost fluid, protein, and nutrients, although the adolescent often perceives these feedings as a punitive measure.

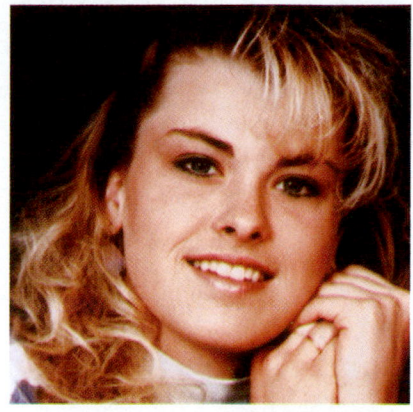

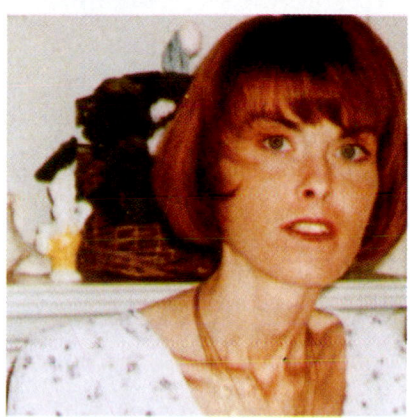

Figure 4–11 ➤ This young woman struggled with anorexia and bulimia from the age of 12 years. Her parents were not aware that she had the disorder until she was 15 years of age. In spite of treatment, her condition worsened and she died in her twenties. These photos show her during her teenage years and then shortly before she died.

BOX 4–8
DSM-IV CRITERIA FOR ANOREXIA NERVOSA

A. Refusal to maintain body weight at or above a minimally normal weight for age and height (e.g., weight loss leading to maintenance of body weight less than 85% of that expected; or failure to make expected weight gain during period of growth, leading to body weight less than 85% of that expected).

B. Intense fear of gaining weight or becoming fat, even though underweight.

C. Disturbance in the way in which one's weight or shape is experienced, undue influence of body weight or shape on self-evaluation, or denial of the seriousness of the current body weight.

D. In postmenarcheal females, amenorrhea, i.e., the absence of at least three consecutive menstrual cycles. (A woman is considered to have amenorrhea if her periods occur only following hormone, e.g., estrogen, administration.)

Note: Reprinted with permission from the *Diagnostic and Statistical Manual of Mental Disorders,* Fourth Edition, Text Revision. Copyright 2000. American Psychiatric Association.

Individual treatment and family therapy are used to address dysfunctional family patterns and assist the family to accept and deal with the adolescent as an independent and less than perfect individual. Family involvement is crucial to effect a lasting change in the adolescent and is most successful with young teens. Nurses, psychologists, family therapists, and dietitians commonly partner to plan and implement therapy.

Long-term outpatient treatment, in either an individual or a group setting, is frequently necessary. Counseling that applies cognitive behavioral therapy may be continued for 2 to 3 years to ensure that weight gain and self-image are maintained. Antidepressant drugs such as imipramine (Tofranil) or desipramine (Norpramin) may be prescribed for coexisting conditions such as depression, anxiety, or obsessive-compulsive disorders. However, they are not generally useful in primary treatment of the disorder (Berkman, Bulik, Brownley et al., 2006).

Indications for hospitalization include loss of 25–30% of body weight, fluid and electrolyte imbalances or arrhythmias, or the need to provide a more intense period of therapy if outpatient treatment fails to produce improvement. Behavior modification techniques are used extensively in combination with counseling and other methods in care of the hospitalized anorectic adolescent.

■ NURSING MANAGEMENT

Nursing Assessment and Diagnosis

Obtain a thorough individual and family history. Ask about usual eating patterns, daily caloric intake, exercise patterns, and menstrual history. Ask about medication use; include prescription, nonprescription, and herbal products. Is there a family history of eating disorders? Assess for signs of malnutrition. Obtain height and weight measurements and compare with norms for the general population. Because the anorectic patient often wears layers of clothes when being weighed, strive to obtain an accurate measurement.

Nursing diagnoses for the adolescent with anorexia nervosa include the following:

- Imbalanced Nutrition: Less than Body Requirements related to inadequate intake
- Risk for Deficient Fluid Volume related to inadequate fluid intake or fluid volume loss from overuse of laxatives and diuretics
- Risk for Imbalanced Body Temperature related to excessive weight loss and absence of subcutaneous fat
- Constipation related to inadequate food intake and overuse of laxatives
- Disturbed Body Image related to distorted perception of body size and shape
- Chronic Low Self-Esteem related to dysfunctional family dynamics
- Compromised Family Coping related to parental tendency to be overcontrolling and perfectionistic

Planning and Implementation

Nursing care centers on meeting nutritional and fluid needs, preventing complications, administering medications, and providing referral to appropriate resources. Specific treatment measures vary depending on physical complications, length and degree of illness, emotional symptoms accompanying the disorder, and family dynamics. Resistance to treatment is common, and nurses who care for anorectic adolescents must deal with their own feelings of frustration and anger.

Meet Nutritional and Fluid Needs

Monitor nutritional and fluid intake, encourage consumption of food, and observe eating behaviors at mealtime. Elimination patterns may be altered as a result of increased intake during hospitalization. Monitor for possible problems, including abdominal distention, constipation, or diarrhea. Daily monitoring of serum electrolytes is necessary.

If TPN is administered, watch for complications such as circulatory overload, hyperglycemia, or hypoglycemia. Use strict aseptic technique when changing tubing or dressings.

SKILL 9–7:
Administering Total Parenteral Nutrition

Administer Medications

Monitor vital signs if the adolescent is receiving antidepressants. Watch for signs of hypertension and tachycardia. Administering medications after meals helps to prevent gastric irritation. Be alert for substance abuse. Anorectics often use products such as excess laxatives or ephedra (also known as ma huang) to induce weight loss. Changes in the central nervous system, vital signs, and other findings may indicate over-the-counter or herbal drug use.

Provide Referral to Appropriate Resources

Refer parents and other family members to the American Anorexia and Bulimia Association, National Anorectic Aid Society, and National Association of Anorexia Nervosa & Associated Disorders for further information about the disorder and a list of support groups in their area.

MediaLink

Eating Disorder Resources/ Support

Evaluation

Expected outcomes for nursing care include weight gain, maintenance of adequate fluid volume, beginning of positive sense of self-esteem, intake of nutritionally balanced diet, and use of psychologic counseling to understand the disorder.

Bulimia Nervosa

Bulimia nervosa is a disorder characterized by binge eating (a compulsion to consume large quantities of food in a short period of time). Usually the episodes of bingeing are followed by various methods of weight control (purging), such as self-induced vomiting, large doses of laxatives or diuretics, or a combination of methods. Bulimia affects 1% of the general population, but 5% or more of young women (Hoek, 2006). Like anorexia, it affects mainly adolescent girls and young women who are White and in the higher socioeconomic classes (Hoek, 2006). The disorder usually begins in middle to late adolescence, frequently emerging during college.

ETIOLOGY AND PATHOPHYSIOLOGY   Causes of bulimia nervosa are similar to those of anorexia nervosa: sensitivity to social pressure for thinness, body image difficulties, and longstanding dysfunctional family patterns. Families may be chaotic and distant from the girl, rather than overinvolved as with the anorectic. Many bulimic individuals experience depression. It is not clear whether the depression is a cause or a result of the bulimic individual's inability to control the bingeing and purging cycles. A bulimic adolescent often binges after any stressful event.

Bingeing usually occurs in secret for several hours until the individual is stopped by abdominal discomfort, by another person, or by vomiting. At first the episodes of binge eating are pleasurable. Immediately following the binge episode, however, feelings of guilt, shame, anger, depression, and fear of loss of control and weight gain arise. As these feelings intensify, the bulimic adolescent becomes increasingly anxious. This usually initiates the purge behaviors.

Purging eliminates the discomfort from bloating and also prevents weight gain. This relieves the feelings of depression and guilt, but only temporarily. Adolescents with bulimia commonly practice the binge–purge cycle many times a day, losing their ability to respond to normal cues of hunger and satiety.

CLINICAL MANIFESTATIONS   Bulimia is often a "silent" disorder since it is easily concealed from healthcare providers. Only about 6% of those with bulimia are believed to receive treatment (Hoek, 2006). Bulimic adolescents, like anorectics, are preoccupied with body shape, size, and weight. They may appear overweight or thin and usually report a wide range of average body weight over the years. Physical findings depend on the degree of purging, starvation, dehydration, and electrolyte disturbance. Erosion of tooth enamel, increased dental caries, and gum recession, which result from vomiting of gastric acids, are common findings. The back of a hand can have calluses from inducing vomiting. Abdominal distention is often seen. Esophageal tears and esophagitis may also occur.

■ COLLABORATIVE CARE

Collaborative care focuses on early diagnosis of the disorder and referral for treatment, with follow-up to ensure continued interventions when needed.

Diagnostic Tests

A comprehensive history is necessary because most bulimic adolescents appear normal in weight or only slightly underweight. Diagnostic tests include hematocrit, hemoglobin, and serum electrolytes; they may identify signs of altered electrolyte and hematologic status. The diagnosis is confirmed by the presence of specific *DSM-IV* criteria (Box 4–9).

Clinical Therapy

Treatment includes management of physiologic problems, and cognitive-behavior therapy. Medications, such as fluoxetine 60 mg/day for adolescents, may be used (Berkman et al., 2006). Management involves a variety of healthcare providers such as physicians, nurses, and therapists. Behavior modification focuses on modifying the dysfunctional eating patterns and restoring a normal pattern. Until the episodes of bingeing and purging are under control, feelings of discouragement and hopelessness prevail. Thus, the focus early in treatment is on initiating an immediate behavioral change. Once initial interventions have been successful, group therapy sessions work well for persons with anorexia or bulimia. Specific treatment measures may include the following:

- Educating the adolescent about good nutrition (including food choice and caloric content)
- Encouraging the adolescent to keep a log or food journal and assisting the adolescent to make connections between emotional states and stress and the impulse to binge or purge
- Setting up a daily dietary routine of three meals and three snacks a day (using the same foods for each meal and snack every day to change misconceptions about the weight-gaining potential of certain foods and to decrease anxiety about what food must be eaten at the next meal)

Once these initial measures have been taken, the underlying psychosocial issues are explored. The goals of therapy are to provide the bulimic adolescent with adaptive coping skills and to improve self-esteem.

Most bulimic adolescents do not require hospitalization. Serious abnormalities in fluid and electrolyte levels caused by uncontrollable cycles of bingeing and vomiting, accompanied by depression or suicidal activity, indicate the need for hospitalization. The prognosis is good with long-term therapy.

BOX 4–9
DSM-IV CRITERIA FOR BULIMIA NERVOSA

A. Recurrent episodes of binge eating. An episode of binge eating is characterized by both of the following:
  1. Eating, in a discrete period of time (e.g., within any 2-hour period), an amount of food that is definitely larger than most people would eat during a similar period of time and under similar circumstances
  2. A sense of lack of control over eating during the episode (e.g., a feeling that one cannot stop eating or control what or how much one is eating)

B. Recurrent inappropriate compensatory behavior in order to prevent weight gain, such as self-induced vomiting; misuse of laxatives, diuretics, enemas, or other medications; fasting; or excessive exercise.

C. The binge eating and inappropriate compensatory behaviors both occur, on average, at least twice a week for 3 months.

D. Self-evaluation is unduly influenced by body weight and shape.

E. The disturbance does not occur exclusively during episodes of anorexia nervosa.

Note: Reprinted with permission from the *Diagnostic and Statistical Manual of Mental Disorders,* Fourth Edition, Text Revision, Copyright 2000. American Psychiatric Association.

■ NURSING MANAGEMENT

Nursing Assessment and Diagnosis

Obtain a thorough individual and family history, including daily dietary intake and weight fluctuations. Inquire about problems such as abdominal pain or distention, which may indicate an abnormal eating or elimination pattern. Assess the oral mucosa for signs of damage to tooth enamel caused by purging; examine hands for evidence of vomiting-induced calluses.

Following are nursing diagnoses that may be appropriate for the adolescent with bulimia nervosa:

- Imbalanced Nutrition: Less than or More than Body Requirements related to disordered eating patterns
- Risk for Deficient Fluid Volume related to fluid volume loss
- Impaired Oral Mucous Membrane related to chemical effects of vomited gastric acids
- Deficient Knowledge (Child) related to health risks of excessive use of laxatives and diuretics
- Anxiety related to discomfort with weight and eating patterns
- Chronic Low Self-Esteem related to dysfunctional family dynamics
- Ineffective Individual Coping related to life stressors

Planning and Implementation

Nursing care includes monitoring nutritional intake and elimination patterns, preventing complications, and providing appropriate referrals.

During hospitalization, the patient should keep a food diary. Be alert to the adolescent who hides, gives away, or discards food from the tray or who exits to use the bathroom after meals. The adolescent should be monitored for at least 30 minutes after meals by remaining in a central area in the company of the nurse or other responsible individuals. Withdrawal from laxatives and diuretics is managed with careful observation for alterations in fluid and electrolyte status. Cardiac monitoring may be necessary if potassium levels are seriously altered. Esophageal tearing or esophagitis is treated to promote mucosal healing. Medications such as antidepressants may be administered. Encourage continuation of group and other therapy sessions.

Bulimic adolescents and their families can be referred to organizations such as those previously listed in the section on anorexia for assistance and information about the disorder.

Evaluation

Expected outcomes for nursing care for the adolescent with bulimia include healthy mucous membranes and skin, adequate intake of fluids and food, balanced food intake, maintenance of normal weight, and absence of bingeing and purging.

Food Reactions

Food reaction encompasses any adverse reaction to foods or substances ingested in foods. The most common food reaction is **food intolerance**, or an abnormal physiologic response to a food that is not IgE mediated. Examples include indigestion or flatulence upon eating certain foods, a sweating reaction to some spices, rhinitis, and hives with urticaria (Burks & Ballmer-Weber, 2006). Milk and grain products are common causes of food intolerance. Chemical additives, antibiotics, preservatives, contaminants in the food, and food colorings also can cause food sensitivity reactions.

The most serious type of food reaction is **food allergy**, an IgE-mediated reaction that is potentially systemic, characteristically rapid in onset, and may be manifested as swelling of the lips, mouth, uvula, or glottis; generalized urticaria; and, in

CULTURE

Lactose Intolerance
Some ethnic groups have a high incidence of lactose intolerance due to low amounts of the enzyme lactase in the gut. Although most members of the group have adequate amounts of lactase in childhood to drink milk products, by adulthood 70–100% of some groups are lactose intolerant. African Americans, Native Americans, and Asians often have lactase deficiency that may begin to emerge during childhood. When intolerance to milk products develops, suggest alternative sources of calcium and other nutrients found in milk. Some people who have mild indigestion are able to eat yogurt with no problem.

COMMUNITY CARE

Food Allergy

Children with food allergies should wear an alert tag and carry an emergency medication such as EpiPen®. Nurses in schools and offices must instruct families, school teachers, and others about the child's allergy and what to do in case of accidental ingestion of the food product.

CLINICAL MANIFESTATIONS OF FOOD ALLERGY

System	Manifestations
Skin and mucous membranes	Urticaria of lips, mouth, throat Hives Reddened cheeks
Circulatory	Hypotension Irregular heartbeat
Respiratory	Sneezing Coughing Congestion Laryngeal edema Recurrent ear infections
Gastrointestinal	Nausea, vomiting, flatulence, diarrhea, bloating
Neurologic	Fatigue Depression, headache Hyperactivity Sleep disturbance Seizures Coma, death

MediaLink

Case Study: Single Parenting and Nutrition Issues

severe reaction, anaphylaxis. Food allergies are the most common cause of anaphylaxis and are most prevalent in children with a family history of allergic reactions to various substances and foods (**atopy**). The foods that most commonly cause a reaction are fish, shellfish, peanuts, tree nuts, eggs, soy, wheat, corn, strawberries, and cow's milk products. About 1% of children have an allergy to peanuts and the incidence is increasing. A majority of the 150 deaths from food allergies that occur annually in the United States are due to peanut allergy (Palmer & Burks, 2006). Children who have both food allergy and asthma are most at risk of death from anaphylaxis due to a food allergy. See the Clinical Manifestations table on page 118 for the child's possible manifestations of allergy. Allergic individuals need to be aware of "hidden" substances in prepared foods. For example, the child who is allergic to nuts will experience a reaction to a food if nut extracts are used in its preparation.

Delayed hypersensitivity reactions are attributed to digestive products of food and require a thorough diet history over several days to identify the offending food. These reactions are more difficult to diagnose, because the reaction can occur up to 24 hours after ingestion of the food. There may also be biphasic reactions that occur 1 to 30 hours after an initial anaphylaxis. Such reactions can be severe and life threatening.

Note that certain foods can cause either allergy or intolerance so accurate diagnosis is needed. An example is cow milk that can cause an allergy with IgE-mediated systemic reactions, or an intolerance from a gastrointestinal response to milk proteins (diarrhea, vomiting, abdominal pain) as a result of lack of the enzyme lactase in the gastrointestinal tract.

Diagnostic tests to identify suspected food allergies include measurement of serum IgE levels, scratch tests, and the **radioallergosorbent test (RAST)**, in which radioimmunoassay is used to measure IgE antibodies to specific allergens (see Chapter 17 ∞). A diet diary helps to track the date, types of foods eaten, and reaction(s), if any. Foods should be eaten singly for several days to determine whether they cause a reaction.

Treatment consists of eliminating the offending foods from the child's diet. Collaborative care involving the child, parents, school, and healthcare providers is needed to ensure that the allergic child does not get exposed to the offending allergen, and that all children with food reactions can avoid contact with foods to which they are allergic or intolerant.

NURSING MANAGEMENT

Prevention is the first step. Instruct parents of infants to introduce new foods at a rate of not more than one new food every 3 to 5 days. If a sensitivity is noted, the causative food can be easily identified. Discuss any changes in diet or preparation of formula. Reassure parents that the child's symptoms will disappear when the offending foods are removed from the diet.

Be alert for skin, respiratory, and other characteristic manifestations of sensitivity or allergy. Refer such cases to an allergist for diagnosis and assist in skin testing and instruction about results. Nursing care of a child with food allergy recognizes that the responsibility for preventing ingestion of an allergenic food for a particular child is shared by the child (when old enough to participate), the family, and the school or other setting (Table 4–8). Recognize that food allergies can be life threatening and plan carefully with the family, childcare facilities, schools, and other community contacts to ensure avoidance of food and emergency treatment, if needed. Help the family identify and eliminate the offending foods. Explain to parents all tests, use of a food diary, and care of the child should a reaction occur. The child and school will need an emergency plan for the child in case of accidental ingestion. Emphasize the importance of reading food labels for hidden foods that can trigger an allergic reaction (Simons, Weiss, Furlong, & Sicherer, 2005). Be sure that the food allergy plan is in place in each setting where the child spends time. Refer the family to the Food Allergy Network.

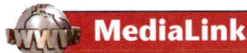

MediaLink

Food Allergy Resources

NUTRITIONAL SUPPORT

Providing adequate nutrition for all children can be a challenge for families. Nutritional needs change as children grow and develop, family patterns must be integrated into the child's intake, and many social influences intervene to influence dietary patterns. Some children require even more careful management to ensure that they receive necessary

Table 4–8	**FOOD ALLERGIES—SHARED RESPONSIBILITY**	
Family Responsibility	**Child Responsibility**	**School Responsibility**
• Notify and work with school to develop an allergy plan for the child • Provide written documentation, instructions, and medications; update and replace as needed (e.g., EpiPen) • Provide a current photo of child for the allergy plan • Educate the child to the level possible depending on age and cognition • Institute review of plan after any reaction	• Do not trade food with other children • Do not eat anything known to contain the allergen or when ingredients are unknown • Notify an adult immediately if an allergen may have been ingested • Know location of emergency medication (e.g., EpiPen)	• Inform all personnel and follow federal, state, and district laws relevant to allergies and sharing medical information • Review health records of all students • Identify core team to work with parents and child to establish prevention plan • Implement treatment upon possible ingestion of allergen; do not wait for a reaction • Teach all staff interacting with child the recognition of food allergy, actions to take in emergency, and elimination measures of allergen from meals, educational tools, arts and craft, incentives, etc. • Allow for safe and accessible storage of emergency medicines; arrange instruction for personnel in administration of medication • Include field trips, transportation on school bus, sports outings in action plan • Ensure emergency communication from all buses, school events, field trips • Be alert for and manage threats or harassment against an allergic child • Institute review of plan after any reaction

Adapted from Food Allergy Network. School guidelines for managing students with food allergies. www.foodallergy.org/school/guidelines.html

nutrients, either due to increased needs or the difficulty in ingesting adequate foods. Several of the particular challenges are discussed in the following text.

Sports Nutrition and Ergogenic Agents

Regular physical activity should be encouraged for all children, with at least 30 to 60 minutes of activity recommended daily. However, during vigorous or prolonged exercise, or during hot weather, there may be special nutritional needs of child and adolescent athletes. A well-balanced diet, reflective of the Food Pyramid, is needed. A wide variety of fresh fruits and vegetables, grains, and complex carbohydrates usually provides for adequate caloric intake. When the child is hungry, extra calories should come from the food groups listed here, rather than from increased intake of fat. When the child or teen is very active, sports bars or drinks can provide the additional needed calories in a nutritionally balanced manner. As always, the height, weight, and BMI percentiles are the best assurance that the individual is growing adequately over time. Adequate energy to perform the sport as well as be attentive and productive at school and for other activities should also be considered.

Water should be increased during activity both to minimize the chance of dehydration and to maximize performance. About 1 hour before vigorous exercise, the child should drink one or two glasses (8 to 16 ounces) of water, and should repeat the same amount of fluid just before the exercise begins. Young children may not feel thirsty, and should be encouraged to drink 6 to 12 ounces of fluid every 15 to 20 minutes during exercise (AAP, Committee on Nutrition, 2004; Cotugna, Vickery, & McBee, 2005). Water is usually the best replacement, but during extended exercise sports drinks may be a good alternative for some of the fluid intake. Additional water is needed after activity. Weight loss of 1 pound indicates a loss of about 0.5 quart of fluid. Be sure the child takes in fluid to replace all losses.

Some common nutrients that may be deficient in all teens, but even more often in the athlete, are calcium and iron. The increased blood volume common in the well-conditioned person necessitates greater intake. Calcium foods such as milk products and dark green vegetables, and iron foods such as adequate meats and grains, can guard against deficiencies. Many adolescents believe that they need extra protein during athletic seasons; however, most Americans ingest adequate protein to meet even the increased needs of sports, although the vegetarian child or adolescent may need assistance to plan a diet with adequate protein.

Many teens ingest a wide variety of dietary supplements, believing that they act as **ergogenic aids**, or products that enhance physical performance by their influence on energy, alertness, or body composition. Adolescents who are athletes may believe that such agents will improve performance during sports. Most of the claims of these products are unproven, and their safety has not usually been investigated, especially in the young. Effects on youth whose bodies are still developing are particularly unknown and the risks are high for permanent interference with some normal growth patterns. Offer guidance and help the family, teen, and school personnel to investigate claims before choosing to use a product. Be sure that if youth choose to use supplements, they know recommended doses, desired effects, and potential side effects of supplements. Be aware that some sports coaches may encourage either small size and/or dieting, or use of dietary supplements to increase weight and muscle. Consider that children and adolescents in activities such as ballet, wrestling, track or running, and horse racing may also have health risks associated with inconsistent or poor intake.

Over 6% of students report taking illegal anabolic steroids and these products can have a wide array of side effects (Centers for Disease Control and Prevention, 2004b). They may stop growth of long bones, lead to endocrine imbalance, and cause increased tendon rupture (Rosenfield, 2005). They are also illegal in sporting events. Andro and DHEA are additional steroidal hormones used by some athletes. Masculinization of females may occur with these hormones and other side effects, such as disruption of glucose balance and insulin sensitivity, and of cholesterol and lipoprotein levels, may occur.

Some common amino acid nutritional supplements include creatine, carnitine, and glutamine. Although side effects to these substances are minimal, their possible en-

COMPLEMENTARY THERAPY

Nutrition and Homeopathy

Many families use food products to promote health and treat diseases. These include herbal products that may be acquired from health food stores or the Internet, and homeopathy, which uses small amounts of natural substances as treatment for conditions such as otitis media and diarrhea in children. Herbs are not tested or regulated by the government, so amounts of ingredients are often not known. However, homeopathy uses dilute amounts of remedies, and prepares them uniformly as described in the *Homeopathic Pharmacopeia*. Some studies have shown effective treatment of minor childhood illnesses by homeopathy. Ask families how they are treating conditions at home and inquire about whether they will give the child a medicine if one is prescribed. Sometimes families use Western medicine to obtain a diagnosis and then treat it at home. Most homeopathy will not harm the child, but in some cases other treatment is needed to prevent dehydration or treat serious disease. Nurses are more able to work effectively with parents using a variety of treatments if questions about home remedies are clear, nonjudgmental, and inserted into every healthcare visit (Kemper & Jacobs, 2003). Are there homeopathic care providers in your community?

hancement of performance is temporary and outcomes of long-term use are unknown. Increasing overall intake to meet needs during high activity is a better alternative. Creatine has been studied more than most supplements; it is made by the body and is present in many protein sources. Supplemental creatine increases the creatine level in muscle and may help to increase performance in short bursts of activity, while not affecting endurance sports. The increase in muscle mass that can occur is largely due to water and the effect will be lost when the supplement is discontinued (Williams, 2006).

Minerals such as chromium, iron, and calcium are used by some youths. Additionally, others use mega-doses of sports supplements and combine a number of drugs, greatly increasing the risk of side effects. The nurse can ask careful and sensitive questions, such as "Many athletes take supplements to aid in performance in sports. What supplements do you take or are you considering?" Information can then be provided to enhance the youth's understanding of nutrition and sports performance. Generally, intake of a balanced diet with adequate carbohydrate, protein, and fat will meet the needs of most athletes and lead to maximal sports performance. School nurses can work with physical education teachers and coaches to plan appropriate programs for youth to prevent use of ergogenic agents (Rosenfield, 2005).

Health-Related Conditions

Many health-related conditions influence the child's nutritional state. Conversely, the child's nutritional state can influence the state of health. The Pathophysiology Illustrated figure below shows some common conditions that influence nutritional needs (Figure 4–12 ➤). These conditions are discussed in various chapters throughout the

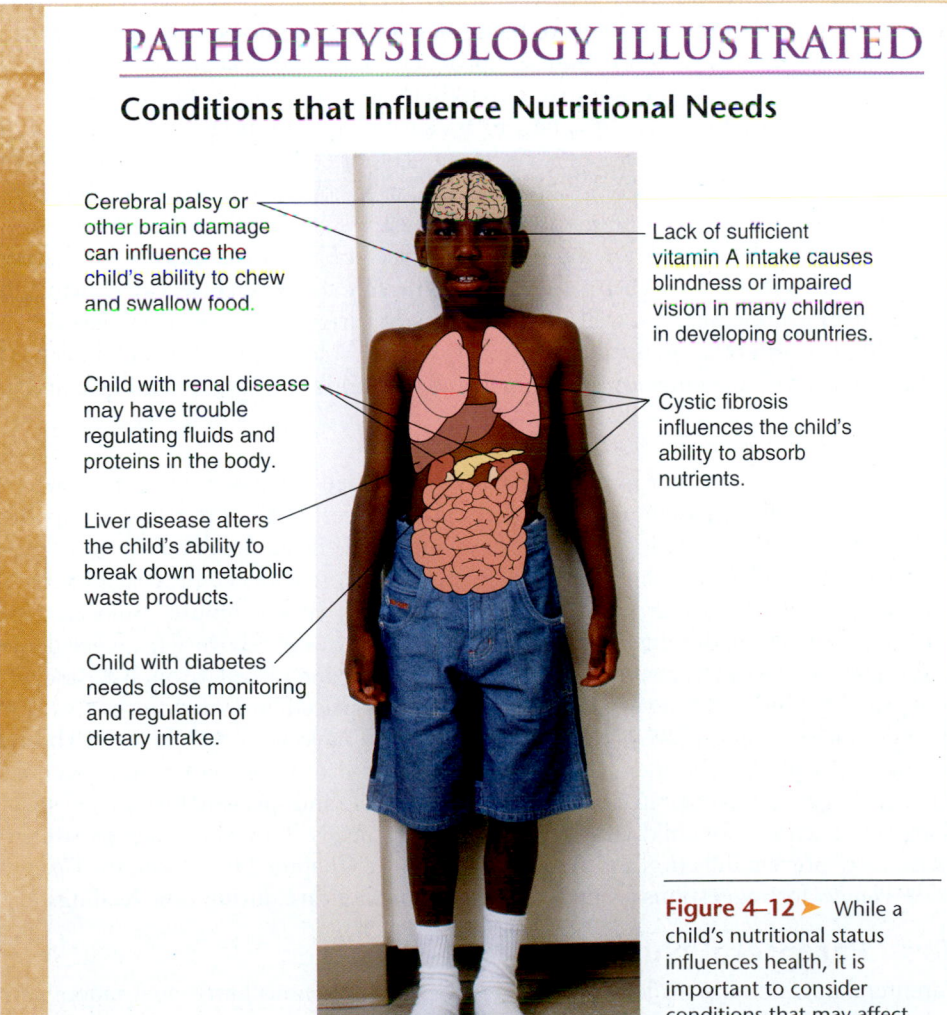

PATHOPHYSIOLOGY ILLUSTRATED

Conditions that Influence Nutritional Needs

Cerebral palsy or other brain damage can influence the child's ability to chew and swallow food.

Lack of sufficient vitamin A intake causes blindness or impaired vision in many children in developing countries.

Child with renal disease may have trouble regulating fluids and proteins in the body.

Cystic fibrosis influences the child's ability to absorb nutrients.

Liver disease alters the child's ability to break down metabolic waste products.

Child with diabetes needs close monitoring and regulation of dietary intake.

Figure 4–12 ➤ While a child's nutritional status influences health, it is important to consider conditions that may affect nutrition in your assessment.

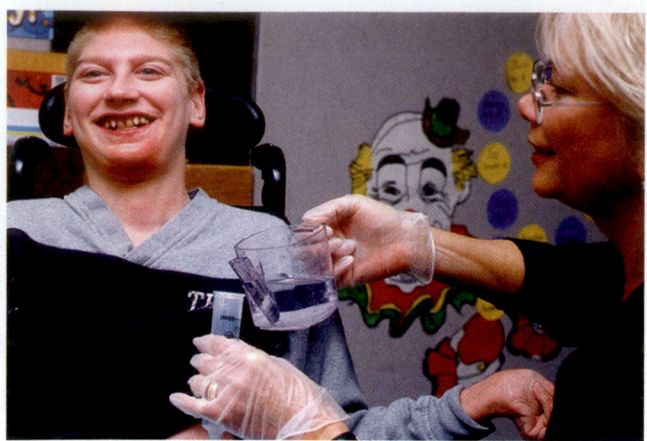

Figure 4–13 ▶ This young boy with cerebral palsy has recently returned to school after surgery on his back. He is limited in his ability to chew and swallow and is receiving tube feedings to supplement the limited diet he can ingest by mouth. The school nurse has instructed the teacher (shown here) in safe administration of tube feedings. What information was in her teaching plan for the school personnel?

text. When you read about them, discuss with classmates how you will adjust normal nutritional assessment and teaching due to the presence of a healthcare concern. Which conditions influence absorption of nutrients? Which cause changes in nutritional intake requirements? Some children benefit from special dietary aids, such as eating utensils and cups that are easy to grasp. Therapists can evaluate and make recommendations about devices that can assist the child at meals.

One example of a child with special nutritional needs is the child with cerebral palsy who may lack the muscular ability to chew and swallow normal foods. Special utensils may be required so the child can grasp them readily. Soft foods or tube feedings may be required to prevent choking on more solid food. Time must be provided within the school day for the child to ingest nutrients. Goals related to self-feeding may be part of the Individualized Education and Health Plans. School nurses play a vital role in educating school personnel about the child's nutritional needs. Partnership and collaboration among the office nurse, school nurse, child, family, and school personnel must occur so that the child is consistently offered nutritious intake in a manner that is conducive with ability to ingest (Figure 4–13▶).

GROWTH & DEVELOPMENT

Vegetarian Diet

When a pregnant teen follows a vegetarian diet, additional help will be needed to encourage adequate nutrition (Johnston & Sabate, 2006). A 24-hour or 2-day diet record will help identify nutritional needs. Consider additional pregnancy needs for energy, protein, n-3 fatty acids, iron, vitamin D, and calcium; note that vitamin B_{12} is recommended as a supplement. Use the Vegetarian Food Guide Pyramid available through the American Dietetic Association.

BOX 4–10

COMMON NUTRITIONAL DEFICIENCIES OF VEGANS

Vitamin D and calcium
Vitamin B_{12}
Minerals: zinc, iron
Fiber
Calories
Protein
Fat

Vegetarianism

Some families choose to eat vegetarian diets and can be helped and encouraged in their endeavors. Several variations of intake occur. **Vegetarians** eat no poultry, meat, or fish. **Lacto-ovovegetarians** eat eggs and dairy products, while **lacto-vegetarians** eat dairy products. In contrast, **vegans** are strict vegetarians and eat no animal products. When people say they are vegetarian, it is best to ask specific questions about what they will and will not eat.

The vegetarian can be very healthy, but may need some additional help to ensure nutritional adequacy. Some common vegan deficiencies are listed in Box 4–10. Completing a 24-hour diet recall for the pregnant or lactating woman, and for vegetarian children, with analysis for RDAs can be helpful. Be sure to routinely assess growth and other nutritional measures as well. Provide ideas of various foods to meet nutritional needs and perform other general nutritional teaching. When a vegetarian child is hospitalized, plan with the nutrition department and the child's family to meet intake needs.

Enteral Therapy

Enteral therapy is a form of nutritional support provided when a child cannot take in enough food orally to sustain health. Since it is the closest form of nutritional support to the natural method of eating, it has the least untoward effects and greatest rate of success. Some of the children who use enteral therapy are those with cerebral palsy or other neurological conditions that lead to weakness of the throat and mouth, children with neoplasm or immune dysfunction, and those in acute states of recovery from accidents or illnesses. A tube can be inserted into the nasal opening and placed through the esophagus into the stomach; however, a tube that is surgically placed into the stomach through an abdominal opening is preferred for long-term use. As long as the child can absorb and use nutrients, enteral therapy can be successful in providing calories and essential nutrients. Commercially prepared formulas are available and specially formulated solutions can be adapted for children with specific dietary needs. The tube and entry site are cared for to prevent infection and skin breakdown. See Chapter 24 ∞ and the *Clinical Skills Manual* for suggestions on management of nursing care during tube feedings.

Total Parenteral Nutrition

Parenteral nutrition has made it possible to provide intravenous nutritional support for individuals who cannot eat or are unable to absorb nutrients from the intestinal tract in

LAW & ETHICS

TPN

Total parenteral nutrition (TPN) is frequently used in the treatment of children who cannot ingest adequate amounts of foods. In many cases, TPN provides nutrients that offer the child nourishment, leading to an improvement in their condition and, therefore, an improved state of health. However, TPN is expensive, complicated to administer, and can have adverse side effects. Is this treatment the best option for all children with inadequate nutrition? How are decisions made about when to institute this type of nutritional support? If someone is unconscious or dying, is this method of nutrition started? These ethical issues are often difficult and have no easy answers. Nurses usually administer TPN in the home and hospital and may feel stressed if families, the patient, and other health professionals do not agree on its use (Breier, 2000; Breier-Mackie & Newell, 2002). Guidelines are available to help healthcare professionals make decisions about treatments, and nurses should seek the guidance of ethics professionals in their agencies when needed.

a normal manner and are at risk of severe malnutrition (Matarese & Gottschlich, 2002). Examples of children who benefit from this method of nutrition are those with congenital malformation of the gastrointestinal tract, head injury, severe burns, or for support after bone marrow transplant, sepsis, or other critical conditions. A catheter is inserted so that a sterile nutrition solution is infused directly into the bloodstream. A central venous catheter is inserted to promote safe infusion. Fluids usually contain glucose; electrolytes such as sodium, potassium, calcium, magnesium, phosphate, and chloride; vitamins; and proteins. Lipid emulsions are another type of TPN used in some children. Meticulous care is needed, whether in the hospital or at home, to ensure safe TPN infusion and treatment. The nurse performs initial assessment and ongoing evaluation and monitoring of treatment, and administers the solutions in the hospital or other settings. See the protocols for TPN management in the *Clinical Skills Manual*.

CRITICAL THINKING IN ACTION

Recall the family introduced in the chapter opener. Yvonne is a 9-month-old infant who is active and healthy. Her mother, Colleen, has brought her to the Women, Infant, and Child (WIC) Nutrition Program clinic, and they are accompanied by Margarita, the grandmother. Colleen feels unprepared to make decisions about what Yvonne should be eating at this age. Yvonne breast-feeds twice daily since Colleen works but wonders if she should continue. The nurse praises Colleen for continuing with these two feedings daily since that ensures the benefits of breast-feeding such as immune protection against some illnesses, and it fosters mother-infant bonding. She reassures Colleen that it is beneficial for her to pump her breasts and suggests that the pumped milk be refrigerated and fed to Yvonne by bottle in the middle of the following day.

1. What fine motor skills would you expect to see in Yvonne at this age that will enable her to perform more self-feeding skills?

2. During the visit, the nurse takes a blood sample for hematocrit. What is the expected level at this age?

What factors put infants in the second half of their first year of life at risk for iron deficiency anemia? What teaching can you do to promote intake of iron? Yvonne has a bottle of regular milk in the middle of the day. How could this contribute to anemia? What is recommended for her intake at this age?

3. Margarita prepares most of Yvonne's meals during the day and speaks Spanish. How will you prepare teaching for this grandmother so that she can benefit from the teaching that the clinic has designed for parents of infants? How can you make that teaching culturally sensitive?

4. As Colleen looks forward now to the next few months, what information will she need to provide nutritious intake for Yvonne? What are expected food patterns at 1 year and 18 months of age?

 Refer to your Prentice Hall Nursing MediaLink DVD-ROM for answers.

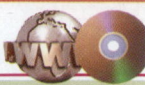

EXPLORE MediaLink

http://www.prenhall.com/ball

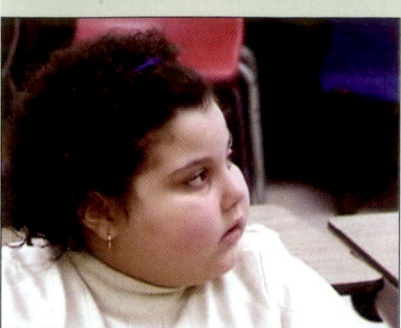

Resources for this chapter can be found on the Prentice Hall Nursing MediaLink DVD-ROM accompanying this textbook, and on the Companion Website at http://www.prenhall.com/ball.

DVD-ROM
Audio Glossary
NCLEX-RN® Review
Videos
   Anorexia Nervosa
   Children and Overweight

COMPANION WEBSITE
Audio Glossary
NCLEX-RN® Review
Care Plan Activity: Childhood Obesity
Case Study: Single Parenting and Nutrition Issues
Critical Thinking
   Comparing Nutrition Labels
   Fast Food Menu Analysis
MediaLink Applications
   Diet and Culture
   Healthy Eating Index
   Managing a Peanut Allergy at School
   Planning a Nutritional Teaching Session
   Vegetarian Teen Diet
WebLinks

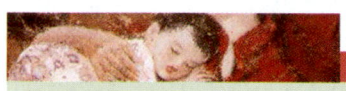

REFERENCES

American Academy of Pediatrics, Committee on Nutrition. (2001). The use and misuse of fruit juice in pediatrics. *Pediatrics, 107,* 1210–1213.

American Academy of Pediatrics, Committee on Nutrition. (2004). *Pediatric nutrition handbook* (5th ed.). Elk Grove Village, IL: American Academy of Pediatrics.

American Academy of Pediatrics, Section on Breastfeeding. (2005). Breastfeeding and the use of human milk. *Pediatrics, 115,* 496–506.

American Dental Association. (n.d.). ADA statement on early childhood caries. Retrieved on August 2, 2006, from www.ada.org/prof/ resources/positions/statements/caries.asp

American Diabetes Association, (2003). Economic costs of diabetes in the U.S. in 2002. *Diabetes Care, 26,* 917–932.

American Diabetes Association (2006). Breastfeeding helps prevent obesity in kids. Retrieved on August 22, 2006 from http://www. diabetes.org/nedocuments.may06final/pdf

American Dietetic Association. (2001). Position of the American Dietetic Association. Breaking the Barriers to Breastfeeding. Journal of the American Dietetic Association 101, 1213–1220.

American Dietetic Association. (2006). Nutrition intervention in the treatment of anorexia nervosa, bulimia nervosa, and eating disorder not otherwise specified (EDNOS). Retrieved on August 3, 2006 from http://www. eatright.org/cps/rde/xchg/ada/hs.xls/advocacy_ adapo701_ENU_HTML.htm

American Psychiatric Association Working Group on Eating Disorders. (2000). Practice

guidelines for the treatment of patients with eating disorders. *American Journal of Psychiatry, 157,* 1–39.

Behrman, R. E., Kliegman, R. M., & Jenson, H. B. (2004). *Nelson textbook of pediatrics* (17th ed.). Philadelphia: Saunders.

Berkman, N. D., Bulik, C. M., Brownley, K. A., Loh, K. N., Sedway, J. A., Rooks, A. & Gartlehnen G. (2006.) Management of eating disorders. Rockville MD: Agency for Healthcare Research and Quality, AHRQ Pub No. 06-E010.

Block, R.W., & Krebs, N. F. (2005). Failure to thrive as a manifestation of child neglect. *Pediatrics, 116,* 1234–1237.

Breier, S. J. (2000). Ethics and total parenteral nutrition. *Journal of Intravenous Nursing, 23,* 52–57.

Breier-Mackie, S., & Newell, C. J. (2002). Home parenteral nutrition: An ethical decision making dilemma. *Australian Journal of Advanced Nursing, 19*(4), 27–32.

Briefel, R. R., & Johnson, C. L. (2004). Secular trends in dietary intake in the United States. *Annual Review of Nutrition, 24,* 401–431.

Burks, W., & Ballmer-Weber, B. K. (2006). Food allergy. *Molecular Nutrition and Food Research, 50,* 595–603.

Centers for Disease Control and Prevention. (2004a). Botulism. Retrieved August 2, 2006, from http://www.cdc.gov/ncidod/aip/research/ bot.html

Centers for Disease Control and Prevention. (2004b). Youth risk behavior surveillance— United States, 2003. *Morbidity and Mortality Weekly Report, 53*(SS-2), 1–28.

Centers for Disease Control and Prevention. (2005a). Bovine spongiform encephalopathy. Retrieved December 26, 2005, from http://www.cdc.gov/ncidod.dvvd.bse/

Centers for Disease Control and Prevention. (2005b). Preventing health risks associated with drinking unpasteurized or untreated juice. Retrieved December 27, 2005, from http:// www.cdc.gov/foodborne/juice.spotlight.htm

Centers for Disease Control and Prevention. (2005c). Variant Creutzfeldt Jakobs Disease (vCJD). Retrieved 2005, from http://www.cdc. gov/ncidod.dvvd/vcjd/epidemiology.htm

Children's Defense Fund. (2004). *The state of America's children.* Washington, DC: Author.

Cotugna, N., Vickery, C. E., & McBee, S. (2005). Sports nutrition for young athletes. *Journal of School Nursing, 21,* 323–328.

Cullen, K.W., & Zakeri, I. (2004). Fruits, vegetables, milk, and sweetened beverages consumption and access to a la carte/snack bar meals at school. *American Journal of Public Health, 94,* 463–467.

Federal Interagency Forum on Child and Family Statistics. (2005). Food security and diet quality. In *America's children: Key national indicators of well-being 2005.* Washington, DC: Author.

Food and Drug Administration. (2004). Backgrounder for the 2004 FDA/EPA consumer advisory: What you need to know about mercury in fish and shellfish. Washington, DC: Department of Health and Human Services. Retrieved on June 8, 2004, from http://www.fda. gov/oc/opacom/hottopics/mercury/ backgrounder.html

Gartner, L. M., & Greer, F. R. (2003). Prevention of rickets and vitamin D deficiency: New guidelines for vitamin D intake. *Pediatrics, 111,* 908–910.

Gentile, D. A., Oberg, C., Sherwood, N. E., Story, M., Walsh, D. A., Hogan, M., &

American Academy of Pediatrics. (2004). Well-child visits in the video age: Pediatricians and the American Academy of Pediatrics' guidelines for children's media use. *Pediatrics, 114,* 1235–1241.

Gluck, M. E. (2006). Stress response and binge eating disorder. *Appetite, 46,* 26–30.

Hagerty, M. A., Schmidt, C., Bernaix, L., & Clement, J. M. (2004). Adolescent obesity: Current trends in identification and management. *Journal of the American Academy of Nurse Practitioners, 16,* 481–489.

Haynes, B. (2005). Creation of a bariatric surgery program for adolescents at a major teaching hospital. *Pediatric Nursing, 31,* 21–23, 59.

Hoek, H. W. (2006). Incidence, prevalence and mortality of anorexia nervosa and other eating disorders. *Current Opinion in Psychiatry, 19,* 389–394.

Institute of Medicine. (2005). *Preventing childhood obesity.* Washington, DC: National Academies Press.

Jenkins, S., & Horner, S. D. (2005). Barriers that influence eating behaviors in adolescents. *Journal of Pediatric Nursing, 20,* 258–267.

Johnston, P. K., & Sabate, J. (2006). Nutritional implications of vegetarian diets. In M. E. Shils, M. Shike, A. C. Ross, B. Caballero, & R. J. Cousins (Eds.), *Modern nutrition in health and disease* (10th ed., pp. 1638–1654). Philadelphia: Lippincott, Williams & Wilkins.

Kazis, K., & Iglesias, M. D. (2003). The female athlete triad. *Adolescent Medicine 14,* 87–95.

Kemper, K. J., & Jacobs, J. (2003). Homeopathy in pediatrics–No harm likely but how much good? *Contemporary Pediatrics 20,* 97–111.

Kramer, M. S. (2001). Promotion of breastfeeding intervention trial (PROBIT). *Journal of the American Medical Association, 285,* 413–420.

Krassas, G. E. (2003). Endocrine abnormalities in anorexia nervosa. *Pediatric Endocrinology Review, 1,* 46–54.

Lee, R. D., & Nieman, D. C. (2007). *Nutrition assessment* (4th ed.). Boston: McGraw-Hill.

Lutz, C., & Przytulski, K. (2006). Nutrition and diet therapy (4th ed.). Philadelphia: F.A. Davis.

Matarese, L. E., & Gottschlich, M. M. (2002). *Contemporary nutrition support practice.* Philadelphia: W. B. Saunders.

MMWR. (2004). Diagnosis and management of foodborne illness: A primer for physicians and other health care professionals. *Morbidity and Mortality Weekly Report, 53,* RR–4, 1–40.

Palmer, K., & Burks, W. (2006). Current developments in peanut allergy. *Current Opinion in Allergy and Clinical Immunology, 6,* 202–206.

Proctor, M. H., Moore, L. L., Gao, D., Cupples, L. A., Bradlee, M. L., Hood, M. Y., & Ellison, R. C. (2003). Television viewing and change in body fat from preschool to early adolescence: The Framingham Children's Study. *International Journal of Obesity and Related Metabolic Disorders 27,* 827–833.

Rideout, V. J., Vandewater, E. A., & Wartella, E. A. (2003). *Zero to six: Electronic media in the lives of infants, toddlers and preschoolers.* Menlo Park, CA: Kaiser Family Foundation.

Rosenfield, C. (2005). The use of ergogenic agents in high school athletes. *Journal of School Nursing, 21,* 333–339.

Sherman, R. T., & Thompson, R. A. (2004). The female athlete triad. *Journal of School Nursing, 20,* 197–202.

Simons, E., Weiss, C. C., Furlong, T. J., & Sicherer, S. H. (2005). Impact of ingredient labeling practices on food allergic consumer. *Annals of Allergy, Asthma and Immunology, 95,* 426–428.

Storey, M. L., Forshee, R. A., & Anderson, P. A. (2004). Associations of adequate intake of calcium with diet, beverage consumption, and demographic characteristics among children and adolescents. *Journal of the American College of Nutrition, 23,* 18–33.

Story, M., Holt, K., & Sofka, D. (Eds.). (2002). *Bright futures in practice: Nutrition* (2nd ed.). Arlington, VA: National Center for Education in Maternal and Child Health.

Urrutia-Rojas, X., & Menchaca, J. (2006). Prevalence of risk for type 2 diabetes in school children. *Journal of School Health, 76,* 189–194.

U.S. Centers for Disease Control and Prevention, U.S. National Center for Chronic Disease Prevention and Health Promotion, U.S. Division of Adolescent and School Health, U.S. Health Resources and Services Administration, U.S. Maternal and Child Health Bureau, U.S. Office of Adolescent Health et al. (2004). *Improving the health of adolescents and young adults: A guide for states and communities.* Atlanta, GA: U.S. Centers for Disease Control and Prevention, National Center for Chronic Disease Prevention and Health Promotion, & Division of Adolescent and School Health.

U.S. Department of Health and Human Services. (2000). *Healthy People 2010.* Washington, DC: U.S. Department of Health and Human Services. Retrieved April 13, 2001, from http://www.health.gov/healthypeople/document.html

U.S. Department of Health and Human Services. (2005). *Dietary guidelines for Americans.* Retrieved from www.healthierus.gov/dietaryguidelines

U.S. Preventive Services Task Force. (2003). Behavioral interventions to promote breastfeeding: Recommendations and rationale. *American Journal for Nurse Practitioners, 7*(11), 23–32.

Viner, R. M., & Cole, T. J. (2005). Television viewing in early childhood predicts adult body mass index. *Journal of Pediatrics, 147,* 429–435.

Waldrop, J. (2005). Early identification and interventions for female athlete triad. *Journal of Pediatric Health Care, 19,* 213–220.

Williams, M. H. (2006). Sports nutrition. In M. E. Shils, M. Shike, A. C. Ross, B. Caballero, & R. J. Cousins (Eds.), *Modern nutrition in health and disease* (10th ed., pp. 1723–1740). Philadelphia: Lippincott, Williams & Wilkins.

5

PEDIATRIC ASSESSMENT

MediaLink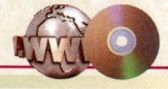

http://www.prenhall.com/ball

See the Prentice Hall Nursing MediaLink DVD-ROM and Companion Website for chapter-specific resources.

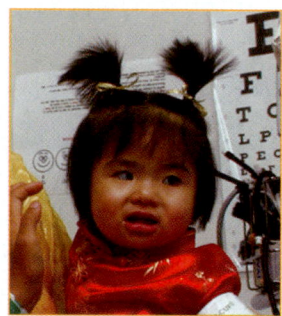

TWO-YEAR-OLD Jasmine was recently adopted into the Porter family. She has been brought to the health clinic for internationally adopted children by her new mother and sister for a comprehensive health assessment. Until 3 weeks ago, Jasmine was living in a center for children eligible for adoption in her native China. She speaks no English and she is very fearful of new and different situations.

Mrs. Porter is anxious to have Jasmine evaluated to identify any health promotion or special healthcare issues that need to be addressed, such as development, growth, nutrition, immunizations, and health conditions. Jasmine had many immunizations before leaving China, and she has never had a major illness or injury. Limited information is available about her biological parents and their health.

Mrs. Porter thinks Jasmine seems small for her age, and she is also concerned that she may have an ear infection. Jasmine's appetite has not been good for the past day, and she has been cranky. She also seems to have a slight fever.

The patient history and physical examination provide a structure and sequence for collecting and analyzing relevant assessment data. The initial physical examination findings provide the baseline for monitoring Jasmine's future growth and development and response to care for any identified health problems. Analysis of the assessment data enables you to form nursing diagnoses and to develop a nursing care plan to guide the nursing care that Jasmine will receive.

LEARNING OUTCOMES

After reading this chapter, you will be able to do the following:

1. Describe the elements of a health history for an infant and child at different ages.

2. Identify communication strategies to improve the quality of historical data collected.

3. Describe strategies to gain cooperation of a young child for assessment.

4. Describe the differences in sequence of the physical assessment for infants, children, and adolescents.

5. Modify physical assessment techniques according to the age and developmental stage of the child.

6. Determine the sexual maturity rating of males and females based upon physical signs of secondary sexual characteristics present.

7. Analyze findings from the assessment of multiple systems and recognize signs indicating the presence of a health condition.

How do examination techniques vary by the age of the child? How does the nurse encourage infants and toddlers to cooperate with the examination? This chapter provides an overview of pediatric assessment, including history taking and examination techniques geared to the unique needs of pediatric patients. Strategies for obtaining the child's history are presented first. The remainder of the chapter then outlines a systematic process for physical examination of the child.

ANATOMIC AND PHYSIOLOGIC CHARACTERISTICS OF INFANTS AND CHILDREN

Children and infants are not only smaller than adults, but also significantly different physiologically. Knowledge of pediatric anatomic and physiologic differences will aid in recognizing normal variations found during the physical examination. It also assists with understanding the different physiologic responses children have to illness and injury. Figure 5–1 ➤ provides an overview of important anatomic and physiologic differences between children and adults.

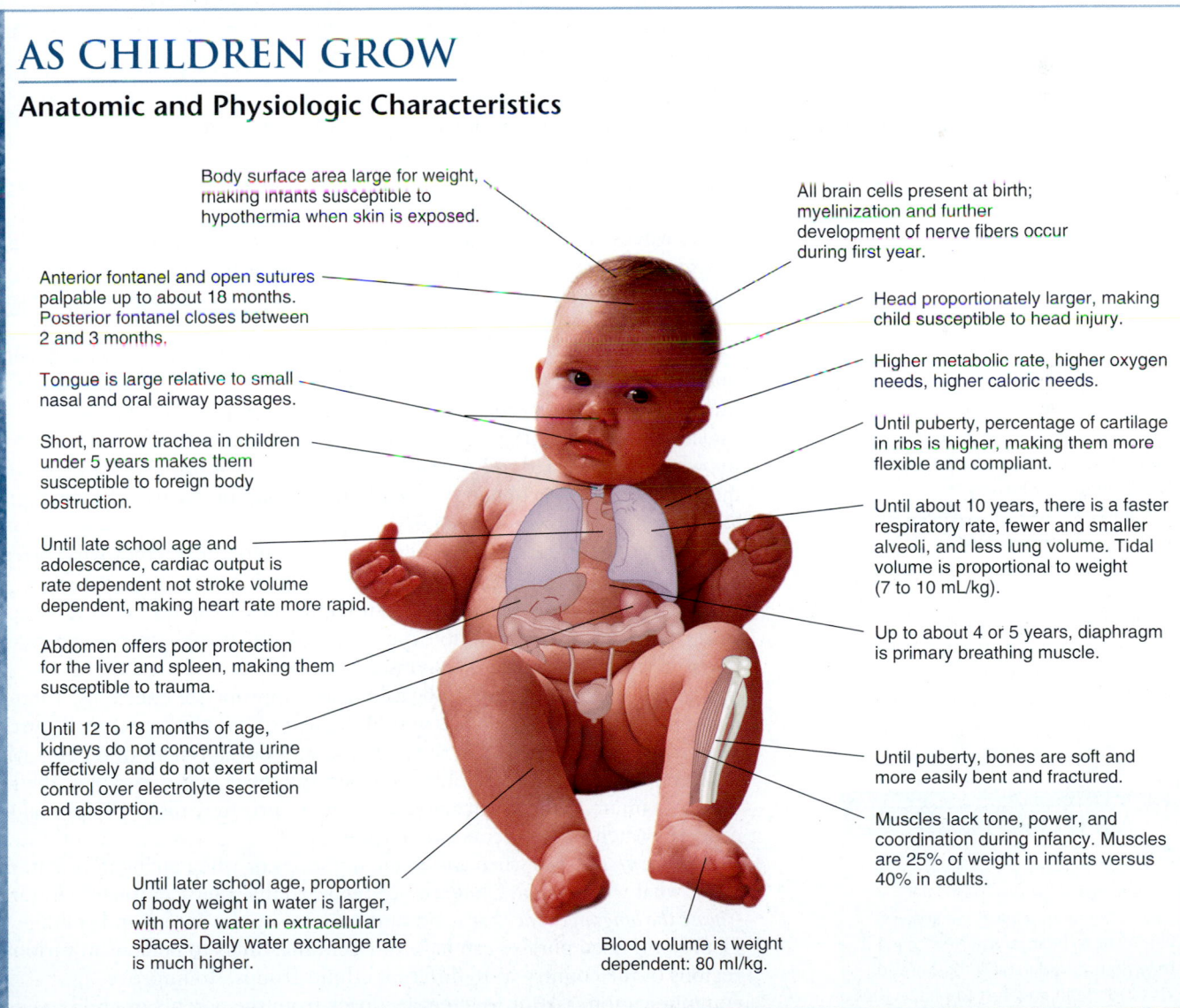

AS CHILDREN GROW

Anatomic and Physiologic Characteristics

Body surface area large for weight, making infants susceptible to hypothermia when skin is exposed.

All brain cells present at birth; myelinization and further development of nerve fibers occur during first year.

Anterior fontanel and open sutures palpable up to about 18 months. Posterior fontanel closes between 2 and 3 months.

Head proportionately larger, making child susceptible to head injury.

Tongue is large relative to small nasal and oral airway passages.

Higher metabolic rate, higher oxygen needs, higher caloric needs.

Short, narrow trachea in children under 5 years makes them susceptible to foreign body obstruction.

Until puberty, percentage of cartilage in ribs is higher, making them more flexible and compliant.

Until late school age and adolescence, cardiac output is rate dependent not stroke volume dependent, making heart rate more rapid.

Until about 10 years, there is a faster respiratory rate, fewer and smaller alveoli, and less lung volume. Tidal volume is proportional to weight (7 to 10 mL/kg).

Abdomen offers poor protection for the liver and spleen, making them susceptible to trauma.

Up to about 4 or 5 years, diaphragm is primary breathing muscle.

Until 12 to 18 months of age, kidneys do not concentrate urine effectively and do not exert optimal control over electrolyte secretion and absorption.

Until puberty, bones are soft and more easily bent and fractured.

Muscles lack tone, power, and coordination during infancy. Muscles are 25% of weight in infants versus 40% in adults.

Until later school age, proportion of body weight in water is larger, with more water in extracellular spaces. Daily water exchange rate is much higher.

Blood volume is weight dependent: 80 ml/kg.

Figure 5–1 ➤ Children are not just small adults. There are important anatomic and physiologic differences between children and adults that will change based on a child's growth and development. Can you identify which of these differences are of greatest concern for the hospitalized child and why?

Obtaining the Child's History
Communication Strategies

What makes communication effective? What does it mean when a parent or caretaker will not look you in the eye when speaking with you? What types of cues indicate that a parent may be withholding historical information?

The health history interview is a very personal conversation with a parent, caretaker, or adolescent during which private concerns and feelings are shared. Try to ensure that this exchange of information with the parent or the child is clearly understood by both parties; that it is an **effective communication**. Effective communication is difficult to accomplish because parents and children often do not correctly interpret what the nurse says, just as the nurse may not understand completely what the parent or child says. People's interpretation of information is based on their life experiences, culture, and education.

STRATEGIES TO BUILD A RAPPORT WITH THE FAMILY When beginning the history, make sure the parents understand the purpose of the interview and that the information will be used appropriately. To develop rapport, demonstrate interest in and concern for the child and family during the interview. This rapport forms the foundation for the collaborative relationship between the nurse and parent that will provide the best nursing care for the child. The following strategies help to establish rapport with the child's family during the nursing history.

- *Introduce yourself* (name, title or position, and role in caring for the child). To demonstrate respect, ask all family members present what name they prefer you to use when talking with them.
- *Explain the purpose of the interview* and why the nursing history is different from the information collected by other health professionals. For example, "The nurses will use this information to plan nursing care best suited for your child."
- *Provide privacy* and remove as many distractions as possible during the interview. If the patient's room does not offer privacy, attempt to find a vacant patient room or lounge.
- *Direct the focus of the interview* with open-ended questions. Use close-ended questions or directing statements to clarify information. Open-ended questions are useful to initiate the interview, develop a rapport, and understand the parent's perceptions of the child's problem; for example, "Tell me what problems led to Roberto's admission to the hospital." Close-ended questions are used to obtain detailed information; for example, "How high was Tommy's fever this morning?"
- *Ask one question at a time* so that the parent or child understands what piece of information is desired and so that it is clear which question the parent is answering. "Does any member of your family have diabetes, heart disease, or sickle cell anemia?" is a multiple question. Ask about each disease separately to ensure the most accurate response.
- *Involve the child in the interview* by asking age-appropriate questions. Young children can be asked "What is your doll's name?" or "Where does it hurt?" Demonstrating an interest in the child initiates development of rapport with both child and parents. Ask older children and teens questions about their illness or injury. Offer them an opportunity to privately discuss their major concerns when their parents are not present.
- *Be honest with the child* when answering questions or when giving information about what will happen. Children need to learn that they can trust their nurse.
- *Choose the language style* that is best understood by the parent and child. Commonly used phrases can have different meanings to persons in various regions of the country or to different ethnic groups. To improve communication, ask for frequent feedback from the parents or child to ensure that their interpretation of phrases is accurate.
- *Use an interpreter to improve communication* when not fluent in the family's primary language (Figure 5–2 ➤).

LAW & ETHICS
HIPPA

Assure the parents and the child that the information provided during the assessment is protected under the Health Insurance Privacy and Portability Act (HIPPA), a federal law that requires written consent to be provided before health information can be shared with healthcare providers outside the facility. To ensure confidentiality of information for parents, avoid using a family member as an interpreter for history taking.

CULTURE
Questioning

Some cultural groups, particularly Asians, try to anticipate the answers you want to hear, or say "Yes" even if they do not understand the question. This is done in an effort to please you or as an expression of politeness. Remember to phrase your questions in a neutral manner.

CAREFUL LISTENING Complete attention is necessary to "hear" and accurately interpret information the parents and child give during the nursing history. Carefully *listen* to the information provided by the parent, as well as how it is expressed, and *observe behavior* during the interaction.

- Does the parent hesitate or avoid answering certain questions?
- Pay attention to the parent's attitude or tone of voice when the child's problems are discussed. Determine if it is consistent with the seriousness of the child's problem. The tone of voice can reveal anxiety, anger, or lack of concern.
- Be alert to any underlying themes. For example, the parent who talks about the child's diagnosis, but repeatedly refers to the impact of the illness on the family's finances or on meeting the needs of other family members, is requesting that these issues be addressed.
- Observe the parent's **nonverbal behavior** (posture, gestures, body movements, eye contact, and facial expression) for consistency with the words and tone of voice used. Is the parent interested in and appropriately concerned about the child's condition? Behaviors such as sitting up straight, making eye contact (if culturally acceptable), and appearing apprehensive reflect appropriate concern for the child. Physical withdrawal, failure to make eye contact, or a happy expression could be inconsistent with the child's serious condition. See Table 5–1 for nonverbal communication patterns used by major cultural groups.

Subtle nonverbal and verbal cues often indicate that the parent has not provided complete information about the child's problem. Observe for behaviors such as avoiding

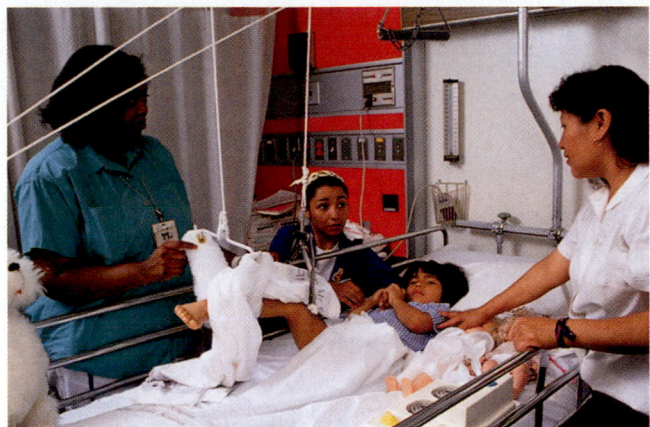

Figure 5–2 ▶ Most hospitals have designated interpreters that you should use. If not, find a professional interpreter whom you have identified beforehand and who knows medical terms and the cultural norms of the family. Avoid using a family member as an interpreter. The interpreter (center) should be positioned to improve communication. Maintain eye contact with the parent or patient, not the interpreter.

Table 5–1	**NONVERBAL COMMUNICATION PATTERNS IN MAJOR CULTURAL GROUPS***
Cultural Group	**Nonverbal Communication Pattern**
African American	Touch common with family members and close friends Close personal space
Chinese	Avoid direct eye contact when listening Distant personal space Prefer not to be touched by strangers
Eastern Indian	Direct eye contact is considered disrespectful Handshake between men only
Hispanic/Latino	Touch used often, especially between members of the same sex Close personal space
Japanese	Direct eye contact is considered disrespectful Handshaking acceptable Not accustomed to intimate physical contact by casual acquaintances Distant personal space
Native American	Limited eye contact during conversation Silence during communication allows thinking and demonstrates respect Close personal space
European (Spanish, French)	Use firm eye contact and look for impact of what has been said

*Behavioral patterns of nonverbal behavior vary within groups, so avoid stereotyping any one group with these communication characteristics.
Data from: Spector, R. E. (2004). *Cultural diversity in health and illness* (6th ed.). Upper Saddle River, NJ: Prentice Hall; Flores, G., Rabke-Verani, J., Pine, W., & Sabharwal, A. (2002). The importance of cultural and linguistic issues in the care of children. *Pediatric Emergency Care, 18*(4), 271–284.

eye contact, change in voice pitch, or hesitation when responding to a question. Being supportive and asking clarifying questions encourage further description or the expression of information that is difficult for the parent or child to share; for example, "It sounds like that was a very difficult experience. How did Latasha react?"

Encourage parents to share information, even if it is private or sensitive, especially when it influences nursing care planning. Often parents avoid sharing some information because they want to make a good impression, or they do not understand the value of the missing information. If parents hesitate to share information, briefly explain why the question was asked—for example, to make their child's hospital experience more pleasant or to begin planning for the child's discharge and home care.

In some cases the parent becomes too agitated, upset, or angry to continue responding to questions. When the information is not needed immediately, move on to another portion of the history to determine whether the parent is able to respond to other questions. Depending on the parent's emotional status, it may be more appropriate to collect the remaining historical data later.

Data to Be Collected

Collect and organize the child's health, medical, and personal-social history to plan the child's nursing care. Health status, psychosocial, and developmental data are organized to help develop the nursing diagnoses and the nursing care plan.

PATIENT INFORMATION   Obtain the child's name and nickname, age, sex, and ethnic origin. The child's birth date, race, religion, address, and phone number can be obtained from the admission form. Ask the parent for an emergency contact address and phone number, as well as work and cell phone numbers. Record the person providing the patient history and that person's relationship to the patient.

HEALTH STATUS   Collect information about the child's health problems and diseases chronologically in a format similar to the traditional medical history.

- The *chief complaint* is the child's primary problem or reason for hospital admission or visit to a healthcare setting, stated in the parent's or child's exact words.
- The *history of the present illness or injury* is a detailed description of the current health problem. This includes the onset and sequence of events, characteristics of and changes in symptoms over time, influencing factors, and the current status of the problem. Each problem is described separately. Table 5–2 lists the specific data to be collected about each illness and injury.
- The *past history* is a more detailed description of the child's prior health problems. It includes the birth history and all major past illnesses and injuries.

Table 5–2	HISTORY OF PRESENT ILLNESS OR INJURY
Characteristic	**Defining Variables**
Onset	Sudden or gradual, previous episodes, date and time began
Type of symptom	Pain, itching, cough, vomiting, runny nose, diarrhea, rash, etc.
Location	Generalized or localized—anatomically precise
Duration	Continuous or episodic, length of episodes
Severity	Effect on daily activities; e.g., interrupted sleep, decreased appetite, incapacitation
Influencing factors	What relieves or aggravates symptoms, what precipitated the problem, recent exposure to infection or allergen
Past evaluation for the problem	Laboratory studies, physician's office or hospital where done, results of past examinations
Previous and current treatment	Prescribed and over-the-counter drugs used, complementary and alternative therapies, other treatments tried (heat, ice, rest), response to treatments

A detailed and complete birth history is obtained when the child's present problem may be related to the birth history (Box 5–1). Record the child's age at the time of each major illness or injury, and remember to include common communicable diseases, surgeries, and hospitalizations. If any transfusions (blood or blood products) have been given in the past, identify the circumstances, type of transfusion, and reaction. Obtain information about each specific diagnosis, treatment, outcome, complication, or residual problem, and the child's reaction to the event.

- The current health status is a detailed description of the child's typical health status.
  - *Health Maintenance*—child's primary care provider, dentist, and other healthcare providers, and the timing of the last visit to each.
  - *Medications*—prescribed and over-the-counter medications taken daily, frequently, or for home management of fever, colds, coughs, cuts, and rashes. Ask about the use of plants, herbs, teas, or other complementary therapies.
  - *Allergies*—to food, medication, animals, insect bites, or environmental exposure, and the type of reaction (e.g., respiratory difficulty, rash, hives, itching).
  - *Immunizations*—review child's record for immunization status, vaccines and dates received, and any unexpected reactions.
  - *Safety Measures Used*—car seat restraint, window guards, medication storage, sports protective gear, smoke detectors, bicycle helmet, firearm storage, and others.
  - *Activities and Exercise*—physical mobility and limitations, adaptive equipment used; play and/or sports activities.
  - *Nutrition*—formula-fed or breast-fed; if breast-fed, for how long, type, and amount of daily formula intake; when solid foods were introduced, enrollment in the WIC (Women, Infants, and Children) Program; eating and snacking habits, variety of foods consumed, "junk foods" eaten, appetite.
  - *Sleep*—length and timing of naps and nighttime sleep; nightmares or night terrors, other sleep disturbances; where the child sleeps, and bedtime rituals.

BOX 5–1
BIRTH HISTORY

Prenatal

Mother's age, health during pregnancy, prenatal care, weight gained, special diet, expected date of delivery
Details of illnesses, radiograph findings, hospitalizations, medications, complications, and timing during pregnancy
Prior obstetric history

Antenatal—Description of Delivery

Site of delivery (hospital, home, birthing center)
Labor induced or spontaneous, length of labor, time/duration or rupture of membranes
Vaginal or cesarean section, forceps or suction used, vertex or breech position
Gestation at birth, single or multiple birth

Condition of Baby at Birth

Weight, Apgar score, cried immediately
Need for incubator, oxygen, suctioning, ventilator
Any abnormalities detected, meconium staining

Postnatal

Difficulties in the nursery—feeding, respiratory difficulties, jaundice, cyanosis, rashes
Length of hospital stay, special nursery, home with mother
Breast- or bottle-fed, weight lost/gained in hospital
Medical care needed in first week—re-admission to hospital

FAMILY HISTORY   The *familial and hereditary diseases* summarize the major familial and hereditary diseases in three generations of family members, including the parents, grandparents, aunts, uncles, cousins, child, and siblings. Collect information about the health status and ethnic background of each parent, and ask if they are related to each other. Label the generations and make a key for relevant diseases. Record information in either a pedigree or a narrative format. Specific diseases to ask about are listed in Table 5–3.

REVIEW OF SYSTEMS   The **review of systems** provides a comprehensive overview of the child's health. This is an opportunity to identify additional signs and symptoms associated with the child's condition. Also, other problems may be revealed that have no direct relationship to the child's significant health problem but could be factors complicating nursing care or home care. For example, asking about any urinary problems may reveal that a child still wets the bed at 7 years of age, although the admission is for a femur fracture. The nurse would then need to consider how bed-wetting might cause problems with the spica cast. For each problem, obtain the treatment, outcomes, residual problems, and age at time of onset. Data-collection guidelines are given in Table 5–4.

PSYCHOSOCIAL INFORMATION   Obtain information about family composition to establish a socioeconomic and sociologic context for planning the child's care in the hospital and at home.

- Family composition, including family members living in the home, their relationship to the child, marital status of parents or other family structure, and people helping to care for the child.
- Household members employed, family income, and financial resources or agencies used such as health insurance, food stamps, or Temporary Assistance for Needy Families (TANF).
- Description of the housing and home environment (atmosphere, emotional stresses, family activities); safe play area; use of city or well water; and availability of electricity, heat, and refrigeration.
- School or childcare arrangements; description of the neighborhood, including playgrounds, transportation, and proximity to stores.
- Changes in family or lifestyle since last seen; number of times the family has moved; how the child and family members have coped with the changes.

Table 5–3	FAMILIAL OR HEREDITARY DISEASES
Infectious diseases	Tuberculosis, HIV, hepatitis, varicella
Heart disease	Heart defects, myocardial infarctions, hypertension, dyslipidemia, sudden childhood deaths
Allergic disorders	Eczema, hay fever, or asthma
Eye disorders	Glaucoma, cataracts, vision loss
Ear disorders	Hearing loss
Hematologic disorders	Sickle cell disease, thalassemia, G6PD deficiency, leukemia, hemophilia
Lung disorders	Cystic fibrosis
Cancer	Type, early age of onset
Endocrine disorders	Diabetes mellitus, hypothyroidism, hyperthyroidism
Mental disorders	Mental retardation, epilepsy, psychiatric disorders
Musculoskeletal disorders	Arthritis, muscular dystrophy
Gastrointestinal disorders	Ulcers, colitis, celiac disease, kidney disease
Metabolic disorders	Phenylketonuria, galactosemia, maple syrup urine disease, Tay-Sach disease
Problem pregnancies	Repeated miscarriages, stillbirths
Learning problems	Attention deficit disorder, Down syndrome

Table 5–4	REVIEW OF SYSTEMS

Body Systems	Examples of Problems to Identify
General	General growth pattern, overall health status, ability to keep up with other children or tires easily with feeding or activity, fever, sleep patterns
	Allergies, type of reaction (hives, rash, respiratory difficulty, swelling, nausea), seasonal or with each exposure
Skin and lymph	Rashes, dry skin, itching, changes in skin color or texture, tendency for bruising, swollen or tender lymph glands
Hair and nails	Hair loss, changes in color or texture, use of dye or chemicals on hair
	Abnormalities of nail growth or color
Head	Headaches
Eyes	Vision problems, squinting, crossed eyes, lazy eye, wears glasses, eye infections, redness, tearing, burning, rubbing, swelling eyelids
Ears	Ear infections, frequent discharge from ears, or tubes in ears
	Hearing loss (no response to loud noises or questions, inattentiveness, was hearing test ever done?), hearing aids or cochlear implant
Nose and sinuses	Nosebleeds, nasal congestion, colds with runny nose, sinus pain or infections
	Nasal obstruction, difficulty breathing, snoring at night
Mouth and throat	Mouth breathing, difficulty swallowing, drooling, sore throats, strep infections, mouth odor
	Tooth eruption, cavities, braces
	Voice change, hoarseness, speech problems
Cardiac and hematologic	Heart murmur, anemia, hypertension, cyanosis, edema, rheumatic fever, chest pain
Chest and respiratory	Trouble breathing, choking episodes, cough, wheezing, cyanosis, exposure to tuberculosis, other infections
Gastrointestinal	Bowel movements, frequency, color, regularity, consistency, discomfort, constipation or diarrhea, abdominal pain, bleeding from rectum, flatulence, nausea or vomiting
	Usual appetite
Urinary	Frequency, urgency, dysuria, dribbling, strength of urinary stream
	Toilet trained—age when day and night dryness was attained, enuresis
Reproductive	For pubescent children
Female	Menses onset, amount, duration, frequency, discomfort, problems; vaginal discharge, breast development
Male	Puberty onset, emissions, erections, pain or discharge from penis, swelling or pain in testicles
Both	Sexual activity, use of contraception, sexually transmitted infections
Musculoskeletal	Weakness, clumsiness, poor coordination, balance, tremors, abnormal gait, painful muscles or joints, swelling or redness of joints, fractures, scoliosis
Neurologic	Brain or head injuries, delayed speech and vocabulary development, problems with articulation
	Seizures, fainting spells, dizziness, numbness
	Learning problems, attention span, hyperactivity, memory problems

Information about daily routines, psychosocial information, and other living patterns forms the basis for many nursing diagnoses as well as the nursing care plan. Collection of information should focus on issues that have an impact on the quality of daily living, even if some data seem to overlap with disease data (Box 5–2).

The psychosocial history for adolescents should focus on critical aspects in their lives (e.g., home environment, education, activities, safety) that may contribute to a less-than-optimal environment for normal growth and development (Goldenring & Rosen, 2004). Possible screening questions to help identify issues for potential intervention are found in Table 5–5.

DEVELOPMENTAL STATUS Information about the child's motor, cognitive, language, and social development will help to plan nursing care. Ask the parent about the child's milestones and current fine and gross motor skills. Obtain the age at which the child first used words appropriately and the current words used or language ability. For children in school, ask about academic performance to assess cognitive development. Ask the parent about the child's manner of interaction with other children, family members, and strangers. Guidelines for a nursing assessment of development can be found in Chapter 3 ∞.

DEVELOPMENTAL APPROACH TO THE EXAMINATION

The sequence and approach to the examination varies by age. Provide a comfortable atmosphere for the examination with privacy so that modesty is respected. Explain the procedures as you begin to perform them. In young children, a foot-to-head sequence is often used so that the least distressing parts of the examination are completed first. In older cooperative children, the head-to-toe approach is generally used.

Newborns and Infants Under 6 Months of Age

Infants are among the easiest children to examine, as they do not resist the examination procedure. Keep the parent present to provide security to the infant. Provide physical comfort during the examination by feeding, using a pacifier, cuddling, or changing the diaper to keep the infant calm and quiet. Distraction such as rocking or clicking noises may help when the infant begins to get distressed. Observe the infant for general level of activity, overall mood, and responsiveness to handling.

Keep the sequence of the examination flexible to take advantage of times the infant is quiet or asleep to auscultate the lungs, heart, and abdomen. If the infant continues to be quiet or can be quieted with a pacifier, palpate the abdomen while the muscles are relaxed. The remainder of the examination can proceed in a head-to-toe sequence. Portions of the examination that will disturb the infant, such as the examination of the hips, should be performed at the end.

Infants Over 6 Months of Age

Because of developing separation and stranger anxiety, it is often best to keep the older infant with the parent. The infant and toddler can be examined on the parent's lap and then held against the parent's chest for some steps, such as the ear examination. The infant will not object to having clothing removed, but make sure the room is warm for the infant's comfort. Observe the infant's general level of activity, mood, and responsiveness to handling by the parent.

Smile and talk soothingly to the infant during the procedure. Use toys to distract the older infant. Use a pacifier or bottle to quiet the child when necessary. Because the infant may be fearful of being touched by a stranger, begin with the feet and hands before moving to the trunk. However, take advantage of opportunities presented when the infant is sleeping or quiet to auscultate the heart and lungs.

Toddlers

Toddlers may be active, curious, shy, cautious, or slow to warm up. Because of stranger anxiety, keep toddlers with their parents, often examining them on the parent's lap. It is possible to create a flat surface for the abdominal and genital examination by sitting close to the parent with knees together. For invasive procedures (ear, eye, and mouth exam) the parent can hold the child closely to the chest with legs between the parent's legs. The cranial nerve assessment or developmental assessment can be used as a method to gain cooperation for other procedures. Much of the neurologic and musculoskeletal assessment can be conducted by observing the child play and walk around in the examining room.

Tell the child what you will do at each step of the examination, using a confident voice that expects cooperation rather than asking. When a choice is possible, let the child have some control. For example, let the toddler choose which ear to examine first or to stand or sit for a certain part of the examination. Let the child hold a security object if it helps.

Table 5–5	ADOLESCENT PSYCHOSOCIAL ASSESSMENT USING THE HEEADSSS SCREENING TOOL

Question Categories	Screening Questions
Home Environment	• Where do you live? Who lives with you? Do you have your own room? • What are relationships like at home? • To whom are you closest at home? • To whom can you talk at home? • Is there anyone new at home? Has someone left recently? • Have you ever had to live away from home? (Why?)
Employment and **E**ducation	• Are you currently in school? • What are your favorite subjects at school? Your least favorite subjects? • How are your grades? Any recent changes? Any dramatic changes in the past? • Have you changed schools in the past few years? • What are your future education/employment plans/goals? • Are you working? Where? How much? • Tell me about your friends at school.
Eating	• What do you like and not like about your body? • Have there been any recent changes in your weight? • Have you dieted in the last year? How? How often? • Have you done anything else to try to manage your weight? • How much exercise do you get in an average day? Week? • What do you think would be a healthy diet? How does that compare with your current eating patterns?
Activities	• What do you and your *friends* do for fun? (With whom, where, and when?) • What do you and your *family* do for fun? (With whom, where, and when?) • Do you participate in any sports or other activities? • Do you regularly attend a church group, club, or other organized activity?
Drugs (Substance Use)	• Do any of your friends use tobacco? Alcohol? Other drugs? • Does anyone in your family use tobacco? Alcohol? Other drugs? • Do you use tobacco? Alcohol? Other drugs? • Is there any history of alcohol or drug problems in your family? Does anyone at home use tobacco?
Sexuality	• Have you ever been in a romantic relationship? • Tell me about the people that you've dated OR Tell me about your sex life. • Have any of your relationships ever been sexual relationships? • Are your sexual activities enjoyable? • What does the term *safer sex* mean to you? • Are you interested in boys? Girls? Both?
Suicide/Depression	• Do you feel sad or down more than usual? • Do you find yourself crying more than usual? • Are you "bored" all the time? • Have you thought a lot about hurting yourself or someone else?
Safety (Savagery)	• Have you ever been seriously injured? (How?) How about anyone else you know? • Do you always wear a seat belt in the car? • Have you ever ridden with a driver who was drunk or high? When? How often? • Do you use safety equipment for sports or other physical activities (for example, helmets for biking or skateboarding)? • Is there any violence in your home? Does the violence ever get physical? • Is there a lot of violence at your school? In your neighborhood? Among your friends? • Have you ever been physically or sexually abused? Have you ever been raped, on a date or at any other time (If not asked previously)?

From: Goldenring, J. M., & Rosen, D. S. (2004). Getting into adolescent heads: An essential update. *Contemporary Pediatrics, 21*(1), 64–90.

Attempt to reduce the child's anxiety by demonstrating the use of instruments on the parent or security object. Begin the examination by touching the feet and then moving gradually toward the body and head. Instruments to examine the ears, eyes, and mouth are usually viewed as the most fearful and should be used at the end of the examination.

Preschoolers

Assess the willingness of the child to be separated from the parent. Younger children will often prefer to be examined on the parent's lap, while older children will be comfortable on the examining table. Most children are willing to undress, but leave the underpants

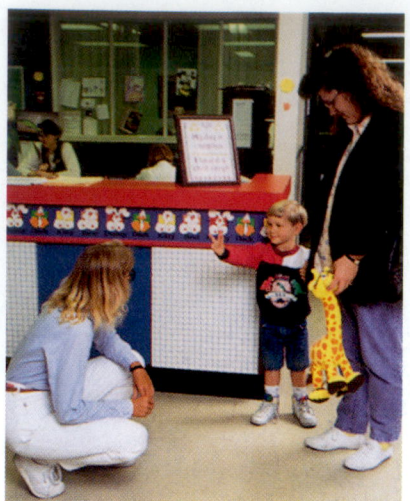

Figure 5–3 ➤ Examination of the child begins from the first contact. You should be observing the behavior of the child and parent by using visual cues to make a proper assessment. Does the child appear well nourished? Does the child appear secure with the parent?

SKILLS 6–1 THROUGH 6–7: *Growth Measurements*

> **CLINICAL TIP**
>
> Special growth curves are available for children with Down syndrome, Turner syndrome, and for children adopted from other countries.

> **CLINICAL TIP**
>
> The palms of the hands and soles of the feet are often lighter than the rest of the skin surface in children with dark skin. In addition, their lips may normally appear slightly bluish.

EQUIPMENT NEEDED

Gloves

on until conducting the genital examination. Most children in this age group are cooperative during the physical examination. Some children will prefer to have the head, eyes, ears, and mouth examined first while others will prefer to postpone them to the end.

Allow the child to touch and play with the equipment. Give simple explanations about the assessment procedures, and offer choice where there is one during the examination. Use distraction to gain the child's cooperation during the examination, such as asking the child to count, name colors, or talk about a favorite activity. Give positive feedback when the child cooperates.

School-Age Children

School-age children willingly cooperate during the examination and sit on the examining table. Anticipate the development of modesty in school-age children and offer a patient gown to cover the underwear. Let the older school-age child determine if the examination will be conducted in privacy or with the parent or siblings present.

A head-to-toe sequence can be used in this age group. Demonstrate how the instruments are used and let the child handle them if he or she wishes. As you perform the examination, tell the child what you are doing and why. Offer as many choices as possible to help the child feel empowered. The examination is a good opportunity to teach the child about how the body works, such as letting the child listen to heart and breath sounds.

Adolescents

Protect the adolescent's modesty before the examination by providing a private place to undress and put on the patient gown, and then during the examination by covering the parts of the body not being assessed. Use the head-to-toe sequence and the same procedures used for adults. Perform the examination in private without parent or siblings unless the adolescent specifically requests the parent's presence. Provide a chaperone when the parent or accompanying adult is not present during the examination.

Adolescents often have lots of concerns regarding their developing bodies. When appropriate, provide reassurance about the normal progression of secondary sexual characteristic development and what further changes to expect.

GENERAL APPRAISAL

The examination begins upon first meeting the child (Figure 5–3 ➤). Measure the infant's weight, length, and head circumference. If the child can stand, substitute a standing height measurement for length. Plot the measurements on the appropriate growth curves (Appendix A ∞). Take the child's temperature, heart rate, respiratory rate, and blood pressure.

Observe the child's general appearance and behavior. The child should appear well nourished and well developed. Infants and young children are often fearful and seek reassurance from their parents. The child may resist interacting with the nurse until rapport is established.

Observe the behavior and tone of voice used by the parent when he or she is talking to the child. Is the child encouraged to speak? Is the child appropriately reassured or supported by the parent? The child should feel secure with the parent and perceive permission to interact with the nurse.

ASSESSING SKIN AND HAIR CHARACTERISTICS

Examination of the skin requires good lighting to detect variations in skin color and to identify lesions. Daylight is preferred when available. Rather than inspecting the child's entire skin surface at one time, examine the skin simultaneously with other body systems as each region of the body is exposed.

Inspection of the Skin

Use gloves to inspect the child's skin for color and the presence of imperfections, elevations, or other lesions.

BOX 5–3
EXAMINATION TECHNIQUES

Following are the specific examination techniques:

- **Inspection.** Purposefully observing the child's physical features and behaviors. Physical feature characteristics include size, shape, color, movement, position, and location. Detection of odors is also a part of inspection.
- **Palpation.** Using touch to identify characteristics of the skin, internal organs, and masses. Characteristics include texture, moistness, tenderness, temperature, position, shape, consistency, and mobility of masses and organs. The palmar surface of the fingers and fingerpads helps determine position, size, consistency, and masses. The ulnar surface of the hand is best to detect vibrations.
- **Auscultation.** Listening to sounds produced by the airway, lungs, stomach, heart, and blood vessels to identify their characteristics. Auscultation is usually performed with a stethoscope to enhance the sounds heard.
- **Percussion.** Striking the surface of the body, either directly or indirectly, to set up vibrations that reveal the density of underlying tissues and borders of internal organs.

Skin Color

The color of the child's skin usually has an even distribution. Check for color variations—such as increased or decreased pigmentation, pallor, mottling, bruises, erythema, cyanosis, or jaundice—that may be associated with local or generalized conditions. Some variations in skin color are common and normal, such as freckles found in the White population and Mongolian spots found on dark-skinned infants (Figure 5–4 ➤). Bruises are common on the knees, shins, and lower arms as children stumble and fall. Bruises on other parts of the body, especially in various stages of healing, should raise a suspicion of child abuse. Bruises often go through various color changes as the body reabsorbs blood over several days. The transition of color often progresses through reddish blue, brownish blue, brownish green, greenish yellow, and yellow-brown before returning to normal skin color. Note any tattoos or body piercings.

When a skin color abnormality is suspected, inspect the buccal mucosa and tongue to confirm the color change. This is especially important in children with darker skin because the mucous membranes are usually pink, regardless of skin color. Press the gums lightly for 1 to 2 seconds. Any residual color, such as that seen in jaundice or cyanosis, is more easily detected in blanched skin. Jaundice may also be noticed in the sclerae of the eyes. Generalized cyanosis is associated with respiratory and cardiac disorders. Jaundice is associated with liver disorders.

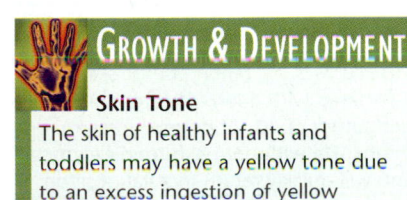

GROWTH & DEVELOPMENT

Skin Tone
The skin of healthy infants and toddlers may have a yellow tone due to an excess ingestion of yellow vegetables.

Palpation of the Skin

Palpation of the skin provides a sense of its characteristics: temperature, texture, moistness, and resilience or turgor. To evaluate these characteristics, lightly touch or stroke the skin's surface. Follow standard precautions by wearing gloves when palpating mucous membranes, open wounds, and lesions. The following list provides details on each of the characteristics of skin palpation.

Temperature

The child's skin normally feels warm to the touch when placing the wrist or dorsum of the hand against the child's skin. Excessively warm skin may indicate the presence of fever or inflammation, whereas abnormally cool skin may be a sign of shock or cold exposure.

Texture

Children have soft, smooth skin over the entire body. Identify any areas of roughness, thickening, or **induration** (area of extra firmness with a distinct border). Abnormalities in texture are associated with endocrine disorders, chronic irritation, and inflammation.

Mongolian spot

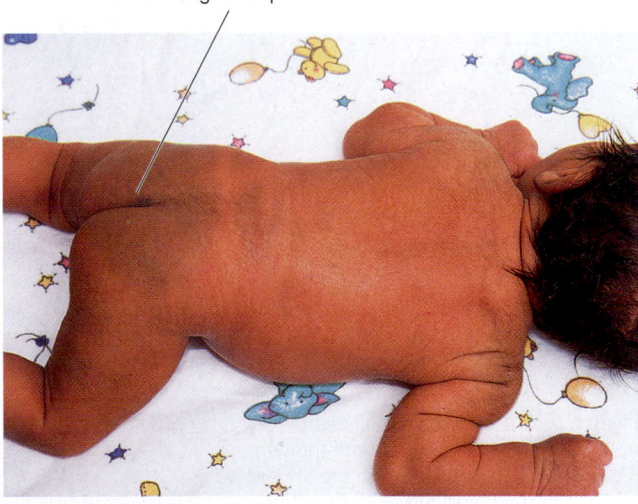

Figure 5–4 ➤ Mongolian spots are large patches of bluish-colored skin with wavy borders and irregular shapes often seen in the sacral area of the back. They are a normal occurrence in a large majority of Native American, Asian, Black, and Hispanic infants, but are sometimes incorrectly thought to be bruises. Mongolian spots usually fade during the first few years of life and disappear by puberty. Mongolian spots covering extensive areas of the posterior and anterior trunk and extremities may be a sign of an inborn error of metabolism (Ashrafi, Shabanian, Mohammadi et al., 2006).

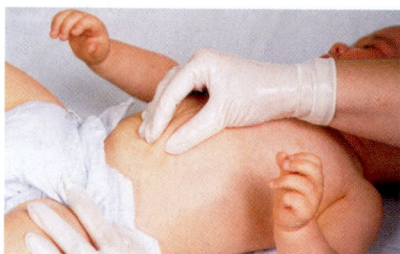

Figure 5–5 ➤ Tenting of the skin associated with poor skin turgor. Assess skin turgor on the abdomen, forearm, or thigh. Skin with normal turgor is elastic and will quickly return to a flat position.

Figure 5–6 ➤ Capillary refill technique: A, Pinch the end of a finger until the skin is blanched. B, Quickly release the finger and watch the blood return to the veins. Count the seconds it takes for the color to return or veins to fill. Slow color return or vein filling time could be related to shock or constriction due to a tight bandage or cast. Small-vein filling time technique: C, Using the index finger, milk a vein on the dorsum of the hand or foot from proximal to distal. D, Release your pressure and color should promptly return.

Moistness

The child's skin is normally dry to the touch. The skin may feel slightly damp when the child has been exercising or crying. Excessive sweating without exertion may be associated with a fever, bronchopulmonary dysplasia, or an uncorrected congenital heart defect.

Resilience (Turgor)

The child's skin is elastic and mobile because of the balanced distribution of intracellular and extracellular fluids. To evaluate skin turgor, pinch a small amount of skin on the abdomen between the thumb and forefinger, release the skin, and watch the speed of recoil (Figure 5–5 ➤). Skin with good turgor rapidly returns to its previous contour. Skin with poor turgor tents or stands up rather than resuming its previous contour. Poor skin turgor is commonly associated with dehydration. Skin that is taut is associated with edema or swelling.

If **edema**, an accumulation of excess fluid in the interstitial spaces, is present, the skin feels doughy or boggy. To test for the degree of edema present, the examiner presses for 5 seconds against a bone beneath the area of puffy skin, releases the pressure, and observes how rapidly the indentation disappears. If the indentation rapidly disappears, the edema is "nonpitting." Slow disappearance of the indentation indicates "pitting" edema, which is commonly associated with kidney or heart disorders.

Capillary Refill and Small-Vein Filling Times

Two techniques can determine the adequacy of tissue *perfusion* (oxygen circulating to the tissues). When capillary refill time or small-vein filling times suggest that tissue perfusion is inadequate, immediately assess the child for shock or a physical constriction such as a cast or bandage that is too tight. The capillary refill time is normally less than 2 seconds (Figure 5–6 A and B ➤). The small-vein filling time is normally less than 4 seconds (Figure 5–6 C and D ➤).

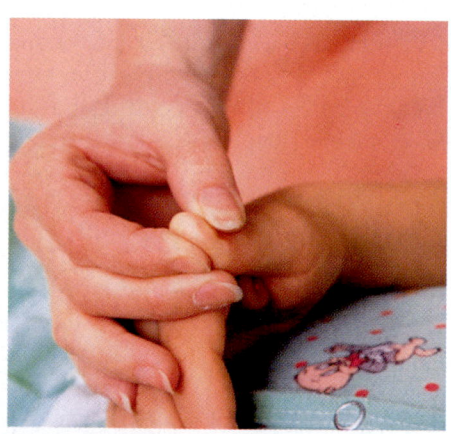

A

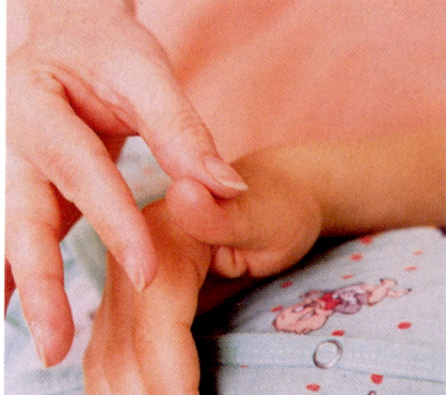

B

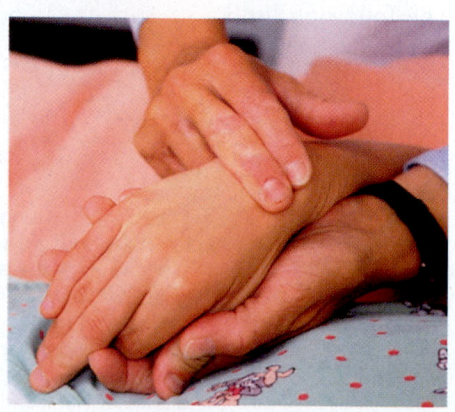

C

D

Skin Lesions

Skin lesions usually indicate an abnormal skin condition. Characteristics such as location, size, type of lesion, pattern, and discharge, if present, provide clues about the cause of the condition. Inspect and palpate the isolated or generalized skin color abnormalities, elevations, lesions, or injuries to describe all characteristics present.

Primary lesions (such as macules, papules, and vesicles) are often the skin's initial response to injury or infection. Mongolian spots and freckles are normal findings that are also classified as primary lesions. Figure 5–7 ➤ describes common primary lesions. *Secondary lesions* (such as scars, ulcers, fissures) are the result of irritation, infection, and delayed healing of primary lesions (see Chapter 30 ∞).

Common patterns of skin lesions are described as follows:

- Annular—circular, begins in center and spreads to periphery
- Polycyclic—annular lesions running together

PATHOPHYSIOLOGY ILLUSTRATED

Common Primary Skin Lesions and Associated Conditions

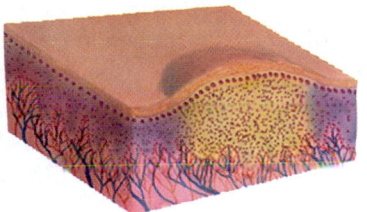

Lesion Name: Papule
Description: Elevated, firm, diameter <1 cm (1/2 in.)
Example: Warts, pigmented nevi

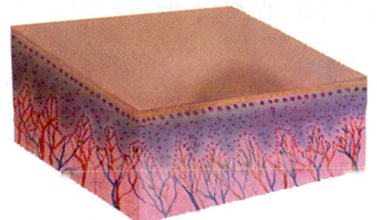

Lesion Name: Macule
Description: Flat, nonpalpable, diameter <1 cm (1/2 in.)
Example: Freckle, rubella, rubeola, petechiae

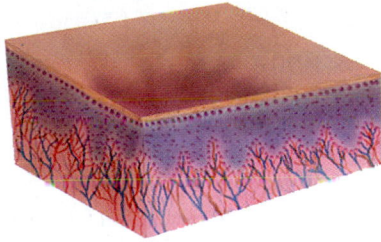

Lesion Name: Patch
Description: Macule diameter >1 cm (1/2 in.)
Example: Vitiligo, Mongolian spot

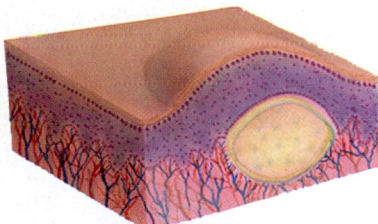

Lesion Name: Nodule
Description: Elevated, firm, deeper in dermis than papule, diameter 1–2 cm (1/2 in.-1 in.)
Example: Erythema nodosum

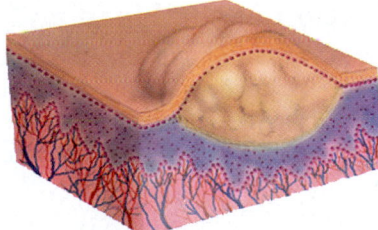

Lesion Name: Tumor
Description: Elevated, solid, diameter >2 cm (1 in.)
Example: Neoplasm, hemangioma

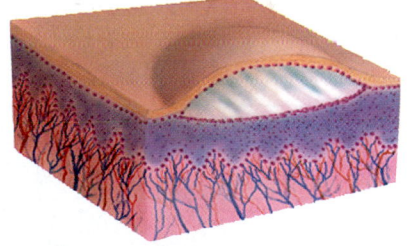

Lesion Name: Vesicle
Description: Elevated, filled with fluid, diameter <1 cm (1/2 in.)
Example: Early chickenpox, herpes simplex

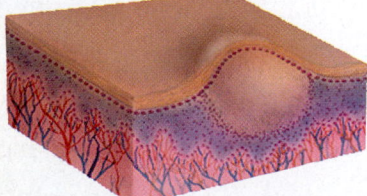

Lesion Name: Pustule
Description: Vesicle filled with purulent fluid
Example: Impetigo, acne

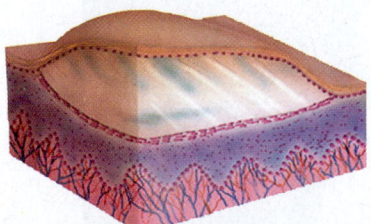

Lesion Name: Bulla
Description: Vesicle, diameter >1 cm (1/2 in.)
Example: Burn blister

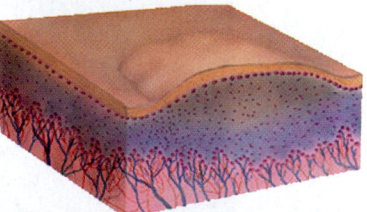

Lesion Name: Wheal
Description: Irregular elevated solid area of edematous skin
Example: Urticaria, insect bite

Figure 5–7 ➤ Common primary skin lesions and associated conditions.

- Linear—in a row or stripe
- Herpetiform—grouped or clustered
- Gyrate—twisted, spiral, coiled

Inspection of the Hair

Inspect the scalp hair for color, distribution, and cleanliness. The hair shafts should be evenly colored, shiny, and either curly or straight. Variation in hair color not caused by bleaching can be associated with a nutritional deficiency. Normally, hair is distributed evenly over the scalp. Investigate areas of hair loss. Hair loss in a child may result from tight braids or skin lesions such as ringworm (see Chapter 30 ∞). Notice any unusual hair growth patterns. An unusually low hairline on the neck or forehead may be associated with a congenital disorder such as hypothyroidism.

Children are frequently exposed to head lice. Inspect the individual hair shafts for small nits (lice eggs) that adhere to the hair (Figure 5–8 ➤). None should be present.

Observe the distribution of body hair as other skin surfaces are exposed during examination. Fine hair covers most areas of the body. Body hair in unexpected places should be noted. For example, a tuft of hair at the base of the spine may indicate a pilonidal cyst. It is important to note the age at which pubic and axillary hair develops in the child. Development at an unusually young age is associated with precocious puberty.

Palpation of the Hair

Palpate the hair shafts for texture. Hair should feel soft or silky with fine or thick shafts. Endocrine conditions such as hypothyroidism may result in coarse, brittle hair. Part the hair in various spots over the head to inspect and palpate the scalp for crusting or other lesions. If scalp lesions are present, describe them using the characteristics in Figure 5–7 or Table 30–3.

ASSESSING THE HEAD FOR SKULL CHARACTERISTICS AND FACIAL FEATURES

What can cause a child's head or face to be asymmetric? How does a normal fontanel feel? What does an unusually large or small head suggest in an infant?

Inspection of the Head and Face

During early childhood the skull's sutures permit expansion for brain growth (Figure 5–9 ➤). Infants and young children normally have a rounded skull with a prominent occipital area. The shape of the head changes during childhood and the occipital area becomes less prominent. An abnormal skull shape can result from premature closure of the sutures.

GROWTH & DEVELOPMENT

Pubic Hair Development
Pubic hair begins to develop in children between 8 and 12 years of age, and axillary hair develops about 6 months later. Facial hair is noted in boys shortly after axillary hair develops.

CLINICAL TIP

Children who were low-birth-weight infants often have a flat, elongated skull because the soft skull bones were flattened by the weight of the head early in infancy. Head flattening is also associated with the recommended sleeping position for infants—on their back. See Chapter 26 ∞ .

EQUIPMENT NEEDED

Tape measure

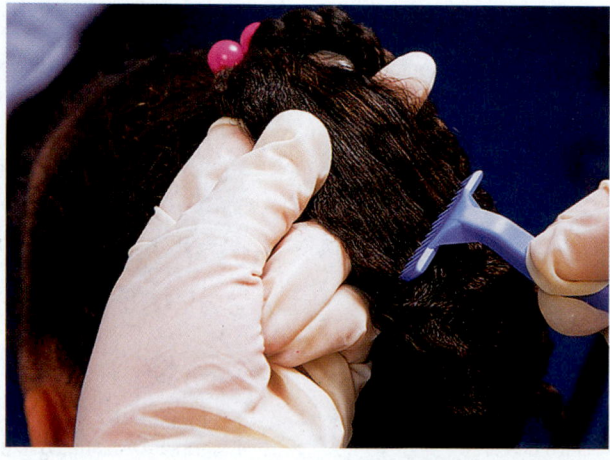

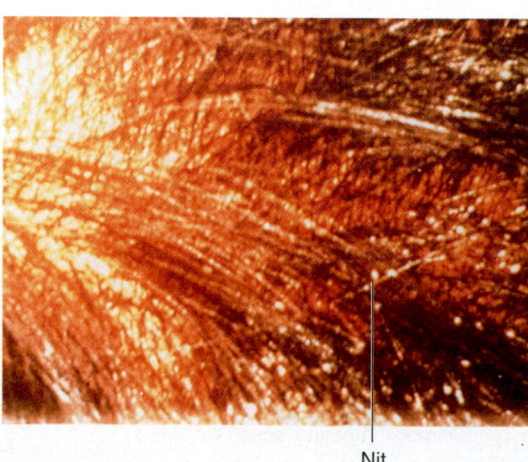

Nit

A   B

Figure 5–8 ➤ A, Inspecting for head lice with a fine-tooth comb. B, Nits on hair. Courtesy of Centers for Disease Control.

AS CHILDREN GROW
Sutures and Fontanels of the Skull

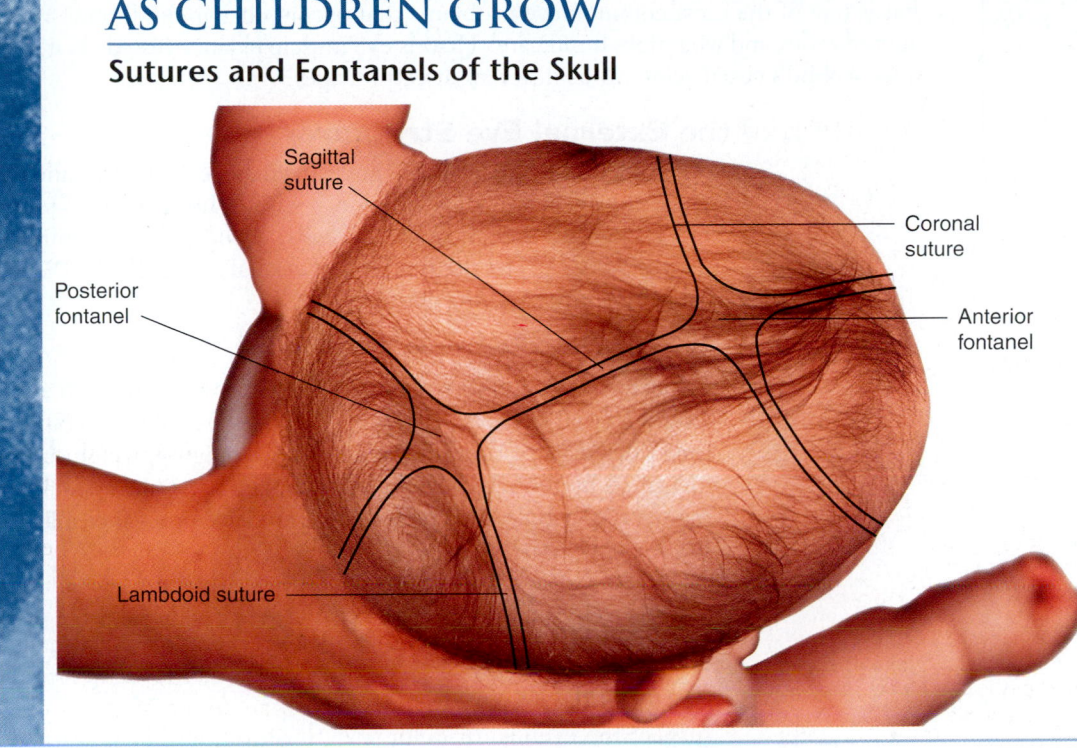

Sagittal suture

Coronal suture

Posterior fontanel

Anterior fontanel

Lambdoid suture

Figure 5–9 ➤ The **sutures** are fibrous connections between the bones of the skull that have not yet ossified. The fontanels are formed at the intersection of these sutures where bone has not yet formed. Fontanels are covered by tough membranous tissue that protects the brain. The posterior fontanel closes between 2 and 3 months. The anterior fontanel and sutures are palpable up to the age of 18 months. The suture lines of the skull are seldom palpated after 2 years of age. After that time, the sutures rarely separate.

The head circumference of infants and young children is routinely measured with a tape measure until 3 years of age to ensure that adequate growth for brain development has occurred. The *Clinical Skills Manual* describes the proper technique. A larger-than-normal head is associated with hydrocephalus, and a smaller-than-normal head suggests microcephaly.

Inspect the child's face for symmetry during several facial expressions such as resting, smiling, talking, and crying (Figure 5–10 ➤). Significant asymmetry may result from paralysis of trigeminal or facial nerves (cranial nerves V or VII), in utero positioning, and swelling from infection, allergy, or trauma.

Next inspect the face for unusual facial features such as coarseness, wide eye spacing, or disproportionate size. Tremors, tics, and twitching of facial muscles are often associated with seizures.

Palpation of the Skull

Palpate the skull in infants and young children to assess the sutures and fontanels and to detect soft bones.

Sutures

Use your fingerpads to palpate each suture line. The edge of each bone in the suture line can be felt, but normally there is no separation of the two bones. If additional bone edges are felt, it may indicate a skull fracture.

Fontanels

At the intersection of the sutures, palpate the anterior and posterior fontanels. The fontanel should feel flat and firm inside the bony edges. The anterior fontanel is normally smaller than 5 cm (2 in.) in diameter at 6 months of age and then becomes progressively smaller. It closes between 12 and 18 months of age. The posterior fontanel closes between 2 and 3 months of age.

A tense fontanel, bulging above the margin of the skull, is an indication of increased intracranial pressure. A soft fontanel, sunken below the margin of the skull, is associated with dehydration.

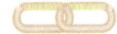

SKILL 6–5:
Measuring Head Circumference

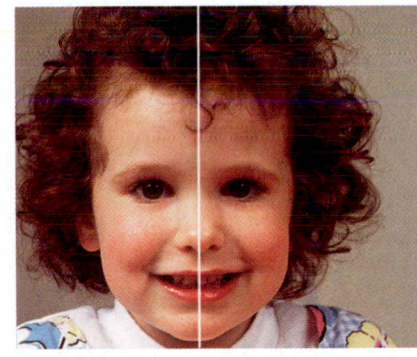

Figure 5–10 ➤ Draw an imaginary line down the middle of the face over the nose and compare the features on each side. Significant asymmetry may be caused by paralysis of cranial nerve V or VII, in utero positioning, and swelling from infection, allergy, or trauma.

CULTURE

Touching the Head
The head is a sacred part of the body to Southeast Asians. Ask for permission before touching the infant's head to palpate the sutures and fontanels (Spector, 2004). When a Hispanic child is examined, however, not touching the head may be considered bad luck.

ASSESSING EYE STRUCTURES, FUNCTION, AND VISION

What is one of the most common eye problems that occurs during childhood? What is the red reflex and what does it indicate? How is eye muscle balance tested? Is it normal for a child's visual acuity to be different at certain ages?

Inspection of the External Eye Structures

The function of the external and internal eye structures and related cranial nerves makes vision possible. Inspect the external eye structures, including the eyeballs, eyelids, and eye muscles (Figure 5–11 ➤). Test the function of cranial nerves II, III, IV, and VI, which innervate the eye structures.

Eye Size and Spacing

Inspect the eyes and surrounding tissues simultaneously when examining facial features. The eyes should be the same size but not unusually large or small. Observe for eye bulging, which can be identified by retracted eyelids or a sunken appearance. Bulging may be associated with a tumor, and a sunken appearance may reflect dehydration.

Next inspect the eyes to see if they are appropriately distanced from each other. **Hypertelorism,** or widely spaced eyes, can be a normal variation in children.

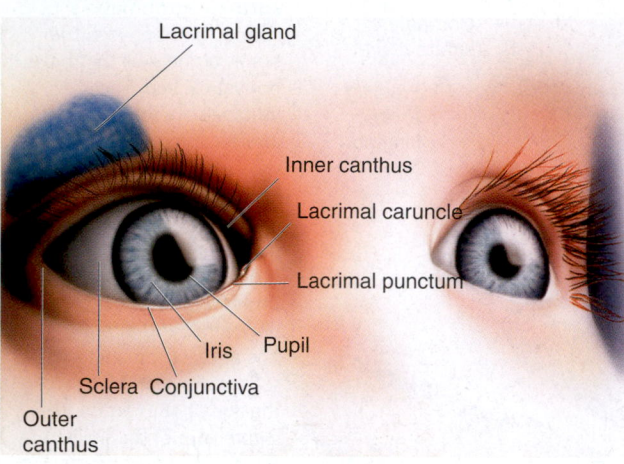

Figure 5–11 ➤ External structures of the eye. Notice that the light reflex is at the same location on each eye.

Eyelids and Eyelashes

Inspect the eyelids for color, size, position, mobility, and condition of the eyelashes. Eyelids should be the same color as surrounding facial skin and free of swelling or inflammation along the edges. Sebaceous glands that look like yellow striations are often present near the hair follicles. Eyelashes curl away from the eye to prevent irritation of the conjunctivae.

Inspect the conjunctivae lining the eyelids by pulling down the lower lid and then everting the upper lid. The conjunctivae should be pink and glossy. The lacrimal punctum, the opening for the lacrimal gland on each lid, is located near the medial canthus. No redness or excess tearing should be present.

When the eyes are open, inspect the level at which the upper and lower lids cross the eye. Each lid normally covers part of the iris but not any portion of the pupil. The lids should also close completely over the iris and cornea. *Ptosis*, drooping of the eyelid that covers some of the pupil, is often associated with injury to the oculomotor nerve, cranial nerve III. *Sunset sign*, in which the sclera is seen between the upper lid and the iris, may indicate retracted eyelids or hydrocephalus.

Inspect the eyes for the palpebral slant (Figure 5–12 ➤). The eyelids of most people open horizontally. An upward slant is a normal finding in Asian children; however, children with Down syndrome also often have an upward slant (Figure 5–13 ➤). A downward slant is seen in some children as a normal variation.

Eye Color

Inspect the color of each sclera, iris, and bulbar conjunctiva. The sclera is normally white or ivory in darker-skinned children. Sclerae of another color suggest the presence of an underlying disease. For example, yellow sclerae indicate jaundice. Typically the iris is blue or light colored at birth and becomes pigmented within 6 months. Inspect the iris for the presence of Brushfield spots, white specks in a linear pattern around the iris circumference, which are often associated with Down syndrome. The bulbar conjunctivae, which cover the sclera to the edge of the cornea, are normally clear. Redness can indicate eyestrain, allergies, or irritation.

Pupils

Inspect the pupils for size and shape. Normally the pupils are round, clear, and equal in size. Some children have a **coloboma**, a keyhole-shaped pupil caused by a notch in the iris. This sign can indicate that the child has other congenital anomalies.

> **CLINICAL TIP**
>
> Children of Asian descent often have an extra fold of skin, known as the epicanthal fold, covering all or part of the medial canthus of the eye.

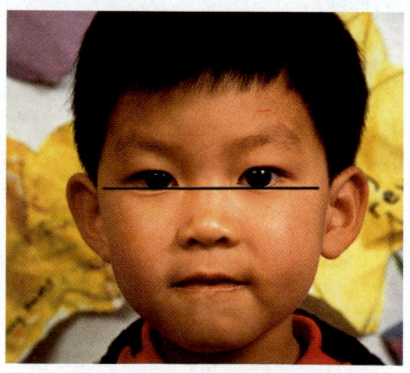

Figure 5–12 ➤ Draw an imaginary line across the medial canthi and extend it to each side of the face to identify the slant of the palpebral fissures. When the line crosses the lateral canthi, the palpebral fissures are horizontal and no slant is present. When the lateral canthi fall above the imaginary line, the eyes have an upward slant. A downward slant is present when the lateral canthi fall below the imaginary line. Epicanthal folds are present when an extra fold of skin partially or completely covers the caruncles in the medial canthi. Which type of slant does this child have?

To test the pupillary response to light, shine a bright light into one eye. A brisk constriction of both the pupil exposed to direct light and the other pupil is a normal finding.

To test pupillary response to accommodation, ask the child to look first at a near object (for example, a toy) and then at a distant object (for example, a picture on the wall). The expected response is pupil constriction with near objects and pupil dilation with distant objects. This procedure tests the optic nerve, cranial nerve II.

Inspection of the Eye Muscles

It is important to detect strabismus, or crossed eyes, because, if uncorrected, visual impairment can result. The evaluation of extraocular movements, the corneal light reflex, and the cover–uncover test are used to detect a muscle imbalance.

Extraocular Movements

Seat the child at eye level to evaluate the extraocular movements. Hold a toy or penlight 30 cm (12 in.) from the child's eyes and move it through the six cardinal fields of gaze as shown in Figure 5–14 ➤. Test a young infant's ability to follow an object from side to side. The child's head may need to be held still until fine motor eye movement develops. Both eyes should move together, tracking the object. This procedure tests the oculomotor, trochlear, and abducens nerves (cranial nerves III, IV, and VI).

Corneal Light Reflex

To test the corneal light reflex, shine a light on the child's nose, midway between the eyes. Identify the location where the light is reflected on each eye. The light reflection is normally symmetric, at the same spot on each cornea. An asymmetric corneal light reflex indicates strabismus (see Figure 5–11).

Cover–Uncover Test

The cover–uncover test can be used to test for eye muscle weakness in older, cooperative children, usually at about 4 or 5 years. See Figure 5–15 ➤ for the technique. Because the eyes work together, no obvious movement of either eye is expected. Unexpected movement of one eye indicates a muscle imbalance.

Vision Assessment

Vision is an important sense for learning, and assessment is essential to detect any serious problems. Vision is evaluated using an age-appropriate vision test, but no simple method exists. It is possible to assess vision in infants and children by observing their behavior in response to certain maneuvers and during play.

Infants and Toddlers

When the infant's eyes are open, test the blink reflex by moving your hand quickly toward the infant's eyes. A quick blink is the normal response. Absence of the blink reflex can indicate that the infant is blind.

To test an infant's ability to visually track an object, hold a light or toy about 15 cm (6 in.) from the infant's eyes. When the infant has fixated on or is staring at the object, move it slowly to each side. The infant should follow the object with the eyes and by moving the head.

Once an infant has developed skills to reach for and then pick up objects, observe play behavior to evaluate vision. The ability to easily find and pick up small toys is a good indicator of vision in children under 3 years of age.

Standardized Vision Charts

Standardized vision charts cannot be used to test vision until the child can understand directions and can cooperate, usually at about 3 or 4 years of age. The Snellen E chart, HOTV chart, and the Picture chart are used to test visual acuity of preschool-age children just as the Snellen Letter chart is used for school-age children and adolescents. The *Clinical Skills Manual* describes the use of these charts.

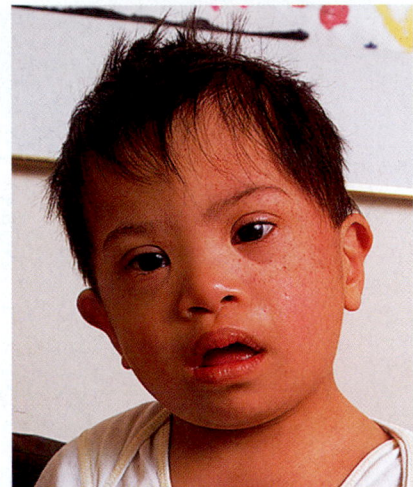

Figure 5–13 ➤ The eyes of this boy with Down syndrome show an upward slant.

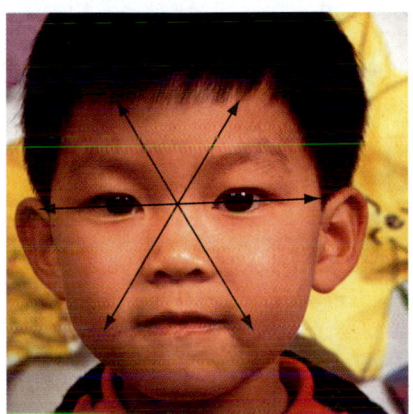

Figure 5–14 ➤ Begin the eye muscle examination with inspection of the extraocular movements. Have the child sit at your eye level. Hold a toy or penlight about 30 cm (12 in.) from the child's eyes and move it through the six cardinal fields of gaze. Both eyes should move together, tracking the object. This procedure tests cranial nerves III, IV, and VI.

GROWTH & DEVELOPMENT

Visual Acuity
Research has revealed that a newborn has vision at birth and prefers faces to other patterns or to following a moving object. The child's visual acuity develops during early childhood.

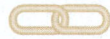

SKILLS 6–18 AND 6–19
Vision Acuity Screening

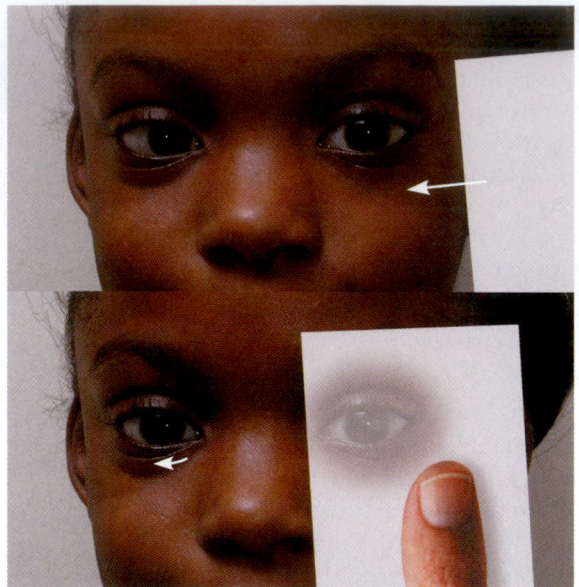
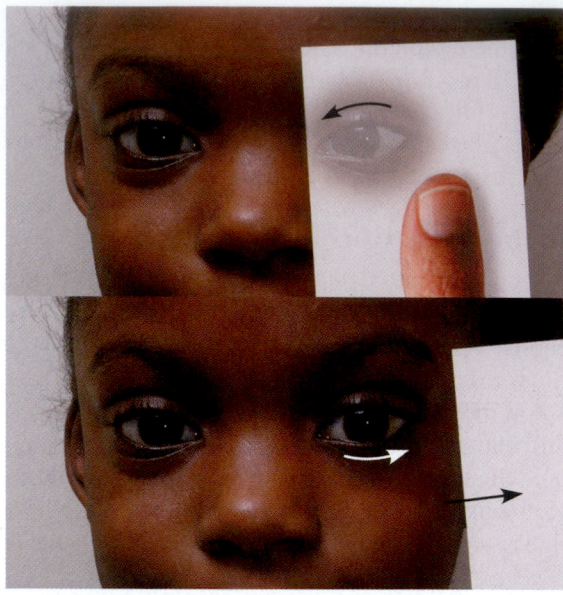

A Right, uncovered eye is weaker   B Left, covered eye is weaker

Figure 5–15 ➤ Cover–Uncover Test. With the child at your eye level, ask the child to look at a picture on the wall. A, As you cover one eye with an index card or paper cup, simultaneously observe for any movement of the uncovered eye. If it jumps to fixate on the picture, the uncovered eye has a muscle weakness. B, As you remove the cover from the eye, simultaneously observe the covered eye for any movement to fixate on the picture. If the eye has a muscle weakness, it drifts to a relaxed position once covered.

CLINICAL TIP

Indications for further evaluation include: visual acuity of 20/40 or less in either eye by 3 to 5 years of age, visual acuity of 20/30 or less in either eye by 6 years of age, or a difference in vision of 2 lines or more on the Snellen eye chart between the eyes, even within the passing range (American Academy of Pediatrics, 2003).

Inspection of the Internal Eye Structures

The fundiscopic examination allows inspection of the internal eye structures—the retina, optic disc, arteries and veins, and macula (Figure 5–16 ➤). The ophthalmoscope is a complex instrument and requires practice to master. The examination is difficult to perform on uncooperative children; it is most often performed by experienced examiners.

Darken the room so the child's pupils dilate. Explain the procedure to the child to gain his or her cooperation. Have a picture on the wall or have the parent or assistant hold a toy for the child to stare at so that the child's eye will not have to be forcibly held open.

Using the Ophthalmoscope

The ophthalmoscope has a lens-and-mirror system and a bright light for inspecting the structures of the internal eye. Different lens powers are arranged on the rotating disk of the ophthalmic head. This system permits compensation for vision differences between the child and examiner. The black numbered plus lenses magnify images, and

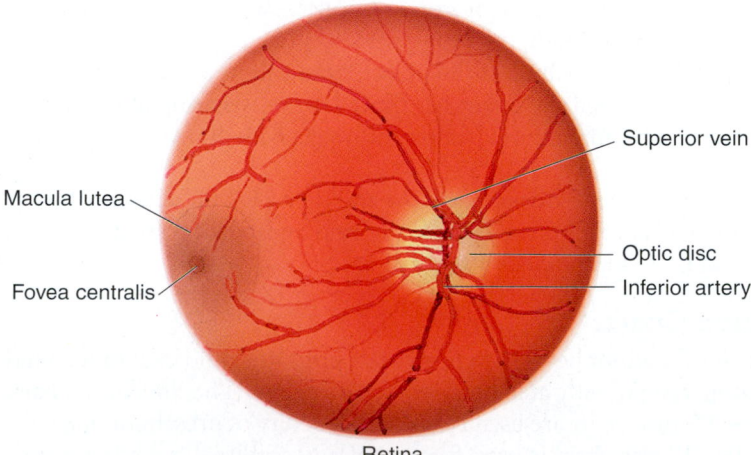

Macula lutea

Fovea centralis

Superior vein

Optic disc

Inferior artery

Retina

Figure 5–16 ➤ Normal fundus.

the red-numbered minus lenses reduce them in a range of powers. The lenses can be changed by rotating the disk with the forefinger.

Turn the ophthalmoscope on and set the lens power at zero. Keep a forefinger on the disk to change the lens power as needed. Look through the lens of the ophthalmoscope, stabilizing it by resting the top against an eyebrow and the handle against a cheek. Use your right eye to examine the child's right eye and your left eye to examine the child's left eye. This position is best for visualizing the eye, and it reduces direct exposure to infection. Place a hand on the child's head for stabilization.

RED REFLEX   Shine the ophthalmoscope light at the child's eye from a distance of 30 cm (12 in.). The first image seen is the red reflex, the reddish glow of the vascular retina. When the red reflex is seen, the light travels through colorless cornea, aqueous humor, lens, and vitreous humor to the retina. The red reflexes should be equal in color, intensity, and clarity. Black spots or opacities within the red reflex are abnormal and may indicate congenital cataracts, hemorrhage, or corneal scars. If a white reflex is seen, the light is reflecting off of a white abnormality, such as a retinoblastoma (McLaughlin & Levin, 2006). The red reflex can also be tested by shining a small flashlight into the eye.

VISUALIZING THE INTERNAL EYE STRUCTURES   Slowly move closer to the child. Deeper levels of the vitreous humor are inspected before the pink retina comes into view. The retina is a deeper pink in dark-skinned children. A blood vessel is the first retinal structure usually seen. Continue moving closer to the child's eye and adjust the plus or minus lenses to focus on this blood vessel. Retinal arteries appear smaller and brighter red than veins. The blood vessels branch to spread and cover the retina.

Inspect and follow the branching of the blood vessels toward the nose until they merge into the optic disc. Dark areas along the blood vessels may indicate retinal hemorrhages. Carefully inspect sites where arteries and veins cross. Notches and indentations at these sites are associated with hypertension.

The optic disc margin is normally sharply defined, round, and yellow to creamy pink. Blurring of the disc margins or bulging of the optic disc is a sign of increased intracranial pressure. Use the diameter of the optic disc to identify the location of other landmarks on the retina.

The macula is located approximately 2 disc diameters lateral to the optic disc. To see the macula, ask the child to look at the light. It appears as a yellow dot surrounded by deep pink. The macula is inspected last because the bright light causes the child to blink and look away.

ASSESSING THE EAR STRUCTURES AND HEARING

How do you identify proper ear placement on the head? What is the significance of low-set ears? Why is otitis media the most common ear problem during early childhood? What play activities can be used to test hearing in young children? How do you evaluate the hearing of an older child?

Inspection of the External Ear Structures

The position and characteristics of the *pinna*, the external ear, are inspected as a continuation of the head and eye examination. The pinna is considered "low set" when the top lies completely below an imaginary line drawn through the medial and lateral canthi of the eye toward the ear. Low-set ears are often associated with congenital renal disorders (Figure 5–17 ➤).

Inspect the pinna for any malformation. The pinna should be completely formed, with an open auditory canal. Next, inspect the tissue around the pinna for abnormalities. A pit or hole in front of the auditory canal may indicate the presence of a sinus. If one of the pinna protrudes outward, there may be swelling behind the ear, a sign of mastoiditis.

Inspect the external auditory canal for any discharge. A foul-smelling, purulent discharge may indicate the presence of a foreign body or an infection in the external

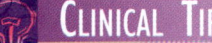

CLINICAL TIP

Keep the red reflex in view to make sure your head and the ophthalmoscope move as one unit. If you lose the red reflex when moving closer to the child, move back, find the red reflex, and start again.

EQUIPMENT NEEDED

Otoscope
Noisemakers (bell, rattle, tissue paper)
Tuning fork, 500–1000 Hz

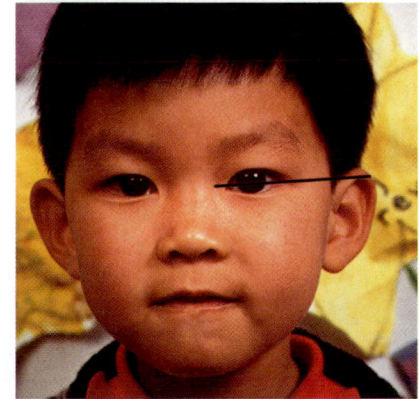

Figure 5–17 ➤   To detect the correct placement of the external ears, draw an imaginary line through the medial and lateral canthi of the eye toward the ear. This line normally passes through the upper portion of the pinna. The pinna is considered "low set" when the top lies completely below the imaginary line. Low-set ears are often associated with renal disorders. Is this a normal ear placement? Yes, it is.

CLINICAL TIP

Choose the largest ear speculum that fits into the auditory canal to form a seal for testing the movement of the tympanic membrane. A large speculum is also less likely to injure the auditory canal if the child moves suddenly.

SKILL 4–3
Positioning a Child for an Otoscope Examination

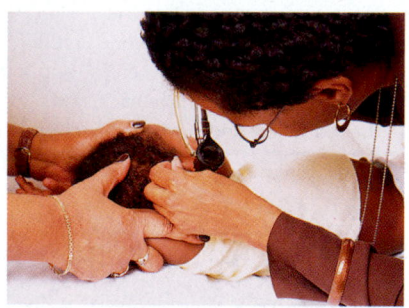

A

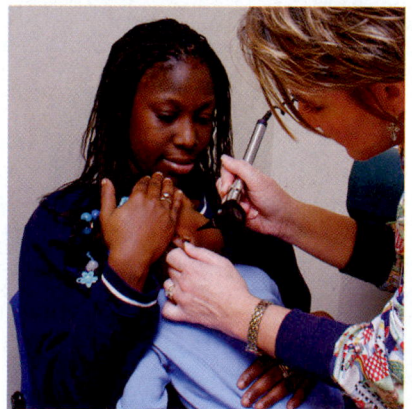

B

Figure 5–18 ➤ A, To restrain an uncooperative child, place the child supine on the examining table. Have an assistant hold the child's arms next to the head to restrain the child's head movements. Restrain the child's body movements by lying across the child's body. Keep your hands free to hold the otoscope and position the external ear. B, An alternate position is to sit the child on the parent's lap with the child's chest and head held firmly against the parent.

canal. Clear fluid or a blood-tinged discharge may indicate a cerebrospinal fluid leak caused by a basilar skull fracture.

Inspection of the Tympanic Membrane

Examination of the tympanic membrane is important in infants and young children because they are prone to acute otitis media, a middle ear infection. The eustachian tubes are shorter, wider, and more horizontally positioned in infants and young children than in older children and adults. This positioning enables bacteria to move from the pharynx, up the eustachian tube, and into the middle ear, causing an infection. See Figure 19–2 ∞.

The otoscope, an instrument with a magnifying lens, bright light, and speculum, is used to examine the internal auditory canal and tympanic membrane. Infants and young children often resist having their ears inspected with the otoscope because of past painful experiences. For that reason it may be wise to delay the otoscopic examination until portions of the assessment requiring cooperation are completed. Use simple explanations to prepare the child. Let the child play with the otoscope or demonstrate how it is used on the parent or a doll. Figure 5–18 ➤ illustrates one method for restraining an uncooperative child. The *Clinical Skills Manual* illustrates another positioning option.

Using the Otoscope

To begin the otoscopic examination, hold the handle of the otoscope in the palm of your hand with the thumb pointed toward the base of the handle. If using a pneumatic squeeze bulb, hold it between the index finger and the handle. Hold the otoscope in the hand closest to the child's face. When the child is cooperative, rest the back of that hand against the child's head to stabilize it. Use the other hand to pull the pinna toward the back of the head and either up or down. Pulling the pinna straightens the auditory canal and improves inspection of the tympanic membrane (Figure 5–19 ➤).

Slowly insert the speculum into the auditory canal, inspecting the walls for signs of irritation, discharge, or a foreign body. The walls of the auditory canal are normally pink, and some cerumen is present. Children often put beads, peas, or other small objects into their ears. If the auditory canal is obstructed by cerumen or a foreign body, warm water irrigation can be used to clean the canal.

The tympanic membrane, which separates the outer ear from the middle ear, is usually pearly gray and translucent. It reflects light, and the bones (ossicles) in the middle ear are normally visible. When the pneumatic attachment is squeezed, the tympanic membrane normally moves in and out in response to the positive and negative pressure applied (Figure 5–20 ➤). Table 5–6 lists the abnormal findings of a tympanic membrane examination and their associated conditions.

Hearing Assessment

Hearing evaluation is important in children of all ages because hearing is essential for normal speech development and learning. Hearing loss may occur at any time during early childhood as the result of birth trauma, frequent acute otitis media, meningitis, or antibiotics that damage cranial nerve VIII. Hearing loss may also be associated with congenital anomalies and genetic syndromes. The hearing of newborns is evaluated at birth. Hearing is also evaluated throughout childhood.

Evaluate hearing by inspection of the child's responses to various auditory stimuli using age-appropriate methods. Use hearing and speech articulation milestones as an initial hearing screen. When a hearing deficiency is suspected as a result of screening, refer the child for audiometry, tympanometry, or evoked response to obtain the most accurate evaluation of hearing.

Infants and Toddlers

Select noisemakers with different frequencies, such as a rattle, bell, and tissue paper, that will attract the young child's attention. Ask the parent or an assistant to entertain the infant with a quiet toy, such as a teddy bear. Stand behind the infant, about 60 cm

Table 5–6	**UNEXPECTED FINDINGS ON EXAMINATION OF THE TYMPANIC MEMBRANE AND ITS ASSOCIATED CONDITIONS**

Characteristics of Tympanic Membrane	Unexpected Findings	Associated Conditions
Color	Redness	Infection in middle ear
	Slight redness	Prolonged crying
	Amber	Serous fluid in middle ear
	Deep red or blue	Blood in middle ear
Light reflex	Absent	Bulging tympanic membrane, infection in middle ear
	Distorted, loss of triangular shape	Retracted tympanic membrane, serous fluid in middle ear
Bony landmarks	Extra prominent	Retracted tympanic membrane, serous fluid in middle ear
Movement	No motility	Infection or fluid in middle ear
	Excess motility	Healed perforation

(2 feet) away from the infant's ear but outside the infant's field of vision, and make a soft sound with the noisemaker. Have the parent or assistant observe the child for any of the following responses when the noisemaker is used: widening the eyes, briefly stopping all activity to listen, or turning the head toward the sound. Repeat the test in the other ear and with the other noisemakers. See Chapter 19 ∞ for more details on hearing testing.

Preschool and Older Children

Use whispered words to evaluate the hearing of children over 3 years of age. Position your head about 30 cm (12 in.) away from the child's ear, but out of the range of vision

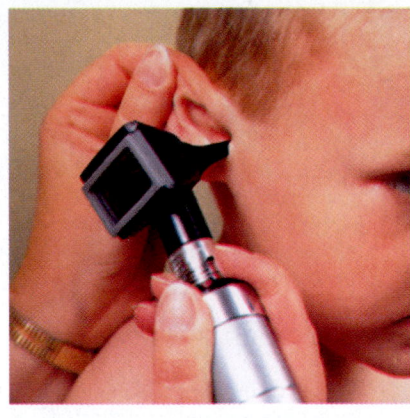

Figure 5–19 ➤ To straighten the auditory canal: pull the pinna back and up for children over 3 years of age; pull the pinna down and back for children under 3 years of age.

NURSING ALERT

Never irrigate the ear canal if any discharge is present, as the tympanic membrane may be ruptured. Water could enter the middle ear and potentially worsen the infection.

SKILLS 6–20 AND 6–21
Hearing Acuity Screening

CLINICAL TIP

An alternative procedure is used to assess hearing when the child will not cooperate by repeating whispered words. In a whisper, direct the child to point to different parts of the body or objects, for example, "Show me your eyes" and "Point to your mouth." Children should point to the correct body part each time.

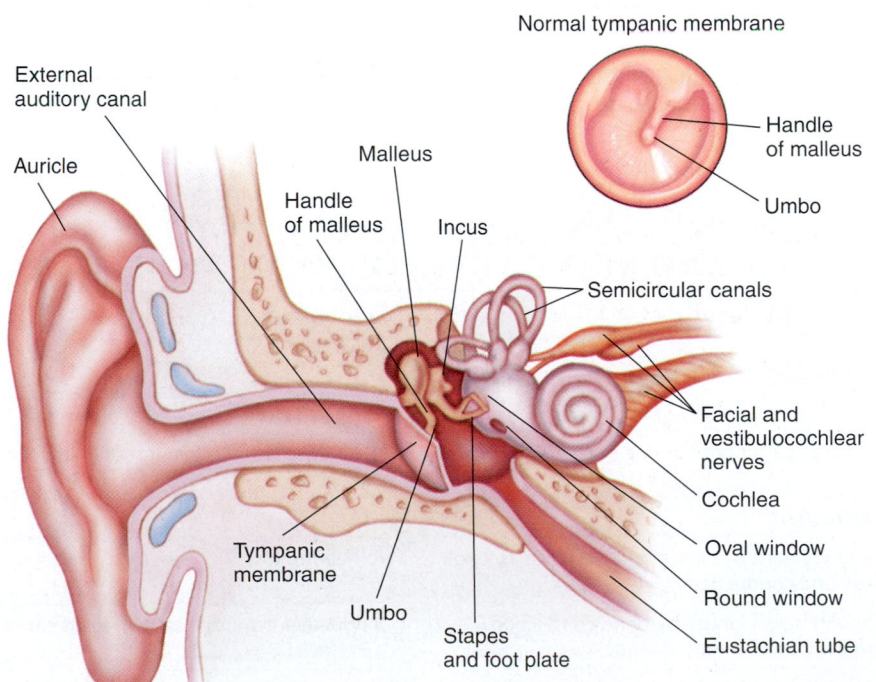

Figure 5–20 ➤ Cross-section of the ear. The tympanic membrane normally has a triangular light reflex with the base on the nasal side pointing toward the center. The bony landmarks, the umbo and handle of malleus, are seen through the tympanic membrane.

GROWTH & DEVELOPMENT

Hearing Loss Indicators

Indicators of hearing loss in an infant:
- No startle reaction to loud noises
- Does not turn toward sounds by 4 months of age
- Babbles as a young infant but does not keep babbling or develop speech sounds after 6 months of age

Indicators of hearing loss in a young child:
- No speech by 2 years of age
- Speech sounds are not distinct at appropriate ages

so the child cannot read your lips. Use words easily recognized by the child, such as *Mickey Mouse*, *hot dog*, and *popsicle*, and ask the child to repeat the words. Repeat the test with different words in the opposite ear. The child should correctly repeat the whispered words.

Bone and Air Conduction of Sound

Use a tuning fork to evaluate the hearing of school-age children who can follow directions. Stroke the tines of the tuning fork to begin the vibration. Avoid touching the vibrating tines, which will dampen the sound. Bone conduction is tested by placing the handle of the tuning fork on the child's skull. Air conduction is tested by holding the vibrating tines close to the child's ear (Figure 5–21 ➤).

To perform the *Weber test*, place the vibrating tuning fork on top of the child's skull in the midline. Ask the child to say where the sound is heard best, either in both ears equally or in one ear. The sound should be heard equally in both ears.

To perform the *Rinne test*, place the vibrating tuning fork handle on the mastoid process behind an ear. Ask the child to say when the sound is no longer heard. Immediately move the tuning fork so that the vibrating tines are held about 2.5 to 5 cm (1 to 2 in.) from the same ear. Again, ask the child to indicate when the sound is no longer heard. The child normally hears the air-conducted sound twice as long as the bone-conducted sound. Repeat the Rinne test on the other ear. Table 5–7 provides an interpretation of the Weber and Rinne tests.

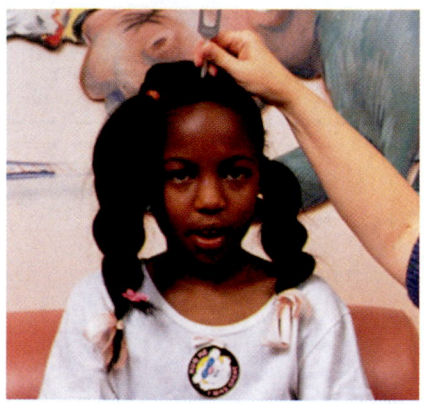
A

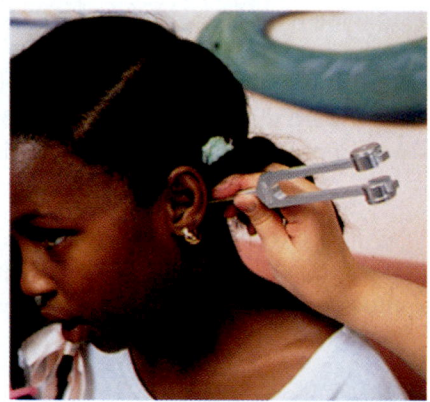
B

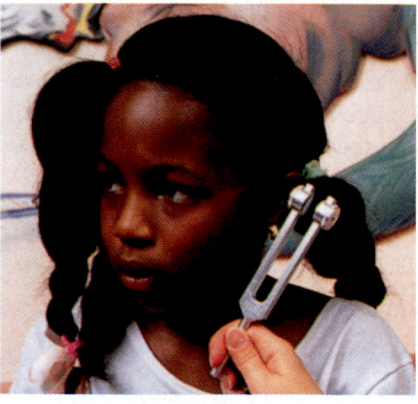
C

Figure 5–21 ➤ A, Weber test. Place a vibrating tuning fork on the midline of the child's head. B, Rinne test, step 1. Place a vibrating tuning fork on the mastoid process. C, Rinne test, step 2. Reposition the still-vibrating tines between 2.5 and 5 cm (1 and 2 in.) from the ear.

Table 5–7	INTERPRETATION OF THE WEBER AND RINNE TESTS OF HEARING
Test and Result	**Associated Condition**
Weber Test	
Sound heard equally in both ears	No hearing loss
Sound heard better in one ear (lateralized)	Conductive hearing loss if sound lateralized to deaf ear
Rinne Test	
Sound heard by air conduction twice as long as bone conduction	No hearing loss
Sound heard longer by bone conduction than air conduction	Conductive hearing loss in affected ear
Sound heard longer by air conduction than bone conduction but less than twice as long	Sensorineural hearing loss in affected ear

ASSESSING THE NOSE AND SINUSES FOR AIRWAY PATENCY AND DISCHARGE

What is the most common cause of nasal obstruction in children? What does nasal flaring indicate? What signs indicate that a foreign body might be lodged in the nose? What does it mean if the child frequently wipes the nose upward with a hand?

Inspection of the External Nose

The external nose characteristics and placement on the face are examined simultaneously with the facial features. Inspect the external nose for size, shape, symmetry, and midline placement on the face. The nose should be proportional in size to other facial features and positioned in the middle of the face. A flattened nasal bridge is the expected finding in Asian and Black children, but may also be seen in children with Down syndrome.

The nasolabial folds are normally symmetric. Asymmetry of the nasolabial folds may be associated with injury to the facial nerve (cranial nerve VII). A saddle-shaped nose is associated with congenital defects such as cleft palate.

Inspect the external nose for unusual characteristics. For example, a crease across the nose between the cartilage and bone is often caused by the allergic child's wiping an itchy nose upward with a hand.

Palpation of the External Nose

When a deformity is noted, gently palpate the nose to detect any pain or break in contour. No tenderness or masses are expected. Pain and a contour deviation are usually the result of trauma.

Nasal Patency

The child's airway must be patent to ensure adequate oxygenation. To test for nasal patency, occlude one nostril and observe the child's effort to breathe through the open nostril with the mouth closed. Repeat the procedure with the other nostril. Breathing should be noiseless and effortless. **Nasal flaring**, an effort the child makes to widen the airway, is a sign of increased respiratory effort or respiratory distress and should not be present.

If the child struggles to breathe, a nasal obstruction may be present. Nasal obstruction may be caused by a foreign body, congenital defect, dry mucus, discharge, polyp, or trauma. Newborns may have respiratory distress because of choanal atresia, a congenital membranous or bony obstruction between the nose and the nasopharynx. Young children commonly place objects up their nose, and unilateral nasal flaring is a sign of such an obstruction.

Assessment of Smell

The olfactory nerve (cranial nerve I) can be tested in school-age children and adolescents. When testing smell, choose scents the child will easily recognize such as orange, chocolate, and mint. When the child's eyes are closed, occlude one nostril and hold the scent under the nose. Ask the child to take a deep sniff and identify the scent. Alternate odors between the nares. The child can normally identify common scents.

Inspection of the Internal Nose

Inspect the internal nose for color of the mucous membranes and the presence of any discharge, swelling, lesions, or other abnormalities. Use a bright light, such as an otoscope light or penlight. For infants and young children, push the tip of the nose upward and shine the light at the end of the nose. The nasal speculum of the otoscope can be used in older children (Figure 5–22 ➤). Avoid touching the septum of the nose with the speculum. Injury to the septum can cause a nosebleed.

Mucous Membranes

The mucous membranes should be dark pink and glistening. A film of clear discharge may also be present. Turbinates, if visible, should be the same color as the mucous membranes and have a firm consistency. When the turbinates are pale or bluish gray, the child may have allergies. A *polyp*, a rounded mass projecting from the turbinate, is also associated with allergies.

EQUIPMENT NEEDED

Otoscope with nasal speculum
Penlight

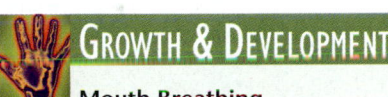

GROWTH & DEVELOPMENT

Mouth Breathing
Infants under 6 months of age will not automatically open their mouths to breathe when their nose is occluded, such as by mucus.

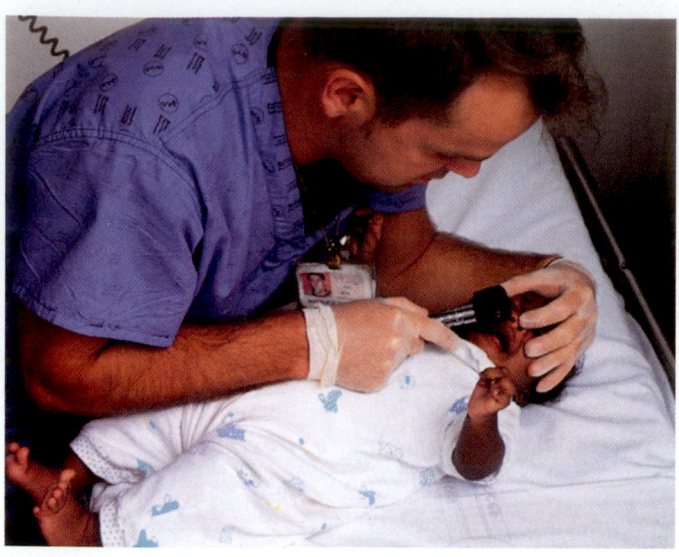
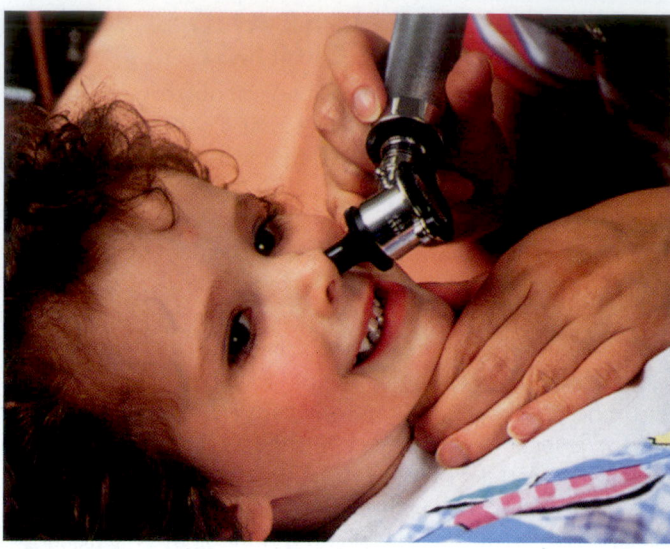

A

B

Figure 5–22 ➤ Technique for examining nose. A, Technique for an infant or small child. B, Technique for an older child.

Nasal Septum

Inspect the nasal septum for alignment, perforations, bleeding, or crusting. The septum should be straight without perforations, bleeding, or crusting. Crusting will be noted over the site of a nosebleed.

Discharge

Observe for the presence of nasal discharge, noting if the drainage is from one or both nares. Nasal discharge is not a normal finding unless the child is crying. Discharge may be watery, mucoid, purulent, or bloody, depending on the condition present. A foul-smelling discharge in only one nostril is often associated with a foreign body. Table 5–8 lists conditions associated with nasal discharge.

Inspection of the Sinuses

The maxillary and ethmoid sinuses develop during early childhood (Figure 5–23 ➤). Sinus infections can occasionally occur in young children. Suspect a sinus problem when the child has a headache or pain and swelling around one or both eyes.

Inspect the face for any puffiness and swelling around one or both eyes that is not normally present. To palpate over the maxillary sinuses, press up under both zygomatic arches with the thumbs. To palpate the ethmoid sinuses, press up against the bone above both eyes with the thumbs. No swelling or tenderness is expected. Tenderness may indicate sinusitis.

Table 5–8	NASAL DISCHARGE CHARACTERISTICS AND ASSOCIATED CONDITIONS
Discharge Description	**Associated Condition**
Watery	
Clear, bilateral	Allergy
Serous, unilateral	Spinal fluid from fracture of cribriform plate
Mucoid or purulent	
Bilateral	Upper respiratory infection
Unilateral	Foreign body
Bloody	Nosebleed, trauma

AS CHILDREN GROW

Sinus Development

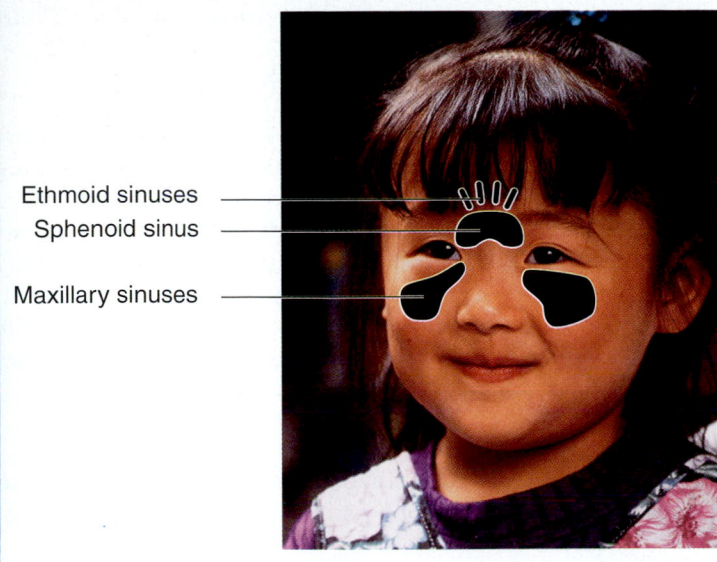

- Ethmoid sinuses
- Sphenoid sinus
- Maxillary sinuses

Figure 5–23 ➤ Sinuses grow and develop during childhood. Maxillary sinuses can be identified in 1-year-old children. Ethmoid sinuses have developed in children by 6 years of age. Sinus problems occur infrequently in children under 7 years.

ASSESSING THE MOUTH AND THROAT FOR COLOR, FUNCTION, AND SIGNS OF ABNORMAL CONDITIONS

What is the best site to evaluate cyanosis in children? What is the expected sequence of tooth eruption? How is it determined that the tongue has adequate movement for all speech sounds? How can the throat be inspected without causing the child to gag?

Inspection of the Mouth

Young children often need coaxing and simple explanations before they will cooperate with the mouth and throat examination. Most children readily show their teeth. If the child resists by clenching the teeth, they can be gently separated with a tongue blade. Wear gloves when examining the mouth because of contact with the mucous membranes (Figure 5–24 ➤).

MediaLink

Mouth and Throat Examination

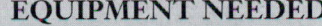

EQUIPMENT NEEDED
Tongue blade
Penlight
Gloves

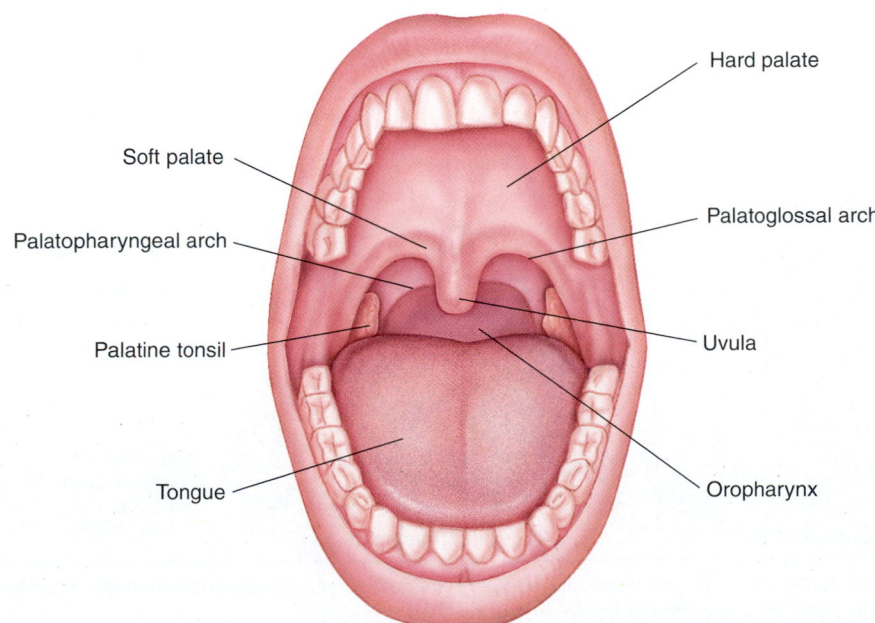

- Hard palate
- Soft palate
- Palatopharyngeal arch
- Palatine tonsil
- Tongue
- Palatoglossal arch
- Uvula
- Oropharynx

Figure 5–24 ➤ The structures of the mouth.

Lips

Inspect the lips for color, shape, symmetry, moisture, and lesions. The lips are normally symmetric without drying, cracking, or other lesions. Lip color is normally pink in white children and more bluish in darker-skinned children. Pale, cyanotic, or cherry-red lips indicate poor tissue perfusion caused by various conditions. Note any clefts or edema.

Teeth

Inspect and count the child's teeth. The timing of tooth eruption is often genetically determined, but there is a regular sequence of tooth eruption. Figure 5–25 ➤ presents the typical sequence of tooth eruption for both deciduous and permanent teeth.

Inspect the condition of the teeth, look for loose teeth, and note any spaces where teeth are missing. Compare empty tooth spaces with the child's developmental stage of tooth eruption. Once the permanent teeth have erupted, none should be missing. Teeth are normally white, without a flattened, mottled, or pitted appearance. Discolorations on the crown of a tooth may indicate caries. Discolorations on the tooth surface may be associated with some medications and fluorosis. See Chapter 19 ∞.

Mouth Odors

During inspection of the teeth, be alert to any abnormal odors that may indicate problems such as diabetic ketoacidosis, infection, or poor hygiene. Be alert for alcohol odors in older children that could signal substance abuse.

AS CHILDREN GROW

Sequence of Tooth Eruption

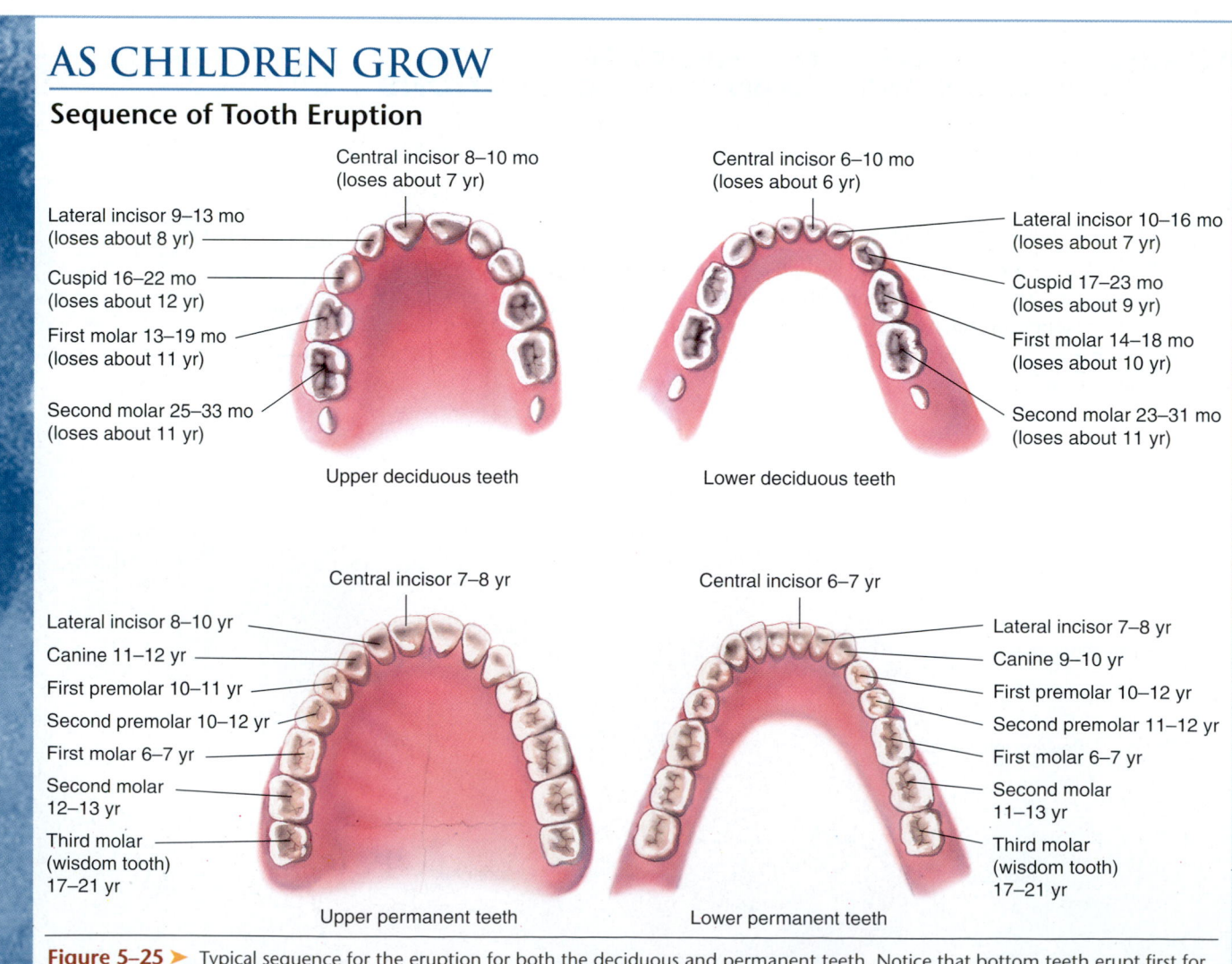

Upper deciduous teeth

Central incisor 8–10 mo (loses about 7 yr)
Lateral incisor 9–13 mo (loses about 8 yr)
Cuspid 16–22 mo (loses about 12 yr)
First molar 13–19 mo (loses about 11 yr)
Second molar 25–33 mo (loses about 11 yr)

Lower deciduous teeth

Central incisor 6–10 mo (loses about 6 yr)
Lateral incisor 10–16 mo (loses about 7 yr)
Cuspid 17–23 mo (loses about 9 yr)
First molar 14–18 mo (loses about 10 yr)
Second molar 23–31 mo (loses about 11 yr)

Upper permanent teeth

Central incisor 7–8 yr
Lateral incisor 8–10 yr
Canine 11–12 yr
First premolar 10–11 yr
Second premolar 10–12 yr
First molar 6–7 yr
Second molar 12–13 yr
Third molar (wisdom tooth) 17–21 yr

Lower permanent teeth

Central incisor 6–7 yr
Lateral incisor 7–8 yr
Canine 9–10 yr
First premolar 10–12 yr
Second premolar 11–12 yr
First molar 6–7 yr
Second molar 11–13 yr
Third molar (wisdom tooth) 17–21 yr

Figure 5–25 ➤ Typical sequence for the eruption for both the deciduous and permanent teeth. Notice that bottom teeth erupt first for each kind of tooth: incisors, cuspids, and molars. Teeth are shed or lost in the same pattern.

Gums

Inspect the gums for color and adherence to the teeth. The gums are normally pink, with a stippled or dotted appearance. Use a tongue blade to help visualize the gums around the upper and lower molars. No raised or receding gum areas should be apparent around the teeth. When inflammation, swelling, or bleeding is observed, palpate the gums to detect tenderness. Inflammation and tenderness are associated with infection, some seizure medications, and poor nutrition.

Buccal Mucosa

Inspect the mucous membrane lining the cheeks for color and moisture. The mucous membrane is usually pink, but patches of hyperpigmentation are commonly seen in darker-skinned children. The Stensen duct, the parotid gland opening, is opposite the upper second molar bilaterally. Normally pink, the duct opening becomes red when the child is infected with mumps. Small pink sucking pads can be present in infants. No areas of redness, swelling, or ulcerative lesions should be present.

Tongue

Inspect the tongue for color, moistness, size, tremors, and lesions. The child's tongue is normally pink and moist, without a coating, and it fits easily into the mouth. A pattern of gray, irregular borders that form a design (geographic tongue) is often normal, but it may be associated with fever, allergies, or drug reactions. Tremors are abnormal. A white adherent coating on an infant's tongue may be caused by thrush, a *Candida* infection.

Observe the mobility of the tongue. Ask the child to touch the gums above the upper teeth with the tongue. This tongue movement is adequate to clearly enunciate all speech sounds. Ask the child to stick out the tongue and lift it so the underside of the tongue and the floor of the mouth can be inspected for distended veins.

Palate

Inspect the hard and soft palate to detect any clefts or masses or an unusually high arch. The palate is normally pink, with a dome-shaped arch and no cleft. The uvula hangs freely from the soft palate. Newborns often have Epstein pearls, white papules in the midline of the palate that disappear in a few weeks. A high-arched palate can be associated with sucking difficulties in young infants.

Palpation of the Mouth Structures

Palpate any masses seen in the mouth to determine their characteristics, such as size, shape, firmness, and tenderness. No masses should be found.

Tongue

To assess the tongue's strength, while simultaneously testing the hypoglossal nerve (cranial nerve XII), place the index finger against the child's cheek and ask the child to push against your finger with the tongue. Some pressure against the finger is normally felt.

Palate

To palpate the palate, insert the little finger, with the fingerpad upward, into the mouth. While the infant sucks against your finger, palpate the entire palate. This procedure also tests the strength of the sucking reflex, innervated by the hypoglossal nerve (cranial nerve XII). No clefts should be palpated.

Inspection of the Throat

Inspect the throat for color, swelling, lesions, and the condition of the tonsils. Ask the child to open the mouth wide and stick out the tongue. A penlight is used to illuminate the throat. A tongue blade can be used, if needed, to visualize the posterior pharynx. The throat is normally pink without lesions, drainage, or swelling. Swelling or bulging in the posterior pharynx may be associated with a peritonsillar abscess.

Tonsils

During childhood the tonsils are large in proportion to the size of the pharynx because lymphoid tissue grows fastest in early childhood. The tonsils should be pink without

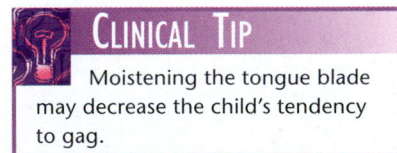

CLINICAL TIP

Moistening the tongue blade may decrease the child's tendency to gag.

PATHOPHYSIOLOGY ILLUSTRATED

Tonsil Size with Infection

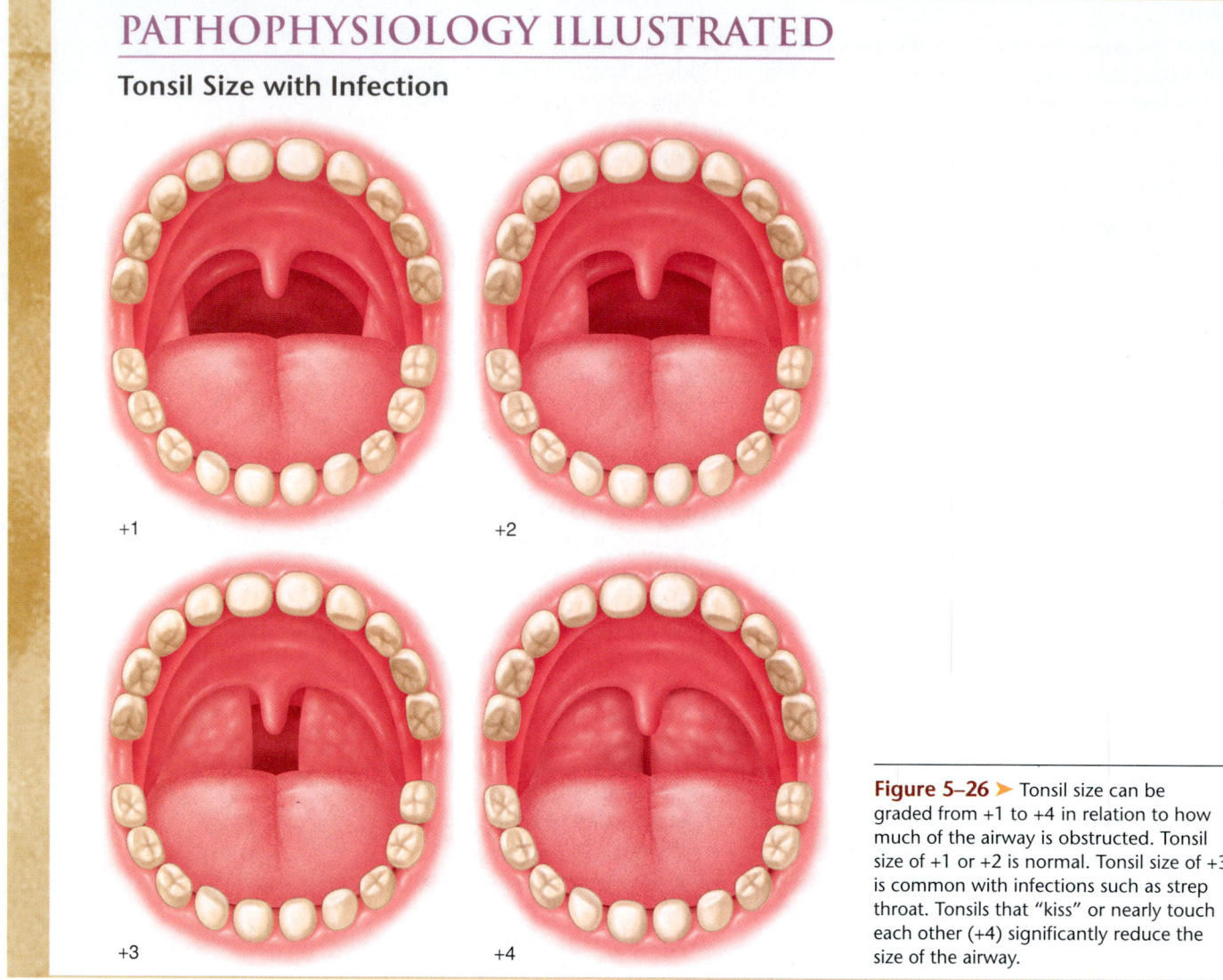

Figure 5–26 ➤ Tonsil size can be graded from +1 to +4 in relation to how much of the airway is obstructed. Tonsil size of +1 or +2 is normal. Tonsil size of +3 is common with infections such as strep throat. Tonsils that "kiss" or nearly touch each other (+4) significantly reduce the size of the airway.

exudate, but *crypts* (fissures) may be present as a result of prior infections. The size of the tonsils can be graded as indicated in Figure 5–26 ➤.

Gag Reflex

Use a tongue blade when you are unable to see the posterior pharynx or need to test the gag reflex. Do this at the end of the examination because children dislike the gagging sensation. Prepare the child for what will happen. Ask the child to say "Ah" and watch for a symmetric rising movement of the uvula. If the uvula does not rise or rises to one side, cranial nerves IX and X may be paralyzed. The epiglottis lies behind the tongue and is normally pink like the rest of the buccal mucosa.

ASSESSING THE NECK FOR CHARACTERISTICS, RANGE OF MOTION, AND LYMPH NODES

What does it mean when a child's head is tilting to one side? By what age should an infant be able to control his or her head? What does a lymph node feel like?

Inspection of the Neck

Inspect the neck for size, symmetry, swelling, and any abnormalities. A short neck with skin folds is normal for infants. The neck is normally symmetric. No swelling should be present. Swelling may be caused by local infections such as mumps or a congenital defect. The neck lengthens between 3 and 4 years of age.

Inspect the child's neck for *webbing*, an extra skin fold on each side of the neck. Webbing is commonly associated with Turner syndrome (see Chapter 29 ∞).

Infants develop head control by 2 months of age. By this age an infant can lift the head up and look around when lying on the stomach. A lack of head control can result from neurologic injury, such as an anoxic episode.

Palpation of the Neck

Face the child and use your fingerpads to simultaneously palpate both sides of the neck for lymph nodes, as well as the trachea and thyroid.

Lymph Nodes

To palpate the lymph nodes, slide your fingerpads gently over the lymph node chains in the head and neck. The sequence for lymph node palpation is as follows: around the ears, and under the jaw, the occipital area, and the cervical chain in the neck (Figure 5–27 ➤). Firm, clearly defined, nontender, movable lymph nodes up to 1 cm (1/2 in.) in diameter are common in young children. Enlarged, firm, warm, tender lymph nodes indicate a local infection.

Trachea

Palpate the trachea to determine its position and to detect the presence of any masses. The trachea is normally in the midline of the neck. It is difficult to palpate in children less than 3 years of age because of their short necks. To palpate the trachea, place your thumb and forefinger on each side of the child's trachea near the chin and slowly slide them down the trachea. Any shift to the right or left of midline may indicate a tumor or a collapsed lung.

Thyroid

As the fingers slide over the trachea in the lower neck, attempt to feel the isthmus of the thyroid, a band of glandular tissue crossing over the trachea. The lobes of the thyroid wrap behind the trachea and are normally covered by the sternocleidomastoid muscle. Because of the anatomic position of the thyroid, its lobes are not usually palpable in the child unless they are enlarged.

Range of Motion Assessment

To test the neck's range of motion, ask the child to touch the chin to each shoulder and to the chest and then to look at the ceiling. Move a light or toy in all four directions

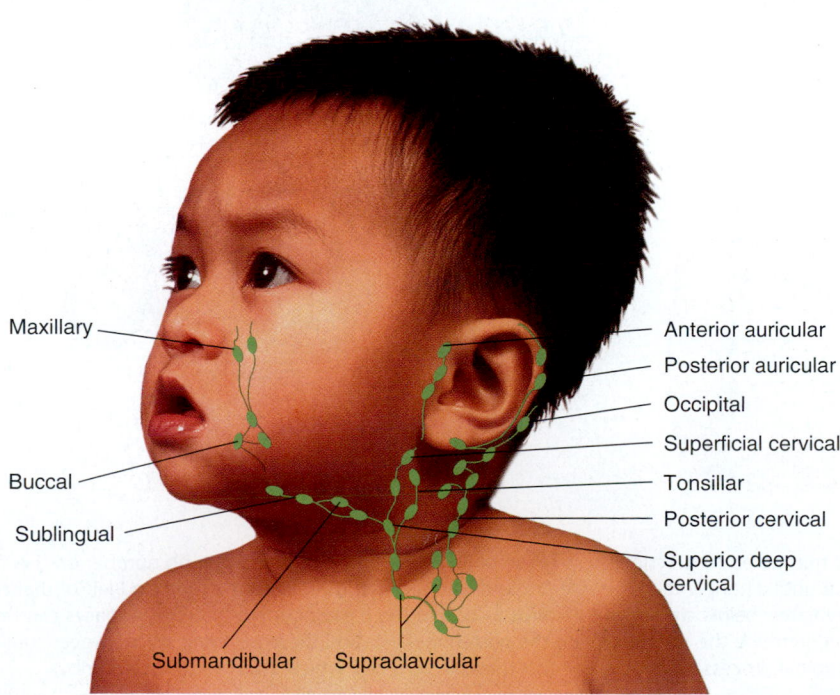

Maxillary
Buccal
Sublingual
Submandibular   Supraclavicular

Anterior auricular
Posterior auricular
Occipital
Superficial cervical
Tonsillar
Posterior cervical
Superior deep cervical

Figure 5–27 ➤ The neck is palpated for enlarged lymph nodes around the ears, under the jaw, in the occipital area, and in the cervical chain of the neck.

when assessing infants. Children should freely move the neck and head in all four directions without pain.

When the child is unable to move the head voluntarily in all directions, passively move the child's neck through the expected range of motion. Limited horizontal range of motion may be a sign of *torticollis*, persistent head tilting. Torticollis results from a birth injury to the sternocleidomastoid muscle or from unilateral vision or hearing impairment. Pain with flexion of the neck toward the chest (Brudzinski's sign) may indicate meningitis. See Chapter 26 ∞.

ASSESSING THE CHEST FOR SHAPE, MOVEMENT, RESPIRATORY EFFORT, AND LUNG FUNCTION

What terms are used to describe the location of specific sounds heard when auscultating the chest? What does it mean when a child's chest is rounded in shape? What are retractions and what do they indicate? How can normal and adventitious breath sounds be distinguished when auscultating the lungs?

Examination of the chest includes the following procedures: inspecting the size and shape of the chest, palpating chest movement that occurs during respiration, observing the effort of breathing, and auscultating breath sounds.

Topographic Landmarks of the Chest

The chest skeleton provides most of the landmarks used to describe the location of findings during examination of the chest, lungs, and heart. The intercostal spaces between ribs are the horizontal markers. The sternum and spine are the vertical landmarks. When both a horizontal and a vertical landmark are used, the location of findings can be precisely described on the right or left side of the patient's chest (Figure 5–28 and Figure 5–29 ➤). Vertical landmarks are described in Table 5–9.

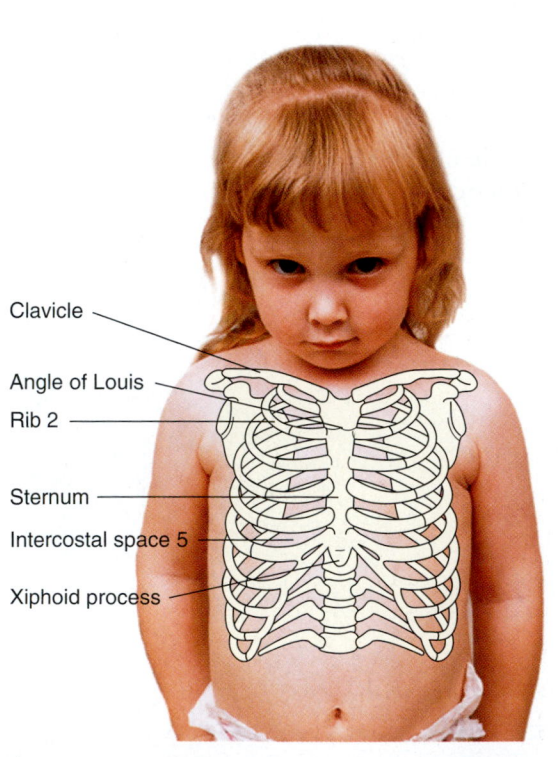

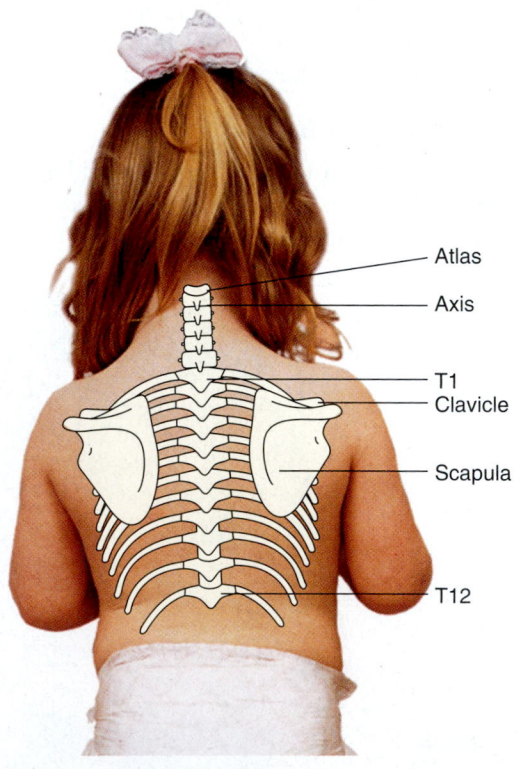

A

B

Figure 5–28 ➤ Intercostal spaces and ribs are numbered to describe the location of findings. A, To determine the rib number on the anterior chest, palpate down from the top of the sternum until a horizontal ridge, the Angle of Louis, is felt. Directly to the right and left of that ridge is the second rib. The second intercostal space is immediately below the second rib. Ribs 3–12 and the corresponding intercostal spaces can be counted as the fingers move toward the abdomen. B, To determine the rib number on the posterior chest, find the protruding spinal process of the seventh cervical vertebra at the shoulder level. The next spinal process belongs to the first thoracic vertebra, which attaches to the first rib.

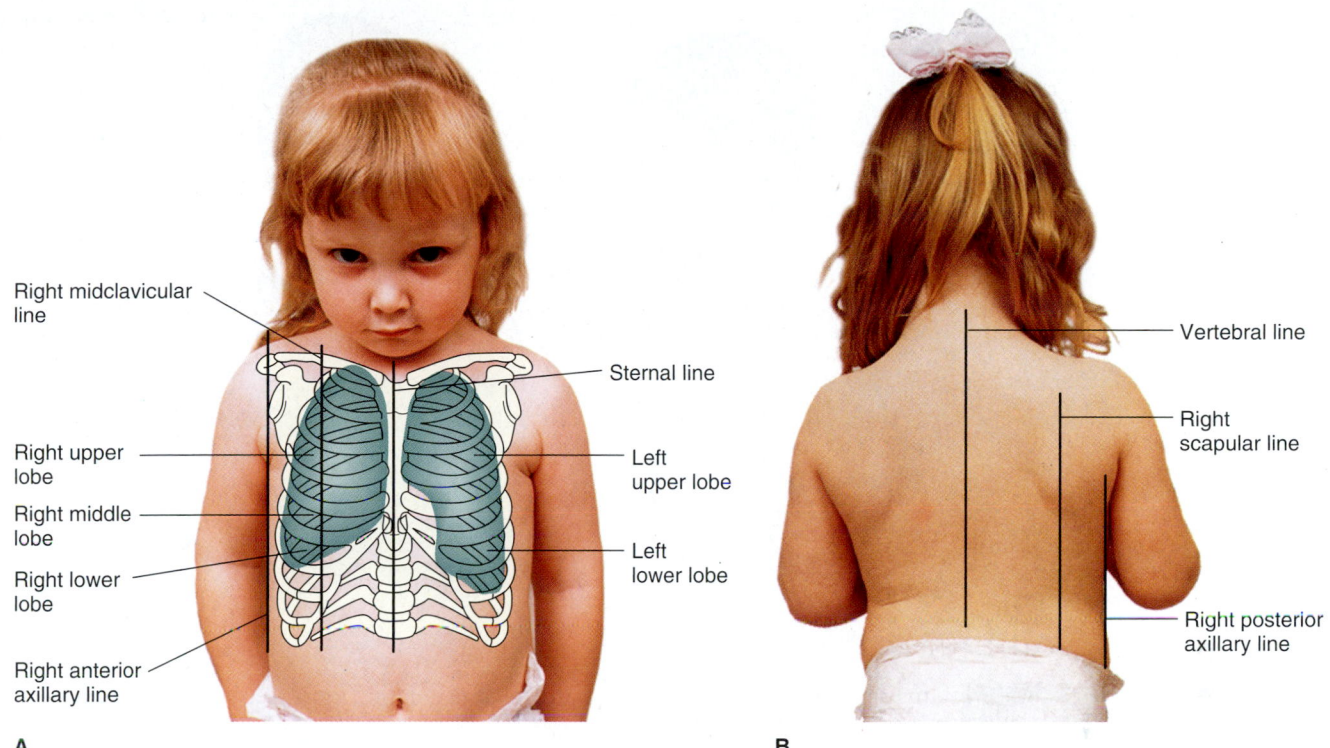

Right midclavicular line

Sternal line

Right upper lobe

Left upper lobe

Right middle lobe

Right lower lobe

Left lower lobe

Right anterior axillary line

A

Vertebral line

Right scapular line

Right posterior axillary line

B

Figure 5–29 ➤ The sternum and spine are the vertical landmarks used to describe the anatomic location of findings. The distance between the finding and the center of the sternum (midsternal line) or the spinal line can be measured with a ruler. Imaginary vertical lines, parallel to the midsternal and spinal lines, are used to further describe the location of findings. A, anterior chest, B, posterior chest.

Table 5–9	VERTICAL LANDMARKS OF THE CHEST
Vertical Lines for Assessing the Chest	**Location of Vertical Lines**
Midsternal	Through the middle of the sternum
Midclavicular	From the middle of the clavicle
Anterior axillary	From the anterior axillary fold
Midaxillary	From the middle of the axilla
Posterior axillary	From the posterior axillary fold
Spinal	Through the spinous processes of the vertebrae

Inspection of the Chest

Position the child on the parent's lap or on the examining table with all clothing above the waist removed to inspect the chest. The thoracic muscles and subcutaneous tissue are less developed in children than in adults, so the chest wall is thinner. As a result the rib cage is more prominent.

Size and Shape of the Chest

Inspect the chest for any irregularities in shape. A chest is considered rounded when the anteroposterior diameter is approximately equal to the lateral diameter. If a child over 2 years of age has a rounded chest, a chronic obstructive lung condition such as asthma or cystic fibrosis may be present.

An abnormal chest shape results from two different structural deformities (Figure 5–30 ➤). If the sternum protrudes, increasing the anteroposterior diameter, pigeon chest (pectus carinatum) may be present. If the lower portion of the sternum is depressed, decreasing the anteroposterior diameter, funnel chest (pectus excavatum)

EQUIPMENT NEEDED

Stethoscope

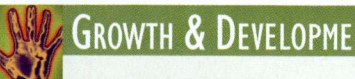

GROWTH & DEVELOPMENT

Chest Diameter

In infants the chest is rounded with the anteroposterior diameter approximately equal to the lateral diameter. The chest becomes more oval with growth. By 2 years of age the lateral diameter is greater than the anteroposterior diameter.

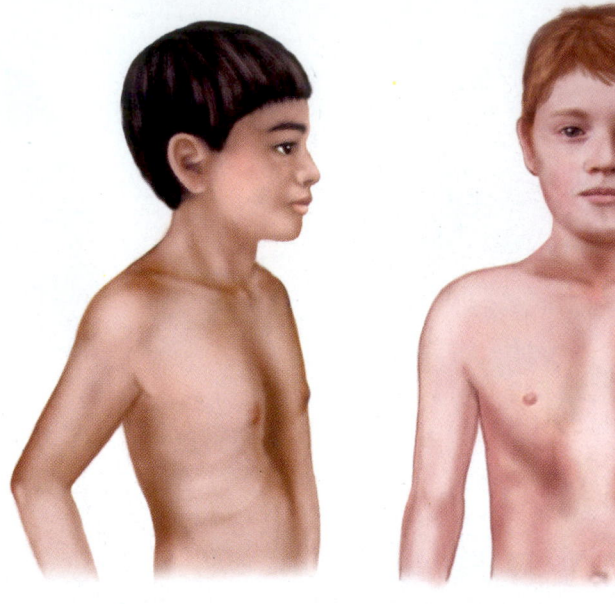

Figure 5–30 ➤ Two types of abnormal chest shape. A, Funnel chest (pectus excavatum). B, Pigeon chest (pectus carinatum).

A   B

GROWTH & DEVELOPMENT

Respiratory Rate

Infants and children have a faster respiratory rate than adults because of a higher metabolic rate and need for oxygen. Infants also tire from the work of breathing when in respiratory distress and begin breathing too slow, a sign of respiratory failure (Dieckmann and American Academy of Pediatrics, 2006).

CLINICAL TIP

To get the most accurate reading of a newborn's and young infant's respiratory rate, wait until the baby is sleeping or quietly resting. Use the stethoscope to auscultate the rate or place your hand on the abdomen. Count the number of breaths for an entire minute, because newborns and young infants can have irregular respirations.

---

may be present. Scoliosis, curvature of the spine, causes a lateral deviation of the chest. See Chapter 28 ∞.

Chest Movement and Respiratory Effort

Inspect for simultaneous chest expansion and abdominal rise. Chest movement is normally symmetric bilaterally, rising with inspiration and falling with expiration. The chest movement of infants and young children is less pronounced than the abdominal movement. The diaphragm is the primary breathing muscle in infants and children under 6 years old. The thoracic muscles are less developed and serve as accessory muscles in cases of respiratory distress. As the thoracic muscles develop, they become primarily responsible for ventilation. On inspiration the chest and abdomen should rise simultaneously. Asymmetric chest rise is associated with a collapsed lung. **Retractions**, depression of sections of the chest wall with each inspiration, are seen when the accessory muscles are used for breathing in cases of respiratory distress.

Respiratory Rate

Because young children use the diaphragm as the primary breathing muscle, observe or feel the rise and fall of the abdomen to count the respiratory rate in children under age 6 years. Table 5–10 gives the normal respiratory rates for each age group. Make every effort to count the respiratory rate when the child is quiet. **Tachypnea**, an elevated respiratory rate, occurs in response to excitement, fear, respiratory distress, fever, and other conditions that increase oxygen needs. **Bradypnea**, an abnormally slow respiratory rate, occurs in response to respiratory failure.

Table 5–10	NORMAL RESPIRATORY RATE RANGES FOR EACH AGE GROUP
Age	**Respiratory Rate per Minute**
Newborn	30–55
1 year	25–40
3 years	20–30
6 years	16–22
10 years	16–20
17 years	12–18

A sustained respiratory rate greater than 60 breaths per minute is an important sign in respiratory distress. At that rate, children develop hypoxemia if treatment is not started. The child's airway is very narrow, resulting in higher airway resistance than occurs in adults. Increased airway resistance means it takes longer for the alveoli to fill with air. The alveoli have a similar problem expiring air with a rapid respiratory rate, so they may become overfilled. This may result in inadequate oxygenation and hypoxemia as less and less air gets to the alveoli for gas exchange (Curley & Thompson, 2001).

Palpation of the Chest

Palpation is used to evaluate chest movement, respiratory effort, deformities of the chest wall, and tactile fremitus.

Chest Wall

To palpate the chest motion with respiration, place the palms and outspread fingers on each side of the child's chest. Confirm the bilateral symmetry of chest motion. Use fingerpads to palpate any depressions, bulges, or unusual chest wall shape that might indicate abnormal findings such as tenderness, cysts, other growths, crepitus, or fractures. None should be found. **Crepitus**, a crinkly sensation palpated on the chest surface, is caused by air escaping into the subcutaneous tissues. It often indicates a serious injury to the upper or lower airway. Crepitus may also be felt near a fracture.

Tactile Fremitus

Crying and talking produce vibrations, known as **tactile fremitus**, that can be palpated on the chest. Place the palms of your hands on each side of the chest to evaluate the quality and distribution of these vibrations. Ask the child to repeat a series of words or numbers, such as *Mickey Mouse* or *ice cream*. As the child repeats the words, move the hands systematically over the anterior and posterior chest, comparing the quality of findings side to side. The vibration or tingling sensation is normally palpated over the entire chest. Decreased sensations indicate that air is trapped in the lungs, as occurs with asthma. Increased sensations indicate lung consolidation, as occurs with pneumonia.

Auscultation of the Chest

Auscultate the chest with a stethoscope to assess the quality and characteristics of breath sounds, to identify abnormal breath sounds, and to evaluate **vocal resonance**. Use an infant or pediatric stethoscope when available to help localize any unexpected breath sounds. Use the stethoscope's diaphragm because it transmits the high-pitched breath sounds better.

Breath Sounds

Evaluate the quality and characteristics of breath sounds over the entire chest, comparing sounds between the sides. Select a routine sequence for auscultating the entire chest so assessment of all lobes of the lungs will be consistently performed. Figure 5–31 ➤ shows one suggested chest auscultation sequence. Listen to an entire inspiratory and expiratory phase at each spot on the chest before moving to the next site.

Three types of normal breath sounds are usually heard when the chest is auscultated. *Vesicular breath sounds* are low-pitched, swishing, soft, short expiratory sounds. They are usually heard in older children but not in infants and young children. *Bronchovesicular breath sounds* are medium-pitched, hollow, blowing sounds heard equally on inspiration and expiration in all age groups. The location of these sounds on the chest is related to the child's developmental status. *Bronchial/tracheal breath sounds* are hollow and higher pitched than vesicular breath sounds.

Breath sounds normally have equal intensity, pitch, and rhythm bilaterally. Absent or diminished breath sounds generally indicate a partial or total obstruction, such as from a foreign body or mucus, that does not permit airflow.

Vocal Resonance

Auscultate the chest to evaluate how well voice sounds are transmitted. Have the child repeat a series of words, either the same as or different from those used for evaluating

---

CLINICAL TIP

Auscultation of breath sounds is difficult when an infant is crying. First, try to quiet the infant with a pacifier, bottle, or toy. If the infant continues to cry, all is not lost. At the end of each cry the infant takes a deep breath, which you can use to assess breath sounds, vocal resonance, and tactile fremitus. Encourage toddlers and preschoolers to take deep breaths by providing a pinwheel to blow or have them blow out a penlight.

When trying to get the child to breathe normally while auscultating the chest, use suggestive language to increase cooperation. "You certainly are good at breathing slowly. Have you been practicing?" The child will often deepen and slow the breathing pattern as you give praise and draw attention to it.

GROWTH & DEVELOPMENT

Lung Auscultation

Infants and young children have a thin chest wall because of immature muscle development. The breath sounds of one lung are heard over the entire chest. It takes practice to accurately identify absent or diminished breath sounds in infants and young children. Because the distance between the lungs is greatest at the apices and midaxillary areas in young children, these sites are best for identifying absent or diminished breath sounds. Carefully auscultate, comparing the quality of breath sounds heard bilaterally.

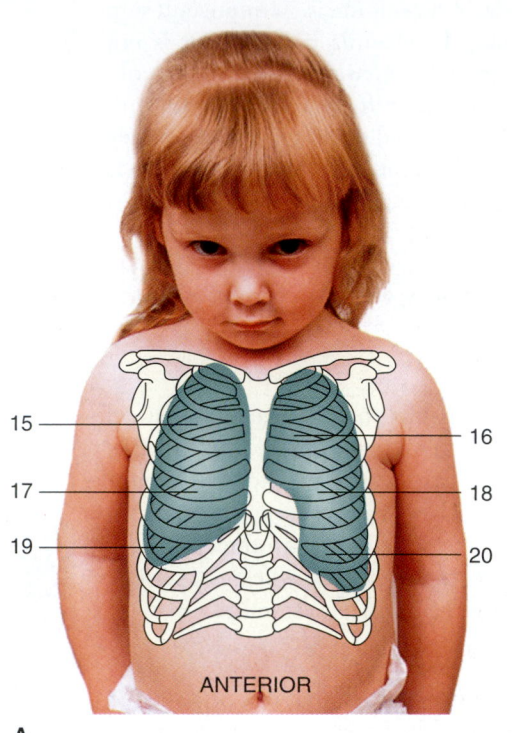
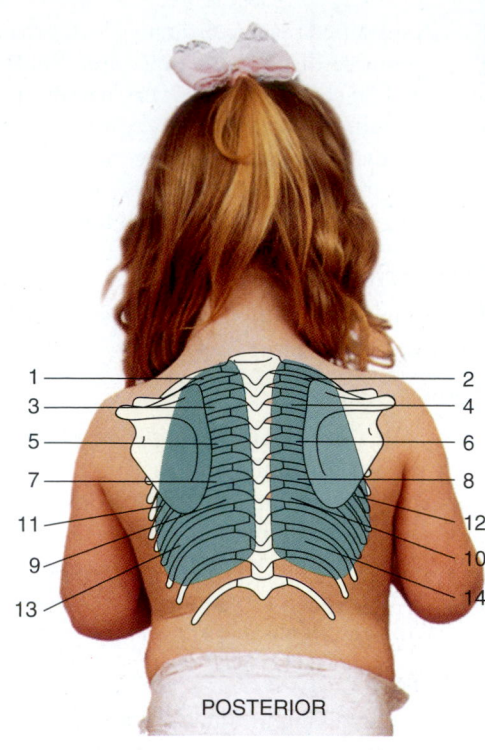

Figure 5–31 ➤ One example of a sequence for auscultation of the chest. A, anterior. B, posterior. **A**

B

ANTERIOR

POSTERIOR

tactile fremitus. Use the stethoscope to auscultate the chest, comparing the quality of sounds from side to side and over the entire chest. Voice sounds, with words and syllables muffled and indistinct, are normally heard throughout the chest.

If voice sounds are absent or more muffled than usual, an airway obstruction condition such as asthma may be present. When a condition causing lung consolidation (e.g., pneumonia) is present, the quality of vocal resonance changes in characteristic ways. These abnormal characteristics are called whispered pectoriloquy, bronchophony, and egophony. **Whispered pectoriloquy** is present when syllables are heard distinctly in a whisper. **Bronchophony** is the increased intensity and clarity of sounds while the words remain indistinct. **Egophony** is the transmission of the "eee" sound as a nasal "ay" sound.

Abnormal Breath Sounds

Abnormal breath sounds, also called *adventitious sounds*, generally indicate disease. Examples of abnormal breath sounds are crackles, rhonchi, and friction rubs. To further assess abnormal breath sounds, the examiner determines their location, the respiratory phase in which they are present, and whether they change or disappear when the child coughs or shifts position. To routinely identify these adventitious sounds takes practice. Table 5–11 describes adventitious sounds.

Abnormal Voice Sounds

Observing the quality of the voice and other audible sounds is also important during an examination of the lungs. Examples of these sounds are hoarseness, stridor, and cough. **Stridor** is a noise resulting from air moving through a narrowed trachea and larynx; it is associated with croup. **Wheezing** is a noise resulting from the passage of air through mucus or fluids in a narrowed lower airway; it is associated with asthma. A *cough* is a reflexive clearing of the airway associated with an allergy or respiratory infection. Hoarseness is associated with inflammation of the larynx.

Percussion of the Chest

Percussion is a method sometimes used to assess the resonance of the lungs and the density of underlying organs, such as the heart and liver. Today there is less reliance on percussion to evaluate the lungs because of the frequent use of radiologic examinations.

Table 5–11	DESCRIPTION OF SELECTED ADVENTITIOUS SOUNDS AND THEIR CAUSE	
Type	**Description**	**Cause**
Fine crackles	High-pitched, discrete, noncontinuous sound heard at end of inspiration *(Rub pieces of hair together beside your ear to duplicate the sound.)*	Air passing through watery secretions in the smaller airways (alveoli and bronchioles)
Sibilant rhonchi	Musical, squeaking, or hissing noise heard during inspiration or expiration, but generally louder on expiration	Bronchospasm or an anatomic narrowing of the trachea, bronchi, or bronchioles
Sonorous rhonchi	Coarse, low-pitched sound like a snore, heard during inspiration or expiration; may clear with coughing	Air passing through thick secretions that partially obstruct the larger bronchi and trachea

When percussing the anterior and posterior chest, choose a sequence that covers the entire chest and permits comparison bilaterally. The same sequence as that used for auscultation is effective. To perform *indirect percussion*, lay the middle finger of the nondominant hand on the child's chest at an intercostal space. Keep the other fingers off the chest. With a springlike motion, use the fingertip of the other hand to tap the finger in contact with the chest (Figure 5–32A ➤). Direct percussion is a technique effective for infants. Tap the chest at an intercostal space with a fingertip to elicit the quality of resonance (Figure 5–32B ➤).

Characteristic patterns of percussion resonance are expected (Figure 5–33 ➤). Characteristic descriptions of sounds heard with percussion of the chest include tympany, flatness, dullness, resonance, and hyperresonance.

ASSESSING THE BREASTS

What does breast tissue feel like? Do boys have breast development during puberty?

Inspection of the Breasts

The nipples of prepubertal boys and girls are symmetrically located near the midclavicular line at the fourth to sixth ribs. The areola is normally round and more darkly

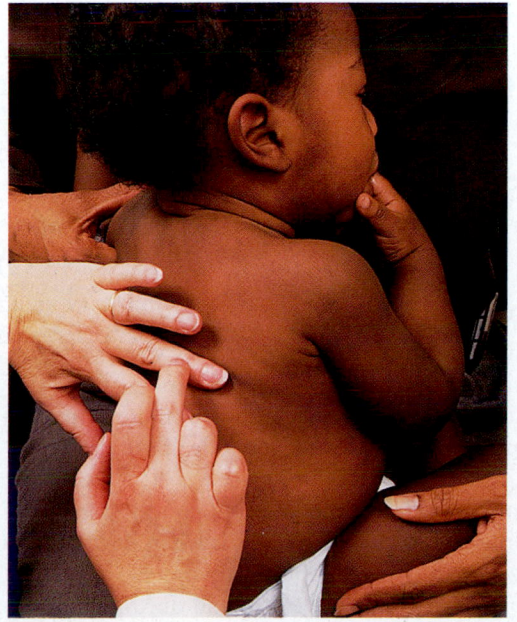

A

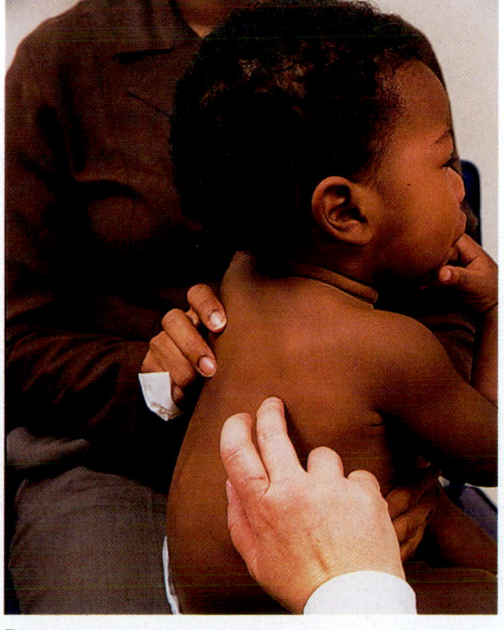

B

Figure 5–32 ➤ A, Indirect percussion. Place the middle finger on the child's chest at an intercostal space with the other fingers off of the chest. Tap the finger with a springlike motion with the fingertip of the other hand. B, Direct percussion. Tap the infant's chest with the fingertip directly at an intercostal space.

Figure 5–33 ➤ Normal resonance patterns expected over the chest. *Tympany* is a loud, high-pitched sound, like a drum. It is usually heard over an air-filled stomach. *Flatness* is a soft, dull sound, like the sound made when percussing your thigh. It is heard over dense muscle and bone. *Dullness* is a moderately loud, thudlike sound. It is heard when percussing over the liver and heart, and at the base of the lungs (at the level of the diaphragm). *Resonance* is a loud, low-pitched, hollow sound, like the sound made when percussing a table. It is heard over the lungs. *Hyperresonance* is a loud, very low-pitched, booming sound. It is usually heard over superinflated lungs. However, because of the thin chest wall in young children, hyperresonance may be a normal finding.

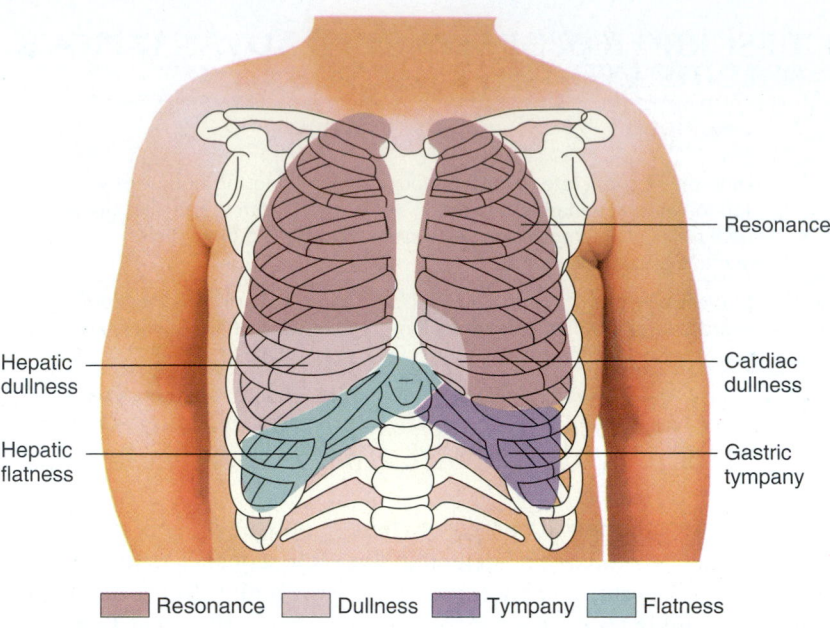

Resonance

Cardiac dullness

Gastric tympany

Hepatic dullness

Hepatic flatness

☐ Resonance ☐ Dullness ☐ Tympany ☐ Flatness

pigmented than the surrounding skin. Inspect the anterior chest for other dark spots that may indicate supernumerary nipples, which are small, undeveloped nipples and areola that may be mistaken for moles. Their presence may be associated with congenital renal or cardiac anomalies.

See page 196 for pubertal development.

Palpation of the Breasts

Palpate the developing breasts of adolescent females for abnormal masses or hard nodules while supine. Use a concentric pattern covering all quadrants of each breast including the axilla, all around the areola, and then around the nipple. Breast tissue normally feels dense, firm, and elastic.

The majority of boys have unilateral or bilateral breast enlargement during adolescence called gynecomastia. It is often most noticeable around 14 years of age and commonly disappears by the time of full sexual maturity. Palpate the tissue to differentiate actual breast tissue from fatty tissue in the pectoral area, and to detect any masses.

ASSESSING THE HEART FOR HEART SOUNDS AND FUNCTION

What is the point of maximum intensity and where is it located? Where are the pulse points to assess pulse quality? Which heart sounds are associated with systole and diastole? What is the normal heart rate for infants and children? What is the difference between heart sounds and murmurs?

EQUIPMENT NEEDED

Stethoscope
Sphygmomanometer

Inspection of the Precordium

Begin the heart examination by inspecting the *precordium*, or anterior chest. Place the child in a reclining or semi-Fowler's position, either on the parent's lap or on the examining table. Inspect the shape and symmetry of the anterior chest from the front and side views. The rib cage is normally symmetric. Bulging of the left side of the chest wall may indicate an enlarged heart.

Observe for any chest movement associated with the heart's contraction. The **apical impulse**, sometimes called the point of maximum intensity, is located where the left ventricle taps the chest wall during contraction. The apical impulse can normally be seen in thin children. A *heave*, an obvious lifting of the chest wall during contraction, may indicate an enlarged heart.

Palpation of the Precordium

Place the entire palmar surface of the fingers together on the chest wall to palpate the precordium. Systematically palpate the entire precordium to detect any pulsations, heaves, or vibrations. Palpating with minimal pressure increases the chance of detecting abnormal findings.

Apical Impulse

The apical impulse is normally felt as a slight tap against one fingertip. Use the topographic landmarks of the chest to describe its location (see Figures 5–28 and 5–29). Any other sensation palpated is usually abnormal.

Abnormal Sensations

A *lift* is the sensation of the heart lifting up against the chest wall. It may be associated with an enlarged heart or a heart contracting with extra force. A *thrill* is a rushing vibration that feels like a cat's purr. It is caused by turbulent blood flow from a defective heart valve and a heart murmur. If present, the thrill is palpated in the right or left second intercostal space. To describe a thrill's location, use the topographic landmarks of the chest (see Figures 5–28 and 5–29) and estimate the diameter of the thrill palpated.

Percussion of the Heart Borders

Percussion of the heart borders is rarely performed during physical examination. The borders of the heart are better identified by radiologic examination.

Auscultation of the Heart

Auscultation is used to count the apical pulse, to assess the characteristics of the heart sounds, and to detect abnormal heart sounds. Use the bell of the stethoscope to detect these lower pitched sounds.

To completely assess heart sounds, auscultate the heart with the child in both sitting and reclining positions. Differences in heart sounds caused by a change in the child's position or by a change in the position of the heart near the chest wall can then be detected. If differences in heart sounds are detected with a position change, place the child in the left lateral recumbent position and auscultate again.

Heart Rate and Rhythm

The apical heart rate can be counted at the site of the apical impulse, either by palpation or by auscultation. Count the apical rate for 1 minute in infants and in children who have an irregular rhythm. The brachial or radial pulse rate should be the same as the auscultated apical heart rate. Table 5–12 gives normal heart rates in children of different ages.

Listen carefully to the heart rate rhythm. Children often have a normal cycle of irregular rhythm associated with respiration called sinus arrhythmia. With *sinus arrhythmia* the child's heart rate is faster on inspiration and slower on expiration. When any rhythm irregularity is detected, ask the child to take a breath and hold it for a few

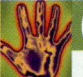

GROWTH & DEVELOPMENT

Apical Impulse

The location of the apical impulse changes as the child's rib cage grows. In children under 7 years old, it is located in the fourth intercostal space just medial to the left midclavicular line. In children over 7 years old, it is located in the fifth intercostal space at the left midclavicular line.

GROWTH & DEVELOPMENT

Heart Rate

The child's heart rate varies with age, decreasing as the child grows older. The heart rate also increases in response to exercise, excitement, anxiety, and fever. Such stresses increase the child's metabolic rate, creating a simultaneous need for more oxygen. Children respond to the need for more oxygen by increasing their heart rate, a response called sinus tachycardia. Because the ventricles have not fully developed in young children under 5 years, they are less able to increase their cardiac stroke volume to deliver more oxygen to the tissues as adults do.

Table 5–12	NORMAL HEART RATES FOR CHILDREN OF DIFFERENT AGES	
Age	**Heart Rate Range (beats/min)**	**Average Heart Rate (beats/min)**
Newborns	100–150	120
Infants to 2 years	80–120	100
2–6 years	70–110	90
6–10 years	60–95	80
10–16 years	60–85	70

seconds while you listen to the heart rate. The rhythm should become regular. Other rhythm irregularities are abnormal.

Differentiation of Heart Sounds

Heart sounds are due to the closure of the valves and vibration or turbulence of blood produced by that valve closure. Two primary sounds, S_1 and S_2, are heard when the chest is auscultated.

S_1, the first heart sound, is produced by closure of the tricuspid and mitral valves when the ventricular contraction begins. The two valves close almost simultaneously, so only one sound is normally heard.

S_2, the second heart sound, is produced by the closure of the aortic and pulmonic valves. Once blood has reached the pulmonic and aortic arteries, the valves close to prevent leakage back into the ventricles during diastole. The timing of the valve closure varies with respirations. Sometimes S_2 is heard as a single sound and at other times as a split sound, that is, two sounds heard a fraction of a second apart.

Sound is easily transmitted in liquid, and it travels best in the direction of blood flow. Auscultate heart sounds at specific areas on the chest wall in the direction of blood flow, just beyond the valve (Figure 5–34 ➤). The sounds produced by the heart valves or blood turbulence are heard throughout the chest in thin infants and children. Both S_1 and S_2 can be heard in all listening areas.

Auscultate heart sounds for quality (distinct versus muffled) and intensity (loud versus weak). First, distinguish between S_1 and S_2 in each listening area. Heart sounds are usually distinct and crisp in children because of their thin chest wall. Muffling or indistinct sounds may indicate a heart defect or congestive heart failure. Document the area where heart sounds are heard the best. Table 5–13 and Figure 5–34 review the location where each sound is normally best heard for assessment of quality and intensity. If the child has a potential murmur, auscultate the heart in the sitting, reclining, and standing positions to see if differences are noted by position change.

Splitting of the Heart Sounds

After distinguishing the first and second heart sounds, try to detect *physiologic splitting*. A split S_2 is more apparent during inspiration when the child takes a deep breath. More blood returns to the right ventricle, causing the pulmonic valve to close a fraction of a second later than the aortic valve. To detect physiologic splitting, auscultate over the pulmonic area while the child breathes normally and then while the child takes a deep breath. Splitting is normally more easily detected after a deep breath. The splitting returns to a single sound with regular breathing. If splitting does not vary with respiration, it is called *fixed splitting*. This is an abnormal finding associated with an atrial septal defect.

CLINICAL TIP

Palpate the carotid pulse when auscultating the heart to distinguish between the two heart sounds. The heart sound heard simultaneously with the pulsation is S_1.

Table 5–13	**IDENTIFICATION OF THE LISTENING SITES FOR AUSCULTATION OF THE QUALITY AND INTENSITY OF HEART SOUNDS**	
Heart Sound	**Locations Best Heard**	**Where Heard Softly**
S_1	Apex of the heart	Base of the heart
	Tricuspid area	Aortic area
	Mitral area	Pulmonic area
S_2	Base of the heart	Apex of the heart
	Aortic area	Tricuspid area
	Pulmonic area	Mitral area
Physiologic splitting	Pulmonic area	
S_3	Mitral area	

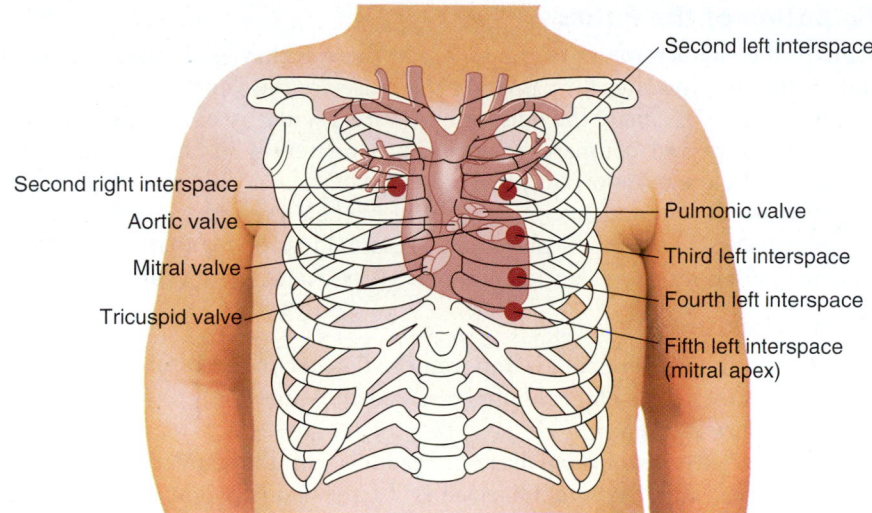

Figure 5–34 ➤ Sound travels in the direction of blood flow. Rather than listen for heart sounds over each heart valve, auscultate heart sounds at specific areas on the chest wall away from the valve itself. These areas are named for the valve producing the sound. *Aortic*: Second right intercostal space near the sternum. *Pulmonic*: Second left intercostal space near the sternum. *Tricuspid*: Fifth right or left intercostal space near the sternum. *Mitral* (apical): In infants—third or fourth intercostal space, just left of the left midclavicular line. In children—fifth intercostal space at the left midclavicular line.

Third Heart Sound

A third heart sound, S_3, is occasionally heard in children as a normal finding. S_3 is caused when blood rushes through the mitral valve and splashes into the left ventricle. It is heard in diastole, just after S_2. It is distinguished from a split S_2 because it is louder in the mitral area than in the pulmonic area.

Murmurs

Occasionally abnormal heart sounds are auscultated. These sounds are produced by turbulence of blood passing through a defective valve, great vessel, or other heart structure. Some murmurs are benign or innocent while others indicate pathology. An experienced examiner must be consulted to distinguish between murmurs.

To hear murmurs in children takes practice. Often, murmurs must be very loud to be detected. For softer murmurs, normal heart sounds must be distinguished before a murmur or an extra sound is recognized. Once a murmur is detected, define the characteristics of the extra sound.

Murmurs are classified by the following characteristics:

- *Intensity.* How loud is it? Can a thrill also be palpated?
- *Location.* Where is the murmur the loudest? Identify the listening area and precise topographic landmarks. Is the child sitting or lying down?
- *Radiation.* Is the sound transmitted over a larger area of the chest, to the axilla, or to the back?
- *Timing.* Is the murmur heard best after S_1 or S_2? Is it heard during the entire phase between S_1 and S_2?
- *Quality.* Describe what the murmur sounds like—for example, machinelike, musical, or blowing.

Venous Hum

Auscultate for a venous hum over the supraclavicular fossa above the middle of the clavicle or over the upper anterior chest with the bell of the stethoscope. A venous hum is heard as a continuous low-pitched hum throughout the cardiac cycle. It may be loudest during diastole or when the child stands, and it does not change with respirations. It may be quieted by having the child turn the neck. A venous hum may be associated with anemia, but it has no pathological significance.

Completing the Heart Examination

A complete assessment of cardiac function also includes palpating the pulses, measuring the blood pressure, and evaluating signs from other systems.

CLINICAL TIP

Following are guidelines for grading the intensity of a murmur:

Intensity	Description
Grade I	Barely heard in a quiet room
Grade II	Quiet, but clearly heard
Grade III	Moderately loud, no thrill palpated
Grade IV	Loud, a thrill is usually palpated
Grade V	Very loud, a thrill is easily palpated
Grade VI	Heard without the stethoscope in direct contact with the chest wall

GROWTH & DEVELOPMENT

Pulses

Infants have a low systolic blood pressure, and detecting the distal pulses is often difficult. Use the brachial artery in the arms and the popliteal or femoral artery in the legs to evaluate the pulses. The radial and distal tibial pulses are normally palpated easily in older children.

SKILL 6–10
Assessing the Blood Pressure

Palpation of the Pulses

Palpate the characteristics of the pulses in the extremities to assess the circulation. The technique and sites for palpating the pulse are the same as those used for adults (Figure 5–35 ➤). Evaluate the pulsation for rate, regularity of rhythm, and strength in each extremity and compare your findings bilaterally. The femoral and brachial pulses are the most important pulses to evaluate.

Palpate the femoral arteries and compare their strength with the strength of the brachial pulse. The femoral pulsations are usually stronger than or as strong as the brachial pulsations. A weaker femoral pulse is associated with coarctation of the aorta.

Blood Pressure

Assessment of blood pressure is important to detect conditions of hypertension or hypovolemic shock. The child should be seated and quiet for 3 to 5 minutes before the blood pressure is taken.

Compare the systolic and diastolic readings with the standard blood pressure values by age, sex, and height in Table 5–14. Use the child's height percentile for age and sex from the standard growth curves to determine the expected blood pressure for the child. A blood pressure value at 50th percentile for the child's age, sex, and height is considered the midpoint of the normal range. A reading above 95th percentile indicates hypertension.

Other Signs

To assess the heart and tissue perfusion, consider other signs, including skin color, capillary refill, and respiratory distress. The mucous membranes are usually pink. Cyanosis is most commonly associated with a congenital heart defect in children. Capillary refill is normally less than 2 seconds, indicating good circulation and perfusion of the tissues. Signs of respiratory distress, such as tachypnea, flaring, and retractions, may be associated with the child's attempts to compensate for hypoxemia caused by a congenital heart defect.

ASSESSING THE ABDOMEN FOR SHAPE, BOWEL SOUNDS, AND UNDERLYING ORGANS

What does a sunken abdomen indicate? What do bowel sounds normally sound like? How frequently should bowel sounds be heard in children? What do the various percussion tones indicate? What does a rigid abdomen indicate?

Topographic Landmarks of the Abdomen

The location of underlying organs and structures of the abdomen must be considered when the abdomen is examined. The abdomen is commonly divided by imaginary lines into quadrants for the purpose of identifying underlying structures (Figure 5–36 ➤).

Inspection of the Abdomen

Begin the examination of the abdomen by inspecting the shape and contour, condition of the umbilicus and rectus muscle, and abdominal movement. Inspect the child's abdomen from the front and side with good lighting. Note any creases, striae, or scars.

Shape

Inspect the shape of the abdomen to identify an abnormal contour. The child's abdomen is normally symmetric and rounded or

> **NURSING ALERT**
>
> In any child in which there is a concern about a heart condition, obtain a blood pressure reading in both an arm and a leg and compare the readings. The blood pressure in the leg should be the same or up to 10 mmHg higher than the arm reading. If the reading in the leg is lower than the arm, coarctation of the aorta may be present.

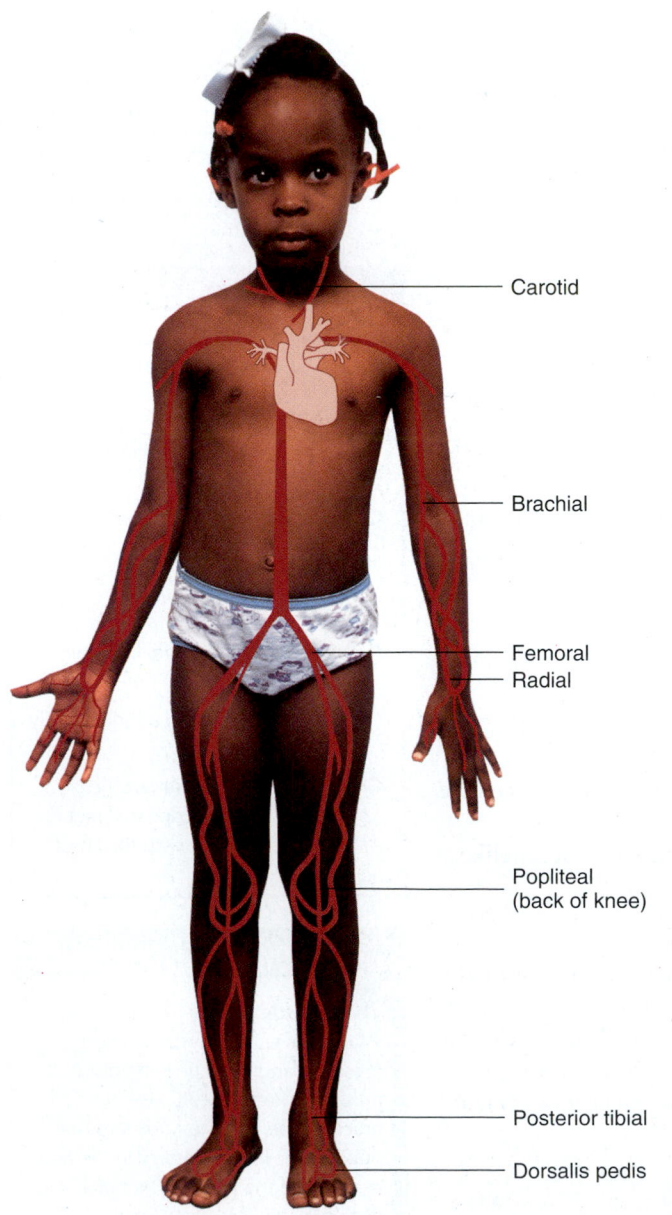

Carotid

Brachial

Femoral
Radial

Popliteal
(back of knee)

Posterior tibial

Dorsalis pedis

Figure 5–35 ➤ The sites used to assess the pulses in children.

flat when the child is supine. A scaphoid or sunken abdomen is abnormal and may indicate dehydration.

Umbilicus

Observe the newborn's umbilical stump for color, bleeding, odor, and drainage. The stump becomes black, dry, and hard within a couple of days after birth. The stump normally falls off between 7 and 14 days after birth. After the stump falls off, inspect the umbilicus for complete healing. Continued drainage may indicate an infection or a granuloma.

Inspect the umbilicus in older infants and toddlers. Children in these age groups often have an umbilical hernia, a protrusion of abdominal contents through an open umbilical muscle ring.

> **CLINICAL TIP**
>
> Perform inspection and auscultation before palpation and percussion because touching the abdomen may change the characteristics of bowel sounds.

> **EQUIPMENT NEEDED**
>
> Stethoscope

Table 5–14	**SYSTOLIC AND DIASTOLIC BLOOD PRESSURE VALUES FOR CHILDREN OF DIFFERENT AGES BY SEX AND HEIGHT PERCENTILE**

GIRLS

Age (Year)	BP Percentile	Systolic BP (mmHg) Percentile of Height							Diastolic BP (mmHg) Percentile of Height						
		5th	10th	25th	50th	75th	90th	95th	5th	10th	25th	50th	75th	90th	95th
1	50th	83	84	85	86	88	89	90	38	39	39	40	41	41	42
	90th	97	97	98	100	101	102	103	52	53	53	54	55	55	56
	95th	100	101	102	104	105	106	107	56	57	57	58	59	59	60
	99th	108	108	109	111	112	113	114	64	64	65	65	66	67	67
2	50th	85	85	87	88	89	91	91	43	44	44	45	46	46	47
	90th	98	99	100	101	103	104	105	57	58	58	59	60	61	61
	95th	102	103	104	105	107	108	109	61	62	62	63	64	65	65
	99th	109	110	111	112	114	115	117	69	69	70	70	71	72	72
3	50th	86	87	88	89	91	92	93	47	48	48	49	50	50	51
	90th	100	100	102	103	104	106	106	61	62	62	63	64	64	65
	95th	104	104	105	107	108	109	110	65	66	66	67	68	68	69
	99th	111	111	113	114	115	116	117	73	73	74	74	75	76	76
4	50th	88	88	90	91	92	94	94	50	50	51	52	52	53	54
	90th	101	102	103	104	106	107	108	64	64	65	66	67	67	68
	95th	105	106	107	108	110	111	112	68	68	69	70	71	71	72
	99th	112	113	114	115	117	118	119	76	76	76	77	78	79	79
5	50th	89	90	91	93	94	95	96	52	53	53	54	55	55	56
	90th	103	103	105	106	107	109	109	66	67	67	68	69	69	70
	95th	107	107	108	110	111	112	113	70	71	71	72	73	73	74
	99th	114	114	116	117	118	120	120	78	78	79	79	80	81	81
6	50th	91	92	93	94	96	97	98	54	54	55	56	56	57	58
	90th	104	105	106	108	109	110	111	68	68	69	70	70	71	72
	95th	108	109	110	111	113	114	115	72	72	73	74	74	75	76
	99th	115	116	117	119	120	121	122	80	80	80	81	82	83	83
7	50th	93	93	95	96	97	99	99	55	56	56	57	58	58	59
	90th	106	107	108	109	111	112	113	69	70	70	71	72	72	73
	95th	110	111	112	113	115	116	116	73	74	74	75	76	76	77
	99th	117	118	119	120	122	123	124	81	81	82	82	83	84	84
8	50th	95	95	96	98	99	100	101	57	57	57	58	59	60	60
	90th	108	109	110	111	113	114	114	71	71	71	72	73	74	74
	95th	112	112	114	115	116	118	118	75	75	75	76	77	78	78
	99th	119	120	121	122	123	125	125	82	82	83	83	84	85	86
9	50th	96	97	98	100	101	102	103	58	58	58	59	60	61	61
	90th	110	110	112	113	114	116	116	72	72	72	73	74	75	75
	95th	114	114	115	117	118	119	120	76	76	76	77	78	79	79
	99th	121	121	123	124	125	127	127	83	83	84	84	85	86	87

(continues)

| Table 5–14 | SYSTOLIC AND DIASTOLIC BLOOD PRESSURE VALUES FOR CHILDREN OF DIFFERENT AGES BY SEX AND HEIGHT PERCENTILE (continued) |

GIRLS

Age (Year)	BP Percentile	Systolic BP (mmHg) Percentile of Height							Diastolic BP (mmHg) Percentile of Height						
		5th	10th	25th	50th	75th	90th	95th	5th	10th	25th	50th	75th	90th	95th
10	50th	98	99	100	102	103	104	105	59	59	59	60	61	62	62
	90th	112	112	114	115	116	118	118	73	73	73	74	75	76	76
	95th	116	116	117	119	120	121	122	77	77	77	78	79	80	80
	99th	123	123	125	126	127	129	129	84	84	85	86	86	87	88
11	50th	100	101	102	103	105	106	107	60	60	60	61	62	63	63
	90th	114	114	116	117	118	119	120	74	74	74	75	76	77	77
	95th	118	118	119	121	122	123	124	78	78	78	79	80	81	81
	99th	125	125	126	128	129	130	131	85	85	86	87	87	88	89
12	50th	102	103	104	105	107	108	109	61	61	61	62	63	64	64
	90th	116	116	117	119	120	121	122	75	75	75	76	77	78	78
	95th	119	120	121	123	124	125	126	79	79	79	80	81	82	82
	99th	127	127	128	130	131	132	133	86	86	87	88	88	89	90
13	50th	104	105	106	107	109	110	110	62	62	62	63	64	65	65
	90th	117	118	119	121	122	123	124	76	76	76	77	78	79	79
	95th	121	122	123	124	126	127	128	80	80	80	81	82	83	83
	99th	128	129	130	132	133	134	135	87	87	88	89	89	90	91
14	50th	106	106	107	109	110	111	112	63	63	63	64	65	66	66
	90th	119	120	121	122	124	125	125	77	77	77	78	79	80	80
	95th	123	123	125	126	127	129	129	81	81	81	82	83	84	84
	99th	130	131	132	133	135	136	136	88	88	89	90	90	91	92
15	50th	107	108	109	110	111	113	113	64	64	64	65	66	67	67
	90th	120	121	122	123	125	126	127	78	78	78	79	80	81	81
	95th	124	125	126	127	129	130	131	82	82	82	83	84	85	85
	99th	131	132	133	134	136	137	138	89	89	90	91	91	92	93
16	50th	108	108	110	111	112	114	114	64	64	65	66	66	67	68
	90th	121	122	123	124	126	127	128	78	78	79	80	81	81	82
	95th	125	126	127	128	130	131	132	82	82	83	84	85	85	86
	99th	132	133	134	135	137	138	139	90	90	90	91	92	93	93
17	50th	108	109	110	111	113	114	115	64	65	65	66	67	67	68
	90th	122	122	123	125	126	127	128	78	79	79	80	81	81	82
	95th	125	126	127	129	130	131	132	82	83	83	84	85	85	86
	99th	133	133	134	136	137	138	139	90	90	91	91	92	93	93

From: National Heart Lung and Blood Institute. (2004). Blood pressure tables for children and adolescents from the fourth report on the diagnosis, evaluation, and treatment of high blood pressure in children and adolescents. Accessed June 11, 2004, from http://www.nhlbi.nih.gov/guidelines/hypertension/child_tbl.htm.

Rectus Muscle

Inspect the abdominal wall for any depression or bulging at midline above or below the umbilicus, indicating separation of the rectus abdominis muscles. The depression may be up to 5 cm (2 in.) wide. Measure the width of the separation to monitor change over time. As abdominal muscle strength develops, the separation usually becomes less prominent. However, the splitting may persist if congenital muscle weakness is present.

Abdominal Movement

Infants and children up to 6 years of age breathe with the diaphragm. The abdomen rises with inspiration and falls with expiration, simultaneously with the chest rise and fall. When the abdomen does not rise as expected, peritonitis may be present.

Other abdominal movements such as peristaltic waves are abnormal. *Peristaltic waves* are visible rhythmic contractions of the intestinal wall smooth muscle, which

Table 5–14	SYSTOLIC AND DIASTOLIC BLOOD PRESSURE VALUES FOR CHILDREN OF DIFFERENT AGES BY SEX AND HEIGHT PERCENTILE (continued)

BOYS

Age (Year)	BP Percentile	Systolic BP (mmHg) Percentile of Height							Diastolic BP (mmHg) Percentile of Height						
		5th	10th	25th	50th	75th	90th	95th	5th	10th	25th	50th	75th	90th	95th
1	50th	80	81	83	85	87	88	89	34	35	36	37	38	39	39
	90th	94	95	97	99	100	102	103	49	50	51	52	53	53	54
	95th	98	99	101	103	104	106	106	54	54	55	56	57	58	58
	99th	105	106	108	110	112	113	114	61	62	63	64	65	66	66
2	50th	84	85	87	88	90	92	92	39	40	41	42	43	44	44
	90th	97	99	100	102	104	105	106	54	55	56	57	58	58	59
	95th	101	102	104	106	108	109	110	59	59	60	61	62	63	63
	99th	109	110	111	113	115	117	117	66	67	68	69	70	71	71
3	50th	86	87	89	91	93	94	95	44	44	45	46	47	48	48
	90th	100	101	103	105	107	108	109	59	59	60	61	62	63	63
	95th	104	105	107	109	110	112	113	63	63	64	65	66	67	67
	99th	111	112	114	116	118	119	120	71	71	72	73	74	75	75
4	50th	88	89	91	93	95	96	97	47	48	49	50	51	51	52
	90th	102	103	105	107	109	110	111	62	63	64	65	66	66	67
	95th	106	107	109	111	112	114	115	66	67	68	69	70	71	71
	99th	113	114	116	118	120	121	122	74	75	76	77	78	78	79
5	50th	90	91	93	95	96	98	98	50	51	52	53	54	55	55
	90th	104	105	106	108	110	111	112	65	66	67	68	69	69	70
	95th	108	109	110	112	114	115	116	69	70	71	72	73	74	74
	99th	115	116	118	120	121	123	123	77	78	79	80	81	81	82
6	50th	91	92	94	96	98	99	100	53	53	54	55	56	57	57
	90th	105	106	108	110	111	113	113	68	68	69	70	71	72	72
	95th	109	110	112	114	115	117	117	72	72	73	74	75	76	76
	99th	116	117	119	121	123	124	125	80	80	81	82	83	84	84
7	50th	92	94	95	97	99	100	101	55	55	56	57	58	59	59
	90th	106	107	109	111	113	114	115	70	70	71	72	73	74	74
	95th	110	111	113	115	117	118	119	74	74	75	76	77	78	78
	99th	117	118	120	122	124	125	126	82	82	83	84	85	86	86
8	50th	94	95	97	99	100	102	102	56	57	58	59	60	60	61
	90th	107	109	110	112	114	115	116	71	72	72	73	74	75	76
	95th	111	112	114	116	118	119	120	75	76	77	78	79	79	80
	99th	119	120	122	123	125	127	127	83	84	85	86	87	87	88
9	50th	95	96	98	100	102	103	104	57	58	59	60	61	61	62
	90th	109	110	112	114	115	117	118	72	73	74	75	76	76	77
	95th	113	114	116	118	119	121	121	76	77	78	79	80	81	81
	99th	120	121	123	125	127	128	129	84	85	86	87	88	88	89

(continues)

move food through the digestive tract. Their presence generally indicates an intestinal obstruction, such as pyloric stenosis.

Auscultation of the Abdomen

To evaluate bowel sounds, auscultate the abdomen with the diaphragm of the stethoscope. Bowel sounds normally occur every 10 to 30 seconds. They have a high-pitched, tinkling, metallic quality. Loud gurgling (*borborygmi*) is heard when the child is hungry. Listen in each quadrant long enough to hear at least one bowel sound. Before determining that bowel sounds are absent, auscultate at least 5 minutes in each quadrant. Absence of bowel sounds may indicate peritonitis or a paralytic ileus. Hyperactive bowel sounds may indicate gastroenteritis or a bowel obstruction.

| Table 5–14 | **SYSTOLIC AND DIASTOLIC BLOOD PRESSURE VALUES FOR CHILDREN OF DIFFERENT AGES BY SEX AND HEIGHT PERCENTILE (continued)** |

BOYS

Age (Year)	BP Percentile	Systolic BP (mmHg) Percentile of Height							Diastolic BP (mmHg) Percentile of Height						
		5th	10th	25th	50th	75th	90th	95th	5th	10th	25th	50th	75th	90th	95th
10	50th	97	98	100	102	103	105	106	58	59	60	61	61	62	63
	90th	111	112	114	115	117	119	119	73	73	74	75	76	77	78
	95th	115	116	117	119	121	122	123	77	78	79	80	81	81	82
	99th	122	123	125	127	128	130	130	85	86	86	88	88	89	90
11	50th	99	100	102	104	105	107	107	59	59	60	61	62	63	63
	90th	113	114	115	117	119	120	121	74	74	75	76	77	78	78
	95th	117	118	119	121	123	124	125	78	78	79	80	81	82	82
	99th	124	125	127	129	130	132	132	86	86	87	88	89	90	90
12	50th	101	102	104	106	108	109	110	59	60	61	62	63	63	64
	90th	115	116	118	120	121	123	123	74	75	75	76	77	78	79
	95th	119	120	122	123	125	127	127	78	79	80	81	82	82	83
	99th	126	127	129	131	133	134	135	86	87	88	89	90	90	91
13	50th	104	105	106	108	110	111	112	60	60	61	62	63	64	64
	90th	117	118	120	122	124	125	126	75	75	76	77	78	79	79
	95th	121	122	124	126	128	129	130	79	79	80	81	82	83	83
	99th	128	130	131	133	135	136	137	87	87	88	89	90	91	91
14	50th	106	107	109	111	113	114	115	60	61	62	63	64	65	65
	90th	120	121	123	125	126	128	128	75	76	77	78	79	79	80
	95th	124	125	127	128	130	132	132	80	80	81	82	83	84	84
	99th	131	132	134	136	138	139	140	87	88	89	90	91	92	92
15	50th	109	110	112	113	115	117	117	61	62	63	64	65	66	66
	90th	122	124	125	127	129	130	131	76	77	78	79	80	80	81
	95th	126	127	129	131	133	134	135	81	81	82	83	84	85	85
	99th	134	135	136	138	140	142	142	88	89	90	91	92	93	93
16	50th	111	112	114	116	118	119	120	63	63	64	65	66	67	67
	90th	125	126	128	130	131	133	134	78	78	79	80	81	82	82
	95th	129	130	132	134	135	137	137	82	83	83	84	85	86	87
	99th	136	137	139	141	143	144	145	90	90	91	92	93	94	94
17	50th	114	115	116	118	120	121	122	65	66	66	67	68	69	70
	90th	127	128	130	132	134	135	136	80	80	81	82	83	84	84
	95th	131	132	134	136	138	139	140	84	85	86	87	87	88	89
	99th	139	140	141	143	145	146	147	92	93	93	94	95	96	97

From: National Heart Lung and Blood Institute. (2004). Blood pressure tables for children and adolescents from the fourth report on the diagnosis, evaluation, and treatment of high blood pressure in children and adolescents. Accessed June 11, 2004, from http://www.nhlbi.nih.gov/guidelines/hypertension/child_tbl.htm.

Next auscultate over the abdominal aorta and the renal arteries for a vascular hum or murmur. No murmur should be heard. A murmur may indicate a narrowed or defective artery.

Percussion of the Abdomen

Use indirect percussion to evaluate borders and sizes of abdominal organs and masses. Percussion is performed with the child supine. Choose a sequence to systematically percuss the entire abdomen (Figure 5–37 ➤).

Different tones are expected when the abdomen is percussed related to the underlying structures. The expected pattern of percussion tones over the abdomen is as follows:

* *Dullness*—found over organs such as the liver, spleen, and full bladder.
* *Tympany*—found over the stomach or the intestines when an obstruction is present or over areas beyond the stomach in infants because of air swallowing.
* *Resonance*—may be heard over other areas.

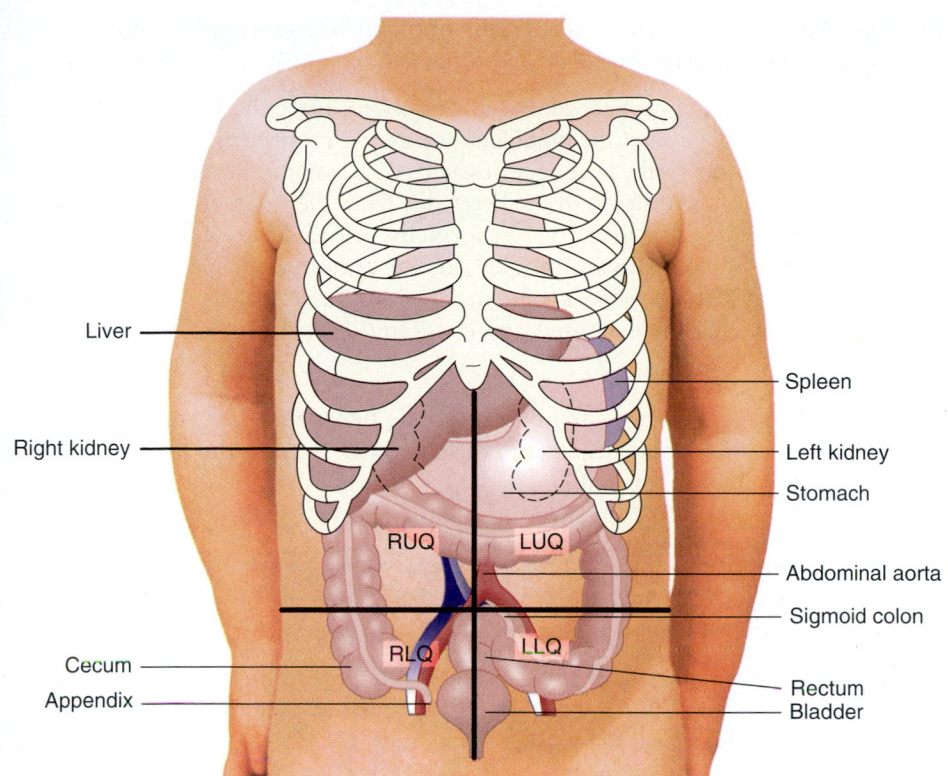

Figure 5–36 ➤ Topographic landmarks of the abdomen. The abdomen is commonly divided by imaginary lines into quadrants for the purposes of identifying underlying structures.

Organ size can be identified by listening for a percussion tone change at the border of an organ. For example, when you percuss down the chest, the upper edge of the liver is usually detected by a tone change from resonant to dull near the fifth intercostal space at the right midclavicular line. The lower liver edge is usually detected 2 to 3 cm (about 1 in.) below the right costal margin in infants and toddlers, but closer to the costal margin in older children.

Palpation of the Abdomen

Both light and deep palpation are used to examine the abdomen's organs and to detect any masses. *Light palpation* is used to evaluate the tenseness of the abdomen (how soft or hard it is), the liver, the presence of any tenderness or masses, and any defects in the abdominal wall. *Deep palpation* is used to detect masses, define their shape and consistency, and identify tenderness in the abdomen.

To make the most accurate interpretation, perform the abdominal examination when the child is calm and cooperative. Organs and other masses are more easily palpated when the abdominal wall is relaxed. Infants and toddlers often feel more secure lying supine across both the parent's and the examiner's laps. A bottle, pacifier, or toy may distract the child and improve cooperation for the examination. Older children often need distraction, especially when there is a question of abdominal tenderness and guarding or when the child is ticklish. Have the child perform a task that requires some concentration, such as pressing the hands together or pulling locked hands apart.

To begin palpation, position the child supine with knees flexed. Stand beside the child and place warmed fingertips across the child's abdomen. Palpate with the edge of the fingers, not just the fingerpads, and palpate in a sequence to examine the entire abdomen. Watch the child's face during palpation for a grimace or constriction of the pupils, which indicates pain.

Light Palpation

For light palpation, use a superficial, gentle touch that slightly depresses the abdomen. Usually the abdomen feels soft and no tenderness is detected. Palpate any bulging along the abdominal wall, especially along the rectus muscle and umbilical ring, which could indicate a hernia. Measure the diameter of the muscle ring, rather than the protrusion,

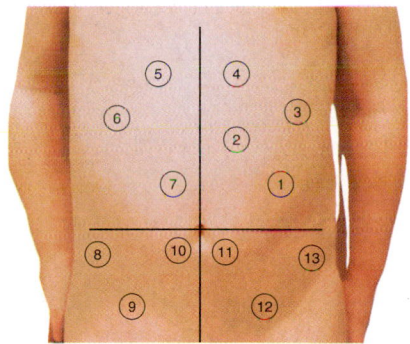

Figure 5–37 ➤ Sequence for indirect percussion of the abdomen.

CLINICAL TIP

Use suggestive words to help the child relax so you can palpate the abdomen. "How soft will your tummy get when my hand feels it? Does it get softer than this? Yes. See, it softens as you breathe out. Will it also be softer here?" In this way, the child learns to relax the abdomen and is challenged to do it better.

to monitor change over time. The muscle ring normally becomes smaller and closes by 4 years of age. An umbilical hernia that persists beyond this age may need surgical repair.

LIVER   Locate and lightly palpate the lower liver edge. Place the fingers in the right midclavicular line at the level of the umbilicus and gently move them toward the costal margin during expiration. As the liver edge descends with inspiration, a flat, narrow ridge is usually felt. Measure the distance of the liver edge from the right costal margin at the right midclavicular line. The liver edge is normally palpated 2 to 3 cm (1 in.) below the right costal margin in infants and toddlers. It may not be palpable in older children. The liver is enlarged when the edge is more than 3 cm (1 in.) below the right costal margin. An enlarged liver may be associated with congestive heart failure or hepatic disease.

Deep Palpation

To perform deep palpation, press the fingers of one hand (for small children) or two hands (for older children) more deeply into the abdomen. Because the abdominal muscles are most relaxed when the child takes a deep breath, ask the child to take regular deep breaths when palpating each area of the abdomen.

SPLEEN   Palpate for the spleen at the left costal margin in the midclavicular line. The spleen tip may be felt when the child takes a deep breath. The spleen is enlarged when it can be easily palpated below the left costal margin.

KIDNEYS   Palpate for the kidneys deep in the abdomen along each side of the spinal column. The kidneys are difficult to palpate in all children, except newborns, because of the deep layer of abdominal muscles and intestines. If a kidney is actually palpated, an abnormal mass may be present.

OTHER MASSES   Occasionally other masses, both normal and abnormal, can be palpated in the abdomen. A tubular mass commonly palpated in the lower left or right quadrant is often an intestine filled with feces. A distended bladder is often palpated as a firm, central, dome-shaped mass above the symphysis pubis in young children. Any fixed mass that moves laterally, pulsates, or is located along the vertebral column may be a neoplasm.

Assessment of the Inguinal Area

The inguinal area is inspected and palpated during the abdominal examination to detect enlarged lymph nodes or masses. The femoral pulse, a part of the heart examination, may be assessed simultaneously with the abdominal examination.

Inspection

Inspect the inguinal area for any change in contour, comparing sides. A small bulge noted over the femoral canal in girls may be associated with a femoral hernia. A bulging in the inguinal area in boys may be associated with an inguinal hernia.

Palpation

Palpate the inguinal area for lymph nodes and other masses. Small lymph nodes, less than 1 cm (1/2 in.) in diameter, are often present in the inguinal area because of minor injuries on the legs. Any tenderness, heat, or inflammation in these palpated lymph nodes could be associated with a local infection.

ASSESSING THE GENITAL AND PERINEAL AREAS FOR EXTERNAL STRUCTURAL ABNORMALITIES

What can a vaginal discharge indicate in a preadolescent girl? Is swelling in a newborn's scrotum normal? Where is the proper location of the urethral meatus on the penis?

Preparation of Children for the Examination

Examination of the genitalia and perineal area can cause stress in children because they sense their privacy has been invaded. To make young children feel more secure, position them on the parent's lap with their legs spread apart. Children can also be

EQUIPMENT NEEDED

Gloves
Lubricant
Penlight

positioned on the examining table with their knees flexed and the legs spread apart like a frog.

In younger children the genital and perineal examination is performed immediately after assessment of the abdomen. The genitals and perineum may be examined last in older children and adolescents.

Inspection of the Female Genitalia

Inspect the external genitalia of girls for color, size, and symmetry of the mons pubis, labia, urethra, and vaginal opening (Figure 5–38 ➤). At that time, determine the stage of pubertal maturation. Simultaneously, look for any abnormal findings such as swelling, inflammation, masses, lacerations, or discharge.

Mons Pubis

Inspect the mons pubis for pubic hair and its characteristics. Preadolescent girls have no pubic hair. See page 197 for guidelines to assess the stage of pubic hair development.

Labia

The labia minora are usually thin and pale in preadolescent girls but become dark pink and moist after puberty. In young infants the labia minora may be fused and cover the structures in the vestibule. These adhesions may need to be separated.

Hymen

Use the thumb and forefinger of one gloved hand to separate the labia minora for viewing structures in the vestibule. The hymen is just inside the vaginal opening. In preadolescents it is usually a thin membrane with a crescent-shaped opening. The vaginal opening is usually about 1 cm (1/2 in.) in adolescents when the hymen is intact. Sexually active adolescents may have a vaginal opening with irregular edges.

Urethral and Vaginal Openings

Inspect the vestibule for lesions. No lesions or signs of inflammation are expected around the urethral or vaginal opening. Redness and excoriation are often associated with an irritant such as bubble bath.

Vaginal Discharge

Preadolescent girls do not normally have a vaginal discharge. Adolescents often have a clear discharge without a foul odor. Menses generally begin approximately 2 years

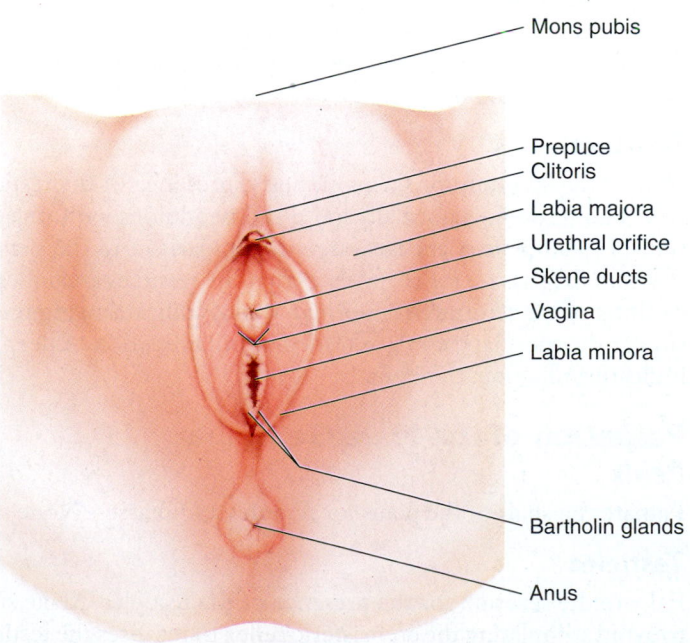

- Mons pubis
- Prepuce
- Clitoris
- Labia majora
- Urethral orifice
- Skene ducts
- Vagina
- Labia minora
- Bartholin glands
- Anus

Figure 5–38 ➤ Anatomic structures of the female genital and perineal area.

after breast-bud development. A foul-smelling discharge in preschool-age children may be associated with a foreign body. Various organisms may cause a vaginal infection in older children.

An internal vaginal examination is indicated when abnormal findings such as a vaginal discharge or trauma to the external structures is noted. Only an experienced examiner should perform the vaginal examination of the child.

Palpation of the Female Genitalia

Palpate the vaginal opening with a finger of your free gloved hand. The Bartholin and Skene glands are not usually palpable. Palpation of these glands in preadolescent children indicates enlargement because of an infection such as gonorrhea.

Inspection of the Male Genitalia

Inspect the male genitalia for the structural and pubertal development of the penis, scrotum, and testicles. Place boys in the tailor position, seated with their legs crossed in front of them. This position puts pressure on the abdominal wall to push the testicles into the scrotum. See page 197 for guidelines to assess the staging of pubic hair and external genital development.

Penis

Inspect the penis for size, foreskin, hygiene, and position of the urethral meatus. The length of the nonerect penis in the newborn is normally 2 to 3 cm (1 in.). The penis enlarges in length and breadth during puberty. The penis is normally straight. A downward bowing of the penis may be caused by a *chordee*, a fibrous band of tissue associated with hypospadias.

When the penis is circumcised, the glans penis is exposed. To inspect the glans penis of an uncircumcised boy, ask the child or parent to pull the foreskin back. Alternatively, the examiner may retract the foreskin. The foreskin of children over 6 years of age normally retracts past the corona easily. If the foreskin is tight and cannot be retracted, phimosis is present.

The glans penis is normally clean and smooth without inflammation or ulceration. The urethral meatus is a slit-shaped opening near the tip of the glans. No discharge should be present. A round, pinpoint urethral meatus may indicate meatal stenosis. Location of the urethral meatus at another site on the penis is abnormal, indicating *hypospadias* (meatus is located on the ventral or undersurface of the penile shaft between the perineum to the tip of the glans) or *epispadias* (meatus is located on the dorsal surface of the penile shaft). Inspect the urinary stream. The stream is normally strong without dribbling. Erythema and edema of the glans (balanitis) may result from infection or trauma. In the uncircumcised penis, purulent discharge and an edematous foreskin may be seen.

Scrotum

Inspect the scrotum for size, symmetry, presence of the testicles, and any abnormalities. The scrotum is normally loose and pendulous with rugae, or wrinkles. The scrotum of infants often appears large in comparison to the penis. A small, undeveloped scrotum that has no rugae indicates that the testicles are undescended. Enlargement or swelling of the scrotum is abnormal. It may indicate an inguinal hernia, hydrocele, torsion of the spermatic cord, or testicular inflammation. A deep cleft in the scrotum may indicate ambiguous genitalia.

Palpation of the Male Genitalia
Penis

Palpate the shaft of the penis for nodules and masses. None should be present.

Testicles

Palpate the scrotum for the presence of the testicles. Make sure your hands are warm to avoid stimulating the cremasteric reflex that causes the testicles to retract. Place your index finger and thumb over both inguinal canals on each side of the penis. This keeps the testicles from retracting into the abdomen (Figure 5–39 ➤).

Gently palpate each testicle with only enough pressure to identify the shape and size. The testicles are normally smooth and equal in size. They are approximately 1 to 1.5 cm (1/2 in.) in diameter until puberty, when they increase in size. A hard, enlarged, painless testicle may indicate a tumor.

If a testicle is not palpated in the scrotum, the examiner palpates the inguinal canal for a soft mass. When the testicle is found in the inguinal canal, try to move it to the scrotum to palpate the size and shape. The testicle is descendable when it can be moved into the scrotum. An undescended testicle is one that does not descend into the scrotum or cannot be palpated in the inguinal canal.

Spermatic Cord

Palpate the length of the spermatic cord between the thumb and forefinger from the testicle to the inguinal canal. It normally feels solid and smooth. No tenderness is expected.

Enlarged Scrotum

When bulging or swelling of the scrotum is present, palpate the scrotum to identify the characteristics of the mass. Try to determine whether the mass is unilateral or bilateral and attempt to reduce the mass by pushing it back through the external inguinal ring. A mass that decreases may indicate an inguinal hernia. A mass that does not decrease may indicate a hydrocele or an incarcerated hernia. To distinguish between a hydrocele and an incarcerated hernia, place a bright penlight under the scrotum and look for a red glow or transillumination through the scrotum. A hydrocele transilluminates; a hernia does not.

Inguinal Canal

Attempt to insert the little finger into the external inguinal canal to determine whether the external inguinal ring is dilated. The inguinal ring is normally too small for the finger to pass into the canal. If the finger passes into the inguinal canal, ask the child to cough. A sensation of abdominal contents coming down to touch the fingertip may indicate an inguinal hernia.

Cremasteric Reflex

Stroke the inner thigh of each leg to stimulate the cremasteric reflex. The testicle and scrotum normally rise on the stroked side. This response indicates intact function of the spinal cord at the T12, L1, and L2 levels.

Inspection of the Anus and Rectum

Inspect the anus for sphincter control and any abnormal findings such as inflammation, fissures, or lesions. The external sphincter is usually closed. Inflammation and scratch marks around the anus may be associated with pinworms. A protrusion from the rectum may be associated with a rectal wall prolapse or a hemorrhoid.

Palpation of the Anus and Rectum

Lightly touching the anal opening should stimulate an anal contraction or "wink." Absence of a contraction may indicate the presence of a lower spinal cord lesion.

Patency of the Anus

Passage of meconium by newborns indicates a patent anus. When passage of meconium is delayed, a lubricated catheter can be inserted 1 cm (1/2 in.) into the anus. Resistance in passage of the catheter may indicate an obstruction.

Rectal Examination

A rectal examination is not routinely performed on children. It is indicated for symptoms of intra-abdominal, rectal, bowel, or stool abnormalities. Only an experienced examiner should perform a rectal examination.

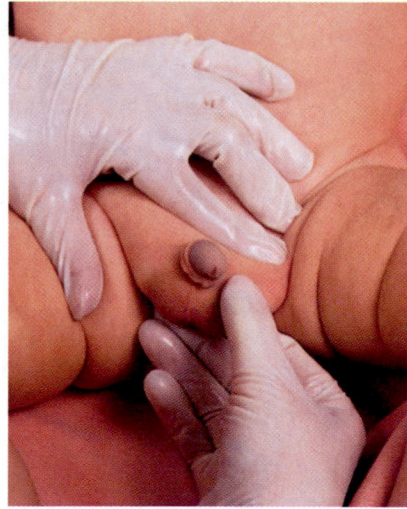

Figure 5–39 ➤ Palpating the scrotum for descended testicles and spermatic cords.

ASSESSMENT OF PUBERTAL DEVELOPMENT AND SEXUAL MATURATION

What is the first stage of breast development in girls? What is the first stage of pubertal development in boys? How is the stage of pubertal development determined in boys and girls?

The age of onset of secondary sexual characteristics can vary with race and ethnicity, environmental conditions, geographic location, and nutrition.

Females

Inspect the child's breasts while the child is sitting. Breast development in girls usually precedes other pubertal changes; however, in 20% of girls, pubic hair may occur first (Pinyerd & Zipf, 2005). Figure 5–40 ➤ shows the Tanner stages of breast development.

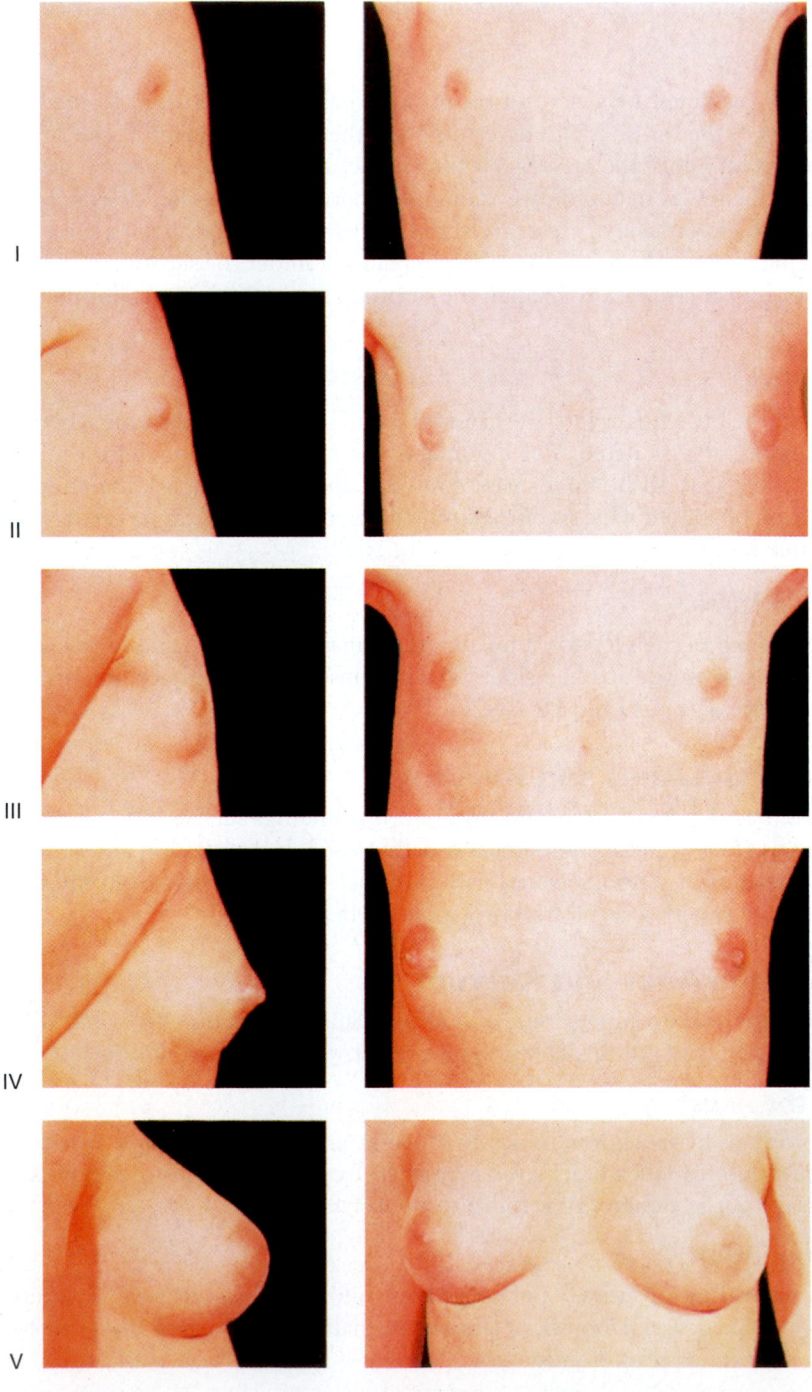

Figure 5–40 ➤ The Tanner stages of breast development.
Used with permission from Van Wieringen et al. (1971). *Growth diagrams 1965 Netherlands.* Groningen: Wolters-Noordhof.

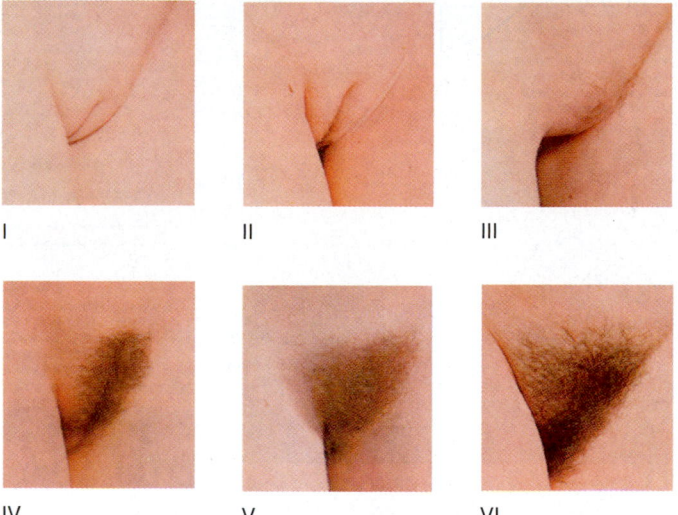

I   II   III

IV   V   VI

Figure 5–41 ➤ The Tanner stages of female pubic hair development with sexual maturation. In Stage II, soft downy hair along the labia majora is an indication that sexual maturation is beginning. Hair grows progressively coarse and curly as development proceeds.
Used with permission from Van Wieringen et al. (1971). *Growth diagrams 1965 Netherlands.* Groningen: Wolters-Noordhof.

Breast budding, the first stage of pubertal development in girls, typically occurs between 8 and 14 years of age. Black girls have a significantly earlier age for the onset of puberty (reaching Tanner stage 2 for breast or pubic hair development) than White girls. Girls with greater body fat may have an increased likelihood for earlier puberty onset (Biro, Huang, Crawford et al., 2006). A girl's breasts may develop at different rates and appear asymmetric.

The presence, amount, and distribution of pubic hair is an indication of the sexual maturation stage in the girl. Preadolescent girls have no pubic hair. Initial pubic hair is lightly pigmented, sparse, and straight. Pubic hair development progresses in consistent stages for all girls. Figure 5–41 ➤ illustrates the normal stages of female pubic hair development. Breast development usually precedes pubic hair development. The presence of pubic hair before 8 years of age is unusual.

Males

Initial signs of pubertal development in males are enlargement of the testicles and thinning of the scrotum. This is followed by straight, downy pubic hair starting at the base of the penis 6 months later. The hair becomes darker, dense, and curly, extending over the pubic area in a diamond pattern by the completion of puberty. The presence of pubic hair before 9 years of age is uncommon, and delayed onset of testicular enlargement after 14 years of age needs evaluation. Penile enlargement generally follows testicular enlargement about 1 year later in genitalia Tanner stage 3. Stages of pubic hair development follow a standard pattern, as seen in Figure 5–42 ➤.

Sexual Maturity Rating

The sexual maturity rating (SMR) is an average of the breast and pubic hair Tanner stages in females and of the genital and pubic hair Tanner stages in males. The rating is the number between 2 and 5, as stage 1 is prepubertal. The SMR is then related to other physiologic events that happen during puberty. Compare the stage of the child's secondary sexual characteristics with information in Figure 5–43 ➤.

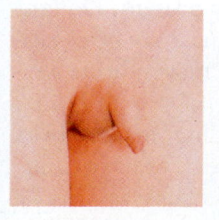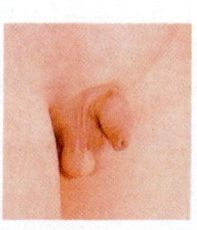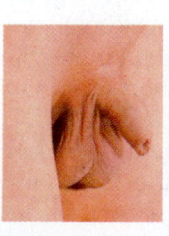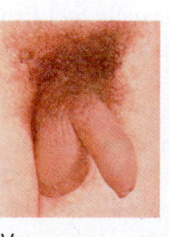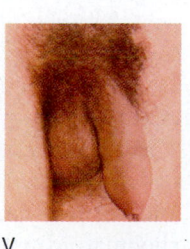

I   II   III   IV   V

Figure 5–42 ➤
The Tanner stages of male pubic hair and external genital development with sexual maturation.
Used with permission from Van Wieringen et al. (1971). *Growth diagrams 1965 Netherlands.* Groningen: Wolters-Noordhof.

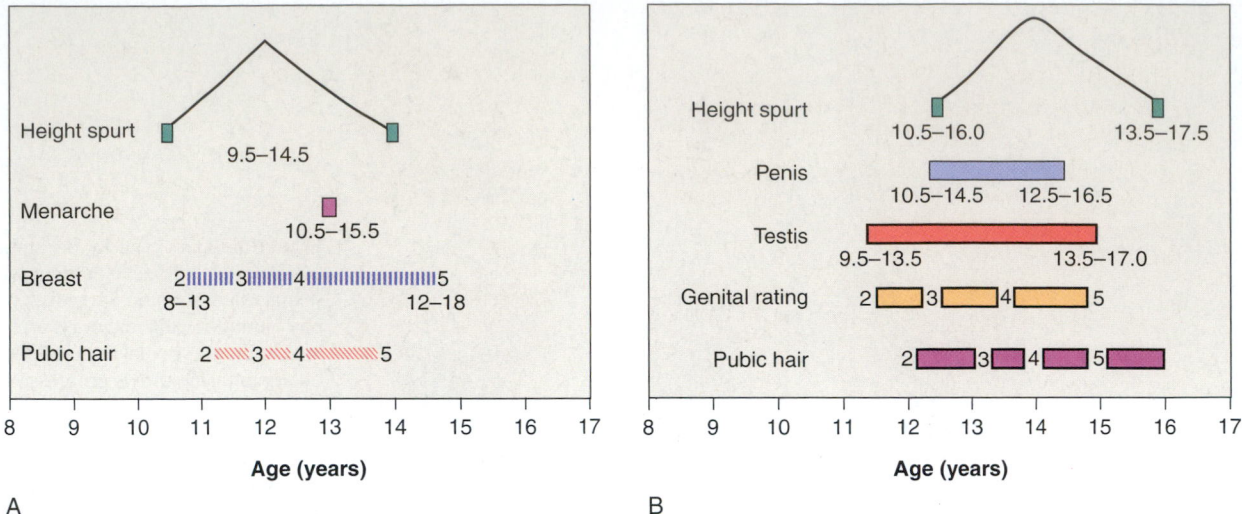

Figure 5–43 ➤ Sexual maturity rating—approximate timing of developmental changes. The numbers indicate stages of development. Range of ages during which some changes occur is indicated by the inclusive numbers below them. A, Females, B, Males.

Used with permission from Marshall W. A., & Tanner, J. M. (1969). Variations in patterns of pubertal changes in girls. *Archives of Disease in Childhood, 44,* 291; and Marshall, W. A. & Tanner, J. M. (1970). Variations in pubertal changes in boys. *Archives of Disease in Childhood, 45,* 13.

In females, menarche generally occurs in SMR 4 or breast stage 3 to 4. The peak height velocity usually occurs before menarche at a mean age of 11.5 years. In males ejaculation usually occurs at SMR 3, with semen noted between SMR 3 and 4. The peak height velocity usually occurs in SMR 4 or genital stage 4 to 5, at about 13.5 years of age.

ASSESSING THE MUSCULOSKELETAL SYSTEM FOR BONE AND JOINT STRUCTURE, MOVEMENT, AND MUSCLE STRENGTH

What do extra skin folds on an arm or leg indicate? What causes poor muscle tone? What condition does a rib hump indicate? At what age is it normal for children to be knock-kneed or bow-legged?

Inspection of the Bones, Muscles, and Joints

Inspect and compare the arms and then the legs for differences in alignment, contour, skin folds, length, and deformities. The extremities normally have equal length, circumference, and numbers of skin folds bilaterally. Extra skin folds and a larger circumference may indicate a shorter extremity.

Inspect and compare the joints bilaterally for size, discoloration, and ease of voluntary movement. Joints are normally the same color as surrounding skin, with no sign of swelling. Children should voluntarily flex and extend joints during normal activities without pain. Redness, swelling, and pain with movement may indicate injury or infection.

Palpation of the Bones, Muscles, and Joints

Palpate the bones and muscles in each extremity for muscle tone, masses, or tenderness. Muscles normally feel firm, and bony masses are not normally present. Doughy muscles may indicate poor muscle tone. Rigid muscles, or hypertonia, may be associated with an active seizure or cerebral palsy. A mass over a long bone may indicate a recent fracture or a bone tumor.

Palpate each joint and surrounding muscles to detect any swelling, masses, heat, or tenderness. None is expected when the joint is palpated. Tenderness, heat, swelling, and redness can result from injury or a chronic joint inflammation such as juvenile rheumatoid arthritis.

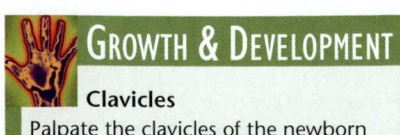

GROWTH & DEVELOPMENT

Clavicles
Palpate the clavicles of the newborn from the sternum to the shoulder. These bones are often fractured during delivery. A mass and crepitus may indicate a fracture.

Range of Motion and Muscle Strength Assessment

Active Range of Motion

Observe the child during typical play activities, such as reaching for objects, climbing, and walking, to assess range of motion of all major joints. Children spontaneously move their joints through the full normal range of motion with play activities when no pain is present. Limited range of motion may indicate injury, inflammation of a joint, or a muscle abnormality.

Passive Range of Motion

When a joint is suspected of having limited active range of motion, perform passive range of motion. Flex and extend, abduct and adduct, or rotate the affected joint cautiously to avoid causing extra pain. Full range of motion without pain is normal. Limitations in movement may indicate injury, inflammation, or malformation. Greater passive than active range of motion may indicate muscle weakness.

Muscle Strength

Observe the child's ability to climb onto an examining table, throw a ball, clap the hands, or move around on the bed. The child's ability to perform age-appropriate play activities indicates good muscle tone and strength. Attainment of age-appropriate motor development is another indicator of good muscle strength (Table 5–15).

To assess the strength of specific muscles in the extremities, engage the child in some games. Compare muscle strength bilaterally to identify muscle weakness. For example, the child squeezes the examiner's fingers tightly with each hand; pushes against and pulls the examiner's hands with his or her hands, lower legs, and feet; and resists extension of a flexed elbow or knee. Children normally have good muscle strength bilaterally. Unilateral muscle weakness may be associated with a nerve injury. Bilateral muscle weakness may result from hypoxemia or a congenital disorder such as Down syndrome. Asymmetrical weakness may be associated with conditions such as cerebral palsy.

When generalized muscle weakness is suspected in a preschool- or school-age child, ask the child to stand up from the supine position. Children are normally able to rise to a standing position without using their arms as levers. Children who push their body upright using the arms and hands may have generalized muscle weakness, known as a positive Gowers' sign. This may indicate muscular dystrophy (see Figure 28–19 ∞).

Posture and Spinal Alignment

Posture

Inspect the child's posture when standing from a front, side, and back view. The shoulders and hips are normally level. The head is held erect without a tilt, and the shoulder

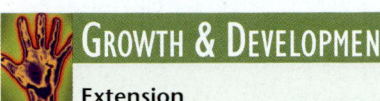

GROWTH & DEVELOPMENT

Extension

Newborns typically have a limited extension of the hips, knees, and elbows, resulting from their flexed fetal position. When the newborn's arms and legs are extended and released, the extremities rapidly return to their flexed fetal position.

CLINICAL TIP

To check the shoulder muscle strength in a newborn, hold the infant upright with your hands under the infant's arms. An infant who is held lightly will normally not slip through the hands. Muscle weakness is present when the infant slides through the hands (Seidel, Ball, Dains et al., 2006, p. 738).

Table 5–15	SELECTED GROSS MOTOR MILESTONES FOR AGE

Gross Motor Milestones	Age Attained
Rolls over from prone to supine position	4 months
Sits without support	8 months
Pulls self to standing position	10 months
Walks around room holding onto objects	11 months
Walks alone well	15 months
Kicks ball	24 months
Jumps in place	30 months
Throws ball overhand	36 months

Note: From Frankenburg, W. K., Dodds, J., Archer, P., Shapiro, H., & Bresnick, B. (1992). The Denver II: A major revision and restandardization of the Denver Developmental Screening Test. *Pediatrics, 89,* 91–97. Reproduced with permission from *Pediatrics*, Figure 2, © 1992.

Table 5–16   NORMAL DEVELOPMENT OF POSTURE AND SPINAL CURVES

2–3 months	6–8 months	10–15 months	Toddler	School-age child
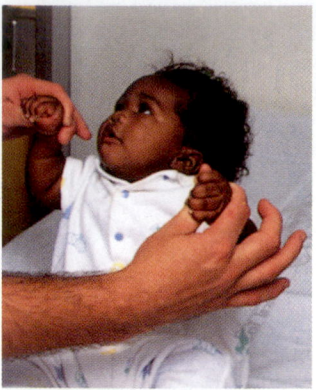	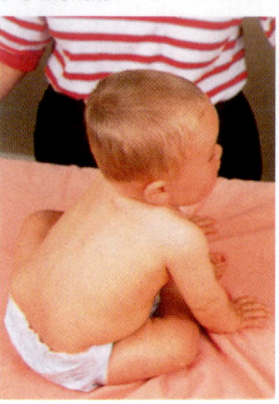	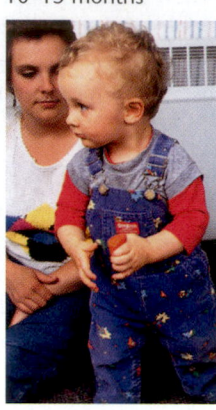	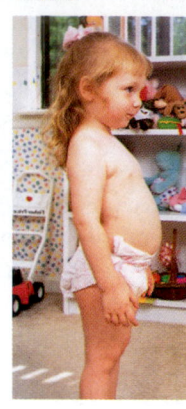	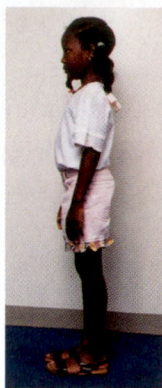
Holds head erect when held upright; thoracic kyphosis when sitting.	Sits without support; spine is straight.	Walks independently; straight spine.	Protruding abdomen; lumbar lordosis.	Height of shoulders and hips is level; balanced thoracic convex and lumbar concave curves.

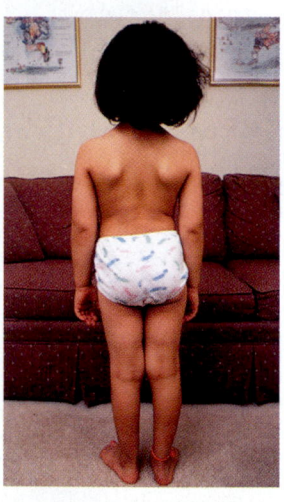

Figure 5–44 ▶ Does this child have legs of different lengths or scoliosis? Look at the level of the iliac crests and shoulders to see if they are level. See the more prominent crease at the waist on the right side? This child could have scoliosis.

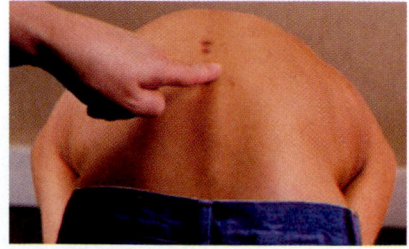

Figure 5–45 ▶ Inspection of the spine for scoliosis. Ask the child to slowly bend forward at the waist, with arms extended toward the floor. Run your forefinger down the spinal processes, palpating each vertebra for a change in alignment. A lateral curve to the spine or a one-sided rib hump is an indication of scoliosis.

contour is symmetric. After beginning to walk, young children often have a pot-bellied stance because of lumbar lordosis. The spine has normal thoracic convex and lumbar concave curves after 6 years of age. Table 5–16 shows normal posture and spinal curvature development.

Spinal Alignment

Assess the school-age child and adolescent for *scoliosis*, a lateral spine curvature. Stand behind the child, observing the height of the shoulders and hips (Figure 5–44 ▶). Ask the child to bend forward slowly at the waist, with arms extended toward the floor. No lateral curve should be present in either position. The ribs normally stay flat bilaterally. The lumbar concave curve should flatten with forward flexion (Figure 5–45 ▶). A lateral curve to the spine or a one-sided rib hump is an indication of scoliosis (see Chapter 28 ∞).

Inspection of the Upper Extremities

Arms

The alignment of the arms is normally straight, with a minimal angle at the elbows, where the bones articulate.

Hands

Count the fingers. Extra finger digits (*polydactyly*) or webbed fingers (*syndactyly*) are abnormal. Inspect the creases on the palmar surface of each hand. Multiple creases across the palm are normal. A single transverse palmar crease that crosses the entire palm of the hand is associated with Down syndrome (Figure 5–46 ▶).

Nails

Inspect the nails for size, shape, and color. Nails are normally convex, smooth, and pink. **Clubbing**, widening of the nailbed with an increased angle between the proximal nail fold and nail, is abnormal (see Figure 21–8 ∞). Clubbing is associated with chronic respiratory and cardiac conditions.

Inspection of the Lower Extremities

Hips

Assess the hips of newborns and young infants for dislocation or subluxation. The skin folds on the upper legs are inspected first. The same number of skin folds should be present on each leg. Uneven skin folds may indicate a hip dislocation or difference in leg length (Allis' sign). Then check for a difference in knee height symmetry (Figure 5–47 ▶).

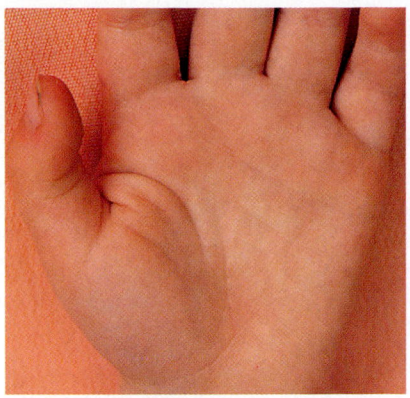
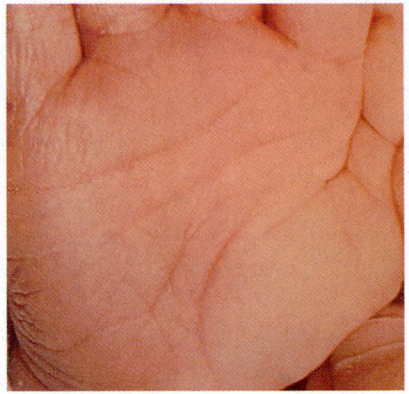

A   B

Figure 5–46 ➤ A, Normal palmar creases. B, Transverse palmar crease associated with Down syndrome.
Used with permission from Zitelli, B. J., & Davis, H. W. (Eds.). (1997). *Atlas of pediatric physical diagnosis* (3rd ed.). St. Louis: Mosby–Year Book.

The Ortolani–Barlow maneuver is used to assess an infant's hips for dislocation or sub-luxation (Figure 5–48 ➤). This maneuver should be performed by a trained healthcare practitioner.

Ask the child to stand on one leg and then the other. The iliac crests should stay level. If the iliac crest opposite the weight-bearing leg appears lower, the hip-bearing weight may be dislocated.

Legs

Inspect the alignment of the legs. After a child is 4 years of age, the alignment of the long bones is straight, with minimal angle at the knees and feet where the bones articulate. As-sess alignment of the lower extremities in infants and toddlers to ensure that normal changes are occurring. To evaluate the toddler with bowlegs, have the child stand on a firm surface. Measure the distance between the knees when the child's ankles are to-gether. No more than 3.5 cm (1.5 in.) between the knees is normal. See Figure 5–49 ➤ for assessment of knock-knees.

Feet

Inspect the feet for alignment, the presence of all toes, and any deformities. The weight-bearing line of the feet is usually in alignment with the legs. Many newborns have a flexible forefoot inversion (metatarsus adductus) that results from uterine posi-tioning. Any fixed deformity is abnormal.

Inspect the feet for the presence of an arch when the child is standing. Children up to 3 years of age normally have a fat pad over the arch, giving the appearance of flat feet. Older children normally have a longitudinal arch. The arch is usually seen when the child stands on tiptoe or is sitting. Inspect the nails of the feet as for the hands.

ASSESSING THE NERVOUS SYSTEM FOR COGNITIVE FUNCTION, BALANCE, COORDINATION, CRANIAL NERVE FUNCTION, SENSATION, AND REFLEXES

What aspects of developmental information are useful for assessment of cognitive function? How are the infant's and child's levels of consciousness evaluated? How are cranial nerves assessed in infants? A scissoring gait is associated with what condition? At what age does a Babinski response become abnormal? What response is expected when a deep tendon reflex is stimulated?

Cognitive Function

Observe the child's behavior, facial expressions, gestures, communication skills, activ-ity level, and level of consciousness to assess cognitive functioning. Match the neuro-logic examination to the child's stage of development. For example, cognitive function

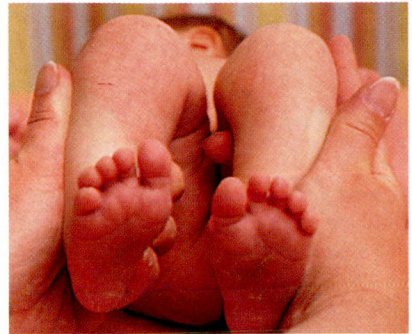

Figure 5–47 ➤ Flex the infant's hips and knees so the heels are as close to the buttocks as possible. Place the feet flat on the examining table. The knees are usually the same height. A difference in knee height (Allis' sign) is an indicator of hip dislocation.
Used with permission from Dee Corbett, RN, Children's National Medical Center, Washington, DC.

GROWTH & DEVELOPMENT

Tibial Torsion

Infants are often born with a twisting of the tibia caused by positioning in utero (tibial torsion). The infant's toes turn in as a result of the tibial torsion. Toddlers go through a skeletal alignment sequence of bowlegs (genu varum) and knock-knees (genu valgum) before the legs assume a straight alignment.

CLINICAL TIP

The neurologic examination provides an opportunity to develop rapport with the child. Many of the procedures can be presented as games that young children enjoy. You can assess cognitive function by how well the child follows directions for the game. As the assessment proceeds, the child develops trust and is more likely to cooperate with examination of other systems.

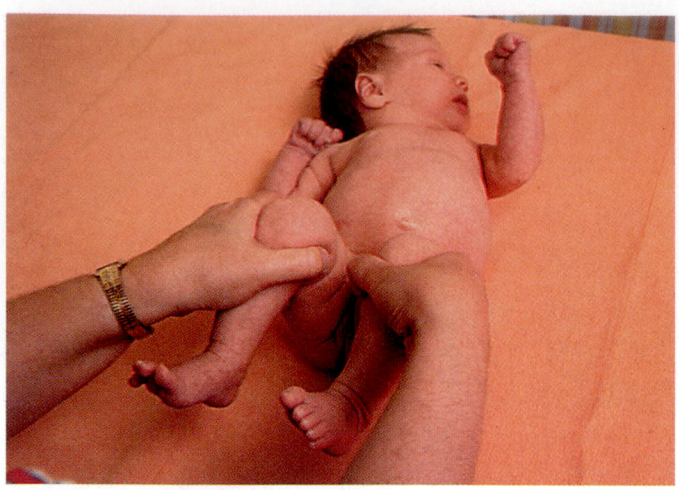

A

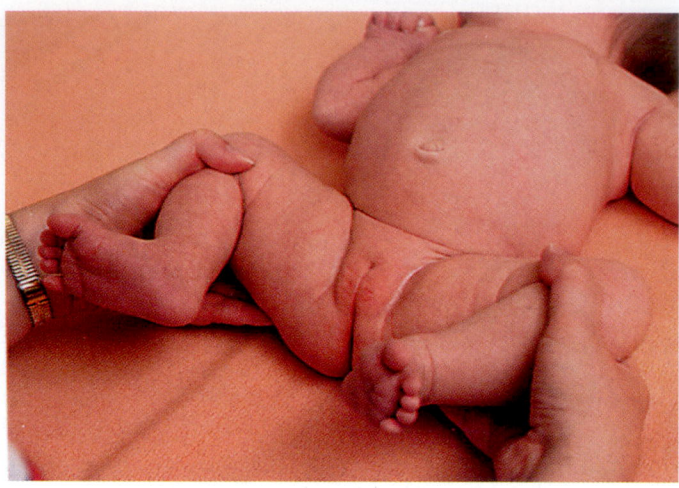

B

Figure 5–48 ▶ Ortolani–Barlow maneuver. A, Place the infant on his or her back and flex the hips and knees at a 90° angle. Place a hand over each knee with the thumb over the inner thigh and the first two fingers over the upper margin of the femur. Move the infant's knees together until they touch, and then put downward pressure on one femur at a time to see if the hips easily slip out of their joints or dislocate. B, Slowly abduct the hips, moving each knee toward the examining table. Keep pressure on the hip joints with the fingers in a lever-type motion. Equal hip abduction, with the knees nearly touching the examining table, is normal. Any resistance to abduction or a clunk felt on palpation can be an indication of a congenital hip dislocation.

EQUIPMENT NEEDED

Reflex hammer
Cotton balls
Penlight
Tongue blades

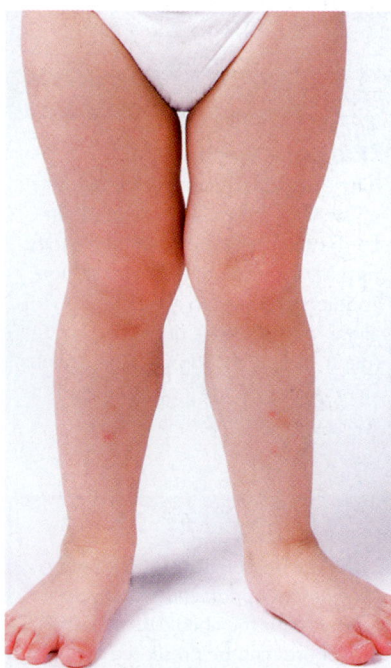

Figure 5–49 ▶ To evaluate the child with knock-knees, have the child stand on a firm surface. Measure the distance between the ankles when the child stands with the knees together. The normal distance is not more than 5 cm (2 in.) between the ankles.

is evaluated much differently in infants than in older children because infants cannot use words to communicate.

Behavior

The behavior of infants and children during the assessment indicates their alertness. Infants and toddlers are curious but seek the security of the parent, either by clinging or by making frequent eye contact. Older children are often anxious and watch all of the examiner's actions. Lack of interest in assessment or treatment procedures may indicate a serious illness. Excessive activity or an unusually short attention span may be associated with an attention deficit hyperactivity disorder.

Communication Skills

Speech, language development, and social skills provide good clues to cognitive functioning. Listen to speech articulation and words used, comparing the child's performance with standards of social development and speech articulation for the child's age (Table 5–17). Toddlers can normally follow simple directions such as "Show me your mouth." By 3 years of age the child's speech should be easily understood. Delay in language and social skill development may be associated with developmental disability.

Table 5–17	EXPECTED LANGUAGE DEVELOPMENT FOR AGE	
Language Milestones	**Age Attained**
Understands Mama and Dada	10 months
Says Mama, Dada, 2 other words; imitates animal sounds	12 months
4–6 word vocabulary, points to desired objects	13–15 months
7–20 word vocabulary, points to 5 body parts	18 months
2-word combinations	20 months
3-word sentences, plurals	36 months

Note: From Capute, A. J., Shapiro, B. K., & Palmer, R. B. (1987). Marking the milestones of language development. *Contemporary Pediatrics, 4,* 24–41.

Memory

Immediate, recent, and remote memory can be tested in children starting at approximately 4 years of age. To evaluate recent memory, ask the child to remember a special name or object. Then 5 to 10 minutes later during the examination, have the child recall the name or object. To evaluate remote memory, ask the child to repeat his or her address or birth date or a nursery rhyme. By 5 or 6 years of age, children are normally able to recall this information without difficulty.

Level of Consciousness

When approaching the infant or child, observe his or her level of consciousness and activity, including facial expressions, gestures, and interaction. Children are normally alert, and sleeping children arouse easily. The child who cannot be awakened is unconscious. A lowered level of consciousness may be associated with a number of neurologic conditions such as a head injury, seizure, infection, or brain tumor.

Cerebellar Function

Observe the young child at play to assess coordination and balance. Development of fine motor skills in infants and preschool children provides clues to cerebellar function.

Balance

Observe the child's balance during play activities such as walking, standing on one foot, and hopping (Table 5–18). The Romberg procedure can also be used to test balance in children over 3 years of age (Figure 5–50 ➤). Once balance and other motor skills are attained, children do not normally stumble or fall when tested. Poor balance may indicate cerebellar dysfunction or an inner ear disturbance.

Coordination

Tests of coordination assess the smoothness and accuracy of movement. Development of fine motor skills can be used to assess coordination in young children (Table 5–19). After 6 years of age the tests for adults (finger-to-nose, finger-to-finger, heel-to-shin, and alternating motion) can be used (Figure 5–51 ➤). The child usually responds enthusiastically when these tests are presented as games. Jerky movements or inaccurate pointing (past pointing) indicate poor coordination, which can be associated with delayed development or a cerebellar lesion.

Gait

A normal gait requires intact bones and joints, muscle strength, coordination, and balance. Inspect the child when walking from both a front and a rear view. The iliac crests are normally level during walking, and no limp is expected. A limp may indicate injury or joint disease. Staggering or falling may indicate cerebellar ataxia. *Scissoring*, in which the thighs tend to cross forward over each other with each step, may be associated with cerebral palsy or other spastic conditions. Persistent walking on the toes may indicate a possible neurologic dysfunction.

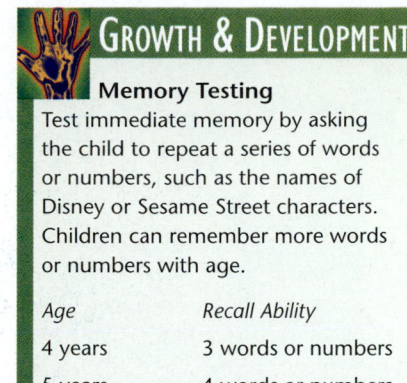

GROWTH & DEVELOPMENT

Memory Testing

Test immediate memory by asking the child to repeat a series of words or numbers, such as the names of Disney or Sesame Street characters. Children can remember more words or numbers with age.

Age	Recall Ability
4 years	3 words or numbers
5 years	4 words or numbers
6 years	5 words or numbers

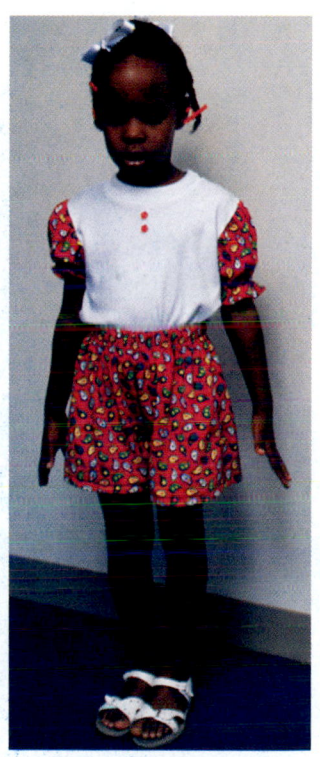

Figure 5–50 ➤ Romberg procedure. Ask the child to stand with feet together and eyes closed. Protect the child from falling by standing close. Preschool-age children may extend their arms to maintain balance, but older children can normally stand with their arms at their sides. Leaning or falling to one side is abnormal and indicates poor balance.

GROWTH & DEVELOPMENT

Gait

Gait is related to the motor development of the child. Toddlers beginning to walk have a wide-based gait and limited balance. With practice the toddler's balance improves and the gait develops a narrower base.

Table 5–18	EXPECTED BALANCE DEVELOPMENT FOR AGE

Balance Milestones	Age Attained
Stands without support briefly	12 months
Walks alone well	15 months
Walks backwards	2 years
Balances on 1 foot for 5 seconds	4 years
Hops on 1 foot, heel-toe walking	5 years
Heel-toe walking backwards	6 years

Table 5–19	EXPECTED FINE MOTOR DEVELOPMENT FOR AGE

Fine Motor Milestones	Age Attained
Transfers objects between hands	7 months
Picks up small objects	10 months
Feeds self with cup and spoon	12 months
Scribbles with crayon or pencil	18 months
Builds 2-block tower	24 months
Builds 4-block tower	30 months
Unfastens front buttons	36 months

Note: From Frankenburg, W. K., Dodds, J., Archer, P., Shapiro, H., & Bresnick, B. (1992). The Denver II: A major revision and restandardization of the Denver Developmental Screening Test. *Pediatrics, 89,* 91–97. Reproduced with permission from *Pediatrics,* Table 2, © 1992.

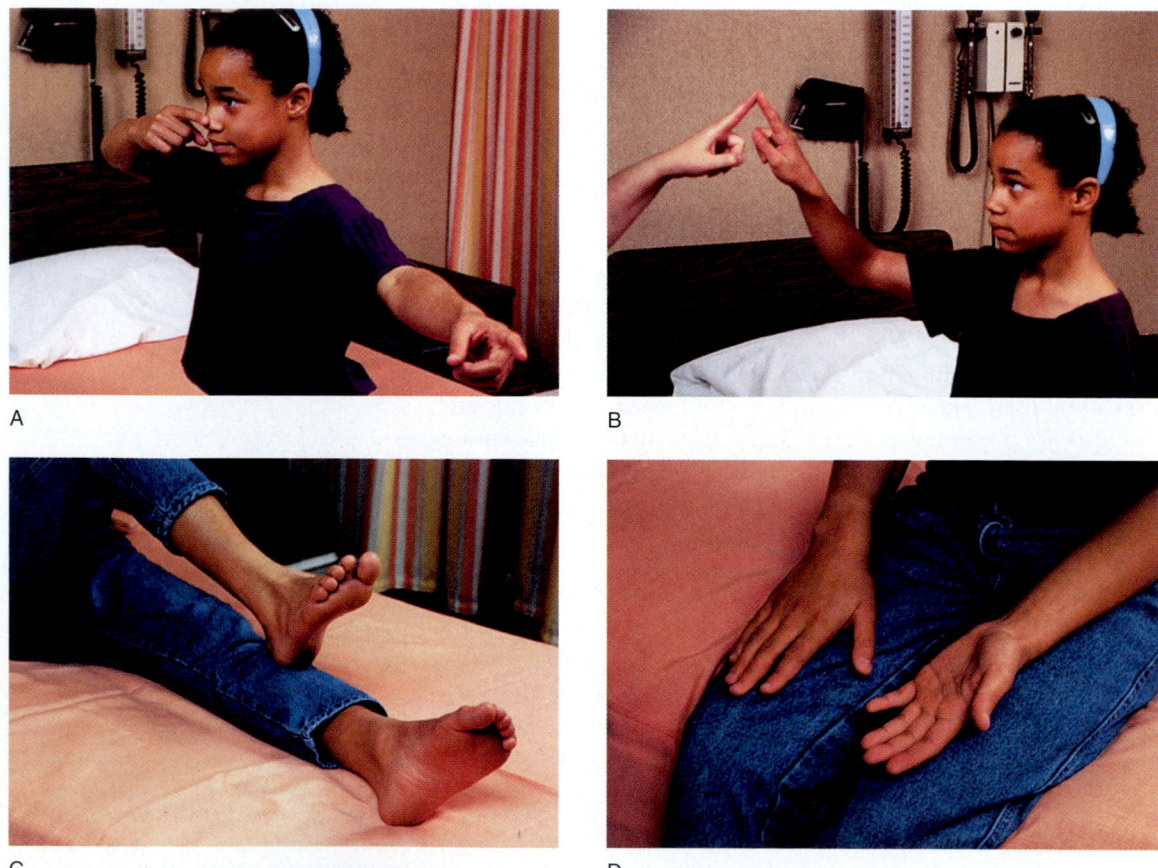

A

B

C

D

Figure 5–51 ▶ Tests of coordination. A, Finger-to-nose test. Ask the child to close the eyes and touch his or her nose, alternating the index fingers of the hands. B, Finger-to-finger test. Ask the child to alternately touch his or her nose and your index finger with his or her index finger. Move your hand to several positions within the child's reach to test pointing accuracy. Repeat the test with the child's other hand. C, Heel-to-shin test. Ask the child to rub his or her leg from the knee to the ankle with the heel of the other foot. Repeat the test with the other foot. This test is normally performed without hesitation or inappropriate placement of the foot. D, Rapid alternating motion test. Ask the child to rapidly rotate his or her wrist so the palm and dorsum of the hand alternately pat the thigh. Repeat the test with the other hand. Hesitating movements are abnormal. Mirroring movements of the hand not being tested indicate a delay in coordination skill refinement.

Cranial Nerve Function

To assess the cranial nerves in infants and young children, modify the procedures used to assess school-age children and adults (Table 5–20). Abnormalities of cranial nerves may be associated with compression of an individual nerve, head injury, or infections.

Sensory Function

To assess sensory function, compare the responses of the body to various types of stimulation. Bilaterally equal responses are normal. Loss of sensation may indicate a brain or spinal cord lesion. Withdrawal responses to painful procedures indicate normal sensory function in an infant.

Superficial Tactile Sensation

Stroke the skin on the lower leg or arm with a cotton ball or a finger while the child's eyes are closed. Cooperative children over 2 years of age can normally point to the location touched.

Superficial Pain Sensation

Break a tongue blade to get a sharp point. After asking the child to close the eyes, touch the child in various places on each arm and leg, alternating the sharp and dull ends of the tongue blade. A paper clip may also be used. Children over 4 years of age can normally distinguish between a sharp and dull sensation each time. To improve the child's accuracy with the test, let the child practice telling you the difference between the sharp and dull stimulation.

An inability to identify superficial touch and pain sensation may indicate sensory loss. Identify the extent of sensory loss, such as all areas below the knee. Other sensory function tests (temperature, vibratory, deep pressure pain, and position sense) are performed when sensory loss is found. Refer to other texts for a description of these procedures.

Infant Primitive Reflexes

Evaluate the movement and posture of newborns and young infants by the Moro, palmar grasp, plantar grasp, placing, stepping, and tonic neck primitive reflexes (Table 5–21). These reflexes appear and disappear at expected intervals in the first few months of life as

GROWTH & DEVELOPMENT

Infant Sensory Function
An infant's sensory function is not routinely assessed. Withdrawal responses to painful procedures indicate normal sensory function.

Table 5–20	AGE-SPECIFIC PROCEDURES FOR ASSESSMENT OF CRANIAL NERVES IN INFANTS AND CHILDREN
Cranial Nerve[a]	**Assessment Procedure and Normal Findings[b]**
I. Olfactory	Infant: Not tested. Child: Not routinely tested. Give familiar odors to child to smell, one naris at a time. *Identifies odors such as orange, peanut butter, and chocolate.*
II. Optic	Infant: Shine a bright light in the eyes. *A quick blink reflex and dorsal head flexion indicates light perception.* Child: Test vision and visual fields if cooperative. *Visual acuity appropriate for age.*
III. Oculomotor IV. Trochlear VI. Abducens	Infant: Shine a penlight at the eyes and move it side to side. *Focuses on and tracks the light to each side.* Child: Move an object through the six cardinal points of gaze. *Tracks object through all fields of gaze.* All ages: Inspect eyelids for drooping. Inspect pupillary response to light. *Eyelids do not droop and pupils are equal sized and briskly respond to light.*
V. Trigeminal	Infant: Stimulate the rooting and sucking reflex. *Turns head toward stimulation at side of mouth and sucking has good strength and pattern.* Child: Observe the child chewing a cracker. Touch forehead and cheeks with cotton ball when eyes are closed. *Bilateral jaw strength is good. Child pushes cotton ball away.*
VII. Facial	All ages: Observe facial expressions when crying, smiling, frowning, etc. *Facial features stay symmetric bilaterally.*
VIII. Acoustic	Infant: Produce a loud sound near the head. *Blinks in response to sound, moves head toward sound or freezes position.* Child: Use a noisemaker near each ear or whisper words to be repeated. *Turns head toward sound and repeats words correctly.*
IX. Glossopharyngeal X. Vagus	Infant: Observe swallowing during feeding. *Good swallowing pattern.* All ages: Elicit gag reflex. *Gags with stimulation.*
XI. Spinal accessory	Infant: Not tested. Child: Ask child to raise the shoulders and turn the head side to side against resistance. *Good strength in neck and shoulders.*
XII. Hypoglossal	Infant: Observe feeding. *Sucking and swallowing are coordinated.* Child: Tell the child to stick out the tongue. Listen to speech. *Tongue is midline with no tremors. Words are clearly articulated.*

[a]Bracketed nerves are tested together.
[b]Italic indicates normal findings.

Table 5–21	TECHNIQUES FOR ASSESSING SELECTED PRIMITIVE REFLEXES, WITH NORMAL FINDINGS AND THEIR EXPECTED AGE OF OCCURRENCE

Primitive Reflex	Technique and Normal Findings[a]	Normal Appearance and Disappearance
Moro 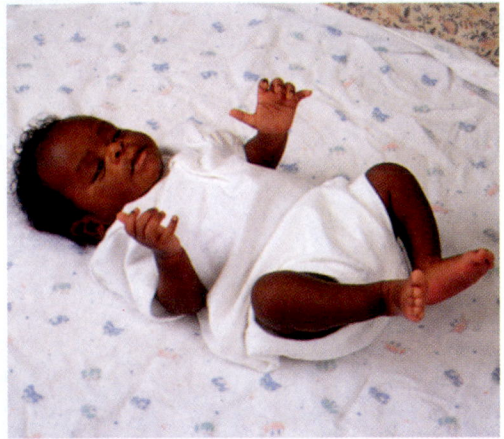	Startle the infant with a sudden noise or change in position. *The arms extend and the fingers form a C as they spread. The arms slowly move together as in a hug. The legs may make a similar motion.*	Present at birth. Decreases in strength by 4 months of age. Disappears by 6 months of age.
Palmar grasp 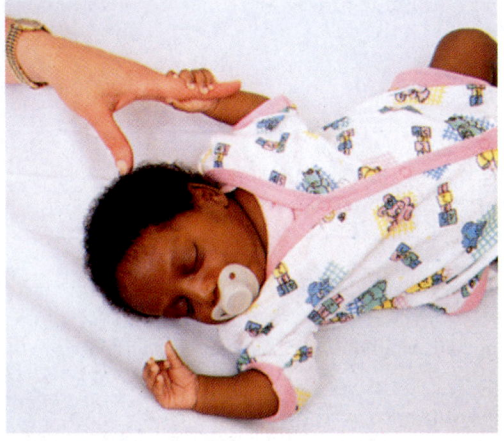	Place finger across the infant's palm and avoid touching the thumb. *A strong grip around the finger is normal.*	Present at birth. Disappears by 3 months of age.
Plantar grasp 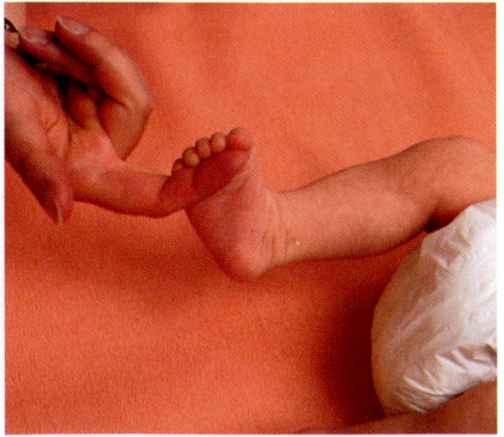	Place finger across the foot at the base of the toes. *The toes normally curl as if gripping the finger.*	Present at birth. Disappears at about 8 months of age.

[a]Italic indicates normal findings.

Table 5–21	TECHNIQUES FOR ASSESSING SELECTED PRIMITIVE REFLEXES, WITH NORMAL FINDINGS AND THEIR EXPECTED AGE OF OCCURRENCE

Primitive Reflex	Technique and Normal Findings[a]	Normal Appearance and Disappearance
Placing 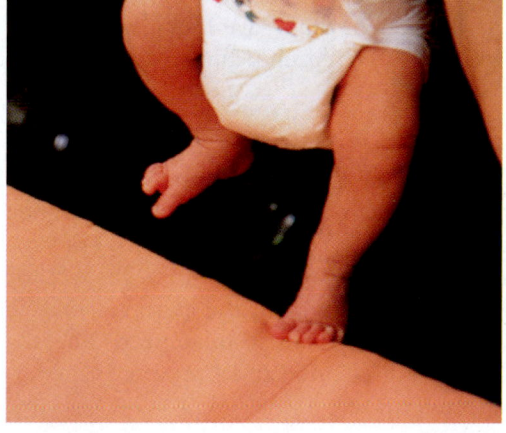	Hold the infant erect and touch the top of one foot with the edge of a table or chair. *The infant normally lifts the foot, as if to step up onto the surface.*	Present within days of birth. Disappears at various times.
Stepping 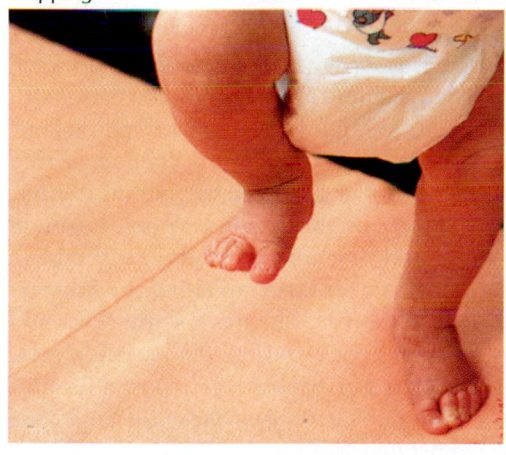	Hold the infant erect and touch the bottom of one foot on the surface of a table or chair. *The feet lift in an alternating pattern as if to walk.*	Present at birth. Disappears between 4 and 8 weeks of age.
Tonic neck 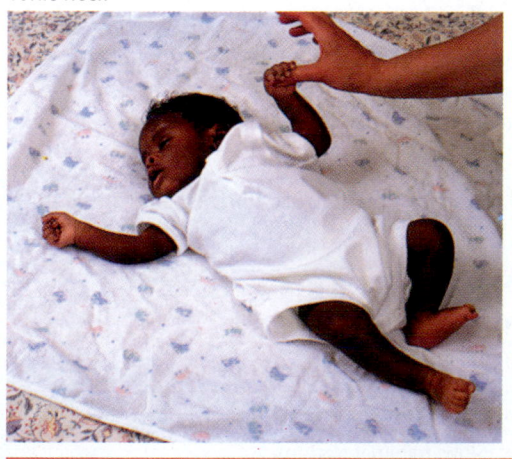	Place the infant in a supine position and, when relaxed, turn the head to one side. Repeat by turning the head to the opposite side. *The arm and leg on the face side normally extend and the opposite arm and leg flex, as if to assume a fencing position.*	Appears about 2 months of age. Decreases by 4 months of age. Disappears no later than 6 months of age. This reflex must disappear before the infant can turn over.

[a]Italics indicates normal findings.

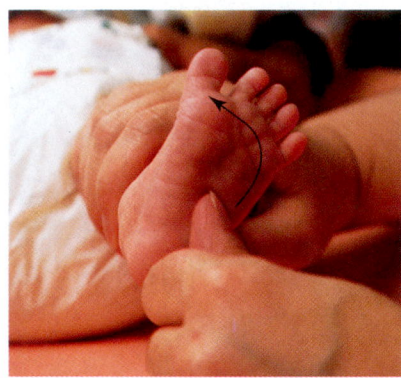

Figure 5–52 ➤ To assess the plantar reflex, stroke the bottom of the infant's or child's foot from the heel, along the lateral sole of the foot and across the ball of the foot. Watch the toes for plantar flexion or the Babinski response, fanning and dorsiflexion of the big toe. The Babinski response is normal in children under 2 years of age. Plantar flexion of the toes is the normal response in older children. A Babinski response in children over 2 years of age can indicate neurologic disease.

the central nervous system develops. Movements are normally equal bilaterally. An asymmetric response may indicate a serious neurologic problem on the less responsive side.

Superficial and Deep Tendon Reflexes

Evaluate the superficial and deep tendon reflexes to assess the function of specific segments of the spine.

Superficial Reflexes

Assess superficial reflexes by stroking a specific area of the body. The plantar reflex, testing spine levels L4 to S_2, is routinely evaluated in children (Figure 5–52 ➤). Assess the cremasteric reflex in boys (see page 195).

Deep Tendon Reflexes

To assess the deep tendon reflexes, tap a tendon near specific joints with a reflex hammer (or with the index finger for infants), comparing responses bilaterally. See Table 5–22 for scoring of deep tendon reflex response. The biceps, triceps, brachioradialis, patellar, and Achilles tendons are usually evaluated in children. Inspect for movement in the associated joint and palpate the strength of the expected muscle contraction (Table 5–23). Responses are normally symmetric bilaterally. The absence of a response is associated with decreased muscle tone and strength. Hyperactive responses are associated with muscle spasticity.

ANALYZING DATA FROM THE PHYSICAL EXAMINATION

Once the physical examination has been completed, group any abnormal findings for each system with those of other systems. Use clinical judgment to identify common patterns of physiologic responses associated with health conditions. Individual abnormal physiologic responses are also the basis of many nursing diagnoses. Be sure to record all findings from the physical assessment legibly, in detail, and in the format approved by your institution.

Let's return to the vignette at the beginning of the chapter. Your thorough physical assessment of Jasmine has revealed a child that appears well nourished and her weight and height when plotted on the growth curve both fall along the 5th percentile. Her head circumference is at the 10th percentile. She has a slight fever and a red right tympanic membrane that has no light reflex and no visible landmarks. The tympanic membrane does not move to positive or negative pressure. Her mucous membranes are moist and skin turgor is good. Based upon these findings, you would be able to select nursing diagnoses appropriate for a child with acute otitis media and being newly adopted into this family. Examples would be the following:

- Acute Pain related to infection and pressure in middle ear
- Readiness for Enhanced Parenting related to newly available information about the child's health status
- Readiness for Enhanced Nutrition related to newly available information about the child's growth pattern

These nursing diagnoses will in turn help direct your nursing care for this child and family.

Table 5–22	NUMERIC SCORING OF DEEP TENDON REFLEX RESPONSES
Grade	**Response Interpretation**
0	No response
1+	Slow, minimal response
2+	Expected response, active
3+	More active or pronounced than expected
4+	Hyperactive, clonus may be present

Table 5–23	**ASSESSMENT OF DEEP TENDON REFLEXES AND THE SPINAL SEGMENT TESTED WITH EACH**

Deep Tendon Reflex	Technique and Normal Findings[a]	Spine Segment Tested
Biceps 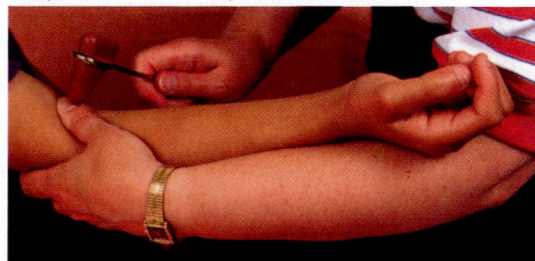	Flex the child's arm at the elbow, and place your thumb over the biceps tendon in the antecubital fossa. Tap your thumb. *Elbow flexes as the biceps muscle contracts.*	C5 and C6
Triceps 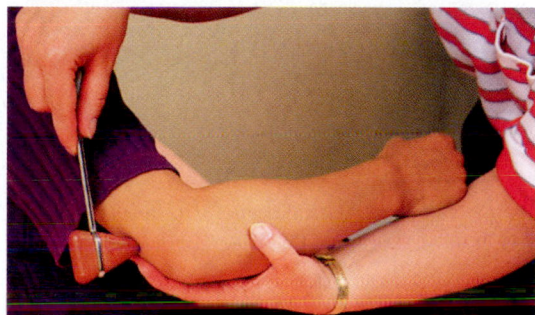	With the child's arm flexed, tap the triceps tendon above the elbow. *Elbow extends as the triceps muscle contracts.*	C6, C7, and C8
Brachioradialis 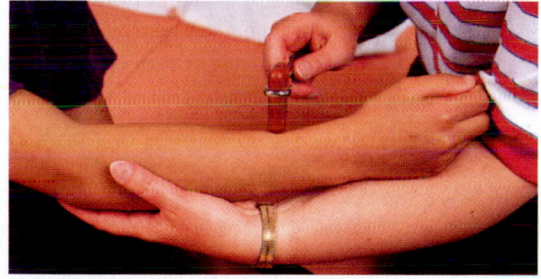	Lay the child's arm with the thumb upright over your arm. Tap the brachioradial tendon 2.5 cm (1 in.) above the wrist. *Forearm pronates (palm facing downward) and elbow flexes.*	C5 and C6
Patellar 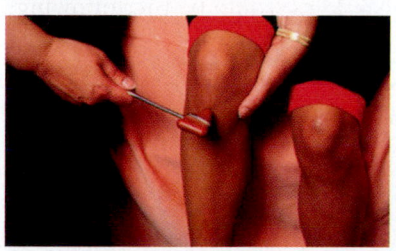	Flex the child's knees, and when the legs are relaxed, tap the patellar tendon just below the knee. *Knee extends (knee jerk) as the quadriceps muscle contracts.*	L2, L3, and L4
Achilles 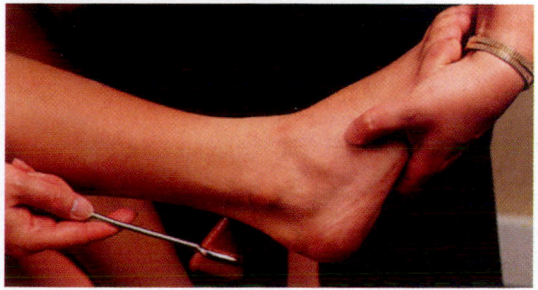	While the child's legs are flexed, support the foot and tap the Achilles' tendon. *Plantar flexion (ankle jerk) as the gastrocnemius muscle contracts.*	S1 and S2

[a]Italic indicates normal findings.

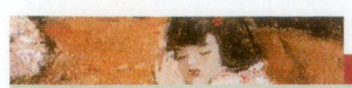

CRITICAL THINKING IN ACTION

ASSESSING A NEWLY ADOPTED CHILD

Recall Jasmine from the opening scenario. She has recently been adopted from China by the Porter family. When Jasmine's length, weight, and head circumference is plotted on a growth curve, she is found to be in the 5th percentile for length and weight, and 10th percentile for head circumference.

1. What behaviors would you look for that might indicate that Jasmine is beginning to develop a relationship with Mrs. Porter?

2. What actions could you take during the physical examination to develop rapport with Jasmine and to reduce her anxiety?

3. What are the physical findings of an ear infection in a child like Jasmine who has been crying during the examination?

4. What is your interpretation of Jasmine's current growth status? Outline a plan to monitor her future growth.

 Refer to your Prentice Hall Nursing MediaLink DVD-ROM for answers.

Explore MEDIALINK 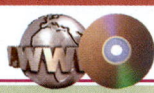 http://www.prenhall.com/ball

Resources for this chapter can be found on the Prentice Hall Nursing MediaLink DVD-ROM accompanying this textbook, and on the Companion Website at http://www.prenhall.com/ball.

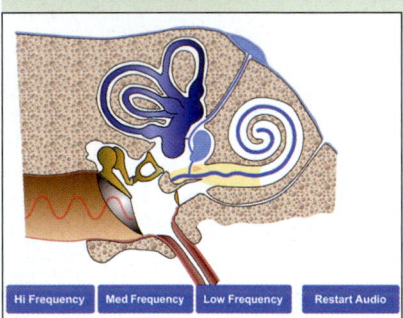

DVD-ROM
Audio Glossary
NCLEX-RN® Review
Animations
  Middle Ear
  Mouth and Throat Examination
  Movement of Joints
  Otoscopic Examination of the Child's Ear

COMPANION WEBSITE
Audio Glossary
NCLEX-RN® Review
Care Plan Activity: Family of a Chronically Ill Child
Case Study: Assessment of a Six-Year-Old Boy
Critical Thinking: Premature Infant Growth
MediaLink Applications
  BMI Calculation
  Blood Pressure Reading
  Assessing Infant Percentiles
  Assessing School-Aged Child Percentiles
WebLinks

REFERENCES

American Academy of Pediatrics. (2003). Eye examination in infants, children, and young adults by pediatricians. *Pediatrics, 111*(4), 902–907.

Ashrafi, M. R., Shabanian, R., Mohammadi, M., & Kavusi, S. (2006). Extensive Mongolian spots: A clinical sign merits special attention. *Pediatric Neurology, 34*(2), 143–145.

Biro, F. M., Huang, B., Crawford, P. B., Lucky, A. W., Striegel-Moore, R., et al. (2006). Pubertal correlates in black and white girls. *Journal of Pediatrics, 148*(2), 234–240.

Curley, M. A. Q., & Thompson, J. E. (2001). Oxygenation and ventilation. In M. A. Q. Curley, & P. A. Moloney-Harmon, *Critical care nursing of infants and children* (2nd ed., pp. 233–308). Philadephia, PA: W.B. Saunders Company.

Dieckmann, R. A. (Ed.) and the American Academy of Pediatrics. (2006). *Pediatric education for prehospital professionals* (2nd ed., p. 55). Sudbury, MA: Jones and Bartlett.

Flores, G., Rabke-Verani, J., Pine, W., & Sabharwal, A. (2002). The importance of cultural and linguistic issues in the care of children. *Pediatric Emergency Care, 18*(4), 271–284.

Goldenring, J. M., & Rosen, D. S. (2004). Getting into adolescent heads: An essential update. *Contemporary Pediatrics, 21*(1), 64–90.

McLaughlin, C., & Levin, A. V. (2006). The red reflex. *Pediatric Emergency Care, 22*(2), 137–140.

National Heart Lung and Blood Institute. (2004). Blood pressure tables for children and adolescents from the fourth report on the diagnosis, evaluation, and treatment of high blood pressure in children and adolescents. http://www.nhlbi.nih.gov/guidelines/hypertension/child_tbl.htm, accessed 6-11-04

Pinyerd, B., & Zipf, W. B. (2005). Puberty—Timing is everything! *Journal of Pediatric Nursing, 20*(2), 75–82.

Seidel, H. M., Ball, J. W., Dains, J., & Benedict, G. W. (2006). *Mosby's guide to physical examination* (6th ed.). St. Louis, MO: Mosby.

Spector, R. E. (2004). *Cultural diversity in health and illness* (6th ed.). Upper Saddle River, NJ: Prentice Hall.

SOCIAL AND ENVIRONMENTAL INFLUENCES ON CHILDREN

6

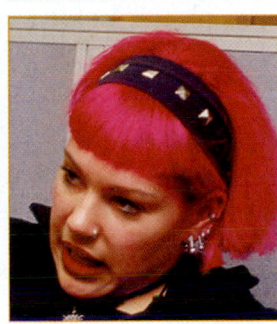

AMY is 15 years old and attends an alternative high school. She recently had an ear piercing and it has become painful. She comes to the health room to ask the school nurse's advice. Upon examination, the nurse notices the area around the piercing is inflamed and mildly edematous. After asking some questions, the nurse learns that Amy's ear was pierced by a friend, using a needle that had been "sterilized" by passing it through a match flame. Amy has had a slight fever, but otherwise feels fine.

In her home state, adolescents under 18 years of age must have a parent's signature for body piercings and tattoos, so Amy chose to have the procedure done by a friend. She believes this is safe since her friend has done many piercings on others. She admits that her parents are not very pleased with her body art, but that they allow her to do it as long as she agrees to stay in high school. She had previously run away and spent several weeks living on the streets.

What healthcare and social needs does Amy have? How can you support both her and her parents? What signs of resilience does Amy show? This chapter examines the complex social contexts in which children live, learn, and grow, and explores the role of nurses in supporting them to reach their potentials. The challenges of providing comprehensive health care for all children and adolescents, no matter their lifestyles, are discussed.

KEY TERMS

branding **230**	hazing **235**
bullying **234**	homosexuality **231**
child sexual	incest **243**
abuse **242**	LGBQ **231**
culture shock **218**	LGBT **231**
cutting **230**	physical abuse **241**
disasters **249**	physical neglect
emotional	**241**
abuse **242**	toxicants **251**
emotional neglect	toxins **251**
242	violence **232**

MediaLink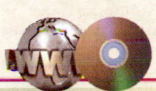

http://www.prenhall.com/ball

See the Prentice Hall Nursing MediaLink DVD-ROM and Companion Website for chapter-specific resources.

LEARNING OUTCOMES

After reading this chapter, you will be able to do the following:

1. Identify major social and environmental factors that influence the health of children and adolescents.

2. List external influences that can affect child and adolescent health.

3. Apply the ecologic model and resilience theory to assessment of the social and environmental factors in children's lives.

4. Examine the effects of substance use, physical activity, and other lifestyle patterns on health.

5. Evaluate the environment for hazards to children, such as exposure to substances and potential for poisoning.

6. Explore the nursing role in prevention and treatment of child abuse and neglect, and other forms of violence.

7. Plan nursing interventions for children related to social and environmental situations.

Many of the major causes of mortality and morbidity in children are closely linked with social influences in the child's environment. The social contexts for young children growing up today are different from those of even a decade ago. Examining the social contexts in which children live and grow can provide insights into the behavior and health of children and adults, and present opportunities for nursing interventions. All nurses must examine the social influences and apply the knowledge gained to plan health care that will benefit youth as they grow into adulthood.

Children and adolescents are also influenced by their environments. The physical setting, exposure to chemical agents, and other environmental factors are increasingly identified as instrumental in determining health. Nurses assess the environment for its risk and protective factors, and then use this information to plan nursing care appropriate to enhance the health status of children and adolescents.

What are the challenges of today's society that children must often face at a very young age? How can nurses help children to face these challenges and to emerge as healthy and contributing members of society? What roles do nurses play in identifying and using the protective factors and in minimizing the risk factors of youth? This chapter will help you to examine and apply these concepts in a variety of nursing settings.

Examine again the major causes of death for children from 1 year of age through adolescence that are presented in Chapter 1 ∞ (Figures 1–6A and 1–6B). Did you notice that most morbidity is related to preventable causes linked to present-day lifestyles? Car crashes, fires, drownings, and homicides are a few examples of common causes of death in children.

Now examine the major reasons for hospitalization (Figure 1–7 ∞). By the time children are 5 years of age, injuries rank as the second cause, and by 10 years, mental disorders and injuries are among the major causes of hospitalization. By the teen years, pregnancy and mental disorders are the most common admitting diagnoses to hospitals. These conditions are related, at least in part, to the environmental settings in which we live. These settings and their influences must be examined in order to understand how to best intervene with children.

THEORETICAL CONCEPTS

In this chapter, two main theories will be used to provide a framework in which to examine societal influences on children. They are the ecological model and the theory of resilience. Both of these theoretical approaches are discussed in Chapter 3 ∞, and should be reviewed now (see Figure 3–5 and Tables 3–5, 3–9, and 3–10).

The ecologic theory views the child and the environment as interacting forces, with children influencing systems around them, even while they are influenced by these systems (Bronfenbrenner, 2005). Close systems providing daily contact are microsystems, but other systems such as parental work and political or cultural environments are also important. Understanding these systems, or the forces in which children function, can provide information that guides care providers. For example, if the parents' employment agencies do not provide healthcare insurance, their children may not obtain necessary health care such as immunizations, treatment for diseases, and growth monitoring.

Resilience theory examines risk and protective factors in the child's environment because they influence the child's adaptation to stressful events, and can often be modified to lead to more productive and healthy outcomes. Families may have protective factors that provide strength and assistance in dealing with crises, and risk factors that promote or contribute to health system challenges. Risk and protective factors can be identified in children, in their families, and in their communities. The combination and interplay of these factors contribute to health status and determine adaptation to a crisis.

Theoretical frameworks are useful when examining social and environmental influences on children because they guide us to assess for certain factors that can be altered. They suggest data to collect and pertinent nursing interventions. They also help

RESEARCH

ADD Health Study

The ADD Health Study (National Longitudinal Study of Adolescent Health) was conducted during the latter 1990s with over 100,000 adolescents and helped to determine the family, school, and individual characteristics associated with risk factors. Parent–family connectedness, school connectedness, a belief in a higher being, and academic success were predictive of youth having the lowest health risks. Attachment to family, school, and parents constitute strong protective factors for adolescence in preventing them from violent behavior such as shoplifting, stealing, fights, and physical injury incidents (Franke, 2003). Nurses can assist adolescents and their families in establishing a sense of attachment to each other. Encourage families to include adolescents in activities, attend their sports and other school events, have meals together regularly, and attend faith-based activities or other community events as a family.

MediaLink

National Health Guidelines and Statistics

foster partnerships with other care providers who use these and similar theories to plan social, psychological, and environmental care for children and their families. For example, nursing strategies can target risk factors, such as encouraging family behaviors to ensure gun safety by teaching the benefits of gun locks and locked gun cabinets in families with firearms. In addition, protective factors can be emphasized, such as when regular exercise is suggested to help maintain normal weight and cardiovascular function.

SOCIAL INFLUENCES ON CHILD HEALTH

Poverty

An important risk factor that influences children's health is poverty. Conversely, basic financial stability is a protective factor that contributes to the general health and well-being of children. One in 6 children is poor. That means he or she lives in a family earning less than $14,128 annually for a family of three persons or less than $18,104 for a family of four (Children's Defense Fund, 2004a). Children are the poorest group in this country; in fact, more children are poor now than at any time in our past. Young children under 6 years are most commonly poor. Single-parent families have a much higher incidence of poverty, but in nearly 80% of poor families at least one parent is working full time (Federal Interagency Forum on Child and Family Statistics, 2003).

Poor children are overrepresented in nearly every health indicator. They are more likely to have unmet health needs, to have difficulty in school, to become teen parents, and to experience multiple health problems. See Table 6–1 for a list of common health problems among poor children and some suggested nursing actions.

Poverty leads to homelessness for some children. Children comprise over 25%, and families represent 39%, of the homeless population (Mullin & Ambrosia, 2005). Families are the fastest growing group of homeless people. In a given year, from 0.9 to 1.3 million children experience homelessness (Haber & Toro, 2004). The reasons for homelessness are also common risks for a number of the other challenges to health discussed in this chapter. Homeless people often have poor finances, may have been abused or victims of other violence, and may have mental instability. Young children tend to be homeless with their parents, while adolescents more often tend to be alone, having run away, been thrown out of a house, or become street youth (Haber & Toro, 2004).

Children who experience homelessness frequently have multiple physical and mental health problems, and lack health insurance to provide care for these problems. Some of the common problems faced by homeless children and families include trauma, alcoholism, respiratory and skin infections, tuberculosis and HIV, and nutritional disorders (Stratigos & Katsambas, 2003). Teens who have been homeless are more likely to engage in other risky behavior, such as unprotected sex with multiple partners and substance abuse. They are more likely to need emergency care, to be depressed, and to become pregnant than other teens (Steele, Ramgoolam, & Evans, 2003).

Health problems related to homelessness and other family characteristics continue even after finding a place to live. Once families leave homeless shelters, children may become separated from their mothers due to parent stress, lack of access to resources, and inability of parents to provide adequate settings for the children (Cowal, Shinn, Weitzman et al., 2002). Complex ongoing care is needed. This may begin in a homeless shelter, but should continue while the family obtains a place to live, accesses other community services, gets the children safely enrolled in school, and attains financial and mental stability. Nurses in all of these settings work with families who are homeless and are instrumental in establishing services where the homeless are located, such as in schools, community clinics, and shelters.

Nursing management for families with children that are poor or homeless focuses on identification of poverty, careful assessment of health risks, and linking the family to resources that can assist with stability and health. There is often no way to identify a poor child from appearance, and children may hide their status when in school or at a healthcare facility. Addresses given may not be accurate, or the address of a shelter might be used. Children living at shelters or in cars and on the street usually do not take the school bus but prefer to walk to avoid stigma. Be alert for children who have

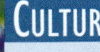

CULTURE

Poverty

Ethnic disparities are striking in poverty rates since 9% of White children are classified as poor, while 27% of Hispanic children and 30% of Black children live in poverty. Additionally, poverty rates are higher in suburban and rural areas than in central cities (Federal Interagency Forum on Child and Family Statistics, 2003).

Table 6–1	COMMON HEALTH PROBLEMS AND NURSING MANAGEMENT OF CHILDREN WHO EXPERIENCE POVERTY OR HOMELESSNESS
Common Health Problems	**Nursing Management**
Lack of immunizations	Check immunization records Provide immunizations at schools and in homeless shelters
Common infectious diseases	Facilitate free clinics in shelters, schools, and community settings Teach hygiene measures Provide resources for disease management Arrange for medications when needed Provide information about resources for bathing, hygiene
Sleep deficits	Inform parents about respite facilities Arrange for children to have quiet sleep time in school if possible
Vision and hearing deficits	Perform screening for deficits Provide resources for eyeglasses, hearing aids, care for ear infections (e.g., service organizations such as Lion's Club)
Nutritional deficits	Perform height and weight checks and nutritional assessment Evaluate family for food security (see Chapter 4 ∞) Be sure child is registered for school breakfast and lunch programs if available Ensure that children are linked to summer food programs at end of academic year Link to Women, Infants, and Children (WIC) Nutrition Program Inform about resources for meals and field gleaning in the community
Dental care problems	Teach oral hygiene Provide toothbrushes and toothpaste Provide bottled water for use if child lives in a car or on the street Perform oral assessment Refer to dental programs for people with low incomes
Injuries	Teach basic safety precautions Visit the living situation if possible to assess for safety hazards Teach "street safe" skills Provide helmets, car seats, or other gear needed
Adolescent pregnancy and sexually transmitted diseases	Provide sexuality teaching Inform about access to family planning services Assess for child abuse and prostitution
Mental illness	Assess for depression Evaluate for suicide potential Provide links to services Plan programs to foster self-esteem Arrange for a Big Brother or Big Sister Refer to extracurricular activities in the school and community Arrange for a school bus stop away from a shelter so other students do not stigmatize the homeless child

multiple health problems and repeated infectious diseases. They are often hungry, and have varying degrees of personal hygiene depending on access to laundry and bathing facilities. See Evidence-Based Practice: Homelessness from the Viewpoint of Children.

Stress

The adverse effect of stress on adults is well documented. More recently, the impact of stress on children has been recognized. Children manifest stress in a variety of ways, including regressive behavior, interrupted sleep, hyperactive behavior, gastrointestinal

EVIDENCE-BASED PRACTICE

Homelessness from the Viewpoint of Children

Problem

Children are the age group showing the fastest growth in homelessness, accounting for about 39% of the homeless population. Due to their ages, children are vulnerable to developmental delays, mental health problems, and effects of violence. Most nurses have not been homeless and do not understand the experience of homelessness for children.

Evidence

A study by four nurses sought to describe the homeless experience from the perspective of children. They interviewed 14 children with an average age of 10 years who were located in shelters in a metropolitan area. The children had been in the shelters from 2 weeks to 6 months, and most had prior periods living in shelters, hotels, or with relatives. The researchers identified five themes common to the children:

- "I'm not homeless."
  The children viewed homelessness as having no resources, and having to live outside. They felt that they had resources and felt they might be ridiculed if people thought they were homeless.
- "I like living in a shelter sometimes."
  While the children had mixed feelings about living in shelters, most were glad to have food, a place to sleep, and a feeling of safety. They described friends in the shelter and were glad to have those relationships.
- "Living in a shelter is hard."
  The children complained about rules and rigid schedules in the shelters. They missed freedom of movement, play space, and privacy.

- "Stop the violence."
  All children described living in violent neighborhoods and the wish that violence would stop. Fighting back was perceived as important to protecting oneself.
- "I need approval."
  Children frequently described how important it was to be noticed and praised by teachers and other adults.

Implications

While this study was small, there were important findings for nurses. The stigma of being homeless should be considered when interacting with children. The researchers suggested reading stories and describing families that lose a home to all children in schools so that the topic is addressed. Nurses can partner with teachers to plan collaborative approaches. The privacy of children should be considered and school buses should not stop directly in front of shelters to pick up children. Integrating positive reinforcement for children into shelter routines, school classrooms, and other settings is important for the child's sense of self-esteem (DeForge, Zehnder, Minick, & Carmon, 2001).

Critical Thinking

Find at least two shelters in your community. Are nurses involved in planning health care? How long do families usually remain? Do the schools know that children are homeless? Do they strive to preserve the privacy of homeless children while supporting their needs for growth, health, and education? What is the nursing role in the shelter, in the school, and in the community?

---

symptoms, crying, and withdrawal from normal events. Common stressful events for children include moving to a new home or school, marital difficulties in the family, abuse, parental deployment in the military, and being expected to achieve at an extremely high level in school or sports (Figure 6–1 ➤). The busy pace of today's lifestyles and the media's impact in encouraging early development of children may put undue stress upon some children and preteens (Elkind, 2007). Adolescents may be stressed by fulfilling many roles, such as student, part-time worker, and active family member. They may also be in school all day, have a sport or music practice for 2 to 3 hours after school, and then have a job for several additional hours. Lack of adequate sleep can add further to stress, in addition to putting the teen at risk for car crashes and poor school performance. For families living in poverty, commonly reported stressors are related to food provision, shelter, transportation, medical care, and personal-time needs.

The child experiencing stress has more frequent respiratory and gastrointestinal illnesses and is more likely to be the victim of an injury. The negative long-term effects of stress on body organs and systems suggest that children under stress are more likely to develop illnesses such as strokes, hypertension, and heart attacks later in life.

Nurses help children to manage stress by assessing what is stressful for each child and then encouraging good coping strategies. Healthy lifestyles including good nutrition, exercise, and plenty of sleep can be emphasized with all children. Integrate these topics into each health promotion/health maintenance visit, using guidelines found in Chapters 8, 9, and 10 ∞ . Parents can be encouraged to provide youth with activities that foster self-esteem and to avoid unrealistic expectations about performance in sports and other activities. Resources to assist with food acquisition, shelter, transportation, and medical care should be provided for families needing the assistance. Assess the family role adaptation needed in military families and provide resources to assist with coping (Murray, 2002). Adolescents may benefit from various approaches for stress management such as massage, rest, physical activity, and yoga.

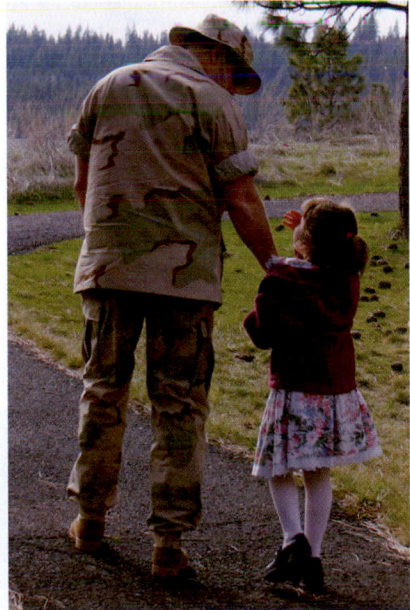

Figure 6–1 ➤ The special relationship between a father about to be deployed in the military and his young daughter is clear. This father has two other children and is spending time with each of them, as well as with the family together, before leaving. The cycle of leaving and returning home can be stressful for families. What are the needs of military families?

RESEARCH

Stressors Identified by Children

Three nurse researchers interviewed 790 children, ages 7 to 12, to identify common stressors, to compare these stressors with those identified 30 years earlier, and to see which ones would not have been evaluated by existing tools on stress (Ryan-Wenger, Sharrer, & Campbell, 2005). Several of their findings were:

- Children and adults may rate stresses differently. For example, children rated fighting in the family as more stressful and the birth of a new sibling as less stressful than parents. Nurses need to assess for recent changes and stresses but then ask the child how these events have affected them.
- Stressors can be grouped into "normative" events such as those related to developmental progression (e.g., being left out at school, wanting more freedom from parents) and "non-normative" stressors due to events related to trauma, illness, disasters, and other uncommon events.
- Stressors that emerged in importance in the 1990s were being made fun of by others, bullying, and general violence. Stressors emerging in the 2000s included being alone, school tests, being overwhelmed with activities after school, and girlfriend/boyfriend problems. Open-ended questions can assist nurses in identifying stressors for individual children. Resources should be offered for common stressors such as being too busy, worrying about violence, and interactions with peers and family.

Family Structure

The families into which children are born profoundly influence them. Children are supported in different ways and acquire different worldviews depending on such factors as whether one or both parents work, how many siblings are present, and whether an extended family is nearby. Note should be made of variations in family structure such as adolescent parent, single parent, gay or lesbian parents, grandparents caring for grandchildren, and stepparents. Societal changes have impacted family life and the needs of children immensely. Working parents often raise children with little time for quality relationships and without the financial resources needed for optimum development (Annie E. Casey Foundation, 2004). All factors influence the physical and mental health of children and can determine their needs for nursing intervention.

Nurses can complete family diagrams during home visits and in other settings to evaluate the people who are important in a child's life. Both the risk factors of the family (e.g., recent separation, parental stress, and limited healthcare coverage) and the strengths manifested (e.g., loving relationships, influential grandparents or other extended family members, and general good health) should be identified and used in planning care. See Chapter 2 ∞ for a thorough discussion of family factors as they relate to family-centered care, and strategies for assessment and intervention with families.

School and Childcare

Once a child is 5 or 6 years of age, several hours daily are spent in a school setting. Physical skills are developed through participation in education and sports. Psychosocial stages are met as the child interacts with children and adults and achieves social interaction patterns and pride in accomplishments. The presentation of concepts that challenge thought processes enhances cognitive development.

Although the primary role of schools is educational, they also perform several health-related functions. School health screening programs play an important role in identifying children with such health problems as hearing loss, visual impairment, and scoliosis. Nurses provide assessment, teaching, and clinical management related to some health problems. Consider the case of Amy in the opening scenario. She went to the school nurse when her body piercing was potentially infected; the nurse examined the site, made suggestions for cleaning, and taught Amy the symptoms she needed to be aware of that could indicate serious infections. Some schools have clinics that examine and provide even more complete health care for children. Many schools teach good nutrition, healthful living, safe sexual practices, and other health-related subjects. A school nurse may be present, at least part time, to plan these classes or to work with teachers. Nurses assist school districts in providing plans for emergency health care when needed. With the increase in mainstreaming, school staff now have the responsibility for administering medications, maintaining urinary catheters, and providing respiratory care and other treatments to ensure the child's proper growth and development. See Chapter 11 ∞ for a further discussion of school nurse activities.

Some children spend part or nearly all of their days in childcare settings (Figure 6–2 ➤). About 19% of children are in childcare up to 9 hours each week, 38% for 10–19 hours each week, 36% for 30–45 hours each week, and 10% for over 45 hours each week (National Institute of Child Health and Human Development, 2003). The closeness of the parent–child relationship, the quality of care, and the length of the childcare day are important in determining childcare effects on children. The mother's sensitivity to her child is the best indicator of child behavior regardless of childcare arrangements (National Institute of Child Health and Human Development, 2003).

Nursing management involves helping parents to explore types of childcare options available and to evaluate programs in their communities (Table 6–2). Care options for young school-age children, either before or after school, can also be shared with

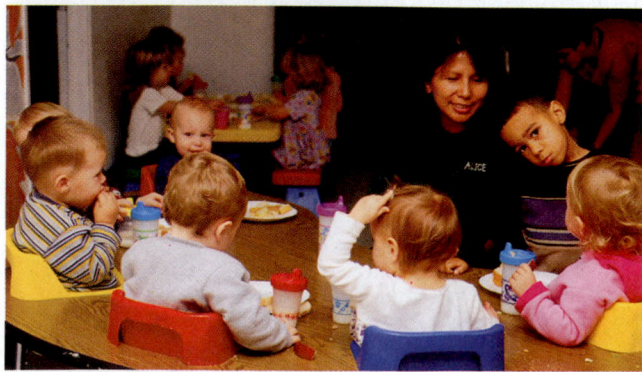

Figure 6–2 ➤ Most children will spend time in childcare settings. It is important to explore options and find the best fit for the child's needs.

Table 6–2 | TYPES OF CHILDCARE

Type of Care	Description	Advantages	Disadvantages
In home	Caretaker comes to home of the child	Child can remain at home Little exposure to infectious diseases No need for alternative care when child is ill	Limited contact with other children to encourage development Most costly
Family childcare	Parent brings child to home of a caretaker	Limited number of children Some exposure to other children and encouragement of development Family-type atmosphere	Little governmental regulation or examination
Center care a. Private, nonprofit (e.g., church, YMCA) b. Public (e.g., Head Start) c. Private proprietary	Parent brings child to a center where many children receive care	A learning curriculum plan is in place Contact with other children can enhance development	Exposure to multiple children increases infectious disease risk

parents. Early intervention programs with at-risk children, such as the Zero to Three Project and Head Start, have been influential in contributing to children's health and welfare and should be recommended when available. Nurses frequently manage the health programs in early intervention, providing for screening and health evaluations and establishing early intervention education plans. Nurses assist families in evaluating childcare centers and share information about accreditation (see Families Want to Know: Evaluation of Childcare). The National Association for the Education of Young Children has established criteria for evaluation of childcare centers for use by centers and parents.

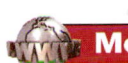

MediaLink

Early Intervention Programs

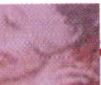

FAMILIES WANT TO KNOW

Evaluation of Childcare

The nurse can help parents to evaluate childcare options and make decisions about placement for their children. Parents should always be welcomed to visit an agency or home childcare—this is essential so they can see the routines in action. Following are suggested questions for them to ask.

Administration

Is the facility licensed?

Who are the administrators? What is their training and experience?

How many staff are employed? What is their training?

Is there a parent board? What part do they play in administering the center?

Physical Environment, Health, and Safety

What is the neighborhood like? Is transportation to the center convenient?

What is the condition of lighting, heat, cooling, ventilation system, play spaces (inside and out), and the building's general condition?

Is playground equipment safe?

Is there a soft material such as bark, sand, or rubber tiles under climbing equipment?

Is there always supervision for the children?

Are there emergency medical forms and signed forms for field trips?

Who may pick up children? How are they signed in and out?

What is the immunization policy and how are records examined and maintained?

Are criminal background checks of staff done for potential child abuse and other problems?

What is the policy for children with infectious diseases and other illnesses?

How are foods prepared? Are staff licensed in food handling?

What is the state of general cleanliness?

Who changes diapers? Are recommendations for standard precautions to prevent pathogen transfer followed?

What arrangements and routines are made for naps and quiet times?

Developmental Approaches

Is the curriculum appropriate for different age groups?

Are there materials and plans for gross motor, fine motor, language, and social development?

How much time do children spend in structured time? Free time?

How is discipline handled?

Do the children appear occupied and happy?

What reading materials are available?

What type and quantity of field trips are planned?

What is the educational level and longevity of the childcare workers?

Is there diversity among the children's backgrounds and experiences?

Community

The community in which a child lives may support the child's development or, conversely, expose the child to hazards. Social programs such as Head Start preschools, sports activities, after-school programs, and child abuse treatment centers offer valuable services that improve the experience of growing children. Conversely, an economically depressed community with scant services and a high homicide rate is unsupportive and hazardous for growing children.

The physical environment is supportive when the child is provided with sidewalks on which to walk to school, open spaces in which to learn and play, and clean air to breathe. Children who must walk to school on unsafe roads, have access to contaminated drinking supplies, or live near polluting manufacturing companies or in crowded housing or old structures are at risk for injuries and health problems such as lead poisoning (see discussions later in this chapter about lead poisoning and exposure to other environmental contaminants).

Nurses should be aware of the types of neighborhoods in the community. Learn about local resources and hazards. Assessment of every child involves information about the community and the health care that the family needs help to obtain. See Chapter 11 ∞ for techniques that supply comprehensive community assessment. Refer children when appropriate for lead poisoning and safe programs after school, and teach them about injury prevention specific to their communities.

Culture

The child's cultural group may influence the use of traditional and contemporary healthcare practices. If the parents or children are recent immigrants, they may still be learning the English language and finding out about healthcare resources. Even in families that have been in this country for some time, a combination of approaches to health care is common. Children of immigrants may feel stress as they combine their family's traditional culture with the new culture in which the family now lives. They may also have responsibility to interpret for the family, since they frequently speak two languages and understand the practices of the new culture.

Recent immigrants may experience **culture shock**, a state of crisis related to the difference in values and lifestyle. This can lead to stress-related symptoms, and create a need for healthcare intervention. Children whose parents immigrated from another country may feel different than peers and develop conflict with their parents, particularly during adolescence.

All cultural groups have rules regarding patterns of social interaction. Schedules of language acquisition are determined by the number of languages spoken and the amount of speech in the home. The particular social roles assumed by men and women in the culture affect school activities and ultimately career choices. Attitudes toward touching and other methods of encouraging developmental skills vary among cultures.

Nurses must become aware of common characteristics of the cultural groups they are serving in order to establish culturally competent nursing care. Arrange for translators when needed. Recognize that traditional and Western health care are often both accepted and used; remain nonjudgmental about traditional healing practices. Provide ethnic foods in healthcare facilities. Evaluate youth in immigrant families for conflict between family and societal expectations.

LIFESTYLE ACTIVITIES AND THEIR INFLUENCE ON CHILD HEALTH

Many of the patterns of daily life play a part in determining the length and quality of one's life. The child's use of tobacco products and controlled substances influences both physical and mental health. Patterns of exercise and use of protective gear help to avoid early disabilities. Media use can influence aggressive behaviors, compete with the need for physical activity, or be a positive force in teaching children new concepts. Body art that can introduce pathogens is an example of a lifestyle pattern that influences mental and physical health, as well as body image.

Substance Use

Substance use and abuse occurs in children and adolescents of all socioeconomic levels and is a growing health problem. About one-half of high school seniors claim to have used drugs in the last 30 days, with alcohol, marijuana, and cigarette use most commonly cited (National Institute on Drug Abuse, 2003). It is important to keep in mind that the use of any substance, such as tobacco, alcohol, or illicit drugs, can pose a serious psychological and physical risk to children and adolescents. Tobacco use and management for the condition is discussed in the following text, followed by sections on alcohol use and drug use, and a management section to address those substances.

Tobacco Use

Tobacco use is the most preventable cause of adult death in the United States. It leads to 430,000 deaths annually, and will be responsible for the premature death of 5 million of today's youth as they reach adult years (U.S. Department of Health and Human Services, 2000). Major health problems linked to tobacco use include cardiovascular disease, cancer, chronic lung disease, low birth weight, and other maternal problems. Even passive smoking or environmental tobacco smoke (ETS) is linked to increased heart disease, blood pressure, and respiratory problems (Leone, 2003). Cigarettes are most common; however, chewing tobacco, snuff, cigars, and bidis may also be used. These all pose significant health hazards.

Many nurses view tobacco use as an adult issue. While sale of tobacco products to children and advertisements aimed at this age group are forbidden by federal law, many youths obtain and use tobacco. After steadily increasing rates of youth smoking for many years, rates began to decrease in 1997. However, a significant number of youths still continue to use tobacco, making this an important health topic. About 30% of high schoolers and 13% of middle schoolers in the United States smoked in the month prior to being surveyed (MMWR, 2003c); about 28% are current users of tobacco, and 16% of students are frequent smokers (use one or more cigarettes/day for at least 30 days) (MMWR, 2004). When including children who have ever smoked, the numbers are even larger. About 54% have tried smoking before high school (MMWR, 2006a). Significant numbers of youth also report using other types of tobacco such as chewing tobacco and cigars in the month prior to being surveyed. Approximately 7.8% of females and 14.8% of males from 13 to 15 years living in the Americas report current use of tobacco other than cigarettes (MMWR, 2006b). It is striking to realize that 3000 youths per day try their first cigarette, and that the major ages for trying tobacco are 9 to 14 years (between sixth and ninth grade). Early initiation of smoking becomes an extremely risky behavior when it is recognized that 80% of current adult smokers began smoking before 18 years of age (MMWR, 2006a). Nicotine is highly addictive; most people who use the substance as an adult become addicted to the substance in adolescent years.

Certain characteristics contribute to the likelihood of tobacco use. They include increasing age, male gender, ethnic group, ease of obtaining tobacco products, and smoking among family members. Low socioeconomic group membership, access to tobacco products, low price of products, advertising, influence of peers, and lack of parental involvement in the youths' lives are also associated with tobacco use (Victoir, Eertmans, Van den Broucke, et al., 2006) (Figure 6–3 ➤).

Several programs have been developed to encourage youths to avoid tobacco use. In addition, smoking cessation programs are available to assist youths who are already regular smokers, and are successful in achieving the goals of cessation or decrease in tobacco. Once a teen is identified as a smoker, using a biological marker such as urine cotinine (a by-product of tobacco) levels can help to identify the frequency of smoking. This information can be used to make suggestions to the teen about the potential outcomes of the behavior and the cessation program that is most likely to be helpful. Successful programs include:

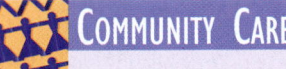

COMMUNITY CARE

Tobacco Products

Forms of tobacco other than traditional cigarettes may be popular among certain groups or in specific parts of the country. *Smokeless tobacco* in forms of chew, snuff, or dip has been used by 6.7% of youth. This type of tobacco is even used by students in school without staff being aware of the behavior. *Bidis* are small, brown, hand-rolled cigarettes that are popular among some youths. *Cigars* have been used by 14.8% of youth (MMWR, 2004). Try to learn what types of tobacco are most common in the local community and plan to integrate history questions during health exams to learn about cigarette and other tobacco use. Never assume a youth is not using tobacco but ask every youth questions about it, without parents in the room.

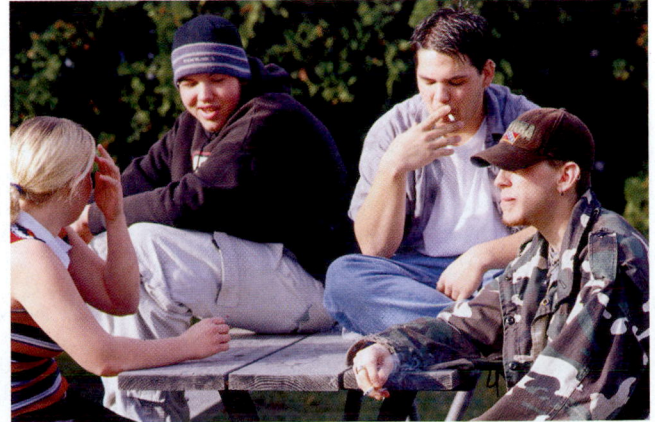

Figure 6–3 ➤ Almost 70% of children have tried smoking by their high school years. Early intervention should begin with assessment for and discussions about smoking hazards starting at 9–10 years of age.

RESEARCH
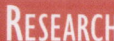

The Youth Risk Behavior Surveillance System

The Youth Risk Behavior Surveillance System is conducted every other year on large representative numbers of youth by the Centers for Disease Control and Prevention. For example, in 2003, 43 states and 15,240 students were included in reported results (MMWR, 2004). The categories of priority health-risk behaviors investigated in each survey are:

- Behaviors contributing to unintentional and intentional injury
- Tobacco use
- Alcohol and other drug use
- Sexual behaviors contributing to unintended pregnancy and sexually transmitted diseases
- Physical inactivity
- Overweight and weight control

CULTURE

Smoking Rates

Among youth in the United States, White youth are significantly more likely to smoke than either Hispanic or Black peers. About 31% of White students reported smoking in the previous month, while 22% of Hispanic and 19% of Black students reported this behavior (MMWR, 2003b; MMWR, 2004). American Indian and Alaska Natives also have high smoking rates, while Asian Americans have low rates (U.S. Department of Health and Human Services, 2000). While Blacks and Hispanics try smoking at rates higher than Whites, they do not as often retain the habit, so Whites surpass other groups when measuring rates of past-year and weekly smoking (Ellickson, Orlando, Tucker, & Klein, 2004). There is also diversity in areas, with overall smoking rates ranging from 10–41% among various states (MMWR, 2004).

- Youth-oriented media campaigns about hazards of tobacco
- Increased tobacco taxes
- Smoke-free policies for schools, restaurants, and other community sites
- Increased regulation of tobacco
- Reduction in youth access to tobacco
- School-based programs in cessation (MMWR, 2002)

NURSING MANAGEMENT

Nursing Assessment and Diagnosis

Nurses are in a unique position to inquire about the incidence of smoking and other tobacco use among youth. Questions should be inserted into all well-child visits, beginning at about 9 to 10 years of age. Inquire about whether family members (especially parents and siblings) smoke or chew, and ask if some of the child's friends have tried smoking. Assess for associated risk behaviors such as alcohol and drug use, sexual activity, and suicidal thoughts. Determine the child's knowledge and beliefs about the benefits and risks of tobacco use. As the child gets older, more direct and detailed questions are necessary. A nonjudgmental approach will be best to obtain a truthful response. School nurses can make observations about numbers of teens smoking and general attitudes about tobacco use. When children come to hospitals and other health facilities for care, use of tobacco should be part of the general admission questions. Remember to include smokeless tobacco use in questioning.

The following nursing diagnoses may apply to youth who smoke or show potential for this behavior:

- Activity Intolerance related to lowered oxygen supply
- Impaired Gas Exchange related to ventilation-perfusion imbalance
- Chronic Low Self-Esteem related to negative self-appraisal
- Deficient Knowledge about Dangers of Tobacco Use related to developmental focus on the present
- Imbalanced Nutrition, Less than Body Requirements related to effects of chemical dependence

Planning and Implementation

The roles of nurses in preventing and intervening in youth smoking are to *inform* youth, *identify* smokers, and *implement* programs for prevention and cessation (Table 6–3). Nurses should provide developmentally appropriate information about the hazards of tobacco use in all settings where youth are present. Posters, flyers, and speakers

Table 6–3	NURSING ROLE IN YOUTH SMOKING PREVENTION

Inform

- Hang posters, provide brochures, and facilitate presentations about smoking risks in all settings where youth are present.
- Target smokers with special information about the effects of nicotine on their bodies.

Identify

- Ask questions about smoking and other tobacco use at every health encounter beginning at about 9–10 years of age.
- For users, ask about the amount and type of tobacco.
- Learn where youth obtain tobacco and be proactive in stopping sales.

Implement

- Encourage young tobacco users to quit.
- Facilitate referral to cessation programs.
- Arrange positive rewards for youth who are successful in cessation.

are particularly useful. Include information about short-term problems such as increased rates of upper respiratory infections and worsening of asthma, as well as long-term effects such as addiction, lung cancer, oral cancer, car crashes, emphysema, and other health problems. Addicted teens who share their stories of difficult withdrawal from tobacco, and adults who have had cancer of the lungs or larynx, may be effective speakers. Find out where teens obtain tobacco products in the community and where they engage in use of the products to target these places. Offer information on available prevention and cessation programs to youth and families in clinics, outpatient surgery centers, community activities, and hospitals. Use opportunities such as adolescent pregnancy and presence of illness to reinforce the hazardous effects of tobacco on the individual and on those nearby. Adolescent mothers should understand the risks for small-for-gestational-age babies when they smoke in pregnancy, and the increased risk of Sudden Infant Death Syndrome (SIDS) when infants are exposed to secondhand smoke (see Chapter 20 ∞ for a detailed discussion of SIDS). Speak to young athletes about the effects of tobacco on athletic performance. Show children the ways in which this product can interfere with their meeting of life goals. Role-play how to tell other youths no when tobacco is offered. Establish programs that increase the sense of self-esteem without tobacco use. Be sure to include parents in the programs so that they see and acknowledge their role in setting an example about tobacco use, and in providing guidelines for the child. Information about the influence of environmental tobacco smoke (ETS or secondhand smoke) should also be provided.

Adopt a nonjudgmental attitude when asking questions about smoking so that those who are using tobacco can be identified. Ask questions without parents present and assure the children that the information will not be shared. Encourage youths to cut back and to quit use of tobacco products. Offer them assistance in these efforts.

Work with the schools and school districts to help establish preventive and cessation programs. There should be clear guidelines about school policies regarding smoking on school grounds. Keeping occasional youth smokers from becoming regular users should be a goal in order to avoid nicotine addiction. Find out what positive incentives can be offered to youth who are successful in quitting smoking. Contract with them to achieve their goals.

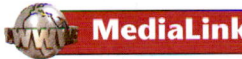

MediaLink

Smoking Cessation Resources and Video

Evaluation

Expected outcomes of nursing interventions regarding tobacco use are lowered rates of regular use, delayed initiation of use, and success of cessation programs. Use the following *Healthy People 2010* (U.S. Department of Health and Human Services, 2000) objectives as guidelines:

- Reduce the proportion of children who are regularly exposed to tobacco smoke at home to 10%.
- Increase smoke-free and tobacco-free environments in schools, including all school facilities, property, vehicles, and school events, to 100%.
- Eliminate tobacco advertising and promotions that influence adolescents and young adults.
- Increase adolescents' disapproval of smoking to 95%.
- Reduce tobacco use by adolescents to 21%.
- Increase the average age of first use of tobacco products from 12 years to 14 years.

Alcohol Use

Alcohol use by the young is very common. An estimated 75% have tried alcohol, which is the drug of choice and convenience for youth. Each day, 7000 children take their first drink. By 12th grade, 83% have had alcoholic drinks (MMWR, 2004). Current use is also common with 45% of high school students admitting to drinking within the last month, and 28% having engaged in binge drinking, or having five or more drinks within a 2-hour period. Even young children are affected since 44% of 8th graders and 66% of 10th graders have tried alcohol, while 20% of 8th graders and 35% of 10th graders have had alcohol in the last month (Johnston, O'Malley, Bachman, & Schulenberg, 2004). Alcohol use frequently starts at an early age since 25.6% of high school students report that their first drink was before age 13 years. Binge drinking is also a problem, as 25.5% of high school students report at least one incidence of having five or more drinks within 2 hours in the 30 days prior to the survey (MMWR, 2006c).

There are numerous health risks associated with drinking by minors. Perhaps the most common and obvious is that of motor vehicle accidents. About 5000 young people annually die from alcohol-related injuries from car crashes, homicides, and suicides (National Institute on Alcohol Abuse and Alcoholism, 2002; 2005). Others experience assault such as alcohol-related date rape. Alcohol affects the developing brain, decreasing intellectual capacity and increasing the chance for future alcohol use. Additionally, early drinking significantly increases the chance that someone will become an alcoholic later in life (Hingson, Heeren, & Winter, 2006). Endocrine problems, liver abnormalities, and decreased bone density can also occur. The neurologic effects of alcohol on the brain are magnified in the young (Alcohol Free Children, 2005; National Institute on Alcohol Abuse and Alcoholism, 2005). Children are much more likely to try alcohol and to become alcoholic when a family member is alcoholic; this is a significant risk as one in five children grow up in a home with an alcoholic adult (American Academy of Child and Adolescent Psychiatry, 2005a).

Many factors influence the child and adolescent who drink alcohol. Patterns in the family, media advertisements, and social environments in high school and college that honor or expect drinking all contribute to the problem. Access is easy for most youth as older siblings or classmates obtain drinks. It is a "rite of passage" for many at teen birthday parties or college events. Alcohol is the most common and accepted drug in today's society and, as such, youth are exposed and often experience its effects without understanding or considering the implications of its use. A risk factor for initiation of alcohol use is a transition time, such as change from middle to high school, or a major family stress, such as parental separation or divorce (Loveland-Cherry, 2006).

Drug Use

In addition to alcohol, a variety of other drugs are used by youth. Almost 40% of students have used marijuana and 20% have used it in the last month. About 7% have used cocaine, with over 3% having used it in the last month. Inhalant use of glue, paints, or other substances is more common, with 12% reporting use and 4% having used in the last month. Approximately 6% report methamphetamine use; and 2.4% used heroin (MMWR, 2004; MMWR, 2006c). Synthetic drugs such as phencyclidine (PCP) (commonly referred to as "designer" drugs) mimic other narcotics, stimulants, and hallucinogens and are also dangerous. Some common contemporary drugs and street names are listed in Table 6–4.

Over-the-counter (OTC) medications are legal substances that are frequently abused. Easily obtainable at grocery stores and drugstores, these drugs include antihistamines, atropine, bromides, caffeine, ephedrine, pseudoephedrine, phenylpropanolamine, and amphetamine-like substitutes. Some youth drink multiple servings of coffee, tea, soda pop, and other beverages with caffeine for the psychoactive effects of caffeine. Super caffeinated beverages, herbal products, and OTC cold and diet medicines may also be used.

Volatile inhalants such as glues are dangerous substances of abuse, and their use appears to be rising among school-age children and adolescents. Each incident of "huffing" or inhaling a substance runs the risk of a serious health problem and death, the latter referred to as sudden sniffing death. Children who "huff" while taking amphetamines such as Ritalin for treatment of attention deficit disorder run an elevated risk of a potentially fatal interaction. See Box 6–1 for common inhalant agents.

Anabolic steroids are the drugs of abuse most commonly used by athletes. About 4% of students report use of illegal steroids. Use is more common in males (4.8%) than females (3.2%) and lifetime use ranges from 2–6.5% (MMWR, 2006c).

| Table 6–4 | COMMON CONTEMPORARY DRUGS |

Drug	Action	Street Names	Route	Time of Action
Methylenediosymethamphetamine (MDMA)	Stimulant; appetite suppressant; Increased pulse, BP, temperature, overhydration, hyponatremia, memory loss	Ecstasy, XTC, X, Adam Clarity, Lover's speed, E	PO (tablets, capsules)	3–6 hours
Gamma-hydroxybutyrate (GHB)	CNS depressant, euphoria, growth hormone release, hypersalivation, hypotonia	Grievous Bodily Harm, G., Liquid Ecstasy, Georgia Home Boy, Date-rape drug	PO (liquid, powder, tablets, capsules)	4 hours
Ketamine	Anesthetic; decreased memory, attention, learning; Increased BP; respiratory collapse	Special K, K, Vitamin K, Cat Valiums	IV, respiratory (injected, snorted or smoked; liquid or powder)	1–2 hours
Rohypnol (benzodiazepine)	Amnesia, sedative; decreased BP, urinary retention; given prior to sexual assault	Roofies, Rophies, Roche, Forget-me Pill	PO, respiratory, (snorted) (tablets)	8–12 hours
Methamphetamine	Stimulant; highly addictive; memory loss, violence, psychosis; cardiac and neurologic damage	Speed, Ice, Chalk, Meth Crystal, Crank, Fire, Glass, Tina, Tweak, Yaba (meth and caffeine)	PO, respiratory, IV (smoked, snorted, injected)	Several hours; long-term permanent effects
Lysergic acid diethylamide (LSD)	Hallucinogen; increased pulse, BP, temperature; psychosis, flashbacks	Acid, Boomers, Yellow Sunshines	PO (liquid, tablets, capsules)	1–2 hours; possible flashbacks later

Note: Data from National Institute of Drug Abuse. (2004). NIDA Community Drug Alert Bulletin—Club Drugs. Bethesda, MD: U.S. Department of Health and Human Services, and Reitman, D. S. (May, 2005). "Club" Drugs 101: Substance use and abuse for 21st century pediatricians. Consultant for Pediatricians, 207–211.

Etiology and Pathophysiology

In most cases, substance abuse represents a maladaptive coping response to the stressors of childhood and adolescence. Individual, peer, family, and community risk factors all contribute to increased incidence of use (American Academy of Child and Adolescent Psychiatry 2005b). A child may begin using alcohol or drugs to deal with stress because family members or peers do so. Children in families with a history of substance abuse are at higher risk of abusing drugs and alcohol. Other risk factors include rebelliousness, aggressiveness, low self-esteem, dysfunctional parental relationships, lack of adequate support systems, academic underachievement, poor judgment, and poor impulse control. Adolescents and young adults use "club drugs" to achieve greater satisfaction during nights of dancing, drinking, and attending clubs. Use of these drugs with alcohol can lead to deadly consequences (see Table 6–4).

Initial experimentation with alcohol or drugs may be unpleasant. With continued use, however, the adolescent learns to "achieve the high," an illusion of power and well-being. The adolescent wants the high more frequently and actively seeks alcohol or drugs. Tolerance to the substance occurs with continued use, and ever-increasing amounts are required to achieve a pleasurable high. Physical and psychologic dependence ensues as the body's tissues require the substance to function properly. Withdrawal symptoms occur when the child or adolescent is deprived of the substance.

Clinical Manifestations

Substance abuse in children and adolescents is commonly overlooked and underdiagnosed by healthcare providers due in part to the wide range of clinical presentations. These vary according to the type of drug abused, the amount, the frequency, the time of last use, and the severity of drug dependence. See the Clinical Manifestations table on page 224 for manifestations of abuse and potential for dependence for several types of drugs.

BOX 6–1
COMMON INHALANT AGENTS

Aerosols

Cooking spray
Whipped cream
Spray paint
Cosmetic sprays

Adhesives

Model glues
Rubber cements

Solvents

Nail polish remover
Paint thinner or cleaner
Lighter fluid
Degreaser

Other

Gasoline
Helium

CLINICAL MANIFESTATIONS COMMONLY ABUSED DRUGS

Drug	Potential For Dependence	Clinical Manifestations
Depressants Alcohol, barbiturates (amobarbital, pentobarbital, secobarbital)	Physical and psychologic: High; varies somewhat among drugs	Physical: Decreased muscle tone and coordination tremors Psychologic: Impaired speech, memory, and judgment; confusion; decreased attention span; emotional lability
Stimulants Amphetamines (e.g., Benzedrine), caffeine, cocaine, MDMA	Physical: Low to moderate Psychologic: High; withdrawal from amphetamines and cocaine can lead to severe depression	Physical: Dilated pupils, increased pulse and blood pressure, flushing, nausea, loss of appetite, tremors, vascular heart disease (with MDMA) Psychologic: Euphoria; increased alertness, agitation, or irritability; hallucinations; insomnia
Opiates Codeine, heroin, meperidine (Demerol), methadone, morphine, opium, oxycodone (Percodan, Oxycontin)	Physical and psychologic: High; varies somewhat among drugs; withdrawal effects are uncomfortable but rarely life threatening	Physical: Analgesia, depressed respirations and muscle tone (may lead to coma or death), nausea, constricted pupils Psychologic: Changes in mood (usually euphoria), drowsiness, impaired attention or memory, sense of tranquility
Hallucinogens Lysergic acid diethylamide (LSD), mescaline, phencyclidine (PCP)	Physical: None Psychologic: Unknown	Physical: Lack of coordination, dilated pupils, hypertension, elevated temperature; severe PCP intoxication can result in seizures, respiratory depression, coma, and death Psychologic: Visual illusions and hallucinations, altered perceptions of time and space, emotional lability, psychosis
Volatile inhalants Glues, typing correction fluid, acrylic paints, spot removers, lighter fluid, gasoline, butane	Physical and psychologic: Varies with drug used	Physical: Impaired coordination, liver damage (in some cases) Psychologic: Impaired judgment, delirium
Marijuana	Physical: Low Psychologic: Usually low; occasionally moderate to high	Physical: Tachycardia, reddened conjunctiva, dry mouth, increased appetite Psychologic: Initial anxiety followed by euphoria; giddiness; impaired attention, judgment, and memory

Common physical manifestations include alterations in vital signs, weight loss, chronic fatigue, chronic cough, respiratory congestion, red eyes, and general apathy and malaise. Lesions in and around the nose and mouth are common. The mental status examination (refer to Chapter 5 ∞) may reveal alterations in level of consciousness, impaired attention and concentration, impaired thought processes, delusions, and hallucinations. Low self-esteem, feelings of guilt or worthlessness, and suicidal or homicidal thoughts are also common. Paraphernalia reported by parents, such as rags, pipes, and canisters, may indicate use, and chemical odors around the clothing and person should be indicative of possible drug use.

Poor school performance and changes in mood, sleep habits, appetite, dress, and social relationships are nonspecific characteristics of the substance-abusing child. These are often the symptoms first noted by family and friends, and should be the subject of questions at each health promotion visit.

■ COLLABORATIVE CARE

Diagnostic Tests

Multiple psychiatric diagnostic criteria exist for each drug class. Children and adolescents who have other psychosocial disorders commonly use or abuse drugs or alcohol. Therefore, assessment and treatment plans should focus not only on the substance use or abuse, but also on the issues underlying the problem. Diagnosis includes assessment of both the family and the substance-abusing child or adolescent. Blood levels of substances and metabolites are sometimes measured.

Clinical Therapy

The primary goal of treatment is to teach the child and other family members to develop and sustain positive coping patterns, and to support them during this process. Most treatment programs offer inpatient and outpatient services, as well as after-care programs. These programs usually consist of peer support focusing on the development of a lifestyle free of drugs or alcohol, healthy family relationships, and positive coping skills. Family involvement is strongly encouraged. Hospitalization is required if the physical dependence is significant and withdrawal places the child at risk for complications such as seizures, depression, or suicidal behavior.

NURSING MANAGEMENT

Nursing Assessment and Diagnosis

Nurses may encounter the substance-abusing child or adolescent in the emergency department or outpatient clinic, in the school and other community settings, or during hospitalization for an injury or other acute problem. Nursing assessment for all children includes taking a thorough history from the parents and child, observing the child's behavior, and performing a physical examination. Assessment tools provide useful information for the healthcare provider. See the PACES tool on this page and the HEEADSS tool in Chapter 5 ∞ (see Table 5–5 on page 155). Maintaining a confidential approach will increase the ability to obtain truthful information about use of substances (American Academy of Child & Adolescent Psychiatry 2005b).

When substance use is known, the history should include the age at which drug use began, the pattern of use, the length of time the drug has been used, the amount of drug used, and the psychologic state while on drugs. A history of parental drug use and noninvolvement in parenting the child puts the child at higher risk for substance abuse, reflecting the combined effects of genetic and environmental influences. Environmental factors such as access to the substance, use with other teens or adults, and resources for treatment are important to consider. Find out what types of addictions are most common in your community so that assessments can be designed to the risks that are highest for youth in those settings (Figure 6–4 ➤).

CLINICAL TIP

PACES provides a framework for areas that should be assessed for each child and teen to identify risk and protective factors related to substance use. How would you phrase questions in each area?
P—Parents, peers
A—Accidents, alcohol/drug use
C—Cigarettes
E—Emotional problems
S—School, sexuality

(Knight, 1997)

CLINICAL TIP

Adolescents who have some or all of the following symptoms may be experiencing alcohol withdrawal: anxiety, headache, tremors, nausea and vomiting, malaise or weakness, insomnia, depressed mood or irritability, and hallucinations. A recurring pattern of these symptoms may indicate youth who have access to alcohol periodically, and then repeatedly experience withdrawal when it is no longer available.

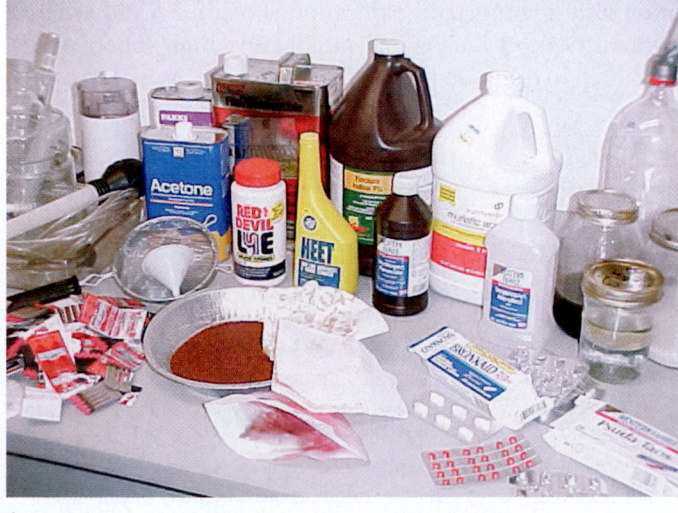

A

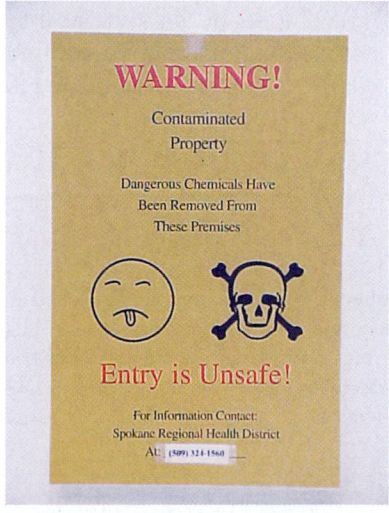

B

Figure 6–4 ➤ A, Methamphetamine is a popular drug because it can be manufactured with items that are available to the lay public such as those shown in the picture on the left. Manufacture of the substance in homes has become a concern of health departments and communities at large. Children can be harmed by the chemicals produced, and may experience neglect and abuse when parents are producing. They may suffer even after the home is found and adults are apprehended as they must be placed in foster homes. B, Homes used for methamphetamine production must be decontaminated before they can be safely used. (Photos courtesy of Spokane Regional Health District.)

Physiologic Assessment

Look for physical signs and symptoms of substance abuse, including bloodshot eyes, dilated pupils, skin and mucous membrane lesions, slurred speech, and weight loss. The adolescent may appear sleepy or restless, or may show signs of clumsiness or inconsistent behavior. Consider all types of substance abuse, including model glue, gasoline, club drugs, herbals, and other sources. Assess for current intoxication effects as well as signs of withdrawal.

Psychologic Assessment

Changes in social habits may indicate substance abuse. Parents may report a drop in the school-age child's or adolescent's grades or decreased interest in school activities. New friends are not introduced to parents, and the adolescent has less contact with parents, teachers, and other adults who were previously important. Conversely, the youth may appear more energetic, always "on a high," have weight loss, and appear to be high achieving. The child's current drug use, potential for violence, and motivation to make changes are noted. Assess the degree of family support available.

Following are possible nursing diagnoses for children and adolescents who abuse drugs or alcohol:

- Impaired Social Interaction related to altered thought processes
- Chronic Low Self-Esteem related to dysfunctional family and social relationships
- Risk for Injury related to altered perceptions and sensorium
- Risk for Violence: Self-Directed or Other-Directed related to physiologic dependence on drugs, alcohol, and other substances

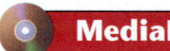

MediaLink

Identifying Youth Who Abuse Drugs and Alcohol Video

Planning and Implementation

Care of children and adolescents who abuse drugs, alcohol, and other substances is challenging and often frustrating. Long-term mental health counseling may be necessary to resolve underlying issues and foster lifestyle and behavioral changes.

Prevention is the most desirable intervention (U.S. Department of Health and Human Services, 2003). The nurse can play a major role in teaching children and their families about substance abuse (see Families Want to Know: Identifying the Youth Who Is Abusing Substances). Parents who set consistent limits and are involved in their children's lives have children with fewer risk-taking behaviors (Tuttle, Melnyk, & Loveland-Cherry, 2002). Assessing parenting styles and enhancing parenting skills during each health promotion visit is important. Education should begin in primary school and continue with intensification during the middle and high school years. Stress reduction resources can help to decrease the need for substance use. Nurses also

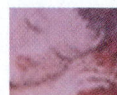

FAMILIES WANT TO KNOW

Identifying the Youth Who Is Abusing Substances

Families are often confused about the behavior of adolescents and unsure whether it represents normal development or abuse of substances. Some characteristics of normal development that help to differentiate these occurrences follow. When concerned about possible substance use, the parent can confront the child or talk with school nurses or counselors.

- Many youth are periodically distant with parents at times, but remain involved with peers in school sports and other activities. Withdrawal from all activities and friends may indicate substance abuse.
- Adolescents often complain about school, but when teachers report that the student meets expectations and is consistently performing in the classroom, this is normal behavior.

- Teens may be weepy on occasion when having a difficult time with friends or not performing as desired. Continued, consistent weepiness is more likely to indicate depression or substance abuse.
- Teens like to stay up late and are frequently tired in the morning, while abusing teens may "nod off" frequently during the day.
- Many adolescents like to achieve a disheveled look in clothing, but the teen who frequently neglects basic hygiene or does not seem to have the energy to wash and dress may be depressed or abusing substances.
- All teens get some infections, but abusing teens may have reddened eyes, oral sores, and constant respiratory discomfort from "snorting" substances.

can play a major role in community education. Various prevention programs have been developed by federal and private organizations.

The child who has begun to use and abuse drugs needs an intensive intervention program. Referral to a psychiatric health specialist is needed for diagnosis and intervention. Group programs and those that integrate the family are most effective. Find out what resources are present in your community to treat youth who are using alcohol or other drugs. Nurses are active in treatment programs as well as sustaining treatment effects and avoiding relapse during visits to community agencies once the youth returns to family, school, and other surroundings. Referral to support organizations may be beneficial for the child, parents, and other family members. Self-help groups, which are available in most communities, include Alcoholics Anonymous, Narcotics Anonymous, Al-Anon, Nar-Anon, and Ala-Teen. Parents may receive support from a group such as Parents Anonymous.

The nurse should be aware of the current substance abuse patterns in specific communities. At the present time, methamphetamine (meth) use is increasing in many areas and represents a severe threat to youth because of its extremely addictive capacity and resistance to treatment. An increasing awareness of meth's dangers has led to legislation that pseudoephedrine can only be sold as a "behind-the-counter" controlled substance since it is used in home laboratories manufacturing meth (Gettig, Grady, & Nowosadzka, 2006).

The youth's protective factors against substance abuse can be identified and used in planning appropriate interventions. For example, a child with goals related to a future career can be helped to see the way in which substance use will interfere with goal attainment. Identifying a strong role model through a program like Big Brothers or Big Sisters can assist children who lack that strength in their families.

Evaluation

Expected outcomes of nursing intervention regarding substance abuse include the following:

- The child abstains from alcohol and street drugs.
- The teen successfully participates in substance abuse programs.
- Developmentally normal social interactions are observed in the child.
- School performance at level of potential is achieved.
- The child is safe from injury.

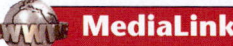

MediaLink

Substance Abuse Resources and Support

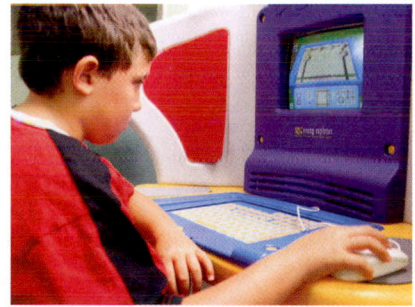

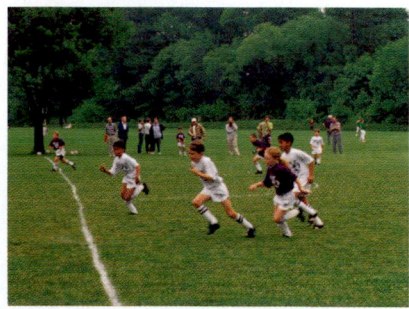

Figure 6–5 ▸ Physical inactivity is a growing problem among children, and can contribute to poor health. It is important to balance sedentary activities, such as playing computer games, with physical and social activities. Sports are an excellent way for children to develop their psychosocial, cognitive, and motor skills. Soccer photo courtesy of Rebecca Scheirer, Kensington, Maryland.

Physical Inactivity/Sedentary Behavior

In the past few decades, children have become increasingly physically inactive. This decrease is a reflection of lifestyles in which car travel is valued, computers and televisions are part of daily life, neighborhoods are sometimes unsafe places for play activities, and schools do not routinely require daily physical education classes (Figure 6–5 ▸).

Children and adolescents are subjected to high amounts of media exposure, including television, movies, radio, magazines, videos, computers (games and Internet), and a variety of other advertising (Escobar-Chaves, 2005). Children spend about 3 hours daily watching television and an additional hour on the computer (Chernin & Linebarger, 2005). This computes to 20 to 30 hours per week for most children, and significantly more for some. It is common for many hours each day to be spent on screen activities. About 37% of high school students watch television over 3 hours each day and about 21% use computer or video games over 3 hours each day (MMWR, 2006a). The effects of screen activities are multiple: (1) physical inactivity while viewing, (2) lack of active cognition, and (3) tendency to eat high fat snacks and excessive calories while viewing. Even at very young ages, children are immersed in various types of media.

Physical inactivity leads to many health concerns. A primary outcome is overweight or obesity (see Chapter 4 ∞). Other outcomes can be an increased rate of type 2 diabetes (see Chapter 29 ∞), increased exposure to television/computer game

MediaLink

Effects of Media on Children Video

RESEARCH

Effects of Media on Young Children

The increasing role of media in children's daily schedules has been known for some time. However, little data examined the issue in very young children. The first study that examined the role of electronic media in the lives of infants, toddlers, and preschoolers found startling results. A nationally representative survey of 1065 parents of children from 6 months to 6 years found the following:

- One in four children under 2 years of age has a television in his or her bedroom; 36% of children under 6 years have a television in their bedrooms, while 27% have a VCR or DVD player, 10% have a video game player, and 7% have a computer.
- Those children who have a television in their bedrooms spend significantly less time reading or playing outside than other children.
- Sixty-five percent of young children live in a household where the television is on at least half of the time; 36% are in homes where the television is nearly always on.
- Young children spend the same amount of time with electronic media as they spend outdoors (about 2 hours each).
- In contrast, these children spend only 39 minutes daily reading or being read to.
- Half of children under 6 years, and 70% of those 4–6 years, have used computers.
- Much new media is targeted at this very young audience.
- Parents have generally positive views of media, with 72% saying computers mostly help child learning, and about half saying that television and videos are very important to the intellectual learning of children (Kaiser Family Foundation, 2003).

These findings are critical for nurses to consider. Physical inactivity and sedentary behavior are linked to obesity, type 2 diabetes, and other chronic disease risk. Children's ready access to media in the home and other settings directly interferes with recommended levels of physical activity. In all settings with parents of young children, ask about exposure to media. Encourage parents to turn off the television in the house except for select and limited viewing times, avoid media use in the child's bedroom, limit exposure to media, and have the child engaged in physical activity for a greater part of the day than in quiet pursuits. Encourage reading and being read to for young children; parents can schedule reading time to at least equal media viewing. Carefully perform developmental testing on children when exposure to media is high (see Chapter 7 ∞).

What other teaching can you identify to address this issue with parents of young children? How can parents integrate media concerns into the evaluation of childcare settings? What might the effects be on child growth and development with excessive use of media?

violence and sexual activity at early ages (see violence discussion later in this chapter), and early progression of cardiovascular disease (see Chapter 21 ∞).

Conversely, patterns of physical activity established in childhood can increase exercise behaviors in adulthood and contribute to lower rates of low back pain, overweight, osteoporosis, heart disease, diabetes, colon cancer, high blood pressure, and a more positive self-image.

Although many children demonstrate low levels of physical activity, a profound decrease in vigorous activity is common in grades 9 through 12. Boys more commonly participate in team sports than girls. Although about 54% of students attend physical education (PE) classes at least once a week, only 33% have daily PE classes (MMWR, 2006c).

Health professionals can integrate assessment of physical activity into all healthcare contacts, and make recommendations to children and families that will help to increase opportunities for physical activity. Nurses assess height, weight, and body mass index to look for signs of overweight (see Chapter 4 ∞). Ask what a typical day is like and include specific questions about television, computers, and video games. Children should be asked about how they like to spend free time. Community and school activities should be encouraged and rewarded. Examples include fun runs, walks of benefit causes, aerobics classes, team sports, roadside cleanups, and fairs and carnivals. Help parents and children learn what they can do for physical fitness. Work with school physical education personnel to plan activities both in and out of physical education class that promote lifelong exercise routines. Work toward the goal of 60 minutes of daily moderate intensity physical activity for all children (U.S. Department of Health and Human Services and U.S. Department of Agriculture, 2005). Help children to gradually increase

FAMILIES WANT TO KNOW

Physical Activity Guidelines for Youth

- Engage in moderate physical activity (bike riding, walking, baseball, roller blading) for 60 minutes at least five times weekly.
- Engage in vigorous physical activity that causes sweating and hard breathing (soccer, running, ice hockey) at least 20 minutes three times weekly.
- Encourage schools to offer physical education to all students, and have students sign up when this is an elective.
- Encourage walking and bike riding to friends' homes and stores when safe.

- Plan physical activities together as a family.
- Get a pet and plan to walk the pet daily.
- Limit television and other similar sedentary activities to no more than 2 hours daily.
- On days home, allow the child to watch television for up to 1 hour, and then insist that 1 hour of reading, 1 hour of physical activity, and 1 hour of socializing with others take place before returning to more television.

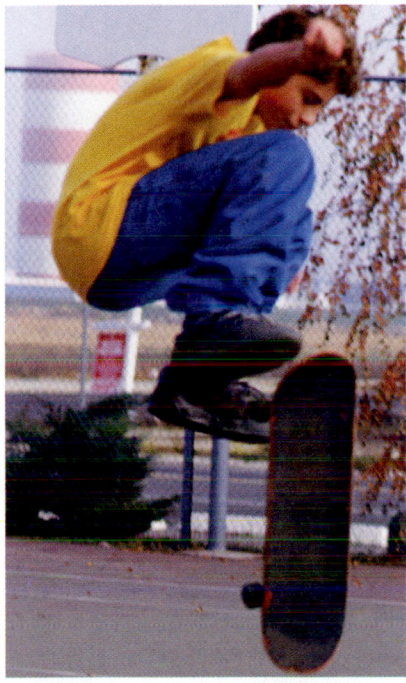

physical activity and decrease sedentary time during regular health promotion visits. See Families Want to Know: Physical Activity Guidelines for Youth.

Injury and Protective Equipment

In the discussion of causes of childhood and adolescent morbidities and mortalities in Chapter 1 ∞, unintentional injuries are listed as a common problem. In fact, 71% of all deaths from age 10 years onward result from four causes—motor vehicle crashes, other unintentional injury, homicide, and suicide (MMWR, 2004). Chapters 8 ∞ through 10 ∞ discuss the frequent injuries seen in children at different developmental ages, and safety precautions to avoid injuries from car crashes, falls, poisonings, and other developmentally related injuries. Many common injuries are preventable with simple use of protective gear and following of safety guidelines (Figure 6–6 ➤).

Nonetheless, 18% of youth rarely or never wear seat belts in automobiles and 38% of those who ride motorcycles do not wear helmets (MMWR, 2004). The use of safe automobile and motorcycle behaviors must be emphasized again in adolescence, with the recognition that risks increase if driving is combined with the use of alcohol and controlled substances. Adolescents sometimes engage in practices that put them at particular risk and nurses should be alert for activities in their communities. Examples include car surfing (standing on the trunk, hood, or roof of a moving vehicle) or street racing (racing cars down a street at extremely high speed).

About 44 million U.S. children ride bicycles, a beneficial physical activity. However, only 15–25% of children are protected by helmet use, even though bicycles are the most common activity connected with injury. Since almost one-half of the U.S. states now have helmet laws, rates are highest in states with helmet legislation. Helmets could prevent up to 88% of serious brain injuries from bicycle crashes (National Safe Kids, 2005). Strategies to make helmet use more attractive to children and adolescents are needed. Nurses can play a major role in programs to educate and reward children for helmet use, and can assist families to find helmets at a price they can afford. Education

Figure 6–6 ➤ What protective gear should children use for skateboarding? How would you convince them to use the protection?

 MediaLink

Extreme Sports Video

NURSING ALERT

A growing number of children engage in "extreme" sports, those that carry a high degree of risk and have not traditionally been common. Some examples are mountain biking, three wheeling, ski racing, snowboarding through trees and on courses with pikes and other challenges, ice climbing, rock climbing, and wakeboarding. While the nurse is probably unable to dissuade youth from engaging in these activities, safety measures should be emphasized. Find out what protective gear the youth wears and what is recommended. Keep at hand examples of stories of youth who have been saved by use of such gear. Encourage the youth to engage in sports activities only when others are present and to have a plan for emergencies, including a working cell phone, leaving information with an adult about plans and expected return, and planning for harsh weather with items such as emergency blankets, gear, and food. Encourage the youth to talk with parents and other adults about the risks and responsibilities of these activities.

CULTURE

Unintentional Injury

Striking ethnic disparity rates exist in the rates of unintentional injury among children. These differences are due mainly to living in impoverished communities rather than any innate biological variations. While the unintentional injury rate in children under 14 years of age declined 39% from 1987 to 2000, the smallest reductions were among American Indian/Alaskan Natives (20% decline) and African American children (36% decline), while higher reductions were seen in Asian/Pacific Islanders (52% decline) and White children (39% decline) (National Safe Kids Campaign, 2005). What are the major causes of unintentional injury in your community and state? What ethnic and age groups are at greatest risk? How can you integrate teaching in your practice that is specific to the findings in your community?

BOX 6–2
SPORTS AND ACTIVITIES REQUIRING SAFETY GEAR

- Rollerblading
- Skateboarding
- Roller hockey
- Ice hockey
- Football
- Soccer
- Baseball
- Scooters
- Skiing or snowboarding

should take place in offices and clinics, in school settings, and throughout the community. Nurses should take an active role in supporting legislation for helmet use, can evaluate proper fits of helmets, and can work for incentives and low-cost helmets (Rezendes, 2006). Other physical activities that require special protective gear are listed in Box 6–2.

Nurses can be active in identifying youth behaviors in communities and working with schools and other community groups to establish educational programs. Efforts should also include adequate conditioning for sports, proper treatment of injuries, prevention of overuse injuries, and assessment of risky activities.

Body Art

Body art in the form of painting, tattooing, and piercing has been donned by humans throughout history. However, there has recently been a resurgence of interest in this decorative art by teens. Many adolescents have multiple body piercings and tattoos and may even resort to performing these decorations on themselves or friends.

About 20% of adolescents and young adults have tattoos, and nearly half have at least one body piercing (Armstrong, 2005; Gold, Schorzman, Murray, Downs, & Tolentino, 2005). In some states, teens must be 18 years of age or have parental permission to obtain body art, but students often report that it is easy to have an adult present who signs and claims to be a parent. Only in some states are tattoo and body piercing businesses required to be licensed and comply with certain regulations (Armstrong, 2005). Remember that Amy, who is described in the opening scenario, had her piercing done by a friend. Amy demonstrates some common characteristics of teens who choose to use body art. It may be seen as a way to establish individualism and independence, and helps some teens to feel part of a peer group. Multiple tattoos and piercings are common, as is the case with Amy (Figure 6–7 ➤).

Body art is a common source of infections with skin pathogens, as well as hepatitis B and C. Body piercing and sharing of hardware is a major method of transmission of hepatitis C, a disease that may not even become manifested until years later (see Chapter 24 ∞ for a discussion of hepatitis). It can be a source of HIV if proper techniques are not followed. Piercings in parts of the body such as the mouth or navel are most prone to bacterial infection and continued redness and irritation. Serious systemic infections such as endocarditis have occurred after some piercings. The pierced site may not appear infected but transfer of organisms causes serious infection and heart damage. When noting signs of systemic infection such as fever, weakness, malaise, and arthralgia (see Chapter 21 ∞ for a full discussion of endocarditis), gather history about body piercings and refer for immediate care to the primary healthcare provider (Goldrick, 2003). Pierced tongues can lead to chipped teeth or even be the cause of choking if dislodged from the site.

One issue that the teen should consider prior to getting a tattoo is the relationship of the tattoo to future lifestyle changes. Advise teens to avoid tattooing the name of a person or musical group since relationships change and tastes in music evolve. Be sure they know the meaning of phrases, foreign words, or Asian symbols. Consider the visibility of the tattoo and its effect on future employment. Tattoos on the face, neck, or other readily visible places may be a detriment during employment interviews. Tattoos should always be considered permanent. Methods for removal may be costly, painful, and unsuccessful (Selekman, 2003).

Another form of body art that is regarded as disfigurement is **branding** or scarification. In this process, the skin is burned to result in a scar. Usually a desired sign, symbol, or word is inscribed. Results are usually not precise and do not adhere to expected designs. This procedure is done on the self or friend, using common household metal implements heated in fires or stoves. Others cut themselves in the form of a desired design, a process called **cutting**. These practices can result in infection, often do not yield the desired result, and may indicate underlying

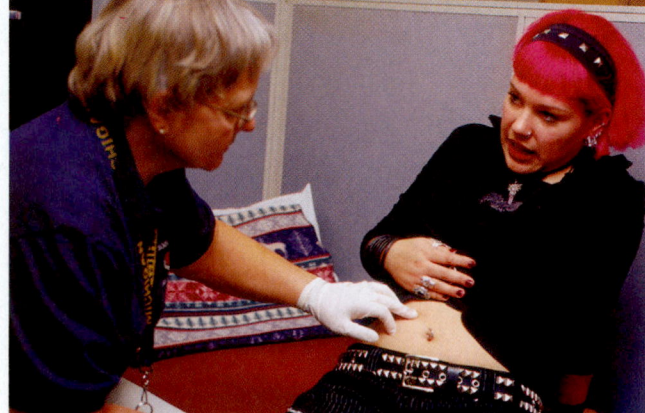

Figure 6–7 ➤ Talk openly with adolescents about their health and teach them to avoid health risks connected with tattoos and piercings.

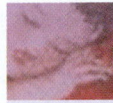

FAMILIES WANT TO KNOW

Care for Tattoos and Body Piercings

Before the Procedure
- Visit several studios to make comparisons of technique, quality, and cleanliness.
- Ask to watch a tattoo or piercing done on someone else.
- Determine the sterilization and hygiene practices of the artist.
- Ask if the artist is licensed and trained.
- Look at pictures of completed art and talk with former clients.
- Insist that new, sterile equipment be opened in front of the person to be decorated.
- Consider if this permanent body decoration is desired for a lifetime.
- Consider what the tattoo or piercing will look like in several years.
- Consider the possible side effects of infection, dislike for the art, or allergy to dyes or metals.
- Be sure that the hepatitis B vaccination is completed before the procedure.
- Be aware that no immunization is available to protect against hepatitis C and HIV.

Care After the Procedure
- Touch the area only after careful handwashing.
- Keep the area elevated and use ice for the first 2 days to minimize swelling.
- Avoid contact with another person's bodily fluids until well healed.
- Turn the piercing jewelry gently several times daily using washed hands.
- Use antibacterial mouthwash, cleaner, or ointment as recommended.
- Avoid pressure and rubbing on the site (such as belts on navel piercings).
- Watch carefully for signs of infection and report them to a healthcare provider:
  - Increased redness
  - Swelling
  - Pain
  - Hot feeling
  - Discharge
- Ask the artist how long healing will take. It varies from 2 months in the mouth to 6–8 months in the navel.
- Metal is dangerous during some medical procedures such as magnetic resonance imaging (MRI) or during surgery. Be sure to tell doctors and nurses about the piercings when hospitalized or receiving medical care, especially if they are not readily visible.
- If you decide to remove a piece of jewelry soon after placement, then the skin may heal with only a slight scar.

problems. They should be discouraged and the youth involved should be referred for further assessment by primary care providers or counselors.

Since teens may choose to obtain body art even if parents object and if there are state laws to prohibit or make it difficult, nursing care must focus on providing information to the teen, assessing sites, identifying infections, and referring if needed (see Families Want to Know: Care for Tattoos and Body Piercings). Care is almost always provided in community settings such as clinics or schools. Ask teens if they are considering body art, because they often do not seek advice before obtaining the art, and may therefore not get adequate teaching (Selekman, 2003). Ask about piercings before all medical procedures since they need to be removed for surgery, magnetic resonance imaging, and some other tests.

Sexual Orientation

Adolescence is a time of identifying emerging sexuality. Most teens establish relationships with members of the opposite sex and learn how to interact in ways that are guided by their peer group, family, and culture. For some youth, the transition into adult sexuality is more challenging, as they feel emotional and sexual attraction to people of the same sex (**homosexuality**). The term *gay* is often used for homosexual males and *lesbian* for homosexual females. Other youth are *bisexual*, or attracted to both men and women, and some are *transgendered*, an imprecise term for individuals who cross gender lines. The initials **LGBT** are sometimes used to refer to these minority sexuality choices, while the acronym **LGBQ** is sometimes used for lesbian, gay, bisexual, or questioning. From 1–10% of youth self-identify as homosexual (Benton, 2003).

Sexual attractions and practices that are different from the mainstream are not deviant, but may be viewed as part of a continuum of sexual expression. No gene, early life experience, or other event directly causes homosexuality.

LGBT/Q youth are at risk for a variety of problems related to emotional and physical health. These include rejection by family members and peers, verbal harassment, sexual abuse and physical assault, a high rate of suicide, depression, substance abuse, high rate of homelessness, and sexual risks of HIV and other sexually transmitted diseases (Benton, 2003). Their health risks need to be identified and appropriate care provided.

Nurses can provide health care for youth who are LGBT in a variety of settings. School nurses and clinics can display a sign to demonstrate that they are accepting of persons with minority sexual preferences. Terminology in assessment should be gender free. Ask the youth, "Do you have one or more sexual partners?" rather than "Do you have a boyfriend?" When youth identify as LGBT, usual care of all kinds should be provided, including preventive care such as immunizations, sports assessments, and injury prevention teaching. Be alert that the youth may have additional health challenges. Ask about peer and parental support; refer to support groups if needed. Provide resources when the teen is homeless, depressed, or suicidal (see Chapter 27 ∞). Perform testing for sexually transmitted diseases if sexual contact is occurring and teach preventive measures. Foster a positive sense of self-esteem through encouraging positive activities such as sports, music, and friendships with peers (Benton, 2003).

VIOLENCE AND ITS EFFECTS ON CHILDREN

Violence is a threatened or actual use of physical force that leads to potential or actual physical or emotional trauma. In the past several years, adults and children alike have been shocked by the violent episodes in homes, schools, and communities. There are many types of violence to which children may be exposed on a regular basis. Children can be the recipients of violence during child abuse and homicides, and they themselves can perform acts of violence on others. They may be touched by violence when parents are killed in gang conflicts, in terrorist attacks, or in wars. The effects of violence are far-reaching and ongoing; they permeate the victim's entire lifetime. This section explores certain types of violence affecting children.

Schools and Communities

At a time when firearm deaths are decreasing overall, unintentional deaths and suicides have increased among children. Many of these deaths are committed with firearms found in the home; about 10% of deaths in children are due to firearm injury (Baxley & Miller, 2006). Forty percent of households with children have guns and in 25% of those homes the firearms are stored loaded or are not secured under lock. Additionally, it is common for parents to report that children do not know firearm locations when the children are actually able to state the locations and have handled the guns (Baxley & Miller, 2006).

Homicide among children has gained attention in past years due to several notable shootings at schools. Although homicide is an extreme example, other types of violence exist. Children report being threatened verbally and with guns or knives at home, in schools, and in neighborhoods. They may be beaten up, bullied, or harassed. They may view domestic violence in their own homes. They may be subjected to dangerous situations in their neighborhoods or during times of homelessness. Date rape or other violence during dating is reported by up to 9% of teens, while 7.5% have been forced to have sexual intercourse (MMWR, 2006c). Several of these types of violence are specifically addressed in the following sections.

Family risk factors have been identified as more commonly seen in situations when violence has been committed against children. In addition, children who commit violence more commonly have ready access to firearms, are exposed to violence in the home or community, engage in violent media viewing, and have poor self-esteem or depression.

Realizing the impact of violence on and by children, several federal healthcare initiatives have begun to assist in lowering violence. Some programs have been helpful, and incidents of homicides and most other violence has begun to decrease. Programs that are most successful include individual children, parents, schools, and communities. Health school professionals are instrumental in identification of signs of violence (Table 6–5). Provide resources for families and children to decrease violence.

NURSING ALERT

When a group of children is attacked or killed in a school shooting, this tragic occurrence gains media attention. However, this tragedy is really part of daily life in many separate settings across the country. About 8 children are killed by a firearm every day in the United States, or about 56 children per week. An additional 200–300 children experience nonfatal firearm injuries (Children's Defense Fund, 2004b). Nurses must intervene in this national tragedy. Become familiar with firearm injury statistics in your community. Teach families about the dangers of firearms. Urge safe storage. Teach children and youth about the danger of firearms. Help schools establish programs to ensure safety for students.

Table 6–5	ASSESSMENT QUESTIONS TO IDENTIFY VIOLENCE RISK AND PROTECTIVE FACTORS

Microsystem
- Have you been hurt by your parents or anyone else at home?
- When was the last time you were teased or bullied at school? What did you do?
- Have you ever brought a gun, knife, or other weapon to school?
- Do you have access to guns and knives at home? At friends' houses?
- What stresses are there in your family now?
- Tell me about school—what do you like and dislike?

Mesosystem
- Do your parents attend school meetings? Talk with your teachers?
- Do you participate in any church, synagogue, or mosque services?
- Do you participate in any community activities?

Exosystem
- What stresses do your parents have at work, in their families, with their health or finances?
- Do you feel like your school helps to keep you safe?
- Are there plans for handling violent episodes at your school if they were to occur?
- Do you feel safe in your neighborhood?
- Where would you go or who would you call if you felt unsafe or were hurt and no one was at home?

War and Terrorism

Internationally, 40 million children experience violence each year and decreasing violence against children has become a focus of both the World Health Organization and the United Nations (World Health Organization, 2002; 2005). Common forms of violence worldwide are war and terrorism. War affects children in several ways: parents leave home to fight in wars, children may be forced to take on adult roles in families when members leave, children become orphans when parents are killed, and some children are trained and forced to fight in battles, carry messages, or otherwise engage in combat themselves (UNICEF, 2006). Children who live through wars or have a parent or sibling die in war can be permanently affected by these events.

Another type of violence is terrorism. The events in the United States of September 11, 2001, and other examples in many countries take a large toll on the mental health of children and adolescents. The response of children to terrorism is not well studied. Disasters such as the World Trade Center attack can lead to sleep and eating problems, fears of entering tall buildings, regression in school performance and other behaviors, and posttraumatic stress disorder (see Chapter 27 ∞). Most children and adolescents experience profound sadness, cling to adults who provide security, and have a variety of somatic complaints (Redlener & Grant, 2002).

Understanding the response of children and adolescents to war and terrorist events can assist healthcare providers in providing interventions to assist children and families. Some key factors include:

- Dose and exposure. Repeated events or more intense experiences, such as being personally involved in a shooting episode, create the greatest psychological trauma. Consider that constant exposure by repeated viewing of war and terrorism in the media magnifies the trauma for viewers.
- Children individualize their experiences related to their developmental levels. Younger children are very affected by physical separation from parents while older children may worry more about repeat events and their future. Much more research is needed to examine the long-term effects of trauma on various age groups.
- In addition to development, the child's prior experiences with stress may contribute both risk and protective factors to new traumatic situations.
- Interventions to assist children can focus on them, their parents, and others in the community, such as teachers. Interventions should be directed at different phases of violence, such as pre-event preparation (emergency preparation and training) and post-event activity (offering special services and resources) (Pine, Costello, & Masten, 2005).

Several resources have been developed to help families and health professionals help children deal with war and violence. See the resources on the National Center for Children Exposed to Violence, Society of Pediatric Nurses, and American Academy of Child & Adolescent Psychiatry Web sites.

> **NURSING ALERT**
>
> **Risk Factors Common in Families with Child Victims of Violence**
> - History of mental illness, domestic violence, incarceration, or substance abuse in the home
> - Family stresses
> - Inadequate childcare or supervision
> - Inadequate family social support
> - Use of corporal punishment for the child
> - Child abuse
> - Access to firearms
> - Gang membership in family or neighborhood
> - High exposure to media violence
> - Child hyperactivity and other developmental behavioral disorders
>
> Note: From Elders, J. (2003). The role of the pediatrician in violence in the school. Accessed January, 30, 2004, from www.schoolhealth.org/reduviol.html. Adapted.

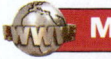 **MediaLink**

Violence Prevention and Support Resources

Bullying

One type of violence that frequently occurs in schools is **bullying**, or aggressive behavior that is intended to cause harm, exists in a relationship with imbalance of power, and occurs repeatedly (Limber, 2003). Bullying behaviors include verbal abuse (taunting, teasing), name calling, threats, spreading rumors, social exclusion, and physical abuse (hitting, shoving, kicking, tripping). About 16% of children in a large national survey had suffered bullying, most commonly in grades 6 through 8, and more frequently among males. Almost 30% of 11- to 15-year-olds have been either victims or perpetrators of bullying. Almost 75% of children from 6 to 13 years report being bullied and 34% report bullying in the past year. Up to 160,000 U.S. children may miss school every day in efforts to avoid bullying (Bauer et al., 2006; Limber, 2003). Although bullying is most commonly reported in schools, it can occur in neighborhoods as children go to and from school, in school buses, sports teams, and other settings.

Bullies are more likely to smoke, drink alcohol, and perform poorly in school, and one in four bullies has a criminal record by 30 years of age (HRSA, 2003). Bullies are more likely to bring weapons to school, putting other children at risk (Fox, Elliot, Kerlikowske, Newman, & Christeson, 2003), and bullying is associated with future delinquent behavior (van der Wal, de Wit, & Hirasing, 2003). They are aggressive, impulsive, and need to dominate others.

However, children who are bullied are more commonly socially isolated and anxious. This social isolation has many negative outcomes, including feelings of depression, low self-esteem, loneliness, and suicidal ideation among those bullied. Health problems such as migraines, stomach pains, suicidal thoughts, and other problems can result. Academic performance commonly deteriorates and rates of school absenteeism increase (Children's Safety Network, National Injury and Violence Prevention Resource Center, 2003; Limber, 2003). Realizing the serious effects of such behaviors, a number of states have now passed legislation that reiterates the rights of all children to attend school in a safe and peaceful manner. Some state education departments mandate school district programs for students about bullying, and clear school policies about dealing with the behavior. The presence of an antibullying school policy is effective in reducing incidence of this form of violence (Fekkes, Pijpers, & Verloove-Vanhorick, 2006).

A campaign by the Health Resources and Services Administration's (HRSA) Maternal and Child Health Bureau targets 9- to 13-year-old youths to prevent bullying. Access their web site for information about dealing with this issue in schools in your state.

MediaLink

Bullying Resources

Incarceration

A growing number of children are entering the judicial system and many are admitted at young ages. Juveniles are responsible for about 12% of arrests for violent crimes, and their lifestyle and environment places them at a four times greater risk of death than the average teen (Snyder, 2003; Teplin, McClelland, Abram, & Mileusnic, 2005). Girls represent an increasing number of children in juvenile justice. Children in detention, courts, and other facilities have frequently been victims as well as perpetrators of violence. They often have multiple risks such as substance abuse, early sexual activity, multiple sexual partners, lack of a healthcare home, and mental health issues (Guthrie, Hoey, Ravoira, & Kintner, 2002). Nurses may work within the juvenile justice system to provide episodic care for children or to partner with others to establish health-related programs within facilities. Youth need:

- Basic physical care such as immunizations, vision and hearing screening
- Nutrition assessment and teaching
- Skin assessment and hygiene practice teaching
- Information about sexuality, sexual practices, and sexually transmitted diseases
- Assessment for substance abuse
- Teaching about hazards of substance use and assistance with quitting
- Mental health services
- Developmental assessment
- Individualized Education Plans to meet cognitive needs

Abandoned Babies

There are no accurate statistics on the number of babies that are abandoned in dumpsters, on doorsteps, and in other locations. This tragedy has been addressed by "Safe Haven" laws in some states that allow women to drop unwanted babies at certain locations such as hospitals and fire stations without legal recrimination. In spite of these laws, babies continue to be randomly abandoned, perhaps because mothers do not know about the laws or because they do not believe they will not be found guilty. Young teen mothers may not want others to know they had a baby. In addition, placement of these babies in adoptive homes is often difficult because of paternity suits. Nurses should know their state's "Safe Haven" law details. Inform adolescents and young women about the law and post information in community sites frequented by women. Partner with young pregnant women to link them to resources such as adoption agencies when they might not want to keep a baby.

Hazing

Hazing is an activity that is forced upon an individual which causes humiliation and is required for membership in an organization or group. It can sometimes be potentially harmful. In the past 30 years, about 60 college students have died from events linked to hazing, and even middle and high school athletes commonly engage in hazing activities (Gershel, Katz-Sidlow, Small, & Zandieh, 2003). Activities might include removing clothes, drinking large amounts of alcohol, using snuff or other substances, being locked in small places, being beaten, and many other behaviors. In spite of its common practice, many coaches are not aware of it, and many students do not know what to do about hazing practices. Ask during health visits if the student has ever had to do something to belong to the group or team. Ask about "scary" things others have had them do. Assist schools and colleges in setting up anti-hazing policies. Encourage students to report hazing. Be aware of the possibility of hazing when seeing children with traumatic injuries.

Domestic Violence

Domestic violence or intimate partner abuse is that which occurs between adult partners in a family. It may involve the parents of a child, or one parent and the significant other. Even teens who are in a sexual relationship with another person can be direct victims in domestic violence. This type of abuse then injures the child or adolescent either by witnessing a loved one being abused, or by being the victim. About 3.3 million U.S. children are annually exposed to violence against their mothers or other female care providers (Regan, 2003). And children who live in homes where intimate partner abuse occurs are 10 times more likely to be abused themselves, so the behavior is often a precursor to child abuse (Regan, 2003). See the additional detailed discussion of child abuse later in this chapter and intimate partner abuse discussions in Chapters 8–10.

Dating Violence

Dating violence is another type of intimate partner abuse; this type occurs in relationships among youth. Most dating violence is directed at females and studies have focused largely on girls. Over 9% of adolescent girls report being victims of dating violence. African American girls report dating violence more commonly than Hispanic or White girls (Howard & Wang, 2003; MMWR, 2006c). Girls who report dating violence were also more likely to report other risk behaviors, such as feeling sad, having attempted suicide, or having used substances such as tobacco and drugs. Early sexual activity, having a higher number of sex partners, and being less likely to use birth control are also associated with higher incidences of dating violence. A cluster risk profile may therefore put adolescents more at risk for dating violence.

Date rape is a term used when dating violence takes the form of rape. This can be particularly harmful to females who often do not want to discuss the event or press charges against the attacker.

■ NURSING MANAGEMENT

Nursing Assessment and Diagnosis

Nurses are in key positions to identify children who are at risk of being recipients and victims of violence. The ecological framework can be used to assess children. Some questions that can be asked are listed in Table 6–5. It is important to detect both the risks that lead to vulnerability and the protective factors that can promote resilience and safety. Questions should be adapted to each age group and inserted in every health-care encounter.

Nurses should screen for violence at each health promotion visit, including gynecologic visits and prenatal care. Ask what is going well and not going well in intimate relationships, and whether the person ever feels unsafe or is forced to do things she does not wish to do. Recognize that while not as common, males may also be victims of violence in close relationships. Recognize that alcohol and other drugs are often connected with violence in relationships, so ask about their use. Organize peer discussion groups about intimacy in order to help youth develop a sense of self-confidence and self-efficacy. This will empower them to refuse relationship activities in which they do not wish to engage.

Nursing care for violence is discussed in the Nursing Care Plan on the following pages. These additional nursing diagnoses may be appropriate:

- Risk for Violence: Self-Directed related to history of violence
- Chronic Low Self-Esteem related to history of abuse
- Interrupted Family Processes related to situational crises
- Delayed Growth and Development related to environmental deficiencies

Planning and Intervention

Nurses intervene with individual children, with families, and in schools and communities to increase safety and decrease violence. Children and families are assisted in meeting basic needs and accessing resources to assist with finances, respite care, domestic violence, and other issues. Education is a key element of intervention.

Providing Information

The nurse can teach family members about the dangers of firearms and the necessity for use of gun locks, locked cabinets, storing guns unloaded, and storing guns and ammunition in separate places. Suggest alternative activities to minimize children's exposure to violence in the media. Inform parents about rating systems for television and other media, and about lockout mechanisms for televisions and computers (see Families Want to Know: Rating Systems for Media). Harmful effects of verbal and physical abuse to the child or other family members are discussed and alternatives explored.

The school-age child and adolescent are presented with information about bullying and strategies for dealing with the problem. School and community resources are provided concerning where the child can go if there are threats of any kind. Date rape and violence are topics for discussion for all teens, as is the importance of reporting the situations when they occur.

Care in the Community

Both in schools and community settings, nurses can plan peer mentoring to provide assistance to children at high risk of experiencing violence. School and community programs for children can be linked and coordinated by nurses to provide for parent involvement and child support. Discuss safety issues, both risks and protective actions, in schools and community groups. Report children who are at risk. Work to establish extended programs for children so that they are safe after school. Help children learn behaviors that will help them to be safe in their communities and at home. Teach positive problem-solving and conflict management techniques to children and parents.

NURSING CARE PLAN   The Child and Violent Behavior

GOAL	INTERVENTION	RATIONALE	EXPECTED OUTCOME
1. Risk for Violence: Other-directed related to history of family violence			
	NIC Priority Intervention— **Environmental Management:** **Violence Prevention:** *Monitoring and manipulation of the environment to decrease the potential for violent behavior directed toward self, others, or the environment*		*NOC Suggested Outcome—* **Impulse Control:** *Ability to restrain compulsive or impulsive behavior in child and others*
The child demonstrates impulse control	• Identify violent behaviors in the child • Provide a safe place for exploration of feelings by referral to school or other counseling, support groups, and other resources • Provide strategies for managing anger, alternative ways for coping with problems	• Violence in the child usually develops over time • The child needs an opportunity to explore feelings and vulnerability • Coping strategies can be learned from others and can help in dealing with a stressful home or community situation	The child expresses ability to manage problems in acceptable ways
The child is secure in a safe environment	• Perform thorough assessment of hazards to physical and emotional state in the child's home, neighborhood, and school • Institute actions that will result in removal of child from unsafe situations • Use community resources to provide respite care, teaching for families, and safety instruction for the child	• Hazards to physical and emotional health promote violence to and from the child • Removal from family, community, or school may be needed to ensure child safety • Stress reduction measures may help to decrease violent behaviors	The child expresses a sense of physical and emotional safety in daily life
2. Impaired Home Maintenance related to insufficient family organization			
	*NIC Priority Intervention—***Home** **Maintenance Assistance:** *Helping the family to maintain the home as a safe place to live*		*NOC Suggested Outcome—* **Role Performance:** *Congruence of an individual's role behavior with role expectations*
Family members are able to meet role expectations	• Provide information on child's developmental needs • Provide ongoing assessment in the home via home healthcare visits • Assist the family in identifying hazards in the environment that can impair the child's growth and development • Evaluate ability of adults to provide a safe, secure, nurturing environment	• Parents needs to understand the developmental progression of their children • Early identification of hazards can lead to proper interventions to protect against harm to the child • Families may need respite care, information about child needs, financial assistance, or other resources in order to meet the needs of the child	Family members meet role expectations, contributing to making the home a safe and secure place for the child
3. Hopelessness related to long-term family stress			
	*NIC Priority Intervention—***Hope** **Instillation:** *Facilitation of the development of a positive outlook in the given situation*		*NOC Suggested Outcome—* **Hope:** *Presence of internal state of optimism that is personally satisfying and life supporting*

(continued)

NURSING CARE PLAN | The Child and Violent Behavior (continued)

GOAL	INTERVENTION	RATIONALE	EXPECTED OUTCOME
3. Hopelessness related to long-term family stress (continued)			
The child will have adequate food, sleep, and express satisfaction with life	• Monitor child's nutritional state and growth and daily patterns • Monitor child's developmental status • Determine adequacy of relationships and support systems	• The child's nutrition, sleep, and other patterns provide clues to the family's ability to perceive hope and provide care for the child • The child needs close personal relationships in order to grow and learn	The child demonstrates normal growth patterns and meets expected developmental outcomes
The family will identify resources to achieve life goals	• Monitor the family's decision making ability • Provide information on community resources • Refer for psychiatric, and other services if needed • Assists in goal setting	• Feeling overwhelmed by events leads to an inability to set goals and make decisions to meet the goals • Resources can assist the family members in setting and achieving realistic goals	The family establishes realistic goals for growth and development of its members, and takes steps to meet the goals
4. Risk for Injury related to physical or psychological conditions in the environment			
	NIC Priority Intervention—**Safety Behavior:** *Family actions to minimize risk of physical or emotional trauma*		*NOC Suggested Outcome*—**Parenting: Social Safety:** *Parental actions to avoid social relationships that might cause harm or injury:* **Risk Control:** *Actions to eliminate or reduce actual, personal, and modifiable health risks*
Risk for physical and emotional injury to the child is decreased	• Identify physical and psychological factors that affect child's safety • Assist family to deal with issues such as mental status challenges, fatigue, financial concern, substance abuse, lack of adequate childcare resources, and other factors • Instruct family on methods of keeping the child safe	• Multiple factors in the family can contribute to risk of violence and lack of safety for the child • Families need information about the impact of unsafe settings on the child and methods that can decrease risk of injury	The child is not injured in emotional ways in the home or other immediate settings
5. Post-Trauma Syndrome related to physical or psychosocial abuse			
	NIC Priority Intervention—**Counseling:** *Use of an interactive helping process focusing on the needs, problems, and feelings of the child who is a victim of abuse or other violence.*		*NOC Suggested Outcome*—**Abuse/Violence Recovery:** *Healing of psychologic and physical wounds of abuse or violence*
The child demonstrates abuse or violence recovery	• Assess the child's affect and behaviors • Evaluate social interactions and sense of trust in others • Assist the child in identifying feelings and coping strategies by providing counseling, art therapy, and other strategies	• Distributed child behaviors can demonstrate a sense of mistrust and insecurity • Establishment of close interactions with others demonstrates reestablishment of a sense of trust • A child who has experienced abuse or other violence needs a therapeutic relationship with a counselor to deal with the trauma and begin to rebuild trust, respect, and to learn coping mechanisms	The child identifies feelings related to violent episode(s) and expresses healing of the self

FAMILIES WANT TO KNOW

Rating Systems for Media

Television Rating	Television Rating—Mature Audience Detail	Video and Computer	Movies	Music
TV-Y: for all TV-Y7: for older children TV-Y7 FV: for older children with fantasy violence content G: general audience TV-PG: parental guidance suggested TV-14: parents strongly cautioned TV-MA: mature audience	FV: fantasy violence L: language V: violence S: sexual situation D: sexual dialogue	EC: for early childhood or those over 3 years E: for everyone over 6 years, mild language E10: for everyone over 10 years, minimal violence T: for teens over 13 years, increased violence and suggestive themes M: for mature viewers over 17 years, intense violence, sexual content, strong language AO: adults only, over 18 years, prolonged violence, sexual scenes, nudity RP: rating pending	G: general PG: parental guidance suggested PG–13: parents strongly cautioned R: restricted to those above 18 years without adult accompaniment NC–17: no one under 18 years admitted, even with adult	Parent Advisory Label: strong language, sex, or substance abuse depicted

Partner with families to assist them in talking to children about war and terrorism. Recognize that youth who have experienced such events themselves are more at risk for mental health disruptions with future events. Answer questions from children honestly but reassure them that many people are trying to make the situation safe. Other suggestions for parents include:

- Limit television viewing and other media exposure because of its constant replaying of the events of terrorism or war. Preschoolers may think the events continue to happen, rather than being a one-time occurrence. Watch with the child and talk about what is happening.
- Continue with structured family events such as meals, recreation, and faith-based activities. Spend time with your child.
- Take cues from the child about how much to discuss. Use words the child or adolescent can understand. Consider having the child draw pictures to assist in expression of feelings about the experience.
- Partner with the school so teachers know what parents have discussed and parents are aware of how events are discussed at school.
- If youth decide to become active by writing letters or joining campaigns, allow them to participate in this way.
- Be alert for regression in behavior, sleep and eating problems, irritability, fear of separation from the family, or other indications of stress (DeRanieri, Clements, Clark, Kuhn, & Manno, 2004). Consider talking with the healthcare provider or a counselor in such situations.
- Expect that even after the child has adjusted, there may be delayed reactions. Anniversaries of events, holidays, and birthdays often bring renewed pain and sadness.

Realize that adults must care for themselves, obtain stress relief, and talk with others in order to have strength and resources available for children.

Nurses can be active in setting up school policies about bullying and integrating assessment and interventions related to bullying into health promotion visits. School programs should:

- Inform all students that bullying is not tolerated.
- Train teachers and other personnel about signs of bullying.
- Ensure adult supervision in hallways and playgrounds, sites where bullying is most common.
- Teach children to promptly report bullying that is experienced or observed.
- Set up peer support for those who are bullied.
- Arrange therapeutic treatment through school counselors and other resources for those who bully; involve parents in the treatment plan.
- Measure incidence of bullying, outcomes of policies, and use data to evaluate policies in schools.

Nurses who are in clinics, offices, and other health promotion settings can also be active in prevention and intervention against bullying:

- Be alert for children with behavior changes (irritability, anxiety, poor self-concept).
- Consider bullying as a potential cause when fear or refusal to attend school is reported by the child or parents.
- Ask questions during visits, such as "Have you ever been afraid to go to school?" or "Tell me the best and worst things about going to your school?" or "What are the other kids in your neighborhood like?"
- Ask parents what they have done about any situations identified. Partner with the parent to act as liaison to the school or other agency.
- Refer identified bullies and victims of bullying to mental health specialists.

Youth with special needs, such as those who are incarcerated, are a special concern of nurses. Jails and detention centers often have a nurse who visits youth on a regular basis or when health problems occur. Health teaching may be provided in some facilities. Halfway houses and homeless shelters are examples of settings where violence prevention and intervention can occur with youth. Mental health centers and other programs have nurses that work with children who are victims of violence (for example, have witnessed domestic violence, have witnessed or had a family member murdered, have been abused at home or school) or perpetrators of violence. See Chapter 27 ∞ for a discussion of posttraumatic stress disorder and its effects on the child and adolescent.

Nurses realize that exposure to violence takes many forms and that assessment for violence should take place in every healthcare encounter, both through observation and questioning. Activity in the community to decrease violence and to provide information and resources for families is an important nursing role.

Evaluation

The expected outcomes of nursing care for violence prevention include:

- A decrease in incidents of homicides, firearm injuries, abuse, date rape, bullying, and other violence is evident among children.
- Programs to decrease violence are established and evaluated.
- Children verbalize what to do if violence occurs, and how to solve problems without becoming violent.
- Youth display personal positive judgment of self-worth.
- Youth are able to make positive choices between alternative behaviors.
- Family functions to provide mutual support for each family member.
- Children exhibit healthy adjustment following violent events.

CHILD ABUSE

One of the most common types of violence against children is child abuse. This type of violence can have implications for both the physical and mental health of children, and can influence their health status long after the abuse has occurred. Awareness of the problem of child abuse is increasing. More cases are being reported; however, these are probably only a small percentage of the total. Approximately 10–20% of children between the ages of 3 and 17 years—about 2.9 million children—are reported as abused each year, with an estimate that three times this number of probable cases may occur. About 1 million of the reported cases are substantiated, while others warrant further assessment and monitoring (U.S. Department of Health and Human Services [DHHS], 2005). More than four children daily (that is about 1500 children annually) die from child abuse in the United States (Childhelp, 2005).

Physical abuse is only one part of a larger problem. The definition of child abuse has expanded over the past 10 years to include physical neglect, emotional abuse and neglect, verbal abuse, and sexual abuse, in addition to physical abuse. Many children who are abused are under the age of 5 years, and some are as young as 3 months. The incidence of abuse is 16/1000 for children under 3 years, 14/1000 for 4–7 years, 12/1000 for 8–11 years, and 6/1000 for 16–17 years (U.S. DHHS, 2005). The average age for sexual molestation is 4 years. The perpetrator is typically the parent (80% of the time) or another legally responsible person who:

- Inflicts or allows another to inflict physical or emotional pain or injury, or
- Creates or allows another to create a significant risk of serious physical or emotional pain or injury, or
- Commits or allows another to commit an act of sexual abuse, as defined by law, against the child.

Abuse generally involves an act of commission, that is, actively doing something to a child physically, emotionally, or sexually, such as hitting, belittling, or molesting. Neglect more often involves an act of omission, such as not providing adequate nutrition, emotional contact, or necessary physical care. Because the evidence is often not visible, emotional abuse and neglect are more difficult to identify and prove than physical abuse or neglect. The major types of abuse and neglect are defined in the following text, with a section on medical maltreatment (Munchausen syndrome by proxy) following. Risk factors for abuse and neglect are listed in Table 6–6.

Physical Abuse

Physical abuse is the deliberate maltreatment of another individual that inflicts pain or injury and may result in permanent or temporary disfigurement or even death. Common methods of physical abuse in children are listed in Table 6–7.

Physical Neglect

Physical neglect is the deliberate withholding of or failure to provide the necessary and available resources to the child. Behaviors constituting physical neglect include failure to provide for the following basic needs: adequate nutrition and hydration, hygiene (e.g., clean diapers and clothes, bathing and toileting facilities), shelter (e.g., warmth in winter), and appropriate health care (e.g., immunizations, dental care, medications, eyeglasses).

Table 6–6	**RISK FACTORS FOR CHILD ABUSE AND NEGLECT**
Factors Increasing Risk for Physical Abuse	**Factors Increasing Risk for Sexual Abuse**
Poverty	Absence of natural father or having a stepfather
Violence in the family	Being female
Prematurity	Mother's employment outside the home
Unrelated male primary caretaker	Poor relationship with parent
Parents who were abused as children	Parental relationship characterized by conflict
Age less than 3 years	Parental substance abuse or social isolation
Handicap or condition that requires a great deal of care (e.g., mental retardation, attention deficit hyperactivity disorder)	
Parental substance abuse or social isolation	

Table 6–7	**METHODS OF PHYSICAL ABUSE IN CHILDREN**

Hitting, slapping, kicking, or punching

Whipping with belts, shoes, or electrical cords **(1)**

Inflicting burns with a lit cigarette or lighter **(2)**

Immersing child or body part in scalding water (commonly legs, perineal area, hands, or feet; see Figure 30–20 ∞)

Shaking the child violently ("shaken child" syndrome)

Tying the child to a fence, bed, tree, or other object

Throwing the child against a wall, down stairs, or against a window

Choking or gagging the child

Fracturing the legs, arms, ribs, or skull

Deliberately administering excessive doses of prescribed or nonprescribed drugs

Deliberately withholding prescribed medication

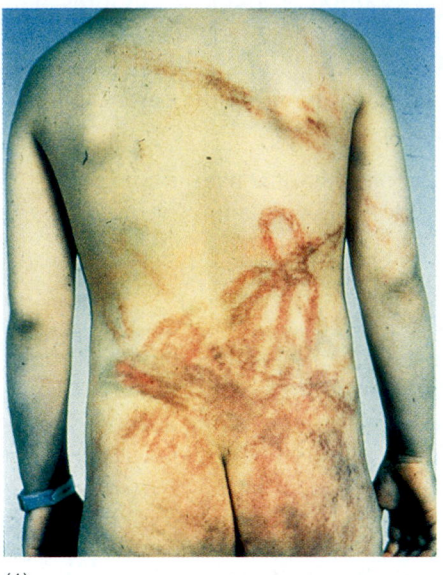

(1)

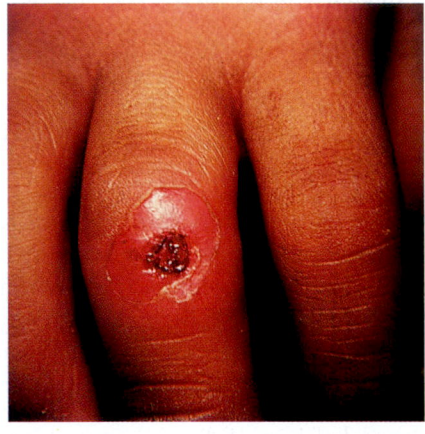

(2)

Used with permission of the American Academy of Pediatrics, Visual Diagnosis of Child Abuse Slide Kit, Photographs Copyright © AAP/Kempe.

Emotional Abuse

Emotional abuse is psychological maltreatment, and usually involves shaming, ridiculing, embarrassing, or insulting the child. It can also include the destruction of a child's personal property, such as tearing up the child's favorite family photographs or letters or harming, killing, or giving away the child's pet. These actions are frequently used as a means of frightening or controlling the child.

Verbal abuse is a common method of emotional abuse. Words can be a violent and volatile weapon against a child, eroding the child's fragile sense of self and destroying self-esteem. Common examples of verbal abuse include yelling obscenities at the child, calling the child names, threatening to "put the child away" or to give away or kill the child's pet, telling the child "I wish you were never born" or "You're worthless," and using words to humiliate, shame, or degrade the child.

Emotional Neglect

Emotional neglect is characterized by the caretaker's emotional unavailability to the child. The usual style of interaction is cold and lacking in sensitive personal attention. The child suffers from a lack of nurturance and failure of the parent or caretaker to meet basic dependency needs.

Sexual Abuse

Child sexual abuse is the exploitation of a child for the sexual gratification of an adult. About 1.2/1000 children (almost 100,000) in the United States are known to be sexually abused each year. Approximately 10% of school children report that they have been sexually abused. Of child sexual abusers, over 80% are immediate family members, other relatives, friends, or neighbors (Saewye, Pettingell, & Magee, 2003; U.S. DHHS, 2005). The word *child* used in conjunction with sexual abuse and molestation refers to anyone who has not reached the age of consent, even if a teenager. **Incest** is sexual activity between close family members, so that marriage would be legally or culturally prohibited. Abusers often threaten to harm or kill the child or another family member if the child discloses the abuse.

Some abusers are pedophiles, people who have sexual impulses toward preadolescent children. The pedophile is at least 16 years of age and at least 5 years older than the victim, who is 13 years of age or younger. Another form of sexual abuse is exhibitionism or obtaining sexual arousal by exposing one's genitals to a stranger. Some children are also victims of prostitution, being forced to offer themselves for money or the pleasures of others, either in person or through videotapes and Internet sources (Thornburgh & Lin, 2002).

In an age of media use the Internet presents children with additional risks. Children may be exposed to material that is inappropriate for them, they may be contacted by pedophiles through chat rooms, and they may provide information such as addresses and phone numbers that allow pedophiles to find them. Absolute control of Internet usage is virtually impossible since about 5 hours daily is spent on electronic media by youth (McColgan & Giardino, 2005). However, strategies can include supervision of Internet use, frequent discussions with youth about Internet sites, blocking some sites and types of software, and teaching all youth about the hazards of Internet conversations. Parents need assistance since most of them are less skilled and knowledgeable about Internet use and often do not understand the risks or believe that their children will be enticed into dangerous activities.

Etiology and Pathophysiology

Regardless of the type of abuse, the most common abuser is the child's parent or guardian or the male friend of the child's mother. Substance abuse is a major contributor to the problem, with about one-half of cases related to parental alcohol or drug abuse (Childhelp, 2005). Risk factors associated with abusive behavior by adults include the following:

- Psychopathology, such as drug addiction or alcoholism, low self-esteem, poor impulse control, and other personality disorders
- Poor parenting experiences, such as abuse in the abuser's own childhood, rejection by the abuser's own parent(s), lack of knowledge of alternative methods of discipline, strong belief in or family tradition of harsh discipline, and lack of parental affection
- Marital stressors and problems with partners, such as hostile-dependent, abusive, or nonsupportive relationships, and one-sided decision making
- Environmental stressors, such as legal, financial, medical, or housing problems
- Social isolation, such as few friends and limited use of sitters, family, or other resources
- Inappropriate expectations for the developmental level of the child

Clinical Manifestations

See the Clinical Manifestations of physical abuse and sexual abuse tables on the next page. Behaviors inconsistent with developmental stage may be apparent. For example, the toddler or preschooler may be indiscriminately friendly with unfamiliar adults, including healthcare providers, rather than demonstrating shyness or anxiety. For the infant or young child with "shaken baby syndrome" or "shaken child syndrome," the symptoms are those of central nervous system injury from repeated coup and contrecoup injury. The high water and gelatinous content of the infants brain makes it highly vulnerable to injury during shaking (see Chapter 26 ∞). Symptoms include vomiting, irritability, fatigue, poor feeding, bradycardia, apnea, enlarged fontanel, and seizures. Bruises are usually not present, but computerized tomography (CT) is often definitive for the diagnosis, with radiographs and magnetic resonance imaging (MRI) used for a thorough diagnostic profile (Carbaugh, 2004; Hymel & Hall, 2005).

CLINICAL MANIFESTATIONS OF CHILD ABUSE

- Multiple bruises in various stages of healing
- Scald burns with clear lines of demarcation and in a glove or stocking distribution (see Figure 30–20)
- Rope, belt, or cord marks, usually seen on the mouth, buttocks, back, legs, and arms (see Figure 1 in Table 6–7)
- Burn scars in various stages of healing
- Multiple fractures in various stages of healing
- Shortness of breath and distress upon being moved, indicating chest contusions and possible rib fractures
- Sedation from overmedication
- Exacerbation of chronic illness (such as diabetes or asthma) because of withholding of medication

CLINICAL MANIFESTATIONS SEXUAL ABUSE IN CHILDREN AND ADOLESCENTS

- Vaginal discharge
- Blood-stained underpants or diaper
- Genital redness, pain, itching, or bruising
- Difficulty walking or sitting
- Urinary tract infection
- Sexually transmitted disease
- Somatic complaints, such as headaches or stomachaches
- Excessively seductive behavior
- Sleeping problems, such as nightmares or night terrors
- Bedwetting
- Unwillingness to go to babysitter, family member, neighbor, or other person
- Fear of strangers
- New or excessive sexual curiosity or play
- Constant masturbation
- Curling into fetal position
- Phobias about particular places, people, or things
- Abrupt changes in school performance and attendance
- Changes in eating habits
- Abrupt changes in behavior (especially withdrawal)
- Child or adolescent female acts like a wife or mother

> ### NURSING ALERT
> **Common Forms of Sexual Abuse**
> - Oral–genital contact
> - Fondling and caressing the genitals
> - Anal intercourse
> - Sexual intercourse
> - Rape
> - Sodomy
> - Prostitution

Manifestations of physical neglect include undernourishment (evidenced by constantly feeling hungry, hoarding or stealing food, and being underweight), unclean clothes and body, poor dental health (extensive cavities or generally poor condition of teeth), and inappropriate clothing for the season.

Manifestations of emotional abuse, verbal abuse, and emotional neglect include fear, poor physical growth, and failure to meet appropriate developmental milestones. The child may have difficulty relating to adults, impaired communication skills, and developmental delays. Behavioral manifestations include anxiety, fear, shame, aggression, delinquency, and depression.

Children who have been sexually abused may exhibit a variety of physical and behavioral signs and symptoms. However, sexual abuse does not always result in apparent injury. Among the many long-term consequences of child sexual abuse are ongoing feelings of shame, guilt, anger, and hostility; decreased self-esteem, which leads to increased self-destructive behavior and risk of suicide; recurrence of victimization experiences; substance abuse; and eating disorders. Factors associated with greater psychological harm to the child include (1) a long period of abuse, (2) use of violent force or threat of violence, (3) abuse involving penetration (intercourse or oral–genital sex), and (4) abuse involving family members, especially the father or stepfather.

■ COLLABORATIVE CARE

The diagnosis and management of child abuse is complicated and requires collaboration among many groups. Often the child is identified in a healthcare setting with an injury and physicians, nurses, and others partner to analyze the situation. Sometimes parents suspect abuse by another care provider and seek assistance, or school officials identify and report suspected abuse. Suspected abuse may be reported so that social service and law enforcement agencies can investigate. Once abuse is verified, treatment may also be complex, involving school counselors, nurses, mental health specialists, physicians, and family members. The child's risk and protective situations are identified in order to build a safety net and to manage the mental health issues.

Diagnostic Tests

Diagnosis of abuse is made on the basis of a careful history and thorough physical examination. Radiographic, CT, and MRI studies may be ordered to identify signs of recurrent abuse such as healed fractures and other damaged tissues. Laboratory studies may involve urine culture for signs of infection or screening for sexually transmitted infections. Genitourinary examination may be performed if sexual abuse is suspected. Some children are admitted directly to the hospital with the diagnosis of suspected abuse or neglect. Less obvious as a victim of abuse is the child admitted with a skull fracture who parents say fell off a chair. A mismatch of the degree of injury and the reported incident, or mismatch of the child's developmental level with the injury, indicate a need to report the incident to authorities for further investigation.

Neglect, which is more difficult to define and identify, frequently requires hospitalization with a comprehensive medical, social, and psychiatric evaluation. Five basic categories must be considered when attempting to diagnose neglect: (1) medical care neglect (lack of necessary medical care), (2) gross safety neglect (lack of appropriate supervision), (3) physical neglect (lack of food and shelter), (4) emotional neglect, and (5) educational neglect.

Interviews by mental health specialists may be performed in cases where the child is old enough to communicate verbally or through play techniques. All 50 U.S. states have extensive statutes regarding the reporting of child abuse and neglect. A specialist must be consulted, especially if the child's testimony will be used in court.

Children do not routinely make false allegations of abuse. If indeed there is reason to believe the allegations are false, a child and adolescent therapist (psychiatrist, psychologist, psychiatric clinical nurse specialist, or social worker) with special expertise should be consulted to determine the truth. Keep in mind that children who withdraw their accusations have often been threatened or coerced into doing so.

Clinical Therapy

Initial therapy focuses on providing safety. Physical injuries are treated and the child is removed from the abusive situation. Children who have been physically, emotionally, or sexually abused are at risk for mental health problems, such as major depression and posttraumatic stress disorder (see Chapter 27 ∞). They require skilled care by mental health professionals who are specially trained in this area. Initially the treatment goals include prevention of self-destructive or other dangerous acts. Children must be encouraged to express their fears and feelings in a safe and supportive environment. Equally important is the child's need to build coping skills and self-esteem. The child must be reassured and convinced that he or she is in no way responsible or to blame for what happened.

Individual treatment with art therapy is often used initially because it is the least threatening method in the early stages of treatment, it can easily be tailored to meet the child's individual needs, and it prepares the child for other forms of treatment such as family and group therapy (Figure 6–8 ➤). Family or group therapy may

LAW & ETHICS

Child Abuse Laws

Every state has a child abuse law specifying the particular behaviors that define every type of abuse. Any professional who works with children and reasonably suspects that a child has been abused is required to report this suspicion to the local agency for child protective services. Reports made in good faith are not liable to countersuits; however, professionals who suspect abuse and do not report it may be held responsible by the courts.

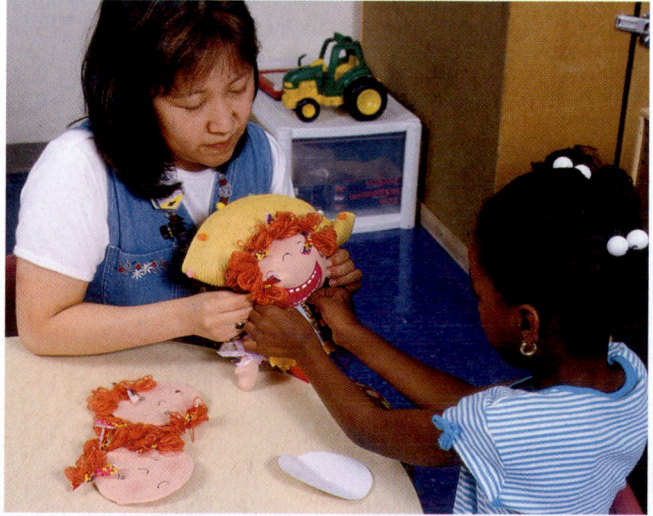

Figure 6–8 ➤ Therapeutic strategies with young children involve various methods of communication, such as dramatic play and art.

be of benefit in exploring the child's concerns and feelings. Anger is common, especially in children who were abused by a trusted adult such as the father or stepfather.

Some children are themselves sexual offenders. An adolescent sexual offender is a minor who commits any sexual act with a person of any age that is against the victim's will, without consent, and/or in an aggressive, exploitive, or threatening manner (Horner, 2003). Some common characteristics of these youth are prior violence, psychological/psychiatric problems, history as a victim of abuse, dysfunctional family, and personal characteristics such as loneliness and low self-esteem.

NURSING MANAGEMENT
Nursing Assessment and Diagnosis

Nursing assessment in instances of suspected child abuse or neglect requires a comprehensive history and physical examination, with documentation of findings. Consultation with social service agencies in the community is important if the family is receiving services.

Obtaining the history can be stressful for both the nurse and the parent. Use of therapeutic communication techniques and a quiet, unhurried environment are helpful. Maintaining a nonjudgmental attitude at all times is essential. Obtaining information about abusive and neglectful behaviors requires the nurse to establish a trusting relationship with parents, who are often afraid to trust any professional.

The health history sequence should include (1) parental concerns, (2) general family history, and (3) specific child history. This sequence begins with nonthreatening topics and allows the nurse to demonstrate concern before asking abuse-related questions. Obtain details about how injuries occurred. The parents' and child's own words should be documented verbatim using quotation marks. Compare reports obtained from each family member for lack of consistency and details that change over time.

It is important to differentiate true child abuse from cultural variations that might inaccurately be assumed to indicate abuse (Figures 6–9A and B ➤). For example, traditional treatment practices are sometimes mistaken for signs of physical abuse. The Chinese practice of cupping, which involves heating a bamboo cup and placing it on the skin, is a traditional treatment for headaches or abdominal pain. The Vietnamese practice of caogio (rubbing out the wind), in which a coin or the fingers are forcefully rubbed on the chest, back, or neck, is used to treat minor ailments. Ask about marks on the skin, how they occurred, and what health practices the family uses.

> ### CLINICAL TIP
> The nurse should communicate in an open manner when dealing with potential child abuse situations. A clear statement of purpose is needed during history taking, for example, "Hello, Mr. S. My name is Joan T. I'm Jonathan's nurse. I will be talking with you and asking you some questions about his overall health."

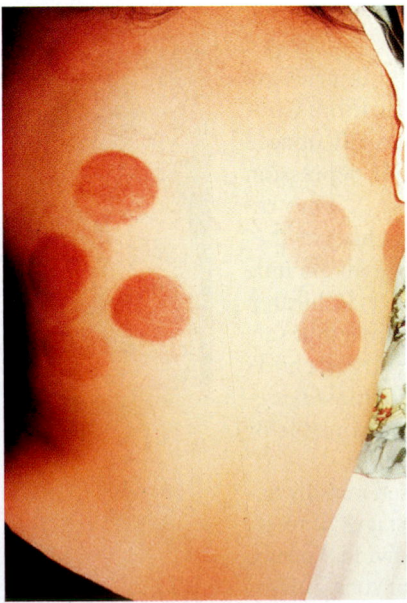

Figure 6–9 ➤ It is important to differentiate cultural practices such as A, cupping and B, coining from signs of child abuse.
Used with permission of the American Academy of Pediatrics, Visual Diagnosis of Child Physical Abuse Slide Kit. Photographs copyright © AAP/Kempe.

A   B

It is desirable to interview the parent and child both separately and together. Parent–child interaction during an intensive history-taking session provides an opportunity to observe the child's behavior and the parent's method of handling and responding to the child.

Data gathered during history-taking are particularly important in light of physical findings. Are there discrepancies between the history and physical assessment data? Do the parents give a history of an uncontrollable, inattentive toddler when the nurse observes a child who is attentive throughout a 15-minute examination? Assess the child's general appearance, including dress and behavior during the assessment. How do the child's affect, behavior, and development compare with those of other children the same age? Be alert for the signs of shaken child syndrome; this most often appears as a subtle neurological condition. Measure head circumference and perform a neurological examination (see Chapter 5).

Be alert for signs of domestic violence; for example, a mother who brings in a child for care displays signs of abuse. Say to the mother, "I see you have a black eye. Can you tell me what happened?" or "You say you are afraid that your boyfriend may hurt Shandra. Has he been hurting you? Do you want to talk about that?" Additionally, use open-ended approaches so that teens who have experienced dating violence know that they can discuss this.

Documentation of findings is important in all situations, but is essential in cases of suspected child abuse and neglect. Record physical findings as observed. Draw diagrams to document skin injuries. Document the location, nature, and extent of injuries with photographs.

Following are nursing diagnoses that may be appropriate for the physically abused or neglected child:

- Defensive Coping related to psychological impairment
- Acute Pain related to inflicted injuries
- Impaired Skin Integrity related to inflicted injuries
- Delayed Growth and Development related to lack of supportive parenting and environment
- Imbalanced Nutrition: Less than Body Requirements related to inadequate caloric intake
- Ineffective Health Maintenance related to lack of parental provision of child's essential needs
- Fear related to actual physical harm or repeated risk of injury
- Risk for Injury related to physical abuse
- Risk for Violence (Parent) related to inability to manage anger

Additional diagnoses that may apply to the emotionally abused or neglected child include the following:

- Defensive Coping related to psychological impairment
- Chronic Low Self-Esteem related to lack of appropriate emotional support from parents
- Disabled Family Coping: Disabling related to dysfunctional family dynamics and pattern of physical abuse

Diagnoses that may apply to the sexually abused child include the following:

- Anxiety related to potential separation from parent
- Rape-Trauma Syndrome related to sexual exploitation
- Ineffective Role Performance related to domestic violence
- Personal Identity Disturbance related to disturbance of usual activities of childhood

Planning and Implementation

Nursing care focuses on helping to remove the child from an abusive environment, preventing further injury, providing supportive care, and reinforcing the importance of follow-up care and counseling.

CLINICAL TIP

When interviewing adolescents, ask questions about dating violence in nonthreatening ways. A suggested approach might be, "Many teens have had sexual experiences that they did not want, where someone forced them to do something sexually. So I ask everyone this: Have you ever had a sexual experience when you didn't want to?" (Saewye, Pettingell, & Magee, 2003, p. 270). Ask about relationships with younger children to identify adolescent sexual offenders (Horner, 2003).

NURSING ALERT

Each person who handles a laboratory specimen or other item (e.g., clothing soiled with semen) in cases of suspected child abuse must be identified in the patient's record, and the specimen must never be left unattended. This documented chain of possession is necessary to ensure the admissibility of the evidence in court.

Prevent Further Injury

Work with social services and community agencies to assess the child's home environment, individuals living in the home, and the actions surrounding the abuse. Assist in removing the child from the home to temporary custody of the court or foster care of another relative, if indicated. Counsel family members about abuse and refer for appropriate therapy. Be sure that all people of childbearing age know the law in your state regarding safe places to leave unwanted babies. Teach all dating youth how to deal with violence during dating. Have domestic violence resources in your community readily available in all settings where care is provided for children.

Provide Supportive Care

Protect and treat the child's injuries (e.g., fractures, burns). Include parents in the child's treatment plan and keep them informed about the child's progress. Even if suspected of inflicting injuries to the child, the parent is still the child's primary caretaker. Talk with the parent as you would with any parent. Be supportive of any guilt expressed. Encourage the parent to assist with the child's care. Observe parent–child interactions and document supportive behaviors and the child's response to the parent versus other care providers.

Interacting nonjudgmentally with a parent suspected of abusing his or her child can be difficult. Talk with a colleague about anger you feel toward the parents or about the child's injuries or specific actions surrounding the abuse. Use team meetings to develop strategies that enable you to work with the parents and child.

Home Care Teaching

If there is any question about the child returning to a potentially dangerous situation, support the child's removal from the situation. The child may receive supervised care in the home by court order. Childcare, home nursing, and social worker visits may need to be arranged. Parents should be referred to parent effectiveness classes, family therapy, and support groups as necessary. If a neighbor or friend is the abuser, then the family may need support and legal advice when a term of incarceration is finished and the perpetrator returns to the community. Some states and communities have sexual offender laws that publicize the presence of an offender on parole within neighborhoods.

Encourage the family to inform other care providers when the child's abuse history may affect a response to care. They should be alert to signs of posttraumatic stress disorder (PTSD) in order to seek assistance if the child has continuing problems (see Chapter 27 ∞).

Evaluation

Expected outcomes of nursing care for the child who has been abused or neglected include maintenance of normal growth and development, establishment of a positive sense of self-esteem, provision of parenting information and stress relief for parents, provision of a nurturing environment for the child, and absence of episodes of abuse.

Munchausen Syndrome by Proxy

Munchausen syndrome by proxy, or medical care abuse, is a potentially deadly form of child abuse that involves the fabrication of signs and symptoms of a health condition in a child. Ninety percent of the time, it is the mother who creates these fictitious signs in her child (the proxy). The victim is usually under 6 years, and commonly under 1 year, of age (Hettler, 2002; Thomas, 2003). Frequently the child's symptoms of illness are used to gain entry into the medical system to meet the abuser's own needs.

The issues of abuse are multidimensional. The child is a victim of the feigned illness, repeated hospitalizations, and invasive procedures. Equally disruptive is the deprivation of the child's daily routine caused by the periodic medical crises.

Munchausen syndrome by proxy should be suspected when unexplained, recurrent, or extremely rare conditions occur; illness is unresponsive to treatment and symptoms change; and the history and clinical findings are inconsistent. The most commonly

---

CLINICAL TIP

When children have been abused, they are often frightened in new situations. Sexually abused children may resist removing clothes for a physical examination or medical test. They may want to wear undergarments to the surgical suite. Members of the gender that abused them may be distrusted. When aware of a history of abuse, ask the parents or guardians how to best facilitate the child's health care. Be sensitive to fears and allow the child to wear clothing, have a support person present, or do whatever may provide a sense of security.

reported signs and symptoms are central nervous system dysfunction, apnea, diarrhea, vomiting, fever, seizures, signs of bleeding (in urine or stool), and rashes. The parent may overdose the child on medications, such as nonprescription drugs and even syrup of ipecac, causing a variety of side effects. Although syrup of ipecac is no longer recommended for home use or sold in pharmacies, it may still be available in some households. The symptoms occur in the presence of the same caretaker and disappear when the child is separated from that caretaker.

The child often appears uncooperative, extremely anxious, fearful, and negative. The caretaker, who in contrast appears very cooperative, competent, and loving, often expresses a desire for the child to recover. The caretaker may even suggest diagnostic procedures to try to determine "what's wrong." Characteristically the caretaker thrives in the healthcare environment.

The cause of Munchausen syndrome by proxy is often complex and rooted in the caretaker's psychiatric illness and own abusive or neglectful childhood. The disorder occurs in all socioeconomic classes. Often the perpetrator has some type of healthcare background, such as nursing or another allied health profession. The abuser is often young, married, and of the middle socioeconomic class. A history of insecure attachment is often present (Adshead & Bluglass, 2005).

A suspicion of Munchausen syndrome by proxy requires a coordinated evaluation by an interdisciplinary team. Team members must organize and communicate a strategic plan regarding collection of evidence, confrontation of the abuser, and management of the hospitalized child. The child's safety is the ultimate concern. When suspected by medical personnel, child protection agencies and law enforcement are informed, and a plan is made for management of the case. The spouse and family members are informed regarding the involvement of law enforcement so that complicity or cooperation can be identified (Thomas, 2003).

Nursing Management

Special care should be taken to maintain a trusting relationship with the caretaker so that he or she does not become suspicious and leave the hospital. Often the best person on the team to function in the role of "trusted other" is a member of the psychiatric consultation team.

Careful documentation of parent–child interactions, presence or absence of symptoms, and other pertinent observations is essential. The child must be closely monitored. If blood is present in the child's urine, stool, or vomitus, careful documentation is needed about whether the nurse was present or whether the sample was provided by the parent. Covert video surveillance may be ordered by the hospital when the syndrome is highly suspected in a particular situation. Expert consultants will be needed to ensure legal requirements for investigation are met. When enough evidence is collected to prove Munchausen syndrome by proxy, the caretaker is confronted by the physician or another member of the psychiatric team in planning with law enforcement officials.

Once diagnosis is made, the child must be placed in a safe setting. Siblings must be examined and their safety considered by social service and law enforcement groups. Only after legal and psychiatric experts determine that the home setting is safe can children be returned to the parent guilty of medical abuse (Hettler, 2002).

ENVIRONMENTAL INFLUENCES ON CHILD HEALTH
Disasters

Disasters are monumental occurrences experienced by people in all countries and cultures. Key elements of disasters are that they involve serious and massive events that impact many people and are beyond the community's ability for management. They may cause death, injury, physical damage, psychological trauma, and economic disruption. Typically, the societal and healthcare infrastructures that deal with community events are totally unable to manage the challenges of the disaster. Most disasters are sudden, such as hurricanes, floods, volcanic eruptions, earthquakes, tsunamis, or mudslides, but some may be slow and insidious, such as drought. Disasters may be natural, such as tornadoes, ice storms, lightning fires, or outbreaks of serious diseases. They may be man-made, such as war and terrorist acts (these were discussed earlier in the chapter). They may be technological or toxicological, such as those caused by nuclear leakage, chemical spills, or contamination (Centers for Disease Control and Prevention [CDC], 2005).

Some major disasters have already been discussed in this chapter, such as school shootings and terrorist acts. The effect of military deployment has also been discussed. This section will summarize important effects of disasters and list psychological support that families and communities can provide in disasters. See Chapters 11 ∞ and 18 ∞ for more specific information about community preparedness and unique physical effects of disasters on children and adolescents.

There are both immediate and delayed responses to the traumatic events of disasters. Disasters are very traumatic for children involved. Further, when they are uprooted from their homes and communities due to such events, they may be in relief centers or temporary housing with increased rates of surrounding violence. See Chapter 18 ∞ for further information about the risks to children in natural disasters, and see Chapter 27 ∞ for mental health effects of such events on children. Initial symptoms include feelings of terror, fear, and dread. Physical symptoms such as nausea, dizziness, tingling, heart palpitations, and sweating may occur. As the impact of the event becomes known, grief and depressive symptoms may emerge. During this phase, sleep and eating disturbances can occur, and people may have difficulty being engaged in other normal life activities. Many people report feeling improved and more like themselves several months after a traumatic event, though they experience episodes when coping is difficult. Other individuals go on to experience posttraumatic stress disorder (PTSD), which involves symptoms that interfere with daily living months or years after the event. See the full discussion on PTSD in Chapter 27 ∞. Characteristic PTSD responses after disasters involve flashbacks and intense emotional responses about the event, avoiding certain places and thoughts because of the intense pain involved with them, and being easily startled or aroused with difficulty controlling anger and other emotions (Centers for Disease Control and Prevention, 2003).

Children have unique responses to disasters, depending on prior life experiences, support of significant others, and their developmental stages. Some general reactions at different ages may include:

Infancy to 6 years—Increased crying and inconsolability; fear of separation from parents and other caregivers; clinging behaviors; regression in developmental tasks

7 to 10 years—Feelings of sadness and/or anger; decreased attention span and concentration that can lead to decreased school performance; focus on details of the disastrous event; disruptive behaviors; somatic complaints; feelings of guilt

11 years and older—Decreased contact with peers and usual activities; increased risk-taking behaviors; increased argumentativeness; refusal to talk about the traumatic events (CDC, 2005)

Nursing Management

Nurses have become important first responders in disasters. They also provide continuing care for individuals and families as a community emerges from the initial trauma. A primary role of nurses is to prevent disasters when possible and to assist communities with emergency preparedness for disasters. Disaster and emergency health care are important components of educational programs and continuing education offerings. Nurses work with schools and community agencies to identify potential hazards and prevent them from causing harm. Examples include establishing standards for storage of hazardous substances in homes, childcare agencies, and communities; working with schools to establish policies related to bullying behaviors and weapons policies; and formulating preparedness plans and crisis responses in homes, schools, and other settings.

When a disaster occurs, nurses are often on the frontline, providing emergency health care for rescued victims, first aid for the walking wounded, and general public health interventions (e.g., vaccines, sanitation, food and water). While physical care is essential (see Chapter 11 ∞), psychological trauma is also addressed. Nurses are well equipped with knowledge of child and adolescent development and can therefore meet the needs of youth in disasters. Nurses can provide a safe place for children, away from media and unfolding traumatic events, such as the rescue of dead and injured. Do not allow children to leave a scene unaccompanied by a parent or other responsible adult. Assess for panic reactions, unexpected behaviors, and changing conditions.

Once the initial disaster is managed and children return to home or other settings, some interventions appropriate with various age groups include:

Infancy to 6 years—Children need support and care by primary caretakers whenever possible. Encourage parents to hold, cuddle, and provide much physical and caring support. Reassurance of their presence, that they will deal with any losses together, and acceptance of the child's clinging behaviors are most supportive to the young child. Avoid repeated exposure of the child to the event by curtailing television and other media coverage.

7 to 10 years—Explain the disaster and answer the child's questions, encouraging parents to do the same. Details such as how dead bodies are managed, how it feels to die in a mine, or what happens when someone bleeds to death are examples of topics that young children may question; prepare parents and schools for this and help them plan for accepting and answering such inquiries. Use techniques such as story telling, drawing, and dramatic play to enable the child to express emotions and understanding of the event (see Chapters 13 ∞ and 27 ∞ for more details on these techniques). Tell the child that feelings of being upset, sad, or angry are normal; allow them to cry and express feelings and be patient for a return to normal sleep and eating patterns. Arrange for increased contact with parents or other significant adults, while gradually returning to peers and normal life activities.

11 years and older—Older children may want to discuss the event with peers although many want increased contact with family members for awhile. Help schools and other community agencies arrange for mental health specialists to assist children in exploring their feelings in safe settings. Provide grief counseling for youth who have lost peers or family members.

Nurses have many roles to play in the immediate and short-term aftermath of a disaster. Additionally, as the days turn into weeks and months, nurses must remain vigilant for children and families who have PTSD and have not returned to normal life patterns. Refer individuals and families for mental health services when anxiety levels remain high; when there is inability to carry out normal life tasks such as eating, working, or attending school; if there are reported incidents of reliving the event; if the child has lasting behavioral changes such as poor school performance, outbursts, and isolation; or when you or the family is concerned about the child (Hanze, 2002). Act as a liaison between all parties, encouraging families to communicate with school personnel and to bring concerns about the child's status to healthcare visits (National Center for Children Exposed to Violence, 2003).

Environmental Contaminants

Earlier in this chapter, the social effects on environments were discussed. Factors like safe neighborhoods for play and access to resources for health care and other services were discussed. In this section, you will examine another important type of environmental exposure—that of contaminants in air, water, and soil. Contaminants are **toxins**, or chemicals produced by metabolism or an organism (e.g., ricin), or **toxicants**, natural or synthetic chemicals not metabolically produced by an organism (Belson, Schier, & Patel, 2005). These products are commonly produced during industrial manufacture, but could be released as a form of terrorism. Children are generally more vulnerable than adults to such exposures because of their developing

GROWTH & DEVELOPMENT

Environmental Risks Unique to Children

Children, especially at young ages, are particularly vulnerable to risks of environmental hazards. Some reasons for these elevated risks include:

- Increased exposure due to being close to the ground so that skin contact and inhalation are magnified
- Increased ingestion due to hand-to-mouth behaviors common in young children
- Increased absorption of products through thin layers of skin
- Decreased metabolism for many products due to developing enzymatic and elimination systems, prolonging exposure in the body
- High metabolic demands that lead to high respiratory and cardiovascular rates, causing increased dangers of poisoning from carbon monoxide and other substances (Etzel, 2004)

bodies. However, it is difficult to measure and draw conclusions about the effects of certain exposures because controlled studies can obviously not be done due to ethical reasons. Therefore, most knowledge about environmental exposure comes from epidemiological studies with large groups of individuals who have experienced an exposure, such as radiation exposure at Chernobyl. Is a type of cancer more prevalent in a certain area? Could that incidence be related to exposure to an environmental contaminant? If the cancer does not arise for many years how can causation be traced? For these reasons, our knowledge of environmental contaminants and their effects on children are limited. A U.S. federal initiative has formed the National Children's Study and Centers, co-sponsored by the National Institute for Environmental Health Sciences and the Environmental Protection Agency, to study health and safety risks to children (Kimmel, Collman, Fields, & Eskenazi, 2005). It is important to examine what is known and to urge families to use some general cautions to minimize potential risks to children.

Contaminants in the environment can influence children in complex ways. Prenatal exposure can affect the developing fetus. Exposure during lactation may bring contaminants to the breast-fed baby. Environmental effects may occur as the child grows through skin contact, inhalation, or food and water ingestion. Since children are exposed to many chemicals on a daily basis, harmful exposures are often difficult to identify. One example of a known harmful agent is environmental tobacco smoke (ETS). The mother who smokes or is exposed to ETS runs an increased risk of having a baby that is small for gestational age or who dies of Sudden Infant Death Syndrome (SIDS, Chapter 20 ∞). The child exposed to ETS has an increased risk of occurrence and severity of asthma and other respiratory diseases.

Some potentially harmful environmental exposures include:

- Pesticides such as organophosphates, organochlorine, chlorpyrifos, dialkylphosphates, carbamates, pyrethroids; children may be exposed through home use, parents who work in pesticide manufacturing, garden/farm/agricultural use, and ingestion through food treated with pesticide
- Outdoor air pollution from automobiles, power plants, and other sources; children spend time outside and therefore have increased exposure
- Indoor air pollution from dust mites, molds, lead particles from old housing, wood smoke, and other sources
- Substances such as polychlorinated biphenyls (PCBs) stored in fatty tissues of the mother and causing fetal exposure, or in animal fats; also present in electrical wiring

Nursing Management

Nurses are instrumental in identifying exposure to environmental toxic agents. Inquire about:

- Parental work with harmful substances such as dust and chemicals
- Age of home (homes built before 1978 or renovated in the last 6 months are at risk for contamination with chemicals)
- Safety items in home such as radon, carbon monoxide, and smoke alarms
- Child and family member with hobby requiring use of toxic materials, such as lead with stained glass work, glue with model building
- Child's consumption of non-food products

When delayed development or behavioral problems are evident, consider the possibility of environmental exposure and refer for blood testing and further evaluation. Test blood levels for contaminants such as lead (see next section). Hair, urine, and other testing may be possible as well. Identification of the toxic exposure and its removal from the environment are critical. Removal from the body by drug treatment is possible for some substances. Instruct the family in prevention of further exposure. Perform periodic growth and developmental measurements on the child and ensure return for further blood tests and other monitoring (Dunn, Burns, & Sattler, 2003).

Poisoning

Young children are at risk for ingestion of foreign substances because of their characteristic behaviors, which involve exploration of the environment. Both ingestion of poisons or toxic substances and ingestion of foreign objects are discussed in this section.

Poisonings are the second leading cause of unintentional home-injury death and account for nearly one-third of all unintentional home injuries (Home Safety Council, 2004). Over 2 million poisonings occur annually in the United States, with over 90% of these in private residences (Watson, Litovitz, Klein-Schwartz et al. 2004). About 39% of poisonings occur in children under 3 years of age and 52% in children under 6 years.

Infants and toddlers commonly place objects in their mouths. Some household items are nontoxic and cause little harm; however, items that contain caustic agents or toxic chemicals can cause irreversible damage or death. The Poison Prevention Packaging Act of 1970 mandates child protective devices for all potentially toxic substances, such as household cleansers and medications. However, many are still ingested by children. Most common causes of pediatric poisonings include cosmetics and personal care products, cleaning agents, analgesics and other medications, foreign bodies, topical agents, and cough/cold preparations. Agents most commonly causing death are analgesics and psychotropic medications (Watson, et al. 2004).

Many other items commonly found in the home are less obvious sources of toxins. The leaves, stems, or flowers of many common household and garden plants are poisonous. Examples include Boston ivy, poinsettia, philodendron, lily-of-the-valley, daffodil (bulbs), azalea, and rhododendron. Nail care products, mothballs, weed and bug killers, and rodent killers are other potential poisons. Although most poisons are ingested, other routes of contamination include dermal, inhalation, and ocular.

Parents who suspect that their child has ingested a poison should immediately call the Poison Control Center (PCC). The PCC will advise parents about treatment to begin at home, and if the child needs treatment in the emergency department. If the child has vomited, the vomitus should be brought to the emergency department. With older children, the possibility of intentional ingestion needs to be considered.

Clinical Manifestations

The manifestations of poisoning depend on the toxin. Some common effects include neurological changes, alterations in vital signs, and gastrointestinal symptoms. Symptoms usually occur within the first 2 hours after exposure, while outcomes can be delayed with controlled release medications, or when a toxic metabolite results from breakdown of the poison (Bryant & Singer, 2003). See Clinical Manifestations of Commonly Ingested Toxic Agents on the following page.

COLLABORATIVE CARE

Collaborative care focuses on identifying the poison and its source; removing the offending agent; stabilizing the child's airway, breathing, and circulation; and reducing the risk of recurrence.

Diagnostic Tests

Blood and urine toxicology screens, as well as arterial blood gas and electrolyte testing, are performed. Testing of vomitus for the presence of medication or other poisonings may be helpful in determining the amount ingested.

Clinical Therapy

In the emergency department the child's vital signs and level of consciousness are assessed and specific information about the poison is obtained from the parent. Box 6–3 summarizes emergency management for poisoning.

The goal of treatment is to prevent further absorption of the poison and to reverse or eliminate its effects. Potential complications of poisoning, depending on the type of poison, include respiratory and/or cardiac arrest, congestive heart failure, liver failure, renal failure, seizures, esophageal or tracheal corrosion with ingestion of caustic substances, and shock.

> **NURSING ALERT**
>
> After numerous years of syrup of ipecac serving as a mainstay in home treatment of poisonings, the American Academy of Pediatrics recommends that "syrup of ipecac should no longer be used routinely as a poison treatment intervention in the home" (American Academy of Pediatrics, 2003.) The nurse informs families to avoid the use of ipecac and encourages disposal of ipecac kept in the home. Instruct the family to pour the ipecac down the drain or toilet and to discard the empty bottle.

Type	Sources	Clinical Manifestations	Clinical Therapy
Corrosives (strong acids and alkaline products that cause chemical burns of mucosal surfaces)	Batteries Household cleaners Clinitest tablets Denture cleaners Bleach Toilet bowl cleaners	Severe burning pain in mouth, throat, or stomach Swelling of mucous membranes; edema of lips, tongue, and pharynx (respiratory obstruction) Violent vomiting; hemoptysis Drooling; inability to clear secretions Signs of shock Anxiety Agitation	Do not induce vomiting! Dilute toxin with water to prevent further damage Give activated charcoal
Hydrocarbons (organic compounds that contain carbon and hydrogen; most are distillates of petroleum)	Gasoline Kerosene Furniture polish Lighter fluid Paint thinners	Gagging Choking Coughing Nausea Vomiting Alteration in sensorium (lethargy) Weakness Respiratory symptoms of pulmonary involvement, tachypnea, cyanosis, retractions, grunting	Do not induce vomiting! (Aspiration of hydrocarbons places child at high risk for pneumonia.) Use gastric lavage if severe central nervous system and respiratory impairment are present Use of activated charcoal is controversial Provide supportive care Decontaminate skin by removing clothing and cleansing skin
Acetaminophen	Many over-the-counter products	Nausea Vomiting Sweating Pallor Hepatic involvement (pain in upper right quadrant, jaundice, confusion, stupor, coagulation abnormalities)	Induce vomiting or perform gastric lavage, depending on amount ingested Administer charcoal or NAC (concentrated form of Mucomyst), which binds with the metabolite, preventing absorption and protecting the liver
Salicylate	Products containing aspirin	Nausea Disorientation Vomiting Dehydration Diaphoresis Hyperpnea Hyperpyrexia Bleeding tendencies Oliguria Tinnitus Convulsions Coma	Depends on amount ingested Induce vomiting Administer intravenous sodium bicarbonate, fluids, and vitamin K
Mercury	Broken thermometers Chemicals Paints Pesticides Fungicides	Tremors Memory loss Insomnia Weight loss Diarrhea Anorexia Gingivitis	Similar to that for lead poisoning (see text discussion)
Iron	Multiple vitamin supplements	Vomiting Hematemesis Diarrhea Bloody stools Abdominal pain Metabolic acidosis Shock Seizures Coma	Induce vomiting Administer intravenous fluids and sodium bicarbonate Desferoxamine chelation therapy

---

BOX 6–3
EMERGENCY MANAGEMENT FOR POISONING

1. Stabilize the child. Assess ABCs (airway, breathing, and circulation). Provide ventilatory support and supplemental oxygen.
2. Perform a rapid physical examination, start an IV infusion, draw blood for toxicology screen, and apply a cardiac monitor.
3. Obtain a history of the ingestion, including substance ingested, where child was found, by whom, position, when, how long unsupervised, history of depression or suicide, allergies, and any other medical problems.
4. Reverse or eliminate the toxic substance using the appropriate method:
   a. Antidotes and agonists
      Mucomyst (for acetaminophen poisoning)
      Digibind (for digoxin poisoning)
      Narcan (for opioid overdose)
      Romazicon (for benzodiazepine overdose)
   b. Gastric lavage
      - A gastric tube is inserted through the mouth.
      - Normal saline solution is instilled and aspirated until the return is clear. This is considered a less effective method of removing ingested substances from the stomach than vomiting. It is reserved for children with central nervous system depression, diminished or absent gag reflex, or unwillingness to cooperate with other measures.
      - This method is contraindicated in children who have ingested alkaline corrosive substances, as insertion of the tube may cause esophageal perforation.
      - Used in children who have ingested acids to decrease continued damage and potential perforation of the stomach and intestines.
   c. Activated charcoal
      - Given to absorb and remove any remaining particles of toxic substances.
        - Usual dosage administration is 1 g/kg of body weight
      - A commercial preparation of activated charcoal is administered orally or through a gastric tube.
        - Available as a ready-to-drink solution in an opaque container.
        - May be mixed with apple juice or soda if protocol allows to encourage consumption.
        - Use a covered cup and straw when giving orally to prevent the child from seeing the black liquid and to minimize spillage.
        - Administer activated charcoal only after the child has stopped vomiting, because aspiration of charcoal is damaging to lung tissue.
        - Should not be administered for ingestion of caustic substances or hydrocarbons.
   d. Cathartics
      - Hastens excretion of a toxic substance and minimizes absorption. The most commonly used cathartic is magnesium sulfate.

Note: Syrup of ipecac: The use of ipecac is no longer recommended because it may not remove all poison and can be harmful in some situations. Encourage parents to remove it from their homes.

5. Perform other measures depending on the child's condition, the nature of the ingested substance, and the time since ingestion. They may include diuresis, fluid loading, cooling or warming measures, anticonvulsive measures, antiarrhythmic therapy, hemodialysis, or exchange transfusions.
6. Constantly evaluate the child's total condition to maintain airway, breathing, and circulation. Therapeutic management is adjusted as needed to treat the evolving condition.
7. Consider the family's emotional status. Provide information about the child, involve them in care when possible, and arrange for support persons and services to be available to them.

NURSING MANAGEMENT

Nursing care focuses on initial emergent care and stabilization of the child with poisoning, followed by family education to reduce the risk of repeated poisoning.

Nursing Assessment and Diagnosis

Take a history from the family about the child's suspected ingestion substance, time, amount, and symptoms. Initial assessment focuses on airway, vital signs, and neurological status. Assess drooling, diaphoresis, and increased or depressed respirations. Assess for wheezing, respiratory distress, or stridor. Assess for decreased responsiveness and seizure activity. Assess heart rate, skin color, capillary refill, peripheral and central pulses, and blood pressure. Assess pupils (abnormally large or pinpoint pupils may be observed). Assess mouth, lips, and tongue for corrosive burns or edema. Assess breath for unusual odor. Assess the child for vomiting and diarrhea. Assess vomitus for presence of medication or other ingested substances. Determine the child's height and weight.

Nursing diagnoses for the child with ingestion of a toxic substance may include:

- Risk for Ineffective Airway Clearance related to effects of toxic substance
- Risk for Impaired Gas Exchange related to effects of toxic substance
- Risk for Aspiration related to depressed neurological status and vomiting
- Risk for Decreased Cardiac Output related to effects of toxic substance
- Risk for Injury related to repeated occurrence of poisoning
- Interrupted Family Processes related to poisoning of a family member

Planning and Implementation

Emergency care focuses on airway and hemodynamic stability, removal of toxic agents, and support of the family. See Box 6–3 for a summary of emergency management for poisoning.

Once immediate care has been provided, nursing care shifts to providing emotional support and preventing recurrence.

Provide Emotional Support

Wait until the child is out of immediate danger before questioning parents in detail about the incident. Encourage parents to express feelings of anger, guilt, or fear about the incident.

Prevent Recurrence

Discuss with parents the need to supervise infants and young children at all times. Ask parents how medicines and cleaning agents are stored and whether the house contains any plants. Teach parents proper methods of childproofing the home. Have the PCC number readily available. Suggest measures for preventing recurrence of poisoning. (See Families Want to Know: Avoiding Childhood Poisoning.)

The toll-free number for the American Association of Poison Control Centers (AAPCC) is **1-800-222-1222**. The number can be accessed from anywhere in the United States and Puerto Rico, and the caller will be connected to the nearest poison control center.

Evaluation

Expected outcomes for nursing care of the child with poisoning include:

- The child maintains ventilatory function.
- The child maintains effective gas exchange and respiratory pattern.
- The child is free from wheezing, coughing, pneumonia, or other signs indicating aspiration.
- The child's heart rate and blood pressure remain stable and appropriate for age.
- Neurological status is appropriate for age.
- The family and child (if older) verbalize understanding of preventive measures and demonstrate measures to improve home environment safety.

FAMILIES WANT TO KNOW

Avoiding Childhood Poisoning

Families with children require instructions for avoiding childhood poisoning. Teach family members these interventions to help avoid childhood poisonings:

- Place household cleaners, medications, vitamins, and other potentially poisonous substances out of the reach of children or in locked cabinets.
- Use warning stickers such as Mr. Yuk on all containers.
- Buy products with child-resistant caps.
- Store products in their original containers.
- Never place household cleansers or other products in food or beverage containers.
- Remove all houseplants from the child's play areas.
- Put the Poison Control Center phone number by every phone in the house.
- Use caution when visiting other settings that are not childproofed (e.g., grandparents' homes). Remember that visitors may have pills in their purses or pockets that are easily reached by children.

Ingestion of Foreign Objects

There are about 100,000 cases of ingestion of foreign objects annually, and approximately 80% of cases of ingestion of foreign objects occur in childhood. The majority of cases present in children between 6 and 36 months of age (Kay & Wyllie, 2005). The most common objects ingested are coins, accounting for 27–70% of cases. Pins, parts of toys, batteries, and bones from foods are some other commonly ingested objects. Adults often witness infants and young children ingesting foreign bodies, and older children will usually report swallowing a foreign object. Most small, round, smooth objects may not cause any clinical distress. However, if the foreign body is lodged in the esophagus, children may present with substernal pain, drooling, and dysphagia. Some children may exhibit respiratory symptoms including wheezing or coughing.

Serious complications can occur following foreign body ingestion. These complications include perforation of the intestinal tract, the most serious sequelae of foreign body ingestion. Sharp objects are associated with a higher perforation rate than dull objects. Approximately 75% of perforations occur in the region of the ileocecal valve. Development of strictures at the site of a retained foreign body may also. Respiratory complications arise if the object becomes lodged in the trachea, bronchi, or lungs. See Chapter 20 ∞ for a discussion of emergency care in these situations.

Since approximately 60–90% of foreign bodies ingested in children are radio-opaque (Kay & Wyllie, 2005), radiographs of the neck, chest, esophagus, and abdomen are useful tools in verifying ingestion and to identify the location of the object. Endoscopic examination and retrieval of the ingested foreign body may be necessary. Approximately 5–10% of children will have the foreign body lodged in the oropharynx, 20% of foreign bodies will be located in the esophagus, 60% will be located in the stomach, and 10% will be located distal to the stomach, usually in the small intestine (Kay & Wyllie, 2005).

Most (80–90%) foreign bodies pass spontaneously through the gastrointestinal system and are eliminated through stool. However, foreign bodies may become lodged in the esophagus and pose a significant risk to the child. Smooth, small, round objects that have passed into the stomach are generally allowed to pass through the bowel without intervention. Esophageal foreign bodies are removed or advanced into the stomach due to the risk for mucosal erosion and catastrophic perforation (Uyemura, 2006). Potentially harmful objects such as batteries, sharp objects, and magnets are removed surgically.

Nursing Management

Nursing care centers on supporting the child, collaborative assistance in the identification and removal of the foreign body, and teaching the child and family measures to reduce reoccurrence. Assess the child for drooling, wheezing, substernal pain, dysphagia, and coughing. Obtain a thorough history from family. Determine, if possible, what was ingested, when the ingestion occurred, and any symptoms that the child experienced. Assess breath sounds.

Prepare the child for radiologic studies. Explain the procedures and reassure the child and family during the studies. Prepare for endoscopic examination and/or retrieval, if necessary. If the foreign object is in the stomach and the child is to be observed for natural excretion of the object, explain monitoring of stools to parents. Suggest the use of tongue blades to examine stools for presence of the foreign body and to report if the object has not been passed within the expected time frame (generally 48 hours). Encourage the family to return for further radiologic examinations to determine the foreign object's progress of passage.

Partner with the family and assist them in establishing a safe home environment for the child. Encourage the family to keep all small items out of the child's reach and to ensure the child is monitored at all times. Expected outcomes for nursing care of the child with ingested foreign body include removal of the foreign body, reduction in risk, and family verbalization of preventative measures to reduce risk of ingestion of foreign bodies.

Lead Poisoning

Lead poisoning has been successfully prevented in many areas of the United States, with a substantial decline in lead levels from the mid-1970s. The average serum lead level for children is now 0.6 µg/dL, down from 15 µg/dL in 1976. About 2.2% of children (434,000) from 1 to 5 years have levels above the recommended upper level of 10 µg/dL. Many of these children are poor and live in older houses in inner cities (MMWR, 2003a). Even children with levels below 10 µg/dL may experience cognitive defects due to lead exposure since there is no known safe level (Bellinger, 2004). Lead in paint is the most common source of lead exposure for preschool children. Children are also exposed to lead when they ingest contaminated food, water, and soil or when they inhale dust contaminated with lead.

Children are at greater risk for lead poisoning because they absorb and retain more lead in proportion to their weight than adults do. Lead is particularly harmful to children under the age of 7 years.

Lead interferes with normal cell function, primarily of the nervous system, blood cells, and kidneys, and adversely affects the metabolism of vitamin D and calcium. Clinical manifestations depend on the degree of toxicity. Neurologic effects include decreased IQ scores, cognitive deficits, impaired hearing, and growth delays. Impaired mental function can occur with blood levels even lower than 10 µg/dL. Lead ingestion by a woman during pregnancy can result in fetal malformations, reduced birth weight, and premature birth. Severe lead poisoning, which can result in encephalopathy, coma, and death, is now rare.

Once in the body, lead accumulates in the blood, soft tissues (kidney, bone marrow, liver, and brain), bones, and teeth. Lead that is absorbed by the bones and teeth is released slowly; thus, exposure to even small doses, over time, can result in dangerously high levels of lead in the body. See Clinical Manifestations of Lead Poisoning below.

The Centers for Disease Control and Prevention now recommend screening children at high risk, with reduced screening for those at low risk (MMWR, 2003a). In addition, all children enrolled in Medicaid should be tested, with follow-up management and care. A blood lead (Pb-B) level is the most useful screening and diagnostic test for lead exposure.

A Pb-B below 10 µg/dL is considered acceptable, although it may still not screen out all children with impaired development due to lead. An environmental history should be obtained for children with Pb-B levels between 10 and 19 µg/dL to identify removable sources of lead. Follow-up testing is required. Children with Pb-B levels between 20 and 69 µg/dL require a full medical evaluation, including a detailed envi-

CLINICAL MANIFESTATIONS	LEAD POISONING
Class I (<9 µg/dL)	Generally asymptomatic although subtle neurological effects may be present with any exposure
Class IIA (10–14 µg/dL) and IIB (15–19µg/dL)	Mild impairment in growth, fine motor skills, and cognition Anemia
Class III (20–44 µg/dL)	General fatigue and motor impairment Difficulty concentrating Paresis or paralysis, tremor Headache Diffuse abdominal pain, vomiting, weight loss, constipation Anemia
Class IV (45–69 µg/dL)	Colic (intermittent, severe abdominal cramps), anorexia, vomiting Hyperirritability Increased lethargy Lead line (blue-black) on gingival tissue
Class V (>70 µg/dL)	Encephalopathy, which may lead abruptly to seizures, changes in consciousness, coma, and death Ataxia

Adapted from Agency for Toxic Substances & Disease Registry (2006). Lead toxicity clinical evaluation. Atlanta: Author.

ronmental and behavioral history, physical examination, and tests for iron deficiency. Interventions to remove sources of lead from the child's environment are necessary. For levels above 25 µg/dL, chelation therapy is also administered. Children with Pb-B levels greater than 70 µg/dL are critically ill from lead poisoning and require immediate chelation therapy and interventions to provide a lead-free environment.

Chelation therapy involves the administration of an agent that binds with lead, increasing its rate of excretion from the body. Calcium disodium ethylenediamine tetraacetate (CaNa$_2$ EDTA), dimercaprol (BAL), d-penicillamine, or succimer (DMSA) may be used. Children with Pb-B levels between 25 and 69 µg/dL receive CaNa$_2$ EDTA for 5 to 7 days, followed by a rest period and then a second chelation treatment. Children with Pb-B levels greater than 70 µg/dL are given both BAL and CaNa$_2$ EDTA, followed by a rest period and a second chelation treatment using CaNa$_2$ EDTA alone. Long-term follow-up of children receiving chelation therapy is essential. The child should never be discharged unless a lead-free home environment has been ensured.

Nursing Management

Nursing care centers on screening, education, and follow-up. Nurses often work with state and local health officials to plan screening for children at high risk of lead exposure. Ask parents about the child's development and eating habits and be alert for risk of lead exposure. Educate parents about sources of lead in the environment and techniques to reduce exposure. Emphasize the importance of housekeeping interventions to reduce exposure to lead dust. These interventions include damp mopping of hard surfaces, floors, window sills, and baseboards; washing the child's hands and face before meals; and frequent washing of toys and pacifiers.

Teach parents the importance of including foods high in iron and calcium in the child's diet to counteract losses of these minerals associated with lead exposure. The child should eat meals at regular intervals, as lead is absorbed more readily on an empty stomach.

Be sure that parents understand the importance of follow-up testing of lead levels. If the child is developmentally delayed, refer the family to an infant stimulation or early intervention program. Referral to social services and either a visiting nurse or home healthcare nurse may also be appropriate.

Expected outcomes of nursing care for the child with lead or other poisoning include the following:

- The child exhibits normal growth and development, including cognition.
- Adequate nutritional intake is ensured for the child.
- Lead or other poisons are removed from the child's environment.
- The family expresses understanding of measures to establish a safe environment for the child.

CRITICAL THINKING IN ACTION

Refer back to 15-year-old Amy, who is described in the chapter opener. She has visited the school nurse due to a painful ear pierced by a friend. The nurse examines all of Amy's piercings on her ears, face, and navel. Amy is talkative and willing to answer the nurse's questions about her body art and her life. She elaborates about the reasons she ran away from home last year and seems to be analyzing her own motives and goals. She now lives at home with her family again.

1. What is Amy's developmental stage according to Erikson? How can the adults in her life encourage her healthy psychosocial development?

2. Amy has clearly demonstrated many risk and protective factors for physical and psychosocial health. What factors place her at risk of disease or developing unhealthy lifestyles? What factors are protective of her health?

3. List at least three nursing diagnoses based on Amy's risk and protective factors. What interventions will increase her protective factors?

4. Exposure to home piercings and to body art presents several health risks. What are they? What immunization should Amy have to prevent her from acquiring a disease transmitted by blood?

 Refer to your Prentice Hall Nursing MediaLink DVD-ROM for answers.

EXPLORE MediaLink

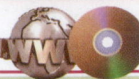

http://www.prenhall.com/ball

Resources for this chapter can be found on the Prentice Hall Nursing MediaLink DVD-ROM accompanying this textbook, and on the Companion Website at http://www.prenhall.com/ball.

DVD-ROM

Audio Glossary
NCLEX-RN® Review
Videos
    The Effects of Media on Children
    Extreme Sports
    Identifying Child Abuse
    Identifying Youth Who Abuse Drugs and Alcohol
    Smoking and Smoking Cessation

COMPANION WEBSITE

Audio Glossary
NCLEX-RN® Review
Care Plan Activity: A Child in the ED
Case Study: Children and Violence
Critical Thinking: Music and Violence
MediaLink Application
    Community Sports
WebLinks

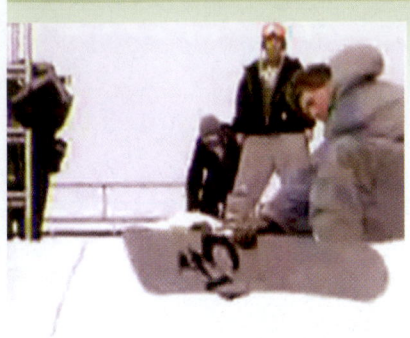

REFERENCES

Adshead, G., & Bluglass, K. (2005). Attachment representations in mothers with abnormal illness behaviour by proxy. *British Journal of Psychiatry, 187,* 328–333.

Alcohol Free Children. (2005). *How does alcohol affect the world of a child?* Washington, DC: National Institutes of Health. NIH Publication #99–4670.

American Academy of Child and Adolescent Psychiatry. (2005a). *Children of alcoholics.* Accessary February 17, 2006, from http://www.aacap.org/publications/factsfam/alcoldc.htm

American Academy of Child and Adolescent Psychiatry. (2005b). Practice parameter for the assessment and treatment of children and adolescents with substance use disorders. *Journal of the American Academy of Child and Adolescent Psychiatry, 44,* 609–621.

American Academy of Pediatrics. (2003). *Poison treatment in the home.* Retrieved August 22, 2006 from www.dap.org/policy/s0/0120.html

Annie E. Casey Foundation (2004). Kids Count 2004. Retrieved August 22, 2006 from http://www.aecf.org/kidscount/databook/ index.htm

Armstrong, M. L. (2005). Tattooing, body piercing, and permanent cosmetics: A historical and current view of state regulations, with continuing concerns. *Journal of Environmental Health, 68*(8), 38–45.

Bauer, N. S., Herrenkohl, T. I., Lozano, P. L., Rivara, F. P., Hill, K. G., & Hawkins, J. D. (2006). Childhood bullying involvement and exposure to intimate partner violence. *Pediatrics, 118,* 235–242.

Baxley, F., & Miller, M. (2006). Parental misperceptions about children and firearms. *Archives of Pediatric and Adolescent Medicine, 160,* 542–547.

Bellinger, D. C. (2004). Lead. *Pediatrics, 113*(Suppl), 1016–1022.

Belson, M. G., Schier, J. G., & Patel, M. M. (2005). Case definitions for chemical poisoning. *Morbidity and Mortality Reports, 54*(RR-1), 1–24.

Benton, J. (2003). Making schools safer and healthier for lesbian gay bisexual and questioning students. *Journal of School Nursing, 19,* 257–259.

Bronfenbrenner, U. (2005). *Making human being human: Bioecologic perspectives.* Thousand Oaks, CA: Sage Publications.

Bryant, S., & Singer, J. (2003). Management of toxic exposure in children. *Emergency Medicine Clinics of North America, 21,* 101–119.

Carbaugh, S. F. (2004). Understanding shaken baby syndrome. *Advanced Neonatal Care, 4,* 105–116.

Centers for Disease Control and Prevention (CDC). (2003). *Coping with a traumatic event.* Accessed February 21, 2006, from http://sss.bt/cdc.gov/masstrauma/copingpub.asp

Centers for Disease Control and Prevention (CDC). (2005). *Maintaining a health state of mind: For parents and caregivers.* Accessed February 21, 2006, from http://www.redcross/org/email/testing/cdc_english/health_parents.asp

Chernin, A. R., & Linebarger, D. L. (2005). The relationship between children's television viewing and academic performance. *Archives of Pediatrics & Adolescent Medicine, 159,* 687–689.

Childhelp. (2005). *National child abuse statistics.* Scottsdale, AZ: Author.

Children's Defense Fund. (2004a). *Basic facts on poverty.* Washington, DC: Author.

Children's Defense Fund. (2004b). *Data. Each day in America.* Accessed August 16, 2004, from http://www.childrensdefense.org/data/ eachday.asp

Children's Safety Network, National Injury and Violence Prevention Resource Center. (2003). *Preventing bullying: The role of the public health professional.* Retrieved January 23, 2004, from http://www/childrenssafetynetwork.org

Chng, C. L., Neill, K., & Fogle, P. (2003). Predictors of college students' use of complementary and alternative medicine. *American Journal of Health Education, 39,* 269–271.

Cowal, K., Shinn, M., Weitzman, B. C., Stojanovic, D., & Labay, L. (2002). Mother-child separations among homeless and housed families receiving public assistance in New York City. *American Journal of Community Psychology, 30,* 711–730.

DeForge, V., Zehnder, S., Minick, P., & Carmon, M. (2001). *Children's perspectives of homelessness.* Pediatric Nursing, 27, 377–383.

DeRanieri, J. T., Clements, P. T., Clark, K., Kuhn, D. W., & Manno, M. S. (2004). War, terrorism, and children. *Journal of School Nursing, 20,* 69–75.

Dunn, A. M., Burns, C., & Sattler, B. (2003). Environmental health of children. *Journal of Pediatric Health Care, 17,* 223–231.

Elkind, D. (2007). *The hurried child: 25th anniversary edition.* Cambridge, MA: Da Capo Lifelong Publishing.

Ellickson, P. L., Orlando, M., Tucker, J. S., & Klein, D. J. (2004). From adolescence to young adulthood: Racial/ethnic disparities in smoking. *American Journal of Public Health, 94,* 293–299.

Escobar-Chaves, S. L. (2005). Impact of the media on adolescent sexual attitudes and behaviors. *Pediatrics, 116* (Suppl.), 297–299.

Etzel, R. A. (2004). Environmental risks in childhood. *Pediatric Annals, 33,* 431–436.

Federal Interagency Forum on Child and Family Statistics. (2003). *American's children: Key national indicators of well-being 2003.* Washington, DC: U.S. Government Printing Office.

Fekkes, M., Pijpers, F. I., & Verloove-Vanhorick, S. P. (2006). Effects of antibullying school program on bullying and health complaints. *Archives of Pediatric and Adolescent Medicine, 160,* 638–644.

Fetro, J. V., Coyle, K. K., & Phaon, P. (2001). Health-risk behaviors among middle school students in a large majority-minority school district. *Journal of School Health, 71,* 30–37.

Fox, J. A., Elliot, D. S., Kerlikowske, R. G., Newman, S. A. & Christeson, W. (2003). *Bullying prevention is crime prevention.* Washington, DC: Fight Crime: Invest in Kids.

Franke, T. M. (2003). The effect of attachment on adolescent violence. *The Prevention Researcher, 10,* 14–16.

Gardiner, P., Breuner, C. C. & Kemper, K. J. (2003). What's the BUZZ? Nonprescription stimulants in the youthful population. *Contemporary Pediatrics, 20*(8), 63–81.

Gershel, J. C., Katz-Sidlow, R. J., Small, E., & Zandieh, S. (2003). Hazing of suburban middle school and high school athletes. *Journal of Adolescent Health, 32,* 333–335.

Gettig, J. P., Grady, S. E., & Nowosadzka, I. (2006). Methamphetamine: Putting the brakes on speed. *Journal of School Nursing, 22*(2), 66–73.

Gold, M. A., Schorzman, C. M., Murray, P. J., Downs, J., & Tolentino, G. (2005). Body piercing practices and attitudes among urban adolescents. *Journal of Adolescent Health, 36,* 352, e17–24.

Goldrick, B. A. (2003). Endocarditis associated with body piercing. *American Journal of Nursing, 103,* 26–27.

Guthrie, B. J., Hoey, E., Ravoira, L.W., & Kintner, E. (2002). Girls in the juvenile justice system: Leave no girls health un-addressed. *Journal of Pediatric Nursing, 17,* 414–423.

Haber, M. G., & Toro, P. A. (2004). Homelessness among families, children, and adolescents: An ecological-developmental perspective. *Clinical Child and Family Psychology Review, 7,* 123–164.

Hanze, D. (2002). How to help children and adolescents deal with the threat of terrorism. *Journal for Specialists in Pediatric Nursing, 7,* 42–44.

Hettler, J. (2002). Munchausen syndrome by proxy. *Pediatric Emergency Care, 18,* 371–374.

Hingson, R. W., Heeren, T., & Winter, M. R. (2006). Age at drinking onset and alcohol dependence. *Archives of Pediatric and Adolescent Medicine, 160,* 739–746.

Home Safety Council. (2004). Retrieved July 4, 2004, from http://www.homesafetycouncil. org/resource_center/resourcecenter.aspx

Horner, G. (2003). Adolescent sexual offenders: A challenge for primary care NPs. *American Journal for Nurse Practitioners, 7*(9), 37–45.

Howard, D. E., & Wang, M. Q. (2003). Risk profiles of adolescent girls who were victims of dating violence. *Adolescence, 38,* 1–14.

HRSA. (2003). *The national bullying prevention campaign.* Washington, DC: Author.

Hymel, K. P., & Hall, C. A. (2005). Diagnosing pediatric head trauma. *Pediatric Annals, 34,* 358–370.

Johnston, L. D., O'Malley, P. M., Bachman, J. G., & Schulenberg, J. E. (2004). *Monitoring the future: National survey results on drug use, 1975–2003.* Bethesda, MD: National Institute of Drug Abuse. NIH Pub # 04–5507.

Kaiser Family Foundation. (2003). New study finds children age zero to six years spend as much time with TV, computers, and video games as playing outside. Accessed February 22, 2006, from http://www.kff.org/entmedia/ entmedia102803nr.cfm

Kay, M., & Wyllie, R. (2005). Pediatric foreign bodies and their management. *Current Gastroenterology Reports, 7,* 212–218.

Kimmel, C. A., Collman, G. W., Fields, N., & Eskenazi, B. (2005). Lessons learned for the National Children's Study from the National Institute of Environmental Health Sciences/U.S. Environmental Protection Agency Centers for children's environmental health and disease

prevention research. *Environmental Health Perspectives, 113,* 1414–1418.

Knight, J. R. (1997). Adolescent substance use: Screening, assessment, and intervention. *Contemporary Pediatrics, 14,* 45, 51–56, 61–72.

Leone, A. (2003). Relationship between cigarette smoking and other coronary risk factors in atherosclerosis: Risk of cardiovascular disease and preventive measures. *Current Pharmacological Design, 9,* 2417–2423.

Limber, S. (2003). *Youth development program: Olweus bullying prevention.* Retrieved from the Clemson University web site at http://www. clemson.edu.scg/youth/IFNLbully.htm

Loveland-Cherry, C. J. (2006). Alcohol, children and adolescents. In J. J. Fitzpatrick (Ed.), *Alcohol use, misuse, abuse, and dependence* (pp. 135–177). New York: Springer Publishing.

McColgan, M. D., & Giardino, A. P. (2005). Internet poses multiple risks to children and adolescents. *Pediatric Annals, 34,* 405–414.

MMWR. (2002). Trends in cigarette smoking among high school students. *Morbidity and Mortality Weekly Report, 51,* 409–412.

MMWR. (2003a). Surveillance for elevated blood lead levels among children—United States, 1997–2001. *Morbidity and Mortality Weekly Report, 52* (SS-10), 1–21.

MMWR. (2003b). Tobacco, alcohol, and other drug use among high school students in Bureau of Indian Affairs—Funded schools, United States, 2001. *Morbidity and Mortality Weekly Report, 52,* 1070–1072.

MMWR. (2003c). Tobacco use among middle and high school students—United States, 2002. *Morbidity and Mortality Weekly Report, 52,* 1096–1098.

MMWR. (2004). Youth risk behavior surveillance—United States, 2003. *Morbidity and Mortality Weekly Report, 53* (SS-2), 1–95.

MMWR. (2006a). Cigarette use among high school students—United States, 1991–2005. *Morbidity and Mortality Weekly Report, 55,* 724–726.

MMWR. (2006b). Use of cigarettes and other tobacco products among students aged 13–15 years—worldwide, 1999–2005. *Morbidity and Mortality Weekly Report, 55,* 553–556.

MMWR. (2006c). Youth risk behavior surveillance—United States, 2005. *Morbidity and Mortality Weekly Report, 55*(SS05), 1–108.

Morris, R. I., & Strong, L. (2004). The impact of homelessness on the health of families. *Journal of School Nursing, 20,* 221–227.

Mullin, K. A., & Ambrosia, T. (2005). Role of the nurse practitioner in providing health care for the homeless. *American Journal for Nurse Practitioners, 9*(9), 37–44.

Murray, J. S. (2002). Helping children cope with separation during war. *Journal for Specialists in Pediatric Nursing, 7,* 127–130.

National Center for Children Exposed to Violence. (2003). *Parents' guide for talking to their children about war.* New Haven, CT: Author.

National Institute of Child Health and Human Development. (2003). *Child care linked to assertive, noncompliant, and aggressive behaviors.* Accessed February 18, 2006, from http://www. nichd.nih.gov.new/releases.child_care.cfm.

National Institute on Alcohol Abuse and Alcoholism (NIAAA). (2002). *Initiative on underage drinking.* Accessed February 17, 2006, from http://www.niaaa.nih.gov.

National Institute on Alcohol Abuse and Alcoholism (NIAAA). (2005). The effects of alcohol on physiological processes and biological development. *Alcohol Research and Health, 28,* 125–132.

National Institute on Drug Abuse. (1999). *Some facts about club drugs.* Bethesda, MD: U.S. Department of Health and Human Services.

National Institute on Drug Abuse. (2003). Teen drug use declined in 2002, report shows. *NIDA News, 17*(5), 12–14.

National Safe Kids. (2005). *Injury facts.* Accessed February 20, 2006, from http://usa. safekids.org/tier3_cd.cfm?folder_ id=540&content_item_id=1213

Pine, D. S., Costello, J., & Masten, A. (2005). Trauma, proximity, and developmental psychopathology: The effects of war and terrorism on children. *Neuropsychopharmacology, 30,* 1781–1792.

Pratt, H. D., & Greydanus, D. E. (2000). Adolescent violence: Concepts for a new millennium. *Adolescent Medicine, 11,* 103–125.

Redlener, I., & Grant, R. (September, 2002). The 9/11 terrorist attack: Emotional consequences persist for children and their families. *Contemporary Pediatrics.* Retrieved August 22, 2006 from www.contemporarypediaties.com/ contpeds/issue/ issueDetail.jsp?id=4760

Regan, K. (2003). When daddy hits mommy. *Advance for Nurses,* October 27–28.

Rezendes, J. L. (2006). Bicycle helmets: Overcoming barriers to use and increasing effectiveness. *Journal of Pediatric Nursing, 21,* 35–44.

Ryan-Wenger, N. A., Sharrer, V. W., & Campbell, K. K. (2005). Changes in children's stressors over the past 30 years. *Pediatric Nursing, 31,* 282–291.

Saewye, E. M., Pettingell, S., & Magee, L. L. (2003). The prevalence of sexual abuse among adolescents in school. *Journal of School Nursing, 19,* 266–272.

Selekman, J. (2003). A new era of body decorations: What are kids doing to their bodies? *Pediatric Nursing, 29,* 77–79.

Silverman, J. G., Raj, A., Mucci, L. A., & Hathaway, J. E. (2001). Dating violence in adolescent girls and associated substance use, unhealthy weight control, sexual risk behavior, pregnancy and suicidiality. *JAMA, 286,* 572–579.

Snyder, H. (December, 2003). Juvenile arrests. *Juvenile Justice Bulletin,* 1–12.

Society for Pediatric Nurses, SPN Public Policy Committee. (2000). Gun accidents, suicides increase among children. *SPN News, 9,* 6.

Spencer, G. A., & Bryant, S. A. (2000). Dating violence: A comparison of rural, suburban, and urban teens. *Journal of Adolescent Health, 27,* 302–305.

Steele, R.W., Ramgoolam, A., & Evans, J. (2003). Health services for homeless adolescents. *Seminars in Pediatric Infectious Diseases, 14,* 38–42.

Stratigos, A. J., & Katsambas, A. D. (2003). Medical and cutaneous disorders associated with homelessness. *Skinmed, 2,* 168–172.

Teplin, L. A., McClelland, C. M., and Abram, K. M., & Mileusnic, D. (2005). Early violent death among delinquent youth: A prospective longitudinal study. *Pediatrics, 115,* 1586–1593.

Thomas, K. (2003). Munchausen syndrome by proxy: Identification and diagnosis. *Journal of Pediatric Nursing, 18*, 174–180.

Thornburgh, D., & Lin, H. S. (2002). *Youth, pornography, and the Internet* (3rd ed.). Washington, DC: National Academies Press.

Tuttle, J., Melnyk, B. M., & Loveland-Cherry, C. (2002). Adolescent drug and alcohol use: Strategies for assessment, intervention, and prevention. *Nursing Clinics of North America, 37*, 443–460.

UNICEF. (2006). *State of the world's children*. Accessed February 20, 2006, from http://www.unicefusa.org/site/c.duLRI80OH/b.262152/k.221E/State-of_the_Worlds_Chil

U.S. Department of Health and Human Services. (2000). *Healthy People 2010*. Washington, DC: Author.

U.S. Department of Health and Human Services. (2003). *Preventing drug use among children and adolescents*. Washington, DC: Author.

U.S. Department of Health and Human Services. (2005). *Summary: Child maltreatment 2003*. Accessed February 20, 2006, from http://www.acf.hhs.gov/programs/cb/pubs/cm03/summary.htm.

U.S. Department of Health and Human Services and U.S. Department of Agriculture. (2005). *Dietary guidelines for Americans 2005*. Washington, DC: Author.

Uyemura, M. C. (2006). Foreign body ingestion in children. *American Family Physician, 72*, 287–291.

Van der Wal, M. F., de Wit, C. A. M., & Hirasing, R. A. (2003). Psychosocial health among young victims and offenders of direct and indirect bullying. *Pediatrics, 111*, 1312–1317.

Victoir, A., Eertmans, A., Van den Broucke, S., & Van den Bergh, O. (2006). Smoking status moderates the contribution of social-cognitive and environmental determinants to adolescents' smoking intentions. Health Education Research 21, 674–687.

Watson, W. A., Litovitz, T. L., Klein-Schwartz, W., Rodgers, G. C., Youniss, J., Redi, N., Rouse, W. G., Rembert, R. S., & Borys, D. (2004). 2003 annual report of the American Association of Poison Control Center toxic exposure surveillance. *American Journal of Emergency Medicine, 22*, 335–404.

World Health Organization (WHO). (2002). *Trauma among children who are victims of violence*. Accessed February 20, 2006, from http://www.afro.who.int/press/2002/pr2002091602.html

World Health Organization (WHO). (2005). Injuries and violence prevention. Accessed http://www.who.int/violence_injury_prevention/media/news/28_06_2005/en/

INTRODUCTION TO HEALTH PROMOTION AND HEALTH MAINTENANCE

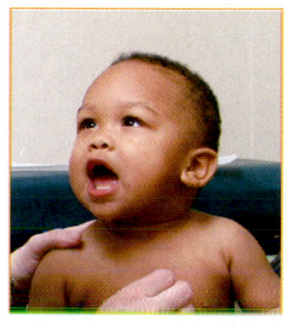

CLARENCE has been brought in for his 15-month-old health supervision visit by his father, Ben, and mother, Karie. Clarence is a healthy but very active toddler and his parents have many questions about his development. They are concerned that Clarence is very active and needs constant supervision. Since both parents work and Clarence is at childcare during the day, they are busy in the evening trying to spend time with him and meet other family obligations. You notice on the record that Clarence missed his 12-month health supervision visit and was last seen when he was 9 months old.

What health promotion activities will be appropriate for this visit? How will you integrate Ben and Karie's questions about Clarence's activity level into the visit? Since Clarence has not been seen in health care for some time, what are some likely health maintenance needs?

KEY TERMS

anticipatory
  guidance 265
health 264
health maintenance
  265
health
  promotion 264
health protection
  265
health
  supervision 266
partnership 267
pediatric health
  care home 266
screening 274
spiritual
  dimension 274

MediaLink
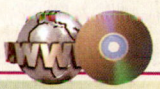

http://www.prenhall.com/ball
See the Prentice Hall Nursing MediaLink DVD-ROM and Companion Website for chapter-specific resources.

LEARNING OUTCOMES

After reading this chapter, you will be able to do the following:

1. Define health promotion and health maintenance.

2. Describe how health promotion and health maintenance are addressed by partnering with families during health supervision visits.

3. Describe the components of a health supervision visit.

4. Explore the nurse's role in providing health promotion and health maintenance for children and families.

5. Describe the general observations made of children and their families as they come to the pediatric healthcare home for health supervision visits.

6. Describe the areas of assessment and intervention for health supervision visits—growth and developmental surveillance, nutrition, physical activity, oral health, mental and spiritual health, family and social relations, disease prevention strategies, and injury prevention strategies.

7. Plan health promotion and health maintenance strategies employed during health supervision visits.

8. Apply the nursing process in assessment, diagnosis, goal setting, intervention, and evaluation of health promotion and health maintenance activities for children and families.

One of the two major goals of *Healthy People 2010* is to help individuals of all ages increase life expectancy and improve their quality of life. The concepts of health promotion and health maintenance provide for nursing interventions that contribute to meeting this goal. Many students in health professions begin their studies with a strong interest in care of ill individuals. However, as time progresses, they learn that "well" people need care also. They need teaching to improve diet, reduce stress, and obtain immunizations. They may seek information about how to exercise properly or ensure a safe environment for their children. These examples of care and teaching are components of health promotion and health maintenance.

Nursing is a holistic profession that examines and works with all aspects of individuals' lives, and has a strong focus on family and community as well. Nurses therefore are uniquely positioned to provide health promotion and health maintenance activities. In fact, these activities should be a part of each encounter with families.

The pediatric nurse applies health promotion and health maintenance in all settings in which children are served—well-child clinics, schools, mobile vans, physician and nurse practitioner offices, and hospitals. This nurse must possess a comprehensive background on all aspects of childcare and an understanding of child growth and development (see Chapter 3 ∞). The family's role in children's health is critical (see Chapter 2 ∞). The impact of contemporary influences on children provides an essential context to realistic nursing care planning (see Chapter 6 ∞). Finally, a thorough understanding of the healthcare conditions that affect children is needed so that health promotion and health maintenance can be integrated within the framework of comprehensive health care. Some children have special healthcare needs and these are integrated into the provision of health promotion and health maintenance.

What is the difference between health promotion and health maintenance? When should nurses engage in activities that focus on health? How can these activities be integrated into health supervision visits for the infant and young child? How do nurses collaborate with other healthcare professionals to offer comprehensive health services in settings accessible to parents and young children? How can nurses help children and their families to maximize the length and quality of life? These questions will be explored in this chapter, along with specific activities that target families with infants and young children.

GENERAL CONCEPTS

In order to understand health promotion and health maintenance, it is important to develop a definition of health. The World Health Organization defines **health** as a state of complete physical, mental, and social well-being and not merely the absence of disease and infirmity (World Health Organization, 1996). Even individuals with chronic disease can be viewed as healthy if they successfully adapt to their conditions. Health is viewed as dynamic, changing, and unfolding; it is the realization of a state of actualization or potential (Pender, Murdaugh, & Parsons, 2006). This basic human right is necessary for development of societies.

Health promotion refers to activities that increase well-being and enhance wellness or health (Pender, Murdaugh, & Parsons, 2006). These activities lead to actualization of positive health potential for all individuals, even those with chronic or acute conditions. Examples include providing information and resources in order to:

- Enhance nutrition at each developmental stage
- Integrate physical activity into the child's daily events
- Provide adequate housing
- Promote oral health
- Foster positive personality development

Health promotion is concerned with developing sets of strategies that seek to foster conditions that allow populations to be healthy and to make healthy choices (World Health Organization, 2001). Improved health requires coherent policies on health

Table 7–1	**LEVELS OF PREVENTIVE HEALTH MAINTENANCE ACTIVITIES**	
Level	**Description**	**Example of Nursing Actions**
Primary prevention	Activities that decrease opportunity for illness or injury	Giving immunizations Teaching about car safety seats
Secondary prevention	Early diagnosis and treatment of a condition to lessen its severity	Developmental screening Vision and hearing screening
Tertiary prevention	Restoration to optimum function	Rehabilitation activities for child after a car crash

Adapted from Murray & Zentner, 2005, p. 44.

promotion, as well as collaboration among governments, international organizations, the society, and private agencies (World Health Organization, 2005). Nurses engage in health promotion by being active in policies that promote health in institutions where they are employed, and by partnering with children and families to promote family strengths in the areas of lifestyles, social development, coping, and family interactions. You will provide **anticipatory guidance** for families when you understand the child's upcoming developmental stages and teach families how to provide an environment to assist in meeting each stage's milestones. Examples of application of this are found in Chapters 8 and 9 ∞.

Health maintenance (or **health protection**) refers to activities that preserve an individual's present state of health and that prevent disease or injury occurrence. Examples of these activities include developmental screening or surveillance to identify early deviations from normal development, providing immunizations to prevent illnesses, and teaching about common childhood safety hazards. Health maintenance activities are commonly preventive in nature and terminology common to community or public health nursing explains the levels and aims of preventive actions. Prevention levels are identified as primary prevention, secondary prevention, and tertiary prevention (Table 7–1).

While it is clear that health promotion and health maintenance activities are closely linked and often overlap, there are some differences. Health maintenance focuses on known potential health risks and seeks to prevent them, or identify them early so that intervention can occur. Health promotion looks at the strengths and goals of individuals, families, and populations, and seeks to use them to assist in reaching higher levels of wellness. It involves partnerships with the family as health goals are set, and with other health professionals and resources to provide for meeting the goals (Figure 7–1 ➤). Apply both health promotion and health maintenance concepts when providing health care, recognizing that the concepts overlap. Health promotion and health maintenance are integrated into healthcare visits for children, with the care provider applying both knowledge of health maintenance concepts and adding information the family has identified that will assist in increasing health or wellness (health

MediaLink

Health Promotion and Health Maintenance Video

Health Promotion and Health Maintenance Overlap

Health Promotion	**Overlap**	**Health Maintenance**
• Nutrition to meet all RDAs and enhance health and well-being, with emphasis on whole grains, fruits, vegetables. • Activities to promote self-concept formation including body image and decision-making skills.	• Nutrition that provides for growth and energy needs also helps prevent chronic diseases. • Integrating positive activities will both promote self-image and decrease potential for injury.	• Nutrition to prevent obesity or growth retardation. • Limiting television viewing to decrease exposure to violence, which may lead to disturbed sleep and aggressive behaviors.

Figure 7–1 ➤ Health promotion and health maintenance overlap. While the focus and goals for health promotion and health maintenance differ, there is often overlap in nursing activities and expected outcomes, as demonstrated in these examples.

LAW & ETHICS

Pediatric Healthcare Home

The American Academy of Pediatrics and the National Association of Pediatric Nurse Practitioners concur that a pediatric healthcare home should offer:

- Family-centered care and trusting partnership
- Sharing of unbiased and clear information
- Provision of primary care to include acute and chronic care, breast-feeding promotion, immunizations, growth and development, screenings, healthcare supervision, counseling about health, nutrition, safety, and parenting and psychosocial issues
- Continuous available care
- Continuity of care
- Referral to specialists as needed
- Referral to early intervention and childcare
- Coordination of services
- Maintenance of a comprehensive central record
- Provision of developmentally appropriate and culturally competent care

(American Academy of Pediatrics, 2002; NAPNAP, 2002)

MediaLink

Health Promotion National Guidelines

promotion). These activities commonly take place at "well child" or health supervision visits.

Health supervision is the provision of services that focus on disease and injury prevention (health maintenance), growth and developmental surveillance, and health promotion at key intervals during the child's life. What health promotion and health maintenance activities are parts of health supervision visits? How can these activities be integrated into all settings where care is provided for children? What are the recommended times for health visits to occur and what care is provided at certain times? How can you organize a health supervision visit to accomplish goals of family and health professionals? These and other questions will be answered in this section and the section that follows on nursing management.

Children all need a medical home, where ongoing health supervision is provided during the developmental years. A medical home or **pediatric health care home** is the site of comprehensive health care by a pediatric healthcare professional in order to ensure optimal health (NAPNAP, 2002). See Chapter 1 ∞ for further description of a medical home or pediatric healthcare home. When a family has an established partnership with a care provider, comprehensive, family-centered health services can be provided based on the family's risks and protective factors. These services may be provided at physician offices, community health clinics, and in the home, schools, childcare centers, shelters, or mobile vans (Figure 7–2 ➤). National guidelines for preventive health services have been developed for infants, children, and adolescents by the U.S. Department of Health and Human Services (DHHS), the American Academy of Pediatrics (AAP), and the American Medical Association. The National Association of Pediatric Nurse Associates and Practitioners supports the list of comprehensive services of a pediatric healthcare home identified by the AAP.

The health supervision visit is individualized to the family and child. Standardized screenings and examinations are included, and time is provided for the family's specific concerns and questions about the child's health. Nurses play an integral part in these comprehensive visits and they partner with other healthcare providers to accomplish health supervision.

A tracking system in the pediatric healthcare home site helps to identify appropriate health supervision activities for each child at every visit. Computers are often used to list appropriate topics for visits at specific ages. If a child misses a visit, the family can be contacted by phone and encouraged to come in for the recommended care. A family may be called if their young child is lacking some immunizations. Recognizing that not all families get into the healthcare home for each visit, every health visit, including an

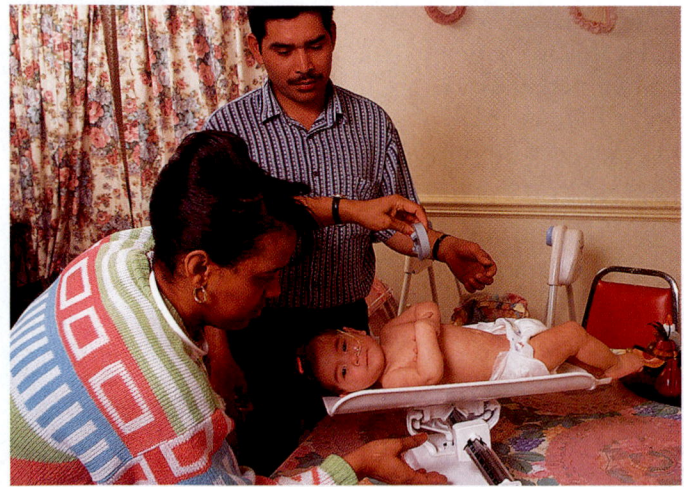

A

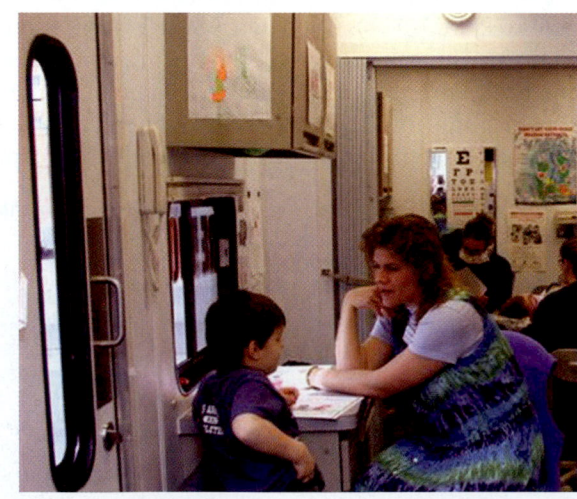

B

Figure 7–2 ➤ A, The nurse is providing a health supervision visit in the child's home after discharge from the hospital for an acute illness. B, A nurse is providing information to a child visiting a mobile healthcare van.

episodic illness visit or care for a chronic illness, is a potential time to complete health promotion and health maintenance activities. For example, immunizations may sometimes be given during a visit for an acute condition such as otitis media (ear infection) if the child has missed a prior health supervision visit. Even when you see children in hospitals, emergency rooms, or other settings, ask about their pediatric healthcare home, and when the last visit occurred. Identify children who need basic health supervision services and provide them or refer to other settings for meeting these needs at another time.

Nurses play an important role in managing health supervision visits. Depending on the setting, the advanced practice nurse may provide all services or support other care providers by obtaining an updated health history, screening for diseases and other conditions, conducting a developmental assessment, and providing immunizations, anticipatory guidance, and health education. And nurses in all settings are instrumental in identifying children who need health supervision and are not obtaining recommended care (Figure 7–3 ➤).

While health supervision visits can address many health-related topics, a limited time generally exists in which to engage a child or family. The nurse needs to direct the encounters and have some ideas for pertinent agendas. *Bright Futures*, an initiative of the United States Maternal and Child Health Bureau, promotes the foundational belief that each child deserves to be healthy and that the community, health professional, family, and child must partner together to achieve this goal. A series of *Bright Futures* booklets on health supervision, nutrition, physical activity, and mental health provide guidance about how the nurse can manage health supervision visits. These publications are now available through the American Academy of Pediatrics and are used throughout Chapters 8–10 ∞ to provide essential guidance for provision of healthcare for children. (Additional resources are also available to assist in implementing the *Bright Futures* concepts in healthcare agencies.) Six concepts should be integrated into child health care and are listed in the following text:

1. The care provider *builds effective partnerships* with the family. A **partnership** is a relationship in which participants join together to ensure healthcare delivery in a way that recognizes each partner's critical roles and contributions in promoting health and preventing illness. The partners in child health include the child, family, health professionals, and the community.
2. The nurse *fosters family-centered communication* by showing interest in the child and family, and effectively conveying information and understanding.
3. The nurse *focuses on health promotion and health maintenance topics during visits*, recognizing that families may not initiate these discussions.

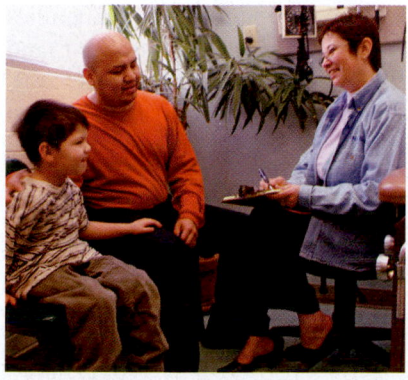
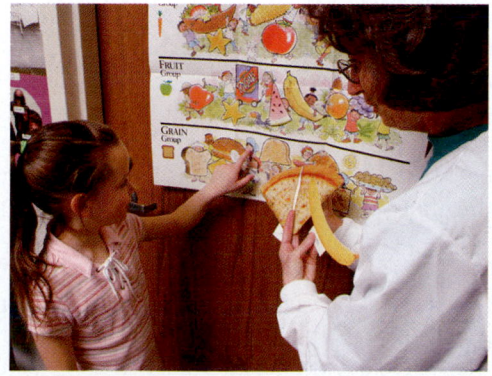
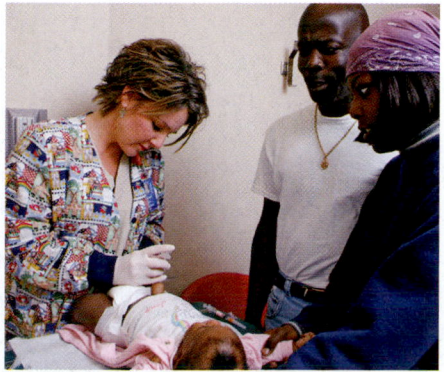

A   B   C

Figure 7–3 ➤ The nurse plays many roles in providing health promotion and health maintenance for children. A, Data are collected from the time a nurse calls the child and family to the examination room and during the history-taking phase. The nurse asks questions while observing the child's behaviors and the relationship between parent and child. The nurse also performs screening tests, including blood pressure, tuberculosis, vision and hearing, and developmental screening. B, Interventions that include teaching may take place. C, A nurse may administer immunizations as parents watch and assist by holding the child. Nurses also play important roles in teaching families information to enhance health.

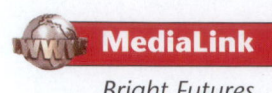

MediaLink

Bright Futures

4. The nurse manages time well to enable health promotion topics to be addressed during visits. This includes reviewing the child's health record and selecting topics pertinent for the child's age and the family's situation.

5. The nurse *educates the family during "teachable moments."* Large teaching plans are not always needed; children and families often learn best when presented with small bits of information based on parent's questions or your observations.

6. The nurse *becomes an advocate for child health issues.* When an issue arises as you care for a child, seek additional data from various sources, talk with others, and strategize how the problem could be solved (Green & Palfrey, 2002).

COMPONENTS OF HEALTH PROMOTION/HEALTH MAINTENANCE VISITS

The nurse identifies and isolates pertinent topics for health promotion and health maintenance during health supervision visits. You will apply your knowledge of areas that need to be addressed with an infant or child of a particular age, and then make general observations of the child and family to guide you to additional topics. While categories to consider vary depending on the child's age, the family's particular needs, and community resources, some common topics generally require attention. Start with the topics described in the following text, integrating general observations as you progress with the visit, and further areas as needed in particular situations.

Contacts with the Family

Healthcare providers work with families in diverse settings and must adapt approaches and interventions dependent on the needs of these families. Prospective parents sometimes interview potential healthcare providers while pregnant with a child in order to choose the pediatric healthcare home that will best meet their needs and approaches to child health. In other situations, parents choose the most convenient setting or a facility that is included in their health insurance coverage. Some families remain with one care provider for years, while others have multiple providers.

Whatever the individual situation, the nurse recognizes that all contacts with family members are a vital link to the child. They are a time to learn about the development of the child, to observe interactions among family members, and to implement effective nursing interventions. Telephone calls, face-to-face meetings, and brief encounters all serve to provide a mutual interaction with the goal of ensuring child health. Consider Clarence's parents, who are described in the opening scenario. They have questions about Clarence's activity level and will likely be receptive to nursing interventions that help them meet parenting challenges.

General Observations

As a pediatric nurse, you will be making *general observations* of infants and their families whenever you encounter them. Be observant during the health supervision visit, and you will have many opportunities for assessing the family. These general observations begin as you call the family in and welcome them to the facility. They continue as you weigh and measure the infant or child, and throughout the visit. Observe the physical contact between the child and other family members, the developmental tasks displayed by the child, and parental level of stress or ease in conducting childcare activities.

Growth and Developmental Surveillance

Growth and developmental surveillance provide important clues about the child's condition and environment. In order to evaluate growth, child height, weight, and body mass index are calculated at each health supervision visit, and results are placed on percentile charts (see Chapters 4 and 5 ∞). Parents are given the information in written form and it is interpreted for them. Physical assessment is performed to be sure the child is growing as expected and has no abnormal or unexplained physical findings (see Chapter 5 ∞). Developmental surveillance is a flexible, continuous process of skilled observations that also provides data about the child's capabilities, allows for early identification of any neurological problems, and helps to verify that the home environment is stimulating. Information may be collected from several sources; for instance, a questionnaire that the parent completes, trigger questions asked during the interview, or observation of the child during the visit. Parents can also be interviewed to identify any developmental concerns they may have about the child or adolescent. When talking with parents, review physical, social, and communication milestones for infants, young children, older children, or adolescents. Detailed milestones for each age group are found in Chapter 3 ∞.

Development is a fragile process determined by both innate conditions and environmental influences. Developmental screening of all children using a regular and organized approach is needed, since about 16% of children have some type of developmental delay or disability (Earls & Hay, 2006). Standardized developmental questionnaires are effective for developmental surveillance of most children, especially when time for health supervision visits is limited (see Tables 7–2 and 7–3). A commonly used test is the Denver II, which can be applied as a developmental chart, like a growth curve, to monitor the child's developmental progress (see Figures 7–4 and 7–5 ➤).

To perform developmental screening with the Denver II or any other standardized screening tools, make sure all directions are followed:

- Choose the proper test for the child's age and desired information.
- Read directions thoroughly or utilize specific training tools available.
- Practice as needed until proficient with the test.
- Calculate the infant's or child's age correctly, especially if premature.
- Attempt to develop rapport with the infant or child to get the best performance.
- Follow directions for administration of items; in some cases, parents can be asked if a child demonstrates specific skills at home, especially if the child is not willing to perform an item during testing.
- Note the child's behavior and cooperativeness during the screening process.
- Analyze the findings using the test instructions to make the correct interpretation.

Failure to perform an item in a single domain does not mean the child has failed the test. The child should be reevaluated at a future visit. Schedule the appointment at a time of day when the child is awake and rested. Failure of multiple items within one domain or across multiple domains is of greatest concern. When poor development patterns in one or more domains are revealed, referral for diagnostic developmental assessment is needed.

CLINICAL TIP

A series of developmental screening tests are available to rate the interaction between caregiver and child. Developed by nurses, the Nursing Child Assessment Satellite Training (NCAST) teaches how to administer screenings of a feeding and a teaching interaction.

Table 7–2	DEVELOPMENTAL SURVEILLANCE QUESTIONNAIRES
Questionnaire	**Guidelines for Administration**
Parent's Evaluation of Developmental Status[a] (birth to 8 years)	Consists of 10 questions for parents to answer in interview; based on research about parents' concerns. Requires less than 5 minutes to complete. English and Spanish forms are available.
Prescreening Development Questionnaire (birth to 6 years)	Parents complete an age-specific form. Helps identify children who need Denver II (PDQ and Revised-PDQ)[b] assessment. Requires less than 10 minutes to complete. PDQ is available in English, Spanish, and French versions; R-PDQ in English only.
Ages and Stages Questionnaire[c] (4–48 months)	Questionnaires for 11 specific ages, with 10–15 items each in areas of fine motor, gross motor, communication, adaptive, personal, and social skills. Parents try each activity with the child. Requires less than 10 minutes to complete. English and Spanish versions are available.
Child Development Inventories[d] (3–72 months)	Consists of 60 yes-no descriptions for three separate instruments to identify children with developmental difficulties. Requires about 10 minutes to complete.

[a]Frances P. Glascoe, Ellsworth & Vandermeer Press Ltd, P.O. Box 68164, Nashville, TN 37206.
[b]Denver Developmental Material, Inc., P.O. Box 371075, Denver, CO 80237-5075.
[c]Brookes Publishing Co., P.O. Box 10624, Baltimore, MD 21285-0625.
[d]Behavior Science Systems, Box 580274, Minneapolis, MN 55458.

Table 7–3	DEVELOPMENTAL SCREENING TESTS FOR INFANTS AND YOUNG CHILDREN
Screening Test	**Guidelines for Administration**
Denver II[a] (birth to 6 years)	Consists of observation of the child in four domains; personal social, fine motor-adaptive, language, and gross motor. Requires 30 minutes to complete. A training video is available.
Bayley Infant Neurodevelopmental Screener (BINST)[b] (3–24 months)	Consists of observation of child with 10–13 items for each of six age-specific scales to assess neurological processes, neurodevelopmental skills, and developmental accomplishments. Requires 10–15 minutes to complete.
McCarthy Scales of Children's Abilities[b] (2.5–8.5 years)	Consists of observation of child in domains of motor, verbal, perceptual-performance, quantitive, general cognition, and memory. Requires 45 minutes to complete.
Denver Articulation Screeening Exam (DASE)[a] (2.5–6 years)	Consists of observation of child's articulation of 30 sound elements and intelligibility. Requires 5 minutes to complete.
Early Language Milestone Scale—2 (ELM)[c] (birth to 36 months)	Consists of observation of child to assess auditory expressive, auditory receptive, and visual components of speech. Requires 5–10 minutes to complete.

[a]Denver Development Materials, Inc., P.O. Box 371075, Denver, CO 80237–5075.
[b]Harcourt Assessment: The Psychological Corporation, 19500 Bulverde Rd., San Antonio, TX 78259.
[c]PRO-ED, Inc., 8700 Shoal Creek Blvd., Austin, TX 78758-6897.

Parents are key participants in their children's developmental screening. They often recognize problems not observed in brief healthcare encounters. Enable them to ask questions and state their observations of the child, provide them with expected developmental tasks and ways to stimulate development, and encourage them to write down observations to form the basis for developmental screening during healthcare visits (Frankenburg, 2004; Williams & Holmes, 2004).

Nutrition

Nutrition is a vital part of each health supervision visit. It makes important contributions to general health and fosters growth and development. Include observations and screening relevant to nutritional intake at each health supervision visit. Eating proper foods for

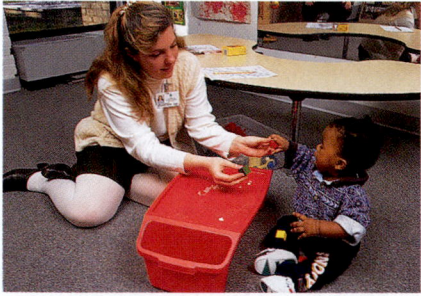

A

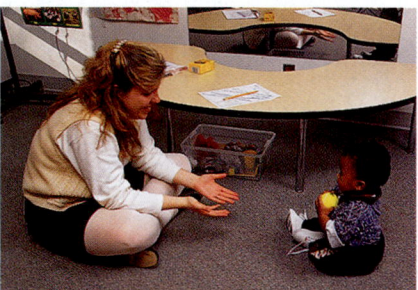

B

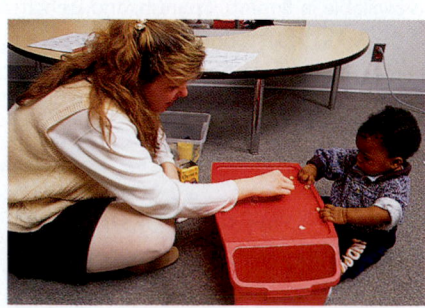

C

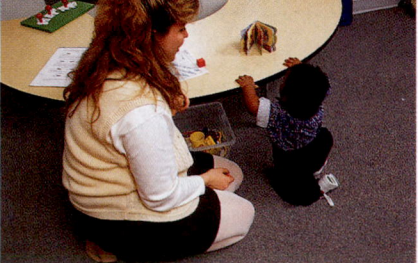

D

Figure 7–4 ▶ Follow all directions for performing the Denver II assessment and for interpreting responses. Use the kit provided with the test to ensure for accuracy of results. For example, yarn is provided to test the infant's ability to follow an object, blocks of a uniform size test fine motor coordination, and pictures on the score sheet are used to test language abilities. Develop rapport with the child and approach the assessment as fun. This often helps the child participate more actively during the entire Denver II assessment. This 9-month-old boy is able to perform the following age-appropriate behaviors: A, Banging two cubes; B, Playing ball with the examiner; C, Using a thumb-finger grasp; and D, Pulling to stand.

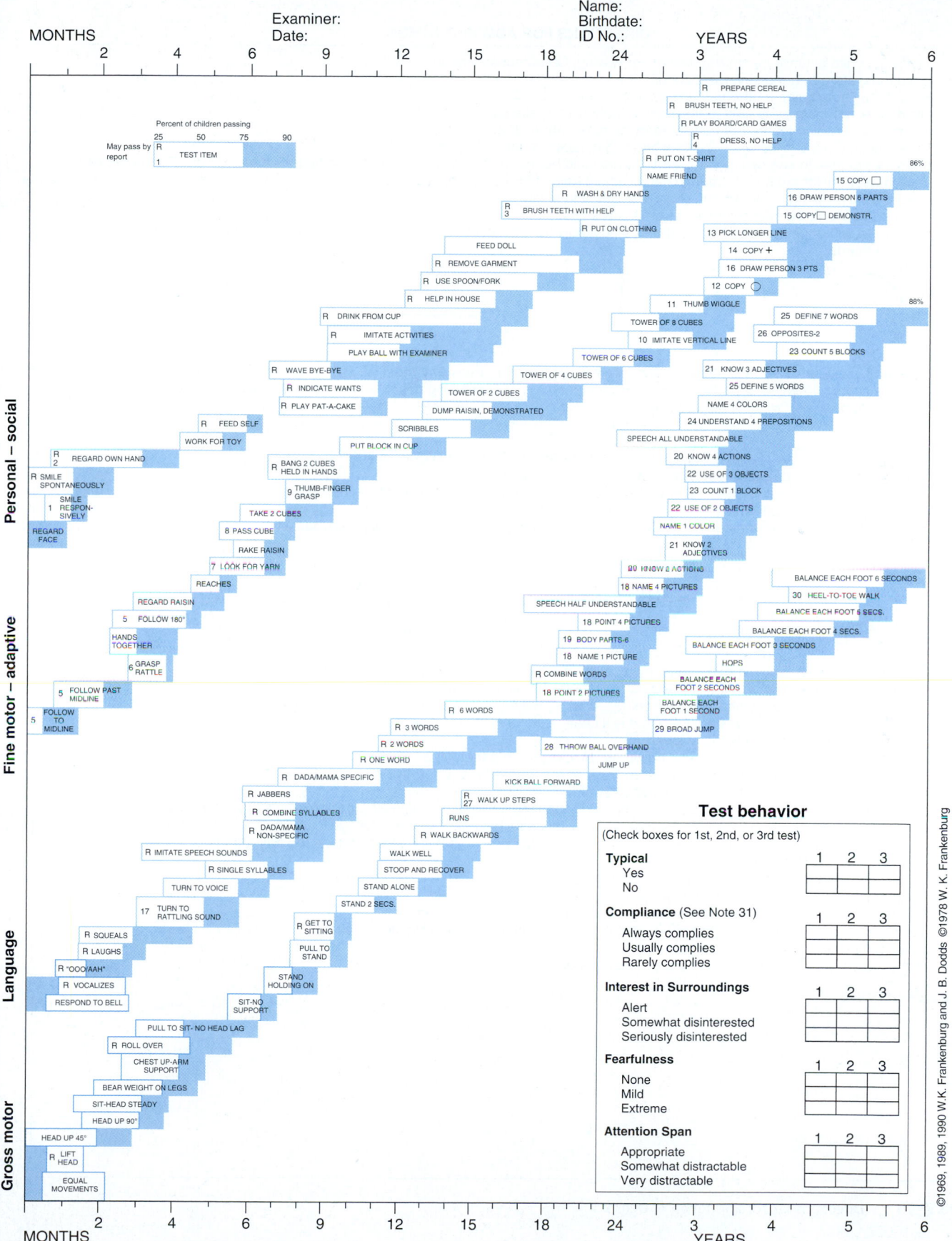

Figure 7–5A ▶ Denver II.

DIRECTIONS FOR ADMINISTRATION

1. Try to get child to smile by smiling, talking, or waving. Do not touch him/her.
2. Child must stare at hand several seconds.
3. Parent may help guide toothbrush and put toothpaste on brush.
4. Child does not have to be able to tie shoes or button/zip in the back.
5. Move yarn slowly in an arc from one side to the other, about 8" above child's face.
6. Pass if child grasps rattle when it is touched to the backs or tips of fingers.
7. Pass if child tries to see where yarn went. Yarn should be dropped quickly from sight from tester's hand without arm movement.
8. Child must transfer cube from hand to hand without help of body, mouth, or table.
9. Pass if child picks up raisin with any part of thumb and finger.
10. Line can vary only 30 degrees or less from tester's line.
11. Make a fist with thumb pointing upward and wiggle only the thumb. Pass if child imitates and does not move any fingers other than the thumb.

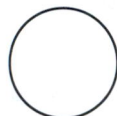 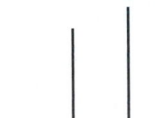 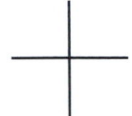 

12. Pass any enclosed form. Fail continuous round motions.
13. Which line is longer? (Not bigger.) Turn paper upside down and repeat. (pass 3 of 3 or 5 of 6).
14. Pass any lines crossing near midpoint.
15. Have child copy first. If failed, demonstrate.

When giving items 12, 14, and 15, do not name the forms. Do not demonstrate 12 and 14.

16. When scoring, each pair (2 arms, 2 legs, etc.) counts as one part.
17. Place one cube in cup and shake gently near child's ear, but out of sight. Repeat for other ear.
18. Point to picture and have child name it. (No credit is given for sounds only.)
    If less than 4 pictures are named correctly, have child point to picture as each is named by tester.

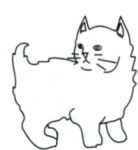 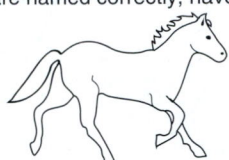 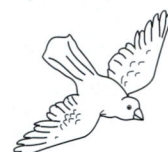 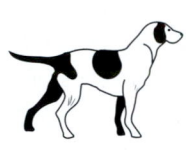 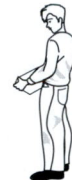

19. Using doll, tell child: Show me the nose, eyes, ears, mouth, hands, feet, tummy, hair. Pass 6 of 8.
20. Using pictures, ask child: Which one flies?... says meow?... talks?... barks?... gallops? Pass 2 of 5, 4 of 5.
21. Ask child: What do you do when you are cold?... tired?... hungry? Pass 2 of 3, 3 of 3.
22. Ask child: What do you do with a cup? What is a chair used for? What is a pencil used for? Action words must be included in answers.
23. Pass if child correctly places <u>and</u> says how many blocks are on paper. (1, 5).
24. Tell child: Put block **on** table; **under** table; **in front of** me, **behind** me. Pass 4 of 4. (Do not help child by pointing, moving head or eyes.)
25. Ask child: What is a ball?... lake?... desk?... house?... banana?... curtain?... fence?... ceiling? Pass if defined in terms of use, shape, what it is made of, or general category (such as banana is fruit, not just yellow). Pass 5 of 8, 7 of 8.
26. Ask child: If a horse is big, a mouse is_____? If fire is hot, ice is_____? If sun shines during the day, the moon shines during the _____? Pass 2 of 3.
27. Child may use wall or rail only, not person. May not crawl.
28. Child must throw ball overhand 3 feet to within arm's reach of tester.
29. Child must perform standing broad jump over width of test sheet (8 1/2 inches).
30. Tell child to walk forward, ⊂○⊂○⊂○ → heel within 1 inch of toe. Tester may demonstrate. Child must walk 4 consecutive steps.
31. In the second year, half of normal children are non-compliant.

OBSERVATIONS:

Figure 7–5B ➤ Directions for administration of Denver II.

age and activity ensures that children have the energy for proper growth, physical activity, cognition, and immune function. Nutrition is closely linked to both health promotion and health maintenance. See Chapter 4 ∞ for detailed nutritional assessment recommendations, and this chapter as well as Chapters 8, 9, and 10 ∞ for specific nutritional questions to ask for each age group. Find out what questions parents have about feeding their children. Integrate the special nutritional needs of children with chronic conditions. Use the information gathered to provide both health promotion and health maintenance interventions.

Physical Activity

Physical activity provides many physical and psychological health benefits. However, there is growing disparity between recommendations and reality among most of our children (Patrick, Spear, Holt, & Sofka, 2001). Research by the Centers for Disease Control and Prevention (CDC) using the Youth Media Campaign Longitudinal Survey (YMCLS) of parents and children found that 61.5% of 9- to 13-year old children report that they do not participate in any organized physical activity during hours outside of school. While organized activities are important and consistent forms of exercise, not all children can participate or desire to do so. However, 22.6% of these children reported that they do not engage in ANY physical activity outside of school. Parents noted that barriers to physical activities included transportation problems, lack of opportunities in area, expenses, lack of parental time, and lack of neighborhood safety (CDC, 2003). The nurse inquires about activities the child prefers and the amount of time for activity during the day. As the child grows older, insert questions about sedentary activities such as number of hours spent watching television or playing computer games. See if the child plays sports at school or in the community. Ask about activities in a typical day to measure amount of activity. Once the nurse gathers data about physical activity, interventions are implemented to enhance activity patterns.

Oral Health

While *oral health* may seem to require the knowledge of a specialist, many implications relate to general health care. Oral health is important because teeth assist in language development, impacted or infected teeth lead to systemic illness, and teeth are related to positive self-image formation. Between 4–5 million children in the United States are affected by tooth decay and pain that interfere with activities of daily living such as eating, sleeping, attending school, and speaking (Ryan, 2003). The nurse applies health promotion to dental health by teaching about oral care and access to dental visits. Health maintenance activities relate to prevention of caries and illness related to dental disease.

Mental and Spiritual Health

Mental and spiritual health are important concepts to address in health promotion and health maintenance visits. Parents can be encouraged to keep a record of mental health issues to bring to health supervision visits. This helps them understand that the healthcare professional is willing to partner with them to assist in dealing with mental health. Suggest topics such as child and parental mood, child temperament, stresses and ways that family members manage stress, or sleep patterns. Make notes in the record as a reminder of questions to ask at the next visit (Jellinek, Patel, & Froehle, 2002). The child and family are both observed for appropriateness of affect and mood. Be alert for signs of depression, stress, anxiety, and child abuse/neglect. The nurse establishes both health promotion and health maintenance goals related to child and family mental health. Health promotion goals relate to adequate resources to meet family challenges, protective factors such as involvement in extended family and the community. Teaching stress reduction techniques such as meditation, relaxation, and imagery, as well as providing resources for yoga or other techniques, is helpful. Health maintenance goals relate to prevention of mental health problems. Examples include providing resources

---

CULTURE

Developmental Testing

Be alert that children who have recently come from other countries and even some born in this country who live in families from minority ethnic groups may have difficulty with some items on developmental tests. For example, children who are not skilled in the English language may not understand some instructions or be able to answer questions about definitions of words. If an item such as "wave good-bye" or "plays patty-cake" represents a practice not common in another culture, the child may not have had exposure to the skill. Be alert for cultural variations, allow the child time to learn a developmental skill, and retest on other occasions.

COMMUNITY CARE

Dental Health

Low-income children are especially prone to poor dental health, so efforts are being extended to help families receive care. Many of the State Children's Health Insurance Programs (SCHIP) offer dental services (VanLandeghen, Bronstein, & Brach, 2003). All children in the Medicaid program are eligible for dental coverage in the Early and Periodic Screening, Diagnostic, and Treatment Services (EPSDT). Private and public clinics in many communities provide low-cost or free care for families with limited financial resources (Ryan, 2003). Many families do not realize their children could receive these services. Find out what resources are available in your state and community, and refer as needed. See Chapter 1 ∞ for further descriptions about available programs.

when domestic violence occurs, or referring cases of suspected child abuse or neglect. The **spiritual dimension** is a connection with a greater power than that in the self, and guides a person to strive for inspiration, respect, meaning, and purpose in life (Murray, Zentner, Pangman, & Pangman, 2005). Spiritual health is seen in the large context as those entities that provide meaning in life. For some, this may be membership in a faith-based group; for others, it may be feeling part of a society with a purpose of greater good, or setting goals for the future. Ask about the family's meaningful activities. Provide links to faith-based groups as needed.

The *relationships* that a child establishes with others begin at birth. The first and most important set of relationships develops with the family. The mother, father, siblings, and perhaps extended family are the contexts in which the baby learns to relate with others. With growth the world widens to encompass other children, friends of the family, peers, school, and the larger community network. In the opening scenario, Clarence spends time each day in childcare. The nurse should inquire about important relationships for Clarence and his parents in that setting. Analyzing the child's relationships at all ages provides important clues to social interactions. From the moment the family is called in from a waiting area, be alert for clues to family interactions. Who is present at the visit, and what roles and interactions can be observed? Likewise, other social interactions are important to evaluate. Does the young infant interact in an age-appropriate manner with the healthcare provider or other children in the area? Ask the parents questions about family and social interactions. Once assessment has taken place, establish goals and interventions related to family and social relationships.

Disease Prevention Strategies

Disease prevention strategies focus mainly on health maintenance, or prevention of disease. Some health disruptions can be detected early and treatment for the condition can begin. **Screening** is a procedure used to detect the possible presence of a health condition before symptoms are apparent. It is usually conducted on large groups of individuals at risk for a condition and represents the secondary level of prevention (Figure 7–6 ➤). Examples include developmental screening (described earlier in this chapter), blood pressure screening, and vision/hearing screening. Most screening tests are not diagnostic by themselves but are followed by further diagnostic tests if the screening result is positive. Once a screening test identifies the existence of a health condition, early intervention can begin, with the goal of reducing the severity or complications of the condition.

Another way to prevent diseases is to immunize children against common communicable diseases. See Chapter 18 ∞ for the complete list of childhood immunizations and schedules for administration; see Chapters 8, 9, and 10 ∞ for the most commonly administered immunizations at specific ages. What immunizations are likely needed by Clarence, described in the opening scenario?

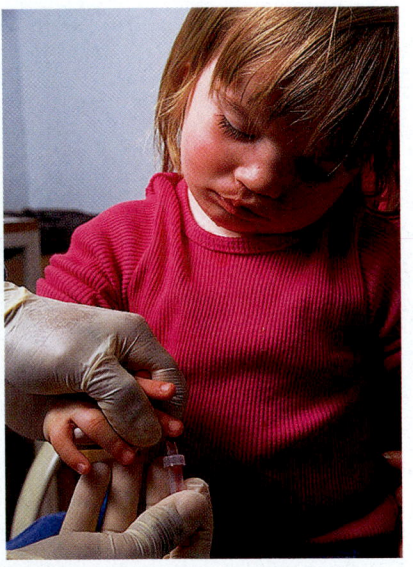

Figure 7–6 ➤ This 18-month-old toddler is having a blood screening test to detect iron deficiency anemia. Children are often screened for adequate levels of iron in later infancy and during toddlerhood.

Injury Prevention Strategies

Most childhood mortality and hospitalization is related to injury (see Chapter 1 ∞). Therefore, it is important for the nurse to integrate *injury prevention* strategies in all health supervision visits. The family is constantly challenged to maintain a safe environment as the child grows older, reaches more advanced developmental levels, is exposed to a widening world outside of the family, and has less supervision. Safety teaching should be integrated with developmental progression. Asking parents to bring their questions about safety to each visit can be a good starting point for discussion. The nurse considers knowledge about the child's age and information from the health supervision visit to plan health maintenance interventions related to injury. Teaching is performed, resources are made available, and parents and children who have experienced injury are invited to present their experiences.

Some common universal injury prevention topics include car safety, pedestrian safety, sports injury prevention, poison prevention, and child abuse prevention.

NURSING MANAGEMENT

Nursing Assessment and Diagnosis

During health supervision visits, a mental portrait of a child and family should be drawn. Observe the parent-child interaction in the waiting room and all throughout the examination. If siblings are present, watch for interactions among all family members. Observe the affect and mood of the child and parents. Nursing assessment of the child and family at each visit for health supervision then focuses on the following:

- Interviewing the family and child to update the health history, to ask about the child's developmental or educational progress, and to identify dietary habits, physical activity, and safety practices
- Eliciting questions and concerns that the parent or child may have
- Conducting developmental surveillance assessments, including review of questionnaires completed by the parent in the waiting room
- Performing age-appropriate screening tests (Table 7–4)
- Performing a physical assessment

Following a thorough assessment, the nurse derives nursing diagnoses that are pertinent for the child's health status and which consider the family needs. Nursing diagnoses are developed jointly with the family as an essential component of the partnership between nurse and family. Examples of nursing diagnoses for an 18-month-old child who is brought by parents for regular health supervision and immunizations may include the following:

- Imbalanced Nutrition: More than Body Requirements related to lack of basic nutritional knowledge
- Risk for Poisoning related to lack of proper precautions with increased mobility to reach and climb
- Health-Seeking Behaviors related to needed immunizations
- Risk for Impaired Parenting related to mother's plans to return to full-time work

Planning and Implementation

Nursing management for health supervision visits begins with collaborative planning with the family. They share their concerns and questions, and the nurse also lists procedures and discussion topics to be addressed. These may include providing immunizations, offering anticipatory guidance about discipline, educating parents and children about healthy behaviors, addressing health promotion regarding nutrition, suggesting ways to prevent disease and injury, and providing referrals for follow-up care. For more information about the recommended schedule for immunizations and the nurse's role in ensuring full immunization status for children, refer to Chapter 18 ∞.

Most parents want to know how to contribute to their child's growth and development. Discussions at the conclusion of the health supervision assessments should focus on building family strengths by promoting the development of competence, confidence, and self-esteem in the growing child. Offering health promotion activities such as these provides a positive ending for the visit. Inquire about the family stresses and strengths in order to plan with them to provide for the child's health promotion.

Although health supervision most likely takes place in an office or clinic setting, most of the nursing management for health supervision can occur in any setting. The nurse recognizes that health promotion and health maintenance activities are key to any nurse-family relationship. For example, if the child is seen in an emergency room for treatment of a fracture, the nurse should ask about immunization status and safety issues. A child with a chronic disorder such as cerebral palsy may obtain most health promotion and health maintenance services in the outpatient clinic at an orthopedic hospital. A child hospitalized for an acute respiratory illness often has a parent present; the nurse should explore the health promotion questions that parent has and perform some teaching about developmental findings. Health promotion is a constant and foundational aspect of all pediatric care. Viewing it as essential ensures that this part of health care, which most closely reflects

Table 7–4	RECOMMENDATIONS FOR PREVENTIVE PEDIATRIC HEALTH CARE, COMMITTEE ON PRACTICE AND AMBULATORY MEDICINE, AMERICAN ACADEMY OF PEDIATRICS, UNITED STATES

Each child and family is unique; therefore, these **Recommendations for Preventive Pediatric Health Care** are designed for the care of children who are receiving competent parenting, have no manifestations of any important health problems, and are growing and developing in satisfactory fashion. **Additional visits may become necessary** if circumstances suggest variations from normal.

These guidelines represent a consensus by the Committee on Practice and Ambulatory Medicine in consultation with national committees and sections of the American Academy of Pediatrics. The Committee emphasizes the great importance of **continuity of care** in comprehensive health supervision and the need to avoid **fragmentation of care**.

AGE[5]	PRENATAL[1]	NEWBORN[2]	2-4d[3]	By 1mo	2mo	4mo	6mo	9mo	12mo	15mo	18mo	24mo	3y	4y
HISTORY Initial/Interval	•	•	•	•	•	•	•	•	•	•	•	•	•	•
MEASUREMENTS Height and Weight		•	•	•	•	•	•	•	•	•	•	•	•	•
Head Circumference		•	•	•	•	•	•	•	•	•	•	•		
Blood Pressure													•	•
SENSORY SCREENING Vision		S	S	S	S	S	S	S	S	S	S	S	O[6]	O
Hearing		O[7]	S	S	S	S	S	S	S	S	S	S	S	O
DEVELOPMENTAL/ BEHAVIORAL ASSESSMENT[8]		•	•	•	•	•	•	•	•	•	•	•	•	•
PHYSICAL EXAMINATION[9]		•	•	•	•	•	•	•	•	•	•	•	•	•
PROCEDURES-GENERAL[10] Hereditary/Metabolic Screening[11]			←—	•	—→									
Immunization[12]		•		•	•	•	•	•	•	•	•			•
Hematocrit or Hemoglobin[13]								→—	—→	★	★	★	★	★
Urinalysis														
PROCEDURES-PATIENTS AT RISK Lead Screening[16]								★—→				★		
Tuberculin Test[17]									★	★	★	★	★	★
Cholesterol Screening[18]												★	★	★
STD Screening[19]														
Pelvic Exam[20]														
ANTICIPATORY GUIDANCE[21]	•	•		•	•	•	•	•	•	•	•	•	•	•
Injury Prevention[22]	•	•		•	•	•	•	•	•	•	•	•	•	•
Violence Prevention[23]	•	•		•	•	•	•	•	•	•	•	•	•	•
Sleep Positioning Counseling[24]	•	•		•	•	•	•							
Nutrition Counseling[25]	•	•		•	•	•	•	•	•	•	•	•	•	•
DENTAL REFERRAL[26]									←————————————			•		

Headers: INFANCY[4,5] (PRENATAL–12mo), EARLY CHILDHOOD[4,5] (15mo–4y)

AGE[5]	5y	6y	8y	10y	11y	12y	13y	14y	15y	16y	17y	18y	19y	20y	21y
HISTORY Initial/Interval	•	•	•	•	•	•	•	•	•	•	•	•	•	•	•
MEASUREMENTS Height and Weight	•	•	•	•	•	•	•	•	•	•	•	•	•	•	•
Head Circumference															
Blood Pressure	•	•	•	•	•	•	•	•	•	•	•	•	•	•	•
SENSORY SCREENING Vision	O	O	O	O	S	O	S	S	O	S	S	O	S	S	S
Hearing	O	O	O	O	S	O	S	S	O	S	S	O	S	S	S
DEVELOPMENTAL/ BEHAVIORAL ASSESSMENT[8]	•	•	•	•	•	•	•	•	•	•	•	•	•	•	•
PHYSICAL EXAMINATION[9]	•	•	•	•	•	•	•	•	•	•	•	•	•	•	•
PROCEDURES-GENERAL[10] Hereditary/Metabolic Screening[11]															
Immunization[12]	•	•	•	•	•	•	•	•	•	•	•	•	•		•
Hematocrit or Hemoglobin[13]	★				←————————— •[14] —————————————→										
Urinalysis	•				←————————————— [15] ——————————————→										
PROCEDURES-PATIENTS AT RISK Lead Screening[16]															
Tuberculin Test[17]	★	★	★	★	★	★	★	★	★	★	★	★	★	★	★
Cholesterol Screening[18]	★	★	★	★	★	★	★	★	★	★	★	★	★	★	★
STD Screening[19]					★	★	★	★	★	★	★	★	★	★	★
Pelvic Exam[20]					★	★	★	★	★	★	★	★	←—[20]—★—→		★
ANTICIPATORY GUIDANCE[21]	•	•	•	•	•	•	•	•	•	•	•	•	•	•	•
Injury Prevention[22]	•	•	•	•	•	•	•	•	•	•	•	•	•	•	•
Violence Prevention[23]	•	•	•	•	•	•	•	•	•	•	•	•	•	•	•
Sleep Positioning Counseling[24]															
Nutrition Counseling[25]	•	•	•	•	•	•	•	•	•	•	•	•	•	•	•
DENTAL REFERRAL[26]															

Headers: MIDDLE CHILDHOOD[4,5] (5y–10y), ADOLESCENCE[4,5] (11y–21y)

| Table 7–4 | RECOMMENDATIONS FOR PREVENTIVE PEDIATRIC HEALTH CARE, COMMITTEE ON PRACTICE AND AMBULATORY MEDICINE, AMERICAN ACADEMY OF PEDIATRICS, UNITED STATES (continued) |

1. A prenatal visit is recommended for parents who are at high risk, for first-time parents, and for those who request a conference. The prenatal visit should include anticipatory guidance, pertinent medical history, and a discussion of benefits of breastfeeding and planned method of feeding per AAP statement "The Prenatal Visit" (1996).
2. Every infant should have a newborn evaluation after birth. Breastfeeding should be encouraged and instruction and support offered. Every breastfeeding infant should have an evaluation 48–72 hours after discharge from the hospital to include weight, formal breastfeeding evaluation, encouragement, and instruction as recommended in the AAP statement "Breastfeeding and the Use of Human Milk" (1997).
3. For newborns discharged in less than 48 hours after delivery per AAP statement "Hospital Stay for Healthy Term Newborns" (1995).
4. Developmental, psychosocial, and chronic disease issues for children and adolescents may require frequent counseling and treatment visits separate from preventive care visits.
5. If a child comes under care for the first time at any point on the schedule, or if any items are not accomplished at the suggested age, the schedule should be brought up to date at the earliest possible time.
6. If the patient is uncooperative, rescreen within 6 months.
7. All newborns should be screened per the AAP Task Force on Newborn and Infant Hearing statement, "Newborn and Infant Hearing Loss: Detection and Intervention" (1999).
8. By history and appropriate physical examination: if suspicious, by specific objective developmental testing. Parenting skills should be fostered at every visit.
9. At each visit, a complete physical examination is essential, with infant totally unclothed, older child undressed and suitably draped.
10. These may be modified, depending upon entry point into schedule and individual need.
11. Metabolic screening (eg, thyroid, hemoglobinopathies, PKU, galactosemia) should be done according to state law.
12. Schedule(s) per the Committee on Infectious Diseases, published annually in the January edition of *Pediatrics*. Every visit should be an opportunity to update and complete a child's immunizations.
13. See AAP *Pediatric Nutrition Handbook* (2004) for a discussion of universal and selective screening options. Consider earlier screening for high-risk infants (eg, premature infants and low birth weight infants). See also "Recommendations to Prevent and Control Iron Deficiency in the United States". *MMWR.* 1998;47 (RR-3):1–29.
14. All menstruating adolescents should be screened annually.
15. Conduct dipstick urinalysis for leukocytes annually for sexually active male and female adolescents.
16. For children at risk of lead exposure consult the AAP statement "Screening for Elevated Blood Levels" (1998). Additionally, screening should be done in accordance with state law where applicable.
17. TB testing per recommendations of the Committee on Infectious Diseases, published in the current edition of *Red Book: Report of the Committee on Infectious Diseases*. Testing should be done upon recognition of high-risk factors.
18. Cholesterol screening for high-risk patients per AAP statement "Cholesterol in Childhood" (1998). If family history cannot be ascertained and other risk factors are present, screening should be at the discretion of the physician.
19. All sexually active patients should be screened for sexually transmitted diseases (STDs).
20. All sexually active females should have a pelvic examination. A pelvic examination and routine pap smear should be offered as part of preventive health maintenance between the ages of 18 and 21 years.
21. Age-appropriate discussion and counseling should be an integral part of each visit for care per the AAP *Guidelines for Health Supervision III* (1998).
22. From birth to age 12, refer to the AAP injury prevention program (TIPP*) as described in *A Guide to Safety Counseling in Office Practice* (1994).
23. Violence prevention and management for all patients per AAP Statement "The Role of the Pediatrician in Youth Violence Prevention in Clinical Practice and at the Community Level" (1999).
24. Parents and caregivers should be advised to place healthy infants on their backs when putting them to sleep. Side positioning is a reasonable alternative but carries a slightly higher risk of SIDS. Consult the AAP statement "Changing Concepts of Sudden Infant Death Syndrome: Implications for Infant Sleeping Environment and Sleep Position" (2000).
25. Age-appropriate nutrition counseling should be an integral part of each visit per the AAP *Handbook of Nutrition* (1998).
26. Earlier initial dental examinations may be appropriate for some children. Subsequent examinations as prescribed by dentist.

Key: • = to be performed   * = to be performed by patients at risk

    S = subjective, by history   0 = objective, by a standard testing method

◄——•——► = the range during which a service may be provided, with the dot indicating the preferred age.

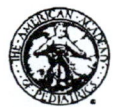

American Academy of Pediatrics

NB: Special chemical, immunologic, and endocrine testing is usually carried out upon specific indications. Testing other than newborn (eg. inborn errors of metabolism, sickle disease, etc) is discretionary with the physician.

Used with permission of the American Academy of Pediatrics (2004).

a partnership with families, will be part of every healthcare encounter. Health maintenance information is included to lessen disease and injury risk (see the Bindler-Ball Pediatric Healthcare Continuum in Chapter 1). Some specific nursing actions for health supervision are described in the following text.

Provide Anticipatory Guidance

Anticipatory guidance involves prediction of the upcoming developmental tasks or needs of a child and gears teaching to those needs. It provides the family with information on what to expect during the child's current and next stage of development. Topics for each visit should include age-appropriate information about healthy habits, prevention of illness and injury, prevention of poisoning, nutrition, oral health, and sexuality. Use health promotional guidance to help the child and family develop strategies that support and enhance social development, family relationships, parental health, community interactions, self-responsibility, and school or vocational achievement.

Because the time for each visit is limited, build upon the parents' current knowledge and care practices, and start with a topic about which they express interest. Time can be used to focus on anticipatory guidance to introduce new information, to reinforce what the family is doing well, and to clear up any poorly understood concepts.

Take advantage of other sources of information in the community to enhance the guidance provided. For example, state and local SAFE KIDS coalitions help inform families about injury-prevention strategies. School health programs such as the National Fire Prevention Association's "Risk Watch" may educate children about injury prevention, and other school programs may educate students about smoking and drug avoidance. Keep informed about the types of health education provided in different community settings so it is easier to reinforce the concepts already being taught.

Encourage Health Promotion Activities

Families often need health education and counseling to promote healthy behaviors in their own child. Examples of focused health education and counseling may be information about environmental control to limit sedentary behaviors, dietary changes to increase fruit and vegetable intake, and switching to low-fat dairy products. Counseling in the case of the 18-month-old toddler for whom nursing diagnoses were previously stated could focus on childcare arrangements and the anticipation and management of potential behavior problems. Collaborate with the parents to learn about their concerns and how they want to improve their parenting.

Patient education and counseling are most effective when the family understands the relationship between a behavior change and the resulting health outcome. When identifying that a family would benefit from a change in health behavior, consider the family members' perceptions about the health change, barriers and benefits to change, and plan interventions to enhance the possibility for change.

Steps in promoting patient education and counseling include:

- Clarifying learning needs of child and family
- Setting a limited agenda
- Prioritizing needs with family
- Selecting teaching strategy (explaining, showing, providing resources, questioning, practicing, giving feedback)
- Evaluating effectiveness (Green & Palfrey, 2002)

Perform Health Supervision Interventions

After all of the information from the interviews, physical assessment, and screening tests is collected and analyzed, specific health and developmental achievements should be summarized for the parents and child. Immunizations are provided as appropriate. Anticipatory guidance may be offered at various points during the health supervision visit.

When a child is found to be at risk for a health condition, integrate health maintenance interventions to lessen the possibility of disease or injury. If an actual health problem is detected, follow-up care must be arranged. The child may need to return for another visit to the primary care provider for further evaluation, or referral to another provider may be needed. The nurse needs to learn about all of the available community resources to make appropriate referrals. The range of such services may include the following:

- Hospital and community-based healthcare specialists from many disciplines (dentists, physicians, physical therapists, speech therapists, nutritionists, social workers)
- Community-based programs (childcare centers, developmental stimulation programs, home visitor programs, early intervention programs, mental health centers, diagnostic and evaluation centers, schools, family support centers, food and nutrition referral centers, public health clinics, churches, and other organizations that support families and children)

Evaluation

Expected outcomes of nursing care include the following:

- The child and family collaborate in a partnership with the healthcare provider in joint problem solving and decision making regarding the management of the child's healthcare needs after appropriate education and counseling.
- The child and family prepare for future health supervision visits by identifying questions or concerns they want to discuss.

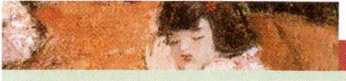

CRITICAL THINKING IN ACTION

Recall the parents of 15-month-old Clarence. They are working parents who are overwhelmed by their son's activity level. They express concern about how to spend time with and ensure safety for Clarence, while having some time to spend with each other.

1. Describe the physical activity skills that you expect to observe in a 15-month-old. Is Clarence typical of this age child?

2. Plan the assessment techniques you will apply to learn more about Clarence's physical activity and social interactions.

3. Clarence's parents are concerned about providing a safe environment for him. List the most important safety precautions that should be taken in the home and during car trips to promote his safety.

4. Plan several interventions that will assist his parents in planning their time so that they have time to spend with Clarence every day and also have some time alone to rest each week.

 Refer to your Prentice Hall Nursing MediaLink DVD-ROM for answers.

EXPLORE MediaLink 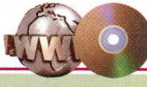 http://www.prenhall.com/ball

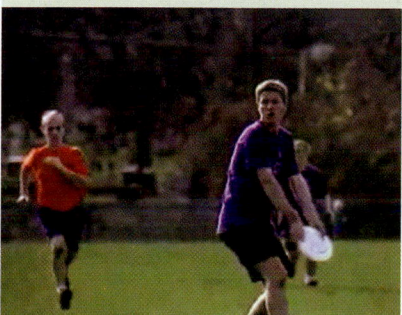

Resources for this chapter can be found on the Prentice Hall Nursing MediaLink DVD-ROM accompanying this textbook, and on the Companion Website at http://www.prenhall.com/ball.

DVD-ROM
Audio Glossary
NCLEX-RN® Review
Videos
  Health Promotion and Health Maintenance
  Healthy People 2010

COMPANION WEBSITE
Audio Glossary
NCLEX-RN® Review
Care Plan Activity: The Child Experiencing Night Terrors
Case Study: Health Promotion
Critical Thinking: Developmental Questionnaires for Toddlers
MediaLink Applications
  Goals of Healthy People 2010
  Outreach Clinics
  Well Child Clinics
WebLinks

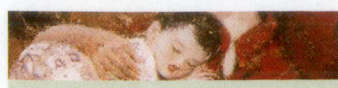

REFERENCES

American Academy of Pediatrics. (2002). The medical home. Policy statement. *Pediatrics 110*, 184–186.

American Academy of Pediatric Dentistry. (2004). *Policy on the dental home*. Chicago, IL: Author.

Centers for Disease Control and Prevention (CDC). (2003). Physical activity levels among children aged 9–13 years—United States, 2002. *Morbidity and Mortality Weekly Report (MMWR), 52,* 785–788.

Earls, M. F., & Hay, S. S. (2006). Setting the state for success: Implementation of developmental and behavioral screening and surveillance in primary care practice—The North Carolina Assuring Better Child Health and Development (ABCD) Project. *Pediatrics 118*, 183–188.

Frankenburg, S. K. (2004). Rethinking well-child care. *Pediatrics 114*, 1736–1737.

Green, M., & Palfrey J. S., (eds.). (2002). *Bright futures: Guidelines for health supervision of infants, children, and adolescents* (2nd ed., rev.). Arlington, VA: National Center for Education in Maternal and Child Health.

Jellinek, M., Patel, B. P., Froehle., M. C. (ed.). (2002). *Bright futures in practice; Mental health Vol II, tool kit.* Arlington, VA: National Center for Education in Maternal and Child Health.

Murray, R. B., Zentner, J. P., Pangman, V. C., & Pangman, C. (2005). *Health promotion strategies through the lifespan.* Newmarket, Ontario: Pearson Education Canada.

NAPNAP. (2002). NAPNAP position statement on the pediatric healthcare home. Retrieved August 25, 2003, from National Association of Pediatric Nurse Practitioners at http://www.napnap.org/practice/positions/healthcarehome.html

Patrick, K., Spear, B., Holt, K., & Sofka, D. (Eds.). (2001). *Bright futures in practice: Physical activity.* Arlington, VA: National Center for Education in Maternal and Child Health.

Pender, N. J., Murdaugh, C. L., & Parsons, M. A. (2006). *Health promotion in nursing practice* (5th ed.). Upper Saddle River, NJ: Prentice Hall.

Ryan, J. (2003). Improving oral health: Promise and prospects. *National Health Policy Forum background paper.* Washington, DC: The George Washington University.

VanLandeghen, L., Bronstein, J., & Brach, C. (2003). *Children's dental care access in Medicaid. The role of medical care use and dentist participation.* CHIRI Issue Brief 2. AHRQ Publication No. 03-0032. Rockville, MD: Agency for Healthcare Research and Quality. Retrieved on June 30, 2003, from http://www.ahrq.gov/about/cods/chirident.htm

Williams, J., & Holmes, C. A. (2004). Improving the early detection of children with subtle developmental problems. *Journal of Child Health Care, 8,* 34–46.

World Health Organization. (1996). *Basic document.* Geneva, Switzerland: WHO.

World Health Organization. (2001). Background information about health promotion. Retrieved June 6, 2003, from http://www.who.int/hpr/backgroundhp/

World Health Organization. (2005). From Bangkok, A new push for health promotion. *Newsletter of the PanAmerican Health Organization.* Retrieved July 11, 2006, from http://www.paho.org/English/DD/PIN/ptoday22_nov05.htm

HEALTH PROMOTION AND HEALTH MAINTENANCE FOR THE NEWBORN AND INFANT

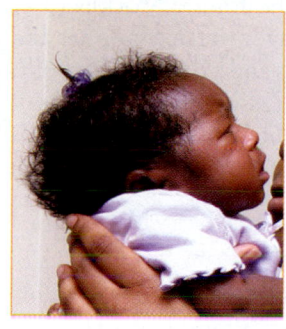

SHANNON comes to the pediatric health services clinic with her 10-day-old daughter, Rhonda. Shannon is a 22-year-old single mother who lives with her 5-year-old daughter and male partner of 2 years, who is the father of their newborn. Shannon had an uncomplicated pregnancy and birth. Rhonda was born at 37 weeks' gestation. She required phototherapy for newborn jaundice and had initial difficulties breast-feeding. Rhonda was discharged at 5 days of age in good health. The nurse weighs and measures Rhonda, and finds that she weighs 1 ounce more than her birth weight. Shannon voices concerns that Rhonda sleeps very little, cries a lot at night, and makes sleep difficult for her boyfriend, who has to get up early for work. The nurse asks Shannon how she knows when Rhonda is ready to feed. Shannon recognizes only Rhonda's crying as a feeding cue. The nurse gives Shannon information on newborn states and cues, and encourages Shannon to notice more subtle feeding cues. The nurse calls the lactation consultant and together they assess Rhonda's breast-feeding effectiveness. The lactation consultant works with Shannon on a feeding plan to ensure that breast feeding is successful. The pediatric nurse then partners with Shannon to strategize how to help Rhonda sleep for longer periods, recognizing that newborns often do not settle into a schedule until well into the second month. What ongoing assessment will Rhonda and her parents need? How can the nurse encourage shared parenting between Shannon and her boyfriend? What coordinated follow-up is required between the pediatric nurse and the lactation consultant?

KEY TERMS

attachment behaviors **284**
dental home **287**
developmental delay **285**
pediatric health care home **294**
self-regulation **288**
separation anxiety **300**
stranger anxiety **300**

MediaLink

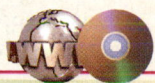

http://www.prenhall.com/ball

See the Prentice Hall Nursing MediaLink DVD-ROM and Companion Website for chapter-specific resources.

LEARNING OUTCOMES

After reading this chapter, you will be able to do the following:

1. Explore the nurse's role in providing health promotion and health maintenance for the newborn, infant, and family.

2. Describe the general observations made of infants and their families as they come to the pediatric healthcare home for health supervision visits.

3. Describe assessment and intervention areas for health supervision visits of newborns and infants—growth and developmental surveillance, nutrition, physical activity, oral health, mental and spiritual health, family and social relations, disease prevention strategies, and injury prevention strategies.

(continued)

Learning Outcomes, continued

4. Plan health promotion and health maintenance strategies employed during health supervision visits of newborns and infants.

5. Apply the nursing process in assessment, diagnosis, goal setting, intervention, and evaluation of health promotion and health maintenance activities for the newborn and infant.

6. Recognize the importance of family in newborn and infant health care, and include family assessment in each health supervision visit.

CLINICAL TIP

Administration of medications can be stressful for the newborn and parents.

- Administer eye prophylaxis before, or at a different time, than the vitamin K injection. The newborn may cry during the vitamin K injection, making it difficult to administer ophthalmic ointment.
- Administer eye prophylaxis when the newborn is calm. Do not attempt to pry the newborn's eyes open when the newborn is crying, or when the infant is supine and facing bright overhead lights. Dim the room, swaddle or contain the newborn's limbs, and hold the newborn semi-upright. If the newborn is awake or drowsy, the eyes will usually open, allowing easier administration of the ophthalmic ointment.
- The newborn is less likely to cry during the vitamin K injection if the nurse lays the newborn on a firm surface and the parent gently holds the newborn's arms across the newborn's chest during the injection. This "containment" helps the newborn stay calm during the procedure.

NURSING ALERT

Cord care practices vary according to region and are often based on institutional tradition rather than evidence-based practice. The objective of cord care is to prevent infection and promote cord separation. Cord care practices include no care, application of triple dye, and application of povidone-iodone, isopropyl alcohol, or antimicrobial ointments. Aseptic cord care decreases bacterial colonization but delays cord separation (Blackburn, 2003, p. 538).

HEALTH PROMOTION AND HEALTH MAINTENANCE FOR THE NEWBORN

For a healthy woman, prenatal care, labor, and birth may be her first experience in an ongoing relationship with healthcare professionals. The quality of that experience is key to ensuring a continuing partnership between her and her child's healthcare providers.

The month following delivery is a time of huge transition for the new mother and her family. Not only is the mother coping with hormonal shifts and a postpartum body, but also changing roles and relationships. The nurse's role is to assess knowledge about self-care and newborn care, teach health promotion and maintenance activities, promote parental confidence in newborn caregiving, and promote a partnership among healthcare professionals and the family.

Contacts with the Family

The nurse who sees the expectant woman during prenatal care has the unique opportunity to help parents prepare for their new roles. The nurse listens attentively and provides information and support. During prenatal visits, parents learn to value health supervision and an active partnership with healthcare professionals. The nurse who interacts with the family in the prenatal period assesses risk and protective factors. Women are often receptive to altering risky behaviors in order to protect the newborn from harm. The motivation to give birth to a healthy newborn is usually strong, and the nurse can use maternal readiness for change to promote behaviors that improve maternal and newborn health.

Most obstetrical care providers encourage the expectant mother to choose her newborn's care provider prior to the baby's birth. Pediatric care providers usually welcome a short office visit, sometimes at no charge, to allow the expectant mother and care provider to assess their "fit" prior to committing to this important relationship (AAP, 2001; Shelov, 2004) (See Families Want to Know: Prenatal Visit to the Pediatric Care Provider). Most pediatric care providers have written information for expectant parents, explaining their professional philosophy of care as well as information about services.

The hospital length of stay for a healthy mother and newborn is short, approximately 48 hours for a vaginal birth and 72–96 hours for an uncomplicated cesarean birth; a hospital stay of less than 48 hours requires that certain criteria be met prior to newborn discharge [American Academy of Pediatrics (AAP), 2004b]. During the hospital stay, the nurse provides ongoing physical assessment of the mother and newborn, while providing education and anticipatory guidance to prepare the mother to care for herself and her newborn following hospital discharge.

Although challenging, the nurse incorporates many newborn health promotion and maintenance activities into this short stay. Starting at the moment of birth, the newborn is continuously assessed and procedures are performed to ensure newborn health. The nurse integrates methods that will help the newborn to adapt to the setting.

For the healthy newborn, early contacts include procedures such as first bath, umbilical cord care (Figure 8–1 ➤), vitamin K and hepatitis B injections, and eye prophylaxis; comprehensive physical assessment (see Chapter 5 ∞ for details); screening procedures such as hearing, metabolic, and maternal syphilis screenings (AAP, 2004b); and observations of newborn feeding and of parent/newborn bonding. See the Medications Used to Treat Newborns on page 284.

FAMILIES WANT TO KNOW

Prenatal Visit to the Pediatric Care Provider

Encourage parents to visit the pediatric healthcare home before the baby is born. This ensures that the home will provide the type of care they want for their infant. Assist parents to prepare questions and make an appointment to visit the provider they are interested in interviewing.

Questions they can ask the provider include:

- How soon after birth will the baby be seen? Can parents be present during the initial physical examination? Will you speak with us again before hospital discharge?
- What is your philosophy about male circumcision? Do you perform circumcision? If not, who does this procedure? Is circumcision performed in the hospital before discharge or in the office after discharge?
- What if our baby needs intensive care? Under what circumstances would our baby need to be transported to a different hospital? Would you continue to provide the baby's care during the hospital stay and after discharge?
- When is our newborn's first office visit? Do we call for that appointment or is it made for us while we are in the hospital?
- As our baby's provider, what can I expect from you? What do you think is your most important job? What do you enjoy most about your work?
- As the parent of a new baby, what do you expect from me? What is my most important job?
- What are the costs of care? Do you accept my method of payment/insurance/government assistance?
- What are office hours? Do you take emergency calls from your own patients at night? What number do we call if we have a question or if we think the baby is sick outside of office hours?

- Who covers your office when you are unavailable? Do you have partners in the office or colleagues in the community who cover for you when you are out? May I have a list of their names and phone numbers?
- Who else answers our questions about routine baby and childcare? What is that person's training? May we meet that person today?
- How much time is usually spent for an office visit? How much time will we have to ask questions?
- If our child needs hospitalization, what hospital do you prefer to use? Would you be our baby's doctor, or would you refer the hospital care to someone else? Why?
- What do you think are the most important things you offer to new families like us? Do you have resources to support breast-feeding mothers? Working mothers?
- If we disagree about a childcare issue or a course of treatment, how would we come to an understanding?

After the interview, parents can ask themselves the following questions:

- Was I comfortable talking with this person? Did this person listen to me?
- Did I get clear answers to my questions?
- Do I feel that I could trust this provider with my child's care?
- Was I comfortable in the office? Did I feel welcome?
- Were all staff members friendly and helpful? Did all staff members seem good at their jobs?
- Did I feel like this provider would be a good "fit" for my family? (AAP, 2001; Shelov, 2004)

At discharge, the family is given an appointment for the first visit in the office or clinic setting; a physician, nurse practitioner, or nurse assessment is recommended at 3–5 days of age, with subsequent follow-up visits for newborns at risk for hyperbilirubinemia or feeding problems (AAP, 2004b). See Families Want to Know: Discharge Teaching for New Parents.

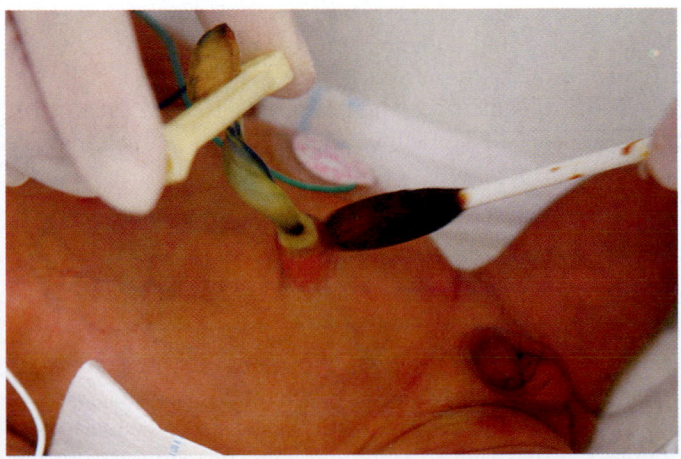

A

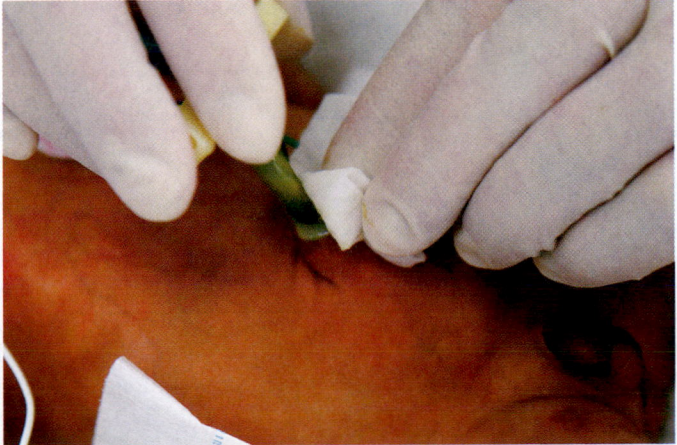

B

Figure 8–1 ➤ Two different methods for cord care: A, Betadine cleaning, and B, Alcohol cleaning.

PROPHYLACTIC MEDICATIONS *Used to Treat Newborns*

Medication	Prophylactic Action/Implication	Nursing Implications
Vitamin K (phytonadione)	To prevent vitamin-K dependent hemorrhagic disease of the newborn.	1.0 mg IM is given within 1 hour of birth. Locate accurate site on ventrogluteal thigh.
Sterile ophthalmic ointment containing tetracycline (1%) or erythromycin (0.5%) or one of a variety of topical agents, including ophthalmic solution of povidone-iodine (2.5%)	As prophylaxis against gonococcal ophthalmia neonatorum.	Place 1–2 cm ribbon along the conjunctival sac of each eye within 1 hour of birth, taking care that the agent reaches all areas of the conjunctival sac.
Hepatitis B virus (HBV) immunoprophylaxis	All women should be screened for hepatitis B as part of routine prenatal care. The first hepatitis B vaccination for the newborn is preferably received prior to hospital discharge; if not received, the newborn should receive the first dose at the initial outpatient visit.	• For babies of HbsAg-negative women, the first dose of HBV vaccine is administered during the newborn period (recommended time) or by age 2 months; second dose 1–2 months later, and third dose by age 6–18 months. • Babies of HbsAg-positive women must receive HBV vaccine within 12 hours of birth AND receive one dose of hepatitis B immune globulin (HBIG) within 12 hours of birth at a second imtramuscular site (opposite thigh). Check the mother's record of hepatitis screening so doses can be given within time recommended.

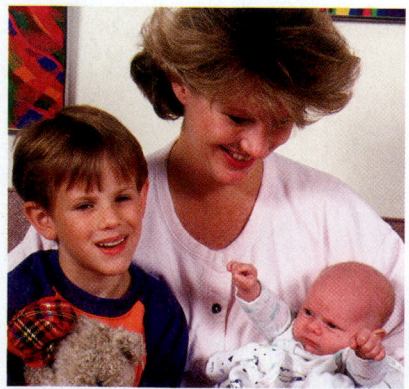

Figure 8–2 ➤ Observation of the newborn and family begins at first contact during the health promotion and health maintenance visit.

General Observations

At the first office visit, the nursing assessment begins with general observations of the newborn and family (Figure 8–2 ➤). This often occurs as the family is called in from the waiting area.

Welcome the family to the facility and comment on the newborn. Ask how the family is adjusting. In the first month of the newborn's life, parents are usually exhausted and experiencing stressful adjustments in their relationship with each other. The nurse gathers information in order to assess the family's needs, to invite discussion, to validate positive parenting efforts, and to promote partnership between the family and the healthcare team.

The nurse assesses development of **attachment behaviors** (behaviors that demonstrate an emotional connection between newborn and caregiver), parental perception of infant temperament, feeding status, safety, family integration, parental mental health, and parental coping mechanisms. Look again at the photo in the chapter opener and identify what attachment behaviors you see Shannon exhibiting toward the baby, Rhonda. The nurse may determine that further assessment is required; for example, if the parent states that breast-feeding is so painful she wants to switch to formula, she is continuously depressed, has started smoking again, or cannot calm her crying baby. The nurse in the pediatric setting is aware that pediatric health is closely connected to the entire family's health. Many concerns require referral for parents out-

FAMILIES WANT TO KNOW

Discharge Teaching for New Parents

Parents should be taught prior to hospital discharge about education materials to help ensure adequate newborn care and instructions regarding how to access healthcare providers for consultation. This information should also be accessible at home. Discharge teaching includes:

- Breast-feeding technique (position, latch, adequacy of urine and stool, lactation referral and resources)
  or
- Formula feeding technique (formula type, preparation, safety, feeding)
- Umbilical cord care
- Bathing and skin care
- How to diaper and dress a newborn
- Temperature assessment using a thermometer
- Signs of newborn illness (Shelov, 2004)
  - Abdominal swelling, especially if accompanied by no bowel movement for 1 or 2 days and/or vomiting
  - Blue skin coloring, especially of the face, lips, or tongue (blue hands and feet are normal in the newborn)

- Persistent coughing or choking during feedings
- Unusually long period of crying that will not stop despite comfort measures
- Jaundice (yellow coloring of the skin) that appears head to toe
- Sleeping through feedings or baby that is too tired or uninterested to eat
- Infected umbilical cord (pus or red skin at base of cord, crying when skin near the cord is touched with your finger)
- Respiratory distress
  - Fast breathing (more than 60 breaths/minute)
  - Retractions (muscles between ribs suck in with each breath)
  - Flaring of nose
  - Grunting while breathing
  - Persistent blue skin color
- Immediate newborn safety
  - Infant car seat use
  - Supine sleeping position

side the pediatric care setting; therefore, the office or clinic should have a system in place and ready access to referrals and resources for parents in need.

Growth and Developmental Surveillance

At this visit, the baby's current weight, length, and head circumference are measured and plotted on a growth chart (see Appendix A ∞), and a basic physical examination is performed (see Chapter 5 ∞).

In the first week of life, most babies lose about 1/10 of their birth weight. For example, a 3500-gram baby (7 pounds, 12 ounces) could lose up to 350 grams (nearly 12 ounces). Growth spurts are evident at around 7–10 days, and again between 3 and 6 weeks of age. By day 10, most babies are back to their original birth weight and gaining about 2/3 of an ounce per day. Length increases by 1–1 ½ inches in the first month, and head circumference increases about 1 inch (Shelov, 2004).

Developmental surveillance includes assessment of the baby's ability to calm when being held or spoken to, and respond to sounds by blinking, crying, quieting, or startling. The baby should be able to fixate on a human face and follow it with his eyes. He or she should be able to lift his or her head momentarily when placed prone, demonstrate a flexed position, and move all extremities. Most babies will sleep for 3 or 4 hours at a time and stay awake for an hour or longer (Green & Palfrey, 2002).

It is normal for parents to compare their newborn's developmental skills with other children of the same age. Every baby develops according to an individual timetable; however, when a baby falls far behind, fails to reach a developmental milestone, or loses a previously acquired skill, the baby requires further evaluation (Shelov, 2004). In the first month of life, signs of **developmental delay** (a delay in mastering functions such as motor coordination and behavioral skills) in a full-term infant usually merit immediate investigation by a pediatrician, pediatric developmental specialist, pediatric neurologist, or a multidisciplinary team of professionals. Parents require additional emotional support, clear and honest communication, and resources to cope with the stress of this situation.

Table 8–1 summarizes some growth and developmental milestones that can commonly be observed during newborn care visits.

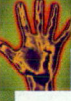

GROWTH & DEVELOPMENT

Signs of Developmental Delay

During the second, third, or fourth week of life, the following signs of potential developmental delay require a complete medical and developmental evaluation to determine if a disability exists and to plan interventions or future management. The pediatric nurse observes the newborn for these signs and may have opportunity to assess for problems through discussing the newborn's abilities and behaviors with the caregiver.

- Sucks poorly and feeds slowly
- Does not blink when shown a bright light
- Does not focus and follow a nearby object moving side to side
- Rarely moves arms and legs; seems stiff
- Seems excessively loose in the limbs, or floppy
- Lower jaw constantly trembles
- Does not respond to loud sounds

(Adapted from Shelov, 2004)

Table 8–1	NEWBORN GROWTH AND DEVELOPMENTAL MILESTONES OBSERVED IN HEALTH PROMOTION AND HEALTH MAINTENANCE VISITS
Growth	• Weight: Baby may lose up to 1/10 of birth weight in the first week of life; birth weight should be re-attained by day 10; weight gain is about 2/3 of an ounce per day thereafter. • Length increases by 1 to 1 1/2 inches. • Head circumference increases by about 1 inch.
Vision	• Focuses 8–12 inches away. • Eyes wander and may cross. • Prefers black and white or high-contrast patterns. • Prefers the human face to all other patterns.
Hearing	• Fully mature hearing. • Recognizes some sounds. • May turn toward familiar sounds and voices.

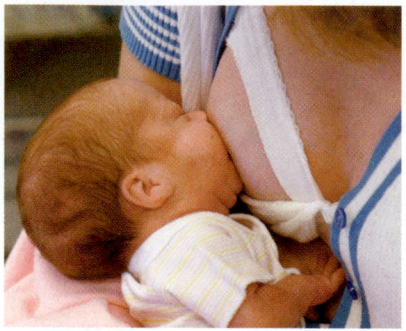

Figure 8–3 ➤ Breast-feeding has lifelong benefits for the mother and child and should be promoted prenatally, in the hospital, and through the first year of health promotion visits.

Nutrition

Healthcare providers in the prenatal setting play a vital role in educating expectant mothers about the health benefits of breast-feeding and providing anticipatory guidance prior to childbirth. The nurse in the birth setting promotes breast-feeding by facilitating nursing in the first 30–60 minutes of life, and providing supportive guidance as the mother begins to develop this skill prior to discharge. Shannon, described in the opening scenario, received breast-feeding information from the nurse and the lactation specialist. Continued assessment, encouragement, and support of breast-feeding are vital to the continued success of breast-feeding mothers, as many mothers initiate breast-feeding and discontinue after a few days or weeks (Committee on Nutrition, 2004). The nurse who encounters breast-feeding mothers should understand the basics of breast-feeding management (Figure 8–3 ➤). Ideally, the pediatric setting has a lactation specialist or resource person who can assess breast-feeding and problem solve with the mother. Referrals to a community lactation specialist or support group may be necessary.

In some cases, mothers choose formula feeding for a newborn. Mothers who use infant formula should feed iron-fortified formula (containing between 4.0–12 mg/L of iron) from birth to 12 months (Committee on Nutrition, 2004). This helps ensure adequate iron stores and very low rates of iron deficiency between 6 and 18 months of age. (See Chapter 4 ∞ for more information about formulas.)

Physical Activity

During the first month of life, the newborn gradually "unfolds" and the body straightens. Movements begin to change from reflexive to purposeful. By the end of the first month, the newborn should be able to:

• Bring hands to eyes and mouth
• Move head side to side when lying on abdomen
• Attempt to lift head when prone

In addition, the newborn's hands are kept in tight fists, and the reflexes are strong (see Chapter 5 ∞) (Shelov, 2004).

Health promotion teaching for the family includes the following activities:

• Position the baby on his or her stomach for supervised play periods. This allows the newborn to lift the head and turn it from side-to-side, make crawling motions, and push up on his or her arms. Allowing supervised "tummy time" is also important for prevention of flat spots on the back of the baby's head caused by constant supine positioning (Persing, James, Swanson, & Kattwinkel, 2003). Be sure to place the baby on his or her back when tired and starting to fall asleep.

- Allow the baby free movement of arms and hands. If the baby is swaddled, allow the hands to be outside the blanket and positioned in midline. This allows flexion and extension of arms, brings hands into the line of vision, and brings hands to mouth (Shelov, 2004).
- Encourage appropriate toys such as a mobile with contrasting colors and patterns; a plastic mirror; music boxes and exposure to soft music on the radio, tape recorder, or CD player; and soft toys with colors, patterns, and gentle sounds.
- Encourage switching positions when bottle-feeding. It may be most comfortable for the mother to hold the baby in a cradle position with the bottle in her right hand (or left hand if left-handed); however, switching arms encourages newborn muscle development and control on each side of the baby's body. Breast-feeding babies automatically feed from both sides. Parents who bottle-feed may need to be reminded to promote this skill in their newborn.
- Beginning at birth, prevent flat spots on the newborn's head from supine positioning by nightly alternating the head position from left to right during sleep and occasionally changing the newborn's orientation in relation to the activity at the room's doorway (Persing, James, Swanson, & Kattwinkel, 2003).

Oral Health

Ideally, pediatric oral health begins with prenatal oral health counseling for parents. If not already established, promotion of healthy oral hygiene practices and routine preventive dental care for parents establishes a foundation for a lifetime of good oral health for their children.

Protective factors for good oral health include good general health, appropriate use of fluoride in family members more than 6 months of age (either topically, in community water systems, or systemically as deemed appropriate by healthcare professionals), high socioeconomic status, family intake of simple sugars occurring primarily at mealtime, and regular use of dental care in an established **dental home**, a specialized dental care provider who manages and facilitates all aspects of oral health care. Risk factors include infant's siblings with dental caries in the past 12 months, active caries present in the mother, suboptimal fluoride exposure, frequent between-meal exposure of family members to simple sugars, low socioeconomic status, no usual source of dental care, and children with special healthcare needs (American Academy of Pediatric Dentistry [AAPD], 2004).

Parents can help prevent decay in their new baby by practicing good oral health habits from birth. In the first month of life, parents should be warned against propping the bottle in the baby's mouth while the baby falls asleep. Babies who sleep with their teeth exposed to juice, formula, or breast milk can develop early childhood caries in primary teeth, even before they emerge. (See Chapter 4 ∞ for further information on early childhood caries.)

Oral disease may be prevented if strategies are applied early enough in the child's life. The nurse plays an important role in assessing risk factors for dental disease, promoting oral hygiene beginning in infancy, and providing anticipatory guidance to help parents ensure good oral health for their children.

Mental and Spiritual Health

Bringing a newborn home can be an overwhelming emotional experience for the mother, her partner, and other family members. An immediate shift in roles and responsibilities must occur within the family. In addition to meeting the newborn's needs, the new mother must also deal with meeting other family members' needs, rapidly shifting emotions, and her postpartum body. At the same time, the family is establishing a secure and healthy atmosphere for the new baby. The nurse assesses signs of a growing secure attachment between parent and child in the first month of life by making observations such as:

- Parent frequently looks at the newborn.
- Parent has specific questions and observations about the newborn's individual characteristics.

RESEARCH

Newborn Self-Regulation

Some newborns and infants have a difficult time learning how to self-soothe, or self-regulate. Particularly affected are those with neurological delays or prematurity. A study was designed to measure the effectiveness of two strategies in assisting babies with brain lesions to quiet when crying. Twelve infants were randomly assigned to receive massage when crying, and 13 were randomly assigned to be swaddled in blankets when crying (Ohgi, Akiyama, Arisawa, & Shigemori, 2004). Parents were instructed in carrying out the prescribed techniques for a 3-week period. Swaddling was found to be the most effective intervention and succeeded in significantly decreasing the infants' crying time. Parents also reported greater satisfaction with this method. While massage therapy may be helpful for some conditions in infants and children, swaddling may be more effective in soothing the crying infant. Teach parents the swaddling technique (place the baby on a blanket and place arms at the sides, bring up the blanket securely around the baby and under one side, bring the other side around so the baby is securely wrapped, bring the bottom up over the feet). Ask about its effectiveness and provide other methods of calming the baby such as rocking, singing, and walking with the baby on the parent's shoulder.

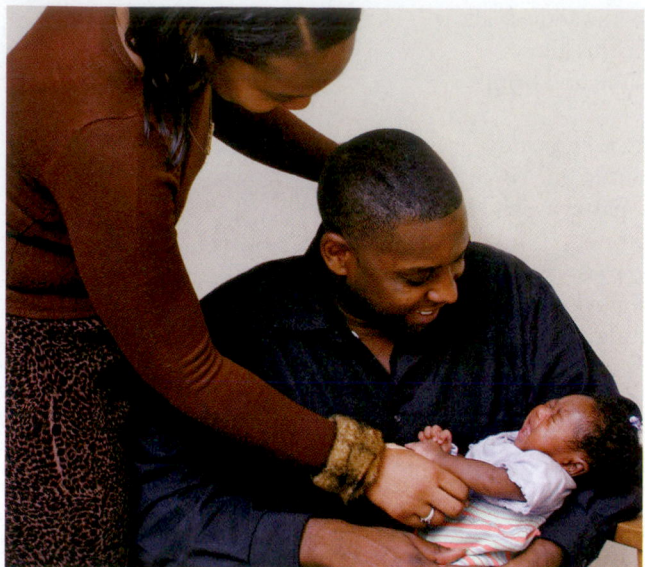

Figure 8–4 ➤ A healthy parent forms strong attachments to the newborn and is motivated to ensure the child's physical and mental health. What observations can you make about these parents' attachment to their newborn infant?

- Parent touches, massages, or gently rubs the newborn.
- Parent attempts to soothe the newborn when the newborn is upset.
- Newborn looks content.
- Newborn signals needs.
- Newborn feeds well.
- Newborn responds to parent's attempts to soothe.

Newborns begin to make their needs known to parents through verbal and nonverbal cues. Engagement cues include looking at, reaching toward, and gazing at the caretaker. Disengagement cues indicate that the baby needs to have some quiet time and include turning away, falling asleep, flailing extremities, and crying. The nurse in this chapter's opening scenario helps the mother, Shannon, to learn her baby's cues of turning toward her, rooting, and engagement, as indicative of a need for feeding or attention. Babies also develop strategies for **self-regulation**, the ability to console the self.

The newborn's mental health and development is highly dependent on the mental and spiritual health of his or her primary caregiver, usually the mother. The mother who is emotionally whole and fully present in her newborn's life is best able to provide the nurturing environment necessary for optimal growth and development (Jellinek, Patel, & Froehle, 2002). Assess for strengths as well as challenges, and offer resources to help the family meet their needs so that attention can be focused on the newborns (Figure 8–4 ➤).

During the health supervision visit, the nurse models behavior for parents that promotes positive infant mental health, such as handling the newborn gently, speaking in a soft voice, noticing attributes ("Look how you hold your head up today! You're really getting strong!"), and noticing likes and dislikes. The nurse strengthens parental confidence by asking the parent what the baby likes, such as, "How does he like to be carried, in your arms or up on your shoulder?" and then following the parent's advice. The nurse also promotes nurturing behavior by parents during procedures, such as allowing the parent to hold the infant on her lap and comforting him while the nurse administers immunizations or draws blood.

Most women experience postpartum "blues" or temporary sadness in the first week after delivery due to hormonal shifts and sleep deprivation. This usually resolves without intervention after a few hours to several days. Postpartum depression is a more serious and debilitating postpartum mood disorder (PPMD) that usually occurs 2–3 months after delivery. Counseling and medication originating from the mother's primary care provider may be necessary interventions. Postpartum psychosis is a serious condition that can occur at any point postpartum and is considered a psychiatric emergency (Jellinek, Patel, & Froehle, 2002).

Relationships

The family is the primary site where the infant learns to interact with other people. Therefore, family dynamics must be examined during health supervision visits. Observations are used to apply strategies that help parents in the relationship with the newborn. Identify both risk and protective factors in the family relationships (Table 8–2).

New parents may need assistance in identifying activities that promote family health and positive parent-newborn interaction. Provide the following suggestions to parents:

- Share newborn care activities. Recognize that you may do things differently than your partner, such as the way you change a diaper or give a bath, but if the baby is cared for, safe and secure, these differences in technique do not matter.
- Compliment one another on newborn caregiving strengths, such as the mother's ability to breast-feed and the partner's ability to calm the crying baby.

Table 8–2	RISK AND PROTECTIVE FACTORS IN NEWBORN AND PARENTS		

Newborn Protective Factors	Newborn Risk Factors
Good health	Preterm birth, congenital disabilities, chronic illness
Normal eating, bowel, and sleep patterns	Feeding and sleep problems
Positive temperament	Fussing, crying, irritability, difficulty consoling
Responds to parent's attention	Diminished social interactions and responsiveness
Normal growth and development	Undernutrition, developmental delay

Parental Protective Factors	Parental Risk Factors
Welcome baby at birth	Baby unplanned and unwanted at birth; potential for neglect and/or rejection
Meet newborn's basic needs for food, shelter, clothing, health care	Financial insecurity, homelessness, lack of knowledge about how to care for newborn
Provide a strong nurturing environment	Cannot promote strong nurturing environment due to serious problems such as abusive behavior, depression, mental illness, substance abuse
Parents have a strong relationship with one another, share care of newborn	Severe marital problems, absent parent, or frequent change of partners
Strong self-esteem, developmental maturity, developing knowledge of infant development	Lack of parenting skills, lack of parenting self-esteem, inability to cope with multiple roles, inappropriate coping strategies
No history of maltreatment as a child	History of maltreatment as a child (risk increases with positive history)

- Attend health supervision visits together as much as possible.
- Be sensitive to when your partner is overstressed and overtired. Ask how you can help and then follow through with suggested activities. Sometimes listening is the most helpful thing you can do.
- Rest and take time for yourself. Make decisions about what must be done (paying bills, laundry, grocery shopping) and what could wait (traveling to visit grandparents, painting the house, cleaning closets). Accept help from family and friends.
- Discuss how you will raise your baby in a loving, supportive, and respectful environment.
- Discuss how you were raised and what you would like to be different in your new family. Learn about parenting strategies and try out what feels comfortable for you.
- Keep in contact with family and friends. Maintain community ties that are important to you, such as social, religious, cultural, or recreational organizations or programs.
- Leave the baby with a trusted friend or family member and take time to be alone once in awhile. Talk about something other than the baby.
- Prepare siblings for the new baby prior to the baby's arrival. Allow siblings to "help" care for the new baby in age-appropriate ways. Praise siblings for positive attention they give to the baby, and allow siblings to express their feelings about the new baby and changes in the family.
- Support one another in seeking and using community resources to strengthen parenting skills, such as classes and parenting groups.

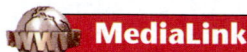

MediaLink

March of Dimes

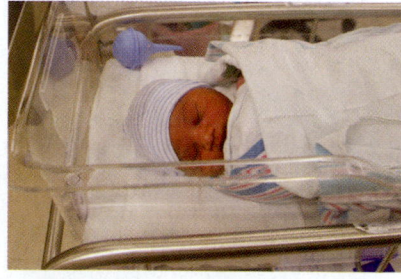

Figure 8–5 ➤ Parents are more likely to place newborns to sleep lying on their backs when they have seen health professionals do this in the hospital. Role model this recommended position for parents when you care for newborns.

- Cuddle, hold, and rock the baby as much as possible. Babies cannot be spoiled by too much attention.
- Take advantage of the baby's awake time to play with the baby. Singing, reading, and simply talking to the baby about what is happening around her or him provides the baby with developmental stimulation.

Disease Prevention Strategies

The newborn period is a critical time for identifying diseases at a time when they can often be successfully treated. Monitoring ensures that the sequelae of diseases can be minimized. For example, identification of a hearing problem may lead to early intervention to maximize the infant's potential for communication development. Disease prevention in the first month of life includes health maintenance activities such as:

- *Metabolic screening* All states require screening for congenital metabolic diseases, such as phenylketonuria. The March of Dimes recommends screening for at least 29 disorders (March of Dimes, 2004).
- *Hearing screening* (see Chapter 19 ∞ for further information about newborn hearing screening).
- *Eye examination* which ensures that the infant's ability to see is developing normally.
- *Immunizations*

See Table 8–3 for immunizations recommended at birth; detailed immunization recommendations can be found in Chapter 18 ∞.

- *Prevention of secondhand smoke exposure* Encourage all parents to avoid smoking near infants, and to stop smoking so that the baby does not inhale smoke from clothing and the environment. About 25% of children live with at least one smoker. Recent research indicates that secondhand smoke (also called environment tobacco smoke or ETS) contains gases and particles that cause Sudden Infant Death Syndrome, acute respiratory infections, slowed lung growth, ear problems, and severe asthma in children (Centers for Disease Control and Prevention, 2006).
- *SIDS risk reduction* (Figure 8–5 ➤) Sudden Infant Death Syndrome is a devastating problem. Chapter 20 ∞ has a detailed description of the condition. Some interventions can lower the risk of SIDS. For information on SIDS risk reduction, see Families Want to Know: SIDS Risk Reduction.
- *Formula safety* (see Chapter 4 ∞) When newborns are fed baby formula, parents need clear instructions about its preparation and storage. These guidelines ensure that the formula is kept free from harmful microorganisms and is prepared in the proper concentration.
- *Handwashing* Handwashing is the key to preventing illness in the newborn and family members. It should be encouraged and modeled at every health promotion and health maintenance encounter. Hand hygiene products can be inserted into diaper bags so that parents always have access to cleansing products.

Table 8–3	IMMUNIZATIONS RECOMMENDED FOR THE NEWBORN	
Immunization	**Recommendation**	
Hepatitis B	Before leaving hospital; for newborn with HBsAg-positive mother, must be given within 12 hours of birth	
Hepatitis immune globulin	Only for newborn with HBsAg-positive mother, must be given within 12 hours of birth	

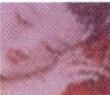

FAMILIES WANT TO KNOW

SIDS Risk Reduction

Sudden Infant Death Syndrome (SIDS) is defined as the sudden unexpected death of an infant less than 1 year of age, with onset of the fatal episode apparently occurring during sleep, that remains unexplained after a thorough investigation, including performance of a complete autopsy and review of the circumstances of death and the clinical history (Krous, Beckwith et al. 2004). SIDS is the major cause of death in infants from 1 month to 1 year of age, with most deaths occurring between 2 and 4 months (Health Resources and Services Administration [HRSA], 2004). See Chapter 20 for further information about SIDS.

Currently, there is no way to prevent SIDS, but parents and caregivers can reduce the risk of a SIDS death. Prenatal behavior and maternal health can influence the occurrence of SIDS. Parents should know the following rules for basic sleep safety to reduce the risk of SIDS.

- Always place the baby on his or her back for sleep.
- Use a safe crib and a firm mattress.
- Remove all fluffy objects from the crib, such as quilts, stuffed animals, and pillows.
- Make sure the baby's face and head stay uncovered during sleep. Use a blanket sleeper instead of blankets in the crib.
- Avoid overheating the baby. A room temperature that is comfortable for the parent is fine for the newborn.
- Never smoke or allow anyone to smoke around the baby.

- *Minimizing the newborn's exposure to disease* Parents should be encouraged to avoid infant exposure to large crowds, especially in cold and influenza season; cover coughs and sneezes; and use good handwashing technique. If the newborn is exposed to varicella, pertussis, herpes, or other serious communicable diseases the caregiver should be alerted.

Injury Prevention Strategies

New parents are sometimes unaware of sources of potential injury for the newborn. Some aspects of injury prevention are pertinent to the newborn's immediate care and other topics promote discussion and provide opportunities for anticipatory guidance. In the immediate newborn period, the nurse should assess the parents' knowledge of injury prevention strategies, and promote healthy and safe habits. Injury prevention strategies include proper and consistent use of an infant car seat, and strategies to prevent falls, burns, choking, drowning, and suffocation (Table 8–4).

Newborn safety awareness begins in the birth setting. Parents should be cautioned against laying the baby on the mother's bed instead of in the bassinet, taught to use the bulb syringe in the event that the baby spits up a large amount of fluid, and instructed to position the baby supine instead of side-lying or prone. Parents should also be oriented to procedures in place to prevent newborn abduction and to their critical role in assuring newborn safety and security. Be sure the parents are equipped to provide the newborn a safe ride home. Refer parents to a local trained Child Passenger Safety Technician for assistance, or use 1-888-327-4236 to find a car seat inspection location. Web sites are also available for car seat safety information.

Following hospital discharge, the nurse promotes safety by encouraging parents to think about the hazards that the child could encounter and how to eliminate them. In the newborn period, the parent or caregiver is uniquely responsible for ensuring that the newborn is not placed in a dangerous situation. The newborn cannot turn on a hot water faucet or run with a sharp object, but it is possible for the parent to inadvertently place the newborn in danger. The newborn is capable of twisting and rolling off any surface higher than the floor, falling out of an infant carrier seat, or drowning while left unattended for a moment in a bathtub filled with only a few inches of water.

Parents might find it helpful to be aware that most pediatric injuries occur when the parents are under stress; for example, when a parent is hungry and tired (the hour before dinner), during pregnancy, during illness or death in the family, when there is tension between parents, and during changes in the environment, such as a change in the child's caregiver or the family's living environment (Shelov, 2004). At these times, the parent should be particularly vigilant and closely supervise children.

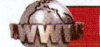

MediaLink

Car Seat Safety Resources

Table 8–4 | INJURY PREVENTION TOPICS FOR NEWBORNS

Topic	Injury Prevention Teaching Topics
Car safety seat	• Choose an infant-only seat or a convertible seat suitable for an infant. • Ensure infant rides rear-facing until at least 1 year of age and more than 20 pounds. • Remember the safest place for all children to ride is in the back seat. Never place a rear-facing car safety seat in the front seat with an active passenger air bag. • Use a car safety seat every time the infant is in the car. • Read and follow the manufacturer's instructions for the car safety seat and the vehicle owner's manual for installation information. • Dress the infant in clothes that allow the straps to go between the legs. Never place blankets under the baby. Buckle the baby into the seat, and place blankets over the baby. • To make sure the car safety seat is installed correctly and the baby is positioned correctly, go to a car seat inspection station. A certified Child Passenger Safety Technician will assist you. Find a list of certified CPS Technicians by state or zip code on the National Highway Traffic Safety Administration web site. Find a car safety seat inspection station online or call 1-888-327-4236.
Shaken Baby Syndrome	Never shake a baby. Recognize that sometimes you will not be able to console your baby. Shaking a baby, even for only a few seconds, can cause serious brain damage and death. One of four shaken babies dies.
Crib	Use a safety approved crib. Slats should be no more than 2 3/8 inches apart. Mattress should be firm and fit snugly into the crib. Keep crib rails raised.
Co-sleeping	Do not co-sleep. The AAP discourages co-sleeping because of the risk of SIDS (with overheating as a possible factor) and the danger of suffocation. Sleep with the baby nearby, but not in the parental bed. If the parent must sleep with the baby, ensure that the infant is supine and separated from any soft surfaces such as pillows; ensure that no blankets will cover the infant's head; beware of spaces between the mattress and the wall, headboard, or footboard; and do not sleep with the baby under the influence of drugs or alcohol. The infant should never sleep in the same bed with siblings due to a significant risk of suffocation.
Baby toys	Use age-appropriate baby toys. Check toys for sharp edges or loose parts. Keep older siblings' toys out of baby's reach. Do not use toys with loops or string cords.
Drowning	Never leave the baby alone in the bathtub. If you must turn your back on the baby or leave the room, take the baby out of the tub.
Suffocation	Keep plastic bags and wrappings away from the baby (take the plastic bag off the crib mattress). Shake baby powder into your hand first and then apply it so the baby does not inhale it. Do not allow a baby or sibling to play with a latex balloon. Keep small objects (such as safety pins, coins, small toys) out of the baby's reach. Do not attach pacifiers, medals, or other objects to the crib or to the baby's body with a string or cord. Do not put the crib near blinds, curtains, or anything with a hanging cord. Do not let the baby wear clothing with strings near the neck (such as a sweatshirt hood that ties with a cord) or a headband that could slip down and wrap around the baby's neck. Use a tight-fitting crib sheet that does not come loose when the corner is pulled.
Burns	Set the hot water heater thermostat lower than 120 degrees F. Do not smoke or drink hot liquids while holding the baby. Do not microwave bottles of formula or breast milk due to uneven heating. Do not expose the baby to direct sunlight.
Falls	Keep a hand on the baby while dressing or diaper changing on a surface other than on the floor. Never leave the baby unsupervised on any high surface such as a bed, changing table, or sofa. Always keep one hand on the baby.
Pet safety	Keep some distance between the newborn and the pet until the pet's initial reaction to the new baby is assessed. Never leave the baby unsupervised with the family dog or cat, or any animal capable of harming the newborn.
Sibling supervision	Never leave your baby alone with a young sibling. When a young child holds the baby, seat the child on a large soft surface, such as the couch and supervise closely. Watch siblings for aggressive behavior toward the newborn, such as hitting or biting. Siblings may take on a caregiving role and imitate adults; watch for "feeding" of non-food items or choking hazards.
Fire safety	Install working smoke detectors on every floor of the house and in every sleeping area. Have a fire escape plan from your house and practice it.
Poisoning	Post the universal phone for U.S. poison control number near your telephone: 1-888-222-1222.
Gun safety	Keep the gun unloaded and locked up. Keep the ammunition locked up separately from the gun. Consider not keeping a gun in the household due to safety hazards for family members.
In case of emergency	• Know when and how to call your pediatric care provider. • Know when it is appropriate to go to the emergency department. • Take a first aid class and learn CPR for children and adults.

Adapted from American Academy of Pediatrics, 2004a; Carbaugh, 2004; *Child Restraints*, 2004; Green & Palfrey, 2002; Shelov, 2004.

NURSING MANAGEMENT

Nursing Assessment and Diagnosis

An essential skill for the nurse in the hospital, clinic, or community setting is the ability to assess the family and newborn and identify potential health promotion and health maintenance activities. Many health promotion and health maintenance activities are pertinent to prenatal health as well as the postpartum period. If maternal and pediatric care providers are located at different agencies, nurses must coordinate and integrate services so that the new mother and family benefit from a seamless continuum of care.

Based on nursing assessments, the nursing diagnoses form the basis for subsequent interventions. Possible nursing diagnoses for the family and newborn in the first month following birth might include:

- Anxiety (Parent) related to change in role status
- Risk for Impaired Attachment related to parental exhaustion or lack of knowledge of infant cues
- Risk for Impaired Parenting
- Effective Breast-Feeding related to basic breast-feeding knowledge
- Ineffective Breast-Feeding related to inadequate sucking by infant
- Infant Feeding Pattern, Ineffective related to newborn's inability to suck effectively
- Readiness for Enhanced Parenting related to lack of information or skills of newborn care

Planning and Implementation

Newborn health maintenance and health promotion begins in the prenatal period. In most cases, the expectant mother is highly motivated to engage in activities that result in a healthy newborn, and the healthcare team has a unique window of opportunity to promote maternal and newborn health.

In the prenatal period, the nurse's goal is to promote an optimal outcome for both mother and newborn. Comprehensive quality prenatal care is outside the scope of this text; however, important health maintenance and health promotion activities include interventions to help ensure healthy diet and exercise; avoid alcohol, tobacco, and drugs; and establish or maintain a dental home. The nurse may assess the need for assistance with food, clothing, and safe housing, which entails numerous referrals and advanced skills to ensure coordinated community services. The nurse provides anticipatory guidance regarding newborn care and safety, and the nurse may assist the woman with choosing a pediatric healthcare provider. The nurse in the prenatal setting plays an important role in educating the woman about breast-feeding's lifelong benefits, and guiding her toward an informed infant feeding decision.

Hospital-Based Care

The hospital length of stay is short for the healthy mother and newborn. The nurse in the birth setting is responsible for assessing and implementing nursing care during a time of dramatic physiologic changes in both mother and newborn, as well as helping the new parents learn basic newborn care skills. Consistent and accurate breast-feeding information is essential to ensure continued efforts at home, and referral to a lactation specialist or support group is helpful. The nurse assesses and refers the mother to community resources as needed for domestic violence and drug, alcohol, or tobacco use. The nurse may coordinate interventions such as WIC to help ensure adequate food and nutritional support. Refer the mother to parenting classes or support groups. Through listening to the family's concerns, providing nurturing responses, respecting cultural differences, and validating parental efforts to learn parenting skills, the nurse further develops the partnership between the family and their healthcare providers.

Prior to discharge the newborn has blood taken for metabolic screening, may have initial hearing screening, and may receive the first hepatitis B vaccination. Follow-up after these interventions requires communication among multiple community agencies and the pediatric care provider to ensure that the newborn receives appropriate continuing care.

Care in the Community

In the outpatient setting, the pediatric healthcare team's goal is to "help the parents gain knowledge and confidence in caring for the physical, intellectual and emotional needs of their infant, and to encourage their personal growth as parents and the family's development as a unit" (Green & Palfrey, 2002). In the first month of the newborn's life, health promotion and maintenance activities may include teaching the parents how to interact with their baby to promote attachment; provide a safe sleeping environment; continue development and validation of baby care activities, especially breast-feeding; and begin to learn about the newborn's temperament in order to respond quickly and correctly to needs in order to promote infant mental health.

The relationship between the family and pediatric healthcare team must be nurtured. Time should be allowed for parents' questions. Cultural differences in perspectives must be considered. Results of screening and testing should be explained. When the nurse involves the parent in the infant's healthcare activities in these ways, it is more likely that parents will be cooperative and interested in promoting and maintaining their child's health.

Evaluation

Expected outcomes for the family and their infant by the end of the first month include:

- The newborn makes a successful transition from intrauterine to extrauterine life.
- Risk factors are identified in the prenatal and newborn period, and nursing assessment coordinates with medical intervention to prevent or manage complications.
- The newborn achieves expected physical and developmental milestones.
- The family begins successful integration of the newborn into the family.
- Parents demonstrate newborn care skills and beginnings of healthy attachment behaviors.
- Parents recognize the importance of health promotion and health maintenance activities and partner with healthcare professionals to promote and maintain the physical and mental health of their newborn and family.

HEALTH PROMOTION AND HEALTH MAINTENANCE FOR THE INFANT

Infancy is a major life transition for the baby and parents. The infant accomplishes phenomenal physical growth and developmental milestones while the family adapts to the addition of a new member and establishes new goals for each of its existing members. Infant health supervision visits are very important to support the health of the baby and the family unit. These visits begin after the newborn period, at about 1 month of age. This is the time when parents establish an ongoing partnership with a healthcare provider. A "medical home" or **"pediatric health care home"** is identified to serve the baby's health needs. The goals of health supervision visits are to identify and address the infant's health promotion and health maintenance needs.

Facilitating breast-feeding, helping parents to understand their infant's temperament, and employing strategies to ensure adequate sleep by the baby and parents are examples of health promotion activities. Health maintenance activities focus on disease and injury prevention. Some examples of these interventions include administering immunizations and teaching about infant car seats.

Establishment of the relationship with a healthcare provider and agency is important so that trust develops and the family will feel comfortable about turning to the professionals for information and guidance as the baby grows. Nurses play a vital role in welcoming new families into office and clinic settings, establishing rapport, and applying principles of communication so that trust and positive partnerships develop between providers and families. Infancy is a time when the child grows in physical, psychological, and cognitive ways; health supervision visits play a key role in fostering healthy growth and development. When should the infant be seen for health supervision visits? What are key components of these visits? How can the nurse best assess and intervene to ensure the infant's health and safety? These are some of the questions that will be answered in this section of the chapter.

Early Contacts with the Family

Health promotion and health maintenance occur in a series of health supervision visits during the first year of life. Schedules vary among facilities, but a common pattern includes visits at about 1 month, 2 months, 4 months, 6 months, 9 months, and 1 year of age. In addition, most children have some episodic illnesses such as gastrointestinal illness or otitis media and visit the facility at other times for treatment of these illnesses. A few children have chronic or serious healthcare problems during the first year, and have extensive contact with the healthcare home and other services.

During these first visits, assess the family for protective factors and risks. Protective factors might include the knowledge level of infant needs, support from family and friends, and the mother's good health and nutritional state during pregnancy. Risk factors could include limited financial resources, lack of preparation for the baby, and illness or other stress among family members. Knowledge of these factors will shape the nursing interventions in the first health supervision in infancy. The nurse applies health promotion principles by building on strengths and fosters health maintenance by intervening to minimize risks.

General Observations

When the family comes to the clinic or office for care with an infant, general observations should begin at first contact (Figure 8–6 ➤). Welcome the family warmly to the facility and comment on the baby. Ask how the family is doing with the baby and how the adjustment is going. Be alert for signs of fatigue or depression in the parents, as these can occur when caring for an infant and can interfere with bonding and positive transition. Upon entering the examination room, it is helpful to explain the plans for the visit, such as "I will weigh and measure your baby now and show you how she is growing. Then I'll ask a few questions about her eating, sleeping, and other things. Then the nurse practitioner will be in to do Rhonda's physical examination. Do you have any questions as we start? Will you undress Rhonda now so we can weigh her accurately?"

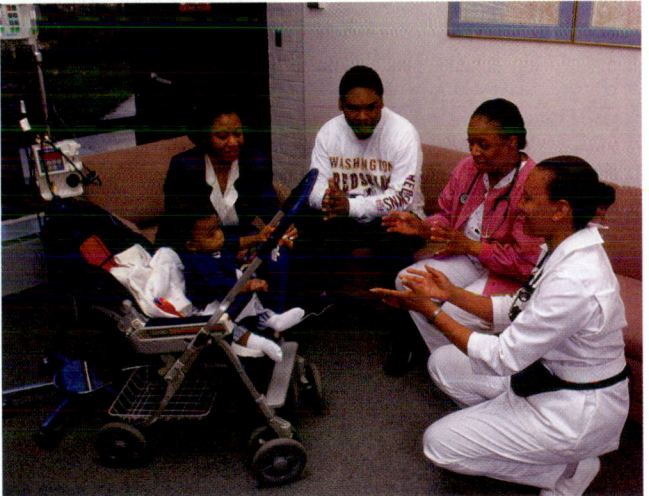

Figure 8–6 ➤ The nurse begins assessment of the infant's family when they are seen in the waiting room and called in for care. What observations can you make of the infant's general appearance? Developmental accomplishments? Interaction of parents with the baby?

Growth and Developmental Surveillance

Physical growth and meeting of developmental milestones provide important information about infants. The baby is measured for accurate length, weight, and head circumference (see *Clinical Skills Manual* and Chapter 5; see Figure 8–7 ➤). The measurements should be placed on growth grids and interpreted. Parents enjoy seeing how the baby is progressing and are usually eager to learn about the child's weight gain and growth percentiles. Be alert for an infant who demonstrates a change in percentile range. For example, if the baby was in the 75th percentile for length and weight at birth, but has fallen to below the 50th percentile for weight, additional assessment will be needed about the baby's feedings. Likewise, if the head circumference is much lower

SKILLS 6–1 THROUGH 6–7:
Growth Measurements

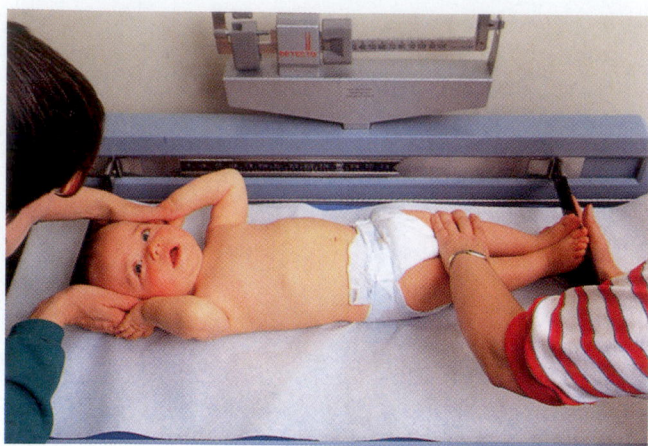

Figure 8–7 ➤ Weighing and measuring length during health supervision visits provides important information about the child's nutrition and general development. This young infant was measured, and then the nurse placed the findings on the growth grid while the parents dressed the child.

CULTURE

Developmental Milestones

Be alert for differences in cultural practices and beliefs that may influence developmental milestones. For example, if a child is kept on a cradleboard for much of the time, the baby may be slow in learning to crawl. This baby may progress directly to standing by furniture without demonstrating as much creeping or crawling as other infants. In addition, when parents do not have English as a primary language and the examiner uses English, common terms might be misinterpreted. Parents might not understand what is meant if you ask "Does your baby have a mobile over the crib at home?" or "Is she starting to be afraid of strangers?" How can you be alert for language differences and become sensitive to miscommunication?

or higher than the length and weight percentiles, further neurological and developmental assessment should be done.

Growth measurement is followed by a physical assessment. The nurse may complete parts of the assessment, with the remainder performed by the physician, nurse practitioner, or other primary care provider. The assessment evaluates each body system, with particular attention paid to heart, skin, musculoskeletal system, abdomen, and neurological status. See Chapter 5 ∞ for a thorough discussion of physical assessment.

Developmental surveillance is integrated into each infant healthcare visit by observing developmental milestones in the infant (see Chapter 3 ∞ for a summary of milestones expected at different ages and see Table 8–5 for specific tasks in infancy). When there is no opportunity to directly observe a skill, ask parents about whether the infant performs the skill. In addition to direct observation, parents are usually requested to fill in a form that asks questions about common developmental tasks. Review the results and determine if additional questions should be asked. When some milestones have not been met, make an appointment for the infant to have a developmental test by a certified examiner. When a child has not been seen as often as recommended, perform a thorough developmental assessment to identify any expected milestones not yet achieved. Reinforce the need to make an appointment for the next visit and plan with the family how to remember the appointment and to ensure the family's ability to bring the child to the healthcare visit.

The nurse establishes health promotion and health maintenance interventions related to growth and development assessment data. Anticipatory guidance related to development is a major component of health promotion. The nurse anticipates the next milestones the infant will be meeting, and recommends ways for the parents to support the infant in progression. Some health promotion activities include:

- Teaching about food introduction that will foster growth
- Encouraging toys and activities that will assist in meeting the next developmental milestones
- Demonstrating gross and fine motor skills that the infant has achieved
- Demonstrating to parents how the child will focus on their faces and mimic their vocal sounds

Other interventions are focused on health maintenance or disease and injury prevention. Safety hazards and ways to avoid them are discussed, and parents are given brochures, web sites, or videotapes to enhance injury prevention information. Can you outline additional health promotion and health maintenance interventions that relate to the infant's growth and development?

Nutrition

The importance of nutrition during the first year of life cannot be overestimated. The baby will triple his or her birth weight by 1 year of age, and has a great need for nutritional balance. From the first sips of breast milk or formula as a newborn, to eating the family meal at 1 year of age, the fast progression of nutritional intake patterns is obvious. See Chapter 4 ∞ for a thorough description of nutritional needs during infancy.

During each visit, the nurse seeks to learn what the baby is eating, and whether the family has any questions or concerns related to intake (Story, Holt, & Sofka, 2002). Open-ended questions are a good way to begin, with more specific questions inserted after the parent's perceptions are known. Once the baby is in the second half of the first year, food patterns of the family become more important. Consider childcare settings as well.

Table 8–5	INFANT DEVELOPMENTAL MILESTONES OBSERVED IN HEALTH PROMOTION AND HEALTH MAINTENANCE VISITS

Age	Developmental Milestones
1 month	• Responds to sound by startle or increased alertness • Follows objects and human face with eyes • Has periods of alertness and restfulness • Comforted by touch or feeding by parent • Has symmetrical movements and generally has arms and legs flexed • Lifts head momentarily when prone
2 months	• Previous characteristics continue • Makes noises such as cooing in response to interaction with adult • Smiles • Lifts head, neck, upper chest when prone • Has increasing head control when held in sitting position
4 months	• Increasing cooing and babbling • Smiles, laughs, makes other noises during interactions • Supports self on hands when prone • Rolls front to back • Touches objects and grasps rattle placed near hand
6 months	• Uses sounds in repeated speech such as bababa, dadadada • Interested in surroundings and toys • When pulled to sitting has no head lag • Sits with support • Grasps objects easily and places them in mouth • Transfers objects from one hand to other • Bears weight on legs when held in standing position
9 months	• Understands simple words and uses more sounds in babbling • Responds to name • Enjoys interactive games with parent • Moves when placed on floor by crawling, creeping, or rolling repeatedly • Sits without support • Stands holding on to support • Plays with toys • Feeds self readily with fingers and tries to use cup
12 months	• Has one or more words • Imitates sounds readily • Increasing interactions and interest in surroundings • Follows directions such as saying or waving bye • Pulls to standing, walks a few steps holding on • Well-developed pincer grasp • Able to drink from cup

Observations from other portions of the visit can provide clues about additional questions to ask. If an infant has not gained weight as expected and has fallen into a lower channel of weight percentile, more specific analysis of intake is needed. Ask for a recall of the baby's intake in the previous day. When the baby does not meet developmental milestones on schedule or is lethargic, intake may be inadequate for age. In these cases support may be needed to ensure adequate intake; a thorough description of feeding may be the first step in analyzing the problem and planning interventions. When the child's ability to take in nutrients or the parent's ability to feed the baby is questioned, an observation of a feeding might take place, either at the healthcare setting or during a home visit.

Additional nutritional assessment measures are used at certain points in the first year. A hematocrit or hemoglobin is generally performed between 9–12 months of age. Lead screening may be needed in certain population groups (see Chapter 6 ∞). Food security screening can be used when appropriate (see Chapter 4 ∞). Each visit includes nutritional teaching about important items. The topics for discussion vary according to age group. See Table 8–6 for suggested teaching topics at specific ages.

Table 8–6	INFANT NUTRITION TEACHING FOR HEALTH PROMOTION AND HEALTH MAINTENANCE VISITS
Age	**Nutrition Teaching**
1 month	• Support breast-feeding efforts • Teach correct formula types and preparation if used • Teach burping and rate of feeding information • Suggest water during hot weather or if family wants to use a bottle at baby's bedtime • Encourage families to view feedings as social interactions; emphasize importance of holding the infant and not propping bottles
2 months	• Continue as previously noted • Review fluid needs of infants • Reinforce food safety for partially used bottles of breast milk or formula • Use warm water for heating bottles rather than microwave to avoid burning • Warn against feeding honey in the first year of life • Begin cleaning of infant gums daily • Provide information about any supplements needed (for example, iron for premature infant, vitamin D for babies not exposed to adequate sunlight)
4 months	• Continue as previously noted • Discuss introduction of first foods between 4–6 months, and surveillance for symptoms of allergy or intolerance • Discuss changing food patterns such as increasing amounts and decreasing numbers of daily milk feedings
6 months	• Continue as previously noted • Reinforce proper introduction of new foods, to include rice cereal, fruits, vegetables • Discuss any unusual food reactions observed • Introduce cup for drinking • Introduce soft finger foods • Serve juice only in a cup and limit to no more than 6 ounces daily • Caution about common choking foods and items • Provide information about fluoride supplement if water supply is not fluoridated
9 months	• Continue as previously noted • If mother does not continue to breast-feed, teach family to use iron-fortified formula for the first year of life • Encourage self-feeding of finger foods, integrating common foods for the family • Introduce source of protein such as tofu, cheese, mashed beans, slivers of meats
12 months	• Continue as previously noted • Support mother who wishes to continue breast-feeding beyond 1 year of age • Encourage cups for all feedings other than breast

Desired outcomes for nutrition in infancy include adequate growth, normal nutritional assessment findings, and knowledge by parents of the infant's nutritional needs.

Physical Activity

Physical activity is needed for adequate development of fine and gross motor skills in infancy. Unlike other times of life, the focus is on providing only the opportunities for activity, without a need to focus on motivation. As long as infants are meeting developmental milestones and have a stimulating environment that provides opportunity for fine and gross motor activity, they will use their motor skills, thus enhancing their performance. Time should be provided each day for the infant to reach for objects, exercise legs and arms freely, and increasingly use head control. Playing with parents or others and being surrounded by toys and other stimulating items will encourage motor behavior in all body parts. Ask the parents for a description of the baby's typical day and listen for these types of play periods.

Observe the infant's physical skills, ask questions about play periods provided, and compose a list of the family protective factors and risk factors in this area. Table 8–7 lists risk and protective factors related to physical activity during infancy.

Table 8–7	RISK AND PROTECTIVE FACTORS REGARDING PHYSICAL ACTIVITY IN INFANCY	
Risk Factors	**Protective Factors**	
• Premature birth • Delayed developmental milestones • Limited stimulation by family or other care providers • Lack of knowledge by family about infant's physical activity needs • Limited community resources for families with infants	• Meets developmental milestones at expected ages • Has contact with parents, siblings, and others for significant time each day • A supportive environment with room to play safely, stimulating surroundings • Physically active family • Family knowledge about infant's physical activity needs • Community programs that promote physical activity in infants and information for families	

Adapted from Patrick, K., Spear, B., Holt, K. & Sofka, D. (Eds.). (2001). *Bright futures in practice: Physical activity.* Arlington, VA: National Center for Education in Maternal and Child Health.

Based on the results of assessment and using the concept of anticipatory guidance, the nurse plans appropriate teaching for the family. Health maintenance deals with prevention of physical development delays. The nurse evaluates success of interventions by the child's progression in physical activity milestones at the next health supervision visit. Adequate parental understanding of the importance of physical activity and the means of supporting the child's activities is an important outcome of care.

Oral Health

The first teeth begin to erupt about midway during infancy. Two front teeth are common at about 6 months of age. However, even before this, parents lay the foundation for good oral health. The mother's intake during pregnancy and breast-feeding are essential to ensuring adequate availability of calcium and other nutrients that will be used as the infant's teeth develop. The nurse in child health supervision settings ensures that the baby has adequate intake of these nutrients via breast-feeding and other foods. A dietary recall of the mother's intake, as well as the infant's, is one way of assessing for nutrients. When the water supply is not fluoridated, inquire about use of fluoride drops.

Help the family establish healthy dental habits. The parents should wipe the infant's gums with soft moist gauze once or twice daily. This helps to clean food residues from the gums and gets the baby accustomed to having something wiping the gums, a practice that may assist when tooth brushing begins. Families are also cautioned to avoid having the baby nurse when sleeping, to avoid use of bottles in bed, and not to allow the baby to drink at will from a bottle during the day. Ask if the child is receiving fluoride drops. These practices are linked to early childhood caries (see Chapter 4 ∞) and can lead to tooth decay. Nurses assess for the presence of teeth and whether patterns are similar to those expected (see Chapter 5 ∞). It is wise to ask if the baby has had any difficulty with teeth eruption. Many babies have increased crying and parents have disrupted sleeping during these periods. Suggest comfort measures such as offering the baby cool beverages and safe "teething toys."

Mental and Spiritual Health

The baby's mental health is related to early experiences, inborn characteristics such as temperament and resilience, and relationships with caregivers. In addition, the first year of life provides opportunities for the infant to develop positive mental health; interventions during this important period can enhance the child's future mental status.

One way to evaluate mental health is to look carefully at the growth and development surveillance data that was previously described. Children who feel secure and have nurturing environments usually grow as expected and perform milestones at usual

> **NURSING ALERT**
>
> Be sure that parents do not give the child excessive fluoride because it can permanently discolor the teeth. For example, this may happen if the parents administer fluoride drops each morning since their water supply has no fluoride, but then have the child at a care center several days each week where the water supply is fluoridated. Fluoride 0.25 mg is recommended for the child who is from 6 months to 3 years in communities with drinking water that contains < 0.3 ppm. Consult drug references for doses recommended at other ages.

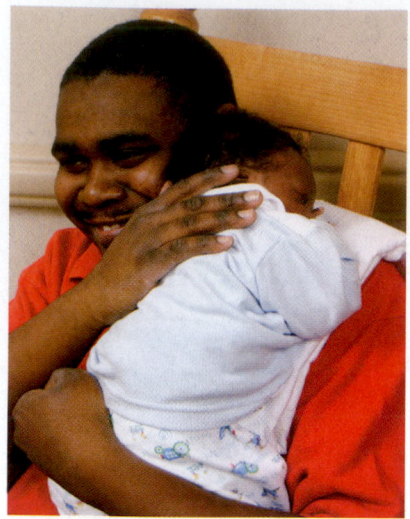

Figure 8–8 ➤ Interactions between the parent and infant provide clues to mental health. Do the adult and child appear comfortable with each other? Is eye contact and vocalization present? Are their bodies soft and relaxed or tense?

GROWTH & DEVELOPMENT

Infant Sleep Patterns

Birth – 3 months
10–16 hours of sleep daily in about five sleep periods of 30 minutes to 3 hours
3–6 months
14 hours of sleep daily with a longer sleep at night plus 2–3 naps daily
By 4–6 weeks, a consistent sleep pattern should emerge
6–12 months
12–14 hours of sleep daily with a longer sleep at night plus 1–2 naps daily

Adapted from Green & Palfrey, 2002.

MediaLink

Helping the Infant Sleep Video

---

times. Slow growth and delayed development are sometimes related to a feeding disorder of infancy and early childhood (see Chapter 4 ∞). In these cases, a disturbed relationship with the primary caregiver influences the infant's psychological state and results in decreased food intake. Another way to assess mental health is to observe the child and parent interacting. Does the parent hold the baby securely and does the child cuddle and settle in to the parent's arms (Figure 8–8 ➤)? Is there eye contact between parent and child? Does the parent appear comfortable in holding and comforting the baby? These interactions indicate bonding or positive attachment.

During the first year, the baby learns to identify parents; beginning at about 6 months of age, infants may cry or protest when another person holds them. This is called **stranger anxiety** and indicates expected attachment to parents. Similarly, infants in the second half of the first year of life may exhibit **separation anxiety** by inconsolable crying and other signs of distress when parents are not present. Recognize that these behaviors are normal, demonstrate healthy attachment to primary caregivers, and indicate mental health. Help parents to recognize them as expected occurrences. Provide them ideas of how to deal with this behavior. They can remain in sight and talk to the baby during health supervision examinations, and they should be encouraged to hold and comfort the baby after painful procedures like immunizations. Once the infant has experienced that the parent leaves and returns, security in the care of others can emerge.

Another important indication of infant mental health is the ability to comfort oneself. Self-regulation is the process of dealing with feelings, learning to soothe self, and focusing on activities for increasing periods of time. Infants learn early how to comfort and calm themselves. Ask parents if the child sucks a finger, softly rocks, or otherwise comforts self when distressed. Some babies prefer to be alone and quiet when tired or distressed; others calm better when held, rocked, or placed in an infant swing. Help the parents to identify and reinforce the infant's methods of self-soothing, and teach swaddling and rocking techniques.

Self-regulation is needed when the infant is learning to go to sleep while tired and agitated. Infants progress into circadian rhythm at 2–3 months and begin to sleep more at night than during the day. By 6 months, the infant commonly sleeps 6 hours without waking, and returns to sleep after one nighttime feeding. A total sleep time of 14 hours/day is common (Davis, Parker, & Montgomery, 2004; Hoban, 2004). Nurses use health promotion principles to teach about sleep patterns in infants, and implement health maintenance when partnering with families to deal with problem sleep behaviors that lead to infant and parent fatigue. See Evidence-Based Practice: Infant Sleep on the following page.

The baby is born into a family with spiritual strengths and limitations. The nurse assesses the family and provides additional resources when needed. While the infant is not mature enough to understand the family's spiritual framework, the atmosphere in the family that relates to nurturing, valuing children, providing a safe and secure environment, and recognizing mental balance is conveyed readily to the infant. The infant's social and psychological health are closely related to these factors. Assess the family's meaningful activities and practices and engagement in faith-based practices. Ask if they have needs or desires for referrals in the community such as to an organized religious body or other meaningful activities.

Many of the nurse's interventions are aimed at healthy mental health development in the baby. Health promotion activities focus on teaching parents the needs of infants for security and interaction. Suggest healthy sleep patterns and how they can be achieved (see Families Want to Know: Helping the Infant Sleep). Teach self-regulation skills so that the parents can help the child become quiet and calm. Health maintenance seeks to identify babies with disruptions in mental health status, often manifested by growth or interaction abnormalities. When the infant has disturbed sleep patterns, difficulty calming self when upset, or the parents do not interpret infant cues related to hunger or discomfort, the nurse plans interventions to help prevent further problems. An expected outcome for these activities is the reestablishment of expected growth and development, and age-appropriate interactions of the infant with others.

EVIDENCE-BASED PRACTICE

Infant Sleep

Problem

Many babies have limited sleeping periods during the night, and their night awakenings disturb parents' sleep. Parents may have busy days and be unable to nap for adequate sleep, and thus cannot perform at a safe and productive level during the day. In an effort to increase sleep, some parents may feed the infant frequently during the day, believing that if the baby has fed well, longer night sleep periods may occur.

Evidence

Infants with more than 11 feeds in 24 hours at 1 week of age were noted to be nearly three times more likely to have night wakenings than infants who had fewer feedings. A group of 316 newborns with more than 11 feedings daily and their families participated in a study and were randomly assigned to receive one of three interventions:

- Three-step behavioral program
- Educational booklet
- Helpline for sleeping problems

After 12 weeks, 82% of babies in the behavioral program slept through the night, compared with 61% for the other two interventions. The behavioral program taught parents to minimize light and social interac-

tion at night, avoid feeding or cuddling at night, and beginning at 3 weeks of age, delay feeding when the baby awoke at night (Nikolopoulou & St. James-Roberts, 2003).

In a similar study with 33 infants, two nurses taught parents of infants with disturbed sleep to gradually decrease their contact with the infants during night awakenings. Night sleep improved significantly at 1 week and at the 2-month follow-up. Infants in turn developed more self-soothing abilities (Skuladottir & Thome, 2003).

Implications

This evidence-based practice provides implications for nursing practice. Ask parents of young newborns to keep track of the number of daily feedings and nighttime awakenings of the infant. For infants with 11 or more feedings, teach parents about how to minimize stimulation and interaction at night, as previously described. Provide opportunities to review results at future health supervision visits.

Critical Thinking

What reasons might working parents have for responding eagerly and interacting with an infant who awakens at night? Do you think there are other reasons why babies awaken at night? What clues help you to decide if an infant sleep problem exists?

Relationships

The infant's social interactions both within and outside the family display enormous growth in the first year. The family is the primary site where the infant learns to interact with other people. Therefore, family dynamics must be examined during health supervision visits. Some factors in the parents' mental health directly affect the home atmosphere, and the baby's resulting health. Depression in parents or other family members is an important condition that can potentially influence the infant's health. Interactions with parents who are depressed will be altered; caretaking, both physical and emotional, can be impaired.

Another challenge to the mental health of families with depressed members is that of domestic violence, a situation in which parents or adult care providers commit violent acts toward one another. Child abuse or maltreatment may also occur in some families with infants. This problem is a serious issue that causes disturbed mental status in the baby. See Chapter 6 ∞ for a detailed description of child abuse and its effect on infants and older children. Suspected child abuse must be reported to legal authorities in order to protect children.

FAMILIES WANT TO KNOW

Helping the Infant Sleep

Helping an infant to self-regulate and be able to sleep for longer periods of time is often a stressful challenge for families. Parents need to have substantial sleep periods themselves in order to be refreshed and able to deal with daily life. When up several times during the night with a baby, parents may become irritable and fatigued. Question the family about the baby's sleep routine. The infant passes into light sleep several times at night and may awaken; self-regulation will assist in helping the infant get back to sleep. Suggestions helpful for the family may involve:

- Place the baby to sleep in a quiet and darkened room
- Have similar bedtime routines each night
- Provide a consistent transitional object, such as a favorite blanket, each night

- Put the baby to bed while still awake rather than after falling asleep nursing so he or she becomes accustomed to getting to sleep without nursing
- Do not try to awaken the baby in NREM (quiet) sleep
- Establish a regular sleep routine and time; routine may involve some cuddling and rocking time but should not be vigorous, stimulating play
- For the baby who has trouble going to sleep, remain in the room for a few minutes but do not establish eye contact; place a hand on the abdomen or chest or gently hold flailing arms and legs (Green & Palfrey, 2002; Jellinek, Patel, & Froehle, 2002; Mindell, 2003)

Table 8–8	ROUTINE IMMUNIZATIONS RECOMMENDED DURING INFANCY

Immunization	Age Recommended
Hepatitis B	After birth up to 2 months (#1) 1–4 months (#2) 6–18 months (#3)
Hepatitis A	12 months (#1) 18 months or at least 6 months after first dose (#2)
Diphtheria, tetanus, acellular pertussis	2, 4, and 6 months (three doses)
Haemophilus Influenzae type b	2, 4, and 6 months (three doses; third dose is not needed if PRP-OMP [Pedvax HIB or ComVax] are used for primary series)
Inactivated poliovirus	2, 4, and 6–18 months (three doses)
Pneumococcal	2, 4, and 6 months (three doses)
Influenza	Annually from 6 months of age
Rotavirus	2, 4, and 6 months (three doses)

The nurse's role related to infant social interactions in health supervision visits is to evaluate the infant's social skills, learn what parents have noticed about the baby's temperament and how it fits with their lives, and make suggestions for positive social development. Desired outcomes for the infant include establishment of close relationships with parents and other family members, a stimulating home environment that is responsive to the baby's temperament, and developmental progression in social interactions.

Disease Prevention Strategies

Infants are prone to many infectious diseases, especially once passive immunity from the mother wanes at about 6 months of age (see Chapters 17 and 18 ∞). Recommended immunizations are administered on schedule to provide the infant protection from some diseases (Table 8–8). Further details on immunizations can be found in Chapter 18. Instruct parents about upcoming immunizations and when the baby should be seen again. Be sure the parent understands the risks and benefits of each immunization. Answer questions truthfully and have resources on hand for interested parents such as brochures and videotapes.

During each health supervision visit, the nurse performs recommended screenings, and counsels the parents about why such screenings are important (Table 8–9). Vision and hearing screening are performed at each healthcare encounter. Screening for anemia and lead poisoning are added at particular times or with certain groups. Families with a history of genetic diseases such as sickle cell disease or cystic fibrosis may choose to have infant screening so that supportive care could begin early if the child has the disease. Parents benefit from teaching about common diseases and conditions of young children and measures for their prevention. Ask about environment tobacco smoke (ETS) and encourage smoking parents to quit. Teach parents to put babies to sleep on their backs to assist in lowering the chance of Sudden Infant Death Syndrome. Be sure parents have a phone number to call when they have questions about conditions or whether the baby should be seen by the healthcare provider. Desired outcomes for disease prevention strategies include adequate management of health problems, integration of immunization and other preventive measures into infant care, and family understanding of preventive measures recommended for infants.

Injury Prevention Strategies

During the first year of life, injury becomes an increasingly common cause of mortality. (See statistics on mortality in children in Chapter 1 ∞.) Strategies must be included in each health supervision visit to lower the risk of injury. Nurses should never assume that

---

NURSING ALERT

Instruct parents to contact a healthcare provider if the infant has:
- Rectal temperature ≥ 100.4°F (38.0°C)
- Seizure
- Skin rash, purplish spots, petechiae
- Change in activity or behavior that makes the parent uncomfortable
- Unusual irritability, lethargy
- Failure to eat
- Vomiting
- Diarrhea
- Dehydration
- Cough

Data from Green and Palfrey, 2002.

Table 8–9	SCREENING DURING HEALTH PROMOTION AND HEALTH MAINTENANCE VISITS

Age	Recommended Screening Tests
1 month	• Vision (follow objects, red reflex) • Hearing (response to sound; screening by machine if not completed in the hospital) • Physical examination with special attention to skin problems, hip dysplasia, foot position and range of motion, mouth, abdomen, cardiac abnormality, tearing of eyes, neurological (including child abuse), anthropometric measurements • Developmental milestones • Dietary screening and stool/urine pattern assessment • Review immunization record
2 months	• As previously noted
4 months	• As previously noted • Vision (add cover–uncover test for strabismus)
6 months	• As previously noted • Vision (add ability to follow object bilaterally, corneal light reflex) • Physical examination with special attention to muscle tone, extremities, appearance of first teeth, tympanic membrane, testicle descent for males
9 months	• As previously noted • Lead exposure and levels if appropriate • Anemia • Physical examination with special attention to symmetry of movement
12 months	• As previously noted • Tuberculosis test if indicated • Physical examination with special attention to condition of teeth

Adapted from Green, M., & Palfrey, J. S. (Eds.). (2002). *Bright futures: Guidelines for health supervision of infants, children, and adolescents,* (2nd ed.). Arlington, VA: National Center for Education in Maternal and Child Health.

parents understand how to insert an infant car seat (Figure 8–9 ➤) correctly or what types of toys and foods can lead to choking. Know the most commons hazards at each age and teach parents methods of avoiding them (see Tables 8–10 and 8–11).

Begin the conversation by asking parents what safety hazards they are aware of in the child's environment. Use this information as the starting point for discussion. Give positive feedback for their awareness of hazards and measures they have taken to prevent them. Consider using a home assessment survey that assists parents in identifying hazards that may be present in their homes. (See Chapter 2 for a description of the Home Observation for Measurement of the Environment.) When infants visit friends, relatives, or neighbors, they may be exposed to other hazardous situations. Grandparents may not have a home that is "babyproofed" and the infant could have access to electrical cords, machinery, medicines in cupboards or purses, or other hazards. Help the parents to evaluate the childcare home or center. Focus on car safety since this is a frequent cause of injury for infants. Provide brochures and other types of information about recommendations. Refer every family for a car seat examination at a certified examination center. Provide resources for car seats if the family is not able to afford one. Discuss other possible safety hazards such as extensions on the parent bicycle and use of baby strollers in areas where cars are present.

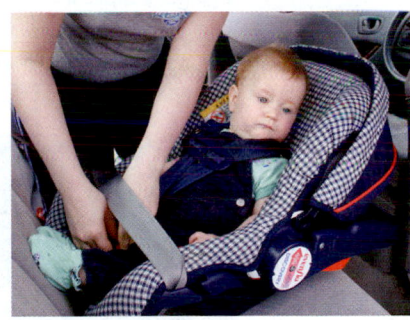

Figure 8–9 ➤ A young mother fastens her infant securely into a backward-facing car seat. Her installation has been evaluated by the local car seat inspector and she has been instructed in proper usage. Locate inspection stations in your community and use them to refer families to verify car seat placement.

NURSING MANAGEMENT
Nursing Assessment and Diagnosis

The nurse working in clinics, offices, and other settings that offer primary care for infants should be skillful in assessing health promotion and health maintenance. The infant's growth, developmental level, general physical health, and mental/social health are assessed. Family interactions and other settings where the infant spends time are

Table 8–10 | INJURY PREVENTION IN INFANCY

Hazard	Development Characteristics	Preventive Measures
Falls	Mobility increases in first year of life, progressing from squirming movements to crawling, rolling, and standing.	Do not leave infant unsecured in infant seat, even in newborn period. Do not place on high surfaces such as tables or beds unless holding child. **(1)** Once mobile by crawling, keep doors to stairways closed or use gates. Standing walkers have led to many injuries and are not recommended.
Burns	Infant is dependent on caretakers for environmental control. The second half of the first year is marked by crawling and increased mobility. Objects are explored by touching and placing in mouth.	Check temperature of bath water and food/liquids for drinking. Cover electrical outlets. Supervise infant so that play with electrical cords cannot occur.
Motor vehicle crashes	Infant is dependent on caretakers for placement in car. On impact with another motor vehicle, an infant held on a lap acts as a torpedo.	Use only approved restraint systems (according to federal Motor Vehicle Safety Standards). The seat must be used for every trip, even if very short. The seat must be properly buckled to the car's lap belt system. **(2)**
Drowning	Infant cannot swim and is unable to lift head.	Never leave infant alone in a bath of even 2.5 cm (1 in.) of water. Supervise when in water even when a life preserver is worn. Flotation devices such as arm inflatables are not certified life preservers.
Poisoning	Infant is dependent on caretakers to keep harmful substances out of reach.	Keep medicines out of reach. Teach proper dosage and administration of medicines to parents. Cleaning products and other harmful substances should not be stored where the infant can reach them. Remove plants from play areas. Have poison control center number by telephone.
Choking	The second half of infancy is marked by exploratory reaching and mouthing objects. Infant explores objects by placing them in the mouth. **(3)**	Avoid foods that commonly cause choking. Keep small toys away from infants, especially toys labeled "not intended for use by those under 3 years."
Suffocation	Young infant has minimal head control and may be unable to move if vomiting or having difficulty breathing.	Position infant on back for sleep. **(4)** Do not place pillows, stuffed toys, or other objects near head. Do not use plastic in crib. Avoid latex balloons.
Strangulation	Infant is able to get head into railings or crib slats but cannot remove it.	Be sure older cribs have slats spaced 6 cm (2⅜ in.) or less apart. The mattress must fit tightly against the crib rails.

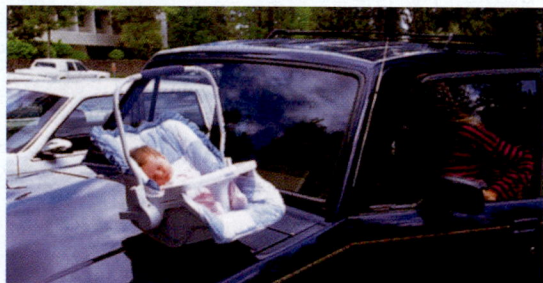

(1) Never leave infant unsecured or on high surface.

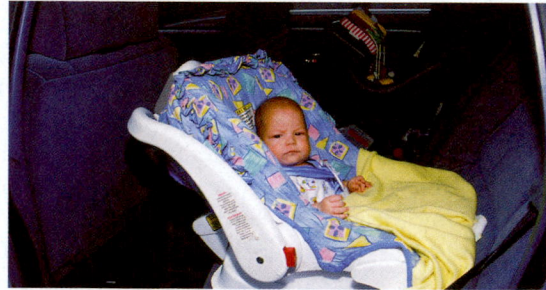

(2) Always use approved restraint system. Place infant in rear-facing seat in backseat of car.

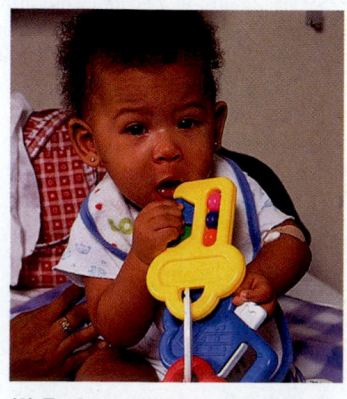

(3) Explores objects with mouth.

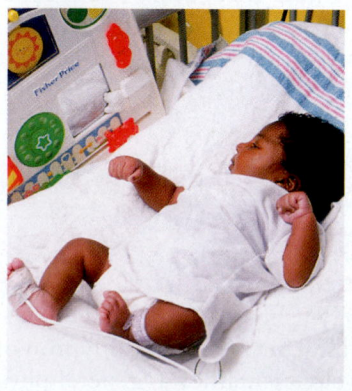

(4) Place infant on back for sleeping, keep toys clear.

Table 8–11	INJURY PREVENTION TOPICS BY AGE

Age	Injury Prevention Teaching Topics
1 month	• Use infant car safety seat • Put baby to sleep on back • Avoid loose bedding and toys in crib • Avoid tobacco use in the environment • Provide adult supervision of the baby at all times by trusted individuals • Test bath water temperature and never leave baby alone in bath • Never place baby on high object such as counter, table, or bed; always keep one hand on the baby during activities like diaper changes to prevent falling • Wash hands correctly and often • Avoid contact with persons with communicable diseases • Have smoke alarms and avoid fire hazards • Learn infant CPR and airway obstruction removal • Never shake the baby • Have plans for emergency care
2 months	• As previously noted • Use only recommended playpens or cribs and keep sides up • Avoid moldy environments • Keep baby toys cleaned • Avoid direct sunlight for the baby • Keep sharp and small objects out of the baby's environment • Keep hot water heater lower than 120°F • Review emergency plan with all care providers
4 months	• As previously noted • Get all poisonous substances out of the baby's view and reach; install locks to keep them inaccessible • Do not use latex balloons or plastic bags near the baby
6 months	• As previously noted • If an infant-only car seat was used, switch to a rear-facing convertible safety seat (intended for babies up to 40 pounds) when baby is 20 to 30 pounds or 26 inches • Empty containers of water immediately after use; be sure pools or other bodies of water are locked and not accessible to baby • Use sunscreen, hat, and long sleeves when baby is in the sun • Keep heavy and sharp objects out of reach; check that all poisons are locked away including in homes visited; keep pet food and cosmetics out of reach • Do not drink hot liquids or eat soup while holding the baby • Have poison control number by phones and programmed into cell phones • Be alert for dangers of hot curling irons and other appliances • Have electrical cords out of reach and not hanging down • Have home and environment checked for lead hazards • Lower infant crib mattress if still in upper position • Install gates and guards on stairs and windows • Never use an infant walker
9 months	• As previously noted • Crawl on the floor and look for hazards at baby's eye level • Pad sharp corners on tables and other furniture • Watch for tables, chairs, and other devices the baby may use for climbing to unsafe places
12 months	• As previously noted • Change to forward-facing car safety seat if baby is at least 20 pounds; install correctly and have installation checked; place in back seat and never in front seat with a passenger air bag • Start teaching the child to wash hands frequently, showing how • Provide own personal items such as clothing and blankets to childcare providers; wash often • Change batteries in home smoke alarms and check system • Turn handles to back of stove; use back rather than front burners; watch for hot liquids • Check care provider setting for safety hazards • Remember that responsible adults should always supervise your infant, not other children • Peruse home once again for hazards now that the child is more active, climbing, and walking

Adapted from Green, M., & Palfrey, J. S. (Eds.). (2002). *Bright futures: Guidelines for health supervision of infants, children, and adolescents* (2nd ed.). Arlington, VA: National Center for Education in Maternal and Child Health.

evaluated for risks and protective factors that influence the child's development. Assess the health of siblings and patterns of integrating the infant into the rest of the family. Particular attention is directed at assessment of risk for diseases and injuries. The data-gathering phase provides parents with the opportunity to ask questions and relay concerns. Further assessment may need to be directed at these areas.

Based on the assessment data, the nurse establishes nursing diagnoses that become the basis for nursing interventions. Both areas of strength and need are included; often the family strengths can be used to further promote health. Some possible nursing diagnoses established during a health supervision visit of an infant might include:

- Effective Breast-Feeding related to the mother's confidence and knowledge
- Interrupted Breast-Feeding related to the mother's resumption of employment outside the home
- Compromised Family Coping related to recent role changes
- Risk for Altered Parent/Child Attachment related to anxiety associated with parenting role
- Sleep Pattern Disturbance (Infant) related to frequently changing sleep routines and cycles
- Impaired Skin Integrity (Infant) related to developmental factors
- Risk for Infection (Infant) related to inadequate acquired immunity
- Risk for Injury (Infant) related to design of environment
- Risk for Altered Growth and Development related to parental substance abuse

Planning and Implementation

The nurse plays a vital role in successful health promotion and health maintenance activities. Explain to parents the procedures being performed and their purpose. Encourage them to ask questions and share their perceptions of the infant's personality, development, and other traits. This will enhance their understanding that health care involves a partnership between them and the care providers. It will lead to trust that promotes their ability to honestly share concerns. Recognize that the first year of the baby's life is a key time for establishing a trusting relationship with health professionals.

Recognize the importance of data provided by simple assessments such as length and weight. Analyze all findings to learn if the child is developing as expected. Much of the visit is spent teaching parents about topics such as safety measures, providing anticipatory guidance related to development, assisting with integration of the new baby into the family, and relaying resources for support of the family in the community, Internet, or other areas. Parenting classes, childcare facilities, and family planning resources are examples of common parental needs. Perform recommended physical and developmental assessment, administer screening tests, and give immunizations. Be sure parents understand the need for tests and treatments, and relay the results of tests to them.

Nurses who work in hospitals, emergency services, and other facilities also are an important link in health supervision. Ask where and how often the child is seen for care. Check immunization schedules to be sure they are up-to-date; administer needed vaccines (Figure 8–10 ➤). When the child is not being regularly seen, find out if the family does not understand the significance of these visits or lacks the resources to obtain them. Refer the family to resources as needed so that they can identify a pediatric healthcare home. Some agencies that provide health supervision are equipped to perform home visits on a regular basis or in case of special need. When nurses make regular home visits to families with many risk factors, health outcomes are improved (Paul, Phillips, Widom, & Hollenbeak, 2004). Seeing the family in the natural setting enables the nurse to tailor interventions to the specific situation. Nutrition, safety, and other teaching is more effective when it matches the family needs. For example, showing how to set up a stimulating environment with safe materials, even if toys are limited, is an effective nursing strategy. Ensure that home visits are performed whenever appropriate and available, either through the pediatric healthcare home or other community agency.

Before the family leaves the facility, be sure they have the next appointment scheduled. Summarize the content of the present visit, emphasizing the family's

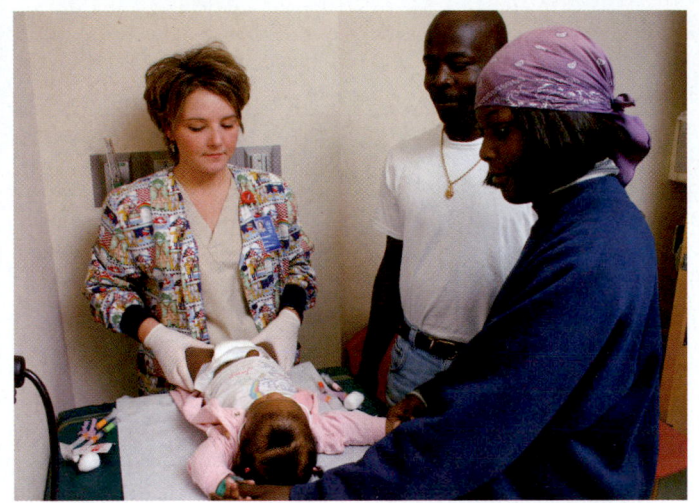
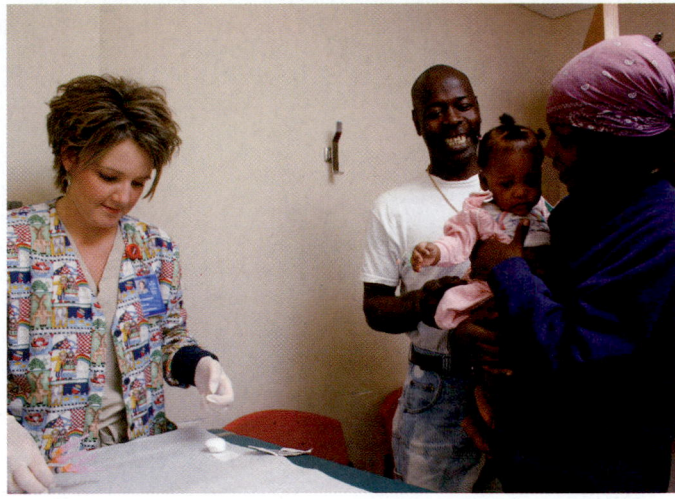

A   B

Figure 8–10 ➤ The nurse positions the baby on the edge of the examination table to isolate the vastus lateralis muscle used for immunization administration. A, The mother holds the baby's arms out of reach. B, After the immunization the parents comfort the infant and are reassured that all is well. Instructions are given for managing side effects and scheduling the next visit.

strengths and the baby's newly acquired developmental skills. Sensitively list any areas that require work in the coming weeks, such as "babyproofing" the home or encouraging the infant to reach for objects. Provide a journal or notebook in which the parents can record the infant's development and write down questions to ask in future visits. Suggest possible topics for the parents to learn about and provide books, brochures, and other printed material.

Evaluation

Expected outcomes of nursing care for the infant and family in health promotion and health maintenance include:

- Parents state common safety hazards at the child's present and upcoming ages.
- The infant demonstrates normal patterns of growth and progression in developmental milestones.
- The infant remains free of disease and injury.
- The infant is well adjusted, showing positive response to the environment and interactions with significant others.

CRITICAL THINKING IN ACTION

Recall 22-year-old Shannon, who is described at the beginning of the chapter. She is a single mother with two daughters, 5-year-old Denise and 10-day-old Rhonda. Shannon lives with her male partner, who is the father of the new baby. Rhonda was born at 37 weeks' gestation, weighed 2800 g (6 lb, 3 oz) at birth, required phototherapy for newborn jaundice, and had initial difficulty breast-feeding. She was discharged from the nursery at 5 days of age.

1. What questions would the pediatric nurse and lactation consultant ask Shannon to assess the adequacy of breast-feeding at this time? What assessments of the newborn will provide clues about the adequacy of intake?

2. Consult Chapter 5 for a description of newborn reflexes. Plan a thorough newborn assessment that includes the reflexes. Why is it important to complete this neurological testing on baby Rhonda?

3. Plan a teaching session for Shannon that describes the sleep patterns of newborns. Integrate suggestions to enable Rhonda and her partner to obtain adequate rest.

4. Denise is Rhonda's 5-year-old sibling. What questions will you ask Shannon about Denise's adjustment to a new sibling?

 Refer to your Prentice Hall Nursing MediaLink DVD-ROM for answers.

EXPLORE MediaLink

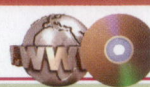

http://www.prenhall.com/ball

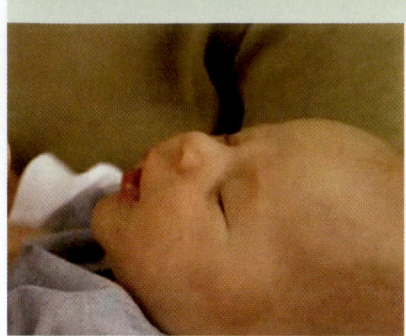

Resources for this chapter can be found on the Prentice Hall Nursing MediaLink DVD-ROM accompanying this textbook, and on the Companion Website at http://www.prenhall.com/ball.

DVD-ROM
Audio Glossary
NCLEX-RN® Review
Video
    Helping the Infant Sleep

COMPANION WEBSITE
Audio Glossary
NCLEX-RN® Review
Care Plan Activity: An Adopted Premature Infant
Case Study: Acceptable Weight Loss of Newborns
Critical Thinking
    Newborn Abduction
    Plot Growth Values
MediaLink Applications
    Baby-proofing the Home
    Determining Gestational Age
    Safety Products
WebLinks

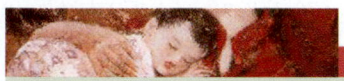

REFERENCES

American Academy of Pediatrics. (2001). The prenatal visit. *Pediatrics, 107,* 1456–1458.

American Academy of Pediatrics. (2002). The medical home. Policy statement. *Pediatrics, 110,* 184–186.

American Academy of Pediatrics. (2004a). *Car safety seats: A guide for families 2004.* Chicago, IL: Author.

American Academy of Pediatrics. (2004b). Hospital stay for healthy term newborns. *Pediatrics, 113*(5), 1434–1436. Also online at http://aappolicy.aappublications.org/cgi/content/full/pediatrics

American Academy of Pediatric Dentistry. (2004). *Policy on the dental home.* Chicago, IL: Author.

American Academy of Pediatrics and The American College of Obstetricians and Gynecologists. (2002). *Guidelines for perinatal care* (5th ed.). Elk Grove Village, IL: Author.

Blackburn, S. T. (2003). *Maternal, fetal, and neonatal physiology: A clinical perspective.* St Louis, MO: Saunders.

Carbaugh, S. F. (2004). Understanding shaken baby syndrome. *Advances in Neonatal Care, 4,* 105–114.

Centers for Disease Control and Prevention. (2006). Secondhand smoke. Retrieved July 12, 2006, from http://www.cdc.gov/tobacco/factsheets/seconhand_smoke_factsheet.htm

Child restraints for newborn infants: A health care provider's guide. (2004). Seattle, WA: Safe Ride News Publications.

Committee on Nutrition. (2004). *Pediatric nutrition handbook,* (5th ed.). Elk Grove Village, IL: American Academy of Pediatrics.

Davis, K. F., Parker, K. P., & Montgomery, G. L. (2004). Sleep in infants and young children: Part one: Normal sleep. *Journal of Pediatric Health Care, 18,* 65–71.

Green, M., & Palfrey, J. S. (Eds.). (2002). *Bright futures: Guidelines for health supervision of infants, children, and adolescents* (2nd ed., rev.). Arlington, VA: National Center for Education in Maternal and Child Health.

Health Resources and Services Administration (HRSA), U.S. Department of Health and Human Services. (2004). *SIDS deaths by race and ethnicity 1995–2001.* Vienna, VA: National Sudden Infant Death Syndrome/Infant Death Resource Center.

Hoban, T. F. (2004). Sleep and its disorders in children. *Seminars in Neurology, 24,* 327–340.

Jellinek, M., Patel, B. P., & Froehle, M. C. (Eds.). (2002). *Bright futures in practice; Mental health vol. II, tool kit.* Arlington, VA: National Center for Education in Maternal and Child Health.

Krous, H. F., Beckwith, B., Byard, R., et al. (2004). Sudden Infant Death Syndrome and unclassified sudden infant deaths: A definitional and diagnostic approach. *Pediatrics, 114,* 234–238.

March of Dimes. (2004). *Newborn screening: March of Dimes newborn screening recommendations: Professionals and researchers.* Online at http://www.marchofdimes.com/printableArticles/580_4043.asp?printable=true

Mindell, J. (2003). *Sleep, infants, and parents. National Sleep Foundation.* Retrieved August 28, 2003, from http://www.sleepfoundation.org/ask/infantsandparents

Nikolopoulou, M., & St. James-Roberts, I. (2003). Preventing sleeping problems in infants who are at risk of developing them. *Archives of Diseases in Children, 88,* 108–109.

Ohgi, S., Akiyama, T., Arisawa, K., & Shigemori, K. (2004). Randomised controlled trial of swaddling versus massage in the management of excessive crying in infants with cerebral injuries. *Archives of Disease in Childhood, 89,* 212–214.

Patrick, K., Spear, B., Holt, K., & Sofka, D. (Eds.). (2001). *Bright futures in practice: Physical activity.* Arlington, VA: National Center for Education in Maternal & Child Health.

Paul, I. M., Phillips, T. A., Widome, M. D., & Hollenbeak, C. S. (2004). Cost-effectiveness of postnatal home nursing visits for prevention of hospital care for jaundice and dehydration. *Pediatrics, 114,* 1015–1022.

Persing, J., James, H., Swanson, J., & Kattwinkel, J. (2003). Prevention and management of positional skull deformities in infants. *Pediatrics, 112,* 199–202.

Shelov, S. P. (Ed.). (2004). *Caring for your baby and young child: Birth to age 5* (4th ed.). Elk Grove, Village IL: American Academy of Pediatrics.

Skuladottir, A., & Thome, M. (2003). Changes in infant sleep problems after a family-centered intervention. *Pediatric Nursing, 29,* 375–378.

Story, M., Holt, K., & Sofka, D. (Eds.). (2002). *Bright futures in practice: Nutrition.* Arlington, VA: National Center for Education in Maternal and Child Health.

HEALTH PROMOTION AND HEALTH MAINTENANCE FOR THE YOUNG AND SCHOOL-AGE CHILD

9

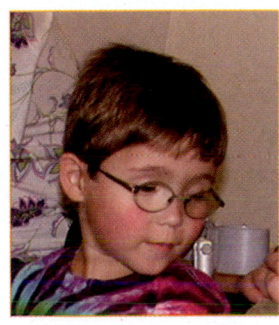

TY is a 10-year-old boy with osteogenesis imperfecta or "brittle bone disease." The disease was diagnosed at 1 year of age when Ty experienced a severe leg fracture while learning to walk although he had his first arm fracture during infancy. Ty's parents encouraged his development and tried to protect him from risks that might lead to fractures. He had about two fractures annually during early childhood, requiring surgery several times. In spite of this, Ty showed steady gains in development. He was home schooled for several years but about 2 years ago his family placed him in a local public school. The school and home healthcare nurse coordinated care to provide Ty with an individualized education plan. He excelled at school, becoming a leader among peers and an honors student. He is a class officer and performs in school plays. Ty has recently had surgery to insert rods to strengthen long bones in his legs and is in a wheelchair during the healing process. His parents believe that Ty's early health care assisted him in successful disease management so that he could continue to develop his social skills. Ty regularly visits his pediatric healthcare home for assessment of growth, monitoring for fractures, and implementation of usual care regarding nutrition, oral health, and injury prevention. Physical activities are suggested that allow for safe exercise, so Ty joined a wheelchair basketball team and swims weekly.

KEY TERMS

body image **333**
deciduous
    teeth **315**
early childhood
    caries (ECC) **315**
individualized
    approach **339**
kinesthesia **314**
latchkey
    children **337**

nightmares **317**
night terrors **317**
population-based
    approach **339**
self-concept **331**
self-esteem **331**
sexuality **333**
spiritual health **334**
stranger
    anxiety **310**

MediaLink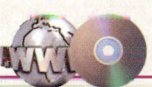

http://www.prenhall.com/ball

See the Prentice Hall Nursing MediaLink DVD-ROM and Companion Website for chapter-specific resources.

LEARNING OUTCOMES

After reading this chapter, you will be able to do the following:

1. State components of growth and developmental surveillance needs for children of toddler, preschool, and school ages.

2. Describe the nutrition, physical activity, and oral health needs of young children.

3. Integrate pertinent mental health care into health supervision visits for young and school-age children.

4. Synthesize data about the family and other social relationships to promote and maintain health of young and school-age children.

5. State components of self-concept for school-age children.

6. Describe the growing importance of peers in planning teaching strategies with school-age children.

7. Plan assessment and interventions appropriate for health promotion and health maintenance during health supervision visits of young and school-age children.

8. Use knowledge of the major injury risks of young and school-age children to plan nursing interventions that contribute to their prevention.

HEALTH PROMOTION AND HEALTH MAINTENANCE FOR THE YOUNG CHILD: TODDLER AND PRESCHOOL AGE

The years following infancy are challenging for parents as the child grows and acquires new developmental skills. The child progresses from the first tentative steps and words at a year of age through the "terrible twos" of toddlerhood and into preschool age when most children attend some type of education program, have well-developed verbal communication, and acquire many gross and fine motor skills. Toddler and preschool ages are often grouped as "young childhood" since the family remains the primary system within which the child interacts, and there are many common health concerns such as nutrition, sleep, and growing independence. Facing consistent changes in development, parents rely on the pediatric healthcare home (medical home) for advice and information. Regular visits are recommended for 12, 15, and 18 months, and at about 2, 3, 4, and 5 years of age. Nurses apply concepts of anticipatory guidance during visits for health promotion and health maintenance to assist parents in the transitions they face.

Recommendations for developmental health supervision of young children includes four main categories. Use this framework to plan these health supervision visits:

1. *Assessment* is performed, using screening tests, evaluations, and observations.
2. *Education* provides information about parent-child interactions, sleep, discipline, and other developmental tasks.
3. *Intervention* includes counseling the parent, making home visits, and ensuring ongoing contacts with health professionals.
4. *Care coordination* between the office setting and community resources ensure that proper referrals occur (Halfon et al., 2003).

General Observations

A collaborative relationship between the family and the healthcare providers should already be established. If, however, the family is new to this care provider, reach out to welcome them warmly and express interest in them as individuals and parents. As families often feel uncomfortable in healthcare settings, it is important to establish positive rapport so they will be able to ask questions and bring up concerns about the child.

While calling the toddler in from the waiting room, it is wise to recall the child just 1 year before. It is amazing that this young child is now able to walk in, even if with a bit of help. Watch for the child's desire for independence or signs of continuing reliance on the parent. By preschool age, the child is totally independent in walking and usually engages in conversations easily. Welcoming the child warmly, the nurse assesses the preschool child's social skills and motor activities. Direct greetings or questions to the child to evaluate **stranger anxiety** and ability to understand simple commands or questions. What verbal skills are observed? Observe the child's general appearance, nutrition, and state of health.

Health supervision visits are adapted for older toddlers and preschoolers to include observations of parental discipline and interaction style. Does the parent respond to the child's questions? Were age-appropriate toys or activities brought to the visit to help occupy the child while waiting? Is the child observant of the environment and alert?

Growth and Developmental Surveillance

An essential assessment skill integrated into the visit is measurement of growth. Weight and length are measured and compared to expected patterns of growth. Once the child can stand to be measured, sometime between 2–3 years of age, charts for standing height rather than recumbent length are used. Body mass index (BMI) is first calculated at 2 years of age and provides information about the relationship of height and weight (see Chapter 4 ∞). Head circumference is usually measured until the child is between 1–2 years of age.

Growth continues to be a primary way of evaluating the child's nutritional status. It may also provide clues about conditions that have not yet been evaluated such as endocrine, cardiac, or other disorders. Depending on the results of growth measurement, additional data may be gathered. For a child under the 5th percentile for weight or BMI, detailed nutritional intake records should begin. Laboratory studies such as hematocrit and hemoglobin can be performed. Patterns of family growth can be examined. What size are the parents and siblings? Ask if the child has had any illness or hospitalization. For children above the 85th percentile for BMI, detailed dietary intake and physical activity history should be taken. Consult the growth grids in Appendix A.

The physical assessment is performed, with some parts conducted by the nurse and others by the primary care provider such as a physician or nurse practitioner. See Chapter 5 ∞ for a thorough discussion of physical examination. The order of the examination and the approaches to the child are particularly important at this age. Leave intrusive procedures such as the ear and eye exam and visualization of genitalia until the end of the exam. Integrate techniques such as allowing the child to play with the stethoscope, "blow out" the light from the otoscope, or make a game of pushing the legs against the examiner to measure symmetry of strength (Figure 9–1 ➤). Preschoolers are generally interested in their bodies so teaching about parts of the examination is helpful. During the physical examination, ask the parents pertinent questions. Consider the young child's expected developmental milestones (see Chapter 3 ∞) and ask questions related to these milestones. Developmental surveillance is integrated throughout the visit and developmental screening and/or testing are performed. Ask if the child has had developmental testing done at a childcare agency or another site.

Nurses generally have in-depth knowledge of child development, through growth and development courses and pediatric nursing curricula, and are thus well positioned to ensure that parental concerns related to child development are addressed (Table 9–1). An accurate developmental screening test should be administered at every well-child visit (Glascoe & Macias, 2003). Fine and gross motor skills, communication methods and social interactions, and language skills are basic components of screening tools. See Chapter 7 ∞ for a list of commonly used tests. Nurses should verify that parents understand and can read the screening tool. Provide assistance and translators as needed.

Additionally, be alert for information that emerges during conversations at the visit and ask further questions as needed. Topics pertinent at health supervision visits of young children include sleep patterns, discipline techniques, toilet training, learning and reading practices, communication, and parental issues and questions. Many children, especially by preschool age, are attending a childcare center. Ask about the

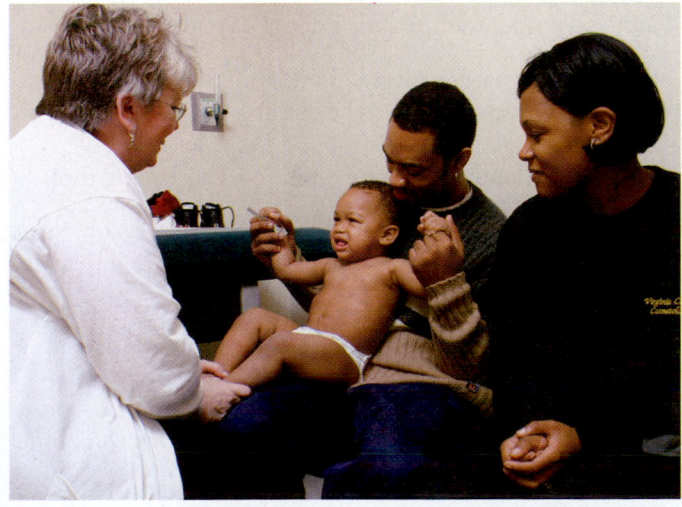

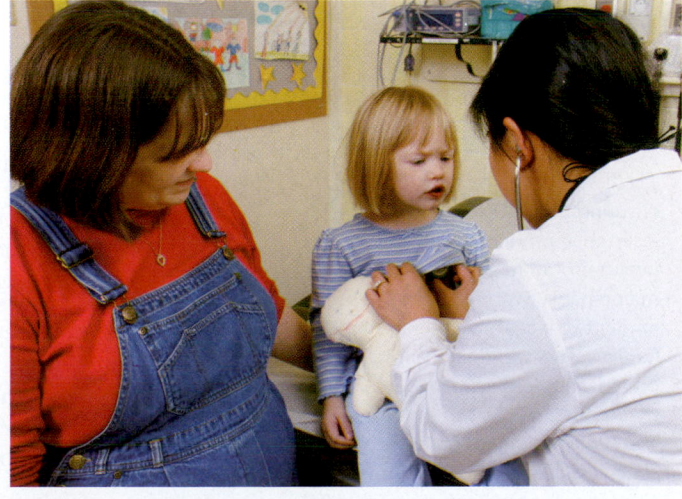

A

B

Figure 9–1 ➤ The approach to examination of the toddler or preschooler is important in order to elicit cooperation. A, The toddler may accept parts of the examination best when seated on the parent's lap such as shown in this photo of a boy with his father. B, The preschooler likes the opportunity to touch and become comfortable with equipment used, or in this case hold a doll that receives the same examinations as the child.

Table 9–1	DEVELOPMENTAL MILESTONES OBSERVED DURING HEALTH PROMOTION AND HEALTH MAINTENANCE VISITS OF TODDLERS AND PRESCHOOLERS
Age	**Developmental Milestones**
12 months	• Walks alone or with help • Enjoys social games and interactions • Speaks one to three words and understands simple commands • Drinks from cup and feeds self
15 months	• Walks by self, crawls or walks up stairs • Stacks two blocks • Points to one or more body parts • Is increasingly interactive • Explores environment
18 months	• Walks with ease • Pushes or pulls toy • Stacks three or more blocks • Uses spoon to eat, spilling often • Follows directions and uses 15–20 words
2–3 years	• Goes up and down steps • Kicks ball • Scribbles and draws lines on paper • Imitates words and actions of adults
3–4 years	• Jumps • Rides tricycle • Draws precise lines on paper; attempts to imitate circle, line, and cross • Always feeds self • Dresses self though sometimes clothes are backwards • Has friends and plays with others
4–5 years	• Recites rhymes and songs • States name • Draws a rudimentary person • Builds tower of blocks and bridges with blocks • Throws ball overhand

RESEARCH

Pediatric Service Satisfaction

Several studies have examined parents' satisfaction with the pediatric services received by their children. These include the 1996 Commonwealth Fund Survey of Parents with Young Children (Young, 1999), the 2000 National Survey of Early Childhood Health (Halfon, 2002; Halfon, Inkelas, Mistry, & Olson, 2004), and the American Academy of Pediatrics survey (AAP, 2000). Topics that have been identified by parents in these surveys as needing more attention in child healthcare visits include:

- Sleep issues
- Discipline
- Toilet training
- Learning/reading
- Child communication
- Parent substance use, emotional state, supports

Nurses can be influential in ensuring that each of these topics is inserted appropriately into each health promotion/health maintenance visit. Additionally, the amount of face-to-face time that families have with healthcare providers is significantly related to their ratings of care, so ensure that you provide time for parents to talk, ask questions, and communicate with all healthcare providers. See Table 9-8 for examples of questions to ask and teaching to perform during the early childhood healthcare visits.

experience and whether developmental skills are a focus of activity. Ask if the parent is pleased with the childcare experience or needs further resources.

Health promotion growth and development issues for toddlers and preschoolers are addressed at each visit. Some common examples include:

- Explaining growth patterns and what is expected in the months ahead
- Providing toys that encourage development of the coming developmental milestones
- Showing parents the child's developmental progression on a screening tool

Likewise, health maintenance activities are included in health supervision visits, with the primary purpose being prevention of disease and injury. Specific examples are included throughout the chapter, but some general areas addressed are:

- Connecting developmental skills with risks for injury such as drowning and car crashes
- Recognizing the possibility of infectious diseases as the child begins a childcare experience and addressing recognition and treatments for common diseases (Glascoe & Macias, 2003)

Expected outcomes for the child include normal growth and development patterns for motor, language, and social skills; parental knowledge of stimulating activities for the child; awareness of the family about risks to growth and development; and healthy body systems for the child.

Nutrition

The child's nutritional status continues to play an important part in promoting health and preventing health disruptions during toddler and preschooler years. Good nutrition fosters normal growth patterns, promotes developmental progression, and helps prevent disorders such as anemia, tooth decay, and immune dysfunction. In addition, intake of food takes on an increasingly social dimension during early childhood as children interact more with adults and other children at mealtimes.

For toddlers, questions for the family focus on introduction of foods, child's eating patterns, and transition from breast or bottle to other liquids. The toddler often consumes small amounts of foods and parents consequently worry about the change in appetite. Showing the parents that the child is growing normally can help allay their anxiety about this common developmental variation. Preschoolers increasingly interact with others during food preparation and meal consumption. Questions focus on the child's likes and dislikes for particular foods, behavior at the table, and establishment of healthy family eating patterns. Ask how often the family eats out, especially at fast food restaurants. When parents are busy and older siblings are in activities, both toddlers and preschoolers may be eating foods such as French fries or milk shakes several times a week. Suggest alternative approaches to the busy lifestyle, such as bringing fresh fruit slices along when an older sibling is at a sporting event, keeping a cooler in the car to maintain cool items, and limiting fast food meals to no more than one or two per week. Encourage the family to set times when they all eat together, even if only a few times per week. If children help prepare this family meal, and then eat together, nutritional knowledge and intake can be positively enhanced. When the child is in a childcare center or home, encourage the parents to find out what food is provided for the child in that setting.

During the toddler and preschool years, children are gaining much more independence about food choices and eating patterns. At the same time, their eating patterns depend mainly on the family; therefore, assessment should involve the entire family unit. Parents can benefit from receiving information about nutrition in young children (Table 9–2).

Health promotion interventions include supporting breast-feeding for young toddlers and ensuring that preschoolers have a role in selecting foods for healthy snacks. Parental education is influential in shaping their young child's diet and should be integrated into all visits (Fuller, Keller, Olson, & Plymale, 2005). Teach the amounts of food that should be offered and frequency of meals. Encourage parents to make food preparation and meals a pleasant experience. See Chapter 4 for additional information about the nutritional needs of young children. An example of an important health promotion item to include with every family is the importance of including "five a day," or five servings of fruits and vegetables into the daily diet. Nurses and parents partner to ensure that the young child establishes healthy eating habits at home and in other daily settings. Health maintenance activities are those that focus primarily on disease and injury prevention, with examples of feeding practices that do not include common choking foods, and limiting daily fruit juice intake to prevent dental caries and excessive caloric intake. Desired outcomes related to nutrition include meeting normal growth and development milestones, maintaining recommended weight, increasing understanding of healthy food patterns, and preventing nutrition-related disorders.

Physical Activity

The toddler and preschooler consistently show gains in fine and gross motor abilities. They move around independently and have more physical activity away from the home base. They commonly visit parks, swim, attend childcare centers, and help with some household tasks. These activities are important, both because they assist the child to continue to develop motor skills, and limit the amount of time spent in sedentary behavior. The toddler and preschool years are an important time for setting the physical activity habits that will continue during childhood.

During toddler years, the main emphasis is on providing experiences that encourage further motor development. The child needs to walk, run, hop, push and pull

Table 9–2	**NUTRITION TEACHING FOR HEALTH PROMOTION AND HEALTH MAINTENANCE VISITS**
Age	**Nutrition Teaching**
1 year	• Support mother who continues to breast-feed • Wean child from bottle by substituting cup • If beginning to use cow milk, use whole milk • Limit juice to 4–6 ounces daily; offer water several times daily • Encourage safety measures—use high chair with strap, secure child and use caution in grocery carts, do not allow foods to be eaten in car • Provide information on choking and airway obstruction removal training • Provide food and water safety guidelines (see Chapter 4 ∞) • Be sure all major food groups have been introduced • Limit high-fat and high-sugar foods • Review amounts of food commonly consumed and frequency of feedings • Review use of fluoride if water supply is not fluoridated
2 years	• Encourage total removal of bottle if still in use • Ensure that all foods common to family have been offered • Offer child-sized eating utensils • Change to low-fat or skim milk if family desires • Limit milk to two servings daily • Teach parents methods for dealing with temper tantrums over food—make food available at meal and snack times only, do not force intake, offer a variety of foods • Teach that child may have days of very low intake due to slowing growth rate
3 years	• Teach normal intake and decreasing number of snacks • Engage child in food preparation and pouring liquids from small pitcher • Recognize that food jags (periods when only 1 or 2 foods are eaten) are common • Recognize importance of social nature of eating; expect child to sit for a short period at meals with family • Meals and snacks should not be eaten while watching television
4 years	• Encourage involving child in snack selection and preparation • Start to teach food groups and importance of nutrition for the body • Alter intake as appropriate depending on weight and BMI • Make dairy products consumed low or reduced fat

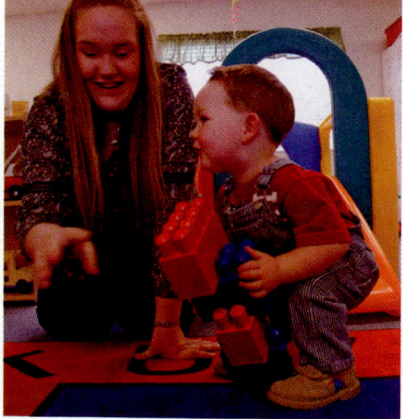

Figure 9–2 ➤ This toddler enjoys motor activity that uses large muscle groups. The preschooler begins to spend increasing amounts of time in coordination of both small and large muscle mass. List several physical activities that you can suggest for the parents of children in each of these age groups.

objects, and throw balls. A minimum of 60 minutes per day of unstructured physical activity is needed (Gunner, Atkinson, Nichols, & Eissa, 2005). Motor activity is a major component in all play times and activities should engage the child's large and small muscle groups (Figure 9–2 ➤). By the preschool years, coordination becomes increasingly important. Physical activity is important for all children, including those with developmental disabilities. The preschooler learns to balance, walk on one foot, skip, and throw and catch with greater accuracy. **Kinesthesia**, or the sense of one's body position and movement, develops during these years. Eye-hand coordination improves at the same time that visual acuity matures (Patrick, Spear, Holt, & Sofka, 2001). The social component plays an important role as children learn to engage in games and activities cooperatively with others.

The nurse applies the concept of resilience by identifying both risk and protective factors related to physical activity (Table 9–3). The assessment becomes the basis for nursing interventions, both to reinforce positive physical activity and to make recommendations for changes where needed.

Since both children and adults are commonly overweight and sedentary in today's society, emphasis on physical activity should be a part of each health supervision visit. Nurses and parents are partners in planning activities for the young child; patterns set in motion at this early age will continue into the rest of childhood and into adulthood. Suggestions for the family may include setting guidelines to limit television and other screen activities to a maximum of 2 hours daily in order to facilitate adequate physical activity time. Children should not have television and computers in their bedrooms. Suggest activities that parents can do with their children. Health promotion teaching

Table 9-3	RISK AND PROTECTIVE FACTORS REGARDING PHYSICAL ACTIVITY IN TODDLERHOOD AND PRESCHOOL

Risk Factors	Protective Factors
• Limited stimulation by family or other care providers • Long work hours by parents • Parents who have little physical activity on a daily basis • Limited social time with other children • Limited access to balls, slides, balance beams, tricycles, and other materials that foster physical activity • Adequate safety gear for activities is not available • Reluctance to try new physical activity • Television or other screen activities are engaged in for more than 2 hours daily • Developmental delay • Slow development of social skills • Lack of knowledge by family about child's physical activity needs • Limited community resources for childcare and physical activity • Unsafe neighborhood and lack of lawns, parks, and other facilities	• Expected developmental progression • Daily contact with other young children • Easily engaged socially with others • Eagerness to try new physical activity • Access to balls, slides, balance beams, tricycles, and other materials that foster physical activity • Adequate safety gear that properly fits child is available • Family members engage in daily physical activity • Family members spend time daily in physical activity with child • Family understands motor developmental milestones and importance of physical activity in childhood • Television and other screen activities are limited to no more than 2 hours daily • Neighborhood contains access to childcare that integrates physical activity • Neighborhood is safe, and contains lawns, parks, and other facilities

Adapted from Patrick, K., Spear, B., Holt, K., & Sofka, D. (Eds.). (2001). *Bright futures in practice: Physical activity.* Arlington, VA: National Center for Education in Maternal and Child Health.

imparts to parents the benefits of activity, such as a healthy immune and cardiovascular system, positive self-concept of the child, and the child's learning of important motor skills. Health maintenance teaching focuses on disease prevention, such as avoidance of overweight, and injury prevention, with use of protective gear for sports.

Expected outcomes of health promotion and health supervision related to physical activity are daily inclusion of at least 60 minutes of activity into life patterns, normal developmental progression of musculoskeletal system, growth in coordination, and appropriate balance between dietary intake and physical activity so that normal weight is maintained.

Oral Health

The early childhood years play an important part in the child's future oral health, and yet dental care remains one of the most preventable and yet commonly unmet health-care needs for children in developed countries (VanLandeghen, Bronstein, & Brach, 2003). **Early childhood caries (ECC)** is defined as one or more decayed, missing, or filled tooth surfaces in a child less than 5 years of age (National Maternal and Child Oral Health Resource Center, 2004). Other terms for this condition include "bottle mouth syndrome" or "baby bottle tooth decay." This condition is caused by inadequate preventive care, which can include poor diet, brushing, and feeding habits. ECC is serious because young children with the condition are more likely to have continuing dental problems that can influence speech, cause pain, and delay development. Teaching prevention at an early age is key to preventing the problem.

The nurse assists the family to ensure oral health for the young child. At about 1 year of age the child should have made a first visit to the dentist. By about 2 years of age, the toddler has a full set of 20 teeth. Evaluate these teeth for condition and number. They help to maintain space for the permanent teeth, foster positive eating habits, and are needed for language development. Inquire about how the family cleans the teeth and ask them to demonstrate if the child has any dental decay. At the end of preschool, the first of these **deciduous teeth** are lost, an important developmental event for most children.

Based on the results of the child's teeth assessment, observation of language skills, and answers to questions directed at parents, plan interventions that will foster maintenance of oral health, thus preventing dental disease. (See Chapter 19 ∞ for emergency treatment of dental injury.) These may include referral to low-cost dental clinics, provision of toothbrush and toothpaste, demonstration to the parents and young child about proper brushing technique, and teaching about limiting sweet snacks and drinks. Remember to positively reinforce health promotion practices such as good oral hygiene for toddlers and preschoolers who brush, visit the dentist, and are careful to limit intake of sweets. Desired outcomes for oral health are eruption of a normal set of deciduous teeth, regular dental care, nutrition and hygiene practices that foster dental health, and child and parent knowledge about oral health.

Mental and Spiritual Health

The family is key in fostering a positive self-image and setting the stage for the young child's mental health. Approximately 13% of preschool children have mental health problems so screening tools and observations can be used to identify children at risk, and to maximize the protective factors in families (Squires & Nickel, 2003). As the family is called in for the visit, begin your assessment of the family's methods of influencing mental health. Observe communication and interactions in the family and the child's ability to interact with healthcare providers. Ask for a description of a typical day or what the child has recently begun to do. The child's sense of self and mental status are related to new accomplishments. Inquire about toilet training, tooth brushing, choosing clothes and getting dressed, using crayons, or other developmental tasks.

Self-regulation by the infant was described as the ability to sooth and comfort the self. By toddler and preschool periods, the young child self-regulates other activities to control anger, desires for objects or foods, and other behaviors. In order to assist the child in developing the ability to control and regulate self, parents often use discipline techniques. Ask about how the parent deals with the child who is having a temper tantrum or showing other undesirable behaviors. Discourage physical punishment and offer alternatives (Ateah, Secco, & Woodgate, 2003). Reinforce positive ways of helping the child set limits for self and make suggestions when parents need assistance (See Families Want to Know: Positive Discipline). The goal of discipline is to help the child develop a sense of right and wrong, and to learn acceptable ways of dealing with other people.

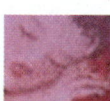

FAMILIES WANT TO KNOW

Positive Discipline

First, provide structure that enhances the possibility of desirable behaviors:

- Limit rules to those that are essential. It will be easier to enforce a few important rules than many that are nonessential.
- Provide an environment where the child is mainly free to explore safely in order to avoid constant cautions. For example, have adequate play space for toddlers with limited fragile glassware in the usual daily environment. It is easier for the toddler to learn not to touch a few objects when adequate objects are provided for play.
- Spend time interacting with the child several times each day. Praise positive behaviors frequently. Preschoolers often like to have charts with stars to record picking up toys, helping a parent, and other positive behaviors. Once a certain number of stars is reached a reward, such as stickers or an outing with the parent, is earned.

When the child shows undesirable behaviors:

- Use distraction as the first approach and praise the child for selecting the new activity suggested by the parent.
- Tell the child one time that the behavior is unsatisfactory and what will happen if the behavior persists.

- Separate the child from a setting in which behavior is undesirable. Place the child in "time-out," a separate place that is safe. Toddlers can be placed in a playpen or crib, while preschoolers are told to sit on a chair. One minute of time-out per year of age is a good length of time. Once time-out is over, provide a positive activity and move the child directly toward the activity.

When undesirable behaviors include other people, such as biting or hitting:

- Tell the child clearly that it is not satisfactory to hurt another person.
- Separate the child immediately from the situation and use time-out.
- If there are repeated episodes, be sure the child is getting adequate sleep and food, has opportunities for active play that releases energy, and has positive attention from many people in the environment. Be sensitive to stresses such as a recent trauma or a new sibling.
- Encourage the child to "use words" instead of hitting or biting. Until able to do so on his or her own, parents can model this behavior. "You feel like saying 'I am really upset that you took my toy away.' Let's use words instead of hitting so your sister knows that."

Adequate sleep and rest are needed for children to master self-regulation. Most toddlers have established regular sleeping patterns with occasional night awakenings. They sleep about 13–14 hours at night with one or two daytime naps (Hoban, 2004). Parents have usually learned to establish clear routines such as reading a story, rubbing a back, and then leaving the child alone. Occasionally parents who work during the day may feel guilty about putting the child to sleep. Help them to spend quality time with the child after arriving home, and then to establish clear sleeping expectations. Transitional objects such as blankets or toys are important for the toddler and can be used during childcare experiences to provide comfort and help maintain normal routines. Some families prefer to have children sleep in the bed with parents. If this is the parents' decision, be sure they are aware of safety hazards such as excessive bedding, falling between the headboard and frame, parental smoking that could lead to fire, or parental alcohol and drug use that can lead to not being alert to the child.

The preschooler sleeps about 11 hours and may have one or no naps each day (Hoban, 2004). Some quiet playtime can be beneficial even for the preschooler who does not nap. At this age, some children develop awakenings at night and may need some assistance in falling back to sleep. **Nightmares** are frightening dreams that awaken the child who is often crying and upset. Parents can reassure the child, rub the child's back, provide some repeat of a bedtime routine such as reading a story, and then allow the child to settle into sleep again. It is not advisable to bring the child to the parental bed since he or she may start to awaken at night in order to continue this practice. **Night terrors** are characterized by a child who cries out and appears frightened. However, in contrast to nightmares, the child having a night terror is not fully awake, and may appear disoriented (Mason & Pack, 2005). Parents should quietly talk to and comfort the child, allowing him or her to return to sleep. There is no recollection of these events the next morning.

The toddler gains more independence in many aspects of life such as mobility and speech. The control over toileting is another milestone that signals greater independence and can lead to a sense of self-control. Ask parents if the toddler has shown interest in toilet training and how they intend to work with the child to attain control over bowel and bladder. Preschoolers are generally well trained for bowel and bladder control with only occasional accidents. These should be treated with understanding rather than blame in order for healthy self-concept to develop. Preschoolers are increasingly aware of gender and sexuality issues. They may ask questions about kissing, love, or their genitals. These questions should be truthfully answered, leaving the child with a positive sense of sexuality. Some exploration of genitals can occur. Children should be told simply that it is something that should occur in private, and then offered other activities to engage them when with other people.

The family's spiritual orientation takes on additional meaning for the toddler and preschooler. They can participate in the family's faith-based practices. This enlarges their microsystem influences to include the religious group, thus reinforcing children's learning about right and wrong. The nurse assesses the family's faith-based or spiritual beliefs and provides support for the family's approach, whether it is in established religious organizations or in the family's other meaningful activities.

Health promotion activities focus on development of a healthy self-concept in the toddler and young child by helping parents to set up successful play experiences, to praise the child for successes, to use effective limit-setting techniques, and to realize and appreciate the child's unique characteristics. Health maintenance seeks to avoid poor self-image that can occur with constant criticism or expectations not in alignment with the toddler's or preschooler's developmental capabilities. Assist the family to spend time together and relax with stress-reducing activities rather than creating an environment where children are overscheduled with commitments (Nelms, 2004). Further examples of the family interactions that can influence the child's self-concept are provided in the following section on relationships.

Desired outcomes for the child related to mental and spiritual health include emergence of a positive self-esteem, ability to self-regulate behaviors, emergence of methods to handle daily stressors, and normal developmental progression in tasks such as toilet training and sleep.

Relationships

Family members are part of the microsystem for the toddler and preschooler; as such, they form a vital part of the child's environment. Families with members who handle stress well and have healthy lifestyle patterns offer security for the young child. When parents are stressed or depressed, the mental status of all family members can be affected. Ask how things are going for the family in general. Inquire about siblings and whether any issues of concern exist that might influence the toddler or preschooler. Illness or behavior problems in a sibling can decrease the parent's ability to deal with other children. The focus on a sibling in need can be confusing to a toddler or preschooler.

Be alert for signs of child abuse and for substance abuse in family members (see Chapter 6 ∞ for a thorough description of child abuse). Have the parents become separated or divorced? Is there a new stepparent?

During questions and observations, the nurse identifies family risk and protective factors. Reinforce strengths and provide services and referrals to deal with risks. Some strengths include:

- Family time together each day
- Parents proud of child's accomplishments and knowledgeable about developmental progression
- Childcare center personnel and family members interact regularly to plan consistent approaches for the toddler and preschooler
- Teen mother of toddler enrolled in high school continuation program with childcare component

Examples of risks to mental health include:

- Mother has been diagnosed with depression
- Uncle in home uses street drugs
- Child awakens with night terrors
- Child was recently in a serious car accident
- Teen mother is estranged from own family and has few goals and resources

Toddlers continue to grow in social abilities, while preschoolers demonstrate large strides in socializing with others. Expect that most toddlers will enjoy playing with other children, although they engage in parallel play, "side by side" with other children. They also engage in play with adults for short periods, such as throwing a ball. However, preschoolers begin to engage in cooperative play activities that directly involve other children. They play "house" where one child plays the mother, and another the child. They engage in simple games where each plays a separate role. Their interactions with adults display similar maturity as they take on tasks such as setting the table for dinner, or picking up books from the floor. Social skills involve getting along with others. Young children exhibit increasing skill in language development, a primary medium for social exchange. From just a few words at 1 year, children progress to stating three-word sentences by 3 years of age. While all parts of speech are not in place, young children certainly have the ability to make needs and thoughts known. Assessment of language skills provides a mirror into this important means of socializing.

Successful social skills involve separating from the parent at times. During toddlerhood, most children spend some time away from parents. Initially they may be fearful and display crying, but gradually they learn to adapt to the new person and place. Preschoolers need to begin developing relationships with other adults and children in order to adapt to the school setting at about 5 years of age. Ask how many people the child has contact with each week, and how he or she manages separation from the parent. Encourage parents to see separation as a skill the child is learning rather than something that is guilt-producing. When they leave the child in a secure setting, they should hug, provide a favorite object, and leave. Short periods initially will teach the child that the parent can be trusted to return. In addition, young children often have tempers and other undesirable behaviors. Assist parents in handling them successfully (see Families Want to Know: Handling Temper Tantrums).

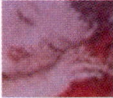

FAMILIES WANT TO KNOW

Handling Temper Tantrums

Temper tantrums are common in toddlers and are manifested as episodes of screaming, crying, pounding objects, kicking, and otherwise showing anger. Toddlers may be expressing frustration with something that has occurred. They have learned that they are independent individuals and have an effect by showing their dismay. Temper tantrums should gradually decrease in number as the child grows into the preschool years. Parents can learn that tantrums are normal but that techniques can assist in handling them successfully. The approaches are similar to those used when the child bites or hits. Some specific suggestions for tantrums include:

- Learn the signals that a tantrum is about to occur. Most toddlers become increasingly agitated and upset. Holding and distracting them at that point may help avoid a tantrum.

- Separate the child from others if possible ("time-out") to eliminate reinforcement by attention given.
- If not possible, be sure the child is safe and not throwing self against objects that could cause injury.
- Remain calm, holding the child firmly still if needed.
- Do not "give in" to the child's demands by giving him or her a food treat or toy; avoid this positive reinforcement of the behavior.
- Talk calmly to the child, verbalizing his or her feelings and what he or she needs to do to calm down.
- Reward the child briefly after control is gained. "It was really good that you could calm down and say you were sorry. Now let's go back to the living room."

Adapted from Colyar, M. R. (2003). *Well-child assessment for primary care providers.* Philadelphia: F.A. Davis Co.

Expected outcomes of health promotion and health maintenance activities with young children include increasing social skills with parents, siblings, and other children and adults; successful management of temperament characteristics; adjustment to time away from the home; and improving language/communication skills.

Disease Prevention Strategies

Toddlers remain prone to many infectious diseases due to immature immune systems. By the preschool age, immune defenses are more mature and communicable diseases are less common. Some immunizations are given during this age period in order to complete the basic series. For children who have not had all immunizations, extra visits to catch them up to recommended levels may be needed. At the end of the preschool period, children have a complete review of the immunization record so any needed injections are given before school entry. See Table 9–4 for immunizations recommended during toddlerhood and preschool. Toddlers and preschoolers also need screening for several health conditions. Earlier visits may have failed to identify a problem due to the child's young age, so areas such as vision, hearing, and developmental milestones are always included.

Recognize that the environment is a powerful influence on children's health. Ask if parents or others in the home smoke. Discourage this practice and describe the health

Table 9–4	IMMUNIZATIONS RECOMMENDED FOR THE YOUNG CHILD

Immunization	Recommendation
Hepatitis B	Series of three doses if not previously completed
Hepatitis A	Series of two doses with first at 12 months and second at least 6 months later
Diphtheria, tetanus, acellular pertussis	Dose #4 in five-dose series from 15–18 months
Haemophilus influenzae type b	Dose #3 in series if using three-dose vaccine
Inactivated poliovirus	Dose #3 given between 6–18 months
Measles, mumps, rubella	Dose #1 from 12–15 months
Varicella	12 months
Pneumococcal	Dose #4 given between 12–15 months
Influenza	Annually from 6–23 months

implications for the child. Is the neighborhood generally safe? Are there air, water, or other toxic exposures? Ask about lead exposure in the home (see Chapter 6 ∞). How much television and other screen time is common in the home? Older siblings who allow the preschooler to play violent video games or watch many hours of inappropriate television can be affecting the young child's mental health. Do parents watch the evening news, even when it involves violence, in front of young children? Do they discuss television shows with the child?

Ask if the child has had any diseases, whether common ones such as middle ear infection, or less common ones such as a serious respiratory infection. Has the child been diagnosed with a chronic disorder like cystic fibrosis or hemophilia? How has that impacted his or her general health and family functioning?

Desired outcomes for disease prevention include integration of prevention methods into the family's daily life, prompt treatment of acute diseases, and individualization of all health supervision topics for the child with a chronic condition or special healthcare need.

Injury Prevention Strategies

Injuries remain a common healthcare problem for children during the toddler and preschooler years. Children's mobility, physical skills, and lack of understanding of the presence of hazards put them at particular risk. In addition, children are generally left to play alone for short periods and toddlers and preschoolers can quickly get into dangerous situations. Every healthcare visit needs to include an assessment of risks and teaching to prevent injuries. Tables 9–5 and 9–6 list injury hazards during these age periods.

Ask parents what they think the most common hazards are for the child's age and add other hazards to their awareness. Car safety always needs reinforcing as the types of seats change when the child reaches 20 and then 40 pounds. Be certain that children from 20–40 pounds:

- Use a convertible forward-facing seat that has been placed in the back seat
- Have harness straps at or above the shoulders

Children over 40 pounds should be placed in a belt-positioning booster seat:

- In the back seat
- That uses both lap and shoulder belts
- With the lap belt low and tight across the lap/upper thigh area and shoulder belt snug across the chest and shoulder

Recommend that parents have their car seat checked by a childcare inspector (Figure 9–3 ➤). Give them the addresses of the closest inspection stations, which you can locate by going through the National Highway Traffic Safety Administration.

Some additional common and serious safety hazards are falls and drowning. In addition to providing general guidelines about safety, these common injuries should be directly addressed. Children often fall down stairs, from counters where they have been placed or have crawled, and from grocery carts. Drowning episodes occur when toddlers and preschoolers are not watched every moment while at a lake or ocean, fall from boats without personal flotation devices on, fall into a backyard pool, or drown in a bathtub or other body of water. While all young children should begin to take swim lessons, this does not guarantee their safety around water. Nursing interventions concentrate on relaying to parents the severity of the risk of falls and drowning for children. Teach them to be aware of the dangers and to avoid them, both at home and in other settings. Refer them to classes on first aid and cardiopulmonary resuscitation.

The child spends increasing time away from the parent. Childcare situations should provide the same supervision the child receives at home. Help parents to ask questions and feel confident in safety at other settings. For example, while parents may be cautious about gun safety at home, few of them inquire if a home the child is visiting has guns and how they are stored.

Preschoolers are generally interested in health and their bodies. This is a time when teaching can become directed both to the parents and to their children. Preschoolers are receptive to practicing street crossing and tricycle/bicycle riding

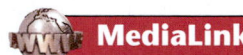

MediaLink

National Highway Traffic Safety Administration

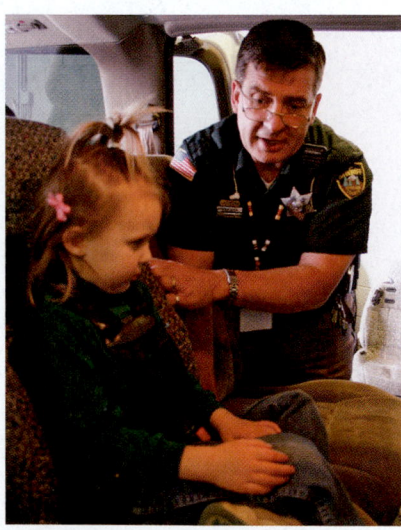

Figure 9–3 ➤ The officer at this police station is certified to examine car seats for children and make recommendations for parents. He is examining a preschooler in a booster seat for proper fit and alignment. Many car seats are improperly installed or not the proper type for a specific age of child, so centers that check seats provide an important service.

Table 9–5	INJURY PREVENTION IN TODDLERHOOD		
	Hazard	**Developmental Characteristics**	**Preventive Measures**
	Falls	Gross motor skills improve: Toddler is able to move chairs to counters and can climb up ladders.	Supervise toddler closely. Provide safe climbing toys. Begin to teach acceptable places for climbing.
	Poisoning	Gross motor skills enable toddler to climb onto chairs and then cabinets. Medicines, cosmetics, and other poisonous substances are easily reached.	Keep medicines and other poisonous material locked away. Use child-resistant containers and cupboard closures. Have poison control center number (1-800-222-1222) by telephone.
	Burns	Toddler is tall enough to reach stove top. Toddler can walk to fireplace and may reach into fire.	Keep pot handles turned inward on stove. Do not burn fires without close supervision. Use a fire screen.
	Drowning	Toddler can walk onto docks or pool decks. Toddler may stand on or climb seats on boat. Toddler may fall into buckets, toilets, and fish tanks and be unable be get top of body out.	Supervise any child near water. Swimming classes do not protect a toddler from drowning. Use child-resistant pool covers. Use approved child life jackets near water and on boats. Empty buckets when not in use.
	Motor vehicle crashes	Toddler may be able to undo seat belt, may resist using car seat, demonstrating characteristic negativism and autonomy.	Insist on safety seat use for all trips. Use approved safety only, such as forward-facing convertible seat. Toddler is not large enough to use car seat belts.

Table 9–6	INJURY PREVENTION IN PRESCHOOL YEARS

	Hazard	Developmental Characteristics	Preventive Measures
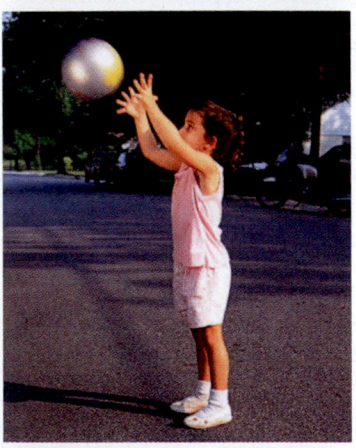	Motor vehicle crashes	Older preschooler independently gets into car and puts on seat belt. Child may forget to belt up or may do so incorrectly.	Verify that child is belted in properly before starting car. Child restraint systems must be used until child weighs 18 kg (40 lb) and is 100 cm (40 in.) tall.
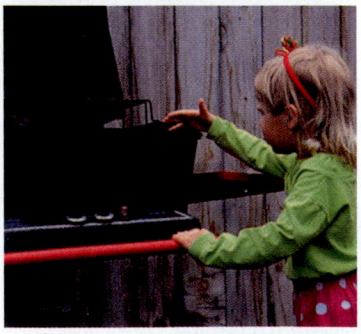	Motor vehicle/ pedestrian accidents	Preschooler increasingly plays outside alone or with friends. Preschooler is unable to judge speed of moving car and assumes driver knows that he or she is present.	Teach child never to go into road. A safe, preferably enclosed, play yard is recommended.
	Drowning	Preschooler who has had swimming lessons may choose to go into a lake or pool.	Teach child never to go into water without an adult. Provide supervision whenever child is near water.
	Burns	Preschooler can understand the hazards of fire.	Teach child to stop, drop, and roll if clothes are on fire. Practice escapes from home are useful. A visit to a fire station can reinforce learning. Teach child how to call 911.
	Needle sticks in hospital	Preschooler can ambulate and is interested in new objects.	Keep needles out of reach. Remove from unit immediately after use.
	Electrical injury in hospital	Preschooler is mobile and may trip over cords and equipment or may choose to examine them.	Avoid use of electrical cords if possible. Keep equipment out of major traffic areas. Keep beds away from electrical outlets. Monitor child closely.

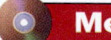
MediaLink

Drowning Prevention Video

skills. It may be helpful to have a place in the clinic or office where they can be taught basic skills such as handwashing or street crossing. Consider the time of year and geographic location and teach appropriately. Spring is often a good time to teach bicycle and water safety, while winter hazards may include woodstoves or other heating devices. See Table 9–7 for further information about toddler and preschooler hazards and safety teaching needed.

Desired outcomes for the child are integration of safe practices into car restraints and other daily activities, progression through toddlerhood and preschool with no serious injuries, prompt care for minor injuries, and increasing understanding by child, parent, and other care providers of the common safety hazards at this age.

Table 9–7	DISEASE AND INJURY PREVENTION TOPICS BY AGE

Age	Injury Prevention Teaching Topics
15 months	• Wash adult and toddler hands frequently • Clean toys with soap and water regularly • Provide child's own bedding for childcare setting and wash weekly • Use forward-facing car safety seat if child is 20 pounds; install correctly and have installation checked; place in back seat and never in front seat with a passenger air bag • Empty containers of water immediately after use; be sure pools or other bodies of water are locked and not accessible • Use sunscreen, hat, and long sleeves in the sun • Keep heavy and sharp objects out of reach; check that all poisons are locked away including in homes visited; keep pet food and cosmetics out of reach • Have poison control number by phones and programmed into cell phones • Be alert for dangers of hot curling irons and other appliances • Have electrical cords out of reach and not hanging down • Keep water temperature from being too hot to touch • Have home environment checked for lead hazards • Secure the child in shopping carts • Do not let child have access to alcoholic drinks • Remember that responsible adults should always supervise your child, not other children • Know CPR, airway obstruction removal, and other first aid
18 months	• As preciously noted • Bolt heavy objects that might be pulled down securely to the wall • Be cautious of the toddler near machinery like lawn mowers or farm equipment in the yard • Use a helmet on the child when taking him or her on the back of a bicycle • Check batteries in home smoke alarms and check system • Ask care providers about discipline methods; do not allow corporal punishment
2–3 years	• As previously noted • When the child is 40 pounds, switch to a belt-positioning booster seat, using vehicle lap and shoulder belt; place in rear seat • Teach handwashing after toileting and other activities • Clean potty chair thoroughly • Keep guns unloaded and locked away in a different locked place than ammunition; install trigger locks • Teach how to cross streets • Provide a helmet for riding tricycles • Check playgrounds for safety hazards and hard surfaces under equipment
3–4 years	• As previously noted • Do not let child play unsupervised • Know CPR, airway obstruction removal, and other first aid for the child who has become a preschooler
4–5 years	• As previously noted • Continue teaching safety skills to the child • Continue supervising when near streets or water sources • Teach safety around strangers (never go with a stranger; find a trusted person like parent or police)

Adapted from Green, M., & Palfrey, J. S. (Eds.). (2002). *Bright futures: Guidelines for health supervision of infants, children and adolescents,* (2nd ed.). Arlington, VA: National Center for Education in Maternal and Child Health.

NURSING MANAGEMENT
Nursing Assessment and Diagnosis

Nurses collaborate with other healthcare professionals such as physicians, nurse practitioners, and speech therapists to assess the health promotion and health maintenance status of young children. The toddler and preschool years are characterized by much developmental progression and strategies need to be constantly adapted to meet the particular needs of the child and family. Once again, it is important to realize that the parents are partners in the child's care. Every health supervision visit should address their questions and concerns, and they should know their observations of the child are an invaluable part of the care process. As the preschooler becomes more verbal, another partner is added to the healthcare team. Ask preschoolers what they want to learn, what questions they have about staying well, and other pertinent questions.

Toddlers and preschoolers are examined for growth, physical health status, and mental/social characteristics. Development is an area that many pediatricians feel ill-prepared to address but which parents commonly want addressed (Halfon et al., 2003). Nurses are adept at describing normal developmental milestones, evaluating children's progression, and using anticipatory guidance to address parental developmental concerns.

Based on a thorough assessment, you will establish nursing diagnoses that are appropriate for the young child and family. Potential nursing diagnoses established during the health supervision of a toddler or preschooler might include:

- Anxiety related to change of environment (new care provider)
- Parental Role Conflict related to lack of support from significant others
- Risk for Delayed Growth and Development related to lead exposure
- Health-Seeking Behaviors related to parental desire for safety information
- Impaired Skin Integrity related to hyperthermia (sunburn)

Planning and Implementation

Based on the established nursing diagnoses, the nurse, in collaboration with other partners, plans strategies to meet the family's needs. Explain that assessment questions are asked in order to provide a picture of the child that can be helpful in partnering with parents to plan health care. Reinforce the importance of the family coming to health supervision visits with their own list of issues. Work with other healthcare professionals to be sure all needs of a particular child and family are addressed.

Some teaching takes place as the examination occurs. Explain the height and weight measurements and what they mean. Relate them to questions about dietary intake and family food patterns. During the physical examination, insert information about common infections such as otitis media (middle ear infection) and share immunization information (see Table 9–8 for a list of potential teaching topics).

If the family has been reluctant to ask questions, reflect on the child's development. "Many children have trouble sleeping through the night; is that the case for Cassandra? What helps her to sleep? What is it like at her bedtime?" Developmental areas such as sleep, discipline, toilet training, and expected developmental milestones should be addressed. If the parents were provided with a journal to record observations and questions in an earlier visit, ask if they have brought it with them.

A key part of the visit involves health promotion activities. It is essential to apply concepts of anticipatory guidance as you address the child's coming developmental progression. If the child will soon be toilet trained, provide information about possible approaches. If the child is learning to swim or has access to water, reinforce safety precautions near water. For the child going to a new childcare center, provide the parents with a list of questions they can ask the care provider, and tips to assist in the transition to a new setting.

Health maintenance activities are added to the visit as you give immunizations and screen for tuberculosis, lead, or problems with language, vision, or hearing. The focus of these activities is to prevent disease or to find it early before there are serious consequences. Whenever you find information that may indicate a problem, be sure to refer the child to the primary care provider, such as a physician or nurse practitioner. You may even recommend that the child be seen by another specialist such as a speech pathologist or dentist. Other health maintenance activities that must be part of each visit with a toddler or preschooler involve teaching about common hazards and how to avoid them. Emergency care in case of injury is also helpful information for parents, so first aid classes can be recommended.

COMMUNITY CARE

Health Hazards

Consult your community-based web sites and national information to learn about common hazards to the health of young children, and include teaching at health maintenance visits to assist parents in prevention techniques. For example, about 10,000 children under 5 years of age have fallen from shopping carts. Most of them stand in the cart's basket, and some climb on the sides (Harrell, 2003). Encourage parents to monitor children carefully in stores and not assume that being in a cart safeguards them. As another example, drowning is the leading cause of unintentional injury death among toddlers, and the second leading cause in all children. Many other children have serious nonfatal submersion events, leaving them with permanent disabilities. The most common characteristic of drowning is inadequate adult supervision (Brenner & the Committee on Injury, Violence, and Poison Prevention, 2003). Teach parents strategies such as having four-sided locked fencing around pools, having constant adult supervision for all children who have access to water, using pools or other sites with lifeguards, using personal flotation devices when boating or near bodies of water, and having parents and other adults prepared to do resuscitation at the scene of submersion.

Table 9–8	SAMPLE QUESTIONS AND TEACHING TOPICS PERTINENT TO EARLY CHILDHOOD VISITS	

Topic	Questions	Teaching
Sleep	How long does Cassandra sleep at night? Does she take naps? Does Jim ever awaken at night crying? Do you have trouble consoling him? Is your daughter able to concentrate on preschool and stay alert during the hours she is there? What concerns do you have about your son's sleep patterns?	Normal amounts of sleep at various ages Establishment of consistent sleep routines Types of sleep disruptions and their treatment
Discipline	Does Cassandra ever misbehave? When it happens, what does she typically do? How do you respond to her behavior? Have you tried using "time-out" when she seems out of control? How does the childcare center deal with inappropriate behavior? Do you agree with their techniques?	Consistency and limit setting Appropriate consequences for behaviors Evaluating methods of discipline Adapting methods to individual children
Toilet training	Have you thought about beginning to toilet train your toddler? How do you think you will do it? What signs have you seen that he might be ready soon? You mentioned that Cassandra has occasional accidents. How often are they and are you concerned about them? What rewards do you use when your son is successful in using the toilet? Do you have a small toilet for him to use?	Readiness cues for toilet training Introducing toilet training Positive reinforcement for children Transitions to childcare and other settings away from home
Learning/reading	Describe the things that Jim is learning now. Is he progressing as you would expect or like? How often do you read to Jim? How does he like reading with you? Have you been able to get books to keep for him at home? Do you ever visit the library together? Does your library have a story time for young children?	Providing stimulating environments for learning Importance of reading to children Importance of providing books for children to look at during play time Pointing out letters to preschool children
Communication	What is Cassandra's language like now? Are you concerned or particularly pleased about any of her ways of communicating? How does she get along with other children in Head Start? What has she been learning about getting along with other children?	Expected language skills Social interaction with adults and other children
Parental issues	How is your life going right now? Do you or anyone else in your family drink more than two drinks per day, smoke, or take street drugs? How is your general mood? Are you often tired, sad, or depressed? Who helps out when you need something? Are there friends or family close to call upon? What resources that you do not have would be helpful to you (e.g., more food, counseling, other parents)?	Effects of parental substance abuse on children Need for healthy mental status to meet child's developmental needs Referrals to needed community resources to meet basic mental status needs

Conclude the visit with some words of praise about the parent and child accomplishments. Provide the date for the next visit. List any resources that are helpful to the family, including the clinic/office contact information and emergency services.

Evaluation

Parents should occasionally be asked to evaluate the care they are receiving at the health promotion and health maintenance site. Use these comments to monitor and adjust procedures as needed. The expected outcomes for nursing care of the toddler and preschooler include:

- The child demonstrates normal patterns of growth and progression in developmental milestones.
- The child remains free of disease and injury.
- Parents relay satisfaction with the pediatric healthcare home.
- The child manifests positive physical, social, and emotional adjustment.

HEALTH PROMOTION AND HEALTH MAINTENANCE FOR THE SCHOOL-AGE CHILD

School-age childhood spans the time when most children enter kindergarten at about 5 years of age, and progresses until about 12–13 years of age when adolescence begins. Even though health promotion and health maintenance needs continue during this time, less-frequent visits to the pediatric healthcare home are recommended. In addition, most children are relatively healthy and need few immunizations, which may lead to only sporadic visits for care. Whenever older school-age children are seen in health care, even for illness or emergency care, it is wise to ask when the last "well child" or health supervision visit was scheduled. Encourage the parents to make an appointment if children are due for a visit. Visits are generally recommended at about 5 years of age, when most children are going to kindergarten, and then at 6–8 years, at 8–10 years, and at 10–12 years. The visits during this time will focus on establishing good health habits related to important issues such as nutrition, physical activity, and mental health; learning the importance of avoiding tobacco and drugs; ensuring success in school, family, and extracurricular activities; and fostering good decision-making and problem-solving skills.

General Observations

The first school-age visit usually occurs just before entry into kindergarten. During this visit the child receives a thorough examination to be certain that physical development is normal, developmental milestones have been met for fine and gross motor skills, school readiness is displayed in social skills and language, and final sets of basic immunizations are completed. The child is often excited about the visit because it is associated with beginning school; however, some anxiety is often felt as it may be the first time the child is aware of getting "shots." As with earlier visits, your observations begin as the child is called in for the visit. It is wise to speak to the child first, introducing yourself and welcoming the child and parents to the office or clinic. Many children of this age actively participate in conversations, making teaching and gathering data easy. For the child who is quiet or looks to the parents, allow more time for him or her to get to know the personnel, directing most initial questions to parents. This may be the first visit where the child is old enough to be a partner in the healthcare visit. Establishing positive rapport with the child will be more likely to enhance efforts designed to teach about health.

Observe if the child brought a book, toy, or some other object to the visit. How are the parents interacting with the child? What types of speech tones are used? Is there mutual respect or are parents and child ignoring each other or having disagreements? The child should walk, showing symmetry and ease of movement; follow instructions about where to go and when to take off shoes for weighing; and demonstrate clear language skills with parent or healthcare personnel.

By the time children come for the 6–8 year and 8–10 year visits, they are expected to be increasingly active in sports, school activities, music, or other interests. Look for clues about their interests as they arrive. Did they bring books, a CD player, or an iPod? What are the book topics or favorite types of music? Ask what they are doing during the summer, or what the two favorite afterschool activities entail. Have them describe a typical day to obtain clues about their lives.

Some children do not commonly come to clinics, offices, or other settings for health supervision visits. School nurses or nurse practitioners in school-based clinics sometimes offer health promotion/health maintenance activities in the school setting. A major focus of school nurses is making the environment conducive to health for groups of children. Schools may offer some parts of the examination to individual children, such as growth and developmental surveillance, or health screening like vision, hearing, or scoliosis. Schools may also work with food service personnel and administration to improve meal and snack quality and minimize unhealthy choices in vending machines, and may work with teachers to integrate concepts such as physical activity and self-esteem into classroom activities. School-based health clinics and school nurses offer healthcare services in schools and are often integral to children's health status (Scully & Hackbarth, 2005). The nurse often links children with healthcare needs to other community services.

During health supervision visits, watch the parents' responses as the child answers questions. Be alert for the parent who interrupts the child or constantly "corrects" what is said. Some comments by the parent should involve praise of the child or looking to the child for opinions on certain topics. This indicates that family members work together and value each other. Ask parents if they came with specific questions or concerns that should be addressed. If the child has an Individualized Education or Health Plan (see Chapter 10 ∞), ask if the parent brought a copy, if the plan is still appropriate, or if it needs updating. Allow the parent an opportunity to meet with the physician, nurse practitioner, or other professional in a private place and without the child present if desired. Be alert for family dynamics that can influence mental health status. Ask if there have been any important changes in the family and how they have influenced the child. During conversations, be alert for reports of separation, divorce, remarriages, ill siblings or grandparents, recent or upcoming moves, parent job changes, substance abuse, incarceration of family members in jail, custody disputes, or other issues. Such topics can be followed up with further questions, as described later in the mental health section, to learn how they influence the child.

Growth and Developmental Surveillance

As the child comes into the health supervision site, height and weight are measured. Be sure to have the child remove his or her shoes and coat. Ask the child and parents if they know the child's current height and weight, and if they have any questions. Plot the percentiles for these measurements, calculate body mass index (BMI) and its percentile, and explain the meaning of these findings later in the visit. Recognize that children do not grow uniformly; they have periods of slow growth followed by fast spurts. Similar to earlier ages, watch for children who have changed channels on a growth grid, and for those above the 85th percentile or below the 3rd percentile for body mass index, and gather additional nutritional data in these cases (see Chapter 4 ∞).

School-age children have logical thought processes and are learning about their bodies. They should be active participants in the physical examination. Explain what you are doing and why. A head-to-toe examination is carried out, with particular attention to systems and skills that influence school success. Vision, hearing, muscular strength, and coordination are examples of areas that impact school performance. (See Chapter 5 ∞ for detailed information about the physical examination.) Remember to provide feedback about the findings; families appreciate knowing that the child's vision is normal and strength is well developed. They should be told what is normal as well as areas that may need more assessment or intervention. Inquire about the child's sleep patterns. During the examination, ask for a description of any illnesses the child has had. Children of school age are generally healthy, with only a few upper respiratory infections or other minor illnesses annually. Unusual complaints may indicate a need for further testing; examples will be discussed in the disease prevention section later in this chapter.

School-age children frequently have minor injuries. These might include falls from bicycles, skin rashes from exposure to plants on a hiking trip, bruises from a ball sport, and other minor mishaps. Be alert for more serious problems that may indicate a need for additional detailed data gathering and teaching. Examples will be discussed in the injury prevention section.

Developmental surveillance continues to be an important part of the examination for school-age children. Some milestones can be observed during the visit while other information is obtained by report of the parent and child. This information is combined with reports about school and other activities in order to establish that the child is developing as desired.

Desired outcomes for growth and developmental surveillance include normal progression with developmental tasks, absence of physical and psychosocial abnormalities or trauma, and integration of safe practices into daily life.

Nutrition

Key concepts related to nutrition in school-age children are independence and formation of habits that influence the future. First, children are increasingly independent in food choices. They usually have strong likes and dislikes for certain foods. They may come home alone and prepare snacks. During school, they choose what to eat from the school lunch or the sack lunch sent by family. They may even have access to vending machines or sales of snacks during school hours. While independence in food choices is growing, the child is greatly influenced in those choices by friends and the media. Foods that may be rejected often include fresh vegetables and fruits, since they get little media attention; and friends may not prefer them. Children with special nutritional needs, such as increased need for calcium described in the opening scenario by Ty, requires individualized attention.

At a time when children choose many of the foods in the daily diet, habits are being formed that will impact nutrition and health in general in the years to come. Good choices will help to promote health—to maintain weight at a recommended level, provide nutrients for adequate growth and activity, and prevent onset of some chronic diseases. However, poor choices can lead to overweight and its accompanying problems, lack of adequate calcium and resultant osteoporosis, eating disorders, or lack of energy for brain growth and optimal performance in school. The patterns established during this period of time are often influential in later nutritional status. Knowledge about foods, family participation in good nutritional practices, and access to healthy foods can all be enhanced by nursing intervention during this critical formative period.

The first nutritional status assessment includes height and weight measurement, body mass index calculation, and examination of percentiles for each measurement on growth grids. Slow, steady growth is the norm during the early school-age years; it will be followed by a growth spurt when the child nears puberty.

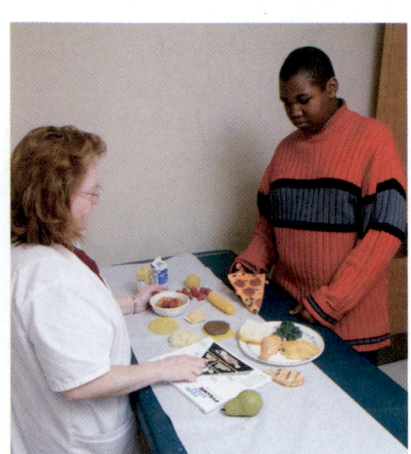

Figure 9–4 ➤ This school-age male is receiving teaching from the nurse about food choices. What benefit do the food models provide in this situation? What other teaching techniques can you suggest?

During the visit, observations provide information about nutritional status. What is the condition of the nails, skin, or hair? What is the energy level and reported physical activity? Does the child look lean or overweight? As the child nears puberty, there may be an increase in fat stores as a preparation for the pubertal growth spurt (Story, Holt, & Sofka, 2002). Integrate some questions for the parent and child into the visit that provide clues about diet. As you observe the child and family and ask dietary questions, list risks and protective factors related to nutrition. Perhaps protective factors relate to adequate access to nutritious foods, a family garden, or weight and height within normal limits. Reinforce the family's positive practices and inform the child of how food choices relate to energy level, school performance, and general health. Risk factors become the basis for teaching and planning with the family for necessary change. It is difficult to tackle several nutritional changes at one time, so concentrate on those most needing attention, and on those the family agrees are important. Provide information about healthy snacks to keep at home, ways to improve calcium intake, the importance of getting at least five fruit/vegetable servings daily, limitation of soda pop to one can daily, and the importance of family meals (Figure 9–4 ➤). Use approaches such as the five-a-day program, which is a coordinated and comprehensive agenda designed to increase the consumption of at least five servings of fruits and vegetables daily. Most children do not consume the goal, so work with the child to compose a list of favorite fruits and vegetables and encourage the parents to have these accessible at home. See if local farmers' markets accept WIC food vouchers if the family uses them and assist in locating sources for favorite fruits and vegetables.

Desired outcomes for health maintenance regarding nutrition include absence of overweight and future chronic disease, adequate intake of all nutrients, and increasing child and family knowledge about nutrition.

Physical Activity

Just as food choices during the school-age years are likely to influence the child's future nutrition, physical activity during these years is often crucial to development of lifelong exercise. During these years, the physically active child continues to refine skills such as eye-hand coordination, muscular strength, agility, and speed. Some children become skilled at ball sports such as basketball, football, soccer, or baseball. Others focus on gymnastics, wrestling, horseback riding, or hockey (Figure 9–5 ➤). Some

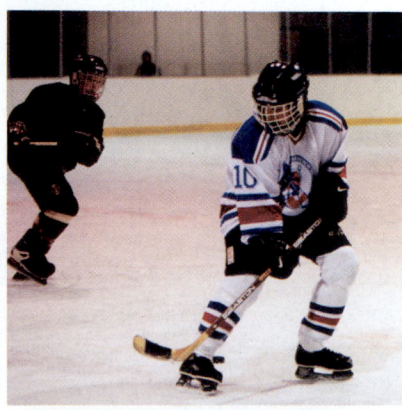

Figure 9–5 ➤ Everyone needs to be physically active. Determine what is enjoyable for a particular child and provide assistance in integrating desirable exercise into daily routines.

do not like team or organized sports but choose skateboarding, skiing, or biking. Whatever the interest, it is important that children identify some physical activity and continue to develop motor skills. The benefits include socialization, positive sense of accomplishment and self-esteem, weight control, and increasing physical ability (Figure 9–6 ➤). Children who do not have an activity of importance often fall behind their peers in agility and skill, making future attempts at an activity very difficult and less likely to be successful.

Similar to earlier periods in life, the nurse lists risk and protective factors related to school-age physical activity (Table 9–9). Families are often significant in promoting physical activity for the child. Find out what the parents do for physical activity and how often. Do they attend a sports club after work or does the child see them engaging in exercise? Most families can include some walking, yard work, or other activity that is done together in order to engage the child. Do they walk to a neighbor's house or a nearby store rather than driving? Do they always take elevators, or choose the stairs in buildings? What is the activity level of siblings? When older siblings are involved in sports, the younger child often is encouraged to develop skills in the same sport.

Children spend much of the day in school, so this setting is important to consider. In an effort to conserve financial resources, some schools have decreased physical education (PE) programs. It is recommended that school-age children have a minimum of 60 minutes daily of physical activity, and that daily physical education classes be integrated into school programs (Strong, Malina, Blimkie et al., 2005). Unfortunately, not all children are enrolled in schools with regular PE classes, and there may be few standards of performance. Additionally, many states and provinces have established tests and standards for performance in certain cognitive areas. In an attempt to increase

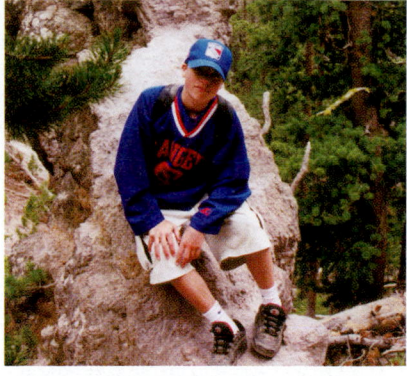

Figure 9–6 ➤ School-age children often enjoy hikes with family, clubs, or other groups. What are the physical and mental health benefits to this physical activity?

Table 9–9	RISK AND PROTECTIVE FACTORS REGARDING PHYSICAL ACTIVITY IN SCHOOL-AGE CHILDREN

Risk Factors	Protective Factors
• Limited role modeling of daily physical activity by parents and other family members • Limited facilities in the neighborhood to encourage activity, such as parks, skateboard facilities, rinks, ball courts • Inadequate financial resources to join clubs or pay for organized sports • School cuts to physical education programs and recess • School tryouts for sports that eliminate all but the best players in certain sports • Reluctance to try new activity • Worry about competence and physical appearance • Television viewing or other screen activities for more than 2 hours daily • Developmental delay and special needs	• Expected developmental skill level • Feels self-confident in ability and physical appearance • Willing to try new activities • Sets goals for learning physical skills • Parents exercise daily and exercise with the child some of this time in a setting the child can see • Parents set expectations that everyone in the family will choose a physical activity and engage in it regularly • Schools provide physical education each day with a variety of offerings; student gets to choose and set goals for some activities • Schools schedule recess or physical activity breaks twice daily • Sports teams are leveled so that all students desiring to play a particular sport, such as soccer, are able to do so • Adequate safety gear that properly fits child is available • Neighborhood provides access to parks, skateboard facilities, rinks, ball courts, and other facilities • Family has adequate financial resources to pay for health club or organized sports • Television viewing and other screen activities limited to no more than 2 hours daily

Adapted from Patrick, K., Spear, B., Holt, K., & Sofka, D. (Eds.). (2001). *Bright futures in practice: Physical activity.* Arlington, VA: National Center for Education in Maternal and Child Health.

teaching time to meet standards, some schools have cut out recess and other breaks. Some schools are located in unsafe areas and outside recreation is not advisable. It is unrealistic to expect children to sit for long periods without physical activity, and such practice reinforces the poor habits of inadequate exercise among children. Nurses are influential members of school committees and can encourage the integration of activity in the school day. You may be able to serve on a school or community committee, informing other committee members of the benefits of 60 minutes of daily exercise to enhance cognitive performance and general health. Teachers and school administrators can be supplied with models of successful school activity programs. Nurses can often be influential in finding community volunteers to work with teams of students. Student nurses, physical education students, senior citizens, and others in the community may be able to help young children play baseball, tennis, or soccer. Other volunteers may teach stretching or warm-up activities. Community partners such as businesses may provide protective gear or uniforms for school sports, especially if the business name can be displayed. In addition, schools can offer alternative activities that some children might prefer to traditional organized sports.

It is essential to consider physical activity for the child who has special healthcare needs. It may be difficult for schools to plan an activity for the child with cerebral palsy, visual impairment, or developmental delay. Search for other community resources and help the family to access them. There may be programs for children to ride horses, swim, ski, and engage in other physical activities. Imagine the thrill that waits for a child who has rarely moved quickly when riding a sled or sliding on skis.

In summary, the nurse plays an important role in meeting desired outcomes of health promotion by suggesting activities that parents can do together, encouraging a plan that includes 60 minutes of daily exercise for the child, becoming active in physical education programs in schools, acting as a positive role model, and helping interested children to partner with community resources for activity. Health maintenance outcomes include use of safety gear and correct techniques to prevent injury from sport participation.

Oral Health

Many changes occur in the mouth during the school-age years, necessitating periodic examination. About 6 years of age, most children lose a tooth, usually in the front. Following that, all 20 of the deciduous or primary teeth will be lost, and the permanent teeth will simultaneously begin to erupt. See Chapter 5 ∞ for the schedule of tooth loss and tooth eruption. In addition, the jawline elongates and teeth move into new positions. Periodic dental visits focus on both the placement of teeth and oral hygiene.

During the health promotion visit, examine the teeth. Look to see how many deciduous and permanent teeth are present. Describe the child's oral hygiene. Ask how often the child brushes, flosses, and visits the dentist. The child should have learned how to brush and floss during preschool years but now independently performs the skills. If there are caries or poor oral hygiene is apparent, ask the child to demonstrate brushing and flossing. Reinforce the need for brushing twice daily and flossing once daily. Provide toothpaste and toothbrushes as gifts during health supervision visits. Local dentists will often provide these supplies so that you can encourage oral hygiene.

Dental visits are recommended every 6 months, so if the child is not visiting on that schedule, ask if finances or transportation are an issue, if the family needs a referral to a dentist, or if there is some other reason. If caries or malocclusion are present, stress the need for a dental appointment soon. Inquire about use of fluoride if the water supply is not fluoridated. Ask if the child has had sealants applied to the permanent teeth; these will help to prevent future caries.

An important risk factor for poor dental health and multiple caries is that of being in a family with low income. Over 50% of the children from low-income homes have no dental care (Kenney, McFeeters, & Yee, 2005). This makes dental caries the most common chronic disease of childhood (Donahue, Waddell, Plough et al., 2005). Learn about dental resources in your community in order to refer families who need these services. Perform thorough oral assessments and teach oral hygiene measures (Guzman-Armstrong, 2005; Tetuan, McGlasson, & Meyer, 2005).

Many children have a high intake of sugared foods and snacks. If this is apparent from the nutritional assessment, discuss the importance of limiting these foods and brushing after their consumption. Frequent brushing is needed when children have braces. Ask them how they are caring for the braces and what the orthodontist has recommended.

The nurse's health promotion activities include positive reinforcement of good hygiene habits, and health maintenance involves teaching about the need for improved care and limiting food that furthers caries formation. Desired outcomes include good oral hygiene, attendance at recommended dental visits, and absence of dental caries.

Mental and Spiritual Health

The school-age years are marked by the emergence of new cognitive skills, ability to interact cooperatively with others, and a feeling of accomplishment in achievements. The child's self-concept and mental health are linked to these important developmental tasks. **Self-concept** is the mental idea that one has of the self. School age is an important period of time in the development of one's self-concept. **Self-esteem** reflects a positive self-concept; it includes the feelings and beliefs of children about their competence and worth as individuals, ability to meet challenges, and opportunities to learn lessons from success and failure (Jellinek, Patel, & Froehle, 2002, p. 90). The aim is to establish a positive sense of self-esteem, even in the face of adversity and challenge. The child who believes in his or her ability to face good times and bad has a lowered chance of mental illness such as depression, eating disorder, and anxiety. Parents are encouraged to evaluate and help to build the child's sense of self-esteem (Table 9–10).

Many of the areas discussed already in this chapter provide clues to the child's self-concept. Are there sports or other physical activities? They may reflect a positive self-concept and body image. However, if the child is forced to do these sports by parents and feels inadequate in their performance, they may promote a negative self-concept and body image. Ask both about the child's activities and how he or she feels about them. Do children enjoy them? How do they rate their performance?

Inquire about school performance and best friends. Is there an increasing independence and responsibility for self? Success in achieving developmental milestones

| Table 9–10 | EVALUATING AND FOSTERING SELF-ESTEEM |

Parents play an important part in fostering the child's self-esteem. The nurse can ask them to evaluate the child and provide suggestions about positive actions.

Evaluation Questions	Positive Actions
What does your child do well?	Build on the child's strengths and talents; point out the child's abilities
How does your child respond to failure?	Assist the child to assess performance; help the child see that mistakes are expected and have lessons to teach
Does your child have close friends?	Arrange structured play times such as going to a movie or cooking with a friend
How does your child respond to new challenges?	Give the child responsibilities at home; encourage your child to try new experiences; help the child feel a sense of control over outcomes
How does your own personality compare to your child's?	Recognize differences in style; appreciate the child's unique qualities; tailor expectations to the child and not to self or other children
Are you setting reasonable and attainable expectations for your child?	Ask the child what is attainable; establish goals for behaviors together

Adapted from Spratt, E. (2002). Assessing and reinforcing your child's self-esteem. In M. Jellinek, B. P. Patel, & M. C. Froehle (Eds.), *Bright futures in practice: Mental health—Volume II. Tool kit.* Arlington, VA: National Center for Education in Maternal and Child Health.

leads to a positive sense of self-esteem in the child. Parents are encouraged to evaluate and help to build the child's sense of self-esteem. A low sense of self-esteem is noted when the child states a disinterest in exercise, school clubs, and family activities. This can lead to loneliness, depression, and mental health problems such as eating disorders (Jellinek, Patel, & Froehle, 2002). When these feelings are noted during a health supervision visit, the nurse should recommend that the child see a counselor at school or another setting, and should recommend that parents be included in the sessions so that they can best help the child.

It is obvious that the family plays a critical part in the child's developing self-esteem and mental health. In order to understand the child, it is necessary to ask questions about and explore dynamics in the family. Several protective factors have been identified for families:

- Communication is open and clear, and parents use problem-solving skills.
- Members are encouraged and appreciated.
- Family is committed to each other, including spending time together.
- Religious or spiritual orientation is present.
- Social connectedness or support is available.
- Resilience or the ability to adapt to new situations is present (Wertlieb, 2003).

Ask about and observe the family's relationships when you are with them. Evaluate the effect of family interactions on children. Model respectful interchanges by listening carefully to children, as well as parents. Gently recognize children if parents answer for them or seem to put them down. Provide brochures and examples of ways to show children their importance. Encourage both parents to come to child health-care visits and support the involvement of both parents in child rearing (Task Force on the Family, 2003). Ask about family stressors such as job changes, financial concerns, illness, substance abuse, and domestic violence. About half of all marriages end in divorce (Task Force, 2003), so be prepared to offer suggestions to deal with this situation (see Chapter 2 ∞ for a discussion of effects of divorce on children and the teaching feature in this chapter). See Families Want to Know: Divorce and the School-Age Child. Ask about and identify risk factors and protective factors. The child's strengths are used to assist the family functioning and will, in turn, give the child a sense of accomplishment. Some examples include:

- A child who is able to act independently can be given responsibility for parts of the home or family function, such as planning the menu for dinner two evenings each week.
- A creative child can be given the task of planning books and other activities for a younger sibling.
- A child with a talent for design can be asked to set the table for dinner guests.

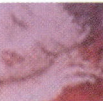

FAMILIES WANT TO KNOW

Divorce and the School-Age Child

Divorce is a common stressful event for school-age children. While parents are engaged in their own stresses, they may benefit from help to plan for ways to lessen the strain on children. They can:

- Be sure the child understands that the divorce is not the child's fault and is only related to the parents' relationship with each other.
- Assert that the child is loved by both parents and will not be abandoned. Spend time with the child regularly to reinforce his or her central role in the family.
- Do not share marital concerns with the child or place the child in a position of having to choose between relationships with one

parent or the other. Conflicts between parents should not take place in front of the child.

- Recognize that the child will feel hurt, sad, and lonely.
- Arrange for support for the child from religious clergy, family, friends, or counselors.
- Maintain child's stability when possible, such as attending the same school, using the same childcare settings, and arranging visits with friends and family members.
- Continue household routines, rules, and discipline.

Adapted from Jellinek, M., Patel, B. P., & Froehle, M. C. (2002). *Bright futures in practice: Mental health—Volume II. Tool kit* (pp. 113–114). Arlington, VA: National Center for Education in Maternal and Child Health.

Self-concept and self-esteem include all aspects of the person, such as cognitive, spiritual, sexual, and physical. **Body image** refers to a specific part of the self-concept: the idea that one forms about one's body. **Sexuality**, another part of the self-concept, refers to the person's view of self as a sexual being, and what that means for one's life. The school-age child is developing a sense of body image and sexuality. Look at the child's appearance and dress. Some children may have poor posture, display a sense of insecurity, and seem uncomfortable with themselves. Others may dress as if they were much older, seem sophisticated, and are clearly assuming the role identification with their gender group. Ask the parents in a private setting what observations they have about the child's body image and sexuality. Inquire about friends of the opposite sex and whether the parent has concerns. Questions related to sexuality will emerge during school years. They should be answered truthfully and fully. Even children who do not ask questions usually need sex education. They may get information in school beginning in about fourth grade, but often still have misconceptions about the bodies of men and women, sexual intercourse, how babies are born, and other topics. Suggest that parents read books with their children that deal with these issues at a level children understand. If books are available at home children will be likely to look at them and ask questions. They should be in the home from third grade on because many young girls may have bodily changes as early as 9 or 10 years of age (see Chapter 5 ∞). This can often put both parent and child at ease and open the door to discussion. Parents should be advised to talk with teachers to learn what is presented in school and be able to supplement and clarify this information. Having discussions at a young age will help open the door to further discussion as the child gets older.

Suggest to parents that the Internet and other media provide information that can confuse children. Encourage them to watch movies with children, encourage frank discussions related to sexuality observed, and answer questions truthfully. Children generally learn about topics such as sexual intercourse, homosexuality, and childbirth from school discussions and the media. It is better to learn from parents than from friends or the media. A few moments alone with parents and children at healthcare visits may help to identify the concerns of each related to sexuality.

By about fourth to sixth grade, most girls have started to have prepubertal body changes and may have begun to menstruate. This provides another opening to discuss mature bodies of men and women and the transformation from childhood to greater maturity. Boys mature about 2 years later than girls, and without an event such as menstruation, parents may be less likely to start discussions with male children. Suggest that parents consciously begin conversations with boys periodically to explain changes they see in themselves and their peers. See Chapter 5 ∞ for further discussion of the body changes seen in the prepubertal period and during puberty.

School-age children continue to develop an ability to self-regulate activities and responses to situations. At this age, the abilities to solve problems and assume more responsibility for self are important. Encourage parents to discuss issues with the child and to seek solutions together when appropriate. The child assumes more responsibility for assisting with meal preparation and home chores, coming home alone after school, and caring for younger siblings. Encourage the parents to praise the child for assuming more family responsibilities and recognize that the child will need some guidance when taking on new tasks.

Sleep is still important for children in order for them to have the energy to perform well in school and other activities. They generally take charge of bedtime routines with reminders about the time to go to sleep, and they sleep through the night. Sleep time varies from 8 to 12 hours, depending on the child and his or her activity level. Busy schedules may interrupt this pattern, leading to irritability, lack of concentration, or even hyperactive behavior (Colyar, 2003). Help children and families plan the appropriate bedtime.

Sleepwalking and sleep talking sometimes occur at this age, but usually decrease as the child nears adolescence. Children who have stress at home, such as parental fighting, ill family members, or inadequate food or shelter, may not get enough sleep and fall asleep at school. Ask the child if falling asleep in class is occurring, and seek additional information about family stressors. This can lead you to interventions such as recommending family counseling or referring to resources to obtain better housing or more stable food sources.

School is a major microsystem influence in the lives of children, and plays a role in self-concept and mental health formation. Ask the child to describe a best friend; if unable to do so, isolation may be occurring. Inquire about what the three best and three worst things are about school. A child with low self-concepts often has trouble talking about and evaluating school. Find out where the child attends school, if the area is generally safe, and how the child gets to school. Encourage the parents to meet the child's teachers, to become active in school activities, and to be available to solve problems with school personnel when needed. Partner with the parents and child when interventions are needed. An office nurse may contact a school nurse when the child needs support in the school environment. This may occur if the child has become ill and missed school, has family stressors, does not get along well with a teacher, or has a condition such as attention deficit disorder. Identify the risk and protective factors in the school environment and plan interventions to support the child when risks are present. Consider the risks and strengths of children with special healthcare needs, such as Ty who is described in the opening scenario.

Certain mental health disorders are commonly seen during the school years. One example includes anxiety problems that result in worries, fears, physical symptoms, stress, and sleep disorders without significantly impairing daily functioning. However, anxiety disorders affect functioning and have more striking characteristics such as clinging, abdominal pain and headache, and refusal to attend school (Hudson, Deveney, & Taylor, 2005). Posttraumatic stress syndrome and depression may also be seen. (See Chapter 27 ∞ for further description of these disorders.) Anxiety disorder, posttraumatic stress, and depression should be referred to a mental health specialist for treatment. However, all children worry at times and this type of anxiety can be helped by learning coping skills and relaxation techniques.

Spiritual health is the ability to develop a spiritual nature, including awareness of a life purpose and fulfillment (Pender, Murdaugh, & Parsons, 2005). School age is a time when children learn more about the people and the world around them, and begin to find their place in that world. Connection with faith-based groups assists some children and families in defining the purpose of life, while others may do so through social activity or a strong moral sense of responsibility. Ask children what brings happiness, how they help other people, or if they are members of a church, synagogue, or mosque. If families seem to have little purpose, parents are withdrawn or depressed, or the child has difficulty answering questions about meaningful activities, suggest methods of engagement in the community. These might include providing contacts at local religious events, posting flyers about community events designed to bring unity to various cultural groups, or suggesting services needing volunteers in the community. Families who spend time together and find meaning in supporting each other nurture the spiritual health of their members. Suggest that every family plan a "family night" weekly when they play games, talk, eat, or engage in other activities together.

The nurse has an important role in fostering the mental and spiritual health of school-age children. Health promotion fosters strengths of families and children, leading to healthy self-concept and positive self-esteem. Health maintenance seeks to prevent mental health disruptions. Be alert for risk factors in families because they represent the need for intervention. Expected outcomes for health promotion and health maintenance activities with school-age children include formation of a positive sense of self-esteem and healthy body image, use of coping skills to deal with stress, sleep patterns that meet needs for rest, and a growing purpose and meaning in life.

Relationships

While the school-age child is gradually moving away from the family as the center of life, the family remains an important anchor. The previous section discussed several areas in which the parents foster development. Ask also about siblings, grandparents, and other extended family members. Sometimes these persons assist in the child's formation of a self-concept. Peers are increasingly important to the school-age child's self-identity. School age is a time of cooperative engagement with others. All children need to be able to learn how to make and maintain friendships and work with others on projects and in recreation.

Inquire about the child's best friends at school and in private, and ask parents if they are comfortable with the child's selection of friends. Find out if the parents facilitate friendships by allowing other children to come to the home and providing transportation as needed. When the child experiences a risk factor such as a move to a new town or school, role-play how to meet new children, and how to make friends. If the child feels like an outcast or outsider among peers at school, explore how the family can create a safe and secure place for the child in extracurricular activities with children who have similar interests. When the child is home schooled, the family may need to plan social events and contacts after usual school hours.

Since peers are important to the school-age child, pressure begins to fit in, to appear like others, and to do what others encourage. Although such pressures are often associated with teen years, they usually begin earlier, at least by 8 or 9 years of age. Ask children what activities friends try to get them to do that they know they should not do, or if friends have tried to get them to smoke. Middle school years are the most common age for beginning to smoke, so always ask children if they have tried smoking, being careful to do this when parents are not present and the children are more likely to be honest. They may tell you about activities when parents are not in the room, such as playing with guns, drinking alcohol or other substances, or other risky behavior. It is best to ask what children do in these situations, what they want to do, and who they can turn to in order to talk about these events. Offer information about the risks connected with behaviors that are described, and suggest people such as parents, teachers, counselors, or clergy who are possible resources. If children's health is at risk, be sure to report the activity to the physician or other healthcare provider so that it can be pursued and the children's safety can be assured. Activities such as playing with firearms or visiting a friend whose parents are making methamphetamine, for example, place children in extreme danger.

School age is often a time when children first experience violence in relationships with others. Some children are bullied, while others are the bullies. Anger and aggression can occur, and children get in fights with each other. Ask children to describe when they last had a disagreement with someone and how the problem was solved. Suggest people like school nurses, teachers, and counselors who can help, and be sure that children feel safe in schools, neighborhoods, and homes. Ask parents how they resolve arguments between children at home and what help they need to help children learn problem-solving skills. Find out what policies the schools have in your community to assist in decreasing harassment of and by children. As you progress in your career, become active on school committees that help children learn how to solve problems peacefully and respond to episodes of violence. See Chapter 6 ∞ for further discussion of violence in children and a detailed discussion of bullying.

The child's temperament still plays a part in response to situations and the ability to self-regulate. (Refer to Chapter 3 ∞ for a detailed discussion of temperament in children.) The "difficult" child may have trouble getting to sleep or in being quiet in the classroom. Have parents plan more physical activity for this child, teach the child that bedtime routines are helpful, and note that sitting near the front of the class can help with concentration. The "slow to warm up" child may need ideas about what to say when meeting new people. Parents can help this child prepare for a new school by visiting with the child, talking about it, and meeting with the teacher so that a warm welcome can occur. The "easy" child is usually adaptable in most situations and is regularly in activities. However, these children may object when other children interrupt them in conversation, fail to take turns, or otherwise "break the rules" of behavior. They might need help to understand differences in temperament in order to be more tolerant of classmates and their behaviors. Often nurses in schools address the issue of individual differences by speaking with classes or small groups of children.

Once again, the nurse takes an active role in promoting the child's health by anticipating developmental issues and preparing parents and children to deal with them. Health maintenance outcomes include preventing problems in interactions.

Disease Prevention Strategies

School-age children are generally healthy. The immune system is mature (see Chapter 17 ∞), personal hygiene practices are more mature than at earlier ages, and immunizations are usually complete. Engage school-age children in active pursuit of their own health. Teach strategies that can enhance disease prevention. Nurses in offices and schools can teach children how to effectively wash hands, how respiratory infections are transmitted, what can cause gastrointestinal illness, and how to best manage their own health problems. Ask children in your settings what topics are of most interest to them and be prepared to suggest common areas of concern such as safety, skin care, athletics, and illnesses. Children are interested in their bodies and can understand the connection between eating well and avoiding illness, maintaining normal weight and preventing type 2 diabetes, avoiding smoking to prevent cancer and other respiratory diseases, and exercising to prevent hypertension.

School-age children are in the concrete stage of intellectual development (see Chapter 3 ∞). This means that teaching is most effective when opportunities are provided to touch, feel, and otherwise become actively engaged in learning. When teaching about smoking, provide models of lungs and have the students breathe through a straw to demonstrate the effects of airway narrowing. These concrete activities will teach them concepts more effectively than simple lecture or reading (Figure 9–7▶). Concepts of health promotion tend to be abstract since they deal with supporting one's highest potential for wellness. Thus, it becomes even more important to provide concrete methods of learning.

Immunizations are generally up-to-date for school-age children. However, some children may have missed earlier doses due to illness or missed healthcare visits. Evaluate the immunization record to be sure it meets all recommendations. Some of the most common immunization needs at this time are:

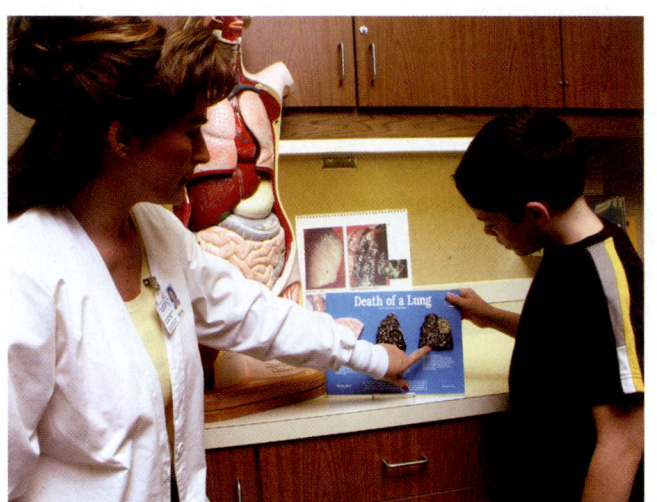

Figure 9–7 ▶ This boy is learning about the effects of smoking on the body through the concrete experience of examining a model of the lungs. Why does this type of hands-on technique help school-age children to learn concepts?

- Hepatitis B (whole series or a missed third shot)
- Hepatitis A (two doses if not previously administered)
- Polio, and measles-mumps-rubella (if booster dose was not given prior to school entry)
- Tetanus and diphtheria and acellular pertussis (Tdap) at the 11-12 year visit
- Varicella if not given earlier and the child has not had the disease
- Meningococcal vaccine (MCV4) at the 11-12 year visit
- Certain vaccines for children at high risk, such as pneumococcal and influenza (see Chapter 18 ∞ for further information on immunizations)

Screening for health risks should occur during the visit. These include hearing and vision screening, blood pressure monitoring, hematocrit for anemia screening, urinalysis, tuberculin skin test, and in some cases screening for hyperlipidemia and lead exposure. Unusual complaints may indicate a need for further testing; examples include:

- Pain other than brief discomfort after an injury
- Headaches
- Bruising
- Lack of coordination
- Repeated infections
- Decreasing vision or hearing
- Problems or changes in school performance or behavior

Children who have an identified health problem or developmental disability may have additional needs for screening and for interventions to assist with health maintenance. For example, the child with cystic fibrosis will need information to lessen the risk of respiratory infection, and the child with diabetes may need additional blood studies. The child who has difficulty reading will need alternative approaches to teaching correct handwashing; demonstration with explanation may be the best approach. A family history of some diseases increases the child's risk and necessitates testing. For example, if a parent has had early cardiovascular disease (before age 55 years), a lipid profile should be performed on the child.

Parents should receive explanations about the screening tests performed and the results obtained. Inform them about vision and hearing results. Send home or call regarding results of blood tests when available. Be sure they understand the findings and have resources to assist in preventing or treating the specific disease in their child. Have them call with questions about health problems the child develops, and provide information about lowering the risks of diseases. Be sure that families know when to keep the child home from school (elevated temperature, active vomiting or diarrhea, coughing up brown or green mucus). Assist schools in setting guidelines for management of infectious diseases in that setting. Contact your local county and state health department for infectious disease guidelines for schools. Desired outcomes for the school-age child include prevention of infectious diseases, prompt treatment for acute infections, and careful management of existing health conditions in order to maximize health potential.

Injury Prevention Strategies

Injuries are a common cause of morbidity and mortality among school-age children, and each health maintenance encounter should include injury prevention strategies. Children have more independence and may be harmed by activities they engage in without adults, such as playing with fire or firearms. They participate in many sports and other physical activities and may suffer related injuries. Some children unfortunately suffer harm due to physical abuse or other forms of violence (see Chapter 6 ∞).

Many common injuries are preventable with the simple use of protective gear and the following safety guidelines. Eighteen percent of youth rarely or never wear seat belts in automobiles (MMWR, 2004). Many children ride bicycles, but only about 16–17% are protected by helmet use, contributing to 23,000 bicycle-related head injuries each year. Bike helmets could prevent up to 88% of serious brain injuries from bicycle crashes (Centers for Disease Control and Prevention, 2006). Strategies to make helmet use more attractive and to ensure correct wearing of helmets are needed (see Evidence-Based Practice: Bicycle Helmet Effectiveness and Use on page 340). Identify youth engaging in risky activities and teach them safe practices. Join with schools and community groups to establish education programs. Provide information about adequate conditioning for sports in order to decrease the chance of overuse injury. Provide a variety of options for physical activity in order to maximize the opportunity for children's participation (Committee on Sports Medicine and Fitness and Council on School Health, American Academy of Pediatrics, 2006). Each visit should contain basic history questions related to injury prevention, and then pursue topics that appear to indicate problems. Once information is collected during the visit, plan two or three health maintenance topics that seem most important for injury prevention in this family. When you have identified a history of injury in the child, collaborate with the family to plan ways to avoid repeated harm. See Table 9–11 for some common injury hazards during the school years. See Table 9–12 for injury prevention teaching.

Children who come home to an empty house after school are called **latchkey children**. The age at which children are ready for this responsibility varies. Parents need help to decide when the child can come home and stay alone and then plan for safety precautions for them. If children have spent increasing periods of short times alone, have displayed good judgment, have several activities and interests that can be pursued alone, and if someone is always directly accessible, then children may be ready to spend 1 or more hours alone after school. Parents can be sure that children have a backup key or entry to the house, should review the schedule for time alone, remove hazards such

Table 9–11	INJURY HAZARDS OF THE SCHOOL-AGE CHILD

	Hazard	Developmental Characteristics	Preventive Measures
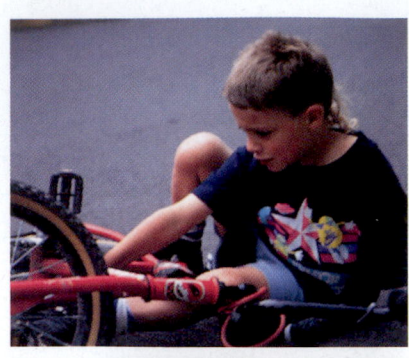	Motor vehicle/ pedestrian/ biking crashes	Child plays outside; may follow ball into road; rides two-wheeler.	Teach child safe outside play, especially near streets. Reinforce use of bike helmet. Teach biking safety rules and provide safe places for riding.
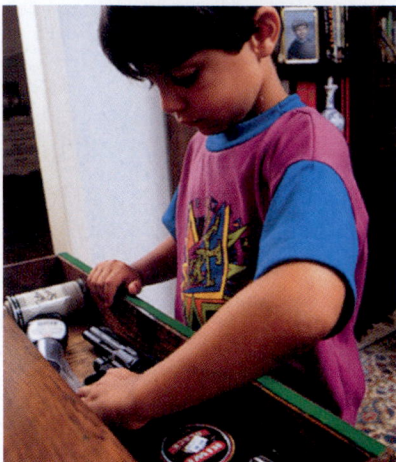	Firearms	Child may have been shown location of guns; is interested in showing them to friends.	Teach child never to touch guns without parent present. Guns should be kept unloaded and locked away. Guns and ammunition should be stored in different locations. Be sure guns have trigger locks.
	Burns	Child may perform experiments with flames or toxic substances.	Teach child what to do in case of fire or if toxic substances touch skin or eyes. Reinforce teaching about 911.
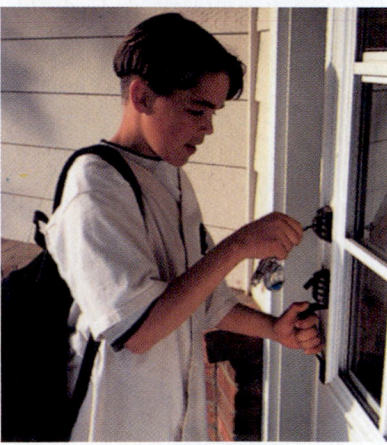	Assault	Child may be left alone after school and may walk, bike, or take public transportation alone.	Provide telephone numbers of people to contact in case of an emergency or if child feels lonely. Leave child alone for brief periods initially, and evaluate child's success in managing time. Teach child not to accept rides from or talk to or open doors to strangers. Teach child how to answer the phone safely. Consider a cell phone and have the child only speak on it with parents.

as firearms, review procedures for emergencies, and arrange for someone that the children can call if lonely.

NURSING MANAGEMENT

Nursing Assessment and Diagnosis

Assessment of health promotion and health maintenance topics occurs in many settings with school-age children. They may be seen in offices or clinics, settings designed to provide such care. They may come for episodic care for a fracture or infection when

Table 9–12	INJURY PREVENTION TOPICS BY AGE
Age	**Injury Prevention Teaching**
5–8 years	• Use a booster seat, properly positioned in the back seat of the car; use lap and shoulder belts • Never place the child in a front car seat with a passenger air bag • Be sure the child knows how to swim and works on these skills regularly • Protect the child with sunscreen when outside • Check smoke alarms and keep them in proper function • Have an escape plan in case of fire in the home • Keep poisons, electrical appliances, and fire starters locked • Keep firearms unloaded and locked; store ammunition in a separate locked location; have trigger locks installed on guns; keep dangerous knives locked • Provide protective gear for bicycling and other activities and insist that it be worn • Teach safety precautions for bicycling and other activities • Teach safety with strangers • Provide a list of people a child can approach if feeling threatened by touch or other experience • Choose care providers carefully; occasionally pick up child earlier than expected; ask policies about discipline and do not leave child with someone who uses corporal punishment • Be sure the child knows emergency numbers, names, and plans • Review carefully any hazardous event that has occurred with the child and summarize what was done correctly and how response could be improved • Limit screen time to 2 hours daily; do not allow violent games or viewing • Review behavior with strangers regularly such as not getting in cars and not engaging in phone or Internet conversations
8–10 years	• Car booster seat used until the child sits upright against the back seat with bent knees over the edge of the seat; insist on use of lap and shoulder belts • Do not place child in front seat of car with a passenger air bag • Do not allow child to operate power tools or machinery • Continue to reinforce other teaching as previously described, include child more fully, and enlarge responsibility to the child with increasing age
10–12 years	• Continue to reinforce teaching as previously described • Parents and child should attend class on cardiopulmonary resuscitation and airway obstruction removal • Avoid high noise levels such as when listening to music through earphones

Adapted from Green, M., & Palfrey, J. S. (Eds.). (2002). *Bright futures: Guidelines for health supervision of infants, children, and adolescents*. (2nd ed.). Arlington, VA: National Center for Education in Maternal and Child Health.

health promotion and health maintenance can be easily integrated. They may be seen in the home or neighborhood center, and are frequently encountered by nurses in schools. Opportunities for assessment and intervention should be used whenever they occur. The individual child is examined, and the family, friends, school, and community are addressed. In addition, these visits provide an opportunity to identify issues early and intervene for health-related problems, including common problems that emerge or become apparent in school age. Inquire about any medications the child uses and perform teaching about these as needed. Use of complementary therapy is common, involving about 33% of families to inquire about these methods of dealing with health in the home. Common techniques involve massage, vitamins, and botanical products (Loman, 2003).

Assessment can be considered on two levels with school-age children. Individual children may be assessed for height and weight, for immunization status, and for use of protective gear during sports. Populations of children may also be assessed since school age is the first time that large numbers of children are together in certain settings. The findings from such assessments will become the basis of an **individualized approach** or a **population-based approach** to health promotion and health maintenance. For example, nurses commonly measure height, weight, and calculate body mass index (BMI) for *individual* children seen in a clinic. The results are shared with the family, and appropriate teaching about weight control and nutritious intake can be

EVIDENCE-BASED PRACTICE

Bicycle Helmet Effectiveness and Use

Problem

About 900 children annually die of bicycle-related injuries in the United States. Although helmets can reduce injury, many times they are not worn correctly.

Evidence

Nearly 500 children visiting a pediatric office were asked to bring their helmet to their health supervision visit, or were supplied with one when they came. Although about 73% of the children claimed to wear a helmet when bicycling, only 4% were able to demonstrate correct fitting and wearing of the helmet. Commonly the helmets were worn too high on the head, were not properly strapped on, or were secured so that they moved around the head excessively. The researchers suggest that helmet assessment be integrated into health supervision visits.

Implications

Nurses should not assume that reports of safety precautions such as wearing helmets or seat belts means that children use these measures correctly. Ask for demonstrations and provide suggestions to improve technique as needed. Common injury causes such as car and bicycle crashes necessitate including at least these evaluations as part of health maintenance activities (Parkinson & Hike, 2003).

Critical Thinking

What are the reasons that children might not wear protective gear during sports? Are there laws in your community about wearing helmets for biking? How can nurses work with parents and schools to increase helmet use? To what incentives would school-age children be most likely to respond?

Reference

Lohse, J. L. (2003). A bicycle safety education program for parents of young children. *Journal of School Nursing, 19,* 100–110; Parkinson, G.W., & Hike, K. E. (2003). Bicycle helmet assessment during well child visits reveals severe shortcomings in condition and fit. *Pediatrics, 112,* 320-323.

addressed. In other settings, nurses may measure a *classroom* of children and use the collective data to plan appropriate interventions. If 40% of children in a school are classified as overweight by BMI percentile, much emphasis should be placed on teaching about dietary intake, physical activity, and the relationship of recommended weight levels to chronic disease risk. However, if only a small number of children are overweight, interventions may not be as extensive about this topic.

Nurses perform growth assessment in school-age children, look for achievement of developmental tasks, and assess physical and mental health and social characteristics. Based on the assessment of individuals or populations of children, nursing diagnoses for children and families are established. Possible nursing diagnoses include:

- Delayed Growth and Development related to abuse
- Impaired Parenting related to lack of knowledge about child health maintenance
- Sleep Deprivation related to sleep terrors
- Risk for Violence Directed at Others related to history of witnessing family violence
- Risk for Loneliness related to long periods alone after school
- Health Seeking Behaviors related to locating swimming classes

Planning and Implementation

The nurse is instrumental in planning interventions to promote and maintain health in school-age children. These interventions may take place in offices, homes, or clinics with an individual child, or in schools and other community settings with groups of children.

When working with individuals, summarize the strengths and needs that you have identified during the visit, and ask children and family members if they concur. Plan together with them to provide the needed information for topics you all have developed. Be sure to emphasize those areas where the family excels. For example, positively reinforce use of car seat belts (see Families Want to Know: Car Safety for the School-Age Child), use of protective sports gear, and being current with immunizations. Summarize the next expected developmental tasks, such as increasing independence and growing self-responsibility for choosing snacks and television shows. Then provide anticipatory guidance to assist with the child's growing independence. As peers are becoming more important, always focus some discussion on maintaining healthy social relationships through school peers, religious or community events, and sibling contacts. A combination of discussion and reading material or pertinent web sites for later exploration are welcomed by most families. Provide telephone numbers of resources for questions and community contacts. Tell the parents when the next health promotion/maintenance visit is recommended. If you come in contact with schoolchildren for episodic care, ask when the last health maintenance visit occurred. If a child is seen for health care after a bicycling accident, the family may be receptive to teaching about safety precautions. When exposed to injuries to the skin, a review of the last tetanus booster may reveal health maintenance needs. Use every opportunity to work with individual children and insert appropriate health promotion/health maintenance topics.

When you are working with groups of children, health promotion focuses on known needs, interests, and risk areas. Nurses in school settings have used a variety of creative approaches to promote the health of youth. Nurses in schools can set up a program to train students in health topics; these students then become peer coaches or health advocates in working with other students. Another activity is evaluating the components of school health programs and making recommendations for additions as needed. The Centers for Disease Control and Prevention (2004) have identified several areas for health policies in schools; they include health education, physical education, health services, mental health and social services, food service, environment, faculty and staff health promotion, and family and community involvement. Bulletin boards, community newspapers, television, and community group membership may all be as effective as teaching in school classrooms. Stress-reduction teaching should be provided on group and individual levels. Nurses can teach or assist in development of progressive relaxation, deep breathing, biofeedback, yoga, or meditation, and can help families to find relaxing activities rather than overscheduling children in multiple activities (Nelms, 2004). Interventions will be most effective if they begin with an understanding of the population served.

Evaluation

Seek evaluation from parents during visits for care. Were their questions answered? Do they know where to turn for advice? Do they know when the child should be seen again for health promotion/maintenance?

The expected outcomes for nursing care of individual school-age children include:

- The child demonstrates normal patterns of growth and development.
- The child, family, and community provide a supportive and nurturing environment for the child.
- The child shows growing independence in directing his or her own health promotion activities.

Expected outcomes of nursing care for groups of children include:

- The children identify lifestyle decisions that influence their health status.
- The school and community offer resources that help to lessen risk factors related to health, and factors of disease/injury prevention.

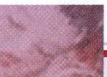

FAMILIES WANT TO KNOW

Car Safety for the School-Age Child

Recommendations include:

- For children over 40 pounds (generally 4–8 years of age), use a belt positioning, forward-facing booster seat located in the back seat. Always use both lap and shoulder belt. Make sure the lap belt fits low and tight across the lap/upper thigh area and the shoulder belt is snug across the chest and shoulder to avoid abdominal injuries.
- Children 4′9″ and taller can sit in a regular car seat restrained with a snug lap and shoulder belt that are correctly located across the lap and chest. The back seat is preferred for all children and necessary for children 12 years and younger.

NOTE: ALL children 12 years and younger should ride in the back seat.

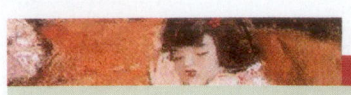

CRITICAL THINKING IN ACTION

Recall the opening scenario which described Ty, a 10-year-old boy with osteogenesis imperfecta. (Consult Chapter 28 for further information about this health condition.) Although he has a health problem, Ty still needs health promotion and health maintenance visits. They need to be adapted to consider his specific needs.

1. Ty spends much of his time in a wheelchair due to his frequent fractures and surgeries. What special dietary needs does he have? What physical activities can be encouraged? Since he swims and recently began wheelchair basketball, what safety needs does he have to prevent injuries during these activities?

2. List the mental health strengths that Ty manifests. How will you use these strengths in planning his care?

3. Plan a teaching session to explain osteogenesis imperfecta to Ty's classmates.

4. Many children with osteogenesis imperfecta have poor dental health due to the disease's effects on teeth. Plan a teaching intervention with Ty to promote good oral hygiene and oral health.

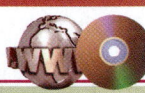 *Refer to your Prentice Hall Nursing MediaLink DVD-ROM for answers.*

EXPLORE MediaLink   http://www.prenhall.com/ball

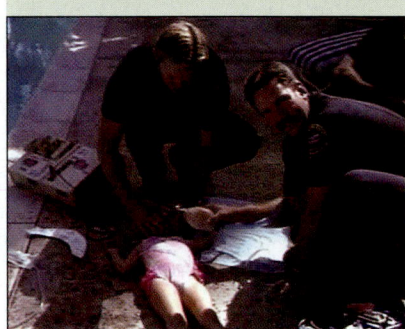

Resources for this chapter can be found on the Prentice Hall Nursing MediaLink DVD-ROM accompanying this textbook, and on the Companion Website at http://www.prenhall.com/ball.

DVD-ROM
Audio Glossary
NCLEX-RN® Review
Video
   Drowning Precautions

COMPANION WEBSITE
Audio Glossary
NCLEX-RN® Review
Care Plan Activity: A Preschooler Needing
   Immunizations
Case Study: Challenges of Single Parenting
Critical Thinking
   Risk Evaluation: Bicycle Riding
   Teaching Plan: Exercise and Blood Pressure
MediaLink Applications
   Childcare Selection Checklist
   Smoking Education Teaching Plans
WebLinks

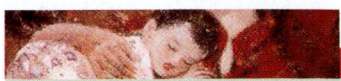

REFERENCES

American Academy of Pediatrics. (2000). *Fellows survey.* Elk Grove Village, IL: Author.

Ateah, C. A., Secco, L., & Woodgate, R. L. (2003). The risks and alternatives to physical punishment use with children. *Journal of Pediatric Health Care, 17,* 126–132.

Brenner, R. A., and the Committee on Injury, Violence, and Poison Prevention. (2003). Prevention of drowning in infants, children, and adolescents. *Pediatrics, 112,* 440–445.

Centers for Disease Control and Prevention. (2004). *School Health Index: A self-assessment and planning guide.* Atlanta: Author.

Centers for Disease Control and Prevention. (2006). Youth Risk Behavior Surveilance – United States, 2005. *Morbidity and Mortality Weekly Report, 55* (55–5), 1–112.

Colyar, M. R. (2003). *Well-child assessment for primary care providers.* Philadelphia: F.A. Davis Co.

Committee on Sports Medicine and Fitness and Council on School Health, American Academic of Pediatrics. (2006). *Active healthy living: Prevention of childhood obesity through increased physical activity.* Retrieved August 3, 2006, from http://www.aap.org/advocacy/releases/may06 physicalactivity.htm

Donahue, G. J., Waddell, M., Plough, A. L., del Aguila, M., & Garland, T. E. (2005). The ABCDs of treating the most prevalent childhood disease. *American Journal of Public Health, 95,* 1322–1329.

Fuller, C., Keller, L., Olson, J., & Plymale, A. (2005). Helping preschoolers become healthy eaters. *Journal of Pediatric Health Care, 19,* 178–182.

Glascoe, F. P., & Macias, M. M. (2003). How you can implement the AAP's new policy on developmental and behavioral screening. *Contemporary Pediatrics, 20*(4), 85–102.

Green, M., & Palfrey, J. S. (Eds.). (2002). *Bright futures: Guidelines for health supervision of infants, children, and adolescents* (2nd ed.).

Arlington, VA: National Center for Education in Maternal and Child Health.

Gunner, K. B., Atkinson, P. M., Nichols, J., & Eissa, M. A. (2005). Health promotion strategies to encourage physical activity in infants, toddlers, and preschoolers. *Journal of Pediatric Health Care, 19*, 253–258.

Guzman-Armstrong, S. (2005). Rampant caries. *Journal of School Nursing, 21*, 272–278.

Halfon, N. (2002). *Child rearing in America: Challenges facing parents with young children.* New York: Cambridge University Press.

Halfon, N., Inkelas, M., Mistry, R., & Olson, L. M. (2004). Satisfaction with health care for young children. *Pediatrics, 113*, 1965–1972.

Halfon, N., Regalado, M., McLearn, K. T., Kuo, A. A., & Wright, K. (2003). *Building a bridge from birth to school: Improving developmental and behavioral health services for young children.* New York: The Commonwealth Fund.

Harrell, W. A. (2003). Effect of two warning signs on adult supervision and risky activities by children in grocery shopping carts. *Psychological Reports, 92*, 889–898.

Hohan, T. F. (2004). Sleep and its disorders in children. *Seminars in Neurology, 24*, 327–340.

Hudson, J. L., Deveney, C., & Taylor, L. (2005). Nature, assessment, and treatment of generalized anxiety disorder in children. *Pediatric Annals, 34*, 97–106.

Jellinek, M., Patel, B. P., & Froehle, M. C. (Eds.). (2002). *Bright futures in practice: Mental health,* Vol I & II. Arlington, VA: National Center for Education in Maternal and Child Health.

Kenney, G. M., McFeeters, J. R., & Yee, J. Y. (2005). Preventive dental care and unmet dental needs among low-income children. *American Journal of Public Health, 95*, 1360–1366.

Lohse, J. L. (2003). A bicycle safety education program for parents of young children. *Journal of School Nursing, 19*, 100–110.

Loman, D. G. (2003). The use of complementary and alternative health care practices among children. *Journal of Pediatric Health Care, 17*, 58–63.

Mason, T. B. A., & Pack, A. I. (2005). Sleep terrors in childhood. *Journal of Pediatrics, 147*, 388–392.

MMWR. (2004). Youth risk behavior surveillance—United States, 2003. *Morbidity and Mortality Weekly Report, 53* (SS02), 1–96.

MMWR. (2006). Youth risk behavior surveillance—United States, 2005. *Morbidity and Mortality Weekly Report, 55* (SS-5). 1–108.

Murray, R. B., Zentner, J. P., Pangman, V. C., & Pangman, C. (2005). *Health promotion strategies through the life span.* Newmarket, Ontario: Pearson Education Canada.

National Maternal and Child Oral Health Resource Center. (2004). Promoting awareness, preventing pain: Facts on early childhood caries (ECC). Retrieved July 12, 2006, from http://www.mchoralhealth.org/PDFs/ECCFactsheet.pdf

Nelms, B. C. (2004). Helping families and communities relax. *Journal of Pediatric Health Care, 18*, 163–164.

Parkinson, G. W., & Hike, K. E. (2003). Bicycle helmet assessment during well child visits reveals severe shortcomings in condition and fit. *Pediatrics, 112*, 320–323.

Patrick, K., Spear, B., Holt, K., & Sofka, D. (Eds.). (2001). *Bright futures in practice: Physical activity.* Arlington, VA: National Center for Education in Maternal and Child Health.

Pender, N. J., Murdaugh, C. L., & Parsons, M. A. (2005). *Health Promotion in Nursing Practice* (5th ed). Upper Saddle River NJ: Prentice Hall.

Scully, J., & Hackbarth, D. (2005). School of nursing sponsorship of a school-based health center: Challenges and barriers. *Nursing Clinics of North America, 40*, 607–617.

Squires, J., & Nickel, R. (2003). Never too soon: Identifying social-emotional problems in infants and toddlers. *Contemporary Pediatrics, 20*(3), 117–125.

Story, M., Holt, K., & Sofka, D. (Eds.). (2002). *Bright futures in practice: Nutrition.* Arlington, VA: National Center for Education in Maternal and Child Health.

Strong, W. B., Malina, R. M., Blimkie, C. J. R., Daniels, S. R., Dishman, R. K., Gutin, B., Hergenroeder, A. C., Must, A., Nixon, P. A., Pivarnik, J. M., Rowland, T., Trost, S., & Trudeau, F. (2005). Evidence based physical activity for school-age youth. *Journal of Pediatrics, 146*, 732–737.

Task Force on the Family. (2003). Family pediatrics: Report of the Task Force on the Family. *Pediatrics, 111* (Supp), 1541–1571.

Tetuan, T. M., McGlasson, D., & Meyer, I. (2005). Oral health screening using a caries detection device. *Journal of School Nursing 21*, 299–306.

VanLandeghen, K., Bronstein, J., & Brach, C. (2003). *Children's dental access in Medicaid. The role of medical care use and dentist participation.* CHIRI Issue Brief 2. AHRQ Publication No. 03-0032, June 2003. Agency for Healthcare Research and Quality, Rockville, MD. Retrieved June 30, 2003, from http://www.ahrq.gov/about/chirident.htm

Wertlieb, D. (2003). Converging trends in family research and pediatrics: Recent findings from the American Academy of Pediatrics Task Force on the Family. *Pediatrics, 111* (Supp), 1572–1587.

Young, K. T. (1999). Listening to parents: A national survey of parents with young children. *Archives of Pediatric and Adolescent Medicine, 152*, 255–267.

10 HEALTH PROMOTION AND HEALTH MAINTENANCE FOR THE ADOLESCENT

KEY TERMS

body image 349
modeling 345
outcome
  expectancy 345
self-concept 349
self-efficacy 345
self-esteem 349
sexuality 349

MediaLink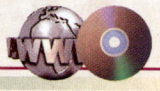

http://www.prenhall.com/ball
See the Prentice Hall Nursing MediaLink DVD-ROM and Companion Website for chapter-specific resources.

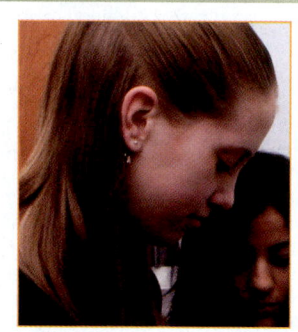

JESSALYN is a 13-year-old seventh grader. She and her friend Kelly both have type 1 diabetes and need to test their blood glucose each day during school. They also both use insulin pumps. When they started using the pumps, the school nurse met with their parents and talked with an endocrinologist in order to be able to help them manage in school. Jessalyn and Kelly's close management of diabetes has enabled them to participate in sports and other school activities. The school nurse performs many of the girls' health supervision activities, such as nutrition assessment, growth monitoring, physical assessment, and relationship fostering with other children. She partners with other healthcare providers to plan comprehensive care for Jessalyn and Kelly.

Youth such as Jessalyn and Kelly require the same health promotion and health maintenance activities as all school-age children. They need teaching about nutrition and physical activity, a review of their immunization records, and to have their safety needs addressed. In addition, due to their chronic disease they need growth monitoring, teaching regarding dietary management, and assistance in monitoring and managing their insulin needs. The chronic disease may also cause mental health challenges due to differences from peers. What health promotion interventions will you plan for Jessalyn and Kelly? Increasing numbers of children and adolescents have diabetes (see Chapter 29 ∞). How will you adapt the usual needs of adolescents when a chronic disease is being managed? How can you integrate the peer group into interventions for the teen with a chronic condition? What adaptations will parents have to make as young children with diabetes become adolescents and begin to manage the disease on their own?

LEARNING OUTCOMES

After reading this chapter, you will be able to do the following:

1. Identify the major health concerns of the adolescent years.
2. Apply communication skills to interactions with adolescents and their families.
3. Apply assessment skills to plan data-gathering methods for nutrition, physical activity, and the mental health status of youth.
4. Intervene with adolescents by integrating activities to promote health and to prevent disease and injury.

HEALTH PROMOTION AND HEALTH MAINTENANCE FOR THE ADOLESCENT

Even more so than with younger children, adolescents are often seen only sporadically for health care, even though annual visits are recommended. They are usually healthy, may not need immunizations, and consequently do not often come for health care. If they have a minor illness, come in for birth control, or need a sports examination, the visit should be viewed as a health supervision opportunity. While the nurse may not perform all components of the usual visit, at least the most important parts are inserted into care. If time is limited, the nurse has to decide which topics to address during a healthcare visit. It is advisable to start with the topic of most interest to the teen and then add some injury prevention teaching, since injury is the greatest risk to teens.

Four lifestyle behaviors are responsible for most of the preventable diseases in adults, and all four typically have their origin in the adolescent years. Assess for them at all visits and insert teaching in the form of verbal information, brochures, or videos or DVDs that can be watched in the healthcare facility. The four behaviors are sedentary lifestyle, unhealthy diet, tobacco use, and risky drinking (Olson, et. al, 2005). These behaviors directly relate to health promotion topics such as dietary and exercise habits, which should be integrated into health encounters. Mental health assessment and teaching are other areas of prime importance. Of course, if the teen suggests he or she is at immediate risk, such as considering suicide in response to depression, this must be dealt with immediately by collaborating with a mental health specialist.

What general principles can guide health promotion programs in adolescents? Some researchers have analyzed theory application and approaches of programs, and others have suggested key elements of programs. Programs that assist adolescents in taking on health promotion behaviors foster a sense of competence, confidence in the youth's own abilities, building of a sense of character and responsibility, connection to other youth and beneficial programs, and the qualities of care and compassion (Lerner & Thompson, 2002). When establishing youth programs, whether with individual adolescents or with groups, the nurse includes evaluation of effectiveness, and plans methods to enlarge and sustain successful approaches.

General Observations

The beginning of an adolescent's visit can be an important source of information, just as it is with younger children. However, the adolescent is at a more advanced stage of development, and the observations you make will relate to this developmental stage.

Ideally, the facility will have a waiting area designed for teens. Teens often dislike waiting for health care with either young children or older adults. Teen waiting areas are popular because they provide a special place, thereby relaying that the teen is important, and can use video and other popular methods to impart health information while the teen waits (Figure 10–1 ➤). As you call the adolescent back for care, observe if parents or friends are present, or if the teen is alone. Young adolescents often come to the facility with parents, who then wait in the waiting room during the examination. Sometimes, if the teen comes in for a special problem, such as a skin lesion or other health concern, the parent follows the adolescent into the examination room. Watch to see if a parent or friend is present, and if that person comes with the teen when called. If someone comes with the teen, be alert that you may need to provide some private time by asking the other person to wait outside for a moment. Reassure the parents that you will talk with them about any of their concerns and questions, and provide them with an opportunity to ask questions and get information as well.

Some teens are comfortable in healthcare settings and actively engage in conversation, while others are nervous and will need more explanations and reassurance as you progress with the first steps of measurement and blood pressure. By adolescence, boys and girls should be assuming more of a partnership role in their own health care. As the visit begins, greet adolescents warmly, ask what concerns and questions they have, and ask for their opinions and reactions throughout the visit. This will show that their thoughts are important and that they play an important role in guiding the

RESEARCH

Applying Theory to Plan for Adolescent Health

A review that analyzed articles describing adolescent health promotion identified the most common theories used by healthcare providers (Montgomery, 2002). A major theory, *social cognitive theory*, was developed by Walter Bandura, who is described in Chapter 3 (Bandura, 1977). The key components of his theory involve **self-efficacy** (the person's belief in his or her ability to perform a behavior) and **outcome expectancy** (what the person expects to get from performing a certain behavior). Learning a new behavior occurs through **modeling,** or imitation of the behavior of someone else. Bandura believes that individuals make decisions about health behaviors based on thought about the consequences and outcomes of those behaviors. The *person's characteristics*, such as self-efficacy and outcome expectancy, interact with the external *environment* and the *behavioral choices* available. All of these components together determine health behaviors, and all can be influenced to promote health. If you were seeking to promote physical activity behaviors in adolescents, some essential components would be:

- Encourage adolescents to believe they can perform the activity (self-efficacy)
- Point out the positive aspects of the behavior (outcome expectancy)
- Show adolescents how to do the activity (modeling)
- Provide a physical setting and opportunity for performing the behavior (environment)
- Allow trial and error, choice in time, and extent of activity (behavioral choices)

Compose a teaching plan to encourage increased physical activity for a teen using all components of the social cognitive theory. List the outcome measures or goals for the teaching, the interventions, and methods of evaluation.

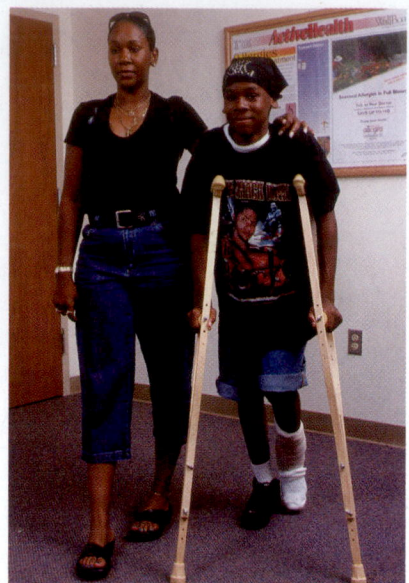

Figure 10–1 ▶ Parents often accompany teens with a healthcare problem in for the examination. Provide an opportunity to see both the teen and parent privately and integrate general health promotion and health maintenance into the visit. What questions can you ask this teen? What teaching might be needed?

healthcare visit. When adolescents are visiting the same office or clinic that they came to during childhood, they usually know and feel comfortable with the care providers. If the setting is new to them, explain the procedures and introduce personnel so they feel more at ease.

Growth and Developmental Surveillance

Adolescence spans several years, and growth and developmental issues vary throughout the period. For young adolescents, or those from about 12 to 13 years of age, growth measurement remains important. Many youth are still growing and use of percentile grids continues to be an important part of care. Growth should remain in the same percentile channel as during childhood, with girls reaching nearly adult height at this age, and boys still continuing to grow. Be alert for youth who have either increased or decreased channels, or are above the 85th percentile or below the 5th percentile for body mass index (BMI). They will need additional assessment of nutritional intake and physical activity.

By middle (14–16 years) and late (17–19 years) adolescence, adult growth is nearly achieved. This occurs earlier for girls than boys. While measurement continues to be performed, nurses assess the BMI more carefully to be sure the height and weight indicate appropriate intake and exercise. Overweight at this age is likely to continue into adulthood, particularly if parents are overweight, so early intervention will be needed to decrease this potential problem. Other youth may have eating disorders and should be referred to a specialist for care. Children from homes without sufficient financial resources may be hungry and lack food. If an adolescent is thin and has little energy, consider this possibility; administer the food security questionnaire found in Chapter 4 ∞. Even the child who is overweight may live in a family with insufficient resources since foods with high fat and caloric content are often less expensive than those with greater nutrient value. For example, a dollar menu at a fast food restaurant meets hunger needs faster and with less expense than fresh fruits, vegetable, and grains.

Few options for measuring the developmental competence of adolescents exist, but observations and questions during care provide information about the adolescent meeting developmental milestones. Key tasks for adolescents involve separating from the parents and establishing positive relationships with peers. The young teen may come to an appointment with a parent and still rely on that parent to answer some questions during the examination. However, the middle and late teen should be increasingly able to come alone, answer questions, and assume responsibility for healthcare decisions. Offer older teens the option of coming into the room alone, stating, "Your mom can wait here and we can come and get her later. Does that sound all right?" During your time with an adolescent, ask questions to learn about peer interactions and activities.

The adolescent receives a physical examination, often by the nurse practitioner or physician. See Chapter 5 ∞ for components of the examination. Some particular parts of the examination to include for teens are scoliosis screening; sexual maturity rating (Tanner stages); breast exam; sexually transmitted disease testing (among those sexually active); pelvic exam and Pap smear (for sexually active females); hematocrit for anemia annually in menstruating adolescents; hearing screening at 12, 15, and 18 years; blood pressure annually; lipid screening for those with a family history of early heart disease or other risk factors; and tuberculosis for those in high risk areas. Most adolescents do not want parents present during the examination, but occasionally they will want a parent for something like a first pelvic examination or a blood draw. Ask them their wishes in a confidential setting so they can freely make the choice. They also may choose to have a healthcare provider of the same gender as them complete the genitourinary examination. Expected outcomes of care include screening and early identification for common health problems, normal patterns of growth, and meeting of developmental milestones.

Nutrition

The young adolescent needs a well-balanced diet to support the growth of this period, and the late adolescent requires intake that supports physical activity and provides nutrients for metabolism and to promote the immune system. While nutritional intake is important, teens often do not eat well. They may be busy and do not want to plan meals, they like to eat high-fat or sugar foods that are popular with other teens, they may diet to achieve weight loss, and some do not have enough financial resources to access proper foods.

Combine the information from the adolescent's measurements with the answers to questions about diet in order to identify possible areas for intervention. Find out what questions the teen has about foods, diet, maintaining desired weight, and topics like vegetarianism or supplements to enhance athletic performance. See Chapter 4 ∞ for further details about these special nutritional topics. Health promotion plans focus on practices that lead to healthy growth and development. They may include teaching about:

- Eating five servings of fruits and vegetables daily
- Including whole grain products to replace refined products whenever possible
- Applying the Food Guide Pyramid in the daily diet (see Chapter 4 ∞)
- Stressing the importance of eating three meals each day including breakfast and lunch
- Eating together as a family several times weekly, which enhances quality food intake
- Planning menus and preparing foods for balanced intake

Health maintenance plans center on those practices that prevent disease including:

- Limiting refined sugar and high fat intake (such as soft drinks and fried foods) in order to maintain weight at the recommended level
- Including two or three servings of dairy products daily to enhance bone formation and decrease chances of osteoporosis as an adult; encourage options that are most enticing to teens such as portable yogurt and pizza with cheese
- Using resources for treatment of eating disorders if they are identified

While much of nutrition teaching should be aimed directly at the adolescent, parents are also included. They can be effective contributors to healthy intake by providing plenty of fruits and vegetables for snacks, having foods attractively prepared and ready for consumption when the teen is hungry, planning several meals together as a family each week, encouraging milk or other forms of calcium intake, and setting a good example for food intake. Help them identify the youth with an eating disorder and provide resources for intervention in these cases. Consider as well the teen with a baby. The adolescent who is pregnant or nursing has even more need for nutritional teaching and may need financial resources to access sufficient food. How will you combine the growth and developmental needs of an adolescent with those of her new baby when planning teaching?

Physical Activity

Many adolescents suffer from the effects of inadequate physical activity. As children get older and enter the teenage years, physical activity decreases, particularly in girls. Only about 36% of adolescents report vigorous activity for 5 days/week. The percentage is lower among certain groups, with only 28% of females reporting that level of activity. The incidence of exercise decreases to about 25% of teens in 12th grade (MMWR, 2006). The recommendation of *Healthy People 2010* (2000) is quite moderate, stating that adolescents should get at least 20 minutes of vigorous activity 3 days weekly, while an expert panel recommends 60 minutes of moderate or vigorous physical activity daily (Strong et al., 2005). At a time when teens are not very active as a group, physical education requirements in school are also decreasing. Only 22% of 12th-grade students regularly attend a PE class (MMWR, 2006). Physical activity levels must therefore be assessed at each health supervision visit or in other contacts with adolescents. Apply resilience theory and assess youth, family, and community for risk and protective factors regarding physical activity (Table 10–1).

Some youth have established regular physical activity programs and their behaviors should be encouraged (Figure 10–2 ➤). Parents who have regular physical activity are important in influencing children, so encourage parental exercise at each pediatric healthcare visit. Be alert for those who exercise but have other health problems. Some

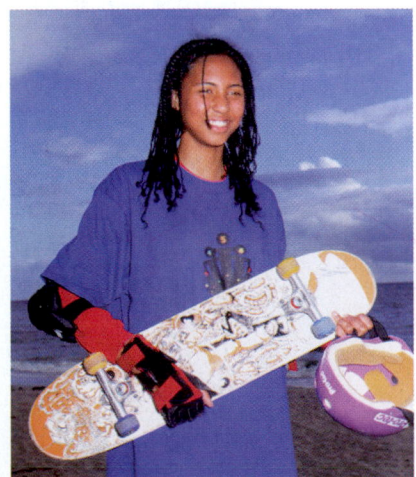

Figure 10–2 ➤ This teen girl is an avid "boarder." How can you encourage and praise her for this activity? What clues do you have that she is using adequate safety measures?

Table 10–1	RISK AND PROTECTIVE FACTORS REGARDING PHYSICAL ACTIVITY IN ADOLESCENCE
Risk Factors	**Protective Factors**
• Lives in isolated setting with little opportunity for contact with other teens • Has a developmental disability that impairs physical movement • Does not like physical activity • Has a pattern and history of low activity levels • Is overweight • Does not feel competent in most sports • Limited financial resources to pay registration fees or buy protective gear for sports • Family members who have little physical activity • Parents who are not active in school sports and committees • Parents who do not like physical activity and have had low levels while their teen was growing up • Parents who have little time or facilities for exercise, or always exercise at a club out of view of their family • Lack of youth and parent knowledge about physical activity needs and benefits • Lack of neighborhood programs for physical activity promotion • Presence of neighborhood hazards and unsafe areas	• Has opportunities for participation in physical activity at home, at school, and in the community • Likes physical activity • Has exercised during all of childhood, often with parents • Knowledgeable about benefits of activity; committed to maintaining exercise patterns • Has many friends living close who participate in physical activity • Youth and parents agree to a 2-hour daily limit of screen time • Availability of financial and other resources for sports gear and protective equipment • Parents participate in regular physical activity and encourage the adolescent to do so • Neighborhood and community provide physical activity options • Public policies maintain parks, green spaces, biking trails, and playgrounds • Programs are available for adolescents with developmental disabilities or other healthcare needs

Adapted from Green & Palfrey (2002). *Bright futures: Guidelines for health supervision of infants, children, and adolescents* (2nd ed.). Arlington, VA: National Center for Education in Maternal and Child Health.

athletes try to eat very little to remain a certain weight for wrestling, running, or other sports. Integrate nutritional teaching that includes the importance of adequate intake for sports performance. Other athletes use nutritional supplements to enhance performance. While most are not harmful, few have proven benefits and their cost is not warranted; some may actually be harmful to adolescents.

Other youth have very little physical activity and feel incompetent in performing many sports. Work with them to find at least one thing they can do on a daily basis—walking their dog in the neighborhood, riding a bike to the store, using stairs instead of elevators when possible, parking on the far side of the school lot and walking farther, swimming at a club their parents belong to or at a local YMCA or YWCA, or saving money to take lessons for something they have always dreamed of doing such as horseback riding or golf. Form interest groups at schools and community centers that provide an outlet for adolescents who cannot "make the team" for school sports. Encourage parents and adolescents to set goals together to integrate some physical activity daily.

The nurse's activities for health promotion concentrate on teaching the health and mental benefits of physical activity such as increased energy, weight control, and a feeling of control and success. Health maintenance focuses on viewing physical activity as a method to prevent disease such as cardiovascular disease and diabetes. Youth who have family members with these diseases or meet adults who have them are more likely to understand the importance of their own activity. Desired outcomes include maintenance of weight within recommended level, daily exercise of 20–60 minutes, and establishment of lifetime exercise routines.

Oral Health

Continued dental care during the adolescent years can ensure oral health. The recommendations remain the same as those for young children. The adolescent should floss daily, brush twice daily with a small amount of fluoridated toothpaste, and visit a dental care provider every 6 months. By about 14 years of age, those students who do not have fluoridated water and have been taking fluoride can stop this supplement. Even the molars have been formed by that age so fluoride tablets are no longer needed. Continue to examine the condition of the teeth and the number of erupted permanent teeth present. Be alert for any unusual growths and ulcers in the mouth and refer for care as needed.

One potential concern that should be addressed includes the availability of dental insurance for the adolescent. The teen whose family does not have dental insurance needs referrals for care to affordable resources. Dental specialists clean off plaque that has formed, apply sealants to erupting molars, examine the teeth for caries, and perform restorative care. Particular groups are more at risk for inadequate dental care. When working with these populations, nurses can question access to care and make recommendations that foster regular checkups. Some teens may wish to whiten the teeth or get orthodontia to improve their appearance. The nurse helps the youth and parents to find resources for needed or desired care. Expected outcomes are dental visits twice annually with recommended follow-up care for problems, resulting in good oral health.

Mental and Spiritual Health

Adolescents have many challenges to their mental health and need support to emerge from adolescence with mental and spiritual strengths. Mental health topics must be addressed at each health supervision opportunity to promote mental health among teens. Mental health is closely linked to developmental tasks such as growing independence, formation of close relationships with peers, becoming confident in accomplishments, and setting goals for the future. Mental health disruptions occur more frequently in adolescents who smoke and engage in other risky behaviors, so assess for all of these risk factors (Chang, Sherritt, & Knight, 2005).

As during other ages, the **self-concept** continues to develop and tailors reactions to the environment. Self-regulation in the form of making decisions to govern oneself is important. **Self-esteem**, or a positive feeling about the self, is a key to meeting life's challenges. Ask what the teen is proud of and has accomplished and what disappointments have occurred as well. Provide resources to deal with disappointments and give praise for the teen's accomplishments. Another part of the self-concept that continues to develop is that of **body image**. Factors such as early or late maturation, overweight or underweight, or the role of the media can influence the teen's body image. A healthy image includes the realization that the body has positive and less positive attributes and that the individual can influence the body by healthy eating and physical activity. Be alert for the teen whose wish for a different body leads to eating disorders and excessive exercise or intake of nutritional supplements.

Sexuality involves both bodily changes that signal mature sexual development, and the mental concept of oneself as a sexual being. Bodily changes and mental concepts do not necessarily mature at the same time, and adolescents may not be ready for sexual maturity and the decisions about sexual behavior simply due to achieving sexual maturation. Most young adolescent girls have begun menstruating; by early to middle adolescence, boys are having nocturnal emissions and ejaculations. Ask teens if they have received information about puberty, body changes, and sexuality. Tell young adolescents that most teens have questions and that you will talk with them about any areas of interest, including contraception and sexually transmitted diseases. Ask older adolescents directly if they have had sexual intercourse and, if so, what they are doing to protect against pregnancy and sexually transmitted diseases. Provide support for adolescents who have decided not to have sexual intercourse. Encourage them to continue this plan, telling them that sexual feelings are normal, but that decisions about sexual intercourse are their right and privilege. Ask teens if they have confusion about sexuality. If teens have identified as homosexual, let them know they are welcome and ask about decisions regarding sexual practices, reinforcing the need for protection against sexually transmitted diseases. Provide community resources to support gay or lesbian teens so that they can develop a social group in which they feel comfortable. Some adolescents are seen for health care at the time they become sexually active. Use

MediaLink

Teen Mental and Spiritual Health Video

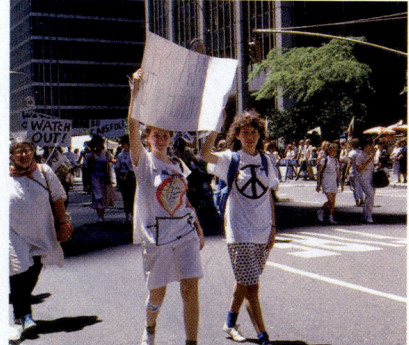

Figure 10–3 ► Teens often become associated with causes. This helps them to feel part of a social group and also provides the opportunities to examine belief systems and to make decisions about meaningful activities.

this opportunity to reinforce and correct prior knowledge about the body and protection against pregnancy and sexually transmitted diseases.

Most adolescents still need discipline or guidance from parents at certain times. Rather than maintain a constant battle over daily events, it is best if parents have just a few important rules that they only rarely have to enforce. Nurses can assist parents to set useful boundaries for teens and offer resources such as parenting groups and web sites for assistance.

Sleep is necessary for anyone to function safely and at a level of one's potential. Unfortunately, many youth do not get the sleep needed for healthy functioning. Teens have an increased need for sleep due to their growth rates and activity levels. At the same time, their internal clocks change, making it more difficult to get to sleep at the usual time. It is thought that a decrease in secretion of melatonin occurs, so the teen does not feel tired in the late evening. However, teens often do not have the number of hours of sleep needed by the time they wake up for school or work. The problem may be worsened if students participate in sports or other activities. They may need to get to school before normal starting hours for music, sports, or other activities, or perhaps stay late into the evenings for practices. Some adolescents then work on weekends or evenings as well. And of course, social activities usually fill much of their time. While about 9 hours of sleep is needed, most adolescents get about 6 hours (Mayo Clinic, 2003).

The effects of sleep deprivation can be serious. Teens cannot perform to their potential in school or at work. Many parents state that adolescents are moody and difficult to communicate with when they are tired. There may be a connection between lack of sleep and substance abuse, and teens commonly use caffeinated beverages to stay awake. Some people tend to eat more when they are tired, and get less physical activity. One of the most serious consequences may be the danger of driving while tired; this is a common cause of accidents. Ask adolescents about what time they go to bed, when they awaken, and whether they are frequently tired. Provide suggestions for regular sleep schedules, avoiding caffeine products in the evening, and planning a day of relaxation into every week.

Temperament or personality-type characteristics continue into adolescence but they generally do not change from earlier years. For example, the active infant and young child is usually an active teenager. The slow-to-warm-up baby may be the adolescent who needs more time to adjust to a new school or teachers. If the adolescent or parent has trouble with personality characteristics, it may be helpful to talk about these traits, help him or her to establish a positive sense about the attributes, and discuss ways to adapt the environment as needed. For example, parents should not expect a slow-to-warm-up teen to be interested in running for a class office. Someone with irregular sleep and eating habits will find it difficult to have a job at a set time and will need to set alarms and other reminders.

Spirituality offers the adolescent comfort and support. Being a member of a teen group in a faith-based home can offer a peer group with similar values and bring meaning to life. Some adolescents reject their parent's faith and seek a different group; others seek to leave religious practices totally while others become more committed to them. Ask them if they have the resources they need to bring meaning to their lives; provide them if needed. Realize that participating in community food kitchens, raising money for causes, and other activities also provide meaning for many adolescents (Figure 10–3 ►).

The nurse actively promotes the mental health of youth by understanding their developmental needs and providing information and resources. Gentle guidance and active partnership with youth help to provide the resources to ensure healthy self-concept, sexuality, and personality development. While most teenagers have many protective factors that can be identified and fostered, a few have risks that can harm mental health. It is important to identify the risks also, and to use health maintenance techniques to lessen the risk factors. Depression and substance use are two common risks to mental health. Depression is discussed in Chapter 27 ∞ and substance use in Chapter 6 ∞. See the quick checklists in Table 10–2 to help in identification of these problems during health supervision visits.

Table 10–2	SIGNS OF DEPRESSION AND SUBSTANCE ABUSE

Depression	Substance Abuse
• Changes in behavior, school performance, sleep, and appetite • Physical complaints • Loss of interest in usual activities • Difficulty in motivating self and setting goals • Change in friends • Feelings of worthlessness • Consideration of death or suicide	• Changes in behavior, school performance, sleep, and appetite • Accidents and other unexplained events • Lack of responsibility • Labile mood and attitude • Hopelessness • Depression • Feelings of ambivalence • A variety of physical changes depending on the substance

Adapted from Chang, Sherritt, & Knight, 2005; Jellinek, Patel, & Froehle, 2002.

Although health promotion and health maintenance activities commonly occur in office or clinic settings, there are many other settings where nurses work with adolescents; mental health activities are often integrated into these settings. Consider offering health promotion/maintenance wherever you might see students. Some nontraditional settings include correctional facilities, school-based health centers, and programs for pregnant teens. Adolescents in these facilities can benefit from services to improve diet, physical activity, and lifestyle behaviors that influence mental health.

The desired outcomes for mental and spiritual health promotion and maintenance include meaningful activities in the adolescent's life, emerging independence, good choices about lifestyle behaviors, and development of successful coping skills.

Relationships

Adolescents form stronger bonds with friends than at any time earlier in development; at the same time they need their parents for guidance and reassurance as they become more independent. As teenagers strive for independence they frequently strike out at parents, test limits, and have conflicts with parents. Interactions in the family provide consistent and important ties at the same time that social interactions become a central part of life. Health promotion helps teens to form strong friendships with peers and continue to value and participate in the family, and helps parents to understand the developmental needs and their role in establishing a new type of relationship with the family's emerging young adult. Partnerships with care providers are important to help families work together to achieve these outcomes.

When adolescents are seen for healthcare visits, assess relationships with others. Provide time alone with both the adolescent and the parents (if they are present) so that everyone has time to talk freely and to ask questions. Some areas already discussed, such as school performance and activities, provide information about the adolescent's friends and how time is spent. Ask teens to describe their best friends and what they do together. Ask parents their opinions of the youth's friends. Inquire about the youth's roles in the family. Does the teen have jobs and responsibilities? What freedom is allowed? What are relationships like with siblings and extended family members such as grandparents and cousins? What activities are done together as a family? Are there differences in the teen's and the parents' answers to these questions? What are the teen's and parents' desires for how the family unit functions together?

Provide an opportunity alone with the teen to talk about issues such as domestic violence. Is the youth abused or is there violence between adults in the family? Are there stressors such as lack of sufficient finances, an ill parent, or a lost job? How have these occurrences affected the adolescent? Minor adjustments can be helped by discussion while some major problems will need referral to mental health specialists.

In their relationships with peers, adolescents often have many of the same issues that emerge with parents. They may have disagreements with friends or feel hurt by things that are said or done. Ask teens about how things are going with friends and what problems they have. Talk about negotiating, joining groups to form new friendships, and the importance of respecting and not making fun of others. Give them strategies for living up to their own standards even when friends are enticing them to do other things. Suggest that having friends one can trust and who have the same ideals can be very supportive and fun in adolescent years. Expected outcomes are the formation of strong relationships both within and outside of the family, along with independence in decision making.

Disease Prevention Strategies

Teenagers typically do not have many diseases and most are minor illnesses like respiratory and gastrointestinal illness. However, some diseases occur, so nurses must always be aware of signs of potential disease. Some common health issues that are described throughout this book include:

- Acne and skin infections
- Body piercing and tattooing
- Sports overuse injuries
- Constipation and diarrhea
- Dental problems

Other observations may signal more serious health concerns and need to be referred for further evaluation. Some examples include:

- Scoliosis
- Anemia
- Excessive tiredness
- Bruising
- Sexually transmitted diseases
- Eating disorder
- Abuse or severe bullying

Several screening tests should be performed during health supervision visits with adolescents, including vision, hearing, smoking, depression, stress, alcohol or other substance use, blood pressure, urinalysis, sexually transmitted infection risk, and in some cases Pap smears and breast examinations. Screening tests with abnormal results require follow-up and intervention. For example, if the adolescent is anemic, iron tablets may be needed and teaching about high iron foods should be done. Vision impairment requires referral to an eye specialist. Presence of sexually transmitted diseases requires teaching and medication treatment. A history of sexual activity will guide you to tests that should be included in the examination.

The adolescent should receive extensive information about ways to protect health and prevent disease. The hazardous outcomes of smoking and other tobacco use are discussed, and cessation programs are encouraged for users. Unprotected sexual activity is presented as a serious health threat. Use of sunscreens to prevent burns and future skin cancer is encouraged. Females are taught breast self-exam and males are taught testicular exam. For youth who are overweight and sedentary, teaching about the possible outcomes such as type 2 diabetes and cardiovascular disease are mentioned. While it would not be advisable to threaten or frighten an adolescent with descriptions of diseases, an understanding of the potential serious outcomes like smoking or diabetes can be motivators for behavior change.

In addition to teaching to prevent disease, the nurse also administers any needed immunizations. Many adolescents have not had immunizations since about school entry time so their record should be carefully reviewed. Some common immunizations needed by adolescents are described in the following list.

- When was the last tetanus-diphtheria booster? A booster of tetanus-diphtheria and acellular pertussis (Tdap) is now recommended at 11–12 years or at 13–18 years for adolescents who did not receive the 11–12 year dose.

COMMUNITY CARE

Sexually Transmitted Infections

Sexually active teens should be screened annually for:

- Chlamydia
- Gonorrhea
- Trichomoniasis
- Human papillomavirus
- Herpes simplex virus
- Bacterial vaginosis

Teens should be screened for syphilis and/or HIV/AIDS if they request testing or meet any of these criteria:

- History of sexually transmitted infection
- More than one sexual partner in past 6 months
- Intravenous drug use
- Sexual intercourse with a partner at risk
- Sex in exchange for drugs or money
- Homelessness
- Males—sex with other males
- Syphilis—residence in areas where disease is prevalent
- HIV/AIDS—blood or blood product transfusion before 1985

Data from: Green, M., & Palfrey, J. S. (2002). *Bright futures: Guidelines for health supervision of infants, children, and adolescents* (2nd ed.). Arlington, VA: National Center for Education in Maternal and Child Health, p. 268.

- Was a second measles-mumps-rubella administered? A second dose may not have been routine when teens were younger so they may need it now.
- Did the teen receive hepatitis A vaccine at a younger age? If not, the vaccine series is needed now.
- Has the youth had hepatitis B vaccine series? This is important for all youth and some may not have received it as infants.
- Did the youth have a clear history of varicella disease? If not, the vaccine is needed.
- Meningococcal vaccine (MCV4) is now recommended for all youth at 11–12 years. If not previously given it is administered at 15 years. All teens who will be college freshman in dormitories should be given meningococcal vaccine.
- Human papillomavirus vaccine is now recommended for all adolescent females at 11–12 years; it may be given as early as 9 years at the clinical judgment of the provider and may be given to all women from 13–26 years as well (Centers for Disease Control and Prevention, 2006).

The results of health screening are shared with the teen and with the parent as appropriate. Teaching and other interventions for disease prevention are examples of health maintenance activities. Expected outcomes are increasing knowledge of common diseases and methods of prevention among teen and parent, use of screening tests by the healthcare provider, and use of the healthcare home by the adolescent for treatment of diseases.

Injury Prevention Strategies

Injury is the greatest health hazard for adolescents, so injury prevention must be integrated into every health contact with youth. The major hazard is automobile crashes (see Chapter 1 ∞). Many teens learn to drive and have a license by 16 years of age. They often transport friends, get distracted by social interactions in the car, have little experience about what to do if a car slides or has mechanical problems, may drink and drive, and are often tired when driving (Figure 10–4 ➤). Several states have instituted graduated driving licensing to help decrease some risks. Commonly, the youth cannot drive other youth for the first few months, cannot drive from about 1 a.m. to 6 a.m., and has serious consequences for speeding or other infractions. Parents in states without these laws may wish to establish them for their own adolescents. Driving should always be presented as a privilege and a responsibility. Serious consequences such as losing the ability to drive for a time after any infraction can be suggested to parents. Because of the great risk of injury and death from car crashes, ask at each health visit if the teen drives, rides with other teens, what rules parents have established about driving, and whether the teen ever drinks and drives or rides with someone who does. Reinforce the need to wear a lap and shoulder belt at all times and to never drink and drive.

Youth are at risk for injury with other motorized vehicles. Motorcycles, four-wheelers, boats, jet skis, farm machinery, and tools are other sources of injury. Ask about the youth's exposure to various machines and teach about avoiding alcohol and drug use, as well as safety gear and precautions to be used. Every health visit should also include other questions that help to identify a wide variety of injury hazards. Once you have asked about common causes of injury, be sure to discuss and provide written material to perform injury prevention teaching. Such measures are important health maintenance activities. See Table 10–3 and Table 10–4. Desired outcomes for nursing care include absence of serious injury, the ability to state sources of risk for injury, and emergency plans for assistance when engaging in any risky activities.

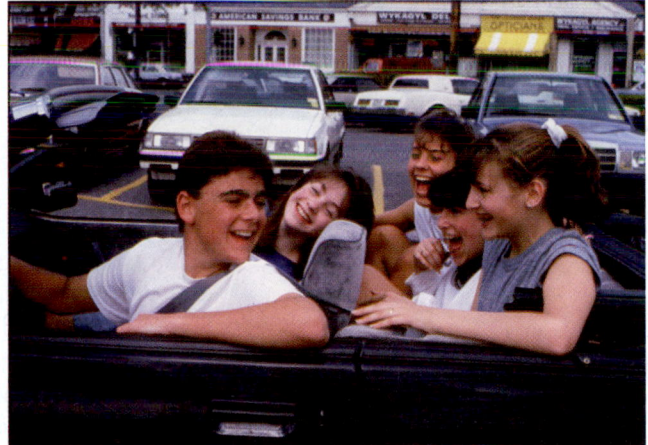

Figure 10–4 ➤ Adolescents often drive motorized vehicles and may be at risk for injury if not properly prepared or protected. What teaching and experience do these youth need for safe enjoyment of the experience of driving and riding with friends? Do schools in your area offer driver education classes? What are the state requirements for youth driver licensure?

Table 10-3	INJURY PREVENTION IN ADOLESCENCE

	Hazard	Developmental Characteristics	Preventive Measures
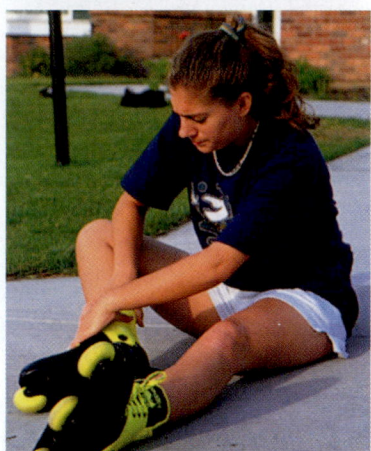	Motor vehicle crashes	Adolescents learn to drive, enjoy new independence, and often feel invulnerable.	Insist on driver's education classes. Enforce rules about safe driving. Seat belts should be used for every trip. Discourage drug and alcohol use. Get treatment for teenagers who are known substance abusers.
	Sporting injuries	Adolescents may participate in physically challenging sports such as soccer, gymnastics, or football. They may be allowed to drive motorboats.	Encourage use of protective sporting gear. Teach safe boating practices. Perform teaching related to hazards of drug and alcohol use, especially when using motorized equipment.
	Drowning	Adolescents overestimate endurance when swimming. They take risks diving.	Encourage swimming only with friends. Reinforce rules and teach them about risks.

■ NURSING MANAGEMENT

Nursing Assessment and Diagnosis

Nurses assess adolescents in a variety of settings, including offices, clinics, schools, home, correctional facilities, extended care facilities, in sports-related endeavors, and family planning clinics. A wide array of health concerns should be included in these assessments. They include measurement of growth; presence of any unusual findings on physical examination; lifestyle choices related to dietary intake, physical activity, and oral hygiene; assessment of mental status, family interactions, and social connections with peers; and any risky behaviors the adolescent engages in such as smoking, unprotected sexual relations, alcohol or drug use, or unsafe driving practices. The people and organizations around the adolescent such as family, school, and neighborhood are all assessed. Remember to list both risks and protective factors. The protective factors can be used during implementation to enhance the youth's resilience.

Based on a thorough assessment, you will establish nursing diagnoses that are appropriate for the adolescent and family. Some possible nursing diagnoses might be:

- Rape-Trauma Syndrome related to date rape
- Impaired Dentition related to ineffective oral hygiene
- Imbalanced Nutrition: More than Body Requirements related to lack of basic nutritional knowledge and obesity in both parents
- Disturbed Sleep Pattern related to frequently changing sleep/wake schedule
- Low Self-Esteem related to situational crisis of friends making fun of adolescent

Table 10–4	INJURY PREVENTION TOPICS FOR ADOLESCENCE

Topic	Teaching
Driving	• Always wear seat and shoulder belt • Do not drink and drive or ride with others who do • Do not talk on a cell phone as you drive • Do not drive when you are tired • Drive with parents or other adults for several months in winter driving conditions if you live where there is snow, ice, or heavy rains • Keep your car in good repair
Sun	• Wear sunscreen • Limit time outside, especially early in summer
Machinery	• Learn how to correctly use power tools • Always have someone near when you use tools or machinery
Emergency care	• Learn first aid, CPR, and airway obstruction removal
Water safety	• Learn to swim well • If you supervise younger children near water, never leave them alone, even for a minute
Fires	• Do not play with fire • Follow guidelines to avoid igniting gasoline • Test smoke alarms in your house every 6 months and annually change batteries
Firearms	• Know and follow rules to keep firearms locked, with ammunition locked in a separate place • Never take out a gun to show a friend unless your parent is also present • Take firearm safety classes if you hunt or target shoot
Hearing	• Avoid loud music, especially for long periods and through ear phones
Sports	• Wear protective gear recommended for your sport
Abuse	• Report any abuse to an adult you trust • Date with other couples whenever possible and report date rape • Do not drink or take drugs

Adapted from Green & Palfrey, 2002.

Planning and Implementation

Whatever the setting, the nurse partners with the adolescent, the parents, and other persons such as teachers or school counselors to plan appropriate goals and related interventions. Nurses work with individual adolescents in offices, schools, and other settings, and often work with groups of adolescents to perform teaching. Apply communication skills effective with teens such as listening to concerns, allowing for discussion, and bringing peers who have had experiences related to the topic being discussed.

Many of your interventions will involve teaching, so it is wise to develop a number of resources for working with teens. Consult the web resources on the Companion Website, and visit agencies in your community to gather appropriate materials. Teaching topics will be directed both at health promotion (providing information to enhance the adolescent's state of health) and health maintenance (sharing tips about how to avoid disease and injury). A good starting point is to have the adolescent identify a personal health goal and begin teaching there. In addition to teaching, you will provide direct care when you administer immunizations, perform vision screening, and examine the spine and posture for scoliosis.

One of the challenges during health supervision for adolescents is including the right mix of teen and parent decision making and involvement. You will again apply communication skills by tactfully allowing time for both parent and adolescent to be seen alone. Realize that you are supporting and providing information for parents, like useful discipline techniques, recognition of common parental feelings about teens, and the need for growing independence by their youth. When you provide teaching to groups of teens in schools, there may be policies about what needs to be sent home to parents. Some schools require that an outline of topics such as sexually transmitted diseases or substance use be sent home for parents to read. Parents may call you with questions about content and approach, or some may choose to attend and sit in on your presentation. This obviously requires that you partner with the school administration, teachers, parents, and others to be effective in your presentation. Collaboration with many individuals and agencies is an important skill.

Whether you see adolescents in offices or other private settings, or in schools, correction facilities, or other places with groups present, leave information about how you or another nurse or care provider can be contacted. Provide brochures, referral numbers, names, and e-mails related to the topics discussed. Encourage annual health supervision visits and suggest a variety of places to obtain this care. For example, if a youth will soon graduate from high school, find out if he or she will be working or attending college and provide links to health insurance or care providers in the new location.

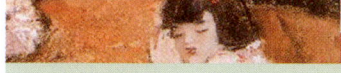

CRITICAL THINKING IN ACTION

Recall the chapter opener describing two young adolescents with type 1 diabetes mellitus. The school nurse meets with Jessalyn and Kelly regularly to monitor their management of diabetes and use of insulin pumps. The school nurse is in close contact with the endocrinologist who treats the girls, and with their parents. Jessalyn was recently hospitalized for an episode of diabetic shock but is presently doing well and is back in school.

DISCUSSION

1. How might the growth patterns of young adolescents affect management of diabetes? Consider the effects of a growth spurt on insulin and glucose needs.

2. The nurse determines that a 24-hour dietary recall might provide information about Jessalyn's diet

that assists in identifying dietary needs. Plan the methods the nurse should use to obtain an accurate recall. See Chapter 4 for nutritional assessment techniques.

3. The nurse will inform classroom teachers about methods of identifying complications of diabetes when Jessalyn and Kelly are in class. What are the signs of hypoglycemia and hyperglycemia?

4. Jessalyn has recently begun practice on the school swim team. Practice is after school, leading to a later-than-usual dinner time for her. Plan a dietary approach to provide adequate snacks and energy for her practice.

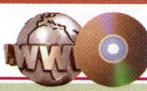 *Refer to your Prentice Hall Nursing MediaLink DVD-ROM for answers.*

EXPLORE MediaLink   http://www.prenhall.com/ball

Resources for this chapter can be found on the Prentice Hall Nursing MediaLink DVD-ROM accompanying this textbook, and on the Companion Website at http://www.prenhall.com/ball.

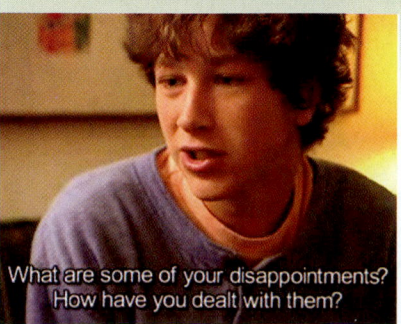

What are some of your disappointments? How have you dealt with them?

DVD-ROM
Audio Glossary
NCLEX-RN® Review
Video
  Teen Mental and Spiritual Health

COMPANION WEBSITE
Audio Glossary
NCLEX-RN® Review
Care Plan Activity: A Teen Who is Overweight
Case Study: Immunization Update
Critical Thinking: Assessment of Adolescent Female
MediaLink Application
  Smoking Education
WebLinks

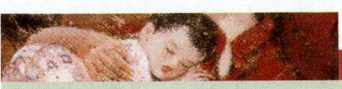

REFERENCES

Bandura, A. (1977). *Self-efficacy in changing societies.* New York: Cambridge University.

Centers for Disease Control and Prevention. (2006). CDC's advisory committee recommends human papillomavirus vaccination. Press Release. Retrieved July 12, 2006, from http://www.cd.gov/od/oc/medi/pressrel/r060629.htm

Chang, G., Sherritt, L., & Knight, J. R. (2005). Adolescent cigarette smoking and mental health symptoms. *Journal of Adolescent Health, 36,* 517–522.

Green, B. L., Person, S., Crowther, M., Frison, S., Shipp, M., Lee, P., & Martin, M. (2003). Demographic and geographic variations of oral health among African Americans based on NHANES III. *Community Dental Health, 20,* 117–122.

Green, M., & Palfrey, J. S. (Eds.). (2002). *Bright futures: Guidelines for health supervision of infants, children, and adolescents,* (2nd ed.). Arlington, VA: National Center for Education in Maternal and Child Health.

Healthy People 2010. (2000). Washington, DC: U.S. Department of Health and Human Services. Retrieved September 1, 2003, from http://www.healthypeople.gov/document/html.volume2/22Physical.htm

Jellinek, M., Patel, B. P., & Froehle, M. C. (Eds.). (2002). *Bright futures in practice: Mental health,* Vol I & II. Arlington, VA: National Center for Education in Maternal and Child Health.

Lerner, R. M., & Thompson, L. S. (2002). Promoting health adolescent behavior and development: Issues in the design and evaluation of effective youth programs. *Journal of Pediatric Nursing, 17,* 338–344.

Mayo Clinic. (2003). Adolescents and sleep. Retrieved September 7, 2003, from http://www.cnn.com/HEALTH/library/CC/00019

MMWR. (2004). Youth risk behavior surveillance—United States, 2003. *Morbidity and Mortality Weekly Report, 53* (SS02), 1–96.

MMWR. (2006). Youth risk behavior surveillance—United States, 2005. *Morbidity and Mortality Weekly Report, 55* (SS 5), 1–108.

Montgomery, K. S. (2002). Health promotion with adolescents: Examining theoretical perspectives to guide research. *Research and Theory for Nursing Practice: An International Journal, 16,* 119–134.

Olson, A. L., Gaffney, C. A., Hedberg, V. A., Gladstone, W., Dugan, S., Mathes, T., & Reiss, P. L. (2005). The Health Teen Project: Tools to enhance adolescent health counseling. *Annals of Family Medicine, 3* (Suppl 2), 563–565.

Qui, Y., & Ni, H. (2003). Utilization of dental care services by Asians and native Hawaiian or other Pacific Islanders: United States, 1997–2000. *Advances in Data, 336,* 1–11.

Simons-Morton, B. G., Hartos, J. L., & Beck, K. H. (2003). Persistence of effects of a brief intervention on parental restrictions of teen driving privileges. *Injury Prevention, 9,* 142–146.

Story, M., Holt, K., & Sofka, D. (Eds.). (2002). *Bright futures in practice: Nutrition.* Arlington, VA: National Center for Education in Maternal and Child Health.

Streng, N. (2000). A student health advocate program. *Journal of School Nursing, 16,* 50–53.

Strong, W. B., Malina, R. M., Blimkie C. J., Daniels, S. R., Dishman, R. K., Gutin, B., Hergenroeder, A. C., Must, A., Nixon, P. A., Pirarnik, J. M., Rowland, T., Trost, S., & Trudeau, F. (2005). Evidence-based physical activity for school-age youth. *Journal of Pediatrics, 146,* 732–737.

Task Force on the Family. (2003). Family pediatrics: Report of the Task Force on the Family. *Pediatrics, 111* (Supp), 1541–1571.

Vargas, C. M., Ronzio, C. R. L., & Hayes, K. L. (2003). Oral health status of children and adolescents by rural residence, United States. *Journal of Rural Health, 19,* 260–268.

11 NURSING CONSIDERATIONS FOR THE CHILD IN THE COMMUNITY

MediaLink

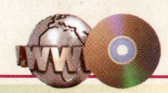

http://www.prenhall.com/ball

See the Prentice Hall Nursing MediaLink DVD-ROM and Companion Website for chapter-specific resources.

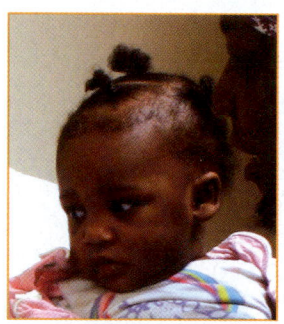

FOUR-MONTH-OLD Kendra has been brought by her parents to the health center for her checkup and next immunizations. Several pediatricians provide care to children at the health center, and nurse practitioners and nurses have an active role in providing health promotion services. The pediatricians in this center also manage many children with chronic health conditions, and they have a close relationship with the local children's hospital. Kendra's parents have selected a primary care provider in the center for her ongoing healthcare services.

Kendra is healthy and growing at an appropriate rate. She has not yet had any illnesses. Her parents have enjoyed watching her grow and gain new developmental skills over the past 4 months. Her mother heard about the benefits of infant massage and spends time each day massaging and interacting with Kendra.

After the pediatrician talks with Kendra's parents and assesses her, the nurse gives Kendra her immunizations and provides additional guidance for the parents regarding Kendra's next stages of growth and development. The focus of her discussion is nutrition, the next skills that Kendra will develop, and methods to promote Kendra's development. Kendra's mother plans to return to work in the next month, so an important discussion involves selecting a childcare provider, and what to observe and ask about when visiting potential care providers. Because the hurricane season is beginning, the nurse also reminds the parents of supplies to have on hand in case a disaster is declared.

What is the role of the nurse in community health settings? What information should be shared with parents about selecting childcare or any special care needed for a child in the school setting? How can families select the complementary and alternative therapies that are safe and effective for children? What information should the nurse share with the parents regarding family preparedness for a natural disaster, and the additional supplies needed for an infant?

LEARNING OUTCOMES

After reading this chapter, you will be able to do the following:

1. List the types of community healthcare settings where nurses provide health services to children.

2. Describe the role of the nurse in each identified community healthcare setting.

3. List at least five ways in which nurses assist families in the home healthcare setting.

4. Describe potential negative consequences of using herbs and other natural products for children.

5. Identify at least four complementary or alternative therapies that have evidence of effectiveness.

6. Describe the roles of nurses in emergency preparedness for children.

7. Identify the roles of nurses in disaster preparedness.

COMMUNITY-BASED HEALTH CARE

Health care for children has been rapidly shifting from the hospital to community settings over the past 15 to 20 years. For example, patterns of healthcare delivery have changed due to technology developments and efforts to reduce healthcare costs. Day surgery in ambulatory surgical centers, newborn discharge after 24 to 48 hours, home care for long-term intravenous antibiotics, and short-stay units associated with emergency departments are common. Options to provide safe, high-quality care with fewer hospitalizations or shorter stays when hospitalization is needed are continually evaluated. Home care services have developed to support families who now care for more acutely ill and chronically ill children in their homes.

This trend in out-of-hospital care is particularly seen among children with chronic health conditions and advanced disease states. Technologic advances, such as portable medical equipment, now make it possible to provide complex healthcare services in the home and other community settings. Strategies to support families who provide home care to their children have developed. Additionally, federal law mandates that education be provided to all children with disabilities, and there are no exceptions based on healthcare status. As a result, schools are now obligated to provide complex health care to children. (See page 391.) See Chapter 12 ∞ for more discussion of care for the child with a chronic illness.

Characteristics of Community-Based Health Care

Today children receive most of their health care in community settings. Depending upon the community and its healthcare resources, as well as the age of the child, this care may be provided in a wide variety of settings, including childcare centers, schools, camps, physician offices, hospital or public health clinics, homeless shelters, and the home.

The nursing role is important in promoting children's health in the community. The range of nursing care provided is quite broad. Examples of nursing care provided in community settings include:

- Monitoring the health and safety of children in childcare centers and schools
- Health promotion and health maintenance
- Episodic health care for acute illnesses and injuries in office settings
- Surgery and diagnostic testing procedures in ambulatory surgical settings
- Home health care
- Care for children in homeless and emergency shelters

Nurses have a variety of positions within these settings, such as: pediatric nurse in an office or clinic setting, community health nurse, home healthcare nurse, school nurse, and nurse practitioner or advance practice nurse. The nurse may assume the role of direct care provider, educator, advocate, or planner in any of these positions. The nurse practitioner and advance practice nurse often assess and manage the care provided to children with acute and chronic health conditions in many health settings.

The nurse working with families in a community setting must use the knowledge of how the larger environment influences the child's health and development and the family's activities. See Chapter 3 ∞ for a discussion of the bio-ecologic model that examines the interactions between the child and the environment, and Chapter 6 ∞ for many examples of environmental influences. Learning about the healthcare resources available within the child's community is important in offering families options for needed healthcare services.

The nurse must assess the family's strengths and needs, evaluate the availability of community resources to match the child's and family's needs, and help families manage the child's health care provided in the home. Developing a partnership with the family is essential as the family will be implementing the care agreed upon by the nurse, other health professionals, and the parents. Education that enables the family and often the child to manage the needed care in a safe and effective manner is essential. For example, the family caring for an infant with a tracheostomy needs to learn how to change the tracheostomy tube and suction the airway when needed, in addition to finding ways to promote the infant's growth, development, and nutrition.

To work effectively in the community, the nurse needs to gain experience and skills in:

- Conducting child and family assessments and working with families to plan individualized healthcare strategies, as well as implementing and evaluating nursing care strategies to match family economic, cultural, and social situations, in addition to available resources.
- Working with community agencies (schools, churches, and other community-based resources) to assess, plan strategies, and implement and evaluate approaches addressed to the healthcare needs of the community's children.

COMMUNITY-BASED HEALTHCARE SETTINGS

Office or Healthcare Center Setting

Every child should have a **healthcare home** or **medical home,** the site of comprehensive health care by a pediatric healthcare professional, in order to ensure the child's optimal health. As noted in the care of Kendra and her parents, the healthcare providers (physicians, nurse practitioners, nurses) in the healthcare home or medical home assume responsibility for coordinating the child's needed health care between all healthcare settings. Important elements of a healthcare home or medical home include the following (American Academy of Pediatrics, 2002):

- Family-centered care that involves a trusting relationship, respecting the diversity and importance of the family in the child's life
- Continuity of care from infancy through adolescence, and transition of adolescents with chronic conditions to adult health care
- Family-centered health promotion and health maintenance care
- Interaction with childcare, school, and community agencies as needed, coordinating care with all health providers

A physician office or health center often serves as the healthcare home. Health promotion and health maintenance services, as well as episodic acute illness and injury care, are provided to the child and family at this location. See Chapters 8, 9, and 10 ∞ for the specific health promotion services provided in the community setting.

Role of the Pediatric Nurse in an Office or Health Center

The nursing process is used when providing care for children in the health center, and in some cases in a mobile health van. The range of assessment responsibilities may vary by setting, as well as the preparation and experience of the nurse (Figure 11–1➤). Specific functions of the pediatric nurse in this setting include:

- Identifying children in need of urgent care or isolation
- Performing nursing assessments including the health history, vital signs, growth and development, nutritional

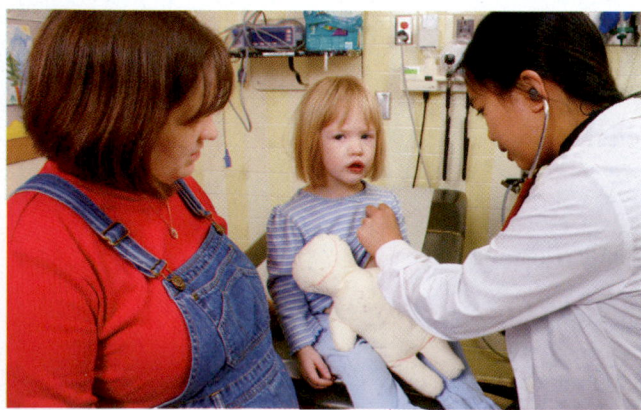

Figure 11–1 ➤ Nurses carefully assess children in the office setting who present with an acute care illness. It is important to identify how serious the child's illness is and to monitor the child for progression of symptoms during the visit. This is also a time to gather information about the child's illness and to identify health information that will be needed for the family to care for the child at home.

status, immunization status, family strengths and challenges, and physical examination

- Performing screening tests to detect health problems such as vision, hearing, anemia, and lead poisoning (see Chapters 8, 9, and 10 ∞)
- Assisting with physician or nurse practitioner examinations and performing diagnostic tests as well as providing information about procedures and offering reassurance
- Developing nursing diagnoses and implementing a plan of care including immunizations, family education for health promotion, or management of a health condition
- Linking families with community resources
- Assuring an office or clinic is a safe environment and that infection control guidelines are followed

An important goal is to develop a positive relationship with the child and family so that optimal health care is provided. This relationship is strengthened over the months and years of providing care to the child and family.

IDENTIFYING SEVERELY ILL AND INJURED CHILDREN   It is important to assess the child with an episodic illness or injury upon arrival in the health center to determine the urgency of care that will be needed. A rapid assessment for changes in mental status, airway patency, breathing, and circulation is used to identify the child that needs immediate medical attention. The child with an urgent condition must be monitored frequently to detect any worsening of the condition and need for emergency care.

Children with serious illnesses often present at a health center or physician office and require emergency care. The nurse collaborates with the physician to develop an emergency response plan for the health center. The nurse is often responsible for teaching the office receptionist to recognize a child that needs immediate assessment by the nurse. The nurse is also often accountable for assuring that all emergency care equipment, supplies, and medications are organized and readily available in the central treatment room. The nurse often assumes a leadership role in promoting basic life support training of office personnel and in coordinating mock drills with all staff in the healthcare setting so that all employees know and perform their designated role when a true emergency occurs.

EDUCATING THE CHILD AND FAMILY   Patient education regarding injury prevention, growth and development, nutrition, healthy lifestyles, and the home care of episodic illnesses and injuries are important nursing roles in the healthcare home or medical home. The nurse also may be responsible for selecting patient education materials for the waiting area and those specifically used to teach families about various conditions. Knowledge of the community and population served by the health center enables the nurse to select appropriate education materials.

Nurses teach families to provide the condition-specific care for the child at home, and assess the need for repeated or additional education. Examples of information provided include:

- Signs that the condition is not improving as expected and when to return to the physician
- How and when to administer prescribed medications and their potential side effects
- Modifications in diet and activity
- Other supportive care for the child's condition
- Education to help the child and family recognize the need to initiate care for a new episode of a chronic condition (e.g., asthma, sickle cell anemia, or hemophilia) that may prevent the need for a healthcare visit or reduce the severity of the episode

IDENTIFYING COMMUNITY RESOURCES   Nurses in the healthcare home are often involved in identifying community resources that are needed by the child and family

---

> **NURSING ALERT**
>
> Nurses have an important role in assuring that a health center is prepared to handle a child with an emergency. Key steps that should be taken to prepare for a patient emergency include the following:
> - Order resuscitation equipment and medications.
> - Check and restock expired and used supplies and medications at least weekly or after each emergency. A log or record should be maintained.
> - Collaborate with the physician to develop triage guidelines and standing orders for common pediatric emergencies.
> - Collaborate with the physician to plan each staff member's role in responding to the emergency.
> - Post the appropriate phone number for calling the local emergency medical services to transport the child to the emergency department.
> - Post the poison control number on all phones.
>
> Data from: Ralston, M. E. (2005). Managing emergencies part 1. *Pediatric Annals, 34*(11), 845–849.

> **CLINICAL TIP**
>
> Essential equipment needed for managing an emergency in an office setting includes the following: oxygen and an oxygen delivery system, bag-valve-mask resuscitator in a pediatric and adult size, clear oxygen masks in various pediatric sizes (both breather and nonrebreather masks with a reservoir), pulse oximeter, oral airways in various sizes, suction devices, peak flow meter, a nebulizer or metered dose inhaler with a spacer/mask, and intravenous needles in various sizes. Examples of essential medications are epinephrine 1:1000 and albuterol (American Academy of Pediatrics Committee on Pediatric Emergency Medicine, 2000). Locate the emergency equipment in every clinical setting where you have assignments.

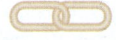

SKILLS CHAPTER 1
Standard and Transmission-Based Precautions

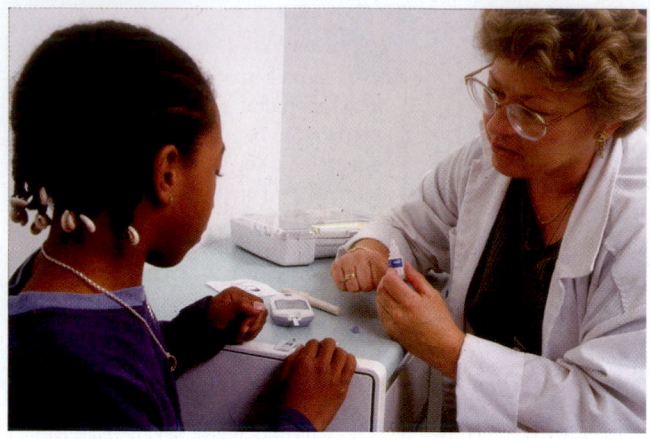

Figure 11–2 ➤ Nurses often assume a larger role in working with children and families with a chronic health condition in the hospital ambulatory setting. Developing a care plan and educating the family to manage the type 1 diabetes is an important role of this pediatric nurse who is also a nationally certified diabetes educator.

COMMUNITY CARE

School-based Health Centers

School-based health centers may exist in some communities. Comprehensive physical, reproductive, and mental health services plus health education are often provided by a multidisciplinary team of nurse practitioners, physicians, physician assistants, mental health providers, and other supporting staff. School-based health centers specifically target children who have difficulty in accessing health care, such as those without insurance or who are underinsured, as well as adolescents (Gustafson, 2005). Since these school-based health centers serve the community where the school is based, the provided services are often better able to integrate community values and culturally appropriate care.

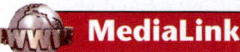 **MediaLink**

Resources for School Nurses

that will help promote the child's health. Compiling a manual of community resources and regularly updating names and phone numbers of contacts will make it easier to provide information efficiently. Examples of community resources that might be included are early intervention programs, support groups, language and translation services, food banks, lead paint abatement services, social services, and mental health services.

ENSURING A SAFE ENVIRONMENT FOR CHILDREN

The health center has many potential hazards such as equipment, cleaning supplies, needles, lancets, medications, and laboratory materials from which the child needs to be protected. The nurse should ensure a safe environment for the child. The child must be attended at all times when in the examination area. Guidelines for infection control must be developed and implemented to reduce the transmission of infectious diseases between child patients and between the healthcare providers and children.

Specialty Healthcare Settings

Pediatric nurses also provide care for children with acute and chronic conditions within hospital outpatient or specialty care ambulatory settings. Children may be referred to physician specialists for diagnostic work-ups or the long-term management of their chronic conditions. In some cases health promotion, health maintenance, and episodic illness care are provided to children with chronic conditions in these settings. With experience pediatric nurses working in a hospital ambulatory setting develop specialized knowledge and skill to meet the specific needs of the population of children receiving care (Figure 11–2➤). The roles for nurses in these settings are similar to those described for the health center.

School Settings

School nurses practice independently as the only licensed healthcare provider in the educational setting. Depending on the community, they serve up to 2000 children in one or more schools. School nursing is a specialized practice of professional nursing that advances the well-being, academic success, and life-long achievement of children. School nurses facilitate positive student responses to normal development; ensure health promotion, health maintenance, and safety; intervene in actual and potential health problems; provide case management services; and actively collaborate with others to build student and family capacity for adaptation, self-management, self-advocacy, and learning (National Association of School Nurses and American Nurses Association, 2005). See Box 11–1 for the Standards of Professional School Nursing Practice.

School nurses work to remove or minimize the health barriers to learning so students can improve school performance. School health services include preventive services, health promotion and health maintenance, health education, emergency care, and the referral and management of acute and chronic health problems. The traditional tasks of screening, first aid, and monitoring immunization status are still performed. Box 11–2 contains *Healthy People 2010* national health objectives that illustrate the breadth of school nursing. Guidelines for health, mental health, and safety in school settings have been developed through the collaboration of multiple national organizations.

Role of the Nurse in the School Setting

Nursing roles in the school setting focus on promoting the health and safety to the population of children enrolled (including faculty and staff) and providing direct care to ill and injured children. Children in the school setting may include infants if childcare is offered for adolescent mothers, as well as preschool-age children attending Head Start, a federally sponsored program to promote child development and educational readiness (Figure 11–3➤). Specific activities include maintaining infection control, monitoring

BOX 11–1
STANDARDS OF PROFESSIONAL SCHOOL NURSING PRACTICE

1. The school nurse collects comprehensive data pertinent to the client's health or the situation.
2. The school nurse analyzes the assessment data to determine the diagnoses or issues.
3. The school nurse identifies expected outcomes for a plan individualized to the client or the situation.
4. The school nurse develops a plan that prescribes strategies and alternatives to attain expected outcomes.
5. The school nurse implements the identified plan by coordinating care delivery, providing health education, employing strategies to promote health and a safe environment, and providing consultation to influence the identified plan, enhance the abilities of others, and effect change.
6. The school nurse evaluates progress toward attainment of outcomes.
7. The school nurse systematically enhances the quality and effectiveness of nursing practice.
8. The school nurse attains knowledge and competency that reflects current school nursing practice.
9. The school nurse evaluates one's own practice in relation to professional practice standards and guidelines, relevant statutes, rules, and regulations.
10. The school nurse interacts with, and contributes to the professional development of, peers and school personnel as colleagues.
11. The school nurse collaborates with the client, the family, school staff, and others in the conduct of school nursing practice.
12. The school nurse integrates ethical provisions in all areas of practice.
13. The school nurse integrates research findings in practice.
14. The school nurse considers factors related to safety, effectiveness, cost, and impact on practice in the planning and delivery of school nursing services.
15. The school nurse provides leadership in the professional practice setting and the profession.
16. The school nurse manages school health services.

Adapted from: National Association of School Nurses and American Nurses Association. (2005). *School nursing: Scope and standards of practice.* Silver Spring, MD: American Nurses Publishing.

LAW & ETHICS

The Child Nutrition and WIC Reauthorization Act

The Child Nutrition and WIC Reauthorization Act of 2004 (P.L. 108-265) improves the effectiveness of the school lunch program, after-school snack program, summer food service program, and the child/adult care food program with goals for nutrition education and physical activity in an effort to address childhood obesity. School nurses may have an important role in the local wellness program that must be implemented in schools seeking federal funds for school lunch programs (Zimmerman, 2005).

CLINICAL TIP

An online School Health Index helps schools perform a self-assessment and plan for improvements in their health and safety policies and programs. This resource was developed by the Centers for Disease Control National Center for Chronic Disease Prevention and Health Promotion (2005). The web site also contains resources to support planning in each of the assessment categories.

health education, assessing conditions that impact health and learning, administering medications, participating on teams to develop individualized education plans (IEPs) and individualized health plans (IHPs), advocating for better nutrition and physical activity to improve overall health, investigating environmental safety hazards, and planning for crisis intervention and support services (Robinson, 2002). See Chapter 12 ∞ for information about IEPs and IHPs. School nurses also have an important role in improving the rate of childhood immunization.

EMERGENCY PREPAREDNESS **Emergency preparedness** is a well-defined plan for emergency medical care response for individual incidents that includes assembling critical equipment and supplies, training to learn essential skills, and identifying roles for individuals involved in the response. School nurses should also take a leadership role in preparing the school to manage life-threatening emergencies by developing a partnership with the local emergency medical services agency, the school administrator and other school personnel, and local primary care physicians (Olympia, Wan, & Avner, 2005). The school nurse is responsible for the direct care of a child with an emergency condition until help arrives. Planning to care for children in the school setting during a disaster event is a further extension of emergency preparedness planning. (See page 374 for more on disaster preparedness.)

Collaboration with the other health professionals in the community is becoming increasingly important to promote health in the school setting. Working with the school's physician consultant or local health district to discuss and update standing orders for the care of children is important so that the nurse can provide care for urgent and emergency health threats that students may potentially experience. Communicating with the child's healthcare provider about the child's specific health conditions makes it possible for the nurse to manage the child's condition in the school setting (Figure 11–4▶). The school

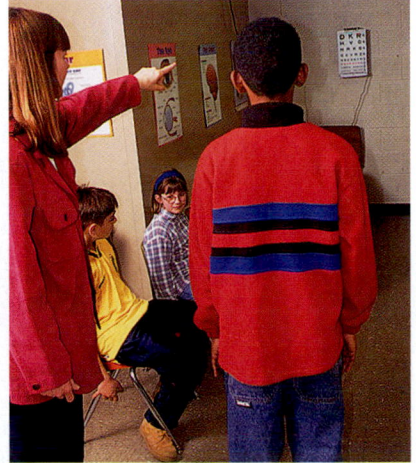

Figure 11–3 ➤ The school often screens large groups of students to identify those that may have a problem that interferes with learning. Screening tests are often organized so all children in a particular grade are assessed, as in this vision screening test.

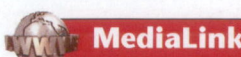
MediaLink

Healthy People 2010

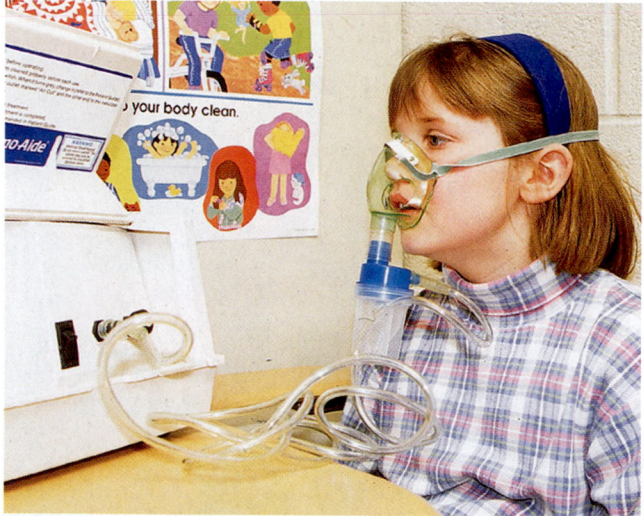

Figure 11–4 ▶ Because some children need medications or other therapies during school hours, the parents and child, school nurse, teacher, and school administrators develop a plan to manage the child's condition during school hours. This document is the child's individual health plan.

nurse often has valuable information to help the child's healthcare providers with their ongoing management.

FACILITATING A CHILD'S RETURN TO SCHOOL The school nurse facilitates the child's return to the classroom following an acute illness or injury, especially when environmental adaptation is required or when a change in health status has occurred. The transition back to school is assisted when the pediatric nurse in the hospital or community setting or the child's healthcare provider contacts the school nurse to coordinate the child's return to school, rather than having the parent take full responsibility for informing the school. Educational materials about the child's condition can be recommended to educate students, faculty, and staff. The school nurse then begins to work with the family to prepare teachers and school administrators for the child's special needs. The child's teacher and classmates can be prepared for the child's physical changes, if appropriate. Sometimes the teacher's expectations of the child need to be modified, as in the case of a child with a mild brain injury who may have decreased ability to concentrate for several weeks during recovery. Often an IHP must be developed or modified. See Chapter 12 ∞.

CHILDREN WITH COMPLEX HEALTHCARE CONDITIONS Previously homebound children, who are **medically fragile** and need skilled nursing care with or without medical equipment to support vital functions, now attend school. See Chapter 12 ∞ for a discussion of these children and their care in the community.

Outcomes of school nursing care may include the following (Selekman & Guilday, 2003):

- Children have increased learning time.
- Students receive first aid, emergency care, and services for their acute healthcare needs.
- Students receive needed, competent, health-related interventions (medications and procedures).
- Students with chronic conditions have their healthcare needs met.
- Students receive appropriate referrals based upon assessments made.
- Children have a safe learning environment.

Childcare Settings

Many young children are cared for in childcare settings while parents are at work. Many types of childcare arrangements exist, such as in-home care by a family member or nanny, a licensed childcare family home setting for up to five children, or a licensed childcare center for six or more children. States establish minimum licensure requirements and guidelines for the safe operation of childcare settings that address the staff qualifications, staff-child ratio, staff training requirements, safe food handling, safe health practices, and environmental safety. Guidelines for the safe operation of childcare centers are available through the National Resource Center for Health and Safety in Child Care.

Nurses often provide information to parents about childcare options and characteristics of high-quality care. Key factors to emphasize for parents include: small infant to caregiver ratios, small size group of children, safe and stimulating environment, well-trained and experienced caregivers, and parent observation time (Youngblade & Carter, 2004). See Chapter 6 .

Role of the Nurse in Childcare Settings

Nurses can assume an important consultant role by assisting in development of the childcare center's policies for health practices, teaching staff about safe health practices, and monitoring and promoting health practices in the setting. The nurse consultant can also teach staff to identify children with illnesses and to provide first aid for injured children. In some cases, especially in childcare centers for ill children, nurses provide health screening and direct care to children (Alkon, Farrer, & Bernzweig, 2004; Evers, 2002). See Evidence-Based Practice: Reducing Injuries in Childcare Centers.

REDUCING DISEASE TRANSMISSION Children in childcare centers are close together in large numbers; they put things in their mouths; they may be contagious before symptoms occur; and they are susceptible to most infectious agents. The nurse can educate and work with the childcare center manager and staff to reduce disease transmission in the following ways:

- Developing guidelines for review of immunizations and plans for exclusion of unimmunized children when a vaccine-preventable disease occurs in the facility (see Chapter 18)
- Checking each child daily for signs and symptoms of illness (e.g., behavior changes, rashes, fever, vomiting, diarrhea, and eye drainage) and developing guidelines for the exclusion and return of children with different infectious conditions
- Teaching staff when and how to perform hand hygiene, manage secretions, sanitize toys and surfaces, and manage cuts and scrapes
- Developing guidelines for diapering infants and toddlers
- Caring for the sick child and reducing exposure to others until the child is picked up by the parent or guardian

HEALTH PROMOTION AND HEALTH MAINTENANCE Health promotion activities are those that will further the child's highest level of functioning and development, such as having activities that stimulate physical development, nutrition that

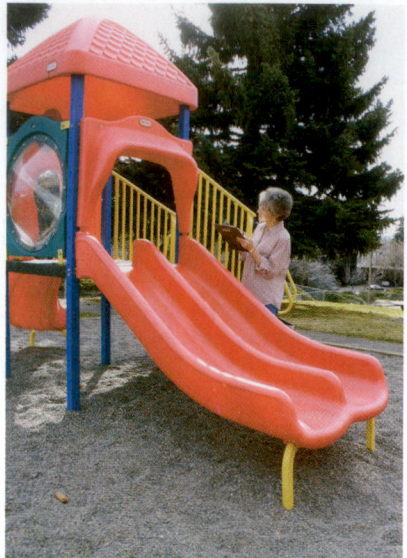

Figure 11–5 ➤ Assess the childcare center's environment for safety hazards. Check the area around playground equipment, making sure there are wood chips or cushioned tiles under the equipment. Inspect the playground equipment for protruding screws, loose nuts and bolts, and instability at least monthly.

fosters growth and ability to perform at a maximum level, and a well-rounded program that considers all types of development, from fine and gross motor, to language, emotional growth, cognition, and social skills. Nurses can design and offer health education programs for the children (tooth brushing, hand hygiene, and blowing the nose into a tissue) to promote healthy habits. Health maintenance activities are those that prevent injury or disease, such as immunization monitoring, infection control, and practices like putting infants on their back to sleep. See Chapter 18 ∞.

ENVIRONMENTAL SAFETY Ensure that the childcare center maintains a current list of which family members may take a child from the facility, and has guidelines for verifying identity when necessary.

The nurse should inspect the childcare environment to identify hazards that could cause injury to the children. Cleaning supplies and other toxins must be stored in a locked cabinet to prevent exposure. Inspect toys used by children to ensure that there are no sharp edges or points, small parts, or pinching parts. Playground equipment should also be checked for safety (Figure 11–5 ➤).

EMERGENCY CARE PLANNING The nurse can help the childcare administrator develop a guideline to assess and identify the child with an emergency health condition and to develop an emergency care plan for instances when a child becomes acutely ill or injured. This plan should include the following elements: giving first aid, calling emergency medical services to transport the child to the emergency department, notifying the parent about the child's condition, and accompanying the child to the emergency department until the parent arrives. A record for each child should include an emergency contact list or preferred health facility should the child need immediate care. Staffing should be adequate to have a staff member accompany the child to the health facility in an emergency.

Childcare centers should also develop an emergency plan for disaster response. An adequate supply of food and water for sheltering in place is important as families may be unable to reach childcare centers to pick up their children during such an event. See page 374.

Other Community Settings

In many other community settings, the nurse's role may be similar to that in a school setting. Promoting health, preventing disease, and preventing injury are equally important in childcare centers, camps, health department clinics, and disaster or homeless shelters. For example, nurses may work with homeless shelter administrators to

---

EVIDENCE-BASED PRACTICE

Reducing Injuries in Childcare Centers

Clinical Question

What are the most common injuries that occur in childcare settings and how do the types of injuries vary by the age of the child?

Evidence

Injury data was collected for a full year from incident reports about the types of injuries occurring to children in two urban childcare centers. A total of 131 children between 6 weeks and 7 years of age (mean age of 24 months) were enrolled full- or part-time in the centers. During the year, a total of 897 incident reports identified 1023 injuries. The distribution of injuries was as follows: bites (39%), falls (23%), bumps and bruises (22%), and scratches, cuts, blisters, and fracture (16%). Only 2 children required medical attention, while the remainder received first aid on site. Infants and toddlers (0 to 36 months of age) had the highest frequency of injury, reflecting in large part the high frequency of biting reported in this age group. Approximately 60% of all injuries occurred in the morning hours (Waibel & Misra, 2003).

Implications

Understanding the type of injuries that happen in childcare centers, the age group most affected, and other information, such as time of day, provides the nurse with important information to help the childcare center to promote the health of enrolled children and make efforts to reduce injuries. Injury prevention strategies can potentially be developed based upon collected data. The number of minor injuries in childcare centers also illustrates the importance of having childcare center staff trained in first aid. It is also important to have guidelines for management of injuries and notification of parents when injuries happen.

Critical Thinking

Consider the distribution of injuries and identify potential strategies that could be used to reduce the number of biting and falling incidents. What actions could the childcare center workers take to reduce the number of incidents that occur during morning hours? Outline the first aid guidelines that a childcare center should have in place to manage each of the most common injuries reported. What guidelines should exist for notifying parents about injuries that occur?

address infection control issues and to assess the safety of the children's environment. See Chapter 6 ∞.

Role of the Nurse in Camp Settings

Nurses in camps function independently and need to use critical thinking skills, much like school nurses. They promote the health of all campers, assess and improve the safety of the children's environment, provide nursing care to children with acute illnesses and injuries, and plan activities to promote health. Some special camps for children with chronic conditions must have trained personnel to provide needed medical and nursing care as well as health education while children are participating in recreational activities. Nurses are responsible for the health care of children attending camp 24 hours a day.

Home Healthcare Setting

Home health care is a component of the continuum of comprehensive community health care provided to children and families in their home. Approximately 300,000 children between birth and 17 years of age received home health care in 2000 (National Association for Home Care and Hospice, 2004). Children with episodic or long-term healthcare conditions can benefit from home healthcare services. Only a small number of these children have conditions serious enough to need continuous (daily, up to 24 hours a day) private duty care in the home. Most children receive intermittent skilled nursing visits to assess the child and examine how family members are managing the child's healthcare needs. Intermittent home healthcare services (one to several visits a week) may be provided to help families during the child's acute recovery, such as a child receiving home antibiotic infusion therapy. Some home healthcare programs visit first-time mothers and their newborns to assess their health and well-being and to offer interventions such as breast-feeding support, newborn metabolic screening, and anticipatory guidance.

Many children needing home health care are medically fragile, and are dependent upon a medical device either for survival or prevention of further disability. Parents and other care providers without backgrounds in health care are given tremendous responsibilities to provide technology-assisted health care to their child. Technology-assisted care in the home may include any of the following: ventilators; tracheostomies; suctioning; nasogastric, gastrostomy, or parenteral feeding with feeding pumps; and intravenous fluids and medications with intravenous pumps. In some cases, families have created mini–intensive care units in their home. Examples of some serious chronic conditions cared for by families in the home include children with congenital heart defects before corrective surgery, bronchopulmonary dysplasia, and cancer in its terminal stage.

The home environment is believed to be optimal for the long-term care of these children so they can participate as family members and have their growth and development promoted. The family gains some control over their lives by having the child in the home rather than coordinating visits to the child and trying to simultaneously maintain a relatively normal family life. However, these families live with significant social, psychological, and physical consequences caused by the child's constant care requirements. They must balance the child's fragility and life-sustaining needs with the needs of the remainder of the family. Parents often feel like they have no choice about providing the ongoing care to their child (Carnevale, Alexander, Davis et al., 2006). See Chapter 12 ∞ for further discussion of support for families of children with chronic conditions.

Health insurers pay many of the costs associated with home care; however, the family may be financially burdened by paying some costs out-of-pocket, such as medications, supplies, and transportation. In some cases a parent must give up employment to provide care to the child. Healthcare systems (healthcare providers and insurers) are challenged to simultaneously address the child's illness and developmental needs while providing the support needed by these families so that children do well in their home environments. The family also needs help to support the growing child in the school and other peer settings.

Role of the Nurse in Home Health Care

Nurses require a variety of skills and knowledge to work in the home healthcare setting, including the following:

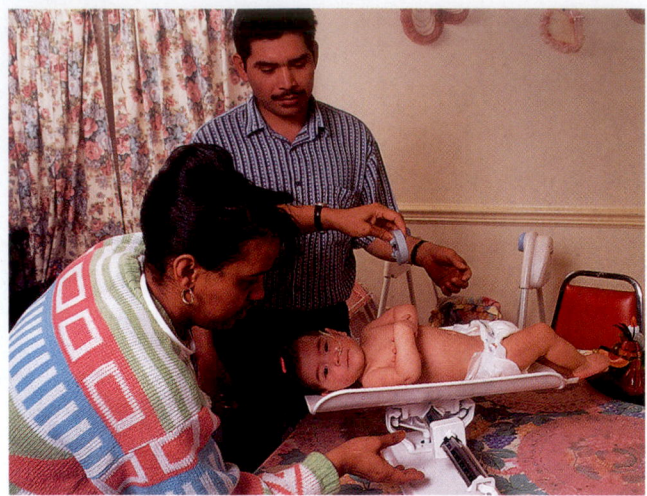

Figure 11–6 ➤ Nurses provide both short-term and long-term services to families in the home setting. In some cases, families need support for a short time after the child is discharged from the hospital following an acute illness. In other cases, families need assistance with complex nursing care for the child dependent on technology for survival.

- Knowledge and experience in acute care practice with various medical technologies used with children. These skills enable nurses to provide direct care, teach the family and child self-care practices, and monitor the child's progress.
- Community assessment skills; an understanding of community resources, financing mechanisms, and multiagency collaboration; and good communication skills.
- An understanding of the community's health resources to better assist families to find the most supportive services to match the child's and family's needs.
- An understanding of the community's cultural diversity and the cultural values of the families served.
- Skill in educating family members to assume care of the child.

Nurses in the home care setting use the nursing process to assess the child, family, and home environment. Then the nurse assists the family to manage the care of a child with a chronic condition more independently while promoting the child's growth and development. A major goal of working with families in the home healthcare setting includes promoting or restoring the child's health while attempting to minimize the effects of the disability and illness, including terminal illness (Figure 11–6➤). The success of home care is also based upon effective cultural communication as described in the accompanying Culture box.

NURSING MANAGEMENT
Nursing Assessment and Diagnosis

Home healthcare nurses assess the home, the child, and the family during intermittent skilled nursing visits. Home assessment is focused on environmental safety for the child and the resources needed for the child's care. When working with the hospital discharge planner to initiate home healthcare services, the following aspects of the home are assessed:

- Home readiness (safe sleeping arrangements, adequate supplies, ability to meet nutritional and fluid needs, telephone access, heat, electricity, refrigeration, lack of any communicable diseases in the home, and safe access into and out of the home).

- Potential hazards related to the child's age, condition, and requirements for technology-assisted care (e.g., when extension cords are needed to reach electrical outlets, the equipment may lose power if someone trips over the cord and disconnects it by mistake).

- Features in the home environment that could cause an acute illness, such as using a woodstove or fireplace that could cause respiratory distress, or renovating a house built before 1960 that could expose the child to lead dust. Additionally, the nurse may identify family members who smoke.

Assessment of the child is focused on the current health status, growth, developmental progress, and social interaction with family members and healthcare providers. Observation of the potential for abuse and neglect is an important ongoing assessment as these children are at a higher risk for abuse.

The family is assessed for parenting skills, as well as their abilities in providing the child's needed medical procedures and monitoring the child's health status. Family strengths and coping abilities are evaluated using the family assessment guidelines in

CULTURE

Assessment

When assessing the child and family in the home, recognize that there are potential conflicts between recommended medical care and the family's preferences. Identify which family member is most influential in decisions about care provided for the child. Use open-ended questions to talk with families and understand the health problem from their point of view. Ask the family to identify the problem, what caused the problem, their concerns with living with the problem, and the impact on the lives of family members. Information gained can then be used to educate the family and to develop a nursing care plan that integrates the family's preferences for the child's care.

Chapter 2 ∞ . The presence of siblings, their developmental and physical status, and their needs should also be assessed. Examples of nursing diagnoses that could apply to the family as the child transitions from the hospital to home setting include the following:

- Impaired Home Maintenance related to ineffective family coping
- Impaired Adjustment (Parents) related to multiple stressors in caring for a child with a complex health condition
- Ineffective Family Therapeutic Regimen Management related to complexity of medical interventions, information misinterpretation, and excessive demands made on the family
- Social Isolation related to demands on family members to care for the child

Planning and Implementation

Nurses help families in the home setting in the following ways:

- Assuring competent care to the child
- Educating parents about the child's condition and physical signs and symptoms that may indicate a change in health status
- Educating parents and demonstrating methods to promote the child's development
- Linking families to community resources, including support groups, respite care, and therapeutic recreation
- Assisting families in time management skills and patient care management
- Advocating for increased insurance coverage or locating other sources of financial assistance

Collaborating with the Family

The nurse and family work in partnership in the home to promote the health of the child and of the family as a unit. Families lose privacy and often find it stressful to have home healthcare nurses in the home for 24 hours a day. Additional stressors exist when the home care nurse is ill or on vacation, often requiring the parent to provide the care or to adjust to a substitute nurse.

The home healthcare nurse must recognize and accept that control belongs to the family in the home care setting. The parents are the employer with the ability to hire and fire, so it is critical for the nurse to develop a respectful and trusting relationship with them. Every interaction is negotiated with the family, or between the family and child, if there are differences in what they want. The nurse must be flexible and able to set aside power. Conflicts may occur when differences in opinion about the child's care become apparent. Open communication is essential so the nurse can learn what is important to the child and family, and then modify the nursing care plan when appropriate. House rules for such things as parking, private areas in the home, and routines may need to be negotiated, but then rules must be followed. Role expectations of the nurse must be clearly understood to reduce stress in the family. The success of home care is also based upon effective cultural communication. For example, some Jewish families follow strict dietary guidelines that do not permit milk and meat to be mixed. The nurse needs to abide by the dietary guidelines and observe the family's food preparation practices.

When nurses provide home care, it is important for a parent to be present and work in partnership with the nurse. Informed consent is needed for invasive treatments and decisions for provision of emergency care to avoid serious risk to life and limb. If parents must leave, a disclaimer protecting the home healthcare nurse from liability may be necessary (Margolan, Fraser, & Lenton, 2004).

The range of nursing care activities that may be included in a child's care plan in the home setting include sensory stimulation, routines of daily living, positioning and skin care with gentle handling, respiratory care, nutrition and elimination, medications, and other supportive therapies. Other providers, such as physical therapists, speech-language therapists, occupational therapists, and social workers, may provide other healthcare services in collaboration with the home healthcare nurse. Nursing

CLINICAL TIP

When working with families in the home make sure house rules are negotiated. Be sure to discuss the following guidelines for the expected behavior and role of the nurse, as well as the family's preferences for involvement in the care of the child (Parra, 2003):

- Access to the home: parking location, door to enter, where to store belongings, refrigerator use, private areas
- Use of the television, VCR, radio, and appliances such as the coffeepot
- Care of child: routines for daily care, feeding, bathing, bedtime, clothing, discipline, division of labor
- Care of child's environment, child's laundry
- Safety: visitors who are permitted to enter the home, arrangement of furniture
- Breaks for meals, where to store food, back-up coverage for the nurse
- Care for and discipline of siblings
- How to communicate (log of key information, meetings with family members at set intervals, schedule of child's appointments, parents' schedule

care should focus on promoting an environment within the home for the child to develop, learn social skills, and gain a sense of identity based on family values.

Emergency Preparedness

Families need to develop an emergency care plan for safe evacuation of the home in case of fire or other emergency. This is even more challenging when the child cannot mobilize independently and requires equipment for continued survival or quality of life. See Families Want to Know: Developing a Fire Escape Plan below for information to help families develop a plan for safe evacuation of the home.

The nurse should help the family develop an emergency care plan for any child whose condition could worsen rapidly and become life threatening, beyond the care that the parents or home healthcare nurse can provide. Examples of health conditions that fall into this category are serious congenital heart defects, tracheostomies, and apnea. Information should provide guidelines for when to call 9-1-1 or the local emergency number. The family should invite the local emergency medical services to visit so emergency medical technicians can become knowledgeable of the child's potential emergency care needs. The emergency care plan should include a written emergency medical history that provides the emergency healthcare provider with enough basic information to understand the child's health condition, to prevent delays in disease-specific treatment, and to minimize unnecessary interventions until the child's personal physician or health record can be consulted.

When the child is dependent upon technology, the family should notify the power company so that high priority can be given to getting resources to the home promptly after power outages. Backup generators may be needed if electrical power for life-sustaining equipment is essential. The child should also be registered for a disaster shelter that can accommodate the child's healthcare needs and at least one caregiver.

MediaLink

AAP Emergency Information Form

Evaluation

Expected outcomes of nursing care include:

- Care of the child's medical needs is integrated into the family's routines when possible.
- The family has an emergency care plan for the child in the event of a disaster, a weather emergency, or if the child's condition suddenly worsens.
- The home healthcare nurse and family work in partnership to promote the child's health, growth, and development.

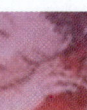

FAMILIES WANT TO KNOW

Developing a Fire Escape Plan

Developing a fire escape plan is important when the family has one or more children with special healthcare needs. Important steps for families to take in developing the plan include:

- Have working smoke detectors in the home and teach children what the alarm means. Make sure batteries are checked at least twice a year.
- Draw a diagram of your house. Mark all windows and doors.
- Plan two routes out of every room. Have a portable ladder to hang out of a second floor window.
- Think about an escape plan if the fire starts in the kitchen, bedroom, or basement.

- Figure out the best way to get infants and young children out of the house. Will you carry them? If there is more than one child who needs to be carried, how will you get them out if you are the only adult?
- Teach preschool and school-age children to follow the escape plan by crawling, touching doors, and going to the window if the door is hot. Show children how to cover their nose and mouth to reduce smoke inhalation.
- Prepare an alternate fire escape plan in case you are alone with the child when the fire begins.
- Keep home exits clear of toys and debris.
- Select a safe meeting place outside the home. Teach children not to go back inside the burning home.

SPECIAL CONCERNS IN COMMUNITY-BASED HEALTH CARE

Complementary and Alternative Medicine

An estimated 20% of families with healthy children use complementary and alternative therapies for their children. In many cases, healthcare providers are not aware of their use (Costello, 2005). Up to 50% of children with chronic conditions are treated with complementary and alternative therapies (Cohen, Kemper, Stevens et al., 2005). Complementary and alternative medicine (CAM) is defined as a group of diverse medical and healthcare systems, practices, and products that are not presently considered to be part of conventional medicine [(National Center for Complementary and Alternative Medicine (NCCAM), 2002b)].

Complementary and alternative medicine use among specific cultural groups has been in practice for thousands of years. The use of CAM therapies in the United States is widespread and is observed in some manner within all cultures.

The terms *complementary* and *alternative* therapies are often used interchangeably, but they have different meanings and applications.

- **Complementary therapy** is a product or treatment used together with conventional medicine. The use of massage therapy in conjunction with a pain medication for a child with a painful condition is a complementary therapy.
- **Alternative therapy** is a product or treatment used in place of conventional medicine. The use of herbal medicines instead of chemotherapy, radiation, and prescribed medications for the treatment of a child's cancer is an alternative therapy.

The NCCAM (2002b) classifies complementary and alternative medicine therapies into five categories, or domains: alternative medical systems, mind-body interventions, biologically based therapies, manipulative and body-based methods, and energy therapies.

- Alternative medical systems are built upon complete systems of theory and practice that evolved separately from conventional medicine in the United States, such as naturopathic, homeopathic, and chiropractic medicine.
- Mind-body interventions use a variety of techniques designed to enhance the mind's capacity to affect body function and symptoms, such as hypnotherapy, biofeedback, prayer, and cognitive-behavioral therapy.
- Biologically based therapies use substances found in nature, such as herbs, foods, and vitamins.
- Manipulative and body-based methods are based on manipulation and/or movement of one or more body parts, such as chiropractic and osteopathic medicine, acupressure, acupuncture, and Tai Chi.
- Energy therapies involve the use of energy fields to surround and penetrate the body, such as Reiki, therapeutic touch, and light therapy.

Descriptions of some common types of complementary and alternative therapies are provided in Table 11–1.

Safety Issues Concerning CAM Therapies

The standards of products, misleading claims of usefulness, safety related to large doses of some products, and standardization of natural products are just a few of the issues raised with the use of herbs and natural products. The same principles and standards of evidence of treatment effectiveness should apply to all treatments, both conventional medicine and complementary and alternative therapies (Ernst, 2006). Parents often believe that herbs and natural products are less likely to be harmful than prescribed medications and do not recognize that safety concerns exist. Examples of problems that may occur with the use of these products include:

- Interaction with the prescribed medications (interferes with metabolism of medication or increases the effect of the prescribed medication, like an overdose)

COMPLEMENTARY THERAPY

Echinacea

Echinacea is one of the most commonly used herbs in the United States and is often used in the treatment of colds. A recent study evaluating the use of Echinacea *(Echinacea purpurea)* for the treatment of colds in children did not find the herb effective. The study comprised of 534 children, ages 2 to 11 years, found that the use of Echinacea did not lessen the number of days the cold lasted or the severity of the symptoms (Taylor, Weber, & Standish, 2003).

Table 11–1	**COMMON TYPES OF COMPLEMENTARY AND ALTERNATIVE MEDICINES**		
Therapy	**Description**	**Potential Use in Children**	**Nursing Implications**
Aromatherapy	Essential oils (extracts or essences) from flowers, herbs, and trees are used to promote health and well-being.	The family may use candles or oils to promote a child's pain relief or to encourage the child's relaxation. Use of aromatherapy in the hospital may reduce nausea due to hospital odors.	Use of aromatherapies for disorders such as asthma and other pulmonary disorders can actually worsen the child's symptoms. Caution these families to avoid aromatherapy.
Dietary supplements	A product (other than tobacco) is taken by mouth that contains an ingredient intended to supplement the diet, such as vitamins, minerals, herbs or other botanicals, amino acids, and substances such as enzymes, organ tissues, and metabolites. Dietary supplements come in many forms, including extracts, concentrates, tablets, capsules, gelcaps, liquids, and powders. They have special requirements for labeling.	Many parents administer daily multiple vitamins to their child. Other therapies used for children include the use of Echinacea for colds.	Assess family's use of dietary supplements for the child. Determine potential interactions between supplements and prescribed medications. Teach parents about safe dosages and safe storage of vitamins for children.
Massage	Therapists manipulate muscle and connective tissue to enhance function of those tissues and promote relaxation, well-being, and relief of pain.	Families may seek massage therapy for children with musculoskeletal disorders or other chronic diseases.	Assess child for benefits of massage. Determine any potential contraindication to massage therapy, such as a fracture.
Therapeutic touch	In therapeutic touch the healing force of the therapist affects the patient's recovery. Healing is promoted when the body's energies are in balance. By passing their hands over the patient, without touching the patient, healers can identify energy imbalances.	The family may enlist a spiritualist or other practitioner to perform therapeutic touch on their child to promote pain relief or a quicker recovery.	Assess the benefits of therapeutic touch on the child (e.g., pain relief). Partner with family to establish other methods of pain relief if therapeutic touch is not effective.
Faith-based therapies	Faith-based practices such as prayer are the most prevalent complementary and alternative therapies in the United States (Barnes, Plotnikoff, Fox, & Pendleton, 2000). Faith-based therapies include faith healing, laying on hands, anointing, prayer, exorcism, pilgrimage, and visits to the sick.	Families may include a variety of faith-based therapies depending on the child's condition.	Provide the child and family a private environment for faith-based ritual practices. Assess for benefits of the therapies. Partner with family to determine alternative methods of therapy if needed.

Data from: National Center for Complementary and Alternative Medicine. (2002b). What is complementary and alternative medicine (CAM)? NCCAM Publication No. D156. Retrieved March 17, 2006, from http://www.nccam.nih.gov, health/whatis.com

- Side effect or allergic reaction directly associated with the product
- Substitution of the product for a prescribed medication that is potentially lifesaving
- Toxic effects occur because of contaminants or other additives in the product, or if the plant used for the herb was incorrectly identified

Not all complementary and alternative therapies should be discouraged. In many cases they should be encouraged and used with traditional medical therapies. The following complementary and alternative therapies have demonstrated effectiveness (Ernst, 2006):

- Acupuncture for nausea and vomiting
- Biofeedback or massage for constipation (Figure 11–7▶)
- Biofeedback or hypnotherapy for headache
- Hypnotherapy for irritable bowel syndrome

Other complementary and alternative therapies are used effectively for relaxation and pain management, such as guided imagery, deep breathing exercises, and meditation.

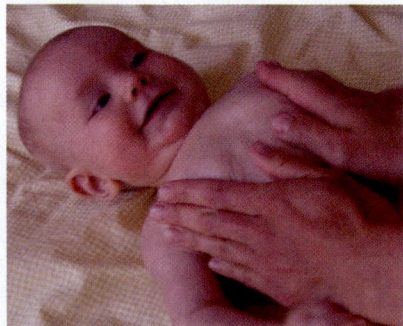

Figure 11–7 ▶ Infant massage is a complementary therapy that promotes relaxation in the infant as well as in the parent performing the massage.

Complementary and alternative medicine practices must be assessed for safety, including positive and negative benefits, cost, efficacy, and clinical usefulness. To date, limited research has been conducted on the safety and effectiveness of complementary and alternative therapies for children. Parents often do not share information about the use of these products because they fear the healthcare provider's disapproval or skepticism. Nurses and other healthcare providers should be respectful of the family's desire to use these therapies, but at the same time be responsible for learning more about them and their effectiveness so that appropriate education and guidance can be provided.

Nursing Management

Use some screening questions to help identify a family's use of complementary and alternative therapies. Ask questions in a nonjudgmental manner to encourage the parent to share the information. Examples of questions to use can be found in the Complementary Therapy box. Also, determine the side effects, risks, and other implications to the child receiving this type of therapy, such as interactions between the herb or other natural product and either foods or prescribed medications.

Partner with the family to promote safe practices with the use of complementary and/or alternative medicines. Educate parents on these important points:

- Little research has been conducted to determine the effectiveness of many therapies.
- Just like prescribed medications, herbs and other natural products may cause a side effect or allergic response.
- In some cases the herb or natural product may be contaminated by heavy metals, drugs, and pesticides that could cause harm.
- Homeopathic products meet important safety guidelines for dosage and preparation standards.
- Encourage parents to share information about complementary and alternative therapies used with the healthcare provider.

See Families Want to Know: Using the Internet to Evaluate Complementary and Alternative Therapies below to assist with further education of parents.

Emergency Medical Services for Children

The emergency medical services (EMS) system is the organized community-based public health response to assure that adults and children with acute illnesses and injuries

CLINICAL TIP

Homeopathic medications are prepared using standardized methods described in the Homeopathic Pharmacopeia of the United States. Standards for the preparation of medications are established within the Food and Drug Administration to ensure that products are of high quality and uncontaminated (Kemper & Jacobs, 2003).

COMPLEMENTARY THERAPY

Screening Questions to Identify a Family's Use of Complementary and Alternative Therapy

- Are you doing anything special to keep your child healthy or to manage a health problem?
- What types of home remedies are used?
- Do you give your child any herb or plant preparations?
- Do you use any homeopathic preparations for your child?
- Do you use any special vitamin therapy for your child?
- Do you use any unconventional or alternative types of care or therapies for your child? What are the benefits to the child when these are used?

Adapted from: Loman, D. G. (2003). The use of complementary and alternative health care practices among children. *Journal of Pediatric Health Care, 17*(2), 58–63.

FAMILIES WANT TO KNOW

Using the Internet to Evaluate Complementary and Alternative Therapies

There are millions of web sites promoting complementary and alternative therapies that are often dangerously misleading. Provide families with guidelines for evaluating complementary and alternative therapies and other medical information on the Internet. Encourage families to use the following questions when looking for health information online to help evaluate the information found.

- Who runs this site?
- Who pays for the site? The source of funding can affect what content is presented and how.
- What is the purpose of the site? The purpose should be clearly stated to help you evaluate how much to trust the information.
- Where does the information come from? The original source of the information should be clearly stated if the organization in charge of the site did not create the information.

- How is the information selected? Determine if evidence is provided about the information rather than just opinions and advice.
- How current is the information? Look for the latest update of information.
- How does the site choose links to other sites? Determine if any criteria are used for decisions about who can link to the site.
- What information about you does the site collect, and why? Does the site ask you to subscribe or become a member? If so, personal information will be collected. Review any privacy policy or similar language before signing up for the site.
- How does the site manage interactions with visitors? Is there a chat room or other online discussion? Review the discussion carefully before joining in.

Data from: NCCAM (2002a). 10 things to know about evaluating medical resources on the Web. NCCAM Publication No. D142. Retrieved March 17, 2006, from www.nccam.nih.gov/health/webresources/.

receive emergency care and timely transport to the hospital emergency department. The EMS system at the local community level is composed of ambulance units and trained emergency medical personnel who respond to emergencies. In some communities, this EMS system is part of the fire department and in others it is a separate organization. Each local EMS service has a medical director who establishes the protocols used by emergency medical personnel when caring for ill and injured individuals. The public accesses the EMS system by placing a call to 9-1-1 or their local emergency phone number. A dispatcher then directs the ambulance unit to respond, takes information, and provides data to the caller about how to manage the ill or injured person until the emergency personnel arrive. State EMS offices set the guidelines for training and certification of emergency medical personnel, equipment to be carried on ambulances, data collection of care provided, and communication systems used. In addition, the State EMS office works closely with hospital emergency departments and trauma centers to coordinate emergency care of patients transported by the EMS system. Federal legislation was enacted in 1984 to assure that children's special needs were integrated into the overall EMS system.

Important Pediatric Physiologic Differences

Children have different physiologic responses to emergencies because of their smaller anatomy and developing organ systems. Small children cannot communicate and describe their health problems, and they are dependent upon family members for security and recognition of the emergency. Due to differences in anatomy, pediatric-sized equipment and supplies are essential. EMS providers need education to assess the child and recognize the signs that the child's condition is a true emergency, and then to provide the appropriate medical intervention before and during transport to the hospital.

Hospitals are part of the EMS system and their emergency departments must be prepared to treat children as well as adults. Emergency departments need to have appropriately sized resuscitation equipment for children of all ages and well-trained emergency department physicians and nurses. Educational programs like Pediatric Advanced Life Support provide opportunities for nurses and physicians to work together effectively to resuscitate a child who is critically ill or injured. In addition, clinical guidelines for a well-orchestrated response to serious trauma and medical emergencies are developed and rehearsed. Urgent care centers and smaller emergency departments need to have agreements with major medical centers to assure that children with life-threatening injuries or illnesses can be transferred and transported to receive a more advanced level of care.

Nurses sometimes work as volunteer EMS providers in their community. Nurses also work as interfacility transport team members, providing care to critically ill children who need to be transferred by ground or air ambulance from a community hospital to a hospital with more advanced care. See Figure 11–8▶ to see the interconnection between the EMS system and hospitals for provision of emergency services.

Disaster Preparedness

Many types of disasters occur each year in the United States. Natural disasters include floods, ice storms, hurricanes, earthquakes, tornados, and fires. Other types of disasters can occur when trains or trucks carrying toxic chemicals and nuclear waste crash or explode. Concerns of terrorism with infectious organisms, toxic chemicals, or radioactive agents have elevated the need for disaster and emergency preparedness. (See Chapter 18 ∞ for information about infectious agents used for bioterrorism.) State agencies, hospitals, and emergency medical services systems are developing community **disaster preparedness** plans for mass casualty events involving both natural and man-made disasters. Efforts to assure appropriate planning and availability of resources during disasters in all communities, including those for children, is ongoing through the funding and coordination of several federal agencies.

Children have special vulnerabilities during a disaster. They have unique psychological vulnerabilities and need special plans for management. (See Chapter 6 ∞ for a discussion of the impact of other disasters on the mental health of children.) The child's size and physiology also leads to special considerations when exposed to chemical, radiological, or biological agents by terrorism (Figure 11–9▶).

MediaLink

EMS for Children Video

GROWTH & DEVELOPMENT

Disaster Planning

Special developmental considerations that must be considered during disaster planning for young children include the following:

- They are unable to flee or take evasive action to escape danger.
- Caregivers or parents may become incapacitated and childcare with mental health support will be needed.
- They are unable to follow the instructions given to adults regarding evacuation or safe actions.
- They cannot distinguish between reality and fantasy.
- Young children may fear emergency responders in protective suits and hoods.

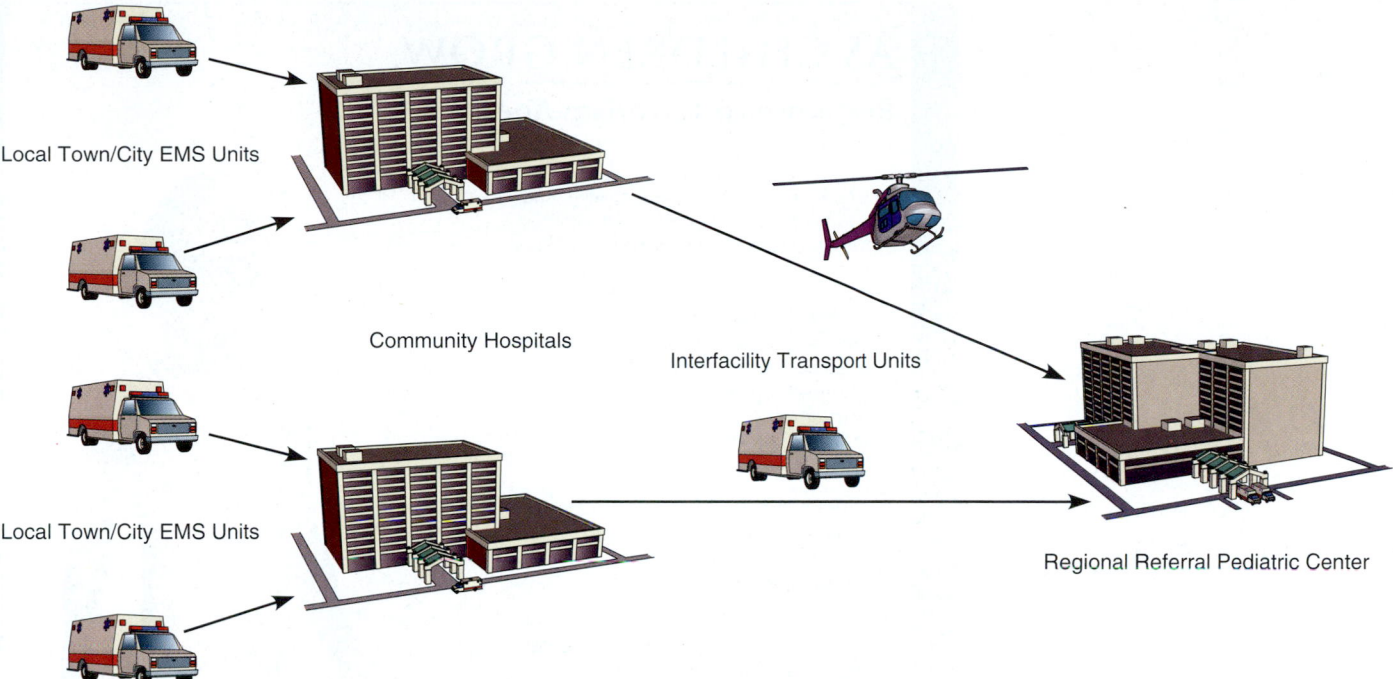

Local Town/City EMS Units

Community Hospitals

Interfacility Transport Units

Local Town/City EMS Units

Regional Referral Pediatric Center

Figure 11–8 ➤ The emergency medical services system is a carefully linked set of resources in the community and region that enables children with serious illnesses and injuries to get the care needed in the most appropriate hospital. The continuum of emergency care includes the child's caregiver at the scene, the communications center taking the call for help, the EMS personnel responding to the scene who provide immediate emergency care and transport the child to the emergency department, and the hospital emergency department. If the child is transported to a community emergency department, but needs more complex care, transfer to a larger hospital or trauma center is then coordinated. A team of specially trained pediatric emergency care providers often manages transfer in an ambulance, helicopter, or small plane. The goal is to get the child to the medical and specialty care resources needed to have the best chance of survival and optimal functional outcome.

Many disasters will cause injuries due to flying debris or building collapse. Health services are needed to treat injuries and potential illnesses caused by contaminated water or other exposures. Terrorist events often involve major injuries due to blast injuries. Clinical manifestations of various chemical and nerve agent exposures are listed in the box on page 377. Clinical manifestations and clinical therapy for infectious agents can be found in Chapter 18 ∞.

The initial response to the scene of a disaster is to get the victims to fresh air and to perform triage to classify all individuals by severity of injury. Responders initiate emergency care and coordinate transport to facilities that can provide needed care. Clinical therapy is focused on determining the type of exposure and providing immediate care to reduce the agent's effects.

Decontamination, the removal of chemicals and nerve agents from the skin, should be performed as soon as possible. Clothing is removed and the child is washed with soap and water. Eye irrigation may be needed to reduce pain and eye damage. Decontamination not only reduces the child's exposure to the toxin, but it helps protect medical personnel who will provide care to the child.

Antidotes such as atropine or pralidoxime may need to be administered for nerve agents. Potassium iodide may be administered for some radiation exposures. Emergency care may involve securing the airway with an endotracheal tube, and providing supplemental oxygen and mechanical ventilation if needed. Treat children with skin exposure to chemicals and blistering agents as if burned. Other therapies are implemented to treat the specific pathophysiology caused by the toxin.

Role of the Nurse in Disaster Preparedness

Pediatric nurses in schools and other community settings play a significant role in preparing families for a disaster. They can help families use developmentally appropriate information to talk with their children about disaster planning and convey

GROWTH & DEVELOPMENT

Decontamination

Decontamination is a challenge with small children. The shower system must use warm water to prevent hypothermia in the child, and water pressure should be low but have high volume. The shower system must be able to accommodate an adult who may be required to hold an infant or young child (Redlener & Markenson, 2003).

Care for children during a disaster in which health professionals must wear personal protective equipment may also be challenging as children may be especially fearful of these strangers. The cumbersome gloves and clothing may make it more difficult to perform essential procedures (Markenson, Reynolds, and American Academy of Pediatrics Committee on Pediatric Emergency Medicine, 2006).

 MediaLink

Disaster Preparedness Resources and Video

AS CHILDREN GROW

Response to Terrorism Agents

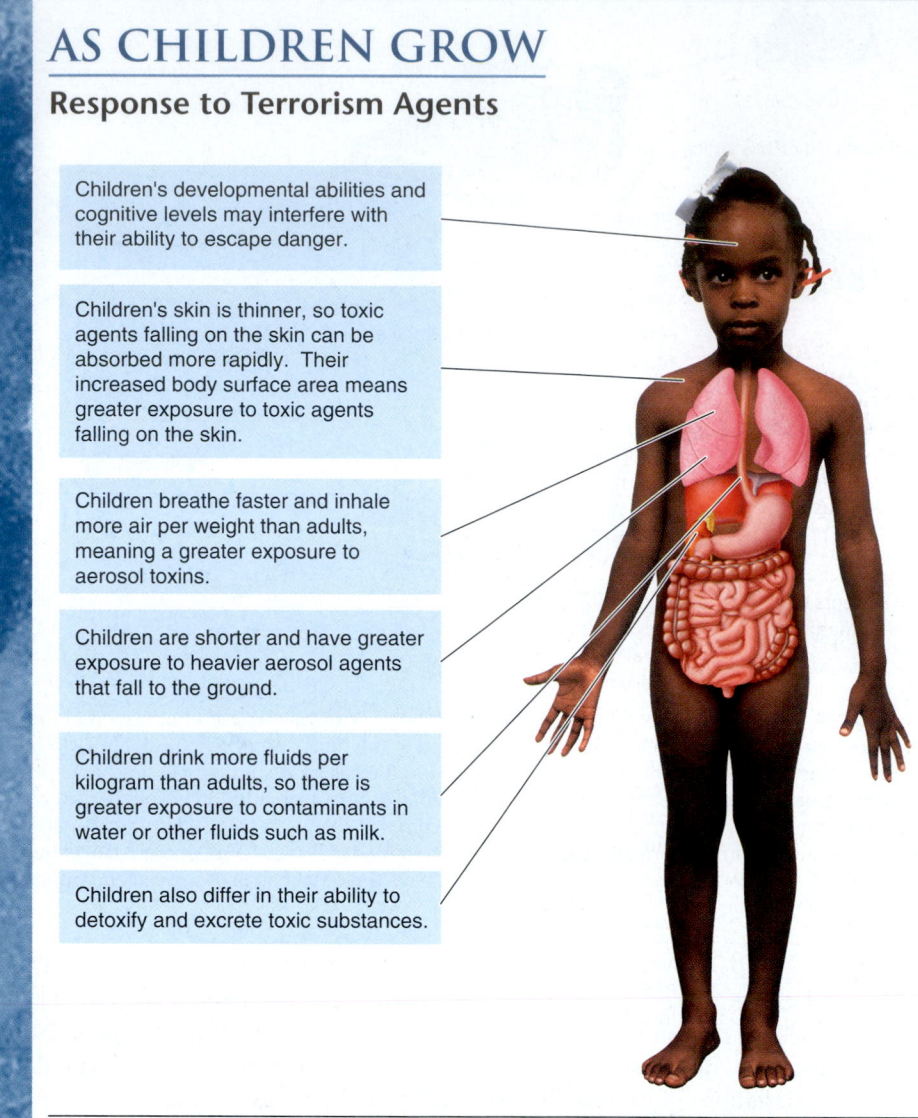

Children's developmental abilities and cognitive levels may interfere with their ability to escape danger.

Children's skin is thinner, so toxic agents falling on the skin can be absorbed more rapidly. Their increased body surface area means greater exposure to toxic agents falling on the skin.

Children breathe faster and inhale more air per weight than adults, meaning a greater exposure to aerosol toxins.

Children are shorter and have greater exposure to heavier aerosol agents that fall to the ground.

Children drink more fluids per kilogram than adults, so there is greater exposure to contaminants in water or other fluids such as milk.

Children also differ in their ability to detoxify and excrete toxic substances.

Figure 11–9 ➤ Children have different physiologic and cognitive vulnerabilities than adults in response to various terrorism agents (Cieslak & Henretig, 2003).

CLINICAL TIP

Because family members are separated many hours a day, an out-of-state family contact should be identified for a rescuer to call and report the child's location and safety. Telephone communication outages in the disaster area may limit the communication between family members. Family members should choose two meeting locations, one at home, and the other outside the neighborhood. All children and family members should memorize the family contact phone number and alternate meeting location address (Florida Institute for Family Involvement, 2006).

information about disasters when they occur. Children need to know what to do in case of a disaster, terrorist event, or other emergency, including who should be approached for help, and what actions to take when at home, at school, or elsewhere in the community (American Academy of Pediatrics, 2006).

Nurses can also help the family develop a disaster plan that anticipates complete disruption of services for several days. Families need to follow guidelines for evacuation when community orders are given. Parents should carry phone numbers of out-of-town contacts, schools, and neighbors at all times. Having a list of medications, clothing, food, water, and other essentials that can be used to quickly pack and respond to the evacuation order is important. Families must be prepared to manage on their own for at least 72 hours following a major disaster (unless the child needs special technology for life support) because it will take at least this long for nationally coordinated help and relief to arrive. See Table 11–2 for a list of emergency supplies to have on hand. A plan for family pets should be made as many shelters will not permit pets to enter.

Additional planning is important when a family has a child with a chronic health condition or is technology assisted (Markenson, Reynolds, & American Academy of Pediatrics Committee on Pediatric Emergency Medicine, 2006).

CLINICAL MANIFESTATIONS | CHEMICAL AND NERVE GAS EXPOSURE

Type of Exposure, Potential Agents	Potential Clinical Manifestation	Clinical Therapy
Chemical inhalation exposure (chlorine, bromine, ammonia, phosgene)	Airway irritation, edema, and obstruction Increased secretions Sensation of choking or suffocation Hoarseness, coughing Bronchospasm, stridor Pulmonary edema Acute respiratory distress syndrome Asphyxia	Get child to fresh air Secure the airway with an endotracheal tube Provide supplemental oxygen Provide assisted ventilation if needed Symptomatic care
Chemical skin and eye exposure (cryogenic liquids, acids, alkalis, corrosives, mustard gas, nitrogen mustard)	Cold injury to skin Chemical burns Erythema, blistering Eye inflammation, pain, blindness Systemic toxicity possible (respiratory distress, bradycardia or tachycardia)	Remove clothing and wash skin with soap and water Airway protection Eye irrigation Treat burns and blisters Fluid resuscitation Analgesia Provide other therapies related to type of exposure
Nerve agents (Tabun, Sarin, Soman, VX)	Cholinergic effects include: Eyes (tearing, pupillary constriction, red conjunctiva, eye pain, dim vision) Headache Respiratory (dyspnea, chest tightness, bronchoconstriction, profuse secretions, respiratory muscle fatigue) Central nervous system (loss of consciousness, seizures, respiratory center depression, apnea, paralysis) Muscle fasciculation, twitching, muscle fatigue Urination Vomiting, diarrhea Sweating	Remove clothing and wash skin and hair with soap and water Antidotes such as atropine or pralidoximine Secure the airway with an endotracheal tube Provide supplemental oxygen Provide assisted ventilation if needed Hydration Seizure control Analgesia
Radiation	May be few signs and symptoms initially Radiation sickness Injuries from a blast	Removal of clothing Potassium iodide Assessment of airway, breathing, and circulation if a blast injury Trauma care for injuries

Data from: Lynch, E. L., & Thomas, T. L. (2004). Pediatric considerations in chemical exposures. *Pediatric Emergency Care, 20*(3), 198–205; Lynch, M. (2005). Atropine use in children after nerve gas exposure. *Journal of Pediatric Nursing, 20*(6), 477–484; Markenson, D., Reynolds, S., & American Academy of Pediatrics Committee on Pediatric Emergency Medicine and Task Force on Terrorism. (2006). The pediatrician and disaster preparedness; *Pediatrics, 117*(2), e340–e362. Redlener, I., & Markenson, D. (2003). Disaster and terrorism preparedness: What pediatricians need to know. *Advances in Pediatrics, 50*, 1–37.

- The utility company needs advance notification when a child is technology assisted to provide emergency power. A contingency plan should be developed by the family when it is anticipated that the power cannot be rapidly restored, such as going to a special shelter that will receive priority service by the utility company.
- An adequate supply of medications, equipment, and supplies should be maintained. Resources to obtain a refill of medication and needed supplies during a disaster should be identified.
- Multiple family members should be trained to provide the needed care for the child as home healthcare providers will not be available.
- Current medical information (emergency medical information forms) should be maintained in case the child's regular healthcare provider is not available.

Many nurses in the affected region, as well as volunteers from other regions, will be actively involved in caring for children injured during the disaster both in the hospital and disaster shelter settings. Physician offices and health centers may become additional sites of care when hospitals become overwhelmed. Nurses can also help after the disaster by assessing children for distress, post-traumatic stress disorder, and promoting security and stability (Ferguson, 2002).

CLINICAL TIP

Resources needed for infants and children in disaster shelters include: diapers, baby wipes, formula, baby food, and oral hydrating fluids. Toys and games are also valuable to provide recreation for older children who may be staying in a shelter for several days. If an emergency and evacuation continues for more than a couple of days, nurses may be effective in planning developmentally appropriate activities for children in shelters. They can plan for and obtain supplies and volunteers to facilitate drawing activities, games, and give parents a respite.

Table 11–2	**RESOURCES FOR SURVIVING A DISASTER FOR 72 HOURS**
Items Needed	**For Sheltering in Place or Evacuation**
Water	One gallon of water per person per day, enough for 3 days. Have extra water for pets.
Food	Three-day supply of foods that do not need refrigeration or cooking (e.g., canned meat, fruits, vegetables, canned or boxed juice, and high-energy foods like raisins, peanut butter, and granola bars). Baby formula and food for infants. Special dietary foods needed by a family member.
First aid kit	One for the home and one for the car.
Nonprescription drugs	Pain reliever, antacid, anti-diarrhea medication, laxative, anti-itch cream.
Prescription medications	Medications should be carried in a purse or hand luggage to keep it accessible.
Tools and supplies	Flashlight and batteries, battery operated radio, paper plates and utensils, needles and thread, whistle, tape, matches in waterproof container, plastic storage containers, manual can opener, and so on.
Sanitary supplies	Soap, waterless alcohol-based cleanser, toilet paper, hygiene products, diapers, baby wipes, plastic garbage bags, disinfectant, household chlorine bleach.
Clothing and bedding	Rain gear, sturdy shoes, warm clothes, hat and gloves, sunglasses, complete change of clothes per person, blankets, sleeping bags.
Family documents	Immunizations, health records, photo of children and other family members (to assist with reunification), passports, will, insurance policies, contracts and deeds, bank account numbers, credit card account numbers, phone book with important numbers, cash, traveler's checks. All should be in a waterproof, portable container.
Special items	Games and books for entertainment.

Data from: Federal Emergency Management Agency. (2000). Are you ready? Retrieved July 5, 2005, from http://www.fema.gov/areyouready/appendix_b.shtm

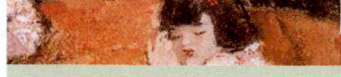

CRITICAL THINKING IN ACTION

Recall 4-month-old Kendra and her parents from the opening scenario, who came to the health center for Kendra's immunizations and health assessment. Kendra's growth and development are occurring as anticipated. Her mother is using a complementary therapy that seems to benefit both Kendra and her mother. Hurricane season is beginning and the family lives in a town near the coast of the Gulf of Mexico.

1. Describe the nursing interventions that should be provided at the time of this visit to Kendra and her family in the health center serving as Kendra's medical home.

2. What is the preparation the health center should have in case Kendra has a serious allergic reaction to a given vaccine?

3. List the key points of discussion to have with Kendra's parents about the use of complementary and alternative therapies in children.

4. List the supplies and resources that Kendra's parents should have on hand to be prepared for a natural disaster.

 Refer to your Prentice Hall Nursing MediaLink DVD-ROM for answers.

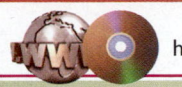

EXPLORE MediaLink   http://www.prenhall.com/ball

Resources for this chapter can be found on the Prentice Hall Nursing MediaLink DVD-ROM accompanying this textbook, and on the Companion Website at http://www.prenhall.com/ball.

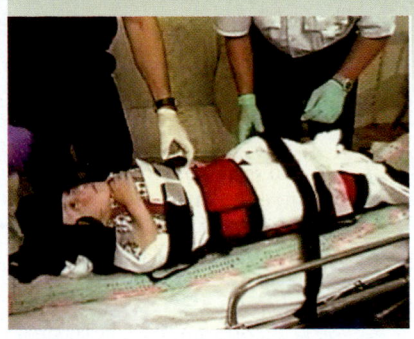

DVD-ROM
Audio Glossary
NCLEX-RN® Review
Videos
  Complementary and Alternative Modalities
  Disaster Preparedness
  EMS for Children

COMPANION WEBSITE
Audio Glossary
NCLEX-RN® Review
Care Plan Activity: School-aged Child with Brain Injury
Critical Thinking
MediaLink Applications
WebLinks

REFERENCES

Alkon, A., Farrer, J., & Bernzweig, J. (2004). Child care health consultants' roles and responsibilities: Focus group findings. *Pediatric Nursing, 30*(4), 315–321.

American Academy of Pediatrics. (2002). The medical home. *Pediatrics, 110*(1), 184–186.

American Academy of Pediatrics. (2006). The pediatrician and disaster preparedness. *Pediatrics, 117*(2), 560–564.

American Academy of Pediatrics Committee on Pediatric Emergency Medicine, Seidel, J. S., & Knapp, J. F. (Eds.) (2000). *Childhood emergencies in the office, hospital, and community: Organizing systems of care.* Elk Grove Village, IL: American Academy of Pediatrics.

Barnes, L. L., Plotnikoff, G. A., Fox, K., & Pendleton, S. (2000). Spirituality, religion, and pediatrics: Interesecting worlds of healing. *Pediatrics, 106*, 899–908.

Carnevale, F. A., Alexander, E., Davis, M., Rennick, J., & Troini, R. (2006). Daily living with distress and enrichment: The moral experience of families with ventilator-assisted children at home. *Pediatrics, 17*(1), e48–e60.

Centers for Disease Control National Center for Chronic Disease Prevention and Health Promotion. (2005). Healthy youth! Welcome to the School Health Index (SHI). Accessed July 11, 2005 from http://apps.nccd.cdc.gov/shi

Cieslak, T. J., & Henretig, F. M. (2003). Ring-a-ring-a-roses: Bioterrorism and its peculiar relevance to pediatrics. *Current Opinion in Pediatrics, 19*, 107–111.

Cohen, M. H., Kemper, K. J., Stevens, L., Hashimoto, D., & Gilmour, J. (2005). Pediatric use of complementary therapies: Ethical and policy choices. *Pediatrics, 116*(4), e568–e575.

Costello, E. (2005). Complementary and alternative therapies: Considerations for families after international adoption. *Pediatric Clinics of North America, 52*, 1463–1478.

Ernst, E. (2006). Complementary and alternative medicine for children: A good or a bad thing? *Archives of Diseases in Childhood, 91*(2), 96–97.

Evers, D. B. (2002). The pediatric nurse's role as health consultant to a child care center. *Pediatric Nursing, 22*(3), 231–235.

Federal Emergency Management Agency. (2000). Are you ready? Retrieved July 5, 2005, from http://www.fema.gov/areyouready/appendix_b.shtm

Ferguson, S. L. (2002). Preparing for disasters: Enhancing the role of pediatric nurses in wartime. *Journal of Pediatric Nurses, 17*(4), 307–308.

Florida Institute for Family Involvement. (2006). Disaster preparedness for families of children with special needs. Retrieved March 17, 2006, from http://www.fifionline/images/PDF%20Files/Disaster%20Planning%20for%20CYSHCN.pdf

Gustafson, E. M. (2005). History and overview of school-based health centers in the US. *Nursing Clinics of North America, 40*, 595–606.

Kemper, K. J., & Jacobs, J. (2003). Homeopathy in pediatrics—no harm likely, but how much good? *Contemporary Pediatrics, 20*(5), 97–111.

Loman, D. G. (2003). The use of complementary and alternative health care practices among children. *Journal of Pediatric Health Care, 17*(2), 58–63.

Lynch, E. L., & Thomas, T. L. (2004). Pediatric considerations in chemical exposures. *Pediatric Emergency Care, 20*(3), 198–205.

Lynch, M. (2005). Atropine use in children after nerve gas exposure. *Journal of Pediatric Nursing, 20*(6), 477–484.

Margolan, H., Fraser, J., & Lenton, S. (2004). Parental experiences of services when their child requires long-term ventilation. Implications for commissioning and providing services. *Child Care, Health & Development, 30*(3), 257–264.

Markenson, D., Reynolds, S., American Academy of Pediatrics Committee on Pediatric Emergency Medicine and Task Force on Terrorism. (2006). The pediatrician and disaster preparedness. *Pediatrics, 117*(2), e340–e362.

National Association for Home Care and Hospice. (2004). Basic statistics about home care. Accessed March 7, 2006, from http://www.nahc.org

National Association of School Nurses and American Nurses Association. (2005). *School nursing: Scope and standards of practice.* Silver Spring, MD: American Nurses Publishing.

National Center for Complementary and Alternative Medicine (NCCAM). (2002a). 10 things to know about evaluating medical

resources on the Web. NCCAM Publication No. D142. Retrieved March 17, 2006, from http://www.nccam.nih.gov/health/webresources/

National Center for Complementary and Alternative Medicine (NCCAM). (2002b). What is complementary and alternative medicine (CAM)? NCCAM Publication No. D156. Retrieved March 17, 2006, from http://www.nccam.nih.gov/health/whatiscam/

Olympia, R. P., Wan, E., & Avner, J. R. (2005). The preparedness of schools to respond to emergencies in children: A national survey of school nurses. *Pediatrics, 116*(6), e738–e745.

Parra, M. M. (2003, May). Nursing and respite care services for ventilator-assisted children. *Caring, 22*, 6–9.

Ralston, M. E. (2005). Managing emergencies part 1. *Pediatric Annals, 34*(11), 845–849.

Redlener, I., & Markenson, D. (2003). Disaster and terrorism preparedness: What pediatricians need to know. *Advances in Pediatrics, 50*, 1–37.

Robinson, J. (2002). The changing role of the school nurse: A partner in infection control and disease prevention. *Journal of School Nursing, 18* (Supplement, October), 12–14.

Selekman, J., & Guilday, P. (2003). Identification of desired outcomes for school nursing practice. *Journal of School Nursing, 19*(6), 344–350.

Taylor, J. A., Weber, W., & Standish, L. (2003). Efficacy and safety of Echinacea in treating upper respiratory tract infections in children. *Journal of the American Medical Association, 290*, 2824–2830.

U.S. Department of Health and Human Services. (2000). *Healthy People 2010* (2nd ed.). Washington, DC: U.S. Government Printing Office. http://www.healthypeople.gov

Waibel, R., & Misra, R. (2003). Injuries to preschool children and infection control practices in childcare programs. *Journal of School Health, 73*(4), 167–172.

Youngblade, L. M., & Carter, C. (2004). Counseling parents on infant day care: How to do it effectively. *Contemporary Pediatrics, 21*(8), 54–72.

Zimmerman, B. (2005, November). What do all these have in common? Linking the Coordinated School Health Program, School Health Council, and the Child Nutrition and WIC Reauthorization Act of 2004—PL 108-265. *NASN Newsletter*, 22–24.

12 NURSING CONSIDERATIONS FOR THE CHILD WITH A CHRONIC CONDITION

KEY TERMS

accommodations
    392
caregiver
    burden **386**
case manager **383**
children with
    special
    healthcare needs
    (CSHCN) **382**
chronic
    condition **381**
chronic sorrow **384**
compassion
    fatigue **389**
developmental
    delay **389**
disability **381**
early
    intervention **391**

handicap **381**
Individualized
    Education Plan
    (IEP) **392**
Individualized
    Family Service
    Plan (IFSP) **392**
Individualized
    Health Plan
    (IHP) **392**
Individualized
    Transition Plan
    (ITP) **392**
normalization **389**
respite care **400**
technology-assisted
    381

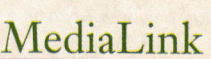 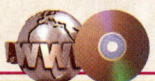

MediaLink

http://www.prenhall.com/ball

See the Prentice Hall Nursing MediaLink DVD-ROM and Companion Website for chapter-specific resources.

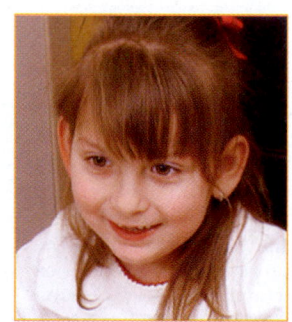

HALEY is an 8-year-old child with cerebral palsy. She had an intraventricular hemorrhage during her neonatal intensive care unit (NICU) hospitalization for very low birth weight. Haley lives with her mother and two older siblings, ages 10 and 13. Her parents divorced when Haley was 3 years old. She does have frequent contact with her father, who visits on weekends. Her father is supportive emotionally, physically, and financially for the care of Haley and her siblings.

Haley's mother is the full-time care provider. Routine care includes hygiene, supplemental enteral tube feedings to promote adequate nutrition in-between oral feedings, range-of-motion (ROM) exercises, and home schooling. Haley uses her motorized wheelchair without any difficulty, and her mother has decided that she would benefit from social interaction and a structured educational environment at the local public school. Her family asks the nurse and case manager at the cerebral palsy clinic for assistance in planning Haley's entry into school.

How can the clinic nurse and case manager assist Haley and her family in this transition? What special arrangements are needed to permit a child to receive care for a chronic condition while at school? What measures can be taken to ensure an effective transition between home and school?

LEARNING OUTCOMES

After reading this chapter, you will be able to do the following:

1. Discuss the various categories of chronic conditions and their etiology.
2. Define the categories of impairment in a child with a chronic condition.
3. Discuss the impact of a child's chronic condition on the family.
4. List the skills and knowledge needed by the nurse to effectively care for the child with a chronic condition in the community.
5. Assess the child with a chronic condition and identify specific nursing interventions for the child at different ages.
6. Discuss the family's role in care coordination.
7. Describe family-centered nursing interventions to assist the family of the child with a chronic condition to effectively care for the child in the home.
8. Describe nursing interventions to support the child with a chronic condition's transition to school and adult living.

THE CHILD WITH A CHRONIC CONDITION

Children with a **chronic condition,** a condition that at the time of diagnosis is expected to last 3 months or more, receive most of their health care in the community. Chronic conditions vary in etiology, manifestations, and their effect on children's physical, psychosocial, and cognitive development. Chronic conditions develop from multiple causes.

- Genetic conditions may result in the child's chronic condition. Examples include muscular dystrophy, hemophilia, sickle cell disease, or cystic fibrosis.
- Conditions resulting from congenital defect or insult to the infant during fetal development may include a neural tube defect, fetal alcohol syndrome, cleft palate, or cerebral palsy.
- Insult or injury associated with birth and care following birth (e.g., sepsis, prematurity, intraventricular hemorrhage) that may lead to conditions such as bronchopulmonary dysplasia, attention deficit disorder, vision or hearing deficit.
- Conditions acquired through injury or acute medical condition such as brain injury, cancer, HIV infection, near drowning, or mental health problem.

This chapter addresses important concepts of care for children with chronic conditions who need more care coordination. Specific chronic conditions are discussed in detail in the chapters addressing body systems.

Technological advancements have improved the survival of children with conditions that were previously associated with high mortality rates, such as very low birth weight, complex cardiac defects, and serious brain injury. Very low-birth-weight infants that survive have increased long-term healthcare needs after experiencing respiratory or cardiovascular disorders, hypoxia, congenital infection, brain injury, prematurity, or intrauterine drug exposure, and they may spend weeks to months in the neonatal intensive care unit (NICU) in order to receive specialized care (Kessenich, 2003).

In most cases, chronic conditions become lifelong disorders. However, the impact on the affected child is variable according to the severity of the condition, the stage of growth and development when the condition occurs, and the child's and family's responses to the condition. While some conditions require intense monitoring and technological support for survival, other conditions cause few limitations and minimal effects on quality of life. See Figure 12–1 ➤ for examples of children with visible and nonvisible disabilities.

Characteristics of Chronic Conditions

Chronic conditions are often defined by diagnostic categories or by functional or social limitations. Examples of these categories include the following (Allen, 2004):

- Limitations in function that would typically be expected for the child's age and development
- Disfigurement
- Dependency on medications or a special diet for control of the condition
- Dependency on medical technology for functioning
- Need for more medical care and related services than typically used by a healthy child of the same age
- Special ongoing treatments at home or school

See Table 12–1 for examples of some chronic conditions by category.

Some children with chronic conditions have a **handicap** or **disability,** a limitation that interferes with their ability to fully participate in society. This can be related to one of the following (Msall, Avery, Tremont et al., 2003): medical impairment (chronic condition); functional limitation (mobility, self-care, communication, or learning-behavior impairment); and difficulty maintaining a social role in school or play.

Some children who are medically fragile are **technology-assisted,** depending on a medical device that is required to sustain life (mechanical ventilators, intravenous nutrition or drugs, tracheostomy, suctioning, oxygen, or nutritional support with tube feedings). Other children depend on medical devices that compensate for vital body

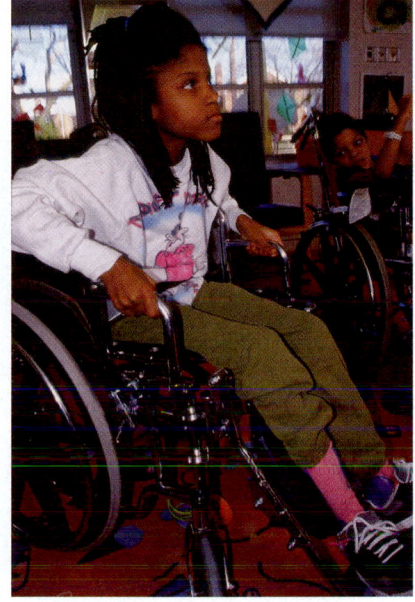

A

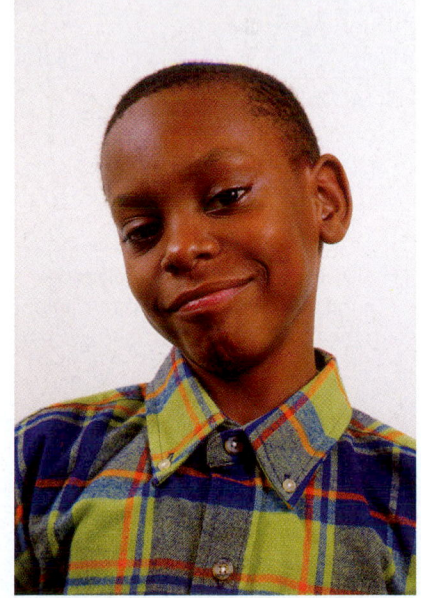

B

Figure 12–1 ➤ A, The child in a wheelchair has a visible disability. B, The child with a seizure may have no visible signs of the condition unless a seizure is witnessed.

Table 12–1	EXAMPLES OF CHRONIC CONDITIONS BY SPECIAL HEALTHCARE NEED CATEGORY
Special Healthcare Need Category	**Chronic Health Condition Examples**
Dependent on prescription medications or special diet	Diabetes mellitus, asthma, seizures, phenylketonuria, organ transplantation
Dependent on medical technology	Renal failure, bronchopulmonary dysplasia
Increased use of healthcare services	Cancer, sickle cell disease, cystic fibrosis
Functional limitations	Down syndrome, brain injury, autism, myelodysplasia, cerebral palsy

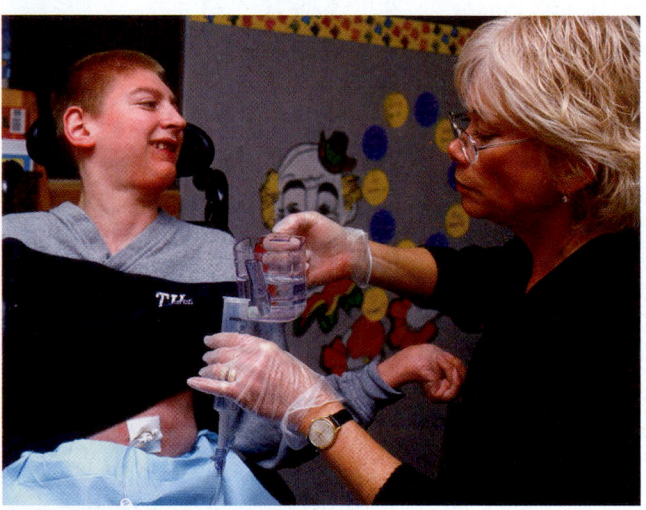

Figure 12–2 ➤ This child needs a gastrostomy tube to ensure adequate nutrition is obtained to support growth and promote resistance to infection.

BOX 12–1
HEALTHY PEOPLE 2010
OBJECTIVES FOR CHILDREN WITH SPECIAL HEALTH CARE NEEDS

- All CSHCN will receive regular ongoing comprehensive care within a medical home.
- All families with CSHCN will have adequate private and/or public insurance to pay for the services they need.
- Services for CSHCN and their families will be organized in ways that families can use them easily.
- Families of CSHCN will participate in decision making at all levels and will be satisfied with the services they receive.

U.S. Department of Health and Human Services. (2000). *Healthy People 2010* (2nd ed.). Washington, DC: U.S. Government Printing Office. www.healthypeople.gov

functions and require nursing care management such as renal dialysis, urinary catheters, and colostomies (Figure 12–2➤).

Children assisted by technology can be cared for at home because equipment has been made small enough to be portable. Home-based equipment used for the child with a chronic condition may include ventilators, enteral feeding tubes, intravenous catheters, infusion pumps, dialysis equipment, and oxygen. With the support of home health services parents can learn to manage the child's care. The benefit to the child is support of physical, emotional, and cognitive growth and development within the home care setting, in a more normal environment. The child who is technology-dependent may, however, be hindered in the ability to participate in normal childhood activities due to the presence of technological equipment (O'Brien & Wegner, 2002).

Many children with a chronic condition and children dependent on technology require specialized health care. The term **children with special healthcare needs (CSHCN)** is applied to "those who have or are at risk for a chronic physical, developmental, behavioral, or emotional condition and who also require health and related services of a type or amount beyond that required by children generally" (Inkelas & Garro, 2005). A national survey revealed that 12.8% (9.3 million) of children in the United States under the age of 18 years have special healthcare needs (van Dyke, Kogan, McPherson et al., 2004). With improved health care and technology, approximately 90% of children with chronic conditions will reach their 20th birthday, and most of these survivors will live on into adulthood (Lindeke, Leonard, Presler et al., 2002).

Children with special healthcare needs use significantly more healthcare resources than those without special healthcare needs, including more visits to clinics, emergency departments, dental visits, inpatient hospital days, and prescription medications. In 2000, children with special healthcare needs represented a small percentage of the nation's children, but they used 41% of the total child health expenditures (Chevarley, 2006). Efforts to reduce health costs have resulted in fewer hospitalizations and more care in the community. Families need considerable assistance for care coordination to ensure that their children have access to the needed care. See Box 12–1 for national health objectives in *Healthy People 2010* that are focused on the health status and healthcare delivery to children with special healthcare needs.

NURSING ROLE IN CARE FOR CHILDREN WITH A CHRONIC CONDITION

Nurses are essential in providing family-centered care to children with a chronic condition and their families. They apply a broad range of knowledge and skills, including the following (Allen, 2004):

- Knowledge of the pathophysiology of the chronic condition and anticipated disease progress
- Family assessment skills to identify the child's and family's strengths, reactions to the stress of the chronic condition, and coping mechanisms
- The ability to work with the family in their efforts to manage the child's normal growth and development, providing culturally sensitive care
- Knowledge of resources (community agencies, tertiary care centers, specialty professionals) appropriate for the child and family with a chronic condition
- The ability to identify a dysfunctional family needing intervention
- The ability to communicate effectively and work collaboratively with other health professionals

Nurses use their knowledge base and skills to provide the health promotion and health maintenance care, as well as condition-specific care needed by the child and family in all healthcare settings. Nurses play a significant role in teaching the parents to manage the child's condition and provide care at home, providing guidelines to promote the child's growth and development, monitoring the child's health status, supporting families during crisis episodes, and referring the family to appropriate community services. Nurses may assume the role of care coordinator or **case manager** to help the family link with appropriate resources, plan care while wisely using health insurance resources, and integrating services needed to promote the best care for the child and family.

THE FAMILY OF A CHILD WITH A CHRONIC CONDITION

Parents of children with a chronic condition report that the time of diagnosis is one of the most stressful times for families (Meleski, 2002). Parents must patiently wait as diagnostic procedures are performed. They are asked repeatedly about the child's health history, and the child is frequently examined. If the condition is potentially life threatening, the parents' anxiety and stress will be increased. This period begins the first transition to becoming a family with a child having special healthcare needs.

Informing the Parents

The way that parents become aware of and informed about their child's chronic condition is as variable as the types of chronic conditions. Chronic conditions present very differently among infants and children.

- Chronic conditions may be detected at birth or early in infancy. Examples include a neural tube defect, a condition like phenylketonuria identified by newborn screening, or a complication of care provided in the NICU, such as bronchopulmonary dysplasia.
- Parents may suspect that their child has a problem and seek a diagnosis, such as in cerebral palsy when the infant does not achieve expected developmental milestones.
- Recurrent illnesses may actually be related to a chronic condition such as asthma or cystic fibrosis. A serious injury, such as a brain injury, can also cause disabilities.
- Some children may start school before their learning or behavior problems are identified.

The manner in which parents are informed of their child's condition and their ability to understand the information influences their ability to cope with the diagnosis. The parents' heightened anxiety level may reduce the comprehension of information heard. Work to ensure that parents learn all important information, individualizing the approach to match the family's level of understanding and communication techniques (Swallow & Jacoby, 2001). See Figure 12–3➤.

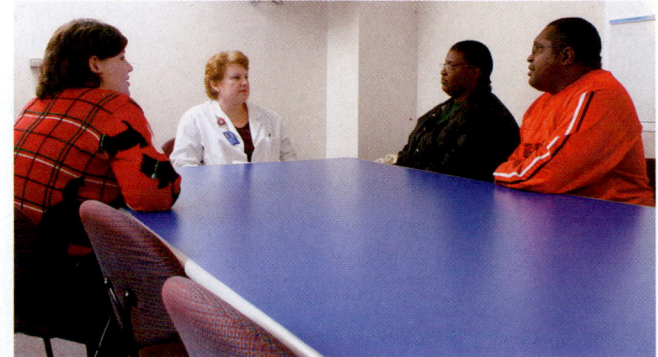

Figure 12–3 ➤ Inform the family about the child's chronic condition in an area with privacy, and be sure to provide adequate time for the family to initially absorb the information and then to ask questions. Offer to meet the next day to review the information and respond to additional questions.

CLINICAL TIP

When discussing a child's chronic condition with family, use the child's name. Avoid labeling the child with a condition, such as "diabetic child"; instead, refer to the situation as "the child with diabetes." This places the emphasis on the *child* rather than the *condition.*

The following guidelines may be considered when the nurse helps inform parents of the diagnosis of a chronic illness or disability in their child:

- Inform parents of their child's diagnosis in person, in a private setting, and free from interruptions. Tell both parents together. Offer parents the opportunity to have a relative or friend as a support person during the discussion.
- Plan and organize the information to be provided. Use simple, direct language without medical jargon. Individualize the pace of the interview and approaches taken to present the explanation, taking into consideration a family's culture and the family's response to the information.
- Share accurate, up-to-date information about the diagnosis, treatment options, specialty referrals, and community resources.
- Talk about the strengths and positive attributes of the child, as well as the child's limitations and characteristics due to the illness or disability.
- Evaluate the discussion with the family to assess whether the family's needs were met and to determine the type of support and/or additional information that should be provided.

Informing the Child

The method for informing the child of a newly acquired chronic condition is individualized and is based on the child's developmental level and age. Questions the child may ask vary but often focus on the cause of the condition, how to make it better, and how it will affect daily life. Provide information tailored to the child's level of understanding and answer questions honestly. See Chapter 13 ∞. The child may also have some guilt feelings because of the changes that will be required in the family to manage his or her condition.

Parental Reactions

Parents need time to comprehend the diagnosis and its meaning to their lives after learning about the child's diagnosis. Some parents may feel relieved that a diagnosis is finally identified after all of the concern, diagnostic testing, and uncertainty. They may feel that their concerns have been validated. For many parents the information may come as a shock or be very distressing, such as may occur at the time of birth. All parents may be challenged by the need to understand medical information and make rapid decisions about treatment (Meleski, 2002). The parents' responses are the same as when the child has a life-threatening illness—shock, disbelief, denial, and anger (see Chapter 14 ∞ for a discussion of grief). Other emotions experienced by parents include sorrow and hopelessness when the permanent nature of the condition is understood (Nuutila & Salanterä, 2006). The nurse should be empathetic and supportive of parental emotional expression.

Parents grieve for the loss of the perfect child and other losses such as the following:

- Loss of family routines and goals
- Loss of the ideal mother-child relationship
- Siblings' loss of normal childhood
- Loss of expectations for the development and life expectancy of the child with the chronic condition
- Child's loss of a normal childhood

Parents may blame themselves or their spouse if the condition is genetic. When the child's condition results in a significant disability, the family has a daily reminder of their losses and how they differ from other families. Parents may have difficulty bonding with the affected infant because of guilt or disappointment, fearing that the infant will not survive or because the infant looks or behaves differently.

Episodes of recurrent sadness are reported by parents, particularly when reminded that their child is different from healthy children (such as when the child starts school). These same parents may deny feeling sad at other times. This pattern of periodic sorrow or grieving interspersed by periods of denial, called **chronic sorrow,** is believed to be a coping mechanism that permits parents to meet their responsibilities in caring for the child (Melnyk, Feinstein, Moldenhouer et al., 2001). The periods of denial allow them to hope so they can function, but it may prevent parents from progressing through the full stages of grieving (Meleski, 2002).

Siblings' Reactions

Siblings of children with a chronic condition may be affected in a variety of ways. Their self-esteem, social support, mood, understanding of the illness, and attitude toward the child's illness are interrelated (Williams, Williams, Graff et al., 2003). They may also experience feelings of jealousy, embarrassment, resentment, and a sense of loneliness and isolation (Beckman, 2002). Some siblings may fear that they themselves will have the same disease or condition as the affected child. Younger siblings may believe, because of magical thinking, that they caused the child's disability (Beckman, 2002). Some siblings are at risk for behavioral problems, lower self-esteem, poor peer relationships, delinquency, depression, anger, excessive worry, and poor school performance (Williams, Williams, Graff et al., 2003). However, some siblings have positive responses and demonstrate increased responsibility, independence, maturity, and a tolerance for differences in other. Siblings who do better are those who are older at the time the illness occurs, have a more cohesive family, and experience better parent-sibling communication (Williams, Williams, Graff et al., 2003).

Siblings of a child with a chronic condition need support from their parents to help with their coping and adjustment. Nurses should help parents to recognize that the sibling needs the following (Ballard, 2004):

- Information and reassurance about the sick child
- Reassurance about his or her own health
- Relief from guilt
- Family communication, inclusion, and emotional support

Nursing actions to help promote improved adjustment for the sibling of a child with a chronic condition include helping parents recognize the need to spend individual time with the sibling (Fanos, Fahrner, Jelveh et al., 2004). Maintenance of family routines is helpful in promoting a sense of the normal. Help the family select appropriate ways the sibling can help with the care for the child with a chronic condition, while also recognizing that the sibling needs a childhood with peer interactions, physical exercise, and recreation.

Family Responses

Having a child with a chronic condition places great demands on parents. Parents worry about many aspects about the child and the care needed, both at the current time and in the future (Coffey, 2006). Many stresses have been reported by families having a child with a chronic condition and the following are commonly reported by families:

- Learning as much as possible about the child's condition and expected progression in severity
- Learning about all the technical aspects of care for the child and how to integrate that care into family routines
- Finding ways each family member can help with the child's care, including extended family members who may live nearby
- Communicating with health professionals and attempting to serve as a full partner in the child's care
- Identifying the most appropriate resources for the child
- Continuing employment and meeting care needs of the child
- Managing a family budget that is drained by expenses for care not covered by health insurance plans and other financial resources
- Attempting to provide siblings as normal a life as possible
- Opening the home to strangers who provide home care to the child
- Coping with episodes when the child's condition worsens and fearing that the child will die
- Working with the child to gradually assume more responsibility for self-care

CULTURE

Communication

The family with English as a second language may experience difficulty in communicating and understanding information in English during stressful situations such as the illness of their child. A translator should be used during these times. Until a translator is available, support the family and promote a calm environment to assist in reducing the family's stress.

English-speaking Mexican American families of children with a chronic condition have reported that they recognize some advantages over Mexican American families who could not communicate easily with nursing staff. Conversely, they also indicated that their lack of Spanish fluency served as a barrier to support from parents of their cultural group that predominantly spoke Spanish (Rehm, 2003).

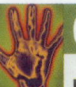

GROWTH & DEVELOPMENT

Environment

The home is often the best environment for children who are technology-assisted or medically fragile as they become more engaged in the family's activities. This leads to improvements in the child's physical, emotional, and psychological health. The child and parents often have reduced anxiety as the focus can be on daily living rather than a focus on the illness and disability (Wang & Barnard, 2004).

Certain transitions or events are more stressful for the family as they disrupt family routines or require adaptation. As mentioned, the time of diagnosis is the first transition or event that changes a family's expectations. Other events or milestones identified as critical times that cause stress or frustration include (Coffey, 2006; Melnyk, Feinstein, Moldenhouer et al., 2001):

- When development milestones do not occur as expected, such as walking at 12 to 15 months and speech delays at 24 to 30 months
- When a younger sibling surpasses the affected child in developmental milestone achievement
- At the time of school entry when differences between the affected child and other children the same age (physical appearance, cognitive ability, or social skills) become very apparent to parents, and at important milestones of school progression (transition to next school and graduation)
- The onset of adolescence
- At the time of transition to adult roles and to adult health services (21 years)
- When parents seriously plan for guardianship of the child
- When the family considers institutionalizing the child

The marriage relationship is at risk for breakdown if the couple is not able to communicate, share in the care for the child and other family members, and have common expectations for the child's condition and abilities to perform self-care. Some families have the strength and resilience to manage the child's healthcare needs and maintain family functioning. However, the burden of caring for the child with special healthcare needs often falls heavily on one parent, usually the mother (Coffey, 2006). Fathers in one study reported strong relationships with their wives, but they missed personal time with their wives as a couple (Goble, 2004). This parental relationship stress may be further increased by concurrent family illnesses, a death in the family, or the presence of a family conflict.

Caregiver Burden

Moving the child who is chronically ill, or a technology-assisted child, to the home setting is a life-changing decision for the family, and it must be done with collaboration between the family and the healthcare team. Preparation for the child's transition to the home requires that the family receive extensive training and instructions on the child's care. Management of the condition involves technological support, medications, and treatment regimens, all potential necessities to maintain the child in the home. Family members must decide who has responsibility for different aspects of the child's care.

This transition is often challenging and intimidating for the family who now must assume the role of independent caregiver. Family members often feel unprepared to handle the complex situation of the chronic condition and/or technological supports. The family may be assuming care of a child who has been hospitalized for months or even years before being discharged home (Harrigan, Ratliffe, Patrinos et al., 2002). The family needs to be highly motivated and possess strength and resiliency factors to overcome the obstacles that will arise. In this way, they will be successful in assuming management responsibility for the child's care.

Caregiver burden is the unrelenting pressure and anxiety of providing care to a child with disabilities day after day while meeting other family obligations. Parents have greater personal strain and caregiver distress when the child has poor functional status, needs extensive care, and the parents have an existing financial burden (Kuster, Badr, Chang et al., 2004). The parents of the child who is medically fragile must perform technical care and complicated procedures, keep records, be vigilant in monitoring symptoms, and make clinical decisions about symptoms detected based upon what is best for the child and family (Figure 12–4▶).

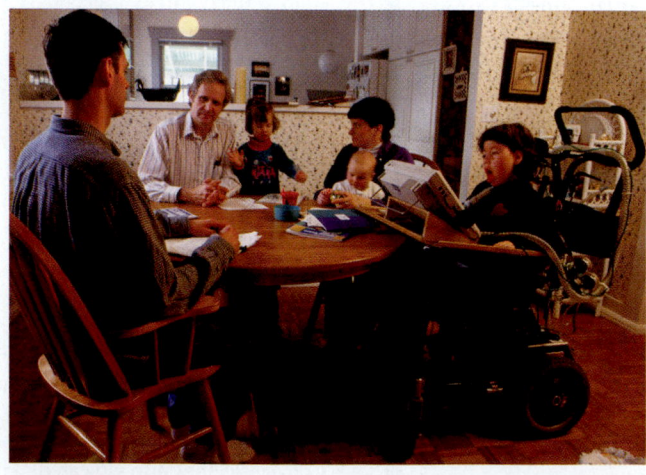

Figure 12–4 ▶   Daily caregiving demands of the child who is medically fragile continues 24 hours a day, 7 days a week. Parents need to identify ways to split the care of the child and other family care management. When the child lives with a single parent, additional healthcare resources are needed so the parent can sleep.

The stressors of parents with a child who is technology-dependent vary by the child's functional status, the extent of care needed, and the financial burden. Some families must give up privacy to have a home healthcare worker provide some of the child's care, sometimes causing conflicts over authority, control, and child-rearing decisions (O'Brien & Wegner, 2002). See Chapter 11 ∞ for the discussion of nursing care in the home. Stress is greater when the family does not trust the care professionals, has unreliable or unskilled care, and must supervise the care professional in the home (Ratliffe, Harrigan, Haley et al., 2002).

Meeting all family obligations may be challenging even when a family support infrastructure exists. There is a constant struggle to keep the needs of the child and the family in balance. Mothers may be unable or not have the energy to meet their own personal needs for health care. Social isolation may be experienced by the parent who remains in the home providing care to the chronically ill child. Spousal support is essential to manage all the family and childcare requirements. Employment responsibilities also must be integrated into the schedule, and hours of work often must be negotiated to ensure parental coverage for the child's care.

Even when parents develop the capacity and skills in care coordination of the child's medical care, the work on behalf of the child remains intensive and must be sustained long term. Administrative work, such as scheduling appointments, keeping records, developing and maintaining lists, completing health insurance claim forms, and appealing denied payments, never stop. Advocacy by seeking resources and opportunities for the affected child continue and change as the child's condition and developmental status change. See Evidence-Based Practice: Identifying and Responding to Unmet Needs.

Parents need to learn to pace themselves to limit fatigue, as limits exist on how much they can do and continue long term. Despite the challenges and despair, some families of children with chronic conditions do lead constructive lives with periods of joy and hope (Kearney & Griffin, 2001). Responses to all these stressors are dependent upon the family's available strengths, resiliency, and resources. See Chapter 2 ∞ for family assessment and nursing interventions for family support. See Table 12–2 for nursing actions to assist families with significant stressors.

Family Financial Issues

The economic impact of caring for a child with a chronic condition is significant. Even with good insurance coverage, the family still incurs a major financial burden (Ratliffe, Harrigan, Haley et al. 2002). While health plans claim that home care of

RESEARCH

Health Needs of Mothers

A study of 38 mothers of children who were ventilator dependent revealed that they rarely participated in health behaviors (planned exercise, balanced nutrition, adequate sleep). Mothers that were able to participate in health behaviors had children functioning at a higher level and the impact of the child's condition on the family was lower. When mothers perceived that the impact of the child's illness on the family was greater, participation in fewer health promotion activities was reported (Kuster, Badr, Chang et al., 2004). Health behaviors can help mothers manage the stress associated with the child's care. Encouraging the use of social supports or respite may enable the mother and other family members to participate in health promotion activities and could improve the mother's overall health.

EVIDENCE-BASED PRACTICE

Identifying and Responding to Unmet Needs

Clinical Question

What are the specific unmet needs reported by families, and do these unmet needs differ by family characteristics or the child's functional level?

Evidence

A study of lower income mothers of 83 children with complex health problems treated in primary care offices revealed that 93% of mothers had at least one unmet need (Farmer, Marien, Clark et al., 2004). The most frequently identified need was information about services for the child and ways to promote the child's health and development. More than 50% of parents also reported a need for caregiver supports, community services, help with family relationships, and financial costs. A greater number of unmet needs were reported when the child functioned at a lower level, and by mothers from minority groups or those who had perceptions of lower social support. Interviews with 30 families (30 mothers and 13 fathers) having one or more children with special healthcare needs helped describe the wide range of responsibilities that parents have in managing their children's health care (Ray, 2002). Findings revealed

that parents spent a large amount of time searching for information, people who could be relied upon for information, and services.

Implications

These studies revealed that families with children having special healthcare needs seek information, but the type of information sought varies by the type of condition, level of function, or special healthcare need. However, ways to promote the child's health and development and community services that match the child's needs are needed by nearly all families. Nurses are in a position to assist families by seeking information about their needs and then attempting to provide needed information, while maintaining current listings of community services for these families.

Critical Thinking

Select a specific pediatric chronic condition that usually requires parents to follow a complex routine to care for the child. Construct a series of questions to ask the family in order to learn about their perceived needs. Consider all the potential supports and services such a family might need and compile a list of local resources that could be recommended to the family.

Table 12–2	NURSING INTERVENTIONS FOR FAMILY STRESSORS
Stressors	**Nursing Implications**
Uncertainty	Be honest in responding to the parents' questions. Serve as an advocate to ensure information from the primary healthcare provider or specialists is being relayed to the family.
Fear of potential loss of their child	If the death of the child is likely or uncertain, support the family and refer to social services or other support to assist the family in anticipatory grieving. Ensure that the family is kept informed about all changes in the child's condition.
High-technology environment of the neonatal or pediatric intensive care unit	Orient the parents to the child's environment. Explain all equipment and procedures. Encourage them to be active participants in the child's care.
Communication with healthcare providers	Partner with the family and serve as their advocate to ensure communication is shared between the multidisciplinary team. Ensure the family understands all communication, and offer clarification if required. Ensure that the parents are fully informed and participate in all decision making regarding the child's care.
Deciding whom to inform about the chronic condition	Assist the family in identifying all individuals who need to know about the child's condition. Extended family members and friends can offer support and may provide assistance with care. Recommend that childcare or school officials (if school age) be informed since the child is in their care for a majority of time.
Increased out-of-pocket expenses	Partner with the family to identify cost-effective measures to reduce expenses. Refer the family to social services to determine any available financial assistance for healthcare services, respite care, meals, or transportation.
Social isolation and role strain	Encourage the family to participate in support groups. Parent-to-parent support groups can offer support and guidance. Encourage the family to take respite time from the child's care. Assist them in determining satisfactory arrangements for respite care (e.g., family member, healthcare or respite provider).
Dividing time between well children and child with chronic condition	Encourage parents to take "special time" with the siblings of the child with a chronic condition. Also encourage the family to include all members in planning family activities and to ensure that each child has an opportunity to plan activities. Identify social supports to help provide opportunities for participation in recreational or peer group activities.

CLINICAL TIP

Child maltreatment is reported to occur more frequently among children who are chronically ill or disabled. Factors that increase the risk of abuse in children with a chronic condition include the following (American Academy of Pediatrics, 2001a):

- Higher emotional, physical, economic, and social demands on the family
- Limited social and community support
- Failure of child to receive medications, appropriate educational placement, adequate medical care
- Increased stress related to the child's behavioral characteristics (e.g., communication problems, aggressiveness)

Assess the family for ineffective coping and the potential for abuse. Make appropriate referrals to support services such as mental health counseling, social services, and respite.

these children costs less, families assume responsibility for many out-of-pocket expenses. An average out-of-pocket expense for the child with a chronic condition to have needed health care is twice what families with healthy children pay. Poor families may pay more than 5% of the family's income for these services (Newacheck & Kim, 2005). Examples of additional expenses that families pay out-of-pocket may include special diets, durable equipment and supplies, transportation to healthcare visits, respite care, and sometimes co-payment for health services. Home health nursing care may be needed if both parents continue to work or to cover the night shift so parents can sleep. The majority of children with chronic conditions have adequate health insurance, but disparities exist in the family's ability to pay for healthcare expenses not covered by insurance among children who live in poverty, are Hispanic, and have the most functional limitations (Honberg, McPherson, Strickland et al., 2005). Impoverished children with chronic illnesses and those who are more severely impaired are the least likely to receive the care or assistive devices they need (Dusing, Skinner, & Mayer, 2004).

Although health insurance payers view the limitation of services as a means to save money, this may not be an effective plan when caring for medically fragile children (Ratliffe, Harrigan, Haley et al., 2002). Because of the rapidly rising cost of health care, all health insurance plans are implementing additional controls to slow the increase in the cost of care. Case management, supported by health insurance payers, is one mechanism used by health plans to contain costs while improving the utilization and distribution of limited resources (Lindeke, Leonard, Presler et al., 2002).

Some families give up employment income when one parent stays home to care for the child. Parents may lose their employment due to excessive absences to provide care for the child or be required to work reduced hours to make sure the child receives adequate care. In other cases the family may have a high incidence of job instability as a direct result of the child's condition. Such job instability further threatens the family's access to health insurance for the remainder of the family as well as the child with a chronic condition.

Promoting Healthy Family Coping

Families often engage in a coping strategy called **normalization.** Through normalization, the family views the care of the child with a chronic condition as a "normal" part of life, rather than an inconvenience or something outside of their routine. The family redefines what is normal for them by adopting a "normalcy lens" that enables them to see that their family follows some normal routines like all other families. The following defining attributes are exhibited by families that experience normalization (Knafl & Deatrick, 2002):

- They acknowledge the child's condition and know that it has the potential to threaten the family's lifestyle.
- Their parenting behaviors and family routines are consistent with how they view other families functioning.
- The child's treatment regimen is integrated into the usual routines of the family and child, in a manner that permits the family to seem normal.
- The parents interact with others based on their view of the child and family as normal.

With normalization, the parents may be able to move the child's condition to the subconscious so that it does not take a dominant place in the family's life and thoughts. They choose to focus on the normal aspects of the child and the family's life. Through normalization, the family perceives success in meeting their needs (Rehm & Rohr, 2002). Threats to sustaining normalization may include worsening of the child's health status that makes the parents more aware of the child's serious condition, changed management routines, new family additions, or other family situational changes.

Some families are unable to achieve or sustain the sense of normalization, even though it may be seen as a desired goal. In many cases these families are still adjusting to their child's condition, the child's condition may have recently changed, or another family stressor is present. In these families, the child's condition may be a major focus of family life or a source of conflict in the family. The child could be viewed as different from peers, leading parents to modify their parenting style to accommodate their dramatically changed view of their child. The child's treatment regimen may also be viewed as a significant burden in ways that make the family different from other families (Knafl & Deatrick, 2002).

Nurses can be effective in working with families by listening to the issues and offering suggestions. Often the opportunity to talk through the child's management plan will help the family consider different strategies that may be effective. The nurse may also provide linkages to community resources that may help the family.

DEVELOPMENTAL CONSIDERATIONS

The child with a chronic condition has the same developmental and emotional needs as the healthy child. The impact of the chronic condition on the child's cognitive, physical, and emotional health may lead to altered developmental achievement expectations. A **developmental delay** results when failure to achieve anticipated developmental milestones exists during specific developmental stages.

Newborn and Infant

Newborns and infants that are medically fragile are at risk for chronic conditions related to brain injury, oxygen deprivation, and respiratory problems. Newborns cared for in the NICU are exposed to an environment of bright lights, loud noises, frequent handling, and painful procedures, all which may negatively affect their neuropsychological development (Kessenich, 2003). See Figure 12–5 ➤.

Nurses should promote development and parent-infant bonding by encouraging the parents to spend time with the infant and engage in face-to-face interaction. When the newborn is stable, provide opportunities for parents to touch, soothe, and care for

LAW & ETHICS

SSI Benefits

The Supplemental Security Income (SSI) program provides social benefits to children with severe mental or physical functional limitations that have lasted or are expected to last at least a year or cause death. Qualification for this program also qualifies the child for Medicaid and a monthly cash payment (American Academy of Pediatrics, 2001b).

COMPLEMENTARY THERAPY

Animal Therapy

Animal-assisted therapy has been helpful in many ways to help ease stresses a child experiences with health care. Introduction of a dog into the home of a child with special healthcare needs may also be beneficial in helping the family with the "normalcy lens." Pets enable family members to express pleasure and affection to the pet, and families may spend more time together around pet-related activities (Gasalberti, 2006).

CLINICAL TIP

While nurses generally describe their role in caring for families and children with a chronic condition as very rewarding, they may develop **compassion fatigue,** an emotion that comes from knowing about the traumatizing events experienced by families and the stress from helping or wanting to help that family. These nurses may experience conflicting feelings, including grief, fatigue, and burnout, particularly if the needs of families and children served are difficult to meet (Maytum, Heiman, & Garwick, 2004). The fatigue and lack of energy associated with compassion fatigue may become more severe and affect the ability to function at work or home (burnout) if the nurse's coping mechanisms are not effective. Self-care activities such as exercise, meditation, recreation, maintaining a sense of humor, and social nonwork relationships are beneficial short-term personal coping strategies.

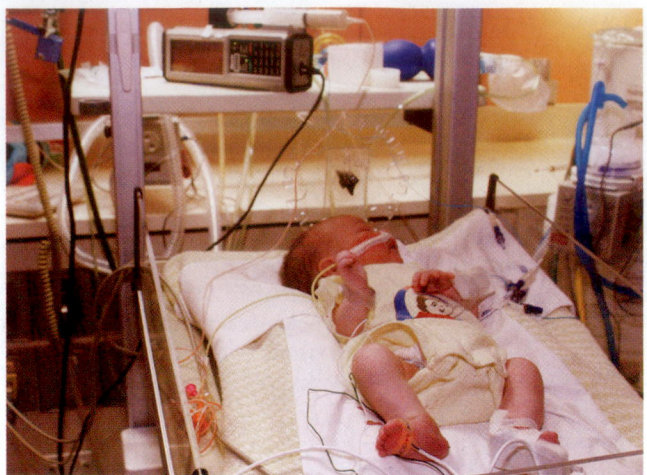

Figure 12–5 ➤ Development of trust may be disrupted for the infant in the NICU or hospital unit when there are multiple caregivers and experiences of painful stimuli. When parents are overwhelmed by the infant's health condition or when frequent hospitalizations prolong separation, parent-infant bonding may be impaired. The infant that experiences a lack of attachment behaviors (cuddling, holding, and talking by the primary caregiver) may not develop the reciprocal communication responses that are important for development of social communication, emotional awareness, and stress regulation (Rees, 2005).

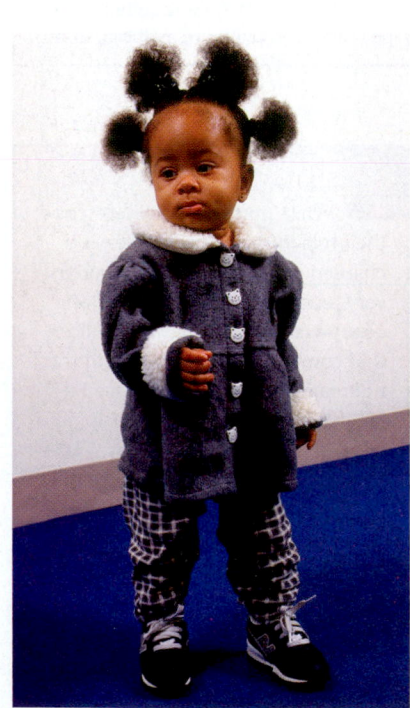

Figure 12–6 ➤ Toddlers may experience difficulty in adapting to constraints of the condition and treatments related to their disorder. Depending on the condition, toddlers may be unable to achieve developmental milestones such as walking, toilet training, and feeding self. Delays in speech also become apparent during this stage.

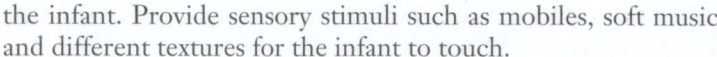

the infant. Provide sensory stimuli such as mobiles, soft music, and different textures for the infant to touch.

Toddler

When the toddler has a chronic condition, parents may need to control and set limits on movement, play, behavior, or social interactions because of the condition. This interferes with the achievement of autonomy and development of self-control. Some parents do more by protecting the child or doing simple tasks they feel the child is incapable of accomplishing, rather than encouraging the child to try to learn to do things independently. The child can lose independence and lack opportunities to meet developmental tasks. Some parents become overprotective, which can lead to vulnerable child syndrome. The child then becomes demanding, dependent, and has disturbed interactions with the parents (Melnyk, Feinstein, Moldenhouer et al., 2001). See Figure 12–6 ➤.

Nurses can promote the development of toddlers with chronic conditions by offering the child choices when possible, such as which color of gown to wear or which food to eat first. Help parents recognize the toddler's capabilities and allow the child to take the time to practice and learn a skill. Identify the next most appropriate developmental tasks for the child to learn and give the parents some strategies they can use to offer learning opportunities.

Preschooler

Preschool children recognize the association between body parts and problems associated with the chronic condition. The preschooler engages in magical thinking during this stage, and the child may believe that his or her thoughts or behaviors caused the condition. The child may also think the condition is a form of punishment. Decreased energy due to the condition may interfere with the preschooler's ability to learn about the environment, develop social relationships, gain a sense of self-confidence, and learn a sense of purpose (Vessey & Rumsey, 2004).

Nurses can promote development by explaining the purpose of treatments and procedures in terms the preschooler can understand, and by emphasizing that treatments are not punishment for any wrongdoing. Look for ways to use play so the child can learn an aspect of self-care, perform an activity, and feel a sense of accomplishment. See Chapter 13 ∞ for ways to use play in the hospital setting. Encourage social interactions with other children when possible. Give positive feedback to the child for appropriate efforts and successes.

School-Age Child

School-age children have an increased understanding of their condition, and they can participate in certain aspects of monitoring and care. Older school-age children begin to understand more about the management of the condition and the long-term needs associated with their condition. They can assume more responsibility of their care such as serum glucose sampling, monitoring the condition of skin under braces, or intermittent self-catheterization.

Some children with chronic conditions have learning difficulties and other limitations that interfere with education and social competence. The child needs to gain social skills, interact with peers, master new information, learn to cope with stress, and acquire skills that lead to self-sufficiency in order to develop a sense of industry. Other children may have functional limitations (self-care, communication, mobility, stamina, and learning) that interfere with participation in school activities and prevent them from gaining a sense of industry (Msall, Avery, Tremont et al., 2003). These children may develop feelings of inferiority and a low self-concept as they recognize differences between themselves and their peers.

Nurses can promote development of school-age children by encouraging their interaction with children in the same age group. When possible, this should occur with children having the same type of chronic condition. Link the child to a peer support group to promote social interaction and to help the child recognize that others also have the same condition. When the child has an extended absence from school because of the chronic condition, encourage contact from school peers and friends through cards and computer messages, as well as the completion of school assignments. Begin to identify aspects of the child's care that the child can learn to assume under the parents' supervision. Inform families of the benefit of special camps for children with the chronic condition (when available) to promote recreation, social interaction, and learning skills of self-care.

Adolescent

Adolescence is a stage of profound physical, psychological, and physiological changes. The adolescent with a chronic condition has numerous challenges with the rapid changes in growth and sexual maturation; ongoing development of identity, body image, and self-concept; and the need to plan for vocational and healthcare transitions. Cognitive development and abstract thinking skills are achieved during this stage, allowing the adolescent to develop an understanding of the short-term and long-term consequences related to the condition (Figure 12–7 ➤).

The adolescent becomes more aware of differences between self and peers. Some adolescents are unable to cope with the recognizable differences between themselves and healthy peers, and they withdraw from social activities and relationships or are drawn to a peer group that may negatively influence behavior. Others may engage in risky behavior (e.g., alcohol, sexual activity, eating incorrect foods) that may be harmful to themselves or to management of their condition, just to be accepted by peers.

Nurses can promote development by providing patient education to help the adolescent learn about the chronic condition, the care needed to manage or control the condition, and teaching problem solving and specific skills for self-care so they can integrate the care management into their daily lives. Coach parents to transition care over to the adolescent and to support the adolescent to make healthy decisions regarding care. Encourage the adolescent to have a safety net of friends who know enough about the chronic condition to assist if a problem occurs, such as a seizure, asthma episode, or insulin reaction. Provide education about sexual maturation and the importance of protected sexual activity. Discourage risky behaviors by the adolescent. Provide the adolescent an opportunity to express concerns regarding self-management, vocational planning, and future independent living.

EDUCATION AND SCHOOLING

Many children with chronic conditions have school activity limitations that can range from inability to attend school, to receiving or needing special education services, to limited school attendance. The majority of children with a functional disability need special education services (Msall, Avery, Tremont et al., 2003). Chronic health impairments by themselves or in combination with other functional disabilities also cause school activity limitations.

All children, including those with chronic conditions and special healthcare needs, are entitled to a free education that is matched to their developmental and functional capabilities by federal law (Individual with Disabilities Education Act and Section 504 of the Rehabilitation Act of 1973). **Early intervention,** special services for infants and toddlers up to age 3 years who have developmental delay or are at risk for developmental delay, is provided through state and local education programs in the hopes that these children will have a lowered total cost of educational services (Blann, 2005). Provisions for adolescent transitional planning for adult living, including vocational training and independent living, are also included in the Individual with Disabilities Education Act.

Attending school is an important transition for children with chronic conditions and their families. Sending the child to school has several benefits for the child and

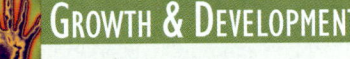

GROWTH & DEVELOPMENT

Sexual Maturation

All adolescents need education about sexual maturation, how to have protected sexual activity, and information about sexually transmitted infections. Even though the child may have functional limitations or chronic conditions, it is important to discuss and discourage risky behaviors, such as alcohol or substance use and sexual activity.

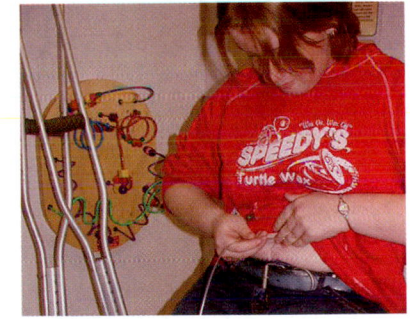

Figure 12–7 ➤ This adolescent is performing a self-catheterization. She needs to learn how to assume responsibility for her personal care and to make good decisions about future life plans. The adolescent with a chronic condition must also learn to independently manage the health condition and to take that condition into consideration when making future life plans. This may be more challenging for adolescents that have a limited life expectancy or when parents are unable to relinquish their control and encourage the child to assume more responsibility for self-care.

LAW & ETHICS

Federal Laws for Providing Education Services for Children with Special Healthcare Needs

- Rehabilitation Act, Public Law (P.L.) 93-112 of 1973, prohibited discrimination against people with a disability. Section 504 specifies that each student who has a physical or mental impairment is entitled to accommodations (e.g., additional time to take a test, strategies that decrease an allergic child's exposure to peanuts, frequent bathroom visits for the child needing intermittent catheterization) needed to attend school and participate as fully as possible in school activities (Moses, Gilchrest, & Schwab, 2005). This act covers many chronic conditions not covered under other education laws.
- The Education for All Handicapped Children Act, Public Law (P.L.) 94-142 of 1975, mandated that all children, even those with handicaps, be provided with public education and related services.
- Education for All Handicapped Children Amendments, P.L. 99-457 of 1986, expanded the scope of P.L .94-142 to include appropriate services for infants and toddlers with disabilities and their families.
- Individuals with Disabilities Education Act (IDEA), P.L. 105-17 of 1997, ensures that all children with disabilities have available to them a free appropriate public education that emphasizes special education and related services designed to meet their unique needs and prepare them for employment and independent living. Every child with a disability must have a written Individualized Education Plan, and parents have the right to question placement decisions and to due process when settling differences.

family. Children have an opportunity for socialization with children and adults beyond the immediate family. Parents gain a sense of normalization as the child attends school like all other children. Parents also benefit by having some respite from the child's care during the school day (Rehm & Rohr, 2002).

Educational System Planning

Careful planning is needed when a child with special needs attends school or receives other education services. Many children have chronic medical conditions that require management during the day in the school environment, such as asthma, diabetes, and attention deficit disorder. Some children just need medications administered regularly or episodically. Other children need more extensive interventions integrated into the school day, such as blood glucose monitoring or intermittent self-catheterization. The education system is obligated to provide reasonable **accommodations** (services or special assistance provided in the school setting to ensure that a student with a physical or mental impairment has access to an appropriate education) to ensure that the child's medical needs are met during the school day. The education system's obligation is negotiated with the family in formalized plans. The school nurse is an active participant on the team that collaborates with the family to develop these formalized plans.

- An **Individualized Family Service Plan (IFSP)** is developed for the early intervention process for infants with special healthcare needs and their families. The IFSP contains information about the services required to support a child's development and enhance the family's capacity to facilitate the child's development. The family and education service providers work as a team to plan, implement, and evaluate services specific to the family's unique concerns, priorities, and resources.
- An **Individualized Education Plan (IEP)** is developed for a child with cognitive, motor, social, and communication impairments who needs special education services. The IEP is jointly planned with the school administrator, school nurse, teacher, parents, and other special support professionals as appropriate for the child's condition. The child is also included in the process when possible. The plan is developed after an assessment of the child's abilities and specific functional limitations.
- An **Individualized Health Plan (IHP)** is developed for the child with medical conditions that needs to be managed within the school setting. An IHP may be developed simultaneously with the IEP for the child with a health problem and a co-existing functional impairment. Some children only need an IHP for management of their chronic medical condition at school, such as daily medication administration or for glucose monitoring and insulin injection. A physician order is required for medication administration and special treatments. Learning may be challenged when the child has frequent acute illness episodes that result in missed days of school, and the IHP often integrates methods to prevent the child from being penalized for those absences.
- An Individualized Section 504 Accommodation Plan may be used rather than an IHP for children with physical or mental impairments. The same process is used for development of the plan.
- An **Individualized Transition Plan (ITP)** is included in the development of an IEP for each child with a chronic disability who is 14 years or older. The ITP focuses on assisting the individual to receive vocational training and in moving successfully from the home into other community living settings as they grow older.

Parents have an important role in advocating for their child to ensure that the child receives the most appropriate educational services. School systems must provide a full range of educational services for the children with special healthcare needs, including services that support cognitive development, self-care skills, mobility, improved communication, and social skills (Figure 12–8 ➤). Because each child's severity and combination of impairments is unique, identifying and matching the specific services for each child requires discussion and negotiation. Parents should make an effort to learn about the different types of educational services that address a child's specific disability in preparation for the IEP meeting. Parents often need a mentor or experienced parent to help with the development of the IEP the first few times. In this way, the parents are better prepared to participate in the educational planning and development of the child's IEP. School nurses are employees of the school system and may be limited in their advocacy role on behalf of individual students. However, school nurses are in a good position to educate the IEP team about specific interventions needed by children with medical conditions and ways to integrate those interventions into the school day. See Box 12–2 for the elements of an IEP.

The Child's Response to Entering School

Children with chronic conditions, whether they cause minimal interference in the child's daily life or are technology-assisted, face certain challenges in the school setting. They may for the first time recognize differences between themselves and other children, such as appearance, abilities, social skills, or special treatment needs. They also may experience social stigma for the first time, experience teasing, or have difficulties forming friendships (Melnyk, Feinstein, Moldenhouer et al., 2001). Some children, particularly adolescents, may attempt to hide their condition or fail to adhere to necessary recommendations, such as dietary restrictions, in order to appear like their peers.

Education for Children Who Are Medically Fragile

Children who are medically fragile or technology-assisted are also entitled to education services in the school setting. The child's need for skilled supportive nursing care

Figure 12–8 ➤ An annual meeting of the school administrator, teacher, school nurse, and other school personnel, as well as the parents and child, is important in identifying the educational goals for the child and the special education resources to help meet those goals for development of the child's IEP.

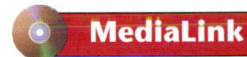

MediaLink

School Reentry Video

BOX 12–2
ELEMENTS OF AN IEP

- Student's name
- Date of meeting to develop or review the IEP
- Statement of transition service needs of student beginning at age 14 years
- Present level of assessments and education performance, including how the child's disability affects the child's involvement and progress in a general curriculum or participation in appropriate activities
- Measurable annual goals that include benchmarks or short-term objectives in meeting the child's needs that enable the child to be involved in or progress in the general curriculum or participate in appropriate activities
- Special education and related services, supplementary aids and services, and program modifications or supports for school personnel needed to enable the child to make advancements toward attaining annual goals
- Explanation to the extent that the child will or will not participate with nondisabled children
- Any specific modification in the administration of state- or district-wide assessments of achievement that are needed for the child to participate in the assessment, or reasons for excluding the child from assessment of achievement
- How the child's progress toward annual goals will be measured
- How the child's parents will be regularly informed of the child's progress toward annual goals and the extent to which the child's progress is sufficient to meet goals by the end of the year.

Data from: U.S. Department of Education. (2000). *A guide to the Individualized Education Program.* Retrieved July 30, 2006, from http://www.ed.gov/parents/needs/speced/iepguide/index.html

must be carefully considered by the parents and the school system. Parents are often anxious about how well the child will be cared for by others during the school day. Risks for the child in the school setting include safety issues related to ventilators, tracheostomy, and medication therapy, as well as exposure to infectious diseases.

The school administration must provide the personnel resources and equipment needed to ensure that care and a care provider are consistently available. Modifications to the school setting for the child, such as wheelchair ramps or an elevator, may be needed. Sometimes the child is placed in a classroom with healthy children, and the teacher is expected to monitor the child with a chronic condition and provide care as needed. Health aides may be assigned to provide care for one or more children with school nurse supervision. Some children are placed in classes composed of children with special healthcare needs where health aides are more available to provide needed care.

Nurses play a key role in assisting the family to understand that a teacher's primary responsibility is to teach, not to provide health care. The teacher is responsible for the health and safety of all children in the classroom. Parents need to have realistic expectations about the level of skilled support services that can be provided to a child who is medically fragile in a classroom. Teachers and education leaders are often challenged to meet the obligations for the child's special education services in balance with the needs of all other children in the classroom.

Home schooling is an option for these children with resources provided through the school system. Home schooling provides education continuity when the child cannot attend school, and it reduces the child's stress and fatigue. Home schooling may be used full time or for periods when the child is too ill to attend school. However, the home-schooled child who is medically fragile loses an important opportunity for peer and social interaction.

Transition to Adulthood

An estimated 21% of adolescents have special healthcare needs resulting from improved survival rates for children with chronic conditions (Scal & Ireland, 2005). When their chronic condition could affect their future ability to work and live independently, customized transition planning is needed in preparation for adulthood and self-determination. An ITP is developed through the IEP process, using a multidisciplinary approach in collaboration with the family to assist in identifying appropriate support programs, community living arrangements away from home, and employment opportunities (Beckman, 2002). Healthy Ready to Work services may be particularly helpful to adolescents and families in planning for the transition to adulthood.

Adolescents need continuous access to health care as young adults to maximize lifelong functioning and potential. Transition planning needs to focus on identifying and moving the adolescent or young adult to adult-oriented healthcare services. Challenges in finding and establishing a healthcare relationship with an adult healthcare provider include the following (Lotstein, McPherson, Strickland et al., 2005):

- The adolescent and parents may be unwilling to end a long-term relationship with present healthcare providers.
- High rates of uninsurance or underinsurance exist (once the young adult reaches 21 years, previous eligibility to the state's child health insurance program (SCHIP) and Medicaid may terminate).
- Adult providers may not be available or willing to see young adults with chronic conditions.

Adolescents with severe developmental or cognitive disabilities may have additional challenges because of their reliance on parents or other caregivers for healthcare decisions (Telfair, Alleman-Velez, Dickens et al., 2005). A *Healthy People 2010* goal is to facilitate healthcare transition for adolescents, and the federal government is working to increase access to resources for this planning (Scal & Ireland, 2005).

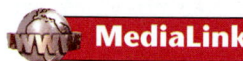

MediaLink

Adolescent Transition Resources

COLLABORATIVE CARE

Care of the child with a chronic condition generally requires a multidisciplinary health professional approach, including physicians, nurse practitioners, nurses, nutritionists, social workers, case workers, physical therapists, occupational therapists, and a case manager.

Hospitalization

Children with chronic disorders are more likely to be hospitalized than children without chronic disorders. Depending on the severity of the condition, frequent hospitalizations or long-term hospitalization for months or years may be required for the child with a chronic condition. The family is an integral part of the plan of care for an ill or hospitalized child. Acute hospitalization resulting from exacerbation of the child's disorder places increased demands and stressors on the child and family. The child and parent may fear worsening of the condition or even death. Refer to Chapter 13 ∞ for a discussion of nursing care of the hospitalized child.

Ethical Issues

Ethical issues often arise for children with chronic conditions or disabilities. Who ultimately makes the decisions—parents or the primary healthcare providers—about withholding treatments, implementing treatments, and other medical care issues is an ongoing debate. Issues regarding clinical ethics related to children with chronic conditions or disabilities include the following:

- Withholding and refusal of treatment
- Advanced directives (Do Not Resuscitate orders) (see Chapter 14 ∞ for further discussion)
- Genetic testing and screening programs
- Prenatal diagnosis, therapeutic abortion, and fetal therapy
- Sexual and reproductive rights, sterilization of adolescents with mental retardation
- Organ donation and rationing of care
- Research involving individuals with disabilities

Additional ethical issues arise from rationing of care, or withholding treatment on the basis of outcome and cost. For example, a child born with a severe congenital malformation may be denied surgical intervention due to increased likelihood of poor outcomes and the cost of treatment. These situations present a challenge to the family and healthcare providers. Most healthcare facilities have an ethics committee with established procedures and guidelines for addressing issues for the child with a chronic disorder or disability.

Health Promotion and Health Maintenance of Children with a Chronic Condition

Most children with a chronic condition are cared for at home with or without home nursing or other healthcare services, and they may rely solely on the family for their support and care. Children with chronic health conditions require regular health promotion, health screening, and health maintenance care, as well as specialized health services to assist the child and family in the condition's management. Parents need education and guidance to reduce risks for further illness and injury and to foster the child's development. The goal is to promote the child's growth and development and permit the child to have as normal a childhood as possible. The child with a chronic condition needs a medical or healthcare home to ensure that all the child's healthcare needs are met. Ideally this healthcare provider is located in the community where the family resides, making it more convenient for the family to obtain health care as well as care for episodic illnesses. Having a regular healthcare provider has many advantages for the family.

- Because the child and family are seen more frequently, a more trusting and family-centered relationship can develop. The healthcare provider learns about the family's strengths and coping abilities.

MediaLink

Health Promotion and Health Maintenance: The Child with a Chronic Condition

- The healthcare provider sees the child and family when things are going well and during exacerbations. This may enable the healthcare provider to identify strategies that help the family to better coordinate the child's care.
- When the provider is based in the same community as the child, information about community resources may be known and reduce the efforts that families make to identify appropriate services needed by the child.

An optimal healthcare arrangement for the child with a chronic condition exists when the medical or healthcare home provider collaborates with a pediatric team or specialist that specializes in the care of children with a specific chronic condition. Pediatric specialists, advanced practice nurses, and other healthcare providers (e.g., physical therapists, social workers, and nutritionists) often function as a team providing coordinated care to the family and child with a chronic condition, such as spina bifida, cystic fibrosis, or cerebral palsy. These specialty teams are often found in major medical centers, requiring travel to the facility. When communication flows from the team to the child's healthcare provider and back to the team, new treatments can be monitored by the child's physician, and consultation can be sought if the child's health status changes.

Sometimes a pediatric specialist serves as the child's medical or healthcare home. While this may seem like a good strategy for care, there are some risks that health promotion services will be minimized. It is important to ensure that regular health promotion and health maintenance services, such as immunizations, are not overlooked during the care of acute exacerbations of the chronic condition.

NURSING MANAGEMENT

In collaboration with the family and a multidisciplinary healthcare team, the nurse assists the family to manage the child's care at home; provides guidelines to promote the child's health, growth, and development; and supports the family by facilitating psychosocial adaptation.

The nurse's role in caring for the chronically ill child includes providing health supervision from infancy to transition into adulthood, collaborating with the multidisciplinary healthcare team, partnering with parents or caregivers to manage the child's care at home, referring the family to appropriate community services, assisting with planning for education services, promoting positive parenting behaviors and psychosocial adaptation and well-being of the child and family, and promoting growth and development of siblings.

Nursing Assessment and Diagnosis

Physiologic and Developmental Assessment

Conduct a physical assessment of the child, noting general health status and focusing on systems affected by the chronic condition. Perform a developmental assessment to help identify future developmental goals.

Family Assessment

Assess individual family members' level of understanding of the condition, treatment, and anticipated outcome of the condition. Parents are often experts in their child's condition, care, and responses to various medical interventions. Determine how well the child's care is integrated into family routines. Evaluate the child's home care environment to determine the presence of abuse, lack of adequate care, or neglect. Assess the family's strengths, coping strategies, stressors, and risk factors (see Chapter 2 ∞).

Nursing diagnoses that may apply to the family of a child with a chronic condition include:

- Compromised Family Coping related to prolonged condition management and inadequate financial resources
- Fatigue related to excessive role demands in caring for the child with a chronic condition and meeting other family obligations
- Anticipatory Grieving related to the child's deteriorating health status

- Deficient Knowledge related to the complex condition management plan
- Risk for Impaired Parenting related to stress with caring for the child with a chronic condition and lack of social support system
- Caregiver Role Strain related to the child's illness chronicity and 24-hour care responsibility

Nursing diagnoses that may apply to a child with a chronic condition are provided on the nursing care plan. Additional nursing diagnoses may be found in the nursing care plans for children with specific chronic conditions in systems chapters. See the Nursing Care Plan on the next page.

Planning and Implementation

The Child with a Newly Diagnosed Chronic Condition

Address the fears and concerns of the family of a child with a newly diagnosed chronic condition. Parents of a newborn or child with a newly diagnosed chronic condition often feel overwhelmed with preparations for home care, the anxiety of caring for the child, grief for the losses associated with expectations for a healthy baby, and supporting the child's growth and development needs.

Discharge Planning and Home Care Teaching

Work with the parents to ensure a smooth transition from hospital to the home environment. Assist the family in the initial discussions with the multidisciplinary team that participates in developing the child's care plan. Ensure that the family understands the role of each care provider.

Provide the condition-specific education to help prepare the family for care at home and begin discharge planning. Education may be initiated by the hospital nursing staff, and then transitioned to special nurse educators or the home healthcare nurses. Care of the technology-dependent child includes educating the family on equipment use and maintenance, medications, specific tasks associated with treatment, and monitoring of the child. Care is taken to ensure that all aspects of management are discussed with the family and that they demonstrate an understanding and ability to perform the required care. Ongoing assistance may be required to help families deal with financial issues, time management, and other challenges. See the systems chapters for condition-specific family education and discharge planning.

During discharge planning the identification of a parent peer or peer support group may be helpful to provide support to the family. Parent peers who have had similar experiences may be very helpful in identifying strategies for the initial care transition in the home and additional issues that arise over time. If the family has a computer, Internet resources for information and family support should be provided.

Collaborate with the family and healthcare team to assure that the child has a medical or healthcare home to provide health promotion and maintenance and to assist with the coordination of local community resources. Promote communication and joint planning of care between the specialty care provider and local healthcare provider. Nurses working in hospital specialty clinics and other community settings can help ensure that children with chronic conditions receive multidisciplinary referrals and appointments. Social services may be called to assist the family with identifying financial resources and other community resources for home management.

Coordination of Care

Care coordination is a process of planning that involves promoting timely access to services, continuity of care, and enhancing the family's well-being (Lindeke, Leonard, Presler et al., 2002). Because numerous healthcare providers and healthcare agencies are often involved in the care of the child with a chronic illness or an injury requiring long-term care, coordination of health services is important to prevent gaps and overlaps, reduction in healthcare costs, and improved family satisfaction (American Academy of Pediatrics, 2005a). A case manager, often a nurse or social worker, may be given responsibility to help the family with care coordination. Case managers are often paid by a healthcare insurer to reduce healthcare costs. The role includes coordinating the

NURSING CARE PLAN The Child with a Chronic Condition

GOAL	INTERVENTION	RATIONALE	EXPECTED OUTCOME
1. Deficient Knowledge (child) related to learning self-care skills			
	NIC Priority Intervention: **Individual Teaching:** *Planning, implementation, and evaluating a teaching program designed to address a patient's particular need.*		*NOC Suggested Outcomes:* **Knowledge:** *Extent of understanding conveyed about the treatment regimen.*
The child will acquire self-care skills for lifetime management.	• Assess the child's developmental level and select an educational approach and self-care activities to match.	• Learning goals for the child must match knowledge and skill expectations appropriate for developmental stage.	The child demonstrates the proper technique in the self-care skill and is able to assume responsibility for that skill with supervision by the parent. Responsibility for self-care increases as new skills are learned.
	• Review with the child all steps involved in the self-care skill and how to perform the skill.	• The child may have watched the routine used by parents many times, and asking the child to list each step helps the nurse identify extra training needed.	
	• Use demonstration/return demonstration until the child is comfortable with procedures.	• Evaluation permits positive reinforcement and guidance for modification of techniques.	
	• Help parents develop a planned sequence of self-care skills to teach the child.	• Parents need guidance to identify appropriate self-care skills that the child is developmentally ready to learn.	
	• Discuss a plan for increased responsibility for self-care with the child and parents.	• Parents often need encouragement to transition responsibility to the child, becoming a supervisor rather than the person controlling care.	
2. Interrupted Family Processes related to management of a chronic disease			
	NIC Priority Intervention: **Normalization Promotion:** *Assisting parents and other family members of children with chronic illnesses or disabilities in providing normal life experiences for their children and families.*		*NOC Suggested Outcomes:* **Family Health Status:** *Overall health status and social competence of the family unit.*
The child and family will manage the required treatments, monitoring, and medications regimen for the child's condition while maintaining family routines and functioning.	• Assess the child's and family's lifestyle and attempt to fit the child's care needs into those schedules.	• Fitting the child's care to the child's and family's life style promotes compliance with the regimen and healthier family processes.	The child and family maintain important family routines and successfully manage the child's condition.
	• Discuss the family's routines for special occasions and vacations and any activities important to the child. Identify ways to modify the child's management for these occasions and activities.	• It is important for the child to participate in special events with the family and peers as a normal child to promote psychological development.	

NURSING CARE PLAN   The Child with a Chronic Condition (continued)

GOAL	INTERVENTION	RATIONALE	EXPECTED OUTCOME
3. Individual Readiness for Enhanced Coping related to self-care management of chronic condition			
	NIC Priority Intervention: **Resiliency Promotion:** *Assisting individuals, families, and communities in development, use, and strengthening of protective factors to be used in coping with environmental and societal stressors.*		*NOC Suggested Outcomes:* **Health-Seeking Behavior:** *Actions to promote optimal wellness, recovery, and rehabilitation.*
The child will develop a support system network.	• Talk with the child about how to tell friends, teachers, and other important persons about the chronic condition.	• These important persons can assist the child in an emergency if they have enough information to assess the problem.	The child identifies the friends, teachers, and other important persons informed about the chronic condition and can provide support when needed.
	• Discuss ways to explain the condition to important persons and how to answer questions. Role-play ways to talk about the condition with friends and teachers.	• Having an opportunity to plan and role-play the conversation will reduce the child's anxiety about condition disclosure. Sharing information about the condition helps others understand changes in lifestyle needed by the child.	
	• Encourage the child to attend peer support groups or camps specific to the child's condition.	• Learning and support networks developed at camp can promote development of problem-solving skills that increase coping abilities.	
4. Health-Seeking Behaviors (Adolescent) related to learning self-management of chronic disorder			
	NIC Priority Intervention: **Self-modification Assistance:** *Reinforcement of self-directed change initiated by the patient to achieve personally important goals.*		*NOC Suggested Outcomes:* **Adherence Behavior:** *Self-initiated action taken to promote wellness, recovery, and rehabilitation.*
The adolescent will develop independent ability to manage his or her condition.	• Allow the adolescent to perform as many self-care procedures as possible at each developmental stage.	• Gradually learning self-care skills helps make this seem a regular expected behavior.	The adolescent performs appropriate daily management of self-care and seeks help to appropriately manage episodic acute problems.
	• Encourage the adolescent to problem solve and make decisions regarding care. Review decisions and provide feedback or appropriate guidance.	• Problem-solving skills and competence in self-care management develop with positive feedback or corrective guidance.	
	• Encourage parents to stay involved even when the adolescent takes primary responsibility for care.	• The adolescent is likely to adhere to a treatment plan when the parents continue to show interest and supervise care.	
	• Encourage the adolescent to discuss the condition and care directly with the healthcare provider.	• The adolescent begins to learn the process for seeking health care and becoming an advocate for his or her own care.	

healthcare team, determining family needs, identifying financial and local support resources, and arranging for needed healthcare services.

The goals of care coordination include (American Academy of Pediatrics, 2005a):

- Gaining access to and integrating services and resources on behalf of the child
- Facilitating communication among multiple professionals
- Preventing duplication of services and unnecessary cost
- Advocating for improved individual outcomes
- Improving the child's and family's quality of life

Care coordination may also include helping the family modify the home to support required technology, such as mechanical ventilation or wheelchair use. Assistance may be required in purchasing or leasing specialized equipment such as ventilators or infusion pumps. The coordination plan also includes determining the potential need for home health nursing or other home health services, such as physical therapy.

Families become very well educated about their child's conditions and the services that would make managing the child's condition easier. Once management goals are established by the multidisciplinary team, the case manager partners with the family to help in the decision making about which healthcare provider or agency is responsible for assisting the child to meet each goal. An important role is helping the family to determine cost-effective strategies to meet healthcare goals and to delay the time when the child reaches the cap on health insurance benefits.

Some families assume the role of care coordinator for their child. It is essential for the family to understand that care coordination is time-consuming and requires ongoing assessment and evaluation of the child's status and anticipated outcomes. Support family members in their decision to lead the care coordination process by helping the parents to become knowledgeable about the child's condition and treatment regimen. Support the parents to take an active role in the treatment planning and decision-making process so that they gain confidence in their abilities. Many hospitals have workshops for parents who are managing the complex care of their children. Parent-to-parent support groups can be valuable to the family by providing advice, support, and suggestions for referrals. Review the care coordination to ensure that the child has access to the most appropriate care and resources. Provide positive feedback to the parents as their advocacy skills increase.

Suggest that the family maintain a log of the healthcare team members, their roles, when the child was seen and any interventions, the results of interventions, and future planned interventions or treatments. The family can use this information when communicating with the healthcare providers, particularly in an emergency, and it may also help eliminate unnecessary duplication of procedures.

Respite Care

Respite care is an important support service to care for the child with a chronic condition while the parents take a short break away from the daily care. An example might be skilled nursing care in a facility or the home so the family can have a weekend away. This support service may help the family to keep the child with a chronic condition in the home. Respite care and other support services (home health services and parent support groups) may also reduce the risk of abuse. Assist the family in identifying respite care that meets the individual family's needs from the services available in the community. Many states have passed legislation for in-home family support services that include respite care. Because many respite services charge for their assistance, the family may require help in identifying respite waiver subsidies available to them. Reliable childcare and enrollment in school are other mechanisms used for families to obtain respite care.

Support the Child with a Chronic Condition

Provide the child with opportunities to express concerns about the condition and the effect the condition has on quality of life. The child who has had the chronic condition since birth or early childhood requires assistance in understanding more about the condition as cognitive development and understanding increase. As the child grows, collaborate with the child and family to include the child in self-care management according

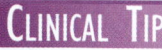
CLINICAL TIP
The ARCH National Resource Center for Crisis Nurseries and Respite Care Services helps parents locate respite care services in their area. The toll-free number is 800-773-5433.

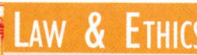
LAW & ETHICS
Katie Becket Act
The Tax Equity and Fiscal Responsibility Act of 1982 (Public Law 97-248), also known as the Katie Becket Act, provides financial assistance so parents can hire trained care providers for respite care (American Academy of Pediatrics, 2005b).

to cognitive and developmental level, and to participate in the decision-making process. Encourage the child to assume a role in the condition's care and management. This may include maintaining a journal, self-administering medications, or monitoring glucose levels. See Families Want to Know: Developmental Strategies for Promoting the Child's Self-Care for more information.

Support the transition of adolescents to adult health services by introducing the adolescent to members of the healthcare team that will eventually assume a role in providing care. Encourage the adolescent to take a more assertive role in healthcare visits with the pediatric healthcare team in preparation for working with a new healthcare team. Ensure that the adolescent understands the role each new member of the team will assume.

Health Promotion

Review the next stage of expected development with parents and provide suggestions and strategies to help the child with a chronic condition achieve developmental milestones. Review the care that other children in the family are receiving to ensure that they obtain appropriate care and stimulation to promote their growth and development. Remind

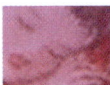

FAMILIES WANT TO KNOW

Developmental Strategies for Promoting the Child's Self-Care

When the child is cognitively able to learn about the chronic condition and begin to take some responsibility for self-care, knowledge of cognitive and psychomotor development help in developing strategies to teach the child about self-care. Ideally such learning should begin early in life, but even when the condition develops at a later age, educating the child can still be based upon knowledge of the child's development. Education and assumption of self-care responsibility should be appropriately matched to the child's developmental abilities. The ultimate goal is to transition all self-care responsibility to an adolescent who has learned all important aspects of the condition, who can manage daily routines and solve problems when an issue with care occurs, and who knows when and how to seek health care in the adult healthcare system (Sawin, Cox, & Metzger, 2004).

- Toddlers (1 to 3 years) can cooperate with the daily routines of care and assist in simple ways, such as holding an item. The toddler can also learn simple concepts such as foods allowed or not allowed. When a routine is established, the toddler learns what to expect through daily repetition.
- Preschoolers (4 to 5 years) are able to imitate some of the parent's behaviors regarding care, and they can learn simple terms that describe their condition and how they feel when the condition is not well controlled (e.g., weak and dizzy with diabetes, difficulty breathing with asthma).

  Parents can help teach the child the simple terms about the condition and have the child practice telling the information to other family members. Help the parent identify a simple task that is part of the management care routine that the child can do to help (holding the spacer during the asthma treatment, washing the hands, taking supplies out of a bag or box).
- Early school-age children (6 to 9 years) are more aware of physical feelings associated with when the condition is and is not well controlled. The child is also capable of performing some aspects of care (fingerstick for glucose monitoring, writing down the glucose reading on a log, controlling inhalation to use aerosol medication, selecting appropriate foods for a meal or snack), having seen it performed by parents repeatedly or after being taught and coached to do it well.

  The parent can support the child's learning by increasing the information provided about the condition and need for

treatment. Give the child an option about which self-care skill to learn first, next, and so on. The parent is then able to select skills appropriate to the child's developmental ability and teach the child to perform them. As the child demonstrates proficiency with a skill, a new skill can be added. The child can take responsibility for learned self-care skills with supervision, and the parent performs other unlearned skills.

- Late school-age children (10 to 12 years) have a greater understanding of how the body works and the impact of the chronic condition. They also have the capability of discussing some aspects of care directly with the healthcare provider. By 12 years of age, the child can learn to perform all the psychomotor skills associated with the condition.

  Parents can support the child in assuming more responsibility for self-care by initially providing a list of all steps in the management plan or other tools that will help with decision making (dose of insulin, adding food to diet on days with soccer practice). Provide corrective feedback as necessary. Continue to be present to answer questions, particularly when problem solving and decisions need to be made about care. Encourage the child to talk independently with the healthcare provider rather than control the discussion.
- Adolescents can, with the prior steps of preparation, become the primary manager of their daily care. They usually have the cognitive ability to problem solve and make adjustments in the care routine for special occasions or illness and to ask for help when a complex care situation develops. The adolescent should have a network of friends and family who are informed about the condition and able to assist in an emergency.

  Parents should monitor the self-care provided without interfering in the adolescent's care routine unless corrective feedback is needed. Encourage the adolescent to take full responsibility for self-care management, but encourage open communication about the condition and other healthcare concerns. Discuss risky behaviors and the potential impact on general health, and specifically the condition. Provide support and assistance during the time the adolescent transitions to adult healthcare providers.

parents of routine health promotion and maintenance needs of all children in the family such as immunizations, dental hygiene, and any screening tests. See Chapters 8–10 ∞.

Discuss parenting approaches for the child with a chronic condition. Encourage a structured environment with limitations that are developmentally appropriate for the child. Assist the family as needed in providing a nurturing environment and offering praise for achievement of tasks.

Facilitate Education Service Planning

Assist the family with school entry of the child with a chronic condition. Discussions with the family can assist them in defining appropriate expectations and goals. The nurse can also take a role in communicating with school personnel about any classroom modifications required by the child, and in educating teachers and other school personnel about the medical or assistive equipment used by the child. This information is then integrated into the child's Individual Health Plan (IHP), which may be a stand-alone plan or tied to an IEP. The school nurse can also play a key role in assisting the family with Section 504 planning activities by serving as a liaison between the school and the child's healthcare team. Key health records that are needed for the planning of the IHP should be assembled after the family provides informed consent. Encourage the family to establish regular communication with the school personnel and school nurse.

In the case of a Do Not Resuscitate (DNR) request for the child at school, encourage collaboration with school personnel, teachers, and other members of the healthcare team as necessary to facilitate an agreement between the school and family. Many school systems do not have a policy that permits honoring a DNR request, and the school nurse is an important liaison in the discussion and development of the policy. Refer to Chapter 14 ∞ for further discussion of DNR requests in school.

Support Family's Psychosocial Adjustment

Collaborate with the child and parents and provide them the opportunity to discuss how the experience of a chronic illness affects their daily lives (Jacobs, 2002). Well siblings may feel neglected by parents due to the time-consuming care process for the child with a chronic condition. Listening and offering strategies to improve the organization of care, as well as the use of community and family supports, can help enhance the family's coping. Help the family see that simple chores performed by the social network can reduce stress, especially during times when the child is hospitalized, such as meals cooked for the family, transportation for well siblings to recreational events, or picking up needed supplies at the supermarket. Referral to a support group for parents, as well as siblings, may assist the family with information, encouragement, and care suggestions (Keefe, 2003). Counseling may be helpful to parents experiencing marital stress.

Assist the family to provide information to the siblings about the child's disability at the appropriate developmental level. Provide instructional materials, videos, books, pamphlets, and other information when available. Inform the parents that siblings of the child with a chronic condition may experience a range of feelings including jealousy, anger, grief, denial, and aggression. Encourage the parents to allow the siblings to express their feelings and concerns. Conflicts or resentment may arise when older siblings are requested to assume increasing responsibility in the care of the child, especially when it interferes with social and recreational activities. Discuss ways of determining the appropriate balance of responsibilities for each family member. If available, referral to support groups for siblings may be beneficial.

Emergency Preparedness

Advance planning is needed to ensure that medically fragile children who need technology for survival or have the potential for life-threatening episodes have the necessary resources in the event of a disaster. The designated shelter for such children, with health professionals and electrical power for the needed equipment, should be identified and known to the family. In the meantime, battery packs for power backup should be available at all times. Additionally, parents need to arrange for durable power of attorney so that consent for emergency medical care can be available as needed. The child and parents may become separated during the disaster, or the parents may become injured and unable to care for the child.

CLINICAL TIP

Special accommodations for the child with disabilities may include extending test-taking times, tutors, note-takers, and the use of technological equipment to assist in the learning environment. Encourage parents to ask questions regarding computer accessibility, arrangements for tutors or note-takers, private-study areas, and individualized attention.

GROWTH & DEVELOPMENT

Siblings of children with a chronic condition may feel overwhelmingly guilty about their feelings of jealousy, shame, and anger. Inform the child that these feelings are normal and that the child is not "bad" for having these feelings.

Evaluation

Expected outcomes for care of the family of a child with a chronic condition may include:

- The child and family establish effective coping mechanisms.
- The child and family experience reduced anxiety.
- The child and family demonstrate understanding and management of the condition.
- Parenting patterns are appropriate and supportive of the child's growth and development.
- Role conflict and caregiver strain are minimized.
- Caregivers achieve adequate rest, sleep, and socialization.
- The child and family adjust to the child's chronic condition.
- The adolescent successfully transitions to adult health services and living arrangements.

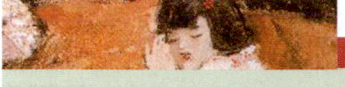

CRITICAL THINKING IN ACTION

Recall Haley, the 8-year-old child with cerebral palsy who will be attending school for the first time. Her mother believes that attending school will help promote her social development and broaden what she can learn. She also thinks that some of the special health services that Haley needs may be available in school, such as physical therapy and speech therapy. Haley's mother has asked for the clinic nurse's advice to help plan her daughter's transition to school. Haley's mother and nurse discuss the potential accommodations that Haley will need for her mobility limitations. The nurse suggests that Haley receive a full educational evaluation so her educational needs can be identified. Once the mother has signed consent, the clinic nurse prepares a summary of Haley's health history for the school nurse that can be used to develop her IEP and IHP.

1. Describe the potential signs and symptoms of cerebral palsy that might be important to consider when Haley's IEP and IHP are developed (see Chapter 26 for more information on cerebral palsy).

2. Based upon Haley's age and developmental stage, what feelings, fears, and concerns might she experience related to entering school?

3. Describe the role of the nurse as Haley's care coordinator.

4. What education does the mother need to prepare her for serving as Haley's advocate with school administrators when her IEP and IHP are developed?

 Refer to your Prentice Hall Nursing MediaLink DVD-ROM for answers.

EXPLORE MediaLink 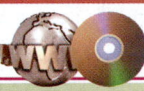 http://www.prenhall.com/ball

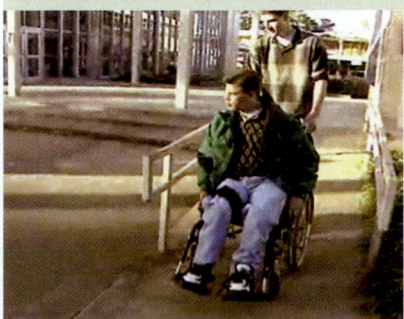

Resources for this chapter can be found on the Prentice Hall Nursing MediaLink DVD-ROM accompanying this textbook, and on the Companion Website at http://www.prenhall.com/ball.

DVD-ROM
Audio Glossary
NCLEX-RN® Review
Video
   School Reentry

COMPANION WEBSITE
Audio Glossary
NCLEX-RN® Review
Care Plan Activity: An Adolescent with Down Syndrome
Case Study: Preschool Entry for a Child with Asthma
MediaLink Applications
   Advocacy and Children with Special Needs
   Health Promotion and Health Maintenance
   IDEA
   IEP
   Individual School Health Plan
   Optimizing Classroom Learning
   Spina Bifida
WebLinks

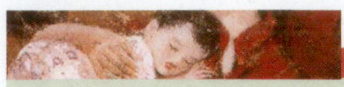

REFERENCES

Allen, P. J. (2004). The primary care provider and children with chronic conditions. In P. J. Allen & J. A. Vessey, *Primary care of the child with a chronic condition* (4th ed., pp. 3–22), St. Louis: Mosby.

American Academy of Pediatrics. (2001a). Policy statement: Assessment of maltreatment of children with disabilities. *Pediatrics, 108*(2), 508–512.

American Academy of Pediatrics. (2001b). The continued importance of supplemental security income (SSI) for children and adolescents with disabilities. *Pediatrics, 107*(4), 790–793.

American Academy of Pediatrics. (2005a). Care coordination in the medical home: Integrating health and related systems of care for children with special health care needs. *Pediatrics, 116*(5), 1238–1244.

American Academy of Pediatrics. (2005b). Helping families raise children with special health care needs at home. *Pediatrics, 115*(2), 507–511.

Ballard, K. L. (2004). Meeting the needs of siblings of children with cancer. *Pediatric Nursing, 30*(5), 394–401.

Beckman, P. J. (2002). Providing family-centered services. In M. L. Batshaw (Ed.), *Children with Disabilities* (5th ed., pp. 683–691). Baltimore, MD: Paul H. Brookes Publishing Co.

Blann, L. E. (2005). Early intervention for children and families with special needs. *Maternal Child Nursing, 30*(4), 263–267.

Chevarley, F. M. (2006). Utilization and expenditures for children with special health care needs (Research Findings #24, Medical Expenditure Panel Survey). Rockville, MD: Agency for Healthcare Research and Quality.

Coffey, J. S. (2006). Parenting a child with chronic illness: A metasynthesis. *Pediatric Nursing, 32*(1), 51–59.

Dusing, S. C., Skinner, A. C., & Mayer, M. L. (2004). Unmet need for therapy services, assistive devices, and related services: Data from the National Survey of Children with Special Health Care Needs. *Ambulatory Pediatrics, 4*(5), 448–454.

Fanos, J. H., Fahrner, K., Jelveh, M., King, R., & Tejeda, D. (2004). The sibling center: A pilot program for siblings of children and adolescents with a serious medical condition. *Journal of Pediatrics, 146*, 831–835.

Farmer, J. E., Marien, W. E., Clark, M. J., Sherman, A., & Selva, T. J. (2004). Primary care supports for children with chronic health conditions: Identifying and predicting unmet family needs. *Journal of Pediatric Psychology, 29*(5), 355–367.

Gasalberti, D. (2006). Alternative therapies for children and youth with special health care needs. *Journal of Pediatric Health Care, 20*(2), 133–136.

Goble, L. A. (2004). The impact of a child's chronic illness on fathers. *Issues in Comprehensive Pediatric Nursing, 27*(3), 153–162.

Harrigan, R. C., Ratliffe, C., Patrinos, M. E., & Alice, T. (2002). Medically fragile children: An integrative review of the literature and recommendations on future research. *Issues in Comprehensive Pediatric Nursing, 25*, 1–20.

Honberg, L., McPherson, M., Strickland, B., Gage, J. C., & Newacheck, P. W. (2005). Assuring adequate health insurance: Results of the National Survey of Children with Special Health Care Needs. *Pediatrics, 115*(5), 1233–1239.

Inkelas, M., & Garro, N. (2005). A picture of needs for children with special health care needs: What we are learning from the national survey. *Journal of Pediatric Nursing, 20*(3), 207–210.

Jacobs, L. A. (2002). Living with a chronically ill child. *American Journal of Nursing, 102*(5), 24A–24C.

Kearney, P. M., & Griffin, T. (2001). Between joy and sorrow: Being a parent of a child with a developmental disability. *Journal of Advanced Nursing, 34*(5), 582–592.

Keefe, S. (2003). Parenting a child with special needs. *Advance for Nurse Practitioners, 11*(10), 73–80.

Kessenich, M. (2003). Developmental outcomes of premature, low birth weight, and medically fragile infants. *Newborn and Infant Nursing, 3*(3), 80–87.

Knafl, K. A., & Deatrick, J. A. (2002). The challenge of normalization for families of children with chronic conditions. *Pediatric Nursing, 28*(1), 49–54.

Kuster, P. A., Badr, L. K., Chang, B. L., Wuerker, A. K., & Benjamin, A. E. (2004). Factors influencing health promoting activities of mothers caring for ventilator-assisted children. *Journal of Pediatric Nursing, 19*(4), 276–287.

Lindeke, L. L., Leonard, B. J., Presler, B., & Garwick, A. (2002). Family-centered care coordination for children with special needs across multiple settings. *Journal of Pediatric Health Care, 16*(6), 290–297.

Lotstein, D. S., McPherson, M., Strickland, B., & Newacheck, P. W. (2005). Transition planning for youth with special health care needs: Results from the national survey of children with special health care needs. *Pediatrics, 115*(6), 1562–1568.

Maytum, J. C., Heiman, M. B., & Garwick, A. W. (2004). Compassion fatigue and burnout in nurses who work with children with chronic conditions and their families. *Journal of Pediatric Health Care, 18*(4), 171–179.

Meleski, D. D. (2002). Families with chronically ill children. *American Journal of Nursing, 102*(5), 47–54.

Melnyk, B. M., Feinstein, N. F., Moldenhouer, Z., & Small, L. (2001). Coping in parents of children who are chronically ill: Strategies for assessment and intervention. *Pediatric Nursing, 27*(6), 548–558.

Moses, M., Gilchrest, C., & Schwab, N. C. (2005). Section 504 of the Rehabilitation Act: Determining eligibility and implications for school districts. *Journal of School Nursing, 21*(1), 48–58.

Msall, M. E., Avery, R. C., Tremont, M. R., Lima, J. C., Rogers, M. L., & Hogan, D. P. (2003). Functional disability and school activity limitations in 41,300 school children: Relationship to medical impairments. *Pediatrics, 111*(3), 548–553.

Newacheck, P. W., & Kim, S. E. (2005). A national profile of health care utilization and expenditures for children with special health care needs. *Archives of Pediatric and Adolescent Medicine, 159*(1), 10–17.

Nuutila, L., & Salanterä, S. (2006). Children with a long-term illness: Parents' experiences of care. *Journal of Pediatric Nursing, 21*(2), 153–160.

O'Brien, M. E., & Wegner, C. B. (2002). Rearing the child who is technology dependent: Perceptions of parents and home care nurses. *Journal of Society of Pediatric Nursing, 7*(1), 7–15.

Ratliffe, C. E., Harrigan, R. C., Haley, J., Tse, A., & Olson, T. (2002). Stress in families with medically fragile children. *Issues in Comprehensive Pediatric Nursing, 25*, 167–188.

Ray, L. D. (2002). Parenting and childhood chronicity: Making visible the invisible work. *Journal of Pediatric Nursing, 17*(16), 424–438.

Rees, C. A. (2005). Thinking about children's attachment. *Archives of Disease in Childhood, 90*, 1058–1065.

Rehm, R. S. (2003). Cultural intersections in the care of Mexican American children with chronic conditions. *Pediatric Nursing, 29*(6), 434–439.

Rehm, R. S., & Rohr, J. A. (2002). Parents', nurses', and educators' perceptions of risks and benefits of school attendance by children who are medically fragile/technology-dependent. *Journal of Pediatric Nursing, 17*(5), 345–354.

Sawin, K. J., Cox, A. W., & Metzger, S. G. (2004). Transitions to adulthood, In P. J. Allen & J. A. Vessey, *Primary care of the child with a chronic condition* (4th ed., pp.137–152). St. Louis: Mosby.

Scal, P., & Ireland, M. (2005). Addressing transition to adult health care for adolescents with special health care needs. *Pediatrics, 115*(6), 1607–1612.

Swallow, V. M., & Jacoby, A. (2001). Mothers' coping in chronic childhood illness: The effect of presymptomatic diagnosis of vesicoureteric reflux. *Journal of Advanced Nursing, 33*(1), 69–78.

Telfair, J., Alleman-Velez, P. L., Dickens, P., & Loosier, P. S. (2005). Quality health care for adolescents with special health care needs: Issues and clinical implications. *Journal of Pediatric Nursing, 20*(1), 15–24.

U.S. Department of Education. (2000). *A guide to the Individualized Education Program.* Retrieved July 30, 2006, from http://www.ed.gov/ parents/needs/speced/iepguide/index.html

U.S. Department of Health and Human Services. (2000). *Healthy People 2010* (2nd ed.). Washington, DC: U.S. Government Printing Office. www.healthypeople.gov

Van Dyke, P. C., Kogan, M. D., McPherson, M. G., Weissman, G. R., & Newacheck, P. W. (2004). Prevalence and characteristics of children with special health care needs. *Archives of Pediatric and Adolescent Medicine, 158*(9), 884–890.

Vessey, J. A., & Rumsey, M. (2004). Chronic conditions and child development. In P. J. Allen & J. A. Vessey, *Primary care of the child with a chronic condition* (4th ed., pp. 23–43). St. Louis: Mosby.

Wang, K. K., & Barnard, A. (2004). Technology-dependent children and their families: A review. *Journal of Advanced Nursing, 45*(1), 36–46.

Williams, P. D., Williams, A. R., Graff, J. C., Hanson, S., Stanton, A., Hafeman, C., et al. (2003). A community-based intervention for siblings and parents of children with chronic illness or disability: The ISEE study. *Journal of Pediatrics, 143*, 386–393.

NURSING CONSIDERATIONS FOR THE HOSPITALIZED CHILD

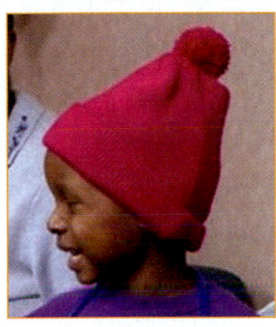 **FIVE-YEAR-OLD** Tiara has a history of obstructive sleep apnea and is scheduled for a tonsillectomy and adenoidectomy (T&A) in the morning. Her mother has brought her in today for pre-op evaluation and instruction. Tiara has no other health problems. Her experience with health care is limited to well-child checkups and immunizations as well as several visits to the otolaryngologist in the past year. She has no prior hospitalizations. Tiara will return in the morning at 6:30 a.m. for surgery. She will be admitted to the pediatric day hospital unit following surgery and plans to spend one night on the unit.

How can the nurse assess what Tiara knows about the surgery? What techniques should be used to teach Tiara about the surgery? What instructions should Tiara's mother receive from the nurse in the pre-op clinic related to care prior to surgery?

KEY TERMS

MediaLink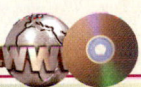

http://www.prenhall.com/ball

See the Prentice Hall Nursing MediaLink DVD-ROM and Companion Website for chapter-specific resources.

LEARNING OUTCOMES

After reading this chapter, you will be able to do the following:

1. Discuss the child's understanding of health and illness according to psychosocial and developmental levels.

2. Discuss the effects of and response to illness and hospitalization on children and their families.

3. Discuss the child's and family's adaptation to hospitalization.

4. Identify nursing strategies to enhance the hospitalization experience for children and their families.

5. Identify nursing strategies to minimize the stressors related to hospitalization.

6. Discuss strategies for preparing children and families for discharge from the hospital setting.

7. Evaluate the effectiveness of teaching strategies used with the hospitalized child and the family.

H ospitalization, whether it is elective, planned in advance, or the result of an emergency or trauma, is stressful for children of all ages and their families. Many pediatric conditions can be managed within the home and community setting; therefore, hospitalization is not necessarily a requirement to manage the child with an illness (Flores et al., 2003) (Box 13–1). However, while fewer children require hospitalization, those who are hospitalized usually have a higher level of illness acuity.

Hospitalized children experience a variety of emotions as they are in an unknown environment, surrounded by strangers, exposed to unfamiliar equipment, and witnessing frightening sights and sounds. These children are subjected to unfamiliar procedures, some of which are invasive or painful, and may even require surgery. For both children and families, routines are disrupted and normal coping strategies are tested.

Nurses today are challenged to provide individualized care for the hospitalized child with complex medical conditions, acute illnesses, or injury. A key role of nurses caring for hospitalized children and their families includes addressing the psychosocial concerns that accompany hospitalization. To minimize the stress of hospitalization, nurses provide support and education to children and their families before, during, and after hospitalization.

During hospitalization, nurses use a family-centered approach and work collaboratively with parents to implement various strategies to promote coping and adaptation and to prepare children for necessary procedures. Nurses are instrumental in ensuring that the developmental and educational needs of children are met, especially when hospitalization is prolonged. Nurses also collaborate with members of a multidisciplinary team and partner with families to assist them in preparation for discharge home or transfer to a long-term care or rehabilitation facility.

MediaLink

A Child's Eye View: Hospitalization

EFFECTS OF HOSPITALIZATION ON CHILDREN AND THEIR FAMILIES

Children's Understanding of Health and Illness

As a child, can you remember thinking that yelling at your mother caused your strep throat? Perhaps as an adolescent you believed that you would never become ill or have an accident. Maybe you feared being in a car crash like that of a friend. Young children have limited knowledge about the body and its relation to health and illness. They do not have the ability to understand how organs work and how they can be affected by illness (Koopman, Baars, Chaplin, & Zwinderman, 2004). Their understanding is based primarily on their cognitive ability at various developmental stages and on previous experiences with healthcare professionals. As children get older they move from having no concept of illness to being able to understand multiple factors related to illness (Koopman et al., 2004). Table 13–1 provides a discussion of childrens' understanding of health and illness according to their developmental level.

BOX 13–1

RESEARCH—CHILD AND PARENTAL EDUCATION TO REDUCE INCIDENCE OF PEDIATRIC HOSPITALIZATIONS

A recent study revealed that many pediatric hospitalizations might be avoided if parents and the child were better educated about the child's condition, medications, importance of avoiding known disease triggers, and the importance of follow-up care. The most frequent conditions for which hospitalization could be avoided through timely and effective outpatient care were asthma, dehydration and gastroenteritis, pneumonia, seizure disorder, and skin infections. Better education can often lead to early treatment at home and decreased need for hospitalization (Flores et al., 2003). Nurses can collaborate with physicians and others to educate parents about the child's condition, proper administration of medications, need for outpatient follow-up, and avoiding known disease triggers. By determining the child and family's level of understanding of the disease/condition, the nurse can directly collaborate with the family to help reduce the number of avoidable hospitalizations.

Table 13–1	**CHILDREN'S UNDERSTANDING OF HEALTH AND ILLNESS ACCORDING TO DEVELOPMENTAL LEVEL**			
Infant	**Toddler and Preschooler**	**School-Age Child**	**Adolescent**	
By approximately 6 months of age, infants have developed an awareness of themselves as separate from their mother or father.	Toddlers and preschoolers are beginning to understand illness, but not its cause.	Understands how germs are spread.	Increasingly aware of the physiologic, psychologic, and behavioral causes of illness and injury.	
Feels anxious when approached by strangers.	May view illness as a form of punishment for bad behavior or as something magical.	Concept of body parts and function is maturing.	Understands how symptoms can be related to certain organ functions in the body.	
Infant is unaware of the effects of illness.	Events that occur just before the onset of the illness may be mistakenly associated with the illness. The child's concept of the body usually is limited to names and locations of some body parts. Preschoolers have a beginning understanding of germs but not how they are spread. Concept of internal organs and bodily functions is vague.	Has a more realistic understanding of the reasons for illness and is able to understand more about the disease and how body organs are affected.	Understands that disease may involve several causes and effects and that multiple organs or body parts may be involved. Concerned with appearance and perceives an illness or injury in terms of its effect on his or her body image.	

Adapted from: Koopman, Baars, Chaplin, & Zwinderman (2004); McQuaid, Howard, Kopel, Rosenblum, & Bibace (2002); Myant & Williams (2005); Peltzer & Promtussananon (2003); Williams & Binnie (2002).

Hospitalization and medical procedures are significant sources of stress for children (Lau, 2002). The child's attempts to deal with these stressors impact both the psychological and physiological well-being of the child (Ryan-Wenger, Sharrer, & Campbell, 2005). Hospitalization disrupts the child's and family's lifestyle. Infants, toddlers, and preschoolers lack the cognitive skills to understand hospitalization and are the most likely age groups to exhibit regression behaviors. Young children have fears and anxieties related to things such as the dark, strangers, and monsters. Hospitalization can exacerbate those anxieties given that the child is in a strange environment. In addition to dealing with these stressors, the child may feel a threat to his or her well-being (Lau, 2002).

Significant stressors for hospitalized children of all ages include:

- Separation from parents or the primary caretaker (or peers)
- Loss of self-control, autonomy, and privacy
- Painful and/or invasive procedures
- Fear of bodily injury and disfigurement

Table 13–2 highlights key stressors of hospitalization for children at each developmental stage. The effects of hospitalization according to developmental stage are discussed in the following section.

Nursing care of the hospitalized child focuses on minimizing the child's fears, anxieties, and disruption of the child's usual routine, and supporting the family. Strategies include minimizing separation anxiety, loss of control, pain related to procedures, and fear of bodily injury and disfigurement.

Infant

By about 6 months of age, infants have developed an awareness of themselves as separate from their mother or father. They are able to identify primary caretakers and to feel anxious when in contact with strangers. Hospitalization can be a traumatic time for an infant, particularly if the parents are not staying with the child. They can sense the anxiety their parents are experiencing during a hospitalization.

The most common stressor of hospitalization for the infant is separation from parents, which is manifested by **separation anxiety**. Bowlby and Robertson identified

Table 13–2	STRESSORS OF HOSPITALIZATION FOR CHILDREN AT VARIOUS DEVELOPMENTAL STAGES	
Developmental Stages	**Responses**	**Nursing Implications**
Infant Separation anxiety Stranger anxiety Painful, invasive procedures Immobilization Sleep deprivation, sensory overload	Sleep-awake cycle disrupted Feeding routines disrupted Displays excessive irritability	Encourage parental presence Adhere to infant's home routine as much as possible Utilize topical anesthetics or pre-procedural sedation as prescribed Promote a quiet environment and reduce excess stimuli
Toddler Separation anxiety Loss of self-control Immobilization Painful, invasive procedures Bodily injury or mutilation Fear of the dark	Is frightened if forced to lie supine Associates pain with punishment Wonders why parents don't come to the rescue	Encourage parental presence Allow parents to hold child in their lap for examinations and procedures when possible Allow choices when possible Utilize topical anesthetics or pre-procedural sedation as prescribed Explain all procedures Provide a "night-light" or flashlight
Preschooler Separation anxiety and fear of abandonment Loss of self-control Bodily injury or mutilation Painful, invasive procedures Fear of the dark	Displays difficulty separating reality from fantasy Fears ghosts and monsters Fears body parts will leak out Fears that tubes are permanent Demonstrates withdrawal, projection, aggression, regression	Encourage parental presence Allow choices when possible Utilize topical anesthetics or pre-procedural sedation as prescribed Explain all procedures Provide a "night-light" or flashlight
School-Age Child Loss of control Loss of privacy and control over bodily functions Bodily injury Separation from family and friends Painful, invasive procedures Fear of death	Displays increased sensitivity to the environment Demonstrates detailed recall of events to self and other patients	Encourage parental participation Allow the child choices when possible Explain all procedures and offer reassurance Utilize topical anesthetics or pre-procedural sedation as prescribed Encourage peer interaction
Adolescent Loss of control Fear of altered body image, disfigurement, disability, and death Separation from peer group Loss of privacy and identity	Displays denial, regression, withdrawal, intellectualization, projection, displacement	Include the adolescent in the plan of care Encourage discussion of fears and anxieties Explain all procedures Ask the adolescent his or her desire for parental involvement Encourage peer interaction

CLINICAL TIP

Parents often feel guilty for leaving their child, especially if the child protests adamantly or cries upon return. Support the parents and reassure them that this protest is a normal behavior and it represents healthy parent-infant attachment. Support them as they leave and provide information for them when they return about what the child's activities have been.

three phases of separation anxiety exhibited in young children who were separated from their mothers for long periods of time (Alsop-Shields & Mohay, 2001). Box 13–2 further describes their work. Characteristic behaviors of children in the three phases of separation anxiety are listed in Table 13–3. Infants, as well as toddlers who are hospitalized, often display some of these behaviors, particularly if parents are unable to remain with the child. In addition to separation anxiety, infants between 6 and 18 months of age may display **stranger anxiety** (wariness of strangers) when confronted with strangers such as healthcare professionals.

Other stressors to the infant include painful procedures, immobilization of extremities, and sleep deprivation caused by disruption of normal sleep patterns and routines.

Because parent-infant attachment is critical to the infant's developmental achievements (see Chapter 3 ∞), the nurse encourages the family to remain with, and be active participants in care of, the hospitalized infant. If parents are unable to remain at the hospital, support visiting the infant as often as possible.

BOX 13–2
THE WORK OF BOWLBY AND ROBERTSON

John Bowlby and James Robertson developed the classic theory of separation anxiety that changed visitation practices in hospitals and pediatric units. While the initial research focused on separation from mother, further work spoke to separation from the parent or primary caregiver. The three stages of separation anxiety were identified as protest, despair, and denial (or detachment). In the initial stage the child resists or protests the parents' departure. This stage may last for several hours or days. After a period of time the child becomes hopeless of the parents return and appears to have "settled in." During this stage of despair the child is quiet and makes little demands on the environment and the hospital staff. This stage is often mistaken for adaptation to the hospital. Before the development of this theory, parents were restricted from visiting their hospitalized child because many viewed this return visit as upsetting to the child, since the child in this stage frequently cries when the parent returns. Robertson and Bowlby viewed this as an opportunity for the child to release his or her emotions. The final stage, denial or detachment, in which the child shows more interest in the environment and little interest in visits from parents, is very rare, especially now that policies in hospitals have changed to allow parents to stay at the bedside. The work of Bowlby and Robertson is an essential component of family-centered nursing care and must continue to be incorporated as policies related to family presence are formulated.

Data from: Alsop-Shields, L., & Mohay, H. (2001). John Bowlby and James Robertson: Theorists, scientists and crusaders for improvements in the care of children in hospital. *Journal of Advanced Nursing, 35*(1) 50–58.

Table 13–3	STAGES OF SEPARATION ANXIETY	
Protest	**Despair**	**Denial (detachment)**
Screaming, crying	Sadness	Lack of protest when parents leave
Clinging to parents	Quiet, appear to have "settled in"	Appearance of being happy and content with everyone
May resist attempts by other adults to comfort them	Withdrawal or compliant behavior	Shows interest in surroundings
	Crying when parents return	Close relationships not established

Adapted from: Alsop-Shields, L., & Mohay, H. (2001). John Bowlby and James Robertson: Theorists, scientists and crusaders for improvements in the care of children in hospital. *Journal of Advanced Nursing, 35*(1) 50–58.

Parents may be hesitant to touch, hold, or provide care for an infant who has tubes and wires attached. They may be afraid of hurting the child or dislodging equipment. Parents may not be aware that it might be okay for them to hold their child. The nurse should advise parents when it is appropriate and assist them as needed.

Toddler

Toddlers are the group most at risk for a stressful experience as a result of illness and hospitalization. This age group is old enough to understand that their routine has been disrupted, but they lack the cognitive ability to understand why. Separation from parents is the major stressor and they protest vigorously when their parents depart. Having activities limited and being confined especially threaten children in this age group. Fear of pain, fear of the dark, fear of invasive procedures, fear of change, and fear of mutilation are additional common stressors for the toddler.

When a parent cannot be present, reminders can be left with the child. These might include a piece of cloth saturated with the mother's favorite perfume or father's cologne (unless the child has a respiratory condition or another contraindication for this intervention), an object belonging to the parent, or an audiotape or videotape with messages from the parents.

Disruption of routine also causes stress for the toddler. The nurse encourages parents to remain present as much as possible for important rituals such as toileting, carrying out bedtime routines, and singing favorite nursery rhymes. Autonomy is the developmental task of the toddler (see Chapter 3 ∞). When possible, maintain the

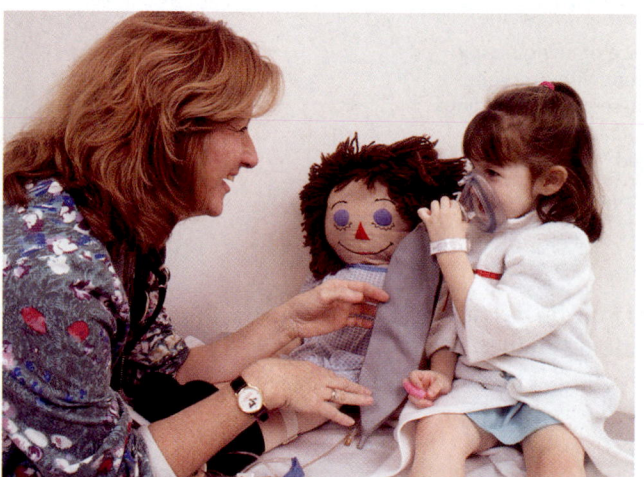

Figure 13–1 ➤ This pediatric nurse wears a colorful uniform to decrease anxiety associated with white uniforms.

toddler's normal home routines for bathing and other activities. Allow the toddler to have choices when possible, such as choosing the color of Jell-o or which gown to wear.

Preschooler

The greatest stressors to preschoolers are the fear of being alone, fear of the dark, fear of abandonment, fear of loss of self-control related to the body and emotions, and fear of bodily injury or mutilation. They may feel guilty about being sick or may view the illness and hospitalization as punishment.

Just as with the toddler, preschoolers desire maintenance of a normal routine. To promote a sense of initiative, the developmental task of the preschool child (see Chapter 3 ∞), the nurse works with the family to maintain routines as much as possible and to encourage the preschool child's independence through offering choices. Nurses who interact with children in this age group should also wear colorful uniforms with familiar designs when possible (Figure 13–1 ➤).

Preschoolers want to know when to expect their parents to return to the hospital. Responding with simple statements such as "after supper" or "before breakfast" gives preschoolers an understanding of the anticipated time since they will not understand "3:00" or "12:00." Encourage parents to make telephone calls to preschoolers if possible. Some parents are able to make calls from work. Hearing their parent's voice and confirming that they will return to the hospital offers preschoolers a sense of security.

Parents often believe that leaving while their children are asleep is better for their children. In actuality, when children do not expect their parents to be absent and they awaken to find their parents gone, they become anxious and may even develop a lack of trust. Encourage parents to tell children when they need to leave and why (e.g., has to go to work or go home). Providing honest information to children gives the assurance that the parent or caregiver can be trusted.

School-Age Child

Major sources of stress for hospitalized school-age children are loss of control related to bodily functions, privacy issues, fear of bodily injury, pain, and concerns related to death. School-age children may also experience separation from family as well as school friends. The child relies on parents and others for support and understanding during stressful events and procedures. School-age children attempt to maintain their composure during painful or invasive procedures but generally still require a great deal of support.

Concepts of time are well-formed, and parents who cannot remain at the bedside are encouraged to tell the child when they will return. Parents are also encouraged to be available for telephone calls to provide support and comfort. As with the toddler and preschooler, stressful procedures can lead to regression or other behavioral changes. Inform the parents that this behavior is normal during stressful situations.

To promote a sense of industry (see Chapter 3 ∞), allow children to participate in their care as much as possible. They should also be encouraged to continue with school work and engage in creative outlets such as art or crafts. Allow the school-age child choices when possible.

Adolescent

Separation from peers, home, and school are major stressors experienced by hospitalized adolescents. Additional stressors for the hospitalized adolescent include fear of bodily injury or changes in body image, disability, pain, and even death. Loss of control, privacy, and independence are also major stressors. Preoccupation with appearance and body image are paramount in this age group. Education and explanations that focus on these issues will provide significant reassurance to the adolescent. Adolescents may experience more dependence on their parents, leading to frustration and anger. Adolescents often try to maintain rigid self-control when undergoing painful and invasive procedures.

The adolescent desires privacy and independence. The nurse who respects these desires and demonstrates interest is often successful in establishing a trusting relationship and assisting the adolescent to cope with the hospitalization and illness. The adolescent is encouraged to discuss thoughts and feelings about experiences. Careful listening by the nurse is essential to establishing a positive rapport.

Educating the adolescent and the family about normal development helps alleviate stress and promote individuation. Treat the hospitalized adolescent as normally as possible, and assist him or her through the developmental tasks of adolescence by fostering learning of appropriate social and coping skills, allowing choices whenever possible, and enhancing self-esteem (Pinckney & Stuart, 2004).

Family Responses to Hospitalization

The illness and hospitalization of a child disrupt a family's usual routines. Parental roles change when a child is being cared for by others in the hospital setting (Simons, 2002). Roles may be altered as one parent remains at the hospital with the child while the other parent or siblings take on additional tasks at home. Family members may experience anxiety and fear, especially when the outcome is unknown or the reason for hospitalization is a potentially serious health condition. Parents who perceive their child is in pain find the experience difficult and require support. Coping is made more difficult by a serious emergency, lengthy illness, chronic condition, poor prognosis, lack of family support, and lack of financial or community services. The burden of missed work, additional expenses, and concern regarding care for children at home compound the stress the family experiences with a hospitalized child. (See Chapter 14 ∞ for a description of nursing support for the family of a child with a life-threatening illness or injury.)

Parents have unique needs and stressors. Nurses should individualize care based on these specific needs (Melynk, Small, & Carno, 2004). Needs that are frequently identified by parents of hospitalized children include the need to be informed, to be seen as a competent parent, to have some control, and to have competent caregivers (Hallström, Runesson, & Elander, 2002). It is essential that nurses assess parental needs and keep parents informed of the child's condition and treatment in order to establish a trusting relationship (Thompson, Hupcey & Clark, 2003). Parents who have support from nursing staff have less anxiety and are better equipped to make decisions and participate in their child's care.

Nurses also need to be alert to cultural patterns in the family that can influence the response to hospitalization and the family's management of the experience, such as views of health and illness and causation of illness. Cultural influences may also determine who the decision maker is in the family regarding healthcare practices, and provide guidelines for acceptable treatments (Spector, 2004).

Siblings' Experience

The siblings of a hospitalized child may receive little attention from the parents who are overwhelmed and anxious about their hospitalized child's health. Parents are preoccupied and may not consider taking the siblings to visit the child in the hospital. It is important for siblings to see the hospitalized child as soon as possible. Often the siblings' perception of what is happening is worse than what is actually going on. How siblings respond is dependent on a variety of factors including age, developmental level, available coping mechanisms, prognosis of the ill child, and perception of the illness (Van Riper, 2003). The siblings may fantasize about the illness or injury and the appearance of their brother or sister. Siblings who are not adequately informed about the hospitalized child's condition may fear that the child will be disabled or die, even when this is unlikely. Younger siblings who do not understand the causes of illness and hospitalization may feel guilty about fighting with or being mean to their brother or sister in the past and believe that they played a role in causing his or her illness. Siblings often have nightmares about the illness or injury their brother or sister has sustained and about the ill child dying (see Chapter 14 ∞ for further discussion of siblings' responses to the dying child).

As family roles and routines continue to change, siblings may feel insecure and anxious. Behavioral problems may develop, or school performance may deteriorate.

Siblings may feel jealous because the ill brother or sister seems to monopolize the parents' attention. Siblings of hospitalized children may demonstrate behaviors ranging from jealousy or envy to resentment, guilt and hostility, anger, insecurity, regression, and fear. Given support and the opportunity to be actively involved, however, the siblings of an ill child can manage well.

As the parents' focus shifts to the hospitalized child, they may need support in dealing with the healthy siblings. Siblings may feel left out when everyone's attention is focused on the ill child. Recognize that siblings may fear becoming ill themselves or believe that they played a role in the child's illness. Siblings need reassurance that they did not cause the illness. Help parents to inform siblings about their brother or sister's condition and hospitalization using language and concepts appropriate to their ages and developmental levels (Ballard, 2004).

As appropriate, encourage siblings to visit. Such a visit is especially encouraged if the child could potentially die; this allows the sibling the opportunity to say good-bye (see Chapter 14 ∞ for further discussion of the dying child). These visits often help to lift the spirits of the hospitalized child and assist siblings to overcome any misconceptions or negative emotions. Because children's fantasies are often worse than reality, unfounded fears may be relieved by a visit.

The nurse prepares the siblings before the visit by explaining sights and sounds likely experienced and by describing how their brother or sister will appear. If the hospitalized child acts, moves, talks, or appears different than usual, provide an explanation beforehand. Describe the hospital environment, including equipment, sounds, and smells. Using a doll, drawing pictures, or showing an actual picture of the child can help prepare the siblings. See Families Want to Know: Strategies for Working with Siblings of a Hospitalized Child.

During the visit, demonstrate how to talk to and touch the ill child and encourage the siblings to do the same. After the visit, discuss with siblings what they saw and felt, and answer any questions they may have. When siblings cannot visit, contact with the hospitalized child can be maintained by sending pictures, drawings, cards, and messages recorded on audiotapes or videotapes, and through e-mail or instant messaging. Collaborate with the family to determine the most appropriate and effective method of communicating if the sibling is unable to visit.

If parents are staying at the hospital with the hospitalized child, help them to establish a routine for the well siblings. For example, encourage them to call the siblings at home at a regular time each night. Allowing the siblings at home the opportunity to share their day, and to receive an update on the hospitalized child, provides a feeling of connectedness and may minimize feelings of jealousy and resentment. The phone call offers siblings a consistent link to their parents as well as the reassurance that they are important and loved.

CLINICAL TIP

Children should be screened prior to visiting a hospitalized sibling on the pediatric unit. Children with fever or other symptoms of infectious disease should not be allowed to visit. The child's hand might be stamped with a smiley face or a sticker might be placed on his or her shirt to indicate the child is okay to visit.

FAMILIES WANT TO KNOW

Strategies for Working with Siblings of a Hospitalized Child

The nurse working with siblings of a hospitalized child can implement the following strategies to assist the siblings in understanding:

- Be truthful. Explain why the child is hospitalized, what the treatment involves, and how long the hospitalization is expected to last.
- Assure siblings that they did not cause the illness and that the hospitalized child did nothing wrong. If a sibling had some involvement in or responsibility for the health crisis, referral for psychological counseling is needed.
- Allow siblings to ask questions and discuss fears and other feelings.

- Encourage siblings to visit if possible. Cover tubes and wires with a sheet. Wash off blood or cover bloody bandages if possible. Prepare them for any equipment, dressing, and procedures they might see, and any sounds they might hear.
- Warn siblings if the hospitalized child is not speaking. Say something like "John can't talk now. He seems to be sleeping deeply. He may be able to hear, though, so you can touch him and talk to him."
- Encourage siblings to express their feelings related to the disruptive effect of the child's hospitalization on family life.

Family Assessment

To support the hospitalized child and provide family-centered care, the nurse develops an understanding of the family dynamics and individualizes the nursing care according to the needs of the child and family. To develop a plan of care that involves all family members, the nurse assesses the impact of the child's illness or hospitalization on the family. Box 13–3 provides a list of questions to guide the nurse in determining the roles of family, knowledge of family, support systems, and effects on siblings. (See Chapter 2 ∞ for a detailed discussion on family assessment.)

Collaborate with the family to determine their resources. These resources include the coping strategies of family members, financial resources, access to health care, and availability of community services. One family may manage quite well with limited financial support because they have effective coping strategies; conversely, another family with greater financial resources may have difficulty caring for an ill child if their coping strategies are ineffective. Staying with a hospitalized child can be a financial drain for parents if they must take a leave of absence from work or miss scheduled work days, and perhaps travel to another location and stay away from home. Additional expenses incurred may include hotel rooms, meals, parking fees, and childcare for other children. Assess the family's ability to manage these additional expenses. A multidisciplinary approach to the burden of hospitalization may provide access to community resources and support for families.

BOX 13–3
FAMILY ASSESSMENT WHEN THE CHILD IS HOSPITALIZED

Family Roles

- What changes will the child's illness create in the family?
- Will household tasks need to be reallocated?
- Will a burden be placed on certain family members?
- Will one parent room in or spend a great deal of time in the hospital?

Knowledge

- What knowledge does the family have about the child's condition and treatment? Do they need further information?
- Is there a need to start discharge planning and teaching early?

Support Systems

- Does the family have health insurance? What percentage of costs will it cover? Will other financial support be needed?
- Are close friends or family available to provide childcare for other children, assist with family tasks, or help in other ways?
- Are there community services such as support groups, camps for children with disabilities, education sessions, or equipment and financial resources to which the nurses can refer the family?

Siblings

- Have siblings been informed of the ill child's condition and the expected outcome?
- Have they been reassured that they did not cause the illness?
- Do they understand the change in roles and family routines?
- Are they able to visit the ill child?
- Have their teachers been informed of the family stress?
- If the hospitalized child's life is threatened, are the siblings involved in a therapy plan to assist them in dealing with that stress?

CULTURE

Traditional Therapies

Many cultural groups, such as Chinese Americans, Mexican Americans, Native Americans, and African Americans, use a combination of Western medicine and traditional or folk medicine (Spector, 2004). This information may not be shared with nurses or physicians, both out of respect and in fear that they will be told not to use these methods. Recognizing and supporting use of traditional practices along with Western medicine can promote health and provide comfort for children and families. Ask the families about the use of traditional, complementary, or alternative therapies.

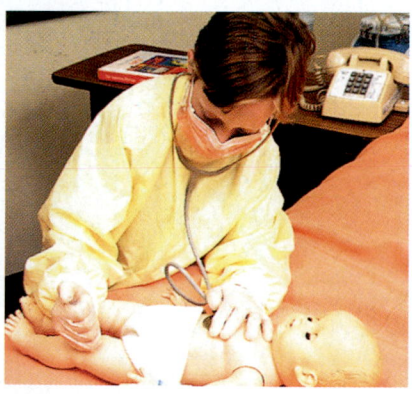

Figure 13–2 ➤ Allowing the child to dress up as a doctor or a nurse helps prepare the child for the hospitalization experience. This helps the child adjust to treatment, care, and the recovery process. Why? What might the child's concerns be? Can you think of any concerns that might be related to cultural background?

The nurse also assesses the family dynamics and evaluates the quality of communication, methods of coping with stress, risk factors, and sources of strength. Collaborate with the family to identify coping mechanisms. Recognize that many children may be hospitalized far from home and their usual support systems. This creates stress for them and for their family members. Find out where family members are staying, how far they are from home, and what normal support systems have been disrupted. Some parents have reported discussing their concerns, praying, information seeking, reading, relaxation, and exercise as common coping mechanisms in these situations (Agazio, Ephraim, Flaherty, & Gurney, 2003). Additional common sources of support include friends, relatives, and pastors as well as hospital chaplains and social workers.

Examine how the family has dealt with the health needs of the child if the child has been hospitalized or required home care in the past. Determine the family members' level of understanding related to the child's hospitalization and anticipated therapy. Collaborate with family members to determine their desired role in the child's care. Assess the family's needs for referral to family service agencies or other community organizations that may be required. Assess the need for support groups or agencies that provide medical equipment or other assistance.

Teaching the child and family, providing support, and referring them to community resources are key elements to providing family-centered care. Additional resources available for the child and family include social workers, child and family mental health professionals, and advanced practice nurses. Additionally, hospital programs and parent support groups are available to assist families in coping with a child's illness.

ADAPTATION TO HOSPITALIZATION

Hospitalization of the child may be planned or unexpected. A child may be hospitalized for any of the following reasons:

- The child develops an acute illness, or exacerbation of chronic illness.
- The child requires diagnostic or treatment procedures or requires elective surgery.
- The child who was previously healthy suffers a serious injury, necessitating unexpected hospitalization.

Planned Hospitalization

When hospitalization is planned, children and their parents have time to prepare for the experience. (See Families Want to Know: Parental Preparation of Children for Hospitalization and Surgery). Through preadmission preparation, children and their families are introduced to the acute care setting. Assess the family's knowledge and expectations and provide information about likely experiences. A variety of approaches can be used to provide information and allay fears:

- Tours of the hospital unit or surgical area are helpful. This activity assists the child and family to become familiar with the environment they will encounter. During tours, preschoolers and school-age children are provided

FAMILIES WANT TO KNOW

Parental Preparation of Children for Hospitalization and Surgery

The nurse can assist the parents in preparing the child for hospitalization and surgery by suggesting the following interventions:

- Read stories to the child about the experience. Numerous books and pamphlets are available. See Table 13–4.
- Talk about going to the hospital, and what it will be like. Talk about coming home.
- Encourage the child to ask questions about the hospital and the surgery.

- Encourage the child to draw pictures of what the hospital will be like.
- Visit the hospital unit before hospitalization, if possible.
- Let the child touch or see equipment, if possible.
- Provide a doctor or nurse kit for the child to play with.
- Let the child dress up like a doctor or nurse, if possible.
- Plan for support via parents' presence, telephone calls, or special items of the parents that the child can keep during the stay.
- Be honest.

opportunities to see and handle items with which they will come in contact.

- The surgical team's attire is less frightening if the child has had a chance to try it on and engage in play while wearing the attire (Figure 13–2 ➤).
- Medical equipment is not as frightening when the child learns what it does and observes how it is used, for example, through demonstration on a doll (Figure 13–3 ➤).
- If a tour is not possible, photographs or a videotape can be used to demonstrate the medical setting and procedures. Puppets and skits are another effective method of explaining procedures to children.
- Many hospitals offer health fairs to explain health procedures to children. During a tour, while hospitalized, or at home, the child can be exposed to books or films that explain in age-appropriate terms what to expect during various procedures (Table 13–4). Coloring books or other methods can also be utilized to reinforce teaching (Figure 13–4 ➤).

Different approaches are useful when adolescents are being prepared for hospitalization. They learn not only from written materials, models, and videotapes, but also from talking with peers who have had similar experiences. To demonstrate respect of privacy, an opportunity for asking questions without parents present is also provided to the adolescent.

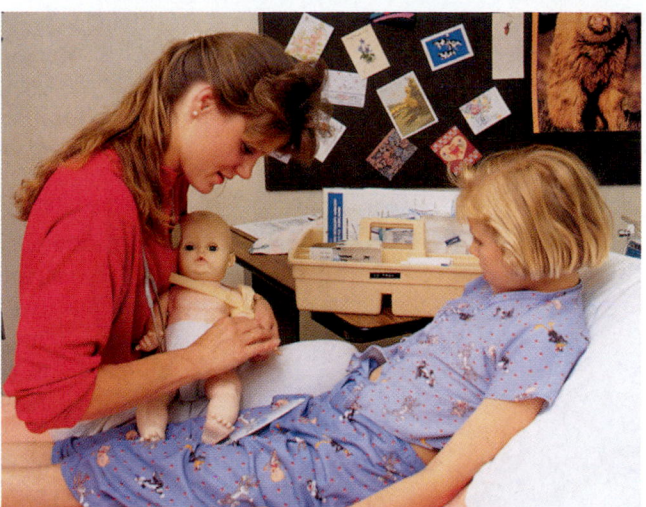

Figure 13–3 ➤ The child's anxiety and fear often will be reduced if the nurse explains what is going to happen and demonstrates how the procedure will be done by using a doll. Based on your experience, can you list five actions you can take to prepare a school-age child for hospitalization?

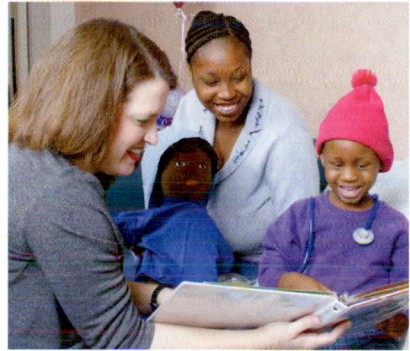

Figure 13–4 ➤ The nurse reads a story to Tiara to reinforce teaching about the hospital.

Table 13–4	SAMPLE TEACHING MATERIALS FOR CHILDREN REGARDING HOSPITALIZATION AND HEALTH CARE

Videotapes	Publishers
Clean Intermittent Catheterization	Learner Managed Designs, Inc.
I Have Epilepsy Too	Epilepsy Foundation
What Do I Tell My Children? How to Help a Child Cope with the Death of a Loved One	Life Cycle Productions

Books	
Barney and Baby Bop Go to the Doctor, by M.Larsen	Lyrick Publishing
The Berenstain Bears Go to the Doctor, by S. Berenstain & B. Berenstain	Random House
Clifford Visits the Hospital, by N. Bridwell	Scholastic, Inc.
Corduroy Goes to the Doctor, by D. Freeman & L. McCue	Viking Penguin, Inc.
Curious George Goes to the Hospital, by M. Rey & H. A. Rey	Houghton Mifflin Company
The Fall of Freddie the Leaf, by L. Buscaglia	Henry Holt & Co.
Franklin Goes to the Hospital, by P. Bourgeois & B. Clark	Scholastic, Inc.
Going to the Hospital, by F. Rogers	Penguin Putnam Books
The Hospital Book, by J. Howe	Crown Publishers
Let's Talk About Going to the Hospital, by M. Johnston	Rosen Publishing Group
A Night Without Stars, by J. Howe	Aladdin Paperbacks
Rita Goes to the Hospital, by M. Davison	Random House
A Visit to the Sesame Street Hospital, D. Hautzig	Random House
When Molly Was in the Hospital: A Book for Brothers and Sisters of Hospitalized Children, by D. Duncan	Rayve Productions

Include the family in preparing the child of any age for hospitalization. Parents can be instrumental in preparing a child for hospitalization by reviewing material presented, being available to answer questions, and being truthful and supportive. Determine the child's normal routine, reactions to stressful situations, and prior experiences with hospitalization to assist in establishing a plan of care for the child.

Unexpected Hospitalization

An unanticipated admission places the child at emotional risk for several reasons, including the lack of preparation for the experience, the uncertainty and unpredictability of events that follow, the unfamiliarity of the environment, and the heightened anxiety of parents. An admission for exacerbation of a disease such as cystic fibrosis or leukemia can provoke feelings of depression or hopelessness.

Assist the child and family who are not prepared for hospital admission to adapt to the experience by orienting them to their immediate environment, providing an opportunity for questions, offering truthful responses, and explaining all procedures and expectations. Discuss the anticipated plan of care for the child and involve the family in the child's care. Provide the family an opportunity to express their fears and concerns. Refer to social services and/or parent support groups if additional support is needed.

NURSING CARE OF THE HOSPITALIZED CHILD

Nursing care of the hospitalized child focuses on providing family-centered care by promoting the child's and family's coping strategies to deal with the stressors of hospitalization, promoting optimal development and safety, and minimizing disruption of the child's usual routine as much as possible.

Special Units and Types of Care

Children admitted to a hospital may be cared for in one or more of the following units: short-stay, outpatient unit, ambulatory surgical unit, general pediatric unit, emergency department, or pediatric intensive care unit. Hospitalized children may require surgical treatment involving preoperative and postoperative care. Children with infectious diseases require isolation precautions. Other children may require rehabilitative care to achieve or restore maximum potential.

Short-Stay, Outpatient, and Ambulatory Surgical Units

Hospitalization stays for children have generally become short, with minor surgery (ambulatory surgical centers), diagnostic tests such as cardiac catheterizations, radiology studies requiring sedation, and treatments such as chemotherapy performed in one day. The child may be admitted in the morning and discharged later that same afternoon. In addition, children who have potentially serious illnesses may be placed on a short-stay or 23-hour observation unit for monitoring or limited treatment, after which a decision is made to either hospitalize the child for additional treatment or discharge the child home if improvement occurs.

These short stays are considered beneficial primarily because they cause minimal disruption of family patterns and are cost effective for the institution, health insurance company, and family. Nurses assist parents to prepare the child properly for planned admissions, monitor the child during the procedures, encourage family participation in care, and keep families well informed (Box 13–4).

Nursing care of the child in short-stay, outpatient, and ambulatory surgical units is the same as for regular hospital admission (see following discussion); however, time for teaching is compressed, requiring the nurse to implement a variety of teaching methods in a minimal amount of time to ensure the family understands discharge instructions. Effective teaching methods include demonstration, videos, pamphlets with verbal review, and informal teaching sessions.

General Pediatric Care Unit

General pediatric units may be subcategorized into medical and/or surgical units, orthopedic units, oncology units, mental health units, and units specific to developmental

CLINICAL TIP

The hospital environment can pose a variety of safety risks for children, especially toddlers and preschoolers. The nurse should dispose of syringe caps, thermometer covers, gloves, and other equipment that children could chew on or swallow. Latex balloons should not be permitted due to the risk of suffocation.

CLINICAL TIP

Continuity in the staff providing care to the child may encourage the child to develop relationships and trust with those persons who can assist and support the child through unfamiliar and strange procedures (Lau, 2002). When possible, the same nurses should be assigned to provide care to the child to establish a sense of routine.

BOX 13–4

NURSING CONSIDERATIONS IN PREPARING PARENTS AND CHILD FOR PLANNED SHORT-STAY ADMISSION

- Are there special requirements, such as not being permitted food or drink or needing extra fluid intake?
- What time and where must the child appear?
- Are any special forms, insurance numbers, or previous records needed?
- How long will the child stay in the hospital?
- Are parents expected or encouraged to be with the child or to stay in the health facility?
- Is there a chance the child may need to remain longer than expected?
- What will the child's condition be for transfer home?
- Will special equipment or care be needed?
- What symptoms can indicate problems?
- Where can the family go or whom can they call in case of problems or questions?

---

levels (e.g., adolescent unit). Whereas some facilities utilize one unit or area (depending on the size of the hospital) that incorporates all of these care specialties, larger medical centers and children's hospitals generally have separate units for specific specialties as previously identified.

Admission to these units may be the result of an acute condition, such as pneumonia or trauma, or as the result of an exacerbation of a chronic condition such as asthma. Other causes for admissions include surgical procedures requiring longer than 24-hour stays and the need for inpatient treatments and services.

Nursing care includes orienting the child and family to the unit and procedures, adhering to the child's normal routine as much as possible, including the child and family in the decision-making process, promoting a safe environment for the child, and promoting the child's growth and developmental needs.

Emergency Care

When a child is brought to an emergency department, the parents are usually frightened and insecure and may even be in a state of shock. The fast pace and critical nature of the unit creates an atmosphere in which parents are hesitant to ask questions and are anxious about the outcome. Anxiety and stress are caused by uncertainties in an emergent environment and the necessity of quick decision making. Numerous procedures, tests, treatments, and fear of pain also lead to stress related to minimal preparation in emergency situations (see Chapter 14 ∞).

The nurse keeps both the child and the family informed about what is being done and when more news may be available. The parents and child are encouraged to remain together as much as possible. Parents who wish to remain with a child during even invasive procedures or resuscitation efforts should be allowed to do so. The Emergency Nurses Association (2005) supports the option of family presence during invasive procedures and resuscitation. The nurse collaborates with the family members to determine their desired presence in critical situations and keeps them informed about the health care provided.

Pediatric Intensive Care Unit

The pediatric intensive care unit (PICU) provides specialized nursing care to infants and children. The patient population includes children with trauma, life-threatening illnesses, acute exacerbations of chronic illness (such as status asthmaticus), or any other condition requiring advanced support and continuous monitoring.

Parents of a child in a pediatric intensive care unit (PICU) are likely to be anxious, particularly since the child's illness may be severe and the prognosis may be guarded. The unfamiliar equipment may create an atmosphere of fear or anxiety. Sensory overload as well as sensory deprivation is a potential problem for the child in the PICU. Numerous healthcare professionals work in the intensive care environment, and without effective and open communication, parents may not know whom to question or even what questions to ask.

Nurses provide comprehensive care to the child, as well as emotional support, explain the purpose of treatments and machines, help parents to hold or touch their child, and provide referral to other services if appropriate. Collaborate with the family and encourage them to write down their questions and direct them to the appropriate source if unable to answer the question. See Chapter 4 ∞ for a discussion of stressors in parents and children in an intensive care unit and the nursing strategies intended to address these stressors.

Isolation

Children who require isolation to prevent spread of infection may experience lack of stimulation due to limited contact with other children and visitors. Frequent family visits are important and should be encouraged. Family members may be reluctant to wear protective garments either out of fear of using them incorrectly or a belief that they are unnecessary. The nurse assures that the family understands the reason for isolation and any special procedures. Having contact with and holding the child are encouraged when possible. (Standard precautions are described in the Clinical Skills Manual.)

Rehabilitation

Rehabilitation units provide children with ongoing care and support to continue recovery beyond the initial period of illness or injury (Figure 13–5 ➤). These may be separate units within a hospital or independent centers. The rehabilitation may be on an inpatient or outpatient basis. Children who experience brain injury, spinal cord injury, near drowning, and burns may require extensive rehabilitation. The rehabilitation process may be lengthy and extensive. Families may need support for adapting to changes in lifestyle, income, finances, and responsibilities.

The objective of rehabilitation is to assist the child with physical, psychosocial, or educational challenges to reach his or her fullest potential and to promote achievement of developmentally appropriate skills. Collaboration with a multidisciplinary team including parental involvement is essential.

Parental Involvement and Parental Presence

Family-centered care recognizes that families are essential to the child's care during illness. The nurse works with the family and multidisciplinary team to involve the parents in the decision-making process and facilitate parental participation in the care of the child (Daneman, Macaluso, & Guzzetta, 2003). Families who feel supported by nursing staff during their child's hospitalization are better equipped to cope with the crisis and thus be open to participating in their child's care and developing skills to provide care for the child after discharge (Miles, 2003).

Integrity of the family unit is fostered through parental involvement during the child's hospital stay. Additionally, parental participation prepares the family for care that will be required when the child goes home. The child benefits greatly from parental presence and participation. The child experiences reduced emotional distress and anxiety if the parents are present. Additionally parent-child attachment is uninterrupted, and the child experiences a decrease in behavioral maladjustments. Parental presence during painful procedures is particularly beneficial in reducing the child's anxiety and stress (Daneman, Macaluso, & Guzzetta, 2003). Parental involvement gives parents control and feelings of being active participants in their child's progress.

Parents experience tremendous stress and anxiety when their child is hospitalized. Expressions of anger are not uncommon, particularly in highly stressful situations such as having a child in the intensive care unit or not knowing or understanding the reason for the child's illness. Parents of hospitalized children may become angry for several reasons including restrictions on visitation and unexpected deterioration in their child's condition, They may also feel that the staff do not value their role in assisting in the care of their child. The lack of complete information and receiving different information from a variety of staff can also provoke anger in parents (Griffin, 2003b). The nurse implements a family-centered approach to develop strategies to reduce sources of parental anger and to handle these stressful situations in a professional and therapeutic manner (Griffin, 2003b).

CLINICAL SKILLS MANUAL
CHAPTER 1
Standard Precautions

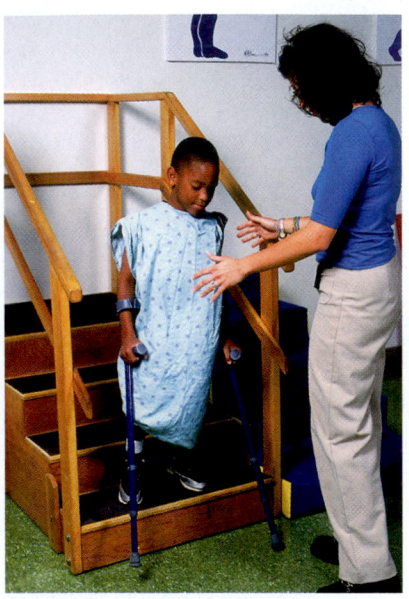

Figure 13–5 ➤ Rehabilitation units provide an opportunity for the child to relearn tasks like walking and climbing stairs. They provide an important transition from hospital to home and community.

CULTURE

Support Systems

There are many cultural influences on health beliefs and practices. For example, Mexican Americans view family as a strong support. Extended family and godparents (compadres) may want to be with a hospitalized child. Although the father of the child is often the spokesperson, mothers commonly are influential in decisions regarding child health care. As another example, Hawaiian families also often wish to have many family members present with a hospitalized child, and may value playing native music and use of aromatherapy (Lassetter & Baldwin, 2005). The nurse should be inclusive of all people the family wishes to have present in the hospital and for explanations about health care.

Hospitals have policies on visitation, including the hours of visitation, who can visit, and how many visitors are allowed at a time. Most children's hospitals or pediatric units state that they allow parents to stay with their child all of the time. Frequently, however, especially in intensive care units, parents are asked to leave during bedside rounds, report, and emergencies. Parents may become upset when these restrictions deny them access and interfere with the amount of time they are able to spend with their hospitalized child (Griffin, 2003a).

Nurses are instrumental in assisting facilities to adapt policies that reflect a family-centered approach (Box 13–5). Collaborate with the family to provide them the opportunity to decide whose presence is most beneficial to the child and family.

Nurses frequently experience changes in a child's condition; however, for parents this change in condition is an alarming event, particularly if the family was not provided anticipatory guidance that the event could occur, and if they were not notified of the change in the child's condition. When parents are not informed in a timely manner or they arrive on a unit and find their child in a different bed or on another unit, or with change in equipment used, they may exhibit confusion and anger (Griffin, 2003b).

Nursing techniques include informing the family of potential problems that may occur. If the child's condition changes, make every effort to inform the family immediately. Identify the best methods of communication with the family such as a cellular telephone, pager, or alternate phone numbers, and have these methods of contact on the child's chart. Determine in advance when parents would like to be notified of common procedures such as blood transfusions, radiologic examinations, and other procedures, to provide them a choice about whether to be present (Griffin, 2003b).

If parents are upset, nurses should acknowledge understanding the situation the parents experienced and collaborate with the family to ensure trust is maintained. Encourage participation in parent-to-parent support groups where other parents of hospitalized children share their experiences and coping mechanisms (Griffin, 2003b).

Parents of hospitalized children may come in daily contact with numerous health-care providers, leading to inconsistent or conflicting information. This causes anger and frustration, particularly where conflict in the diagnosis or discharge planning exists (Griffin, 2003b). The nurse acts as family advocate by listening to family members, answering their questions, and collaborating with the multidisciplinary team to ensure continuity of care and consistent communication (Simons, 2002).

Parents of a hospitalized child may feel that staff do not value their involvement in the child's care, especially in high-technology intensive care units. Feeling unable to provide care to their child may lead the parents to express anger toward the staff. In applying a family-centered approach, nurses should collaborate with the parents to determine their desired level of involvement in the infant's or child's care. Simple tasks, such as weighing the child, feeding, holding, and bathing, provides the parent opportunities to participate in the care of the child (Griffin, 2003b).

Working with parents who are angry presents a challenge to pediatric nurses. It is essential that nurses support each other when these situations arise. Nurses implement a variety of techniques to handle these challenges, including education such as inservice training on managing anger in the clinical setting, support through peers, mentoring, or debriefing opportunities. Additionally, the nurse's own feelings in response to parental anger can also be addressed by use of these techniques (Griffin, 2003b).

Preparation for Procedures

Numerous procedures may occur during hospitalization, from collection of urine or blood specimens to lumbar punctures and surgery. Special techniques can help the child to understand and cope with feelings about these procedures. Techniques used to prepare the child depend on developmental age, coping abilities, and previous experience.

Psychological Preparation

Preparation may begin a few moments to several days before the procedure, depending on the child's age. In providing sensitive care to the child, nurses assume that a procedure can potentially be traumatic for the child. Even providing urine in a specimen

---

BOX 13–5

TAKING "VISITATION" OUT OF THE PEDIATRIC CARE SETTING

A family-centered approach to pediatric hospitalization recognizes that the family is an integral part of the child's life and care. Parents and family members *should not* be made to feel as though they are visitors to their child. A better approach to policy would be to use terms such as *family time* rather than *visiting hours* or *visiting policy*. Nurses can be the impetus for this movement by encouraging a change in policy and the language used (Griffin, 2003a).

CULTURE

Use of Interpreters

Nurses in the pediatric acute care environment frequently encounter patients and parents who do not speak English. It is imperative that nurses use appropriate interpreter services to communicate with these families. Use of children and family members to obtain patient history, provide explanations of illness and treatment, and to obtain informed consent can lead to concerns related to accuracy of the information. In some situations, the family member providing the interpretation might actually withhold information to protect the ill child and/or the parents (Lehna, 2005).

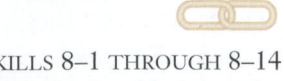

SKILLS 8–1 THROUGH 8–14
Medication Administration

cup or undergoing radiologic examination can be frightening if the child does not understand the reason for the procedure or what to expect. Administration of medication can also be frustrating or anxiety inducing for the child. The nurse prepares the child for medication administration and uses techniques appropriate to the developmental level of the child, assuring that the medication is safely given (Table 13–5).

Use techniques appropriate for the child's developmental level to assess the child's knowledge and feelings about the procedure. Use of drawings, stories, body outline

Table 13–5	VARIATIONS IN MEDICATION ADMINISTRATION TO CHILDREN	
Route	**Developmental Considerations**	**Techniques**
Oral	Children under 5 years cannot generally swallow pills and capsules. Children may not want to take medicine.	• Medications are usually given in liquid form (elixir, syrup, or suspension). • Sometimes tablets are crushed or capsules are opened and mixed with one spoon of food. Crushed pills may also be mixed in a small amount of liquid such as cherry syrup. Check with the pharmacy to be sure this does not inactivate the drug. Never crush enteric-coated or timed-release medicine. • When choosing a vehicle for crushed tablets, use only one spoonful of applesauce, pudding, jelly, or similar food or 1–2 mLs of liquid. • Use a 1 mL oral syringe for amounts less than 1 mL to increase accuracy. • Position young children upright to avoid choking and aspiration. • Give liquid medicines slowly by oral syringe aimed at the inside of the cheek. A preschooler may prefer to drink the medicine from a medicine cup, but the medication must first be measured using a syringe to ensure accuracy. • Have the expectation that the medicine will be taken. Let children choose the type of fluid to drink after, but do not ask if they will take their medicine now.
Rectal	Colon is small in size.	• For children under 3 years, the nurse's gloved fifth finger is used for insertion. After this age, the index finger can usually be used. • Lubricate the tip of the suppository. The nurse may need to hold the buttocks together for a few minutes to keep the medication from being expelled.
Ophthalmic and Otic	Young children may be fearful of medicines placed in the eyes or ears.	• Adequate immobilization is needed to avoid injury. • The nurse's hand can be stabilized by resting the wrist on the child's head. • Explanations and therapeutic play can be used with children old enough to explain the process of administration. • Have medication at room temperature.
Topical	Skin of infants is thin and fragile.	• Only prescribed doses and medicines appropriate for young children should be used on the skin. • Covering the area or keeping the child's hands occupied may be necessary to ensure adequate contact of medication with the skin.
Intramuscular	Anatomy and physiology of children differ from that of adults.	• Gluteus maximus muscle (dorsal gluteal site) must not be used until the child has been walking for at least 1 year. • Vastus lateralis site is preferred for young children. • Amounts to be administered should be limited to no more than 1–2 mL for ventrogluteal site depending on muscle size. • The deltoid muscle is rarely used in young children except for the small amounts injected in some vaccines.
Intravenous	Veins are small and fragile. Fluid balance is critical.	• Careful maintenance of sites is needed. • Common infusion sites include hands and feet, although scalp veins are sometimes used in infants. • Infusion pumps require frequent monitoring. • Syringe pumps are often used when minimal fluid is to be given over an extended period of time. • Central lines are commonly used for long-term intravenous medication therapy.

See *Clinical Skills Manual* for further medication administration techniques. Adapted from: Bindler, R., & Howry, L. (2005). *Pediatric drug guide*. Upper Saddle River, NJ: Prentice Hall Health.

dolls, anatomically correct dolls, and conversation with the child are examples of techniques the nurse can use depending on the age of the child. When assessing the child's perception about procedures, the nurse should consider the following:

- Does the child know the purpose of the procedure?
- Has the child experienced this procedure before? Was the experience painful, frightening, or reassuring?
- What does the child think will happen? Are the child's beliefs accurate?
- Is the procedure painful?
- What techniques does the child use to gain control in challenging situations?
- Will the parents or other caregiver be present to provide support?

When explaining a procedure, use words that the child understands to describe the procedure and its purpose. Many words have more than one meaning and may be misinterpreted by young children (Fleitas, 2003) (Table 13–6). Older children require explanations geared to their cognitive level and previous experiences. They will want to know what is happening, why, and what they can do to cope during the procedure (Table 13–7).

Provide written information, videos, and other available media for adolescents and schedule time for questions and discussions. Adolescents can make many choices about their own health care. For example, they can be asked such questions as "Do you want your hand numbed for the intravenous start?" Some adolescents desire their parents to be involved in their care, while others prefer to minimize their parents' role. The nurse collaborates with the adolescents to assure that their wishes are known regarding parental presence. Parental presence can provide comfort and support to the child during procedures. Parents should be allowed to choose whether they want to stay for the procedure. Some parents may feel that they will be too upset to support the child, while others will choose to stay.

Physical Preparation

Physical preparation depends on the age of the child and the procedure. Preprocedural sedation may be required. If sedation is required the child will have to be NPO (nothing by mouth) for a period of time. Infants might be provided sucrose for procedures (see Chapter 15 ∞ for pain management). Procedural checklists are often utilized.

Performing the Procedure

Procedures on young children are generally performed in a **treatment room** (a room designated for performing treatments such as intravenous starts, blood drawing, and lumbar punctures) in order to promote the child's sense of security that the room is a "safe" and relatively pain-free site (Box 13–6). After the procedure, the child is returned

> **CLINICAL TIP**
> When a potentially painful procedure will be occurring, an anesthetic cream such as EMLA, ELA-MAX, or Numby Stuff is applied before the planned procedure. This can lessen discomfort and, therefore, fear in the child.

> **CLINICAL TIP**
> Procedures should never be performed in a playroom or during a play activity. The nurse acts as the child's advocate by ensuring that treatments by other healthcare professionals (such as blood drawing or respiratory treatments) are not performed in the playroom. Assist the child back to his or her own room for treatment, and reassure the child he or she may return to the playroom after the treatment is completed.

Table 13–6	LANGUAGE ALTERNATIVES WHEN COMMUNICATING WITH YOUNG CHILDREN
Potentially Confusing or Ambiguous Words or Statements	**Alternate Communication Choice**
"We will give you some dye in your arm."	"We will put some warm medicine into your arm."
"I will give you a shot."	"I will give you some medicine through a small needle."
"This will hurt or burn."	"It might feel sore or very warm."
"The doctor will make a small cut/incision."	"The doctor will make a small opening."
"You are going to have some anesthesia."	"You'll get some medicine that you breathe or get through your arm to make you sleep."
"The medicine tastes bad."	"Some children say the medicine tastes different to them."

Table 13–7 | ASSISTING CHILDREN THROUGH PROCEDURES

Developmental Stage	Before Procedure	During Procedure
Infant	None for infant. Explain to parents the procedure, the reason for it, and their role. Allow parents the option of being present for the procedure.	Nursing staff should immobilize the infant securely and gently. Parents should not be asked to hold the child down. Perform the procedure quickly. Use touch, voice, pacifier, and bottle as distractions. Ask parent to hold, rock, and sing to the infant after the procedure.
Toddler	Give explanation just before the procedure, since toddler's concept of time is limited. Explain that the child did nothing wrong; the procedure is simply necessary. Allow parents the option of being present for the procedure.	Perform in treatment room. Nursing staff should immobilize the child securely. Give short explanations and directions in a positive manner. Avoid giving choices when none are available. For example, "We are going to do this now" is better than "Is it okay to do this now?" Allow child to cry or scream. Comfort child after the procedure. Give child a choice of favorite drink or special sticker.
Preschool child	Give simple explanations of the procedure. Basic drawings may be useful. While providing supervision, allow the child to touch and play with equipment to be used if possible. Since any entry into the body is viewed as a threat, state that the child's body will remain the same, and use adhesive bandages to reassure the child that the body is intact and parts will not "fall out."	Perform in the treatment room. Nursing staff should immobilize the child securely. Give short explanations and directions in a positive manner. Encourage control by having the child count to 10 or spell name. Allow child to cry. Give positive feedback for cooperation and getting through procedure. Encourage the child to draw afterward to explore the experience.
School-age child	Clear, thorough explanations are helpful. Use drawings, pictures, books, and contact with equipment. Teach stress-reduction techniques such as deep breathing and visualization. Offer a choice of reward after procedure is completed.	Be ready to immobilize the child if needed. Allow the child to remain in position by self if child is able to be still. Explain throughout procedure what is happening. Facilitate use of stress-control techniques. Praise cooperative efforts.
Adolescent	Give clear explanations orally and in writing. Teach stress-reduction techniques. Explore fear of certain procedures, such as staple removal or venipuncture.	Assist adolescent in self-control. Assist with use of stress-control techniques. Explain expected outcome and tell when results of test will be completed.

BOX 13–6
TREATMENT ROOM

The treatment room is a special room utilized for the pediatric population for procedures such as intravenous starts, lumbar punctures, and blood drawing. The treatment room is utilized rather than the child's own hospital room so that the child always has a "safe" environment and comfort zone by knowing that no unpleasant or painful procedures will occur in his or her room.

Pediatric hospitals and large medical centers generally provide treatment rooms on each unit. Smaller hospitals and community hospitals may not provide a specific treatment room designated for pediatrics; however, any room other than the child's own room is an appropriate alternative. If smaller hospitals do not have a treatment room or provide an alternative, nurses acting as a child advocate should be vigilant in encouraging the establishment of such a room to minimize the stressors the hospitalized child experiences.

to his or her room for comfort and reassurance. A choice of reward often soothes the young child. Older children can be given the option of having a procedure performed in the treatment room or in their own hospital room. Older school-age children and adolescents may prefer to remain in their room for the procedure.

The procedure is performed as quickly and efficiently as possible. Parents may wish to be involved or may prefer to be available afterward to comfort the child. If the parents wish to participate, ask them to hold the child's hand or stand close by for comfort. Utilize nursing staff instead of parents to immobilize the child as needed. Following the procedure, no matter how the child responded, the child should be praised.

Maintain a positive attitude when preparing the child and reassure the child that it is normal to be frightened of unknown experiences. The parents or nurse can be designated to support the child by way of a gentle touch, talking, singing, reassurance, or stress-reduction techniques. Refer to Chapter 15 ∞ for discussion of pain management and sedation for procedures.

Preparation for Surgery

A child's surgical experience may be elective, planned in advance, or the result of an emergency or trauma. How a child responds to the experience depends on the psychological and physical preparation he or she receives. The accompanying Nursing Care Plan summarizes key elements of preoperative and postoperative care.

Preoperative Care

Preoperative care of the child includes both psychosocial and physical preparation for surgery. The goal of preoperative teaching is to reduce the fear associated with the unknown and decrease stress and anxiety associated with surgery.

NURSING CARE PLAN   The Child Undergoing Surgery

GOAL	INTERVENTION	RATIONALE	EXPECTED OUTCOME
Preoperative Care			
1. Deficient Knowledge related to preoperative and postoperative events			
	NIC Priority Intervention: **Teaching, Preoperative:** *Assisting a patient to understand and mentally prepare for surgery and postoperative recovery.*		*NOC Suggested Outcome:* **Knowledge:** *Extent of understanding conveyed about treatment regimen.*
The child and family will acquire knowledge related to the operation.	• Ask questions of the parent and child about surgery.	• Prior knowledge and understanding can be reinforced and used to guide your presentation.	The child and family are able to verbalize details about expected preoperative and postoperative events. They ask questions that demonstrate understanding.
	• Teach about preoperative and postoperative events using appropriate developmental methods such as dolls, drawings, stories, and tours.	• Developmental level determines the cognitive approach that works best for teaching.	The child demonstrates skills needed in the postoperative period.
	• Reinforce information the family has received about the purpose of surgery.	• The physician may have explained operation.	
	• Have the child demonstrate postoperative events that pertain to his or her case such as deep breathing, putting bandage on doll, taping intravenous line on doll, and pressing patient-controlled analgesia button.	• Concrete experience promotes learning.	
	• Allow the parents and child to ask questions.	• Learners must have opportunity to ask questions.	
2. Anxiety related to change in health status			
	NIC Priority Intervention: **Anxiety Reduction:** *Minimizing apprehension, dread, foreboding, or uneasiness related to an unidentified source of anticipated danger.*		*NOC Suggested Outcome:* **Coping:** *Actions to manage stressors that tax an individual's resources.*
The child and family will show decreased behavior indicating anxiety.	• Question the child about expectations of hospitalization and previous experiences.	• Previous experiences can influence present anxiety level.	The child and family demonstrate less anxiety. They verbalize understanding and comfort in hospital routines.
	• Orient the child to the hospital setting, routines, staff, and other patients.	• Familiarity with the setting and people can decrease anxiety by removing unknown factors.	Parents support the child for traumatic procedures.
	• Institute age-appropriate play and interactions with the child.	• Play can increase trust level and decrease anxiety.	
	• Explain procedures and prepare for those that might cause trauma. Encourage parents to support the child.	• The child is more likely to trust caregivers if they are truthful and if parents are present.	
	• Allow the parents and child to ask questions.	• Questioning provides an opportunity to explain the unknown, which decreases anxiety.	

(continued)

NURSING CARE PLAN The Child Undergoing Surgery (continued)

GOAL	INTERVENTION	RATIONALE	EXPECTED OUTCOME
3. Risk for Infection and Injury related to exposure to nosocomial infection and use of preoperative medication			
	NIC Priority Intervention: **Infection Control and Fall Prevention:** *Minimizing the acquisition and transmission of infectious agents, and instituting special precautions with patient at risk of falling.*		*NOC Suggested Outcome: Actions to eliminate or reduce actual, personal, and modifiable health risks.*
The child will show no signs of infection.	• Monitor vital signs at least every 4 hours. Inspect skin and respiratory status each shift.	• Increase in vital sign levels, skin lesions, nasal drainage, or adventitious breath sounds can indicate signs of infection in the child.	The child's vital signs and assessment are within normal limits.
The child will remain free of injury.	• Report any variations from expected vital signs.	• Symptoms are reported so surgery can be canceled if necessary.	The child is transported safely to the operating room.
	• Keep side rails up after preoperative medication is given. Maintain NPO status when ordered. Transport the child to the operating room safely secured.	• Preoperative medication can alter level of consciousness. NPO status prevents aspiration.	
Postoperative Care			
4. Impaired Skin Integrity related to disruption of skin surface			
	NIC Priority Intervention: **Wound Care:** *Prevention of wound complications and promotion of wound healing.*		*NOC Suggested Outcome:* **Wound Healing:** *The extent to which cells and tissues have regenerated following intentional closure.*
The child will be free of infection.	• Monitor vital signs per hospital routine. Record and report changes from baseline.	• Changes in vital signs, especially increased temperature and pulse, can indicate infection.	The child shows no signs of infection.
	• Monitor surgical dressing and drains every hour.	• Excess drainage may indicate infection.	The surgical wound heals without infection.
	• Change or reinforce dressings when wet.	• Wet dressing can allow organisms to come into contact with surgical wound.	
	• Check the intravenous site every 2 hours for redness, swelling, pain, or pallor.	• Intravenous lines may become infiltrated or cause thrombophlebitis.	The intravenous line remains patent without signs of infection.
	• Teach parents signs of infection before discharge. Teach parents aseptic technique for dressing change and wound care.	• Parents report signs of infection and perform home care as needed.	The child continues to demonstrate no signs of infection at home.
5. Risk for Constipation related to surgical procedure and anesthetics			
	NIC Priority Intervention: **Constipation Management:** *Establishment and maintenance of regular bowel elimination.*		*NOC Suggested Outcome:* **Bowel Elimination:** *Ability of the gastrointestinal tract to form and evacuate stool effectively.*
The child will achieve and maintain normal bowel functioning by the fourth postoperative day.	• Auscultate bowel sounds every 4 hours. Offer liquids only when bowel sounds are present. Assess the abdomen for distention.	• Restricting fluids avoids distention if peristalsis is not normal.	The child has bowel movement within 2 to 3 days after surgery with normal pattern by the fourth postoperative day.

NURSING CARE PLAN	The Child Undergoing Surgery (continued)		
GOAL	**INTERVENTION**	**RATIONALE**	**EXPECTED OUTCOME**
5. Risk for Constipation related to surgical procedure and anesthetics (continued)			
	• Document the character and frequency of bowel movements.	• Knowledge of bowel status ensures early identification of constipation.	
	• Advance the diet as tolerated.	• Fluids and roughage promote normal bowel functioning.	
	• Increase activity as ordered and tolerated.		
6. Risk for Fluid Volume Imbalance related to intravenous infusion and NPO status			
	NIC Priority Intervention: **Fluid Management:** *Promotion of fluid balance and prevention of imbalance complications.*		*NOC Suggested Outcome:* **Fluid Balance:** *Balance of water in intracellular and extracellular components.*
The child will achieve and maintain proper circulating volume.	• Monitor vital signs per hospital routines.	• Changes in vital signs, especially pulse or blood pressure, can indicate fluid imbalance.	The child remains in fluid balance with no vomiting in postoperative period.
The child will tolerate oral intake when started, with no nausea, vomiting, or dehydration present.	• Record intake and output. Be alert for fluid loss via dressings or watery stools. Evaluate hydration status by skin turgor and mucous membranes.	• Intake and output are roughly equivalent. Urinary retention sometimes occurs postoperatively as a result of anesthesia. Fluid status can be assessed by skin and mucous membrane hydration.	
	• Monitor laboratory values of hematocrit and hemoglobin.	• Increased hematocrit and hemoglobin can indicate hemoconcentration and underhydration. Decreased serum values can indicate hemodilution or overhydration.	
	• Begin oral intake after assessment of bowel sounds. Record vomiting. Administer antiemetics if indicated.	• Vomiting can cause fluid loss.	
7. Impaired Gas Exchange related to anesthetics and pain			
	NIC Priorty Intervention: **Airway Management:** *Facilitation of patency of air passages.*		*NOC Suggested Outcome:* **Respiratory Status:** *Ventilation: Movement of air in and out of lungs.*
The child will maintain adequate ventilation with no respiratory impairment.	• Auscultate lungs every 2 hours. Record rate, rhythm, and quality of respiration. Evaluate respiratory rate after analgesics.	• Early identification of respiratory difficulty aids early treatment. Analgesics, especially morphine, may slow respiratory rate.	The child moves adequate air in and out of lungs.
	• Administer oxygen if ordered.	• Oxygen may facilitate breathing status postoperatively.	
	• Reposition the child every 2 hours.	• Repositioning ensures expansion of all lung fields.	
	• Encourage deep breathing and coughing every 2 hours. Use incentive spirometer, pinwheels, or other blow toys appropriate for the development level of the child.	• All areas of the lungs must be expanded. Mucus is expectorated.	
	• Ensure proper intake and output.	• Balanced fluid status ensures liquefication of secretions and prevents excess fluid accumulation.	

(continued)

GOAL	INTERVENTION	RATIONALE	EXPECTED OUTCOME
8. Pain related to surgical procedure			
	NIC Priority Intervention: **Pain Management:** *Alleviation of pain or a reduction in pain to a level of comfort that is acceptable to the patient.*		*NOC Suggested Outcome:* **Pain Control Behavior:** *Personal actions to control pain.*
The child will maintain an adequate comfort level.	• Assess behavioral cues (e.g., crying, movement, guarding).	• Behavior of preverbal children provides clues to pain experience.	The child's pain is controlled as demonstrated by a low number on the pain control scale (behavioral or verbal).
	• Use an appropriate pain scale with verbal children.	• Pain scales allow children to quantify the amount of pain	
	• Administer prescribed pain medications on a regular basis.	• Narcotics and nonnarcotic analgesics alter pain perception.	
	• Use age-appropriate non-pharmacologic methods of pain control (e.g., distraction, repositioning).	• Nonpharmacologic interventions interfere with pain perception.	
9. Risk for Impaired Skin Integrity related to limited mobility after surgery			
	NIC Priority Intervention: **Skin Surveillance and Pressure Management:** *Collection and analysis of patient data to maintain skin integrity and minimize pressure to body parts.*		*NOC Suggested Outcome:* **Risk Control:** *Actions to eliminate or reduce actual personal and modifiable health threats.*
The child's skin will remain intact.	• Turn and reposition the child every 2 hours.	• Repositioning takes pressure off the skin and allows increased circulation.	The child develops no pressure areas.
	• Keep linens clean and dry.	• Clean linen decreases the chance of skin breakdown.	The wound heals without complication.
	• Check pressure areas when turning and rub erythematous areas with lotion.	• Rubbing increases circulation.	
	• Get the child up and ambulating when ordered.	• Movement decreases pressure on skin.	
	• Check the incision for drainage, redness, and intactness of staples or stitches every 4–8 hours.	• Early identification of infection or problems with wound healing can ensure fast treatment.	
10. Anxiety (Child and Family) related to equipment and surgical outcome			
	NIC Priority Intervention: **Anxiety Reduction:** *Minimizing apprehension, dread, foreboding, or uneasiness related to an unidentified source of danger.*		*NOC Suggested Outcome:* **Coping:** *Actions to manage stressors that tax an individuals' resources.*
The child and family will verbalize comfort with postoperative care and outcome.	• Explain monitors, drainage dressings, intravenous lines, and procedures.	• Knowledge of purpose decreases anxiety.	The child and family demonstrate coping skills to deal with hospitalization.
	• Reassure the child and family that anxiety is a normal response to the stressful event of surgery.	• Knowledge of what is expected decreases anxiety.	
	• Encourage parental presence and care of the child.	• The child's anxiety decreases with parental presence.	
	• Use touch and other nonverbal and verbal communication with the child and family.	• Effective communication reassures child and family.	

NURSING CARE PLAN	The Child Undergoing Surgery (continued)		
GOAL	**INTERVENTION**	**RATIONALE**	**EXPECTED OUTCOME**
11. Knowledge Deficit (Child and Family) related to needed home care			
	NIC Priority Intervention: **Teaching, Postoperative:** *Health System Guidance: Facilitating a patient's location and use of appropriate health services.*		*NOC Suggested Outcome:* **Knowledge:** *Home Care: Extent of understanding conveyed about home care.*
The child and family will verbalize self-care required at home.	• Provide oral and written home care instructions regarding surgical wound care, medications, activities, and diet.	• Teaching regarding home care is necessary early in hospitalization.	The child and family demonstrate skills needed for home care following discharge. They verbalize plans for future care.
	• Provide a number to call for questions or concerns. Instruct on follow-up visits.	• Parents need to know emergency information and that follow-up care is required.	

Psychosocial Preparation

Preoperative teaching is geared to the child's developmental level. If child-life specialists (discussed later in the chapter) are available, they can also play an important role in preparing the child for surgery. When the child will be transferred to an intensive care unit or recovery room after surgery, a visit to the area before surgery can reduce the fear and anxiety associated with waking up in a strange environment filled with frightening sights, sounds, and smells. The use of tapes, puppets, body outline dolls, anatomically correct dolls, drawings, and models is encouraged to teach the child about the surgical procedure. For example, a doll was used as a teaching aid in preparing Tiara, the 5-year-old described in the opening vignette, for surgery. Playing with stethoscopes, gowns, masks, and syringes without needles also helps the child feel more in control (see discussion about therapeutic play later in this chapter). Children are reassured that their parents can accompany them to the operating room floor and will be waiting when they awaken from surgery. Parents should be allowed to carry infants and young toddlers to the pediatric holding area or have them ride in one parent's lap in a wheelchair. Older toddlers and preschoolers should be allowed to ride in a special wagon if possible. Special teddy bears and blankets are generally allowed in the pre-op holding area and provide comfort to the child. The nurse should make sure that the item is labeled with the child's name. Prepare family members for what to anticipate and what is expected of them. Special equipment such as intravenous setups and monitoring devices are explained. In some hospitals, only one or two immediate family members are allowed to visit the child at one time. Visitors may be required to wear special gowns, shoes, or hats, and they may be restricted to certain areas.

Parental Presence During Anesthesia Induction

Many hospitals now allow parents to be present with their child during anesthesia induction and again in the post-anesthesia recovery area. Parents often want to support their child before and immediately after a surgical procedure, and their presence offers reassurance and comfort to the child. The decision to allow parents to be present during induction of anesthesia must be made on an individual basis. Nurses should be open to change in practice and realize that incorporating the option of parental presence during anesthesia induction supports the principles of family-centered care (Romino, Keatley, Secrest, & Good, 2005). The nurse explains expectations, such as surgical gown, cap, shoe covers, and the parent's role in presence during induction. The nurse offers the parents an opportunity to ask questions and voice concerns.

Physical Preparation

Preparation for surgery may occur in designated preoperative areas. Procedures generally conducted in preoperative areas include premedication, intravenous start (if not

SKILL 9–5
Administering IV Fluids

BOX 13–7
PREOPERATIVE CHECKLIST

✓ Check that consent forms are witnessed and signed and in the patient's chart.
✓ Be sure the child's name band is in place.
✓ Be sure any allergies are prominently noted in the child's chart.
✓ Remove any prosthetic devices, including orthodontic appliances.
✓ Check the child's mouth for loose teeth and tongue piercings.
✓ Remove eyeglasses or contacts and jewelry.
✓ Bathe and cleanse the operative site if ordered.
✓ Put the child in a hospital gown, allowing the child to wear underwear.
✓ Check that all special tests have been completed and the results are in the child's chart.
✓ Have the child void before surgery.
✓ Keep the child NPO before surgery.
✓ Give the child prescribed medications.
✓ Transport the child safely to the operating room.

performed following general anesthesia), and preparation of the surgical site. If urinary catheterization is necessary, it is usually not performed until the child has been anesthetized.

Preoperative procedures and guidelines vary among hospitals and outpatient surgical centers. Preoperative checklists are used in ambulatory and acute care settings to ensure proper physical preparation of patients for surgery. A sample preoperative checklist is provided in Box 13–7. Weigh the preoperative child accurately, measure vital signs, and ask about last fluid intake amount and type. Monitor urinary output. NPO status in an infant and young child is distressing to both the child and the parents. Reinforce teaching regarding necessary NPO status as needed and provide support to the child and the family. See Families Want to Know: Waiting for the Child to Go to Surgery.

Nursing management during the preoperative period includes establishing accurate baseline data, administering prescribed fluids, and performing assessments of fluid status. When an intravenous infusion is prescribed, start the infusion (see the Skills Manual), ensuring that the type of fluid and flow rate match those that are ordered and that would be expected for the weight of the child.

Of necessity, the young child who undergoes surgery usually is restricted from consuming oral foods and fluids just before, during, and for a period after surgery. The length of time the child is kept without oral intake prior to surgery varies. Recommendations from the American Society of Anesthesiologists indicate that clear liquids may be given up until 2 hours prior to surgery, breast milk until 4 hours prior to surgery, and infant formula 6 hours prior. Milk and a light meal may be consumed until 6 hours prior to surgery. In general, older children will have a longer time without intake, infants much shorter (Crenshaw & Winslow, 2002). Infants will generally have very specific orders related to what time they should be made NPO for breast milk, formula, and clear liquids. This time will depend on what time the infant is scheduled for surgery. Because children beyond infancy do not usually eat or drink during the night, orders are usually written for NPO after midnight. If surgery is not scheduled for the morning, however, more specific orders should be written, especially for the toddler and preschool-age child, who will not be as tolerant of an extended NPO status. The ultimate decision on how long the child is NPO lies with the anesthesiologist and may vary depending on personal experiences and beliefs.

Infants are especially unable to conserve fluids; therefore, even a short time of NPO status for a diagnostic test may lead to imbalance. Surgery often causes fluid loss from bleeding, which can further compromise fluid balance. In addition, the child may experience third-spacing, a loss or pooling of fluid in a body space such as the abdomen, either in response to surgery or the child's condition. While decisions about the total amount of fluid required is determined by anesthesiologists during the surgery, the nurse needs an understanding of the amount of fluid generally required during the perioperative period. If a child is NPO prior to surgery and no intravenous line has been started, the child requires additional fluids during and after surgery to compensate for those not taken in during the period of fasting. See Chapter 16 ∞ for fluid requirements for children.

The decisions regarding the types of fluids administered before, during, and after surgery are determined based on the child's condition, length of surgery, and clinical

FAMILIES WANT TO KNOW

Waiting for the Child to Go to Surgery

Waiting for the child to go to surgery can be a very stressful time for both the family and the child. The major stressor for the infant and young child is the need to be NPO. Having a child who is upset because of hunger is very stressful for parents. Other stressors for parents include the risks of the surgery, pain the child will experience after the surgery, and in some cases what diagnosis may be made during or following the operation. Nurses must be sensitive to the concerns of the parents and provide support to these families. If the scheduled time for surgery has passed and no one has come to transport the child to the pediatric holding area, the nurse should call the operating room and see when they might expect that someone will come to get the child for surgery. While this takes a few minutes, it is an essential aspect of a trusting family-centered environment.

condition. During surgery, nurses continue to administer fluids and measure fluid losses, and assess the child continuously.

Postoperative Care

Post-anesthesia care units (PACU) are the receiving areas for children following surgery. In the PACU, the child is recovered from anesthesia and is either discharged home or transferred to the unit specified.

Postoperative care of the child includes both physical and psychologic care. In the immediate postoperative period, perform baseline monitoring of vital signs; evaluate evidence of fluid loss via dressings, vomiting, or drainage tubes; and record hourly urinary output. Maintain effective airway clearance and monitor for evidence of respiratory depression or distress. Examine the postoperative orders and ensure that the child receives the type and amount of intravenous fluid indicated.

The child's level of consciousness is evaluated, and vital signs are assessed frequently according to agency protocol. The surgical site is observed for drainage, and dressings are monitored for bleeding. The nurse monitors the child's intake and output hourly and provides comfort and pain relief. See Chapter 15 ∞ for details concerning pain management. Administer medications in a developmentally appropriate manner (see Table 13–5). Resumption of oral intake is dependent on the surgical procedure, the child's condition, and surgeon protocol. When the child resumes intake of oral fluids, small amounts of clear liquids should be given first. The child should be monitored for nausea and vomiting. If the child tolerates clear liquids, the diet can be progressed per physician's orders.

Parents are encouraged to visit with the child as soon after surgery as possible (Figure 13–6 ➤). The child may be discharged home directly from an outpatient surgical procedure or, depending on the child's condition, may be transferred to a general pediatric unit or intensive care unit. (See accompanying nursing care plan.)

> ### CLINICAL TIP
> If surgery is postponed for an infant or young child who is NPO and does not have IV access, the nurse should consult with the physician to see if the child needs to have an IV started.

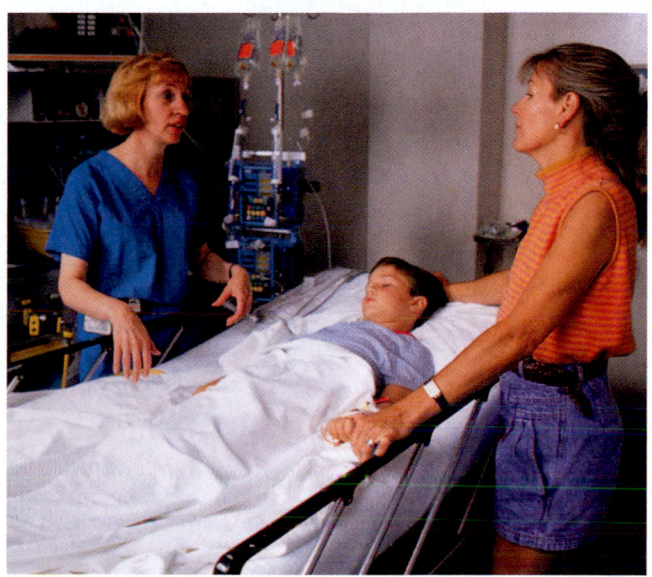

Figure 13–6 ➤ This child has just undergone surgery and is in the post-anesthesia care unit (PACU). Although the child's physical care is immediate and important, remember that both the child and the family have strong psychosocial needs that must be addressed concurrently. It is important to reunite the family as soon as possible after surgery.

Postoperative Home Care Instructions

Routine postoperative instructions for the family of the child undergoing outpatient or one-day-stay surgical procedures include monitoring for signs of infection, such as drainage, redness, or swelling of the surgical incision, fever, and change in behavior. Instructions for follow-up visit, medications, other treatments, and wound care, as well as signs and symptoms that require medical attention, are also provided. Additional instructions are tailored according to the surgical procedure and the child's condition. The nurse ensures the family understands home care instructions through their return demonstration and verbalization of understanding.

STRATEGIES TO PROMOTE COPING AND NORMAL DEVELOPMENT OF THE HOSPITALIZED CHILD

During hospitalization, care of the child focuses not only on meeting physiologic needs, but also on meeting psychosocial and developmental needs. Several strategies may be used to help children adapt to the hospital environment, promote effective coping, and provide developmentally appropriate activities. These strategies include child-life programs, rooming in, therapeutic play, and therapeutic recreation.

Rooming In

The practice of **rooming in** involves a parent staying in the child's hospital room during the course of the child's hospitalization. Some hospitals provide cots, while others have special built-in beds on pediatric units. In some institutions, a parent is provided

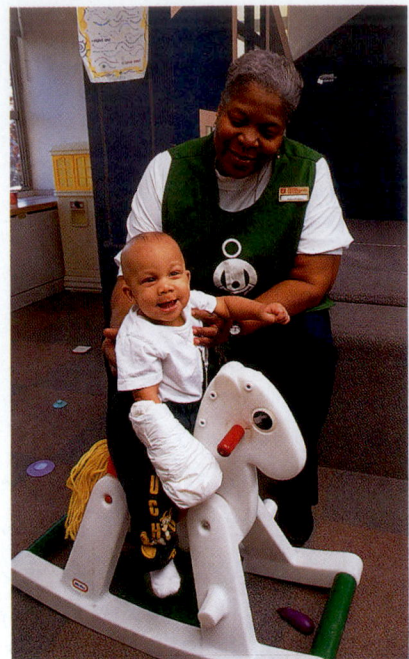

Figure 13–7 ➤ Volunteers such as this foster grandmother can provide stimulation and nurturing to help young children adapt to lengthy hospitalizations.

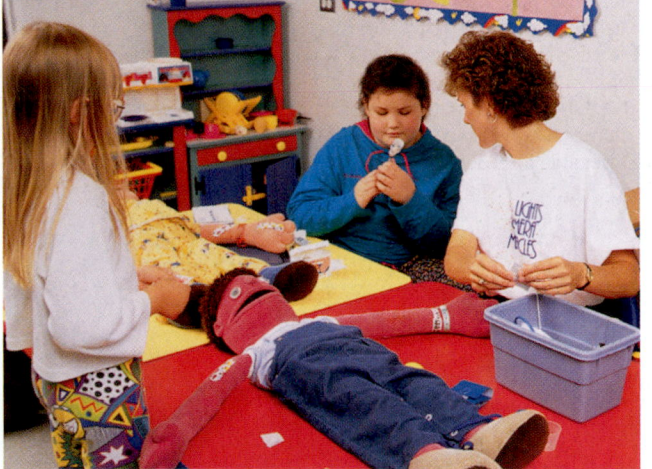

Figure 13–8 ➤ A child-life specialist works with children being treated for cancer. Special dolls are used to familiarize children with the procedures they undergo.

a separate room on the unit. Parents who stay at the bedside usually want to help care for their child (Dudley & Carr, 2004). Communication between the nurse and family is important so that the parent's desire for involvement is understood and supported.

Rooming in provides the child with the comfort and security of parental presence. Parents may feel more comfortable staying with their child and participating in care, while others may experience more stress if they are missing work and are away from home and other children. Collaborate with the parents to assist them in establishing a rooming-in plan that is beneficial to both the child and family. For example, parents may alternate turns staying with the child, and even grandparents, aunts and uncles, and grown siblings may be included in the plan.

Some facilities offer free or reduced-cost meals to the parent rooming in. The parent who does not receive these meals may often skip many meals due to the financial impact on an already over-burdened budget related to illness and hospitalization. The nurse should be alert to parents who never leave the bedside and make sure the parent is eating. Emphasize the importance of the child's need for a healthy parent. Social services or other departments in the hospital may be able to assist the family in obtaining meals while rooming in with the hospitalized child.

Parents rooming in with their child for an extended hospitalization can be encouraged to take advantage of facilities such as the Ronald McDonald house, or other housing available for parents, at some point during the stay as a respite for a few hours. This will provide them with an opportunity for needed rest and privacy.

Child-Life Programs

Many hospitals have child-life programs that focus on the psychosocial needs of hospitalized children. Professional child-life specialists, paraprofessionals, and volunteers staff these departments (Figure 13–7 ➤). A **child-life specialist** plans activities to provide age-appropriate play for children either in the child's room or in a specialized playroom. Some of the planned activities are designed to assist children in working through feelings about illness. Examples include playing with medical equipment, acting out procedures or treatments on dolls, using games to act out feelings, or drawing pictures about hospital treatments (Figure 13–8 ➤).

Both the child-life department and the nursing staff focus on the emotional needs of hospitalized children. Child-life specialists and nurses collaborate to formulate a plan together to assist children with particular needs. Before engaging in activities, attention is given to the child's level of mobility, fatigue, readiness to participate, and other barriers such as pain. The nurse and child-life specialist can work together to determine appropriate methods to use to promote coping with painful procedures.

Therapeutic Play

Play is a significant component of childhood. The stress of illness and hospitalization increases the value of play. Not only is normal development facilitated by play, but play sessions can provide a means for the child to learn about health care, to express anxieties, to work through feelings, and to achieve a sense of mastery or control over frightening or little-understood situations. In the present era of cost containment, play programs may be minimized in hospitals; therefore, nurses should document the need for and benefits of play.

Play that presents an opportunity to deal with the fears, concerns, and stressors of health experiences is called **therapeutic play**. Therapeutic play has many benefits both for the child and the health professional. It allows the child an opportunity to relive, understand, and integrate fearful healthcare experiences. The child can achieve a sense of mastery by being in control of the occurrences during play. This helps to lower the child's stress and anxiety about the events. In addition, the healthcare professional can observe the child's play to learn more about the type of events that cause anxiety to the child. The child's coping methods can be observed and additional techniques offered to the child. *Play therapy* is a mental health technique used to treat children with mental health problems. It is not used to treat anxiety caused by normal life events.

Through therapeutic play, the child's knowledge of his or her illness or injury can be assessed. A common technique involves using an outline drawing of the body (Figure 13–9 ➤) or having the child draw a picture about the hospitalization. Drawings can be used to determine what the child knows and understands about the hospitalization. They can also give an indication regarding the anxiety and stress the child is feeling (Lukash, 2002; Tielsch & Allen, 2005). In addition to assessment, drawing can be used as a nursing intervention. Demonstrate to the child on a drawing what will occur during surgery or a treatment. The child's drawings of healthcare experiences allow him or her to express fears and gain mastery over the situation.

Dramatic play, in which medical situations encountered are reenacted by the child, often assist the child to cope with painful treatments and intrusive procedures. Safe medical equipment such as bandages and syringes without needles, and scrubs and uniforms for dress up, are effective materials for encouraging dramatic play. These activities allow the child the opportunity to become familiar with the hospital environment and procedures. Through observation of dramatic play the nurse assesses the child's perception of the illness and procedures and then clarifies those misconceptions. Dramatic play also offers an outlet for anxiety in children trying to deal with stressful and confusing situations.

A variety of techniques may be used to promote therapeutic and dramatic play (Table 13–8). Specific techniques are chosen to reflect the child's developmental stage.

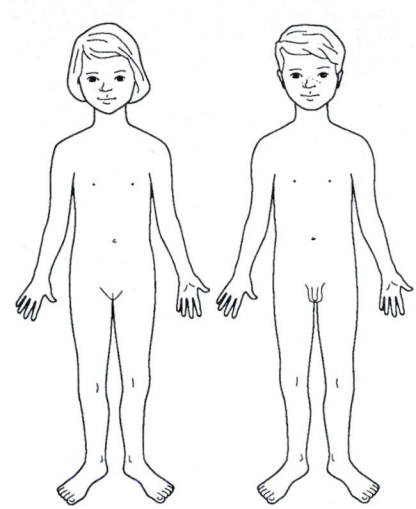

Figure 13–9 ➤ The nurse can use a simple gender-specific outline drawing of a child's body to encourage children to draw what they think about their medical problem. Such drawings reveal a child's interpretation, which the nurse can work with to provide enhanced teaching.

Table 13–8	**THERAPEUTIC PLAY TECHNIQUES**	
Technique	**Assessment**	**Interventions**
Stories	Have the child make up a story about a picture. Analyze content and emotional clues in the story. Have children tell a story about an important experience in a group of other children.	Read or make up stories to explain illness, hospitalization, or other specific aspects of health care. Emotions such as fear can be included.
Drawings	Ask the child to draw a picture about being in the hospital. Consider subject matter, size and placement of items in drawings, colors used, presence or absence of physical barriers, and general emotional feeling.	Use the child's drawings or outlines of the body to explain care, procedures, or conditions. Provide an opportunity for the child to draw pictures of his or her choice or directed topics such as a picture of the child's family or healthcare encounter. Ask the child: "Tell me about your picture." Be alert to the child's emotions: "This child must be frightened by the big radiograph machine."
Music	Observe types of music chosen and effects of played music on behavior.	Encourage parents and children to bring favorite tapes or CDs to the hospital for stress relief. Have tapes playing during tests and procedures. Parents can record their voices to play for infants and young children during separations. During longer hospitalizations children can tape messages for siblings or classmates, who are then encouraged to record their responses. Playtime can include the opportunity to play instruments and sing.
Puppets	The puppets can ask questions of young children, who are often more likely to answer the puppet than a person.	Perform short skits to teach children necessary healthcare information. Include emotional content when appropriate.
Dramatic play	Provide dolls and medical equipment, and analyze the roles assigned to dolls by the child, the behavior demonstrated by the dolls in the child's play, and the apparent emotions. Dolls with illnesses or health problems like those of the child are especially helpful (see Figure 13–10).	Provide dolls and equipment for play sessions. To ensure safety, supervise closely when actual equipment is used. Respond to emotions and behavior shown. Use dolls and equipment such as casts, nebulizer, intravenous apparatus, and stethoscope to explain care. Use dolls with problems or illnesses similar to those of the child when available. Provide toys that foster expression of emotion, such as a pounding board and indoor darts.
Pets	Provide pet therapy. Watch the interaction between child and animal (see Figure 13–11).	Respond to emotions the child shows. Facilitate touch and stroking of animals.

Additional techniques, such as sand or water play, may be appropriate in specific situations.

BOX 13–8
PRIZE BASKET

A "prize" basket is an effective method of providing rewards and distraction to the toddler, preschooler, and even school-age child. The basket contains age-appropriate toys, games, and items that the child may choose from as a reward for participating in a procedure. For example, bubbles, stuffed animals, small dolls, coloring books, balls, and books are inexpensive (they may also be donated) items that the child can choose from. Of importance, even if the child is uncooperative, once the procedure is completed, the child should be praised and offered the opportunity to choose from the prize basket.

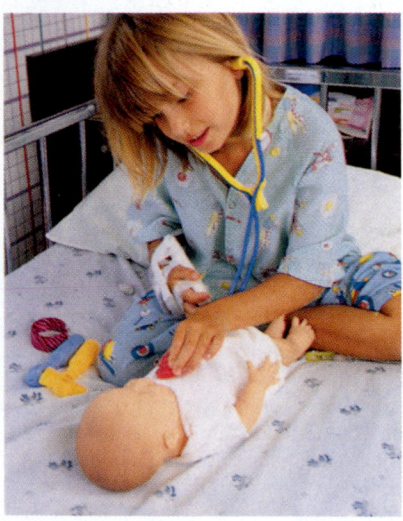

A

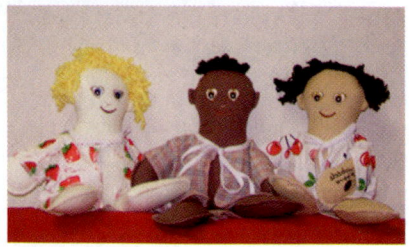

B

Figure 13–10 ➤ A, Age-appropriate play will help the child to adjust to hospitalization and care. B, Having the child play with dolls, like these Shadow Buddies, that have "conditions" similar to his or her own will help the child adjust. Such play helps the child realize what activities are possible.
Used with permission of The Shadow Buddies Foundation, http://www.shadowbuddies.org.

The nurse assures that a variety of age-appropriate toys and distraction materials (stress balls, bubbles, music) and "prizes" are available (Box 13–8). Families are encouraged to bring the child's favorite age-appropriate toys from home.

Many hospitals, particularly children's hospitals, provide playrooms on each of the units to allow children a place to play and socialize with same-age peers. These rooms are generally brightly decorated in children's themes, and provide numerous opportunities for play, such as board games, video games, supplies for painting or drawing, and age-appropriate toys for each developmental level. There may be options for computer communication with children in other hospitals. Many electronic play stations are portable for children on isolation or unable to come to a playroom. Specific interventions according to developmental level are discussed in the following text.

Infants

Infants require external stimuli for growth. The use of mobiles, music, mirrors, and other stimulation helps to promote stimulation and offer comfort to the infant. Parents and family are encouraged to cuddle or rock the infant and sing lullabies. Talking to the infant encourages interaction and play.

Toddler

Through play, toddlers explore the environment and learn to identify with significant people in their lives. Play is also an acceptable way for toddlers to release tensions caused by stress or aggressive impulses.

Approach toddlers slowly and make the initial approach in their parents' presence, if possible, to decrease feelings of stranger anxiety (wariness of strangers). Playing a variation of peek-a-boo or hide-and-seek using the curtain surrounding the toddler's crib or bed helps promote the realization that objects that are out of sight, such as parents, do return. The use of objects, such as a familiar blanket or stuffed animal, can temporarily substitute for the security of parents. The toddler can be read familiar stories. Repetition of stories promotes a sense of stability in the unfamiliar hospital environment.

A doll is a familiar toy that can be used to re-create a stressful environment, thereby providing an opportunity for the child to express and work through feelings. Other developmentally appropriate toys for toddlers include familiar objects from home such as measuring cups or spoons, wooden puzzles, building blocks, and push-and-pull toys. Playing with safe hospital equipment (bandages, syringes without needles, and stethoscopes) helps toddlers to overcome the anxiety associated with these items. Supervise these play sessions and remove hospital equipment when you leave.

Preschooler

The nurse can intervene to reduce the stress produced by preschoolers' fears through the use of certain kinds of play. A simple outline of the body or a doll can be used to address the child's fantasies and fears of bodily harm. Playing with safe hospital equipment may help preschoolers to work through feelings such as aggression (Figure 13–10 ➤). Both preschool and school-age children may enjoy playing with a toy hospital.

Preschoolers prefer crayons and coloring books, puppets, felt and magnetic boards, play dough, books, and recorded stories. Preschoolers and older children often enjoy **pet therapy** (Figure 13–11 ➤). Children's hospitals and units can have visits from pets, to provide diversion and physical contact (Kaminski, Pellino, & Wish, 2002).

School-Age Child

Although play begins to lose its importance in the school-age years, the nurse can still use some techniques of therapeutic play to help the hospitalized child cope with stress. Age-appropriate crafts and activities provide diversion and a sense of accomplishment for the school-age child. School-age children often regress developmentally during hospitalization, demonstrating behaviors characteristic of an earlier state, such as separation anxiety and fear of bodily injury. Outlines of the body and anatomically correct dolls or condition-specific dolls (see Figure 13–10b) can be used to illustrate the cause and treatment of the child's illness. Terms for body parts that are suitable for older children are used. Drawings provide an outlet for expression of fears and anger.

School-age children enjoy collecting and organizing objects and often ask to keep disposable equipment that has been used in their care. They may use these items later to relive the experience with their friends. Games, books, school work, crafts, tape recordings, and computers and video games provide an outlet for stress and increase self-esteem in the school-age child. The type of play used should promote a sense of mastery and achievement.

Adolescent

Many of the special play techniques used with younger children are not suitable for adolescents. However, adolescents do require a planned **therapeutic recreation** program to assist them in meeting developmental needs during hospitalization. Peers are very important to the adolescent, and the isolation of hospitalization can be difficult. Telephone contact with other teenagers and visits from friends should be encouraged. Interactions with other hospitalized teenagers at a pizza party, video game, movie night, or during other activities can help adolescents feel a sense of normalcy (Figure 13–12 ➤). Physical activities that provide an outlet for stress are recommended. Even adolescents on bed rest or in wheelchairs can play a modified form of basketball. Some hospitals provide a teen room or teen lounge with age-appropriate activities such as a pool table, video games, and computers.

The independence of adolescence is interrupted by illness. Nurses can provide choices for teenagers to assist them in regaining control. Providing the adolescents with options and encouraging them to choose an evening of recreational activity can promote their feelings of independence.

Adolescents and school-age children also prefer to wear their own clothing while hospitalized. Depending on the adolescent's condition, passes to leave the hospital for special activities and recreation may be possible.

Strategies to Meet Educational Needs

Some hospitalizations are so short that the absence of the child or adolescent from school and peers is of minimal concern. However, if hospitalization is expected to last longer than a few days or if the child's condition will change, necessitating special school arrangements, the nurse assesses the effects of hospitalization on the child's education.

When an elective procedure occurs, collaborate with families to assist in the arrangement of the extended school absence with teachers. The child can then be provided with school work to complete in the hospital or at home when capable. This minimizes educational deficits and future problems for the child. Pencils, paper, comfortable work areas, computers, and quiet work times are provided to meet the child's educational needs. Telephone calls and Internet connections can be arranged as needed. Pediatric hospitals generally provide in-house teachers to meet the child's educational needs. The hospital teachers collaborate with the child's school teachers to ensure the child is meeting the educational objectives to avoid deficits upon return to school.

The social aspects of school and peers are also considered. Peers are encouraged to visit a hospitalized classmate, send cards and letters, call on the telephone, or communicate via the Internet. Classmates may even want to videotape a class session, allowing everyone the opportunity to send a message to the child. When the child returns to school, the nurse can visit the classroom to provide classmates with information about the child's medical condition or assist the child in creating his or her own presentation about the hospital experience and medical condition.

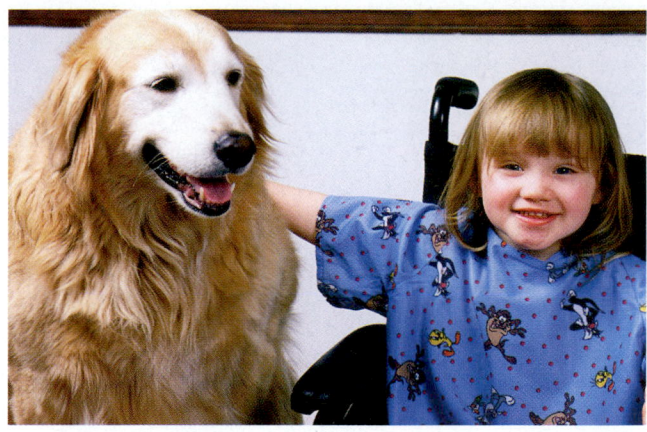

Figure 13–11 ➤ Hospitals may have pet therapy from specially trained animals to provide comfort and distraction during health care. Both the child and the dog seem to be smiling!

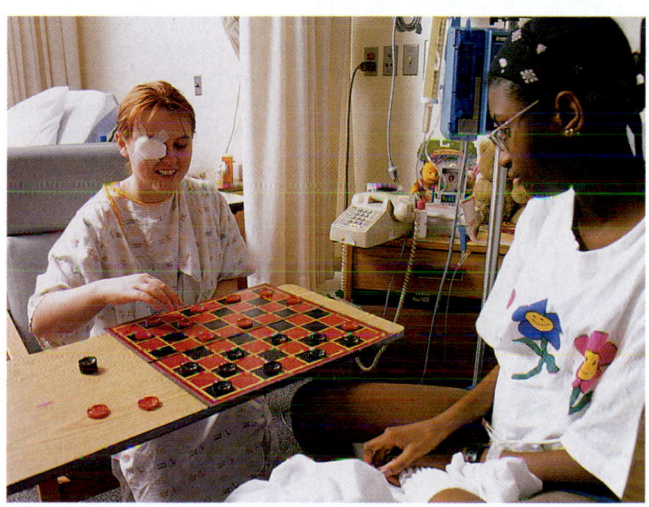

Figure 13–12 ➤ Having interaction with other hospitalized adolescents and maintaining contact with friends outside the hospital are very important so that the teenager does not feel alone. A friendly yet competitive checkers game helps to stimulate these teenagers and allows for self-expression. What are the other benefits?

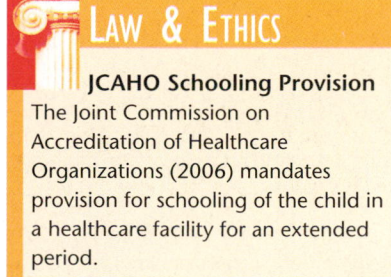

LAW & ETHICS

JCAHO Schooling Provision
The Joint Commission on Accreditation of Healthcare Organizations (2006) mandates provision for schooling of the child in a healthcare facility for an extended period.

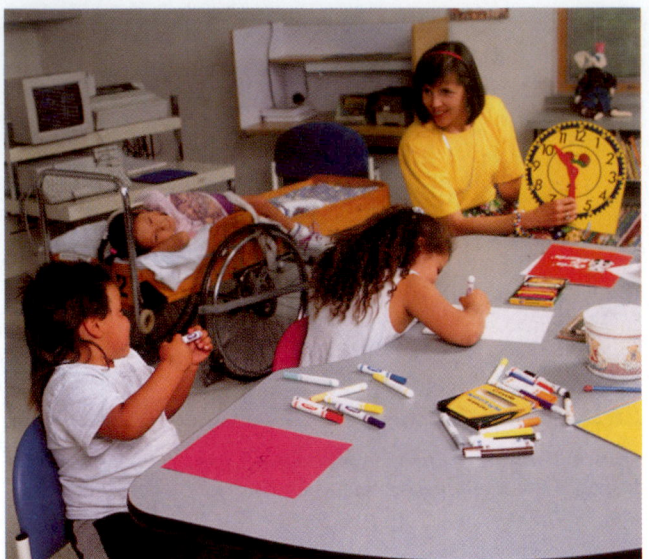

Figure 13–13 ➤ Shriner's Hospital in Spokane, Washington, has a special classroom and teacher for children undergoing a lengthy hospital stay, enabling them to remain current with their schoolwork. The child who falls behind other students might not fit in when he or she returns to school or might be required to repeat a grade. What are the potential consequences of these situations?

The hospital nurse may contact the child's school nurse when special arrangements are necessary for situations such as mobility challenges. For example, the child who is wearing a large cast or who requires medications or other treatments, such as tracheostomy care, may offer challenges in a traditional school setting. Refer to Chapter 11 ∞ for further discussion of caring for the child in the community.

The child with chronic health problems or requiring long-term hospitalization has additional needs with regard to school. Hospitals or rehabilitation units may have classrooms, teachers, and facilities to promote learning (Figure 13–13 ➤). Many school districts provide tutors or computer connections for students who are hospitalized or receiving home care for extended periods. Teachers can visit children at the hospital or at home. Parents are often pivotal in making arrangements to meet the child's educational needs, since they interact with the child, the school, and the healthcare team. Further discussion of meeting the educational needs of the child with a chronic condition is provided in Chapter 12 ∞.

Child and Family Teaching

Teaching is an essential part of the nurse's role in the care of hospitalized children and their families and begins with the initial contact between the family and healthcare providers. The American Nurses Association's and Society of Pediatric Nurses' statement on the scope and standards of pediatric clinical nursing practice mandates teaching as a component of pediatric nursing care (American Nurses Association & Society of Pediatric Nurses, 2003).

Teaching may be informal, as when the nurse integrates an explanation during routine care, or structured, as when the nurse plans and implements a formal teaching program. However, with shorter hospitalization stays few group interactions are possible, necessitating that most teaching be conducted during conversations and patient care (London, 2004).

Nurses emphasize to the family that most teaching will occur in informal sessions rather than in formalized programs. The family should be aware of the teaching process to encourage active listening and participation. Actively involve the family in the learning process to assure their understanding. The nurse and family partner together to identify the family's learning needs and appropriate teaching method to best convey the information. Recall that different family members may be at various cognitive and anxiety levels and therefore have needs for different types of teaching. Develop a plan with both the family and other healthcare professionals to facilitate learning among the child and family members.

Teaching about the behaviors observed in hospitalized children and the strategies to deal with these behaviors is helpful for parents. For instance, providing information for parents of hospitalized toddlers on the typical behaviors of hospitalized children, and on the strategies to assist children, leads to less anxiety on the part of the parents and to greater parental involvement and support of the child during the hospitalization.

Teaching directed at children that takes into account their developmental level and cognitive abilities will facilitate a deeper understanding of the illness (McQuaid, Howard, Kopel, Rosenblum, & Bibace, 2002). Learning is achieved more successfully when teaching involves more than one sense (such as hearing, vision, and touch). Teaching directed at parents must be geared to their level of understanding. If English is not spoken or is the parents' second language, then a translator may be necessary. If translators are needed to facilitate understanding, be sure they are arranged for and available for teaching sessions.

Timing is a critical factor in teaching. Parents and children are less receptive to teaching when they are preoccupied with stress or activities. Collaborating with the parents in scheduling specific times for teaching sessions may be most effective in maximizing the experience.

Depending on the information to be presented, teaching may use the cognitive, psychomotor, or affective domains of learning. Teaching that includes all three domains is more effective than simply using one. Explanations or reading materials are tailored to a level the parent can understand. The choice of tools used varies depending on the child's diagnosis and available materials. The tools include pamphlets, booklets, videos, and models.

Teaching Plans

A teaching plan is a written document that includes goals and expected outcomes, interventions needed to achieve the specified goals, and a method and time for evaluation of the expected outcomes. The teaching plan may also specify teaching methods and types of materials to be used. Multidisciplinary teaching plans provide clear communication for all health team members in the teaching process. Documentation of teaching allows for continuity of care between nurses and other disciplines. Developing a teaching plan helps to ensure that all the necessary information is included and makes teaching more efficient.

The child's primary caretaker is an active participant in the development of the teaching plan as well as the implementation. The primary caretaker is most often a parent but may be a close family member (uncle, aunt, or grandparent). Multiple members of the household with caregiving roles will ideally be involved in the educational process. The first step in establishing a teaching plan is to assess the child's or parent's knowledge, skills, and feelings by asking the following questions:

- What does the parent/caretaker or child know about the health issue?
- What are the expectations of the child and family?
- What is the cognitive level or ability to learn?
- Is there a desire to learn?
- What previous experiences affect the learning experience, either positively or negatively?
- What previous interventions have been the most useful for the child and family?
- What resources are available to the parents, child, and nurse that enhance understanding of the health condition?
- Are there feelings or beliefs that might interfere with the learning process?
- What complementary care does the family use, and how does this relate to the teaching plan?

The second step involves deciding what knowledge, skill, or change in attitude is desired. Outcome criteria or objectives are established with the parent and child.

Possible teaching methods and a range of approaches are explored. A variety of resources, including written materials (books, pamphlets, handouts, and stories), computer software, audiovisual presentations, and others, are available to encourage interest from the child and family. See Box 13–9 for a sample teaching plan, and Box 13–10 for teaching methods.

Teaching for Children with Special Healthcare Needs

Children who have disabilities may have special learning needs (Allen & Vessey, 2004). If the child has a visual impairment or perceptual difficulty, material is presented in auditory and tactile ways. Children who have hearing deficits require visual and tactile presentations. When psychomotor skill performance is needed, special aids and devices may be necessary for the child with neuromuscular conditions to allow the child to hold a syringe, draw up a liquid, or perform other tasks. Children who have learning disabilities may require more frequent reinforcement and shorter teaching sessions. These children are evaluated often for comprehension in order to adjust teaching as necessary.

Nurses individualize teaching plans and sessions according to the child's ability and needs. Adequate assessment of the child's strengths and abilities, along with collaboration

BOX 13–9
STANDARDIZED TEACHING PLAN: PREPARING THE CHILD FOR SURGERY

Surgery may be planned or unexpected. Whether the child is encountered in the clinic, pre-op admissions clinic, emergency room, or pediatric unit, the nurse should prepare the child for surgery as much as possible. While younger children should be told about a planned operation the day before the surgery, school-age children and adolescents should be told as soon as the operation is scheduled. Age-specific guidelines should be followed. (See Table 13–7, Assisting Children Through Procedures, and the accompanying Nursing Care Plan, The Child Undergoing Surgery).

General Principles
- Ask the child's parents what they have told their child about the operation.
- Assess the child's perception of the operation using developmentally appropriate activities.
- Teach the child about the operation and what to expect during the pre- and postoperative period, clarifying any misconceptions.
- Reassess the child's perception of the operation.

Sample Teaching Plan for Tiara, the 5-Year-Old Girl in the Opening Scenario, Scheduled for a Tonsillectomy and Adenoidectomy

When: At the preadmissions visit the day prior to surgery

Where: In a quiet room, without distraction

How:
- Ask Tiara's mother what she has told her daughter about the surgery.
- Ask Tiara to draw a picture about going to the hospital.
- Ask Tiara why she needs the operation.
- Using a body outline doll or picture of a body outline, ask Tiara to show you what part is going to be fixed.
- Use pictures, books, dolls, and safe medical equipment to clarify misconceptions and teach Tiara about the operation. Allow Tiara the opportunity to dress up in scrubs and play with safe medical equipment.
- Reassess Tiara's understanding of the operation by allowing her to dress up in scrubs and "operate" on a doll. Include what she will see, hear, taste, smell, and feel in both the preoperative and postoperative period.

BOX 13–10
LEARNING THROUGH SENSES

For children who can hear, touch, see a model or equipment, read, look at pictures, or even smell things like alcohol swabs, learning is more complete. This is particularly important for the school-age child in the stage of concrete operational thought, who must be able to manipulate materials in order to learn.

with parents and other members of the multidisciplinary team, can assist the nurse to establish an individualized plan to establish the most effective teaching methods for the child.

Children who have chronic conditions or special healthcare needs may have been hospitalized numerous times and have received other health care at home and in the community. They usually have adapted coping mechanisms that help them deal with the chronic illness. Nurses can talk with the child to determine what has helped in the past, provide information about what to expect during the current hospitalization, assign staff members who are familiar when possible, and follow each child's lead in assisting his or her coping.

Nurses do not assume that children with a history of numerous hospitalizations understand all activities since each hospitalization is different. Even the most routine activities are explained. The updated plan of care is regularly reviewed with parents and children. Provide children with opportunities to ask questions and express concerns and fears. Assess each child's individual learning needs. Older children can be asked how they best like to learn. Determine the necessity for special equipment or teaching methods.

PREPARATION FOR HOME CARE

Nurses play an important role in preparing the child and family for discharge home; this preparation starts early during the hospitalization. The nurse works with the social service department, home care agencies, and the family to plan for equipment, procedures, and other home care needs. Parents of very young infants who have been hospitalized will need assistance to bond with and learn interaction skills with the baby in addition to assistance with physical care (Whitfield, 2003). Home care nurses collaborate with the hospital nurse and assist families to meet the child's healthcare needs.

Assessing the Child and Family in Preparation for Discharge

The discharge process is best started on admission to the hospital. The healthcare team, including the primary healthcare provider, nurse, social worker, and discharge planner, works with the family to ensure a smooth transition. Assess the family's ability to manage the child's care and if any special adaptation of the home environment is necessary.

When a child who has been hospitalized for an extended time period is to be discharged home, the school district is contacted and plans for education or re-entry into school are made. This involves an assessment of the child by the school district and formulation of an *Individualized Education Plan* (IEP). The IEP may include home tutors, specialized services from persons such as physical or speech therapists, or arrangements for transport of the child with a disability to the school and provisions for special medical care as needed. An *Individualized Health Plan* (IHP) may also be required. See Chapter 11 ∞ for a detailed discussion on Individualized Education Plans and Individualized Health Plans.

Some common problems that interfere with successful discharge planning include financial concerns, the family's unavailability for teaching and planning, lack of equipment or site, and lack of teamwork among involved healthcare disciplines. Nurses who assess for these potential problems from the initial contact with the child and family can intervene and assist the family to resolve these problems as soon as possible.

Preparing the Child and Family for Discharge

The family may need to learn physical and rehabilitative procedures for the child's care. Short-term care may be necessary until the child regains full function. In other situations, care may be required throughout the child's life. This may involve measuring vital signs or assessing blood glucose levels. For the child requiring complex long-term care, parents may need to learn about intravenous lines, medications, oxygen administration, or ventilators (Figure 13–14 ➤). Some facilities provide families with the opportunity to provide 24-hour care to the child prior to discharge in order to help them gain confidence in providing care and allow the nurse to assess for areas requiring further teaching. See Chapter 12 ∞ for discussion of the child with a chronic condition.

Collaborate with the parents to teach them treatment procedures and proper equipment use as needed for the child's care. The goals of teaching include parents' ability to demonstrate care technique, their appropriate use of equipment, and their ability to identify symptoms requiring report to the healthcare provider (Meleski, 2002)

Parents of children at risk for respiratory or cardiac arrest are encouraged to learn cardiopulmonary resuscitation (CPR) (refer to the *Clinical Skills Manual*). Arrangements for individual sessions to teach the family CPR can be arranged. Some families require support and assistance to become providers of end-of-life care (see Chapter 14 ∞ for end-of-life care).

Not all children discharged after hospitalization will require any additional care. However, these families still have need of support and education, as they may continue to be anxious or stressed over their child's hospitalization. Standard discharge plans for routine hospital discharge include the follow-up appointment date, phone number to call for questions, medication instructions, signs and symptoms to monitor specific to the condition, and care at home. Ensure that the family understands these instructions and has ample opportunity for questions before discharge home.

Preparing the Child and Family for Home Health Care

Children discharged from the hospital may require short-term or long-term home health care. Children with multisystem conditions may require home care involving specialized equipment and personnel. Early planning provides the family time to investigate health insurance benefits, support services in the community, and other needs before discharge. The education provided and the parents' ability to perform care is discussed with a visiting nurse or individual who manages the home care program. See the Evidence-Based Nursing box on page 438.

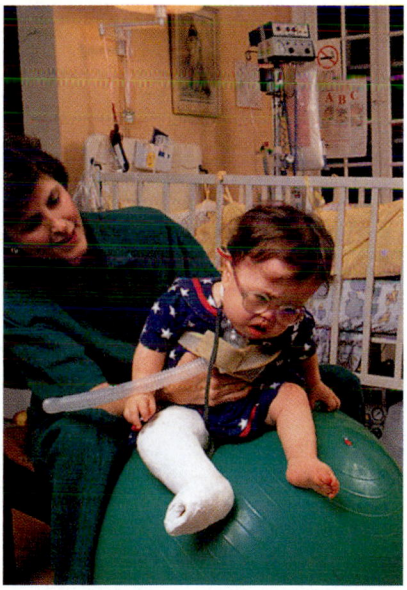

Figure 13–14 ➤ This child with chronic medical problems is being cared for at home. Are there any legal implications for the hospital and the nurse associated with the preparation of the child and family for home care?

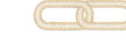

SKILL 11–18
Performing Cardiopulmonary Resusitation

EVIDENCE-BASED PRACTICE

Preparing Families to Provide Health Care for Children at Home

Problem

Children are often discharged from hospitals while still requiring complicated healthcare procedures, so parents need to learn how to perform these procedures safely. Parents may not be able to be in the hospital consistently during the hospitalization or they may not be as involved in the child's care as would be helpful for learning the needed skills.

Evidence

Using a qualitative approach, researchers interviewed families of 14 children hospitalized for a variety of chronic illnesses. Parents identified a lack of support by personnel when they were present in the hospital; they often felt in the way and did not want to disturb the routines of the unit. Parents reported that they were frequently not included in decision making about the child, and yet felt responsibility for managing the multiple needs of the child's condition once they returned home (Ygge & Arnetz, 2004). Other authors have noted that teaching families is often viewed as a short-term task, but in reality it is ongoing and needs to be integrated into all interactions in order to adequately prepare the family for discharge (London, 2004).

Implications

Preparing families for care of their children is a complex task and the situation in the hospital is sometimes not conducive to teaching and learning. Nurses can support parents during rooming in by making them comfortable and integrating them into discussions and decisions about the child's care; they are collaborators in all of the care involved. Nurses can also view every interaction as a teachable moment and constantly include teaching whenever a parent is present. Explain medications, what assessments are being performed, and how this will be adapted in the home situation. Provide resources for the responsibility the parent takes on as the child returns home, including phone numbers, parent support groups, reading material, and Internet sources. Ask parents what care they feel comfortable with and what they need more assistance to perform. Involve them in the decision about referral to home health care or school nurse.

Critical Thinking

What conditions in the hospital will assist parents to feel welcome and part of the hospital routine? How can parents become a part of rounds to their own child? What questions can they be asked? How can the nurse help to explain to parents the meaning of conversations that take place near the child by healthcare personnel? How can you adapt your teaching plan to include integration of home care into every interaction with the parents? How can you record the teaching needs of parents so that other nurses can continue with needed information, demonstrations, and assessments? What techniques need to be part of discharge care so that parents leave with resources to get future questions answered as they take over total care of the child?

The nurse collaborates with the social service department, home care agencies, and the family to plan for equipment, procedures, and other home care needs. Home care nurses then assume the child's care and assist families to meet the child's healthcare needs. See Chapter 11 ∞ for further discussion of home health care.

Preparing the Child and Family for Long-Term Care or Rehabilitation

When ill or injured children require long-term care, they are often transferred from an acute care hospital to a rehabilitation center or other long-term care facility. Like discharge planning, the rehabilitation phase of the treatment does not begin at the time of discharge from the acute care hospital but, instead, early in the hospitalization phase. The plan of care is instituted in the hospital, interventions and therapies are begun, and plans are made for continued care. A multidisciplinary team, including the nurse, social worker, and case manager, coordinates the process and collaborates with the family to ensure a transition that causes the least disruption to the child and family.

When it becomes apparent that a child will require long-term care, the healthcare team explores with the family the options and resources available to provide such care:

- Home care with support services such as visiting nurses and physical therapists
- A long-term care facility
- A specialized rehabilitation center that can provide care for an extended period

The nurse supports the family during the decision-making process about which option will be the most beneficial, considering the needs of the child, the financial implications, the roles and supports available to the family unit, and the resources available in the community. Guidelines to assist parents in evaluating rehabilitation centers are available from the Brain Injury Association of America (Brain Injury Association of America, 2006).

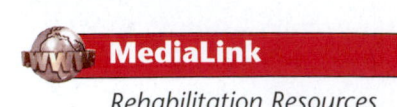

MediaLink

Rehabilitation Resources

Families often require assistance in determining the insurance coverage for long-term care or rehabilitation because coverage for these services may be limited. Social services can play an important role in assisting the family in identifying insurance coverage. If a parent must take a leave of absence from work to provide care for the child, inform the parent about the coverage provided by the Family Medical Leave Act (U.S. Department of Labor, 2004). Collaborate with social services to assist the family to understand and complete the applications, if needed.

Nurses in acute care hospitals frequently coordinate services when transfer to another facility occurs. This involves providing information about the child's history, plan of care, treatment, and current status to the new facility. Forms are available to assist the person responsible for coordinating the transfer. Copies of nursing and medical care plans are often provided to ensure continuity of care.

Families require support and assistance in dealing with the transfer from the acute care setting to another facility. The family may benefit from a visit to the facility before the child is transferred. Meeting the staff and becoming familiar with the environment can assist the family in preparing the child for a new environment. The family can then provide the child with brochures, pictures, and other materials from the facility and explain what the child can anticipate experiencing upon transfer. If possible, visits from a rehabilitation center or long-term care facility nursing staff to the child before transfer can also be beneficial to the child.

Regardless of the needs of the child after discharge, whether discharged home without need for further care, or with the need for home health care or rehabilitative care, the nurse maintains a family-centered approach to provide the child and family with information and support during the discharge process. The nurse ensures that the family is prepared for the discharge and that any treatments and monitoring are understood by the family. Contact information is provided and any support services required are arranged before the child is discharged.

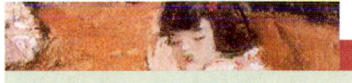

CRITICAL THINKING IN ACTION

THE CHILD UNDERGOING T & A

Recall Tiara, the child described in the chapter opening vignette. She is a 5-year-old girl who was admitted to the hospital for a tonsillectomy and adenoidectomy (T&A). Following Tiara's operation, she refused to drink liquids because she was afraid it would hurt when she swallowed. Because of her initial reluctance to drink liquids and her mother's concern about caring for her at home, Tiara spent the night in the hospital. After receiving intravenous pain medication, Tiara realized that she could swallow without too much pain and began to eat Popsicles and drink liquids. She was then switched to oral pain medication. The next morning Tiara was drinking liquids well enough that she was to be discharged home.

1. What information should the nurse include in the discharge teaching plan for Tiara's mother?

2. As Tiara and her mother are preparing to leave the hospital, Tiara states "I am going to be good so I do not have to come to the hospital anymore!" How should the nurse respond?

3. Tiara's mother states that she is worried that her daughter will not drink enough at home. What can the nurse suggest to Tiara's mother to encourage her to drink fluids? What are symptoms of dehydration that Tiara's mother should watch for over the next few days?

4. Children Tiara's age have many fears and stressors related to the hospital and surgery. How can Tiara's mother assist her daughter to express her feelings about the hospital experience once she is home?

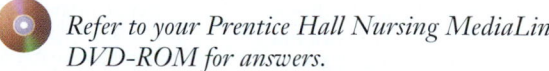

Refer to your Prentice Hall Nursing MediaLink DVD-ROM for answers.

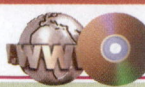

EXPLORE MediaLink

http://www.prenhall.com/ball

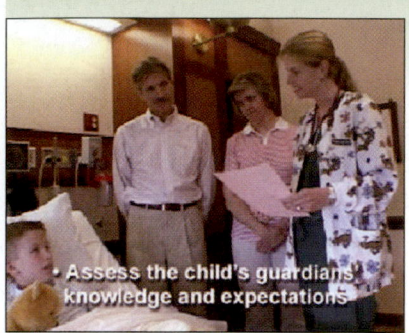

Resources for this chapter can be found on the Prentice Hall Nursing MediaLink DVD-ROM accompanying this textbook, and on the Companion Website at http://www.prenhall.com/ball.

DVD-ROM
Audio Glossary
NCLEX-RN® Review
Videos
A Child's Eye View: Hospitalization
Preparing A Child for Hospitalization

COMPANION WEBSITE
Audio Glossary
NCLEX-RN® Review
Care Plan Activity: A Hospitalized Toddler
Case Study: Preparing the Child for Surgery
MediaLink Applications
Children's Hospitals
Child Life Specialist
Drawing Blood from a Toddler
Hospitalization by Age Group
WebLinks

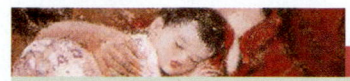

REFERENCES

Agazio, J. B., Ephraim, P., Flaherty, N. J., & Gurney, C. A. (2003). Effects of nonlocal geographically separated hospitalizations upon families. *Military Medicine, 168*(10), 778.

Allen, P. J., & Vessey, J. A. (2004). *Primary care of the child with a chronic condition,* (4th ed.). St. Louis: Mosby.

Alsop-Shields, L., & Mohay, H. (2001). John Bowlby and James Robertson: Theorists, scientists and crusaders for improvements in the care of children in hospital. *Journal of Advanced Nursing, 35*(1), 50–58

American Nurses Association & Society of Pediatric Nurses. (2003). *Scope and standards of pediatric nursing practice.* Washington, DC: nursebooks.org.

American Society of Anesthesiologists. (2005). Practice guidelines for fasting and the use of pharmacologic agents to reduce the risk of aspiration: Application to healthy patients undergoing elective procedures. Accessed September 9, 2005, from http://www.asahq.org/publicationsAndServices/NPO.pdf.

Ballard, K. L. (2004). Meeting the needs of siblings of children with cancer. *Pediatric Nursing, 30*(5), 394–401.

Bindler, R., & Howry, L. (2005). *Pediatric drug guide.* Upper Saddle River, NJ: Prentice Hall Health.

Brain Injury Association of America. (2006). A Guide to Selecting and Monitoring Brain Injury Rehabilitation Services. Accessed July 2, 2006 from http://www.biausa. org/Pages/splash.html

Crenshaw, J. T., & Winslow, E. (2002). Preoperative fasting: Old habits die hard: Research and published guidelines no longer support the routine use of "NPO after midnight," but the practice persists. *American Journal of Nursing, 102*(5), 36–44.

Daneman, S., Macaluso, J., & Guzzetta, C. (2003). Healthcare providers' attitudes toward parent participation in the care of the hospitalized child. *Journal for Specialists in Pediatric Nursing, 8*(3), 90.

Dudley, S. K., & Carr, J. M. (2004). Vigilance: The experience of parents staying at the bedside of hospitalized children. *Journal of Pediatric Nursing: Nursing Care of Children and Families, 19*(4), 267–275.

Emergency Nurses Association. (2005). Position statement: Family presence at the bedside during invasive procedures and/or resuscitation. Retrieved March 12, 2006, from http://www.ena.org/about/position/.

Fleitas, J. (2003). The power of words. *MCN, 28*(6), 384–388.

Flores, G., Milagros, A., Chaisson, C. E., & Donglin, S. (2003). Keeping children out of hospitals: Parents' and physicians' perspectives on how pediatric hospitalization for ambulatory care-sensitive conditions can be avoided. *Pediatrics, 112*(5), 1021–1030.

Griffin, T. (2003a). Facing challenges to family-centered care I: Conflicts over visitation (Family Matters). *Pediatric Nursing, 29*(2), 135–137.

Griffin, T. (2003b). Facing challenges to family-centered care II: Anger in the clinical setting. *Pediatric Nursing, 29*(3), 212.

Hallström, I., Runesson, I., & Elander, G. (2002). Observed parental needs during their child's hospitalization. *Journal of Pediatric Nursing, 17*(2), 140–148.

Joint Commission on Accreditation of Healthcare Organizations. (2006). Comprehensive Accreditation Manual for Hospitals, PC.6.40 http://www. jointcommission.org

Kaminski, M., Pellino, T., & Wish, J. (2002). Play and pets: The physical and emotional impact of child-life and pet therapy on hospitalized children. *Children's Health Care, 31*(4), 321–335.

Koopman, H. M., Baars, R. M., Chaplin, J., & Zwinderman, K. H. (2004). Illness through the eyes of the child: The development of children's understanding of the causes of illness. *Patient Education and Counseling, 55,* 363–370.

Lassetter, J. H., & Baldwin, J. H. (2005). Improving the experience of hospitalization for Hawaiian children on the mainland through cultural sensitivity to Hawaiian ways of healing. *Journal of Pediatric Nursing, 20,* 170–176.

Lau, W. K. (2002). Stress in children: Can nurses help? *Pediatric Nursing, 28*(1), 13–19.

Lehna, C. (2005). Interpreter services in pediatric nursing. *Pediatric Nursing, 31*(4), 292–296.

London, F. (2004). How to prepare families for discharge in the limited time available. *Pediatric Nursing, 30*(3), 212.

Lukash, F. (2002). Children's art as a helpful index of anxiety and self-esteem with plastic surgery. *Plastic and Reconstructive Surgery, 109*(6), 1777–1786.

McQuaid, E. L., Howard, K., Kopel, S. J., Rosenblum K. & Bibace, R. (2002). Developmental concepts of asthma: Reasoning about illness and strategies for prevention. *Applied Developmental Psychology, 23,* 179–194.

Meleski, D. D. (2002). Families with chronically ill children. *American Journal of Nursing, 102*(5), 47–54.

Melnyk, B. M., Small, L., & Carno, M. (2004). The effectiveness of parent-focused interventions in improving coping/mental health outcomes of critically ill children and their parents: An evidence base to guide clinical practice. *Pediatric Nursing, 30*(2), 143–148.

Miles, M. S. (2003). Support for parents during a child's hospitalization. *American Journal of Nursing, 103*(2), 62–64.

Myant, K. A., & Williams, J. M. (2005). Children's concepts of health and illness: Understanding of contagious illnesses, non-contagious illnesses and injuries. *Journal of Health Psychology, 10*(6), 805–819.

Peltzer, K., & Promtussananon, S. (2003). Black South African children's understanding of health and illness: Colds, chicken pox, broken arms and AIDS. *Child: Care, Health & Development, 29*(5), 385–393.

Pinckney, R. B., & Stuart, G. W. (2004). Adjustment difficulties of adolescents with sickle cell disease. *Journal of Child and Adolescent Psychiatric Nursing, 17*(1), 5–12.

Romino, S. L., Keatley, V. M., Secrest, J., & Good, K. (2005). Parental presence during anesthesia induction in children. *AORN Journal, 81*(4), 780–792.

Ryan-Wenger, N. A., Sharrer, V. W., & Campbell, K. K. (2005). Changes in children's stressors over the past 30 years. *Pediatric Nursing, 31*(4), 282–291.

Simons, J. (2002). Parents' support and satisfaction with their child's postoperative care. *British Journal of Nursing, 11*(22), 1442–1449.

Spector, R. E. (2004). *Cultural diversity in health and illness* (6th ed.). Upper Saddle River, NJ: Prentice Hall.

Thompson, V. L., Hupcey, J. E., & Clark, M. B. (2003). The development of trust in parents of hospitalized children. *Journal for Specialists in Pediatric Nursing, 8*(4), 137–147.

Tielsch, A. H., & Allen, P. J. (2005). Listen to them draw: Screening children in primary care through the use of human figure drawings. *Pediatric Nursing, 31*(4), 320–327.

United States Department of Labor. (2004). Family and medical leave act. Accessed September 9, 2005, from http://www.dol.gov/esa/whd/fmla/

Van Riper, M. (2003). The sibling experience of living with childhood chronic illness and disability. *Annual Review of Nursing Research, 21,* 279–302.

Whitfield, M. F. (2003). Psychosocial effects of intensive care on infants and families after discharge. *Seminars in Neonatology, 8,* 185–193.

Williams, J. M., & Binnie, L. M. (2002). Children's concept of illness: An intervention to improve knowledge. *British Journal of Health Psychology, 7,* 129–147.

Ygge, B. M., & Arnetz, J. E. (2004). A study of parental involvement in pediatric hospital care: Implications for clinical practice. *Journal of Pediatric Nursing, 19,* 217–223.

14

THE CHILD WITH A LIFE-THREATENING CONDITION AND END-OF-LIFE CARE

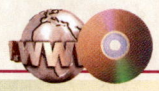

MediaLink

http://www.prenhall.com/ball

See the Prentice Hall Nursing MediaLink DVD-ROM and Companion Website for chapter-specific resources.

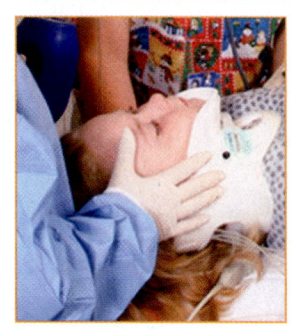

ALEXA, 6 years old, was a passenger in the back seat of her parents' car when another car struck them broadside, pushing in the back passenger door. Even though Alexa was wearing a lap belt, her head struck the car window. She was unconscious at the scene, and she had a bruise across her abdomen where the lap belt restrained her. The emergency medical technicians responded and decided Alexa had injuries serious enough to transport her to the trauma center. A cervical collar was applied in case her cervical spine was also injured. Upon arrival at the trauma center, Alexa's airway, breathing, circulation, and responsiveness were assessed. She was breathing spontaneously and her heart rate was strong and regular, but more rapid than normal. Her blood pressure was appropriate for her age. Because she was still not fully responsive, an endotracheal tube was inserted and oxygen was administered. An intravenous line was started to administer lactated Ringer's solution. Alexa's abdomen was slightly distended, and she flinched and withdrew to touch when her abdomen was palpated in the left upper quadrant. Further evaluation will determine the extent of Alexa's head injury and if she has a spleen laceration or other injury in the abdomen. She was admitted to the pediatric intensive care unit so she could be monitored carefully for changes to her physiologic status and be provided needed treatment.

LEARNING OUTCOMES

After reading this chapter, you will be able to do the following:

1. Describe the child's responses to having a life-threatening illness or injury by developmental level.

2. Discuss the responses of parents and siblings when the child has a life-threatening illness or injury.

3. Describe the coping mechanisms used by the child and family in response to stress.

4. Develop a nursing care plan for the child with a life-threatening illness or injury.

5. Identify the physiologic and psychologic changes that occur in the dying child.

6. Develop a nursing care plan to provide family-centered care for the dying child and his or her family.

7. Describe the development of the child's concept of death.

8. Describe the responses of nurses caring for children who die.

What do children like Alexa face after admission to the pediatric intensive care unit (PICU)? What nursing strategies can help a critically ill or injured child cope with the experience? What stressors will families face during the child's hospitalization? What interventions could help them in this crisis? What interventions are needed when the child is dying? This chapter offers guidance about providing supportive care to critically ill and injured or dying children like Alexa and to their families.

The intense emotional and physical demands placed on the critically ill or injured child present a challenge to nurses' attempts to provide developmentally appropriate care. The child's parents and siblings are confronted with a stressful situation. A family-centered model of nursing practice offers a framework for performing interventions that help to minimize stress and enhance coping by parents, siblings, and the ill or injured child.

LIFE-THREATENING ILLNESS OR INJURY

A **life-threatening condition** is one in which there is a substantial probability of death even though treatment may be successful in curing the condition or prolonging life (Institute of Medicine, 2003, p. 37). A threat to a child's life may be expected, as in a chronic illness or progressive disabling disease. More often though, the death is unexpected due to an unintentional injury—the leading cause of death in children—or an acute illness. See Chapter 1 ∞ for the leading causes of death in children in different age groups. How children, parents, and siblings cope with the threat will depend on the anticipated or unanticipated nature of the event and the conditions surrounding the child's admission to the hospital.

When death results from a chronic disease or terminal illness, the child and family have time to adjust to the impending death. Parents can become involved in the child's therapy as integral members of the treatment team. Emergency admission for an acute illness or unintentional injury, however, brings with it sudden stressors as the child and family are thrust into an unfamiliar environment, confronted with frightening or invasive procedures, and faced with an uncertain outcome.

Nursing care of children and families coping with specific chronic diseases or terminal illnesses such as cancer, cystic fibrosis, or muscular dystrophy is discussed elsewhere in this book. The following discussion focuses on the concepts of nursing care for children with life-threatening illnesses or injuries and nursing care of the dying child.

THE CHILD'S EXPERIENCE

Admission to the hospital, emergency department, or pediatric intensive care unit (PICU) is one of the most frightening experiences a child can have. The critically ill child may appear extremely anxious and fearful, or withdrawn, solemn, and preoccupied with his or her physical condition. The illness or injury often brings pain, decreased energy, and changes in the child's level of consciousness. Younger children may be unable to understand what is happening to them (Figure 14–1 ➤). The PICU environment appears overwhelming, fast paced, and frightening. The child's normal sleep patterns can be disrupted because of the lack of day-night patterns in many intensive care units. Being cared for by strangers contributes to the child's anxiety. The child's limited ability to move intensifies feelings of powerlessness and vulnerability. Children admitted to a PICU are at risk for posttraumatic stress disorder (Melnyk, Small, & Carno, 2004). See Chapter 27 ∞ .

Children's responses to stress are influenced by their developmental levels, past experiences, types of illness, coping mechanisms, and available emotional support. Nurses need to take into consideration how the child's developmental level and coping skills will influence his or her ability to deal with the PICU

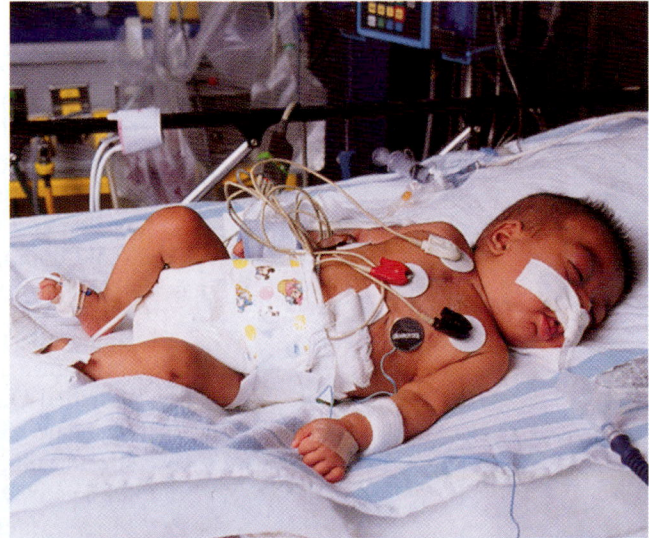

Figure 14–1 ➤ Jooti feels pain, hears noises, has her sleep disrupted, and has limited mobility because of all the equipment attached to her.

experience. Successful coping can provide the child with the skills to handle difficult situations in the future.

Stressors to the Child

An unanticipated admission places the child at emotional risk for several reasons, including the lack of preparation for the experience, the uncertainty and unpredictability of events that follow, the unfamiliarity of the environment, and the heightened anxiety of parents. An admission for exacerbation of a disease such as cystic fibrosis or leukemia can provoke feelings of depression or hopelessness. See Chapter 13 ∞ for the stressors and responses of children to hospitalization by age group.

The child cared for in the pediatric intensive care unit will experience all the stressors of a child who is hospitalized. Children in the PICU are likely to be at greater risk for short- and long-term psychological and behavioral problems (Board, 2005; Melnyk, Alpert-Gillis, Feinstein et al., 2004). These children are more ill and experience more invasive procedures. They are restricted to their bed and attached to equipment and monitors associated with their care. However, they are also more often treated with sedation and analgesia, and this may lessen memories of stressful experiences (Board, 2005).

Coping Mechanisms

Coping consists of cognitive and behavioral responses to manage specific internal and external demands that exceed a person's resources, enabling the person to solve problems and to respond emotionally. The child may mirror the parents' behaviors and responses, which may help or hinder the child's response to stress. The child's temperament, previous coping experiences, and availability of support systems all combine to influence his or her ability to cope with the current experience.

The nature and severity of the illness and an emergency admission to the hospital stress a child's coping capabilities. Defense mechanisms displayed by children in these situations include regression, or return to an earlier behavior (a common reaction to stress), denial, repression (involuntary forgetting), postponement, and bargaining. Within the PICU, coping strategies reported by school-age children include sleeping or taking a nap, which is a behavior avoidance strategy. Talking with someone such as a nurse or family member, and sometimes praying, were other reported coping strategies (Board, 2005).

■ NURSING MANAGEMENT

Nursing Assessment and Diagnosis

Nursing assessment involves, in addition to physiologic parameters, skilled observation of the child's psychosocial and emotional needs. It is important for the nurse to understand normal psychosocial and cognitive development in order to plan developmentally appropriate interventions. Assessment should include the child's response to illness, the environment, coping strategies, and the need for information and support.

The Nursing Care Plan on pages 445–446 includes common nursing diagnoses for the child coping with a critical illness or injury. The following nursing diagnoses may also be appropriate:

- Impaired Verbal Communication related to the effects of endotracheal intubation and mechanical ventilation
- Spiritual Distress related to the crisis of illness or suffering
- Disturbed Sleep Pattern related to circadian asynchrony, excessive stimulation, pain, and anxiety caused by the critical care unit environment
- Deficient Diversional Activity related to forced inactivity
- Hopelessness related to critical illness, deteriorating physical condition, or prolonged activity restrictions creating isolation
- Anticipatory Grieving related to potential loss of body function or impending death of self

NURSING CARE PLAN	The Child Coping with a Life-Threatening Illness or Injury		
GOAL	**INTERVENTION**	**RATIONALE**	**EXPECTED OUTCOME**
1. Anxiety (Child) related to separation from parents, foreign environment, strangers as caretakers, invasive procedures			
	NIC Priority Intervention: **Anxiety Reduction:** *Minimizing apprehension, dread, foreboding, or uneasiness related to an unidentified source of anticipated danger.*		*NOC Suggested Outcome:* **Anxiety Control:** *Ability to eliminate or reduce feelings of apprehension and tension from unidentified source.*
The child will exhibit or express an increased sense of security.	• Encourage parents to remain at the bedside (open visitation) and to participate in the child's care by touching, talking to, reading to, and singing to the child.	• Presence of parents is comforting to the child.	The child appears more relaxed and acknowledges parents' presence. Behavioral manifestations of anxiety are absent.
	• Talk with the child. Avoid discussions at the bedside that the child should not overhear.	• The child may overhear and remember, even if unconscious.	
	• Offer to arrange a visit from the chaplain or other spiritual support.	• Spiritual support often provides comfort and sustenance in a time of crisis.	
	• Provide the child with developmentally appropriate explanations when possible. Encourage the child to ask questions and express concerns.	• Information reduces anxiety and builds trust.	
	• Prepare child in advance for procedures using developmentally appropriate techniques.	• Preparation decreases anxiety related to the unknown.	
	• Make the child's bedside more personal and familiar by encouraging parents to bring in security objects, family photos, and favorite toys from home.	• Security objects decrease the foreignness of the hospital environment. The child derives comfort from the presence of personal items.	
	• Involve the child in play appropriate to developmental age (see Chapter 13 ∞).	• Play provides familiarity, decreases fantasy, and provides motor activity.	
	• Provide care using a primary nursing care model.	• Consistency in caregivers helps to build the child's trust.	
2. Powerlessness (Moderate) related to inability to communicate, and control relinquished to the healthcare team			
	NIC Priority Intervention: **Mutual Goal Setting:** *Collaborating with patient to identify and prioritize care goals, then developing a plan for achieving those goals.*		*NOC Suggested Outcome:* **Participation: Healthcare Decisions:** *Personal involvement in selecting and evaluating healthcare options.*
The child or adolescent will have an increased sense of control over the situation.	• Provide opportunities for choices when possible. Encourage participation in self-care.	• Such opportunities provide a sense of control and autonomy through decision making.	The child or adolescent expresses satisfaction over the ability to control some elements of the situation.
	• Prepare the child or adolescent in advance (timing dependent on developmental level) for procedures. Describe the sensations that will be experienced. Allow some choice in timing or method of pain relief.	• Information reduces anxiety and fear associated with the unknown and helps the child maintain self-control.	

(continued)

NURSING CARE PLAN	The Child Coping with a Life-Threatening Illness or Injury (continued)		
GOAL	INTERVENTION	RATIONALE	EXPECTED OUTCOME
2. Powerlessness (Moderate) related to inability to communicate, and control relinquished to the healthcare team (continued)			
	• Perform procedures efficiently. Tell the child before (timing dependent upon developmental level), repeat explanation of why procedure is necessary, complete procedure in consistent manner, and offer praise or a special story when completed.	• Information and reward or praise allows child to maintain some self-control during procedures.	
	• Provide routines for the child both within a 24-hour period and for scheduled care. When possible, incorporate rituals from home.	• Self-control is maintained through rituals.	
	• Encourage play as a means of expressing feelings.	• Play is a normal activity for children and provides freedom of expression.	
	• Provide other means of communication to the intubated child (e.g., a word board or finger board).	• Maintaining communication provides the child autonomy and independence.	
	• For the child requiring immobilization to prevent him or her from pulling out lines or injuring self, have a person hold the child as often as possible rather than use a physical immobilizer. Wrapping IV lines well and using armboards can help maintain lines and avoid the need for immobilization.	• Release from a physical immobilizer helps diminish the sense of powerlessness that accompanies their use.	
3. Acute Pain related to injuries, invasive procedures, surgery			
	NIC Priority Intervention: **Pain Management:** *Alleviation of pain or a reduction in pain to a level of comfort that is acceptable to the patient.*		*NOC Suggested Outcome:* **Comfort Level:** *Feelings of physical and psychologic ease.*
The child will experience reduced pain and improved comfort.	• Frequently assess the child's pain: location, intensity, what makes it better or worse.	• Assessment provides baseline information from which a plan of care can be developed.	The child experiences a perceived or actual improvement in comfort level.
	• If appropriate, use pain assessment scale (see Chapter 15 ∞).	• Use of scale provides continuity and consistency in monitoring of the child's pain.	
	• Provide optimal pain relief with prescribed analgesics 24 hours a day during the acute phase of care. Provide comfort measures—position changes, backrubs, and so on. Provide diversional activities as appropriate or possible. Incorporate the family in pain relief modality.	• Providing analgesia around the clock promotes comfort and healing. Physiologic and psychologic methods of pain control can be used in combination to maximally improve outcomes.	

Planning and Implementation

Nursing care focuses on promoting a sense of trust, providing education about the illness or injury, preparing the child for procedures, facilitating the use of play, and promoting a sense of control. Physiologic care for the child in the PICU may include the following: frequent physiologic assessment, pain and sedation management, nutritional support, medication administration, managing multiple IV lines and pumps, maintaining ventilatory and hemodynamic monitoring equipment, and wound care.

Provide Psychosocial Care for the Child

Children admitted to a PICU need support for the stressful experience. Children often feel and hear even when unconscious, so touch and verbal interchanges are important. Nurses play a key role in providing the child with developmentally appropriate support. Nursing interventions are directed at building a trusting relationship, minimizing the stressors experienced by the child, and promoting coping. Ongoing reassessment of progress in meeting the child's needs is critical. The accompanying Nursing Care Plan on pages 445–446 summarizes care for the child coping with a life-threatening illness or injury.

Promote a Sense of Security

For children of all ages, feeling secure depends on a sense of physical and psychologic safety. A sense of physical security is difficult to attain within the PICU because of the frequent procedures that are part of the child's treatment plan. The parent's presence provides the best sense of psychologic safety and reduces anxiety (American Academy of Pediatrics, 2003). An open visitation policy that enables parents to be at the bedside is optimal. Including parents as partners in the child's care provides the child comfort and reassurance. Children whose parents have high anxiety levels pick up their parents' emotional cues and become more anxious. Consistency of staff is invaluable in developing familiarity and a trusting relationship with the child.

Personalizing the child's bedside can promote comfort and a sense of security. Pictures from home, a favorite blanket or toy, music tapes or CDs, or posters can make the environment friendlier and more familiar to the child (Figure 14–2 ➤). Religious or spiritual icons may also provide psychological support.

Provide Education and Prepare the Child for Procedures

A child's ability to understand the cause of the illness and its therapy depends on his or her cognitive abilities. Help younger children to understand that illness and hospitalization are not a punishment. Preparation for procedures is important at all ages, even for the unconscious or sedated child. Toddlers will benefit from being talked to, soothed, and touched during and after the procedure. Provide preschoolers, school-age children, and adolescents with an explanation of the sensations they can expect to experience (temperature, vibrations, sounds, smells, tastes, sight). See Chapter 13 ∞ for further information about preparation and support of the child during procedures.

Facilitate the Use of Play

The use of play is important in alleviating stress and helping children to prepare for procedures. It is also another way for the nurse to assess the child's developmental level. Even within the PICU, therapeutic play diminishes fantasies, provides motor activity, and helps the child cope with stressors (see Chapter 13 ∞). Children who have limited mobility due to tubes and immobilizers can still feel a sense of accomplishment, for example, by completing a puzzle, even if the nurse points to each piece and the child responds through nods and gestures where it should be placed. Play can help children work through a painful situation, making it more tolerable.

Promote a Sense of Control

Children between toddlerhood and adolescence experience a loss of control during a life-threatening illness. This loss of control may be related to the body, emotions, normal routines, or privacy. Nursing interventions should promote a sense of control over these areas.

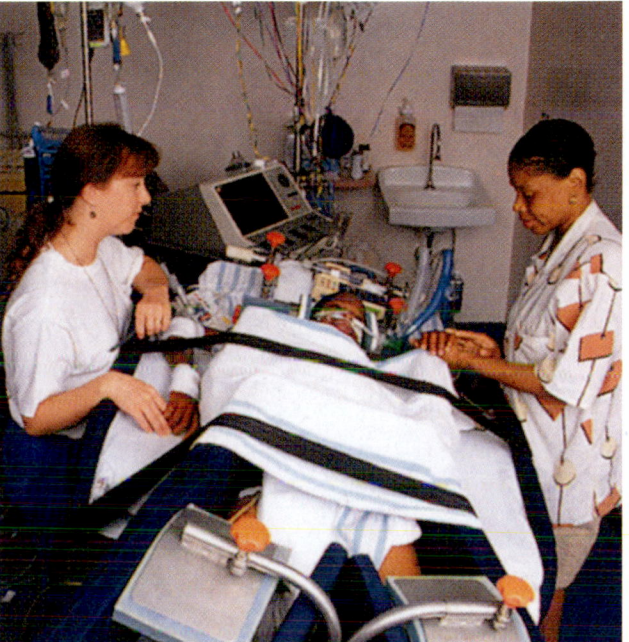

Figure 14–2 ➤ By their very nature, PICUs are ominous and sterile. To lessen this effect, it can help to personalize the child's space. Being there with the child and parent, answering questions, or just talking can be a comfort to both.

Give the child choices whenever possible. Even the simple choice of which color gown to wear can help the child feel in control. Scheduling routine activities and treatments at the same time each day adds predictability and lessens anxiety. Limited mobility and the use of immobilizers, although sometimes necessary, contribute to the child's sense of powerlessness.

Physical immobilizers are sometimes used in children with altered consciousness to prevent the unintentional removal of technological devices or equipment. The Joint Commission on Accreditation of Healthcare Organizations requires that hospitals have policies and procedures for the use of restraints or immobilizers. If immobilizers must be used, plan to release them regularly for short periods. Restrain all children as little as possible, and explain the rationale for immobilizers, emphasizing that they are not a punishment (see Skills 4–1 to 4–6). Provide the child diversional activities, for example, by reading stories, playing music, or watching videotapes. Seek input from the family about the child's preferences and family values regarding music, television, and videotapes or DVDS (see Chapter 13 ∞).

Enhance the child's coping skills by teaching the child and family a combination of relaxation, visual imagery, or distraction techniques, and comforting self-talk phrases, such as "This will be over soon. If I stay calm, it will be all right. It will be over faster and then I can do something fun." Help the parents become the child's coping coaches. Additional information about these techniques is provided in Chapter 15 ∞.

Evaluation

Expected outcomes of nursing care include:

- A trusting relationship is developed with the child and family.
- The child is given preparation and support for procedures.
- The child's coping is promoted by family presence and therapeutic play.

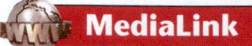

SKILLS 4–1 TO 4–6
Positioning and Restraint Therapies

MediaLink

JCAHO Restraint Policy

THE PARENTS' EXPERIENCE

The uncertainty and unpredictability of a child's life-threatening illness or injury challenge a family's coping and stability. The sudden loss of the parenting role with the emergency admission of their child causes stress. Families will display many different reactions and coping strategies, such as crying, emotional outbursts, fear, and demanding information. Parents are at risk for development of posttraumatic stress disorder, depression, and anxiety disorders when the child is hospitalized in an intensive care unit (Melnyk, Alpert-Gillis, Feinstein et al., 2004). Children who are hospitalized for a critical illness cannot be adequately cared for if their families' needs are not met. Not only will parents find it difficult to support the child if their own needs are not met, but they also can transmit their anxiety to the child, who then becomes even more anxious.

What Makes a Problem a Crisis?

A **family crisis** occurs when a family encounters a problem that seems insurmountable and with which the family cannot cope in its usual ways. The critical care environment and the implications of a life-threatening illness or injury are far removed from the everyday experiences of most families. The unfamiliarity of the environment and the uncertainty and seriousness of the illness or injury create a crisis for the family.

Unexpected illness or injury adds another dimension of stress, since families have little time to prepare for the experience. A sudden admission threatens family integrity, causing enormous stress and separation from loved ones. The interruption of the unique parent-child relationship can be more stressful to parents than the physical PICU environment. Stresses are intensified when divorce, separation, and stepparenting are being experienced. Other current family stresses such as financial problems, long distance from home to hospital, or another family member with an illness can add to the state of crisis. See Chapter 2 ∞ for a discussion on family assessment and family resiliency.

Reactions to Life-Threatening Illness or Injury

Parents typically progress through stages that might include shock and disbelief; anger and guilt; deprivation and loss; anticipatory waiting; and readjustment or mourning.

Shock and Disbelief

The universal reaction of parents to a child's life-threatening illness is shock and disbelief. As the familiar is disrupted, parents experience a loss of control, an inability to regain their bearings, and feelings of immobility. The hospital environment, emergency department, or PICU may seem unreal. The emotions parents experience initially are intensified by the physical appearance of their child (particularly after a major injury); the presence of monitors, tubing, and equipment; and the actual injury or illness. As the mother of a 5-year-old trauma patient said, "I felt distanced, in a daze, in and out of it that first day after the accident."

Shock and disbelief begin in the first few moments after hearing the "news" and can last for days. The shock helps postpone the full impact of the crisis. During this period, parents grope for answers and explanations about the illness or injury. Information must be repeated many times to parents, because in this stage they are often unable to easily assimilate information.

Anger and Guilt

Anger and guilt surface as parents become more aware of their child's illness or injury. Their anger may be directed toward themselves or each other because they could not protect their child. Other individuals may be blamed, such as the driver of a motor vehicle involved in the crash injuring the child. Parents may also be angry with their child. This anger may be a result of injuries the child sustained when breaking known rules such as drinking and driving, playing with matches, or riding a bike without a helmet. Lastly, the anger may not be directed at anyone specifically. Injuries caused by natural disasters such as an earthquake, flood, or hurricane provoke just as much anger as those that result from the actions of people. This may create a challenge to the parents' spiritual beliefs.

Parents typically react to their child's illness or injury with some degree of guilt. This reaction may be magnified in the PICU environment. The fact that the guilt usually has no basis in real events does not lessen the feeling. A question parents frequently ask at this stage is, "Why not me instead of my child?" Parents' feelings of guilt may have one of two causes:

1. *They may feel responsible for causing the illness or injury.*   Statements such as, "If only I hadn't sent him to the store on his bike, this wouldn't have happened," or, from the father of a 2-year-old who nearly drowned, "Maybe if I hadn't been working, he would have been in my care and this wouldn't have happened," reflect feelings of guilt for causing or failing to prevent the injury.
2. *They may feel guilty about not noticing the onset of an illness or disregarding earlier symptoms of an illness.*   The mother of a 1-year-old with meningitis repeatedly said, "I shouldn't have waited so long to take her to the doctor!"

Deprivation and Loss

As the shock associated with the child's life-threatening condition slowly recedes, new stressors emerge. Within minutes or hours, parents are deprived of their familiar role of being a parent of a healthy child and have an unexpected and unfamiliar role of being a parent of a critically ill child. The difficulty and ambivalence parents feel in releasing a part of their responsibility as the child's primary caretakers to strangers can threaten their self-esteem and self-control. If parents cannot participate in the child's care, they may feel helpless or worthless.

Anticipatory Waiting

Once the child's condition is stabilized and survival seems likely, parents often move into a period of anticipatory waiting. This stage is characterized as "life suspended in time." Parents spend a great deal of time waiting: for test results, for explanations, for their child to become conscious, or for surgery to be over. Parents may fear leaving the area because they may miss an important procedure, physician visit, or decision or change in treatment. Lack of mobility decreases the parents' ability to use typical coping mechanisms, so anxiety and the sense of powerlessness may increase. Pagers or cellular phones provided to family members of critically ill children allow them to take breaks away from the child's bedside while knowing they can be quickly reached when needed (Gavaghan & Carroll, 2002). The use of pagers or cellular phones can decrease feelings of frustration and anger associated with arriving at the bedside and not being notified that there has been a change in the child's condition (Griffin, 2003).

Parents may have a preoccupation with medical details. During this period, parents may ask questions about the long-term effects of the illness or injury on the child, about the potential for brain damage, or about the need for additional surgeries. Parents may place demands on staff and be frustrated when the child's progress is slow.

Readjustment or Mourning

The last stage that parents experience is readjustment or mourning. Readjustment is experienced as the child recovers, improves steadily, and prepares for transfer and discharge. In contrast, parents of the child who dies reenter the cycle of emotions characteristic of grief. Parents also mourn when the child remains seriously ill or unresponsive, when the outcome remains uncertain for an extended period, or when long-term care is required.

Table 14–1 lists the most important needs of parents during a child's critical illness or injury.

MediaLink

Resources and Support for Parents

■ NURSING MANAGEMENT

Nursing Assessment and Diagnosis

Nurses who work with families of critically ill children have a unique opportunity to help them adapt and to promote family functioning. Begin by assessing the family's reaction to the illness, coping skills, stressors, and needs. See Chapter 2 ∞. This initial assessment provides a baseline of information for developing a care plan and strategies to meet the family's psychosocial as well as physiologic needs.

Several nursing diagnoses may apply to parents who are dealing with their child's critical illness or injury. Examples include:

- Interrupted Family Processes related to the impact of a critically ill child on the family system
- Spiritual Distress related to the child's critical illness, suffering, or death
- Disabed Family Coping related to the child's severe or fatal illness
- Fatigue related to extreme stress, sleep deprivation, and crisis
- Anticipatory Grieving related to potential death of the child or loss of body functions
- Readiness for Enhanced Family Coping related to constructive crisis management

Planning and Implementation

Nursing care focuses on providing information and building trust, promoting parental involvement, providing for parents' physical and emotional needs, facilitating positive staff-parent relationships and communication, and maintaining or strengthening family support systems. A family-centered approach will help meet the needs of families, minimize stress, and enhance family coping. See Table 2–1 ∞. The challenge to nurses is to blend and balance technology with caring.

Provide Information and Build Trust

Orient parents to the hospital, as well as to the unit routines, to help them adapt to their surroundings. Parents will gain a sense of control and independence if they know where to get supplies, and how to find the lounge, cafeteria, and restrooms.

Table 14–1	NURSING INTERVENTIONS TO MEET PARENTAL NEEDS DURING THEIR CHILD'S CRITICAL CARE HOSPITALIZATION

Parental Needs	Nursing Interventions
Information is the most important identified need	• Provide information and frequent updates about the child's condition. Repeat the information and provide other materials frequently as parents forget or cannot concentrate on details with all their stress. • Explain about the child's condition, equipment being used, and procedures of care. • Facilitate a discussion with the physician at least daily. • Provide general information about unit policies, team members, phone numbers, and so on.
Proximity to their child	• Provide permission for the parents to remain at the bedside. • Encourage parents to touch and speak with the child and demonstrate ways if parents are hesitant. • Work within the unit to provide open, flexible visiting hours.
Reestablishment of their parental role and control	• Implement family-centered care so parents feel recognized as important to their child's recovery and as the decision maker for the child's treatment options.
Participation in their child's care	• Encourage parents to participate in care (e.g., bathing and hair care, diaper changes, feeding, range of motion exercises, massages). • Encourage parents to help with diversional activity (e.g., reading, singing, telling stories). • Let the parents explain equipment and procedures to the child to reduce the child's fears.
Confidence in the treatment plan and caregivers	• Try to maintain continuity in staffing and healthcare contacts. • Demonstrate caring for the child. • Provide assurance that the child is receiving appropriate treatment and pain management.
Psychologic support	• Acknowledge that the situation is difficult. • Help parents to focus on the positive or unchanged aspects of the child's appearance. • Encourage parents to get rest and nutrition to help them maintain physical resources necessary for coping. • Provide space and privacy as needed. • Give hope—an essential component of coping. • Offer the choice of other family members to be present. • Discuss the possible responses of siblings and the long-term emotional responses of the child patient.

The information given to parents must be provided frequently and accurately. Deliver information on the child's illness, condition, and plan of care in a manner and language readily understandable to parents. Upon admission, parents need to be given an idea of what to expect in the days ahead and be prepared for special procedures or major changes in therapy that may become necessary. Parents and siblings also need to be prepared before they see the child the first time. Tell them what tubes and monitors are present and how the child will look and react.

Honesty in discussions with parents is extremely important. If parents feel misled or that information is being withheld, a trusting relationship will be impossible. Informed parents, however, will feel that they are active participants in decision making and care planning for their child. Trust is facilitated when parents believe that the staff truly cares about the child and sees him or her as an individual, special child.

Parents also need a sense of hope regarding their child's illness to help them cope. Focus on the positives as the child progresses through the different phases of the critical illness.

CLINICAL TIP

Explain to the child and parents, in easy-to-understand terms, the purpose of equipment that is being used. Answer alarms quickly. Follow with an explanation of why alarms sound.

Promote Parental Involvement

An important role of nurses is to encourage and support parents in their parenting role. The parents' place when possible is at the bedside—their very presence can comfort the child, minimize fears, and reduce the child's distress during invasive procedures. They provide continuity and may notice subtle condition changes that a newly assigned nurse may miss. Throughout the child's hospitalization, parents will continue to need reassurance and encouragement. Open visitation by parents is important to maintain their parenting role.

Participation in care of the child helps parents cope with the child's life-threatening illness or injury (Katz, 2002). Providing information about behaviors and emotions the child is likely to exhibit as well as guidelines about what physical care they can provide helps the parents gain a sense of control over the situation and a sense of empowerment (Melnyk, Alpert-Gillis, Feinstein et al., 2004). Parents who do not remain with their child at the bedside may feel undervalued (Griffin, 2003). Giving parents a role at the bedside, such as providing personal care, is one way to promote involvement.

Family Presence During Resuscitation and Invasive Procedures

Many hospitals are implementing policies that permit families to be present during resuscitation and invasive procedures. Some parents who choose to witness a child's resuscitation note that it was important to know that everything possible was done to help the child. When parents are permitted to be present a support person is with them and these steps are usually followed (Levetown, 2004):

- Prior to entering the room, the parents are informed about the environment, equipment near to and on the child and its purpose, and who is in the room and caring for the child.
- The parents are told that if they feel uncomfortable or get in the way of the resuscitation team, they will be escorted out.
- The parents are positioned so they can see the child's face and hold his or her hand. Encourage the parents to tell the child how much he or she is loved.
- If the parents are looking around, explain what is being done for the child and why.
- If the child is declared dead, reassure the parents that they were present at the child's last moment and that the child (use child's name) felt loved.

Provide for Physical and Emotional Needs

The experience of having a child with a critical illness drains parents' physical and emotional reserves. Parents often need encouragement to take care of themselves and to periodically take a break. A statement such as "It is important for you to eat and rest because Alexa is really going to need you when she wakes up" helps parents to realize that becoming exhausted benefits neither them nor the child. Provision of a pager or cellular phone may help reduce the parents' anxiety. Record the parents' cellular phone numbers on the medical record and at the bedside.

Many communities have a residence for families of hospitalized children. This is often an inexpensive but warm and supportive environment for families. The Ronald McDonald Children's Charities support many of these residences. Computer resources for families in the hospital and at these residences may make it possible for parents to stay in contact with concerned family and friends. When financial burdens are a consideration, parents may need family support and social service referrals.

Parents are often at different levels of coping during a crisis. The child's critical illness may foster cohesion between the couple and build a stronger relationship. Unfortunately, the reverse may also be true—differences in styles or levels of coping may foster a sense of isolation, placing a strain on the couple's relationship. Nurses should be alert to family dynamics and refer the family for support or counseling, if indicated.

Facilitate Positive Staff–Parent Relationships and Communication

Given the intensity of the parents' experience when their child is critically ill, it is easy to see how problems can arise between staff and parents. Each healthcare team member

CLINICAL TIP

If parents choose not to witness the resuscitation, regular updates (5- to 10-minute intervals) should be provided to the parents as they wait in a private area. A designated support person (chaplain or family support team member) should be present with the parents as they wait.

MediaLink

Ronald McDonald Children's Charities

must be aware of the child's current status so that parents receive the same information from all staff. Consistency in the message can instill confidence. Provide explanations geared to the parents' level of understanding, using language the parents can understand.

Parents need to know who has the overall responsibility for their child's care. They should be introduced to the nurse and physician responsible for the child's care. This is especially important in teaching hospitals that have rotating staff. The staff physician with the overall responsibility should meet with parents as often as necessary to talk about changes in the child's condition or treatment plan and to allow time for parents to ask questions (Figure 14–3 ➤). Encourage parents to keep a daily log or notebook to record information on the child's care, progress, and needs, as well as questions they want to ask the healthcare team. Family care conferences can be helpful when a large number of team members provide care. Arrange for daily visits by an interpreter if the family does not speak or understand English well. Have information about the child's condition and care summarized for communication at that time.

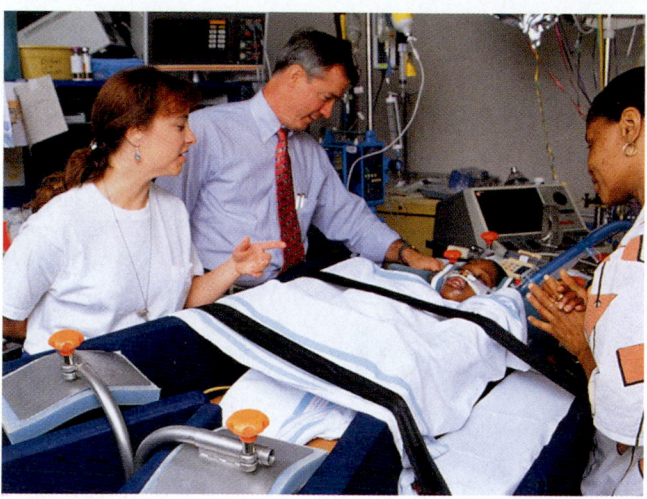

Figure 14–3 ➤ In times of crisis, everyone likes to know that someone is in charge and who that person is. The parents should meet and talk with the staff physician in charge and the nurses as often as possible. Parents need to know that someone is responsible, even if different people are providing care.

Maintain or Strengthen Family Support Systems

Support systems are the extended network of family, friends, and religious and community contacts that provide nurturance, emotional support, and direct assistance to parents, enabling them to cope with overwhelming problems and crises. Most parents indicate that having family or friends nearby is crucial as a support system.

Parents may need to be reassured that it is all right to ask for help from family, friends, or community services. They may be uncomfortable asking for help, and instead attempt to handle multiple responsibilities themselves, often to the point of exhaustion. Some parents are unable to respond to offers of help because it requires too great a mental effort on their part.

Nurses may need to intervene on parents' behalf when they have inappropriate support. Parents may be frustrated by people who come to visit unannounced, stay too long, or visit too often. They may find it difficult to tell well-meaning but insensitive friends that they cannot deal with visitors right now. In these situations, the nurse can offer to serve as a gatekeeper. Suggest that parents inform family and friends about a specific time for visits or phone calls to allow for rest periods. An extended family member may be given the responsibility of relaying information to others.

Families of critically ill or dying children often have emotional needs beyond the support capabilities of the nurse caring for the child. Referrals to family and support services or pastoral care may be beneficial in these instances.

Evaluation

Expected outcomes of nursing care include:

- The nurse establishes a trusting relationship and effective communication with the family.
- Parents participate in their child's care as much as desired.
- Family members receive emotional support and nurturance needed to sustain them through their child's illness.

THE SIBLINGS' EXPERIENCE

As the parents' focus shifts to the critically ill child, they may need support in dealing with the healthy siblings. Siblings also need care and may feel left out when everyone's attention is focused on the ill child. Siblings of critically ill children may demonstrate behaviors ranging from jealousy or envy to resentment, guilt and hostility, anger, insecurity, regression, and fear. Recognize that siblings may fear becoming ill themselves or believe that they played a role in the child's illness. Siblings often have nightmares about the illness or injury their brother or sister has sustained and about the ill child dying.

Inform siblings about their brother's or sister's condition using language and concepts appropriate to their ages and developmental levels. As appropriate, siblings should be allowed to visit. Such a visit should be encouraged if the child could potentially die, to allow the sibling to say good-bye. Because children's fantasies are often worse than reality, unfounded fears may be relieved by a visit. These visits often also help to lift the ill child's spirits.

Preparation for the visit is important. Before the visit, talk with the siblings about what to expect and describe how their brother or sister will look. If the ill child acts, moves, talks, or looks different than usual, provide an explanation beforehand. Describe the hospital environment, including equipment, sounds, and smells. Using a doll, drawing pictures, or showing an actual picture of the child can help prepare the siblings. Box 14–1 summarizes strategies for working with siblings of an ill or injured child.

During the visit, the nurse should demonstrate how to talk to and touch the ill child and encourage the siblings to do the same (Figure 14–4 ➤). The length of the visit should be relatively short, based on the child's developmental age. After the visit, discuss with siblings what they saw and felt, and answer any questions they may have. When a sibling cannot visit, contact with the ill child can be maintained by sending pictures, drawings, cards, and messages recorded on audiotapes or videotapes (Figure 14–5 ➤).

If parents are staying at the hospital with the ill child, encourage them to call the siblings at home daily. Allowing the siblings at home the opportunity to share their day as well as to receive an update on the ill child provides a feeling of connectedness. The phone call offers siblings a consistent link to the parent as well as the reassurance that they are important and loved. Internet contact may also allow for instant messaging and a way to communicate with older siblings. Arrange for access to a computer or the Internet if possible for families that will find this contact supportive.

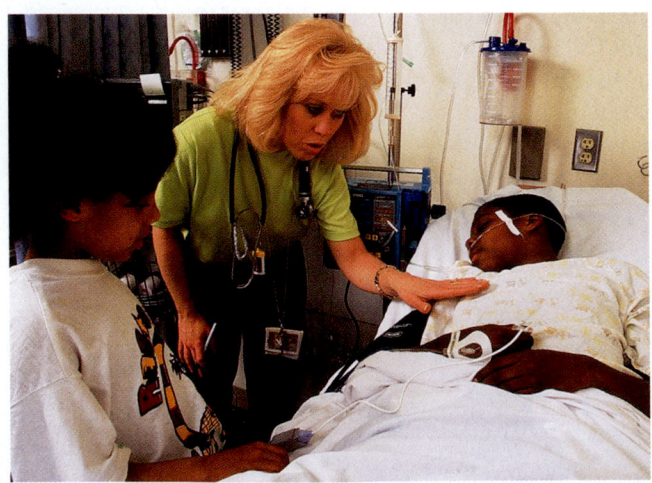

Figure 14–4 ➤ During the sibling's visit to the ill child, it is important to talk with the sibling and answer any questions asked in an honest manner at a level the child can understand.

END-OF-LIFE CARE

When the family is faced with end-of-life decision making and care because of a child's chronic condition or multiple acute care episodes, the family relies on the nurse and other members of the healthcare team to provide honest information about various treatment options and potential outcomes. Depending on cognitive abilities, developmental stage, physical and mental status, and prior experiences with health care, the child should also participate in the decision-making process (Beale, Baile, & Aaron, 2005). The family may need to consider issues such as palliative care, hospice care, Do-Not-Resuscitate requests, continuation of schooling, organ/tissue donation, and autopsy. See Box 14–2.

Palliative Care

The World Health Organization defines **palliative care** as the total care of patients whose disease is not responsive to curative treatment (Ferrell & Coyle, 2002). It combines active and compassionate therapies intended to sooth, comfort, and relieve persons with life-limiting conditions while maintaining quality of life (Institute of Medicine, 2003). These therapies may be combined with other therapies aimed at reducing or curing the illness and treating symptoms more aggressively than hospice care. Palliative care is appropriate for some conditions that may possibly be cured, but treatment failure is also possible, such as in cases of advanced or progressive cancer or severe congenital heart defects. In some cases care is palliative from the time of diagnosis, such as in cases of severe forms of *osteogenesis imperfecta* or certain chromosomal disorders. Other conditions that should be considered for palliative care include muscular dystrophy, severe immune deficiency, cystic fibrosis, and severe respiratory failure (Himmelstein, Hilden, Boldt et al., 2004). About 8600 children each day could benefit from palliative care that acknowledges their limited life expectancy and severity of illness. Unfortunately, they do not receive it (Rushton, 2005). A significant barrier to palliative care for children is the technological advances that give parents hope that death can be avoided and the cultural denial of the fact that children actually die. In some cases, a child with a progressive chronic condition could have repeated life-threatening experiences, making it difficult to determine when the child might actually die. The inability to predict when death might occur often results in poor access to healthcare support and services that could improve the quality of life (Rushton & Catlin, 2002). An integrated strategy that combines services from the palliative care team with the medical team working to cure the child of a serious condition such as cancer can help the family and child participate more actively in the planning process (Rushton, 2005).

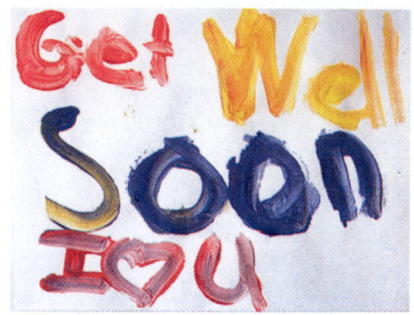

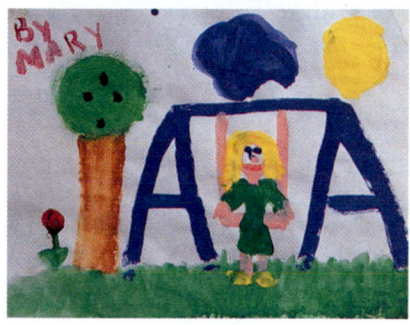

Figure 14–5 ➤ It is important that parents and siblings feel comfortable communicating with the seriously ill child. If siblings cannot visit, they should be encouraged to paint or record messages. They need to be able to express themselves and to feel that they are helping.

MediaLink

Guidelines for Quality Palliative Care

BOX 14–2

NURSING ROLES IN IMPROVING PEDIATRIC PALLIATIVE, END-OF-LIFE, AND BEREAVEMENT CARE

The nurse and other members of the healthcare team work collaboratively to improve end-of-life care for children and their families through the following actions:

1. Plan nursing care for children with life-threatening medical conditions and their families that matches the child's physical, cognitive, emotional, and spiritual level of development.
2. Implement family-centered care, ensuring that families are part of the care team and their beliefs, feelings, and desires are respected.
3. Plan and provide compassionate care for children with life-threatening conditions and for their families beginning at the time of diagnosis through death and bereavement.
4. Seek information, education, and mentoring to gain proficiency and skill in working effectively with children who are dying and their families.
5. Work within the healthcare facility to promote needed changes that will improve the palliative, end-of-life, and bereavement care for children and their families.
6. Participate in research designed to increase healthcare professional understanding of clinical, cultural, organizational, and other practices or perspectives that can improve palliative, end-of-life, and bereavement care for children and their families.

Data from: Institute of Medicine. (2003). *When children die: Improving palliative and end-of-life care for children and their families.* Washington, DC: National Academies Press, p. 7.

RESEARCH

Advance Care Planning

When the child has a progressive condition that will result in the child's death, advance care planning was valued by a small number of parents interviewed about their experiences. Parents felt the process of advance care planning benefited the children and the family because it assured the best care for the child by focusing on the child's quality of life and prevented unnecessary suffering (Hammes, Klevan, Kempf et al., 2005).

Advance care planning for a child's death should include the following (Himmelstein et al., 2004):

- Identify the decision makers and make sure all on the care team are aware
- Describe the expected changes in the child's functional ability and quality of life as the disease progresses
- Determine whether the family's and child's goals are curative, comfort, or not known at the time
- Help the family make decisions about medical interventions that are desired and how intervention decisions should be modified as the child's health status changes
- Provide anticipatory guidance about changes to expect when the child is near death and identify who will help the family manage the child's symptoms.

Hospice Care

Hospice care helps patients who are terminally ill to live their remaining time to the fullest—alert, without pain, and with choices and dignity. Hospice care may be provided in the home, a special unit in the hospital, or in a free-standing facility. Families and children receive emotional, spiritual, and medical support from the care team that may include nurses, physicians, religious leaders, social workers, and mental health professionals. It is estimated that less than 1% of dying children receive hospice services (Himmelstein et al., 2004). However, an estimated 5000 children in their last 6 months of life could potentially benefit from hospice care on any given day (Institute of Medicine, 2003). Some families do not see hospice as an acceptable alternative because it requires them to accept the child's impending death and may imply that they are giving up hope (Klopfenstein & Young-Saleme, 2002). Families may need assistance to see that hospice is an opportunity to focus on the time left with the child. Home hospice care allows the family to spend time with the terminally ill infant or child without technical equipment and the presence of strangers. The hospice nurse provides anticipatory guidance to the child and family so they are not alarmed by the signs and symptoms of impending death, such as nausea and respiratory difficulty. Appropriate pain management is also provided. Grief counseling and support may also be available to families following the child's death.

When a child receives palliative and/or hospice care the family and healthcare providers collaborate to determine which treatments are appropriate to continue with the child's end-of-life care, such as total parenteral nutrition, intravenous fluids, gastric or nasogastric feedings, and certain medications. Nurses participate on the multidisciplinary team to assure comprehensive care to the dying child and family. Health plan coverage for pediatric palliative/hospice care services or alternate financial assistance is investigated.

Ethical Issues Surrounding a Child's Death

Because a child's death is so emotionally charged, many potential misunderstandings and conflicts can develop between families and healthcare providers. The more common ethical issues that need to be addressed include withdrawal or withholding treatment, parental treatment refusal, and Do-Not-Resuscitate orders. See Chapter 1 ∞ for ethical decision-making principles and terminology.

Withdrawal of or Withholding Treatment

The decision to withdraw or withhold life-sustaining treatments from the dying child is very difficult and emotional for parents. Withholding nutrition and hydration may be especially difficult because parents often associate food with nurturing and love, or the fear that death will be hastened. Other treatments such as medications, mechanical ventilation, and dialysis may be withdrawn if the child's outcome is inevitable death and continuing treatment causes more suffering than benefit or prolongs the active dying process. (See Evidence-Based Practice: Improving the Quality of Pediatric End-of-Life Care in the PICU.)

The nurses may feel conflicted when parents are unable to discontinue aggressive therapies that the nurse feels are extending the child's suffering. Consultation with a

EVIDENCE-BASED PRACTICE

Improving the Quality of Pediatric End-of-Life Care in the PICU

Clinical Question

The majority of children who die because of life-limiting conditions die in the hospital setting, and many times in the pediatric intensive care unit (PICU). What are the parents' perspectives with regard to improving their child's quality of care?

Evidence

A study involving parents of 56 children who had died in the pediatric intensive care unit focused on care provided to the child and parental end-of-life decision making. Parents struggled with issues such as how adequate the information was about particular aspects of the child's care and loss of control. The study results indicated that when parents considered withdrawal of life support, they placed the highest priorities on quality of life, likelihood of improvement, and their perception of their child's pain and discomfort (Meyer, Burns, Griffith et al., 2002). Another study was conducted by interviewing parents of 44 children who had died at one children's hospital. Themes emerging from the interviews included the following: parents appreciated being highly involved in decision making, difficult news should be delivered by a familiar person, one caregiver should be in charge throughout all phases of treatment, improved services for siblings was needed, and pain management was critical. Characteristics of caregivers who were described as effective included honest, clinically accurate, compassionate, and available. Language barriers with Spanish-speaking families compromised the ability of these families to fully understand the child's care and made them feel isolated (Contro, Larson, Scofield et al., 2002).

Implications

Identifying the specific care valued by parents when a child is dying in the PICU, using interpreters as needed, is important for planning nursing care and multidisciplinary palliative care. Nurses can assist the family through the decision-making process by providing honest, factual responses to the family's questions. Communication and nursing care planning should ensure that family-centered care is provided by integrating values important to the family.

Critical Thinking

Consider the special needs of parents of a newborn with a cardiac congenital anomaly that cannot be corrected by surgery. Identify the family-centered palliative care plan for the infant who is expected to die within the next few days.

---

member of the hospital ethics committee can help clarify the issues involved and reduce the emotions associated with the conflict. During the consultation an unbiased professional collects facts about the child's condition, clarifies the beliefs and values of parents and health professionals, and improves communication while investigating options for compromise (Rushton, 2004). Consider that in some cases the parents may wish to prolong a pain-free death until an important family member has had a chance to say good-bye (Jacobs, 2005).

Conflicts Regarding Parental Treatment Refusal

Parents and healthcare providers sometimes disagree over what, if any, medical interventions should be provided when the child is dying. Parents may refuse treatments based on religious convictions or because they wish to avoid prolonging the child's life in order to provide a peaceful death (Institute of Medicine, 2003). Initiating highly technical, but possibly futile, interventions may cause emotional and financial stress that overwhelms parents.

Court intervention may be initiated by the healthcare team to have a surrogate legal guardian appointed in certain situations when recommended care is refused. Intervention is based on the legal principle that failure to obtain adequate medical care for a child violates the state child neglect laws (Institute of Medicine, 2003). Consultation with the hospital's ethics committee should also be obtained to help resolve the conflict. The nurse is sometimes in the uncomfortable position of trying to provide care to the infant or child while an adversarial rather than a supportive relationship exists with the parents. The nurse should demonstrate proper concern and care of the child in these cases, and seek support and guidance to work with the family as needed.

Do-Not-Resuscitate Orders

Parents faced with a child's inevitable death may be asked to consider a Do-Not-Resuscitate or Do-Not-Intubate (DNR or DNI) order. The family and healthcare providers must decide if a resuscitation attempt would be in the best interest of a child with an end-stage condition. Factors considered are allowing the child to die with dignity and the possibility of causing more harm and suffering if resuscitative measures are implemented. Parents need ongoing support as they may feel they are "giving up" on their child. Make sure that the family understands that the child will receive further care and interventions such as oxygen, suctioning, pain control, and supportive nursing care in the presence of a DNR order.

CLINICAL TIP

Some healthcare facilities are replacing the Do-Not-Resuscitate (DNR) order with the phrase "allow natural death" (AND). This phrase may be more acceptable to families, as they are allowing the child to die peacefully rather than requesting that intervention be withheld. This helps them consider the option as being in the child's best interest, rather than "giving up" (Ramer-Chrastek, Brunnquell, & Hasse, 2002).

The Americans with Disabilities Act of 1990 and the Education for All Handicapped Children Act mandate that all children with disabilities—including those with terminal illnesses—are entitled to the same education as other students. Children with a chronic or terminal illness may be at high risk of dying while at school. School officials have many concerns about accepting a DNR order, including the effect of the student's death on a classmate, liability issues, and the potential misinterpretation of the DNR order for an emergency such as choking. The majority of school districts (80%) do not have policies, regulations, or protocols for dealing with a student's DNR order, and most states have no laws providing liability to school personnel for honoring a student's DNR order or for withholding CPR (Kimberly, Forte, Carroll et al., 2005).

CARE OF THE DYING CHILD

Care of the dying child presents one of the greatest challenges to the nurse, requiring the utmost sensitivity and compassion. Children as young as 5 years of age can sense when they are seriously ill. A child's awareness of death develops more rapidly when he or she is experiencing the progression of a disease and related medical treatment. Children with life-threatening illnesses often learn about death and their own illness from exposure to other seriously ill and dying children during hospitalization or clinic visits.

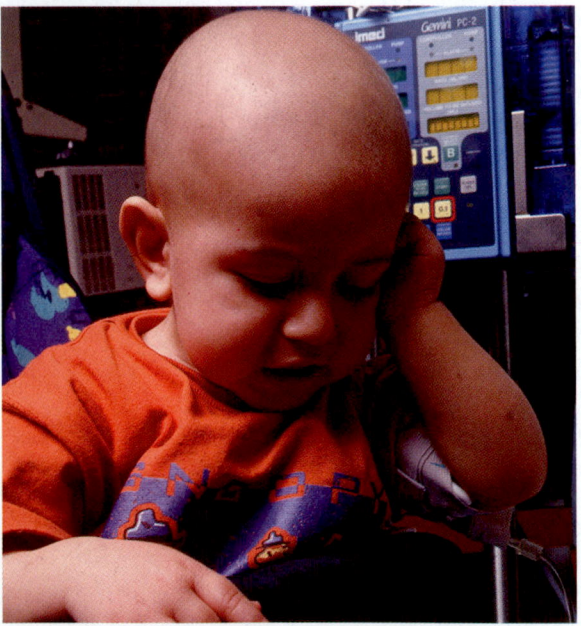

Figure 14–6 ➤ The toddler with a life-limiting condition recognizes that he feels bad and that routines are different. His anxiety may increase due to the concern and feelings of sadness exhibited by his parents.

Awareness of Dying by Developmental Age

Infants and toddlers are not actually aware of death, but they are aware of and react to changes in normal routines and the behavior of parents. Toddlers may know they feel bad, but they do not understand that their physical symptoms are associated with impending death. See Figure 14–6 ➤.

Preschool children can see their bodies deteriorate and feel the effects of medications used during disease progression and treatment. Changes in self-concept occur as they perceive these body changes. They often describe their illness in terms of mutilation to their body. They may realize that they are dying because of these physical changes, as well as the reactions of parents and hospital staff.

School-age children also have subtle fears about body integrity and anxieties about the seriousness of their illness. This greater preoccupation with illness is considered by many professionals as the child's version of **death anxiety**, a feeling of apprehension or fear of death. Children may express death anxiety as a concern with treatments that invade the body or interfere with normal body functions.

Adolescents have a mature understanding of death, but the normal developmental milestones of adolescence add to their problems in facing a terminal illness. They are struggling to establish their own identity and plans for the future. At a time when body image is extremely important, they may be faced with the possibility of mutilation and disfigurement. Dying adolescents are often isolated from their peers during a period when peers are the most essential social group. Adolescents with terminal illnesses may be angry because they recognize their loss when the whole world is opening up to them.

Do not expect adolescents to handle feelings in the same way that adults do. Adolescents often avoid expressing anger, an expected stage of grieving, against the family by seeking to control and direct these feelings elsewhere. They often become angry at changes in treatment procedures, lack of explanations, and threats to their independence. As death nears, the adolescent may permit comforting and support and may accept care from warm and loving family members, as long as he or she is not treated in a condescending manner.

NURSING MANAGEMENT

Nursing care of the dying child and family focuses on providing family-centered support for their physical and psychosocial needs.

Nursing Assessment and Diagnosis

Assess the child's physiologic status and comfort level. Physiological changes in the dying chld may be directly related to the child's disease process or injury. Signs and symptoms of approaching death are provided in the Clinical Manifestatons of the Dying Child table below.

Assess the child's awareness of impending death. Examples of questions the child may ask include: What will death be like? Will I be able to breathe? What happens after I die? Will an angel come to take me away? When will I be with [person closest to child] again? Will my parents be all right? Will you remember me? Assess the ability of the parents to talk with the child about dying.

Assess the family for coping skills and need for social supports. Identify any cultural or spiritual traditions, rituals, and beliefs related to loss and grieving that are important to the family.

CULTURE

Assessing Cultural Differences in Dealing with Death

Consider the customs and attitudes that might reflect the family's cultural heritage and affect their response to death. Discussion of each of these beliefs that a family may have will help plan culturally appropriate nursing care to families.

- How much to reveal to a child about the diagnosis and prognosis
- How much to participate in medical decision making
- The degree of trust in the medical system
- The amount of emotional display that is appropriate
- The role of children, women, and the elderly
- The concept of an afterlife and how to prepare for it
- Whether death should take place alone, with the family, or with an extended group
- Whether death should take place in the home or the hospital
- Funeral and burial customs
- The length of the mourning period

From: Lewis, L., Brecher, M., Reaman, G. H., & Sahler, O. J. (2002). How can you help meet the needs of dying children? *Contemporary Pediatrics, 19*(4), 147–159.

CLINICAL MANIFESTATIONS | THE DYING CHILD

Body System	Clinical Manifestations
Cardiovascular system	• The heart rate may initially increase as hypoxia develops, then the heart rate and blood pressure decrease, resulting in decreased cardiac output. • A change in pulse pressure and a decrease in the volume of Korotkoff's sounds indicate imminent death. • Peripheral circulation decreases, leading to diaphoresis, clammy cool skin, and changes in skin coloring (mottled to cyanotic). Mottling is a sign of imminent death.
Respiratory system	• Impaired cardiac function leads to pulmonary congestion, tachypnea, diminished breath sounds, and hypoxia. • Dyspnea; **air hunger**, the most severe form of dyspnea, may cause the child to look panicked, gasp for breath, and sit upright. • **Cheyne-Stokes breathing** (periods of shallow breathing alternating with apnea) is a sign of imminent death. • As muscles relax, secretions accumulate in the oropharynx and bronchi. The "death rattle" is caused by air passing through these secretions. • Moaning or grunting with breathing is not uncommon.
Neurological system	• Decreased cerebral perfusion, hypoxemia, metabolic acidosis, the influences of disease-related factors, and an accumulation of toxins from renal and liver failure lead to neurological dysfunction. • Agitation or restlessness, withdrawal, increasing drowsiness, confusion may occur; the child may be unconscious during final hours. • The child may speak of visions (persons or objects) not visible to others. • Hearing and vision acuity may deteriorate, but remember that hearing is considered to be the last of the senses to diminish before death.
Musculoskeletal system	• Extreme muscle weakness and fatigue, difficulty with swallowing. • May be unable to reposition self, toilet self, or effectively cough and clear secretions.
Renal system	• Decreased kidney function and urine production. • Sphincters relax and incontinence can occur.
Gastrointestinal system	• Decreased oral fluid intake and anorexia are common. • Parenteral fluids may cause edema and increased respiratory secretions leading to shortness of breath and cough. • Sphincters relax and bowel incontinence can occur.

Examples of nursing diagnoses that apply to the dying child and family include the following:

- Fear (Child) related to unanswered questions and concerns of abandonment
- Death Anxiety (Child) related to impending death
- Anticipatory Grieving (Parents) related to imminent death of child
- Hopelessness (Parents) related to failure of therapies to prolong life

Planning and Implementation

Nursing care for the dying child and the family includes providing comfort, assisting the child in a peaceful death, assisting the child and family with coping strategies, and facilitating grief.

Physiologic Care

A major goal in care of the dying child is to promote comfort and keep the child pain free. Provide analgesia to promote optimal pain relief. Oral, transdermal, or rectal analgesia is available for families who choose to withhold intravenous fluids. Complementary care for comfort and pain management as described in Chapter 15 ∞ can be used by the nurse and family members.

If air hunger occurs, elevate the head of the bed, open a window, or use a circulating fan. An opioid may be prescribed for air hunger or tachypnea as its action dilates the pulmonary vessels, reduces oxygen consumption, and decreases pulmonary congestion.

Other physiologic care includes keeping the airway clear of secretions, bathing and keeping the skin dry and intact, changing the child's position frequently, and encouraging favorite foods and liquids as tolerated. Involve the parents in physical care and encourage them to hold and comfort the child.

Psychological Care

Parents may prefer not to talk with the child about the seriousness of the illness and potential for death out of a desire to protect the child from bad news, and a fear that the child will lose hope (Mazanec & Tyler, 2003). Even when children are not told they are dying, they know their condition is worsening. They are undergoing treatments, not feeling well, and picking up cues from their parents. They usually do not have the same fears about dying that adults do. Kübler-Ross (1983) noted that children are more fearful of abandonment than death. When children are not informed, they may have more fears and feel more isolated. Providing information and talking with the child about his or her concerns can reduce the child's anxiety, remove the sense of secrecy they feel, and enable them to focus on the time remaining (Beale et al., 2005).

Some children keep most of their thoughts about death to themselves. If they have not been told that they are dying, they may feel isolated and get the message not to discuss their condition. They may fear that the family members will abandon them emotionally. Children often avoid displaying anger, since they fear desertion more than death. They may also believe that expressing their awareness of death and their fears will place added emotional burdens on family members that could be unbearable to the family.

Provide the child with opportunities for fantasy play, drawings, and storytelling, without emphasizing or reinforcing death themes. Listen to what children tell you about themselves and their lives. **Death imagery**, the child's references to death or death-related topics (going away, separation, funerals), may be themes of their stories. Strategies for talking with a dying child are described in Box 14–3.

When caring for adolescents, remember that outbursts of anger are common but not personally directed at the nurse. Provide activities to help adolescents channel their feelings. Continue providing support in spite of their behavior. This approach may encourage adolescents to accept comforting without losing face. Be available to listen when the adolescent wants to talk and express feelings and frustrations. Promote friendships with other adolescents who have similar interests or problems.

Parents may not recognize the child's death anxiety because of their own fears, concerns, and feelings of helplessness. Depending on the family's cultural and religious beliefs, a chaplain or other healthcare professional who specializes in working with

---

CLINICAL TIP

Some parents ask that their child not be told he or she is dying. Do you abide by their wishes when the child asks you if he or she is dying? Tell the parents that the child asked the question. Offer to set up a meeting with the healthcare team to discuss their fears and concerns about telling their child the truth. Offer parents words and phrases they can use to talk with their child about his or her death at a developmentally appropriate level. Some parents may prefer that the child's questions be answered honestly by another professional. A professional who has special bereavement counseling training can assist children and families with discussions.

RESEARCH

Talking about Cancer

Investigators in Sweden asked 449 parents whose child had died from cancer if they had talked with their child about death. Nearly one-third of the parents had talked with their child about death, and none of the parents regretted having the discussion. Parents were more likely to talk with their child if they sensed the child was aware of his or her imminent death, if they were religious, or if the child was older at the time of diagnosis (Kreicbergs, Valdimarsdóttir, Onelöv et al., 2004).

BOX 14–3
STRATEGIES FOR TALKING TO THE DYING CHILD

- Make sure an agreement is reached early on with parents and child about open communication.
- Be receptive when children initiate a conversation. Recognize that behavior changes (disruptive behavior, withdrawal, anger, hyperalert state, sleeping more than usual) may indicate a struggle with emotions and an opportunity to engage the child in discussion.
- Identify how much the child knows and wants to know. Identify any fantasies and concerns, and then provide correct information, matching the amount of information the child wants.
- Allow the child to express his or her feelings and to be upset, even if this is a difficult discussion.
- Reassure the child that you will be available to listen and give support.
- Recognize that some children communicate best through nonverbal means, (i.e., art and music). The child may be willing to talk through a puppet or a stuffed animal.
- Acknowledge that the child's life can be complete, even if it is short. Let dying children know they will always be loved and remembered.
- Empower children as much as possible in circumstances concerning their deaths. Reassure them of continued love and physical closeness.

Note: Adapted from Beale, E. A., Baile, W. F., & Aaron, J. (2005). Silence is not golden: Communicating with children dying from cancer. *Journal of Clinical Oncology, 23*(15), 3629–3631.

---

terminally ill children and families may help reduce a child's spiritual fears and promote peace and comfort among family members.

Family Support

Work closely with the family when the child's death is imminent, because they will remember the experience and words spoken for the rest of their lives. Prepare the family for changes in the child's appearance and behavior. Providing the parents with a room to be alone with the child ensures privacy at this extremely personal time. Ask the family in a nonjudgmental, supportive manner what is important to them in the final moments and hours of their child's life and what will be important to them in the grief process. Certain religious or cultural practices may need to be planned and should be accommodated when possible. Holding the child is a universal request and should be permitted, along with touching, stroking, kissing, and talking soothingly (Figure 14–7 ➤) Many families find that saying good-bye as a group is helpful. Families need to cry together and to tell each other how much they will miss each other. They need to be assured that the vigil with the child is important so the child does not feel isolated or abandoned as death approaches. See Table 14–2 for common mourning and after-death rituals.

Tissue and/or Organ Donation

Families may be asked about making an anatomical gift. Information about organ and tissue donation is usually shared with families by specially trained personnel who identify the appropriate time to talk with families. Nurses can become better prepared to serve the family of the dying child and potential organ recipients by becoming familiar with the healthcare facility's criteria for organ and tissue procurement. Generally an organ procurement organization coordinator will collaborate with the nurses and healthcare team to support the process.

Need for Autopsy

When the exact cause of death is not clear, an autopsy may be suggested. In the event of an unnatural or unexpected death (suicide, homicide, Sudden Infant Death Syndrome), an autopsy may be required by state law. Parents may be hesitant to consent to autopsy when they have a choice because they are uneasy about the child's body being further invaded. Support is provided to the family during decision making by explaining that the autopsy will likely reveal the cause of death. This information may be especially important if the death is potentially due to a genetic disorder, affecting future childbearing decisions.

CULTURE

Hmong Rites
Many culturally influenced rules and customs surround dying. For instance, the Hmong belief system holds that children will live in eternity in the same state in which they existed at the time of death. Therefore, it is important that the child's body be intact at death.

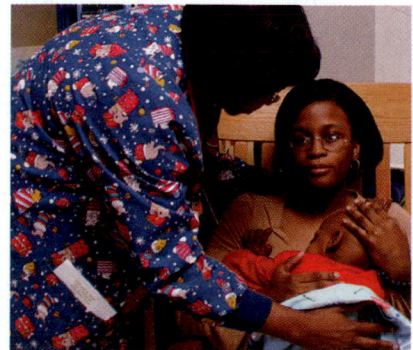

Figure 14–7 ➤ In the final days of a child's life, emphasis is on promoting the child's comfort and supporting the family. The parents are encouraged to hold the child to give comfort and a sense of security and love.

Table 14–2	CULTURAL TRADITIONS IN MOURNING AND AFTER-DEATH RITES	
Religious Group	**Rituals You Might Observe**	**Organ Donation or Autopsy Beliefs**
American Indians	• Beliefs and practices vary widely • Navajo do not touch the deceased or their belongings	Varies among tribes
Buddhism	• Last-rite chanting at bedside • Cremation common	Organ donation considered act of mercy, autopsy individual choice
Catholicism	• Sacrament of the sick • Obligated to take ordinary but not extraordinary means to prolong life • Burial is common	Autopsy, organ donation acceptable
Christian Science	• Unlikely to seek medical help to prolong life • Disposal of body and parts decided by family	Individual decides about organ donation
Hinduism	• No restrictions to right-to-die issue • Religious prayers chanted before and after death • Cremation common • Men and women display outward grief • Thread tied around wrist signifies a blessing; do not remove	Autopsy, organ donation acceptable
Islam	• Attempts to shorten life prohibited • Body is washed only by Muslim of same gender	Organ donation acceptable Autopsy only for medical or legal reasons
Jehovah's Witness	• Use of extraordinary means to prolong life is individual choice • Burial determined by family preference	Autopsy if required by law Organ donation forbidden
Judaism	• If death is inevitable, no new procedures needed, but must continue those ongoing • Body ritually washed • Burial as soon as possible; all body parts must be buried together • Seven-day mourning period	Autopsy permitted in certain circumstances, organ donation is complex issue
Mennonite	• Do not believe life must be continued at all cost	Autopsy and organ donation acceptable
Mormonism	• If death is inevitable, promote a peaceful and dignified death • Burial in "temple clothes"	Autopsy permitted with permission of next of kin, organ donation is permitted
Protestantism	• Burial or cremation is individual decision	Organ donation, autopsy are individual decisions
Seventh Day Adventist	• Follow ethic of prolonging life • Disposal of body and burial are individual decisions	Autopsy, organ donation acceptable

Note: From Spector, R. E. (2005). *Cultural diversity in health and illness* (6th ed., pp. 128–133). Upper Saddle River, NJ: Prentice Hall Health. Adapted.

Postmortem Care and Family Support

Offer ongoing support after the child dies. Questions like the following may help begin the conversation: " I am sorry for your loss. How can I help?" "What are your traditions when an infant or child dies?" "Is there someone I can call for you?"

Identify the family's wishes for postmortem care before performing any care. Ask before removing any jewelry or other item from the child because cultural and spiritual practices may specify that the article remain on the child after death. The nurse should follow the healthcare facility's guidelines for postmortem care. The child should be positioned according to guidelines or cultural/religious practices, the room should be cleaned, and medical equipment should be removed.

After the child's death, allow the family to spend as much time as they need with the child's body. Never rush family members who are saying good-bye to the child. Save all of the child's personal items—especially in the case of an infant, whose parents may have few mementos. A lock of hair, handprint or footprints, the infant's identification band, the child's weight and height, the last clothes or patient gown worn by the child sealed in a plastic bag to retain the child's scent, or a picture of the infant can be sources of comfort and remembrance for families. It may be traumatic for the family to receive the child's possessions, so when possible, use a special remembrance box or container for this purpose.

When a newborn or young infant has died, wrap the baby in a blanket and offer the mother and other family members the opportunity to hold the baby. Parents may want to bathe and dress the infant. The family experiencing the death of a newborn may appreciate an offer to take pictures of the baby and family together, if picture taking is not prohibited by religious or cultural traditions. However, some families may feel uncomfortable taking pictures with their dead baby and refuse the offer. Ask for permission before cutting a lock of the baby's hair as some cultural and religious groups prohibit it, such as Native Americans. Handprints and footprints may be captured using ink pads or clay and be given to the parents. Some parents may initially refuse to accept any of the baby's personal items or pictures. These items should be stored to allow the parents the opportunity to obtain them later.

Parents may need information about resources available to help with a memorial service or funeral. Later, acknowledge with parents that certain dates—such as the day of the week the child died, the child's birthday, or family holidays—will be difficult and may trigger intense sadness again. Provide grief counseling resources and encourage the family to continue to use them for at least the first year after the death. Parents may benefit from keeping a journal of their thoughts and memories, or writing letters or poems to or about their child.

Evaluation

Expected outcomes of caring for the dying child and family may include the following:

- The child is pain free and comfortable, and the child's physiologic needs are met.
- The cultural and spiritual needs of the dying child and family are met.
- The dying child and family receive support during the dying process.
- The family receives continued support after the child's death.

BEREAVEMENT

Parents' Reactions

The death of one's child is probably a parent's most painful experience. **Grief**, an individual's feelings and behaviors in response to death, is painful, individualized, and exhausting. Many factors influence the parents' grief responses, including their perception of the preventability of the illness or injury, the suddenness and other circumstances of the death, the nature of their attachment to the child, previous losses, spiritual or religious orientation, and culture.

Although parents progress through distinct stages of grief, as described on page 449, the time line and nature of the grief process differ for each individual. The intense pain and shock initially felt by parents gradually give way to feelings of anger, guilt, depression, and loneliness. Very slowly, and with much support, energy returns and parents again begin to enjoy life experiences. Spouses may need additional support when they are at different levels of grieving to prevent a sense of loneliness and isolation.

Emphasize to parents that although the period surrounding their child's death is difficult, caring for themselves physically and mentally is important. Parents may experience friction due to differing rates and intensity of grief. The nurse can give a list of appropriate support groups, books, and articles to parents for later use. Parents can be referred to national organizations, such as the Candlelighters Foundation or Compassionate Friends, and to local support groups for bereaved parents or siblings. Some institutions have formal follow-up programs for bereaved parents to encourage a healthy progression through the grieving process.

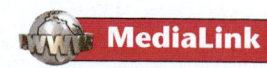

MediaLink

Grief Resources

Sudden Death of a Child

Although many children die because of chronic illness or terminal condition, more than 40% of child deaths between 1 and 19 years of age are caused by unexpected injuries

(Health Resources and Services Administration, 2002). The sudden and unexpected death that results from Sudden Infant Death Syndrome, injury, illness, suicide, or violence can lead to more intense grief that takes longer to resolve than grief experienced after an expected death (Menke, 2002). Parents have not had time to prepare for the child's death. Parents need support to deal with the death of the child and to deal with their surviving children. See Box 14–4 for nursing care strategies to provide comfort and support for the dying child and the family.

Death of a Newborn or Young Infant

Approximately 15,000 infants are born each year who are dying at birth or have conditions that are incompatible with prolonged life beyond the first year (Catlin & Carter, 2002). The death of a newborn forces parents to experience their child's entire life in a short period of time, and they are faced with overwhelming grief at a time when they anticipated the experience of joy. Unique experiences may occur with multiple births, such as the death of one or more of the infants, leading to conflicting emotions for the parents. While they mourn the death of one child, they must parent and bond with the survivor. Concerns arise as the parents fear losing the other infant (Lundqvist, Nilstun, & Dykes, 2002). Refer parents to a perinatal bereavement program or support group. They often feel guilty and a failure for having a child die.

Siblings' Reactions

Siblings experiencing the death of a brother or sister require supportive and compassionate care. In the course of the child's illness the siblings probably will have received less attention from parents. They may fear that they caused their brother or sister to be injured or become ill, or worry that bad thoughts on their part brought on the illness. Siblings have reported feeling loneliness, anxiety, anger, and jealousy during the dying process (Nolbris & Hellstrom, 2005). Nurses and other support personnel can assist the surviving children to adapt to their parent's distraction, grief, and increased

---

BOX 14–4
STRATEGIES FOR WORKING WITH PARENTS WHOSE CHILD DIES SUDDENLY

- Provide private space with telephone access.
- Identify a spokesperson for the medical team to stay with the family and keep them informed during resuscitation efforts. Have both parents present if possible.
- During the discussion, speak plainly and directly about the condition. Assess the family's understanding of the information.
- Allow as much time as possible for the family to understand the seriousness and worsening of the child's status. Provide several updates during the resuscitation (two or three times over 15 minutes) or by allowing them to be present during the resuscitation. Prepare them for what is to come.
- Offer to telephone clergy, family, and friends.
- After the death, prepare the body for viewing by covering disfiguring wounds and explaining any tubes or lines that must remain because of legal or medical examiner requirements.
- Provide the time and place for the family to be with the child after death. Depending upon cultural preferences, the family may wish to bathe the child or hold and rock the child.
- Sit close and make eye contact. Let the parents know that everything possible was done for the child. If the child was not in pain or did not suffer, share that information. Share your emotions with the family. Accept whatever emotions family members express.
- Convey information to the family about the cause of death, requirements for or value of an autopsy with a sudden death, funeral preparations, and the normal grief process.
- Arrange for family follow-up to see how they are responding to the child's loss and to review autopsy findings.

Data from: Knapp, J., Mulligan-Smith, D., and the Committee on Pediatric Emergency Medicine. (2005). Death of a child in the emergency department. *Pediatrics, 115*(5), 1432–1437.

protectiveness of them. The siblings need to hear that the parents' grief in no way diminishes the love felt for them. Table 14–3 highlights children's understanding of death at different developmental stages and some of the possible behavioral responses.

When talking to the siblings of a dying child, honesty is most important. Provide explanations in language that is developmentally appropriate. Reassure siblings that they did not cause their brother or sister to die (unless they did contribute to the

Table 14–3	A CHILD'S UNDERSTANDING OF DEATH AND POSSIBLE BEHAVIORAL RESPONSES WHEN A FAMILY MEMBER DIES
Understanding of Death	**Possible Behaviors**
Infant	
• Lacks understanding of concept of death • May sense caregivers are tense, routines are altered	• May show sadness by turning away from your gaze • Resists cuddling and eats less • Excessive crying, clingy • Sleeping more than usual
Toddler	
• Unable to distinguish fact from fantasy • No understanding of true concept of death • Aware someone is missing—separation anxiety • Unable to distinguish death from temporary separation or abandonment	• Clingy, refuses to let parent out of sight • Stops walking and talking, regression from previously achieved milestones • Shows distress by biting, hitting, tears • Fearfulness • Problems eating and sleeping • Sleep disturbances
Preschooler	
• Believes death is temporary • Magical thinking—believes dead person can be brought back to life • Believes bad thoughts cause death • Believes magical thinking can bring dead person back or can cause death to occur with thoughts • Has beginning experience with death of animals and plants	• May fear going to sleep, has nightmares, afraid of dark • Out-of-control behavior, hyperactivity, tantrums, regression • Problems with bowel and bladder control • Crying spells • Seems morbidly fascinated with death • Asks lots of questions • Displays anger at failure to keep person "alive," breaks toys, aggressive to friends • Regression to baby talk or thumb-sucking • Complaints of abdominal pain
School-Age Child	
• Acquires more realistic understanding of death • By 8–10 years, understands that death is permanent and irreversible, and that people die from internal and external causes • Believes that death is universal and will happen to him or her • May have exaggerated concerns about death	• May deny sadness by hiding tears and acting more like adults • Difficulty concentrating on school work • Psychosomatic complaints—stomachache or headache • Acting-out behavior, aggression, anger at being abandoned • May try to comfort parents by taking over tasks • May fear someone else they love will die
Adolescent	
• Intellectually capable of understanding death • Has a better grasp of association between illness and death • Sense of invincibility conflicts with fear of death • Able to recognize effect of death on others	• Same as school-age child • May have severe depression • Acting-out behavior—risk-taking behavior, delinquency, suicide attempts, promiscuity, pseudo-indifference

Adapted from: Menke, E. M. (2002). Handling children's grief at the first anniversary. *Journal of Pediatric Health Care, 16*(5), 267–270.

child's death) and that death was not a punishment for wrongdoing. Allow the siblings to ask questions. Acknowledge the emotions they are feeling, and emphasize that it is all right for them to be sad, angry, frightened, or tearful. The nurse should use the same amount of energy and concern in acknowledging their grief as acknowledging that of adults. Ask how they feel about saying good-bye to the dying child, and provide physical and emotional support. Preparation of the siblings before seeing the dying child involves a brief explanation of what they will see, feel, hear, and smell. Answer questions truthfully. Siblings may have to hear information several times.

As appropriate and comfortable, siblings should be permitted to participate in planning the child's memorial or funeral service. Being able to grieve as a family provides siblings with a sense of connectedness to parents and provides security at a vulnerable time. If siblings attend the funeral, prepare them for what to expect, such as an open casket or behaviors of mourners. Provide a support person, such as a family member or close friend, who can monitor the siblings' needs while the parents attend to other matters. Keep the family together as much as possible.

As with parental bereavement, sibling bereavement is a lifelong process. The nurse should encourage parents to make sure other caregivers and teachers know about the sibling's loss. Let the child express feelings other than sadness (e.g., guilt and anger). Encourage them to express grief through art, stories, and writing. Children can be encouraged to celebrate their sibling's life by preparing collages of photographs, collecting the child's favorite toys, and making a keepsake box.

STAFF REACTIONS TO A CHILD'S DEATH

Children are highly valued by society because of their potential future contributions. Children are expected to have a normal life span, and the death of a child is often viewed as a tragedy. Caring for dying children is especially stressful and demanding for health-care professionals. Health professionals caring for the dying child may feel a sense of helplessness, that they have failed the child, and sadness for the child's short life (Beale,

---

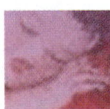

FAMILIES WANT TO KNOW

Strategies to Help Children and Adolescent Siblings Handle Grief

Nurses can share the following information with families when a child has died. Suggested strategies according to developmental level include:

Infants to Age 3 Years

- Encourage parents to hold and cuddle their child. This may alleviate the child's fear of separation.
- Speak to the child in a soft and comforting voice.
- As much as possible, follow familiar routines.
- Be tolerant of regressive behaviors.
- Talk and answer questions in terms that the child will understand.

Preschoolers

- Listen to the child and answer questions honestly.
- Try to follow usual routines and provide play activities.
- Assure the child that he will not be alone.
- Be tolerant of regressive behaviors; provide play activities.
- Reassure the child that his thoughts or actions in no way contributed to the death.
- Keep memories alive with pictures and other things that remind the child of the loved one Allow the child to participate in rituals such as going to the cemetery, releasing helium balloons, and planting flowers.

School-Age Children

- Listen to the child and answer questions honestly, as the school-age child will cope by gathering as much information as possible.
- Return to usual routines and activities.
- Keep memories alive through activities such as art, music, creating a memory book, sewing a quilt, and planting a garden.
- Share Internet resources.
- Use coping support groups.

Adolescents

- Be available and foster open communication.
- Share grief and feelings with the adolescent.
- Keep memories alive with pictures and other things that remind the child of the loved one. Access counseling and support groups.
- Share Internet resources.
- Facilitate contact with friends through cellular phones and the Internet.

Adapted from: Menke, E. M. (2002). Handling children's grief at the first anniversary. *Journal of Pediatric Health Care, 16*(5), 267–270.

Baile, & Aaron, 2005). Nurses involved in long-term relationships with children experience grief when these children die. Some nurses cope by distancing themselves socially from the dying child and family to maintain composure and a professional demeanor.

Caring for the dying child may be especially difficult for nurses with young children of their own. They tend to identify with the child, making it more likely that they will have difficulty dealing with the death in a professional manner. Nurses may not be able to recognize the dying child's anxiety and fears because of their own personal defenses against their sense of helplessness to alter the course of the child's disease.

Nurses who work with terminally ill children and their families need special preparation to meet the needs of these individuals and to simultaneously manage personal stress. Mentorship with experienced hospice nurses, as well as additional educational experiences, may help promote professional nursing care. Nurses who work with dying children and families must learn to cope effectively with grief and develop empathy, competence, and confidence in their ability to provide more humane and effective nursing care. Although crying with families was once considered unprofessional to some, it is now recognized as an expression of caring and empathy. Nurses should feel free to express their sorrow and grief for the child and family. Some nurses attend funeral and memorial services when invited by the patient's family.

Nurses working in emergency departments caring for children who die suddenly or in hospice settings and hospital units that care for terminally ill children need support systems to help balance the stresses of working with dying children. The workplace should acknowledge the stress nurses experience when working with terminally ill children. Support systems may include discussions with peers or debriefing group sessions with mental health professionals that provide an opportunity to discuss their feelings and concerns (Figure 14–8 ➤). Participating in team decisions regarding the dying child's plan of care (palliative rather than curative) helps many nurses manage their distress. Some hospitals conduct an annual memorial service for pediatric patients that staff may attend.

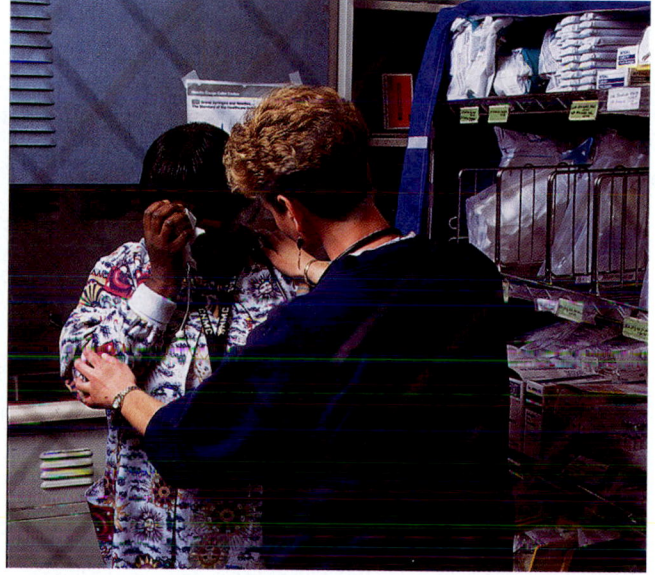

Figure 14–8 ➤ Nurses need to express grief in a supportive environment after a child's death. Sharing the sadness and grief or futility of resuscitation efforts with colleagues can often help nurses continue to provide supportive care to the next families who need compassionate care.

CRITICAL THINKING IN ACTION

Recall Alexa in the opening scenario. She is unconscious from hitting her head and has a serious abdominal injury following a motor vehicle crash in which she was a passenger. She is being cared for in the pediatric intensive care unit, so that she can be monitored and her injuries prevented from becoming life threatening. The abdominal CT scan has revealed a spleen laceration that is bleeding, so she is being carefully monitored for hypovolemia. She has regained consciousness, but drifts off to sleep frequently. Alexa's mother is at her bedside. Her father, who was driving the car, is being evaluated at another hospital, and Alexa's 8-year-old sister Sharon is temporarily staying with a neighbor.

1. What are the developmentally appropriate nursing interventions to address Alexa's stressors related to this sudden hospitalization?

2. What physical assessment procedures are used to monitor Alexa's condition?

3. What nursing interventions should be implemented to support Alexa's family?

4. What information should be provided to Sharon to help her understand what has happened to Alexa?

 Refer to your Prentice Hall Nursing MediaLink DVD-ROM for answers.

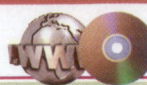
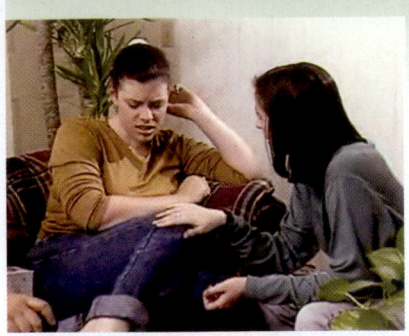

Resources for this chapter can be found on the Prentice Hall Nursing MediaLink DVD-ROM accompanying this textbook, and on the Companion Website at http://www.prenhall.com/ball.

DVD-ROM
Audio Glossary
NCLEX-RN® Review
Video
Parental Reaction to the Death of a Child

COMPANION WEBSITE
Audio Glossary
NCLEX-RN® Review
Care Plan Activity: The Grieving Family
Case Study: A Premature Infant
Critical Thinking
The Dying Child's Experience
Nursing Interventions for Parents Experiencing Distress
MediaLink Applications
WebLinks

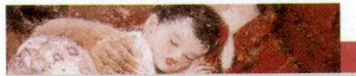

REFERENCES

American Academy of Pediatrics, Committee on Hospital Care and the Institute of Family Centered Care. (2003). Family-centered care and the pediatrician's role. *Pediatrics, 112*(3), 691–696.

Barnes, L. L., Plotnikoff, G. A., Fox, K., & Pendleton, S. (2000). Spirituality, religion, and pediatrics: Intersecting worlds of healing. *Pediatrics, 106*(4) Part 2, 899–909.

Beale, E. A., Baile, W. F., & Aaron, J. (2005). Silence is not golden: Communicating with children dying from cancer, *Journal of Clinical Oncology, 23*(15), 3629–3631.

Board, R. (2005). School-age children's perceptions of their PICU hospitalization. *Pediatric Nursing, 31*(3), 166–175.

Catlin, A., & Carter, B. (2002). Creation of a neonatal end-of-life palliative care protocol. *Neonatal Network, 21*(4), 37–49.

Contro, N., Larson, J., Scofield, S., Sourkes, B., & Cohen, H. (2002). Family perspectives on quality of pediatric palliative care. *Archives of Pediatric and Adolescent Medicine, 156*(1), 14–19.

Ferrell, B. R., & Coyle, N. (2002). An overview of palliative care. *American Journal of Nursing, 102*(10), 18.

Gavaghan, S. R., & Carroll, D. L. (2002). Families of critically ill patients and the effect of nursing interventions. *Dimensions of Critical Care Nursing, 21*(2), 64–71.

Griffin, T. (2003). Facing challenges to family-centered care II: Anger in the clinical setting. *Pediatric Nursing, 29*(3), 212–214.

Hammes, B. J., Klevan, J., Kempf, M., & Williams, M. S. (2005). Pediatric advance care planning. *Journal of Palliative Medicine, 8*(4), 766–773.

Health Resources and Services Administration, Maternal and Child Health Bureau. (2002). *Child health USA, 2002.* Rockville, MD: U.S. Department of Health and Human Services.

Himmelstein, B. P., Hilden, J. M., Boldt, A. M., & Weissman, D. (2004). Pediatric palliative care. *New England Journal of Medicine, 350*(17), 1752–1762.

Holbrook, T. L., Hoyt, D. B., Coimbra, R., Potenza, B., Sise, M., & Anderson, J. P. (2005). Long-term posttraumatic stress disorder persists after major trauma in adolescents: New data on risk factors and functional outcomes. *Journal of Trauma, Injury, Infection, and Critical Care, 58*(4), 764–771.

Institute of Medicine (2003). Patterns of childhood death in America. In M. J. Field & R. E. Behrman. *When children die: Improving palliative and end-of-life care for children and their families* (pp. 41–71). Washington, DC: National Academy Press.

Jacobs, H. H. (2005). Ethics in pediatric end-of-life care: A nursing perspective. *Journal of Pediatric Nursing, 20*(5), 360–369.

Katz, S. (2002). When the child's illness is life-threatening: Impact on parents. *Pediatric Nursing, 28*(5), 453–464.

Kimberly, M. B., Forte, A. L., Carroll, J. M., & Feudtner, C. (2005). Pediatric do-not-attempt-resuscitation orders and public schools: A national assessment of policies and laws. *American Journal of Bioethics, 5*(1), 59–65.

Klopfenstein, K. J., & Young-Saleme, T. (2002). Your role in the spectrum of adolescent cancer: Diagnosis through the treatment to care at life's end. *Contemporary Pediatrics, 19*(8), 105–127.

Knapp, J., Mulligan-Smith, D., and the Committee on Pediatric Emergency Medicine. (2005). Death of a child in the emergency department. *Pediatrics, 115*(5), 1432–1437.

Kreicbergs, U., Valdimarsdóttir, U., Onelöv, E., Henter, J. I., & Steineck, G. (2004). Talking about death with children who have severe malignant disease. *New England Journal of Medicine, 351*(12), 1251–1253.

Kübler-Ross, E. (1983). *On children and death.* New York: Macmillan.

Levetown, M. (2004). Breaking bad news in the emergency department: When seconds count. *Topics in Emergency Medicine, 26*(1), 35–43.

Lewis, L., Brecher, M., Reaman, G. H., & Sahler, O. J. (2002). How can you help meet the needs of dying children? *Contemporary Pediatrics, 19*(4), 147–159.

Lundqvist, A., Nilstun, T., & Dykes, A. (2002). Experiencing neonatal death: An ambivalent transition into motherhood. *Pediatric Nursing, 28*(6), 621–626.

Mazanec, P., & Tyler, M. K. (2003). Cultural considerations in end-of-life care. *American Journal of Nursing, 103*(3), 50–58.

McCaffrey, A. M., Eisenberg, D. M., Legedza, A. T. R., Davis, R. B., & Phillips, R. S. (2004, April 26). Prayer for health concerns: Results of a national survey on prevalence and patterns of use. *Archives of Internal Medicine, 164,* 858–862.

Melnyk, B. M., Alpert-Gillis, L., Feinstein, N. F., Crean, H. F., Johnson, J., Fairbanks, E., et al. (2004). Creating opportunities for parent empowerment: Program effects on the mental health/coping outcomes of critically ill young children and their mothers. *Pediatrics, 113*(6), e597–e607.

Melnyk, B. M., Small, L., & Carno, M. (2004). The effectiveness of parent-focused interventions in improving coping/mental health outcomes in critically ill children and their parents: An evidence base to guide clinical practice. *Pediatric Nursing, 30*(2), 143–148.

Menke, E. M. (2002). Handling children's grief at the first anniversary. *Journal of Pediatric Health Care, 16*(5), 267–270.

Meyer, E. C., Burns, J. P., Griffith, J. L., & Truog, R. D. (2002). Parental perspectives on end-of-life care in the pediatric intensive care unit. *Critical Care Medicine, 30*(1), 226–231.

Nolbris, M., & Hellstrom, A. L. (2005). Siblings' needs and issues when a brother or sister dies of cancer. *Journal of Pediatric Oncology Nursing, 22*(4), 227–233.

Ramer-Chrastek, J., Brunnquell, D., & Hasse, S. (2002). Letting nature take its course. *American Journal of Nursing, 102*(10), 24CC–24JJ.

Rushton, C. H. (2004). Ethics and palliative care in pediatrics. *American Journal of Nursing, 104*(4), 54–63.

Rushton, C. H. (2005). A framework for integrated pediatric palliative care: Being with dying. *Journal of Pediatric Nursing, 20*(5), 311–325.

Rushton, C. H., & Catlin, A. (2002). Pediatric palliative care: The time is now? *Pediatric Nursing, 28*(1), 57–70.

Ryan-Wenger, N. A. (1996). Children, coping, and the stress of illness: A synthesis of research. *Journal of the Society of Pediatric Nurses, 1*(3), 126–138.

Spector, R. E. (2005). *Culture Diversity in Health and Illness* (6th ed, pp. 128–133). Upper Saddle River, NJ: Prentice Hall Health.

Winston, F. K., Baxt, C., Kassam-Adams, N. L., Elliott, M. R., & Kallan, M. J. (2005). Acute traumatic stress symptoms in child occupants and their parent drivers after crash involvement. *Archives of Pediatric and Adolescent Medicine, 159*(11), 1074–1079.

PAIN ASSESSMENT AND MANAGEMENT

15

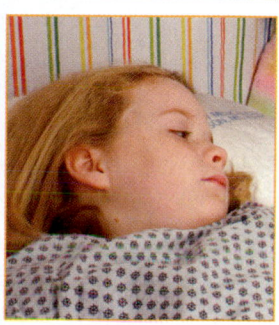

SUSIE, 6 years old, is being prepared to undergo an adenoidectomy because of obstructive sleep apnea. During her preoperative teaching the nurse shows Susie how to use a pain scale, explaining what each of the faces means. The nurse tells Susie that she will be asked to point to the face that matches how much she hurts several times after her operation. Susie is asked what is the most amount of pain she has ever felt, and what caused that pain. The nurse will use this information to help Susie identify the amount of pain she has during future pain assessments. Susie is encouraged to tell the nurse or her parents when she has pain after the operation because she will be given medicine for the pain to make her feel better.

The nurse also discusses the importance of assessing and treating pain with Susie's parents as Susie will go home the day after surgery. The nurse lets them know that keeping Susie's pain level low will make it easier for her to swallow liquids after surgery and promote her healing.

KEY TERMS

acute pain 470
anxiolysis 491
chronic pain 470
deep sedation 491
distraction 487
electroanalgesia 488
equianalgesic dose 479
iontophoresis 491
light sedation 491
nociception 470
nociceptors 471

nonsteroidal anti-inflammatory drugs (NSAIDs) 479
nurse-controlled analgesia 482
opioids 479
pain 470
patient-controlled analgesia (PCA) 481
sedation 491
tolerance 486
withdrawal 480

MediaLink

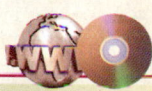

http://www.prenhall.com/ball

See the Prentice Hall Nursing MediaLink DVD-ROM and Companion Website for chapter-specific resources.

LEARNING OUTCOMES

After reading this chapter, you will be able to do the following:

1. Describe the physiologic and behavioral consequences of pain in children.
2. List behavioral indications that an infant or a child has pain.
3. Identify when to use a behavioral pain scale and a self-report pain scale.
4. Identify when opioids should be given to children and how they should be administered.
5. Explain why nonpharmacologic (complementary) methods of pain management are effective.
6. Develop a nursing care plan for an infant and for a child in acute pain that integrates pharmacologic interventions and developmentally appropriate nonpharmacologic (complementary) therapies.
7. Develop a nursing care plan for assessing and monitoring the child having sedation and analgesia for a medical procedure.

LAW & ETHICS

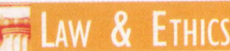

Standards for Pain

In 2001, the Joint Commission on Accreditation of Health Care Organizations introduced standards for the assessment and management of pain in patients. All patients have the right to assessment and management of pain, and patient education includes managing pain as a part of treatment.

GROWTH & DEVELOPMENT

Newborn and Infant Pain

Neonates and infants also remember pain. By 6 months of age, children demonstrate anticipatory fear of pain to immunizations and pin pricks (Hall & Anand, 2005).

CULTURE

Pain Experiences

Think about your personal pain experiences during childhood and how your family members encouraged you to be stoic or to express pain. These types of experiences often contribute to a health professional's attitudes about pain experienced by children. For example, healthcare workers may believe that being in pain for a little while is not so bad or that pain helps build character. Be aware that subtle nonverbal and verbal differences in expression of pain by different cultures exist and need to be accepted.

Every child has his or her own perception of pain. A neurologic response to tissue injury, **pain** is an unpleasant sensory and emotional experience associated with actual or potential tissue damage (Young, 2005). See Figure 15–1 ➤ for the pathophysiology of the pain response. The perception of pain, **nociception**, involves not only the actual tissue injury, but also the child's understanding, emotions, and past history of pain (Huether & Defriez, 2006). Effective pain management is every child's right.

ACUTE AND CHRONIC PAIN

Pain may be either acute or chronic. **Acute pain** is sudden and of short duration; it may be associated with a single event, such as surgery or injury, that can be linked to the pain discomfort. The inflammatory response following the initial tissue injury helps sustain the pain response. The pain often disappears as healing occurs. **Chronic pain** is persistent, lasting longer than 6 months; it is often associated with a prolonged disease process such as juvenile rheumatoid arthritis or cancer.

Misconceptions About Pain in Children

Healthcare professionals once believed that children feel less pain than adults. Undertreatment of pain was based on these attitudes about pain, the difficulty and complexity of pain assessment in children, and inadequate research. Despite improvements in pain management, some nurses still undertreat pain, either by not giving pain medication even when a child reports pain, giving less pain medication than ordered, or having a lack of awareness of the value of nonpharmacologic interventions (Van Hulle-Vincent, 2005; Vincent & Denyes, 2004). For a review of past myths and the contrasting reality, see Table 15–1.

Research has shown that past beliefs about children's perception of pain were incorrect. Even neonates feel pain. All the necessary peripheral and central nervous system anatomical structures and functional ability to process pain are present by 20 weeks' gestation (Pasero, 2002). Pain impulses are transmitted along the nonmyelinated C fibers and the pain signal is less precise. Pain conduction may be slower in neonates, but the distance the pain stimuli must travel is much shorter than in adults. Because the descending neurotransmitters are less developed, newborns are less able to reduce the pain impulses. Premature and newborn infants may be even more sensitive to pain than older children.

Clinical Manifestations

Physiologic Indicators

Acute pain stimulates the adrenergic nervous system and results in physiologic changes, including tachycardia, tachypnea, hypertension, pupil dilation, pallor, increased perspiration, and increased secretion of catecholamines and adrenocorticoid hormones. Changes in these signs demonstrate a complex stress response. These signs are not specific to pain, so they cannot be used for monitoring pain.

Chronic pain of long duration that is persistent or continuous permits physiologic adaptation, so normal heart rate, respiratory rate, and blood pressure levels are often seen (Huether & Defriez, 2006).

Behavioral Indicators

Children in acute pain display a variety of behaviors, such as the following:

- Short attention span (child is difficult to distract)
- Irritability (child is difficult to comfort)
- Facial grimacing, biting, or pursing lips; see Figure 15–2 ➤ for facial expressions of newborns and infants
- Posturing (guarding a painful joint by avoiding movement), remaining immobile, or protecting the painful area
- Drawing up knees, flexing limbs, massaging affected area
- Lethargy, remaining quiet, or withdrawal
- Sleep disturbances

PATHOPHYSIOLOGY ILLUSTRATED

Pain Perception

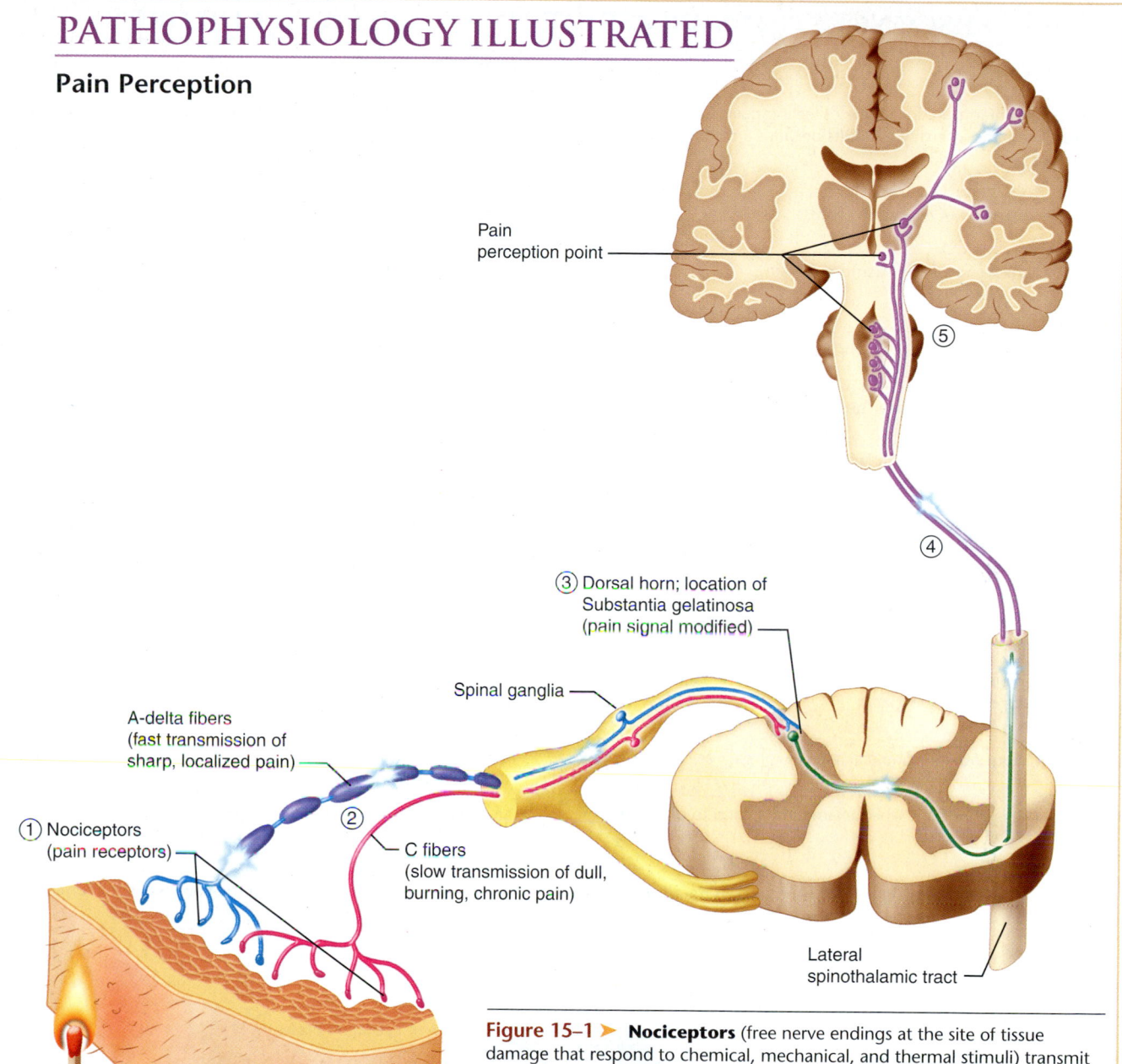

Pain perception point

⑤

③ Dorsal horn; location of Substantia gelatinosa (pain signal modified)

Spinal ganglia

④

A-delta fibers (fast transmission of sharp, localized pain)

① Nociceptors (pain receptors)

②

C fibers (slow transmission of dull, burning, chronic pain)

Lateral spinothalamic tract

Figure 15–1 ➤ **Nociceptors** (free nerve endings at the site of tissue damage that respond to chemical, mechanical, and thermal stimuli) transmit pain information by specialized nerve fibers to the gate at the posterior part of the spinal cord. Unmyelinated C fibers slowly transmit dull, burning, diffuse pain as well as chronic pain. Large, myelinated A-delta fibers quickly transmit sharp, well-localized pain. Nociceptors are stimulated by mechanical, thermal, and chemical injury. Biochemical mediators (bradykinin, prostaglandins, leukotrienes, serotonin, histamine, catecholamines, and substance P) are produced in response to tissue damage. These substances help move the pain impulse from the nerve endings to the spinal cord. After the sensory information reaches the substantia gelatinosa in the dorsal horn of the spinal cord, the pain signal may be modified depending on the presence of other stimuli, from either the brain or the periphery. The pain signal is then transmitted to the thalamus of the brain primarily through the lateral spinothalamic tract and reticulospinal and spinomesoencephalic nerve pathways, where perception occurs. The thalamus is the main relay station for sensory information. Pain information is then transmitted to the cerebral cortex as well as the reticular and limbic systems for the processing and interpretation of pain. Once the sensation reaches the brain, emotional responses may increase or decrease the intensity of the pain perceived (Huether & Defriez, 2006).

Since there is two-way control of nociceptive transmission within the spinal tracts, pain perception can be modulated when a competing nonpain impulse is sent along the same pathways that pain transmission uses. This simple explanation of the Gate Control Theory of pain helps explain how the pain impulses to the brain are transmitted and inhibited at the level of the dorsal horn of the spine. The brain also has a significant role in inhibiting the perception of pain. Endogenous opioids (endorphins) are produced in response to painful stimuli to help inhibit pain impulses in the spinal cord and the brain (Huether & Defriez, 2006).

Table 15–1	MISCONCEPTIONS ABOUT PAIN IN INFANTS AND CHILDREN
Myth	**Reality**
Neonates and infants are incapable of feeling pain. Children do not feel pain with the same intensity as adults because a child's nervous system is immature.	By 20 week's gestation, a fetus has most of the anatomic and functional requirements for pain processing. Term infants have the same level of sensitivity to pain as older infants and children. Preterm infants may actually have greater sensitivity.
Infants are incapable of expressing pain.	Infants express pain with both behavioral and physiologic cues that can be assessed.
Infants and children have no memory of pain.	Preterm infants have been noticed to associate the smell of alcohol with heel sticks and to try to pull the foot away to avoid the pain. Infants cry in anticipation of immunizations.
Parents exaggerate or aggravate their child's pain.	Parents know their child and are able to identify when the child is in pain.
Children are not in pain if they can be distracted or they are sleeping.	Children use distraction to cope with pain, but they soon become exhausted when coping with pain and fall asleep.
Repeated experience with pain teaches the child to be more tolerant of pain and cope with it better.	Children who have more experience with pain respond more vigorously to pain. Experience with pain teaches how severe the pain can become.
Children tolerate discomfort well. They become accustomed to pain after having it for a while.	Children do not tolerate pain any better than adults, and may have less tolerance with prior painful experiences. They do not become accustomed to pain or cope with it better than adults.
Children recover more quickly than adults from painful experiences such as surgery.	Children heal quickly from surgery, but they have the same amount of pain from surgery as an adult.
Children tell you if they are in pain. They do not need medication unless they appear to be in pain.	Children may be too young to express pain or afraid to tell anyone other than a parent about the pain. The child fears the treatment for pain may be worse than the pain itself.
Children without obvious physical reasons for pain are not likely to have pain.	The cause of pain cannot always be determined. The feeling of pain is subjective and should be accepted by nurses.
Pain response is important when examining a child to diagnose a condition.	Giving pain medication does not hinder the evaluation of a child with a surgical condition in the emergency department (Zempsky, Cravero et al., 2004).
Children run the risk of becoming addicted to pain medication when used for pain management.	Addiction is extremely rare when the child is treated for an acute condition.

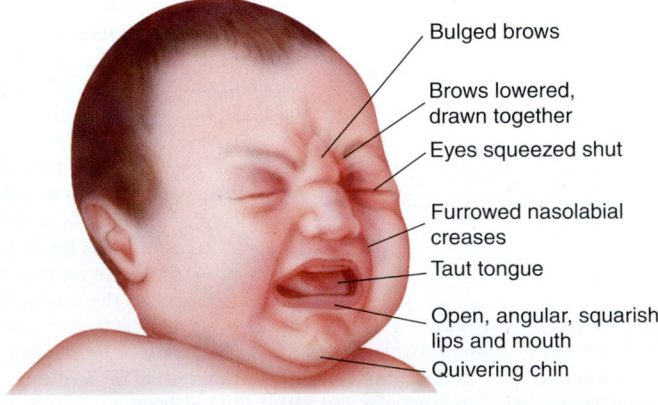

Figure 15–2 ➤ Neonatal characteristic facial responses to pain include bulged brow, eyes squeezed shut, furrowed nasolabial creases, open lips, pursed lips, stretched mouth, taut tongue, and a quivering chin.
Note: Redrawn from Carlson, K. L., Clement, B. A., & Nash, P. (1996). Neonatal pain: From concept to research questions and the role of the advanced practice nurse. *Journal of Perinatal Neonatal Nursing, 10*(1), 64–71.

Labels (from figure): Bulged brows; Brows lowered, drawn together; Eyes squeezed shut; Furrowed nasolabial creases; Taut tongue; Open, angular, squarish lips and mouth; Quivering chin

Preverbal children may show conflicting signs of pain (restlessness, agitation or withdrawal, hyperalert or vigilant, grimacing, crying, or anger), making pain assessment and management more challenging.

Children often suffer additional emotional distress and fear that the discomfort will worsen. Depression and/or aggressive behavior are frequently overlooked as indicators of pain.

Consequences of Pain

Unrelieved pain is stressful and has many undesirable physiologic consequences (Table 15–2). For example, the child with acute postoperative pain takes shallow breaths and suppresses coughing to avoid more pain. These self-protective actions increase the potential for respiratory complications. Unrelieved pain may also delay the return of normal gastric and bowel functions and cause a stress ulcer. Anorexia associated with pain may delay the healing process. The long-term effects of pain on the child's physical or psychologic condition are unknown.

PAIN ASSESSMENT

The goal of pain assessment is to provide accurate information about the location and intensity of pain and its effects on the child's functioning. No laboratory tests are routinely used to assess pain. Prolonged, severe pain produces a physiologic stress response that includes the chemical release of catecholamines, cortisol, aldosterone, and other corticosteroids. Insulin secretion also decreases, resulting in hyperglycemia. The immune and anti-inflammatory responses of the body are also diminished (McCance, Forshee, & Shelby, 2006).

Pain History

Parents can provide a great deal of information about the child's response to pain, such as the following:

- How the child typically expresses pain, both verbally and behaviorally. Children and parents use similar terms to describe pain. Some examples of words used are *a hurt, owie, boo-boo, stinging, sore, cutting, burning, itching, hot,* and *tight.* Knowing the appropriate word to use makes communicating with the child easier. The parent can often provide signs to help recognize the child's pain.
- The child's previous experiences with painful situations and reactions.
- How the child copes with and manages pain. The child with several past pain experiences may not exhibit the same types of stressful behaviors as the child with few pain experiences.
- What works best to reduce the child's pain.
- The parent's and child's preferences for analgesic use and other pain interventions.

CULTURE

Pain Terminology

The terms *pain, hurt,* and *ache* have been found to describe pain intensity across cultures. Pain is most intense, hurt is less severe, and ache is least severe (Gaston-Johansson, Albert, Fagan et al., 1990). Similarly, pain and hurt mean greater pain than ache in school-age children and adolescents (LaFleur & Raway, 1999). The term *tender* or *tenderness* may be confusing for some families in which English is a second language. Tender or tenderness is more commonly associated with caring or romance or with meat than with soreness or pain.

RESEARCH

Frequently Used Words

A recent study investigated the initial words used by children to describe pain and the age at which these words were first used. The most frequently used words by young children were *hurt, ouch,* and *ow.* Some children began using one of these words indicating pain as young as 18 months. Use of these words may help with pain assessment of young children (Stanford, Chambers, & Craig, 2005).

Table 15–2	PHYSIOLOGIC CONSEQUENCES OF UNRELIEVED PAIN IN CHILDREN

Responses to Pain	Potential Physiologic Consequences
Respiratory Changes	
Rapid shallow breathing	Alkalosis
Inadequate lung expansion	Decreased oxygen saturation, atelectasis
Inadequate cough	Retention of secretions
Neurologic Changes	
Increased sympathetic nervous system activity	Tachycardia, change in sleep patterns, increased blood glucose and cortisol levels
Metabolic Changes	
Increased metabolic rate with increased perspiration	Increased fluid and electrolyte losses
Immune System Changes	
Depression of immune response	Increased risk of infection
Gastrointestinal Changes	
Increased intestinal secretions and smooth muscle sphincter tone	Impaired gastrointestinal functioning, ileus

Data from: McCaffrey, M., & Pasero, C. (1999). *Pain: Clinical manual* (2nd ed., pp. 24, 27). St. Louis: Mosby; and Mitchell, A., & Boss, B. J. (2002). Adverse effects of pain on the central nervous systems of newborns and young children: A review of the literature. *Journal of Neuroscience Nursing, 34*(5), 228–236.

Older children may be able to give a history of painful episodes. When attempting to obtain information about the child's pain experiences and present level of pain, keep in mind that many children modify their pain descriptions depending on the type of questions asked and what they expect will happen as a result of their response. Examples of questions to ask the child include the following:

- What kinds of things caused hurt in the past and what made the hurt feel better?
- What do you tell your mother (or other significant person) when you hurt (are in pain)? What do you want your mother to do for the hurt?
- What would you like the nurse to do when you hurt? What should the nurse or anyone else do when you hurt?
- Where is the hurt, and what does it feel like? What could be causing the hurt?

Cultural Influences on Pain

Children's culture and social learning have a tremendous influence on their expression of pain. Children learn directly and indirectly from their parents about how to respond to pain. They observe family members in pain and try to imitate their responses. By showing approval and disapproval, parents teach their children how to behave when in pain. This instruction includes the following:

- Self-control and coping if a certain level of pain should be tolerated and how much discomfort justifies a complaint
- How to express the complaint to get assistance and when to stop complaining
- Whom to approach for pain relief

For example, boys in the United States are usually encouraged to hide their pain by acting brave and not crying. Girls are often encouraged to openly express their pain.

Developmental Responses to Pain

A child's responses to and understanding of pain depend on the child's age and stage of development. See Table 15–3 to learn more about the child's responses at each age. A child's responses to acute or chronic pain are also influenced by other factors (Anthony & Schanberg, 2005):

- Cognitive-behavioral factors—stress, mood, coping skills, psychological adjustment
- Biological factors—genetics, disease activity, medications, pain processing
- Environmental factors—parent pain experience, parent coping and adjustment, family relationships, school and social relationships

Young children are unable to give a detailed description of their pain because of their limited vocabulary and pain experiences. Depending on their developmental stage, children use different coping strategies, such as escape, postponement or avoidance, diversion, and imagery, to deal with pain. Healthcare providers now recognize that children do not complain of pain for several reasons:

- Some children believe they need to be brave.
- Preschoolers and adolescents may assume the nurse knows they have pain.
- Some children are afraid that an injection to relieve pain will hurt more than the pain they have.

Pain Assessment Scales

Various pain scales are used to assess pain in children.

Nonverbal Children

Physical and behavioral indicators are used to quantify pain in nonverbal children and rely on the nurse's observation of the child. Pain behavior scales involve assessing behaviors that have been identified as indicators of pain. It is important to make sure the

CULTURE

Expression of Pain

Some ethnic groups do not openly express pain while other cultural groups use verbal and nonverbal methods to express pain freely. Remember that children have individualized responses, and younger children have had less time to acquire culturally learned behaviors.

GROWTH & DEVELOPMENT

Exhibiting Stress

School-age children and adolescents may not exhibit distress in direct proportion to their pain intensity. Thus, behavioral measures (e.g., facial expression, limited movement) may not match the child's self-report of pain intensity. Because children in these age groups can accurately report pain intensity with a pain assessment tool, use and believe this self-report of pain as a valid pain assessment.

Table 15–3	CHILDREN'S UNDERSTANDING OF PAIN, THEIR BEHAVIORAL RESPONSES, AND VERBAL DESCRIPTIONS OF PAIN BY CHILDREN OF DIFFERENT DEVELOPMENTAL STAGES		
Age Group	**Understanding of Pain**	**Behavioral Response**	**Verbal Description**
Infants < 6 months	No apparent understanding of pain; neonates exposed to repeated painful experiences in ICU demonstrate memory of pain by holding their breath when approached by care providers	Generalized body movements, chin quivering, facial grimacing, poor feeding	Cries
6–12 months	Anticipate a painful event such as an immunization with fear; responsive to parental anxiety	Reflex withdrawal to stimulus, facial grimacing, disturbed sleep, irritability, restlessness	Cries
Toddlers 1–3 years	Do not understand what causes pain and why they might have pain; demonstrate fear of painful situations; use common words for pain such as *owie* and *boo-boo*	Localized withdrawal, resistance of entire body, aggressive behavior, disturbed sleep	Cries and screams, cannot describe intensity or type of pain
Preschoolers 3–6 years (preoperational)	Pain is a hurt; have language skills to express pain and skills increase with age; do not relate pain to illness but may relate pain to an injury; often believe pain is punishment; do not understand why a painful procedure will make them feel better or why an injection takes pain away	Active physical resistance, directed aggressive behavior, strikes out physically and verbally when hurt, low frustration level	Can identify location and intensity of pain, denies pain, may believe his or her pain is obvious to others
School-Age Children 7–9 years (concrete operations)	Can understand simple relationships between pain and disease but have no clear understanding of the cause of pain; can understand the need for painful procedures to monitor or treat disease; may associate pain with feeling bad or angry; may recognize psychologic pain related to grief and hurt feelings	Passive resistance, clenches fists, holds body rigidly still, suffers emotional withdrawal, engages in plea bargaining	Can specify location and intensity of pain and describe its physical characteristics in relation to body parts
10–12 years (transitional)	Better able to understand the relationship between an event and pain; have a more complex awareness of physical and psychologic pain, such as moral dilemmas and mental pain	May pretend comfort to project bravery, may regress with stress and anxiety	Able to describe intensity and location with more characteristics, able to describe psychologic pain
Adolescents 13–18 years (formal operations)	Have a sophisticated understanding of the causes of physical and mental pain; relate to the pain experienced by others; pain has both qualitative and quantitative characteristics	Want to behave in a socially acceptable manner (like adults), show a controlled behavioral response	More sophisticated descriptions as experience is gained; may think nurses are in tune with their thoughts, so they don't need to tell the nurse about their pain

infant or child can have all of the scale's behavioral indicators assessed to obtain an accurate score. For example, if the child is sedated, a relaxed facial expression may be observed even though pain is present and skew results. The number identified using a pain behavior scale, such as the Neonatal Infant Pain Scale (NIPS) and the FLACC Behavioral Pain Assessment Scale (FLACC), provides a pain-behavior score, not a pain-intensity score (Pasero & McCaffery, 2005).

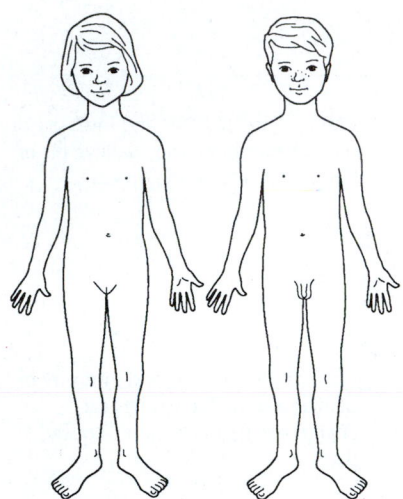

Figure 15–3 ➤ Use a body outline for children to identify all the locations of pain either with a marker or crayon. Different color crayons can be used to identify different levels of pain. This tool can be used independently or as a part of the Adolescent Pediatric Pain Tool.

NEONATAL INFANT PAIN SCALE   The NIPS is designed to measure procedural pain in preterm and full-term neonates up to 6 weeks after birth. The neonate's facial expression, cry quality, breathing patterns, arm and leg position, and state of arousal are observed. This tool has high inter-rater reliability and validity. See Table 15–4.

FLACC BEHAVIORAL PAIN ASSESSMENT SCALE   The FLACC is designed to measure acute pain in infants and young children following surgery, and it can be used until the child is able to self-report pain with another pain scale. FLACC is an acronym for the five categories that are assessed: Face, Legs, Activity, Cry, and Consolability. To use FLACC, the nurse observes the child during routine care for 5 or more minutes, and then selects the score that most closely matches each behavior noted. The scores for the five categories are added together for the total score. The tool has validity and reliability for evaluation of postoperative pain (Manworren & Hynan, 2003; Willis, Merkel, Voepel-Lewis, & Malviya, 2003). See Table 15–5. The FLACC has also been used as a tool for parents to provide proxy pain ratings for children with cognitive impairments. A recent study revealed that parents' estimates of their child's postoperative pain correlated well with the nurse's estimate of the child's pain (Voepel-Lewis, Malviya, & Tait, 2005).

PAIN LOCATION   Young children (3 years and older) can localize pain if given an outline of the front and back of the body (Figure 15–3 ➤). The child can mark where the pain is located or color the areas of pain with crayons. The child should use one color for the place where it hurts the most, and another color for areas with less pain.

Self-Report Pain Scales

Other scales depend on the child's self-report of pain intensity. To use pain scales the child must be developmentally ready and understand the concept of a little or a lot of pain well enough to tell the nurse. Children 2 to 3 years of age are usually able to un-

Table 15–4	NEONATAL INFANT PAIN SCALE (NIPS)
Characteristic	**Scoring Criteria**
Facial Expression 0 = Relaxed muscles 1 = Grimace	• Restful face with neutral expression • Tight facial muscles; furrowed brow, chin, and jaw (Note: At low gestational ages, infants may have minimal facial expression)
Cry 0 = No cry 1 = Whimper 2 = Vigorous cry	• Quiet, not crying • Mild moaning, intermittent cry • Loud screaming, rising, shrill, and continuous (Note: Silent cry may be scored if infant is intubated, as indicated by obvious mouth and/or facial movements)
Breathing Patterns 0 = Relaxed 1 = Change in breathing	• Relaxed, usual breathing pattern maintained • Change in drawing breath; irregular, faster than usual, gagging, or holding breath
Arm Movements 0 = Relaxed/restrained (with soft restraints) 1 = Flexed/extended	• Relaxed, no muscle rigidity, occasional random movements of arms • Tense, straight arms; rigid; or rapid extension and/or flexion
Leg Movements 0 = Relaxed/restrained (with soft restraints) 1 = Flexed/extended	• Relaxed, no muscle rigidity, occasional random movements of legs • Tense, straight legs; rigid; or rapid extension and/or flexion
State of Arousal 0 = Sleeping/awake 1 = Fussy	• Quiet, peaceful, sleeping; or alert and settled • Alert and restless or thrashing; fussy

Note: From Lawrence, J., Alcock, D., McGrath, D. P. et al. (1993). The development of a tool to assess neonatal pain. *Neonatal Network, 12*(6), 61.

Table 15–5	FLACC BEHAVIORAL PAIN ASSESSMENT SCALE		
Categories	**Scoring**		
	0	**1**	**2**
Face	No particular expression or smile	Occasional grimace or frown; withdrawn, disinterested	Frequent to constant frown, clenched jaw, quivering chin
Legs	Normal position or relaxed	Uneasy, restless, tense	Kicking or legs drawn up
Activity	Lying quietly, normal position, moves easily	Squirming, shifting back and forth, tense	Arched, rigid, or jerking
Cry	No cry (awake or asleep)	Moans or whimpers, occasional complaint	Crying steadily, screams or sobs; frequent complaints
Consolability	Content, relaxed	Reassured by occasional touching, hugging, or being talked to; distractable	Difficult to console or comfort

How to Use the FLACC

In patients who are awake: observe for 1 to 5 minutes or longer. Observe legs and body uncovered. Reposition patient or observe activity. Assess body for tenseness and tone. Initiate consoling interventions if needed.

In patients who are asleep: observe for 5 minutes or longer. Observe body and legs uncovered. If possible, reposition the patient. Touch the body and assess for tenseness and tone.

Whenever feasible, behavioral measurement of pain should be used in conjunction with self-report. When self-report is not possible, interpretation of pain behaviors and decisions regarding treatment of pain require careful consideration of the context in which the pain behaviors are observed.

Interpreting the Behavioral Score
Each category is scored on the 0–2 scale, which results in a total score of 0–10.

0 = Relaxed and comfortable   **4–6** = Moderate pain
1–3 = Mild discomfort   **7–10** = Severe discomfort or pain or both

Merkel, S. I., Voepel-Lewis, T., Shayevitz, J. R., & Malviya, S. (1997). The FLACC: A behavioral scale for scoring post-operative pain in young children. *Pediatric Nursing, 23*(3), 293–297.

derstand the concept of "more or less." These children cannot be given more than three choices on a pain scale (none, some, a lot) when assessing pain. When children can understand rank order and are able to classify, match, and estimate, a numerical scale can be used. A child who correctly responds to either of the following items is developmentally ready for a numerical scale (Merkel, 2002):

- Which number is larger, 5 or 9? Which number is smaller, 7 or 4?
- The child places several blocks or pieces of paper of different sizes in a row from biggest to smallest.

OUCHER SCALE Examples of self-report pain scales include the Oucher Scale and the FACES Pain Rating Scale. The Oucher Scale presents a series of six photographs of a child expressing increased intensity of pain in combination with a vertical Visual Analog Scale. See Figure 15–4 ➤. The child selects a face that best fits his or her level of pain; an older child can select a number between 0 and 10. The nurse should *not* compare the photos with the child's facial expression to determine pain level. The tool has been developed for three cultural groups in the United States with validity and reliability for children between 3 and 12 years of age. In addition, an Asian version of the Oucher was recently developed and validated with Taiwanese children (Yeh, 2005).

FACES PAIN RATING SCALE The FACES Pain Rating Scale has a series of six cartoon-like faces with expressions from smiling to tearful that can be used by children starting at 3 years of age. See Figure 15–5 ➤. The nurse explains the meaning of each face and asks the child to select the face that is the closest match to the pain felt. As with the Oucher Scale, the nurse should *not* compare the faces with the child's facial expression to determine pain level. Comparison of pain scales with faces revealed that those scales with a smiling face as the indicator of no pain resulted in higher pain

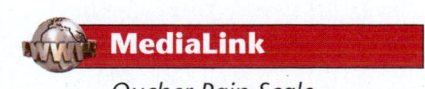

MediaLink

Oucher Pain Scale

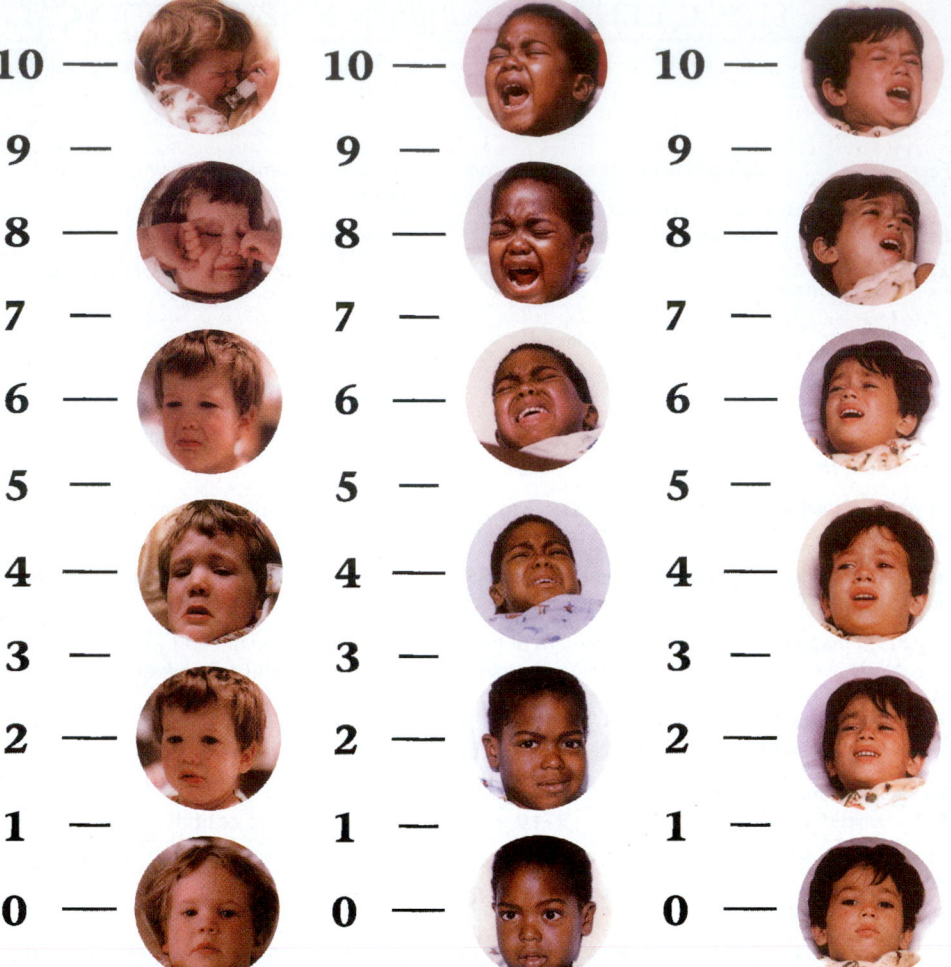

Figure 15–4 ➤ Use the Oucher Scale that is the best match for the child's ethnicity. After determining that the child has an understanding of number concepts, teach the child to use the scale. Point to each photo and explain that the bottom picture is "no hurt," the second picture is a "little hurt," the third picture is "a little more hurt," the fourth picture is "even more hurt," the fifth picture is "a lot of hurt," and the sixth picture is the "biggest or most hurt you could ever have." The numbers beside the photos can be used to score the amount of pain the child reports. The Caucasian version of the Oucher was developed and copyrighted by Judith E. Beyer, RN, PhD, 1983. The African American version of the Oucher was developed and copyrighted by Mary J. Denyes, RN, PhD, and Antonio M. Villarruel, RN, PhD, 1990. The Hispanic version of the Oucher was developed and copyrighted by Antonio M. Villarruel, RN, PhD, 1990.

ratings by children, their parents, and their nurses than scales using a neutral expression face as an indicator of no pain (Chambers, Hardial, Craig et al., 2005).

School-age children and adolescents have better number concepts and language skills, so additional tools can be used to assess their pain intensity. The nurse should ask the child to describe the pain and give its location. Providing some words such as *sharp*, *dull*, *aching*, *pounding*, *cold*, *hot*, *burning*, *throbbing*, *stinging*, *tingling*, or *cutting* can help the child describe his or her pain.

NUMERIC PAIN SCALE   The Numeric Pain Scale or Visual Analog Scale is a single 10-cm horizontal or vertical line that has descriptors of pain at each end (no pain, worst possible pain). Marks and numbers are placed at each centimeter on the line.

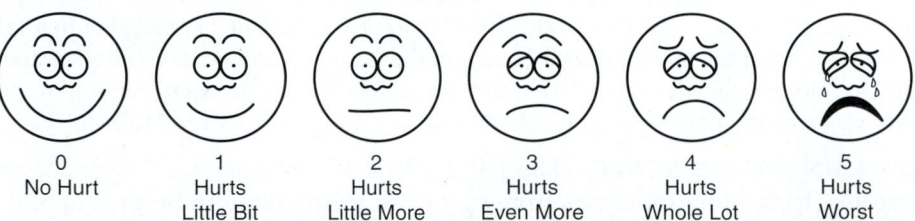

0	1	2	3	4	5
No Hurt	Hurts Little Bit	Hurts Little More	Hurts Even More	Hurts Whole Lot	Hurts Worst

Figure 15–5 ➤ The FACES Pain Rating Scale is valid and reliable in helping children to report their level of pain. Make sure the child has an understanding of number concepts and then teach the child to use the scale. Point to each face and use the words under the picture to describe the amount of pain the child feels. Then ask the child to select the face that comes closest to the amount of pain felt.
From: Wong, D. L., & Baker, C. M. (1988). Pain in children: Comparison of assessment scales. *Pediatric Nursing*, *14*, 9–16.

POKER CHIP TOOL   The Poker Chip Tool uses four checkers or poker chips to quantify pain. The child is asked to pick the number of chips that best matches the pain felt, with one chip being a little pain and four being the most pain he or she could have.

WORD-GRAPHIC RATING SCALE   The Word-Graphic Rating Scale has words describing increasing pain intensity across a horizontal line. The child marks the line that is closest to the level of pain felt. A millimeter ruler can be used to quantify the pain and record the pain score. See Figure 15–6 ➤.

ADOLESCENT PEDIATRIC PAIN TOOL   The Adolescent Pediatric Pain Tool includes a human figure drawing, the Word-Graphic Rating Scale, and a choice of descriptive words. Adolescents indicate pain sites on the human figure outline, use the Word-Graphic Rating Scale as described, and use the word choices to characterize the pain felt.

CLINICAL THERAPY FOR PAIN

Pain management includes both analgesia and complementary therapies. Children need adequate pain medication, but complementary therapies can be particularly helpful in reducing the unpleasantness and the anxiety of painful episodes (Howard, 2003).

Pain Medications

Medication interventions include the use of opioids, **nonsteroidal anti-inflammatory drugs (NSAIDs)**, and non-narcotic analgesics (acetaminophen).

Opioids

Opioids are analgesics commonly given for severe pain, such as after surgery or for a severe injury. Opioids (e.g., morphine and codeine) may be administered by oral, subcutaneous, intramuscular, and intravenous routes. Administration of opioids by an oral route is as effective as by intramuscular and intravenous routes when the drug is given in an **equianalgesic dose** (the amount of drug, whether given by oral or parenteral routes, needed to produce the same analgesic effect) (Table 15–6). Oral and intravenous routes are preferred for children. The intramuscular route causes pain at the time of the injection. Titration of the dosage to achieve a desired response level, as can occur with the intravenous route, is not possible (Zempsky, Cravero et al., 2004). Rectal preparations of some opioids are also available. The optimal analgesic dose varies widely among patients in all age groups (American Pain Society, 2003b).

Common side effects include sedation, nausea, vomiting, constipation, and itching. Potential complications of opioids include respiratory depression, cardiovascular collapse, and addiction. When the child's condition is unstable, as in trauma or critical illness, the dosage of opioids must be carefully calculated to match the child's cardiorespiratory status. Safety guidelines for frequent assessments and cardiorespiratory monitoring or pulse oximetry (when the infant or child has a condition that puts him or her at risk for respiratory depression) should be followed when using opioids in children (Greco & Berde, 2005). Addiction is a rare complication in adults and children treated for painful conditions.

> ### ➤ NURSING ALERT
>
> Respiratory depression (unresponsiveness and a respiratory rate less than 12 breaths/min in children less than 2 years of age) may progress to respiratory arrest and is the major life-threatening complication of opioid administration. Clinical signs that predict the development of respiratory depression include sleepiness, small pupils, and shallow breathing. Children at particular risk for respiratory depression induced by an opioid are those with an altered level of consciousness, an unstable circulatory status, a history of apnea, or a known airway problem such as obstructive sleep apnea. Some hospitals use continuous pulse oximetry when children at risk for respiratory depression receive opioids.
>
> Respiratory depression is most likely to occur when the child is sleeping. This augments the depressant effect on the respiratory center and potential airway obstruction by the tongue (American Pain Society, 2003b). Identify the time interval before drug-specific peak respiratory depression occurs, and then carefully monitor the child's vital signs during that period to detect respiratory depression. Naloxone is the drug used for reversal of opioids' adverse effects.

No Pain	Little Pain	Moderate Pain	Large Pain	Worst Possible Pain

Figure 15–6 ➤   The Word-Graphic Rating Scale has words rather than numbers under the line. It may be used by itself or with the Adolescent Pediatric Pain Tool. Teach the child to use the tool by pointing to the side of the line that is no pain. Then run your finger along the line and tell the child that this location is the worst possible pain. If the child has some pain, ask the child to make a mark along the line that is the best match for the amount of pain felt. Use a millimeter ruler to measure from the "no pain" end of the line to the marked location to identify the pain score. Make sure the line is the same length each time pain is assessed so comparisons can be made.
Data From: Sinkin-Feldman, L., Tesler, M., & Savedra, M. (1997). Word placement on the Word-Graphic Rating Scale by pediatric patients. *Pediatric Nursing, 23*, 31–34.

| Table 15–6 | OPIOID ANALGESICS AND RECOMMENDED DOSES FOR CHILDREN AND ADOLESCENTS* |

| Drug | Approximate Equianalgesic Oral Dose | Approximate Equianalgesic Parenteral Dose | Recommended Starting Dose (Adults >50 kg) | | Recommended Starting Dose (Children[a] & Adults <50 kg) | |
			Oral	Parenteral	Oral	Parenteral
Morphine	30 mg	10 mg	15–30 mg every 3–4 hr	5–8 mg every 2–4 hr	0.3 mg/kg every 3–4 hr	0.1 mg/kg every 2–4 hr
Codeine	120 mg	75 mg IV or subcutaneous	30–60 mg every 3–4 hr	60 mg every 2 hr	0.5–1 mg every 3–4 hr[b]	NR
Hydromorphone (Dilaudid)	7.5 mg	1.5 mg	4–8 mg every 3–4 hr	1.5 mg every 3–4 hr	0.06 mg/kg every 3–4 hr	0.015 mg/kg every 3–4 hr
Levorphanol (Levo-Dromoran)	4 mg (acute) 1 mg (chronic)	2 mg (acute) 1 mg (chronic)	2–4 mg every 6–8 hr	2 mg every 6–8 hr	0.04 mg/kg every 6–8 hr	0.02 mg/kg every 6–8 hr
Meperidine (Demerol)	300 mg	75 mg	NR	75 mg every 3 hr	NR	NR
Methadone (Dolophine, others)	10 mg 2–4 mg (chronic)	5 mg 2–4 mg (chronic)	5–10 mg every 4–8hr	10 mg every 4–8 hr	0.2 mg/kg every 4–8 hr	0.1 mg/kg every 4–8 hr
Oxycodone (Roxicodone)	30 mg	NA	15–20 mg every 3–4 hr	NA	0.1–0.2 mg/kg every 3–4 hr[a]	NA
Fentanyl	0.1 mg	0.01 mg	5 mcg/kg lozenge	50–100 mcg every 1–2 hr	5–15 mcg/kg Oralet[c]	0.5–1 mcg/kg every 1–2 hr

NR = Not recommended; NA = Not available

* For all parenteral opioids, start with the low dose and titrate to effective pain control.

[a] Infants under 6 months of age should receive a lower per kilogram dose.

[b] Caution: Doses of aspirin and acetaminophen in combination with opioid/NSAID preparation must also be adjusted to the patient's body weight.

[c] The Oralet is not widely used because of nausea and vomiting side effects.

Data from: American Pain Society. (2003b). *Principles of analgesic use in the treatment of acute pain and cancer pain* (5th ed., pp. 14–17). Glenview, IL; and Greco, C., & Berde, C. (2005). Pain management for the hospitalized pediatric patient. *Pediatric Clinics of North America, 52*(4), 995–1027.

MediaLink

Morphine Animation

When given opioids over an extended period of time, children may experience **withdrawal**, the physical signs and symptoms that occur when a sedative or pain drug is stopped suddenly in a patient with physical dependence. An example would be a child in an intensive care setting who experienced life-threatening injuries, multiple surgeries, and invasive procedures for long-term treatment. Slowly weaning the child off of the opioid over 2 to 4 weeks will prevent withdrawal symptoms. See Table 15–7 for signs and symptoms of withdrawal.

| Table 15–7 | SIGNS AND SYMPTOMS OF OPIOID OR SEDATIVE WITHDRAWAL |

System	Signs and Symptoms
Central nervous system	Irritability, increased wakefulness, tremulousness, hyperactive deep tendon reflexes, clonus, inability to concentrate, frequent yawning, sneezing, delirium, hypertonicity, visual or auditory hallucinations
Gastrointestinal system	Feeding intolerance with vomiting, diarrhea, uncoordinated suck and swallow
Sympathetic nervous system	Tachycardia, tachypnea, increased blood pressure, nasal stuffiness, sweating, fever

Data from: Tobias, J. D. (2000). Tolerance, withdrawal, and physical dependency after long term sedation and analgesia of children in the pediatric intensive care unit. *Critical Care Medicine, 28*(6), 2122–2132.

Table 15–8	**ACETAMINOPHEN, NSAIDs, AND RECOMMENDED DOSES FOR CHILDREN AND ADOLESCENTS**			
Oral NSAID Peak Action Time	**Usual Adult Dose**	**Usual Pediatric Dose**	**Comments**	
Acetaminophen 0.5–2 hr	650–1000 mg every 4 hr	10–15 mg/kg every 4 hr	Lacks the peripheral anti-inflammatory activity of other NSAIDs; rectal suppository available	
Aspirin 1–2 hr	650–1000 mg every 4–6 hr	10–15 mg/kg every 4 hr	Do not use in children under 12 years with possible viral illness due to link with Reye syndrome; may cause gastric upset and bleeding; rectal suppository available	
Choline magnesium trisalicylate (Trilisate) 2 hr	1000–1500 mg every 12 hr	25 mg/kg every 12 hr	Does not increase bleeding time like other NSAIDs; also available as oral liquid	
Ibuprofen 0.5 hr	200–400 mg every 4–6 hr	6–10 mg/kg every 6–8 hr	Available as oral suspension	
Naproxen (Naprosyn) 2–4 hr	250–500 mg every 6–8 hr	5 mg/kg every 12 hr	Available as oral liquid	

Data from: American Pain Society. (2003b). *Principles of analgesic use in the treatment of acute pain and cancer pain* (5th ed., pp. 4–5). Glenview, IL; and Greco, C., & Berde, C. (2005). Pain management for the hospitalized pediatric patient. *Pediatric Clinics of North America, 52*(4), 995–1027.

Acetaminophen and Nonsteroidal Anti-Inflammatory Drugs

Nonsteroidal anti-inflammatory drugs (NSAIDs) such as aspirin, primarily given orally, are medications with analgesic properties effective for the relief of mild to moderate pain and chronic pain. Table 15–8 presents recommended dosages of these drugs. They are most commonly used for bone, inflammatory, and connective tissue conditions. An NSAID may be prescribed in combination with an opioid to increase its effectiveness, and also reduce the amount of opioids needed.

Acetaminophen is a non-narcotic analgesic that is used like an NSAID. It works by raising the pain threshold and is equal to aspirin in analgesic properties.

Drug Administration

Pain from surgery, major trauma, or cancer is present for predictable periods because of the effects of tissue damage. Pain relief should be provided around the clock. Every effort should be made to give the child analgesics without causing more pain. The preferred routes of administration are intravenous, local nerve block, and oral.

Continuous-infusion analgesia is recommended for children with continuous or persistent severe pain because constant drug levels eliminate peaks and valleys in pain control. Analgesics may also be given intravenously on a scheduled basis (e.g., every 3 to 4 hours). Delays in giving analgesics increase the chances of breakthrough pain and the subsequent anticipation of pain. Giving analgesics on an as-needed (PRN) basis for acute pain also results in the loss of pain control. More medications are often needed to restore pain control than would have been required for continuous infusion analgesia.

Patient-Controlled Analgesia

Patient-controlled analgesia (PCA) is a method of administering an intravenous analgesic, such as morphine, using a computerized pump programmed by the healthcare professional and controlled by the child. After initial pain control has been achieved with a continuous IV infusion by the nurse, the child presses a button to receive a smaller analgesic dose for episodic pain relief (Figure 15–7 ➤). A continuous infusion of an opioid prevents a recurrence of pain during long sleeping periods. Safety

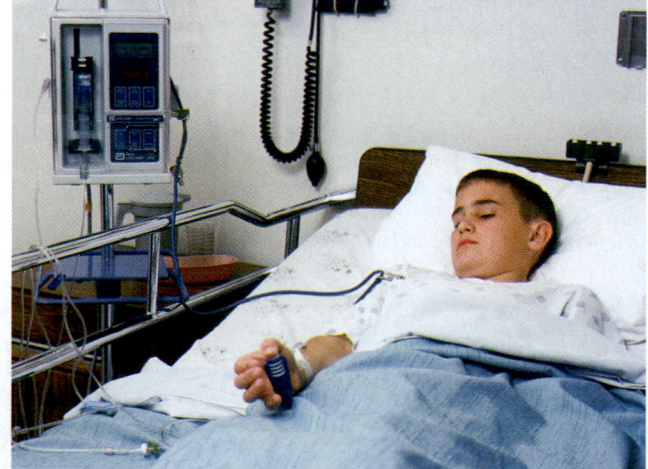

Figure 15–7 ➤ By using patient-controlled analgesia, the older child is able to regulate the intake of an intravenous analgesic such as morphine.

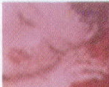

FAMILIES WANT TO KNOW

Patient-Controlled Analgesia (PCA)

- What is PCA? Analgesia means pain relief: you get to control the amount of medicine you receive by using the machine.
- The machine gives the medicine by passing it through the tube that is connected to your intravenous line. When you push the button, the machine pumps pain medicine into the intravenous line to make you feel better.
- The machine limits the amount of medicine you can get to what the doctor orders. You can get any amount up to the maximum by repeatedly pushing the button. The push button will not let you make a mistake if you drop it or roll on it.

- Whenever you feel pain, hurt, or discomfort, push the button to get more medicine. You should be the only one to push the button.
- No needles for pain shots are needed as long as the intravenous line is in place.
- The PCA may not relieve all of your pain, but it should make you feel comfortable. Let the nurse know if you think your PCA is not working.
- The PCA will be used until you can take pills or drink liquid pain medicine.

CLINICAL TIP

Nurse-controlled analgesia is becoming more common for children who are too young for PCA. In nurse-controlled analgesia, nurses provide small boluses of morphine in addition to the continuous IV infusion to treat breakthrough pain using a computerized pump with calibrated dosing administered by pushing a button (Greco & Berde, 2005; Howard, 2003).

features to prevent overdoses include the ability to set the maximum number of infusions per hour and the maximum amount of drug received in a given time period. Additional pain medication may be ordered as needed to supplement the continuous and patient-administered infusion when pain control is not maintained.

Children selected for PCA should be able to push the injection button and understand that pushing the button will give them a small amount of additional medication to relieve pain. This method of pain management is especially useful for pain control in the first 48 hours after surgery when oral pain management is not possible. PCA is prescribed mostly for children 5 years old and older. Parents are sometimes given responsibility for pushing the injection button for younger children or those with disabilities; however, safety concerns regarding overmedication of children with parent-controlled analgesia have been reported (Greco & Berde, 2005). See Families Want to Know: Patient-Controlled Analgesia (PCA).

Children and adolescents benefit from PCA by receiving continuous pain control and having the ability to control their comfort level with no trauma from injections. Once children can take oral analgesics, PCA is discontinued.

Regional Pain Management

Epidural pain control provides selective analgesia and has become more common for postoperative pain management. A catheter is inserted into either the lumbar or the caudal space (Figure 15–8 ➤). Only minute doses of drugs are needed because of the high concentration achieved at the opioid receptors in the spinal cord's dorsal horn (Pasero, 2003).

Local nerve blocks, such as a popliteal block for anesthesia and analgesia of an extremity, are used more frequently for pain control after surgery. A subcutaneous catheter is inserted into the local area for infusion of the analgesia. Pain control is achieved without systemic side effects from the medication. Tingling felt in the fingers or toes of the affected extremity is the first sign that the nerve block is receding.

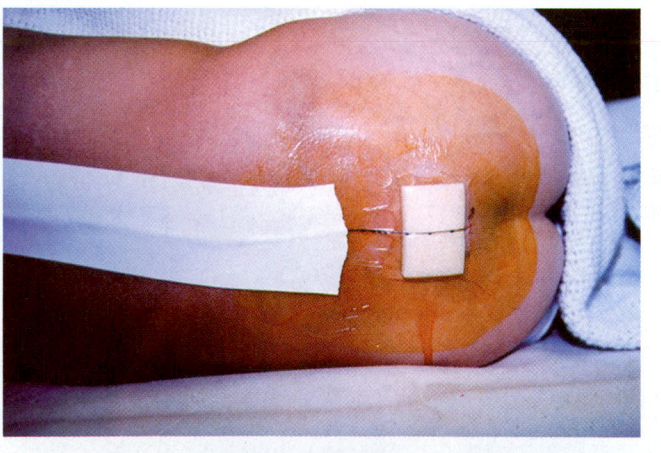

Figure 15–8 ➤ An epidural pain block is one example of a regional anesthesia used for postoperative pain management. Once the epidural catheter is placed, it is securely taped and wrapped. Small doses of pain medication may be continuously infused by a pump. Courtesy of Shriner's Hospital for Children, Spokane, WA.

■ NURSING MANAGEMENT
Nursing Assessment and Diagnosis

Nurses have an ethical obligation to relieve a child's suffering not only because of the consequences of unrelieved pain but also because appropriate pain management may have benefits such as earlier mobilization, shortened hospital stays, and reduced costs. To provide effective nursing management of children in pain, anticipate the presence of pain and recognize the child's right to pain control.

When assessing pain in children, keep the following questions in mind:

- What is happening in tissues that might cause pain? Assume that children who have had surgery, injury, vaso-occlusive episode, or illness are experiencing pain, since these events also cause pain in adults. Are there multiple injury sites?
- What external factors could be causing pain? For example, is the cast too tight or is the child poorly positioned in bed?
- Are there any indicators of pain, either physiologic or behavioral?
- How is the child responding emotionally?
- How does the child or parent rate the pain?

Physiologic symptoms such as nausea, fatigue, dyspnea, bladder and bowel distention, and fever may influence the intensity of pain felt by a child. Fear, anxiety, separation from parents, anger, culture, age, or a previous pain experience may also affect the child's behavior or responses to pain stimuli.

When working with an infant or child, determine which pain scale is the most appropriate for the circumstance and developmental stage. When using a self-report pain assessment tool, use the same tool each time you assess for pain or for the evaluation of pain management. This makes comparison of assessment results possible. Maintain a chronological record of the child's pain assessments along with actions taken to relieve pain and follow-up assessments to determine the effectiveness of those actions.

Remember that surgery and trauma can result in multiple sites of pain (incision or laceration, cut or bruised muscles, interrupted blood supply, nasogastric tube placement, insertion sites of intravenous lines). When using pain scales in the assessment of a verbal child, attempt to identify all sites of pain. Then evaluate the intensity of pain at each site. Examples of nursing diagnoses for children in pain include the following:

- Chronic Pain related to chronic condition and disability
- Ineffective Coping related to inadequate level of perception of control
- Nausea related to opioids
- Impaired Physical Mobility related to pain

Planning and Implementation

Nursing management involves the following actions to increase and maintain patient comfort once the assessment is completed and nursing diagnoses are developed: pain medication; complementary therapies; monitoring, evaluating, and documenting the effectiveness of pain-control measures to provide optimal comfort; and patient education.

The accompanying Nursing Care Plan summarizes nursing care for the child with postoperative pain.

Pharmacologic Intervention

Give analgesics as ordered by the physician, ensuring that the dose is appropriate for the child's weight. When administering an opioid by intravenous infusion, PCA, or nurse-controlled analgesia, monitor the flow rate and the site for infiltration. Follow institutional guidelines for monitoring vital signs and use of a pulse oximeter or cardiorespiratory monitor in children at risk for respiratory depression. Vital signs (heart rate and blood pressure) may not change in response to effective analgesia when infection, trauma, or other stressors keep them elevated. Make sure analgesic antagonists such as naloxone are available should complications develop.

Check for and report the presence of other side effects of analgesics, such as sedation, nausea, vomiting, itching, urinary retention, and constipation. An alternative opioid or medications to treat the side effects may be ordered when analgesia is needed long term.

When a regional nerve block is used, the analgesic effect does not recede for several hours after the catheter is removed. Be careful when ambulating a child with a regional nerve block in an extremity. Protect the extremity from injury because the child has reduced feeling in the limb. Monitor the child for tingling of fingers or toes, an indication that the analgesic effect is receding. Begin oral analgesia to maintain pain control.

CLINICAL TIP

Naloxone may be used to treat respiratory depression caused by an opioid drug at a dose and slow infusion rate that does not reverse the narcotic's pain-control effects. A continuous infusion or repeated doses may be needed for severe overdoses.

NURSING CARE PLAN   The Child with Postoperative Pain

GOAL	INTERVENTION	RATIONALE	EXPECTED OUTCOME
1. Severe Acute Pain (Abdominal) related to surgery and injury			
	NIC Priority Intervention: **Pain Management:** *Alleviation of pain or a reduction in pain to a level of comfort that is acceptable to the patient.*		*NOC Suggested Outcome:* **Comfort Level:** *Feelings of physical and psychologic ease.*
The child will report pain relief (to a level acceptable to the child on a pain scale).	• Give analgesic by a pain-free method.	• The child may deny pain to avoid analgesia by painful route.	The child reports pain relief after administration of analgesia.
	• Have the child select a pain scale and rate the amount of pain perceived before and 30–60 minutes after analgesia is given to ensure pain relief.	• The child's pain rating is the best indicator of pain. Maintenance of pain control requires less analgesia than treating each acute pain episode.	
	• Assess pain control each hour to assure that the child's pain is relieved.	• Frequent monitoring identifies inadequate pain control before it becomes significant.	
	• Reposition the child every 2 hours to maintain good body alignment.	• New positions decrease muscle cramping and skin pressure.	
	• Provide therapeutic touch or massage. Encourage the parents to read a story or play favorite music.	• Complementary therapy reduces stress and enhances the analgesic action.	
2. Disturbed Sleep Pattern related to inadequate pain control			
	NIC Priority Intervention: **Sleep Enhancement:** *Facilitation of regular sleep/awake cycles.*		*NOC Suggested Outcome:* **Sleep:** *Extent and pattern of sleep for mental and physical rejuvenation.*
The child will experience fewer disruptions of sleep by pain.	• Give analgesia by continuous infusion or every 3–4 hours around the clock.	• Pain breakthrough occurs even during sleep and disturbs the healing effects of sleep.	The child's sleep is undisturbed by pain. The child sleeps for the age-appropriate number of hours per day.
3. Ineffective Therapeutic Regimen Management related to self-management of pain control and use of nondrug pain-control measures			
	NIC Priority Intervention: **Self-Modification Assistance:** *Reinforcement of self-directed change initiated by the patient to achieve personally important goals.*		*NOC Suggested Outcome:* **Treatment Behavior: Illness or Injury:** *Personal actions to palliate or eliminate pathology.*
The child and family will effectively use patient-controlled analgesia (PCA) and complementary therapy pain-control measures.	• Teach the child how the PCA works and when to push the button.	• The child must know that pushing the PCA button will keep pain under control.	The child's pain rating stays low.
	• Teach the family and the child how to use age-appropriate imagery, distraction, relaxation techniques, and other complementary therapy pain-control measures.	• Complementary therapy pain-control measures reduce the amount of analgesia needed.	The child and family independently use complementary therapies for pain control.
The child and family will use appropriate analgesia after discharge.	• Discuss appropriate pain control to use at home after discharge.	• The family and child may be anxious about pain management at home.	The family understands pain-relief measures for use at home and knows where to call if help is needed.

NURSING CARE PLAN | The Child with Postoperative Pain (continued)

GOAL	INTERVENTION	RATIONALE	EXPECTED OUTCOME
4. Risk for Ineffective Breathing Pattern related to opioid overdose			
	NIC Priority Intervention: **Respiratory Monitoring:** *Collection and analysis of patient data to ensure airway patency and adequate gas exchange.*		*NOC Suggested Outcome:* **Vital Signs Status:** *Temperature, pulse, respirations, and blood pressure within expected range for the individual.*
The child will maintain adequate ventilations.	• Verify that correct dose of opioid analgesia is given for the child's weight.	• Respiratory depression is a significant complication of opioid analgesia when too much analgesia is given.	There is no episode of respiratory depression associated with analgesia.
	• Monitor vital signs and depth of inspirations before analgesic is administered and at time of peak drug action.	• Respiratory depression episode must not progress to respiratory arrest. All opioids act on brainstem center, which decreases responsiveness to CO_2 tension.	
	• Calculate agonist dose ordered by physician to be sure it will reverse respiratory depression, but not counteract effect of analgesia.	• Valuable time will be saved if an agonist is needed for an episode of respiratory depression. Complete reversal of analgesia will cause the child to have significant pain.	
5. Constipation related to opioid administration and decreased motility of gastrointestinal tract			
	NIC Priority Intervention: **Constipation Management:** *Prevention and alleviation of constipation.*		*NOC Suggested Outcome:* **Bowel Elimination:** *Ability of gastrointestinal tract to form and evacuate stool effectively.*
The child will have minimal constipation.	• Palpate the abdomen, and assess bowel sounds and abdominal distention.	• Signs of constipation must be anticipated and identified.	The child has bowel movements at least every 2 days while on opioid pain control.
	• Request physician order for stimulating laxative and stool softener.	• Opioids increase the transit time of feces and interfere with bile enzymes needed for evacuation.	
	• Provide fluids of choice to increase fluid intake when IV fluids are decreased. Encourage fruit juices for some of the fluids.	• Extra fluids will counteract opioid action of increasing the absorption of water from the large intestine. Fruit juices such as prune and pear juice have a laxative effect.	
	• Inform family and child that constipation is a side effect of pain medication.	• Parents can become partners in managing fluid intake and monitoring bowel movements.	

Oral NSAIDs are generally ordered for less severe pain or chronic pain. These medications may mask fever. Be alert to the potential complication of gastrointestinal hemorrhage in critically ill children who have increased gastric acids as a physiologic stress response to pain.

Assess the child for pain 15 to 30 minutes following intravenous pain medication and 1 hour after oral pain medication to determine if adequate pain control was achieved. Evaluate the child's level of pain frequently to identify any increase in pain intensity. Use information collected from the child and parent, as well as from an appropriate pain scale. Dramatic reductions in pain should occur, although not all pain may disappear. Use a flowsheet to document assessments, medication administration, and results of pain-control measures to guide ongoing nursing actions.

Many children sleep after receiving an analgesic. This sleep is not a side effect of the medication or a sign of an overdose, but the result of pain relief. Pain interrupts sleep, and once pain is relieved, the child can sleep comfortably. However, sleep does not always indicate pain control. A child in pain may fall asleep in exhaustion. Look for signs of disturbed sleep such as excess movement or moaning that may indicate pain.

Become an advocate for children when the dose or type of analgesic ordered is inadequate or breakthrough pain occurs due to wide variations in pain intensity. **Tolerance** is a decrease in a drug's effect over time or the need for increasing amounts of the drug to produce or maintain the same level of pain relief or sedation effect. This may occur when children with severe pain have been taking opioids or sedatives for several days. Breakthrough pain occurs, and an increase in dosage is needed to achieve the previous level of pain relief. Tolerance can be delayed with effective use of pain scales to allow appropriate drug dosing, and often less analgesia is needed.

Before asking the physician to change the analgesia dosage, review the child's record for documentation that the prescribed drug has been given at the appropriate dose and frequency and that the child's pain relief is ineffective despite these actions. After verifying the record, provide the physician with information about the characteristics of the child's pain and ask that the medication be changed. See Evidence-Based Practice: Giving Children Adequate Pain Medication.

Nonpharmacologic Intervention

Complementary therapies are the nonpharmacologic methods of pain control that can be used with or without analgesics (Figure 15–9 ➤). The Gate Control Theory helps explain why complementary pain management techniques are effective in helping to control pain. Inhibitory neurons in the dorsal horn of the spinal cord regulate pain transmission to the brain. Stimulation of the inhibitory neurons by sensations such as nonpainful touch and pressure or massage trigger the substantia gelatinosa in the dorsal horn of the spinal cord to "close the gate" and decrease the transmission of pain impulses to the brain (Huether & Defriez, 2006). Psychologic interventions with other complementary therapies are another mechanism for closing the gate.

One or more of these methods may provide adequate relief of low levels of pain. When used with analgesics, nonpharmacologic techniques often increase the analgesic's effectiveness or reduce the dosage required. When used in association with a medical procedure, remember to use an intervention before, during, and after the pro-

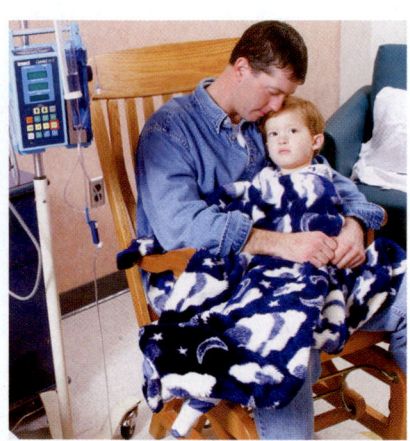

Figure 15–9 ➤ The presence of the parent is an important part of pain management. Children often feel more secure telling their parents about their pain and anxiety.

EVIDENCE-BASED PRACTICE

Giving Children Adequate Pain Medication

Clinical Question

In several recent studies researchers found that some children continue to be undermedicated for moderate and severe pain despite continuing efforts to promote effective pain management for children (Vincent, 2001; Vincent & Denyes, 2004). Why does adequate management of children with acute pain continue to be a problem?

Evidence

A study by Vincent and Denyes in 2004 explored factors related to the actions 67 nurses took to relieve children's pain in actual clinical situations in a children's hospital. The 132 children were experiencing pain from surgery, burns, vaso-occlusive episodes, and trauma. Nurses studied had a moderately high level of knowledge and attitudes about relieving children's pain. Behavioral manifestations of pain led more nurses to believe a child's self-report of pain. Nurses did tend to give more analgesia to children reporting higher pain levels, meaning that the child's pain level is what triggered the nurses to administer analgesia.

Implications

Surprisingly 26% of children reporting pain received no analgesia, and the 51% of children with moderate to high levels of reported pain received markedly less than the recommended and ordered amounts of analgesia. Pediatric nurses have an obligation to ask children to report their pain levels and then to accept that this pain rating is accurate. Behavioral cues that pain exists should not be necessary to evaluate pain in children who can self-report pain. Crying and grimacing in pain are not the only pain behaviors to look for. Pain behaviors vary among children. For example, children use play as a distraction to self-manage pain, and they sleep after becoming fatigued from dealing with pain. Children are entitled to comfort and pain relief, so all information that informs the nurse that the child is experiencing pain should be used in making decisions to relieve pain.

Critical Thinking

What could be some reasons for undermedication of children by nurses? What is your role in improving children's pain management in all settings?

cedure to have the full effect of the distraction. See Families Want to Know: Helping a Child Cope with Pain.

Assemble a pain management kit to promote distraction, imagery, and relaxation in children. Items that might be included are magic wands, pinwheels, bubble liquid, a slinky spring toy, a foam ball, party noisemakers, and pop-up books. It may also be helpful to include items for therapeutic play such as syringes, adhesive bandages, alcohol swabs, and other supplies from a medical kit. The pain management kit may be especially helpful for distracting children who are being prepared for surgery or for painful procedures.

Application of Heat and Cold

Heat application promotes dilation of blood vessels. The increased blood circulation permits the removal of debris of cell breakdown from the site. Heat also promotes muscle relaxation, breaking the pain–spasm–pain cycle. To reduce edema, do not apply heat in the first 24 hours after an injury.

The application of cold is believed to slow the ability of pain fibers to transmit pain impulses. Cold also controls pain by decreasing edema and inflammation, and by causing partial or complete anesthesia or numbness of the skin. When cold is applied, assess the skin for redness or signs of irritation. Take care to avoid causing thermal injury. Discontinue cold applications immediately if the skin alternately blanches and reddens afterwards or if blisters or redness do not subside between applications.

Sucrose Solution

Concentrated sucrose solutions (24%) with a pacifier may be used as a pain relief measure in preterm and term newborns up to 1 month of age. Contact of the sucrose with the oral mucosa promotes natural pain relief by activating endogenous opioids (Morash & Fowler, 2004). The analgesic effect of sucrose lasts approximately 3 to 5 minutes, with a peak action in 2 minutes (Mitchell & Waltman, 2003). The pacifier may be dipped into the prepared solution or a moistened pacifier may be dipped into a packet of sugar (Greenberg, 2002). Allow the infant to continue sucking on the pacifier during the procedure to enhance the effectiveness of the sucrose solution (Morash & Fowler, 2004).

Distraction

Distraction involves engaging a child in a wide variety of activities to help him or her focus attention on something other than pain and the anxiety associated with the procedure. Examples of distracting activities are listening to music; singing a song; playing a game, including virtual reality games; watching television or a video; and focusing on a picture while counting. Select activities that are developmentally appropriate for the child. Children in severe pain cannot be distracted, but do not assume the pain is gone if a child can be distracted.

Cutaneous Stimulation and Massage

Cutaneous stimulation involves gently rubbing the painful area, massaging the skin gently, and holding or rocking the child. Touching and massage provide a stimulus to

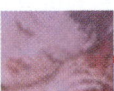

FAMILIES WANT TO KNOW

Helping a Child Cope with Pain

Parents are the single most powerful nonpharmacologic method of pain relief available to children. A parent's presence greatly reduces the anxiety associated with pain and hospitalization (Broome, 2000). Children often feel more secure telling their parents about their pain and anxiety. When parents are actively participating in the child's care during hospitalization, teach them about how complementary therapies can be used to enhance the child's pain management. Help the parent select the age-appropriate complementary therapy for the child:

- Infants: holding, cuddling, sucking a pacifier, massage

- Toddlers: massage, stories, bubbles, touch, holding and rocking, music
- Preschoolers: engaging in play, stories, music, imagine being a superhero, watching television or a video
- School-age children: rhythmic breathing, muscle relaxation, guided imagery, talking about pleasant experiences, playing games, listening to radio, watching television or a video
- Adolescents: rhythmic breathing, muscle relaxation, guided imagery, having visitors, playing games, watching television, listening to radio or tape player

compete with the pain stimuli transmitted from the peripheral nerves to the spinal cord. These actions may reduce the pain felt by the child. Swaddling and blanket rolls may calm a distressed neonate.

Relaxation Techniques

Relaxation techniques are used to reduce muscle tension, which aggravates pain. Relaxation methods include rhythmic breathing and alternately tensing and relaxing selected muscle groups for 10 seconds each. Progressively move from specific muscle groups to more central muscles. Enhance relaxation by focusing the child's attention on something pleasant.

Guided Imagery

Imagery is a cognitive process that encourages the child to focus concentration on an event or place unrelated to the pain process. The focus can be on exploring a favorite place, doing a favorite activity, remembering a funny story, or being a superhero. This method is most effective in children over 6 years of age. Ask the child to think about all the sights, sounds, smells, tastes, and feelings that will help him or her to experience the favorite place, activity, or story. Guided imagery is a form of self-hypnosis, and it is most effective when preceded by a relaxation exercise.

Hypnosis

An altered state of consciousness occurs when appropriate suggestions distort perception, memory, and mood. Children who respond to hypnotic suggestions are often more relaxed and experience less pain.

Cognitive Behavior Therapy

Various psychological techniques such as preparation with dolls, role-playing, role modeling, and practicing desirable behavior may be combined with relaxation, hypnosis, and guided imagery to promote coping with multiple invasive procedures in children with cancer and chronic illnesses.

Electroanalgesia

Also known as transcutaneous electrical nerve stimulation (TENS), **electroanalgesia** delivers small amounts of electrical stimulation to the skin by electrodes. This electrical stimulation is stronger than the pain impulses; because of the Gate Control Theory, it is thought to interfere with the transmission of pain from the peripheral nerves to the spinal cord. TENS may be used for both acute and chronic pain management. The only known side effect is skin irritation at the electrode site.

Discharge Planning and Home Care Teaching

Children are frequently discharged from the hospital with oral analgesics following surgery, injury, or treatment of acute medical conditions. Parents have the responsibility to provide adequate pain control for their child after day surgery. The child usually leaves the surgical center pain free, and the parents may not anticipate pain. Take the time to discuss

---

COMPLEMENTARY THERAPY

Hypnotherapy for Children

Hypnotherapy, the most widely studied of the complementary/alternative therapies, is often successfully prescribed for pain and a variety of other conditions such as bed-wetting, asthma, stool-withholding, habit disorders, anxiety and fears, migraine headaches, nausea from chemotherapy, needle phobias, warts, insomnia, tics, and other problems (Anbar, 2003; Thompson, 2004).

Children have a great capacity to use their imaginations and fantasy worlds for therapeutic gain and are actually more successful than adults in attaining a hypnotic state. Children entering a healthcare environment are often fearful. As the nurse, you can induce a more relaxed state in children by speaking quietly, focusing them on their breathing, and suggesting they imagine something pleasant—the ingredients of hypnotic induction.

Hypnosis is an altered state of awareness facilitating heightened concentration, decreased awareness of external stimuli, increased relaxation, and increased suggestibility. Hypnotherapy can be as simple as teaching a child to blow on a pinwheel while getting an injection. This diminishes the pain and fear of the needle by focusing the child's heightened attention elsewhere. More formal hypnotherapy is done by a therapist trained in pediatric hypnotherapeutic techniques that use the images and language of the child to induce relaxation and give posthypnotic suggestions. Language such as, "You are the boss of your body and you can help make this headache not bother you anymore" is used to help children gain mastery over their physical symptoms.

the importance of pain management and its benefits in promoting the child's healing. Make sure parents know that a sudden increase in pain intensity may indicate the development of a complication requiring medical attention when efforts to manage the child's pain have been made.

Provide guidance to help parents assess their child's pain, and for school-age children and adolescents to assess their own pain. Teach parents and children about the dosage and frequency of administration and the side effects of the analgesic ordered. Review nonpharmacologic methods of pain control with parents and children. Encourage children and parents to use the techniques that work best for them.

Evaluation

Expected outcomes of nursing care include:

- The child's pain level is assessed frequently and pain management is effective in improving the child's comfort.
- The child successfully uses a PCA pump to control acute pain.
- Age-appropriate nonpharmacologic methods of pain management enhance the comfort provided by medications.

Nursing Management of Chronic Pain

Some children have medical conditions that cause chronic pain and episodic acute pain, such as rheumatoid arthritis, cancer, sickle cell anemia, headaches, recurrent abdominal pain, and HIV infection. Children and adolescents have reported that chronic and recurrent pain has an impact on the quality of their life and restrictions in daily activities such as school attendance, sleep, appetite, social interactions, and recreation (Ross-Isigkeit, Thyen, Stöven et al., 2005).

Chronic pain may be nociceptic or neuropathic, which is caused by abnormal functioning of the nervous system. The sympathetic nervous system is not aroused in the same way it is with acute pain. Physical and psychological signs and symptoms, as well as behavior, should be viewed together. Behavioral indicators of chronic pain and pain of long duration include inactivity to avoid pain, depression, difficulty sleeping, and an inability to concentrate (Huether & Defriez, 2006).

No tools have been developed to assess chronic pain for any child age group, and effective management strategies for children with chronic pain need to be identified. Assessment and evaluation of chronic pain in children should include the following aspects (American Pain Society, 2003a):

- Approach pain as the present problem and obtain the history of pain onset, its development over time, intensity, duration, location, what makes it worse or relieves it, and its impact on daily life (sleeping, appetite, school, and social interactions).
- Identify the amount of distress the child and family experience with pain, including anxiety, depression, and hopelessness.
- Determine what the family and child believe causes the pain and their response to it.
- Identify past pain problems in the family and the current methods of treatment.
- Observe the child's appearance, posture, gait, and emotional and cognitive state.
- Assess muscle spasms, trigger points, areas sensitive to light touch, and perform a complete neurologic examination.

Older children with recurrent episodes of pain can be encouraged to keep a diary or log to describe the characteristics, timing, activities, and potential triggers of their pain, as well as their response to pain treatment measures. A pain assessment scale should be used to rate the pain intensity before and after medications and other pain control measures are used. This record can help improve pain management.

CLINICAL TIP

Many common health problems (otitis media, pharyngitis, and urinary tract infection) have pain as one of the presenting symptoms. Often the only medication prescribed is an antibiotic to clear the infection. This may leave the child in pain for 48 to 72 hours until the antibiotic brings the infection under control. Give parents recommendations for pain control and comfort measures during this period.

- Make sure parents have acetaminophen or ibuprofen in an appropriate formulation (drops, elixir, tablets) for the child's age, and that the medication's expiration date has not passed.
- Inform the parents about the correct amount of the pain medication to use and how frequently it can be given.
- Suggest complementary therapies appropriate for the child's age to help manage the child's pain.

Examples of nursing diagnoses for children with chronic pain include:

- Chronic Pain related to arthritic joint inflammation and degeneration
- Sleep Pattern Disturbed related to ineffective management of chronic pain
- Impaired Physical Mobility related to ineffective management of chronic pain

Children with chronic conditions (arthritis, sickle-cell disease, hemophilia, cancer, recurrent headaches, etc.) often need long-term pain management. NSAIDs and acetaminophen are often ordered for pain management. Transdermal fentanyl patches may be used for some children with more severe chronic pain. Strategies for chronic pain management include the following:

- Explain and validate pain and its causes
- Encourage the use of a pain diary (see Figure 15–10 ➤).
- Discuss treatment goals with the child and family and jointly develop a care plan that integrates pharmacologic and nonpharmacologic (complementary) methods
- Develop a care plan for recurrent painful episodes associated with acute flare-ups of their condition
- Provide effective preventive pain management for procedural pain, as many of these children have numerous medical procedures

Parents should be actively engaged in pain control for their child. Teach parents the importance of pain control and how to use a variety of complementary therapies with their child to supplement the pain medications administered. Refer children with long-term pain to a pediatric pain program, where they can be evaluated for customized strategies to manage pain.

SEDATION AND PAIN MANAGEMENT FOR MEDICAL PROCEDURES

Children undergo a wide variety of painful diagnostic and treatment procedures in the hospital and in outpatient settings. Procedures such as chest tube insertion, arterial puncture, lumbar puncture, bone marrow aspiration, fracture reduction, laceration repair, insertion of a central or peripheral intravenous line, and burn debridement cause significant pain in children. The anticipation of these procedures causes anxiety and emotional distress that can lead to greater intensity of pain. Children who have experienced severe pain in the past may be unwilling to cooperate with healthcare personnel.

Clinical Therapy
Minor Medical Procedures

Topical anesthetics can be used to reduce the pain associated with the first needlestick. Various mechanisms for topical anesthesia include the following:

- Vapocoolant sprays can be used for injections.
- Eutectic mixture of local anesthetics (EMLA) cream, a mixture of 2.5% lidocaine and 2.5% prilocaine in an emulsion, is effective if applied 60 minutes before a needlestick procedure on intact skin (Rogers & Ostrow, 2004). It is approved for use in infants as young as 3 months of age (Weise & Nahata, 2005). See Figure 15–11 ➤.

Figure 15–10 ➤ A pain diary is an important tool to help record the painful episodes a child experiences with a chronic condition such as rheumatoid arthritis or recurrent painful episodes as occurs with sickle cell anemia. A pain scale should be used to record pain intensity at the time of intervention and 1 hour later.

Date	Time	Pain Intensity	Pain Medication Taken	How Much	Other Pain Relief Methods	Amount of Pain 1 Hour Later

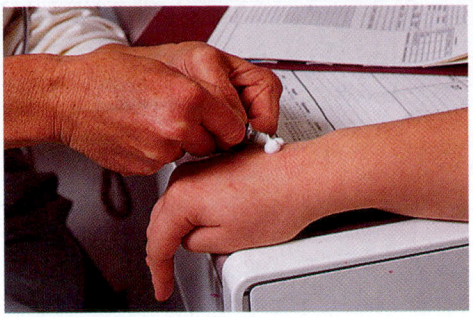
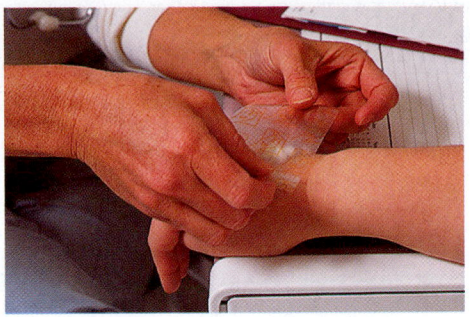

A   B

Figure 15–11 ➤ When painful procedures are planned, use EMLA cream to anesthetize the skin where the painful stick will be made. A, Apply a thick layer of cream over intact skin (one half of a 5-g tube). B, Cover the cream with a transparent adhesive dressing, sealing all the sides. The cream anesthetizes the dermal surface in 45–60 minutes.

- L-M-X4, 4% lidocaine, formerly called ELA-Max, is effective if applied 30 minutes before a needlestick (Eichenfield, Funk, Fallon-Friedlander et al., 2002). L-M-X4 is available without a prescription.
- **Iontophoresis**, the use of a small machine that generates electric current to transport lidocaine hydrochloride and epinephrine into the skin, works in about 10 to 15 minutes (Schultz, Strout, Jordan et al., 2002). Some children do not tolerate the sensations of the procedure or may rarely develop a partial-thickness burn.
- Lidocaine-epinephrine-tetracaine gel applied to the skin can be used for laceration repair (Young, 2005).
- A local anesthetic such as lidocaine buffered by sodium bicarbonate is often injected to provide analgesia for emergency invasive procedures, such as laceration repair. Lidocaine can also be injected subcutaneously in a small area to reduce the pain of deeper needle insertion.

Sedation

Sedation is a medically controlled state of depressed consciousness (light to deep) used for painful diagnostic and therapeutic procedures. Procedures such as burn debridement, laceration repair, bone marrow aspiration, and fracture reduction are associated with so much pain and anxiety that children need premedication with analgesia and **anxiolysis** (mild sedation). Sedation is often used to gain the child's cooperation for the medical procedure. Drugs for sedation include the following (Boswinkel & Litman, 2005):

- Chloral hydrate
- Benzodiazepines such as Diazepam (Valium) and Midazolam (Versed)
- Pentobarbital
- Ketamine
- Propofol (Diprivan)
- Analgesics such as Fentanyl

When sedatives are given in lower doses, **light sedation** occurs during which the child maintains protective reflexes, maintains a patent airway, and appropriately responds to verbal stimuli. **Deep sedation** is a controlled state of depressed consciousness or unconsciousness in which the protective reflexes are lost. See the Clinical Manifestations feature for characteristics of light and deep sedation. Analgesia must be given in association with sedation because the sedated child can still feel pain but not communicate its presence.

Guidelines should exist in every healthcare facility where pediatric sedation is performed to ensure safe healthcare practices. These guidelines often require that the health professionals monitoring the child have specific qualifications, such as pediatric advanced life support training. With the combined effects of analgesia and sedatives,

MediaLink

Care Plan Activity: Pain Management for a Preschooler

CLINICAL MANIFESTATIONS	LIGHT AND DEEP SEDATION	
Assessment Factors	**Light Sedation**	**Deep Sedation**
Airway	Able to maintain airway independently and continuously	Unable to maintain airway independently or continuously
Cough and gag reflexes	Reflexes intact	Partial or complete loss of reflexes
Level of consciousness	Easily aroused with verbal or gentle physical stimulation	Not easily aroused, may not respond purposefully to verbal or gentle physical stimulation

Data from: Proudfoot, J. (2002). Pediatric procedural sedation and analgesia (PSA): Keeping it simple and safe. *Pediatric Emergency Medicine Reports, 7*(2), 1–2.

> ### ▶ NURSING ALERT
>
> Whenever sedation is given, be sure to have the resources available to monitor the child's vital signs and to provide advanced life support if the child should progress to deep sedation. If case complications occur, the following equipment should be immediately available: suction apparatus, a bag-valve mask for assisted ventilation with capability of delivering 90–100% concentration oxygen, an oxygen supply (5 L/min for more than 60 minutes), and antagonists to sedative medication that are premeasured and ready to administer.

the child must be carefully monitored for respiratory depression and signs of deep sedation. Antagonist agents are available for opioids and benzodiazepines when the effects of sedation and respiratory depression need to be reversed (Coté, 2005).

Nursing Management

Increase Comfort During Painful Procedures

Help the child cope with a painful procedure by telling the child what sensations to expect and what will happen during the procedure. This reduces stress more effectively than just providing information about the procedure. See Chapter 13 ∞ for methods of preparing children of different developmental ages for procedures.

Drugs may not be used for quick procedures, such as a dressing change, or an unexpected intravenous insertion, injection, or venipuncture. Complementary therapies, especially guided imagery, relaxation techniques, and distraction, may reduce the anxiety associated with the anticipation of the procedure. Teach parents and children to use these interventions before procedures. Help children control their anxiety through therapeutic play.

Patient Monitoring

When pharmacologic pain management is used for a procedure, the nurse's responsibilities include the following:

- Treat anticipated procedure-related pain prophylactically. For example, give an analgesic before a bone marrow aspiration or fracture reduction. Permit time for the drug to become effective.
- Manage preexisting pain before beginning a procedure such as scrubbing a burn.
- Whenever possible, administer drugs by a nonpainful route (oral, transmucosal, intravenous). Avoid intramuscular or subcutaneous injections.
- When procedures must be repeated (for example, bone marrow aspirations for children with leukemia), give optimal analgesia for the first procedure to reduce anxiety about future procedures.
- To prevent increased anxiety, avoid delays in performing procedures.
- Document the results of pain management.

When the child receives sedation, monitoring the child's status is important. Children may easily transition between light and deep sedation. Nursing assessments include *visual* confirmation of respiratory effort, color, and vital signs. Pulse oximetry and other technology may be used for monitoring, but the equipment must not replace visual assessment. Vital signs must be checked every 15 minutes until the child regains full consciousness and level of functioning. If light sedation progresses to deep sedation, advanced airway management skills are essential and vital signs should be checked every 5 minutes.

Criteria for discharge after sedation include the following (Bindler & Ball, 2003):

- Satisfactory and stable cardiovascular function and airway patency
- Easily arousable, protective reflexes intact
- Adequate hydration
- Infant is able to hold the head up and sit up unassisted if old enough to do so, or the child can stand and walk without assistance
- Discharge status is the same as admission status

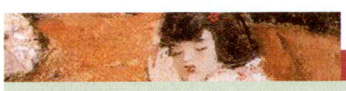

CRITICAL THINKING IN ACTION

Recall Susie, the 6-year-old at the beginning of the chapter who is to have an adenoidectomy for obstructive sleep apnea. She will spend one night in the hospital to make sure she has no airway complications. Susie received a dose of IV morphine in the postanesthesia unit at 2 p.m. She has an order for IV morphine every 4 hours, until she is able to swallow and keep fluids down. Once she has good oral intake her pain medication order is for acetaminophen every 4 hours.

1. What are the most appropriate pain assessment scales for Susie to use to report her level of pain to the nurse?

2. What complementary pain therapies are of value for Susie's condition and age?

3. Susie weighs 25 kg. What is the appropriate dose of morphine for Susie and the calculated volume to be administered?

4. Describe the important nursing assessments for Susie following morphine and acetaminophen administration.

5. Develop a teaching plan for Susie's mother for pain management once Susie is discharged.

 Refer to your Prentice Hall Nursing MediaLink DVD-ROM for answers.

EXPLORE MediaLink

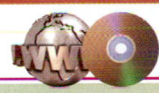 http://www.prenhall.com/ball

Resource for this chapter can be found on the Prentice Hall Nursing MediaLink DVD-ROM accompanying this textbook, and on the Companion Website at http://www.prenhall.com/ball.

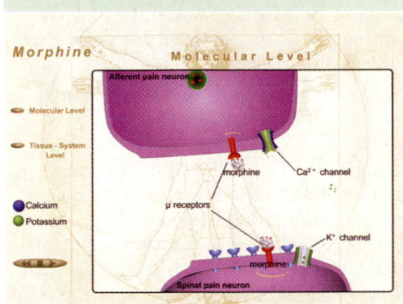

DVD-ROM
Audio Glossary
NCLEX-RN® Review
Animations/Videos
  Morphine
  Pain Management Kit

COMPANION WEBSITE
Audio Glossary
NCLEX-RN® Review
Care Plan Activity: Pain Management for a Preschooler
Critical Thinking: Postoperative Pain Assessment
MediaLink Applications
  Calculating Morphine Dosage for a Toddler
  Conscious Sedation Management
  Pain and Distraction Techniques
WebLinks

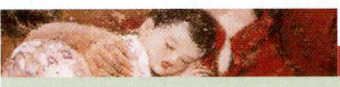

REFERENCES

American Pain Society. (2003a). Pediatric chronic pain: A position statement from the American Pain Society. Retrieved October 22, 2003, from www.ampainsoc.org/cgi-bin/print/print/pl

American Pain Society. (2003b). *Principles of analgesic use in the treatment of acute pain and cancer pain* (5th ed.). Glenview, IL: Author.

Anbar, R. D. (2003). Self-hypnosis for anxiety associated with severe asthma: A case report. *BMC Pediatrics, 3*(1), 3–7.

Anthony, K. K., & Schanberg, L. E. (2005). Pediatric pain syndromes and management of pain in children and adolescents with rheumatic disease. *Pediatric Clinics of North America, 52,* 611–639.

Bindler, R. C., & Ball, J. W. (2003). *Clinical skills manual for pediatric nursing: Caring for*

children (3rd ed.). Upper Saddle River, NJ: Prentice Hall.

Boswinkel, J. P., & Litman, R. S. (2005). The pharmacology of sedation: How to determine the best agent for each procedure and patient. *Pediatric Annals, 34*(8), 607–613.

Broome, M. E. (2000). Helping parents support their child in pain. *Pediatric Nursing, 26*(3), 315–317.

Chambers, C. T., Hardial, J., Craig, K. D., Court, C., & Montgomery, C. (2005). Faces scales for the measurement of postoperative pain intensity in children following minor surgery. *Clinical Journal of Pain, 21*(3), 277–285.

Coté, C. J. (2005). Strategies for preventing sedation accidents. *Pediatric Annals, 34*(8), 625–633.

Eichenfield, L. F., Funk, A., Fallon-Friedlander, S., & Cunningham, B. B. (2002). A clinical study to evaluate ELA-MAX (4% liposomal lidocaine) as compared with eutectic mixture of local anesthetics cream for pain reduction of venipuncture in children. *Pediatrics, 109*(5), 1093–1099.

Gaston-Johansson, F., Albert, M., Fagan, E., & Zimmerman, L. (1990). Similarities in pain descriptions of four different ethnic-culture groups. *Journal of Pain and Symptom Management, 5*(2), 94–100.

Greco, C., & Berde, C. (2005). Pain management for the hospitalized pediatric patient. *Pediatric Clinics of North America, 52*(4), 995–1027.

Greenberg, C. S. (2002). A sugar-coated pacifier reduces procedural pain in newborns. *Pediatric Nursing, 22*(3), 271–277.

Hall, R. W., & Anand, K. J. S. (2005). Short- and long-term impact of neonatal pain and stress: More than an ouchie. *NeoReviews, 6*(2), e69–e74.

Howard, R. F. (2003). Current status of pain management in children. *JAMA Journal of the American Medical Association, 290*(18), 2464–2469.

Huether, S. E., & Defriez, C. B. (2006). Pain, temperature regulation, sleep, and sensory function. In K. L. McCance & S. E. Huether (Eds.), *Pathophysiology: The biologic basis for disease in adults and children* (5th ed., pp. 447–462). St. Louis, MO: Mosby–Year Book.

Joint Commission on the Accreditation of Health Care Organizations. (2001). *Pain standards for 2001*. Oakbrook Terrace, IL: Author.

LaFleur, C. J., & Raway, B. (1999). School-age child and adolescent perception of the pain intensity associated with three word descriptors. *Pediatric Nursing, 25*(1), 45–55.

Lawrence, J., Alcock, D., McGrath, D. P., et al. (1993). The development of a tool to assess neonatal pain. *Neonatal Network, 12*(6), 61.

Manworren, R. C. B., & Hynan, L. S. (2003). Clinical validation of FLACC: Preverbal patient pain scale. *Pediatric Nursing, 29*(2), 140–146.

McCaffrey, M., & Pasero, C. (1999). *Pain: Clinical manual* (2nd ed., p. 24, 27). St. Louis: Mosby.

McCance, K. L., Forshee, B. A., & Shelby, J. (2006). Stress and disease. In K. L. McCance & S. E. Huether (Eds.), *Pathophysiology: The biologic basis for disease in adults and children* (5th ed., pp. 447–462). St. Louis, MO: Mosby–Year Book.

Merkel, S. (2002). Pain assessment in infants & children: The finger span scale. *American Journal of Nursing, 102*(11), 55–56.

Merkel, S. I., Voepel-Lewis, T., Shayevitz, J. R., & Malviya, S. (1997). The FLACC: A behavioral scale for scoring post-operative pain in young children. *Pediatric Nursing, 23*(3), 293–297.

Mitchell, A., & Boss, B. J. (2002). Adverse effects of pain on the central nervous systems of newborns and young children: A review of the literature. *Journal of Neuroscience Nursing, 34*(5), 228–236.

Mitchell, A., & Waltman, P. A. (2003). Oral sucrose and pain relief in preterm infants. *Pain Management Nursing, 4*(2), 62–69.

Morash, D., & Fowler, K. (2004). An evidence-based approach to changing practice: Using sucrose for infant analgesia. *Journal of Pediatric Nursing, 19*(5), 366–370.

Pasero, C. (2002). Pain assessment in infants and young children: Neonates. *American Journal of Nursing, 102*(8), 61–65.

Pasero, C. (2003). Epidural analgesia for postoperative pain. *American Journal of Nursing, 103*(10), 62–64.

Pasero, C., & McCaffery, M. (2005). No self-report means no pain-intensity rating. *American Journal of Nursing, 105*(10), 50–53.

Proudfoot, J. (2002). Pediatric procedural sedation and analgesia (PSA): Keeping it simple and safe. *Pediatric Emergency Medicine Reports, 7*(2), 1–2.

Rogers, T. L., & Ostrow, C. L. (2004). The use of EMLA cream to decrease venipuncture pain in children. *Journal of Pediatric Nursing, 19*(1), 33–39.

Ross-Isigkeit, A., Thyen, U., Stöven, H., Schwarzenberger, J., & Schmucker, P. (2005). Pain among children and adolescents: Restrictions in daily living and triggering factors. *Pediatrics, 115*(2), e152–162.

Schultz, A. A., Strout, T. D., Jordan, P., & Worthing, B. (2002). Safety, tolerability, and efficacy of iontophoresis with lidocaine for dermal anesthesia in ED pediatric patients. *Journal of Emergency Nursing, 28*(4), 289–296.

Sinkin-Feldman, L., Tesler, M., & Savedra, M. (1997). Word placement on the Word-Graphic Rating Scale by pediatric patients. *Pediatric Nursing, 23*, 31–34.

Stanford, E. A., Chambers, C. T., & Craig, K. D. (2005). A normative analysis of the development of a pain-related vocabulary in children. *Pain, 114*(1-2), 278–284.

Thompson, N. L. (2004). *Hypnotherapy for children*. Frederick, MD: Publish America.

Tobias, J. D. (2000). Tolerance, withdrawal, and physical dependency after long term sedation and analgesia of children in the pediatric intensive care unit. *Critical Care Medicine, 28*(6), 2122–2132.

Van Hulle-Vincent, C. (2005). Nurses' knowledge, attitudes, and practices regarding children's pain. *MCN American Journal of Maternal Child Nursing, 30*, 177–183.

Vincent, C. V. (2001). Nurses' analgesic practices with hospitalized children. *Journal of Child and Family Nursing, 4*(2), 79–89.

Vincent, C. V., & Denyes, M. J. (2004). Relieving children's pain: Nurses' abilities and analgesic practices. *Journal of Pediatric Nursing, 19*(1), 40–50.

Voepel-Lewis, T., Malviya, S., & Tait, A. R. (2005). Validity of parent ratings as proxy measures of pain in children with cognitive impairment. *Pain Management Nursing, 6*(4), 168–174.

Weise, K. L., & Nahata, M. C. (2005). EMLA for painful procedures in infants. *Journal of Pediatric Health Care, 19*(10), 42–47.

Willis, M. H. W., Merkel, S. I., Voepel-Lewis, T., & Malviya, S. (2003). FLACC behavioral pain assessment scale: A comparison with the child's self-report. *Pediatric Nursing, 29*(3), 195–198.

Wong, D. L., & Baker, C. M. (1988). Pain in children: Comparison of assessment scales. *Pediatric Nursing, 14*, 9–16.

Yeh, C. H. (2005). Development and validation of the Asian version of the Oucher: A pain intensity scale for children. *Journal of Pain, 6*(8), 526–534.

Young, K. D. (2005). Pediatric procedural pain. *Annals of Emergency Medicine, 45*(2), 160–171.

Zempsky, W. T., Cravero, J. P., and the Committee on Pediatric Emergency Medicine and Section on Anesthesiology and Pain Medicine. (2004). Relief of pain and anxiety in pediatric patients in emergency medical systems. *Pediatrics, 114*(5), 1348–1356.

ALTERATIONS IN FLUID, ELECTROLYTE, AND ACID-BASE BALANCE

16

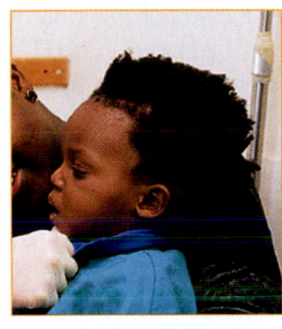

VERNON is 18 months old. Several days ago he developed vomiting and diarrhea. His parents tried to get him to eat, but he had little appetite. He drank a little water and a few sips of juice, but the next morning he was listless and would not drink anything. The diarrhea continued.

Vernon's mother brought him to the urgent care center. Vernon is irritable on arrival, and his mother reports that he has been alternately irritable and lethargic. His mucous membranes and tongue appear dry, and skin turgor over the abdomen is slightly decreased. His mother notes that Vernon has had only two wet diapers today and says the urine in his diapers was dark in color. She also reports that he weighed 12 kg (26 lb) at the clinic last week. However, when the nurse weighs him, the scale reads only 11 kg (24 1/2 lb). Vernon is moderately dehydrated. He needs rapid replacement of the proper type of fluids.

What happens inside the body when dehydration occurs? How can a nurse recognize dehydration? What types of fluid does Vernon need? What nursing management is important for his recovery? Why are young children at greater risk for dehydration than adults? What do parents need to be taught to prevent and manage dehydration? This chapter presents information that will enable you to answer these questions.

LEARNING OUTCOMES

After reading this chapter, you will be able to do the following:

1. Describe normal fluid and electrolyte status for children at various ages.
2. Identify regulatory mechanisms for fluid and electrolyte balance.
3. Recognize threats to fluid and electrolyte balance in children.
4. Analyze assessment findings to recognize fluid and electrolyte problems and acid-base imbalance in children.
5. Describe appropriate interventions for children experiencing fluid and electrolyte problems and acid-base imbalance.

KEY TERMS

acidemia 496	hypotonic
acidosis 497	fluid 518
alkalemia 496	interstitial fluid 496
alkalosis 497	intracellular
anion 521	fluid 496
body fluid 496	intravascular
body surface	fluid 496
area 499	isotonic
buffer 497	dehydration
cation 517	(or isonatremic
dehydration 501	dehydration)
diffusion 496	501
electrolytes 496	isotonic fluids 518
extracellular	Kussmaul
fluid 496	respirations 542
filtration 496	oncotic
hypertonic	pressure 513
dehydration (or	osmolality 516
hypernatremic	osmosis 496
dehydration) 501	Pco_2 497
hypertonic	pH 496
fluid 520	pitting edema 515
hypotonic	Po_2 497
dehydration (or	saline 512
hyponatremic	
dehydration) 501	

MediaLink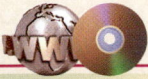

http://www.prenhall.com/ball
See the Prentice Hall Nursing MediaLink DVD-ROM and Companion Website for chapter-specific resources.

FOCUS ON

Fluid, Electrolyte, and Acid-Base Balance

ANATOMY AND PHYSIOLOGY

Physiology of Fluid and Electrolyte Balance

Fluid in the body is in a dynamic state. In persons of all ages, fluid continuously leaves the body through the skin, in feces and urine, and during respiration. Much of the human body is composed of water. **Body fluid** is body water that has solutes dissolved in it. Some of the solutes are **electrolytes**, or charged particles (ions). Electrolytes such as sodium (Na^+), potassium (K^+), calcium (Ca^{++}), magnesium (Mg^{++}), chloride (Cl^-), and inorganic phosphorus (Pi) ions must be present in the proper concentrations for cells to function effectively.

In persons of all ages, body fluid is located in several compartments. The two major fluid compartments contain the **intracellular fluid** (fluid inside the cells) and the **extracellular fluid** (fluid outside the cells). The extracellular fluid is made up of **intravascular fluid** (the fluid within the blood vessels) and **interstitial fluid** (the fluid between the cells and outside the blood and lymphatic vessels). Extracellular fluid accounts for about one third of total body water, while intracellular fluid accounts for about two thirds. The concentrations of electrolytes in the fluid differ depending on the fluid compartment. For example, extracellular fluid is rich in sodium ions; intracellular fluid, by contrast, is low in sodium ions but rich in potassium ions (Table 16–1).

Fluid moves between the intravascular and interstitial compartments by a process called **filtration**. Water moves into and out of the cells by the process of **osmosis**. These processes are discussed later in the chapter. Electrolytes move over cell membranes both by **diffusion** of particles from a location of greater to less concentration and by active transport that is effective even against the concentration gradient.

Physiology of Acid-Base Balance

Normal acid-base balance is necessary for proper function of the cells and the body. The number of hydrogen ions (H^+) present in a fluid determines its acidity. Increasing the hydrogen ion concentration makes a solution more acidic. Because the hydrogen ion concentration in body fluids is very low, acidity is expressed as **pH** (the negative logarithm of the hydrogen ion concentration) rather than as the hydrogen ion concentration itself. The range of possible pH values is 1 to 14. A pH of 7 is neutral. The lower the pH, the more acidic the solution. A pH above 7 is basic or alkaline. The higher the pH, the more basic the solution. Body fluids are normally slightly basic.

The pH of body fluids is regulated carefully to provide a suitable environment for cell function. The pH of the blood influences the pH inside the cells. **Acidemia** is a term that refers to a blood pH below normal levels, whereas **alkalemia** is an increased blood pH. For the enzymes outside the cells to function optimally, the pH must be in the normal range. If the pH inside the cells becomes too high or too low, then the speed of chemical reactions becomes inappropriate for proper cell function. Cell protein function relies on the correct level of hydrogen ions. Thus, acid-base imbalances result in clinical signs and symptoms. In severe cases, they may cause death.

In the course of their normal function, all cells in the body produce acids. Cells produce two kinds of acids: carbonic acid (H_2CO_3) and metabolic (noncarbonic) acid. These acids are released into the extracellular fluid and must be neutralized

Table 16–1	ELECTROLYTE CONCENTRATIONS IN BODY FLUID COMPARTMENTS		
	Extracellular Fluid (ECF)		**Intracellular Fluid (ICF)**
Components	**Vascular**	**Interstitial**	
Na^+	High	High	Low
K^+	Low	Low	High
Ca^{++}	Low	Low	Low (higher than ECF)
Mg^{++}	Low	Low	High
Pi	Low	Low	High
Cl^-	High	High	Low
Proteins	High	Low	High

or excreted from the body to prevent dangerous accumulation. They can be neutralized to some degree by the buffers in body fluids. Carbonic acid is excreted by the lungs in the form of carbon dioxide and water. Metabolic acids are excreted by the kidneys. Examples of metabolic acids are pyruvic, sulfuric, acetoacetic, lactic, hydrochloric, and beta-hydroxybutyric acids.

Buffers

The maintenance of hydrogen ions within the normal range relies heavily on buffers. A **buffer** is a compound that binds hydrogen ions when their concentration rises and releases them when their concentration falls (Figure 16–1 ➤). Several kinds of buffers are present in the body (Table 16–2). Various body fluids have buffers to meet their special needs. The bicarbonate buffer system neutralizes metabolic acids (Figure 16–2 ➤); however, it cannot neutralize carbonic acid.

All buffer systems have limits. For example, if there are too many metabolic acids, the bicarbonate buffers become depleted. The acids then accumulate in the body until they are excreted by the kidneys. Clinically, this is seen as a decreased serum bicarbonate concentration and decreased blood pH.

Role of the Lungs

The lungs are responsible for excreting excess carbonic acid from the body. A child breathes out carbon dioxide and water, the components of carbonic acid, with each breath. With faster and deeper breaths, more carbonic acid is excreted. Since carbonic acid is converted in the body to carbon dioxide and water by the enzyme carbonic anhydrase, an indirect

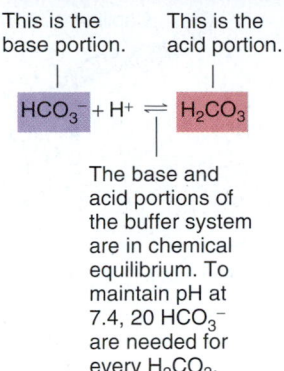

This is the base portion.   This is the acid portion.

$$HCO_3^- + H^+ \rightleftharpoons H_2CO_3$$

The base and acid portions of the buffer system are in chemical equilibrium. To maintain pH at 7.4, 20 HCO_3^- are needed for every H_2CO_3.

Figure 16–2 ➤ The bicarbonate buffer system.

Table 16–2	**IMPORTANT BUFFERS**
Buffer	**Major Locations in the Body**
Bicarbonate	Plasma; interstitial fluid
Protein	Plasma; inside cells
Hemoglobin	Inside red blood cells
Phosphate	Inside cells; urine

laboratory measurement of carbonic acid is **Pco$_2$**, the partial pressure of carbon dioxide in arterial blood.

Although a child can voluntarily increase or decrease the rate and depth of respirations, they are usually involuntarily controlled. The **Po$_2$** (partial pressure of oxygen in arterial blood), Pco$_2$, and pH of the blood are monitored by chemoreceptors in the hypothalamus of the brain and in the aorta and carotid arteries. The input from the chemoreceptors is combined with other neural input to change breathing according to needs. Rate and depth increase or decrease according to the amount of carbonic acid that needs to be excreted.

If a child has a condition that decreases the excretion of carbonic acid or causes breathing to be too slow or shallow (such as overmedication following surgery), carbonic acid accumulates in the blood. Clinically, this is seen as an increased blood Pco$_2$ and is a form of respiratory **acidosis**. The reverse will also be true in the child breathing excessively or deeply. This leads to decreased Pco$_2$ and respiratory **alkalosis**.

Role of the Kidneys

The kidneys regulate metabolic acids from the body in two ways: They reabsorb filtered bicarbonate to prevent its loss in the urine, and they regenerate bicarbonate when needed to restore balance (Yucha, 2004). Bicarbonate is formed when acids and ammonium combine with extra ions. The blood bicarbonate concentration is an indicator of the amount of metabolic acids present, because bicarbonate is used in buffering the acids. When the concentration is normal, metabolic acids are present in usual amounts (Figure 16–3 ➤).

In a healthy child, the result of these renal processes is excretion of metabolic acids and maintenance of blood bicarbonate concentration within normal limits. These processes

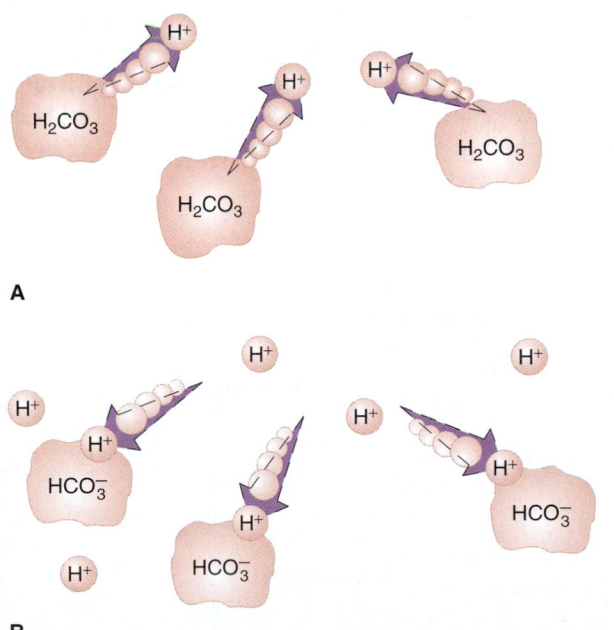

A

B

Figure 16–1 ➤ A, How buffers respond to an excess of base. If the blood has too much base, the acid portion of a buffer pair (e.g., H_2CO_3 of the bicarbonate buffer system) releases hydrogen ions (H^+) to help return the pH to normal. B, How buffers respond to an excess of acid. If the blood has too much acid, the base portion of a buffer pair (e.g., HCO_3^- of the bicarbonate buffer system) takes up hydrogen ions (H^+) to help return the pH to normal.

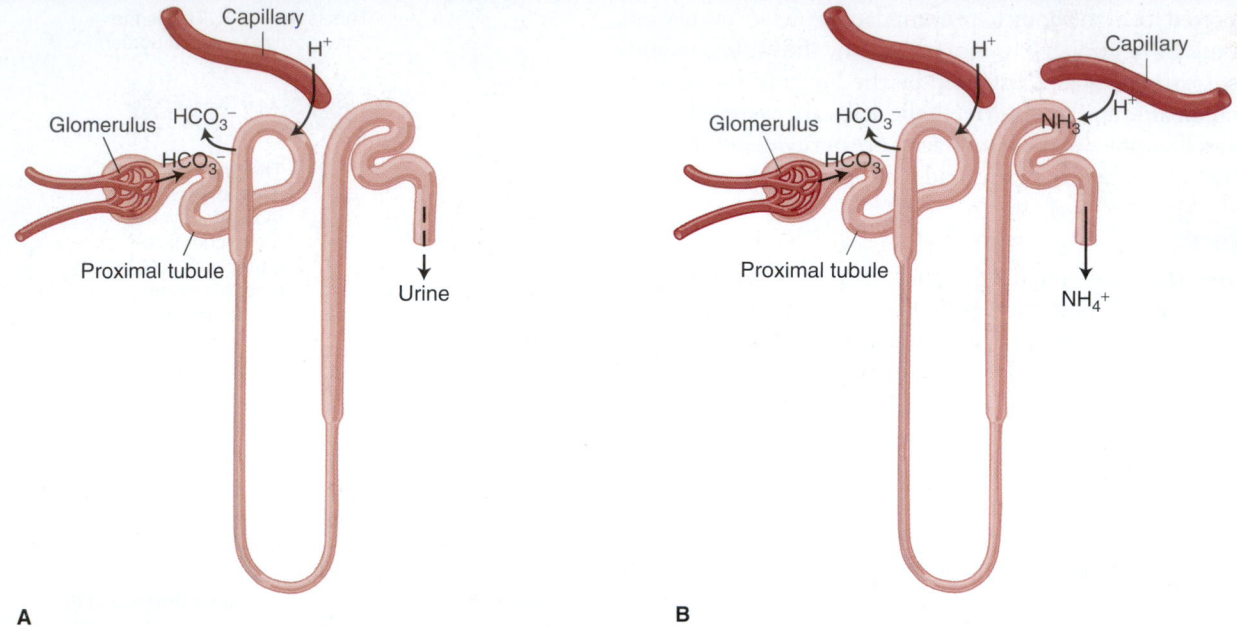

Figure 16–3 ➤ A, Recycling of bicarbonate by the kidneys. Bicarbonate ions that are in the blood are filtered into the renal tubules at the glomerulus. In the proximal tubules, bicarbonate ions are reabsorbed into the blood at the same time that hydrogen ions are transported from the blood into the renal tubular fluid. B, Secretion and buffering of hydrogen ions in the kidneys. If the urine is too acidic, the cells that line the urinary tract could be damaged. To prevent this problem, hydrogen ions secreted into the distal tubules are neutralized by phosphate buffers or bound to ammonia and excreted in the form of ammonium

may take several hours to days to be effective in restoring balance when acidosis occurs. In the child whose kidneys are not producing enough urine, metabolic acids may not be effectively excreted. Accumulation of these acids uses up many of the available bicarbonate buffers, resulting in a decreased serum bicarbonate concentration and metabolic acidosis.

Role of the Liver

The liver also plays a role in maintaining acid-base balance by metabolizing protein, which produces hydrogen ions. It also synthesizes proteins needed to maintain osmotic pressures in the fluid compartments.

PEDIATRIC DIFFERENCES

Infants and young children differ physiologically from adults in ways that make them vulnerable to fluid, electrolyte, and acid-base imbalances. The percentage of body weight that is composed of water varies with age (Figure 16–4 ➤). The percentage is highest at birth (and higher in premature than in

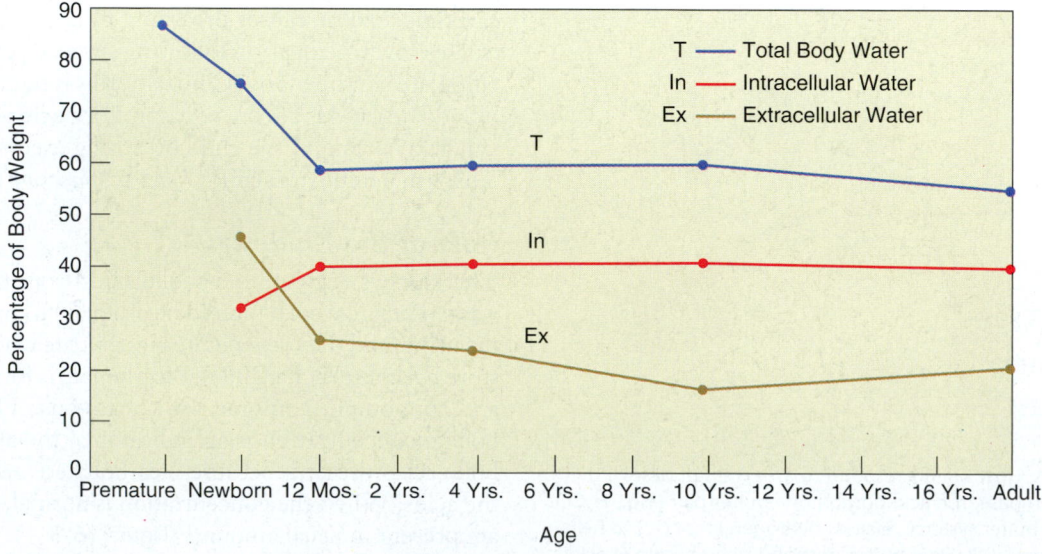

Figure 16–4 ➤ The major body fluid compartments at various ages. *Extracellular fluid* is composed mainly of vascular fluid (fluid in blood vessels) and interstitial fluid (fluid between the cells and outside the blood and lymphatic vessels). *Intracellular fluid* is that within cells.
From Bindler, R., & Howry, L. (2005). *Pediatric drug guide.* Upper Saddle River, NJ: Prentice Hall.

full-term infants) and decreases with age (see As Children Grow, Figure 16–5 ➤). Neonates and young infants have a proportionately larger extracellular fluid volume than older children and adults because their brain and skin (both rich in interstitial fluid) occupy a greater proportion of their body weight. Much of our extracellular fluid is exchanged each day. During infancy, there is a high daily fluid requirement with little fluid volume reserve; this makes the infant vulnerable to dehydration. As an infant grows, the proportion of water inside the cells increases, extracellular amount decreases in comparison, and the risk of fluid imbalance begins to decrease.

Infants and children under 2 years of age lose a greater proportion of fluid each day than older children and adults and are thus more dependent on adequate intake. They have a greater amount of skin surface or **body surface area** (BSA; relationship between height and weight measured in squared meters) and thus have greater insensible water losses through the skin. Because of this large BSA, they are also at greater risk when burned.

In addition, respiratory and metabolic rates are high during early childhood. These factors lead to greater water loss from the lungs and greater water demand to fuel the body's metabolic processes (Figure 16–6 ➤). Due to these factors, the

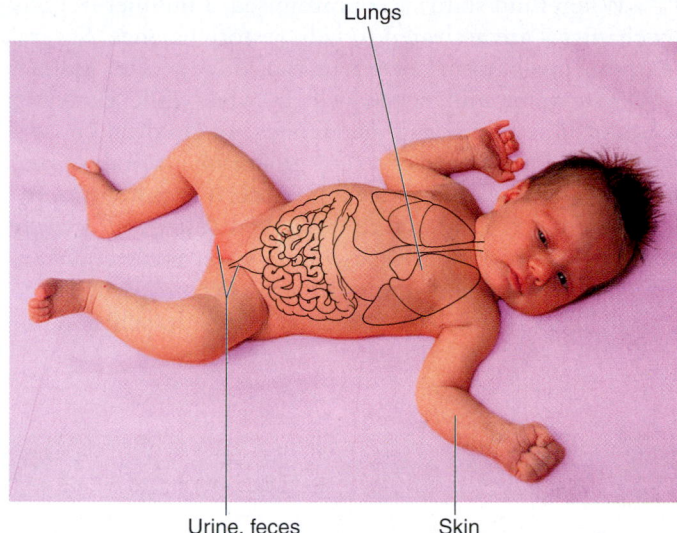

Figure 16–6 ➤ Normal routes of fluid excretion from infants and children.

exercising child dehydrates easily and must consume more fluid during physical activity, particularly during hot weather (Committee on Sports Medicine and Fitness, 2000).

AS CHILDREN GROW

Fluid and Electrolyte Differences

Newborn

75% Total body water
• ECF 45%
• ICF 30%

Brain and skin occupy a greater proportion of body weight and are high in interstitial fluid

Infant

65% Total body water
• ECF 25%
• ICF 30–40%

High BSA promotes fluid loss

Little fluid reserve in intracellular fluid

5–6x greater fluid exchange daily

High metabolic rate requires generous fluid intake

Child/Adolescent

50% Total body water
• ECF 10–15%
• ICF 40%

Kidneys are immature until 2 years and unable to conserve water and electrolytes or fully assist in acid–base balance

Figure 16–5 ➤ The newborn and infant have a high percentage of body weight comprised of water, especially extracellular fluid, which is lost from the body easily. Note the small stomach size which limits ability to rehydrate quickly.

When fluid status is compromised, a number of body mechanisms are activated to help restore balance. Several of these mechanisms occur in the kidney. The kidneys conserve water and needed electrolytes while excreting waste products and drug metabolites. In children under 2 years of age, however, the glomeruli, tubules, and nephrons of the kidneys are immature. They are thus unable to conserve or excrete water and solutes effectively (see Chapter 25 ∞). Because more water is generally excreted, the infant and young child can become dehydrated quickly or develop electrolyte imbalances. In addition, infants have a weaker transport system for ions and bicarbonate, placing them at greater risk for acidosis and acid-base imbalances. Children under 2 years of age also have difficulty regulating electrolytes such as sodium and calcium. Renal response to high solute loads is slower and less developed, with function improving gradually during the first year of life.

Examples of diagnostic and laboratory tests used to evaluate fluid, electrolyte, and acid-base balance are provided in the accompanying table. Use the guidelines below to perform a nursing assessment for these functions.

DIAGNOSTIC AND LABORATORY TESTS FOR FLUID, ELECTROLYTE, AND ACID-BASE BALANCE

Laboratory Test	Purpose	Nursing Implications
Arterial blood gases	Arterial blood can be analyzed for pH, partial pressure of carbon dioxide (Pco_2), partial pressure of oxygen (Po_2), or serum bicarbonate (HCO_3^-). Levels are analyzed for information about acid-base balance.	Arterial blood gases are commonly obtained from an existing arterial line. Prepare the child and family for the procedure. Obtain necessary supplies and be certain the child is restrained adequately so that the line is safely accessed. Label and transport the sample to the laboratory on ice.
Serum electrolyte panel	The variety of electrolytes measured in the serum can reflect imbalances in water and electrolyte values. They provide the basis for further assessment and diagnosis of the condition and for the types of fluids needed during management to reestablish balance.	Prepare the child for the blood test. Perform the test in a treatment room. An existing intravenous line may be used for access if it is available.
Urinary specific gravity	This measure of urine's density is used to assess its concentration. An increasing number indicates higher concentration of molecules, signifying lower levels of hydration.	A very small amount of urine is needed to complete a specific gravity test. Obtain the sample and perform the refractometer test.

ASSESSMENT GUIDELINES FOR THE CHILD WITH A FLUID, ELECTROLYTE, OR ACID-BASE ALTERATION

Assessment Focus	Assessment Guidelines
Body weight	• Has weight decreased since last measurement or weight reported by family? • If so, how much? What percent of body weight is the weight loss?
Skin and mucous membranes	• What are the temperature, turgor, and moistness of the skin? • Describe moistness of oral mucous membranes. • Describe moistness of the eyes and presence of tears. • Is edema present in any body parts?
Cardiovascular and respiratory systems	• What are pulse and blood pressure? • Test capillary refill and small-vein filling times. • What is the respiratory rate? Is the rate regular?
Gastrointestinal system	• Does the child have nausea, vomiting, or diarrhea? If so, how often and for how long has it continued? • Is the child eating and drinking? How much and what types of foods and fluids?
Urinary system	• What is the child's urinary output? • What is the urine specific gravity?
Musculoskeletal system	• Describe muscle tone and symmetry.
Neurological system	• Describe the child's state of alertness and any changes observed. • What is the level of consciousness? • Is the anterior fontanel at the skin surface or does it appear sunken?

A thorough understanding of fluid, electrolyte, and acid-base homeostasis and imbalances is essential when providing nursing care to pediatric patients, like Vernon in the preceding scenario. This chapter presents information about the processes that maintain fluid and electrolyte balance, and describes the common imbalances that may occur in children. It also describes how the body regulates acid-base status and explains the management of acid-base imbalances.

Many health conditions cause changes in body fluids that must be regulated and managed. Sometimes management of fluid status in the home or in a short-term ambulatory facility can prevent more serious illness or hospitalization. Examples of conditions that commonly require fluid, electrolyte, or acid-base balance include gastroenteritis, burns, kidney disorders, oral fluid restriction for surgery, anorexia or bulimia, or dehydration and electrolyte imbalances that can result from athletics in hot weather.

FLUID VOLUME IMBALANCES

When fluid excretion and losses are balanced by the proper volume and type of fluid intake, fluid balance will be maintained. If, however, fluid output and intake are not matched, fluid imbalance may occur rapidly. In addition to the immaturity of physiologic processes, many health conditions make young children more vulnerable to fluid deficit. The major types of fluid imbalances are extracellular fluid volume deficit (dehydration), extracellular fluid volume excess, and interstitial fluid volume excess (edema).

Extracellular Fluid Volume Imbalances
Extracellular Fluid Volume Deficit (Dehydration)

Extracellular fluid volume deficit occurs when there is not enough fluid in the extracellular compartment (vascular and interstitial). Depending on the cause of dehydration, sodium may be at a normal, low, or elevated level. (Hyponatremia and hypernatremia are described later in the chapter, on pages 517–521.) The state of body water deficit is called **dehydration**. The three major types of dehydration are:

- **Isotonic dehydration** (or **isonatremic dehydration**). This occurs when fluid loss is not balanced by intake and the losses of water and sodium are in proportion. The serum sodium is therefore within normal limits even though the circulating blood volume is lowered. Most of the fluid lost is from the extracellular component. This type of dehydration is commonly manifested in the illnesses of young children through such symptoms as vomiting and diarrhea.
- **Hypotonic dehydration** (or **hyponatremic dehydration**). This occurs when fluid loss is characterized by a proportionately greater loss of sodium than water. Serum sodium is below normal levels. Compensatory fluid shifts occur from the extracellular to intracellular components in an attempt to establish normal proportions, thus leading to even greater extracellular dehydration. Severe and prolonged vomiting and diarrhea, burns, and renal disease can lead to this condition, as well as administration of intravenous fluid without electrolytes in treatment of dehydration.
- **Hypertonic dehydration** (or **hypernatremic dehydration**). This occurs when sodium loss is proportionately less than water loss. Serum sodium is above normal levels. Compensatory fluid shifts occur from the intracellular to extracellular components in an attempt to establish normal proportions. The extracellular component therefore remains fairly normal, delaying the onset of signs and symptoms of dehydration until the condition is quite serious. Neurological symptoms reflecting intracellular imbalance may occur simultaneously with more common symptoms of dehydration. The condition may be caused by health problems such as diabetes insipidus (see Chapter 29 ∞) or administration of intravenous fluid or tube feedings with high electrolyte levels.

The body continuously attempts to compensate for fluid and electrolyte imbalance by shifting fluid and electrolytes from one component to another. Therefore, it is rare for

NURSING ALERT

Health conditions contributing to fluid imbalance include:
- Radiant heat (phototherapy) used to treat hyperbilirubinemia increases insensible water loss through the skin.
- The increased respiratory rate in some illnesses leads to excessive water loss from lungs.
- Fever increases the metabolic rate and, therefore, water demands of metabolism (for each degree of Celsius increase above 37 degrees, 0.42 mL/kg/hr of additional fluid is needed).
- Vomiting and diarrhea increase fluid and electrolyte losses from the gastrointestinal system.
- Fistulas, blood loss, and drainage tubes contribute to fluid deficits.
- Renal disease can influence rates of fluid excretion.

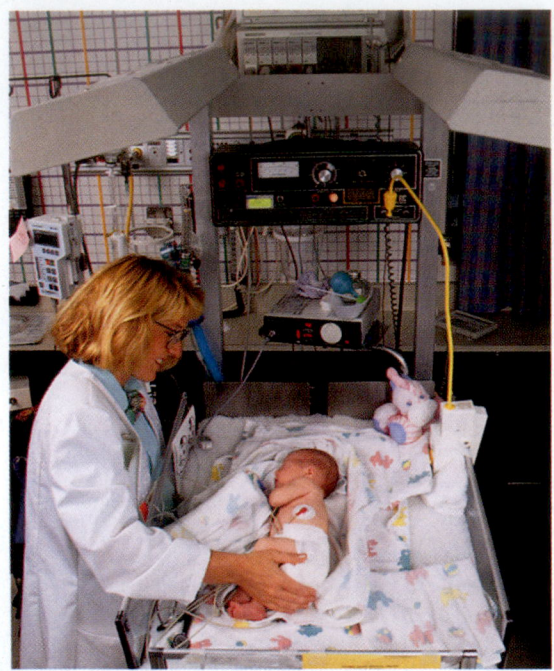

Figure 16–7 ➤ Use of an overhead warmer or phototherapy increases insensible fluid excretion through the skin, thus increasing the fluid intake needed.

only one type of dehydration to occur; the child's fluid and electrolyte status and symptoms are constantly changing. Ongoing assessment and management will be needed.

ETIOLOGY AND PATHOPHYSIOLOGY   Extracellular fluid volume deficit is usually caused by the loss of sodium-containing fluid from the body. The situations that most often cause loss of fluid containing sodium are vomiting, diarrhea, nasogastric suction, hemorrhage, and burns. Vomiting and diarrhea are common manifestations of disease in children throughout the world, and each year up to 5 million children die from dehydration related to diarrhea. About 300 to 500 die annually in the United States from this problem; about 220,000 are hospitalized (9% of pediatric hospitalizations); and about 1.5 million receive care on an outpatient basis (Dale, 2004; Dennehy, 2005; Nager & Wang, 2002).

Another cause of extracellular fluid volume deficit in infants is increased water loss in low-birth-weight infants who are kept under radiant warmers to maintain heat (Figure 16–7 ➤). Their high BSA puts them at risk of dehydration due to insensible fluid loss through the skin. Less frequently, adrenal insufficiency, accumulation of extracellular fluid in a "third space" such as the peritoneal cavity, and overuse of diuretics may be the cause. The latter etiology is most often seen in bulimic adolescents for weight control (see Chapter 4 ∞).

Excessive exercise during very hot weather without sufficient fluid replacement can lead to fluid and electrolyte imbalance. Children are more likely than adults to experience imbalance from exercise, because of the physiological differences explained earlier in this chapter. Because children have a larger BSA, they can gain more heat from the environment when it is hot, and lose more when it is cold (Binkley, Beckett, Casa et al., 2002). In addition, the high metabolic rate of children is further increased during exercise so that fluid lost in metabolism is significant. Children may not feel thirsty and so fail to drink even when dehydrated (Committee on Sports Medicine and Fitness, 2000).

Burns involve complex health problems that are described in Chapter 30 ∞. Burns of the skin usually involve huge loss of body fluids, including water and electrolytes, particularly sodium. Hypotonic dehydration is the type most commonly seen in the initial period after a burn. Serum proteins are also lost, so body fluid is more likely to leak into interstitial spaces, causing edema and further contributing to the fluid deficit. The kidneys decrease urine production because of their decreased blood flow, which leads to lowered urinary output. While the fluid imbalance of burns is therefore very complicated, the first imbalance encountered is often that of dehydration with accompanying hyponatremia.

For burns, gastroenteritis, and other illnesses, initial dehydration in the first 3 days reflects a high loss of extracellular fluid. About 80% of the fluid loss is extracellular, and only about 20% intracellular. However, with time the relationship begins to change, so that in illnesses over 3 days, about 60% of fluid loss is extracellular while 40% is intracellular (Johns Hopkins Hospital, 2005). Because the electrolyte composition of extracellular and intracellular fluids differs (see Table 16–1), electrolyte management will need to be adapted in long-term conditions.

CLINICAL MANIFESTATIONS   The signs of dehydration relate to the severity or degree of the body water deficit (Table 16–3). They are a result of both the decreased fluid (e.g., diminished turgor and mucous membrane moisture) and the body's response to the fluid deficit (e.g., pulse and blood pressure changes). See the Clinical Manifestations of Extracellular Fluid Volume Deficit on the next page. Clinical Manifestations of Exertional Heat Illness are listed on page 504.

Mild dehydration is hard to detect, because children appear alert and have moist mucous membranes. Infants may be irritable and older children are thirsty. In moderate dehydration, the child is often lethargic and sleepy, but there may be periods of

Table 16–3	SEVERITY OF CLINICAL DEHYDRATION		
Clinical Assessment	Mild	Moderate	Severe
Percent of body weight lost	Up to 5% (40–50 mL/kg)	6–9% (60–90 mL/kg)	10% or more (100 mL/kg or more)
Level of consciousness	Alert, restless, thirsty	Irritable or lethargic (infants and very young children); alert, thirsty, restless (older children and adolescents)	Lethargic to comatose (infants and young children); often conscious, apprehensive (older children and adolescents)
Blood pressure	Normal	Normal or low; postural hypotension (older children and adolescents)	Low to undetectable
Pulse	Normal	Normal or rapid	Tachycardia or bradycardia
Skin turgor	Normal	Poor	Very poor
Mucous membranes	Moist	Dry	Parched
Urine	May appear normal	Decreased output (< 1 mL/kg/hr) dark color; increased specific gravity	Very decreased or absent output
Thirst	Slightly increased	Moderately increased	Greatly increased unless lethargic
Fontanel	Normal	Sunken	Sunken
Extremities	Warm; normal capillary refill	Delayed capillary refill (> 2 sec)	Cool, discolored, delayed capillary refill (> 3–4 sec)
Respirations	Normal	Normal or rapid	Changing rate and pattern
Deep	Normal	Slightly sunken, decreased tears	Deeply sunken, absent tears

restlessness and irritability, especially in infants. Skin turgor is diminished, mucous membranes appear dry, and urine is dark in color and diminished in amount. Pulse rate is usually increased and blood pressure can be normal or low. Vernon, described at the beginning of this chapter, was displaying symptoms of moderate dehydration. His urine output was decreased, and he had lost about 8% of his body weight. What other signs and symptoms of moderate dehydration can you identify in the opening scenario? What additional assessments would you want to perform on Vernon?

Severe dehydration is manifested by increasing lethargy or nonresponsiveness, markedly decreased blood pressure, rapid pulse, poor skin turgor, dry mucous membranes, seizure activity, and markedly decreased or absent urinary output.

CLINICAL MANIFESTATIONS	EXTRACELLULAR FLUID VOLUME DEFICIT
Etiology	Clinical Manifestations
Decreased fluid volume	Weight loss Sunken fontanel (infant)
Inadequate circulating blood volume to offset the force of gravity when in upright position	Postural blood pressure drop (older children) Dizziness
Decreased intravascular volume	Increased small-vein filling time Delayed capillary refill time Flat neck veins when supine (older children)
Inadequate circulation to the brain	Dizziness, syncope
Inadequate circulation to the kidneys	Oliguria
Cardiac reflex response to decreased intravascular volume	Thready, rapid pulse
Decreased interstitial fluid volume	Decreased skin turgor

CLINICAL MANIFESTATIONS	EXERTIONAL HEAT ILLNESS	
Condition	**Etiology**	**Manifestations**
Heat cramps	Dehydration Electrolyte imbalance Neuromuscular fatigue	Acute, painful muscle cramps Thirst Fatigue
Heat syncope	Peripheral vasodilation Reduced cardiac output Cerebral ischemia	Tunnel vision Pale, sweaty skin Decreased pulse Dizziness, faintness
Heat exhaustion	Elevated core body temperature Sodium loss	Sweating, pallor Dehydration Muscle cramps Nausea, anorexia, diarrhea Decreased urinary output Weakness, fainting, dizziness
Heat stroke	Elevated core temperature (>104°F) Temperature regulation overwhelmed by heat production or absence of adequate heat loss Organ system failure from overheating	Tachycardia Hypotension Sweating Hyperventilation Altered mental status, seizures, coma Vomiting, diarrhea Death can occur from severe acidosis, hyperkalemia, renal failure, and disseminated intravascular coagulation
Exertional hyponatremia	Serum sodium <130 mmol/L Exercise over 4 hours with water or other low-solute fluids for replenishment	Disorientation, headache, lethargy Swollen extremities Vomiting Pulmonary or cerebral edema Death can occur from sodium imbalance

Adapted from Binkley, Beckett, Casa, Kleiner, & Plummer, 2002.

■ COLLABORATIVE CARE

Diagnostic Tests

The diagnosis of dehydration is best accomplished by clinical observations (see Table 16–3). A major observation that provides clues about the degree of dehydration is percent of weight loss. A synthesis of studies on dehydration showed that abnormal capillary refill time, skin turgor, and abnormal respirations were the most useful clinical signs of dehydration to assist in identifying the disorder (Steiner, DeWalt, & Byerly, 2004). The serum electrolyte panel may be helpful in severe and continuing dehydration that is complicated by electrolyte imbalance or acidosis. The tests include serum electrolytes, creatinine, and glucose. Elevated blood urea nitrogen (>17 mg/dL) and low serum bicarbonate (<16 mmol/L) are also useful to identify moderate and severe dehydration (Wathen, MacKenzie, & Bothner, 2004). The results can be used to target the fluid type and amount to best meet the imbalances identified. Urine specific gravity may provide useful information.

Clinical Therapy

Medical management depends on accurate identification of the degree of dehydration. The treatment of extracellular fluid volume deficit is administration of fluid containing sodium. This may be accomplished by oral rehydration therapy or by intravenous fluids.

Oral rehydration therapy has been used for a number of years in developing countries without an accessible supply of intravenous fluids. More recently, the benefits of using this therapy early to prevent severe dehydration and to treat mild and

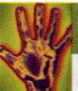

GROWTH & DEVELOPMENT

Urine Specific Gravity

Urine specific gravity may increase in older children who are dehydrated. However, due to the inability of the child under 2 years of age to concentrate urine effectively, a rising specific gravity may not be seen as definitively in the younger dehydrated child.

moderate dehydration in children in developed countries has been recognized. The therapy is successful in treating the dehydration caused by many gastrointestinal illnesses and prevents hospitalization for many infants and young children. It is the treatment of choice for children with diarrhea who have mild to moderate dehydration (King, Glass, Bresee, & Duggan, 2003). Solutions are available commercially that contain water, carbohydrate (glucose), sodium, potassium, chloride, and lactate. Some clinicians allow lactose-free milk, breast milk, or half-strength milk to be given in addition to oral rehydration therapy solution. A WHO/UNICEF solution was developed for use with cholera and is not generally used for diarrhea treatment in the United States, as its sodium and chloride loads are higher than that of other commercial solutions (Box 16–1).

When the child is severely dehydrated, intravenous fluid will be given, often accompanied with oral rehydration. The intravenous fluid is often Ringer's lactate followed by or accompanied with dilute saline, such as one half or one quarter normal saline. The fluid combination replenishes the extracellular fluid volume and adds solutes to return the body fluid to normal. The child may be hospitalized or treated with intravenous fluids in a short-stay unit until the dehydration is controlled. Once hydration is completed, the child may resume an age-appropriate diet.

BOX 16–1
ORAL REHYDRATION AND MAINTENANCE FLUIDS FOR MILD AND MODERATE DEHYDRATION

Pedialyte	Nutralyte
Ricelyte	ReVital
Infalyte	Hydralyte
KaoLectrolyte	Rehydralyte
Cerealyte	Equalyte
Lytren	Resol
Pediatric Oral Maintenance Solution (ORS)	
WHO/UNICEF oral rehydration solution	

NURSING MANAGEMENT
Nursing Assessment and Diagnosis

Weigh the child daily with the same scale and without clothing. Compare to past weights and calculate weight loss. Carefully measure intake and output, urine specific gravity, level of consciousness, pulse rate and quality, skin turgor, mucous membrane moisture, quality and rate of respirations, and blood pressure (Figure 16–8 ➤). Compare the blood pressure when the child is supine with the pressure when the child is sitting with legs hanging down or standing. If the child is dehydrated, the sitting or standing blood pressure will be lower than the supine blood pressure, because blood accumulates in the dependent legs. The nurse will obtain samples of urine and blood as needed for dehydration evaluation. Evaluate the alertness of the child and any signs of lethargy or weakness.

The nursing diagnosis of Deficient Fluid Volume applies to all children who have an extracellular fluid volume deficit. Other diagnoses depend on the severity of the condition and the age of the child. Several nursing diagnoses that might be appropriate for the mildly to severely dehydrated child are included in the accompanying nursing care plans. Additional care of the child with dehydration from gastroenteritis can be found in Chapter 24 ∞. Specific examples of nursing diagnoses include the following:

- Fluid Volume (Deficient) related to fluid volume loss or failure of regulatory mechanisms
- Risk for Ineffective Peripheral Tissue Perfusion related to hypovolemia
- Risk for Injury related to postural hypotension

Planning and Implementation

Nursing care of the dehydrated child focuses on preventing dehydration when possible, providing oral rehydration fluids, teaching parents oral rehydration methods, and, if necessary, administering intravenous fluids to restore fluid balance. The accompanying Nursing Care Plans summarize care of the child with mild to severe dehydration.·

Prevent Dehydration

Nursing care can often prevent dehydration. Carefully monitor temperature probes in radiant warmers and isolettes for newborns to prevent overheating and resulting dehydration. Teach parents to use proper clothing for infants to prevent overheating. Nurses play an important role in educating parents, youth, school personnel, and

CLINICAL TIP

To calculate the percentage of weight loss:
- Subtract the child's present weight from the original weight to find the loss.
- Divide the loss by the child's original weight.

EXAMPLE: In the opening scenario, Vernon weighed 12 kg (26 lb) at the clinic last week. However, when he is weighed today, the scale reads only 11 kg (24 1/2 lb). In this case, subtracting 11 kg from 12 kg yields 1 kg of weight loss. Dividing 1 kg by his original weight of 12 kg reveals that he has lost approximately 8% of his body weight, which indicates moderate dehydration.

CLINICAL TIP

To obtain urine from an infant for testing specific gravity, place two cotton balls in the diaper. When they are wet, push them into a 10-mL syringe and squeeze out the urine with the plunger.

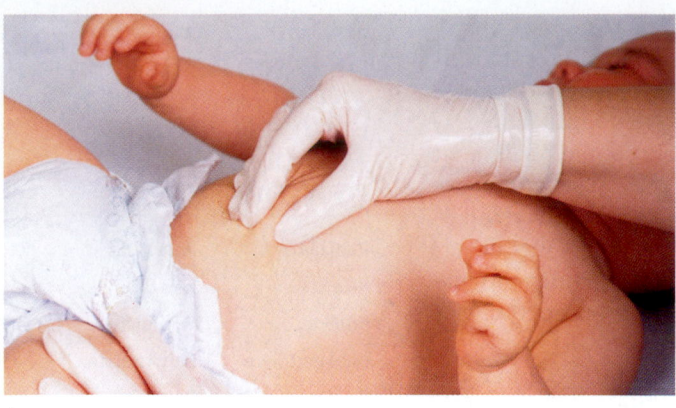
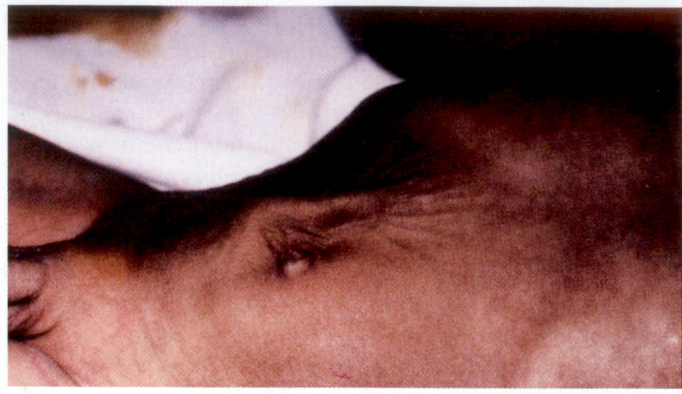

A   B

Figure 16–8 ➤ Assessing skin turgor takes skill and practice. A, In moderate dehydration the skin may have a doughy texture and appearance. B, In severe dehydration, "tenting" of the skin is observed. Diminished turgor is most easily assessed in infants or children with little subcutaneous fat; it is more difficult to assess in those with larger amounts of fat. The chest, abdomen, and upper thighs are locations to measure turgor.

NURSING CARE PLAN   The Child with Mild or Moderate Dehydration

GOAL	INTERVENTION	RATIONALE	EXPECTED OUTCOME
1. Ineffective Management of Therapeutic Regimen related to family knowledge deficit diarrhea and vomiting			
	NIC Priority Intervention: **Family Involvement:** *Facilitate family participation in care of the child.*		*NOC Suggested Outcome:* **Participation:** *Healthcare Decisions: Personal involvement in selecting healthcare options.*
Parents will describe appropriate home management of fluid replacement for diarrhea and vomiting.	• Explain how to replace body fluid with an oral rehydration solution. Encourage parents to keep the solution at home and begin use with the first sign of diarrhea.	• Use of an oral rehydration solution can enable successful treatment of vomiting and diarrhea at home.	Parents are successfully able to treat the child's diarrhea and vomiting at home. Child is adequately hydrated.
	• Teach parents to continue the child's normal diet in addition to providing replacement fluids for diarrhea.	• Diet plus fluid supplementation leads to faster recovery.	
	• Provide verbal and written instructions to parents at each well-child visit.	• Parents are provided with a reference for late use.	
2. Knowledge Deficient (Parent) related to causes of dehydration			
	NIC Priority Intervention: **Teaching:** *Teach causes of dehydration.*		*NOC Suggested Outcome:* **Knowledge:** *Extent of understanding conveyed about treatment regimen.*
Parents will state common causes of childhood dehydration.	• Teach parents childhood conditions that commonly lead to dehydration.	• If parents recognize situations that can lead to dehydration, they will be more alert to its appearance.	Parents recognize conditions of risk for dehydration in children.
3. Risk for Fluid Volume, Deficient related to worsening of child's condition			
	NIC Priority Intervention: **Fluid Management:** *Promote fluid balance.*		*NOC Suggested Outcome:* **Fluid Balance:** *Balance of water in extra- and intracellular compartments of body.*
Parents will seek health care for the child's worsening condition.	• Teach parents to seek care when the child's vomiting or diarrhea worsens, or the child's mental alertness changes.	• Severe dehydration may occur if milder forms are not successfully treated.	Parents seek prompt attention for the child's worsening condition, preventing the development of severe dehydration.

NURSING CARE PLAN   The Child with Severe Dehydration

GOAL	INTERVENTION	RATIONALE	EXPECTED OUTCOME
1. Fluid Volume, Deficient related to excess losses and inadequate intake			
	NIC Priority Intervention: **Fluid Management:** *Promote fluid balance.*		*NOC Suggested Outcome:* **Fluid Balance:** *Balance of water in extra- and intracellular components of the body.*
The child will return to normal hydration status and will not develop hypovolemic shock.	• Monitor weight daily. Assess intake and output every shift. Assess heart rate, postural blood pressure, skin turgor, small-vein filling time, capillary refill time, fontanel (infant), and urine specific gravity every 4 hours or more frequently as indicated.	• Frequent assessment of hydration status facilitates rapid intervention and evaluation of the effectiveness of fluid replacement.	The child has signs of normal hydration.
	• Administer intravenous fluids as ordered. Monitor for crackles in dependent portions of the lungs.	• Replace fluid lost from the body. Excessive replacement of sodium-containing fluids could cause extracellular fluid volume excess.	
2. Risk for injury related to decreased level of consciousness			
	NIC Priority Intervention: **Fall Prevention:** *Institute special precautions.*		*NOC Suggested Outcome:* **Fall Prevention:** *Minimize risk factors that precipitate falls.*
The child will not experience injury.	• Raise the side rails of the bed. Ensure that a small child does not become tangled in bedcovers.	• Safety measures protect the child.	The child does not fall or suffer other injury.
	• Monitor level of consciousness every 2–4 hours or more often as indicated.	• Frequent assessment provides evidence of the need for safety interventions and of the effectiveness of therapy.	
	• Monitor serum sodium concentration daily or more often.	• Elevated serum sodium concentration causes brain cell shrinkage and decreased level of consciousness.	
	• Have the child sit before rising from bed and assist to stand slowly.	• Slow adjustment to upright posture reduces light-headedness from decreased blood volume.	
3. Activity Intolerance related to bed rest/immobility			
	NIC Priority Intervention: **Activity Therapy:** *Plan activities to meet child's developmental needs.*		*NOC Suggested Outcome:* **Energy Conservation:** *Manage energy to sustain activity.*
The child will engage in normal activity for age.	• Plan activities appropriate for the age of the child that can be done in bed.	• Activities will provide distraction and promote recovery.	The child engages in normal developmental activities and receives adequate rest.
	• Group nursing interventions to provide time for the child to rest.	• The child will require more rest than usual.	
	• Provide assistance during meals and other activities as needed.	• Prevention of overexertion will conserve body fluid and promote healing.	

coaches about the dangers of heat-related illness. Prevention is key, so that children can exercise safely. Prior to a new exercise regime, perform assessment for risk factors. This includes medical conditions that put the child at high risk, such as cystic fibrosis, diabetes, obesity, or mental retardation. Prior history of heat-related illness or recent change from a cooler to hotter environment increases risk. Long exercise periods increase the stress upon the body. The major nursing interventions are partnering with families and athletic coaches to prevent problems and to recognize and treat them promptly. See Families Want to Know: Preventing Heat-Related Illness. Recognize that heat syndromes can result in death, so prevention, prompt recognition, and treatment are essential.

Provide Oral Rehydration Fluids

In mild or moderate dehydration, oral rehydration fluid is the first intervention (see Box 16–1) (Fonseca, Holdgate, & Craig, 2004; Spandorfer, Alessandrini, Joffe, Localio, & Shaw, 2005). It is given in frequent small amounts; for example, 1 to 3 teaspoons of fluid every 10 to 15 minutes is a useful guideline for starting oral rehydration. For the first 2 to 4 hours of treatment, 50 mL of fluid for each kilogram of the child's weight should be the target intake. Instruct parents to continue to administer 1 teaspoon every 2 to 3 minutes even if the child vomits, as small amounts of the fluid may still be absorbed. Children are often treated in special sections of emergency departments or outpatient clinics for several hours to begin hydration. Oral or nasogastric tube feedings of oral rehydration are administered while monitoring occurs.

Teach Parents Oral Rehydration Methods

Instruct parents about the types of fluids and amounts to be given. See Families Want to Know: Oral Rehydration Therapy Guidelines. Begin teaching parents of all newborns and reinforce teaching at each well-child visit. Advise parents to continue the child's normal diet in addition to providing the rehydration solution. Cereals, starches, soups, fruits, and vegetables are allowed. Tell parents to avoid simple sugars, which can worsen diarrhea because of osmotic effects, including soft drinks (if used, they should be diluted with equal parts of water), undiluted juice, Jell-O, and sweetened cereal.

▶ NURSING ALERT

Sugar facilitates the absorption of sodium in oral rehydration fluids. Teach parents not to give diet beverages for oral rehydration, because they contain no sugar and will not be effectively absorbed. However, if an oral rehydration solution is too concentrated, it can worsen the diarrhea. Juice and cola are highly concentrated and should be diluted to half strength when given to a child who has diarrhea. Encourage parents to keep an oral rehydration solution in liquid or powder form on hand at all times and to use these solutions rather than juice or soda when the child first develops diarrhea.

FAMILIES WANT TO KNOW

Preventing Heat-Related Illness

Teach parents, coaches, and youth the following preventive techniques:

- Precede exercise programs with physical examination designed to identify risks.
- Reduce intensity of activity when temperature or humidity is high.
- Allow a 10- to 14-day period of acclimation to higher temperatures before reaching usual exercise level.
- Ensure hydration before activity begins.
- During activity, stop for fluids every 15–20 minutes. Children up to 90 pounds should drink 150 mL (5 ounces) and over 90 pounds should drink 250 mL (9 ounces). A combination of water and sports drink is best.
- Recognize low urine volume or dark color as a sign of dehydration.
- Wear light-colored, light clothing. Never use rubber clothing designed to promote weight loss through sweating.
- Maintain adequate sleep and nutritional status.

Additional tips for coaches:

- Weigh all children before and after events to evaluate if weight, and therefore fluids, are maintained.

- Be familiar with signs of heat-related illness.
- Have cell phones or other mechanisms to call for emergency assistance.
- Have at least two adults present at exercise sessions.
- Keep adequate fluids and sports drinks readily available.
- During all-day practices, allow 2–3 hours rest during the middle of the day with fluids and food provided.
- Practice in shade or use fans, if possible.
- Obtain and use a wet-bulb globe temperature (WBGT) risk measurement that considers humidity (70% of heat stress), radiation (20% of heat stress), and temperature (10% of heat stress). For WBGT < 75°F, activities are allowed with monitoring for heat-related problems; for 75–79°F, enforce longer rest periods in the shade every 15 minutes; for 79–84°F, limit activities for all children and eliminate activity for those not acclimated; and >85°F, cancel all athletic activity.
- Understand symptoms for recognition of all heat-related problems.
- Obtain prompt first aid treatment for any heat-related problems.

Adapted from Binkley, Beckett, Casa, Kleiner, & Plummer, 2002; and Committee on Sports Medicine and Fitness, 2000.

RESEARCH

Use of Oral Rehydration Therapy

In spite of the recommendation of the American Academy of Pediatrics (Provisional Committee on Quality Improvement, 1996) and other groups to use outpatient oral rehydration therapy (ORT) for mild and moderate dehydration, many healthcare providers continue to hospitalize these children and administer intravenous therapy (Nager & Wang, 2002). Hospitalization is expensive and disruptive for families, while care providers state that it seems easier than keeping a child in an outpatient setting for several hours to institute ORT.

Several analyses of studies performed with children have demonstrated the success and efficacy of ORT (Fonseca et al., 2004). In order to study the possibility of decreased treatment time, a study with 96 children from 3 to 36 months of age randomly assigned the moderately dehydrated children to receive either rapid nasogastric hydration or rapid intravenous (IV) hydration. Both methods were accomplished within 3 hours in an emergency department, and were effective in treating children for dehydration. However, the nasogastric rehydration was significantly less expensive. The authors offer the possibility of rapid rehydration as a cost-effective management technique for moderately dehydrated children (Nager & Wang, 2002). In another study of 18 moderately dehydrated children with gastroenteritis, half were given ORT and half were started on intravenous therapy. The length of treatment in the emergency department was significantly lower for the ORT group than the IV group, and ORT required significantly less staff time. Parents reported greater satisfaction with ORT therapy, and the outcomes for the children were comparable (Atherly-John, Cunningham, & Crain, 2002).

Nurses can support ORT for children with mild or moderate dehydration. Teach parents to keep appropriate fluids at home and to institute the therapy early during vomiting and diarrhea episodes. Monitor children receiving the therapy in outpatient settings, whether by traditional oral therapy or rapid nasogastric hydration.

Repeated vomiting of large volumes of fluid or a worsening of the child's condition can indicate the need for intravenous therapy. Teach parents when to seek further medical care. If the child's condition worsens or does not improve after 4 hours of oral rehydration therapy, parents should contact a healthcare professional.

Monitor Intravenous Fluid Administration

The hospitalized child usually requires administration of intravenous fluids. The nurse is usually responsible for starting the intravenous line and administering the prescribed fluids (see Evidence-Based Practice: Intravenous Starts). Be sure that the amount of fluid administered corresponds with the diagnosed dehydration state of the child (Box 16–2).

CLINICAL TIP

A normal saline solution is a salt solution that has the same percentage of salt as the human body. This is a 0.9% solution of sodium chloride. The term *normal* indicates that there is the same weight, in grams, of sodium and chloride in the solution. There are 154 mEq/L of sodium and 154 mEq/L of chloride in normal saline. Normal saline or Ringer's lactate (Ringer's lactate contains carbohydrate and additional electrolytes) may be used for early rehydration. Often more dilute sodium solutions follow such as 1/2 normal saline or 1/4 normal saline. If the child is not taking in oral fluids or food, dilute saline solutions with glucose may be prescribed.

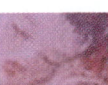

FAMILIES WANT TO KNOW

Oral Rehydration Therapy Guidelines

Calculate the specific amounts required for individual children based on the guidelines below and instruct parents in terminology they understand. Provide measuring devices with proper amounts marked.

- Children with diarrhea and no dehydration should be continued on age-appropriate diets.
- For mild dehydration, give 50 mL/kg oral rehydration therapy in the first 4 hours in addition to replacing fluids lost in stool and emesis. (Measure emesis and give 10 mL/kg of fluid for each diarrheal stool.)
  - Start slowly, administering 3–5 mL in a small cup or spoon every few minutes. Increase amounts gradually if no vomiting occurs.
  - Recommend or provide samples of ORT solutions. Suggest ready to feed or powdered forms for choice by parents.

- For moderate dehydration, give 100 mL/kg oral rehydration therapy in first 4 hours in addition to replacing fluids lost as previously described.
- For severe dehydration, the child is hospitalized and treated with intravenous fluids. When hydrated adequately or concurrently with intravenous rehydration, begin oral rehydration therapy with 50–100 mL/kg of fluid in 4 hours and stool replacement as previously described.
- Recalculate fluid needs after first 4 hours and adjust as needed. If the child is not taking increased fluids and otherwise improving by this time, contact the healthcare provider.
- When rehydration is complete, resume normal diet.

Note: Adapted from Provisional Committee on Quality Improvement, Subcommittee on Acute Gastroenteritis. (1996). Practice parameter: The management of acute gastroenteritis in young children. *Pediatrics, 97,* 424–436.

EVIDENCE-BASED PRACTICE

Intravenous Starts

Problem

Parents often voice dissatisfaction with the number of intravenous starts to which their young hospitalized children are subjected, as children experience pain and anxiety when intravenous lines are started.

Evidence

The Children's Hospital of Denver created a task force to address problems of venous access. Co-chairs in this collaborative project included a nurse from the neonatal intensive care unit, a general surgeon, and a radiologist. Additional nurses from units using peripheral intravenous lines served as committee members. A tracking tool was developed to collect information on intravenous placements for a 1 month period. Other children's hospitals were also surveyed for their practices regarding venous access policies and procedures (The Venous Access Task Force, 2002).

Implications

Based on the analysis of internal and external data, the task force developed recommendations to (1) develop a group of specially trained nurses to act as resources for other staff nurses, (2) create an algorithm to provide guidelines for decisions about peripheral vs. peripherally inserted central venous catheters vs. central venous catheter insertion, (3) use the specially trained nurses to educate staff members about the new algorithm, and (4) develop a tracking/evaluation mechanism for the new algorithm and trained nurse group.

Critical Thinking

This clinical situation is an example of partnership among healthcare specialists in order to improve care for hospitalized children. What were the benefits of having an interdisciplinary group to examine the topic of intravenous starts? How would you suggest that parent satisfaction before and after a program like this be measured? What could be the benefits of having a nursing resource group and an intravenous start guideline to positively influence the hospitalization of young children requiring intravenous infusion for dehydration?

Verify that the type of fluid administered is that which is prescribed. Usually, about half of the 24-hour total maintenance and replacement needs will be given in the first 6 to 8 hours, with a slower rate infused for the remainder of the 24 hours. During the first 1 to 3 hours, the infusion rate may be highest to rapidly expand the vascular space. Rapid infusion of 20 to 30 mL/kg over 1 to 2 hours is sometimes used in outpatient settings, followed by oral fluids. When oral fluids are maintained, the decision for discharge can be made and hospitalization avoided.

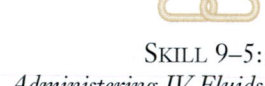

SKILL 9–5:
Administering IV Fluids

Maintain the intravenous line carefully so fluid infusion can be kept on schedule (refer to the *Clinical Skills Manual*). Use a pump to prevent inadvertent, rapid infusion, which can lead to fluid overload and electrolyte imbalance. Play with the toddler and preschool child frequently and use diversionary methods, as necessary, to distract the child from the intravenous line. Monitor the child carefully and implement safety

---

BOX 16–2

CALCULATION OF INTRAVENOUS FLUID NEEDS

1. First, calculate the maintenance fluid needs of the child, according to the following guideline:

Usual Weight	Maintenance Amount
Up to 10 kg	100 mL/kg/24 hr
11–20 kg	1000 mL + (50 mL/kg for weight above 10 kg)/24 hr
>20 kg	1500 mL + (20 mL/kg for weight above 20 kg)/24 hr

   Example: Vernon's weight is 12 kg. He needs 1000 mL + (50 × 2), or 1100 mL/24 hr for maintenance fluid.

2. Next, calculate replacement fluid for that lost:
   Example: Vernon has lost 1 kg (8%) of his body weight. Multiplying the percentage of body weight x 10 yields the mL/kg/24 hr required:

   $$8 \times 10 = 80 \ \text{mL/kg/24 hr}$$
   $$80 \ \text{mL/kg} \times 12 \ \text{kg} = 960 \ \text{mL}$$

   Thus, Vernon's replacement fluid needs are 960 mL/24 hr.
   It is also helpful to know that 1 liter of fluid weighs about 1 kilogram. The amount of fluid deficit can be roughly estimated using this formula. In Vernon's case, since he has lost 1 kg of weight, his replacement fluid need is roughly equivalent to 1 L (1000 mL). This is very close to the 960 mL calculated in the previous formula.

3. Finally, calculate continued losses and add to the total maintenance and replacement needs.

precautions as necessary. Even when an intravenous infusion is used, the child is started on oral rehydration simultaneously. As more oral fluids are tolerated, the intravenous infusion is decreased.

Maintain Safety

The child who is dehydrated is often dizzy and lethargic. Keep side rails up and supervise and assist the child when getting up. Have parents stay at the bedside while the child is being treated in ambulatory units and urge them to maintain safety precautions as they take the child home.

Discharge Planning and Home Care Teaching

Prevention of dehydration is the best approach when possible. Encourage breast-feeding because it is associated with a decreased incidence of gastroenteritis. During health promotion and health maintenance visits, encourage all parents to keep oral rehydration fluids at home in case they are needed. Address the need for increasing fluids in hot weather and when the child is exercising. Reinforce safety teaching to decrease incidence of burns, an important cause of dehydration. Teach the signs and symptoms of gastroenteritis. Indications for bringing a child in for care include:

- Under 6 months or weight of < 8 kg
- Other health problems, premature birth
- Fever of 38°C (100.4°F) for infants < 3 months or 39°C (102.2°F) for child 3–36 months
- Visible blood in stool
- Persistent vomiting and substantial volumes of diarrhea
- Report of symptoms indicative of dehydration
- Change in mental status
- Inability of child to take in ORT or of parent to feed ORT (King, Glass, Bresee, & Duggan, 2003).

Prior to discharge from the hospital or outpatient facility after treatment for dehydration, parents need instructions about types of fluids and amounts to encourage. Teach the signs of dehydration (see Table 16–3) so that if the child does not take in adequate fluids, parents can seek help immediately. Instruct them to begin the child's normal diet once hydration is complete, as determined by adequate urinary output and normal behaviors. Review methods of minimizing the child's chance of acquiring gastrointestinal infections (e.g., avoiding contact with other children who are infected; using careful handwashing and dishwashing procedures when a child in the home is affected).

Nurses should be alert for children in the community who have other health conditions that predispose them to fluid and electrolyte imbalance. Examples include those with cancer, AIDS, cystic fibrosis, and renal disease. When these children are seen for health promotion and health maintenance visits, or because of a health complication, they should be evaluated for fluid and electrolyte imbalance.

Evaluation

Expected outcomes of nursing care for the child with dehydration include the following:

- Water and electrolytes are balanced in intracellular and extracellular compartments.
- Urinary output is within normal limits.
- Adequate fluid intake meets maintenance needs.
- Vital signs are within normal limits.

Extracellular Fluid Volume Excess

Extracellular fluid volume excess occurs when there is too much fluid in the extracellular compartment (vascular and interstitial). This imbalance may also be called saline excess or extracellular volume overload. If this disorder occurs by itself (without saline

COMMUNITY CARE

Dehydration

Dehydration is commonly viewed as an acute care health problem, and in many cases this is the case. Children acquire dehydration from an illness such as gastroenteritis or following surgery or other illness. However, sometimes chronic conditions can lead to dehydration and electrolyte imbalance. The problem may arise over a long period of time and the child's deteriorating condition may not be easily recognized. For this reason, whenever children with conditions that can influence hydration status are seen for health care, such as during health promotion visits, they should have a thorough assessment of nutritional status, fluid intake, and other measures of hydration status (Sarhill, Mahmoud, Christie, & Tahir, 2003). Be alert in particular for children with conditions such as cancer, AIDS, renal disease, and other health problems that influence either intake or output of body fluid.

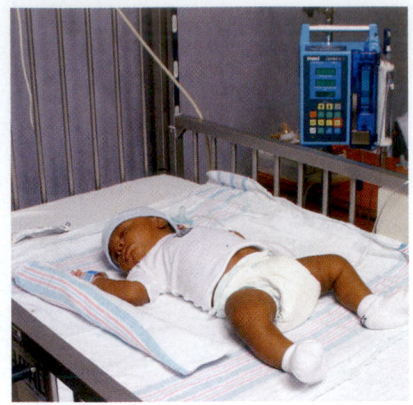

Figure 16–9 ➤ If isotonic fluid containing sodium is given too rapidly or in too great an amount, an extracellular fluid volume excess will develop. It is important to monitor fluid intake, excretion, and retention in infants and children.

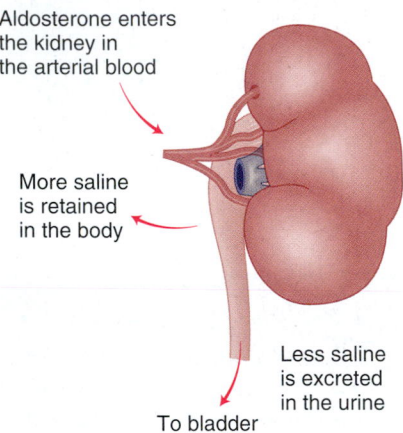

Aldosterone enters the kidney in the arterial blood

More saline is retained in the body

Less saline is excreted in the urine

To bladder

Figure 16–10 ➤ Aldosterone has a saline-retaining effect. Increased aldosterone secretion can be caused by adrenal tumors or congestive heart failure.

> ### CLINICAL TIP
>
> You can tell if a child's weight gain is due to normal growth or to the development of extracellular fluid volume excess by looking at the speed with which the increase develops. Sudden weight gain (e.g., 0.5 kg [1 lb] in 1 day) is due to the accumulation of fluid. Gain of 0.5 kg overnight is due to retention of about 500 mL of saline.

disturbance), the serum sodium concentration is normal. There is simply too much extracellular fluid, even though it has a normal concentration.

Infants and children who develop an extracellular fluid volume excess have a condition that causes them to retain **saline** (sodium and water) or they have been given an overload of sodium-containing isotonic intravenous fluid (Figure 16–9 ➤). What conditions cause retention of saline? The hormone aldosterone is secreted by the adrenal cortex. One of its normal functions is to cause the kidneys to retain saline in the body (Figure 16–10 ➤). Saline excess can be caused by any condition that results in excessive aldosterone secretion, such as adrenal tumors that secrete aldosterone, congestive heart failure, liver cirrhosis, and chronic renal failure (Figure 16–11 ➤). Most glucocorticoid medications (such as prednisone) have a mild saline-retaining effect when taken long term. Intravenous fluid volume regulation is important, especially in young children. Either inaccurate calculation of needed fluid or inadvertent infusion of excess fluids can cause overload.

Because fluid has weight, extracellular fluid volume excess is characterized by weight gain. An overload of fluid in the blood vessels and interstitial spaces can cause clinical manifestations such as bounding pulse, distended neck veins in children (not usually evident in infants), hepatomegaly, dyspnea, orthopnea, and lung crackles. Edema is the sign of overload of the interstitial fluid compartment. In an infant, edema is often generalized. Edema in children with extracellular fluid volume excess occurs in the dependent parts of the body, that is, in the parts closest to the ground. Thus, edema is evident in sacral areas in a child supine in bed. Edema that develops from other causes is described in the next section of this chapter.

Diagnosis of extracellular fluid volume excess is determined by clinical evaluation of weight gain and other manifestations. Serum electrolyte panels aid in diagnosis, and studies of liver or renal function may provide information about the cause of the condition.

Clinical therapy for extracellular fluid volume excess focuses on treating the underlying cause of the disorder in order to reduce the extracellular fluid volume excess. For example, a child who has congestive heart failure is given medications to strengthen the heart's ability to contract (see Chapter 21 ∞). Diuretics may be given to remove fluid from the body, thus reducing the extracellular fluid volume directly.

NURSING MANAGEMENT

Rapid weight gain is the most sensitive index of extracellular fluid volume excess. Therefore, daily weighing is an important nursing assessment. Measure the child's intake and output and weigh the diapers of infants. When treatment is successful, output is greater than intake. Assess the character of the pulse and observe for neck vein distention when the child is sitting (usually visible only in older children). Monitor for signs of pulmonary edema (an indication of severe imbalance) by listening to lung sounds in the dependent lung fields (crackles) and assessing for respiratory distress (rapid respiratory rate, use of accessory muscles of respiration). Observe for edema.

The potential for a child to develop a fluid overload is present whenever an isotonic intravenous solution containing sodium is being administered. Examples of these types of solutions include normal saline (0.9% NaCl), Ringer's solution, and lactated Ringer's solution. Therefore, monitor the infusion rate frequently and carefully and use a pump when possible to aid in accurate administration (Figure 16–12 ➤).

If an excess of fluid has already developed, administer the medical therapy as prescribed and monitor for any complications of the therapy. For example, many diuretics increase potassium excretion in the urine, an increase that may lead to an abnormally low plasma potassium concentration unless potassium intake is increased. (Refer to the discussion of hypokalemia later in this chapter.) It is also important to monitor for the development of extracellular fluid volume deficit as a result of diuretic therapy.

If edema is present, provide careful skin care and protection for edematous areas. Teach parents how to provide skin care and perform position changes at home. See the following section for additional interventions related to edema.

If a child has a long-term condition such as chronic renal failure that predisposes him or her to extracellular fluid volume excess, a dietary sodium restriction may be prescribed (see Chapter 25 ∞ for further details). Teach parents how to manage sodium restriction. Plan low-sodium meals that fit the family's cultural practices. If the child is old enough to participate, incorporate games into the teaching. If a scale is available, teach parents to take and record an accurate daily weight.

Expected outcomes include electrolyte balance, maintenance of intact skin, and dietary intake as prescribed.

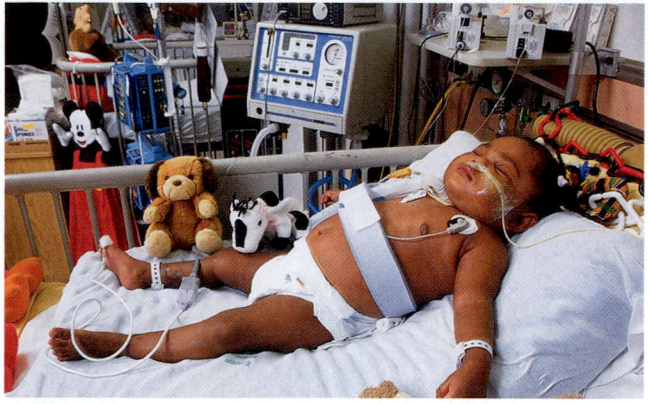

Figure 16–11 ➤ This infant with congenital heart disease has signs of generalized edema. Note the fluid retention in the face and abdomen.

Interstitial Fluid Volume Excess (Edema)

Edema is an abnormal increase in the volume of the interstitial fluid. It may be caused by an extracellular fluid volume excess or it may be due to other causes.

The causes of edema are best understood in the context of normal capillary dynamics. Fluid moves between the vascular and interstitial compartment by the process of filtration. Filtration is the net result of forces that tend to move fluid in opposing directions. The strongest forces will determine the direction of fluid movement.

At the capillary level, two forces (blood hydrostatic pressure and interstitial osmotic pressure) tend to move fluid from the capillaries into the interstitial fluid, while two other forces (blood colloid osmotic pressure and interstitial fluid hydrostatic pressure) tend to move fluid in the opposite direction (from the interstitial fluid into the capillaries). The net result of these forces usually moves fluid from the capillaries into the interstitial compartment at the arterial end of the capillaries and fluid from the interstitial compartment back into the capillaries at the venous end of the capillaries. This process brings oxygen and nutrients to the cells and removes carbon dioxide and other waste products.

Edema occurs if the balance of these four forces is altered so that excess fluid either enters or leaves the interstitial compartment (Pathophysiology Illustrated, Figure 16–13 ➤). This may occur through (1) increased blood hydrostatic pressure, (2) decreased blood colloid osmotic pressure, (3) increased interstitial fluid osmotic pressure, or (4) blocked lymphatic drainage. Various clinical conditions are associated with these altered forces (Box 16–3), as described here.

1. *Increased blood hydrostatic pressure.* When extracellular fluid volume excess occurs, the increased fluid volume in the vascular compartment congests the veins. The pressure against the sides of the capillary is increased and more fluid then enters the interstitial compartment.
2. *Decreased blood colloid osmotic pressure.* Much of the osmotic pressure that pulls fluid into the capillaries is due to the presence of albumin and other plasma proteins made by the liver. The part of the blood osmotic pressure that is due to plasma proteins is often called **oncotic pressure** or blood colloid osmotic pressure. Any condition that decreases plasma proteins will decrease blood colloid osmotic pressure and cause edema. For example, if a clinical condition causes large amounts of albumin to leak into the urine, the liver will not be able to make albumin fast enough to replace it. As a result, the plasma protein level will fall, decreasing the blood osmotic pressure. Without this pulling force to return fluid to the capillaries, edema will occur. This is the cause of the edema that occurs in children who have nephrotic syndrome (see Chapter 25 ∞). Another cause in children is

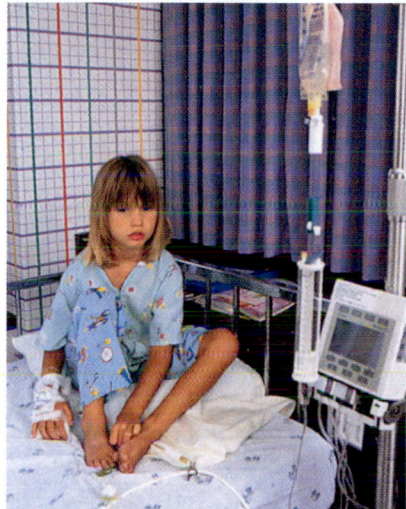

Figure 16–12 ➤ The use of a volume control device with an intravenous saline infusion is important to prevent a sudden extracellular fluid volume overload.

CLINICAL TIP

An infant's urine output is important in monitoring both dehydration and edema. Weigh the diaper before and after use. A 1 g weight increase in the diaper equals approximately 1 mL of urine volume. Change the diaper frequently to minimize loss from evaporation.

PATHOPHYSIOLOGY ILLUSTRATED

Capillary Dynamics and Edema

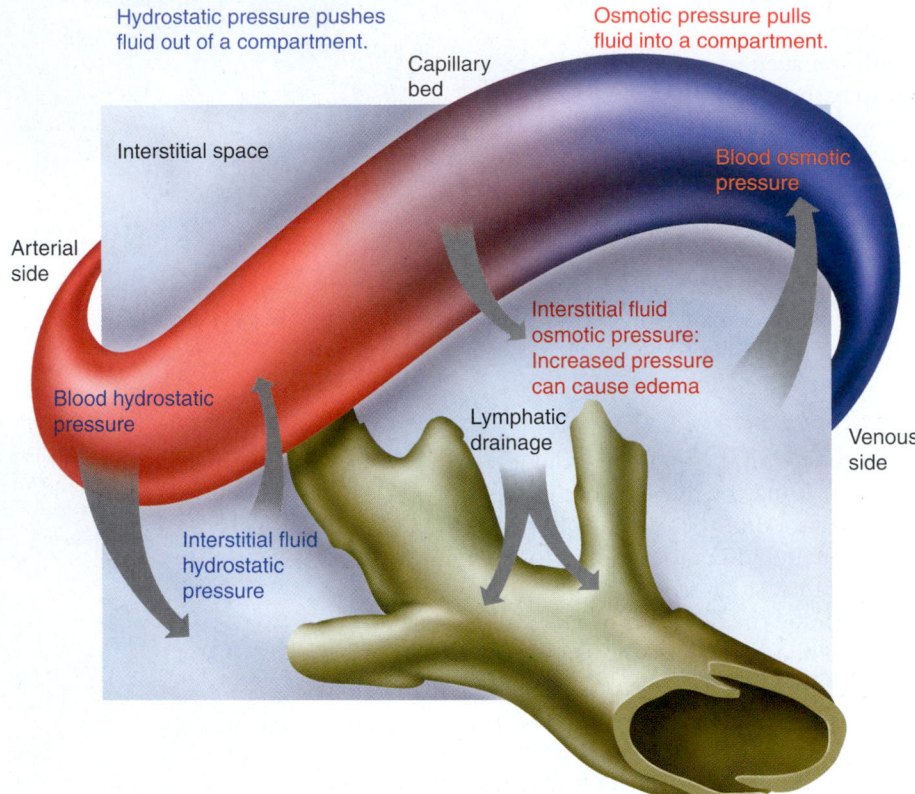

Hydrostatic pressure pushes fluid out of a compartment.

Osmotic pressure pulls fluid into a compartment.

Capillary bed

Interstitial space

Blood osmotic pressure

Arterial side

Interstitial fluid osmotic pressure: Increased pressure can cause edema

Blood hydrostatic pressure

Lymphatic drainage

Venous side

Interstitial fluid hydrostatic pressure

Normally, lymphatic drainage removes small proteins and excess interstitial fluid. Blocked lymphatic drainage can cause edema.

Figure 16–13 ➤ With normal capillary dynamics, fluid moves out of the compartment by the force of hydrostatic pressure in the blood vessel and is pulled out by interstitial osmotic pressure. Fluid is forced into the compartment by interstitial hydrostatic pressure and pulled in by compartment osmotic pressure. Abnormal capillary dynamics cause edema.

NURSING ALERT

Occasionally intravenous fluid is infused too rapidly, endangering the fluid and electrolyte status of a young child. The nurse can take the following measures to minimize this risk:

- Use small bags of fluid, so if the fluid were to infuse quickly, the amount infused would be limited.
- Always use infusion pumps when available so that the rate is programmed and monitored.
- Check and double-check the machine after setting to be sure it was properly programmed.
- Have another nurse check your calculation of rates and total fluid to be infused until you are certain of your skill in this area.
- Finally, remember that even mechanical pumps can have faulty performance, so check the intravenous line, bag, and rate frequently.

prolonged surgical procedures with significant blood loss. Intravenous fluids and blood may be infused during surgery to replace these losses, but plasma proteins are lost and not fully restored by infusion, causing edema in the postoperative period.

3. *Increased interstitial fluid osmotic pressure.* Ordinarily, only a few small proteins enter the interstitial fluid, and the interstitial fluid osmotic pressure is small. If the capillary becomes abnormally permeable to proteins, however, the influx of large amounts of proteins into the interstitial fluid causes a dramatic increase in interstitial fluid osmotic pressure. This increased pulling force keeps an abnormal amount of fluid in the interstitial compartment. This mechanism plays an important part in the edema caused by a bee sting or a sprained ankle. It occurs to a greater extent in burns, leading to swelling at the same time that there is a great loss of fluid volume through the burned skin (see Chapter 30 ∞).

4. *Blocked lymphatic drainage.* The lymph vessels normally drain small proteins and excess fluid from the interstitial compartment and return them to the blood vessels. If this process is blocked, fluid accumulates in the interstitial compartment. This may occur when a tumor blocks lymphatic drainage.

BOX 16–3

CLINICAL CONDITIONS THAT CAUSE EDEMA

Edema Due to Increased Blood Hydrostatic Pressure

Increased Capillary Blood Flow

- Inflammation
- Local infection

Venous Congestion

- Extracellular fluid volume excess
- Right heart failure
- Venous thrombosis
- External pressure on vein
- Muscle paralysis

Edema Due to Decreased Blood Osmotic Pressure

Increased Albumin Excretion

- Nephrotic syndrome (albumin leaks into urine)
- Protein-losing enteropathies (excess albumin in feces)

Decreased Albumin Synthesis

- Kwashiorkor (low-protein, high-carbohydrate starvation diet provides too few amino acids for liver to make albumin)
- Liver cirrhosis (diseased liver unable to make enough albumin)

Edema Due to Increased Interstitial Fluid Osmotic Pressure

Increased Capillary Permeability

- Inflammation
- Toxins
- Hypersensitivity reactions
- Burns

Edema Due to Blocked Lymphatic Drainage

- Tumors
- Goiter
- Parasites that obstruct lymph nodes
- Surgery that removes lymph nodes

CULTURE

Sodium Use

To adapt teaching about low-sodium diets to the cultural practices of a family, ask them what types of food they usually eat. Help them to choose low-sodium foods from their diets and to avoid high-sodium foods. This approach is more effective than giving the same list of restricted foods to each family.

For example, some Asians may use monosodium glutamate to flavor foods and can be encouraged to add this at the table for family members who can have extra sodium rather than during cooking. Many Hispanic groups use large amounts of cheese that can provide significant sodium. Encourage them to look for low-sodium cheese and substitute cottage cheese for other types since it is lower in sodium. Low-sodium milk is available and a good option for young children. Canned foods tend to have high sodium, so teach all families to use fresh or frozen produce rather than canned when possible.

Edema causes swelling, which may be localized or generalized. The swelling of tissue may cause pain and restrict motion. Edema that is due to extracellular fluid volume excess or right-sided heart failure usually occurs in the dependent portion of the body. In a child who is walking, dependent edema is observed in the ankles; in a child who is supine in bed, it is seen in the sacral area. The skin over an edematous area often appears thin and shiny.

The main focus of clinical therapy for edema is to treat the underlying condition that caused the edema. Such conditions are discussed throughout this book. The edema from inflammation of an injury is initially treated with cold to reduce capillary blood flow and thus reduce blood hydrostatic pressure.

■ NURSING MANAGEMENT

A child or parent may make comments that alert the nurse to the development of edema. Shoes may become tight by the end of the day (dependent edema); the waistband of pants or a skirt may be "outgrown" suddenly (generalized edema or ascites, which is accumulation of fluid in the peritoneal cavity); the eyes may be puffy (periorbital edema); a ring may be too tight; fingers may "feel like sausages." In many cases visual inspection is sufficient to recognize edema. Observe for the presence of **pitting edema**, a "pit" or concave indentation that remains after an edematous area is pressed downward by the examiner's fingers. To detect changes in the amount of swelling, measure around the

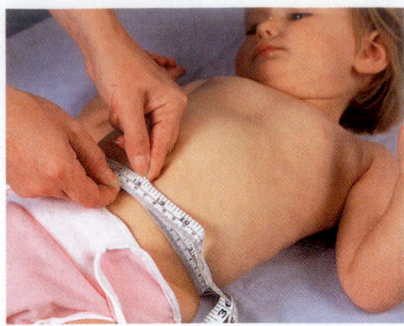

Figure 16–14 ▶ Finding the same location each day for measuring circumference to assess edema can be accomplished by use of a reference point. An indelible marker may be used to mark the measurement location on the skin, if this is acceptable to the child and parents.

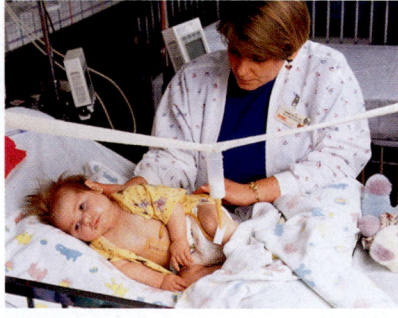

Figure 16–15 ▶ Edematous tissue is easily damaged. It must be kept clean, dry, and free of pressure.

edematous part (Figure 16–14 ▶). If the edema is caused by extracellular fluid volume excess, daily measurements of weight and intake and output are a necessary part of the daily assessment. Nursing assessment should also focus on the integrity of the skin, presence of pain, restricted motion, and alterations in the child's body image.

Elevation of an area of localized edema helps to reduce the swelling. The skin over an edematous area needs extra care because it is fragile (Figure 16–15 ▶). Carefully position an infant or child who is on bed rest and turn frequently to prevent pressure sores (see Chapter 30 ∞ for further information on pressure sores). Turning must be performed carefully to avoid skin abrasion by rubbing against the sheets. Pat the skin dry after cleansing rather than rubbing it. Trim the child's fingernails smooth to prevent scratching. Teach parents skin care for the child at home. Teach older children to inspect their skin carefully to identify areas needing special care.

If restricted mobility is a problem, specific plans to help the child manage activities are needed. For example, if an edematous finger restricts the motion of a hand, food can be cut into bite-size portions before the meal is served, so that the child can still eat independently.

Discomfort from edema may require creative interventions by the nurse. If the child has a fluid restriction, access to fluids needs to be planned to provide satiety. Distraction with toys or activities appropriate to the child's developmental level can be useful. Interventions to treat the underlying problem can also reduce the edema and its accompanying discomfort. Interventions for edema should be added to the nursing management of the underlying condition that causes the edema. Administration of the prescribed medical therapy and observation for the complications of therapy are nursing responsibilities.

Discuss with school-age children and adolescents feelings of embarrassment about the edematous appearance. They need to understand the reason for edema and be able to explain it to peers. Arrange for the child to meet other children with similar concerns.

Desired outcomes of care include maintenance of intact skin, normal respiratory sounds and effort, and normal weight patterns.

ELECTROLYTE IMBALANCES

All body fluids contain electrolytes, although the concentration of those electrolytes varies, depending on the type and location of the fluid. When a serum electrolyte value is reported from the laboratory, it provides information about the concentration of that electrolyte in the blood. It may not necessarily reflect the concentration of the electrolyte in other body compartments. Refer to Table 16–1 to see which electrolytes are of highest and lowest concentration in the blood and other fluid compartments.

Electrolytes are normally gained and lost in relatively equal amounts so the body remains in balance. However, when a child has an abnormal route of loss, such as vomiting, wound drainage, or nasogastric suction, electrolyte balance can be disturbed. Monitoring for signs of imbalance becomes important.

Sodium Imbalances

The serum sodium concentration reflects the **osmolality** of body fluids, that is, their degree of concentration or dilution. It refers to the number of moles of the substance per kilogram of water in the solution. Serum sodium concentration reflects the proportion of water and sodium in the extracellular compartment. When the osmolality of body fluids becomes abnormal, the cells shrink or swell. These cell size changes are due to osmosis, the movement of water across a semipermeable membrane into an area of higher particle concentration. Sodium levels are maintained at high extracellular and low intracellular levels by the sodium-potassium pump, which moves these electrolytes against their expected concentration gradients (Figure 16–16 ▶).

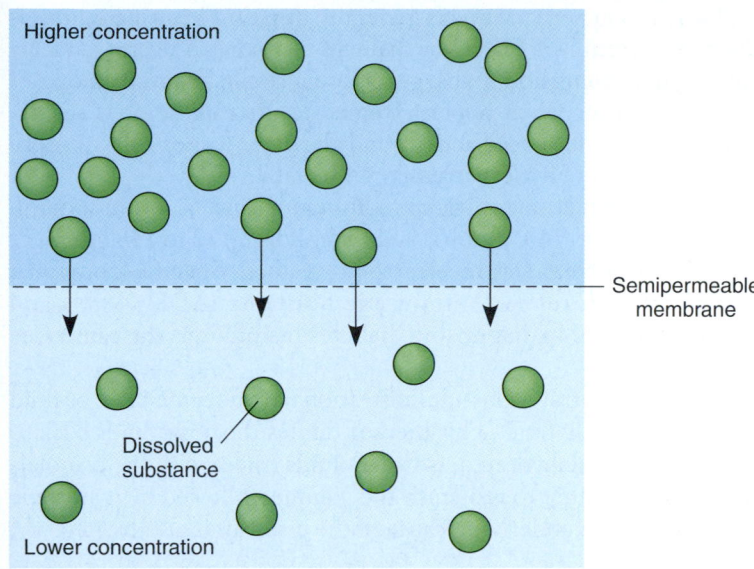

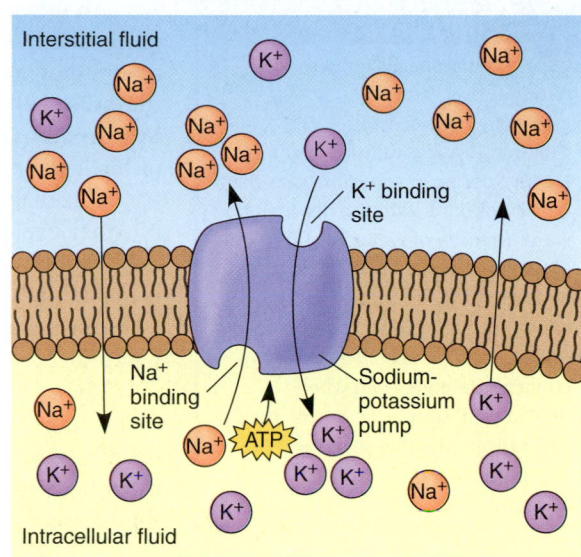

A   B

Figure 16–16 ➤ A, Water balance is maintained by the simple passage of molecules from greater to lesser concentration across cell membranes. B, Sodium levels are maintained by an active transport system, the sodium-potassium pump, which moves these electrolytes across cell membranes in spite of their concentrations. At times, a pathophysiologic condition causes the pump to not function as quickly and efficiently as needed to maintain balance.

Sodium plays several important roles in the body and is an important **cation** (positively charged particle). It is important in blood pressure regulation and maintenance of fluid volume.

Hypernatremia

Hypernatremia is a condition of increased osmolality of the blood. The body fluids are too concentrated, containing excess sodium relative to water. A serum sodium level above 148 mmol/L in children (146 mmol/L in newborns) is diagnostic of hypernatremia.

Hypernatremia results from conditions that cause the body to lose relatively more water than sodium or to gain relatively more sodium than water (Table 16–4). Examples include children who do not have access to adequate water or are developmentally delayed and do not perceive thirst. Special circumstances in which a high solute intake may occur without adequate water include an infant formula that is too concentrated or one that is prepared with salt instead of sugar. A breast-fed baby not receiving adequate breast milk who has normal water loss may develop hypernatremic dehydration. This is a particular risk at 2 to 3 days of age, when babies generally have a diuresis, if the baby does not feed well or the mother does not yet produce an adequate amount of breast milk (Moritz, Manole, Bogen, & Ayus, 2005).

Table 16–4	CAUSES OF HYPERNATREMIA	
Loss of Relatively More Water than Sodium	**Gain of Relatively More Sodium than Water**	
Diabetes insipidus (not enough antidiuretic hormone)	Inability to communicate thirst	
Diarrhea or vomiting without fluid replacement	Limited or no access to water	
Excessive sweating without fluid replacement	High solute intake without adequate water (e.g., tube feedings)	
High solute intake without adequate water (causes kidneys to excrete water)	Intravenous hypertonic saline	

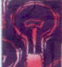
An infant or child who has hypernatremia is generally thirsty. The urine output is diminished unless the hypernatremia is caused by diabetes insipidus. A decreased level of consciousness manifested by confusion, lethargy, or coma results from shrinking of the brain cells. Seizures can occur when hypernatremia occurs rapidly or is severe. Symptoms in the neonate include decreased activity and alertness, loss of 10% or more of birth weight, and seizures. Severe hypernatremia can be fatal.

The major laboratory test that is diagnostic of sodium imbalance is serum sodium. Normal level for newborns is 131 to 146 mmol/L and for children 132 to 148 mmol/L. See Table 16–5 for a list of normal serum electrolyte values. Specific gravity of urine is concentrated in hypernatremia. Antidiuretic hormone (ADH) levels and 24-hour urinary output are helpful in diagnosing diabetes insipidus as the cause (see Chapter 30).

Hypernatremia is treated by intravenous administration of **hypotonic fluid**, or fluid that is more dilute than normal body fluid. This therapy dilutes the body fluids back to normal concentration. If a child is dehydrated, **isotonic fluids** (those with the osmolality of body fluids) may be ordered first to replenish the volume, followed by hypotonic fluid to correct the osmolality. The underlying cause of the disorder is also treated.

■ NURSING MANAGEMENT

Teaching can prevent many cases of hypernatremia. Be sure the breast-feeding mother has instruction and resources about lactation before discharge after delivery. If discharged soon after birth, be sure the infant has an appointment to have weight and alertness checked within the first few days, and instruct the parents about normal output of four to six wet diapers daily. By about 10 days, infants should have regained the birth weight. Assess the infant's alertness and general neurological status.

When an infant is sick or developing slowly, parents sometimes want to feed the infant more concentrated formula to build the child's strength. Parents and caregivers of bottle-fed babies should be taught never to give undiluted formula concentrate or evaporated milk due to the high sodium content.

Children with delayed development are at risk for hypernatremia since they may not be able to recognize thirst or obtain fluids when dehydrated. Teach parents about the child's fluid requirements and ensure that nursing staff offers adequate fluids when the child is hospitalized.

Parents should be cautioned to keep salt out of reach, because eating handfuls of salt has caused hypernatremia. Teach parents to offer extra fluids during hot weather. See Families Want to Know: Preventing Heat-Related Illness on page 508. Teach oral rehydration therapy for use at home during mild vomiting and diarrhea (see page 509).

Table 16–5	**NORMAL SERUM VALUES FOR ELECTROLYTES IN INFANTS AND YOUTH**	
	Newborn	**Infant and Child**
Sodium	131–144 mmol/L	132–141 mmol/L
Potassium	Premature 4.5–7.2 mmol/L Term 3.2–5.7 mmol/L	3.3–4.7 mmol/L
Calcium	Premature 3.5–4.5 mEq/L (1.7–2.3 mmol/L) Term 4–5 mEq/L (2–2.5 mmol/L)	4.4–5.3 mEq/L (2.2–2.7 mmol/L)
Magnesium	1.3–2.7 mg/dL (0.5–1.1 mmol/L)	1.6–2.7 mg/dL (0.7–1.1 mmol/L)

*Note: Laboratories may have slightly different levels of normal depending on assays performed. Always consult the normal values for your particular laboratory.

When a child is hospitalized for hypernatremia, monitor serum sodium level and measure intake and output and urine specific gravity. Specific gravity changes toward normal levels as therapy progresses. Frequently assess responsiveness to monitor the effect of hypernatremia on brain cells. As the concentration of body fluids returns to normal, the child will become more alert and responsive. Watch for rebound hyponatremia while monitoring the fluid replacement. Implement safety interventions such as raised bed rails for protection. Ensure adequate rest and introduce developmentally appropriate activities when the child is alert.

Water deprivation is a form of child neglect or abuse. In neglect, the parents simply do not provide adequate water for the child. A form of child abuse that sometimes includes water deprivation is Munchausen syndrome by proxy (see Chapter 6 ∞). A small child who is hospitalized with hypernatremia that does not have a detectable cause may be subject to water deprivation. Assess the child's general condition, developmental tasks, the family dynamics, and the parent's understanding of formula preparation and the child's fluid intake needs.

Nurses can prevent hypernatremia in hospitalized infants and children by administering water between tube feedings, keeping water available, and offering it frequently. Offering frequent small amounts and using Popsicles and other creative interventions can increase children's intake.

Desired outcomes of treatment for hypernatremia include balance of electrolytes and fluid in the intracellular and extracellular compartments, as well as alert level of consciousness.

Hyponatremia

In hyponatremia, the osmolality of the blood is decreased. The body fluids are too dilute, and contain excess water relative to sodium. Hyponatremia is the most common sodium imbalance in children (Greenbaum, 2004). A serum sodium level below 135 mmol/L in children (133 mmol/L in newborns) is diagnostic of hyponatremia.

ETIOLOGY AND PATHOPHYSIOLOGY   Hyponatremia results from conditions that cause gain of relatively more water than sodium or loss of relatively more sodium than water (Table 16–6). Oral intake of water causes hyponatremia in unusual conditions such as forced fluid intake. More commonly, parents feed an infant only water or dilute formula to save money instead of regular-strength formula or breast milk. Excessive swallowing of swimming pool water by an infant can have the same effect. Infants are vulnerable to the type of hyponatremia caused by water intoxication, because they have a poorly developed thirst mechanism and may continue to drink, and then are unable to excrete excess water quickly due to immature kidney function (Chamley, Carson, Randall, & Sandwell, 2005). Exercise-associated hyponatremia can occur when persons in prolonged physical activity such as marathon running consume hypotonic fluids in the form of water or sports drinks above the levels lost in respiratory,

Table 16–6	**CAUSES OF HYPONATREMIA**	

Gain of Relatively More Water than Sodium	**Loss of Relatively More Sodium than Water**
Excessive intravenous D_5W (5% dextrose in water) rather than isotonic fluids for hospitalized children	Diarrhea or vomiting with replacement by tap water only instead of fluid containing sodium
Excessive tap water enemas	Excessive sweating such as in cystic fibrosis
Irrigation of body cavities with distilled water	Diuretics, especially thiazides
Excessive antidiuretic hormone	
Forced excessive oral intake of tap water	
Excessive intake of water during exercise	
Congestive heart failure	

gastrointestinal, skin, and urinary routes (Exercise-Associated Hyponatremia Consensus Panel, 2005). Hospitalized children who are treated with hypotonic saline rather than isotonic solutions can also acquire hyponatremia. Young children are at particular risk because they commonly respond to surgery with increased levels of antidiuretic hormone (ADH) for 3 to 5 days postsurgery, causing decreased excretion of urine; use of hypotonic solutions during this period can cause hyponatremia. Additionally, they have a high brain-to-skull mass and are therefore at high risk of developing the neurologic complications of hyponatremia (Moritz & Ayus, 2003).

CLINICAL MANIFESTATIONS The child who has hyponatremia has a decreased level of consciousness, which results from edema of brain cells. Manifestations include anorexia, nausea, vomiting, confusion, headache, respiratory distress, muscle weakness, decreased deep tendon reflexes, agitation, lethargy, or confusion. The condition can progress to respiratory arrest, dilated pupils, decorticate posturing, and coma. If hyponatremia arises rapidly or is extreme, seizures may occur, and is a frequent cause of seizures in infants under 6 months of age. Severe hyponatremia can be fatal.

■ COLLABORATIVE CARE

Laboratory analysis of plasma or serum demonstrates a low sodium level.

Hyponatremia should be prevented in hospitalized children receiving intravenous solutions (particularly postoperatively) by administering isotonic rather than hypotonic solutions. In cases of improper formula preparation or fluid intake, hyponatremia is treated by feeding proper formula or restricting the intake of water. This therapy allows the kidneys to correct the imbalance by excreting excess water from the body. Intravenous **hypertonic fluid** (more concentrated than body fluid) may be administered for severe cases. Use of this concentrated saline is a way to rapidly increase body fluid concentration, but it must be monitored carefully because it can easily cause rebound hypernatremia. For exercise-associated hyponatremia, intravenous access is established at the first-aid site, hypertonic saline is administered, and oxygen is delivered (Exercise-Associated Hyponatremia Consensus Panel, 2005). In cases of diabetes insipidus, treatment for the condition is needed (see Chapter 29 ∞).

■ NURSING MANAGEMENT
Nursing Assessment and Diagnosis

Monitor serum sodium level and measure intake and output. If an infant with hyponatremia has normal antidiuretic hormone (ADH) levels, and other causes have been ruled out, careful questioning about proper preparation of formula and feeding practices is needed. A toddler or school-age child may be subjected to forced fluid intake as a form of child abuse. Sensitive interviewing and a caring manner on the part of the nurse can help identify such problems in a family.

Because hyponatremia is characterized by a decreased level of consciousness, frequent assessment of responsiveness will be necessary to monitor the response to therapy. The child will become more alert and responsive as the concentration of body fluids returns to normal. Carefully monitor hospitalized children and those exercising for signs of hyponatremia.

The highest priority nursing diagnosis for hyponatremia addresses the risk for injury related to the child's decreased level of consciousness and cerebral edema. The following nursing diagnoses might also apply:

- Self-Care Deficit related to weakness and fatigue
- Altered Health Maintenance related to parental information misinterpretation about infant formula
- Ineffective Breast-Feeding related to inadequate sucking by infant or inadequate milk production

Planning and Implementation

Nurses can prevent hyponatremia in hospitalized children by using normal saline instead of distilled water for irrigations and by avoiding tap water enemas. Verify intravenous types and amounts and question use of hypotonic fluids in a child with no intake of sodium. Teach parents to replace body fluids lost through diarrhea or vomiting with oral electrolyte solutions (see discussion of oral rehydration therapy earlier in this chapter). Teach the person with prolonged exercise to slowly increase exercise times, rehydrate according to thirst, and ensure intake of sodium-containing fluids. The child with diseases such as cystic fibrosis or who is taking thiazide diuretics needs intake above that recommended for usual maintenance needs.

Evaluation

Expected outcomes of nursing care for hyponatremia include the following:

- The child remains safe from injury.
- Balance of fluid and electrolytes is maintained.
- Proper intake of formula, breast milk, and other fluids is established.

Potassium Imbalances

Potassium is an essential **anion** (negatively charged particle) that performs many necessary functions in the body. It is present in high levels in intracellular fluids and is active in enzyme performance in cells. It is needed for contractility of heart and skeletal muscle. Potassium intake in healthy children comes from potassium-rich foods such as fruits and vegetables. Potassium is absorbed easily from the intestine.

A potassium imbalance arises when the serum potassium concentration rises or falls outside the normal range. Potassium imbalances are caused by alterations in potassium intake, distribution, or excretion; or by loss of potassium through an abnormal route such as burns, emesis, or renal failure.

Most of the potassium ions in the body are found inside the cells. The sodium-potassium pump in cell membranes moves potassium ions into cells to maintain the high intracellular potassium concentration (see Figure 16–13). In addition, potassium ions can be shifted into or out of cells by various physiologic factors (Figure 16–17 ➤). Potassium is excreted from the body through urine, feces, and sweat. The hormone aldosterone increases potassium excretion in the urine.

Hyperkalemia

Hyperkalemia, an excess of potassium in the blood, is reflected by a level above 5.8 mmol/L in children or above 5.2 mmol/L in newborns.

ETIOLOGY AND PATHOPHYSIOLOGY   Hyperkalemia is caused by conditions that involve increased potassium intake, shift of potassium from cells into the extracellular fluid, and decreased potassium excretion. Renal insufficiency is a primary cause

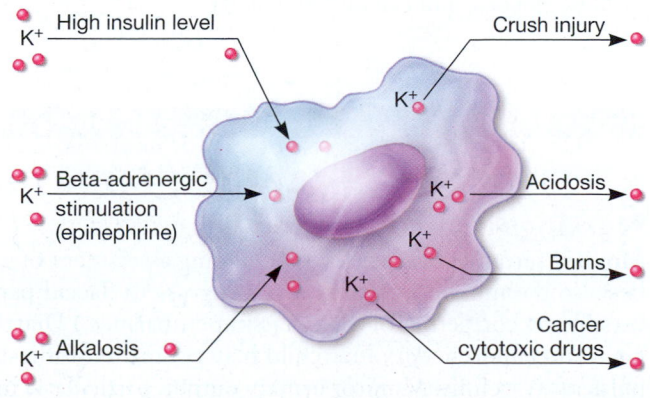

Figure 16–17 ➤ Factors that shift potassium ions into or out of cells.

NURSING ALERT

Drugs that may cause hyperkalemia:

Potassium-containing preparations
Cytotoxic agents
Potassium-sparing diuretics
Angiotensin-converting enzyme inhibitors
Nonsteroidal anti-inflammatory analgesics
Beta-blockers
Heparin
Nonsteroidal anti-inflammatories
Trimethoprim-sulfamethoxazole antibiotic

CLINICAL TIP

If an infant's hyperkalemia was diagnosed using blood obtained from a heel stick, intracellular fluid may have contaminated the sample. A venous sample should be obtained. Additionally, it is possible for a blood sample to be damaged and show increased potassium when tested. If there is an absence of symptoms in the child, obtain a repeat sample for analysis to verify results.

of hyperkalemia (Burger, 2004a). Increased potassium intake is usually due to intravenous potassium overload. Excessive or too rapid intravenous administration of potassium-containing solutions can occur if the potassium requirement is overestimated or if the intravenous infusion runs in too quickly.

Blood transfusion is another source of potassium intake that may cause hyperkalemia. Potassium ions leak out of red blood cells that are stored in a blood bank. The longer the blood is stored, the more potassium leaks out of cells and accumulates in the fluid portion of the transfusion. Hyperkalemia from administration of stored blood arises when multiple units are transfused, as when infants receive exchange transfusions or children receive multiple blood transfusions after a serious injury or in surgery.

Shift of potassium from cells into the extracellular fluid occurs when there is massive cell death, as with a crush injury, in sickle-cell anemia (hemolytic crisis), or when chemotherapy for a malignancy is rapidly effective. In these situations, the dead cells release their high-potassium contents into the extracellular fluid. Potassium ions also shift out of cells in metabolic acidosis caused by diarrhea and in diabetes mellitus when insulin levels are low.

Decreased potassium excretion occurs with acute or chronic oliguria during renal failure, severe hypovolemia, and conditions that decrease the secretion of aldosterone by the adrenal cortex (lead poisoning, Addison's disease, hypoaldosteronism). Several medications can cause hyperkalemia.

CLINICAL MANIFESTATIONS   All clinical manifestations of hyperkalemia are related to muscle dysfunction because potassium plays a vital role in muscle activity. Hyperactivity of gastrointestinal smooth muscle causes intestinal colic, cramping, and diarrhea in some children. The skeletal muscles become weak, beginning typically with leg weakness and then ascending up the body. Weakness can progress to flaccid paralysis. The child is often lethargic. Dysfunction of cardiac muscle causes cardiac arrhythmias such as tachycardia and may result in heart failure and cardiac arrest. Abnormalities in the electrocardiogram include a prolonged QRS complex, a peak in T waves, and prolonged PR intervals. Renal signs include oliguria and anuria (Burger, 2004a).

COLLABORATIVE CARE

The major diagnostic tool is the serum laboratory test for potassium. In addition, observations of symptoms and abnormal electrocardiograph are indicative of hyperkalemia. Hyperkalemia is treated by management of the underlying condition that caused the imbalance. For mild cases, intake of potassium is restricted, and loop or thiazide diuretics may be administered. If the serum potassium concentration is very high or is causing dangerous cardiac arrhythmias, treatment to decrease the serum potassium level may be ordered. These treatments may remove potassium from the body or drive it from the extracellular fluid into the cells. Potassium is removed from the body by peritoneal dialysis or hemodialysis, and with a cation exchange resin (Kayexalate) or 70% sorbitol, both of which can be administered orally or rectally. Medical treatments that drive potassium ions into cells are intravenous sodium bicarbonate, intravenous insulin, glucose, and calcium gluconate.

NURSING MANAGEMENT
Nursing Assessment and Diagnosis

Monitor serum potassium levels. Ongoing assessment of muscle strength is important, because the muscle weakness may progress to flaccid paralysis. (This paralysis is reversible on correction of the potassium imbalance.) Diarrhea or colic can occur in infants and children. An older child may complain of intestinal cramping. Monitor the pulse rate carefully. Monitor urinary output, particularly in children with renal disease.

Nursing diagnoses for a child who has hyperkalemia depend on the severity of the clinical manifestations. The cause of the imbalance may also lead to useful diagnoses that guide teaching for the child and the parents regarding safety measures and accurate medication administration. The following nursing diagnoses may apply:

- Activity Intolerance related to decreased cardiac output secondary to cardiac arrhythmias
- Risk for Injury related to muscle weakness
- Self-Care Deficit: Hygiene and Dressing related to neuromuscular impairment
- Anxiety related to change in health status
- Ineffective Health Maintenance related to parental lack of exposure to potassium intake in chronic renal failure
- Ineffective Management of Therapeutic Regimen related to complexity of therapy

Planning and Implementation

Nursing care includes measures to prevent hyperkalemia from developing in hospitalized children. If hyperkalemia does develop, care shifts to administering intravenous solutions, monitoring cardiopulmonary status continuously, ensuring safety, promoting adequate nutrition, and preparing the child and family for discharge. For the child in the community, potassium levels are monitored when the child is taking a drug that can cause hyperkalemia, such as those used for cancer treatment.

Prevent Hyperkalemia

Any child who is receiving an intravenous infusion that contains potassium is at risk for hyperkalemia. Check that urine output is normal before administering intravenous potassium solutions. Observe the child closely and perform cardiorespiratory monitoring.

Be sure blood or packed red blood cells are fresh, especially for the child receiving multiple transfusions and for all neonates. Use a cardiac monitor during infusion of these products to watch for arrhythmias.

Administer Intravenous Solutions

Once a child is diagnosed as hyperkalemic, ensure that any infusions with added potassium are stopped. Several infusions may need to be managed, including glucose, bicarbonate, and calcium gluconate. Maintain the infusion at the ordered rate and monitor the child's condition frequently.

Monitor Cardiopulmonary Status

Upon diagnosis of hyperkalemia, an electrocardiogram is performed and a cardiac monitor is applied. Monitor for any changes in cardiac status and for cardiac arrhythmias. Report abnormal rate and character of pulse as well as shortness of breath.

Ensure Safety

Since the child is weak, side rails should be raised. Position the child carefully. Assist the child with activities requiring leg muscle strength, such as going to the bathroom, climbing into bed, or pushing up in bed. Encourage quiet activities appropriate for developmental level with frequent rest periods. Document and report any change in muscle weakness.

Promote Adequate Nutritional Intake

Adequate caloric intake is necessary to prevent tissue breakdown and the resultant potassium release from cells. Offer the child nourishing snacks if his or her appetite is decreased. Restrict potassium-rich foods.

Discharge Planning and Home Care Teaching

If the child has chronic renal failure or another condition that decreases aldosterone secretion, parents and the child need to be taught to restrict foods that are high in potassium (Families Want to Know: Potassium-Rich Foods). Most oral rehydration solutions, including Pedialyte, contain potassium and should not be used to provide fluid

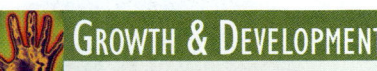

GROWTH & DEVELOPMENT

Hyperkalemia
The nursing diagnoses for children with hyperkalemia will prompt a nurse to provide safety measures appropriate to the child's developmental level and to assist the child with activities that muscle weakness makes difficult. It is important to provide play and diversional activities that take into account both the child's degree of muscle strength and the appropriate developmental level.

for the child. Instruct the family not to use salt substitutes, which commonly contain potassium. Parents should check with the care provider and pharmacist before giving even over-the-counter products to the child, as some of these medications contain potassium. Management of renal failure at home with frequent visits for dialysis and other treatments can be challenging. Refer to Chapter 25 ∞ for further suggestions to help parents handle this condition.

Evaluation

Expected outcomes of nursing care for hyperkalemia include the following:

- The child returns to a state of fluid and electrolyte balance.
- Safety is maintained.
- The child receives adequate nutritional intake to provide essential potassium.
- Normal cardiac rate and rhythm is maintained.

Hypokalemia

Hypokalemia occurs when the serum potassium concentration is too low. Total body potassium may be decreased, normal, or even increased when the serum level is low, depending on the cause of the imbalance. Serum potassium levels below 3.5 mmol/L in children (3.7 mmol/L for newborns) are diagnostic of hypokalemia.

Etiology and Pathophysiology

Hypokalemia is caused by conditions that involve increased potassium excretion, decreased potassium intake, shift of potassium from the extracellular fluid into cells, and loss of potassium by an abnormal route.

Increased potassium excretion through the gastrointestinal tract is the major cause of hypokalemia in children (Burger, 2004b). Loss of potassium occurs through vomiting and diarrhea (gastroenteritis). In the chapter opening vignette, Vernon had increased potassium excretion through diarrhea. Self-induced vomiting in bulimia is another example of this cause. Nasogastric suctioning (Figure 16–18 ➤) and intestinal decompression can cause potassium loss.

Causes of increased urinary potassium excretion are osmotic diuresis (glucose present in urine), hypomagnesemia, hypercalcemia, increased aldosterone (hyperaldosteronism, congestive heart failure, nephrotic syndrome, cirrhosis), and increased cortisol (Cushing's disease and syndrome). Eating large amounts of black licorice made from the root of *Glycyrrhiza glabra* increases renal retention of sodium and excretion of potassium (Burger, 2004b).

Decreased potassium intake will lead to hypokalemia slowly, or more rapidly if combined with increased excretion or loss of potassium. Hospitalized children may be placed on NPO status and receive prolonged intravenous therapy without potassium.

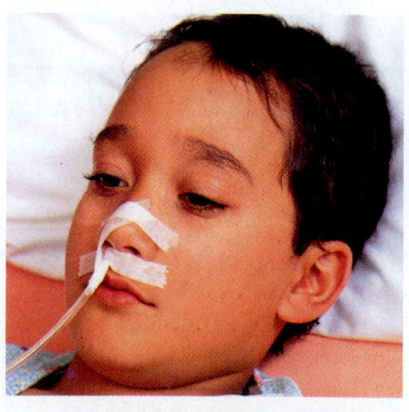

Figure 16–18 ➤ Because this child has a nasogastric tube in place that requires suctioning, it is important to monitor his potassium levels.

Adolescents concerned about weight loss or those with anorexia nervosa may embark on diets low in potassium and may take medications that induce diuresis or diarrhea.

Shift of potassium from the extracellular fluid into cells occurs in alkalosis and hypothermia (unintentional or induced for surgery). Hyperalimentation often causes hypersecretion of insulin, which also shifts potassium into cells. Hypokalemia can also be caused by several medications.

Clinical Manifestations

Since the ratio of intracellular to extracellular potassium determines the responsiveness of muscle cells to neural stimuli, it is not surprising that the clinical manifestations of hypokalemia involve muscle dysfunction. Gastrointestinal smooth muscle activity is slowed, leading to diminished bowel tones, abdominal distention, constipation, or paralytic ileus. Skeletal muscles are weak and unresponsive to stimuli, deep tendon reflexes are diminished, and weakness may progress to flaccid paralysis. The respiratory muscles may be impaired. Cardiac arrhythmias can occur, particularly a prolonged QT interval, depressed ST segment, and flat or inverted T waves. Polyuria, polydipsia, and decreased urine specific gravity result from changes in the kidney caused by hypokalemia (Burger, 2004b; English, 2002).

■ COLLABORATIVE CARE

The major diagnostic tool is the serum laboratory test for potassium. In addition, observations of symptoms and an abnormal electrocardiograph are indicative of hypokalemia. Medical management of hypokalemia focuses on replacement of potassium while treating the cause of the imbalance. Potassium replacement may be given intravenously or orally.

■ NURSING MANAGEMENT
Nursing Assessment and Diagnosis

Monitor serum potassium levels. Observe for muscle weakness, which is frequently detected first in the legs. Parents may report that muscle weakness restricts the child's activities and impairs interactions with peers. Skeletal muscle strength can be difficult to assess if the child is lethargic, as shown with Vernon at the beginning of the chapter.

Muscle weakness may affect the respiratory muscles. Assess the child frequently to determine the need for assisted ventilation. Cardiac monitoring is important for continued assessment of hypokalemia-associated arrhythmias.

Assess for diminished bowel sounds. Ask the parents if the child has recently been awakening to use the toilet at night or has begun bedwetting after previously being dry at night. These may be symptoms of polyuria associated with chronic hypokalemia.

The most important nursing diagnoses in the child with severe hypokalemia relate to cardiac arrhythmias and respiratory muscle weakness. The following nursing diagnoses may apply:

- Risk for Activity Intolerance related to decreased cardiac output secondary to cardiac dysrhythmias
- Ineffective Breathing Pattern related to respiratory musculoskeletal impairment
- Risk for Injury related to muscle weakness
- Self-Care Deficit: Hygiene and Dressing related to neuromuscular impairment
- Constipation related to decreased motility
- Anxiety related to change in health status
- Ineffective Health Maintenance related to management of potassium supplements or high-potassium diet

---

NURSING ALERT

Drugs that may cause hypokalemia:
Beta-adrenergic agonists
Insulin
Potassium-wasting diuretics
Parenteral penicillins
Glucocorticoids
Aminoglycoside antimicrobials
Systemic antifungals
Antineoplastics
Laxatives, especially when abused
Osmotic diuretics (mannitol)

- Ineffective Management of Therapeutic Regimen related to complexity of potassium therapy
- Imbalanced Nutrition: Less than Body Requirements related to lack of basic nutritional knowledge regarding safe weight-loss diet

Planning and Implementation

Nursing care of the child with hypokalemia focuses on ensuring adequate potassium intake, monitoring cardiopulmonary status, promoting normal bowel function, ensuring safety, providing dietary counseling, and preparing the child and family for discharge.

Ensure Adequate Potassium Intake

Since potassium is excreted from the body every day, daily potassium intake is necessary to prevent hypokalemia. A hypokalemic child who is able to eat should be given a high-potassium diet. Teach parents (and the child if old enough) which foods are high in potassium and how to incorporate them into the daily diet (see Families Want to Know on page 524).

Children who have no oral intake for a period of time should receive intravenous fluids that contain potassium. Calculate the dosage to ensure accuracy, and be sure that the infusion runs on schedule. Sometimes the child will complain of burning along the vein when potassium is infused. The infusion may need to be slowed temporarily to relieve pain and maintain the intravenous line. Remain vigilant to maintain patency of the vein in order to avoid infiltration, which can cause phlebitis and pain. A central line is a better choice than a peripheral line in order to decrease side effects of administration. Consult the hospital formulary for dilution and administration guidelines; it must be administered slowly to avoid arrhythmias and cardiac arrest. Ensure adequate fluid output for the child's age to avoid hyperkalemia from potassium infusion.

Check serum potassium for high or low potassium levels. Analyze other electrolytes and acid-base balance. Monitor urine output. An oliguric child can develop hyperkalemia when receiving supplements.

Monitor Cardiopulmonary Status

Hypokalemia potentiates digitalis toxicity. A hypokalemic child who is receiving digitalis needs careful surveillance for digitalis toxicity, which is manifested as anorexia, nausea, vomiting, and bradycardia. Observe for these effects. Take the pulse rate and rhythm regularly. Monitor respirations and ease of breathing to watch for decreased respiratory muscle activity.

Promote Normal Bowel Function

Ensure adequate fluids and fiber in the diet. Monitor and record the number of stools and report inadequate stools.

Ensure Safety

Keep side rails up. Assist the child as needed to move into and out of bed. Reposition the child frequently to preserve the skin integrity of limbs that are not moved regularly. Perform passive range of motion if the child is not moving. Use supportive pillows to position the child properly.

Provide Dietary Counseling

The adolescent who is trying to lose weight and not consuming a nutritious diet needs dietary teaching. More intensive treatment will be needed for teens who are anorexic or bulimic (see Chapter 4 ∞ for interventions in these cases).

Discharge Planning and Home Care Teaching

Teach parents how to give potassium supplements, if prescribed. Liquid or powdered potassium supplements can be mixed with juice or sherbet to improve the bitter taste. The parent should call the mixture "medicine" so that the child does not learn to dislike all juices. Teach the parents signs of both hypokalemia and hyperkalemia and whom to call to report these symptoms. The signs must be reported promptly so medications can be adjusted.

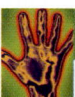

GROWTH & DEVELOPMENT

Bradycardia

Bradycardia occurs at a different level for children of various ages.

For infants, a pulse rate below 100 is considered bradycardia. For young children, 80 may be the identified number, whereas for adolescents, a pulse below 60 is bradycardia. Look at the child's age and normal pulse range to find changes that indicate bradycardia.

Evaluation

Expected outcomes of nursing care during hypokalemia include the following:

- Normal rate and rhythm of heart and respiratory system is maintained.
- Regular bowel movements are established.
- The child is free from injury.
- The child and family have adequate knowledge regarding food sources of potassium.

Calcium Imbalances

A normal serum calcium concentration is important for many physiologic functions, including muscle and nerve function, secretion of hormones, bone formation and strength, and clotting of the blood. Calcium is the most abundant mineral in the body, and about 98% of it is located in the bones (Roberts, 2005). There are three forms of calcium in plasma—calcium bound to protein, calcium bound to small organic ions (e.g., citrate), and free ionized calcium (Ca^{++}), the only physiologically active form. A discussion of dietary calcium intake and its importance for bone formation can be found in Chapter 4.

Calcium imbalances are caused by alterations in calcium intake, absorption, distribution, or excretion. Calcium absorption requires vitamin D for maximum efficiency and is greatest in the duodenum. Calcium distribution involves calcium entry into and exit from bones and the distribution of different forms of calcium in the plasma. Excretion of calcium occurs in urine, feces, and sweat (Figure 16–19 ➤).

Parathyroid hormone is the major regulator of the plasma calcium concentration. It increases this concentration by increasing calcium absorption, increasing calcium withdrawal from bones, and decreasing calcium excretion in the urine. The plasma calcium

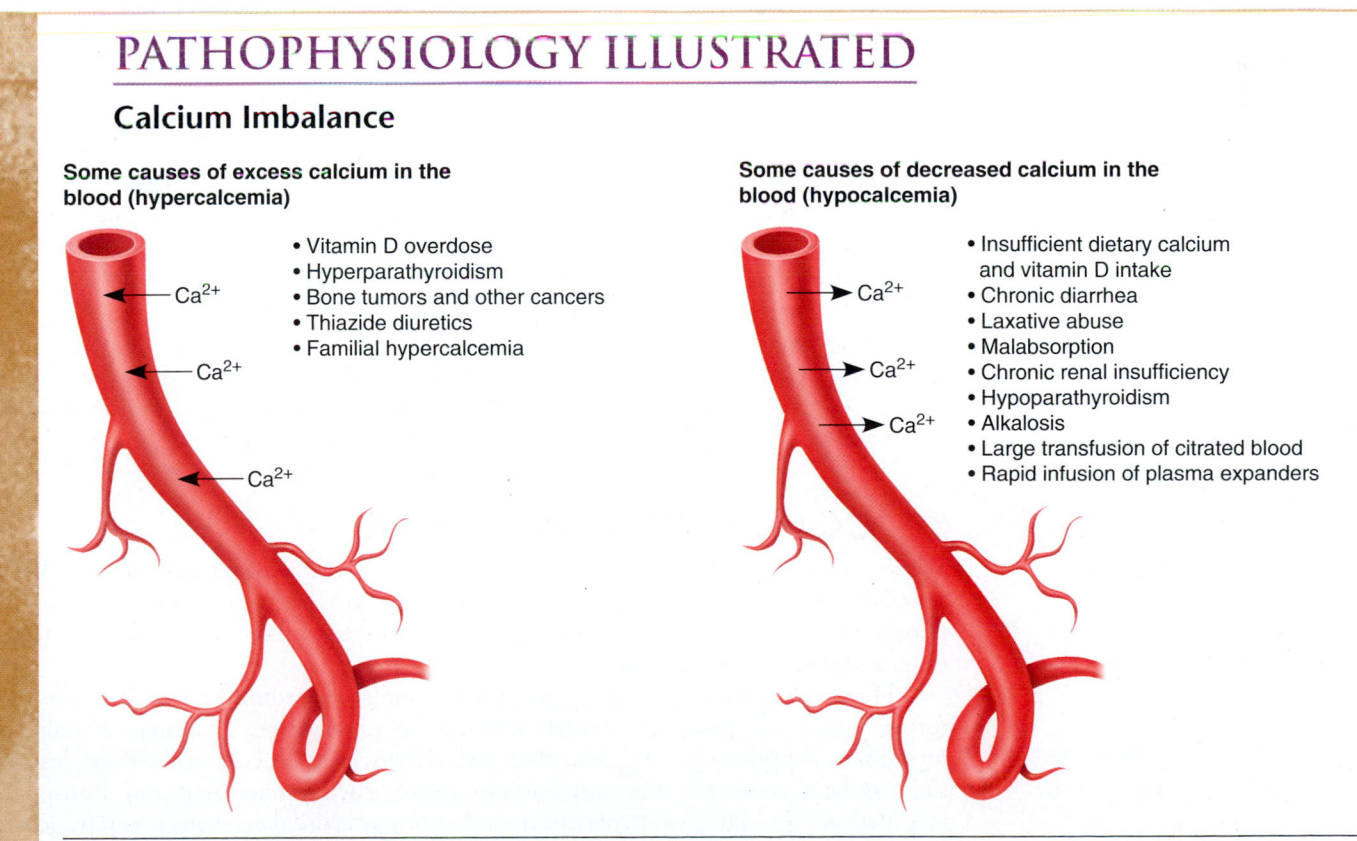

PATHOPHYSIOLOGY ILLUSTRATED

Calcium Imbalance

Some causes of excess calcium in the blood (hypercalcemia)

Ca^{2+}
Ca^{2+}
Ca^{2+}

- Vitamin D overdose
- Hyperparathyroidism
- Bone tumors and other cancers
- Thiazide diuretics
- Familial hypercalcemia

Some causes of decreased calcium in the blood (hypocalcemia)

Ca^{2+}
Ca^{2+}
Ca^{2+}

- Insufficient dietary calcium and vitamin D intake
- Chronic diarrhea
- Laxative abuse
- Malabsorption
- Chronic renal insufficiency
- Hypoparathyroidism
- Alkalosis
- Large transfusion of citrated blood
- Rapid infusion of plasma expanders

Figure 16–19 ➤ A variety of conditions can lead to hypercalcemia and hypocalcemia.

concentration has an important influence on cell membrane permeability and influences the threshold potential of excitable cells. For this reason, calcium imbalances alter neuromuscular irritability.

Hypercalcemia

Hypercalcemia refers to a plasma excess of calcium (above 5.3 mEq/L [2.7 mmol/L] in children or 5 mEq/L [2.5 mmol/L] in newborns). Because so much calcium is stored in the bones, however, the serum levels of calcium may not reflect body stores.

ETIOLOGY AND PATHOPHYSIOLOGY Hypercalcemia is caused by conditions that involve increased calcium intake or absorption, shift of calcium from bones into the extracellular fluid, and decreased calcium excretion. Hypercalcemia due to increased calcium intake or absorption may occur if an infant is fed large amounts of chicken liver (source of vitamin A), is given megadoses of vitamin D or vitamin A, or if a child or adolescent consumes large amounts of calcium-rich foods concurrently with antacids (milk-alkali syndrome). Infants with very low birth weight can develop hypercalcemia if they have inadequate phosphorus intake, as bone phosphorus and calcium will be resorbed. Hypercalcemia may also occur when children receiving total parenteral nutrition are given doses of calcium that are too high.

Most cases of hypercalcemia in children are due to a shift of calcium from bones into the extracellular fluid. The excessive amounts of parathyroid hormone produced in hyperparathyroidism cause calcium withdrawal from bones. Prolonged immobilization also causes withdrawal of calcium from bones. Often, the excess calcium ions are excreted in the urine. However, if calcium is withdrawn from bones faster than the kidneys can excrete it, hypercalcemia results. Hypercalcemia also occurs with many types of malignancies such as leukemias. The malignant cells produce substances that circulate in the blood to the bones and cause bone resorption. The calcium from the bones then enters the extracellular fluid, causing hypercalcemia. Bone tumors and chemotherapy destroy bone directly, leading to the release of calcium. Familial hypercalcemia and infantile hypercalcemia are rare congenital disorders.

Thiazide diuretics (e.g., thiazide and hydrochlorthiazide) decrease calcium excretion in the urine and may contribute to development of hypercalcemia. Other drugs that can cause hypercalcemia include lithium and theophylline (Carmichael & Alper, 2004).

CLINICAL MANIFESTATIONS Hypercalcemia may have nonspecific symptoms, making diagnosis difficult. Many of the signs and symptoms of hypercalcemia are manifestations of decreased neuromuscular excitability. Constipation, anorexia, nausea, and vomiting can occur. Fatigue and skeletal muscle weakness predominate. Confusion, lethargy, and decreased attention span are common, and polyuria develops. Severe hypercalcemia may cause cardiac arrhythmias and arrest. Neonates with hypercalcemia have flaccid muscles and exhibit failure to thrive. Hypercalcemia increases sodium and potassium excretion by the kidneys and can lead to polyuria and polydipsia.

▪ COLLABORATIVE CARE

Serum calcium is tested although the blood levels may not reflect bone stores. Additional diagnostic laboratory analyses to assist in diagnosis of the cause include albumin, phosphate, magnesium, alkaline phosphate, electrolytes, blood urea nitrogen, creatinine, and parathyroid hormone.

Hypercalcemia is treated by increasing fluids and administering the diuretic furosemide (Lasix) to increase excretion of calcium in the urine. Treatment to decrease intestinal absorption of calcium involves effective use of glucocorticoids. Bone resorption can be decreased by administration of glucocorticoids and calcitonin. Phosphate is sometimes given to treat hypercalcemia, but it may cause dangerous precipitation of calcium phosphate salts in body tissues. Dialysis may be used, if necessary. Treatment of the underlying cause for the disorder is needed as well.

NURSING MANAGEMENT

Nursing Assessment and Diagnosis

Nursing assessment of a child with hypercalcemia includes monitoring serum calcium levels, level of consciousness, gastrointestinal function, urine volume, specific gravity, cardiac rhythm, and pH. With chronic hypercalcemia, assessment of activity tolerance and developmental level becomes important.

Many nursing diagnoses are appropriate for children who have hypercalcemia. Diagnoses that address cardiac and neuromuscular manifestation are especially important. The following nursing diagnoses may apply:

- Risk for Activity Intolerance related to decreased cardiac output secondary to cardiac arrhythmia
- Risk for Injury related to decreased level of response
- Risk for Injury related to neuromuscular impairment
- Risk for Injury related to possibility of spontaneous fractures
- Self-Care Deficit: Hygiene and Dressing related to neuromuscular impairment
- Anxiety related to change in health status
- Constipation related to decreased motility
- Risk for Imbalanced Nutrition: Less than Body Requirements related to anorexia and nausea
- Risk for Impaired Urinary Elimination related to renal calculi

Planning and Intervention

Carefully calculate calcium in total parenteral nutrition and other solutions, administer these solutions with caution, and use cardiac monitoring to prevent hypercalcemia in hospitalized children.

Interventions to increase fluid intake are important for children with hypercalcemia or those who are immobilized. A generous fluid intake, appropriate to the child's age, is necessary to keep the urine dilute and to help reduce constipation (a common symptom of hypercalcemia). An acidic urine helps to keep calcium from forming stones. Because urinary tract infections may cause the urine to be alkaline, nursing interventions to prevent urinary tract infection are necessary. Thiazide diuretics, which decrease calcium excretion, should not be given to the hypercalcemic child. Provide a high-fiber diet to help reduce constipation.

Increasing mobility through assisted weight bearing helps to decrease the withdrawal of calcium from bones that is caused by immobility. If the hypercalcemia is caused by withdrawal of calcium from bones, the child is at risk for fractures with minor trauma and must be handled with special care. See Chapter 28 ∞ for further discussion of care following fractures and prolonged casting.

Teach parents to avoid giving calcium-rich foods and calcium antacids (e.g., Tums) to children with hypercalcemia. Vitamin D supplements should be avoided as they increase calcium absorption from the gastrointestinal tract.

Evaluation

Expected outcomes of nursing care include the following:

- The cardiac pump effectively maintains perfusion.
- The child is free from injury.
- Normal bowel excretion is maintained.
- Adequate nutritional status is maintained.

> **CLINICAL TIP**
> To decrease calcium intake in hypercalcemia, restrict intake of milk, ice cream, and other dairy products. Nondairy fruit-based desserts are acceptable alternatives.

Hypocalcemia

Hypocalcemia is a serum deficit of calcium (below 4.4 mEq/L [2.2 mmol/L] in children or 4 mEq/L [2 mmol/L] in newborns). Remember that serum calcium levels may not reflect body stores of this mineral, as most of the body's calcium is stored in bone.

ETIOLOGY AND PATHOPHYSIOLOGY   Hypocalcemia is caused by conditions that involve decreased calcium intake or absorption, shift of calcium to a physiologically unavailable form, increased calcium excretion, and loss of calcium by an abnormal route.

Decreased calcium intake or absorption causes hypocalcemia in children with chronic generalized malnutrition, or with a diet that is low in vitamin D and calcium. Female adolescents trying to lose weight or maintain a low weight often decrease foods that contain calcium and may develop chronic hypocalcemia. In these cases, premature bone loss and inadequate bone formation occur. (See Chapter 4 ∞ for further discussion of calcium intake during adolescence.) This deficit cannot be made up later in life, thus increasing the risk of osteoporosis.

Even with a normal calcium intake, hypocalcemia occurs if the mineral is not absorbed. If a child does not have enough vitamin D, calcium is not absorbed efficiently from the duodenum. Sunlight speeds formation of vitamin D in the skin. Children who are institutionalized without access to sunlight (e.g., severely developmentally delayed children), those with very dark skin, or children kept well covered when outside may become hypocalcemic because of the lack of vitamin D (see Chapter 4 ∞). Uremic syndrome is another cause of vitamin D deficiency. It interferes with the kidney's ability to activate vitamin D. High phosphate intake can cause hypocalcemia. Chronic diarrhea and steatorrhea (fatty stools) also reduce calcium absorption from the gastrointestinal tract.

The shift of calcium into a physiologically unavailable form occurs when calcium shifts into bone or free ionized calcium in plasma binds to proteins or small organic ions in the plasma. Too much calcium shifts into bones in various types of hypoparathyroidism, including DiGeorge syndrome (congenital absence of the parathyroid glands). Hypomagnesemia impairs parathyroid hormone function and may cause hypocalcemia. Some types of neonatal hypocalcemia are associated with delayed parathyroid hormone function or hypomagnesemia. Calcium shifts rapidly into bone when rickets is treated. A high plasma phosphate concentration causes plasma calcium to decrease. Alkalosis causes more calcium to bind to plasma proteins. The ionized hypocalcemia persists until the alkalosis resolves or the citrate is metabolized by the liver. Citrate in transfused blood products may bind with calcium so it is inactive. Children who receive liver transplants are hypocalcemic for several days because of impaired citrate metabolism.

Increased calcium excretion occurs in steatorrhea, when calcium secreted into the gastrointestinal fluid binds to the fecal fat in addition to the dietary calcium that is bound in the feces. A similar situation occurs in acute pancreatitis.

Loss of calcium by an abnormal route may contribute to hypocalcemia as calcium is lost from the body through burn or wound drainage or sequestered in acute pancreatitis. Many different medications can cause hypocalcemia.

CLINICAL MANIFESTATIONS   The signs and symptoms of hypocalcemia are manifestations of increased muscular excitability (tetany). In children they include twitching and cramping, tingling around the mouth or in the fingers, carpal spasm, and pedal spasm. Laryngospasm, seizures, and cardiac arrhythmias are the more severe manifestations of hypocalcemia and may be fatal. Hypocalcemia may cause congestive heart failure, especially in neonates.

Although these symptoms are diagnostic of acute calcium deficiency, a more common state in children and adolescents is chronic low intake of calcium. This may be manifested by spontaneous fractures in infants and in adolescents who exercise excessively.

■ COLLABORATIVE CARE

Laboratory measurement of calcium is the most useful diagnostic tool. Cardiac monitoring may be performed to observe for cardiac arrhythmias.

Hypocalcemia is treated by oral or intravenous administration of calcium. The original cause of the imbalance is also treated. If the hypocalcemia is due to hypomagnesemia, the magnesium must be replenished before the calcium replacement can be successful. When the cause is chronic low dietary intake, counseling is needed about high-calcium foods, and perhaps the necessity for vitamin D intake or supplements.

NURSING ALERT

Drugs that may cause hypocalcemia:
Antacids (if overused)
Laxatives (if overused)
Oil-based bowel lubricants
Anticonvulsants
Phosphate-containing preparations
Protein-type plasma expanders during rapid infusion
Antineoplastics

GROWTH & DEVELOPMENT

Hypocalcemia
Hypocalcemia in infants is more frequently manifested as tremors, muscle twitches, and brief tonic-clonic seizures.

NURSING MANAGEMENT
Nursing Assessment and Diagnosis

Carefully assess growth in the young female who is trying to diet. When an adolescent female is very thin, be sure to ask about excessive sports and other activities, and about regularity of menstrual periods. If periods are irregular or not occurring, collect additional dietary information to help determine whether the girl is lacking in intake of calcium, calories, and other nutrients. These assessments are needed even if serum calcium values are normal. Look for signs of inadequate nutrition such as fat and muscle wasting, dry hair, and cold hands and feet.

In those who have acute hypocalcemia, assess for muscle cramps, stiffness, and clumsiness; grimacing caused by spasms of facial muscles and twitching of arm muscles; and laryngospasm. Increased neuromuscular excitability may be detected by testing for Trousseau's sign or Chvostek's sign. Many healthy newborns have a positive Chvostek's sign; however, this assessment should be reserved for children over several months of age.

The effects of increased neuromuscular excitability in the child with hypocalcemia are the basis for the following nursing diagnoses:

- Risk for Injury related to potential for fractures
- Risk for Ineffective Breathing Pattern related to laryngospasm
- Risk for Activity Intolerance related to decreased cardiac output secondary to cardiac arrhythmias
- Disturbed Sensory Perception related to electrolyte imbalance
- Imbalanced Nutrition: Less than Body Requirement related to lack of basic nutritional knowledge of sources and recommended amounts of calcium intake

Planning and Implementation

To correct calcium deficiency in the hospitalized child, give oral or intravenous calcium as ordered. Monitor for complications of calcium supplementation. A 10% calcium gluconate solution should be readily available for emergency use in severe hypocalcemia. Calcium is never given intramuscularly because it causes tissue necrosis. See Medications Used to Treat Acute Hypocalcemia on page 532.

Take measures to ensure safety for the child who is hospitalized with hypocalcemia. Seizure precautions may be necessary. Explain the cause of muscle cramps to parents and older children.

Counsel the family about dairy products and nondairy foods rich in calcium (Families Want to Know: Calcium-Rich Foods). For the adolescent female whose weight and menstrual patterns show irregularities, total calories and calcium intake should be increased. Teaching may also be needed about proper calcium intake and its importance both to athletic performance and to prevention of osteoporosis. Encourage three glasses of nonfat milk per day. Teach ways to use milk in the diet. For example, sprinkle nonfat dry milk on cereal and other foods. If the child is lactose intolerant, emphasize nondairy sources of calcium and advise parents to purchase special milk treated with lactase. As this milk is more costly, inadequate family finances may be an impediment to its use. If a child has a health condition leading to chronic diarrhea, encourage increased intake of calcium-rich foods. Calcium supplements in the form of calcium carbonate tablets may be used.

Evaluation

Expected outcomes of nursing care for hypocalcemia include the following:

- Ingestion of recommended dietary allowances for calcium is maintained.
- The child displays calcium balance.
- The child is free from injury.

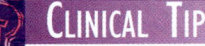

MEDICATIONS USED TO TREAT *Acute Hypocalcemia*

Medication	Action	Nursing Implications
10% calcium gluconate IV	Calcium is a normal body electrolyte and may need to be infused in infants or young children with health problems leading to low calcium. It is also used during exchange transfusion in neonates since citrate in the blood transfusion can bind body calcium. In the form of CaCl, calcium may be used during resuscitation. Calcium regulates excitability of muscles and nerves, and therefore affects cardiac function (inotropic effect); is necessary for blood clotting; plays a role in storage and release of neurotransmitters, in renal function, and in maintaining cell membranes; antidote to excessive magnesium infusion.	Verify dose carefully with the prescriber and another nurse. Monitor heart rate and rhythm—hypotension and bradycardia can occur. Use extreme caution if given to a child with cardiac or renal disease. Maintain IV carefully to avoid extravasation; do **not** administer by peripheral infusion, scalp vein, IM, or SC. Precipitates when given in infusion with bicarbonate.

Magnesium Imbalances

Magnesium is necessary for enzyme function in cells, acetylcholine release, glycolysis, stimulation of ATPases, and bone formation. Magnesium is a component of chlorophyll; thus, magnesium intake is aided by eating dark green leafy vegetables. Nuts and grains are also good sources of this mineral. Magnesium is absorbed primarily from the terminal ileum. It is distributed among the extracellular fluid (small amounts), the cells (larger amounts), and the bones (largest amounts). Magnesium excretion occurs in urine, feces, and sweat.

Magnesium imbalances are caused by alterations in magnesium intake, distribution, or excretion; by loss through an abnormal route; or by a combination of these factors. The plasma magnesium concentration influences the release of acetylcholine at neuromuscular junctions. Thus, magnesium imbalances are characterized by alterations in neuromuscular irritability.

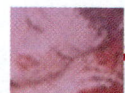

FAMILIES WANT TO KNOW

Calcium-Rich Foods

When a child needs to increase sources of calcium, parents may be unfamiliar with the variety of foods that contain calcium. Although they are aware that dairy products have high calcium, there are many other foods that add a significant amount of calcium to the diet, and which may be more acceptable to families in certain cultures. Some possible sources of calcium include the following.

Milk	Figs
Cheese	Chicken
Yogurt	Salmon (canned with bones)
Pudding	Grains (Cream of Wheat, farina, bran muffins)
Egg yolks	Sardines (canned)
Legumes	Tofu
Nuts	Fruit drinks with added calcium

Hypermagnesemia

Hypermagnesemia occurs when the plasma magnesium concentration is too high (above 2.4 mg/dL [0.99 mmol/L]). Keep in mind that the serum levels measured in the laboratory may not reflect body magnesium stores, because most of the magnesium in the body is located in the bones and inside the cells.

Hypermagnesemia is caused by conditions that involve increased magnesium intake and decreased magnesium excretion. Impaired renal function leading to decreased magnesium excretion is the most common cause of hypermagnesemia in children. In both oliguric renal failure and adrenal insufficiency, magnesium ions that cannot be excreted in the urine accumulate in the extracellular fluid.

Less frequently, increased magnesium intake may cause hypermagnesemia. Magnesium sulfate ($MgSO_4$) given to treat eclampsia in the mother before delivery causes hypermagnesemia in the newborn. Abnormally high amounts may also be taken in magnesium-containing enemas, laxatives, antacids, and intravenous fluids. Epsom salt is a readily available product and is a nearly pure magnesium sulfate preparation; its use as an enema has caused death in children. It has been used as a cathartic in the treatment of poisoning in the past but due to its potential for overdose, sorbitol is now preferred (Tofil, Benner, & Winkler, 2005). Aspiration of seawater, as in near-drowning, is an uncommon but potentially serious source of excessive magnesium intake. Children with Addison's disease can have abnormally high magnesium levels.

Clinical manifestations of hypermagnesemia include decreased muscle irritability, hypotension, bradycardia, drowsiness, lethargy, and weak or absent deep tendon reflexes. In severe hypermagnesemia, flaccid muscle paralysis, fatal respiratory depression, cardiac arrhythmias, and cardiac arrest occur.

Hypermagnesemia is managed primarily by increasing the urinary excretion of magnesium. This is usually accomplished by increasing fluid intake (except in oliguric renal failure) and by the administration of diuretics. Dialysis may sometimes be necessary.

■ NURSING MANAGEMENT

Monitor serum magnesium levels. Take the child's blood pressure (to watch for hypotension), heart rate and rhythm (to monitor for bradycardia and cardiac arrhythmias), respiratory rate and depth (to watch for respiratory depression), and deep tendon reflexes (to check muscle tone and paralysis or movement). Keep the side rails of the bed raised. Children with hypermagnesemia or oliguria should not be given magnesium-containing medications or sea salt.

Teach parents of children with chronic renal failure that these children should never be given milk of magnesia, antacids that contain magnesium, or other sources of magnesium; teach them to read labels and recognize ingredients. Caution all parents to avoid use of Epsom salts for children. When hypermagnesemia is treated with diuretics, monitor potassium levels to watch for hypokalemia.

Expected outcomes of nursing care include maintenance of electrolyte balance, normal neuromuscular tone, safety, and regular heart rate and rhythm.

Hypomagnesemia

Hypomagnesemia refers to a plasma magnesium concentration that is too low (below 1.5–1.7 mg/dL [0.62–0.70 mmol/L]). Remember that the serum levels of magnesium may not reflect body stores, as most of the magnesium in the body is found in cells and bones.

Hypomagnesemia is caused by conditions that involve decreased magnesium intake or absorption, shift of magnesium to a physiologically unavailable form, increased magnesium excretion, and loss of magnesium by an abnormal route. Hypocalcemia often accompanies and contributes to hypomagnesemia.

Neonates whose mothers are diabetic sometimes develop hypomagnesemia in the newborn period. Decreased magnesium intake or absorption can occur if a child who is not eating has prolonged intravenous therapy without magnesium. Chronic malnutrition

NURSING ALERT

Oral Magnesium

Magnesium tablets, capsules, solution, and suspension are available for relief of acid indigestion and to stimulate peristalsis. Popular products contain magnesium citrate, magnesium hydroxide, magnesium oxide, and magnesium salicylate. When used as a cathartic, administer the recommended amount of water to ensure bowel evacuation. The most common side effect is abdominal cramping accompanied by diarrhea; other side effects are dehydration, respiratory depression, and electrolyte imbalance.

Intravenous Magnesium

Intravenous magnesium is administered in the form of magnesium sulfate to treat severe hypomagnesemia, refractory hypocalcemia, and intractable seizures. Intravenous magnesium has side effects of hypermagnesemia, respiratory depression, hypotension, and CNS depression. This form of therapy requires close monitoring of body systems and electrolyte status.

is another cause of decreased magnesium intake. Magnesium absorption is decreased in chronic diarrhea, short bowel syndrome, malabsorption syndromes, and steatorrhea.

A shift of magnesium to a physiologically unavailable form may occur after transfusion of many units of citrated blood products, because magnesium bound to the citrate is not physiologically active. Such transfusions cause prolonged hypomagnesemia in liver transplant patients who have impaired citrate metabolism. Magnesium shifts rapidly into bones that have been deprived of adequate stores.

Increased magnesium excretion in the urine occurs with diuretic therapy, the diuretic phase of acute renal failure, diabetic ketoacidosis, and hyperaldosteronism. Chronic alcoholism, occasionally seen in adolescents, increases urinary magnesium excretion. Magnesium contained in gastrointestinal secretions is bound to fat and excreted in the stool.

Loss of magnesium by an abnormal route occurs with prolonged nasogastric suction and through sequestration of magnesium in acute pancreatitis. Several medications may cause hypomagnesemia, such as magnesium-wasting diuretics, some antineoplastic agents, systemic antifungals, aminoglycoside antibiotics, and laxatives without magnesium.

Hypomagnesemia is characterized by increased neuromuscular excitability (tetany). The clinical manifestations are hyperactive reflexes, skeletal muscle cramps, twitching, tremors, and cardiac arrhythmias. Seizures can occur with severe hypomagnesemia. Hypomagnesemia is associated with high mortality for children in the pediatric intensive care unit (Singhi, Singh, & Prasad, 2003).

Magnesium serum levels are measured, along with serum calcium and potassium, since these electrolyte disturbances often occur together. Hypomagnesemia is managed by administering magnesium and treating the underlying cause of the imbalance.

NURSING MANAGEMENT

In addition to monitoring serum magnesium levels, nursing assessment of hypomagnesemia includes monitoring deep tendon reflexes, testing for Trousseau's and Chvostek's signs (see page 531), monitoring cardiac function, and observing for muscle twitching. Children who are able to talk will report muscle cramping. Because magnesium levels are not routinely measured in many settings, request the test for any child who has risk factors and early manifestations of hypomagnesemia. When intramuscular or intravenous magnesium is ordered, administer carefully as directed and monitor vital signs. Electrocardiogram and renal studies may precede drug administration. Have resuscitative drugs and equipment readily available during drug administration.

Teach parents of a child with hypomagnesemia or continuing risk factors such as chronic diarrhea to include foods containing magnesium in the diet (see Families Want to Know: Magnesium-Rich Foods). Before administering magnesium supplements, verify that the child's urine output is adequate. Monitor deep tendon reflexes if intravenous magnesium is given, and observe for complications of magnesium supplementation.

Expected outcomes for nursing care include restoration and maintenance of electrolyte balance.

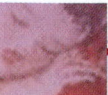

FAMILIES WANT TO KNOW

Magnesium-Rich Foods

Magnesium is a mineral with which most families are not familiar. When a child needs to increase magnesium intake, families can be encouraged to add two to three of the following foods to the child's daily diet:

Whole-grain cereal	Almonds
Dark-green vegetables	Peanut butter
Soy	Egg yolk

Table 16–7	RISK FACTOR ASSESSMENT FOR FLUID IMBALANCES	
Isotonic Fluid (Extracellular Fluid Volume Imbalances)		**Water**
• Source of increased intake?		• Source of increased intake?
• Aldosterone secretion increased or decreased?		• Antidiuretic hormone secretion increased or decreased?
• Source of loss from the body?		• Source of unusual loss from the body?

Clinical Assessment of Fluid and Electrolyte Imbalance

How can you assess children appropriately for fluid and electrolyte imbalance without thinking through the clinical manifestations of every possible disorder one after the other? First, perform a rapid risk factor assessment on each child to see which factors are present (Tables 16–7 and 16–8). Remember that most imbalances influence other factors so it is common to find more than one type of fluid and electrolyte problem. Examining several body systems such as cardiovascular, respiratory, and neurologic will be necessary to get a comprehensive picture of the child.

A risk factor assessment may be performed mentally during routine tasks. Look for factors that alter the intake, retention, and loss of isotonic fluid and water. This information is used to evaluate which fluid imbalance is most likely to occur in a particular child. Next, look for factors that alter electrolyte intake and absorption, distribution between plasma and other electrolyte pools, excretion, and abnormal routes of electrolyte loss. This information is used to evaluate which electrolyte imbalances are most likely to occur in the child. A review of pathophysiology is important to understand the role of the other electrolytes and substances, such as phosphorus, in the body. Apply growth and development to realize what types of problems might be most common in various age groups. For example, the newborn is more likely to be dehydrated due to lack of adequate intake, while the toddler more commonly has fluid loss from nausea and vomiting.

After evaluating possible imbalances for the child, perform a clinical assessment. Assessment of fluid imbalances is performed by assessing weight changes, vascular volume, interstitial volume, and cerebral function (Table 16–9). Assessment of electrolyte imbalances is performed by assessing serum electrolyte levels, skeletal muscle strength, neuromuscular excitability, gastrointestinal tract function, and cardiac rhythm (Table 16–10). Next, check for other manifestations that are specific to a particular high-risk imbalance (e.g., polyuria in hypokalemia). Evaluate any serum laboratory values available. This method of risk factor assessment followed by clinical assessment provides a rapid yet thorough approach to assessment for fluid and electrolyte imbalances.

Table 16–8	RISK FACTOR ASSESSMENT FOR ELECTROLYTE IMBALANCES		
Electrolyte Intake and Absorption	**Electrolyte Shifts**	**Electrolyte Excretion**	**Electrolyte Loss by Abnormal Route**
• Increased? • Decreased?	• From electrolyte pool to plasma? • From plasma to electrolyte pool?	• Increased? • Decreased?	• Vomiting? • Diarrhea? • Nasogastric suction? • Wound? • Burn? • Excessive sweating?

Table 16–9	SUMMARY OF CLINICAL ASSESSMENT OF FLUID IMBALANCES	
Assessment Category	**Specific Assessments**	**Changes with Fluid Imbalances**
Rapid changes in weight	Daily weights	Weight gain—extracellular volume excess Weight loss—extracellular volume deficit; clinical dehydration
Vascular volume	Small-vein filling time Capillary refill time Character of pulse Postural blood pressure measurements Lung sounds in dependent portions Central venous pressure Tenseness of fontanel (infants) Neck vein filling (older children)	Increased—extracellular volume deficit; clinical dehydration Increased—extracellular volume deficit; clinical dehydration Bounding—extracellular volume excess Thready—extracellular volume deficit; clinical dehydration Postural drop—extracellular volume deficit; clinical dehydration Crackles—extracellular volume excess Increased—extracellular volume excess Decreased—extracellular volume deficit; clinical dehydration Bulging—extracellular volume excess Sunken—extracellular volume deficit; clinical dehydration Full with upright—extracellular volume excess Flat when supine—extracellular volume deficit; clinical dehydration
Interstitial volume	Skin turgor Presence or absence of edema	Skin tents—extracellular volume deficit; clinical dehydration Edema—extracellular volume excess
Cerebral function	Level of consciousness	Decreased—clinical dehydration

Table 16–10	SUMMARY OF CLINICAL ASSESSMENT OF ELECTROLYTE IMBALANCES	
Assessment Category	**Specific Assessments**	**Changes with Electrolyte Imbalances**
Skeletal muscle function	Muscle strength	Weakness, flaccid paralysis—hyperkalemia; hypokalemia
Neuromuscular excitability	Deep tendon reflexes Chvostek's sign (not infants) Trousseau's sign Paresthesias Muscle cramping or twitching	Depressed—hypercalcemia; hypermagnesemia Hyperactive—hypocalcemia; hypomagnesemia Positive—hypocalcemia; hypomagnesemia Positive—hypocalcemia; hypomagnesemia Digital or perioral—hypocalcemia Present—hypocalcemia; hypomagnesemia
Gastrointestinal tract function	Bowel sounds Elimination pattern	Decreased or absent—hypokalemia Constipation—hypokalemia; hypercalcemia Diarrhea—hyperkalemia
Cardiac rhythm	Arrhythmia Electrocardiogram	Irregular—hyperkalemia; hypokalemia; hypercalcemia; hypocalcemia; hypermagnesemia; hypomagnesemia Abnormal—hyperkalemia; hypokalemia; hypercalcemia; hypocalcemia; hypermagnesemia; hypomagnesemia
Cerebral function	Level of consciousness	Decreased—hyponatremia; hypernatremia Examples of Metabolic Acids Pyruvic acid Sulfuric acid Acetoacetic acid Lactic acid Hydrochloric acid Beta-hydroxybutyric acid

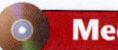

MediaLink

Acid-Base Balance Animation

ACID-BASE IMBALANCES

There are four acid-base imbalances. Two are the result of processes that cause too much acid in the body and are referred to as acidosis. The other two imbalances are the result of processes that cause too little acid in the body and are called alkalosis. An acid-base disorder caused by too much or too little carbonic acid is called a respiratory acid-base imbalance. A disorder caused by too much or too little metabolic acid is

Table 16–11	NORMAL BLOOD pH AND GASES		
	Infants	**Children**	**Adolescents**
Arterial blood pH	7.18–7.50	7.27–7.49	7.35–7.41
Arterial blood Po_2	60–70 mmHg (8.0–9.3 pKa)	80–108 mmHg (10.7–14.4 pKa)	80–100 mmHg (10.7–13.3 pKa)
Arterial blood Pco_2	27–41 mmHg (3.6–5.5 pKa)	32–48 mmHg (4.3–6.4 pKa)	32–48 mmHg (4.3–6.4 pKa)
Arterial blood HCO_3^- (bicarbonate)	19–24 mmol/L	18–25 mmol/L	20–29 mmol/L

called a metabolic acid-base imbalance (Box 16–4). See Table 16–11 for normal blood pH and blood gas levels.

Arterial blood gas measurements (ABGs) provide a laboratory evaluation of a child's current acid-base status. In addition to the four components of acid-base balance listed in Table 16–12, oxygenation saturation, or the percentage of hemoglobin saturated with arterial blood, is normally 95–100% (Pruitt & Jacobs, 2004). Box 16–5 provides a method that can help to interpret the pH, Po_2, Pco_2, and bicarbonate concentrations, which are the most important acid-base measures. End-tidal CO_2 can provide a continuous noninvasive measurement. (Remember that Pco_2 reflects carbonic acid status and bicarbonate concentration reflects the metabolic acid status.)

Respiratory Acidosis

Respiratory acidosis is caused by the accumulation of carbon dioxide in the blood. Since carbon dioxide and water can be combined into carbonic acid, respiratory acidosis is sometimes called carbonic acid excess. The condition can be acute or chronic. It is controlled by the lungs.

Etiology and Pathophysiology

Any factor that interferes with the ability of the lungs to excrete carbon dioxide can cause respiratory acidosis. These factors may interfere with the gaseous exchange within the lungs, may impair the neuromuscular pump that moves air in and out of the lungs, or may depress the respiratory rate (Table 16–13; Figure 16–20 ➤).

As the Pco_2 begins to increase, the pH of the blood begins to decrease. Compensatory mechanisms begin to act in the form of nonbicarbonate buffers, additional

---

BOX 16–4
ACID-BASE IMBALANCES

Acidosis: Relatively too much acid in the body
- Respiratory acidosis: Relatively too much carbonic acid
- Metabolic acidosis: Relatively too much metabolic acid

Alkalosis: Relatively too little acid in the body
- Respiratory alkalosis: Relatively too little carbonic acid
- Metabolic alkalosis: Relatively too little metabolic acid

Table 16–12	LABORATORY VALUES IN ACID-BASE IMBALANCE		
Imbalance	P_{CO_2}	pH	HCO_3^-
Respiratory Acidosis			
Uncompensated	Increased	Decreased	Normal
Partially compensated	Increased	Decreased but moving toward normal	Increasing
Fully compensated	Increased	Normal	Increased
Respiratory Alkalosis			
Uncompensated	Decreased	Increased	Normal
Partially compensated	Decreased	Increased but moving toward normal	Decreasing
Fully compensated	Decreased	Normal	Decreased
Metabolic Acidosis			
Uncompensated	Normal	Decreased	Decreased
Partially compensated	Decreasing	Decreased but moving toward normal	Decreased
Fully compensated	Decreased	Normal	Decreased
Metabolic Alkalosis			
Acute condition; uncompensated	Normal	Increased	Increased
Partially compensated	Increasing	Increased but moving toward normal	Increased
Fully compensated	Full compensation limited by the need for oxygen	Full compensation limited by the need for oxygen	Full compensation limited by the need for oxygen

---

BOX 16–5
HOW TO INTERPRET ARTERIAL BLOOD GAS MEASUREMENTS

Ask the following questions to analyze blood gas results.

1. **What is the pH?** If the pH is normal, the child has no imbalance or has compensated for an imbalance. If the pH is below normal, the child has acidosis. If the pH is above normal, the child has alkalosis.

2. **What are the P_{O_2} and oxygenation saturation?** Lowered levels of both demonstrate hypoxemia. Administering oxygen may help to reverse the hypoxemia and prevent further acid-base imbalance.

3. **What is the P_{CO_2}?** If the P_{CO_2} is normal, the child does not have an acid-base imbalance. If the P_{CO_2} is above normal, the child has respiratory acidosis. This may be the primary disorder or may be a compensatory response to metabolic alkalosis. Looking at the bicarbonate concentration helps you decide. If the P_{CO_2} is below normal, the child has respiratory alkalosis. Again, this can be the primary disorder or may be a compensatory response to metabolic acidosis.

4. **What is the bicarbonate concentration?** If the bicarbonate concentration is within normal range, the child does not have a metabolic acid-base imbalance. If the bicarbonate is above normal, the child has metabolic alkalosis. This can be a primary disorder or can be compensatory in respiratory acidosis. When bicarbonate is below normal, the child has metabolic acidosis, either as a direct disorder or as a compensatory response to respiratory alkalosis.

5. **What do the results together tell you?** If the pH is abnormal and either the P_{CO_2} or bicarbonate concentration is normal, there is an uncompensated acid-base disorder. If all three values are abnormal, the child has a partially compensated disorder and the pH will provide the definitive answer. If P_{CO_2}, pH, and bicarbonate are all decreased, then partially compensated metabolic acidosis is most likely. If pH is normal and P_{CO_2} and bicarbonate are abnormal, there is a fully compensated acid-base disorder.

6. **What are the child's history and clinical signs?** Does your interpretation fit with what you know about the child's medical condition and with assessments you are making? This last step helps you to integrate laboratory data with the clinical picture to strengthen your nursing care of the child with an acid-base imbalance.

---

hydrogen ion excretion by the kidneys, and formation and decreased bicarbonate excretion by the kidneys. These compensatory mechanisms take several days to become active so the child manifests a changing clinical situation, depending on the underlying cause and the amount of compensation occurring (see Table 16–12).

Clinical Manifestations

Acidosis in the brain cells causes central nervous system depression, manifested by confusion, lethargy, headache, increased intracranial pressure, and even coma. Acute re-

---

Table 16–13	CAUSES OF RESPIRATORY ACIDOSIS

Factors Affecting the Lungs	Factors Affecting the Neuromuscular Pump	Factors Affecting Central Control of Respiration
Aspiration	Flail chest	Sedative overdose
Spasm of the airways	Pneumothorax or hemothorax	General anesthesia
Laryngeal edema	Mechanical underventilation	Head injury
Epiglottitis	Hypokalemic muscle weakness	Brain tumor
Croup	High cervical spinal cord injury	Central sleep apnea
Pulmonary edema	Botulism	
Atelectasis	Tetanus	
Severe pneumonia	Kyphoscoliosis	
Cystic fibrosis	Poliomyelitis	
Bronchopulmonary dysplasia	Muscular dystrophy	
Pulmonary embolism	Congenital diaphragmatic hernia	
	Guillain-Barré syndrome	

spiratory acidosis can lead to tachycardia and cardiac arrhythmias. The child's arterial blood gases always show an increased P_{CO_2}, the laboratory sign of increased carbonic acid. Serum pH can be decreased or normal.

COLLABORATIVE CARE

Laboratory tests involve arterial blood gases, as described previously. Treatment of respiratory acidosis requires correction of the underlying cause. For example, treatment may include bronchodilators for bronchospasm, mechanical ventilation for neuromuscular defects, decreasing sedative use, or surgery for kyphoscoliosis.

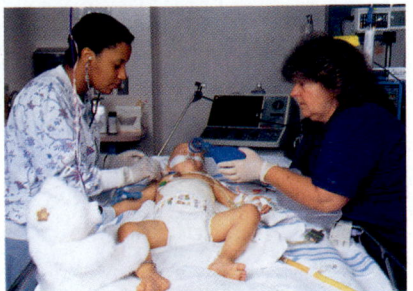

Figure 16–20 ➤ This child may develop respiratory acidosis or respiratory alkalosis. If the tidal volume is set too low during mechanical ventilation, carbon dioxide (carbonic acid) will accumulate in the body (respiratory acidosis) because it is not being excreted by the lungs. If the tidal volume is set too high, carbon dioxide will be depleted in the body (respiratory alkalosis) because it is being excreted in great quantities.

NURSING MANAGEMENT
Nursing Assessment and Diagnosis

Nursing assessment plays a pivotal role in decisions about interventions for respiratory acidosis, especially in chronic conditions such as cystic fibrosis and kyphoscoliosis. Assess respiratory rate, rhythm, and depth carefully. Take the apical pulse and be alert for tachycardia or arrhythmia. A cardiac monitor may be used. Obtain serial arterial blood gas measurements in acute conditions to evaluate changing status. Assess the level of consciousness and energy. Observe for chronic fatigue, headache, or decreased level of consciousness.

Several nursing diagnoses may apply to the child with respiratory acidosis. The most important of these addresses the child's risk for injury. Other nursing diagnoses depend on the specific clinical manifestation and the particular cause of the acidosis. Examples include:

- Risk for Injury related to decreased level of consciousness
- Activity Intolerance related to decreased cardiac output secondary to cardiac dysrhythmias
- Ineffective Breathing Pattern (Hypoventilation) related to neuromuscular impairment
- Acute Pain (Headache) related to cerebral vasodilation
- Ineffective Family Management of Therapeutic Regimen related to complexity of bronchodilator therapy

Planning and Implementation
Care in the Community

Teach children at risk for respiratory acidosis and their parents preventive measures to use at home. For the child with a chronic condition such as cystic fibrosis, muscular dystrophy, or kyphoscoliosis, demonstrate deep breathing and encourage its use several times each day. Teach the family signs of infection—including fever, increased respiratory secretions, and discomfort with breathing—so the problems can be treated promptly to prevent further respiratory involvement. Position the child to facilitate chest expansion (Figure 16–21 ➤). Teach parents about proper administration of any necessary medications. For example, the child with cystic fibrosis may receive antibiotics to prevent respiratory infections. Teach parents and older children about home respirator use (Figure 16–22 ➤).

Hospital-Based Care

For the hospitalized child, the focus is on ensuring safety. Keep side rails raised, and turn and position the child frequently. Evaluate mental status and document and report any changes in alertness. When laboratory values of blood pH and P_{CO_2} are available, evaluate them promptly and report any changes or abnormalities. Administer medications as ordered. Carefully watch the doses of sedatives to avoid further respiratory depression. Provide suctioning and encourage deep breathing.

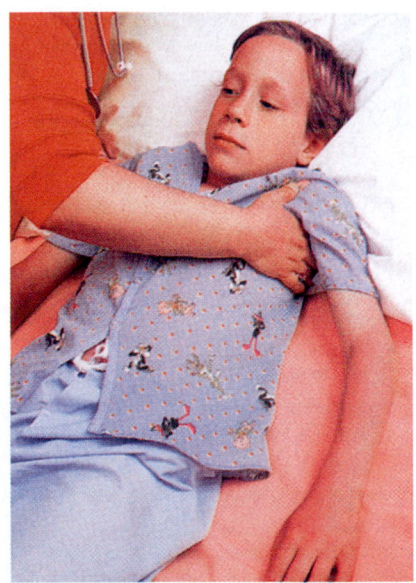

Figure 16–21 ➤ Positioning to facilitate chest expansion. If the child is positioned to avoid chest compression or slumping to the side, this will help correct respiratory acidosis.

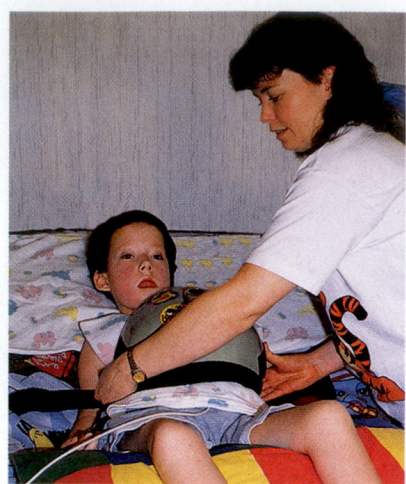

Figure 16–22 ▶ This child, who has muscular dystrophy, uses a "turtle" respirator at home to assist with breathing. His parents required instructions from the nurse on use of the respirator. The family has a generator to provide electricity for the respirator during power outages.

GROWTH & DEVELOPMENT

Deep Breathing

It is usually difficult to get a young child to do deep breathing or to use the "blow bottle" that is often given to older children and adults. To make deep breathing fun, use a pinwheel and have the child turn it during play. Alternatively, give a child a straw and have him or her blow bubbles in a glass of water, or have the child use the straw to blow scraps of paper across the bedside table.

BOX 16–6

CAUSES OF HYPERVENTILATION

Hypoxemia
Anxiety
Pain
Encephalitis
Septicemia caused by gram-negative bacteria
Mechanical overventilation
Fever
Salicylate poisoning
Meningitis

Evaluation

Expected outcomes of nursing care for the child with respiratory acidosis include the following:

- Safety is maintained for the child.
- Adequate rate and rhythm of respirations are manifested.
- Disorders that have contributed to the imbalance are corrected.

Respiratory Alkalosis

Respiratory alkalosis occurs when the blood contains too little carbon dioxide. It is sometimes called carbonic acid deficit.

Excess carbon dioxide loss is caused by hyperventilation, in which more air than normal is moved into and out of the lungs. Common causes of hyperventilation are listed in Box 16–6. Some of the most common causes in young children are hypoxia such as that from severe asthma, salicylate poisoning, and sepsis (Schwaderer & Schwartz, 2004).

In many cases, respiratory alkalosis only lasts for several hours. Renal compensation does not occur, as these compensatory mechanisms take several days to begin action. An example is the hyperventilation that occurs with acute anxiety. If the condition persists, however, the kidneys will begin to retain more acid and excrete more bicarbonate. Hydrogen ions will be released from body buffers to decrease plasma bicarbonate. While the imbalance continues, cellular function is thus protected by returning pH to normal levels.

Arterial blood gas measurements show a decreased P_{CO_2} in respiratory alkalosis. Blood pH is generally elevated. The lack of carbon dioxide causes neuromuscular irritability and paresthesias in the extremities and around the mouth. Muscle cramping and carpal or pedal spasms can occur. The child may be dizzy or confused.

Diagnosis is made by complete arterial blood gas measurements and thorough physical assessment. Clinical therapy focuses on correcting the condition that caused the hyperventilation so that the body's compensatory mechanisms can return carbon dioxide levels to normal. Oxygen therapy may be helpful in cases of hypoxia, salicylates are removed from the body when poisoning is the cause (see Chapter 6 ∞ for further information on poisoning), drugs that have interfered with breathing are changed, sepsis is treated with effective medication, and anxiolytic medications may be used to treat anxiety.

■ NURSING MANAGEMENT

Assess the child's level of consciousness and ask if the child feels light-headed or has tingling sensations or numbness in the fingers, toes, or around the mouth. Assess the rate and depth of respirations. Monitor the hospitalized child's P_{O_2} with serial arterial blood gas measurements to evaluate changes in status. A careful assessment is needed regarding the cause of hyperventilation. Did an occurrence cause anxiety for the child? Is pain present (see Chapter 15 ∞)? Has the child received salicylates in any form? Is the child mechanically ventilated? Is there a central nervous system infection such as meningitis?

Nursing care for the child with respiratory alkalosis centers on teaching stress management techniques, maintaining pain control, promoting respiratory function, ensuring safety, maintaining fluid status, and providing health supervision and home care.

Teach Stress Management Techniques

When anxiety is the cause of respiratory alkalosis, instruct the child to breathe slowly, in rhythm with your own breathing. Teach stress control techniques such as relaxation and imagery for situations that cause anxiety (Table 16–14).

Table 16–14	TECHNIQUES FOR REDUCING ANXIETY IN CHILDREN WITH PARETHESIAS		
Infant	**Toddler or Preschooler**	**Young School-Age Child**	**Older School-Age Child or Adolescent**
Calming touch Quiet voice Swaddling Holding quietly	Stuffed toy to hug Singing familiar quiet nursery songs Acknowledging the child's feelings Holding calmly	Talking quietly about a happy event Telling a familiar story Reading a familiar book together Explaining that the tingling will go away Use of simple guided imagery Supportive listening	Explaining the reason for the tingling and that it will go away Use of guided imagery Familiar music on tape or radio Asking what the child does when anxious or "scared" Talking about coping strategies

Maintain Pain Control

Use medications, imagery, distraction, positioning, massage, and other techniques to decrease pain and maintain pain management. Chapter 15 ∞ describes these and other measures to assist with pain control.

Promote Respiratory Function

Have the child cough, or suction as needed. Be certain that mechanical ventilation systems are working properly. Oxygen saturation is usually monitored continuously; observe and record results.

Ensure Safety

Provide a safe environment for the child who has a decreased level of consciousness. Be sure the child is supervised when sitting or standing up. Keep bed rails raised.

Regulate Fluid Status

Renal compensation to manage ongoing respiratory alkalosis requires adequate urinary output. Regulate fluid intake to ensure urine output unless fluids are restricted due to medical condition.

Care in the Community

Teach parents to keep aspirin and other salicylate products out of reach of children, preferably in a locked medicine box. Instruct parents to call the Poison Control Center immediately in case of poison ingestion.

Evaluation

Expected outcomes of nursing care for the child with respiratory alkalosis include the following:

- Normal respiratory rate and rhythm are manifested.
- Safety is maintained for the child.
- Fluid status is appropriately regulated.

> **NURSING ALERT**
>
> The Po_2 must be checked before any therapy for respiratory alkalosis is started, because it is dangerous to stop hyperventilation if oxygenation is poor. When Po_2 is low, the child's hyperventilation may be a protective mechanism to increase blood oxygenation. Other measures such as oxygen therapy or mechanical ventilation may need to start first, followed by treatment for the cause of respiratory alkalosis.

Metabolic Acidosis

Metabolic acidosis is a condition in which there is an excess of any acid other than carbonic acid. For this reason, it is sometimes called noncarbonic acid excess.

Etiology and Pathophysiology

Metabolic acidosis is caused by an imbalance in production and excretion of acid or by excess loss of bicarbonate (Table 16–15). Excess accumulation occurs by one of two mechanisms. First, a child can eat or drink acids or substances that are converted to acid in the body. Examples include aspirin, boric acid, and antifreeze. Second, cells can make abnormally high amounts of acid that cannot be excreted. This is the case in ketoacidosis of untreated diabetes mellitus, untreated growth hormone deficiency, in children with bladder construction that uses part of the bowel, or the starvation that

Table 16–15 | CAUSES OF METABOLIC ACIDOSIS

Gain of Metabolic Acid	Loss of Bicarbonate
Ingestion of acids (e.g., aspirin)	Diarrhea
Ingestion of acid precursors (e.g., antifreeze)	Intestinal or pancreatic fistula
Oliguria (e.g., renal failure)	Proximal renal tubular acidosis
Distal renal tubular acidosis	
Hyperalimentation	
Diabetic ketoacidosis	
Starvation ketoacidosis	
Some inborn errors of metabolism (e.g., maple syrup urine disease)	
Tissue hypoxia (lactic acidosis)	

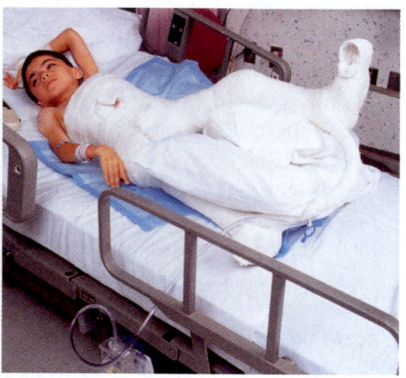

Figure 16–23 ➤ With any postoperative or immobilized child, it is important to monitor urine output to detect oliguria. If the kidneys do not produce very much urine, the metabolic acids accumulate in the body and cause metabolic acidosis. Inadequate fluid intake in the postoperative or immobilized child can lead to oliguria and, potentially, metabolic acidosis. Note this child's urine collection device.

can occur in anorexia or bulimia. A disorder of excretion occurs in conditions such as oliguric renal failure (Figure 16–23 ➤).

Bicarbonate can be lost from the body through the urine or through excessive loss of intestinal fluid. Diarrhea, fistulas, and ileal drainage are all possible sources. Carbonic anhydrase inhibitors can cause loss of excess bicarbonate in the urine.

When the pH of the blood decreases below normal, the chemoreceptors in the brain and arteries are stimulated and respiratory compensation begins. The child's rate and depth of breathing increase and carbonic acid is removed from the body. The blood pH shifts to a more normal range even though the cause is not corrected. The underlying condition and the degree of compensation will alter the clinical laboratory values observed.

Clinical Manifestations

Laboratory values show decreased blood pH and decreased HCO_3^- and Pco_2. An attempt at respiratory compensation causes one of the most important signs of metabolic acidosis, increased rate and depth of respirations (hyperventilation) or **Kussmaul respirations.** Severe acidosis can cause decreased peripheral vascular resistance and resultant cardiac arrhythmias, hypotension, pulmonary edema, and tissue hypoxia. Confusion or drowsiness may result, as well as headache or abdominal pain.

■ COLLABORATIVE CARE

Laboratory tests include blood pH and arterial blood gases. Treatment of metabolic acidosis depends on identification and treatment of the underlying cause. For example, renal failure is treated with medications of dialysis, an intestinal fistula is repaired, and hyperalimentation formula is regulated to decrease acidosis. In severe metabolic acidosis, intravenous sodium bicarbonate may be used to increase the pH and to prevent cardiac arrhythmias. This treatment is difficult to manage, because renal excretion can cause excess retention of bicarbonate; therefore, intravenous sodium bicarbonate is used only in severe situations, such as prolonged cardiac arrest.

■ NURSING MANAGEMENT
Nursing Assessment and Diagnosis

When families bring a young child in for a health promotion visit, assess the risk of poisoning in the home and the family's knowledge of prevention techniques. For the child being treated for acidosis, assess the rate and depth of respirations. Evaluate the child's level of consciousness frequently. Be alert for signs or complaints of headache and abdominal pain. Serial arterial blood gas measurements will usually be obtained to evaluate changes in status.

The following nursing diagnoses can apply to the child with metabolic acidosis:

- Risk for Injury related to confusion/drowsiness or decreased responsiveness
- Risk for Decreased Cardiac Output related to cardiac dysrhythmias
- Ineffective Tissue Perfusion (Cerebral) related to tissue hypoxia
- Ineffective Family Management of Therapeutic Regimen related to complexity of management of diabetes mellitus

Planning and Implementation

Ensure safety, taking into account the child's level of consciousness and alertness. Turn the child and change his or her position to prevent pressure on the skin. Limit the child's activities to decrease cardiac workload.

Position the child to facilitate chest expansion. Provide oral care during rapid respirations because the mouth may become dry. Monitor intravenous solutions and laboratory values indicating acid-base balance. Report changes promptly.

Once the child is stabilized, provide teaching to compensate for knowledge deficits. This teaching for home prevention should take place at each health promotion visit for all children. Teach parents of young children to keep medications and acids locked in a secure place and out of reach to prevent poisoning (Figure 16–24 ➤). This includes medicines with aspirin as well as substances commonly kept in the garage for car maintenance. Teach about home management of diabetes and about early identification and treatment to avoid diabetic ketoacidosis. Expected outcomes of nursing care relate to prevention of acidosis and restoration of normal body balance during disease processes.

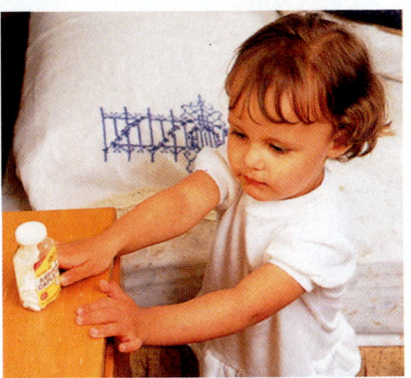

Figure 16–24 ➤ Teaching parents to use safety latches on cabinets to keep aspirin away from small children can prevent one cause of metabolic acidosis.

Metabolic Alkalosis

Metabolic alkalosis occurs when there are too few metabolic acids. It is sometimes called noncarbonic acid deficit.

A gain in bicarbonate or a loss of metabolic acid can cause metabolic alkalosis (Table 16–16). Bicarbonate is gained through excessive intake of bicarbonate antacids or baking soda or through metabolism of bicarbonate precursors such as the citrate contained in blood transfusions. Increased renal absorption of bicarbonate can occur in profound hypokalemia, primary hyperaldosteronism, or extreme deficit in extracellular fluid volume. Acid can be lost through severe vomiting, such as that seen in infants with pyloric stenosis and in continued removal of gastric contents through suction.

When the chemoreceptors in the brain and arteries detect the rising pH of metabolic alkalosis and respirations decrease, carbonic acid is retained in the body. This carbonic acid can neutralize the bicarbonate and return pH toward normal.

Blood pH, bicarbonate, and Pco_2 are usually elevated in metabolic alkalosis. Hypokalemia often occurs simultaneously (refer to discussion of hypokalemia earlier in this chapter). Respiratory rate and depth usually decrease. Increased neuromuscular

Table 16–16	CAUSES OF METABOLIC ALKALOSIS
Gain of Bicarbonate	**Loss of Metabolic Acid**
Ingestion of baking soda	Prolonged vomiting (e.g., pyloric stenosis)
Ingestion of large quantities of bicarbonate antacids	Nasogastric suction
Exchange transfusion or massive transfusion (citrate is metabolized to bicarbonate)	Cystic fibrosis
Increased renal absorption of bicarbonate	Hypokalemia
	Diuretic therapy
	Hyperaldosteronism
	Adrenogenital syndrome
	Cushing's syndrome

irritability, cramping, paresthesia, tetany, seizures, and excitation can occur. Finally, this state can progress to weakness, confusion, lethargy, and coma.

Laboratory tests include blood pH and arterial blood gases. Clinical therapy is directed at treating the underlying cause of the condition. Increasing the extracellular fluid volume with intravenous normal saline is used to facilitate renal excretion of bicarbonate. Medications such as acetazolamide increase renal excretion of bicarbonate as well.

NURSING MANAGEMENT

Assess the child's level of consciousness frequently. Alertness may decrease after an initial period of excitement, so regular assessments are needed. Monitor neuromuscular irritability. Observe for nausea and vomiting. Assess the rate and depth of respirations carefully. Obtain serial arterial blood gas measurements as ordered.

Facilitate ease of respirations. Ensure safety by keeping bed rails elevated and by turning the child frequently. Position the child on the side to avoid aspiration of vomitus.

If antacids were the cause of the alkalosis, teach the child and parents about correct use of these medications.

MIXED ACID-BASE IMBALANCES

It is possible for two acid-base imbalances to occur simultaneously. For example, a child with cystic fibrosis can develop respiratory acidosis from lung problems and concurrent metabolic alkalosis from vomiting during an illness. Treatment with diuretics may cause concurrent metabolic alkalosis resulting from extracellular volume depletion and hypokalemia in a child with congestive heart failure and chronic respiratory acidosis. In these cases, all underlying causes must be identified and treated. Care of children with mixed acid-base imbalances is often complicated, requiring hospitalization and careful management. Upon discharge, the nurse can teach parents about signs of imbalance that need to be reported and treated to prevent further complications. Evaluation of care is based on outcomes of adequate respiratory ventilation and metabolic balance.

CRITICAL THINKING IN ACTION

Consider the scenario involving Vernon at the beginning of this chapter. He is an 18-month-old who has had vomiting and diarrhea for several days. Assessment of body weight loss, skin turgor, and level of activity suggest moderate dehydration. Vernon refuses attempts at feeding him orally, his pulse becomes rapid, and his blood pressure decreases. Voiding is decreased and capillary refill is slow. Vernon is admitted to the short-stay unit and an intravenous infusion is started.

DISCUSSION

1. Based on his age, what oral fluids might be best to offer to Vernon? What questions will you ask his mother about his normal fluid intake at home?

2. What additional assessment will you perform on Vernon to gather further information about his state of dehydration?

3. Since Vernon has had vomiting and diarrhea, he is probably deficient in an electrolyte present in high quantities in these body fluids. What electrolyte, in addition to sodium, is likely deficient?

4. A major nursing role is to plan care for Vernon while he is in the unit to rehydrate him. Calculate his replacement and maintenance fluid needs. Formulate a plan of care to include the amounts of oral rehydration therapy he should be offered over the next several hours.

 Refer to you Prentice Hall Nursing MediaLink DVD-ROM for answers.

EXPLORE MediaLink

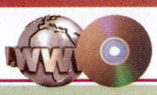

http://www.prenhall.com/ball

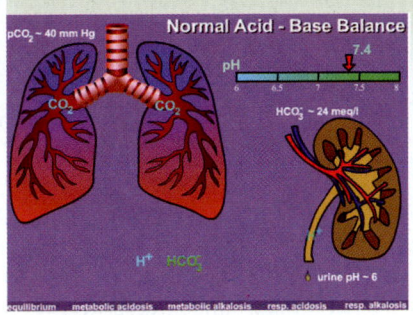

Resources for this chapter can be found on the Prentice Hall Nursing MediaLink DVD-ROM accompanying this textbook, and on the Companion Website at http://www.prenhall.com/ball.

DVD-ROM
Audio Glossary
NCLEX®-RN Review
Animations
   Acid-Base Balance
   Hyperkalemia

COMPANION WEBSITE
Audio Glossary
NCLEX®-RN Review
Care Plan Activity: Infant Feeding
Case Study: Lab Panels
Critical Thinking: Formula Preparation at a Home Visit
MediaLink Applications
   Acute Diarrhea
   Fluids Intake for Children Who Exercise
   Hyponatremic Dehydration
   Identifying Intravenous Fluids
   Understanding and Interpreting Blood Gases
WebLinks

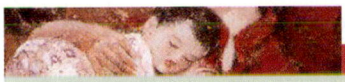

REFERENCES

Atherly-John, Y. C., Cunningham, S. J., & Crain, E. F. (2002). A randomized trial of oral vs intravenous rehydration in a pediatric emergency department. *Archives of Pediatric and Adolescent Medicine, 156,* 1240–1243.

Bindler, R., & Howry, L. (2005). *Pediatric Drug Guide.* Upper Saddle River, NJ: Prentice Hall.

Binkley, H. M., Beckett, J., Casa, D. J., Kleiner, D. M., & Plummer, P. E. (2002). National Athletic Trainers' Association position statement: Exertional heat illnesses. *Journal of Athletic Training, 37,* 329–343.

Burger, C. M. (2004a). Hyperkalemia. *American Journal of Nursing, 104*(10), 66–70.

Burger, C. M. (2004b). Hypokalemia. *American Journal of Nursing, 104*(11), 61–65.

Carmichael, K. A., & Alper, B. S. (2004, December). Hypercalcemia. *The Clinical Advisor,* 67–69.

Chamley, C. A., Carson, P., Randall, D., & Sandwell, M. (2005). *Developmental anatomy and physiology of children.* Edinburgh: Elsevier.

Committee on Sports Medicine and Fitness. (2000). Climatic heat stress and the exercising child and adolescent. *Pediatrics, 106,* 158–159.

Dale, J. (2004). Oral rehydration solutions in the management of acute gastroenteritis among children. *Journal of Pediatric Health Care, 18,* 211–212.

Dennehy, P. H. (2005). Acute diarrheal disease in children: Epidemiology, prevention, and treatment. *Infectious Disease Clinics of North America, 19,* 585–602.

English, M. (2002). Challenges in managing profound hypokalemia. *British Medical Journal, 324,* 269–270.

Exercise-Associated Hyponatremia Consensus Panel. (2005). Consensus statement of the 1st International Exercise-Associated Hyponatremia Consensus Development Conference, Cape Town, South Africa 2005. *Clinical Journal of Sports Medicine, 15,* 208–213.

Fonseca, B. K., Holdgate, A., & Craig, J. C. (2004). Enteral vs. intravenous rehydration therapy for children with gastroenteritis. *Archives of Pediatrics & Adolescent Medicine, 158,* 483–490.

Greenbaum, L. A. (2004). Pathophysiology of body fluids and fluid therapy. In R. E. Behrman, R. Kliegman, & H. B. Jenson, *Nelson textbook of pediatrics* (17th ed., pp. 191–242). Philadelphia: Saunders.

Johns Hopkins Hospital. (2005). *The Harriet Lane handbook* (17th ed.). St. Louis: Mosby.

King, C. K., Glass, R., Bresee, J. S., & Duggan, C. (2003). Managing acute gastroenteritis among children. *MMWR, 52*(RR16), 1–16.

Moritz, M. L., & Ayus, J. C. (2003). Prevention of hospital-acquired hyponatremia: A case for using isotonic saline. *Pediatrics, 111,* 227–230.

Moritz, M. L., Manole, M. D., Bogen, D. L., & Ayus, J. C. (2005). Breastfeeding-associated hypernatremia: Are we missing the diagnosis? *Pediatrics, 116,* 3343–3347.

Nager, A. L., & Wang, V. J. (2002). Comparison of nasogastric and intravenous methods of rehydration in pediatric patients with acute dehydration. *Pediatrics, 109,* 566–572.

Provisional Committee on Quality Improvement, Subcommittee on Acute Gastroenteritis. (1996). Practice parameter: The management of acute gastroenteritis in young children. *Pediatrics, 97,* 424–436.

Pruitt, W. C., & Jacobs, M. (2004). Interpreting blood gases: Easy as ABC. *Nursing 2004, 34*(8), 50–53.

Roberts, K. E. (2005). Pediatric fluid and electrolyte balance: Critical care case studies. *Critical Care Nursing Clinics of North America, 17,* 361–373.

Sarhill, N., Mahmoud, F. A., Christie, R., & Tahir, A. (2003). Pain and symptom management: Assessment of nutritional status and fluid deficits in advanced cancer. *American Journal of Hospice and Palliative Care, 20,* 465–473, 480.

Schwaderer, A. L., & Schwartz, G. J. (2004). Back to basics: Acidosis and alkalosis. *Pediatric Review, 25,* 350–357.

Singhi, S. C., Singh, J., & Prasad, R. (2003). Hypo- and hypermagnesemia in an Indian pediatric intensive care unit. *Journal of Tropical Pediatrics, 49,* 99–103.

Spandorfer, P. R., Alessandrini, E. A., Joffe, M. D., Localio, R., & Shaw, K. N. (2005) Oral versus intravenous rehydration of moderately dehydrated children: A randomized, controlled trial. *Pediatrics, 115,* 295–301.

Steiner, M. J., DeWalt, D. A., & Byerly, J. S. (2004). Is this child dehydrated? *JAMA, 291,* 2746–2754.

Tofil, N. M., Benner, K. W., & Winkler, M. K. (2005). Fatal hypermagnesemia caused by an Epsom salt enema: A case illustration. *Southern Medical Journal, 98,* 253–256.

The Venous Access Task Force. (2002). Using evidence-based practice to create a venous access team. *Journal of Pediatric Nursing, 17,* 450–454.

Wathen, J. E., MacKenzie, T., & Bothner, J. P. (2004). Usefulness of the serum electrolyte panel in the management of pediatric dehydration treated with intravenously administered fluids. *Pediatrics, 114,* 1227–1234.

Yucha, C. (2004). Renal regulation of acid-base balance. *Nephrology Nursing Journal, 31,* 201–208.

17

ALTERATIONS IN IMMUNE FUNCTION

KEY TERMS

MediaLink

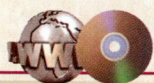

http://www.prenhall.com/ball

See the Prentice Hall Nursing MediaLink DVD-ROM and Companion Website for chapter-specific resources.

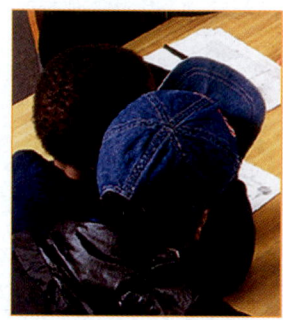

RAYMOND, a 2-year-old child, has had recurrent infections since he was born. In the last 3 months, he has had bronchitis twice, otitis media three times, and several colds. Raymond has had a fever, vomiting, and diarrhea for several days, and does not appear to be improving. His mother brings him to an ambulatory clinic for evaluation.

After a thorough history is taken, blood tests are performed to assess Raymond's immune function. On the basis of an evaluation of Raymond's clinical symptoms and the results of the laboratory tests, he sees a specialist and is diagnosed with acquired immunodeficiency syndrome (AIDS). Raymond is admitted to a special unit of the hospital for children with AIDS so that his treatment can begin. Like many of the other children, Raymond is often irritable and difficult to console. Because he vomits frequently, the nurses pay particular attention to Raymond's nutritional problems, giving him frequent small feedings.

Raymond is diagnosed as having failure to thrive, a common sequela of AIDS. Broad-spectrum antibiotics are given, and he is assessed frequently for the development of new infections. Drugs for treatment of human immunodeficiency virus (HIV) are initiated. A multidisciplinary team, including nurses, physicians, nutritionists, and social services professionals, are involved in planning Raymond's care.

LEARNING OUTCOMES

After reading this chapter, you will be able to do the following:

1. Describe the structure and function of the immune system.
2. Apply knowledge of the immune system to the care of children with immunological disorders.
3. Explain the differences between primary and secondary immunodeficiency.
4. Identify infection control measures to prevent the spread of infection in children with an immunodeficiency.
5. Develop a nursing care plan in partnership with the family for a child with human immunodeficiency virus (HIV).
6. Describe the differences between immune deficiency diseases and autoimmune diseases.
7. Describe nursing management for the child with an autoimmune condition such as systemic lupus erythematosus or juvenile rheumatoid arthritis.
8. Describe exposure prevention measures for the child with latex allergy.
9. Apply nursing interventions and prevention measures for the child experiencing other hypersensitivity reactions.

FOCUS ON
The Immune System

ANATOMY AND PHYSIOLOGY

The function of the immune system is to recognize any foreign substances within the body—in simple terms, to distinguish "nonself" from "self"—and to eliminate foreign substances as efficiently as possible. When the body recognizes the presence of a substance that it cannot identify as part of itself, the body protects itself through the immune response. Normally, the immune system responds to an invasion of foreign substances, or antigens, in numerous ways. It produces **antibodies**, or proteins that work against **antigens**, the foreign substances that trigger the immune response. There are many types of antibodies, which are described later in this section. The immune system also produces other types of cells, such as T lymphocytes and natural killer (NK) cells.

Immunity is either natural or acquired. Natural immune defenses are those an infant has at birth, such as intact skin, body pH, natural antibodies from the mother, and inflammatory and phagocytic properties. Acquired immunity consists of humoral (antibody-mediated) and cell-mediated immunity and is not fully developed until a child is about 6 years of age.

Humoral immunity is responsible for destroying bacterial antigens. B lymphocytes, produced in the bone marrow, gut, and other lymphoid tissue, are the central factor in humoral immunity, and develop into plasma cells that produce antibodies. Antibodies are a type of protein called **immunoglobulins**, of which there are five types: IgM, IgG, IgA, IgD, and IgE (Table 17–1). IgM, IgG, and IgA act to control a number of body infections, whereas IgE is useful in combating parasitic infections and is part of the allergic response. The role of IgD is unknown.

Antibodies are found in serum, body fluids, and certain tissues. When a child is first exposed to an antigen, the B-lymphocyte system begins to produce antibodies that react specifically to that antigen (Figure 17–1 ➤). It takes approximately 3 days for this process, known as **primary immune response**, to occur. Subsequent encounters with the antigen trigger memory cells, resulting in a **secondary immune response** within 24 hours.

Cellular immunity or *cell-mediated immunity* uses T lymphocytes, produced mainly in the thymus, to provide cellular immunity and protect against most viruses, fungi, slowly developing bacterial infections such as tuberculosis, and tumors. In addition, they control the timing of the response in delayed hypersensitivity reactions, such as the purified protein derivative (PPD) test, and they are responsible for the rejection of foreign grafts, such as transplants. Specialized types of T lymphocytes include killer T cells, suppressor T cells, and helper T cells. Suppressor T cells inhibit B lymphocytes from differentiating into plasma cells. Helper T cells aid in the proliferation and immunologic function of other cells. T lymphocytes have proteins on their surfaces that attract and trap receptors; they can be used to measure the immune activity of these cells. For example, some of the common proteins are CD2, CD3, CD4, CD5, CD7, and CD8. Natural killer (NK) cells (also known as non-B/non-T lymphocytes) originate in the bone marrow and thymus and migrate to the blood and spleen. They play a role in control of viral infection, tumors, and autoimmune disease.

Complement is a component of blood serum consisting of 11 protein compounds. It is an inactive enzyme that activates in response to antigen-antibody functions, resulting in a generalized inflammatory reaction that kills foreign cells. It also plays a role in causing some autoimmune diseases.

Immune cells also secrete proteins called **cytokines** that carry messages for immune system function. Lymphocytes, monocytes, and macrophages all secrete cytokines that have a variety of effects on the target cells. Effects may include stimulation of growth through proliferation of cells, differentiation of cellular actions, production of inflammation, sensitization to pain, and other actions. Interleukins, a type of cytokine, were first identified in white blood cells but now are known to be present in many cells. Many types of interleukins have been identified and some are known to influence the function of the immune system.

PEDIATRIC DIFFERENCES

Immune system development is a complex and multifactorial process. Early in-utero experiences, environmental exposures after birth, and other factors influence this important feedback system. It protects children from harmful diseases but also leads to conditions such as asthma (Chapter 20), food allergy (Chapter 4), or skin atopy (Chapter 30) ∞.

Table 17–1	CLASSES OF IMMUNOGLOBULINS
IgM	Present in intravascular spaces
IgG	Present in all body fluids
IgA	Present in secretions of gastrointestinal, respiratory, and genitourinary tracts
IgD	Presence and function not yet described
IgE	Present in internal and external body fluids

PATHOPHYSIOLOGY ILLUSTRATED

Primary Immune Response

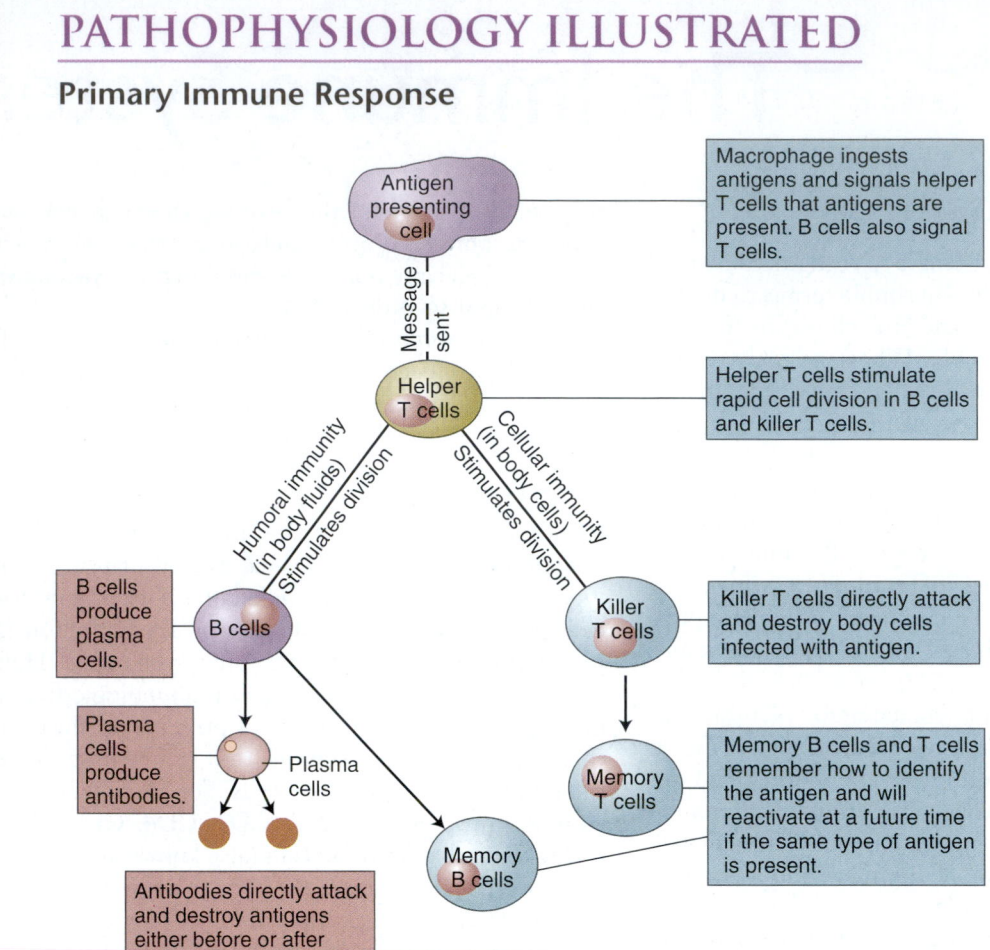

Figure 17–1 ➤ The primary immune response encompasses a cascade of events that involve humoral and cellular immunity.

Infants and children have differing amounts of some immunoglobulins. IgG is the only immunoglobulin that crosses the placenta; as a result, a newborn's levels are similar to those of the mother's. This maternal IgG disappears by 6 to 8 months of age. The infant's IgG then increases gradually until mature levels are reached at 7 to 8 years. IgM levels are low at birth, rise markedly at 1 week of age, and continue to increase until adult levels are reached at about 1 year. IgA and IgE are not present at birth. Manufacture of these immunoglobulins begins by 2 weeks of age; however, normal values are not achieved until 6 to 7 years. It is thus easy to see why children under 6 years of age become ill so often—they do not have a full complement of immunoglobulins.

In contrast, cell-mediated immunity achieves full function early in life. Early in fetal life, the thymus begins producing T cells and by birth many of these cells are present. The thymus is large at birth, grows during childhood and adolescence, and decreases in size in adulthood (Chamley, Carson, Randall, & Sandwell, 2005). Other lymphoid tissues, such as the spleen and tonsils, are also comparatively large in young children. Because of the well-developed cellular immunity, any blood infused into newborns is generally irradiated to prevent **graft-versus-host disease** (a series of immunologic reactions in response to transplanted cells) from transfused lymphocytes (see As Children Grow, Figure 17–2 ➤).

Newborns have somewhat lower numbers of NK cells than older children and adults, decreasing their ability to respond to certain antigens. The levels of some complement proteins are lower in newborns than in older children and adults, thus delaying and hampering response to certain infections. Levels of monocytes and macrophages are low (Marodi, 2006). Newborns are most prone to development of infection, particularly when born as prematures, since they both have lower levels of their own immune protections, as well as less IgG obtained from the mother. Feeding of human milk is protective against newborn infections. Nurses also play an important role in following infection control practices in newborns and to promptly identify infections in children of all ages.

Examples of diagnostic and laboratory tests used to evaluate immune system function are provided in the accompanying table. Use the guidelines on page 550 to perform a nursing assessment of the immune system.

AS CHILDREN GROW

Immunoglobulins Throughout Childhood

Figure 17–2 ▶ Different types of immunoglobulins mature at variable times throughout childhood. Children have high levels of some types of immunoglobulins, while others may be low at certain periods during development.

DIAGNOSTIC AND LABORATORY TESTS FOR THE IMMUNE SYSTEM

Diagnostic Test	Purpose	Nursing Implications
Enzyme immunoassay (EIA) and enzyme-linked immunosorbent assay (ELISA)	Commonly used test to identify HIV; detects antibodies to the virus. Positive results are verified by the Western blot test.	• Collect a sample in the recommended tube and arrange prompt transport to the laboratory. • Perform collection from the child in a treatment room or laboratory rather than in the hospital or clinic room.
Immunoglobulins	Alterations in IgG, IgA, IgM, IgD, and IgE can signify a variety of immune system disorders such as deficiency disease and allergy.	• See nursing implications for EIA + ELISA.
Polymerase chain reaction	A test that makes copies of a DNA sequence that can then be analyzed; useful to detect HIV or other conditions with only small amounts of blood.	• See nursing implications for EIA + ELISA.
Rapid HIV tests	Rapid HIV tests using saliva and urine produce results in 60 minutes or less. They are useful for quick screening but results must be confirmed with serum tests as false positives can occur.	• See nursing implications for EIA + ELISA.
RAST	Measures the amount of IgE in serum; specific antibodies to certain substances can indicate an allergy to specific allergens.	• See nursing implications for EIA + ELISA.
Skin reactions	Pin prick intradermal testing can be performed for a wide variety of substances. Local reactions indicate allergic response to the substances injected.	• Cleanse skin and label in order to ensure proper reading of skin reactions to various substances. • The extensive group of tests required can be challenging for the young child; the upper back is sometimes used so that the child can lie prone on the table or bed and a parent can offer distraction during the procedure.

(continued)

DIAGNOSTIC AND LABORATORY TESTS FOR THE IMMUNE SYSTEM (continued)

Diagnostic Test	Purpose	Nursing Implications
Western blot test	The definitive and confirmatory test for HIV. Allows visualization of particular antibodies to each viral protein.	• See nursing implications for EIA + ELISA

Laboratory Test	Purpose	Nursing Implications
Complete blood count (CBC)	The CBC measures types of all cells in the serum. It includes all leukocytes (white blood cells) that are important in immune function. If the test is a CBC with differential, the various levels of all types of WBCs are listed, a necessary laboratory test in diagnosing and managing immune system disorders. Numbers of T and B cells and their ratios provide diagnostic information.	• Collect a blood sample in the recommended tube and arrange prompt transport to the laboratory. • Perform blood collection from the child in a treatment room or laboratory rather than in the hospital or clinic room.
Complement	Serum complement levels assist in diagnosis of immune system disorders.	• See nursing implications for complete blood count.

ASSESSMENT GUIDELINES FOR THE CHILD WITH AN IMMUNE SYSTEM ALTERATION

Assessment Focus	Assessment Guidelines
Family History	• Does a family member have a history of allergy? Does the mother or other family member have a history of HIV or other immune system disorder? • Has the child been treated prophylactically for HIV due to the mother's positive status?
Growth and Development	• Growth should be regular and remain in approximately the same channels. The child should have a healthy appetite and consume normal amounts of food for age. Developmental milestones should emerge at expected times. Delayed growth and development, as well as lethargy and lack of energy, can indicate immune system malfunction.
Skin and Mucous Membranes	• Is the skin intact? Are there lesions of the mucous membranes? • Are infections or allergic responses commonly occurring? • Do lesions heal quickly without additional infection?
Evidence of Disease	• Frequently recurring infections and unusual infectious agents may signify immune system malfunction. Respiratory system infections, as well as frequent and untreatable ear infections, are common signals of problems.

MediaLink

Immune Response Animation

What are the signs and symptoms of immunologic disorders in children? Many times they are nonspecific. Raymond's admitting signs and symptoms, described in the opening scenario, are characteristic of several different immunodeficiency disorders. The immune system is one of the few body systems that regulates, either directly or indirectly, all other body functions. Thus, a problem with the immune system can have multisystem consequences and may be life threatening. Allergic reactions to food or frequent episodes of otitis media may indicate a disorder of immune function. Immune conditions can be mild to severe and life threatening. Congenital abnormalities sometimes signal a defect in cellular immunity. In this chapter, we will examine some of the more common disorders of immune function and discuss nursing care of both children who have these diseases and their families.

IMMUNODEFICIENCY DISORDERS

Immunodeficiency, a state of decreased responsiveness of the immune system, can occur to varying degrees in response to any number of events. Children with congenital immunodeficiency, or **primary immune deficiency**, are born with a failure of humoral antibody formation (B-cell disorder), a deficient cellular immune system (T-cell disorder), or a combination of both defects. Approximately 50,000 new cases of primary immunodeficiency are diagnosed each year in the United States (Cooper, Pommering, & Koranyi, 2003). In these congenital disorders, the immune deficiency is not caused by another condition. However, immunodeficiency may also be acquired, as in human immunodeficiency virus (HIV) infection. Acquired immunodeficiency is also called **secondary immune deficiency**.

B-Cell and T-Cell Disorders

In B-cell disorders, immunoglobulins may be present in inadequate numbers or nearly absent. X-linked hypogammaglobulinemia, selective IgA deficiency, and common variable immunodeficiency are examples of such disorders. Because newborns are protected from infection by maternal antibodies in the first months after birth, symptoms of B-cell disorders usually become apparent after 3 months of age. Infants with these disorders have frequent recurrent bacterial infections and failure to thrive. With treatment, consisting of intravenous immunoglobulins and antibiotics, most children survive into adulthood. Prognosis depends on the degree of antibody deficiency.

T-cell disorders are characterized by inadequate numbers of T lymphocytes or absence of T-cell functions. Isolated T-cell disorders are rare, usually accompanied by a B-cell disorder, and may be associated with congenital abnormalities (as in DiGeorge syndrome) or of unknown cause. Table 17–2 compares laboratory values for selected congenital immunodeficiency disorders.

DiGeorge syndrome is caused by abnormalities in chromosome 22 (it is known as 22q.11 deletion syndrome), and is often diagnosed soon after birth. The syndrome is characterized by the absence of parathyroid or thymus glands, resultant hypocalcemia, cardiac defects, low-set ears, hypertelorism (widely set eyes), palate abnormalities, renal dysfunction, tetany 48 hours after birth, lymphadenopathy, viral and fungal infections in the neonatal period, and neurocognitive and psychiatric disorders (Goldmuntz, 2005; Connell & Hodgson, 2005). Pneumonia and failure to thrive are common, and T-lymphocyte counts are usually low or very low for age. However, great variability is seen in the

Table 17–2	LABORATORY FINDINGS FOR SELECTED CONGENITAL IMMUNODEFICIENCY DISORDERS
Disorders	**Laboratory Findings**
B cell	
X-linked hypo-gammaglobulinemia	Reduced IgA, IgM, IgE, IgG (<100 mg/dL), absence of B cells in peripheral blood, normal T cells
Selective IgA deficiency	IgA <10 mg/dL
Common variable immunodeficiency	IgA, IgM reduced; IgG <250 mg/dL
T cell	
DiGeorge syndrome	Lymphopenia; absent T-cell functions, decreased T cells, normal B cells
Immunodeficiency with hyper-IgM	Reduced IgG, IgA; elevated IgM; mutations in T-cell surface proteins
Combined	
Severe combined immunodeficiency syndrome (SCID)	Complete absence of T- and B-cell and NK immunity
Wiskott-Aldrich syndrome	Thrombocytopenia, low platelet volume, nonfunctional B cells, normal IgG, decreased IgM, increased IgA, increased IgE; inability to respond to polysaccharide antigens

syndrome so that some children display considerable T-cell abnormalities and others, even with severe disease, have only moderately low numbers of T-cell abnormalities (Markert, Alexieff, Sarzotti et al., 2004). Children diagnosed with the disorder are treated with antibiotics for prophylaxis against pneumonia from *Pneumocystis carinii*, oral calcium, thymus transplantation, and HLA-identical bone marrow transplantation.

Immunodeficiency with hyper-IgM is a T-cell disorder that mainly affects males and causes decreased T-cell function, variable abnormal levels of immunoglobulins, and high titers of some antibodies. It is usually X-linked but is autosomal in some cases. Pulmonary and sinus bacterial infections generally occur in the first 2 years of life (Koleilat, Williams, & Ryan, 2003). Treatment with intravenous immune globulin (IVIG) therapy is helpful although later malignancies and liver disease can occur.

Severe Combined Immunodeficiency Disease

Severe combined immunodeficiency disease (SCID) is a congenital condition characterized by absence of both humoral and cellular immunity. SCID occurs in X-linked recessive, autosomal recessive, and sporadic forms. The disorder is more common in males than females (Cooper, Pommering, & Koranyi, 2003). Without appropriate treatment, children born with SCID usually die within the first 2 years of life.

Etiology and Pathophysiology

Severe combined immunodeficiency disease is caused by genetic mutations of cellular receptors to interleukin. The mutations lead to impaired lymphoid development in children with low T and NK cells. B lymphocytes may be absent or, if present, are defective in performance (Bonilla & Geha, 2006).

Clinical Manifestations

Symptoms in a child born with SCID develop early in life. The neonate often demonstrates a susceptibility to infection by 3 months of age. Often the first infection seen is a resistant oral candidiasis. Manifestations in addition to oral candidiasis include failure to thrive, chronic diarrhea, sepsis, and chronic infections such as otitis media or pneumonia. Additionally, failure to completely recover from infection, frequent reinfection, and infection with viruses such as cytomegalovirus and the bacterium *Pneumocystis carinii* are characteristic. Children are also highly susceptible to serious infections such as meningitis, skin or organ infection, osteomyelitis, or sepsis.

Some infants experience graft-versus-host disease as a result of placental transfer of maternal T lymphocytes. The reaction may be manifested by a perinatal rash that resembles measles or atopic dermatitis (Koleilat, William, & Ryan, 2003). If the child receives foreign tissue, for example, in a blood transfusion, signs such as skin rash, fever, hepatosplenomegaly, and diarrhea may occur.

■ COLLABORATIVE CARE

A marked reduction in lymphocyte counts is indicative of SCID. B and T lymphocytes are generally few in number or absent from the peripheral blood and lymphoid tissues. In some cases, the B-lymphocyte count may be elevated, although these cells do not function normally. NK cells are few in number. Immunoglobulin levels are significantly reduced. Refer to Table 17–2 for laboratory findings in SCID. Diagnosis is usually made only after extensive laboratory testing. In addition to a complete blood count, erythrocyte sedimentation rate, and B- and T-cell lymphocyte counts, other studies including IgA, IgG, and IgM antibody titers; neutrophil count; and titer levels of immunizations received and neutrophil count may be performed (Table 17–3). A chest radiograph is conducted to assess thymus size.

The goal of medical management is to restore immune function. Intravenous immune globulin (IVIG) is administered to provide protection until humoral immunity can be established. Hematopoietic stem cell transplantation offers the best hope for children with SCID (see Chapter 22 ∞). T-cell function is restored with the transplantation, and new cells appear 3 to 4 months after infusion of the donor stem cells. Prognosis for the child is poor without aggressive therapy and transplant.

Table 17–3	CELLS EVALUATED IN LABORATORY STUDIES FOR IMMUNE CONDITIONS	
Test and Type of Cell Evaluated	**Action**	**Implication of Increased or Decreased Levels**
White blood cell (WBC) count		
Neutrophil	Phagocytic cell that defends against bacteria	Increased in bacterial infection, inflammatory processes, and some malignancies
Eosinophil	Associated with antigen–antibody reaction	Increased in allergic reaction; decreased in children receiving corticosteroids
Lymphocytes (T, B, non-B/non-T [NK])	Major components of immune system	Increased in many infections; decreased in children with immune deficiency
Immunoglobulins		
(IgM, IgG, IgA, IgD, IgE)	Many roles in a number of immunologic reactions	Increased in presence of infection or allergic response; decreased in children with immune deficiency

With the identification of the various genetic defects for SCID in recent years, gene transfer has been successfully attempted to treat a small number of children. This experimental therapy is expected to be used more often in the future, particularly for certain defects (Bonilla & Geha, 2006; Champi, 2002).

Prevention and prompt treatment of infection are essential. Antibiotic therapy is targeted at infectious agents. Antibiotic prophylaxis and specific immunization recommendations for immunodeficiency are needed (see Chapter 18 ∞ for a thorough discussion of, and resources about, immunization for children with special needs). Children with T-cell deficiencies should receive cytomegalovirus-negative irradiated blood products due to the risk of infection and graft-versus-host disease from lymphocytes in donor blood (Cooper et al., 2003).

NURSING MANAGEMENT

Nursing Assessment and Diagnosis

Obtain a thorough history of infections, including age of onset, type of causal organism, frequency, and severity. Take a family history, and find out if the child has had any unusual reactions to vaccines, medications, or foods. Measure the child's height and weight accurately to identify failure to thrive. Assess the child's nutritional intake and fluid and electrolyte balance. Assess for evidence of infections involving the skin, subcutaneous tissues, respiratory system, and mucous membranes. Palpate the abdomen for hepatomegaly and the lymph nodes for lymphadenopathy. Perform a developmental assessment and assess for delays in achievement of developmental milestones. Assess family support systems and coping mechanisms when a child is diagnosed with the disorder.

The primary nursing diagnosis for a child with SCID is Risk for Infection related to immunodeficiency. Other nursing diagnoses may include the following:

- Imbalanced Nutrition: Less than Body Requirements related to chronic illness
- Risk for Impaired Skin Integrity related to immunologic deficit
- Risk for Caregiver Role Strain related to a child with a chronic, life-threatening illness
- Risk for Delayed Growth and Development related to physical disability and chronic illness

Planning and Implementation

Nursing care of the immunodeficient child focuses on preventing infection. However, even with the use of environmental controls, such as keeping children inside special units to maintain a sterile environment, these children are prone to **opportunistic infections** (those caused by organisms that are usually nonpathogenic, but can cause infections in persons who lack normal immunity).

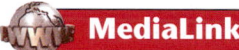

SKILLS CHAPTER 1
Protective Methods

MediaLink

The National Immunization Program

Prevent Systemic Infection

Frequent and thorough hand hygiene is important. Standard precautions are always used, with transmission-based precautions when indicated. Implement sterile aseptic technique when caring for all sites where needles, catheters, central lines, endotracheal tubes, pressure-monitoring lines, and peripheral intravenous lines enter the child's body. The child should be placed in a negative pressure room, and contact with infectious individuals should be avoided. Food and other items entering the hospital room may need special treatment. The child should be placed in a private room, and contact with infectious individuals should be minimized. Live vaccines for the child and family members are avoided. See Chapter 18 ∞ and the CDC web site for information about immunization recommendations in the immunocompromised child.

Promote Skin Integrity

The skin is the only intact defense that many immunodeficient children have. Provide thorough and frequent skin care, and observe all possible pressure areas closely for signs of breakdown or infection. Implement measures to avoid skin trauma. Reposition the child frequently and encourage range of motion exercises.

Promote Nutritional Balance

Encourage adequate fluid and nutritional intake. Provide foods that the child prefers and those with high nutritional value. Offer small frequent feedings of high-calorie, protein-rich foods. Protein intake can be increased by adding dried milk powder to foods. Energy intake can be increased by adding small amounts of fats and special nutritional formulas to the diet. Only pasteurized milk and juice products should be used to avoid the chance of infection. Refer to a dietitian as needed to plan with parents the best individualized diet for the child.

Manage Medication Therapy

Many of the medications used in the long-term treatment of children with SCID have numerous side effects. Monitor closely for side effects of antibiotics, such as overgrowth of resistant organisms (e.g., thrush infections in the mouth, *Clostridium difficile* infections of the gastrointestinal tract) and administer IVIG safely. See Medications Used to Treat Immune Disorders.

Provide Emotional Support and Referral

SCID is a life-threatening and devastating disease. Even with aggressive therapy, the prognosis is poor for children who do not receive hematopoietic stem cell transplant. Evaluate the family's knowledge about the disease and provide education on infection control measures and signs of infection. Involve the parents by encouraging them to assist in and manage care for their child (see Families Want to Know: Reducing Risk of Infection). The parents may be experiencing guilt because of the genetic nature of the disease and the difficulties of treatment. Listen closely to their concerns and encourage them to discuss their fears. Refer them to an appropriate support group or counselor if needed. Genetic counseling should be encouraged.

Evaluate the family's ability to care for the child at home. Provide opportunities for the child to have contact with other children when it is safe to do so. Suggest activities that will foster development. Offer financial resources and other referrals as needed. See Chapter 14 ∞ for information about assisting the family in care of the child with a life-threatening illness.

The family of a child who undergoes hematopoietic stem cell transplantation requires additional support and referrals. The transplantation procedure involves surgery for both the ill child and the donor, often another child in the family (refer to the discussion in Chapter 22 ∞). After the infusion of the donor cells, the ill child will be hospitalized for several months until T-lymphocyte levels are sufficient to provide

MEDICATIONS USED TO TREAT *Immune Disorders*

Medication	Action/Indication	Side Effects	Nursing Implications
Immune Globulin	Intravenous immune globulin (IVIG) is prepared from pools of multiple samples of human plasma and contains globulin (primarily IgG). It is used after exposure to diseases such as hepatitis B, in idiopathic thrombocytopic purpura, in Kawasaki disease, AIDS, and other disorders. Specific types of immune globulin are effective against specific diseases. For example, RespiGam helps to decrease incidence of respiratory syncytial virus, and HBIG is effective to prevent infection after exposure to hepatitis B.	Local inflammatory reaction, malaise, fever, nausea, vomiting, arthralgia; hypersensitivity reaction with fever, chills, anaphylactic shock; infusion reaction with nausea, flushing, chills, headache, difficulty breathing, pain in back or abdomen.	• Have emergency drugs and equipment readily available to treat hypersensitivity reaction or infusion reaction. • Child may be treated with antipyretic or antihistamine before the infusion. Follow manufacturer directions for reconstitution, dilution, and intravenous infusion rates. Do not mix with other medications for infusion. • Monitor vital signs throughout infusion. Stop infusion immediately and notify physician when any signs of hypersensitivity occur. • Activate emergency system as needed. • Have family instruct healthcare providers about IVIG therapy as immunization recommendations will be altered.

Data from Bindler, R.M., & Howry, L.B. (2005). Pediatric Drug Guide with Nursing Implications. *Upper Saddle River, NJ Prentice Hall.*

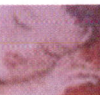

FAMILIES WANT TO KNOW

Reducing Risk of Infection

- Wash all bottles, nipples, and pacifiers with hot water and soap, or in the dishwasher.
- Do not allow the child to share utensils, cups, bottles, or pacifiers.
- Use safe food preparation practices such as peeling fruit and vegetables and using different surfaces and utensils for preparing meats and other foods.

- Change diapers frequently. Cleanse skin with mild soap and dry thoroughly.
- Wash hands before handling the child, after changing diapers, and before feeding the child.
- Maintain clean pets and keep the pet's environment clean.
- Avoid exposing the child to illnesses in others, such as respiratory and skin infections.

resistance to infection. During this period, parents may need to rely on social services to help manage the family situation, particularly if the child is hospitalized at a medical center far from the family's home. Assess the family's situation and make appropriate referrals to social services and to support groups. Introduce parents to other families with a child undergoing transplantation.

Evaluation

Expected outcomes of nursing care include the following:

- The child will be free from infection.
- The child will demonstrate adequate nutritional status as determined by normal growth patterns.
- Intact skin will be maintained.
- The family will demonstrate adaptive coping to the demands of a chronic illness.
- The child will demonstrate developmental performance within normal level for age.

Wiskott–Aldrich Syndrome

A combined congenital immunodeficiency syndrome, Wiskott–Aldrich syndrome is an X-linked disorder that causes mutation in the WAS gene and changes in the WAS protein (Ochs & Thrasher, 2006). The gene resides on Xp11.22-Xp11.3. The incidence is 4 in 1 million live male births (Dibbern & Routes, 2004). In this condition the IgG levels are normal or elevated, IgM levels are decreased, and IgA and IgE levels are increased. The condition is characterized by thrombocytopenia, eczema, hemorrhagic tendencies, recurrent infections, and malignancy such as lymphoma in adolescence and early adulthood (Ochs & Thrasher, 2006). Thrombocytopenia with bleeding tendencies appears during the neonatal period. Eczema appears by 1 year of age. Infections involve the middle ear and often lead to chronic otitis media. Meningitis may be caused by organisms such as *H. influenzae*, *P. carinii*, *S. pneumoniae*, and varicella. Children are particularly susceptible to infections from herpes viruses and lymphoreticular malignancies, especially of the lymphatic system.

The diagnosis is made in the early neonatal period on the basis of the thrombocytopenia, which leads to petechiae and bleeding (refer to Table 17–2). Manifestations of Wiskott–Aldrich syndrome vary; some children maintain normal lymphocyte levels for years. Treatment is supportive and includes antibiotic prophylaxis, platelet infusions, monthly intravenous immune globulin infusions, and sometimes splenectomy. Treatment for the syndrome often involves hematopoietic stem cell transplantation, which is preferred early in life before repeated infections have occurred (Conley, Saragoussi, Notarangelo et al., 2003; El-Alfy & El-Sayed, 2004).

Nursing Management

Nursing care is similar to that for the child with SCID. Assess for splenomegaly, cervical lymphadenopathy, and hepatomegaly. Observe for excessive bleeding from wounds or the gastrointestinal tract.

Refer the parents for genetic counseling to help them understand the transmission of the disease and the probability of having another child with the same disorder. Arrange for psychologic support for those parents who may be overwhelmed with guilt from learning that the illness is inherited.

Help the parents and family cope with the knowledge that the child has a chronic and potentially fatal illness. Referral to family counseling may be appropriate. Provide support during the process of transplantation. Expected outcomes are a return to normal immunologic function or successful coping with a life-threatening illness.

Acquired Immunodeficiency Syndrome

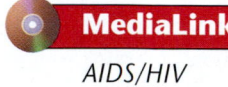

AIDS/HIV

Acquired immunodeficiency syndrome is caused by the human immunodeficiency virus (HIV-1). HIV destroys the body's ability to fight infection. Opportunistic infections that would normally not affect healthy people attack the HIV-infected person, and AIDS (or the advanced stage of HIV) is diagnosed.

Soon after acquired immunodeficiency syndrome (AIDS) was recognized in homosexual adults and intravenous drug abusers, cases of AIDS were seen in children. Increasing numbers of children have been diagnosed with the human immunodeficiency virus (HIV), making HIV infection a leading cause of immune disease in infants and children and a major cause of death in children.

A significant number of HIV cases in children are the result of perinatal transmission. The Centers for Disease Control and Prevention (CDC) estimates that approximately 300 infants are born with HIV infection each year in the United States (CDC, 2003). These numbers have decreased from the previously reported estimates of 1000 to 2000 infants born annually with HIV infection during the 1990s, primarily because of more effective identification and treatment of infected mothers and babies.

A major cause of HIV infection in teens is unprotected sexual intercourse. While rates of HIV have remained the same or decreased from 2000–2004 in other age groups, they have increased in 15- to 19-year-olds. Less common causes of HIV infection include blood and other transfusions and injection drug use (CDC, 2005). For the four years from 2001–2004, 15,338 U.S. children and teens from birth to 19 years were diagnosed with HIV/AIDS (Box 17–1).

The virus affects multiple systems and eventually destroys the child's immune system. An understanding of the natural history of HIV disease is still evolving, as there are several important differences in the disease progression and clinical manifestations of pediatric and adult HIV infection.

Etiology and Pathophysiology

Children can acquire HIV in a form of **vertical transmission** (perinatal transmission) from their mothers transplacentally or during delivery. Transmission can occur during birth from blood, amniotic fluid, and exposure to genital tract secretions, and after birth through breast milk from HIV-positive mothers. However, risk for perinatal transmission has been significantly reduced since mothers identified as infected receive zidovudine (AZT) during pregnancy and are delivered by c-section. In addition, the baby is given drug therapy after birth (Ramstead, 2003). Due to the high rate of transmission from mother to infant, HIV counseling and voluntary testing are encouraged for all pregnant women.

HIV has also been transmitted to children through transfusions of infected blood before mandatory screening of blood and blood products was instituted in 1985. Most of these children were infected during treatment of hemophilia. Although some adolescents with AIDS also have hemophilia, with infected blood the expected etiology, adolescents now most commonly acquire the virus through unprotected sexual activities or occasionally through intravenous drug use.

HIV selectively targets and destroys T cells, thereby decreasing and eventually eliminating cellular immunity. HIV destroys the CD4 T cells (helper cells) that are crucial to normal function of the immune system. HIV selectively targets T cells, decreasing cellular immunity, and affecting humoral immunity as well. Thus, the child is left unprotected against a myriad of bacterial, viral, fungal, and opportunistic infections, which are ultimately fatal. Every organ system can be affected (see Figure 17–3 ➤).

Clinical Manifestations

The neonate is asymptomatic at birth. The time period for development of opportunistic infections varies; however, the interval from HIV infection to the onset of overt AIDS is shorter in children than in adults, and shorter in children infected perinatally than in those infected through transfusion. Most children with AIDS have non-specific findings, including lymphadenopathy, hepatosplenomegaly, nephropathy, oral candidiasis, failure to thrive and weight loss, diarrhea, chronic eczema and dermatitis,

---

CULTURE

HIV/AIDS Worldwide

While major inroads have been made in the United States and several other developed countries to stem the numbers of HIV/AIDS cases in children, developing countries have not been able to afford testing or treatment. Subsequently, they have large numbers of affected children. The countries most acutely affected are in Africa: in Botswana, 57.7% of childhood deaths are due to AIDS; in Zimbabwe, 42.2%; in Swaziland, 40.6%; in Namibia, 36.5%; and in Zambia, 33.6%. In contrast, the world rate of child deaths that are related to AIDS is 4% (Kline, 2006).

LAW & ETHICS

HIV Screening in Prenatal Care

The 2001 CDC recommendations for pregnant women included HIV screening as a routine part of prenatal care. In 2006, the CDC recommended screening for patients in all healthcare settings unless the patient declines such testing. Pregnant women should be offered repeat HIV screening in the third trimester in areas with elevated HIV rates (Centers for Disease Control and Prevention, 2006).

BOX 17–1
PEDIATRIC HIV/AIDS STATISTICS

By the end of 2004, 15,338 HIV/AIDS cases had been identified in U.S. children. Of these, 9443 were in children under 13 years, 959 were in 13- to 14-year-olds, and 4936 were in 15- to 19-year-olds. However, the rates of infection have slowed dramatically for children under 13 years (61% since 2000). In 2004, the last year with complete calculated data, there were 174 new cases in this age group. In contrast, rates are increasing in 15- to 19-year-olds, as demonstrated by the 1080 new cases in that age group in 2004.

However, the incidence of disease is only part of the story. Some children continue to live with the disease, while others are deceased. At present there are 3713 children under 13 years, 1239 children from 13 to 14 years, and 3683 children from 15- to 19 years living with HIV/AIDS. By 2004, many children had died from AIDS: 5094 children under 13 years, 266 13- to 14-year-olds, and 1055 15- to 19-year-olds had died of the disease (Centers for Disease Control and Prevention, 2005).

Nurses are involved in administering HIV tests and counseling pregnant women, teaching youth about measures to decrease risk of the disease, and providing care for the children affected by the disease. Care during the chronic illness is provided to maintain and promote health, end-of-life care is administered when needed, and nurses provide solace and assistance for families managing the complex disease of HIV/AIDS.

PATHOPHYSIOLOGY ILLUSTRATED

Human Immunodeficiency Virus

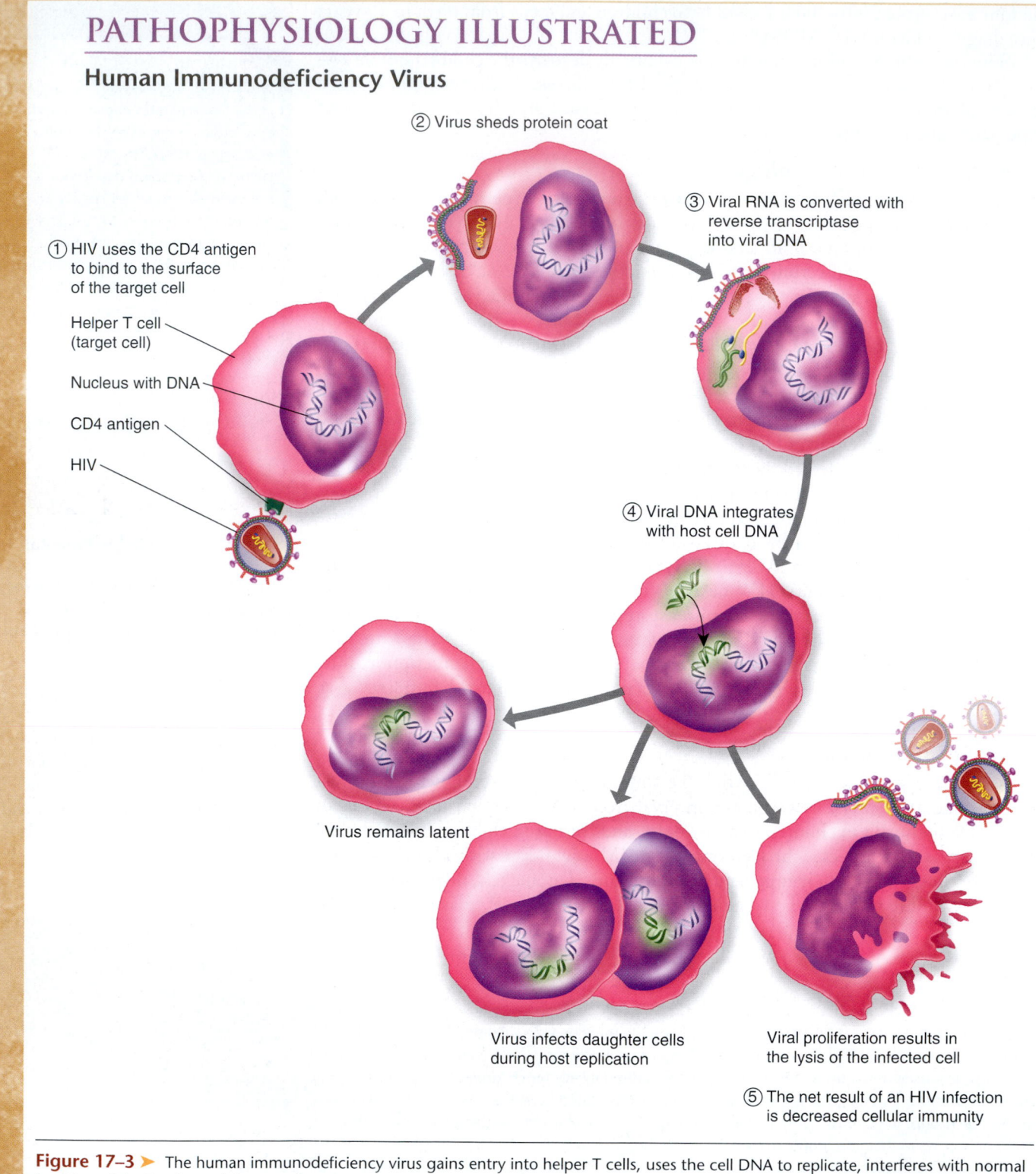

② Virus sheds protein coat

③ Viral RNA is converted with reverse transcriptase into viral DNA

① HIV uses the CD4 antigen to bind to the surface of the target cell

Helper T cell (target cell)

Nucleus with DNA

CD4 antigen

HIV

④ Viral DNA integrates with host cell DNA

Virus remains latent

Virus infects daughter cells during host replication

Viral proliferation results in the lysis of the infected cell

⑤ The net result of an HIV infection is decreased cellular immunity

Figure 17–3 ▶ The human immunodeficiency virus gains entry into helper T cells, uses the cell DNA to replicate, interferes with normal function of the T cells, and destroys the normal cells.

and fever. Specific symptoms often appear within about 2 years of infection, and include conjunctivitis, ear infections, and tonsillitis. Raymond, described at the beginning of this chapter, had several of these findings, such as a history of recurrent, acute infections (bronchitis, otitis media, and upper respiratory infections). See Clinical Manifestations of Human Immunodeficiency Virus in Children on the next page.

| HUMAN IMMUNODEFICIENCY VIRUS IN CHILDREN

Etiology	Clinical Manifestations	Clinical Therapy
Frequent, chronic, or unusual infections due to poor immune response	Chronic bilateral otitis media Oral candidiasis *Pneumocystis carinii* pneumonia (PCP) Skin disorders Fever	Vigorous antimicrobial therapy for treatment of infections Limit exposure to groups of people Obtain recommended immunizations
Poor nutritional intake due to lack of appetite caused by disease and medications	Failure to thrive (eating disorder of childhood) Weight and body mass index below 10th percentile Chronic diarrhea Skin irritation	Monitor growth Supplemental intake such as enteral feedings at night, and TPN if needed Meticulous skin care to prevent breakdown
Immune system overgrowth to compensate for lack of proper immune response	Hepatosplenomegaly and lymphadenopathy	Assess abdomen frequently Teach about safe transport to avoid injury to liver and spleen

Note: Be alert for the possibility of HIV infection in infants with combinations of listed clinical manifestations, especially in infants known to be at risk.

Bacterial and opportunistic infections, such as *Streptococcus*, *Haemophilus influenzae*, *Salmonella*, and *Pneumocystis carinii* pneumonia (PCP), as well as malignancies such as lymphoma, frequently occur as the disease progresses. Lymphocytic interstitial pneumonitis is a common manifestation of pediatric AIDS. Frequently children develop encephalopathy, resulting in developmental delay or a deterioration of motor skills and intellectual functioning. About 75% of new cases of HIV in adolescents occur in minority populations such as Blacks and Hispanics, so teaching about methods to avoid infection must be strongly emphasized in these groups (Rangel, Gavin, Reed, Fowler, & Lee, 2006).

COLLABORATIVE CARE

Diagnostic Tests

Most children with AIDS are diagnosed early in life. Serologic tests for detection of the virus, performed within 48 hours of birth, are monitored in infants born to HIV-positive mothers. Infants with initially negative tests should be retested at 1 to 2 months. Tests are again repeated at 3 and 6 months, and then again at 15 and 18 months. The preferred test is the polymerase chain reaction (PCR); other tests include p24 antigen, or HIV culture (which is not universally available). Any positive result is confirmed by retesting. When the infant has had two negative tests, testing with enzyme-linked immunosorbent assay (ELISA; HIV antibody) should be done at 12, 15, and 18 months. After two consecutive negative results with ELISA, the child is considered free of HIV. In addition, a complete blood count (CBC) and CD41 T-cell subset is performed at 3 to 6 months. A quick response HIV test using saliva is available for use in certain circumstances. Positive results are checked with blood studies (Box 17–2). The Centers for Disease Control and Prevention (CDC) considers children under 13 years of age to be infected if their symptoms meet the CDC criteria for AIDS, if they have HIV in the blood or tissues, or if they have antibodies to HIV. The CDC criteria address two issues: the diagnosis of HIV and the clinical classification of children infected with HIV (Table 17–4).

Laboratory tests are used to determine the severity of disease. The viral load is the number of circulating HIV particles per millimeter.

- Viral loads of less than 10,000 are low risk.
- Viral loads of 10,000 to 100,000 are moderate risk.
- Viral loads greater than 100,000 are high risk.
- A T4 (CD4) count of >500 cells/mm^3 for 6–12 years of age, 71,000 cells/mm^3 for 1–5 years of age, and 71,500 cells/mm^3 for 12 months of age represents a competent immune system.

BOX 17–2
HIV TESTING

Many people who are at risk of HIV infection may not have HIV testing readily available. To reduce barriers to early detection of the virus, rapid HIV tests have been made available. Specimens are obtained from saliva or fingerstick for a blood sample. Oral fluids are obtained by gently swabbing both the upper and lower outer gum of the mouth. Results are available in 1 hour or less and some do not require blood draws. Some options include OraQuick Rapid HIV-1/2 Antibody Test, Reveal Rapid HIV-1 Antibody Test, Uni-Gold Recombigen HIV Test, and Multispot HIV-1/HIV-2 Rapid Test. They require preparedness for counseling in the same session as the test is administered and confirmation for positive tests by traditional methods (Centers for Disease Control and Prevention 2004b; Greenwald, Burstein, Pincus, & Branson, 2006).

Table 17–4	CLINICAL STAGING OF PEDIATRIC HIV INFECTION

Diagnosis of HIV Infection in Children

- HIV infected (two or more positive tests for HIV or demonstrates AIDS)
- Perinatally exposed (born to a mother known to be infected with HIV)
- Seroconverter (born to a mother known to be infected with HIV but has had two negative HIV tests)

When Infected, the Child with HIV is Classified as

- Category N—not symptomatic
- Category A—mildly symptomatic with two or more of the following:
  - Lymphadenopathy
  - Hepatomegaly
  - Splenomegaly
  - Dermatitis
  - Parotitis
  - Recurrent or persistent upper respiratory infection, sinusitis, or otitis media
- Category B—moderately symptomatic with additional symptoms to those previously listed, such as:
  - Anemia
  - Bacterial meningitis, pneumonia, sepsis
  - Candidiasis
  - Cardiomyopathy
  - Cytomegalovirus
  - Diarrhea
  - Hepatitis
  - Herpes simplex virus, herpes zoster
  - Leiomyosarcoma
  - Nephropathy
  - Persistent fever
  - Toxoplasmosis
- Category C—severely symptomatic, manifested by
  - Multiple, recurrent infection
  - Encephalopathy
  - Kaposi's sarcoma
  - Lymphoma
  - Wasting syndrome

Note: From American Academy of Pediatrics, 2006.

- A T4 count of 200–499 cells/mm^3 for 6–12 years of age, 500–999 cells/mm^3 for 1–5 years of age, and 750–1,499 cells/mm^3 for 12 months of age indicates a moderately suppressed immune system.
- A T4 count of <200 cells/mm^3 for 6–12 years of age, 500 cells/mm^3 for 1–5 years of age, and 750 cells/mm^3 for 12 months of age indicates a severely suppressed immune system. (AIDSInfo, 2005).

Clinical Therapy

Medical management begins with prevention of the spread of HIV from mother to newborn. Due to the rapidity of disease progression in perinatally transmitted HIV infection, early identification of infected infants is important to ensure the most effective treatment. HIV-infected mothers should be identified during pregnancy, and their infants should undergo periodic laboratory testing, as previously described. Pregnant women infected with HIV who are treated with zidovudine (AZT) and deliver their babies by cesarean section reduce the chance of transmission to 1%. All infected mothers should receive oral zidovudine (AZT) after the first trimester of pregnancy and intravenous AZT during labor and delivery; in addition, the newborn of an infected mother should receive 6 weeks of oral AZT after birth.

All infants of infected mothers should start prophylaxis against PCP (a commonly serious or fatal outcome in infants) by the age of 4 to 6 weeks of age and continue to 12 months, or until two negative HIV tests have been documented (at 1 and 4 months of age). Drugs used for PCP prophylaxis include trimethoprim-sulfamethoxazole (Bactrim or Septra), dapsone, or aerosolized pentamidine. A CBC with differential is performed at birth, 4 to 6 weeks, and 12 weeks to monitor for drug side effects.

Treatment for the child diagnosed with HIV involves drugs to boost the immune response, and highly active antiretroviral therapy (HAART). Intravenous immune globulin (IVIG; see page 555) has been used to prevent bacterial infections in children. Prompt therapy with anti-infectives is used for bacterial and viral opportunistic infections.

Children as young as 3 months are given antiretroviral drugs, including nucleoside reverse transcriptase inhibitors such as zidovudine (AZT), didanosine (DDI), zalcitabine (DDC), lamivudin (3TC), and stavudine (D4T). The protease inhibitors (PIs), ritonavir, and nelfinavir have now been approved for use in children over 2 years, and other PIs are currently under investigation (AIDSinfo, 2005; Edmunds & Mayhew, 2004). The protease inhibitors are most effective when used in combination with nucleoside reverse transcriptase inhibitors, which slow replication of the virus. Drug trials have demonstrated reduction of serum HIV load in infants who acquired the infection from their mothers and were treated with a combination of several antiviral drugs. See Medications Used to Treat HIV below.

The earlier the child develops AIDS, the poorer the prognosis. However, as treatment improves, more children are living longer with the disease. Younger children are more

CLINICAL TIP

Use of AZT as a single agent is appropriate only when used in infants of unknown HIV status during the first 6 weeks of life to prevent perinatal HIV transmission. Combinations of drugs are commonly used for all other cases. For children on HAART therapy, CBC with differential is performed at birth, at 4 to 6 weeks, at 12 weeks, and regularly during therapy to monitor for drug effects.

MEDICATIONS USED TO TREAT *HIV*

Medication	Action	Nursing Implications
Nucleoside Analogs or Nucleoside Reverse Transcriptase Inhibitors (NRTIs)		
Examples: Zidovudine (AZT) Didanosine Zalcitabine Stavudine Lamivudine Abacavir	Inhibits action of viral reverse transcriptase, an enzyme in the conversion of RNA to DNA	• Baseline data include physical assessment, laboratory studies (especially measurement of white and red blood cell counts); monitored at least monthly for changes. • Common side effects include fever, headache, insomnia, myalgia, nausea, vomiting, diarrhea, anorexia, bone marrow suppression with resulting granulocytopenia and anemia, dyspnea, cough, skin rash. • Teach signs and symptoms of infection. • Be sure family realizes that the drug neither cures HIV nor prevents transfer from the person infected to others.
Protease Inhibitors		
Examples: Saquinavir Ritonavir Indinavir Nelfinavir Kaletra (lopinavir/ritonavir combination) Fosamprenavir	Blocks the function of the enzyme protease needed for viral formation and growth	• Baseline data include physical assessment and laboratory studies (such as serum electrolytes, CBC, liver function studies, blood glucose, hemoglobin A_{1c}, serum amylase, CPK); monitored at least monthly for changes. • Side effects include CNS, CV changes, life-threatening hematologic changes, respiratory distress, and allergy; monitor for specific side effects of the particular drug administered. • Oral forms taken within 2 hours of a full meal. • Be sure family realizes that the drug neither cures HIV nor prevents transfer from the person infected to others.
Nonnucleoside Reverse Transcriptase Inhibitors		

Examples: nevirapine, delavirdine	Bind to viral reverse transcriptase and disrupt the conversion of RNA to DNA	• Baseline data include physical assessment and laboratory studies (such as liver and kidney function tests, CBC and differential); monitored at least monthly for changes.
		• Side effects include fever, headache, nausea, diarrhea, hepatitis, altered liver function, anemia, neutropenia, drowsiness and fatigue, rash, Stevens-Johnson syndrome.
		• Be sure family realizes that the drug neither cures HIV nor prevents transfer from the person infected to others.
		• Teach the family to:
		  • Notify healthcare provider immediately if rash appears.
		  • Use caution in driving or other hazardous activity due to fatigue.
		  • Avoid St. John's wort, which may decrease the medication's activity.

Note: The average cost of annual therapy with a combination of drugs as recommended is about $10,000 (Burpo, 2000). What special financial needs will families have when someone is treated for HIV?

likely to die of pulmonary diseases or infection, while those who survive past 10 years of age are more likely to die of cardiac disease, wasting syndrome, encephalopathy, and infection with *Mycobacterium* avium complex. Many children who acquired HIV in perinatal transmission (before frequent testing during pregnancy and treatment during pregnancy and in neonates) are now entering the adolescent age group (Rangel et al., 2006).

■ NURSING MANAGEMENT
Nursing Assessment and Diagnosis

For infants at risk of HIV infection, obtain the HIV test results of the mother, if available. When these are positive, the infant will need to be screened numerous times during infancy for HIV infection, as described in the previous section. Facilitate the screening and explain the necessity to the family.

Physiologic Assessment

Assessment centers on observation and evaluation of potential sites of infection. Assess breath sounds, respiratory status, arterial blood gases, level of consciousness, and mental status. Any evidence of lymphocytic interstitial pneumonitis or neurologic abnormalities should be reported. Assess the child's height and weight frequently. Observe for signs of failure to thrive and assess for anemia. Look for *Candida* infections in the mouth and the diaper area. Note any developmental delays in motor skills or intellectual functioning, which could result from encephalopathy and poor nutrition, and can signal an increasing severity in symptom level. These should be reported so that further medical evaluation can be carried out.

Psychosocial Assessment

Assess family support systems and coping mechanisms, as the stress of caring for a child with AIDS may overwhelm parents. Assess the family's ability to care for the child. If the mother is infected, inquire about the extended family's ability to provide daily care as well as emotional support. Support the family when they decide to inform a school-age child or adolescent of the diagnosis (see Families Want to Know: Informing the Child of HIV Status). When assessing an adolescent with AIDS, evaluate the teen's understanding of how AIDS is transmitted and the response to the diagnosis.

The accompanying Nursing Care Plan includes common nursing diagnoses that may apply to a child hospitalized with AIDS. Other nursing diagnoses may include the following:

- Diarrhea related to gastrointestinal infection, malignancy, or drug reactions
- Impaired Gas Exchange related to pulmonary disease
- Delayed Growth and Development related to chronic infection and poor nutrition
- Risk for Compromised Family Coping related to life-threatening illness

FAMILIES WANT TO KNOW

Informing the Child of HIV Status

The American Academy of Pediatrics Committee on Pediatric AIDS recommends that school children and adolescents with HIV be informed of their diagnosis. Because telling the child is difficult for parents, they often avoid doing so. Since parents usually want to be the ones to tell the child, however, they need help to plan how to discuss the issue and ongoing support in the process of communication (Instone, 2000). Nurses can assist in the following ways:

- Help parents understand the need to discuss the diagnosis with the child.

- Provide information about how to tell the child. Role-play with the parents how to talk with the child; assist parents to be honest.
- Provide sources of hope—successes of treatment, children living with HIV and maintaining an active life.
- Refer the family to support groups and web-based discussion groups.
- Help the family plan for respite care as needed.
- Provide emotional support for this difficult work and allow for ongoing opportunities to express concerns, fears, and anxieties.

NURSING CARE PLAN   The Child with Acquired Immunodeficiency Syndrome

GOAL	INTERVENTION	RATIONALE	EXPECTED OUTCOME
1. Risk for infection related to immunosuppression			
	NIC Priority Intervention: **Infection Control:** *Minimizing the acquisition and transmission of infectious agents.*		*NOC Suggested Outcome:* **Risk Control:** *Actions to eliminate or reduce actual, personal, and modifiable health threats.*
Risk factors for infection will be eliminated as evidenced by infection control.	• Assess the child every 2–4 hours for fever; lesions in the mouth; redness, inflammation, soreness, and lesions on the skin or around intravenous lines.	• Fever is one of the few signs of infections in the immunosuppressed child who does not have a sufficient number of white blood cells.	The child has no fever and shows no other signs of infection.
	• Auscultate for changes in breath sounds every 2 hours. Perform pulmonary treatment (coughing, deep breathing, incentive spirometry) every 2–4 hours.	• Pneumonia is a likely infection in the child with AIDS.	
	• Enforce strict hand hygiene. Allow no fresh flowers, fruits, or vegetables in child's room. Screen visitors for colds or recent exposure to varicella. Use blood and body fluid precautions (refer to the *Clinical Skills Manual*). Practice strict asepsis for dressing changes and suctioning.	• Control of environmental factors helps prevent infection.	
	• Coordinate patient care assignments to avoid exposing the child to individuals with recent infections, varicella immunization, or children not fully immunized.	• Preventing exposure to diseases minimizes chances for infection.	
	• Organize patient care activities to allow for adequate periods for rest.	• Rest periods allow the child to regain energy.	
	• Follow recommendations of CDC and AAP for immunizing immunosuppressed children. Avoid varicella vaccine. Perform annual TB testing.	• Special recommendations consider the child's decreased immune response and the danger of acquiring disease from certain live virus vaccines.	
2. Imbalanced Nutrition: Less than Body Requirements related to loss of appetite and decreased absorption of nutrients			
	NIC Priority Intervention: **Nutrition Management:** *Assistance with or provision of a balanced dietary intake of food and fluids.*		*NOC Suggested Outcome:* **Nutritional Status:** *Nutrient value: adequacy of nutrients taken into the body.*
The child will demonstrate adequate nutritional status to meet metabolic needs.	• Encourage frequent small meals to promote nutritional and fluid intake. • Maintain nasogastric tube feeding, if ordered. Hyper-alimentation may be necessary to ensure adequate nutrition.	• Additional nutrition is required to rebuild the immune system.	The child eats frequent meals of adequate nutritional content.
	• Eliminate unpleasant stimuli and odors from the environment during meals.	• Unpleasant stimuli decrease the desire for food.	
	• Monitor skin turgor every shift.	• Skin turgor reflects hydration status.	
	• Involve a nutritionist in planning a diet for the child that includes favorite foods.	• Including favorite foods encourages intake.	

(continued)

NURSING CARE PLAN **The Child with Acquired Immunodeficiency Syndrome** (continued)

GOAL	INTERVENTION	RATIONALE	EXPECTED OUTCOME
3. Risk for impaired skin integrity related to skin infection, immobility, or diarrhea			
	NIC Priority Intervention: **Skin Surveillance:** *Collection and analysis of patient data to maintain skin integrity.*		*NOC Suggested Outcome:* **Risk Control:** *Actions to eliminate or reduce actual, personal, and modifiable health threats.*
The child will have structural intactness and normal physiologic function of skin.	• Observe all pressure areas closely for signs of infection or breakdown.	• Skin care is important in the immunocompromised child. The skin may be the only intact defense the child has.	The child is free of preventable skin breakdown.
	• Keep skin clean and dry. Provide perineal care to minimize irritation from diarrhea.	• Prevents breaking or cracking of skin.	
4. Risk for Impaired Oral Mucous Membrane related to infection			
	NIC Priority Intervention: **Oral Health Restoration:** *Promotion of healing for a patient who has an oral mucosal lesion.*		*NOC Suggested Outcome:* **Tissue Integrity:** *Structural integrity and normal physiologic function of mucous membranes.*
The child will have intact oral mucous membranes.	• Inspect mouth for sign of blistering or lesions.	• Candidal infection is frequently associated with immunodeficiency.	The child has intact oral mucous membranes.
	• Provide mouth care with normal saline solution of lemon-glycerine swabs every 2–4 hours.	• Provides comfort and promotes healing.	
5. Pain related to infections			
	NIC Priority Intervention: **Pain Management:** *Alleviation of pain or a reduction in pain to level of comfort that is acceptable to the patient.*		*NOC Suggested Outcome:* **Comfort Level:** *Feelings of physical and psychologic ease.*
The child will be free of pain or experience only mild pain/discomfort.	• Observe for signs of pain and discomfort. • Medicate for pain as ordered, monitor and document results. • Implement general comfort measures (e.g., holding, rocking).	• Pain relief adds to comfort of the child and family.	The child demonstrates evidence of pain relief.
6. Deficient Knowledge (Parent) related to home care of child with AIDS			
	NIC Priority Intervention: **Teaching, Treatment:** *Preparing a patient and family to understand and mentally prepare for a treatment.*		*NOC Suggested Outcome:* **Knowledge, Treatment Regimen:** *Extent of understanding conveyed about AIDS treatment.*
The parent(s) will demonstrate knowledge about home care, measures to prevent infection, and signs and symptoms to report to healthcare providers.	• Explain the importance of optimizing the child's health status and reducing risk of complications through diet, rest, and meticulous personal hygiene. Be sure that parents and other family members understand how AIDS is spread and appropriate precautions.	• Knowledge about the disorder and preventive measures is necessary to provide safe and effective home care for the child.	The parent describes appropriate home care and preventive measures for a child with AIDS.
	• Discuss with parents and child reasons for protective measures.	• Knowledge of rationale increases compliance.	
	• Inform family about signs and symptoms of infection that should be reported promptly to the physician or nurse (fever, chills, cough, mild erythema).	• Prompt treatment improves outcome.	

Planning and Implementation

The first step in dealing with HIV infection is prevention. Nurses must be active in evaluating test results and instituting measures to prevent vertical transmission of HIV to the infants of infected mothers. Adequate testing, prophylaxis for HIV and PCP, and follow-up visits for evaluation of general health and development for all infants at risk of the disease is advised. Guidelines from the American Academy of Pediatrics recommend that pediatricians offer HIV testing and counseling to adolescents who are sexually active or involved in substance abuse (American Academy of Pediatrics, Committee on Pediatric AIDS, 2001). Recommendations also have been made for inclusion of HIV and AIDS education into comprehensive health education for students from kindergarten through 12th grade (American Academy of Pediatrics, Committee on Pediatric AIDS, 1998) (Box 17–3). Nurses can implement these policies and counsel teens about the dangers and prevention measures for HIV.

If the child is diagnosed with HIV, close health supervision is needed to ensure medications and examinations are carried out. When HIV progresses to AIDS, nursing care is similar to that of a child with any serious, chronic, life-threatening disease. It centers on preventing infection, managing pain, promoting respiratory and other organ function, promoting adequate nutritional intake, and providing emotional support to the parents and child, while promoting the child's growth and development. The accompanying nursing care plan summarizes nursing care for the child hospitalized with acquired immunodeficiency syndrome.

Prevent Infection

Immunosuppressed children become infected with bacteria as well as other organisms that are common in the environment. Protect the neonate from HIV-infected maternal secretions. Bathe the newborn as soon as possible after delivery and wash the eyes and face before administration of prophylactic eyedrops or ointment. Avoid invasive procedures in the newborn and encourage the mother to formula feed the baby rather than breast-feed (Luxner, 2003).

Frequent hand hygiene and limiting exposure of the child to individuals with upper respiratory or other infections are the best interventions to protect the child with HIV from acquiring other infections. The child with HIV should be immunized as soon as he or she is at the recommended age for diphtheria, tetanus, and acellular pertussis; inactivated poliovirus, *Haemophilus influenzae* type b, hepatitis B, pneumococcal vaccine, and annual influenza vaccine. Live measles-mumps-rubella vaccine is administered at 12 months unless the child is severely immunocompromised, because the risk of serious outcomes for measles is great. Live varicella vaccine should be administered if the child has no or mild symptoms of HIV. Tuberculosis is more common in children with AIDS, so annual skin tests that are read by health professionals are recommended (American Academy of Pediatrics, 2006). See Chapter 18 ∞ for further recommendations about the child who is immunocompromised and immunization recommendations.

> ### ➤ NURSING ALERT
>
> Healthcare workers who come in contact with blood or other body fluids of children infected with HIV are at risk for exposure to the virus. Standard precautions should be used in caring for all children, as HIV status and presence of other infections may not be known (refer to the *Clinical Skills Manual*).
>
> Because children with HIV or other bloodborne infections may be enrolled in childcare centers, staff in these centers should use standard precautions in handling blood and body fluids. Instruct childcare center personnel in the use of these precautions. Assist childcare centers in establishing procedures to notify all parents when a child with an infectious disease has been at the center. Parents of immunocompromised children can then take any necessary precautions to minimize the chances of their children becoming ill. Parents of HIV-infected children must be very cautious to limit the exposure of their children to infectious diseases.

BOX 17–3
TEACHING ABOUT AIDS

The American Academy of Pediatrics recommends that HIV and AIDS education be part of health education in kindergarten through 12th grade. School nurses should be educated about HIV/AIDS, ethics, testing, and counseling. The particular roles defined for nurses in school settings include:

1. Participate in education programs for teachers
2. Assist schools and other organizations to develop education programs
3. Review, adapt, and develop educational materials
4. Participate in public discussions about HIV/AIDS
5. Take part in meetings with school administrators, staff, and parents
6. Facilitate networking among parents and AIDS community groups

Note: Adapted from American Academy of Pediatrics, Committee on Pediatric AIDS. (1998). Human immunodeficiency virus/acquired immunodeficiency syndrome education in schools. *Pediatrics, 101*, 933–935.

HIV/AIDS and Hispanics

Hispanics account for a disproportionate 18% of the total AIDS cases diagnosed. These high rates are due to poverty and inadequate access to quality health care. In addition, women may be reluctant to ask male partners to wear a condom due to the machismo behavior of some males; this can increase the risk of heterosexual spread of disease. Nurses need to be aware of these cultural concerns in the Hispanic population and provide clients an opportunity to discuss their knowledge and concerns about HIV/AIDS. CDC-funded programs are now providing community-based free health clinics and other bilingual services (Centers for Disease Control and Prevention, 2004a).

Educate sexually active adolescents about the importance of practicing safe sex and the ramifications of high-risk sexual behaviors and intravenous drug use.

Promote Medication Regimen Adherence

The treatment regimen with the use of antiretroviral therapies for the child with HIV or AIDS may be complex and time consuming, presenting an overwhelming challenge to the child and their family. Non-adherence to the prescribed antiretroviral treatment regimen will likely result in increased morbidity and mortality. Some common reasons for nonadherence include frequent dosing, child's displeasure with medication (large pills, gritty powders, bitter taste), and associated side effects including nausea and rashes (Brackis-Cott, Mellins, Abrams, Reval, & Dolezal, 2003).

Strategies for achieving optimal management of the treatment regimen include educating the parent and/or care provider, as well as the child when old enough to understand, regarding the purpose of the medication, the benefits of adhering to the regimen, and the potential consequences of failure to adhere to the regimen. Behavior modification techniques, using positive reinforcement, can be very effective in promoting the child's adherence. Support should be provided to the family and the medication regimen should be tailored to the family's routine. Praise should be offered to the child and parent for adhering to the regimen. If problems exist in the management of the treatment regimen, carefully listen to the family to help determine the cause. Collaborate with the family in establishing goals to help meet the prescribed treatment regimen. Consider the effect of cultural beliefs on medication adherence (see Evidence-Based Practice: Adolescents with HIV Infection and Medication Regimen Adherence). If further intervention is required, other options include direct observational therapy or home visits.

Promote Respiratory Function

Because many children with AIDS develop pneumonia, encourage the child to cough and deep breathe every 2 to 4 hours. In the community, regular physical activity encourages lung aeration. When in the hospital, blowing cotton balls with a straw, blowing bubbles, or other games may engage the interest of a younger child. Reposition infants frequently so all areas of the lungs can aerate. Rest periods to conserve energy and lower the body's demand for oxygen are important.

EVIDENCE-BASED PRACTICE

Adolescents with HIV Infection and Medication Regimen Adherence

Problem

Medication adherence is a major problem in the HIV-infected adolescent.

Evidence

An increase in incidence of human immunodeficiency virus has been seen in the United States, particularly among young people ages 13 to 19 years. Adherence to highly active antiretroviral therapy (HAART) has been shown to decrease morbidity and mortality. However, medication adherence in this age group is often poor. The REACH (Reaching for Excellence in Adolescent Care) project has conducted studies evaluating medication adherence in the HIV-positive adolescent.

In face-to-face interviews of HIV-infected adolescents enrolled in REACH from several U.S. cities, only 41% ($n = 171$) reported consistently taking their medication as prescribed. Depressed mood was a major factor in nonadherence.

Another REACH study of 114 HIV-positive adolescents prescribed HAART were interviewed regarding barriers associated with medication adherence. Participants reported simply forgetting to take their medication, not having medication available to take (e.g., left medication at

home), and variations in their daily routine as key reasons for not taking the prescribed medications as directed.

Implications

In these studies, adherence to medication regimes was noted to be closely tied to depressed mood and lack of understanding of the importance of strictly following medication directions, as well as to daily routine. This suggests that improving organizationsl skills, better education, and treatment for depression could have a positive impact on medication adherence.

Critical Thinking

1. What are some barriers that may lead to medication nonadherence in the HIV-positive adolescent?
2. What support does the adolescent need to improve medication adherence?
3. What measures can the nurse take to improve medication adherence in the adolescent?

Reference

Murphy, D. A., Wilson, C. M., Durako, S. J., Muenz, L. R., & Belzer, M. (2001). Antiretroviral medication adherence among the REACH HIV-infected adolescent cohort in the USA. *AIDS Care, 13*(1), 27–41.

Promote Adequate Nutritional Intake

Because many children with AIDS have failure to thrive, nutrition is an important part of their care. (See Chapter 4  for information to include in a detailed nutritional assessment.) A nutritionist should be involved in planning an appropriate diet for the child that provides necessary calories, protein, and other nutrients. Vitamins may be especially lacking in the diets of infected children. Antioxidants (vitamin A, vitamin E, zinc, and selenium) are known to enhance general immune system function and should be consumed at recommended levels. Periodic dietary analysis and teaching are needed. Adequate nutrition is sometimes provided by hyperalimentation, nasogastric, or gavage feeding.

Diarrhea resulting from gastrointestinal infection and lactose intolerance is a common finding in children with HIV infection and complicates other nutritional disturbances. Antidiarrheal medications may be prescribed, or alternative formulas tried. Keep the child's lips and mouth moist and pay close attention to hydration status. Monitor the skin turgor and urine output, and provide careful perineal skin care to prevent infection.

The frequency of *Candida* infections leads to blisters, cracking, and discharge involving the oral mucous membranes. Mouth care with a non-alcohol-based solution such as normal saline or lemon-glycerine swabs should be performed every 2 to 4 hours. Precautions to guard against food-borne illness are particularly important for the child infected with HIV (see Families Want to Know: Food Safety and HIV).

Provide Emotional Support

The family of the child with AIDS is under emotional stress; this is compounded if the mother and others in the family are also infected. Integrate social services and support groups into the care of the child as soon as the diagnosis is made. Spend time talking with the family about their fears and feelings. In many communities and social groups, AIDS still carries a tremendous stigma, and the family may not be able to discuss their feelings outside of the healthcare environment. Safeguard the family's wishes regarding the privacy of the diagnosis.

Clarify any misconceptions the older child with AIDS may have about the transmission of the disease. Routes of transmission and the need for safe sexual practices must be clearly discussed with adolescents. Providing support for adolescents is particularly important, as the dependence that this chronic and terminal disease brings can make it difficult to meet the developmental task of independence. Adolescents may benefit from contact with other infected peers.

Discharge Planning

The diagnosis of AIDS is surrounded by strong emotions and fears. Be honest and direct. Education is essential. Explain that there is no evidence that casual contact among family members can spread the infection. For the child who has been hospitalized, home care needs should be identified well in advance of discharge.

Discuss the family's finances as well as health insurance coverage for the child's care. Assess the family's ability to provide nutritious food, required medications, and a

---

LAW & ETHICS

Confidentiality

Disclosure of patient information is a breach of confidentiality that may subject a nurse to legal action. Disclosure of confidential information occurs when a patient's condition—for example, a diagnosis of AIDS—is discussed inappropriately with any third party.

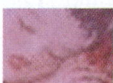

FAMILIES WANT TO KNOW

Food Safety and HIV

The child with HIV infection is more prone to food-borne disease. Instruct parents to practice the following:

1. Use a separate cutting board for meats, and wash it with hot soapy water after use.
2. Wash all utensils with hot soapy water between any uses.
3. Wash and peel fresh fruits and vegetables.
4. Use a disposable cloth or cloth that is washed after each meal to clean dishes. A sponge can harbor organisms and should not be used.
5. Have well water checked for contaminants regularly if that is the source of drinking water.
6. Do not allow the child to eat raw or undercooked meats, fish, eggs, or cookie dough.
7. Use bleach solution for cleaning surfaces in the kitchen.

supportive environment. Refer to services as needed to ensure provision of quality care for the child after discharge.

Support groups, home healthcare nursing services, financial assistance, respite care, and psychological counseling are usually needed at some point during the child's illness, and the family should be aware of the availability of such services. Help the family deal with feelings of guilt about the child's condition.

Care in the Community

Much of the care of the child with HIV infection or AIDS takes place in the community. Evaluate the family and community support systems and provide resources and referrals as needed. Many children with HIV infection are placed in foster homes, and these families need careful instruction to manage this multifaceted illness.

School attendance guidelines for children with AIDS by the American Academy of Pediatrics (AAP) and the CDC recommend unrestricted school attendance for children with AIDS as long as their physician approves. Contraindications to school attendance include lack of control of body secretions, biting, and open wounds that cannot be covered. The nurse often prepares the school personnel with training related to care for children with known and unknown cases of HIV. The nurse also may be responsible for providing medicines or other care for the child with HIV at school. It is recommended that children with HIV take part in school sports. While injuries are possible, it is unlikely that large quantities of blood will be present in sports injuries; thus, risk to others in contact with the injured child will be low. Additionally, coaches and others should be instructed in how to follow universal precautions for all injuries that happen in sports events (Kukka, 2004).

Assist the family to alter the home environment in order to provide standard precautions during care. Make sure the child and family understand that HIV is transmitted through blood, urine, stool, and other body secretions. Dispel myths about HIV transmission. Teach family members the importance of careful hygiene. Encourage careful hand hygiene and tell parents to use precautions when handling body fluids. Explain that they should wear gloves when changing diapers; disposing of urine, stool, and emesis; or treating the child's cuts and scrapes. Instruct parents to use a bleach solution for disinfection of objects when necessary and to avoid contact with persons with infectious illnesses. Precautions to guard against food-borne illness are particularly important for the HIV-infected child. Parents will also need instruction on correct administration and side effects of any medications the child is taking. Giving a child a complicated combination of drugs can be challenging for all families, so use teaching that is tailored to the particular family and perform repeated evaluation of the family's success with medication administration.

Emphasize the importance of promoting the child's development. Frequent developmental screening should be performed. Teach the parents how to support the child in achieving developmental milestones. Encourage contact with other children and adults, provide for appropriate toys, teach parents how to encourage the child's communication, and praise the family for what the child has already accomplished. Children who manifest decreasing developmental milestones or other neurologic symptoms should be assessed for HIV-induced encephalopathy by the primary care provider. The nurse's record of development will be of great importance in this situation.

The child must receive regular health promotion and health maintenance care, such as child health supervision visits, immunizations, and care for any other health conditions.

Evaluation

There are many desired outcomes of care for the child with HIV infection or AIDS. Expected outcomes of nursing care include the following:

- Decreased numbers of cases of pediatric HIV due to vertical transmission from known infected mothers will be demonstrated.
- Interventions will be successful in preventing infectious diseases in children with the virus.

COMMUNITY CARE

Dispelling Myths About HIV Transmission

- Although HIV has been found in saliva and tears, it does not necessarily mean that HIV can be transmitted by those body fluids. HIV has not been recovered from the sweat of HIV-infected individuals. Furthermore, contact with saliva, tears, or sweat has not been shown to result in transmission of the virus.
- Casual, closed-mouth, or "social" kissing is not a risk for transmission of HIV. The risk of transmission through open-mouthed kissing is low.
- Human biting is not a common method of transmitting HIV. In cases of HIV transmission by a bite, severe trauma with extensive tissue tearing and damage and the presence of blood were documented.
- There is no evidence that HIV is transmitted through insect bites.

Adapted from Centers for Disease Control and Prevention. (2006b). HIV and its transmission. Retrieved January 30, 2007, from http://www. cdc.gov

MediaLink

Health Promotion and Health Maintenance Overview: AIDS

- Children will have adequate respiratory function and perfusion.
- Nutritional intake of affected children will support normal growth patterns and prevent malnutrition.
- The family who has a child with HIV will demonstrate adequate coping with the stress of chronic disease.
- The child will be able to attend school and receive other supports in the educational process.

AUTOIMMUNE DISORDERS

In an immune system damaged by pathologic changes, an immune response may occur to some of the body's own proteins, resulting in the production of autoantibodies. These pathologic conditions in which the body directs the immune response against itself—identifying "self" as "nonself"—are called autoimmune disorders.

The primary feature of autoimmune disorders is tissue injury caused by a probable immunologic reaction of the host with its own tissues. Structural or functional changes occur as immune cells attack other cells in the body.

The autoimmune disorders are grouped into systemic and organ-specific diseases. Systemic diseases, which largely involve more than one organ, include systemic lupus erythematosus and juvenile rheumatoid arthritis. Organ-specific diseases, which primarily affect a single organ, include insulin-dependent diabetes mellitus (IDDM; see Chapter 29 ∞) and thyroiditis. Idiopathic (or immune) thrombocytic purpura, an immune disease affecting blood platelets and clotting, is discussed in Chapter 22 ∞.

Systemic Lupus Erythematosus

Systemic lupus erythematosus (SLE), a generalized disorder seen mainly in females, is a chronic inflammatory disease of unknown origin that involves many organ systems, and is characterized by remissions and exacerbations. The disorder affects 7 per 100,000 individuals and is more common in African Americans, Hispanics, and Asians than in Caucasians. Females are affected more than males, with a 9:1 ratio (Pullen, Cannon, & Rushing, 2003; Stichweh, Arce, & Pascual, 2004). The majority of cases are diagnosed in the teenage and early adult years.

Etiology and Pathophysiology

The exact etiology of SLE is unknown. A genetic component is suspected as the disease is often more common in certain families. It is believed that an outside environmental agent causes the body to initiate an abnormal immune system response to its own tissues (Lupus Foundation of America, 2004; Pongmarutani, Alpert, & Miller, 2006). The body produces autoantibodies and combines with antigens to form immune complexes. These antigen-antibody complexes are then deposited in the connective tissue, leading to widespread inflammation and tissue damage. The tissues most likely to be affected are the small blood vessels, glomeruli, joints, spleen, and heart valves. Because many systems can be affected simultaneously, organ damage with subsequent system failure may occur.

Clinical Manifestations

The three major classifications of systemic lupus erythematosus are:

- *Systemic lupus.* This involves one or more of the following systems: cardiovascular, central nervous, hematological, kidneys, lungs, musculoskeletal.
- *Drug-induced lupus.* This is associated with some antineoplastic drugs, isoniazid (INH), hydralazine (Apresoline), and others. The symptoms generally subside after the drugs are discontinued.
- *Discoid lupus.* This disorder is limited to the skin.

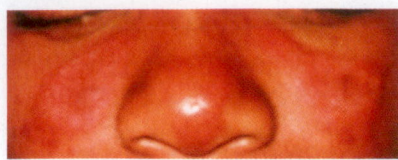

Figure 17–4 ➤ This child displays a "butterfly" rash across the cheeks and bridge of the nose. It is often seen in the child with SLE.
From Zitelli, B. J., & Davis H. W. (Eds.). (1997). *Atlas of pediatric physical diagnosis* (3rd ed., p. 192). St. Louis, MO: Mosby, Inc.

Manifestations may be acute, with onset of nephritis, arthritis, or vasculitis; or may be gradual with nonspecific symptoms. Symptoms depend on the organ involved and the amount of tissue damage that has occurred. Initial symptoms include recurrent fever, chills, fatigue, malaise, and weight loss. The most common symptoms are arthritis and skin rash. A butterfly rash on the face, consisting of a pink or red rash over the bridge of the nose extending to the cheeks, is a characteristic finding (Figure 17–4 ➤). Children with SLE may have hemolytic anemia, with a low white blood cell and platelet count; bleeding disorders; hypergammaglobulinemia; and vasculitis. See Clinical Manifestations of Systemic Lupus Erythematosus below for a comprehensive list of possible manifestations.

Systemic lupus erythematosus is characterized by periods of remission and exacerbation (flares). Flares are triggered by a variety of causes including sun exposure, a cold or other infection, and stress. The child or family may be able to identify other triggers to flares, such as particular events, activities, or situations.

■ COLLABORATIVE CARE

Blood tests reveal anemia, an elevated blood urea nitrogen (BUN), abnormal plasma proteins, abnormal erythrocyte sedimentation rate (ESR), presence of antinuclear antibodies, and a positive lupus erythematosus (LE) cell reaction, which indicates nonspecific inflammation. The Coombs test is positive. Radiologic examinations include chest radiographs and CT scans, as well as an MRI of the affected joints. A 24-hour urine collection and imaging studies, as well as renal biopsies, may be performed to evaluate lupus nephritis. Urinalysis may reveal proteinuria.

The goals of medical management are to create a remission of symptoms and to prevent complications. Corticosteroids, such as prednisone, are prescribed to control in-

CLINICAL MANIFESTATIONS	SYSTEMIC LUPUS ERYTHEMATOSUS
System	**Clinical Manifestations**
Integumentary	A butterfly rash on the face, consisting of a pink or red rash over the bridge of the nose extending to the cheeks, is a characteristic finding Photosensitivity Alopecia Mouth or nose ulcers
Hematologic	Hemolytic anemia Leukopenia (low white blood cells) Thrombocytopenia (low platelet count) Bleeding disorders
Musculoskeletal	Joint pain Raynaud's phenomenon (fingers turning white and/or blue in the cold) Arthritis Arthralgia
Neurological	Chorea Dizziness Seizures Cerebral vascular accident (CVA) and resultant quadriplegia
Pulmonary	Pleural effusions Pleuritis
Cardiac	Pericarditis Vasculitis
Renal	Glomerulonephritis Renal failure Lupus nephritis
Other	Hypergammaglobulinemia Extreme fatigue

flammation. Antimalarial preparations, such as hydroxychloroquine and chloroquine, are used to treat symptoms associated with skin lesions and renal and arthritic problems. Although the exact action of these drugs on SLE is not known, they often permit continued remission with a lowered dose of steroids. Nonsteroidal anti-inflammatory drugs (aspirin, ibuprofen, naproxen) are used to relieve muscle and joint pain. Immunosuppressant drugs, such as cyclosporin and methotrexate, have been used to help control SLE (see Medications Used to Treat SLE below). Diet may be restricted if the child has excessive weight gain or fluid retention from steroids and renal damage.

Prognosis depends on the severity of the internal organ involvement; however, while systemic lupus erythematosus was once considered a fatal disease, the survival rate now is more than 97% (American College of Rheumatology, 2003). Kidney failure is managed by hemodialysis or peritoneal dialysis. Renal transplantation has been very successful for treatment of renal failure secondary to lupus nephritis.

NURSING MANAGEMENT

Nursing management focuses on thorough assessments due to the multitude of systems that can be affected by SLE, and teaching to enhance general health practices.

Nursing Assessment and Diagnosis

Thorough assessments are needed, as symptoms are widespread. Based on the combination of symptoms that are manifested, a unique group of nursing diagnoses is identified.

MEDICATIONS USED TO TREAT *Systemic Lupus Erythematosus*

Medication	Action/Indication	Nursing Implications
Corticosteroids prednisone	To control inflammation	• Monitor for side effects including weight gain, mood changes, insomnia, and elevated serum glucose. • Caution must be taken with corticosteroids as they may interfere with normal growth and increase susceptibility to infection.
Topical steroids fluocinonide cream (Lidex)	To treat dermatologic symptoms	• Apply to clean, dry skin. • Apply thin layer.

Antimalarial preparations
  hydroxychloroquine (Plaquenil)
  chloroquine
	To treat symptoms associated with skin lesions and renal and arthritic pain. Although the exact action of these drugs on SLE is not known, they often permit continued remission with a lowered dose of steroids.	• Administer with milk or meals to reduce gastric irritation.
		• Teach family to report the following serious side effects:
		  • Weakness
		  • Visual symptoms
		  • Hearing loss
		  • Bruising
		  • Unusual bleeding
		  • Skin eruptions

Nonsteroidal anti-inflammatories (NSAIDs)
  aspirin
  ibuprofen
  naproxen
	To relieve muscle and joint pain	• Monitor for side effects including abdominal pain, bleeding, and gastrointestinal complications.
		• Teach family to monitor for side effects and to avoid administration of additional NSAIDs.

Immunosuppressants
  cyclosporine
  methotrexate
	To help control systemic lupus erythematosus during acute exacerbations	• Monitor for infection.
		• Implement measures to reduce risk of infection.
		• Monitor for thrombocytopenia.
		• Teach family that child should avoid exposure to sunlight; wear sunscreen and sunglasses.

Physiologic Assessment

Assess the child's nutritional status including baseline weight and history of recent weight loss or weight gain. The skin is assessed for rashes, ulcers, photosensitivity, ecchymosis, petechiae, cyanosis, and hair loss. Respiratory assessment includes breath sounds and respiratory rate and assessing for pleural effusion or pleuritis. Cardiovascular assessment includes vital signs, heart tones, and symptoms of pericarditis or friction rub. Musculoskeletal assessment includes joint pain, joint deformity, pain, weakness, and ability to perform activities of daily living. Neurological assessment includes changes in affect or cognitive abilities and seizure activity. Gastrointestinal assessment includes splenomegaly.

Psychosocial Assessment

Because SLE is a chronic disease that affects primarily adolescents, psychosocial assessment is indicated. Assess family interactions, exploring stressful situations such as divorce or trauma. Treatment-related restrictions and changes in appearance can lead to withdrawal, depression, and suicidal tendencies. Perform psychological assessments periodically as the child grows and adapts to the disorder or faces new developmental challenges with a chronic disease. The following nursing diagnoses may apply to the child with SLE:

- Risk for Ineffective Management of Therapeutic Regimen (family) related to complexity of therapeutic regimen
- Risk for Ineffective Tissue Perfusion (Renal) related to interrupted blood flow in kidneys
- Risk for Impaired Skin Integrity related to immunologic deficit
- Risk for Activity Intolerance related to chronic disease
- Risk for Disturbed Body Image related to side effects of medications and skin alterations
- Risk for Infection related to immunosuppressive medications
- Chronic Pain related to joint inflammation and injury
- Disturbed Body Image related to changes from the disease and medication treatment
- Compromised Family Coping related to demands of chronic illness with unknown outcome

Planning and Implementation

The goals of nursing care are to assist the child to manage and cope with a chronic disease, prevent infection, promote nutrition, facilitate a remission, and recognize and avoid triggers for flares.

Prevent Infection

Infections are a leading cause of death for patients with systemic lupus erythematosus. Prophylactic antibiotics may be required for dental work and surgical procedures. Instruct the patient and family to inform all healthcare providers of the disease in order to plan for prophylactic measures. Educate the patient and family on the importance of adhering to the immunization schedule, and to obtain a yearly influenza vaccine to prevent infection. Instruct the family on hand hygiene and infection control measures in the home, and warn adolescents about the dangers of tattooing and body piercing because of the risk of infection.

Maintain Fluid Balance

Because most children with SLE have renal involvement, it is important to monitor intake and output and frequently evaluate the child's fluid and electrolyte status. Renal dysfunction can manifest itself by edema, muscle cramps, diarrhea, tetany, and convulsions.

Promote Adequate Nutrition

Currently, there are no specific dietary plans for the child with systemic lupus erythematosus; however, the diet may be restricted according to renal involvement, weight gain, weight loss, or other complications. The child is at risk for weight gain associated with treatment with steroids and a decreased activity level during exacerbations of this disease. A well-balanced, nutritious diet as well as appropriate fluid intake for age should be encouraged.

Promote Skin Integrity

Presence of the rash on mucous membranes can cause weakening of the tissues, placing the child at increased risk for infection. Encourage the use of good hygienic measures and a mild soap. Recommend that adolescents limit their use of cosmetics. Reinforce the importance of avoiding sunlight as much as possible, as well as the use of sun protection factor (SPF) of 15 or higher at all times when in the sun. Encourage the child to wear protective clothing to limit exposure to sunlight. (See Chapter 30 for a discussion of sun exposure.) Avoidance of fluorescent lighting is recommended since exacerbations of systemic lupus erythematosus have been reported following this exposure (Mulvihill, 2003). Encourage the adolescent to avoid the use of tanning beds. Provide instructions on oral care to maintain intact oral mucosa. Provide instructions on the care of the head if alopecia occurs.

Promote Rest and Comfort

Because of fatigue and joint pain, the child has little energy reserve during acute episodes of the disease. Encourage frequent rest periods and a nutritious diet to maximize energy stores. A physical therapist can plan a program to encourage mobility and increase muscle strength.

Manage Side Effects of Medications

Observe for side effects of medications used for treatment, and teach the child and family about these effects. For example, immunosuppressant drugs can promote infection anywhere in the body; and nonsteroidal anti-inflammatory drugs commonly cause gastric distress and bleeding of the gastrointestinal tract. The antimalarial drug hydroxychloroquine can cause serious vision changes; thus, frequent eye examinations are needed.

Provide Emotional Support

Adolescents may have an altered body image as a result of rash, alopecia, arthritic changes in the joints, and chronic disease. Referral to a lupus support group, social services, or counseling may be helpful. The American Lupus Society and the Lupus Foundation of America can provide information to help parents and children adjust to the disease. The Arthritis Foundation also publishes a useful pamphlet: *Meeting the Challenge: A Young Person's Guide to Living with Lupus*. The family needs ongoing support and information to deal with the complexity of the disease.

Avoidance of Triggers for Disease Flares

Many children and their parents can recognize the signs of an impending flare and the triggers that precede them. Partner with the parents and child to implement measures to avoid these triggers. Discuss preventive behaviors such as avoiding sun exposure and avoiding stressors. Adolescents should be warned that alcohol, smoking, and drugs also pose an increased risk due to the potential to stimulate flares. Female adolescents who are sexually active should avoid birth control pills that contain the hormone estrogen since the extra estrogen may exacerbate symptoms. In addition, alternate birth control methods should be discussed with the adolescent.

Evaluation

Successful outcomes of nursing care involve management of this chronic disease. Expected outcomes of nursing care include the following:

- Normal intake and output levels, with demonstrated fluid and electrolyte balance.
- Intact skin is maintained.
- A balance of rest and activity is maintained to promote development.
- Medications are managed to promote health and prevent side effects.
- The child or adolescent develops a positive body image.

MediaLink

Lupus Resources

Juvenile Rheumatoid Arthritis

Juvenile rheumatoid arthritis (JRA) is a chronic autoimmune inflammatory disease characterized by joint inflammation resulting in decreased mobility, swelling, and pain that occurs slightly more often in girls than in boys. Juvenile rheumatoid arthritis is the most common type of arthritis in children and adolescents, and usually occurs in children between 2 and 5 or between 9 and 12 years of age. It may enter remission or occasionally continue as a chronic disease. Approximately 5 to 18 of every 100,000 children develop juvenile rheumatoid arthritis each year (Ilowite, 2002).

Remission may last for months, years, or a lifetime. Juvenile rheumatoid arthritis affects joints and surrounding tissues in addition to possibly affecting other organs such as the heart, lungs, liver, and eyes. During its course, the child may experience pain, impaired mobility, and interference with normal growth and development. However, 70% of children with juvenile rheumatoid arthritis experience permanent remission of the disease by adulthood. In rare cases, the disease is unresponsive to treatment or the child may suffer lasting impairment such as bone and joint changes. Children with early onset have a better prognosis for complete recovery.

Etiology and Pathophysiology

The cause of JRA is unknown, but it is thought to have an autoimmune basis. Inflammation begins in the joint and leads to pain and swelling (Figure 17–5 ➤). Scar tissue eventually develops, resulting in limited range of motion. There are three types of JRA: pauciarticular, systemic, and polyarticular. *Pauciarticular arthritis* primarily affects the knees, ankles, and elbows, and occurs more frequently in females. *Systemic arthritis* affects males and females equally and characteristically is manifested by high fever, polyarthritis, and rheumatoid rash. Systemic arthritis also affects internal organs and joints. *Polyarticular arthritis* involves many joints (five or more), particularly the small joints of the hands and fingers. It may also affect the hips, knees, feet, ankles, and neck.

Clinical Manifestations

JRA may be restricted to a few joints or be systemic with involvement of multiple joints. Symptoms can include fever, rash, lymphadenopathy, splenomegaly, and hepatomegaly. The child may develop a limp or obviously favor one extremity over the other. A slow rate of growth or uneven growth of extremities may also be noted. Pain, stiffness, loss of motion, and swelling occur in the large joints such as the knees. Older children may develop symmetric involvement of the small joints of the hand. The disease is frequently chronic, extending over several years after an initial manifestation with pain and other symptoms. However, remissions and exacerbations are characteristic.

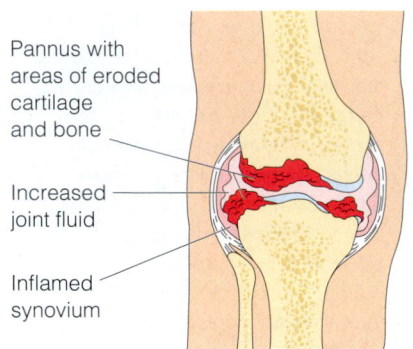

Pannus with areas of eroded cartilage and bone

Increased joint fluid

Inflamed synovium

Figure 17–5 ➤ Joint inflammation and destruction in rheumatoid arthritis.

■ COLLABORATIVE CARE

Diagnosis is made primarily on the basis of the history and assessment findings, in particular, arthritis having an onset before 17 years of age and persisting for at least 6 weeks, with no other identifiable cause. The disease may occur for a limited time and then improve (monophasic), may recur periodically (polycyclic), or may last for 3–6 months or longer (persistent) (Singh-Grewal, Schneider, Bayer, & Feldman, 2006). There are no specific laboratory tests for the disease. In some children, rheumatoid factor, human leukocyte antigen (HLA) B27, and antinuclear antibody (ANA) tests are positive, and the erythrocyte sedimentation rate (ESR) may be elevated.

Medical management involves drug therapy, physical therapy, and, when necessary, surgery. The goals of treatment are to relieve pain and prevent contractures. Salicylates (aspirin) or nonsteroidal anti-inflammatory drugs (tolmetin sodium, naproxen, diclofenac, ibuprofen) are prescribed to reduce inflammation. Steroids may be used with children who have moderately active disease. Children who do not respond to aspirin or nonsteroidal anti-inflammatory drugs may be treated with sulfasalazine and methotrexate. Physical therapy is performed to increase the strength and mobility of joints while protecting them from injury. Surgery is occasionally performed to relieve pain and maintain or improve joint function in children with joint contractures.

Complications such as eye chronic uveitis, which results from chronic inflammation, may occur in children with JRA, especially those with pauciarticular arthritis. Children with polyarticular and systemic juvenile rheumatoid arthritis should be examined by an ophthalmologist for uveitis every 6 months, and children with pauciarticular arthritis should be examined every 3 months.

Growth interference for the child with JRA is a potential complication. The specific disorder may result in bone growth disturbance such as contractures or effusions. The administration of corticosteroids can also inhibit growth.

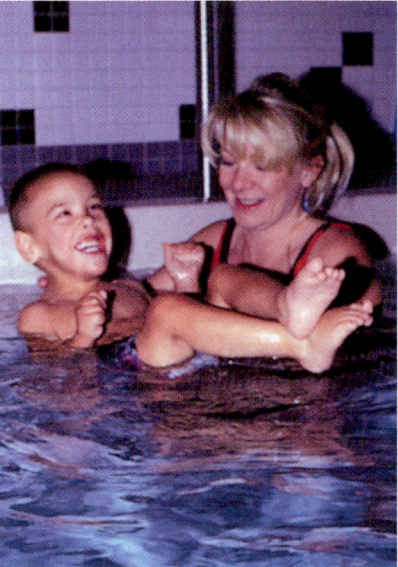

Figure 17–6 ➤ The physical therapist uses hydrotherapy to help maintain joint function in a child who has juvenile rheumatoid arthritis.

NURSING MANAGEMENT

Nursing Assessment and Diagnosis

A careful history is important, as it is sometimes the primary mode of diagnosis. Assess for joint swelling and deformities, fever, nodules under the skin, growth delays, and enlarged lymph nodes.

The following nursing diagnoses may apply to the child with JRA:

- Activity Intolerance related to chronic pain
- Impaired Physical Mobility related to joint stiffness
- Anxiety (Child and Family) related to stress of chronic illness
- Chronic Pain related to joint inflammation
- Disturbed Body Image related to illness

Planning and Implementation

Nursing care focuses on promoting mobility, encouraging adequate nutrition, and teaching the parents and child about the disease and its management. Most care will occur in the community, including physical therapy, with only occasional hospitalizations at the time of an exacerbation of the disease.

Promote Improved Mobility

Physical therapists play an essential role in the child's treatment. The goals of physical therapy are to maintain joint function, strengthen muscles, increase tone, maintain body alignment, and prevent permanent deformities such as contractures. Range-of-motion exercises, stretching, hydrotherapy, and swimming help to prevent deformities (Figures 17–6 ➤ and 17–7 ➤). Encourage the child to perform activities of daily living. Medications may be given to reduce joint swelling and inflammation. In addition, warm compresses to the involved joints are soothing.

Encourage Adequate Nutrition

Promote general health by encouraging a well-balanced diet. Children with decreased mobility may have reduced metabolic needs, and excess weight causes additional muscle strain. Periodically perform diet recalls and nutritional assessments. Plot growth carefully and watch for changes in growth percentiles. (See Chapter 4 ∞ for additional information regarding nutritional assessment.)

Care in the Community

The child with JRA may never, or rarely, be hospitalized. Most care takes place during visits to healthcare offices, clinics, and physical therapy. Teach parents about the child's condition and prognosis, and answer their questions about the child's treatment. The child and family may need support to adjust to the diagnosis of a chronic illness. Encourage the child to maintain contact with peers and to attend school when possible. Explain to the child and parents that overexertion may lead to exacerbation of the disease. Inform parents about possible complications of JRA, such as altered growth related to early closure of epiphyseal plates, small joint contractures, and synovitis. Teach parents about signs of infection, encourage recommended immunizations, and encourage health promotion activities such as nutritious diet and adequate rest. Parents and children can be referred to the Arthritis Foundation and the American Juvenile Arthritis Foundation for further information and support.

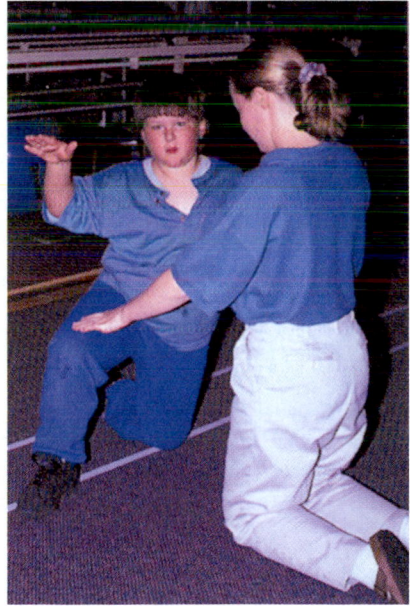

Figure 17–7 ➤ Stretching exercises are an important part of physical therapy for a child who has juvenile rheumatoid arthritis.

> **NURSING ALERT**
>
> Infants and children with juvenile rheumatoid arthritis who are receiving aspirin therapy are at risk of developing Reye syndrome if they contract influenza or chickenpox. These children are immunized with varicella vaccine and should receive influenza vaccine in the fall of each year.

RESEARCH

Increasing Incidence of Allergy

Atopic diseases such as rhinitis, dermatitis, asthma, and gastrointestinal allergy affect over 20% of the population of the United States. This represents a significant increase in incidence over the last two decades. Researchers are attempting to identify why there is such an increase in allergic diseases and presently are exploring two major theories (McGeady, 2004). They are:

1. Nutritional patterns and environmental exposures have changed, exposing children to different potential allergens than those previously encountered.

2. Modern life has removed children from exposure to infectious agents early in life. They are generally not exposed to organisms commonly found on farms. This has favored response by IgE to common substances in the environment, a Th2 response leading to atopy, rather than a Th1 response, which diverts the T-cell response toward responses to more harmful organisms.

Researchers continue to study incidence of allergy and exposure to environmental characteristics to determine the causes of increased allergy. How would you design studies to determine which theory of allergy answers the question about increase in incidence?

Partner with the family and school officials to meet the child's needs. Accommodations at school may include providing a set of books for the home so that the child is not required to carry the books home daily. Be aware that additional time may be required for the child to move from class to class. Adaptive computers and tutors during exacerbations may also be helpful. School nurses work with the child, family, and school personnel to establish the child's Individualized Education Plan (IEP).

Evaluation

Expected outcomes of nursing care for the child with JRA include the following:

- The child maintains joint mobility.
- The child expresses comfort and freedom from pain.
- The child develops a positive body image.
- The child is free from infection.
- Parents express adequate understanding, support, and management of the therapeutic regimen.

Allergic Reactions

Allergy is one of the major chronic illnesses of children today. Why are some children allergic to cats, for instance, although no one else in the family has allergies? To answer this question, the nurse requires a basic understanding of the mechanisms of allergy.

An allergy is an abnormal or altered reaction to an antigen. Antigens responsible for clinical manifestations of allergy are called **allergens**. Allergens can be ingested in food or drugs or injected or absorbed through contact with unbroken skin. Common allergens in children include medications such as penicillin; animal dander; dust mites, mold, and plant pollens; and foods such as nuts, seafood, or egg white. Having a family member with an allergy increases the chance that a child will be affected, even to different allergens or by showing different bodily manifestations. Prevalence of allergy is rising and has been called the "epidemic of atopy" (McGeady, 2004). An allergic reaction is an antigen-antibody reaction and can manifest itself as anaphylaxis, atopic disease, serum sickness, or contact dermatitis. Therefore, the symptoms can be mild to severe or life threatening, and they can be localized or systemic. Characteristic findings in children with allergies are summarized in Table 17–5.

The **hypersensitivity response**, an overreaction of the immune system, is responsible for allergic reactions. Hypersensitivity reactions have been classified into four types (Table 17–6). Type I hypersensitivity reactions are immediate reactions that occur within seconds or minutes of exposure to the antigen. Symptoms can include a wheal and flare in the skin, edema, spasm of smooth muscle, wheezing, vomiting, diarrhea, or anaphylaxis. The release of chemical substances such as histamine is responsible for the signs and symptoms exhibited. The first time a child is exposed to the

Table 17–5	CHARACTERISTIC FINDINGS IN CHILDREN WITH ALLERGIES
System	**Clinical Manifestation**
Respiratory	Asthma, rhinitis (seasonal and perennial), serous otitis media, cough, pneumonia, croup, edema of glottis
Gastrointestinal	Abdominal pain and colic, stomatitis, constipation, diarrhea, bloody stools, geographic tongue, vomiting
Skin	Angioedema, urticaria, eczema, atopic dermatitis, erythema multiforme, purpura, drug and food rashes, contact dermatitis
Nervous	Headache, tension, fatigue, convulsions, Ménière's disease, tremor
Eye	Conjunctivitis, cataract, ciliary spasm, iritis
Blood	Thrombocytopenic purpura, hemolytic anemia, leukopenia, agranulocytosis
Musculoskeletal	Arthralgia, myalgia, rheumatoid arthritis, torticollis
Genitourinary	Dysuria, vulvovaginitis, enuresis
Miscellaneous	Anaphylactic shock, serum sickness, autoimmune diseases

Table 17-6	TYPES OF HYPERSENSITIVITY REACTIONS		
Type	**Etiology**	**Clinical Manifestations**	**Examples**
Type I Localized or systemic reactions (anaphylaxis)	Antibodies bind to certain cells, causing release of chemical substances that produce an inflammatory reaction.	Hypotension, wheezing, gastrointestinal or uterine spasm, stridor, urticaria	Extrinsic asthma, hay fever
Type II Tissue-specific reactions	Antibodies cause activation of a complement system, which leads to tissue damage.	Variable; may include dyspnea or fever	Transfusion reaction, ABO incompatibility, hemolytic disease of the newborn
Type III Immune-complex reactions	Immune complexes are deposited in tissues, where they activate complement, which results in a generalized inflammatory reaction.	Urticaria, fever, joint pain	Acute glomerulonephritis, serum sickness
Type IV Delayed reactions	Antigens stimulate T cells that release lymphokines, which cause inflammation and tissue damage.	Variable; may include fever, erythema, itching	Contact dermatitis, tuberculin skin test, graft-versus-host disease, allograft rejection

NURSING ALERT

Anaphylaxis is an exaggerated hypersensitivity reaction that may manifest with itching; localized or generalized hives on the hands, feet, or mucosa; soft-tissue swelling; cough; dyspnea; pallor; sweating; and tachycardia. Severe reactions may lead to respiratory distress or death. Nursing roles involve preventing anaphylactic reactions by teaching families how to minimize exposure and by alerting all healthcare personnel in hospitals and clinics to the child's allergy. In addition, knowledge of emergency procedures is important in all facilities such as schools, homes, and hospitals.

allergen, there is no reaction. With every exposure thereafter, however, the allergic child may have a reaction to the allergen.

Type II reactions are cytotoxic antibody reactions that occur when IgG or IgM antibodies recognize a drug or cell membrane and cause a hypersensitivity reaction. Drug-induced reactions such as anemia or thrombocytopenia result. Type III reactions are immune complex reactions when soluble complexes of drugs or their metabolites cause a deposit with the walls of blood vessels.

Type IV reactions are delayed responses that do not appear until several hours after exposure and require 24 to 72 hours to develop fully. A type IV reaction, which is not confined to any specific tissue, is elicited by relatively complex antigens such as those of bacteria and viruses and by simple antigens such as drugs and metals. Symptoms include contact dermatitis, itching, and blistering. (See Chapter 30 ∞ for a description of contact dermatitis.)

Assessment of the child with allergy includes a complete physical examination; laboratory, radiograph, and pulmonary function studies; tests of nasal function; and skin testing. Treatment generally involves avoidance of the allergen, such as substitution of a different drug when the child has a drug allergy. Desensitization may sometimes be used, with increasing doses of the allergen administered intradermally in an office where resuscitation is readily available. This treatment is useful for allergy to bees or some pollens. For skin allergies, the allergen is avoided, skin is kept well lubricated, and topical steroids may be used. Oral antihistamines are sometimes used to treat allergy. When exposure to an allergen occurs, medical care may require treatment of anaphylaxis.

Nursing Management

The child with allergies requires a thorough assessment, including a complete past medical history, family history, personal and social history, and review of symptoms. The history focuses on the following areas:

- What symptoms does the child experience? Encourage the child to describe the difficulty in his or her own words.
- Are the symptoms continuous or intermittent? What are the frequency and duration of episodes?
- When did the child first begin to experience symptoms? Did the child have eczema or a feeding problem in infancy or childhood? Did the infant have frequent episodes of colic or skin problems when new foods were introduced? Was there a change in symptoms at puberty? Are the symptoms becoming worse or spontaneously improving?

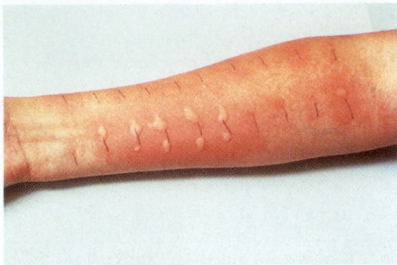

Figure 17–8 ➤ Results of intradermal skin testing on the forearm. Injections are given on each side of the markings. Note the positive results marked by induration and erythema in response to certain antigens.
Note: From VU/Southern Illinois University/Visuals Unlimited.

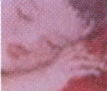

SKILL 11–18
Performing Cardiopulmonary Resuscitation

• What known agents in the environment cause difficulties?
• Are there seasonal variations in symptoms? At what time of the day or night do symptoms usually occur?

The nurse may be responsible for performing intradermal skin tests for allergies (Figure 17–8 ➤). Nursing care focuses on treating the symptoms, alleviating the anxiety of the child and parents, and identifying the allergens. Teaching the child and family how to minimize or avoid exposure to allergens is important. Parents of children who have had severe reactions to bee or wasp stings should be taught how to take precautions and how to provide emergency treatment if the child is stung.

Instruct the family on proper use of epinephrine (see Families Want to Know: Using an EpiPen®). Families may also need instructions on allergy-proofing the home. Pets, dust, carpets, fabrics, feather pillows and bedding, and cigarette smoke can all cause allergic reactions (see Families Want to Know: Removing Common Allergens from the Home). If families are reluctant to give up pets, frequent baths can reduce dander, which is the usual allergen.

When the child has type I reactions to an environmental substance, avoidance of the allergen is most critical. In addition, care providers, families, and school personnel must be able to treat anaphylaxis if exposure to the allergen occurs. Be sure to label the child's chart, bed, and apply a red armband to alert others to allergies when the child is hospitalized. School nurses keep records about children's allergies and inform school personnel about the allergies and cautions that need to be followed. See Chapter 4 ∞ for more information about serious allergies to food such as peanut allergy. Nurses must be aware of the resuscitation procedures and equipment in all facilities such as hospital units, offices, childcare centers, and schools. See Chapter 20 ∞ for information on airway maintenance and refer to the *Clinical Skills Manual* for resuscitation procedures.

Latex Allergy

Latex allergy is common among certain occupations, including healthcare workers, and among patients with certain health conditions. For example, about 7% of healthcare workers, 50% of children with spina bifida, and 34% of children with three or more surgeries are sensitive to latex (Bousquet, Flahault, Vandenplas et al., 2006; Reines & Seifert, 2005). Among healthcare workers, sensitization to gloves is most prevalent (22%), 3.6% report contact urticaria, and 2.3% have asthma or rhinitis (Filon & Radman, 2006). Many healthcare products, such as gloves, drains, catheters, and intravenous ports, contain latex, which is a sap from the rubber tree. Latex allergy is caused by an IgE-mediated response that develops after repeated exposure to latex. In some cases, intraoperative deaths have occurred when allergic individuals were exposed to latex products during surgery. A reaction to latex products can be manifested as an irritant reaction of the skin, type IV of delayed hypersensitivity, with redness, inflammation, and blisters on the skin; or type I hypersensitivity, which is immediate and often has systemic manifestations (itchy eyes, asthma, or anaphylaxis).

Children most at risk for latex allergy include those with myelodysplasia and congenital urinary tract anomalies. Up to 70% of children with spina bifida have im-

FAMILIES WANT TO KNOW

Using an EpiPen®

If the child has had a severe or systemic reaction in the past, ensure that the parents know how to handle an anaphylactic reaction if the child experiences another reaction.

• Kits with syringes of premeasured epinephrine are available by prescription.
• Ensure that family members understand how to use the kit.
• Encourage the child to wear a medical alert bracelet.

• Instruct the family on proper storage of the kit and to avoid exposing the kit to sun or high temperature.
• Instruct the family to frequently check the expiration date of the adrenaline.
• Emphasize to the family that a kit should be readily available at school, camp, childcare, or other settings, with someone instructed in its use.

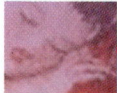

FAMILIES WANT TO KNOW

Removing Common Allergens from the Home

Exposure to the known allergens in the home setting is important. Several measures that families can take to minimize contact with allergens are as follows:

- Remove household pets.
- Control dust by frequent cleaning.
- Clean with moist cloths and mops to remove dust.

- Use plastic covers on mattresses and pillows.
- Avoid carpeting when possible.
- Avoid toys that collect dust (plastic and wood toys are better alternatives than stuffed fabric toys).
- Use high-efficiency air filters.
- Repair homes to prevent entry of water and subsequent molds.
- Consider dehumidification in moist climates.

---

munoglobulin E (IgE) antibodies to latex, and other at-risk groups include children with bladder exstrophy (Hourihane, Allard, Wade, McEwan, & Strobel, 2002). Persons who have had repeated surgeries are also at higher risk due to high exposure to latex during surgery. Healthcare personnel are also at risk for latex allergy because of exposure in the workplace (Box 17–4). Persons who are allergic to latex also have a high incidence of allergy to certain foods, most commonly kiwi fruit, bananas, and avocadoes (Taylor & Erkek, 2004).

Children and adolescents at high risk should receive allergy testing for latex; the radioallergosorbent test (RAST) is most often used. It measures circulating IgE antibodies to many allergens and generally correlates well with specific skin test results. Healthcare personnel must use alternative products when caring for those persons at risk.

When a positive skin test has occurred or when the person has had a reaction to latex, all latex products must be removed from the allergic individual's environment. Alternative products, such as nonlatex gloves and catheters, must be used when providing health care. These individuals should also wear a medical identification bracelet at all times, and should have an epinephrine kit readily available at home and school. Be alert for any signs of hypersensitivity when the child is receiving health care, and be prepared with drugs and equipment to treat anaphylaxis. This is especially important in operative settings when acute anaphylaxis is often life threatening. Emphasize to parents and children that many everyday products contain latex, including latex balloons and condoms (Table 17–7). Also consider exposure to earphones for music, phones, and mouse pads for the computer (Paskawicz, 2005).

GRAFT-VERSUS-HOST DISEASE

Graft-versus-host disease can occur when organs are transplanted or when bone marrow or stem cells are transfused into a recipient, typically as treatment for leukemia or severe combined immunodeficiency disease. The donated cells attach to the recipient child's

MediaLink

Latex Allergy Resources

NURSING ALERT

Starting in September 1998, the Food and Drug Administration ordered that medical products with latex carry a warning label that reads: "Caution: This product contains natural rubber latex, which may cause allergic reactions." Check on the labels of products in your healthcare facility to find this label. What products do you expect to need the label? When children have latex allergy, have the family investigate all medical supplies for the warning label.

BOX 17–4

MEASURES TO PROTECT AGAINST LATEX ALLERGY

Healthcare personnel are at high risk of developing latex allergy because of intense exposure to products containing latex. An estimated 8–12% of healthcare workers are latex sensitive. You can protect yourself by using the following measures.

- Decrease exposure by using alternative products when available (use synthetic rubbers, polyethylene, nitrile, neoprene, vinyl gloves).
- Use powder-free gloves if using latex gloves (the powder has high amounts of latex, which can be inhaled).
- Avoid use of oil-based hand creams and lotions before putting on latex gloves, as these preparations break down the latex.
- When symptoms of sensitivity to latex occur on exposure (rash, hives, nasal congestion, conjunctivitis, cough, or wheeze), contact the employee health department of your facility.
- If diagnosed as latex allergic, avoid all contact and wear a medical identification bracelet.

Contact the National Institute for Occupational Safety and Health (NIOSH) at 800-346-4647 or the American Nurses Association at 800-637-0323 for more information.

Table 17–7 | LATEX IN THE HOSPITAL ENVIRONMENT

Frequently Contain LATEX	Examples of LATEX-SAFE Alternatives/Barriers
Adhesives, skin (Smith+Nephew)	Mastisol (Ferndale)
Anesthesia circuits, bags, oxygen masks	Neoprene (Anesthesia Associates, Ohmeda adult), *some* Vital Signs
Bandaids	Active Strip (3M), CURAD Neon, Readi-Bandages, NHP, *some* Airstrip
Blood pressure cuff, tubing (J&J)	Cleen Cuff (Vital Signs), nylon (*some* Trimline)
Bulb syringe	*selected* Davol, Medline, Rusch, Premium, Baxter
Casts: Delta-Lite Podiatry, Orthoflex (J&J)	Scotchcast soft, Delta-Lites, *recent* Conformable (J&J), Caraglas Ultra, liners (Gore)
Catheters, condom	Clear Advantage, ProSys NL, *selected* Coloplast, Rochester, PolyTech (Hollister)
Catheters, indwelling & systems, UDS	*some* Am BioMed, Argyle, Bard, Cook, Dale, Kendall, Lifetech, Mentor, Rochester, Rusch, Vitaid. Adapters & plug (Addto)
Catheters, cardiac, vascular, pulmonary	*some* World Medical, Am BioMed
Catheters, straight, coude	Mentor, RobNel (Sherwood), Coloplast, *selected* Bard, Rusch catheters
Catheters, feeding	Accumark feeding catheter (Sims Portex)
CPR manikins & Medical training aids	*most* Laerdal products
Dressings: Dyna-flex, butterfly closures (J&J) BDF Elastoplast, Action Wrap, Coban (3M) Lyofoam (Acme), Spandage (Medi-tech), Telfa	Duoderm, Reston foam (3M), Opsite, Venigard, Comfeel, Sorbaview, Telfa(some) Xeroform, PinCare, Bioclusive, Montg'ry strap (J&J), Webril, Metalline, Selopor, Opraflex, Centurion brief, *some* Airstrips, Rainbow Net (Surgilast), VAC
NOTE: latex in package only: Steri-strip wound closure system, Tegaderm, Tegasorb, Active Strips (3M), Nu-Derm (J&J), CURAD	
Ear Plugs	Grainger (5F767)
Elastic wrap: ACE, Esmarch, Zimmer Dyna-flex, Elastikon (J&J)	E-Cotton, CEB elastic(coNco), Champ (Carolon), Adban Adhesive, X-Mark (Avcor) Co-Flex, PowerFlex (Andover), Comprilan (Jobst), Esmark (DeRoyal, NHP)
Electrode bulbs, pads, grounding	*some* Baxter, Dantec EMG, Conmed, ValleyLab, Vermont Med, Staodyn, Neotrode
Endotracheal tubes, airways	*selected* Berman, Mallinckrodt, Polamedco, Portex, Rusch, Sheridan, Shiley
Enemas	BabyLax, Theravac, Bowel Man't Tube (MIC), Pharmaseal set, all Fleet Ready-to-use, cone irrigation set (Convatec), silicone retention cuff tip (Lafayette)
G-tubes, buttons	Silicone (Bard, Flexiflo, MIC, Rusch, Stomate)
Gloves: sterile, clean, surgical, orthodontic	Allergard (J&J), dermaprene (Ansell), N-DEX (Best), Safeskin Nitrile, Neolon, SensiCare, Tru-touch (Maxxim), Nitrex, Tactyl 1,2 (SmartPractice), Duraprene, (Allegiance Healthcare), Elastyren (Hermal, Center Labs), Boston Medical, Masel, Neotech
Incentive deep breathing exerciser	Voldyne 5000 (Sherwood David & Geck), Triflo II
IV access: injection ports, Y-sites, bags, pumps, buretrol ports, PRN adapters, buretrol ports, PRN adapters, needleless systems	**Cover Y-sites and bag ports—do not puncture. Use stopcocks for meds.** Polymer injection caps + burettes + Safsite (Braun), Abbot systems, Walrus, Gemini (IMED), *selected* Baxter (InterLink), Statlock, Ready Med, ConMed, Clave, Alaris, Hudson, *select* Sims, IV boards (Avcor), Terumo Pumps: Mach II, ADS 100; Clic-Open (vial top remover - Sepha Pharm.)
OR/Infection Control masks, hats, shoe covers	*some* by Kimberly Clark, TECNOL; OR & sterile packs (CML, DeRoyal) twill ties
Medication vial stoppers	*some* AmRegent, Astra, Bedford Labs, Fujisawa, Gensia, Glaxo, Lilly, Roche
Miscellaneous items	Soft-Grip fabric clamp covers(Scanlan), Precision Dynamics I.D. bracelets
Penrose drains	Jackson-Pratt, Zimmer Hemovac
Pulse oximeters, thermometer probes	Nonin oximeters, *selected* Nellcor sensors, Diatec probe covers
Reflex hammers	Cover with plastic bag
Respirators	Advantage (MSA), HEPA-Tech (Uvex), PFR 95 (Tecnol), 3M 1860
Resuscitators, manual	*certain* Ambu, Armstrong, Laerdal, Puriton Bennett, Vital Blue, Respironics, Rusch
Spacer (for metered dose inhalers)	ACE spacer (Center Labs), OptiHaler (HealthScan)
Stethescope tubing	PVC (*some* Littman) cover with ScopeCoat or latex-free stockinette (**Alba**health)
Suction tubing	PVC (Davol, Laerdal, Mallinckrodt, Superior, Yankauer) Medline, Ballard
Syringes, disposable	Terumo Medical, Abbott PCA Abboject, Norm-Ject (Air-Tite), EpiPen, *selected* BD syringes, AdvantaJet (Activa)
Tapes: pink, Waterproof (3M), Zonas, Moleskin, cloth, Waterproof (J&J), adhesive felt (Acme)	Dermicel (J&J), Durapore, Microfoam, Micropore, Transpore (3M) Cath-Strip (Genetic Labs), Ice Tape (P.O.Pak), All-Felt (Universal Foot Care)
Tonopen disposable covers (glaucoma tester)	
Tourniquets	Children's Medical, Grafco, VelcroPedic, X-Tourn straps(Avcor), Free-Band(Kent)
Theraband (also strip, tube), Other OT supplies	REP Bands & Cords (OPTP), Exercise putty (Rolyan), new Thera-Band Exercisers plastic
Tubing, sheeting	tubing-Tygon LR-40 (Norton), elastic thread, sheets (JPS Elastomerics)
Vascular stockings (Jobst)	Compriform Custom (Jobst)

Table 17–7	LATEX IN THE HOSPITAL ENVIRONMENT (continued)	

Frequently Contain LATEX	Examples of LATEX-SAFE Alternatives/Barriers
Latex in the Home and Community	
Art supplies: paints, glue, erasers, fabric paints	Elmers (School Glue, Glue-All, GluColors, Carpenters Wood Glue, Sno-Drift paste) FaberCastel erasers, Crayola (**except** stamps, erasers), Liquitex paints, DickBlick Tempera & acrylic paints & soap erasers, Play-Doh
Balloons	Mylar balloons, self-sealing *Myloons*
Balls: Koosh balls, tennis balls, bowling balls	PVC (Headstrom Sports Ball), Nerf Foam Balls
Carpet backing, gym floor, basement sealant	Provide barrier - cloth or mat
Chewing gum	Bubblicious, Trident (Warner-Lambert), Wrigley gums (check new products)
Clothes: applique on Tees, elastic on socks, underwear, sneakers, sandals	Cloth-covered elastic, neoprene (Decent Exposures, NOLATEX Industries) Buster Brown elastic-free socks (Vermont Country Store)
Condoms, contraceptive sponges, diaphragm	Polyurethane (Avanti), female condom (Reality), Wideseal Silicone Diaphragms (Milex), Trojan Supra Condom
Crutches: tips, axillary pads, hand grips	Cover with cloth, tape
Dental dams, cups, bands, root canal material orthodontic rubber bands	PURO/M27 intraoral elastics (Midwest Orthodontic), wire springs, sealant (Delton) dams (Meer Dental, Hygenic Corp), John O Butler, Earloop masks (Richmond)
Diapers, Incontinence pads, rubber pants	Huggies, First Quality, Gold Seal, Tranquility, Always, *some* Attends, Drypers Diapers (not training pants), Confidence (Paper-Pak), Pampers, Luvs
Feeding nipples	Silicone, vinyl (**selected** Gerber, Evenflo, MAM, Ross, Mead Johnson)
Food handled with latex gloves	Synthetic gloves for food handling
NOTE: Associated allergies are reported to banana, avocado, chestnut, kiwi and other fruits	
Handles on racquets, tools, bicycles	Vinyl, leather handles, or cover with cloth or tape
Infant toothbrush-massager	Soft bristle brush or cloth, Gerber/NUK
Kitchen cleaning gloves	PVC MYPLEX (Magla), cotton liners (Allerderm)
Miscellaneous items	*some* medical stickers by MediBadge, UAL, Cushie Tushie Potty Seat
Newsprint, ads, coupons, lottery scratch tickets	
Pacifiers	Soothies (Children's Med Ventures), **selected** Binky, Gerber, Infa, Kip, MAM
Rubber bands, bungee cords	Plasti bands
Toys - Stretch Armstrong, old Barbies	Jurassic Park figures (Kenner), 1993 Barbie, Disney dolls (Mattel), many toys by Fisher Price, Little Tikes, Playschool, Discovery, Trolls (Norfin), Silly-putty
Water toys & equipment: beach thongs, masks, bathing suits, caps, scuba gear, goggles	PVC, plastic, nylon, Suits Me Swimwear
Wheelchair cushions, tires	Jay, ROHO cushions, Use leather gloves, Sof Care bed/chair cushions (Gaymar)
Zippered plastic storage bags	Waxed paper, plain plastic bags, Ziploc bags

Note: From the Spina Bifida Association of America, www.sbaa.org, 4590 MacArthur Blvd NW, Suite 250, Washington, DC 20001–4226. Used with permission.

bone marrow and begin production. The child's lymphocyte production increases and immune response develops. However, despite prior blood and tissue typing, sometimes the donor cells are incompatible with the recipient cells and the new cells being to mount a type IV hypersensitivity/immunologic response in the child who has received the transplant (Behrman, Kliegman, & Jenson, 2004; Vogelsang, Lee, & Bensen-Kennedy, 2003).

Graft-versus-host disease may be either acute or chronic. Acute disease occurs in the first 100 days after transplant. The skin manifests a pruritic and macular-papular rash that begins on the extremities and progresses to the trunk. Gastrointestinal effects include nausea, vomiting, anorexia, diarrhea, cramping, and abdominal pain. Impaired liver function tests and jaundice often occur. However, chronic graft-versus-host disease occurs after the first 100 days. Recurrent infections, skin reactions, and thrombocytopenia are evidenced, with mouth, throat, and esophageal ulcers, gastrointestinal disorders, cholestasis, and eye irritation (Higman & Vogelsang, 2004).

Careful physical examination and laboratory tests are used to diagnose and stage the disease. Early identification is key to beginning therapy and stopping progression of the life-threatening condition. Several immunosuppressant drugs are used in treatment. Nursing care focuses on careful assessments of all children who have received transplants and partnering with other health professionals for treatment. Skin, gastrointestinal system, nutrition and growth, and eye examinations are commonly stressed during the therapeutic phase. Children and their families need information and support about this immune system complication of transplantation of bone marrow or stem cells.

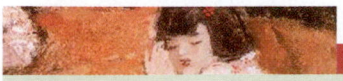

CRITICAL THINKING IN ACTION

Recall Raymond, the 2-year-old introduced at the beginning of this chapter, who, after repeated infections, was diagnosed with AIDS. Raymond had no other risk factors for HIV and AIDS, so the healthcare team recommended that Raymond's mother be tested for the infection. She was subsequently diagnosed with HIV while Raymond's 5-year-old sister tested negative for HIV. The family is dealing with the diagnosis for both Raymond and his mother as well as learning to care for Raymond.

DISCUSSION

1. Raymond is having difficulty eating. After you consider his age of 2 years and the recommended intake at this age, plan a daily menu for him with several small feedings.

2. You have just been assigned to care for Raymond during a day shift. Organize your morning assessment of Raymond. Plan to observe the systems constituting the most frequent sources of infection in children with HIV.

3. What is the most common cause of Raymond's infection with HIV? How might the family react when they learn about perinatal transmission?

4. Dealing with the challenges of HIV in a young child taxes the family's resources. Plan nursing care that involves HAART medication administration and interventions to promote Raymond's development.

 Refer to your Prentice Hall Nursing MediaLink DVD-ROM for answers.

EXPLORE MediaLink 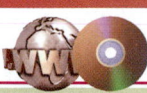 http://www.prenhall.com/ball

Resources for this chapter can be found on the Prentice Hall Nursing MediaLink DVD-ROM accompanying this textbook, and on the Companion Website at http://www.prenhall.com/ball.

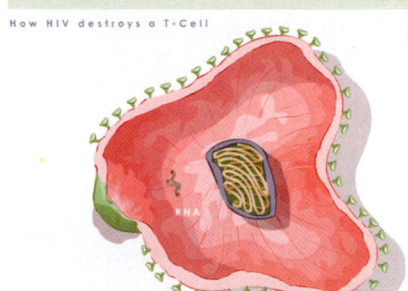

How HIV destroys a T-Cell

DVD-ROM
Audio Glossary
NCLEX-RN® Review
Animations/Videos
 AIDS/HIV
 HIV Infection and Transmission
 Primary and Secondary Immune Response

COMPANION WEBSITE
Audio Glossary
NCLEX-RN® Review
Care Plan Activity: Severe Combined Immune
 Deficiency Syndrome
Case Study: Needle-stick Injury
Critical Thinking: Discussing HIV with Adolescents
MediaLink Application: Peanut Allergy
WebLinks

REFERENCES

AIDSInfo. (2005). Guidelines for the use of antiretroviral agents in pediatric HIV infection. Retrieved September 25, 2006, from http://aidsinfo.nih.gov

American Academy of Pediatrics, Committee on Pediatric AIDS. (1998). Human immunodeficiency virus/acquired immunodeficiency syndrome education in schools. *Pediatrics, 101,* 933–935.

American Academy of Pediatrics, Committee on Pediatric AIDS and Committee on Adolescence. (2001). Adolescents and human immunodeficiency virus infection: The role of the pediatrician in prevention and intervention (RE0031). *Pediatrics, 107*(1), 188–190.

American Academy of Pediatrics. (2006). *Red book: Report of the committee on infectious diseases.* (27th ed.). Elk Grove Village, IL: Author.

American College of Rheumatology. (2003). Retrieved December 22, 2003, from http://rarediseases.about.com/gi/dynamic/offsite .htm?site=http%3A%2F%2Fwww.rheumatolog y.org%2Fpatients%2Ffactsheet%2Fsle.html

Behrman, R. E., Kliegman, R. M., & Jenson, H. B. (2004). *Nelson textbook of pediatrics* (17th ed., pp. 738–741). Philadelphia: Saunders.

Bindler, R., & Howry, L. (2005). *Pediatric drugs and nursing implications.* Upper Saddle River, NJ: Prentice Hall Health.

Bonilla, F. A., & Geha, R. S. (2006). Update on primary immunodeficiency diseases. *Journal of Allergy and Clinical Immunology, 117,* S435–S441.

Bousquet, J., Flahault, A., Vandenplas, O., Amielle, J., Duron, J. J., Pecquet, C., Chevrie, K., & Annesi-Maesano, I. (2006). Natural rubber latex allergy among health care workers: A systematic review of the evidence. *Journal of Allergy and Clinical Immunology, 118*, 447–454.

Brackis-Cott, E., Mellins, C. A., Abrams, E., Reval, T., & Dolezal, C. (2003). Pediatric HIV medication adherence: The views of medical providers from two primary care programs. *Journal of Pediatric Health Care, 17*, 252–260.

Burpo, R. H. (2000). Common antiviral agents used in women's and children's care. Journal of Obstetric, *Gynecologic and Neonatal Nursing, 29*, 181–200.

Centers for Disease Control and Prevention. (2003). Rapid HIV testing of women in labor and delivery. Retrieved April 22, 2006, from http://www.cdc.gov/hiv/pubs/vt-women.htm

Centers for Disease Control and Prevention (2004a). HIV/AIDS among Hispanics. Retrieved December 5, 2004, from http://www.cdc.gov/hiv/pubs/facts/hispanic.htm

Centers for Disease Control and Prevention. (2004b). OraQuick rapid HIV test for oral fluid. Frequently asked questions. Retrieved December 4, 2004, from http://www.cdc.gov

Centers for Disease Control and Prevention (2005). Cases of HIV infection and AIDS in the United States, 2004. Retrieved April 22, 2006, from http://www.cdc.gov/hiv/topics/surveillance/resources/reports/2004/report.htm

Centers for Disease Control and Prevention (2006a). Revised recommendations for HIV testing of adults, adolescents and pregnant women in health-care settings. *Morbidity and Mortality Weekly Report, 55*(RR14), 1–17.

Centers for Disease Control and Prevention (2006b). HIV and its transmission. Retrieved January 30, 2007 from http://www.cdc.gov

Chamley, C. A., Carson, P., Randall, D., & Sandwell, M. (2005). *Developmental anatomy and physiology of children*. St. Louis: Elsevier.

Champi, C. (2002). Primary immunodeficiency disorders in children: Prompt diagnosis can lead to lifesaving treatment. *Journal of Pediatric Health, 17*, 17–21.

Conley, M. E., Saragoussi, D., Notarangelo, L., Elzioni, A., & Asanova, J. L. (2003). An international study examining therapeutic options used in treatment of Wiskott-Aldrich syndrome. *Clinical Immunology, 109*, 272–277.

Connell, F., & Hodgson, S. (2005). Our evolving understanding of 22q.11 deletion syndrome. *Developmental medicine and child neurology, 47* 796.

Cooper, M. A., Pommering, T. L., & Koranyi, K. (2003). Primary immunodeficiencies. *American Family Physician, 68*, 2001.

Dibbern, D. A., & Routes, J. M. (2004). Wiscott–Aldrich syndrome. Retrieved June 20,

2004, from http://www.emedicine.com/med/topic1172.htm

Edmunds, M. W., & Mayhew, M. S. (2004). *Pharmacology for the primary care provider* (2nd ed.). St. Louis: Elsevier Mosby.

El-Alfy, M. S., & El-Sayed, M. H. (2004). Overwhelming postspenectomy infections: Is quality of patient knowledge enough for prevention? *Hematology Journal, 5*, 77–88.

Filon, F. L., & Radman, G. (2006). Latex allergy: A follow up study of 1040 healthcare workers. *Occupational and Environmental Medicine, 63*, 121–125.

Goldmuntz, E. (2005). DiGeorge syndrome: New insights. *Clinical Perinatology, 32*, 963–978.

Greenwald, J. L., Burstein, G. R., Pincus, J., & Branson, B. (2006). A rapid review of rapid HIV antibody tests. *Current Infectious Disease Reports, 8*, 125–131.

Higman, M. A., & Vogelsang, G. B. (2004). Chronic graft-versus-host disease. *British Journal of Haematology, 125*, 435–454.

Hourihane, J. O., Allard, J. M., Wade, A. M., & McEwan, A. I., & Strobel, S. (2002). Impact of repeated surgical procedures on the incidence and prevalence of latex allergy: A prospective study of 1263 children. *The Journal of Pediatrics, 140*, 479–482.

Ilowite, N. T. (2002). Current treatment of juvenile rheumatoid arthritis. *Pediatrics, 109*, 109–115.

Instone, S. L. (2000). Perceptions of children with HIV infection when not told for so long: Implications for diagnosis disclosure. *Journal of Pediatric Healthcare, 14*, 235–243.

Kline, M. W. (2006). Perspectives on the pediatric HIV/AIDS pandemic: Catalyzing access of children to care and treatment. *Pediatrics, 117*, 1388–1393.

Koleilat, M. A., Williams, L. W., & Ryan, M. E. (2003). Read the warning signs of primary immunodeficiency. *Contemporary Pediatrics, 20*, 65–81.

Kukka, C. (2004). Bloodborne infections: Should they be disclosed? Is differential treatment necessary? *Journal of School Nursing, 20*, 324–330.

Lupus Foundation of America. (2004). Retrieved December 4, 2004, from http://www.lupus.org/education/types/html

Luxner, K. L. (2003). The complicated prenatal experience. In M. H. Hogan & R. S. Glazebrook, (Eds.), *Material Newborn Nursing*. Upper Saddle Creek, NJ: Prentice Hall.

Markert, M. L., Alexieff, M. J., Li, B., Sarzotti, M., Ozaki, D. A., Devlin, B. H., Sempowski, G. D., Rhein, M. E., Szabolcs, P. L., Hale, L. P., Buckley, R. H., Coyne, K. E., Rice, H. E., Mahaggey, S. M., & Skinner, J. A. (2004). Complete DiGeorge syndrome: Development of rash, lymphadenopathy, and oligoclonal T cells

in 5 cases. *Journal of Allergy and Clinical Immunology, 113*, 734–741.

Marodi, L. (2006). Innate cellular immune response in newborns. *Clinical Immunology, 118*, 137–144.

McGeady, S. J. (2004). Immunocompetence and allergy. *Pediatrics, 113*, 1107–1113.

Morbidity and Mortality Weekly Report (2003). Advancing HIV prevention: New strategies for a changing epidemic—United States. *MMWR, 52*, 329–332.

Mulvihill, K. (2003). Systemic lupus erythematosus: Early identification, co-management are key KP contributions. *Advances for Nurse Practitioners, 11*, 32–36.

Murphy, D. A., Wilson, C. M., Durako, S. J., Muenz, L. R., & Belzen, M. (2001). Antiretroviral medication adherence among the REACH HIV infected adolescent who are in the USA. *AIDS Care, 13*(1), 27–41.

Ochs, J. D., & Thrasher, A. J. (2006). The Wiskott–Aldrich syndrome. *Current Review of Allergy and Clinical Immunology, 117*, 725–738.

Paskawicz, J. (2005). Latex allergy revisited. *Clinician Reviews, 15*(11), 66–75. Retrieved January 15, 2002, from http://www.pediatrics.org/cgi/content/full/106/6/e76

Pongmarutani, T., Alpert, P. T., & Miller, S. K. (2006). Pediatric systemic lupus erythematosus: Management issues in primary practice. *Journal of the American Academy of Nurse Practitioners, 18*, 258–267.

Pullen, R. L., Cannon, J. D., & Rushing, J. D. (2003). Managing organ-threatening lupus erythematosus. *Medsurg Nursing, 12*, 368–379.

Ramstead, C. (2003). HIV counseling, testing, and referral: Putting revised guidelines to use. *Clinician Reviews, 13*, 58–64.

Rangel, M. C., Gavin, L., Reed, C., Fowler, M. G., & Lee, L. M. (2006). Epidemiology of HIV and AIDS among adolescents and young adults in the United States. *Journal of Adolescent Health, 39*, 156–163.

Reines, H. D., & Seifert, P. C. (2005). Patient safety: Latex allergy. *Surgical Clinics of North America, 85*, 1329–1340.

Singh-Grewal, D., Schneider, R., Bayer, N., & Feldman, B. M. (2006). Predictors of disease course and remission in systemic juvenile idiopathic arthritis. *Arthritis & Rheumatism, 54*, 1595–1601.

Stichweh, D., Arce, E., & Pascual, V. (2004). Update on pediatric systemic lupus erythematosus. *Current Opinion in Rheumatology, 17*, 577–587.

Taylor, S., & Erkek, E. (2004). Latex allergy: Diagnosis and management. *Dermatology Therapeutics, 17*, 289–301.

Vogelsang, G. B., Lee, L., & Bensen-Kennedy, D. M. (2003). Pathogenesis and treatment of graft-versus-host disease after bone marrow transplant. *Annual Review of Medicine, 54*, 29–54.

18

INFECTIOUS AND COMMUNICABLE DISEASES

KEY TERMS

acellular pertussis
    vaccine **589**
active immunity
    588
antibodies **588**
antigen **588**
communicable
    disease **585**
direct transmission
    585
disease surveillance
    587
endogenous
    pyrogens **605**
indirect
    transmission **585**
infectious disease
    585

killed virus vaccine
    588
live virus vaccine
    589
nosocomial
    infections **623**
opisthotonos **617**
pandemic **587**
passive immunity
    588
phagocytosis **604**
prostration **611**
toxic appearance
    622
toxoid **588**
transplacental
    immunity **589**
zoonosis **605**

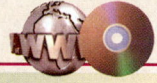

MediaLink

http://www.prenhall.com/ball

See the Prentice Hall Nursing MediaLink DVD-ROM and Companion Website for chapter-specific resources.

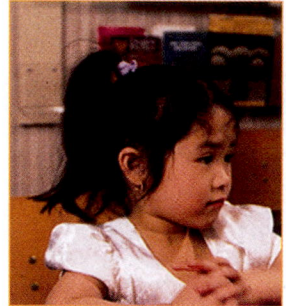

LIAN, 5 years old, has accompanied her mother and 2-year-old brother, Joe, to the pediatric clinic. The primary purpose of the health visit today is because Joe is sick. He has had a fever of 38.3°C (101°F) for the past 3 days and his mother is concerned. Joe has been to this office several times in the past few months for health care related to minor illnesses, but this is the first time Lian has come along.

When the nurse asks about Lian's last visit to the doctor and the status of her immunizations, her mother says Lian has not been seen for about 2 years. Lian will start school soon, and her mother is not sure whether Lian has had all of her shots. In checking Lian's health records, the nurse notes that she is in need of several immunizations, including DTaP, polio, MMR, PCV7, varicella, and hepatitis A. Joe needs polio, MMR, PCV7, Hib, and hepatitis A vaccines.

Should Lian be given any of these immunizations today, even though her brother is ill? Can immunizations be given at the same time? Should Joe also receive any immunizations today?

LEARNING OUTCOMES

After reading this chapter, you will be able to do the following:

1. Describe why children are more vulnerable than adults to infectious and communicable diseases.

2. Describe the process of infection and modes of transmission.

3. Understand the role that vaccines play in reduction and elimination of infectious and communicable diseases.

4. Develop a nursing care plan for children of all ages needing immunizations.

5. Recognize common infectious and communicable diseases.

6. Describe the medical and nursing management of common infectious and communicable diseases.

INFECTIOUS DISEASE AS A HEALTH PROBLEM

An **infectious disease** is any communicable disease caused by microorganisms that are commonly transmitted from one person to another or from an animal to a person. A **communicable disease** is an illness that is **directly transmitted** from one person or animal to another by contact with body fluids, **indirectly transmitted** by contact with contaminated objects, or by vectors (ticks, mosquitoes, other insects). Infectious and communicable diseases are a major cause of morbidity in infants and children in the United States, and in some cases result in death.

For a communicable disease to occur, all of the following need to be present (Figure 18–1 ➤).

- An infectious agent, or pathogen
- An effective means of transmission or spread of the infectious agent
- A susceptible host

Infants and young children are often susceptible hosts. Their immune systems are not fully developed and they have not yet developed antibodies to many agents (see Chapter 17 ∞). Therefore, they cannot defend themselves against infectious and communicable diseases as well as older children and adults. Other characteristics, such as immunodeficiency and poor health, may increase a child's risk of contracting an infectious disease.

Young children such as Lian and Joe are particularly susceptible to illnesses that are transmitted among close contacts or through exposure to microorganisms in various settings. Children can develop complications or secondary infections resulting from the infectious disease that require healthcare intervention and may be an economic burden to families. Nurses have an important health promotion role in reducing the transmission of infectious diseases by immunization and in partnering with families to interrupt the transmission of infection in other ways, such as quarantine or hand hygiene.

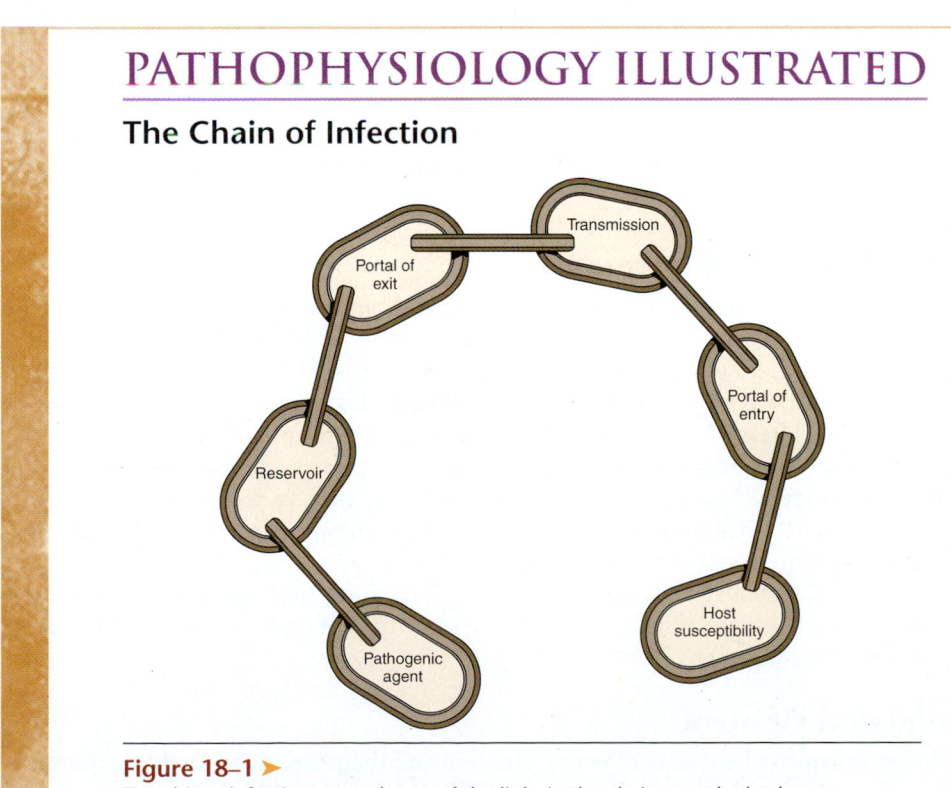

PATHOPHYSIOLOGY ILLUSTRATED

The Chain of Infection

Figure 18–1 ➤
To achieve infection control, one of the links in the chain must be broken.

Reducing the number of preventable childhood illnesses is a major national goal in *Healthy People 2010*, and nurses are important partners in this effort. Specific objectives are targeted at the reduction or elimination of the following infectious diseases (Department of Health and Human Services, 2000):

- *Elimination.* Rubella and congenital rubella syndrome, diphtheria, *Haemophilus influenza* type b, measles, mumps, polio, and tetanus.
- *Reduction.* Pertussis, hepatitis B, varicella, food-borne pathogens, and HIV infection.

Common preventable infectious diseases are a significant public health problem. The national health objectives are a reflection of how significant these preventable diseases are as a public health problem. When these infectious diseases are not prevented, there is an impact on the family and the healthcare system. Parents may accrue costs for medications and treatments for what could have been prevented; health insurers must also cover the cost of conditions that might have been prevented. Excessive healthcare resources are used when the infectious disease becomes widely transmitted and treatment is required by infected children and their families. Parents miss work while caring for the child and may become ill as well. Children are directly impacted when they miss time from school and interrupt their learning.

Special Vulnerability of Newborns and Young Infants

The capability and function of the immune system of newborns and young infants is becoming more clearly understood. Infants are particularly vulnerable to infectious diseases. See Focus on the Immune System in Chapter 17 ∞.

The immune system is not fully mature at birth, although passively acquired maternal antibodies provide limited protection. Immunoglobulin G (IgG) is transferred through the placenta so that full-term infants have levels comparable to their mother, but the half-life of IgG provided through the placenta is about 20 days. Placental transfer of antibodies for gram-negative organisms is minimal, and the newborn has protection only for viruses and gram-positive organisms to which the mother has been exposed. Other immunoglobulins (IgA, IgE, IgD, and IgM) do not transfer through the placenta. In addition, preterm infants may have fewer maternal antibodies as most of the placental transfer of IgG occurs during the third trimester (Lott & Kenner, 2003). Breast-feeding does provide some continuing passive protection, but many infants are not breast-fed. Since immunizations have not been given, disease protection is incomplete.

Development of Immunity

As children grow, they develop immunity through immunization or exposure to the natural disease. As children mature and become more active, they interact more frequently with other children and adults and also increase their exposure to infectious agents (Figure 18–2 ➤). Young children in childcare, for example, are in close contact with other children who are susceptible to most infectious organisms.

In some cases, it is not possible to limit exposure to certain organisms as a child may be contagious before symptoms appear, such as with varicella (chickenpox) and parvovirus B-19 (fifth disease). See the table beginning on page 607 for more information about these and other communicable diseases.

As healthy children are exposed to more infections, they naturally develop antibodies. Thus, subsequent infections with the same type of organism may be less severe or avoided (see Chapter 17 ∞).

Infection Control

The poor hygiene behaviors of young children and their caregivers facilitate transmission of infectious diseases among young children in childcare settings and other environments such as hospitals, clinics, and physician offices. The fecal-oral and respiratory

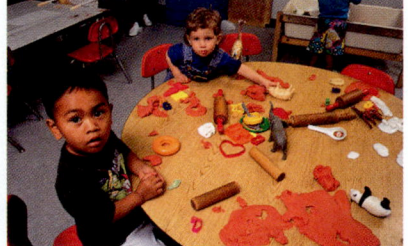

Figure 18–2 ➤ Infectious diseases are easily transmitted in settings such as childcare centers where children handle common objects.

CULTURE

Beliefs About Disease Causation

In some cultures, infectious diseases are seen as punishment or the result of curses or evil spirits. For example, Native Americans traditionally view illnesses as the result of disharmony or displeasing the spirits. They may not believe in the germ theory of disease causation.

routes are the most common sources of transmission in children. Children usually do not wash their hands after toileting unless they are closely supervised. They put toys and their hands in their mouths, and then rub their nose and eyes. They often are unable to care for a runny nose without help. Diapers may leak stool and provide exposure to fecal organisms. In addition, caregivers in childcare centers, other persons caring for children, and healthcare professionals may not use proper hand hygiene techniques (Figure 18–3 ➤). All of these behaviors promote the transmission of infection. See Families Want to Know: Reducing the Transmission of Infection.

Preventing the spread of infectious diseases is a process that involves several strategies that must be well coordinated. Proper hand hygiene is one of the most important health promotion strategies for all age groups of children as well as childcare providers.

Nurses have a very significant role in this process and are responsible for implementing several infection control strategies.

- Use standard and transmission-based precautions.
- Wash hands with soap and water when visibly dirty or contaminated by blood or other body fluids (Centers for Disease Control, 2002a, p. 32).
- Use alcohol-based hand sanitizers to decontaminate the hands in all other clinical situations as recommended (Centers for Disease Control, 2002a, p. 32).
- Separate or quarantine ill children from well children. Perform triage of children frequently in clinics and physician offices to identify children who should be isolated from other children in the waiting room. Separate hospitalized children with infections from those at great risk for infection, such as children with compromised immune systems.
- Promote and provide immunizations. See the immunization schedule on page 596.
- Eliminate the habitat or reservoir of the host (e.g., eliminating standing water where mosquitoes breed, killing mosquitoes that carry malaria).
- Kill the pathogen (e.g., sanitize toys and contact surfaces).
- Educate parents and caregivers of children about the need for hand hygiene and standard precautions, safe food preparation and storage, taking action to avoid exposure to certain organisms (e.g., ticks that cause Lyme disease), and the importance of immunizations.

Public health authorities conduct **disease surveillance**, monitoring patterns of disease occurrence from the cases of infectious and communicable diseases reported by healthcare workers to state health officials. While many infectious and communicable diseases have decreased in occurrence, they remain a significant source of morbidity and mortality in infants and children, especially in developing countries. National disease surveillance efforts have increased in response to concerns of bioterrorism or a **pandemic**, the emergence and worldwide spread of an influenza or other viral or bacterial organism that causes significantly increased morbidity and mortality. An example is pandemic flu.

IMMUNIZATION

The development and widespread availability of vaccines has been one of the great breakthroughs of modern medicine. The average infant born in 2006 receives immunizations for 13 diseases by the age of 6 years. The diseases for which vaccines are routinely recommended include the following: measles, mumps, rubella, polio, pertussis (whooping cough), diphtheria, tetanus, *Haemophilus influenzae* type b, hepatitis A and B, pneumococcus, varicella (chickenpox), and influenza. The new rotavirus vaccine was approved for administration to infants in 2006. In addition, vaccines have been developed recently for older children, adolescents, and adults to protect against pertussis, meningococcus, and the human papillomavirus. Administering these vaccines greatly improves the health of children and reduces the parental burden of caring for ill children.

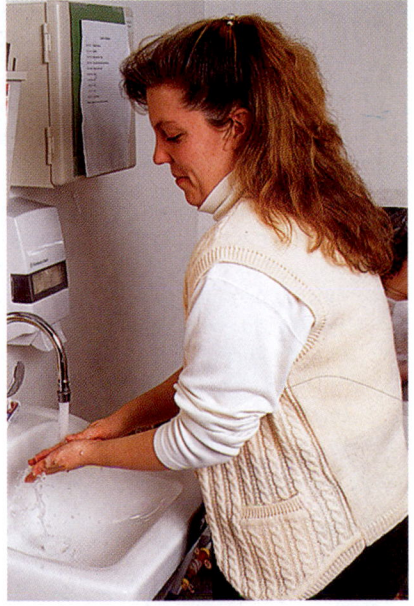

Figure 18–3 ➤ Proper handwashing is one of the most effective measures in preventing transmission of microorganisms.

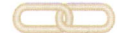

SKILLS CHAPTER 1
Standard Precautions

RESEARCH

Family Hand Hygiene

A recent study was conducted among 208 ethnically diverse families (837 people) that had children enrolled in a childcare setting with 5 or more children. One purpose of the study was to see if alcohol-based gels (purchased on the family's initiative) or handwashing for hand hygiene was effective in reducing respiratory and gastrointestinal illness transmission between the child who acquired an illness while in childcare and the child's family members. Based on surveys of family hand hygiene practices and data collected on family illnesses over a 4-week period, the use of alcohol-based gels was associated with reduced transmission of respiratory illness in the home (Lee, Salomon, Friedman et al., 2005).

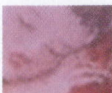

FAMILIES WANT TO KNOW

Reducing the Transmission of Infection

Teach families to reduce the transmission of infection among family members with the following practices:

- Use disposable tissues and discard immediately after use.
- Wash hands thoroughly with soap and water or alcohol-based gels after all contact with the child's diaper, runny nose, and mucous membranes.
- Teach children to cough or sneeze into their elbow rather than into their hands.
- Teach children to wash their hands with soap and water after toileting and before eating.
- Do not allow children to share dishes and utensils.

- Wipe kitchen counters and surfaces where food is prepared and eaten with a disinfectant such as Lysol® or a bleach solution.
- Wash hands well before preparing food. Follow guidelines for safe food preparation and storage.
- Wash dishes in warm soapy water or use the sanitizing cycle on the dishwasher.
- Wipe counters and surfaces that are used for diaper change or that the child touches with a disinfectant such as Lysol®, a bleach solution, or isopropyl alcohol. Make sure the diaper changing area is well away from food preparation areas.
- Dispose of diapers in closed containers.

RESEARCH

Hand Hygiene at Home

A study was conducted in 292 families (1053 persons) with a child in childcare on the effect of alcohol-based hand sanitizers on transmission of gastrointestinal illness in the home. Half of the families were given alcohol-based gels and education materials on hand hygiene and the remaining families (control group) received materials on nutrition and were asked not to use an alcohol-based gel. Families reported the same pattern of handwashing prior to the study. Families were contacted weekly for 5 months about infections in the home. Families using the hand sanitizer had a 59% lower incidence of secondary gastrointestinal illness (Sandora, Taveras, Shih et al., 2005).

MediaLink

Infectious and Communicable Diseases Resources

Before the 1950s when infant and childhood immunization programs were initiated, the annual impact of infectious and communicable diseases in the United States was staggering. Thousands of children died or had permanent disabilities as a result of being infected from diseases such as polio, rubella, measles, diphtheria, pertussis, and *Haemophilus influenza* type b (Children's Hospital of Philadelphia, 2006).

Etiology and Pathophysiology

Immunization introduces an **antigen** (a foreign substance that triggers an immune system response) into the body, allowing immunity against a disease to develop naturally. The person produces **antibodies**, which are proteins capable of responding to specific antigens. In **active immunity** (in which antibody production is stimulated without causing clinical disease), an antigen is given in the form of a vaccine.

When a child needs antibodies faster than the body can develop them, **passive immunity** may be induced, with antibodies produced in another human or animal host and given to the child. This approach is also used with at-risk children after a single exposure to a disease to prevent the disease from occurring or to reduce its severity. For example, if a child who has never had a tetanus immunization steps on a rusty nail, the child needs immediate protection (passive immunity) from tetanus. Tetanus immune globulin is given by injection to combat the tetanus toxin produced when bacterial spores are introduced by the nail. Passive immunity does not confer lasting immunity, so the tetanus toxoid vaccine is administered to start the process of antibody development (active immunity).

Since the first vaccines were developed in the late 1800s, many diseases have decreased dramatically in incidence. The introduction of vaccines against childhood diseases such as measles, mumps, rubella, polio, pertussis, diphtheria, *Haemophilus influenzae* type b, hepatitis B, and chickenpox has greatly improved the quality of life for children and adults. Since the introduction of the pneumococcal conjugate vaccine in 2000 there has been a 35% reduction in invasive disease (meningitis and pneumonia) caused by pneumococcal strains resistant to penicillin, and a 78% reduction in disease caused by strains targeted in the vaccine among children less than 2 years of age (Peters & Edwards, 2002; Whitney, Farley, & Hadler, 2003).

Types of vaccines against childhood illnesses used in the United States include the following:

- **Killed virus vaccine**. A vaccine that contains a microorganism that has been killed but is still capable of inducing the human body to produce antibodies. Example: inactivated poliovirus vaccine.
- **Toxoid**. A toxin that has been treated (by heat or chemical) to weaken its toxic effects but retain its antigenicity. Example: tetanus toxoid.

- **Live virus vaccine**. A vaccine that contains a microorganism in live but attenuated, or weakened, form. Example: measles and varicella vaccines.
- **Recombinant forms**. An organism that has been genetically altered for use in vaccines. Examples: hepatitis B and **acellular pertussis vaccine** (a vaccine that uses proteins from pertussis rather than the whole cell to stimulate the process of active immunity).
- **Conjugated forms**. An altered organism joined with another substance to increase the immune response. Example: The *Haemophilus influenzae* type b (Hib) vaccine is conjugated with a protein-carrier like tetanus toxoid (PRP-T); however, this specific vaccine brand confers no immunity to tetanus.

Improvements in vaccine technology continue to increase the safety and efficacy of immunization against an increasing number of diseases. Today's vaccines are often produced synthetically by means of recombinant DNA technology or genetic engineering.

Clinical Manifestations

Children receiving vaccines can have a variety of responses as the body responds to the injected antigen stimulating the immune response. Depending on the specific immunization, up to 50% of vaccine recipients have a local reaction that includes erythema, swelling, pain, and induration at the site of the injection. Systemic reactions that often occur include fever, fussiness or irritability, malaise, and anorexia. With some vaccines, other systemic reactions include a rash or arthralgia.

Allergic reactions to vaccines do occur; however, the rate is low, with only 2281 allergic reactions in 1.9 billion doses (0.012%) in the United States between 1991 and 2001 (Schuval, 2003). This is in contrast to the incidence of allergic reactions to food (6–8%) and antibiotics (7.3%) in children (Schuval, 2003). Local allergic reactions, such as a wheal and urticaria, can occur in minutes to hours after the injection. A severe local allergic reaction is manifested by warmth, erythema, edema, petechiae, or ulceration occurring 2 to 8 hours after vaccination. A non-life-threatening systemic allergic reaction, such as generalized urticaria or transient petechiae, may occur within minutes. Anaphylaxis is a life-threatening reaction that is manifested by hypotension, generalized urticaria, and angioedema. Laryngeal edema has occurred in rare cases with nearly every vaccine. The reactions to specific vaccines can be found on the medications table listing common pediatric immunizations on pages 590–594.

Other serious reactions to vaccines occur in rare instances, for which the National Vaccine Injury Compensation Program was established. The range of illnesses and disabilities that may occur include anaphylaxis, encephalopathy, bacterial neuritis, chronic arthritis, thrombocytopenia purpura, and death. Each of these reactions is a reportable event. The significant reactions eligible for compensation specific to each vaccine are listed in Table 18–1 on page 595.

■ COLLABORATIVE CARE

Vaccines should be administered at specific ages and intervals. The timing for first immunizations is determined by the age at which **transplacental immunity** (passive immunity transferred from mother to infant) decreases or disappears, and when the infant or child develops the ability to make antibodies in response to the vaccine. Scientists continue to study the duration of protection from vaccines. Some vaccines do not confer lifelong immunity. For example, it was recently determined that a second dose of varicella vaccine is necessary for immunity (Centers for Disease Control and Prevention, 2006a).

Immunization Schedule

The recommended schedule for immunization is updated at least annually to reflect new vaccines and the need for repeat immunization. The Advisory Committee on

---

CLINICAL TIP

Thimerosol, a bacteriostatic agent that contains ethyl mercury, was previously used to prevent contamination of vaccines in multidose vials. Because of the possible association between mercury poisoning and nerve and brain damage, vaccine manufacturers worked to remove thimerosol from vaccines. Many vaccines now have either no thimerosal or only trace amounts (American Academy of Pediatrics, 2006, p. 48).

NURSING ALERT

Preparation for Emergencies

Be prepared for potential vaccine anaphylaxis. Keep epinephrine 1:1000 and resuscitation equipment immediately available. The dose for epinephrine (aqueous 1:1000) is 0.01 mL/kg per dose up to 0.5 mL intramuscularly. The dose can be repeated every 10–20 minutes for up to a total of three doses until symptoms subside or other emergency care interventions are initiated (American Academy of Pediatrics, 2006, p. 65).

LAW & ETHICS

National Childhood Vaccine Injury Act

The National Childhood Vaccine Injury Act of 1986 provides compensation for a family if a link between a child's immunization and a serious adverse effect is found. The Vaccine Adverse Event Reporting System (VAERS) was established in 1988 to track serious vaccine reactions. Follow-up of the patient's condition occurs at 60 days and 1 year after the adverse event. Follow guidelines for reporting according to the Vaccine Adverse Event Reporting System detailed in Table 18–1 on page 595.

MEDICATIONS USED FOR *Pediatric Immunizations*

Immunization Type	Side Effects	Contraindications	Nursing Implications
Diphtheria and pertussis vaccines and tetanus toxiod (DTaP, Tdap) *Type:* Inactivated. *Route:* Intramuscular. *Dosage:* 0.5 mL. *Age(s) given:* DTaP at 2, 4, 6, 15–18 months; 4–6 years (five doses); 11–12 years (Tdap). May give at same time as all other vaccines, in a separate site. *Storage:* Store in body of refrigerator at 2°–8°C (35°–46°F). Do not freeze. Tripedia and Infanrix are licensed for all 3 doses. Daptacel is licensed for the first 4 doses. Pediarix is composed of DTaP, Hep B, and IPV and can be given as the primary series. TriHiBit is composed of DTaP and Hib. PENTACEL[a] is composed of Hib, DTaP, and IPV. BOOSTRIX[a] and Adacel[a] (Tdap vaccines) are approved for children over 10 years and adults.	*Common:* Redness, pain, swelling, nodule at injection site; temperature up to 38.3°C (101°F); drowsiness, irritability, fussiness; anorexia within 2 days of injection. Increase in frequency and magnitude of local reactions with fourth and fifth doses, (e.g., entire limb swelling). *Serious:* Allergic reaction, anaphylaxis; shock or collapse (hypotonic-hyper-responsive episode—sudden loss of muscle tone, pallor, fever, and unresponsiveness), fever above 38.8°C (102°F); febrile seizure; persistent inconsolable crying; coma or permanent brain damage.	Hypersensitivity to vaccine component; for gelatin hypersensitivity do not use tripedia. Occurrence of a serious side effect after previous administration of DTaP, such as anaphylaxis or encephalopathy within 7 days after DTP or DTaP. Precautions in additional DTaP doses should be considered in children with the following reactions within 48 hours of the previous dose: • Fever ≥ 40.5°C (105°F) • Continuous inconsolable crying lasting ≥ 3 hours • Pale or limp episode or collapse • Convulsion within 3 days of dose. Administration should be delayed for 1 month after immunosuppressive therapy and until moderate to severe febrile illnesses have resolved. Administration of immune serum globulin within last 90 days. Tdap is contraindicated in adolescents with a history of coma or prolonged seizures within 7 days of prior vaccine with pertussis.	Use same brand for all doses where feasible. Prior to immunization, ask about previous reactions to immunization. DTaP may coincide with or hasten the recognition of a seizure disorder. In children with a history of seizures with or without fever, give acetaminophen at the time of vaccine and then every 4 hours for 24 hours. Shake vaccine before withdrawing. Solution will be cloudy. If it contains clumps that cannot be resuspended, do not use. Daptacel stopper vial contains latex. Pediarix stopper vial is latex-free. When required, simultaneous administration of tetanus immune globulin or diphtheria antitoxin should be given in separate sites with a new needle and syringe. Inform parents of the chance of increased reaction to the third and fourth doses. Defer the vaccine when the child has a progressive neurologic problem until the child is stable. DT is given to children <7 years of age who have had a serious reaction to the pertussis component of the DTP or DTaP vaccine. Td is given to children ≥7 years. Adolescents 11 to 18 years who received Td, but not Tdap, are encouraged to get a dose of Tdap to gain protection against pertussis (Centers for Disease Control, 2006b). Carefully check vials of DTaP, DT, Td, and Tdap to ensure that the proper vaccine is administered for the child's age. The series does not need to be restarted, no matter how long since the previous dose was given. After the primary series of three is completed, a tetanus booster may be given in the case of a contaminated wound or burn if five or more years have passed since the last dose (American Academy of Pediatrics, 2006, p. 650).
Haemophilus influenza type B (Hib) *Type:* Inactivated. *Route:* Intramuscular. *Dosage:* 0.5 mL. *Age(s) given:* 2, 4, 6, 12–15 months; (Four doses for HbOC[a] [HibTITER] and PRP-T[a] [ActHIB]). or 2, 4, 12–15 months (three doses for PRP-OMP[a] [PedvaxHIB]). May give at same time as all other vaccines in a separate site.	*Common:* Pain, redness, or swelling at site *Serious:* Allergic reaction of anaphylaxis (extremely rare); fever	Prior anaphylactic reaction to this vaccine.	Prior to immunizations, ask if child is immunosuppressed. Solution is clear and colorless. Refrigerate reconstituted PedvaxHIB and discard within 24 hours. Use or discard reconstituted ActHIB and OmniHIB within 30 minutes. Since schedules for product preparations of different companies vary, it is important to read package inserts carefully. If the first dose is given between 7 and 11 months of age, three doses are needed. If the first dose was given at 12 to 14 months of age, give a booster dose in 8 weeks. If the first dose is given when the child is over 15 months or under 5 years, only one dose is needed (American Academy of Pediatrics, 2006, p. 317). Second and third doses can be given 4 to 8 weeks after the first.

(continued)

Immunization Type	Side Effects	Contraindications	Nursing Implications
Haemophilus influenza, type B (Hib) (continued) *Storage*: Store in body of refrigerator at 2°–8°C (35°–46°F). Do not freeze. HibTITER, ActHIB, and PedvaxHIB are single vaccine preparations. Comvax is a combination of PRP-OMP plus HepB. TriHIBit is composed of DTaP and Hib.			Use the same vaccine preparation for all doses of the primary series, if possible. The series does not need to be restarted, no matter how long since the previous dose was given.
Hepatitis A *Type*: Inactivated. *Route*: Intramuscular. *Dosage*: 0.5 mL (1.0 mL over 18 years). *Age(s) given*: 12–23 months; 2–18 years, 6–12 months after first dose (two doses) in areas with increased incidence. May give at same time as all other vaccines in a separate site. *Storage*: Store in body of refrigerator at 2°–8°C (35°–46°F). Do not freeze; do not use if has been frozen. Havrix and Vaqta are single vaccine preparations.	*Common*: Pain, tenderness, soreness, redness, swelling, and warmth at injection site; rash, fever. Rare reports of anaphylaxis/ anaphylactoid reactions.	Known hypersensitivity to any vaccine component. Prior hypersensitivity reaction to the vaccine.	Shake well, slightly opaque white suspension. No reconstitution is needed. Can be given for post-exposure prophylaxis against hepatitis A. Immune globulin and vaccine can be given at the same time in different sites. Do not restart the series, no matter how long since the previous dose. Vaccine brands can be interchanged. Vaqta vials have a latex stopper.
Hepatitis B Vaccine (HB) *Type:* Inactivated. *Route*: Intramuscular. *Dosage*: Engerix-B[a]: 10 mcg or Recombivax HB[a]: 5 mcg. *Age(s) given*: Birth–2 months, 1 month after first dose; 6 months after first dose. or Birth–2 months, 1–4 months, 6–18 months (three doses). May give at same time as all other vaccines in a separate site. *Storage*: Store in body of refrigerator at 2°–8°C (35°–46°F). Do not freeze. Engerix-B and Recombivax HB are single vaccine preparations. Comvax is a combination of Hib and Hep B. Newborn dose should be monovalent (single vaccine) preparation.	*Common*: Pain or redness at injection site. *Serious*: Allergic reaction or anaphylaxis; fever.	Prior anaphylaxis, liver abnormalities. Serious hypersensitivity reaction to past dose. Yeast hypersensitivity.	Prior to immunization, check status of mother's hepatitis B test and presence of other liver disease. If mother has HBsAg+ or unknown status, give vaccine to infant within 12 hours of birth along with hepatitis B immune globulin in another site. Shake vaccine before withdrawing. Solution will appear cloudy. Various formulations (pediatric, adult, dialysis) are available in different strengths. Read package insert carefully to determine proper dosage for age for the formulation used. A three-dose series can be started at any age. Minimum spacing for children and teens is 4 weeks between #1 and #2, and 8 weeks between #2 and #3. The last dose in an infant series should not be given before 6 months of age. Infants of HBsAG+ mothers should have anti-HBs levels checked after vaccine completion and be reimmunized if anti-HBs levels are less than 10 milli International Units/mL (American Academy of Pediatrics, 2006, p. 347). Vaccine brands can be interchanged for three-dose series. The series does not need to be restarted, no matter how long since the previous dose was given.

(continued)

MEDICATIONS USED FOR *Pediatric Immunizations* (continued)

Immunization Type	Side Effects	Contraindications	Nursing Implications
Human Papillomavirus Vaccine (Quadravalent) *Type:* Recombinant. *Route:* Intramuscular. *Dosage:* 0.5 mL. *Age(s) given:* Girls 11–12 years, second dose 2 months later, third dose 4 months later (over a 6-month period). May be administered with hepatitis B vaccine in separate site. *Storage:* Store in body of refrigerator at 2°–8°C (35°–46°F). Do not freeze. GARDASIL[a] is a single vaccine preparation.	*Common:* Pain, swelling, erythema at the injection site, pruritus, and fever. *Potential serious reactions:* Headache, gastroenteritis, bronchospasm, asthma, arthritis.	Hypersensitivity to any vaccine substances. Not recommended for pregnant women. Should not be given to individuals with bleeding disorder. Use caution when administering to lactating women as it is not known if vaccine is excreted in human milk.	Shake well before use. Solution is a white cloudy liquid. No dilution or reconstitution is needed. Protect vaccine from light to protect its potency. Vaccine is licensed for girls as young as 9 years old and for women up to 26 years old. Testing is ongoing for potential use of the vaccine in males. Vaccine should be administered before onset of sexual activity. Discuss this new vaccine and its potential with parents to prevent cervical cancer as well as human papillomavirus infections. The fact that human papillomavirus is transmitted by sexual activity may reduce acceptance of vaccine by some parents in preteen years.
Influenza *Type:* Inactivated (TIV), live attenuated for intranasal use (LAIV). *Route:* Intramuscular (all ages), intranasal (5 years and older). *Dosage:* 0.25 mL in infants 6 to 35 months, 0.5 mL beginning at 3 years. *Age(s) given:* 6 to 59 months (all children), older high-risk children. May give at same time as all other vaccines in a separate site. *TIV storage:* Store in body of refrigerator at 2°–8°C (35°–46°F). Do not use if it has been frozen. *LAIV Storage:* Keep frozen. May be thawed and kept in refrigerator at 2°–8°C (35°–46°F) for no more than 24 hours before use. Flu Shield[a] (Trivalent, inactivated vaccine). Flu Mist[a] (LAIV).	*Common after TIV:* May have soreness or swelling at injection site, fever, aches. Life-threatening allergic reactions are rare. *Common after intranasal vaccine:* Runny nose or nasal congestion, fever, headache or muscle aches, abdominal pain, and occasional vomiting. No life-threatening problems were detected during clinical trials.	Contraindicated in children with history of anaphylactic reaction to egg or chicken protein, hypersensitivity to thimerosol, known hypersensitivity to gentamicin or other aminoglycosides. LAIV is contraindicated in children on long-term aspirin therapy; have reactive airway disease or other conditions considered high risk for influenza; close contacts with severely immuno-suppressed person; known or suspected immune deficiency disorders. Should not be given within 3 days of pertussis vaccine (*Mosby's Drug Consult,* 2004). Postpone vaccine when child has acute febrile illness until symptoms abate, but may be given with minor illness, with or without fever.	Thawed intranasal vaccine is pale yellow, clear to slightly cloudy. Administered annually in autumn at the time recommended by the CDC. Intranasal dose is split (0.25 mL) with a dose divider clip. Administer in each nostril while child is sitting in an upright position. Insert the tip of the sprayer inside the nose and depress the plunger to spray. Breast-feeding is not a contraindication for use of either vaccine in infants. Children younger than 9 years of age who are receiving the influenza vaccine for the first time should get two doses separated by at least 4 weeks (injectable) and 6 weeks (intranasal). Children at high risk are those on long-term aspirin therapy, have chronic disorders of the cardiovascular or pulmonary system (including asthma), have a condition that increases risk for aspiration, chronic metabolic disease, renal dysfunction, hemoglobinopathies, or immunodeficiency (Centers for Disease Control, 2006c, p. 2). Must be re-immunized each year (one dose) as immunity wanes.
Measles, Mumps, Rubella Vaccines (MMR) *Type:* Live attenuated. *Route:* Subcutaneous. *Dosage:* 0.5 mL. *Age(s) given:* 12–15 months; 4–6 years (two doses).	*Common:* Elevated temperature 1–2 weeks after immunization; redness or pain at injection site; noncontagious rash; joint pain.	Prior anaphylactic reaction to vaccine. Hypersensitivity to neomycin or gelatin. Severely impaired immune system due to malignancy, immune deficiency disease, immunosuppressive therapy.	Reconstituted vaccine is a clear, yellow solution. Give entire contents of reconstituted vial even if more than 0.5 mL. Prior to immunization, ask if child has allergy to neomycin or gelatin. Observe the child with an egg allergy for 90 minutes after injection. Egg allergy is not a contraindication for the vaccine (Cox, 2006).

(continued)

Immunization Type	Side Effects	Contraindications	Nursing Implications
Measles, Mumps, Rubella Vaccines (MMR) (continued) May give at same time as all other vaccines in a separate site. *Storage:* Store in body of refrigerator at 2°–8°C (35°–46°F). When reconstituted, keep refrigerated and away from light; discard if unused within 8 hours. Diluent is stored at room temperature or in refrigerator. Do not freeze. ProQuad[a] combines varicella vaccine with MMR.	*Serious:* Allergic reaction or anaphylaxis; febrile seizure; meningitis (usually mild); encephalopathy; thrombocytopenia purpura; and rare cases of coma and permanent brain damage.	Wait at least 3 to 11 months after administration of immune globulin or blood products (time determined by the type) before giving vaccine. Pregnancy or possibility of pregnancy within 4 weeks. Thrombocytopenia or history of thrombocytopenic purpura. Tuberculosis or positive PPD.	Inquire about immunosuppression. MMR vaccine is recommended for those infected with HIV. Instruct adolescent girls of childbearing age to avoid pregnancy for 3 months after immunization. Give tuberculosis (TB) test at same time as MMR or 4–6 weeks later. If MMR and Varivax are not given on the same day, space them ≥ 28 days apart. As college students are at greater risk due to decreasing immunity, make sure they have received a second MMR dose.
Meningococcal Tetravalent Conjugate Vaccine (MCV4) *Type:* Inactivated. *Route:* Intramuscular. *Dosage:* 0.5 mL in children 11–12 years and older. May be given at same time as typhoid or Td vaccine. *Storage:* Store in body of refrigerator at 2°–8°C (35°–46°F) until use. Do not freeze. Menactra[a] is a single vaccine preparation.	*Common:* Pain at injection site, headache, and fatigue. Less than 5% experienced a severe systemic reaction in vaccine trials (Bilukha & Rosenstein, 2005). A possible association between MCV4 (Menactra) and Guillain Barré syndrome occurring 2 to 4 weeks after vaccination has been reported (Food and Drug Administration, 2005).	Hypersensitivity to any component of vaccine, including diphtheria toxoid. Patients at risk for hemorrhage should not receive vaccine. Pregnant women should receive vaccine only if clearly needed.	Protect vaccine from light. May be given to children 11 years or older who are immunosuppressed by disease or medication. Use MPSV4 for younger children (see table on page 598). Recommended for control of meningococcal outbreaks caused by serogroups A, C, W-135, and Y. Until adequate supply exists, recommended for preadolescents and adolescents wishing to reduce health risks, such as those going to boarding school or college. Vial stopper contains latex.
Pneumococcal Conjugate Vaccine (Heptavalent) (PCV7) *Type:* Inactivated. *Route:* Intramuscular. *Dosage:* 0.5 mL. *Age(s) given:* 2, 4, 6, 12–15 months *Storage:* Store in body of refrigerator at 2°–8°C (35°–46°F). Do not freeze. Prevnar[a] is a single vaccine preparation.	*Common:* Soreness, swelling, redness at injection site; mild to moderate fever; irritability, drowsiness, restless sleep, decreased appetite, vomiting and diarrhea, rash or hives. *Severe:* Allergic reaction or anaphylaxis.	Hypersensitivity to diphtheria toxoid.	Clear, colorless, or slightly opalescent liquid. May be given to children up to 9 years. Use PPV23 for children 2 years and older at high risk for aquiring pneumococcal infection (see table on page 598). The series does not need to be restarted, no matter how long since the previous dose was given.
Poliovirus Vaccine (IPV) *Type:* Inactivated. *Route:* Subcutaneous or intramuscular depending upon vaccine used. *Dosage:* 0.5 mL. *Age(s) given:* 2, 4,12–18 months; 4–6 years (four doses). May give at same time as all other vaccines in a separate site.	*Common:* Swelling and tenderness, irritability, tiredness. *Serious:* Allergic reaction or anaphylaxis	Hypersensitivity to vaccine components: neomycin, streptomycin, polymyxin B. Anaphylactic response. Pregnancy.	Prior to immunization, ask if the child has an allergy to neomycin, streptomycin, or polymyxin B (whichever of these antibiotics the specific vaccine to be used contains). Clear, colorless suspension. Do not use if it contains particulate matter, becomes cloudy, or changes color. Recommended for use in all vaccine doses. All doses must be separated by at least 4 weeks. The series does not need to be restarted, no matter how long since the previous dose was given.

(continued)

MEDICATIONS USED FOR *Pediatric Immunizations* (continued)

Immunization Type	Side Effects	Contraindications	Nursing Implications
Poliovirus Vaccine (IPV) (continued) *Storage:* Store in body of refrigerator at 2°–8°C (35°–46°F). Do not freeze Pediarix includes IPV, DTaP, and HepB. PENTACEL[a] is composed of Hib, DTaP, and IPV. IPV may be given as single vaccine preparation.			There is no contraindication to giving IPV to an infant or child when a family member is immunocompromised.
Rotavirus Vaccine (PRV) *Type:* Live. *Route:* Oral. *Dosage:* 2 mL. *Age(s) given:* 2, 4, and 6 months (three doses) May give at same time as all other vaccines. *Storage:* Store in body of refrigerator at 2°–8°C (35°–46°F). Do not freeze. RotaTeq[a] is a single vaccine preparation.	Data from vaccine trials. *Common:* Vomiting, diarrhea, irritability. *Potential serious adverse reactions:* Seizures, bronchiolitis, gastroenteritis, pneumonia, fever, urinary tract infection.	Hypersensitivity to vaccine components. Hypersensitivity after receiving a dose of vaccine. Should not be given to infants with a known or suspected weakened immune system.	Pale yellow clear liquid in single dose tube for direct oral administration. Protect vaccine from light. Squeeze the liquid into the infant's mouth toward the inner cheek until the dosing tube is empty. No restrictions on the infant's intake of formula, breast milk, or food before or after vaccine. Discard the empty tube and cap into approved biological waste container. All three doses of vaccine should be completed by 32 months of age.
Varicella Virus Vaccine *Type:* Live attenuated. *Route:* Subcutaneous. *Dosage:* 0.5 mL. *Age(s) given:* 12–15 months; and 4–6 years (two doses). 13 years or older (two doses 4–8 weeks apart) *Storage:* Frozen at –15°C (5°F) or colder. May be stored in refrigerator at 2°–8°C (35°–46°F) up to 72 hours before reconstitution. Do not refreeze. Varivax[a] is a single vaccine preparation. ProQuad[a] combines varicella vaccine with MMR.	*Common:* Pain or redness at injection site; fever up to 38.8°C (102°F) in children or up to 37.7°C (100°F) in adults. Less commonly a vaccine-related rash (mild exanthem of 6 to 10 lesions that last for 2 to 3 days) may occur during first month after the injection. *Severe:* Allergic reaction or anaphylaxis; thrombocytopenia; febrile seizure; CNS manifestations.	Prior anaphylactic reaction to vaccine. Hypersensitivity to neomycin or gelatin. Immunodeficiency or receiving immunosuppression therapy. Administration of immune serum globulin or blood products in last 3–11 months. Active untreated TB. Pregnancy. Moderate or severe febrile illness.	Prior to immunization, ask if child is immunodeficient or on immunosuppression treatment or had an allergy to neomycin or gelatin. Determine if a family member is immunocompromised. Clear, colorless to pale yellow liquid when reconstituted. Once reconstituted, vaccine must be used within 30 minutes or discarded. Give the entire contents of the vial even if more than 0.5 mL. Instruct adolescent girls of childbearing age to avoid pregnancy for 3 months after immunization. The vaccine is effective. Only very mild cases of breakthrough varicella occurred in children who were immunized, primarily caused by wild type virus (American Academy of Pediatrics, 2006, p. 719).

[a] Trade names

Data from: American Academy of Pediatrics. (2006). *Red book: Report of the committee on infectious disease* (27th ed.). Elk Grove Village, IL: Author; Immunization Action Coalition; Mosby (2004). *Mosby's drug consult 2004.* St. Louis: Mosby, Inc.; Bindler, R. M., & Howry, L. B. (2005). *Pediatric drugs and nursing implications* (3rd ed.). Upper Saddle River, NJ: Prentice Hall Health; and Buck, M. L. (2005). Meningococcal conjugate vaccine. *Pediatric Pharmacology, 11*(5), Retrieved June 7, 2005, from http://www.medscape.com/viewarticle/505508_print; Merck & Co. Inc. (2006). Gardasil, Retrieved June 13, 2006, from http://www.fda.gov/cber/label/hpvmer060806LB.pdf

Table 18–1	NATIONAL VACCINE INJURY COMPENSATION PROGRAM—VACCINE INJURY TABLE, JULY 1, 2005[a]

Vaccine	Adverse Event	Time Interval
I. Tetanus toxoid-containing vaccines (e.g., DTaP, Tdap, DTP-Hib, DT, Td, TT)	A. Anaphylaxis or anaphylactic shock B. Brachial neuritis C. Any acute complication or sequela (including death) of above events	0–4 hours 2–28 days Not applicable
II. Pertussis antigen-containing vaccines (e.g., DTaP, Tdap, DTP, P, DTP-Hib)	A. Anaphylaxis or anaphylactic shock B. Encephalopathy (or encephalitis) C. Any acute complication or sequela (including death) of above events	0–4 hours 0–72 hours Not applicable
III. Measles, mumps and rubella virus-containing vaccines in any combination (e.g., MMR, MR, M, R)	A. Anaphylaxis or anaphylactic shock B. Encephalopathy (or encephalitis) C. Any acute complication or sequela (including death) of above events	0–4 hours 5–15 days Not applicable
IV. Rubella virus-containing vaccines (e.g., MMR, MR, R)	A. Chronic arthritis B. Any acute complication or sequela (including death) of above event	7–42 days Not applicable
V. Measles virus-containing vaccines (e.g., MMR, MR, M)	A. Thrombocytopenic purpura B. Vaccine-Strain Measles Viral Infection in an immunodeficient recipient C. Any acute complication or sequela (including death) of above events	7–30 days 0–6 months Not applicable
VI. Polio live virus-containing vaccines (OPV)	A. Paralytic polio —in a non-immunodeficient recipient —in an immunodeficient recipient —in a vaccine associated community case B. Vaccine-strain polio viral infection —in a non-immunodeficient recipient —in an immunodeficient recipient —in a vaccine associated community case C. Any acute complication or sequela (including death) of above events	 0–30 days 0–6 months Not applicable 0–30 days 0–6 months Not applicable Not applicable
VII. Polio inactivated-virus containing vaccines (e.g., IPV)	A. Anaphylaxis or anaphylactic shock B. Any acute complication or sequela (including death) of above event	0–4 hours Not applicable
VIII. Hepatitis B antigen-containing vaccines	A. Anaphylaxis or anaphylactic shock B. Any acute complication or sequela (including death) of above event	0–4 hours Not applicable
IX. Hemophilus influenzae type b polysaccharide conjugate vaccines	A. No condition specified for compensation	Not applicable
X. Varicella vaccine	A. No condition specified for compensation	Not applicable
XI. Rotavirus vaccine	A. No condition specified for compensation	Not applicable
XII. Vaccines containing live, oral, rhesus-based rotavirus	A. Intussusception B. Any acute complication or sequela (including death) of above event	0–30 days Not applicable
XIII. Pneumococcal conjugate vaccines	A. No condition specified for compensation	Not applicable
XIV. Any new vaccine recommended by the Centers for Disease Control and Prevention for routine administration to children, after publication by Secretary, HHS of a notice of coverage[b]	A. No condition specified for compensation	Not applicable

[a]Effective date: July 1, 2005
[b]As of **December 1, 2004**, hepatitis A vaccines have been added to the Vaccine Injury Table (Table) under this category. As of **July 1, 2005**, *trivalent* influenza vaccines have been added to the Table under this category. Trivalent influenza vaccines are given annually during the flu season either by needle and syringe or in a nasal spray. All influenza vaccines routinely administered in the United States are trivalent vaccines covered under this category. See *News* on the VICP web site for more information (www.hrsa.gov/osp/vicp).
Retrieved 10/24/2005

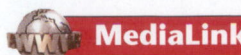

MediaLink

CDC Recommended
Immunization Schedule

Immunization Practices (ACIP) of the Centers for Disease Control, the American Academy of Pediatrics (AAP), and the American Academy of Family Practitioners (AAFP) collaborate to provide a uniform vaccination schedule. See Figure 18–4 ➤ for the recommended schedule of immunizations in the United States. As the vaccine schedule changes at least annually, visit the CDC web site for the most current recommendations.

Schedules and recommendations vary for children who begin immunizations later in childhood or need catch-up doses. See the alternate schedule for catch-up immunizations on the Centers for Disease Control and Prevention web site. Immunization recommendations vary for children who have recently received immune globulin or immunosuppressive agents. Supplemental immunizations for meningococcal and pneumococcal infections are recommended for certain children, as noted in the table on page 598.

Figure 18–4 ➤ Recommended Childhood Immunization Schedule, United States, 2006.

DEPARTMENT OF HEALTH AND HUMAN SERVICES • CENTERS FOR DISEASE CONTROL AND PREVENTION

Recommended Childhood and Adolescent Immunization Schedule — UNITED STATES • 2006

Vaccine ▼ / Age ▶	Birth	1 month	2 months	4 months	6 months	12 months	15 months	18 months	24 months	4–6 years	11–12 years	13–14 years	15 years	16–18 years
Hepatitis B[1]	HepB	HepB		HepB[1]		HepB					HepB Series			
Diphtheria, Tetanus, Pertussis[2]			DTaP	DTaP	DTaP		DTaP			DTaP	Tdap	Tdap		
Haemophilus influenzae type b[3]			Hib	Hib	Hib[3]	Hib								
Inactivated Poliovirus			IPV	IPV		IPV				IPV				
Measles, Mumps, Rubella[4]						MMR				MMR		MMR		
Varicella[5]						Varicella					Varicella			
Meningococcal[6]									MPSV4		MCV4	MCV4 / MCV4		
Pneumococcal[7]			PCV	PCV	PCV	PCV				PCV	PPV			
Influenza[8]						Influenza (Yearly)					Influenza (Yearly)			
Hepatitis A[9]										HepA Series				

Vaccines within broken line are for selected populations

Range of recommended ages — Catch-up immunization — 11–12 year old assessment

This schedule indicates the recommended ages for routine administration of currently licensed childhood vaccines, as of December 1, 2005, for children through age 18 years. Any dose not administered at the recommended age should be administered at any subsequent visit when indicated and feasible. ▨ Indicates age groups that warrant special effort to administer those vaccines not previously administered. Additional vaccines may be licensed and recommended during the year. Licensed combination vaccines may be used whenever any components of the combination are indicated and other components of the vaccine are not contraindicated and if approved by the Food and Drug Administration for that dose of the series. Providers should consult the respective ACIP statement for detailed recommendations. Clinically significant adverse events that follow immunization should be reported to the Vaccine Adverse Event Reporting System (VAERS). Guidance about how to obtain and complete a VAERS form is available at **www.vaers.hhs.gov** or by telephone, **800-822-7967**.

1. **Hepatitis B vaccine (HepB).** *AT BIRTH:* All newborns should receive monovalent HepB soon after birth and before hospital discharge. **Infants born to mothers who are HBsAg-positive** should receive HepB and 0.5 mL of hepatitis B immune globulin (HBIG) within 12 hours of birth. **Infants born to mothers whose HBsAg status is unknown** should receive HepB within 12 hours of birth. The mother should have blood drawn as soon as possible to determine her HBsAg status; if HBsAg-positive, the infant should receive HBIG as soon as possible (no later than age 1 week). **For infants born to HBsAg-negative mothers,** the birth dose can be delayed in rare circumstances but only if a physician's order to withhold the vaccine and a copy of the mother's original HBsAg-negative laboratory report are documented in the infant's medical record. *FOLLOWING THE BIRTHDOSE:* The HepB series should be completed with either monovalent HepB or a combination vaccine containing HepB. The second dose should be administered at age 1–2 months. The final dose should be administered at age ≥24 weeks. It is permissible to administer 4 doses of HepB (e.g., when combination vaccines are given after the birth dose); however, if monovalent HepB is used, a dose at age 4 months is not needed. **Infants born to HBsAg-positive mothers** should be tested for HBsAg and antibody to HBsAg after completion of the HepB series, at age 9–18 months (generally at the next well-child visit after completion of the vaccine series).

2. **Diphtheria and tetanus toxoids and acellular pertussis vaccine (DTaP).** The fourth dose of DTaP may be administered as early as age 12 months, provided 6 months have elapsed since the third dose and the child is unlikely to return at age 15–18 months. The final dose in the series should be given at age ≥4 years.
   Tetanus and diphtheria toxoids and acellular pertussis vaccine (Tdap – adolescent preparation) is recommended at age 11–12 years for those who have completed the recommended childhood DTP/DTaP vaccination series and have not received a Td booster dose. Adolescents 13–18 years who missed the 11–12-year Td/Tdap booster dose should also receive a single dose of Tdap if they have completed the recommended childhood DTP/DTaP vaccination series. Subsequent **tetanus and diphtheria toxoids (Td)** are recommended every 10 years.

3. ***Haemophilus influenzae* type b conjugate vaccine (Hib).** Three Hib conjugate vaccines are licensed for infant use. If PRP-OMP (PedvaxHIB® or ComVax® [Merck]) is administered at ages 2 and 4 months, a dose at age 6 months is not required. DTaP/Hib combination products should not be used for primary immunization in infants at ages 2, 4 or 6 months but can be used as boosters after any Hib vaccine. The final dose in the series should be administered at age ≥12 months.

4. **Measles, mumps, and rubella vaccine (MMR).** The second dose of MMR is recommended routinely at age 4–6 years but may be administered during any visit, provided at least 4 weeks have elapsed since the first dose and both doses are administered beginning at or after age 12 months. Those who have not previously received the second dose should complete the schedule by age 11–12 years.

5. **Varicella vaccine.** Varicella vaccine is recommended at any visit at or after age 12 months for susceptible children (i.e., those who lack a reliable history of chickenpox). Susceptible persons aged ≥13 years should receive 2 doses administered at least 4 weeks apart.

6. **Meningococcal vaccine (MCV4).** Meningococcal conjugate vaccine (MCV4) should be given to all children at the 11–12 year old visit as well as to unvaccinated adolescents at high school entry (15 years of age). Other adolescents who wish to decrease their risk for meningococcal disease may also be vaccinated. All college freshmen living in dormitories should also be vaccinated, preferably with MCV4, although **meningococcal polysaccharide vaccine (MPSV4)** is an acceptable alternative. Vaccination against invasive meningococcal disease is recommended for children and adolescents aged ≥2 years with terminal complement deficiencies or anatomic or functional asplenia and certain other high risk groups (see *MMWR* 2005;54 [RR-7]:1-21; use MPSV4 for children aged 2–10 years and MCV4 for older children, although MPSV4 is an acceptable alternative.

7. **Pneumococcal vaccine.** The heptavalent **pneumococcal conjugate vaccine (PCV)** is recommended for all children aged 2–23 months and for certain children aged 24–59 months. The final dose in the series should be given at age ≥12 months. **Pneumococcal polysaccharide vaccine (PPV)** is recommended in addition to PCV for certain high-risk groups. See *MMWR* 2000; 49(RR-9):1-35.

8. **Influenza vaccine.** Influenza vaccine is recommended annually for children aged ≥6 months with certain risk factors (including, but not limited to, asthma, cardiac disease, sickle cell disease, human immunodeficiency virus [HIV], diabetes, and conditions that can compromise respiratory function or handling of respiratory secretions or that can increase the risk for aspiration), healthcare workers, and other persons (including household members) in close contact with persons in groups at high risk (see *MMWR* 2005;54[RR-8]:1-55). In addition, healthy children aged 6–23 months and close contacts of healthy children aged 0–5 months are recommended to receive influenza vaccine because children in this age group are at substantially increased risk for influenza-related hospitalizations. For healthy persons aged 5–49 years, the intranasally administered, live, attenuated influenza vaccine (LAIV) is an acceptable alternative to the intramuscular trivalent inactivated influenza vaccine (TIV). See *MMWR* 2005;54(RR-8):1-55. Children receiving TIV should be administered a dosage appropriate for their age (0.25 mL if aged 6–35 months or 0.5 mL if aged ≥3 years). Children aged ≤8 years who are receiving influenza vaccine for the first time should receive 2 doses (separated by at least 4 weeks for TIV and at least 6 weeks for LAIV).

9. **Hepatitis A vaccine (HepA).** HepA is recommended for all children at 1 year of age (i.e., 12–23 months). The 2 doses in the series should be administered at least 6 months apart. States, counties, and communities with existing HepA vaccination programs for children 2–18 years of age are encouraged to maintain these programs. In these areas, new efforts focused on routine vaccination of 1-year-old children should enhance, not replace, ongoing programs directed at a broader population of children. HepA is also recommended for certain high risk groups (see *MMWR* 1999; 48[RR-12]1-37).

The Childhood and Adolescent Immunization Schedule is approved by:
Advisory Committee on Immunization Practices www.cdc.gov/nip/acip • American Academy of Pediatrics www.aap.org • American Academy of Family Physicians www.aafp.org

Increasing the Number of Children Immunized

Efforts to increase the numbers of children protected from vaccine preventable diseases and to monitor immunization status is a national public health initiative. *Healthy People 2010* states important goals for reduction of vaccine preventable diseases.

- Adequately immunize 90% of U.S. children by their second birthday.
- Adequately immunize 95% of children in kindergarten and first grade.
- Have 95% of children less than 6 years of age participating in a fully operational population-based immunization registry. Once fully operational, the registries should meet 13 functional standards that will enable states or managed care organizations to monitor the immunization status of their population (Centers for Disease Control, 2002b; Department of Health and Human Services, Office of Disease Prevention, 2000).

Many missed opportunities to immunize children have been identified. Children (and siblings present) should have their immunization status assessed during all healthcare visits, hospitalizations, and in schools. Efforts to increase immunization levels

Recommended Immunization Schedule for Children and Adolescents Who Start Late or Who Are More Than 1 Month Behind

UNITED STATES • 2006

The tables below give catch-up schedules and minimum intervals between doses for children who have delayed immunizations. There is no need to restart a vaccine series regardless of the time that has elapsed between doses. Use the chart appropriate for the child's age.

CATCH-UP SCHEDULE FOR CHILDREN AGED 4 MONTHS THROUGH 6 YEARS

Vaccine	Minimum Age for Dose 1	Minimum Interval Between Doses			
		Dose 1 to Dose 2	Dose 2 to Dose 3	Dose 3 to Dose 4	Dose 4 to Dose 5
Diphtheria, Tetanus, Pertussis	6 wks	4 weeks	4 weeks	6 months	6 months[1]
Inactivated Poliovirus	6 wks	4 weeks	4 weeks	4 weeks[2]	
Hepatitis B[3]	Birth	4 weeks	8 weeks (and 16 weeks after first dose)		
Measles, Mumps, Rubella	12 mo	4 weeks[4]			
Varicella	12 mo				
Haemophilus influenzae type b[5]	6 wks	4 weeks if first dose given at age <12 months / 8 weeks (as final dose) if first dose given at age 12-14 months / No further doses needed if first dose given at age ≥15 months	4 weeks[6] if current age <12 months / 8 weeks (as final dose)[6] if current age ≥12 months and second dose given at age <15 months / No further doses needed if previous dose given at age ≥15 mo	8 weeks (as final dose) This dose only necessary for children aged 12 months–5 years who received 3 doses before age 12 months	
Pneumococcal[7]	6 wks	4 weeks if first dose given at age <12 months and current age <24 months / 8 weeks (as final dose) if first dose given at age ≥12 months or current age 24–59 months / No further doses needed for healthy children if first dose given at age ≥24 months	4 weeks if current age <12 months / 8 weeks (as final dose) if current age ≥12 months / No further doses needed for healthy children if previous dose given at age ≥24 months	8 weeks (as final dose) This dose only necessary for children aged 12 months–5 years who received 3 doses before age 12 months	

CDC

CATCH-UP SCHEDULE FOR CHILDREN AGED 7 YEARS THROUGH 18 YEARS

Vaccine	Minimum Interval Between Doses		
	Dose 1 to Dose 2	Dose 2 to Dose 3	Dose 3 to Booster Dose
Tetanus, Diphtheria[8]	4 weeks	6 months	6 months if first dose given at age <12 months and current age <11 years; otherwise 5 years
Inactivated Poliovirus[9]	4 weeks	4 weeks	IPV[2,9]
Hepatitis B	4 weeks	8 weeks (and 16 weeks after first dose)	
Measles, Mumps, Rubella	4 weeks		
Varicella[10]	4 weeks		

1. **DTaP.** The fifth dose is not necessary if the fourth dose was administered after the fourth birthday.
2. **IPV.** For children who received an all-IPV or all-oral poliovirus (OPV) series, a fourth dose is not necessary if third dose was administered at age ≥4 years. If both OPV and IPV were administered as part of a series, a total of 4 doses should be given, regardless of the child's current age.
3. **HepB.** Administer the 3-dose series to all children and adolescents <19 years of age if they were not previously vaccinated.
4. **MMR.** The second dose of MMR is recommended routinely at age 4–6 years but may be administered earlier if desired.
5. **Hib.** Vaccine is not generally recommended for children aged ≥5 years.
6. **Hib.** If current age <12 months and the first 2 doses were PRP-OMP (PedvaxHIB® or ComVax® [Merck]), the third (and final) dose should be administered at age 12–15 months and at least 8 weeks after the second dose.
7. **PCV.** Vaccine is not generally recommended for children aged ≥5 years.
8. **Td.** Adolescent tetanus, diphtheria, and pertussis vaccine (Tdap) may be substituted for any dose in a primary catch-up series or as a booster if age appropriate for Tdap. A five-year interval from the last Td dose is encouraged when Tdap is used as a booster dose. See ACIP recommendations for further details.
9. **IPV.** Vaccine is not generally recommended for persons aged ≥18 years.
10. **Varicella.** Administer the 2-dose series to all susceptible adolescents aged ≥13 years.

Report adverse reactions to vaccines through the federal Vaccine Adverse Event Reporting System. For information on reporting reactions following immunization, please visit **www.vaers.hhs.gov** or call the 24-hour national toll-free information line **800-822-7967**. Report suspected cases of vaccine-preventable diseases to your state or local health department.

For additional information about vaccines, including precautions and contraindications for immunization and vaccine shortages, please visit the National Immunization Program Website at **www.cdc.gov/nip** or contact **800-CDC-INFO (800-232-4636)** (In English, En Español — 24/7)

Figure 18–4 ➤ *continued*

> **NURSING ALERT**
>
> Immune globulin inhibits the response to live virus vaccines such as measles, mumps, rubella, and varicella. Ask about recent administration of immune globulin or immunosuppression therapy. Refer to the most current guidelines to identify the appropriate interval (3 to 12 months) between administration of immune globulin or completion of immunosuppression therapy and live virus vaccine administration.
>
> Similarly, if immune globulin must be given within 14 days after administration of a live virus vaccine, the vaccine should be administered again after the period specified in the most current guidelines, unless serologic testing determines that the child developed adequate serum antibodies (American Academy of Pediatrics, 2006, p. 36).

MEDICATIONS USED FOR *Supplemental Immunizations*

Vaccine	Recommendation
Meningococcal (MPSV4)	For children 2 to 10 years of age with asplenia. It can be given concurrently with other vaccines in a different site. In school-age children, protection with this vaccine against group A and C polysaccharides is thought to last 3 to 5 years (American Academy of Pediatrics, 2006, p. 457). At 11 years, the MCV4 vaccine may be used. See the vaccine information on page 593.
23-valent Pneumococcal (PPV23)	For children older than 2 years of age with sickle-cell disease, asplenia, chronic heart and lung disorders, diabetes mellitus, nephrotic syndrome, renal failure, HIV infection, cochlear implant, cerebrospinal fluid leaks, or other immune compromised status. American Indians and Alaskan Native children residing in areas with high rates of invasive pneumococcal disease are also recommended to receive PPV23. An additional dose is given 3 to 5 years after the first dose (American Academy of Pediatrics, 2006, page 533). Give a second dose 3 to 5 years after the first dose of PPV23.

among children are also supported by managed care organizations that require contracted healthcare providers to comply with the pediatric immunization standards, and patient records are audited to ensure compliance.

The reported level of full immunization for children between 19 and 35 months of age in 2004 was 81%. Full immunization was defined as four doses of DTP/DT/DTaP, three doses of poliovirus vaccine, one measles-containing vaccine, three doses of Hib vaccine, and three doses of hepatitis B vaccine. National coverage of varicella vaccine was 87.5% and for three or more doses of pneumococcal (PCV7) was 73.2% (Centers for Disease Control, 2005c). Adolescents are now a group to target for immunization with the new recommended vaccines for this age group, such as MCV4, HPV, second dose of varicella, and hepatitis A and B if not previously immunized.

Immunization of Immigrants

Children less than 10 years of age who are internationally adopted are not required to have proof of immunizations prior to entry into the United States; however, adoptive parents are required to indicate their intent to have the child become fully immunized (American Academy of Pediatrics, 2006, p. 183). For other child immigrants, such as refugees, vaccines should be administered according to a catch-up schedule when no written record of immunizations is available or there is doubt about the potency of vaccines given. Alternatively, antibody titers can be measured for the various vaccines to determine the child's need for additional immunizations (American Academy of Pediatrics, 2006, p. 36). Many vaccines on the United States recommended schedule may not be available in countries of the child's origin.

Challenges in Achieving Optimal Immunization Rates

Lower immunization rates of children are often associated with economic factors, limited access to health care, lack of healthcare services at hours convenient for working parents, inadequate education regarding the importance of immunization, and religious prohibitions. The federal Vaccine for Children program provides free vaccines for qualified children and adolescents less than 19 years of age and has resolved some of the economic factors associated with vaccine coverage.

An increasing number of parents are choosing not to immunize their children for philosophical reasons. Some of these reasons include the following (Benin, Wisler-Scher, Colson et al., 2006):

- Concerns that too many vaccines are dangerous and they can harm their child.
- Belief that vaccines do not work—even some vaccinated children get the infectious disease, so the vaccines are not completely protective.

LAW & ETHICS

Vaccines for Children Program

The Vaccines for Children program was established in 1994 through the amendment of the Social Security Act by Section 1928. This program provides immunizations to children who are uninsured, Medicaid recipients, Native Americans, and Alaska Natives in their physician's office. This program also helps children whose insurance does not cover vaccination when they receive their immunizations in a federally qualified health center or rural health clinic. The Vaccines for Children program also makes sure that eligible children are able to receive newly recommended vaccines to improve immunization rates (Centers for Disease Control, 2004).

- Disagreement with government regulation and monitoring of immunizations.
- Belief that their child is not at risk because the disease threat is low due to so many other children being immunized.
- Realization that the number of adverse events to vaccines now exceeds the number of cases of vaccine preventable diseases, and the public has increased access to this information.
- Belief that they can control their child's susceptibility to disease and the outcome if they become infected.
- Belief that it is better to get the disease to develop immunity.

All healthcare providers should be consistent in their message about the value of vaccines and provide parents with an opportunity to have their questions answered prior to giving consent for immunization. It is important to understand that parents want to protect their child from diseases or from the potential harm of the vaccines. A trusting relationship between the healthcare provider and the parents is also an important factor in obtaining consent for immunizations (Benin, Wisler-Scher, Colson et al., 2006). See Families Want to Know: Vaccine Safety.

MediaLink

Frequently Asked Questions About Immunizations

NURSING MANAGEMENT
Nursing Assessment and Diagnosis

Inquire about the health status of the child or adolescent and identify any contraindications to giving the needed immunizations. Questions to ask parents include the following (Immunization Action Coalition, 2005):

- Is the child sick today?
- Does the child have allergies to medications, food, or any vaccine?
- Has the child had a serious reaction to a vaccine in the past?
- Has the child had a seizure or brain problem?
- Does the child have cancer, leukemia, AIDS, or another immune system problem?
- Has the child taken cortisone, prednisone, or other steroids, or anticancer drugs, or had radiograph treatments in the past 3 months?
- Has the child received a transfusion of blood or blood products or been given a medicine called immune (gamma) globulin in the past year?
- Is the child/teen pregnant or is there a chance she could become pregnant during the next month?
- Has the child received vaccines in the past 4 months?

Contraindications may include an acute illness with high fever, hypersensitivity reaction to specific vaccine components, immune globulin therapy in the last 3 to 6 months, cancer treatment, and pregnancy (American Academy of Pediatrics, 2006, pp. 45–50). See the vaccine table for specific vaccine contraindications on pages 590–594.

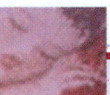

FAMILIES WANT TO KNOW

Vaccine Safety

Parents often have questions about vaccines if given the chance to ask. Potential explanations that can be given to parents in response to their questions include (Tenrreiro, 2005):

- Immunization is one of the most important ways you can protect your child. Vaccines stop diseases that children used to get. These diseases either killed children or made them very sick.
- If children were no longer immunized, the diseases would come back. If your child is not immunized, he or she could get very sick or die if he or she gets one of the diseases. Then your child could infect other children, who could get very sick or die.
- There are risks with every vaccine, but most risks are mild. Your child might have a fever, redness, or pain in the leg. Each vaccine can cause an allergic reaction or a seizure, but they are rare events.
- The safety of vaccines is improving with new information from research and new methods to make vaccines.
- Trustworthy information about immunizations can be found on the Internet.

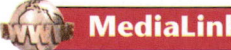

MediaLink

Vaccine Administration Record

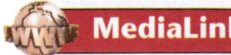

MediaLink

Vaccine Information Statement (VIS)

Nurses are responsible for reviewing a child's immunization record and determining whether the child needs immunization. Make sure you use the most current guidelines for comparison with the child's record as new vaccines may be approved or the schedule may be modified each year. If the child is behind in appropriate immunizations for age, determine the best combination of vaccines to give at this visit to better protect the child. Also take advantage of opportunities to give needed immunizations to siblings accompanying the family on the visit. A minor illness should not deter immunization.

Many missed opportunities to immunize children have been identified. To avoid missed opportunities in administering immunizations, be sure to evaluate the child's immunization record (as well as the record of siblings present) in all healthcare settings: on acute care units in the hospital, in the emergency department, in health clinics, and in school. To reduce the number of missed opportunities for full immunization of children, use the following guidelines (American Academy of Pediatrics, 2006):

- Reminders should be placed in the child's health record to remind healthcare providers of the child's need for immunizations.
- A call-back system should be established or reminders should be sent to parents about the child's need for immunizations when due or overdue.
- Immunizations can be given when the child has a minor illness with or without a low-grade fever, and with antibiotic treatment. Recent exposure to an infectious disease is not a reason to defer a vaccine.
- Several vaccines—diphtheria, tetanus, and acellular pertussis (DTaP); measles, mumps, and rubella (MMR); hepatitis B (HBV); *Haemophilus influenzae* type b (Hib); inactivated polio (IPV); varicella; and heptavalent pneumococcal vaccines—can be given at the same visit.
- Combination vaccines, such as Pediarix (combining DTaP, HepB, and IPV) can reduce the overall number of injections needed in the first 2 years from 20 to 14.
- Two injections can be given in different sites on the same extremity.
- Medically stable premature infants and low birth weight infants should receive the same immunizations as full-term infants starting at 2 months of age.
- Immunizations can be given even when there was a local reaction to a prior vaccine or a family member had an adverse response.

The accompanying Nursing Care Plan explores three potential nursing diagnoses that may apply to the child needing immunizations. Additional nursing diagnoses may include the following:

- Ineffective Airway Clearance related to an airway obstructed by swelling
- Risk for Impaired Skin Integrity related to vaccine response
- Ineffective Health Maintenance related to cultural beliefs regarding routine immunization

Planning and Implementation

Nurses should be strong advocates for immunization. Being well informed about immunizations, their potential side effects, and recommended schedules assists immunization efforts.

Family Education and Informed Consent

Federal legislation requires consent to be obtained before administering a vaccine. In most healthcare settings, the nurse is responsible for informing the parents or the child's legal guardian, supplying literature, and obtaining written consent before the vaccine is administered. It is also the nurse's responsibility to make sure that the most current Vaccine Information Statement (VIS) is provided to the parents about the vaccines to be administered. When teaching about immunizations, make sure that the parents understand the information in the VIS and answer any questions the parents might have. Identify the vaccines due to be given at this visit and on the next visit so that the parents know their child's immunization status. It may save time to give parents the VIS for the next vaccines to take home and review prior to the next visit.

Discuss vaccine risks and benefits with parents. They have often heard sensational stories about the consequences of vaccines, so correct information is needed to help them make informed decisions. For example, studies have repeatedly failed to find a relationship between the measles-mumps-rubella vaccine and the development of autism (DeStefano, Bhasin, Thompson et al., 2004; Smeeth, Cook, Fombonne et al., 2004). Other studies have not revealed a relationship between vaccines and disorders such as asthma (Destefano, Gu, Kramarz et al. 2002), inflammatory bowel disease

NURSING CARE PLAN The Child Needing Immunizations

GOAL	INTERVENTION	RATIONALE	EXPECTED OUTCOME
1. Risk for Infection related to inadequate acquired immunity			
	NIC Priority Intervention: **Immunization/Vaccination Management:** *Monitoring immunization status, facilitating access to immunizations, and provision of immunizations to prevent communicable disease.*		*NOC Suggested Outcome:* **Immune Status:** *Adequacy of natural and acquired appropriately targeted resistance to internal and external antigens.*
The child will become adequately protected from disease-preventable illnesses.	• Review the child's immunization record for needed vaccines at each healthcare visit.	• Assessment identifies the children who have missed needed immunizations.	The child is adequately protected from vaccine-preventable illnesses.
	• Identify all due vaccines that can be provided simultaneously.	• Many vaccines can be given at the same visit to more adequately protect the child. This also saves healthcare trips for families.	
	• Identify potential contraindications to needed vaccines. Review past reactions to vaccines.	• Reduces the risk for the child and other caretakers to have adverse reactions to vaccines.	
2. Effective Therapeutic Regiment Management			
	NIC Priority Interventions: **Decision-Making Support:** *Providing information and support for a patient who is making a decision regarding health care.*		*NOC Suggested Outcome:* **Knowledge Treatment: Regimen:** *Extent of understanding conveyed about a specific treatment regimen.*
Parents will sign consent for vaccines to be given.	• Educate the parents about the need for specific vaccines and the risk if not given. Provide Vaccine Information Statements. Obtain signed consent before giving vaccines.	• Informed consent is required for all treatments.	The parent(s) complete(s) the consent form, which is placed in the child's file.
	• Review past reactions to vaccines and describe common potential reactions and why they occur.	• Parents should expect common reactions and know they indicate the child's body is building protection to the illness.	
Parents will state the side effects of vaccines given.	• Describe serious side effects that should be reported to the healthcare provider.	• Parents need to be prepared for potential serious side effects so they can obtain care.	Parents report all serious side effects to the healthcare provider.
Parents will manage common side effects of vaccines.	• Teach parents general comfort measures for children's common side effects; for example: • Cool pack to tender legs • Acetaminophen for fever and discomfort • Rocking and holding the infant • Gentle movement of affected extremity	• Parents will know how to make the child more comfortable during the 24–48 hours after the vaccines are given.	The child is given comfort measures after vaccine administration.

(continued)

NURSING CARE PLAN The Child Needing Immunizations (continued)

GOAL	INTERVENTION	RATIONALE	EXPECTED OUTCOME
3. Risk for Injury related to vaccine reaction			
	NIC Priority Intervention: **Risk Identification:** *Analysis of potential risk factors, determining health risks, and prioritization of risk reduction strategies for an individual or group.*		*NOC Suggested Outcome:* **Risk Control:** *Actions to eliminate or reduce actual, personal, and modifiable health threats.*
The child's potential vaccine reactions will be safely managed.	• Prepare for life-threatening reactions by having resuscitation drugs and equipment immediately available.	• Anaphylactic reactions must be managed quickly and effectively.	The child has no reaction or has a severe reaction to a vaccine that is managed effectively.
	• Monitor the child for 15 minutes after the vaccines are given before letting the child go home.	• A life-threatening response will usually become apparent within this time frame.	
	• Assess the child for extreme anxiety and injection fearfulness.	• These are potential signs the child may have a vasovagal response to the injection.	
	• Have the fearful child or adolescent sit or lie down until symptoms of vasovagal response have disappeared.	• The child who faints may sustain a head injury.	
	• Report all serious vaccine-related reactions to the appropriate agency using the standard form.	• This is a legal requirement for all healthcare providers.	

CLINICAL TIP

Select the correct needle length for intramuscular injections for infants so that medication does not get into the subcutaneous tissue. When the medication reaches the muscle mass, local reactions to immunizations are reduced. A needle 5/8-inch long can be used in term infants for injections in the anterolateral thigh. Between 2 and 12 months of age, use a needle 1-inch long. For toddlers and children, the needle should be 1- to 1¼-inch long for the anterolateral thigh site (American Academy of Pediatrics, 2006, p. 20).

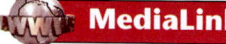

MediaLink

Immunization Refusal Form

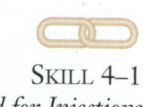

SKILL 4–1
Positioning a Child for Injections

(Taylor, Miller, Lingram et al., 2002), Sudden Infant Death Syndrome (Institute of Medicine, 2003), and type 1 diabetes (Hviid, Stellfeld, Wohlfahrt, & Melbye, 2004).

The nurse is required to record the (1) month, day, and year of administration; (2) vaccine given; (3) manufacturer; (4) lot number and expiration date of the immunization given; (5) site and route of administration; and (6) name, title, and address of the person who administers the vaccine. Obtain written consent to give the needed vaccines on the healthcare facility's standardized form from the parent or guardian. Provide parents with a record of the child's immunizations, and record the vaccines given in the healthcare agency's official records.

Parents have the right to refuse immunizations, but if there is a disease outbreak, the nonimmunized child must be kept out of childcare or school. If the parent chooses not to have the child receive a particular vaccine, document an informed refusal. A form for documentation of informed refusal is available online.

Provide guidelines for managing expected mild reactions at home. Make sure parents have the correct dosage information for the acetaminophen or ibuprofen formulation that is in the home. Schedule the child's next appointment for a health supervision visit to complete needed immunizations for age. See Families Want to Know: Care of the Child After Immunizations.

Reducing Pain and Anxiety

Prepare the parent to help reduce the anxiety and pain of the immunizations. Show the parent how to hold the child still or use an assistant to hold the child. Let them know it is okay to be anxious, but have them try to stay calm for the child. Some techniques that may reduce pain and anxiety associated with injections include the following:

• Coach the parent to hold and talk with the child during the injections.
• Give infants up to 2 months of age 25% sucrose water to suck (mix 1 packet of sugar in 10 mL of tap water) immediately before the injection. Sucrose water has been demonstrated to reduce pain in newborns. See Chapter 15 ∞.

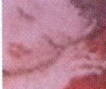

FAMILIES WANT TO KNOW

Care of the Child After Immunizations

After your child receives an immunization, observe for any reactions that might occur (Schuval, 2003).

- Check the injection site. Local pain, redness and swelling are common. Ice can be put on the site to help reduce swelling and pain. Acetaminophen or ibuprofen may be given to reduce a fever and pain. The symptoms disappear in a day or two.
- The child may have a fever, joint pain, muscle aches, or fatigue within hours to days after the vaccine is given. Give acetaminophen or ibuprofen for pain, and call your healthcare provider if you are concerned about the symptoms.

- If your child has a mild allergic reaction to the vaccine, you might notice a few hives around the injection site.
- A severe allergic reaction is indicated by a flushed face; swelling of the face, mouth, or throat; wheezing or other difficulty breathing; or shock (confusion, lack of movement or response, or unconsciousness). If these symptoms occur, call 9-1-1 or your emergency number so your child can be taken to the emergency department for treatment. While waiting for the ambulance to arrive, lie the child down on his or her back and raise the legs to promote blood return to the vital organs.

- Apply pressure at the site for 10 seconds before the injection.
- Instruct parents how to apply EMLA cream to the site for an hour before the injection.
- Use vapocoolant spray immediately before the injection.
- Give two injections simultaneously in different extremities using two different providers.
- Use age-appropriate distraction techniques. See Chapter 15 ∞.
- Encourage the parent of an infant to comfort the child after the injection.

Give the appropriate immunizations to the child as efficiently as possible, while providing support to the child (Figure 18–5 ➤). Nurses should make efforts to reduce the pain associated with vaccine injections, especially since infants and children must return for more injections in the future. Reducing pain will also lessen the anxiety associated with future visits for health care. See Evidence-Based Practice: Nursing Care During Immunizations.

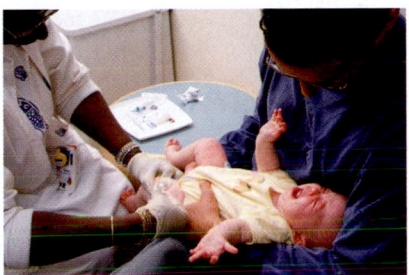

Figure 18–5 ➤ Give immunizations quickly and efficiently. Do not prolong the wait and let fear grow. The child will be anxious, especially if more than one injection must be given.

EVIDENCE-BASED PRACTICE

Nursing Care During Immunizations

Clinical Question

How can nurses reduce the pain and anxiety associated with injections?

Evidence

A study about the use of distraction to reduce the distress of immunizations was conducted with 90 infants ages 2 months to 3 years in a rural health department. Nurses performing injections were trained in the use of appropriate behaviors and distraction techniques (an age-appropriate toy and a popular cartoon movie) to use with the study children. Infants and children in the control group could be provided with comfort, reassurance, and empathy, but no toy or movie. Interactions were videotaped and scored by researchers. Infants in the distraction group displayed less distress than the control group. In many cases the parents helped supplement the distraction provided by the nurse (Cohen, 2002). Another study explored methods to reduce the pain stress associated with four immunization injections provided to 116 infants between 6 and 16 weeks of age. The intervention group received a bottle with 10 mL of 25% sucrose 2 minutes before the injections. They were then allowed to suck on a pacifier or bottle of formula throughout the injections and afterwards. Parents were asked to hold the infants on their lap with their upper bodies close to the parent, making the legs available for injection. The control group received immu-

nizations on the examining table with no specific comfort measures provided. Infants in the intervention group cried less, and parents expressed the desire for the same procedure to be used in future visits (Reis, Roth, Syphan et al., 2003).

Implications

Infants and young children often receive several injections for immunizations at health promotion visits. This makes parents distressed by the number of injections and associated pain. Nurses can use simple comfort measures and distraction to reduce the pain and distress associated with immunizations. By assembling a toolkit of distraction devices for infants and children of various ages, the nurse can be quickly prepared to provide age-appropriate distraction. Sucrose solution can be prepared in advance, anticipating the number of young infants that will need immunizations in a morning or afternoon. Nurses can also provide guidance to parents about how they can hold and comfort the infant during the injections.

Critical Thinking

Identify the different methods nurses use for comforting infants receiving immunizations in a busy clinical setting. Compare the effectiveness of those methods with distraction and sucrose solution to help you identify your future nursing care interventions for immunizations.

CLINICAL TIP

Store vaccines properly in the refrigerator or freezer to ensure the vaccine's potency. Read the package inserts of vaccines to determine proper storage conditions. Refrigerators should have separate doors for the refrigerator and freezer units. Check the temperature of each unit twice daily and record the temperatures on a log to make sure a consistent temperature range is maintained (refrigerator at 35° to 46°F (2° to 8°C) and freezer at 5°F (−15°C) or lower). Jugs of water in the refrigerator and trays of ice in the freezer help maintain a consistent temperature in the units. Store the vaccines in the middle of the units, placing the older vaccines in the front. Make sure the facility has an emergency plan for safe storage of vaccines in case of a power outage or natural disaster.

Maintaining Vaccine Potency

Assure the effectiveness of the vaccines administered. An improperly stored or poorly administered vaccine may be rendered ineffective, thus preventing the child from developing immunity.

Check the expiration of vaccines prior to use. When reconstituting vaccines, it is important to use the solution provided and follow the manufacturer's directions. Write the date and time on the bottle if it is a multidose vial. Some reconstituted vaccines (varicella and MMR) have a short shelf life and are available only in single-dose vials. See vaccine-specific information in the medication table on pages 590–594.

Evaluation

Expected nursing outcomes include the following:

- Parents are fully informed and give consent for immunizations.
- All age-appropriate immunizations are provided for the child at each health visit or catch-up immunizations are provided as needed.
- The parents are prepared to manage mild reactions to immunizations at home.
- Parents are able to identify and report serious reactions to immunizations.

INFECTIOUS AND COMMUNICABLE DISEASES IN INFANTS AND CHILDREN

Infectious and communicable diseases cause acute illnesses. These diseases are caused by bacterial, viral, protozoan, or fungal organisms. As noted earlier, infants and children develop infectious and communicable diseases more frequently than adults do. Active immunity to microorganisms does not occur until there is natural exposure or immunization that leads to the development of antibodies. Therefore, infants and children are more susceptible to the large number of infectious organisms to which they have no resistance.

Epidemiology and Pathophysiology

Microorganisms (bacterial, viral, fungal, and protozoan) use the human body to reproduce. Many microorganisms are pathogens that cause infectious and communicable diseases. They enter the body through direct contact with mucous membranes and injured skin, inhalation, and ingestion. Biting insects or animals (vectors) also inject organisms into the skin and blood. The microorganisms spread through the lymph and blood to other tissues and organs where they multiply. The initial response of the body to invasion by bacteria is inflammation. Endotoxins increase capillary permeability and trigger fever.

When antibodies have developed to a specific microorganism to which the child is exposed, they protect the child by

- Preventing bacterial toxins from binding with the tissues
- Preventing the initial attachment and entrance of viruses into the cells
- Producing a substance (opsonin) that makes the bacterial outer capsule susceptible to **phagocytosis** (the engulfment and destruction of microorganisms, dead cells, and foreign particles), and
- Activating the inflammatory response when a microorganism succeeds in invading the body through its defenses.

Antimicrobials also prevent the growth of or destroy microorganisms that have not developed antibiotic resistance. See Chapter 17 ∞ for more information about the inflammatory and immune response.

Viruses are the most common cause of infections in humans. They are parasitic organisms that invade the cells and take them over for their own survival and reproduction. As they reproduce cell to cell, eventually the body's immune response to the virus overwhelms it and the infection is cured. In some cases the virus reproduces at such a slow rate that the infected person is asymptomatic and becomes a carrier of the virus. Secondary bacterial infection can occur in virus-damaged cells. See Chapter 17 ∞ for more information about the immune response and viral infections such as HIV.

Fever

Fever is an increased body temperature of 38°C (100.4°F) taken by the rectal or tympanic route or 37.8°C (100°F) by the oral route. In response to an infection, **endogenous pyrogens** (interleukins, interferons, and tumor necrosis factor) are released by macrophages in response to an invasive infectious organism. These pyrogens travel through the circulatory system to the hypothalamus, the control center for the regulation of body temperature. In the hypothalamus, the pyrogens trigger the production of prostaglandins that are believed to raise the body's thermoregulatory set-point, thus causing the fever to occur (Crocetti & Serwint, 2005). See Figure 18–6 ➤.

A rise in the hypothalamus's set-point leads to a cold response with shivering and chills, vasoconstriction, and decreased peripheral perfusion. Heat loss from the body is reduced and the body temperature rises to the new temperature set-point. When the temperature is elevated, the heart rate increases. One degree of temperature elevation causes an increase in respiratory rate by four breaths per minute and increases the metabolic need for oxygen by 7%. Vasodilation occurs and the skin flushes, becoming warm to the touch.

Infectious and communicable diseases differ in their epidemiology, transmission, and incubation period. Many infectious diseases are communicable between humans, but many are vaccine-preventable. The epidemiology, clinical manifestations, treatment, prevention, and nursing care of selected infectious and communicable diseases of childhood are detailed in the Clinical Manifestations table that follows and Table 18–2. Some infectious diseases are transmitted by insects or animals (**zoonosis**) and are not communicable from person to person. See Table 18–3. See Chapter 30 for information about impetigo, scabies, and lice. See Chapter 19 for information about conjunctivitis. See Chapter 25 for information on sexually transmitted infections.

PATHOPHYSIOLOGY ILLUSTRATED

Fever

Figure 18–6 ➤ The hypothalamus functions as the body's thermostat, directing the body to conserve or dissipate heat. When microorganisms invade the body, endogenous pyrogens are released into the bloodstream. These substances travel to the hypothalamus, where they trigger the production and release of prostaglandins, which initiate the fever response. Blood is diverted from the extremities to more central vessels. This helps increase the core body temperature by decreasing heat loss. Shivering increases both metabolic action and heat production. The hypothalamus then maintains the temperature at the new set-point.

CLINICAL MANIFESTATIONS | INFECTION IN INFANTS AND CHILDREN BY AGE GROUP

System	Infants	Children
Central nervous system	Irritable Decreased responsiveness Lethargy Bulging anterior fontanel High-pitched cry Muscle weakness *Additional Signs in Newborns:* Seizures Subtle changes in muscle tone or hypotonia	Irritable or combative Stiff neck Back pain Decreased responsiveness Photophobia Brudzinski sign Kernig sign Malaise
Cardiovascular	Tachycardia Decreased perfusion Weak peripheral pulses Pallor or mottled skin Flushed, dry skin Delayed capillary refill time *Additional Signs in Newborns:* Cyanosis Hypotension Bradycardia	Tachycardia Decreased perfusion Weak peripheral pulses Pallor or flushed, dry skin Delayed capillary refill time
Respiratory	Tachypnea Increased work of breathing with retractions, nasal flaring Crackles Cough Stridor Decreased oxygen saturation Irregular breathing *Additional Signs in Newborns:* Apnea (new onset or increased episodes) Increased or new-onset oxygen requirement Grunting	Tachypnea Dyspnea Retractions Nasal flaring Crackles Cough Stridor Decreased oxygen saturation
Gastrointestinal	Vomiting Diarrhea Abdominal distention Poor feeding *Additional Signs in Newborns:* Abdominal wall discoloration Paralytic ileus Bloody stool Jaundice or hepatosplenomegaly	Nausea and vomiting Diarrhea Abdominal discomfort Abdominal distention Poor appetite
Renal	WBCs and bacteria in urine *Additional Signs in Newborns:* Decreased urine output Hematuria, proteinuria	WBCs and bacteria in urine
Hematopoietic (see Appendix C ∞ for expected laboratory values by age)	Neutropenia Increased immature WBCs (bands) in bacterial infections Lymphocytosis in viral infections *Additional Signs in Newborns:* Fraction of band cells > 0.2 Thrombocytopenia	Leukocytosis Increased immature WBCs (bands) in bacterial infections Lymphocytosis in viral infections
Metabolic	Hyperthermia or hypothermia Hypoglycemia or hyperglycemia	Hyperthermia Chills Hypothermic in septic shock
Other	Rash Dry mucous membranes Poor skin turgor Sunken anterior fontanel Petechiae and/or purpura	Rash Petechiae and/or purpura Dry mucous membranes Poor skin turgor

Table 18–2	SELECTED INFECTIOUS AND COMMUNICABLE DISEASES IN CHILDREN

Disease	Clinical Manifestations	Clinical Therapy	Nursing Management
Chickenpox (Varicella)*+ *Causal agent*: Varicella-zoster, human herpesvirus 3. *Epidemiology*: Humans are the source of infection. Peak occurrence is in the late fall, winter, and spring. Maternal antibodies disappear 2–3 months after birth. *Transmission*: Direct contact of the virus to the mucous membranes or conjunctiva primarily through airborne spread of secretions and occasionally with lesion contact. *Incubation period*: 14–21 days. *Period of communicability*: Most contagious 1 to 2 days before the rash to shortly after onset of rash. Contagious state continues until all lesions are crusted over. This period may be prolonged after passive immunization or in immunodeficient children.	Acute onset of mild fever, malaise, anorexia, headache, mild abdominal pain, and irritability occurs before and with eruption. The rash begins as a macule on an erythematous base and progresses to a papule, then to a clear, fluid-filled vesicle. The rash may erupt for 1–5 days and is itchy. Up to 250 to 500 lesions of all stages may be present at any one time. Crusts may remain for 1–3 weeks. The lesions begin on the trunk, scalp, and face, and then spread to the rest of the body. Ulcerative lesions may be seen in the mucous membranes. Lesions in the mouth may lead to decreased fluid intake and dehydration. *Complications*: Complications are rare but can include secondary infection (cellulitis, local abscesses, sepsis, meningitis, encephalitis, pneumonia), thrombocytopenia, and Reye's syndrome. Chickenpox can be fatal in newborns of infected mothers and immunocompromised children. Children undergoing chemotherapy, steroid treatment, or transplant therapy should be carefully monitored after exposure to the disease.	Fluid from vesicle or scab can be tested using polymerase chain reaction for diagnosis. Medical management is supportive. Oral and IV acyclovir is used within 24 hours (oral or IV) for immunocompromised patients, children treated with chronic salicylate therapy, and oral or aerosol corticosteroids. Acyclovir is not recommended for healthy children with uncomplicated chickenpox (American Academy of Pediatrics, 2006). Varicella-zoster immune globulin or immune globulin IV is given as soon as possible to newborns of infected mothers and exposed immunocompromised, unimmunized children up to 4 days after exposure. *Prognosis*: Most children recover fully. Children who are immunocompromised or who were treated with corticosteroids during the incubation period must be treated aggressively. *Prevention*: Varicella is vaccine preventable. See the medication table on page 594. Between 1995 and 2004, the rate of disease decreased by 85% (American Academy of Pediatrics, 2006). The vaccine may be given within 72 hours after exposure to prevent or significantly modify the disease. Wild virus cases occur in vaccinated children.	• Use airborne and contact precautions while children are contagious. • Upon admission to the hospital, inquire about Varicella immunization or recent exposure. Place all exposed children in isolation to protect newborns and immunocompromised patients. • Nurses caring for the exposed or infected child should have documented immunity. • When treated at home, isolate the child from all susceptible individuals, especially medically fragile and immunocompromised children or adults, and women early in pregnancy. Notify the school or childcare facility of the child's illness. • Secondary cases are often more severe than the primary case. • The child with eczema or sunburn may have a more severe rash. • Give nonaspirin antipyretics to control fever. • Give oral antihistamines for relief of itching. Oatmeal and Aveeno baths are soothing. Caladryl lotion applied to lesions may also provide relief. • Keep the child's fingernails short and clean. Young children may need to wear soft cotton mittens when itching cannot be controlled. • Change bed linens frequently. Wash linen in mild soap and rinse well. • Reassure the child that the lesions are temporary and will go away. • Observe the child closely for symptoms of complications such as drowsiness, meningeal signs, respiratory distress, and dehydration. Disorientation and restlessness may indicate viral encephalitis. • Monitor for acyclovir side effects: nausea, vomiting, diarrhea, abdominal pain, as well as allergic skin reactions or headache. Monitor renal function if the child has renal insufficiency.

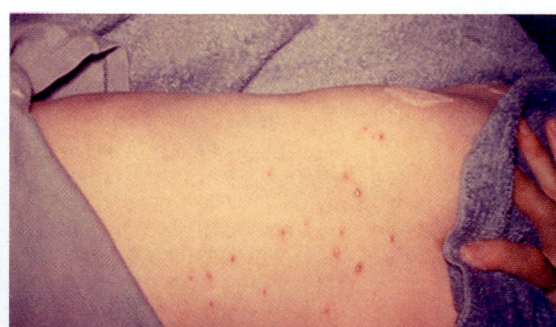

Skin lesions of chickenpox. CDC

*Indicates that a vaccine or antitoxin is available for use in high-risk or as-needed situations.
+Indicates that the disease has a safe and effective vaccine.

(continued)

Table 18–2	SELECTED INFECTIOUS AND COMMUNICABLE DISEASES IN CHILDREN (continued)		
Disease	**Clinical Manifestations**	**Clinical Therapy**	**Nursing Management**
Coxsackievirus *Causal Agent*: Coxsackievirus A16 and Enterovirus 71. *Epidemiology*: Occurs worldwide, most commonly in summer and early fall. Sporadic outbreaks are seen, especially among children in out-of-home settings. Immunity probably occurs after clinical or subclinical infection, but duration of the immunity is unknown. *Transmission*: Fecal-oral and respiratory routes. *Incubation period*: 3–6 days. *Period of communicability*: 2 days before rash to 2 days after it disappears.	Each of the coxsackieviruses causes a different set of manifestations. Herpangina is an acute, self-limiting viral disease characterized by the sudden onset of fever, sore throat, and small, discrete grayish papulovesicular ulcerative pharyngeal lesions that gradually increase in size. In hand, foot, and mouth disease, the lesions are more diffuse and may occur on the buccal surfaces of the cheeks, gums, and sides of the tongue. Papulovesicular lesions occur on the hands and feet and last for 7–10 days. Children may be irritable and have a fever, anorexia, dysphagia, malaise, and a sore throat. *Complications*: Children with immune deficiencies may have persistent central nervous system infections for several months (American Academy of Pediatrics, 2006).	Diagnostic tests include a cell culture to detect the virus. Medical care is supportive. Immune globulin IV may be used in life-threatening neonatal infections and in immunodeficient children with chronic meningoencephalitis (American Academy of Pediatrics, 2006). *Prognosis*: Recovery is generally good with supportive care. *Prevention*: Avoid contact with infected persons early in the disease.	• Isolate the child while contagious. Use standard contact precautions if the child is hospitalized. • Use good hand hygiene. • Apply topical lotions and give systemic medications as ordered to lessen the pain and relieve the irritation. • Offer cool drinks and soft, bland foods (no citrus, salty, or spicy foods). Swallowing may be painful. • Offer warm saline mouth rinses. • Observe for dehydration. • Provide reassurance and support to parents. • Give nonaspirin antipyretics for fever. Keep the child out of school or childcare while the child is febrile.
*Diphtheria**[*+]* *Causal agent:* Corynebacterium diphtheriae. *Epidemiology:* Occurs mostly in colder months in unimmunized, partially immunized, and immunized children with waning immunity. Cases of cutaneous and wound diphtheria occur sporadically in the tropics. Maternal immunity lasts up to 6 months after birth. The disease is endemic in areas where immunization is no longer routine, such as Russia. *Transmission:* Contact with nasal or eye discharge, or skin lesion; or less commonly by indirect contact with contaminated items. Unpasteurized milk has served as a vehicle. *Incubation period:* 2–7 days or longer. *Period of communicability:* Usually 2–4 weeks or until 4 days after antibiotics are started.	Symptoms can be mild or severe with a gradual onset over 1–2 days. Low-grade fever, anorexia, malaise, rhinorrhea with a foul odor, cough, sore throat, hoarseness, stridor or noisy breathing, cervical lymphadenitis, and pharyngitis may be present. In more severe cases, the membranes of the tonsils, pharynx, and larynx are affected. The characteristic membranous lesion is a thick, bluish white to grayish black patch that covers the tonsils. It can spread to cover the soft and hard palates and the posterior portion of the pharynx. Attempts to remove the membrane result in bleeding. *Complications:* Produces an endotoxin that causes myocarditis and peripheral neuropathy (diplopia, slurred speech, difficulty swallowing, or paralysis of the palate) or ascending paralysis similar to Guillain-Barré syndrome.	Diagnostic tests include a culture from any mucosal or cutaneous lesion. Administration of IV antitoxin and antibiotics within 3 days of onset of symptoms. The child must be tested for sensitivity to horse serum before giving the antitoxin. When diphtheria is suspected, antibiotic therapy (penicillin G or erythromycin) should be initiated without waiting for laboratory results. Removal of membrane may be needed to treat airway obstruction. *Prognosis*: With treatment, prognosis is good. If untreated, death may occur due to airway obstruction. *Prevention*: Diphtheria is a vaccine-preventable disease. Booster doses are needed every 10 years after primary series. See the medication table on page 590. This is a reportable disease.	• Use droplet precautions for pharyngeal disease and contact precautions for cutaneous disease. • Monitor closely for signs of increasing respiratory distress, as well as cardiac and neurologic complications. Provide humidified oxygen as necessary. • Have emergency airway equipment available. • Administer antibiotics. Give no medications containing caffeine or other stimulants. • Use oral suction gently as necessary. • Allow children to use mouthwash if desired. Gargling is not permitted because it can irritate the pharyngeal surfaces. • Encourage liquids as tolerated. Intravenous fluids may be necessary. • Provide emotional support to the family. • Initiate the search for patient contacts to give antibiotics and immunization boosters.

Table 18–2	SELECTED INFECTIOUS AND COMMUNICABLE DISEASES IN CHILDREN (continued)		
Disease	**Clinical Manifestations**	**Clinical Therapy**	**Nursing Management**
Erythema Infectiosum (Fifth Disease) *Causal agent*: Human parvovirus B-19. *Epidemiology:* Occurs worldwide, most often in winter and spring. The disease also occurs in epidemics, with peak activity every 6 years. The incidence is highest in children between the ages of 5 and 14 years. *Transmission:* Respiratory secretions and blood. *Incubation period:* 6–21 days. *Period of communicability:* Believed to be the highest the week before symptom onset. 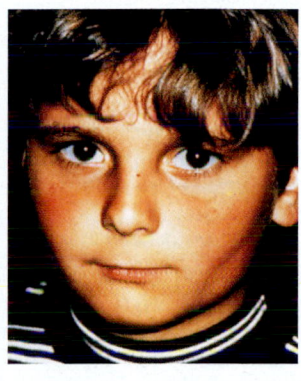 Characteristic facial rash of erythema infectiosum (fifth disease). Courtesy of Centers for Disease Control and Prevention, Atlanta, GA.	Stage 1 begins as a flu-like illness (headache, chills, malaise, nausea, body ache) lasting 2–3 days. A symptom-free period of 1 to 7 days follows. Stage 2 occurs 1 week later with a fiery-red rash on the cheeks giving a "slapped face" appearance. Circumoral pallor is seen. In 1 to 4 days a lace-like symmetric, erythematous, maculopapular rash appears on the trunk and limbs, spreading proximal to distal but sparing the palms and soles. Stage 3 lasts 1–3 weeks as the rash fades but can reappear if the skin is irritated or exposed to sunlight. The rash may be mildly pruritic. *Complications*: Children with hemolytic conditions may have transient aplastic crisis. Arthritis and arthralgia may occur.	Diagnosis is made by physical signs, or a serologic test for immunoglobulin (Ig) M parvovirus B-19-specific antibody. Medical treatment is supportive and recovery is usually spontaneous. Children with hemolytic conditions may need blood transfusions if an aplastic crisis occurs. Immunodeficient patients may develop a chronic infection for which IV immune globulin therapy is often effective (American Academy of Pediatrics, 2006). *Prognosis*: Fetal infection may occur, resulting in fetal hydrops or spontaneous abortion. *Prevention*: Avoid contact with infected persons.	• Children with aplastic crisis are often hospitalized. • Use standard and droplet precautions. Isolation is needed only for children with aplastic crisis or when immunosuppressed. • Nonaspirin antipyretics may be given to control fever. • Use soothing oatmeal or Aveeno baths if the rash is pruritic. Antipruritics may also help to relieve itching. • Encourage rest and offer frequent fluids. • Keep children out of direct sunlight if possible. Provide protective, light, loose clothing if exposure to sunlight cannot be avoided. • Provide quiet diversionary activity. There is no reason to keep the immune competent child out of school or day care once he or she is no longer infectious. • Explain the three stages of rash development to parents.
Haemophilus Influenzae, Type B[+] *Causal agent*: Coccobacilli *H. Influenzae* bacteria, which has several serotypes and can be encapusulated or nonencapsulated. *Epidemiology:* Occurs most often in the spring and summer. Most commonly affected are infants and young children in childcare centers. Low-birth-weight children and children with chronic illnesses have an increased susceptibility. *Transmission:* Direct contact or droplet inhalation. The organism is frequently asymptomatically colonized in the respiratory tract. *Incubation period*: Unknown. *Period of communicability*: 3 days from onset of symptoms.	Begins with a viral upper respiratory infection. The organism passes through the mucosal barrier to directly invade the bloodstream. It can cause several severe invasive illnesses, including meningitis, epiglottitis, pneumonia, septic arthritis, and cellulitis. It is also a cause of sepsis in infants. Other illnesses include sinusitis, otitis media, bronchitis, and pericarditis. Each disease has very specific clinical manifestations. Invasive disease has decreased 99% since the introduction of the vaccine (American Academy of Pediatrics, 2006). *Complications*: Illness caused by *H. influenzae* type B responds to antibiotic therapy. Left untreated, severe sequelae and death, especially in young infants, can occur from conditions such as meningitis, epiglottitis, sinusitis, pneumonitis, and cellulitis.	Diagnosis by culture of blood, cerebrospinal fluid, or middle ear aspirate. Treatment consists of antibiotic therapy. Rifampin may be given to unprotected household contacts (not pregnant women), if another child has not completed immunizations, within 1 week after diagnosis. *Prognosis:* With rapid diagnosis and treatment, recovery is good but highly dependent on the disease the organism has caused. When treatment is delayed, the prognosis for full recovery becomes much more guarded. *Prevention*: Immunization for *H. influenzae* type B. See the medication table on page 590.	• Use droplet precautions until 24 hours after the initiation of antibiotics. • Antibiotic therapy is administered intravenously for severe infections. Infections such as otitis media can be managed with oral antibiotics. • Unimmunized children under the age of 4 years are at increased risk for developing disease from *H. influenzae*. Specific prophylactic measures for susceptible children may be ordered by the physician. • Administer antipyretics to help the child feel more comfortable. • Closely monitor IV sites for patency and infiltration. • Perform nursing care measures specific to the illness. • Inform family members that rifampin turns urine and other body fluids orange, and it will cause stains.

For Hepatitis A, Hepatitis B, and Hepatitis C, see Chapter 24 ∞ .

(continued)

Table 18–2	SELECTED INFECTIOUS AND COMMUNICABLE DISEASES IN CHILDREN (continued)		
Disease	**Clinical Manifestations**	**Clinical Therapy**	**Nursing Management**
Influenza *Causal agent:* Orthomyxoviridae, types A and B. *Epidemiology:* Prevalent in the United States from October to March, but the virus is active in other parts of the world year-round. During annual epidemics, 10–40% of healthy children are infected, and 1% are hospitalized (American Academy of Pediatrics, 2006). *Transmission:* Spreads by aerosolized particles and direct contact with respiratory secretions. *Incubation period:* 1 to 4 days. *Period of communicability:* One day before symptoms until 5 days after onset of illness.	Abrupt onset of fever (38° to 40°C), chills, cough, runny nose, sore throat, malaise, aches, headache, and anorexia. Children may have nausea and vomiting, diarrhea, and abdominal pain. Children may also present with croup, bronchiolitis, conjunctivitis, or other nonspecific febrile illness. *Complications:* Otitis media, exacerbations of chronic lung conditions such as asthma and cystic fibrosis. Pneumonia, croup, bronchiolitis, and wheezing may occur in up to 25% of children. Myositis, myocarditis, encephalitis, transverse myelitis, Reye's syndrome, and Guillain-Barré syndrome are all potential complications.	Diagnostic tests may include viral culture, rapid antigen testing from throat or nasopharynx, polymerase chain reaction, and immunofluorescence. Treatment is supportive. Antiviral therapy (oseltamivir, and zanamivir) may be given to children 1 year of age or older at high risk of complications. Relenza is approved for children 5 years and older (Food and Drug Administration, 2006). Amantadine and rimantadine should not be used due to viral resistance (Centers for Disease Control, 2006c, pp. 2–3). Follow updated antiviral therapy guidelines on http://www.cdc.gov/flu. When antiviral medication is initiated within 2 days of symptoms, the duration of symptoms may be reduced by 1 to 1½ days. *Prevention:* Influenza vaccine is now recommended for infants and children over 6 months of age. See the medication table on page 592.	• Use droplet and contact precautions for hospitalized infants and children. • The child is usually cared for at home. Encourage parents to wash hands frequently and to reduce exposure of other family members to the infected child. • Provide fluids to keep nasal secretions moist and to prevent dehydration. • Provide acetaminophen or ibuprofen for fever management and mild pain. • If antiviral medications are given, be alert for nausea and vomiting. Zanamivir can exacerbate asthma. • Provide rest and quiet diversional activities. • Teach parents to be alert to signs of complications from the viral infection. • Nurses should be familiar with pandemic influenza plans for the local area and state (http://www.pandemicflu.gov)
Measles (Rubeola)*[+] *Causal agent:* Mobillivirus, a member of the paramyxovirus group. *Epidemiology:* Occurrence peaks in the late winter and early spring. In developed countries, measles occurs mostly in outbreaks among unimmunized children, or possibly those with declining immunity. Spreads by direct contact with droplets or by airborne route. Passive maternal immunity lasts until the infant is age 12–15 months. In developing countries, measles remains an endemic disease and is a significant cause of infant and child morbidity and mortality.	Children are quite ill in the 3–5 day prodromal phase, with symptoms including high fever, conjunctivitis, coryza, cough, anorexia, and malaise. Koplik's spots (small, irregular, bluish white spots on a red background) appear on the buccal mucosa about 2 days before and after the rash appears. The characteristic red, blotchy, maculopapular rash that becomes confluent usually appears 2–4 days after onset of prodromal phase. The rash begins on the face and spreads to the trunk and extremities. Symptoms gradually subside in 4–7 days. Other symptoms include anorexia, malaise, fatigue, and generalized lymphadenopathy.	Diagnosis can be made by a serologic test for immunoglobulin (Ig) M measles antibody. Treatment is supportive. No antiviral therapy is available. Antibiotics are used for secondary bacterial infections. *Prognosis:* Recovery is generally good with supportive care. *Prevention:* Measles is a vaccine-preventable disease. See the medication table on page 592. Immune globulin, administered up to 6 days after exposure, may be helpful in preventing the disease in susceptible persons (immunocompromised children, infants less than 1 year of age, pregnant women). All healthcare workers should have documented immunity.	• If the child is hospitalized, maintain airborne precautions during the contagious period. • Use a cool-mist vaporizer to help clear respiratory passages. • Suction nose and oral cavity very gently as necessary. • Give nonaspirin antipyretics for fever and antipruritics for itching. • Assess lungs carefully, especially in young children, in whom pneumonias are a common complication. • Antitussives may be ordered to control coughing. • Keep lights dim, and cover windows if the child has photophobia. • Elevate the head of the bed. Keep the room cool with good air circulation. Provide light, nonirritating blankets. • Keep skin clean and dry. No soaps should be used.

Table 18–2	SELECTED INFECTIOUS AND COMMUNICABLE DISEASES IN CHILDREN (continued)

Disease	Clinical Manifestations	Clinical Therapy	Nursing Management
Measles (Rubeola) *[+]—Cont.* *Transmission:* Airborne, respiratory droplets and contact with infected persons. *Incubation period:* About 8–12 days. *Period of communicability:* Begins 3–5 days before the rash until 4 days after the rash appears. 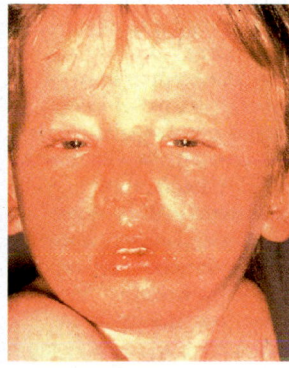 Measles facial rash, third day of rash. Courtesy of Centers for Disease Control and Prevention, Atlanta, GA.	*Complications:* Diarrhea, otitis media, pneumonia, bronchitis, laryngotracheobronchitis, encephalitis, and death. Complications and sequelae occur most often in children who are malnourished, medically fragile, and immunosuppressed. The younger the child, the greater the risk for complications.	This is a reportable disease. A total of 37 cases were reported in the United States in 2004, and many were imported from another country or secondary exposures to these infected children (Centers for Disease Control, 2005b).	• Maintain fluid intake. Offer cool liquids frequently in small amounts. Blended, pureed, and mashed foods are most easily tolerated. • Maintain bed rest. Visitors should be immune to measles. • Provide diversions such as music, stories, and favorite toys.
Meningococcus *Causal agent: Neisseria meningitides,* a gram-negative diplococcus. *Epidemiology:* Most often in winter or early spring. Spread by respiratory droplets from human carriers. Majority of infections in the United States are caused by serogroups B, C, and Y. Highest rates are in children under 2 years and in 11 years and older (Bilukha & Rosenstein, 2005). African Americans and persons of low socioeconomic status are at higher risk. Outbreaks have occurred in childcare centers, college dormitories, and military recruit camps. *Transmission:* Direct contact with droplet respiratory secretions. *Incubation period:* 1 to 10 days. *Period of communicability:* until 24 hours after antibiotic started.	Abrupt onset of flu-like symptoms of fever, chills, malaise, muscle aches, vomiting, and **prostration** (extreme exhaustion). Meningitis neurologic signs include drowsiness, disorientation, hallucinations, and convulsions. Meningococcemia: An urticarial, maculopapular, or petechial rash also appears that may progress to purpura. The condition may further deteriorate to shock, hypotension, disseminated intravascular coagulation, and coma. *Complications:* Loss of digits or limbs due to necrosis, hearing loss, arthritis, myocarditis, pericarditis, ataxia, seizures, hemiparesis, cranial nerve palsies, and obstructive hydrocephalus. Up to 10% of children and 25% of adolescents with invasive meningococcal disease die (American Academy of Pediatrics, 2006).	Diagnostic tests include cultures of the blood and cerebrospinal fluid culture. A Gram stain of petechial skin scrapings may also be done. *Treatment:* Penicillin G is given IV (cefotaxime, ceftriaxone, and ampicillin are alternate antibiotics). Chloramphenicol is used for children allergic to penicillin. The child is managed aggressively in the intensive care unit to maintain the airway, assist ventilation, and manage shock with IV fluids and vasopressers. Plasma, blood, or platelets are used to treat the disseminated intravascular coagulation. *Prevention:* A vaccine has been approved for adolescents 11 years and older. A vaccine is available for children over 2 years old with asplenia and other high-risk conditions. See the medication tables on pages 593 and 598. Close contacts are given medication (rifampin, ceftriaxone, or ciprofloxacin) for prophylaxis. Health professionals exposed to oral secretions need prophylaxis (American Academy of Pediatrics, 2006). This is a reportable disease.	• The child will be hospitalized. Use standard precautions and droplet precautions until the antibiotic has been administered for 24 hours. • Disease onset is abrupt and rapidly progresses to life threatening. Be alert for development of shock and respiratory compromise. Have emergency equipment available and be prepared to perform resuscitation. • When giving IV fluids and blood products, make sure the child does not get overloaded with fluids, and monitor for evidence of increased intracranial pressure. • Keep the family informed of the child's status and treatment as the disease progresses. Help the family to mobilize its support system. • The surviving child will likely need rehabilitation. Work with the social worker or case manager to transition the child to long-term care. • Help identify close contacts that should receive prophylactic antibiotics and educate them about the expected side effects (i.e., orange urine with rifampin). • Teach close contacts to be observant for signs of illness and to seek health care promptly if they occur.

(continued)

Table 18–2	SELECTED INFECTIOUS AND COMMUNICABLE DISEASES IN CHILDREN (continued)		
Disease	**Clinical Manifestations**	**Clinical Therapy**	**Nursing Management**
Mononucleosis *Causal agent*: Epstein-Barr virus (EBV), a member of the herpesvirus group. *Epidemiology*: Occurs worldwide in no seasonal pattern. Infection commonly occurs early in life, and spread among family members is common. *Transmission*: Direct contact with infected oropharyngeal and genital tract secretions. EBV can survive in saliva for several hours outside the body. EBV can also be transmitted by blood transfusion. *Incubation period*: estimated to be 30–50 days. *Period of communicability*: Indeterminate, asymptomatic carriage is common (American Academy of Pediatrics, 2006).	In very young children, mononucleosis may cause irritability, but be otherwise asymptomatic. A maculopapular rash may be seen in a few cases. In other children, the disease is characterized by malaise, headache, anorexia, abdominal pain, fatigue, and fever for 2–3 days, followed by lymphadenopathy and a sore throat. Hepatosplenomegaly may occur. Pain from swelling of the tonsils and lymph nodes may be significant. The syndrome typically lasts 2–3 weeks and is self-limited. Weakness and lethargy may continue for several months. *Complications*: Rare side effects include central nervous system symptoms such as encephalitis, aseptic meningitis, and Guillain-Barré syndrome. Splenic rupture, respiratory failure, and hematologic complications such as thrombocytopenia can also occur. In immunodeficient children, fatal infections or lymphomas can develop.	Diagnostic tests include the serologic monospot test or a heterophil antibody response test. Greater than 10% atypical lymphocytes and a positive heterophil antibody response test are diagnostic (American Academy of Pediatrics, 2006). Treatment is supportive. Corticosteroids may be used to control tonsillar swelling and pain when there is impending airway obstruction, massive splenomegaly, myocarditis, or hemolytic anemia. Ampicillin and amoxicillin should be avoided as a nonallergic rash often develops (American Academy of Pediatrics, 2006). *Prognosis*: After recovery, the virus remains latent in the lymphoid system. It can be reactivated during periods of immunosuppression. *Prevention*: No known prevention.	• Children are usually treated at home. Standard precautions should be used. • Give antipyretics and analgesics for fever and sore throat. Offer warm salt water for gargling. Offer soft foods and encourage fluids. • Maintain bed rest during acute phase. • Give adolescents a sense of responsibility by involving them in decisions about care whenever possible. Be sure to include parents and adolescents in discussions. • Reassure adolescents who may be worried about keeping up with schoolwork that they can return to school when the fever is gone and swallowing is normal. • Teens should avoid kissing until the fever has been gone several days. • Contact sports should be avoided until the liver and spleen are normal, usually in about 4 weeks. • If splenomegaly is present, alcohol should be avoided for 3 months after liver function test results return to normal.
Mumps (Parotitis) + *Causal agent:* Rubulavirus in the paramyxoviridae family. *Epidemiology:* Occurs worldwide in unvaccinated children, most often in winter and spring. Infection and vaccination induce lifelong immunity. Maternal antibodies begin to disappear in infants at the age of 12–15 months. *Transmission:* Contact with respiratory tract secretions. *Incubation period:* 12–25 days. *Period of communicability:* 1–2 days before parotid swelling until 9 days after swelling occurs.	Malaise; low-grade fever; and earache, headache, pain with chewing, decreased appetite and activity; followed by bilateral or unilateral parotid gland swelling. Swelling peaks around the third day. Meningeal signs (stiff neck, headache, and photophobia) occur in about 15% of patients. *Complications*: Orchitis (inflammation of the epididymis, pain on testicular palpation, and scrotal swelling—most often unilateral) may occur in postpubertal males; sterility is relatively rare (American Academy of Pediatrics, 2006). Oophoritis, pancreatitis, glomerulonephritis, myocarditis, thrombocytopenia, cerebellar ataxia, and hearing impairment are sometimes seen.	Diagnostic tests include a viral culture from a throat washing, urine, or cerebrospinal fluid. Serum mumps immunoglobulin (Ig) M antibody titer may also be performed. Therapy is supportive, focused on symptom relief. *Prognosis*: Mumps is usually self-limiting. *Prevention*: Mumps is a vaccine-preventable disease. See the medication table on page 592. This is a reportable disease. In 2006 an outbreak of more than 2500 cases of mumps in 11 states occurred in the United States. The infection was originally imported from Britain (Centers for Disease Control, 2006d).	• Use standard and droplet precautions for hospitalized children while contagious. • Children are usually cared for at home. They are generally uncomfortable but are rarely very ill. • Avoid exposure to immunocompromised or susceptible individuals. • Give nonaspirin analgesics and antipyretics to control fever and pain. • Encourage fluid intake. Swallowing and chewing may be painful. Offer soft and blended foods. Avoid foods and beverages that increase salivary flow (citrus, spices, and candies) because they cause pain. • Talking may be painful. Provide a bell or other attention-getting device. • Apply warm or cool compresses, whichever is preferred, to the parotid area.

Table 18–2	SELECTED INFECTIOUS AND COMMUNICABLE DISEASES IN CHILDREN (continued)		
Disease	**Clinical Manifestations**	**Clinical Therapy**	**Nursing Management**

Mumps (Parotitis) [+]—cont.

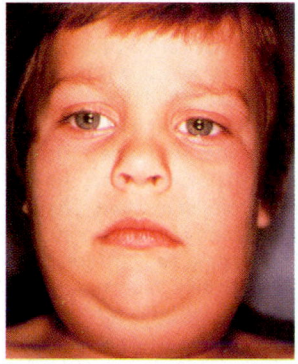

This child has mumps with diffuse lymphedema of the neck.
Courtesy of Centers for Disease Control and Prevention, Atlanta, GA.

Nursing Management:
- Be alert for signs of complications. Headache, stiff neck, vomiting, and photophobia may indicate meningeal irritation.
- Provide scrotal supports if testicular swelling occurs.
- Reassure children that the facial swelling will go away.
- Keep children out of school or childcare until 9 days after parotid swelling occurs. Encourage diversional activities.

Pertussis (Whooping Cough) [+]
Causal agent: Bordetella pertussis.
Epidemiology: Occurs worldwide. Most common in children under 6 months of age. Epidemic cycles occur every 3–4 years. Pertussis may occur in healthcare workers, adolescents, or adults who have waning immunity, and these individuals can spread the disease to unimmunized children. Neither pertussis infection nor vaccine immunity is long lasting (Cherry, 2005).
Transmission: Respiratory droplets and direct contact with discharge from the respiratory membranes.
Incubation period: 7–10 days.
Period of communicability: Begins about 1 week after exposure. Communicable for 5–7 days after antibiotic therapy is initiated. The disease is most contagious before the paroxysmal cough stage.

The onset is insidious.
Catarrhal stage: The disease begins with nasal congestion, a runny nose, low-grade fever, and a mild nonproductive cough, lasting about 2 weeks.
Paroxysmal stage: The cough is more severe at night with coughing spasms when the child attempts to expel a thick mucoid plug. A forceful inspiration through a narrowed glottis and stridor, or "whooping," follows. Young infants may have apnea rather than the "whooping." Sucking on a bottle may trigger the coughing spell. Coughing may be accompanied by flushing; cyanosis; vomiting; and profuse drainage from the nose, eyes, and mouth. Paroxysmal coughing may last 1–6 weeks or more. Dehydration may result from decreased oral intake.
Convalescent stage: Up to 6 weeks when paroxysms gradually subside.
Adolescents and adults often have symptoms of an upper respiratory infection with persistent coughing spasms lasting longer than 7 days.
Complications: Pneumonia, atelectasis, otitis media, encephalopathy, seizures, and death. Highest mortality rate and complication rate is in infants under 1 year.

Diagnostic tests include culture and polymerase chain reaction (PCR) testing.
Treatment with macrolide antibiotics (erythromycin, azithromycin, and clarithromycin); corticosteroids, if ordered; and supportive care.
Prognosis: The disease is most severe in infants under 1 year of age, and most deaths occur in this age group.
Prevention: Pertussis is a vaccine-preventable disease. See the medication table on page 590. Close contacts should be treated with macrolide antibiotics for prophylaxis (Tiwari, Murphy, & Moran, 2005). Vaccine protection wanes after 5 to 10 years.
This is a reportable disease. An estimated 800,000 to 3.3 million cases occur in the United States per year in a cyclic pattern (Cherry, 2005).

- Use droplet precautions until 5–7 days after antibiotics are initiated. Most hospitalized cases occur in children under the age of 5 years.
- Use a cardiac monitor and pulse oximetry to continuously assess respirations and oxygen saturation. The smaller the child, the greater the risk for respiratory distress and apnea.
- Remain with the child during coughing spells, when hypoxic and apneic episodes are most likely. Give oxygen if ordered. Have emergency equipment available.
- Provide humidification. Gentle suctioning may be necessary.
- Give nonaspirin antipyretics as needed for fever.
- Encourage frequent rest periods.
- Allow the child to eat desired foods in small frequent feedings.
- Encourage the child to take fluids. The child may need IV hydration if oral intake is not tolerated.
- Provide emotional support to parents.
- Teach parents to watch for signs of respiratory failure and dehydration if the child is managed at home.

(continued)

Table 18–2	SELECTED INFECTIOUS AND COMMUNICABLE DISEASES IN CHILDREN (continued)

Disease	Clinical Manifestations	Clinical Therapy	Nursing Management
Pneumococcal infection [+] *Causative agent:* Streptococcus pneumoniae, a gram-positive diplococcus. *Epidemiology:* The organism is found in the nasopharynx of healthy people. Outbreaks occur in the winter and spring among people in more crowded settings. In temperate climates, 8 of 90 serotypes account for most of the invasive pediatric infections. The disease is more common in infants, young children, African Americans, American Indians, and Alaskan Natives. Of particular concern is the development of penicillin- and multi-antibiotic-resistant strains. *Transmission:* Respiratory secretions and droplets. *Incubation period:* 1–3 days. *Period of communicability:* Unknown. Probably less than 24 hours after beginning effective antibiotic therapy.	The signs and symptoms are related to the focal area of infection. The organism causes otitis media, sinusitis, pharyngitis, laryngotracheobronchitis, pneumonia, meningitis, and bacteremia. In otitis media, upper respiratory infection, fever, ear pain, and decreased appetite are seen. In bacteremia, there is unexplained fever and no localized infection site. In pneumonia, fever, chills, chest pain, dyspnea, malaise, and a productive cough are seen. In meningitis, inconsolable crying, increased irritability, lethargy, refusal to eat, nausea, vomiting, diarrhea, myalgia, photophobia, and seizures are seen. *Complications:* Prior to the introduction of a vaccine it caused 30–50% of acute otitis media, and was a major cause of sinusitis, meningitis, bacteremia, and pneumonia (Durbin, 2004). Other complications include septic arthritis, osteomyelitis, endocarditis, and brain abscess.	Diagnostic tests include bacterial culture from site of infection. Symptomatic care is provided. Antibiotic selection is based upon susceptibility of organism to penicillin, macrolides, and others. Up to 50% of pneumococcal strains are penicillin resistant. Third-generation cephalosporins (cefotaxime or ceftriaxone) may be used. Vancomycin and rifampin are used in combination when strains are resistant to antibiotics listed above (American Academy of Pediatrics, 2006). *Prevention:* Many serotypes are preventable with immunization. See the medication tables on pages 593 and 598. Significant reduction in invasive disease and antibiotic-resistant strains caused by serotypes in the vaccine have occurred since initiating vaccination of infants (Durbin, 2004).	• If the child is hospitalized, maintain standard precautions. • Provide nonaspirin antipyretics for control of fever and comfort. • Encourage fluids, and monitor intake and output. • Monitor vital signs and level of consciousness to identify signs of worsening condition. • Educate parents about the need for the vaccine, as the unimmunized child could become infected repeatedly with different serotypes. • Many children with mild disease will be treated at home. Educate parents about signs indicating a need to seek additional medical care, the need for proper medication administration, and comfort measures for the child. • Individuals with congenital asplenia or traumatic splenectomy, malignancy, sickle cell disease, and nephrotic syndrome are at higher risk for invasive disease with this organism. • Additional factors that increase risk of pneumococcal disease include poverty, crowded housing, homelessness, and exposure to tobacco smoke.
Poliomyelitis [+] *Causal agent:* Poliovirus is an enterovirus with three serotypes. *Epidemiology:* Occurs worldwide. Polio primarily affects children and immunocompromised or unimmunized adults caring for infants who received live poliovirus vaccine. The vaccine induces lifelong immunity. Since live poliovirus vaccine was discontinued in the United States, no vaccine-associated paralytic poliomyelitis has been reported since 2000 (American Academy of Pediatrics, 2006, p. 543). *Transmission:* Primarily by the fecal-oral route, but also the respiratory route.	Affects the central nervous system. Less severe infections may be limited to fever and stiffness in the neck and back, headache, vomiting, and sore throat. In other cases, fever, headache, stiff neck, Kernig or Brudzinski sign, decreased deep tendon reflexes, and progressive weakness occur. With cranial nerve involvement, there may be respiratory tract muscle paralysis. An increased respiratory rate may interfere with the ability to talk because frequent pauses are needed. Onset of paralysis may be sudden, in hours, or gradual over 3–5 days. Paralysis results from damage to motor neurons.	Diagnosis is made by cell culture from stool or throat swabs. Treatment is supportive. No chemotherapeutic agents that directly kill the poliovirus are available. *Prognosis:* Respiratory complication is life threatening and involves 5–10% of all cases. Respiratory paralysis may lead to death. Motor paralysis may result in long-term disability. *Prevention:* Poliomyelitis is a vaccine-preventable disease. See the medication table on page 593. This is a reportable disease.	• Use standard and contact precautions in the hospital and keep the child on strict bed rest. • Observe closely for respiratory paralysis (ineffective cough, talking with frequent pauses, shallow and rapid respiratory rate). Have emergency equipment at bedside. Assist ventilations as needed until mechanical ventilation is set up. • Administer sedatives and nonaspirin analgesics as ordered to allow for rest and comfort. Moist hot packs may relieve discomfort. • Encourage fluids. • Position the child to promote body alignment. • Perform range-of-motion exercises to prevent contractures after the acute phase.

Table 18–2	SELECTED INFECTIOUS AND COMMUNICABLE DISEASES IN CHILDREN (continued)

Disease	Clinical Manifestations	Clinical Therapy	Nursing Management
Poliomyelitis [+]**—cont.** *Incubation period*: Usually 7–10 days (range 3–21 days). *Period of communicability*: Greatest shortly before and right after clinical symptoms develop when the virus is in the throat. Excreted in the feces for several weeks.	*Complications*: Permanent motor paralysis, respiratory arrest, myocardial failure, aseptic meningitis, and post-polio syndrome.		• Provide emotional support. • Patients are alert and aware. Tell them what is happening to them. • Long-term orthopedic (physical therapy) support may be needed by some children.
Roseola (Exanthem Subitum, sixth disease) *Causal agent:* Human herpesvirus type 6 (HHV-6). *Epidemiology:* Occurs worldwide, primarily in children 6–24 months of age (after maternal antibodies decline). No seasonal pattern. *Transmission:* Likely to be from respiratory secretions of healthy individuals. *Incubation period:* Appears to be 9–10 days. *Period of communicability*: Lifelong persistent viral shedding in healthy individuals (American Academy of Pediatrics, 2006).	Sudden, high fever up to 40.5°C (105°F) for 3–8 days, during which the child does not appear toxic (normal appetite and behavior). The fever phase is followed by a characteristic pale pink, discrete, maculopapular rash, which starts on the trunk and spreads to the face, neck, and extremities. The rash can last for 1–2 days. The child's appetite is normal. *Complications*: Children may have febrile seizures during high fever stage. Encephalopathy may develop in rare cases.	Roseola is self-limiting, and treatment is supportive. *Prognosis*: Roseola is benign in most cases. Nearly all children over 2 years of age have an antibody titer to HHV-6 (American Academy of Pediatrics, 2006).	• Children are rarely hospitalized, but if they are, use standard precautions. • Give nonaspirin antipyretics to control fever. • Observe closely for any seizure activity, especially during the acute febrile periods. • Encourage fluids. • Reassure parents that the rash will disappear in a few days.
Rotavirus *Causal agent:* Group A, B, and C Rotaviruses *Epidemiology:* Occurs during late fall to early spring in yearly diarrhea epidemics in the United States. Most common cause of severe diarrhea in children under 5 years. *Transmission:* Fecal-oral route. *Incubation:* 2 to 4 days. *Period of communicability:* Virus is present in stool before onset and may persist up to 21 days after onset of symptoms.	Acute onset of low-grade fever and vomiting followed by watery diarrhea 1 to 2 days later. Up to 10–20 diarrheal stools a day. Symptoms lasting 3 to 8 days. *Complications*: Dehydration and electrolyte disturbances. Death in rare circumstances.	Diagnosis by enzyme immunoassay or latex agglutination assay to detect group A rotavirus antigen. Treatment involves adequate fluid and electrolyte replacement with oral rehydration solution. Introducing a regular diet within a few hours of rehydration shortens the duration of the disease (Dennehy, 2005). If severely dehydrated, IV fluid resuscitation is performed. No antiviral therapy is available. *Prevention*: Naturally acquired infection protects against reinfection that causes severe diseases. A new vaccine has been approved for infants. See the medication table on page 594.	• Use standard and contact precautions. • Hand hygiene with soap and water removes 75% of virus from contaminated hands. Use of alcohol-based hand sanitizers after washing with soap and water increases effectiveness (Dennehy, 2005). • Clean contaminated surfaces and follow by disinfecting with an alcohol-containing disinfectant (Dennehy, 2005). • Assess hydration status frequently. • Breast-feeding is continued during oral rehydration therapy. Formula feeding can begin 12 to 24 hours after starting oral rehydration therapy. • Older children can be fed complex carbohydrates and lean meats, yogurt, fruits and vegetables 12 to 24 hours after starting oral rehydration therapy.

(continued)

Table 18–2	SELECTED INFECTIOUS AND COMMUNICABLE DISEASES IN CHILDREN (continued)		
Disease	**Clinical Manifestations**	**Clinical Therapy**	**Nursing Management**

Disease	Clinical Manifestations	Clinical Therapy	Nursing Management
Rubella (German Measles) [+] *Causal agent:* An RNA virus, member of the family Togaviridae, genus *Rubivirus.* *Epidemiology:* Occurs worldwide and is most prevalent in the winter and spring. Maternal antibodies disappear about 6–9 months after birth. Most U.S. cases occur among foreign-born children and adults from countries that do not have rubella vaccination programs. Congenital rubella syndrome is thought to occur due to lack of immunization. Four cases were reported from 2001 to 2004 in the United States (Centers for Disease Control, 2005a). *Transmission:* Droplet spread, direct contact with infected persons, or contact with articles soiled by nasal secretions. *Incubation period:* 14–21 days (most commonly 16–18 days). *Period of communicability:* 7 days before until 7 days after the rash onset. Infants with congenital rubella may shed the virus for months after birth.	Rubella is generally a mild disease with a characteristic pink, nonconfluent, maculopapular rash. The rash appears on the face; progresses to the neck, trunk, and legs; and disappears in the same order. Prodromal symptoms occur 1–5 days before the rash and include low-grade fever, headache, malaise, coryza, sore throat, and anorexia. Forschheimer spots (discrete, erythematous pinpoint or larger lesions on the soft palate) are seen during the prodromal phase. Generalized lymphadenopathy involving the postauricular, suboccipital, and posterior cervical areas is common up to 7 days before the rash. Many cases are asymptomatic. Neonatal signs of congenital rubella syndrome include growth retardation, radiolucent bone disease, hepatosplenomegaly, thrombocytopenia, and purpuric skin lesions (giving a "blueberry muffin" appearance). *Complications:* Complications are rare, but include arthritis in adolescents, encephalitis.	Diagnostic tests include cell culture from a nasal swab, and detection of IgM or IgG antibodies. Treatment is supportive. Rubella is generally self-limiting in children. *Prognosis:* Disease is usually mild and benign. Major risk is for fetus if the mother is infected in the first trimester. Congenital rubella syndrome is associated with ophthalmologic, cardiac, auditory, and neurologic anomalies. *Prevention:* Rubella is a vaccine-preventable disease. See the medication table on page 592. Females of childbearing age need to be immunized to reduce the risk for congenital rubella syndrome. All healthcare workers should have documented immunity. 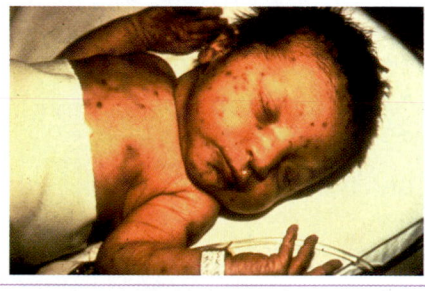 Congenital rubella syndrome. Courtesy of Centers for Disease Control and Prevention, Atlanta, GA.	• Maintain standard and droplet precautions for contagious children. • Maintain contact precautions for infants with congenital rubella syndrome until 1 year of age unless nasopharyngeal and urine cultures are repeatedly negative after 3 months of age (American Academy of Pediatrics, 2006). • Children are usually treated at home. They should be isolated from pregnant women. • Give nonaspirin analgesics and antipyretics for any pain and fever. • Allow children to choose what they would like to eat and drink. Encourage fluids. • Provide quiet activities. • Exclude children from childcare or school for 7 days after onset of rash. School and childcare facilities should be notified of the child's illness.
Streptococcus A *Causal agent:* Group A streptococci (GAS). *Epidemiology:* The illness is caused by various M-protein groups of group A beta-hemolytic streptococci. Different strains are associated with pharyngeal and pyodermal infections, and also rheumatic fever and acute glomerulonephritis (American Academy of Pediatrics, 2006). Pharyngeal infections tend to occur more in late fall, winter, and spring. Pyodermal infections tend to occur in warmer seasons because of the association with minor skin trauma and insect bites.	*Pharyngeal:* Abrupt onset with a sore throat, dysphagia, malaise, high fever, chills, headache, abdominal pain, anorexia, and vomiting. A beefy red pharynx with exudate (strep throat) and tender cervical nodes are seen. Palatal petechiae may be seen. Absence of cough or rhinitis in most cases. *GAS respiratory tract infection:* Children under 3 years may develop serous rhinitis and a respiratory illness with moderate fever, irritability, and anorexia rather than pharyngitis.	Diagnosis can be made by a rapid strep antigen test or culture of secretions from the pharynx and tonsils. Cultures of skin lesions are not indicated (American Academy of Pediatrics, 2006). Prompt antibiotic treatment is effective. Penicillin V is the drug of choice. Erythromycin is used if the child is allergic to penicillin. Uncomplicated impetigo is treated with mupirocin ointment. Invasive strains causing necrotizing fasciitis or myositis need IV antibiotics and surgical intervention (exploration and debridement of dead tissue).	• Children with uncomplicated infections are usually cared for at home. • Promote bed rest during the febrile stage. • Give nonaspirin antipyretics to control fever. Teach parents important signs of a worsening condition. • For pharyngeal infections, offer warm salt water for gargling, a soft diet, and nonacidic beverages. Encourage fluids. Provide cool, clear liquids. Swallowing may be difficult. • Explain to parents the importance of giving the child the full course of antibiotics. • Encourage family members with sore throats to have throat cultures taken.

Table 18–2	SELECTED INFECTIOUS AND COMMUNICABLE DISEASES IN CHILDREN (continued)

Disease	Clinical Manifestations	Clinical Therapy	Nursing Management
Streptococcus A—Cont. *Transmission:* Contact with respiratory secretions for pharyngitis or skin lesions for pyoderma. *Incubation period:* Pharyngeal: usually 2–5 days; Pyodermal: usually 7–10 days. *Period of communicability:* For weeks in untreated pharyngeal infections. Noncontagious within 24 hours of starting antibiotics.	*Scarlet fever:* A characteristic erythematous, sandpaper rash that blanches with pressure appears in some cases 12–48 hours after onset of symptoms, concentrates in flexor skin creases, and spares the circumoral area. In 3–4 days, the rash begins to fade and the tips of the toes and fingers begin to peel. The classic strawberry tongue is seen on day 4- 5. *Pyodermal:* Lesions (impetigo) are honey-colored crusts at the site of open lesions. *Complications:* If untreated, acute otitis media, sinusitis, peritonsillar or retropharyngeal abscess, cervical lymphadenitis, acute rheumatic fever, acute glomerulonephritis. Invasive disease with toxic shock syndrome, bacteremia, and necrotizing fasciitis or myositis can be fatal.	*Prognosis:* Recovery is usually good with antibiotic therapy. Up to 15% of healthy children become chronic carriers (American Academy of Pediatrics, 2006). *Prevention:* None. 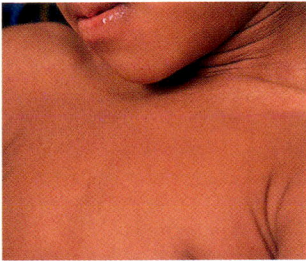 Skin rash of scarlet fever.	• For impetigo, teach the parents to wash the skin, remove crusts, and apply antibiotic ointment. • If the child is hospitalized, maintain droplet precautions for pharyngeal infections and contact precautions for skin lesions for 24 hours after beginning antibiotics. Monitor vital signs, especially temperature. Administer antibiotics as ordered. • If the child develops invasive streptococcal infection, use standard precautions. The child with toxic shock syndrome will need intensive care to manage shock and fluid and electrolyte imbalances.
Tetanus *Causal agent:* Clostridium tetani or tetanus bacillus. *Epidemiology:* The bacillus is common and exists as a spore in soil, dust, and animal excretions. The organism produces an endotoxin that affects the central nervous system. *Transmission:* The organism is transmitted to humans through puncture wounds or broken skin. Newborns can acquire tetanus via the umbilical cord if they are born in an unclean area, a contaminated implement is used to cut the cord, or clay is applied to the umbilical cord as a ritual in some Middle Eastern cultures. *Incubation period:* 3 days–3 weeks (average 8 days). *Period of communicability:* Not communicable to other individuals except through skin wounds.	Stiffness of the neck and jaw, with painful facial spasms and difficulty chewing and swallowing over a few days, and headache. Noise or sudden movement may stimulate spasms. Spasms of facial muscles may produce a grinning expression (risus sardonicus). Localized prolonged and painful muscle contraction may occur at the site of the wound. Eventually rigidity of the abdomen and trunk produce **opisthotonos** (rigid hypertextension of the entire body). Spasms and fever occur along with difficulty swallowing the increased oral secretions. Respiratory muscles can be affected and cause airway obstruction and suffocation. Newborns have difficulty with sucking, progressing to an inability to suck, irritability, and nuchal rigidity. *Complications:* Laryngospasm, respiratory distress, death.	Tetanus immune globulin is given to unimmunized persons as soon as possible. Tetanus toxoid is given at the same time in a separate site. Medications are provided to treat muscle spasms. Intensive care is provided with cardiorespiratory monitoring, assisted ventilation, IV metronidazole or penicillin G, nutrition, and supportive care. Wound cleansing and debriding is performed. Survival beyond 4 days indicates an increased chance of recovery. Paroxysms become less frequent and complete recovery may take weeks. *Prognosis:* 30% mortality; much higher in newborns. Intensive care has improved mortality. *Prevention:* Tetanus is a vaccine preventable disease. See the medication table on page 590. Tetanus boosters are updated every 10 years, or, if a potentially contaminated wound occurs, in 5 years. Proper surgical debridement of wounds decreases the chance of infection.	• Prevent disease by checking immunization records and administering immunizations as necessary. • Give immune globulin to unimmunized persons. • Assist with wound debridement. • Use standard precautions, as the child with tetanus is hospitalized. • Monitor the child's condition. Handle as little as possible. Reduce stimulation by placing the child in a quiet, darkened room. • Offer skin and respiratory care. The child may need an endotracheal tube, suctioning, and supplemental oxygen for airway support. • Provide feedings via total parenteral nutrition or feeding tube. • Maintain hydration with IV fluids and electrolytes. • Try to reduce the child's anxiety, as mental status may be unaffected. • Prepare the family for a possible poor prognosis.

Tuberculosis, see Chapter 20 ∞.

Table 18–3	SELECTED INFECTIOUS DISEASES TRANSMITTED BY INSECT OR ANIMAL HOSTS (ZOONOSIS)		
Disease	**Clinical Manifestations**	**Clinical Therapy**	**Nursing Management**
Lyme Disease* *Causal agent:* Borrelia burgdorferi, a spirochete. *Epidemiology:* Occurs in 49 states and the District of Columbia. Most cases occur in the Northeastern, Mid-Atlantic, and North Central states (American Academy of Pediatrics, 2006). Exposure occurs in any outdoor setting where ticks are endemic. Lyme disease occurs year round, with the highest risk of infection in the summer. Incidence is highest in U.S. children between 5 and 9 years of age. *Transmission:* The tick transmits the infected spirochete after feeding for 36 hours. Lyme disease is the most common vector-borne illness in North America. *Incubation period:* 1–55 days after an infected tick bite. A rash in 48 hours is an allergic reaction or infection, not Lyme disease. *Period of communicability:* The infection is not contagious from person to person.	Stage 1 (localized): malaise, fatigue, headache, stiff neck, mild fever, and muscle and joint aches. Erythema migrans, a slowly expanding red rash, starts as a red macule or papule that expands over days or weeks to become a large annular red area, sometimes with partial central clearing; usually at least 5 cm in diameter. The rash may look like a bruise in dark-skinned patients. Only 50% of patients have the rash (Savely, 2006). Stage 2 (early disseminated) occurs 1–4 months after the bite in untreated children. The most common symptoms are multiple erythema migrans, cranial nerve palsies, arthralgia, headache, fatigue, and meningitis. Stage 3 (late disseminated) occurs months later and includes recurrent Lyme arthritis and central nervous system changes that may become chronic problems. *Complications:* Left untreated, Lyme disease can cause significant neurologic deficits, including arm and leg weakness, Bell's palsy, encephalopathy, optic neuropathy, meningitis, severe headaches, and cognitive and behavioral changes as well as chronic arthritis, and disorders of the peripheral nerves.	Diagnosis is by presence of erythema migrans. An enzyme-linked immunosorbent assay (ELISA) plus the Western blot test may be used in Stage 2. Treatment for localized disease is a 2–3 week course of oral antibiotics (amoxicillin or cefuroxime in children 8 years and younger, doxycycline or tetracycline in children over 8 years). For disseminated disease, oral or IV antibiotics (depending upon body system involved) may be given for up to 4 weeks. *Prognosis:* Lyme disease does not cause acute life-threatening illness, but it may result in significant morbidity, especially when chronic. *Prevention:* Avoid areas that are heavily tick infested, and wear protective clothing. Check for ticks (especially hidden in hair) after every outing. Check pets because they can carry home ticks that are then transferred to the child. Remove ticks as soon as possible. There is no acquired immunity. No vaccine is currently available.	• Children with early disease are usually treated at home. Children with progressive symptoms may be hospitalized. Use standard precautions. • Educate parents about the need for the long course of medications, informing them that the spirochete can go dormant. • Tell parents to have the child avoid sun exposure when taking doxycycline. • Nonaspirin analgesics and antipyretics may provide relief of mild fevers, headaches, and muscle and joint aches. • Children with Lyme disease may tire easily. Promote rest and avoid vigorous activities that may be difficult. • Educate parents and children about the disease and early recognition of the symptoms. • Teach parents to safely remove ticks. To remove a tick, grasp it gently but firmly with a fine-point tweezers where the mouthparts are attached. Pull gently—avoid squeezing the tick's body—until it releases. Clean the area with soap and water (American Academy of Pediatrics, 2006). • Tell parents to mark the date of tick bite on the calendar and monitor the child's health for flu-like symptoms over the next 30 days. Encourage them to seek medical attention promptly if symptoms develop. • Provide emotional support.

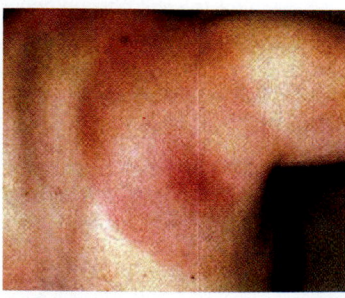

The appearance of the erythema migrans rash may vary in early Lyme disease.
From Pfizer Central Research (1989). Lyme disease. Grofon, CT: author.

Table 18–3	SELECTED INFECTIOUS DISEASES TRANSMITTED BY INSECT OR ANIMAL HOSTS (ZOONOSIS) (continued)		
Disease	**Clinical Manifestations**	**Clinical Therapy**	**Nursing Management**
Malaria *Causal agent:* Plasmodium, 4 species (P. falciparum, P. vivax, P. ovale, P. malariae). *Epidemiology:* Occurs in tropics and subtropics in Africa, Americas, Asia, and Oceana. Children have the highest mortality. The disease is acquired during travel to an endemic area. P. falciparum causes the most serious disease. *Transmission:* The saliva of an infected female Anopheles mosquito introduces the parasite to the person when feeding between dusk and dawn. The parasite infects the hepatic cells and reproduces. When the hepatic cell ruptures, parasites are released and infect the red blood cells. Transmission can occur by blood transfusion or transplacentally. *Incubation period:* Varies by type. P. falciparum in 7 to 10 days, and up to 1 year for other types. *Period of communicability:* Communicable by blood or blood product transfusion, or the transplantation of organs from an infected person.	Nonspecific signs include high fever alternating with chills, profuse diaphoresis, and fatigue. Periods of symptomatic improvement may be seen between cycles lasting 48 or 72 hours, depending upon the type of infection. Children may also have fever, anorexia, vomiting, splenomegaly, and anemia. Additional symptoms include myalgia, malaise, headache, abdominal pain, back pain, pallor, diarrhea, nausea, and vomiting. Attacks may recur over the course of the year after infection, but the parasites die out gradually if reinfection does not occur. Children who live in endemic areas and survive the first 5 years of life develop immunity to the severe effects of the disease as long as they have frequent re-exposure to the infection. *Complications:* Severe anemia in young children. Cerebral malaria occurs in children 3 to 6 years of age. Older children and adolescents more commonly have pulmonary edema, respiratory failure, renal failure, spontaneous bleeding, and shock. Children with asplenia are at high risk for death. This causes 1–2 million deaths worldwide annually (Agrawal & Teach, 2006).	Diagnostic tests include blood smears for parasites, or a plasmodium HRP2 antigen enzyme-linked immunosorbent assay (ELISA). Laboratory tests often reveal anemia and thrombocytopenia. The child is hospitalized for fluid replacement, anemia management, and antipyretics. The blood is regularly monitored for parasite density. Antimalarial medications include: chloroquine, quinine sulfate and tetracycline, clindamycin, doxycycline, mefloquine, and atovaquone-poguanil. The medication selected is based upon drug resistance by the type of Plasmodium species. Medications may be given orally or by IV. Hypoglycemia may result from quinine treatment. ICU care is needed in severe disease to monitor for mental status changes, severe anemia, renal failure, and pulmonary edema. Children may need blood transfusions for severe anemia. *Prevention:* While in endemic areas, minimize contact with mosquitoes, use DEET insect repellent, screened rooms, DEET-treated mosquito netting, and cover the body with light-colored clothing. Antimalarial chemoprophylaxis is recommended when traveling to an endemic region. There is no vaccine.	• Use standard precautions for the hospitalized patient. • Maintain fluid intake. Monitor intake and output. • Monitor blood glucose level and be prepared to respond to sudden hypoglycemia. • Observe for signs of increasing illness severity such as confusion, seizures, and shock. Be prepared to protect the patient from injury and provide emergency support with an airway and oxygen supplementation until the child can be transferred to the ICU. • Monitor the hematocrit and hemoglobin levels. • Administer antipyretics to control the fever and promote comfort. • Provide education and emotional support to parents. • Educate families traveling to endemic areas about the importance of antimalarial chemoprophylaxis. Explain the need to take the medication correctly despite the common side effects of nausea and vomiting. • Discuss the need to protect children during nocturnal feeding times of mosquitoes with protective clothing, mosquito repellent, and mosquito netting around the bed. • Inform adolescents and parents that mefloquine may cause vivid dreams and a sense of "feeling odd" (Laufer, 2006).
*Rabies (Hydrophobia)** *Causal agent:* Rhabdoviridae, two types (urban, in dogs; wild, in wildlife). *Epidemiology:* Occurs worldwide. Urban rabies is generally controlled by vaccination of dogs and cats. Rabies can occur in many wild animals, particularly bats, foxes, skunks, and raccoons.	Children may be free of symptoms during the long incubation period. Illness may begin with mild respiratory or gastrointestinal symptoms, fever, headache, chills, and malaise. Initial acute symptoms may also include pain or paresthesia at the site of exposure.	No diagnosis is possible during incubation. Diagnosis is confirmed by fluorescent antibody staining of the dead animal's brain tissue or patient saliva or reverse transcriptase-polymerase chain reaction of saliva or brain tissue (Mani & Murray, 2006).	• Work with family members and local animal control to find and quarantine any animal suspected of having rabies, if possible. • Administer HRIG and HDCV as ordered. • Provide emotional support to the family while reinforcing the urgency for the vaccine and the need for a series of injections. • Ensure that the vaccine is injected into the muscle to prevent vaccine failure.

Table 18–3	SELECTED INFECTIOUS DISEASES TRANSMITTED BY INSECT OR ANIMAL HOSTS (ZOONOSIS) (continued)		
Disease	**Clinical Manifestations**	**Clinical Therapy**	**Nursing Management**
Rabies (Hydrophobia)—cont. *Transmission:* Infected saliva from bite of rabid animal. Virus enters the wound and travels along the nerves from point of entry to the brain, where it multiplies and migrates along the efferent nerves to the salivary glands. Human-to-human transmission is rare with corneal or other organ transplant (Mani & Murray, 2006). *Incubation period:* Highly variable; average 30 to 90 days. This period depends on the amount of virus in the saliva, how close the bite is to the brain or major nerves, the number of bites, and how deeply the saliva penetrated the skin.	Acute neurologic signs include furious rabies (anxiety, agitation, hallucinations, and other bizarre behavior) or paralytic rabies (paresthesia or weakness that progresses to paralysis and complete respiratory paralysis) (Mani & Murray, 2006). Painful contractures in the muscles used for swallowing lead to hydrophobia (50% of patients), a reflex contraction at the sight of liquid. The patient progresses to coma and respiratory failure. *Complications:* Usually results in death.	Immediately wash animal bites thoroughly with soap and water and irrigate well with a virucidal agent such as povidone iodine (Mani & Murphy, 2006). Suturing should be avoided if possible. Post-exposure prophylaxis with human rabies immune globulin (HRIG) and human diploid cell rabies vaccine (HDCV) should be given as soon as possible to all persons bitten by animals that may be rabid. Half of the HRIG is infiltrated around the wound and the remainder is given IM. HDCV is repeated on days 3, 7, 14, and 28 after the bite (five doses). The HDCV series may be stopped if the animal is found free of rabies. Expert advice on the administration of these vaccines is available from state and local health officials. The vaccine is of no value once rabies symptoms are present. *Prognosis:* If symptoms develop, no drug improves the prognosis *Prevention:* Immunize all domestic animals against rabies.	• Inform parents and the child about the side effects of the vaccine—irritation at the injection site, itching, headache, muscle aches, nausea, and dizziness. • If the child acquires rabies, he or she will be hospitalized. • Institute contact and droplet precautions. The virus is transmitted primarily in the saliva and cerebrospinal fluid. • Make the child as comfortable as possible. • Keep liquids out of sight of the hydrophobic child. • Use caution in the late stages of the disease when children are usually combative. Various medications, paralyzing agents, and sedatives may be used to provide relief. Coma and death occur after an exhaustive period of excitement and agitation that may last for days. • Provide emotional support to the family of the dying child. • Participate in local education about rabies and safe interactions with dogs. See Chapter 30 ∞ . • Teach children to avoid contact with all unknown animals, dead or alive.
Rocky Mountain Spotted Fever (Tickborne Typhus Fever, Sao Paulo Typhus) *Causal agent:* Rickettsia rickettsii. *Epidemiology:* Rocky Mountain spotted fever (RMSF) occurs in most of the United States, southwestern Canada, and Mexico. More than half of all U.S. cases occur in Arkansas, Oklahoma, North Carolina, South Carolina, and Tennessee. Generally occurs between April and September. Most infections occur in children who are less than 15 years of age. Infection induces immunity. *Transmission:* Transmitted by bites of ticks, principally dog and wood ticks. Ticks need to feed for 12–24 hours to transmit the organism. *Incubation period:* 2–14 days (most commonly 7 days) after bite of an infected tick.	Onset may be gradual or rapid with vague signs. Children may be very ill. Sudden onset is characterized by a moderate to high fever (40°C) that lasts for 2–3 weeks, significant malaise, abdominal pain, nausea, vomiting, deep muscle pain, persistent headache, chills, and conjunctival injection. The characteristic rash, red macules, and papules that blanch usually appear between the second and fifth days. It starts on the wrists and ankles and often involves the palms and soles before becoming widely disseminated. The rash may not be easily seen in children with dark skin. The rash becomes petechial on the fifth or sixth day, and purpura may occur. It is rarely pruritic. Up to 10% of children do not	Diagnostic tests are not always reliable, but immunofluorescent or immunoperoxidase staining of biopsied lesions is used (Cohen, 2004). Treatment of choice is doxycycline regardless of patient age for 5–7 days or until the child has been afebrile for 3 days (Chapman, 2006). Hospitalization is often necessary. *Prognosis:* Delay in treatment can cause a more severe disease. A mortality rate of 2–4% is associated with delayed treatment (Razzaq & Schutze, 2005).	• Use standard precautions. • Children may require prolonged hospitalization, including monitoring in the ICU. • Have hemodynamic monitoring equipment and emergency supplies readily available. • Administer antibiotics as prescribed. • Observe for any abnormal bleeding. • Make the child as comfortable as possible. If the child is unconscious, support the extremities and keep the eyes closed and lubricated. • Provide quiet diversion activities. • Provide emotional support, and keep parents informed about the child's condition.

Table 18–3	SELECTED INFECTIOUS DISEASES TRANSMITTED BY INSECT OR ANIMAL HOSTS (ZOONOSIS) (continued)		
Disease	**Clinical Manifestations**	**Clinical Therapy**	**Nursing Management**
Rocky Mountain Spotted Fever—cont. *Period of communicability*: There is no evidence of person-to-person transmission.	develop a rash (Cohen, 2004). The child may have splenomegaly, hepatomegaly, and jaundice. *Complications:* Disseminated intravascular coagulation (DIC) and acute respiratory distress syndrome. Partial paralysis of lower extremities may occur. Gangrene may require amputation of digits or extremities.	*Prevention*: Avoid areas that are heavily tick infested, and wear protective clothing. Check children for ticks and, if found, remove promptly.	

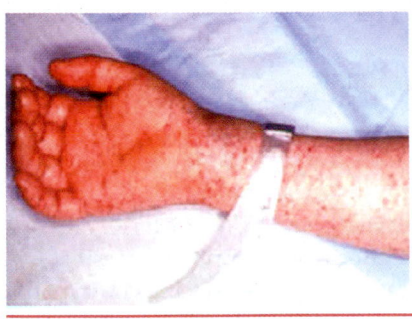

Rash of Rocky Mountain spotted fever.
From Pfizer Central Research. (1989). *Lyme disease*, CT: Author

Clinical Manifestations

The child with an infectious or communicable disease has several symptoms. Initially there may be nonspecific symptoms such as fatigue, malaise, weakness, and decreased responsiveness or a lowered ability to concentrate. Skin rash, poor appetite, malaise, vomiting and/or diarrhea, and body aches are some common signs and symptoms. Fever is the most common sign of infectious disease in infants and children. Signs and symptoms of infection in newborns, infants, and children are associated with the system involved.

COLLABORATIVE CARE

Diagnostic Tests

Diagnostic tests include cultures from sites where the infection may potentially be located, such as the skin, pharynx, blood, urine, feces, and cerebrospinal fluid. See the *Clinical Skills Manual* for guidelines related to collection of specimens. In some cases, radiographs or special imaging may be used to identify localized infection in an organ such as the lungs.

Clinical Therapy

A fever can be a beneficial physiologic response, helping to slow the growth of organisms that thrive at lower body temperatures. A fever helps to mobilize the immune response by increasing neutrophil production and T-cell proliferation (Crocetti & Serwint, 2005). Fever is not inherently harmful until it reaches 41°C (105.9°F). For this reason, medical management may include postponing treatment of low-grade fevers under 38.9°C (102°F) in otherwise healthy children to promote the body's natural defenses against an infection.

Fevers are often treated, especially if associated with discomfort. Acetaminophen and ibuprofen are the preferred antipyretics for children. Aspirin is no longer recommended for children because of its association with Reye's syndrome. Antipyretics reduce fever by inhibiting prostaglandin synthesis, which results in lowering of the body's temperature set-point.

COMPLEMENTARY THERAPY

Hot and Cold Theory

Many cultures subscribe to the hot and cold theory of disease causation. "Hot" and "cold" do not refer to temperature, but to categories. Fever, a hot condition, is treated by giving the patient cold substances (foods or medicines). Cold foods include vegetables, fruits, and fish. Cold medicines include orange flower water, linden, and sage.

COMMUNITY CARE

Community-Acquired Methicillin-Resistant *Staphylococcus aureus*

Community-acquired methicillin-resistant *Staphylococcus aureus* is an organism that causes aggressive infection in healthy children that has occasionally been fatal. Necrotizing fasciitis (an advancing soft-tissue infection), abscess formation, scalded skin syndrome, and toxic shock-like syndromes have occurred. Risk factors include participation in team sports, crowded living conditions, childcare center attendance, recurrent skin infections, and similar lesions in a family member. Transmission occurs by direct contact with an infected person or contact with contaminated objects (Tufts & Hardman, 2006). Prevention and management among athletes includes showering with soap and water after competitions, avoiding the practice of sharing towels and personal items, covering all wounds, encouraging athletes to care for wounds and report those that are potentially infected, and regularly cleaning shared athletic equipment.

Administration of antibiotics may also be used for infectious diseases. Antibiotics have been responsible for decreases in morbidity and mortality from infections among children. However, strains of bacteria have developed resistance to many antibiotics. Children with chronic illnesses such as cystic fibrosis, sickle-cell disease, and acquired immunodeficiency syndrome (AIDS) are particularly susceptible to infection by drug-resistant pathogens.

Antiviral medications, such as acyclovir, may be ordered for certain types of viral infections, such as varicella (chickenpox), herpes simplex virus type I and II, Influenza, and others. If the child is immunocompromised, the antiviral medication needs to be provided very early in the infectious period to minimize the potentially life-threatening consequences of the infection.

Some infectious or communicable diseases must be reported to the state health department for disease surveillance and to determine the effectiveness of certain preventive measures such as vaccines. Cases can be reported on standardized state forms or on designated web sites.

NURSING MANAGEMENT

Nursing Assessment and Diagnosis

Assess the child's hydration status and fluid intake, vital signs, comfort level, and appetite and observe for seizures and for a **toxic appearance** (lethargy, poor perfusion, hypoventilation or hyperventilation, and cyanosis). The child with a fever may be irritable and restless, sleep fitfully, and have nonspecific muscular pain. Identify those children who may be at higher risk for a serious illness in association with a fever, in particular:

- Infants and children having a toxic appearance
- Neonates less than 28 days of age with a temperature over 38°C (100.4°F)
- Children less than 4 years of age with a temperature over 41°C (105.8°F)
- Children with conditions such as a ventriculoperitoneal shunt, congenital heart disease, asplenia, and sickle-cell disease

Observe the child for other signs of infection, such as a rash, nausea and vomiting, and/or diarrhea, as well as generalized symptoms of a poor appetite and malaise.

Examples of nursing diagnoses that may be appropriate for children with infectious and communicable diseases include:

- Hyperthermia related to infectious disease process
- Risk for Deficient Fluid Volume related to hypermetabolic state
- Impaired Skin Integrity related to hyperthermia and self-mutilation of skin lesions
- Impaired Oral Mucous Membrane related to infectious disease process
- Deficient Fluid Volume related to repeated episodes of vomiting and diarrhea
- Ineffective Therapeutic Regimen Management (family) related to complexity of care required by the child

Planning and Implementation

Most children with infectious diseases are cared for at home; however, children may be evaluated in various healthcare settings. Nursing care includes assisting with the collection of cultures, treating infection, administering antibiotics on schedule, monitoring antibiotic blood levels if indicated, monitoring the response to therapy, staying alert for signs that the infection is worsening, and educating parents.

Prevent Disease Transmission

In the clinic setting, isolate children with suspicious rashes from other children. All items with which the infected child comes into contact are considered contaminated (linens, toys, medical equipment, etc.). When possible, hard surfaces and toys in the waiting and examining rooms where the child was seen should be wiped down with

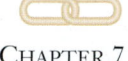

SKILLS CHAPTER 7
Specimen Collection

antiseptic solution before another child uses the room. Dispose of linens in appropriately marked linen bags.

Children are often admitted to the hospital for treatment of severe infections. In addition, countless numbers of **nosocomial** (hospital-acquired) **infections** occur each year. Implement transmission-based precautions, including isolation, to reduce exposure of other children and staff to the infectious agent. Follow your facility's standard precautions and transmission-based precautions to reduce the spread of infectious diseases to staff and other patients. Bring any questions and concerns to your hospital's infection control nurse.

Managing Fevers

Nursing care for treatment of fever includes administering antipyretics, removing unnecessary clothing, and careful continued monitoring of temperature progression. Identify clear fluids the child prefers to drink, and encourage the intake of extra fluids.

Care in the Community

Teach parents to care for their child at home, including how and when to give antipyretics, over-the-counter medications, and antibiotics, if ordered; what foods and beverages are appropriate; and how to care for rashes and other topical symptoms. Provide guidelines about the types of fluids to encourage.

Parents often fear a fever, believing it is a disease rather than a symptom of an illness. Their greatest fears about the harmful effects of fever include seizure, brain damage, and death (Nativio, 2005). Provide information and reassurance. Help them to recognize signs of the child's worsening condition in association with the child's specific disease. See Families Want to Know: Evaluating and Treating Fever in Children.

> 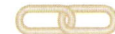 **NURSING ALERT**
>
> The practice of alternating acetaminophen with ibuprofen in the care of children with fever is not based upon scientific evidence. Each medication is effective in managing fever. However, because the medications have different durations of action (4 hours for acetaminophen and 6 hours for ibuprofen) and many different preparations, there is risk for overdosing the child if the administration schedule is not strictly adhered to. In addition, there are potentially synergistic effects on the kidneys by the two medications when given in an alternating schedule that can cause renal tubular toxicity. An important patient safety initiative is to use only one antipyretic for fever management of children (Carson, 2003).

SKILLS CHAPTER 1
Standard Precautions

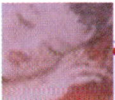

FAMILIES WANT TO KNOW

Evaluating and Treating Fever in Children

About Fevers

- A fever is not a disease; it is the body's response to an infection. It means the child's body is using natural defenses to fight an infection.
- If the child has a fever and does not look sick, it may be better to let the child use the body's natural defenses to fight off the virus or bacteria causing the fever, but follow guidelines about when to contact the child's healthcare provider.

Treating the Fever

- Use a thermometer to check the child's temperature every 4 to 6 hours.
- Use either acetaminophen or ibuprofen to lower a fever. Check the label to make sure to give the correct dose—drops and syrups do not have the same concentration. Do not alternate medications.
- Remove all but a light layer of the child's clothing.
- Monitor the child's behavior and response to fever medication. The fever medication will reduce the child's temperature, but the temperature may not return to normal until the child is recovering from the illness.
- If sponging the child, give fever medication first, and then use tepid water to sponge the child. Cool water may increase shivering and discomfort. Alcohol should not be used.
- The temperature may rise again 4 hours after giving acetaminophen or 6 hours after ibuprofen. Check the temperature and give another dose of fever medicine. Follow the recommendations on the bottle for the maximum number of doses allowed per day.

Call Your Healthcare Provider Immediately if Any of the Following Occur

- The infant is under 2 months old and has a fever over 38.0°C (100.4°F).
- The child has a fever over 40.1°C (104.2°F) and any of the symptoms below are present:
  - The child is crying inconsolably or whimpering. The child cries when moved or otherwise touched by the parent or other family members.
  - The child is difficult to awaken.
  - The child's neck is stiff.
  - There are purple spots present on the skin.
  - Breathing is difficult and no better after the nose is cleared.
  - The child is drooling saliva and is unable to swallow anything.
  - The child has a convulsion or seizure.
  - The child acts or looks very sick.

Call Your Healthcare Provider within 24 Hours if:

- The child is 2 to 4 months old (unless fever occurs within 48 hours of a DTaP shot and the infant has no other serious symptoms).
- The fever is higher than 40.1°C (104.2°F) (especially if the child is under 3 years old).
- The child complains of burning or pain with urination.
- The fever has been present for more than 24 hours without an obvious cause or location of infection.
- The fever went away for more than 24 hours and then returned.

RESEARCH

Medicating for Fever

A recent study in Israel of 464 children ages 6 to 36 months compared the treatment of fever with acetaminophen (12.5 mg/kg) every 6 hours, ibuprofen (5 mg/kg) every 8 hours, or alternating doses of acetaminophen (12.5 mg/kg) and ibuprofen (5 mg/kg) every 4 hours. The group of children receiving the alternating therapy had a more rapid reduction of fever and a lower mean temperature than the two other groups (Sarrell, Wielunsky, & Cohen, 2006). This study did not effectively compare alternating doses of antipyretics with single antipyretics because the alternating medications were given more frequently than the single medication, and more antipyretic medication was in the bloodstream at one time. More study is needed before parents are routinely encouraged to alternate acetaminophen and ibuprofen for treating a fever.

Teach parents the importance of proper use of antibiotics when ordered to help reduce the development of antibiotic-resistant bacteria:

- Give all the antibiotic dosages as prescribed for the full number of days ordered. Spread the doses around the clock to keep blood levels constant, as much as possible. This will help ensure that the bacteria causing the infection are eradicated, rather than having some bacteria left alive to mutate and resist the antibiotic in the future.
- Make sure parents know to give the antibiotic with food or without food to promote optimal absorption.
- Discard the antibiotic when all the doses have been given. Antibiotics have an expiration date and lose potency after that date.
- Do not share the antibiotic with any other family member. If that family member is ill, there will not be enough antibiotic to fully treat the infection, even if the same bacteria is causing the infection.

Educate parents about methods to reduce disease transmission in the home such as hand hygiene. Encourage parents to limit the exposure of elderly family members and infants to the ill child. Make sure that the ill child's dishes and utensils are washed in hot soapy water or sanitized in a dishwasher.

Evaluation

Expected outcomes of nursing care include the following:

- Opportunities for spread of infection are minimized between patients and family members.
- The child's fever is effectively managed with antipyretics.
- The full treatment with antibiotics, if ordered, is completed.

EMERGING INFECTION CONTROL THREATS

Special attention is now directed at disease surveillance associated with infectious agents. Weapons of terrorists (anthrax, smallpox, plague, botulism, hemorrhagic fever, or tularemia) or the emergence of rare infectious diseases, such as severe acute respiratory syndrome (SARS), need to be identified as early as possible so that public health measures can be initiated.

Specific biological agents that could potentially be used for terrorism, along with signs, symptoms, and clinical therapy, are described in the Clinical Manifestations table on page 625. The state public health system is activated to identify cases, to control the spread of infection, and to prepare the mass casualty response to care for the potential large numbers of ill adults and children (see Chapter 11 ∞).

Nursing Management

Nurses have responsibility for maintaining a high level of suspicion when numerous individuals with similar signs and symptoms seek care in any healthcare facility. Initiating infection control measures such as airborne and contact precautions may help reduce the transmission of infection. Instituting isolation before a definitive diagnosis is made is appropriate when the level of suspicion is high. Assess children and provide supportive nursing care for the identified infection.

Nurses should regularly review guidelines posted by the Centers for Disease Control and Prevention about the management of specific health threats. They should also participate in planning for the healthcare facility's preparedness to respond to potential epidemics as a partner in the state and local emergency preparedness planning (see Chapter 11 ∞).

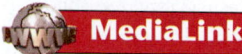

MediaLink

Emerging Infection Control Threats

Organisms	Clinical Manifestations	Clinical Therapy
Anthrax *Causal agent:* Bacillis anthracis	• Cutaneous—papule that progresses to a vesicle that develops into a skin ulcer with a depressed black scab area in the center. Not painful. Child may have fever, malaise, headache, and regional lymphadenopathy. • Gastrointestinal—nausea, loss of appetite, bloody diarrhea, hematemesis, fever, stomach pain, severe abdominal pain followed by fever and septicemia. • Inhalation—brief prodrome with respiratory symptoms like a sore throat, mild fever, malaise, muscle aches followed by development of dyspnea, cough, chest pain, shortness of breath, and systemic symptoms. Shock, pleural effusion, and meningitis may develop without treatment.	• IV ciprofloxacin or doxycycline for patients over 12 years. For children under 12 years, IV ciprofloxacin plus clindamycin and penicillin G. • For postexposure prophylaxis: vaccine approved for those over 18 years (three doses at 0, 2, and 4 weeks) and oral ciprofloxacin or amoxicillin for 30 days (Markenson, 2005).
Botulism *Causal agent:* Clostridium botulinum	• Ptosis, diplopia, blurred vision. Sluggishly reactive pupils. • Speech and swallowing problems, dysarthria, dysphonia, and dysphagia, loss of gag reflex. • Acute, afebrile symmetric descending flaccid paralysis, progressing to loss of head control, hypotonia, generalized weakness, deep tendon reflexes diminish or disappear. Constipation. • May be preceded by abdominal cramps, nausea, vomiting, or diarrhea. • May become confused or obtunded.	• Slow IV infusion of equine antitoxin diluted in normal saline may halt symptoms, but symptoms may not be reversed. • Epinephrine and diphenhydramine for serum sickness or urticaria.
Hemorrhagic Fever *Causal agent:* Ebola or Marburg virus	• Abrupt onset of fever, myalgia, headache, nausea, vomiting, abdominal pain, photophobia, diarrhea, chest pain, cough, pharyngitis. • Maculopapular rash prominent on trunk soon after fever, bleeding into skin (petechiae, ecchymosis, subconjunctival hemorrhages, shock, and circulatory collapse in short period). • Ghostlike appearance, looks critically ill.	• Management of hypotension and shock and maintenance of fluid and electrolyte balance. • Replacement of blood, platelets, and plasma for severe hemorrhage. • Ribavarin may be helpful, but not approved by the FDA for this purpose.
Plague *Causal agent:* Yersinia pestis	Pneumonic plague with aerosol route of transmission • Severe respiratory illness with high fever, chills, headache, cough, breathing difficulty. • May have gastrointestinal symptoms, such as nausea, vomiting, diarrhea, and abdominal pain. • Rapidly developing pneumonia, bloody or watery sputum. • May lead to respiratory failure and shock. Bubonic plague with release of infected fleas • Swollen, tender lymph gland that is painful • Fever, chills, headache, fatigue. • May be fatal if untreated.	• Gentamicin IV or streptomycin IM. Alternate antibiotics include IV doxycycline, ciprofloxacin, or chloramphenicol. • Prophylaxis with doxycycline or ciprofloxacin.
Smallpox *Causal agent:* Variola major virus	• Prodrome 2 to 4 days before rash: abrupt onset with fever (101°F or higher), malaise, headache, muscle pain, prostration, nausea and vomiting, and backache. • Rash begins as red spots in mouth and on tongue that develop sores and break open. Then a few macules known as herald spots appear on the forehead, face, and extremities. Over the next few days a generalized rash develops, progressing from macules to papules, to tense vesicles, to tense deep pustules with an umbilicated appearance. Most cases have discrete, semi-confluent to confluent vesicles with a depression in the center. Lesions are firm, all in the same stage of development, more concentrated on the extremities than the trunk. The temperature usually falls and the patient feels better. • The pustules form scabs by the end of the second week, and the scabs fall off after 3–4 weeks.	• Supportive care. • Antibiotics for secondary infection. • Vaccine can be effective if given within first few days after exposure.
Tularemia *Causal agent:* Francisella tularensis	• Febrile illness, fatigue, chills, headache, malaise, body aches. • Cough, substernal pain, dyspnea, chest pain. • May develop hemorrhagic inflammation of airways that progresses to bronchopneumonia, pleuritis, and hilar lymphadenopathy. • May also have pharyngitis, bronchiolitis, and pneumonia with systemic symptoms.	• Supportive care in the intensive care unit. • Gentamicin IV or streptomycin IM. Alternate antibiotics include IV doxycycline, ciprofloxacin, or chloramphenicol. • Prophylaxis with doxycycline or ciprofloxacin.

Data from: Markenson, D. (2005). The treatment of children exposed to pathogens linked to bioterrorism. *Infectious Disease Clinics of North America, 19,* 731–745; Yetman, R. J., Parks, D., & Taft, E. (2002). Management of patients exposed to biologic weapons. *Journal of Pediatric Health Care, 16*(5), 256–261; Centers of Disease Control. (2003). Retrieved September 24, 2003, from http://www.bt.cdc.gov

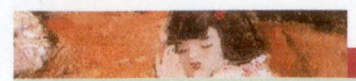

CRITICAL THINKING IN ACTION

Recall 5-year-old Lian and her 2-year-old brother Joe in the opening scenario. The pediatric clinic they visit has recently implemented guidelines to increase the number of children who are fully immunized. Nurses in the clinic are expected to look for opportunities to review records for immunizations needed. In this case, the nurse also looked at Lian's record, even though she was not the scheduled patient for the visit. Lian has been healthy, has no allergies, and is taking no medications.

DISCUSSION

1. Which vaccines should Lian receive today? When should she return for the remaining needed vaccines?

2. Should Joe receive all his needed vaccines on this visit even though he has a fever?

3. What are some potential methods to reduce the pain associated with immunizations for both Lian and Joe?

4. What is the patient education that should be given to Lian's and Joe's mother about the expected reactions to the vaccines given to each of them?

 Refer to your Prentice Hall Nursing MediaLink DVD-ROM for answers.

EXPLORE MediaLink 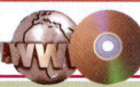 http://www.prenhall.com/ball

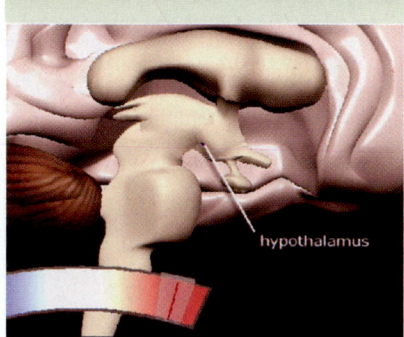

hypothalamus

Resources for this chapter can be found on the Prentice Hall Nursing MediaLink DVD-ROM accompanying this textbook, and on the Companion Website at http://www.prenhall.com/ball

DVD-ROM
Audio Glossary
NCLEX-RN® Review
Animation
   Fever

COMPANION WEBSITE
Audio Glossary
NCLEX-RN® Review
Care Plan Activity: Immunization Schedule for an Infant
Case Study: Flu Shot Immunizations for Siblings
MediaLink Application: Vaccine Shortages
WebLinks

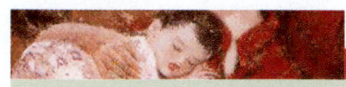

REFERENCES

Agrawal, D., & Teach, S. J. (2006). Evaluation and management of a child with suspected malaria. *Pediatric Emergency Care, 22*(2), 127–133.

American Academy of Pediatrics Committee on Infectious Disease. (2006). *Red book: 2006 Report of the Committee on Infectious Disease* (27th ed.). Elk Grove Village, IL: Author.

Benin, A. L., Wisler-Scher, D. J., Colson, E., Shapiro, E. D., & Holmboe, E. S. (2006). Qualitative analysis of mothers' decision-making about vaccines for infants: The importance of trust. *Pediatrics, 117*(5), 1532–1541.

Bilukha, O. O., & Rosenstein, N. (2005). Prevention and control of meningococcal disease. *Morbidity and Mortality Weekly Report, 54*(RR-7), 1–21.

Bindler, R. M., & Howry, L. B. (2005). Pediatric drugs and nursing implications (3rd ed.). Upper Saddle River, NJ: Prentice Hall Health.

Buck, M. L. (2005). Meningococcal conjugate vaccine. *Pediatric Pharmcology, 11*(5). Retrieved June 7, 2005, from http://www.medscape.com/viewarticle/505508_print

Carson, S. M. (2003). Alternating acetaminophen and ibuprofen in the febrile child: Examining the evidence regarding efficacy and safety. *Pediatric Nursing, 29*(5), 379–382.

Centers for Disease Control and Prevention. (2002a). Guidelines for hand hygiene in health-care settings. *Morbidity and Mortality Weekly Report, 51*(RR-16), 1–56.

Centers for Disease Control and Prevention. (2002b). Immunization registry use and progress—United States, 2001. *Morbidity and Mortality Weekly Report, 51*(3), 53–56.

Centers for Disease Control and Prevention. (2004). Vaccines for Children program. Retrieved May 12, 2006, from http://www.cdc.gov/PROGRAMS/IMMUN10.HTM

Centers for Disease Control and Prevention. (2005a). Achievements in public health: Elimination of rubella and congenital rubella syndrome—United States, 1969–2004. *Morbidity and Mortality Weekly Report, 54*(11), 279–282.

Centers for Disease Control and Prevention. (2005b). Measles—United States, 2004. *Morbidity and Mortality Weekly Report, 54*(48), 1229–1231.

Centers for Disease Control and Prevention. (2005c). National, state, and urban area vaccination coverage among children aged 19–35 months—United States, 2004. *Morbidity and Mortality Weekly Report, 54*(29), 717–721.

Centers for Disease Control and Prevention. (2006a, June 29). CDC's advisory committee recommends changes in varicella vaccinations, Retrieved July 5, 2006, from http://cdc.gov/od/media/pressrel/r060629-b.htm

Centers for Disease Control and Prevention. (2006b, February 23). Preventing tetanus, diphtheria, and pertussis among adolescents: Use of tetanus toxoid, reduced diphtheria toxoid, and acellular pertussis vaccines. *Morbidity and Mortality Weekly Report, 55*, 1–34.

Centers for Disease Control and Prevention. (2006c, June 28). Prevention and control of influenza: Recommendations of the Advisory Committee on Immunization Practices (ACIP). *Morbidity and Mortality Weekly Report, 55*, 1–44.

Centers for Disease Control and Prevention. (2006d, May 18). Update: Multistate outbreak of mumps—United States, January 1-May 2, 2006, *Morbidity and Mortality Weekly Dispatch 55*, 1–5.

Chapman, A. S. (2006). Diagnosis and management of tickborne rickettsial diseases: Rocky Mountain spotted fever, ehrlichioses, and anaplasmosis—United States. *Morbidity and Mortality Weekly Report, 55*(RR-4), 1–27.

Cherry, J. D. (2005). The epidemiology of pertussis: A comparison of the epidemiology of the disease pertussis with the epidemiology of *Bordatella pertussis* infection. *Pediatrics, 115*(5), 1422–1427.

Children's Hospital of Philadelphia. (2006). Vaccine education. Retrieved July 13, 2006, from http://www.chop.edu/consumer/jsp/division/generic.jsp?id=75697

Cohen, B. A. (2004). Papular rash on hands and feet after 3 days' fever and headache. *Contemporary Pediatrics, 21*(7), 15–17.

Cohen, L. L. (2002). Reducing infant immunization distress through distraction. *Health Psychology, 21*(2), 207–211.

Cox, J. E. (2006). Egg-based vaccines. *Pediatrics in Review, 27*(3), 118–119.

Crocetti, M. T., & Serwint, J. R. (2005). Fever: Separating fact from fiction. *Contemporary Pediatrics, 22*(1), 34–41.

Dennehy, P. H. (2005). Update on a high-morbidity infection: Rotavirus. *Contemporary Pediatrics, 22*(12), 34–40.

Department of Health and Human Services, Office of Disease Prevention and Promotion. (2000). *Healthy People 2010*. Washington, D.C., http://www.healthypeople.gov

DeStefano, F., Bhasin, T. K., Thompson, W. W., Yeargin-Allsopp, M., & Boyle, C. (2004). Age at first measles-mumps-rubella vaccination in children with autism and school-matched control subjects: A population-based study in metropolitan Atlanta. *Pediatrics, 113*(2), 259–266.

DeStefano, F., Gu, D., Kramarz, P., Truman, B. I., Iademarco, M. F., Mullooly, J. P., et al.

(2002). Childhood vaccinations and risk of asthma. *Pediatric Infectious Disease Journal, 21*(6), 498–504.

Durbin, W. J. (2004). Pneumococcal infections. *Pediatrics in Review, 25*(12), 418–423.

Food and Drug Administration (2005). FDA and CDC issue alert on Menactra meningococcal vaccine and Guillain Barré Syndrome. Retrieved January 6, 2006 from http://www.fda.gov/bbs/topics/NEWS/2005/NEW1238.htm

Food and Drug Administration. (2006). FDA approves a second drug for prevention of influenza A and B in adults and children. Accessed April 3, 2006, from http://www.fda.gov/bbs/topics/news/2006/new01231.html

Hviid, A., Stellfeld, M., Wohlfahrt, J., & Melbye, M. (2004). Childhood vaccination and type 1 diabetes. *New England Journal of Medicine, 350*(14), 1398–1404.

Immunization Action Coalition. (2005). Screening questionnaire for child and teen immunization. Retrieved July 3, 2006, from http://www.immunize.org

Institute of Medicine Board of Health Promotion and Disease Prevention. (2003). Immunization safety review: Vaccinations and sudden unexpected death in infancy. Washington, DC: National Academy Press. Retrieved September 25, 2003, from http://books.nap.edu/books/0309088860/html/1.html

Laufer, M. K. (2006). Hitting the dirt road: How to prep families for travel to developing countries. *Contemporary Pediatrics, 23*(3), 45–54.

Lee, G. M., Salomon, J. A., Friedman, J. F., Hibberd, P. L., Ross-Degnan, D., et al. (2005). Illness transmission in the home: A possible role for alchol-based gels. *Pediatrics, 115*(4), 852–860.

Lott, J. W., & Kenner, C. (2003). Assessment and management of the immune system. In C. Kenner & J. W. Lott, *Comprehensive neonatal nursing* (3rd ed., pp. 550–579). Philadelphia: Saunders.

Mani, C. S., & Murray, D. L. (2006). Rabies. *Pediatrics in Review, 27*(4), 129–135.

Markenson, D. (2005). The treatment of children exposed to pathogens linked to bioterrorism. *Infectious Diseases of North America, 19*, 731–745.

Merck & Co. Inc. (2006). Gardasil, retrieved June 13, 2006 from http://www.fda.gov/cber/label/hpvmer060806LB.pdf

Mosby. (2004). *Mosby's drug consult 2004*. St. Louis: Mosby, Inc.

Nativio, D. G. (2005). Understanding fever in children. *American Journal for Nurse Practitioners, 9*(11/12), 47–52.

Peters, T. R., & Edwards, K. M. (2002). Pneumococcal vaccines: Present and future. *Pediatric Annals, 31*(4), 261–268.

Pichichero, M. E., Rennels, M. B., Edwards, K. M., Blatter, M. M., Marshall, G. S., et al. (2005). Combined tetanus, diphtheria, and 5-component pertussis vaccine for use in

adolescents and adults. *Journal of American Medical Association, 293*(24), 3003–3011.

Razzaq, S., & Schutze, G E. (2005). Rocky Mountain spotted fever: A physician's challenge, *Pediatrics in Review, 26*(4), 125–129.

Reef, S. E., Frey, T. K., Theall, K., Abernathy, E., Burnett, C. L., Iscnogle, J., et al. (2002). The changing epidemiology of rubella in the 1990s: On the verge of elimination and new challenges for control and prevention. *Journal of the American Medical Association, 287*(4), 464–472.

Reis, E. C., Roth, E. K., Syphan, J. L., Tarbell, S. E., & Holubkov, R. (2003). Effective pain reduction for multiple immunization injections in young infants. *Archives of Pediatrics & Adolescent Medicine, 57*, 1115–1120.

Sandora, T., Taveras, E., Shih, M., Resnick, E. A., Lee, G. M., et al. (2005). A randomized controlled trial of a multifaceted intervention including alcohol-based hand sanitizer and hand-hygiene education to reduce illness transmission in the home. *Pediatrics, 116*(3), 587–594.

Sarrell, E. M., Wielunsky, E., & Cohen, H. A. (2006). Antipyretic treatment in young children with fever. *Archives of Pediatric and Adolescent Medicine, 160*(2), 197–202.

Savely, G. R. (2006). Update on Lyme disease. *Clinician Reviews, 16*(4), 45–50.

Schuval, S. (2003). Avoiding allergic reactions to childhood vaccines and what to do if they occur. *Contemporary Pediatrics, 20*(4), 29–53.

Smeeth, L., Cook, C., Fombonne, E., et al. (2004). MMR vaccination and pervasive developmental disorders: A case-control study. *Lancet, 364*(9438), 963–969.

Taylor, B., Miller, E., Lingram R., et al. (2002), Measles, mumps, and rubella vaccination and bowel problems or developmental regression in children with autism: Population study. *British Medical Journal, 324*, 393.

Tenrreiro, K. N. (2005). Time-efficient strategies to ensure vaccine risk/benefit communication. *Journal of Pediatric Nursing, 20*(6), 469–476.

Tiwari, T., Murphy, T. V., & Moran, J. (2005). Recommended antimicrobial agents for the treatment and postexposure prophylaxis of pertussis: 2005 CDC guidelines. *Morbidity and Mortality Weekly Report, 54*(RR-14), 1–16.

Tufts, G., & Hardman, M. E. C. (2006). Community-acquired methicillin-resistant *Staphylococcus aureus. Clinician Reviews, 16*(1), 52–57.

Whitney, C. G., Farley, M. M., & Hadler, J. (2003). Decline in invasive pneumococcal disease after introduction of protein-polysaccharide conjugate vaccine. *New England Journal of Medicine, 348*(18), 1737–1746.

Yetman, R. J., Parks, D., & Taft, E. (2002). Management of patients exposed to biologic weapons. *Journal of Pediatric Health Care, 16*(5), 256–261.

19

ALTERATIONS IN EYE, EAR, NOSE, AND THROAT FUNCTION

KEY TERMS

audiography **659**

binocularity **636**

conductive hearing loss **658**

decibels **657**

esotropia **629**

mixed hearing loss **658**

myringotomy **653**

nystagmus **629**

sensorineural hearing loss **658**

tinnitus **658**

tympanogram **659**

tympanostomy tubes **653**

vision **630**

visual acuity **629**

MediaLink

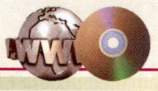

http://www.prenhall.com/ball

See the Prentice Hall Nursing MediaLink DVD-ROM and Companion Website for chapter-specific resources.

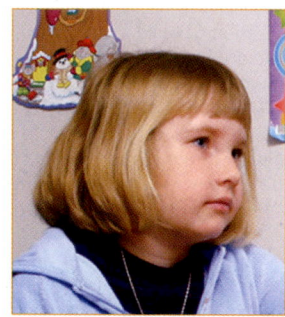

KATE is 5 years old and has had decreased hearing ability from birth. Once Kate's hearing loss was diagnosed, her family explored options to assist her with communication. Kate's parents learned sign language and began using it as she learned language. Once Kate was 2 years of age, they decided to have a cochlear implant placed in her inner ear. Kate was slowly introduced to sounds over time and adjusted to her new sense of hearing. She started to make sounds in response to sounds in the environment, and a speech therapist assisted in helping the family introduce her to speech.

Kate communicates verbally now. Each week she visits a speech therapist who helps her learn how to listen for sounds, solve problems, and respond verbally. Both Kate's mother and father attend the therapy sessions so they can learn how to best communicate with Kate at home. The nurse in the office plays an integral part in fostering Kate's development. Ongoing developmental assessments and teaching to enhance Kate's environment so that she learns social and communication skills have been important nursing interventions. In addition, safety teaching and immunizations have been addressed by the nurse in the pediatric healthcare home.

As Kate begins kindergarten, the school nurse can collaborate with the office nurse and then work with Kate's family to plan for establishment of an Individualized Education Plan to enhance Kate's learning. Assisting the family to cope with the transition to school and facilitating Kate's continued acquisition of skills are key nursing functions.

LEARNING OUTCOMES

After reading this chapter, you will be able to do the following:

1. Describe abnormalities of the eyes, ears, nose, throat, and mouth in children.

2. Plan for screening programs and identification of children with vision and hearing abnormalities.

3. Plan nursing care for children with vision or hearing impairments.

4. Use the latest recommendations when implementing care and teaching for children with abnormalities of the eyes, ears, nose, throat, and mouth.

5. Integrate preventive and treatment principles when implementing care for children related to the eyes, ears, nose, and throat.

FOCUS ON
Eye, Ear, Nose, and Throat

ANATOMY AND PHYSIOLOGY

Sight, hearing, taste, and smell depend on proper functioning of receptor organs and interpretation by the brain. Thus, certain cranial nerves are also an integral part of the anatomy and physiology of the eye, ear, nose, throat, and mouth. Children are prone to both inborne and acquired sensory alterations, as well as a wide array of infections and injuries that can affect the eye, ear, nose, throat, mouth, and upper respiratory system.

Eye

The eye is a complex structure composed of the eyeball and its supporting structures. The *sclera*, or white part of the eye, is the outermost layer. It is transparent in the anterior eye to form the *cornea*, which allows light to enter. The *iris*, or colored part of the eye, is muscular, allowing it to change the size of the *pupil* and regulate the light that enters the eye. The *lens* is located behind the pupil and focuses light onto the retina. The *anterior chamber*, or the space between the cornea and iris, is filled with a fluid called *aqueous humor*. The *posterior chamber* is located behind the lens and is filled with *vitreous humor*. The innermost, posterior section of the eye is the *retina*, which has an inner layer that receives light impulses and an outer neural layer that transports visual images to the brain by the optic nerve (cranial nerve II). The *rods* in the retina perceive vision in dim light and allow for peripheral vision; the *cones* perceive vision in bright light and are responsible for color discernment. See As Children Grow, Figure 19–1 ➤, for normal structures of the child's eye.

The eye has several supporting structures that assist in the sensation of vision. *Eyebrows*, *eyelids*, and *eyelashes* protect the eye and add touch sensation. The *conjunctiva* lines the cornea and the inside of the eyelids, lubricating the eye and keeping it viable. The lacrimal apparatus and ducts bathe the eye and produce tears. A series of six muscles allow the eye to move to all planes and maintain the shape of the eyeball. They are innervated by the oculomotor, trochlear, and abducens nerves (cranial nerves III, IV, V).

Ear

The ear is responsible for the sensory ability of hearing and it establishes the sense of equilibrium. The *external ear* contains the *auricle*, which is visible outside the body; the *external canal*; and the *tympanic membrane*. These structures collect sound waves and direct them to the middle and inner ear. The *middle ear* lies behind the tympanic membrane and contains three bones necessary for sound vibrations: the *incus*, *malleus*, and *stapes*. Another part of the middle ear, the *eustachian tube*, connects to the nasopharynx and equalizes ear pressure. The *inner ear* contains the bony labyrinth, which in turn houses the *vestibule*, *semicircular canals*, and the *cochlea*. The vestibule and semicircular canals are responsible for the sense of equilibrium. The cochlea contains the *organ of Corti*, which contains sensory hair cells that are innervated by the acoustic nerve (cranial nerve VIII).

Nose, Throat, and Mouth

The structures of the nose, throat, and mouth are important to all humans. Mucous membranes bathe these body parts and have a high rate of growth. They help to maintain hygiene and protect the body from infectious agents. Salivary apparatus and taste buds are essential parts of the mouth and tongue. The nasal passages contain external nostrils, the sinuses, and the pharynx (or throat). The olfactory, facial, glossopharyngeal and vagus nerves (cranial nerves I, VII, IX, X) are responsible for the sense of smell, taste, coordinated swallowing, and the gag reflex, respectively.

PEDIATRIC DIFFERENCES
Eye

How are the eyes of children different from those of adults? Chapter 5 ∞ provides a detailed discussion of the assessment of the eyes and **visual acuity**, the ability to discriminate letters or other objects. The eyes of neonates differ from the eyes of adults in several ways. Visual acuity in neonates ranges between 20/100 and 20/400. The lens is more spherical and cannot accommodate to both near and far objects, which means that the neonate sees best at a distance of about 20 cm (8 in.). Because the optic nerve is not yet completely myelinated, the ability to distinguish color and other details is decreased. If the infant is preterm, especially less than 32 weeks' gestation, retinal vascularization, particularly in the periphery of the retina, may be incomplete. Pupillary reflex reaction is detected by about 28 to 30 weeks' gestation and so may be sluggish in preterm infants. The rectus muscles that control binocular vision may be somewhat uncoordinated at birth. The eyes should be aligned and movement coordinated by the age of 3 months. Transient **nystagmus** (involuntary rapid eye movement) and **esotropia** (momentary turning inward of eyes) are common in neonates, but decrease in incidence during the first few months of life. Conjunctival and retinal hemorrhages may be observed in the newborn as a result of the trauma of birth; they usually

AS CHILDREN GROW

The Eye

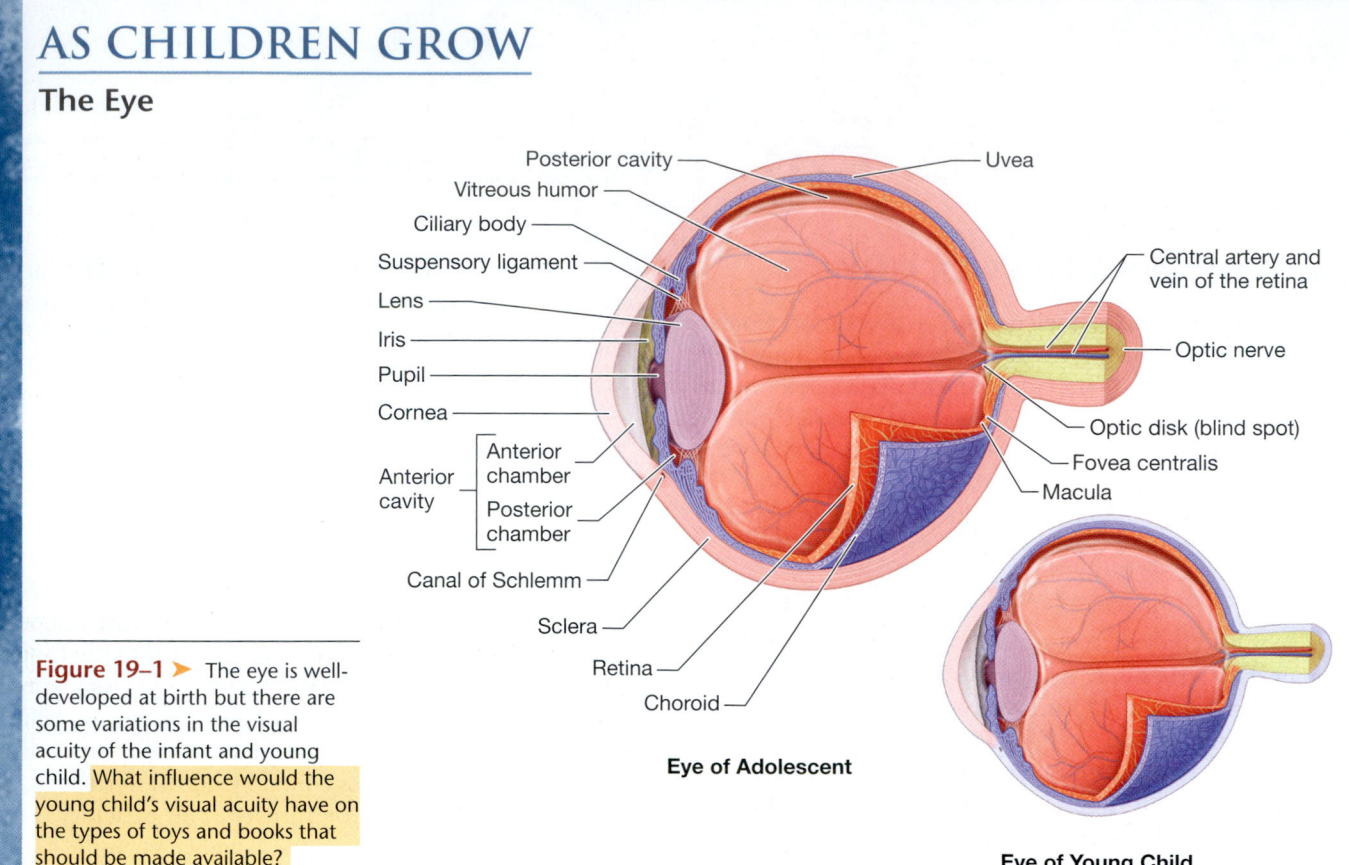

Figure 19–1 ➤ The eye is well-developed at birth but there are some variations in the visual acuity of the infant and young child. What influence would the young child's visual acuity have on the types of toys and books that should be made available?

Labels on diagram: Posterior cavity, Vitreous humor, Ciliary body, Suspensory ligament, Lens, Iris, Pupil, Cornea, Anterior cavity (Anterior chamber, Posterior chamber), Canal of Schlemm, Sclera, Retina, Choroid, Uvea, Central artery and vein of the retina, Optic nerve, Optic disk (blind spot), Fovea centralis, Macula

Eye of Adolescent

Eye of Young Child

improve gradually and have no lasting effects. The red reflex is examined in children because it is a key method for identifying the presence of retinoblastoma (see Chapter 5 ∞ for the method to evaluate red reflex and Chapter 23 ∞ for a description of retinoblastoma).

The cornea of the infant and young child occupies a larger portion of the orbit than in the adult; the eyeball is about 3/4 of its adult size (Chamley, Carson, Randall, & Sandwell, 2005). Because the eyeball is relatively unprotected laterally, it is more easily injured. The sclera of the neonate is thin and translucent with a bluish tinge, and the iris is blue or gray. Eye color changes during the first 6 months of life. Infants produce tears to nourish and oxygenate the outer layers of the cornea. However, parents do not see tears when a young infant cries because the infant's lacrimal system drains them efficiently into the nasal cavity.

As infants grow, their eyes mature and their vision improves. The eyeball grows until the third year, when growth slows, until normal adult size is reached by 14 years (Chamley, et. al, 2005). By the age of 2 or 3 years, most children have a visual acuity of 20/50, and by the age of 6 or 7 years, it is 20/20. See Figure 19–1 for a summary of pediatric differences of the eye. Visual acuity is measured using standardized letter or picture charts (see Chapter 5 ∞ and the *Clinical Skills Manual*). **Vision** refers to the complex process of acquiring meaning from what is seen, involving the eye, brain, and related neurologic and physiologic structures.

Cognitive development interacts with a child's maturing physiologic system to bring increasing meaning to objects in sight (Table 19–1). The first few years of life are considered critical for the formation of normal vision. As acuity improves, the brain learns to interpret messages received from the eyes. Disturbances in vision, even in one eye, can affect the retinal nerve function, muscle function in the eye, or the brain's ability to interpret visual input.

Ear

Why do infants and young children have more ear problems than adults? The eustachian tube, which connects the nasopharynx to the middle ear, is proportionately shorter, wider, and more horizontal in infants than in older children or adults (As Children Grow, Figure 19–2 ➤). During sucking, yawning, and other movements, the tube opens for milliseconds, allowing free passage of air between the nasopharynx and the middle ear. These factors predispose young children to development of otitis media or middle ear infection.

The fetus can hear at about 20 weeks' gestation while the auditory nerve function is mature at about 5 months of age in the infant. Before 34 weeks' gestation, the external ear is soft with little cartilage apparent. The external ear canal is small at birth, although the internal ear and middle ear are relatively large. As a result, the tympanic membrane is close to the surface and can be easily injured.

Table 19-1	VISUALLY RELATED DEVELOPMENTAL MILESTONES	
Age	**Milestone**
Term neonate	Demonstrates alertness to visual stimulus presented 8–12 in. (20–30 cm) from eyes
1 month	Follows an object 60 degrees horizontally and 30 degrees vertically; blinks at an approaching object
2 months	Follows a person from 6 ft (2 m) away; smiles in response to a face; raises head 30 degrees from prone
3 months	Tracks an object through 180 degrees; regards own hand; begins visual-motor coordination
4–5 months	Social smile; reaches for a cube 12 in. (30 cm) away; notices a raisin 12 in. (30 cm) away
7–8 months	Picks up a raisin by raking
8–9 months	Pokes at holes in a peg board; neat pincer grasp; crawling
12–14 months	Stacks blocks; places a peg in a round hole; stands and walks

Note: From Scheiner, A. P. (1996). Vision problems: Impairment to blindness. In A. M. Rudolph, J. I. E. Hoffman, & C. D. Rudolph (Eds.), *Rudolph's pediatrics* (20th ed., p. 167). Stamford, CT: Appleton & Lange.

Nose, Throat, and Mouth

Up to the age of 6 months, infants are primarily nasal breathers. Edema and nasal discharge may interfere with adequate air intake and feeding. Mucosal swelling and exudate may block the small nasal passages of young children. The immature immune system of young children (see Chapter 17 ∞ for further description) and the frequent exposure to other children with illnesses causes a high rate of upper respiratory infections in this population.

The palatine tonsils, which are visible on oral examination, are located on each side of the oropharynx. The method for examining a child's throat is discussed in Chapter 5 ∞. Although tonsils vary in size considerably during childhood, they are normally large, especially in school-age children. The nasopharyngeal tonsils (adenoids) lie in the posterior wall of the nasopharynx, just above the oropharynx. In children, the adenoids may become enlarged, harboring bacteria and interfering with breathing.

The mouth is an important organ for the infant as strong muscles are needed for sucking and thereby receiving nutrients. Sucking is an important developmental skill that promotes the muscles needed for later speech development. Taste sensation is present before birth, as evidenced by increased swallowing of amniotic fluid that has been sweetened (Chamley, et. al, 2005). Taste sensations increase during childhood. By about 6 months of age the first tooth emerges, and by about 2 years the full set of 20 primary teeth is present. Tooth loss of the primary set begins about 5–6 years, and gradually the secondary teeth (32 total) erupt during childhood. See Chapter 5 ∞ for a further description of teeth eruption.

Examples of diagnostic and laboratory tests used to evaluate the eye, ear, nose, and throat are provided in the accompanying table. Use the guidelines on the following page to perform a nursing assessment for the child with an alteration of the eye, ear, nose, and throat.

AS CHILDREN GROW

Eustachian Tube

Position of eustachian tube is at less of an angle (more horizontal) in the young child, resulting in decreased drainage.

End of eustachian tube in nasal pharynx opens during sucking.

Eustachian tube equalizes air pressure between the middle ear and the outside environment and allows for drainage of secretions from middle ear mucosa.

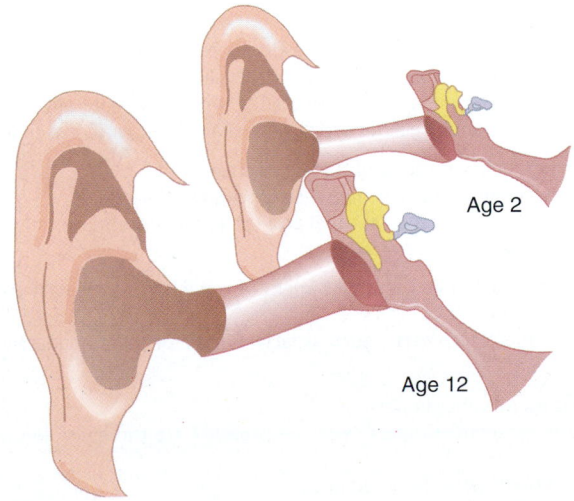

Age 2

Age 12

Figure 19–2 ➤ Of the three anatomical differences in the eustachian tube between adults and small children (shorter, wider, more horizontal), which do you think could cause more problems for the child and why? Answer: More horizontal. Small children who are bottle-fed in a supine position have a greater probability of developing otitis media because the eustachian tube opens when the child sucks and the horizontal angle provides easy access to the middle ear. In older children, the increased angle helps keep foreign substances and infectious agents away from the middle ear.

DIAGNOSTIC AND LABORATORY PROCEDURES/TESTS FOR THE EYE, EAR, NOSE, AND THROAT

Diagnostic Test	Purpose	Nursing Implications
Audiologic screening	A sweep screening of various tones (generally 500, 1000, 2000 Hertz) at the 20 or 25 decibel level. Each ear is tested separately.	Perform a practice session with the sound louder than will be tested, giving feedback when the child understands and follows the directions. Then direct the child away from the machine and screener so that he or she gets no clues about when the sound is being delivered. Ask the child to raise a hand when the sound is heard. Vary the length of time between sound delivery. The young child can be taught to place a block in a container each time a sound is heard.
Newborn hearing screening	• Otoacoustic emission test measures response of cochlear hair cells to clicks from a probe placed in the ear canal. • Auditory brainstem response test measures response of the cochlea, cranial nerve VIII, and auditory brainstem pathways via electrical response of surface scalp electrodes.	Administer tests as directed. Consult results as soon as available. Report abnormalities promptly to primary care provider and follow-up with infant and family as needed.
Tympanogram	Measures movement of the tympanic membrane and pressure in the middle ear, thereby affecting the ability of the middle ear to transmit sound.	Conduct test as directed. Report abnormalities promptly to primary care provider.

Laboratory Test	Purpose	Nursing Implications
Complete blood count (CBC)	The CBC measures types of all cells in the serum. It includes all leukocytes (white blood cells) that are important in identifying infections in the eye, ear, nose, or throat.	Collect the sample before administering the first dose of antibiotic. Transfer to laboratory via agency protocol and examine results promptly.
Culture and sensitivity	Cultures are taken to isolate microorganisms causing infection and to establish the antibiotics to which the microorganisms are sensitive. Cultures of the nasopharynx are used to diagnose streptococcal throat infection, cultures of sinus fluid assist in diagnosis of sinus infections, and eye cultures assist in identifying bacterial conjunctivitis.	Collect sample before administering the first dose of antibiotic. Consult the results of sensitivity once available to determine if the antibiotic ordered is effective.

Data from: Corbett, J. V. (2004). *Laboratory tests and diagnostic procedures with nursing diagnoses* (6th ed.). Upper Saddle River, NJ: Prentice Hall.

ASSESSMENT GUIDELINES FOR THE CHILD WITH AN ALTERATION OF THE EYE, EAR, NOSE, OR THROAT

Assessment Focus	Assessment Guidelines
Eyes	• Describe eye structures and symmetry. • Describe visual acuity using screening test appropriate for age. • Measure extraocular movements to all quadrants. Evaluate corneal light reflex, cover-uncover test, and visual fields. • Using the ophthalmoscope, elicit and evaluate the red reflex bilaterally. • Observe for and report abnormalities such as eye drainage, cloudiness of lens, or abnormal movement.
Ears	• Describe placement and symmetry of the external ear. • Describe auditory acuity using screening test appropriate for age. • Using the otoscope, evaluate the ear canal and tympanic membrane. • Ask about pain and discomfort from the ear.
Nose	• Describe the nose for symmetry and placement. Are the nares bilaterally patent? Are there lesions or drainage? • Are several smells identified? • Are signs of sinus infection present, such as facial edema or pain, headache, and tenderness upon palpation over sinus areas?
Mouth and throat	• Are oral mucous membranes intact? • How many primary/secondary/loose teeth are present? Are there visible caries? Are there broken or chipped teeth present? • Evaluate soft and hard palate for intactness. • Describe the throat and size/appearance of tonsils. • Palpate cervical lymph nodes, noting size and tenderness.

How are conditions of the eye, ear, nose, and throat related? Which conditions have the potential to affect a child's growth, development, and behavior? In what settings do children with eye, ear, nose, and throat conditions receive care?

Because the eye, ear, nose, and throat are connected, a malformation, infection, or other condition in one of these structures may affect them all. Intact sensory structures support the attainment of developmental milestones; thus alterations, especially to the eye and ear, may delay a child's development. (See Chapter 3 ∞ for expected developmental milestones at each age.) In the chapter opening scenario, Kate's condition was diagnosed when she was very young, and she received a cochlear implant and speech therapy to enhance her development. Most children with eye, ear, nose, and throat disorders are treated at home or in the community rather than in the hospital. Infections of the eye, ear, and upper respiratory system are common abnormalities and most pediatric nurses will need to be experts in assessment and interventions for these conditions. Health promotion and health maintenance settings provide an opportunity for screening to identify alterations, for teaching to prevent injuries, and for applying interventions that capitalize on sensory capabilities to enhance development.

DISORDERS OF THE EYE

Infectious Conjunctivitis

Conjunctivitis is an inflammation of the conjunctiva, the clear membrane that lines the inside of the lid and sclera. There are several types of conjunctivitis, depending on the cause of inflammation. Bacteria, viruses, allergies, trauma, or irritants cause the conjunctiva to become edematous and reddened with a yellow or white discharge (Figure 19–3 ➤). Parents commonly refer to all conjunctivitis as "pink eye."

Conjunctivitis in an infant under 30 days of age is called *ophthalmia neonatorum*. These infections are usually acquired from the mother during vaginal delivery as a result of contact with infected vaginal discharge containing bacterial organisms such as *Chlamydia trachomatis* and *Neisseria gonorrhoeae*. Antibiotics are instilled into the eyes of newborns in most states soon after birth as a prophylactic measure.

In infants who have frequent tearing and mattering (eyelid discharge that has formed a crust) on awakening, a plugged lacrimal duct may mimic conjunctivitis. Treatment involves massaging the tear duct every 4 hours when the infant is awake. Lacrimal ducts that remain plugged after the age of 1 year may have to be opened surgically.

Bacterial conjunctivitis is common in older children. It is characterized by edema of the eyelid, reddened conjunctiva, and enlarged preauricular lymph glands. Mucopurulent discharge causes matting and makes the eyes difficult to open upon awakening. Older children with conjunctivitis complain of itching or burning, mild photophobia, and a feeling of scratching under the lids.

Common infectious organisms include *Staphylococcus aureus*, *Haemophilus influenzae*, *Streptococcus pneumoniae*, *Moraxella catarrhalis*, and *Escherichia coli* (Mah, 2006; Stephenson, 2003). Most cases are caused by hand-to-eye contact and the disease can rapidly spread when groups of youth spend time together, such as among young children and adolescents in schools and childcare centers, and among college students in dormitories or on sports teams. The infection can be bilateral but is more commonly unilateral.

Other infections in newborns and children can be caused by viruses. Viral conjunctivitis is commonly bilateral. Adenovirus is a common cause and spreads from respiratory adenovirus infection in a hand-to-eye manner.

Herpes simplex virus (HSV) can also cause infections, either by transfer from a mother with herpes infection to a neonate during birth or by contact with an infected person in infants or children of any age. Ophthalmic herpes infection is often accompanied by characteristic vesicular lesions on the skin of the face. A culture of the lesion is performed for diagnosis and any accompanying conjunctivitis is assumed to be caused by herpesvirus. For the infection caused by HSV, prompt and vigorous treatment is needed to prevent eye injury or blindness, which can occur in children with recurrent herpesvirus infections as a result of antibody reaction to the viral antigen.

Swollen eyelid

Inflamed conjunctiva

Purulent discharge

Figure 19–3 ➤ Acute conjunctivitis. The major difference between bacterial and viral conjunctivitis is that bacterial conjunctivitis has a purulent discharge that may result in crusting whereas the discharge from viral conjunctivitis is serous (watery). Allergic conjunctivitis produces watery to thick drainage and is characterized by itching.
Adapted from: Newell, F. W. (1996). *Ophthalmology: Principles and concepts* (8th ed.). St. Louis: Mosby Year-Book.

LAW & ETHICS

Prophylactic Eye Treatment

By federal law, all infants born in the United States are given prophylactic eye treatment soon after delivery to help prevent ophthalmia neonatorum. The nurse is responsible for administering this eye ointment. Penicillin, tetracycline, erythromycin, or povidone–iodine ointments are most commonly used.

Sometimes an infant can develop chemical conjunctivitis due to the prophylactic eye ointment. A chemical reaction should be considered as a possible cause when conjunctivitis develops within 24–48 hours after instillation of the medication.

Herpesvirus infections commonly recur, so periodic treatment and sometime prophylaxis may be needed.

Allergic conjunctivitis is a common cause of eye discomfort (Abelson & Granet, 2006). When conjunctivitis is caused by an allergy, the child complains of intense itching. Examination reveals reddened eyes with watery discharge and the conjunctivae have a "cobblestone" appearance. The eyes may also appear edematous.

Collaborative Care

In most cases, a diagnosis of the cause of conjunctivitis is made based on the history and symptoms. Cultures can be taken, especially in infants or in cases suspected of being unusual bacterial illness or herpesviruses. A Gram stain of discharge and conjunctival scraping for potential Chlamydia or herpes are performed. Infants and children must be promptly referred to primary care providers or eye specialists for treatment of possible eye infections. When diagnosed in an infant in the neonatal intensive care unit, the infant is isolated to prevent the disease's spread to other infants.

Antibiotic eye medication is prescribed in droplet or ointment form if a bacterial infection is suspected. Treatment may be started after a laboratory sample is obtained but before the results are known. Fluoroquinolones are now frequently used to treat bacterial conjunctivitis; drops or ointment can be used. When gonococcal conjunctivitis occurs in newborns, ceftriaxone is recommended; the disease is resistant to penicillin. Chlamydial infections are treated with oral erythromycin or tetracycline. Careful total evaluation of the newborn with any conjunctivitis is also performed to watch for other signs of infection. Instructions for instilling eye medications are given in the *Clinical Skills Manual*.

Adenoviral conjunctivitis may be treated with comfort measures such as cleaning drainage away with a warm clean cloth, avoiding bright lights, and avoiding reading. Ophthalmic antibiotics are sometimes given to prevent bacterial invasion due to frequent rubbing of the eyes. Herpes simplex virus infections of the eye are treated promptly by an ophthalmologist, neonatologist, or others who are trained in this serious disease. Topical drugs are used, and often are combined with a systemic antiviral agent such as acyclovir (Teoh & Reynolds, 2003). Neonatal herpes simplex virus is treated vigorously with parenteral acyclovir for 14 days (or longer if central nervous system involvement is found upon lumbar puncture), and with topical ophthalmic medication (trifluridine, iododeoxyuridine, or vidarabine). Recurrent lesions may necessitate suppressive or prophylactic treatment with oral acyclovir (American Academy of Pediatrics, 2006).

If an allergen is believed to be the cause of conjunctivitis, systemic or topical antihistamines may be prescribed. Topical steroids and vasoconstrictors may also be used (Abelson & Granet, 2006). Decongestants can be combined with systemic antihistamines for short-term therapy. More current treatment involves use of mast-cell stabilizers to decrease the activation of mast cells that accompanies allergic reactions. Most mast-cell stabilizers have been tested and found to be safe in children 3 years of age and older (Alexander, 2003). See Medications Used to Treat Conjunctivitis for types of medications used to treat eye conditions.

Nursing Management

Nurses routinely instill prophylactic antibiotics into the eyes of newborns after birth. A careful examination should occur so that any cases of ophthalmia neonatorum are referred promptly to an ophthalmologist. Women infected with gonococcus or Chlamydia should be identified so their babies can receive attention and medication at birth to prevent infection. Babies born at home should have ocular examinations soon after birth.

Nurses also perform assessments of the eyes of infants and children in many settings and refer for care those with identified redness, edema, and discharge. Because bacterial infectious conjunctivitis is extremely contagious, tell parents that children should not return to childcare or school until they have been using an antibiotic for 24 hours. Teach parents the importance of careful hand hygiene and the avoidance of

CLINICAL TIP

During assessment, place a gloved index finger on the child's nose next to the inner corner of the eye and apply gentle pressure for several seconds. If mucopurulent drainage is discharged from the eye, bacterial conjunctivitis may be present.

MEDICATIONS USED TO TREAT *Conjunctivitis*

Medication	Action/Indication	Nursing Implications
Fluoroquinolones (e.g., norfloxacin, ciprofloxacin, ofloxacin, levofloxacin, sparfloxacin)	Antibiotic effective against a broad spectrum of gram-positive and gram-negative organisms; generally interfere with enzymes needed for DNA replication in bacteria causing eye infections.	• If a culture and sensitivity test is ordered, perform the test before beginning the antibiotic. • Teach parents correct administration of drops or ointment. • Be alert for signs of reactivity to medication that might be manifested as local burning, crusting, itching, and edema.
Acyclovir	Anitviral drug effective against herpes simplex virus (HSV).	• Most viral conjunctivitis infections are not treated; good hygiene practices are followed and the infection clears without treatment by medication. However, herpes simplex virus infections must be treated because they can harm vision. Acyclovir is administered intravenously to neonates and some children with HSV; ongoing suppressive oral therapy is used for recurred infections. • Teach family to recognize characteristic herpes skin lesions and report them and all eye redness immediately. Ensure that family and other care providers understand the possible chronic nature of HSV and engage in careful hygiene to prevent spread when infections are active. • Prepare and administer IV form as ordered, over at least 1 hour. Shake oral suspension when that form is used for children.
Mast-cell stabilizers (e.g., cromolyn, nedocromil, olopatadine)	Inhibit release of histamine from mast cells, thereby decreasing allergic response. Used to treat itching and other symptoms of allergic conjunctivitis.	• Teach family the correct installation of medication. Encourage other methods to decrease itching such as cool compresses several times daily to the eyes. Avoid rubbing eyes, which can introduce bacteria or virus to the already inflamed eyes. If medication does not provide relief or additional eye symptoms appear, consult again with healthcare provider.

shared towels. Tell parents that children should not rub their eyes; mittens may help prevent infants from doing so. Toddlers may be distracted by activities that keep their hands busy. Teach parents the proper techniques for instilling eye medications (see Families Want to Know: Instilling Eye Medications). For children with allergies, alert parents to signs of infection so that if the child develops conjunctivitis, prompt treatment will be obtained. The pruritis of allergic conjunctivitis may be relieved by lying clean washcloths with very cold water over the eyes for several minutes two to three times daily. Avoid use of contact lenses during periods of allergic conjunctivitis since they can further exacerbate the condition.

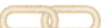

SKILLS 8–5 AND 8–6
Administering Ophthalmic Medications

Periorbital Cellulitis

Periorbital cellulitis is an infection of the eyelid and surrounding tissues that is usually caused by bacteria and is an uncommon complication of sinusitis in some children. The average age for occurrence is 7.5 years (Nageswaran, Woods, Benjamin, & Shetty, 2006). Children present with edematous, tender, and red or purple eyelids; restricted, painful movement of the area around the eye; and fever. Periorbital cellulitis should be treated promptly to prevent the spread of the infection to the posterior orbit, which could lead to serious outcomes such as brain abscess or decreased vision. Clinical therapy includes

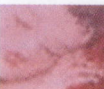

FAMILIES WANT TO KNOW

Instilling Eye Medications

It can be challenging to safely instill eye medication into the eyes of young children. Give parents the following suggestions:

- Wash hands well.
- Be sure the medicine is warmed at least to room temperature.
- Remove any drainage from the eye with a clean or sterile moist, warm cloth or gauze.
- Wash hands again.
- Place the child on the back with eyes closed.

- Gently pull the lower lid down to form a small pocket.
- Apply a thin string (for ointment) or drops of the medicine.
- Allow the eyelid to return to its normal position.
- Have the child keep the eye closed for several seconds.
- Help prevent spread of the infection by keeping the child's hands clean.
- Enhance comfort by keeping the head elevated to decrease swelling and by avoiding exposure to bright light.

hospitalization for intravenous administration of antibiotics, drainage of infection in some cases, and the application of hot packs. Children usually respond favorably within 48 to 72 hours.

Nursing management of periorbital cellulitis begins with identification of potential cases and prompt referral for treatment. When the child is hospitalized, the nurse administers antibiotics, provides supportive care, monitors vital signs, and teaches the family about the infection. Desired outcomes are rapid resolution of the infection and return to normal daily activities with no impairment in eye function.

Visual Disorders

Vision, the complex process of acquiring meaning from what is seen, depends on many factors. The eyes must move quickly and in a coordinated manner (see Chapter 5 ∞ for discussion of eye movement assessment). They must function together for clear, single vision to occur. If this ability, called **binocularity**, is not present (perhaps due to strabismus or amblyopia), the child cannot make sense of the images the brain receives. Normally, the objects seen are integrated with other senses through eye-hand coordination, and with the brain through visual imagery and discrimination of objects seen. Although visual acuity is essential, the child's movements, mental processes, and other senses all interact to give meaning to objects that are viewed. About 5–10% of young children have some type of vision impairment, with amblyopia present in 1–4% and refractive errors in 5–7%. If uncorrected, early visual impairment interferes with learning, developmental progression, and school performance; it may even lead to further deterioration of vision and to total blindness (U.S. Preventive Services Task Force, 2005).

Etiology and Pathophysiology

Several common visual disorders involve errors of refraction (see Figure 19–4 ➤). As light enters the eye, it is bent or refracted to fall on the retina. Variations in the shape of the eyeball are often genetic in nature and can cause light rays to fall in another area of the eye, where they cannot be interpreted. Common refractive errors include:

- *Hyperopia (farsightedness).* Light rays focus posterior to the retina, resulting in an inability to focus on nearby objects. All children have some degree of hyperopia until 9 to 10 years of age. However, their eyes can accommodate sufficiently to enable them to see near objects clearly. Blurring of vision occurs only in children with excessive hyperopia, or a difference in accommodation between the two eyes. Amblyopia, or a weakening of the poorer eye, can occur in these children if treatment is not obtained.
- *Myopia (nearsightedness).* Light rays focus anterior to the retina, resulting in an inability to see far-off objects. Although children of any age can manifest myopia, it most commonly develops at about 8 years of age. The child may complain of headaches and often squints to improve distance vision.

PATHOPHYSIOLOGY ILLUSTRATED

Visual Abnormalities

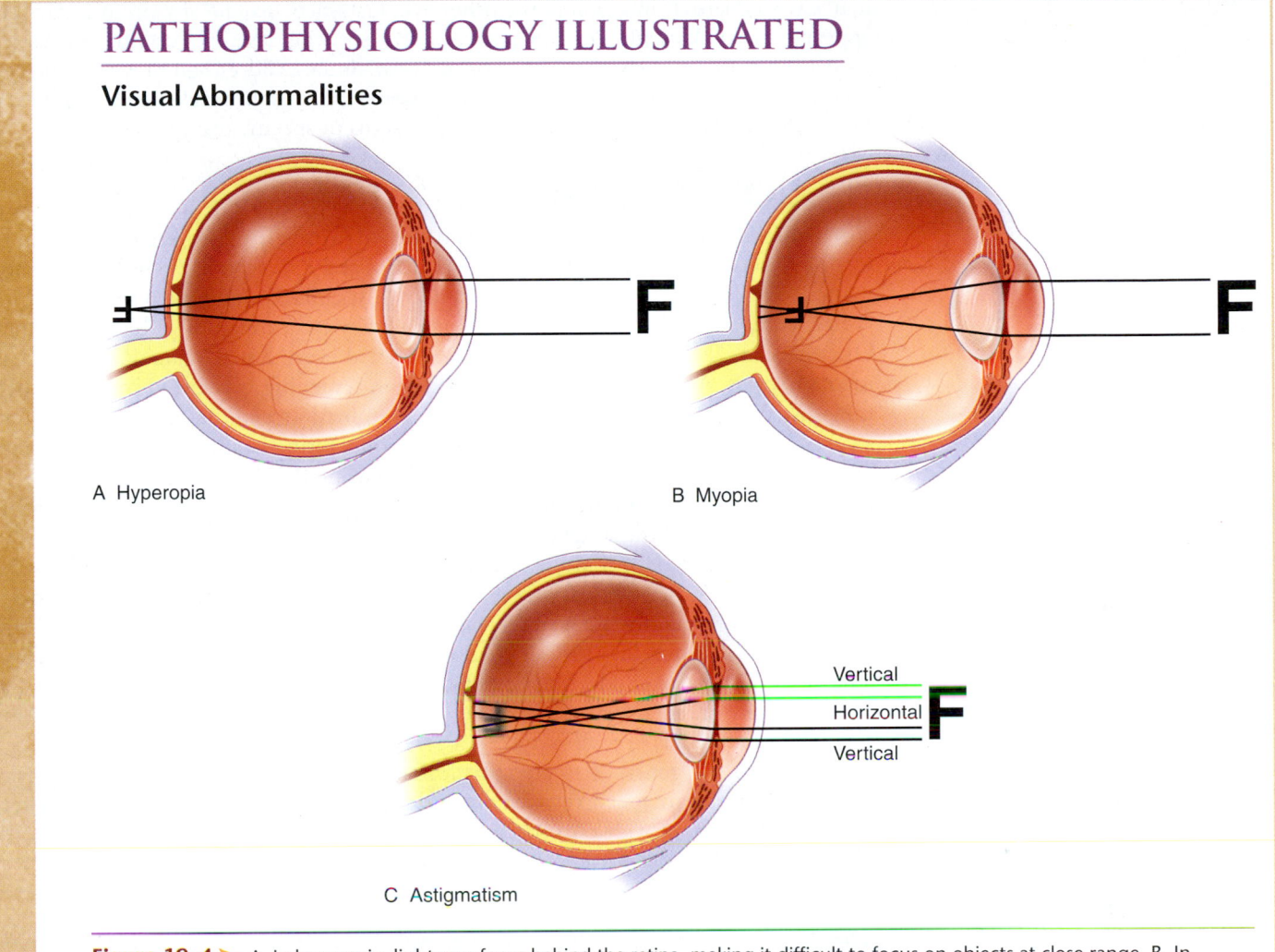

A Hyperopia

B Myopia

C Astigmatism

Figure 19–4 ➤ A, In hyperopia, light rays focus behind the retina, making it difficult to focus on objects at close range. B, In myopia, light rays focus in front of the retina, making it difficult to focus on objects that are far away. C, In astigmatism, light rays do not uniformly focus on the eye due to abnormal curvature of cornea or lens.

- *Astigmatism.* Light rays are refracted differently depending on their place of entry to the eye. The curvature of the cornea or lens is not uniformly spherical, causing blurred images. The child with astigmatism often holds pages very close to the face to obtain the best visual image.

Other common visual disorders in children are characterized by abnormal musculature that causes asymmetric eye movement and by other anatomic abnormalities. They include:

- Strabismus
- Amblyopia
- Cataracts
- Glaucoma
- Retinoblastoma

Strabismus, amblyopia, cataracts, and glaucoma are described in the Clinical Manifestations of Visual Disorders table on pages 639–640, while retinoblastoma is discussed in Chapter 23 ∞.

Clinical Manifestations

Children with eye abnormalities may demonstrate a variety of behaviors. An infant who notices objects only on one side or consistently holds the head more to one side may have a decrease in vision in the other eye. Cataracts may be visualized as the lens appears cloudy. Muscular problems may be evident when the eyes do not move symmetrically or one eye deviates inward or outward. Some children squint, cover one eye, hold toys or books close to the face, or have watering eyes. See the clinical manifestations table on the following pages for further signs of specific disorders.

■ COLLABORATIVE CARE

Visual disturbances must be diagnosed and treated promptly to prevent impairment or loss of visual acuity (Centers for Disease Control and Prevention, 2004; U.S. Department of Health and Human Services, 2000). Most children undergo a simple test for visual acuity during healthcare visits as soon as they can cooperate with the examiner. Once in school, children's visual acuity is screened every 2 to 3 years during the elementary years. A child who does not pass vision screening is referred to an ophthalmologist or optometrist for more detailed examination of near and far vision, eye structure and movement, and color discrimination. During health promotion visits, infants and young children should be examined by using the cover-uncover test, and the red reflex should be examined with an ophthalmoscope. See Chapter 5 ∞ for thorough descriptions of these tests.

Compensatory lenses are prescribed for many visual disorders, particularly refractive disorders. See the section on visual impairment later in this chapter for more details. A significant difference in visual acuity between the eyes is often a result of amblyopia or strabismus, and further treatment by patching or surgery may be needed. The visual acuity of a child with compensatory lenses should be reevaluated every 1 to 2 years. More frequent visits to an eye specialist are needed when a child is being treated for amblyopia or strabismus.

Cataracts are generally treated surgically with removal of the lens, placement of lens transplant, or use of corrective contact lenses. Glaucoma frequently requires surgery in children to provide outflow for fluid and resultant decrease in intraocular pressure. A variety of cancers are treated with surgery and chemotherapy.

■ NURSING MANAGEMENT

The nurse plays an important role in identifying eye disorders in children. Ask questions that will help to identify the child with a decrease in visual acuity (Table 19–2). You will perform careful eye examinations of newborns and children. Observe for symmetry of placement and movement, ability to follow objects with each eye, and any abnormalities in appearance. The corneal light reflex, cover-uncover test, and visual acuity testing are essential tests for every child. See Chapter 5 ∞ for a description of eye examination and the *Clinical Skills Manual* for visual acuity tests. Vision screening should be conducted at birth and at all well-child visits (Ottar-Pfeifer, 2005).

Nurses in schools also plan and carry out regular visual acuity screening on children. Generally certain grades (such as kindergarten, 2, 5, and 8) are screened annually along with any children new to a district. The nurse performs and records the screening results, and informs the school and families of any children with abnormal results who are referred to an eye specialist for care. An important part of the screening process is following up on referrals to be certain that children receive the diagnostic care they need. (See Chapter 11 ∞.)

When abnormalities are found on screening, nurses refer families to the care of an eye specialist. When prescriptive lenses are used, the nurse instructs the parent and child on correct wear practices and care. If surgery is needed, surgical and postoperative follow-up are needed, including pain control, observing for signs of infection (ophthalmic or systemic), and administering needed eye medications. Sterile technique is used postoperatively to provide eye care. Promptly report deviations from normal such as increased pain, redness, discharge, or edema of the eye; increased temperature

NURSING ALERT

Some youth are using decorative contact lenses and some even "trade" their lenses with other youth. Contact lenses should only be prescribed and fitted by a qualified eye professional. There have been reports of bacterial conjunctivitis, corneal damage, and allergic reactions to cosmetic lenses. The U.S. Food and Drug Administration (FDA) has issued a press release about the dangers of improperly obtained lenses.

CLINICAL MANIFESTATIONS | VISUAL DISORDERS

Etiology	Clinical Manifestations	Clinical Therapy
Strabismus Can be congenital or acquired. Seen in 5% of all children Most common types: Esotropia: inward deviation of eyes ("crossed eyes") Exotropia: outward deviation of eyes ("wall-eyes")	Eyes appear misaligned to observer. May occur only when child is tired. Symptoms include squinting and frowning when reading; closing one eye to see; having trouble picking up objects; dizziness and headache. Corneal light reflex and cover-uncover tests confirm diagnosis. Child may have no other abnormalities but certain conditions such as cerebral palsy, hydrocephalus, Down syndrome, and seizure disorder are more commonly accompanied by strabismus.	Occlusion therapy (patching the fixating or good eye to force use of the weak eye) Compensatory lenses Surgery of the rectus muscles to correct muscle imbalance Eyedrops to cause blurring of the good eye Prisms Vision therapy (eye exercise) If treatment is begun before 24 months of age, amblyopia (reduced vision in one or both eyes) may be prevented.

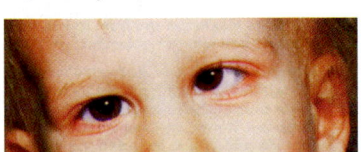

Strabismus.
Reprinted from Paediatrics, *2e, Thomas & Harvey, p. 130, 1997, by permission of the publisher Churchill Livingstone.*

Etiology	Clinical Manifestations	Clinical Therapy
Amblyopia ("lazy eye") Reduced vision in one or both eyes; affects 7% of children. Amblyopia can result from anything that causes visual deprivation to one eye. The most common causes are untreated strabismus, with the child "tuning out" the image in deviating eye, congenital cataract, or visual differences between eyes.	Symptoms are the same as for strabismus. Vision testing can be used to diagnose condition.	Compensatory lenses Occlusion therapy for 2–6 hours daily Occasionally vision therapy (eye exercises) is used in an attempt to improve the weaker eye. Atropine 1% 1 gtt/day in unaffected eye. Treatment is discontinued when visual acuity no longer improves; 20/20 acuity rarely attained. Treatment is most successful if received by 5–6 years of age.
Cataracts Occur when all or part of the lens of the eye becomes opaque, which prevents refraction of light rays onto the retina Seen in 1 of every 250 newborns	Can affect one or both eyes and may be congenital or acquired. Clouding of lens indicates presence of cataract, however, cataracts are not always visible to naked eye. Symptoms include distorted red reflex, symptoms of vision loss (see strabismus), white pupil. May be present alone but sometimes associated with fetal alcohol syndrome and Down syndrome.	Must be diagnosed at a young age for successful treatment; many cases are missed. Specific treatment depends on whether one or both eyes are affected, extent of clouding, and presence of other ocular abnormalities. Surgical removal of lens and corrective lenses; contact lenses frequently used; results of surgery are good; surgery before the age of 2 months is associated with the best results; visual acuity in 55% of children is 20/40 or better. Lens implant may be used. Eye protectors and restrains are used postoperatively to prevent injury; antibiotic or steroid drops may be used for several weeks; treatment for amblyopia may be necessary.

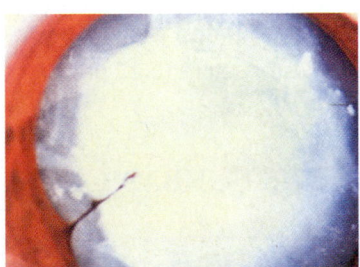

Congenital cataract.
From Vaughan, D., Asbury, T., & Riordan-Eva, P. (1992). General ophthalmology *(13th ed., p. 172). New York: McGraw-Hill Companies.*

Etiology	Clinical Manifestations	Clinical Therapy
Glaucoma Increased intraocular pressure damages eye and impairs visual function; ciliary body of eye produces aqueous fluid that flows between iris and lens into anterior chamber; if enough fluid accumulates, blindness results; affects 1 in 100,000 newborns.	Symptoms of congenital glaucoma include tearing, blinking, corneal clouding, eyelid spasms, and progressive enlargement of eye; photophobia (extreme sensitivity to light). Symptoms of acquired glaucoma include constant bumping into objects in child's periphery (painless visual field loss); seeing halos around objects.	Surgery to reduce intraocular pressure is treatment of choice, since medications used to combat glaucoma in adults are not as effective in children. Compensatory lenses used following surgery.

(continued)

Etiology	Clinical Manifestations	Clinical Therapy
May be congenital (primary) or acquired (secondary) and affect one or both eyes.	Diagnosis is made using tonometer, which measures intraocular pressure.	Treatment is not always successful, especially if the child has congenital glaucoma, so parents' feelings regarding care of a visually handicapped child should be explored.

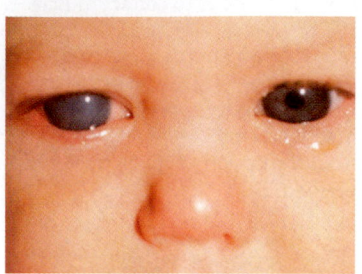

Congenital glaucoma.
From Vaughan, D., Asbury, T. & Riordan-Eva, P. (1992) General ophthalmology. *(13th ed., p. 172). New York: McGraw-Hill Companies.*

Data from Alterneier W. A. (2000). Preschool vision screening: The importance of the two-line difference. *Pediatric Annals, 29,* 264–267; Bacal, D. A., & Wilson, M. C. (2000). Strabismus: Getting it straight. *Contemporary Pediatrics, 17,* 49–60; Start, N.B. (2000). Vision therapy for learning disabilities and dyslexia. *Journal of Pediatric Health Care, 14,* 32–33.

SKILLS 6–18 AND 6–19
Visual Acuity Screening

or pulse, which may indicate infection; increased sensitivity to light; or other abnormalities. Children are usually discharged home with instructions to minimize certain vigorous activities for a certain period of time. Perform postoperative and discharge teaching and emphasize the importance of follow-up visits.

Color Blindness

Color blindness is an X-linked recessive disorder found in 10% of males and less than 0.05% of females (Swanson & Cohen, 2003). The most common form affects the ability to distinguish between the colors red and green, but there are other variations. Preschool boys are tested for color blindness in some clinics to identify those with the disorder. The Ishihara color blindness test is often used and consists of numbers embedded in a background that are difficult for a person with color blindness to see. Color blindness is not treatable and management focuses on issues of safety (e.g., problems

Table 19–2	ASSESSMENT QUESTIONS FOR IDENTIFYING VISUAL DISTURBANCES IN CHILDREN

Infant	Young Child	School-Age Child
Ask the parents: Does your baby follow an object from one side to the other? What is your baby's reaction when you are directly in front and close? Does the baby seem to notice an object to the right and left sides? Do your baby's eyes ever appear to move asymmetrically? What is your baby learning to do right now?	Ask the parents: Does your child follow you with his or her eyes as you come into a room? Are other objects followed with ease? Do both eyes work together or does one seem to wander off? At what age did your baby sit, stand, walk? Does your child have any difficulty picking up objects?	Ask the parents: Does your child like to look at pictures and read? Does your child hold toys or books close, or sit very close to the television? Does your child squint or rub the eyes? Is he or she performing at grade level in all subjects? Has your child demonstrated any learning difficulties? Does he or she use a computer, watch television, or play computer games? Does your child play sports and games at the same level of ability as peers?

in distinguishing red–green traffic signals) and techniques to improve discrimination of colors in the affected color groups.

Retinopathy of Prematurity

Retinopathy of prematurity (ROP) occurs when immature blood vessels in the retina constrict and become necrotic. This condition, which may occur in infants of low birth weight or of short gestation, can heal completely or lead to mild myopia or retinal detachment and blindness.

Etiology and Pathophysiology

Retinopathy of prematurity results from injury to the developing capillaries of the retina. Oxygen therapy is associated with the development of ROP (Figure 19–5 ➤), but other factors such as respiratory distress, mechanical ventilation, apnea, bradycardia, heart disease, multiple blood transfusions, infection, hypoxia, hypercarbia, acidosis, shock, and sepsis have also been linked with the disorder. Cerebral palsy is sometimes an associated factor and more cases are seen in multiple births. It is most common in infants born before 28 weeks' gestation and weighing under 1600 g (3 lb, 8 oz) at birth. A genetic link may be present as White infants are more commonly affected than those of African heritage, and Alaska Natives have a high rate of the disorder. In developed countries ROP is the second most common cause of blindness, occurring in 12.5% of infants born from 23–26 weeks' gestation (Tasman, Patz, McNamara et al., 2006; Wheatley, Dickinson, Mackey, Craig, & Sale, 2002).

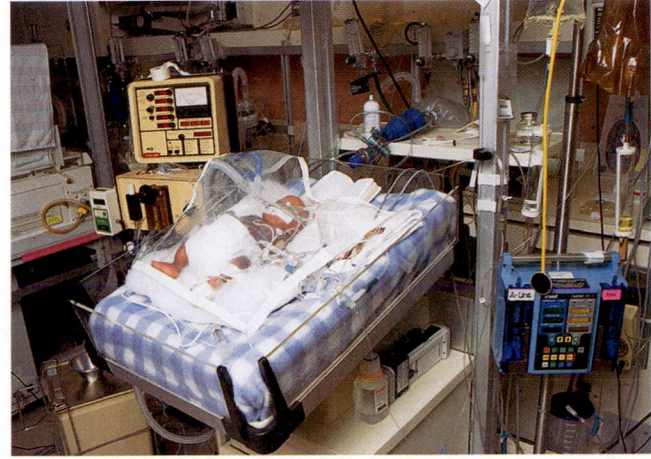

Figure 19–5 ➤ This premature infant in the neonatal intensive care unit is receiving artificial ventilation—a risk factor for retinopathy of prematurity. The infant will need careful management of oxygen exposure and periodic eye examinations.

The retina is normally vascularized by about 8 months' gestation. For the premature infant, however, this process must continue after birth. The environmental and other conditions listed in the preceding paragraph appear to affect its course. Arteriole constriction, followed by vascular proliferation of abnormal vessels, occurs. In most cases, the abnormal vessels gradually regress and normal vascularization takes place. Sometimes, however, the abnormal vascularization continues into the vitreous cavity, causing abnormalities of the retina, optic disc, and macula. It is not known why the disease progresses in some cases, but progression is directly linked to lower birth weight, greater prematurity, and duration (not necessarily concentration) of oxygen therapy.

Although the developing capillaries are lost, in up to 90% of cases some degree of revascularization occurs later (Tasman et al., 2006). The degree of visual loss, varying from slight to total, is determined by the degree of revascularization that occurs.

Clinical Manifestations

Retinopathy of prematurity is characterized by progressive changes in the retinal blood vessels, and, in severe disease, by retinal detachment. Premature and low-birth-weight infants at risk for the disease are given frequent ocular examinations to ensure early detection of these changes. For infants who do not receive ophthalmologic examinations, the resulting visual impairment may be detected only later in infancy when the child progresses slowly in meeting developmental milestones, fails to reach for objects, and does not follow objects or faces with the eyes. When visual impairment is present, the child usually manifests myopia. Total loss of vision can occur in the child who suffers a retinal detachment.

■ COLLABORATIVE CARE

Diagnostic Tests

Diagnosis is made by ophthalmologic examination. A classification system is used to describe the location, extent, and severity of the disease (American Academy of Pediatrics, Section on Ophthalmology, 2001; Tasman et al., 2006). See Table 19–3. All infants at risk, particularly those under 2000 g (4 lb, 3 oz) at birth or born before 33 weeks' gestation,

Table 19–3	DIAGNOSIS OF RETINOPATHY OF PREMATURITY

Zone (Area of Retina Involved with Abnormal Vasculature)	Stage (Severity of ROP Wherever It Is Present)	Plus Disease (Vascular Dilation and Tortuosity Is Noted in Posterior Pole in Area Near Optic Nerve)	Threshold (Measure of Severity of Disease; Used to Judge When Treatment Is Needed)
Zone I (most posterior and near optic nerve head)	Stage 1 (line divides vascular and avascular retina)	Presence	Threshold I (stage 3 ROP in Zone I or II and five continuous or eight cumulative "clock hour" areas with plus disease; treatment is required)
Zone II (outside or area anterior to Zone I)	Stage 2 (line of demarcation is elevated)	Absence	
Zone III (only present on temporal side of eye; nasal quadrants are adequately vascularized)	Stage 3 (New vascularization is present in the demarcation area)		

Data from Good, W. V., & Gendron, R. L. (2001). Retinopathy of prematurity. Ophthalmology Clinics of North America, 14, 513–519.

RESEARCH

Retinopathy of Prematurity and Reduction of Light Exposure

Several groups have studied whether retinopathy of prematurity is associated with exposure to bright lights in neonatal intensive care units. It has been hypothesized that since babies would normally be in a dark womb and their retinal vessels are still developing, damage might be done by environmental light. In a meta-analysis of five studies, pooled data provided no support for this hypothesis. Placing premature infants in goggles or other eye covers does not appear to lower the incidence of retinopathy of prematurity (Phelps & Watts, 2003). Goggles may have other benefits such as helping the infant to sleep better, and they are also routinely used during treatment of hyperbilirubinemia by light therapy.

are assessed frequently by an ophthalmologist who is experienced with the condition. The disease does not manifest itself before 4 to 6 weeks after birth, so it is important that the infant receive regular eye examinations until the risk is discounted. If the infant shows signs of disease, eye examinations continue every 1 to 2 weeks. Involvement of blood vessels in the periphery of the retina rarely leads to visual impairment. With involvement in other areas of the retina, risk of visual problems is more common (Quinn, 2005).

Clinical Therapy

Treatment of infants with severe retinopathy of prematurity involves using cryotherapy or laser therapy to stop progression of the disease process. Other surgical procedures such as a scleral buckle procedure and vitrectomy have been used in retinal detachments. Associated problems such as strabismus, amblyopia, and myopia should be managed to promote maximal development.

NURSING MANAGEMENT

Nursing Assessment and Diagnosis

Assessment of the infant at risk for retinopathy of prematurity begins at birth by identification of infants who may require oxygen therapy. Look for risk factors such as prematurity and low birth weight. Assess the infant's breathing efforts and report any changes. Be certain the ventilation equipment is properly set to deliver the correct amount of oxygen. Ventilatory equipment is meticulously monitored. The nurse weans the infant from oxygen as indicated by an oxygen saturation reading in concordance with standing orders in the neonatal intensive care unit. Note the cumulative risks in a particular case (longer exposure to oxygen increases risk) and ensure referral to an ophthalmologist for evaluation and monitoring.

The accompanying Nursing Care Plan outlines several nursing diagnoses for a child with a visual impairment secondary to retinopathy of prematurity. Following are other nursing diagnoses that may be appropriate for an infant with the potential to develop ROP or a child with resulting visual impairment:

- Sensory/Perceptual Alteration (Visual) related to altered transmission of impulses

- Potential Impaired Gas Exchange related to ventilation-perfusion imbalance
- Delayed Growth and Development related to effects of visual impairment
- Altered Family Processes related to a child with a visual impairment

Planning and Implementation

The nurse plays an important role in preventing retinopathy of prematurity. Encourage early and regular prenatal care to prevent unnecessary premature births. Administer oxygen only to newborns who need it, and in the amount specified by the physician. Ensure that the proper ventilatory settings are used. Be alert for infants with multiple risk factors and refer them, when appropriate, for ophthalmologic examination. Parents of infants at risk for ROP require information about the disorder, as well as support, as the long-term effects on the child's vision are often identified only after subsequent examinations as the child grows. Families may be frustrated that a prognosis cannot be made at the time of the first eye examination. Explanations and consistent updates on the infant's condition can be reassuring.

The accompanying Nursing Care Plan summarizes care for the child with a visual impairment resulting from retinopathy of prematurity. The nurse is instrumental in case management for such children. Reinforce to parents the importance of follow-up eye examinations. Teach methods of stimulating development for the visually impaired child (refer to the next section).

Evaluation

Expected outcomes of nursing care for the child with retinopathy of prematurity include:

- Visual impairment will be identified early in the child's life and an intervention program will be established.
- The child will achieve normal developmental milestones. The child's visual condition will be effectively managed by the family.

Visual Impairment

Low vision, or the inability to correct vision to a normal level, is present in 1.2 to 1.4 children per 1000 (Centers for Disease Control and Prevention, 2004). Amblyopia is the most common cause of low vision in children, affecting 2–3% of children (Hartmann, Bradford, Chaplin et al., 2006). While overall 2.5% of children have visual impairment or blindness, the rate rises to 3.3% for children from 6–17 years of age. There is considerable ethnic disparity as 3.6% of Hispanic children, 2.6% of Black children, and 2.3% of non-Hispanic White children are affected by visual impairment (MMWR, 2005).

Many conditions discussed earlier in this chapter lead to temporary or permanent visual impairment. Infants who are premature; whose mothers were infected prenatally with rubella, toxoplasmosis, or other viruses; and who have certain congenital and hereditary conditions have a high risk of visual problems (Table 19–4). Fetal alcohol syndrome (FAS) is a major cause of visual disturbance; see Chapter 27 ∞ for a further description of FAS.

The signs of visual impairment depend on the cause and degree of the problem and the age of the child (Table 19–5). The child's eyes may appear crossed or watery, and the lids may be crusty. Verbal children may complain of itching; dizziness; headache; or blurred, double, or poor vision.

■ COLLABORATIVE CARE

The American Optometric Association and American Public Health Association recommend comprehensive vision examination starting at 6 months of age, while the American Academy of Ophthalmology and American Academy of Pediatrics recommend screening by 3 years of age (Center for Health and Health Care in Schools, 2004). The United States Preventive Services Task Force (USPSTF) recommends

NURSING CARE PLAN The Child with a Visual Impairment Secondary to Retinopathy of Prematurity

GOAL	INTERVENTION	RATIONALE	EXPECTED OUTCOME
1. Disturbed Visual Sensory Perception related to altered reception, transmission, and integration resulting from retinopathy of prematurity			
	NIC Priority Intervention: **Visual Deficit Enhancement:** *Assistance in accepting and learning alternate methods for living with diminished vision.*		*NOC Suggested Outcome:* **Developmental Progression:** *Compensate for sensory deficits by maximizing use of impaired senses.*
The child will receive adequate sensory input	• Provide kinesthetic, tactile, and auditory stimulation during play and in daily care (e.g., talking and playing). Provide music while bathing an infant using bells and other noises on each side of infant. Verbally describe to a child all actions being carried out by adult.	• Because visual sensory input is not present, the child needs input from all other senses to compensate and provide adequate sensory stimulation.	The child demonstrates minimal signs of sensory deprivation.
2. Risk for Injury related to impaired vision			
	NIC Priority Intervention: **Fall Prevention:** *Instituting special precautions with patients at risk for injury.*		*NOC Suggested Outcome:* **Risk Control:** *Actions to eliminate or reduce modifiable health threats.*
The child will be protected from safety hazards that can lead to injury.	• Evaluate environment for potential safety hazards based on age of child and degree of impairment. Be particularly alert to objects that give visual cues to their dangers (e.g., stoves, fireplaces, candles). Eliminate safety hazards and protect the child from exposure. Take the child on a tour of new rooms (e.g., schools, hotel room, hospital room).	• The child may be at risk for injury related both to developmental stage and inability to visualize hazards.	The child will experience no injuries.
3. Risk for Altered Growth and Development related to Impaired vision			
	NIC Priority Intervention: **Developmental Enhancement:** *Facilitating or teaching parents and caregivers to facilitate optional growth and development of children.*		*NOC Suggested Outcome:* **Child Growth and Development:** *Milestones of developmental progression.*
The child has experiences necessary to foster normal growth and development.	• Help parents plan early, regular social activities with other children. • Provide opportunities and encourage self-feeding activities. • Provide an environment rich in sensory input. • Assess growth and development during regular examinations to identify the child's strengths and needs.	• The visually impaired child benefits developmentally from contact with other children. • To obtain adequate nutrients, the child needs to feel comfortable feeding self. • Sensory input is needed for normal development to occur. • Regular examinations aid in early identification of growth problems or developmental delays, so that appropriate interventions can be planned.	The child demonstrates normal growth and development milestones.

NURSING CARE PLAN — The Child with a Visual Impairment Secondary to Retinopathy of Prematurity

GOAL	INTERVENTION	RATIONALE	EXPECTED OUTCOME
4. Risk for Compromised Family Coping related to child's prolonged disability from sensory impairment			
	NIC Priority Intervention: **Family Mobilization:** *Utilization of family strengths to influence child's health positively.*		*NOC Suggested Outcome:* **Positive Coping:** *Extent to which family can mobilize resources to deal with the child's needs.*
The family identifies methods for coping with their visually impaired child.	• Provide explanation of visual impairment as appropriate. • Refer parents to organizations, early intervention programs, and other parents of visually impaired children. • Assist parents to plan for meeting developmental, educational, and safety needs of their visually impaired child. Offer resources for changing home environment to assist visually impaired child.	• The parents may feel guilt about the child's visual impairment, which can be allayed by knowledge of the cause. • The parents will receive needed information and support from others. • The child may require an enhanced environment in order to foster developmental progress.	The family successfully copes with the experience of having a visually impaired child.

Table 19–4   COMMON CAUSES OF VISUAL IMPAIRMENT IN CHILDREN

Congenital or Hereditary
• Cataracts
• Glaucoma
• Tay-Sachs disease
• Marfan syndrome
• Down syndrome
• Fetal alcohol syndrome
• Prenatal infections (maternal infection)
  • Rubella
  • Toxoplasmosis
  • Herpes simplex
• Retinoblastoma

Acquired
• Injury to eye or head
• Infections
  • Rubella
  • Measles
  • Chickenpox
• Brain tumor
• Retinopathy of prematurity
• Cerebral palsy

Table 19–5   SIGNS OF VISUAL IMPAIRMENT

Infants
• May be unable to follow lights or objects
• Do not make eye contact
• Have a dull, vacant stare
• Do not imitate facial expressions

Toddlers and Older Children
• May rub, shut, or cover eyes
• Tilt or thrust head forward
• Blink frequently
• Hold objects close
• Bump into objects
• Squint

screening to detect amblyopia, strabismus, and defects in visual acuity in children younger than 5 years (United States Preventive Services Task Force, 2004). Despite differences in recommendations, it is clear that all young children should have vision examinations in order to identify vision problems early in life.

Clinical therapy depends on the child's condition and may include surgery, medication, and supportive aids. In the case of a disorder that results in permanent visual impairment, an interdisciplinary team of specialists works with the child and family. Nurses have an important role in this team, collaborating with not only families but with other healthcare professionals to plan appropriate interventions.

NURSING MANAGEMENT
Nursing Assessment and Diagnosis

Prevention of low vision, early identification of the condition, and interventions to enhance development of children with low vision provide the focus for nursing care. (See Evidence-Based Practice: Nursing Role in Vision Screening and Follow-up.) Vision screening facilitates early detection and treatment of conditions that can lead to vision loss. Visual testing can be done at any age, including immediately after birth. Developmental milestones that require vision, such as following bright lights, reaching for objects, or looking at pictures in a book, can be used to assess vision. For children over the age of 3 years, visual acuity is most frequently measured by means of an age-appropriate acuity test (see Chapter 5 ∞ and the *Clinical Skills Manual*). The photoscreener is a device that can be used to take a photo of the child's eyes and is useful for infants, toddlers, and preschoolers. The photo can be used to diagnose refraction errors, eye opacities, and misalignment (Donahue, Baker, Scott et al., 2006). Visual fields and the ability to discriminate colors are tested at school age, when children can cooperate.

EVIDENCE-BASED PRACTICE

Nursing Role in Vision Screening and Follow-up

Problem/Clinical Question

Screening for visual ability is important in order to identify children with impairments. The American Academy of Pediatrics recommends that children be screened at every well-child visit, beginning in the newborn period, to include vision history, vision assessment, external inspection of the eyes and lids, eye movement assessment, pupil examination, and elicitation of red reflex. Once the child can cooperate, usually by about 3 years, a vision test such as HOTV or tumbling E, along with ophthalmoscopic examination, should be added to the examination (American Academy of Pediatrics, Committee on Practice and Ambulatory Medicine, 2003; U.S. Preventive Services Task Force, 2005). Nurses are often the health professionals that conduct vision examinations, evaluate results, and provide follow-up care. They participate in well-child health visits and often perform assessments of vision in schools. What evidence is available to assist nurses in this important role?

Evidence

A study of 1677 children in preschool, kindergarten, and first grade applied the HOTV acuity test and two types of photoscreening devices. (See the *Clinical Skills Manual* for a further description of these types of screening.) Photoscreening was found to be significantly more effective in identifying children with visual impairment, and was faster to perform (Leman, Clausen, Bates et al., 2006).

Once visual impairment is identified, an essential nursing role is to refer for appropriate care and to follow-up to determine if that care is received. A study attempted to determine the contributing factors to lack of follow-up care after a failed vision screening. An interview was conducted with 66 families who had a child referred for eye examination after school screening. The researchers found that 85% of the families had low incomes. The barriers to eye care they identified included financial reasons, logistical problems (no ability to get to appointments), social or family issues (large family with adults all working or recent change in residence), and perceptual barriers (did not believe results or perceive the importance of the referral) (Kimel, 2006). Another study focused on the school nurse-to-student ratio and its influence on care for students. While the National Association of School Nurses recommends a ratio of 1 nurse for 750 students, many schools do not achieve that recommendation. The schools in the study had ratios of 1:451 to 1:7440. While student vision screening and referral rates were similar for all of the schools, the schools with lower ratios (less students served per nurse) had significantly greater numbers of referred students who received further care (Guttu, Engelke, & Swanson, 2004).

Implications

Nurses play a vital role in ensuring that children receive early, periodic, and regular visual and eye screening. Evidence that suggests the most accurate methods should be closely examined. Photoscreening machines represent an important new addition to the tools that nurses can use. While identification of problems is important, the nursing roles of referral for care, identifying barriers to care, and ensuring that follow-up care has been received are also integral to vision care.

Critical Thinking

What vision screening methods are available in the offices, clinics, and schools in your community? How could you perform vision screening in the hospital setting if a child did not demonstrate expected visual ability for age? Design a follow-up program for a school that screens all kindergarten and first graders for visual acuity. What questions will you ask parents during a well-child visit for a 2-year-old to determine if vision is normal? How will you combine your knowledge of developmental milestones with screening for vision?

References

American Academy of Pediatrics, Committee on Practice and Ambulatory Medicine, Section on Ophthalmology. (2003). Eye examination in infants, children, and young adults by pediatricians. *Pediatrics, 111*, 902–907.

Guttu, M., Engelke, M. K., & Swanson, M. (2004). Does the school nurse-to-student ratio make a difference? *Journal of School Health, 74*, 6–9.

Kimel, L. S. (2006). Lack of follow-up exams after failed school vision screenings: An investigation of contributing factors. *Journal of School Nursing, 22*, 156–162.

Leman, R., Clausen, M. M., Bates, J., Stark, L., Arnold, K. K., & Arnold, R. W. (2006). A comparison of patched HOTV visual acuity and photoscreening. *Journal of School Nursing, 22*, 237–243.

U.S. Preventive Services Task Force. (2005). Screening for visual impairment in children younger than five years: Recommendation statement. *American Family Physician, 71*, 333–336.

Children who are visually impaired may lag in development of cognitive and other skills. Sighted children learn the word *cup* using four senses—sight, touch, hearing, and taste—to obtain the information necessary to connect words with the objects they represent. In contrast, children with visual impairments rely on only three senses—touch, hearing, and taste. They learn concepts through differences in sounds, textures, and shapes. Many visual disorders are linked with conditions that influence development. Thus, a child with cerebral palsy or fetal alcohol syndrome should be assessed frequently to identify a visual disorder, as well as to evaluate normal developmental milestones.

Nursing diagnoses for the child with impaired vision may include the following:

- Disturbed Sensory Alteration (Visual) related to altered sensory perception
- Risk for Injury related to poor vision
- Risk for Delayed Growth and Development related to visual impairment
- Risk for Ineffective Family Coping related to demands of a child with a sensory impairment

Planning and Implementation

The first intervention used by nurses in all settings is prevention of visual impairment when possible, both in children with normal sight and those with some visual impairment in order to prevent further damage. Teach safety in activities that can injure the eye. Encourage protective eyewear in sports such as hockey, handball, and football. Work with school personnel to establish guidelines for protective eyewear for chemistry or other science or industrial education courses that may present a risk to eyes. Keep laser pointers away from children since they can cause retinal damage, especially when stared at for 10 seconds. Young children do not blink as often as adults or older children and so are at greater risk of retinal damage from lasers.

Several interaction strategies can be used by nurses who work with visually impaired children. Nursing care focuses on encouraging the child's use of all senses, promoting socialization, helping parents to meet the child's developmental and educational needs, and providing emotional support to parents. Refer the parents to an early intervention program upon diagnosis. Be sure that a regular series of developmental screenings is performed either in the early intervention program or during healthcare visits. Developmental screening should be done about every 2 months during infancy, and every 6 months from 1 to 5 years. As the child grows, assess for physical activity, since children with visual impairment are less likely than sighted children to achieve physical activity milestones. Suggest exercise that is safe and continues to challenge physical development. Dancing, balance and coordination activities, as well as running, can all be encouraged. Nearly all care will occur in community and home settings.

Encourage Use of All Senses

Children who are partially sighted or blind use other senses to a great extent. Encouraging the use of the eyes as much as possible is important even if a child has poor vision (Figure 19–6 ➤). See Families Want to Know: Enhancing Development of the Visually Impaired Child.

Promote Socialization

The child's interactions and socializations should be as normal as possible (similar to those of sighted children of the same age and development).

- Stroke, rock, and hug infants and children who are visually impaired. Sing and talk to them. These infants do not make eye contact and have rather blank expressions.
- Teach parents to read body language and vocalization as expressions of emotion. Facial expressions give a great deal of information, but infants and children with poor vision do not have the ability to learn by visual imitation. Show parents how to use tactile means to teach appropriate facial expressions. For example, a touch on the arm can be soft and stroking to indicate a smile, but firmer to indicate dismay or frown.

GROWTH & DEVELOPMENT

Visual Impairment

Infants with visual impairment use kinesthesia, touch, and language to socialize. They will appreciate and use touch more than other children and will respond to verbal explanations when others use nonverbal communication. Vision affects both fine and gross motor skills, so skills such as hand-to-mouth coordination and walking may be delayed in children who are visually impaired.

CLINICAL TIP

Strategies for nurses working with visually impaired children:

- Call the child's name and speak before touching the child.
- Tell the child when you are leaving the room.
- Describe what each procedure will feel like (e.g., blood pressure cuff, otoscope).
- Let the child touch the equipment to establish familiarity.
- Describe what foods are present and their locations on the food tray.

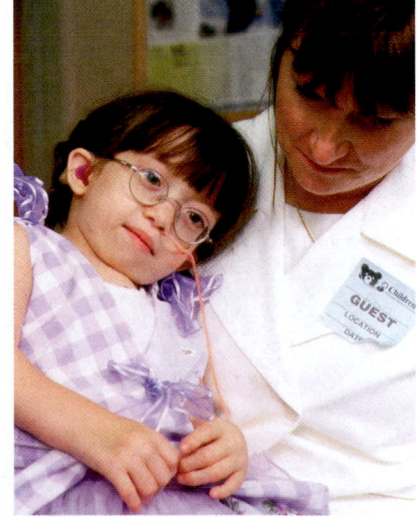

Figure 19–6 ➤ This child with a visual impairment needs ongoing developmental assessment and a comprehensive Individualized Education Plan. As is true with many children, she has several healthcare needs. Note that she is receiving tube feedings.

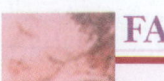

FAMILIES WANT TO KNOW

Enhancing Development of the Visually Impaired Child

- Encourage a toddler or preschooler who is visually impaired to look at pictures in well-lit settings. Have a school-age child read large-print books. Computers designed for the visually impaired are also available. The Optacon (a device that raises print so it can be felt by the child) and View Scan (which magnifies print) are instruments that improve the ability to read.
- Expose the infant and child to everyday sounds.
- Encourage the infant to use the sense of touch to explore people and objects. Have the parents purchase toys with sound and texture in mind. Directional concepts can be taught using games. Responding to the infant's and child's vocalizations encourages the use of speech.
- Teach specific techniques for toileting, dressing, bathing, eating, and safety.
- When the child becomes mobile, furniture and other objects in the environment should be kept in the same positions so the

child can safely move around independently. Extra care must be taken to prevent injuries when a child does not see.
- Emphasize the child's abilities. Adolescents can use seeing-eye dogs or a white cane to function independently.
- Encourage the child to function independently within normal developmental parameters.
- If in the hospital or another strange environment, orient the child to the placement of objects and do not rearrange them.
- Teach those around the child to:
  - Announce their presence to the child when approaching.
  - When walking with a blind child, walk slightly ahead of the child so he or she can sense your movements.
  - Let the child hold the seeing person's arm rather than the reverse.
  - Identify the contents of meals and encourage the child to feed self.

CLINICAL TIP

Clean the child's glasses daily with warm water and a clean, soft dry cloth. Follow the prescriber's and family's directions for care of contact lenses. General guidelines include:
- Allow the child to wear the lenses for the recommended time only.
- Store each lens in the right or left containers as labeled.
- Wash hands carefully before contact with the child's eyes or lenses.
- Use a cleaning solution on the lens after its removal.
- Rinse the lens with the recommended rinsing solution.
- Keep the lenses in the case with the disinfecting solution.
- Note on the chart that the child wears lenses.

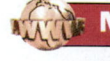

MediaLink

Resources for the Visually Impaired

- Explain to parents that discipline and rewards for children with poor vision should be the same as those for other children in the family. The child should be given age-appropriate tasks.
- Encourage contact with peers as the child grows older. Teach the child to look directly at persons who are talking to him or her. Play, sports, and other activities can be modified to give the visually impaired child the same social experiences as a sighted child.
- Foster physical activity for children with visual impairment by encouraging involvement in early intervention programs; recommending programs that increase cardiovascular strength, endurance, upper body strength, and flexibility; and facilitating participation in and reward for sports and athletics.

Care in the Community

Public laws require that each state provide educational and related services for children with disabilities (see Chapter 11 ∞). Parents and professionals should develop an Individualized Education Plan (as discussed in Chapter 11) that maximizes the child's learning ability. If possible, the child with a vision problem should attend childcare and preschool with children who have normal visual acuity. While some developmental skills such as feeding and dressing may develop slower than in sighted children, plans for encouraging development tailored to the child's needs can assist in learning skills. Provide parents with information about educational options before their child reaches school age. Education should take place in a setting that allows the child to have contact with other children and to participate in social activities. Familiarize the child with each new environment and allow time for adjustment. The child may be mainstreamed with a tutor, be partially mainstreamed in a resource room, attend special classes, or be tutored at home. If the child is to attend public school, suggest to parents that they contact the school well before enrollment to ensure that school personnel understand the child's disability.

Make sure that items such as large-print books, Braille materials, audio equipment, or an Optacon (described earlier) is available. Ensure that frequent eye examinations are performed and assist with proper use and care of prescribed glasses or contact lenses, as necessary.

Provide Emotional Support

Family members often need help to understand the child's abilities and disabilities. Support them as they learn about the child's visual problems, tell friends and family, and then adjust to support the child.

- Encourage habilitation as soon as realistically possible. Make the adjustment easier by providing information about the child's specific type of visual impairment, available community services, and groups or associations for children with similar vision conditions. Suggest resources to families of children with visual disorders.
- Be supportive and listen to the family's concerns regarding the child's visual deficit.
- Ensure that parents meet their own physical and emotional needs so they are better able to care for and provide support to their child.

Evaluation

Expected outcomes of nursing care for the child with a visual impairment include:

- The child will remain safe from injury.
- The child will achieve growth and developmental milestones to maximum potential.
- An Individualized Education Plan will be established and followed for the child.
- The family members will express effective stress management.

Injuries of the Eye

In the United States, eye injuries are common in boys 11 to 15 years of age and in all children ages 9 to 11 years. Boys from 11–15 years have four times more eye injuries than girls. About 42,000 sports injuries occur annually with about half of these in children (Committee on Sports Medicine and Fitness, 2004). Sports, darts, fireworks, air-powered BB guns, blunt and sharp objects, chemical and thermal burns, physical irritants, and abuse may cause eye trauma (Behrman, Kliegman, & Jenson, 2004). Recreational activities such as sports and projectile toys are common causes. Older children may be injured by chemicals in school science laboratories.

Some injuries can be treated at home, but many necessitate a trip to the emergency department or require hospitalization. Personnel take a careful history of the injury, perform, assessment of the eye, and measure visual acuity. Clinical Manifestations and Emergency Treatment of Eye Injuries on page 650 summarizes emergency treatment of common eye injuries.

Nursing Management

Promoting prevention of injury is an important nursing intervention. Nurses perform teaching at each health promotion examination about ways to avoid eye injuries in children. Protective eyewear should be used by participants in all sports with a risk of eye injury, with extreme caution in those with diminished vision or only one functional eye. The most common injuries occur in baseball, basketball, swimming, bicycling, and football (Center for Health and Health Care in Schools, 2004).

Nurses should also be informed about emergency treatment of eye injuries, inform parents and school personnel of care, and manage transfer to medical facilities when eye injury occurs. See the clinical manifestations table for emergency care.

DISORDERS OF THE EAR

Otitis Media

Otitis media, or inflammation of the middle ear, is sometimes accompanied by infection. This condition is one of the most common childhood illnesses. About 70% of infants have at least one case of acute otitis media during the first year of life, and 93% have been diagnosed with the problem by age 7 years. Peak incidence is in the first 2 years of life, particularly from 6–20 months of age (Bernius & Perlin, 2006). Otitis media occurs more frequently among boys and in children who attend childcare centers, in those with allergies, in children exposed to tobacco smoke, and in those who use pacifiers several hours daily. It is most common during the winter months. Children with conditions such as cleft lip and palate or Down syndrome more often experience otitis media.

COMMUNITY CARE

Sports Requiring Eye Protection

Inform parents, children, coaches, teachers, and others that many sports require eye protection:

- Badminton
- Baseball
- Basketball
- Bicycling
- Fencing (requires face cage)
- Handball
- Hockey (field, ice, roller, street)
- Lacrosse
- Racquetball
- Soccer
- Squash
- Swimming (requires swim goggles)

NURSING ALERT

Be sure to check the immunization status of the child with an eye injury. If the child has not had a tetanus booster within 5 years, this immunization should be given.

CLINICAL MANIFESTATIONS   EMERGENCY TREATMENT OF EYE INJURIES

Condition and Etiology	Clinical Manifestations	Clinical Therapy
Subconjunctival hemorrhage (caused by coughing, mild trauma, or increased physical activity)	Reddened area in conjunctiva	Usually heals spontaneously; child should see ophthalmologist if most of sclera is covered or if condition does not clear up in 1–2 weeks
Periorbital ecchymosis	"Black eye" or bruising of the skin around the eye	Apply ice to eye area (both eyes) for 5–15 minutes every hour for the first 1–2 days after injury (even if only one eye is affected, both eyes may discolor); then apply warm compresses beginning the second day after injury
Foreign body on conjunctiva	Intense pain or feeling of something in the eye	Do not let child rub eye; remove material on surface of eye by closing upper lid over lower lid, irrigating or everting upper lid, visualizing material, and removing it with a slightly damp handkerchief; patch eye and transport child to emergency department if foreign body cannot be removed
Corneal abrasion	Intense pain and redness	Superficial corneal abrasions are diagnosed by touching a sterile fluorescein strip to lower conjunctiva; dye remains where corneal epithelial cells are disrupted; most corneal abrasions heal spontaneously or antibiotic ointment may be prescribed and eyes patched in some children
Burns (alkaline burns readily penetrate cornea and are more serious than acid burns)	Pain and/or complaints of "blindness" or vision loss	For child with chemical burn, irrigate eye for 15–30 minutes; transport child to emergency department, where irrigation should continue (see Clinical Skills Manual); pupils are dilated to reduce pain and prevent adhesions; after irrigation is complete, eyes are patched and antibiotics are prescribed
Penetrating and perforating injuries	Pain	Obtain medical assistance immediately; never try to remove an object that has penetrated the child's eye; such objects should be removed by an ophthalmologist; prevent the child from rubbing the injured eye; cover both eyes with shield before transportation to emergency department
Eye injuries caused by severe blows to head and eye (blunt trauma can seriously injure all eye structures, including orbit, which can be fractured)	Pain and redness	Transport immediately to ophthalmologist's office or emergency department for evaluation and treatment. Personnel should be aware that retinal hemorrhage is a common presentation of the type of child abuse called "shaken child syndrome" (see Chapter 6 ∞ for further discussion of child abuse)

Breast-feeding appears to be protective against otitis media. In the past decade, an increased number of cases have been observed, and recent changes have been made in recommendations for treatment (American Academy of Pediatrics, 2004; Pelton, 2005).

Etiology and Pathophysiology

The specific cause of otitis media is unknown, but it appears to be related to eustachian tube dysfunction. Often an upper respiratory infection precedes the development of otitis media. This infection causes the mucous membranes of the eustachian tube to become edematous. As a result, air that normally flows to the middle ear is blocked, and the air in the middle ear is reabsorbed into the bloodstream. Fluid is pulled from the mucosal lining into the former air space, providing a medium for the rapid growth of pathogens. The tympanic membrane and fluid behind it become infected. The most common causative organisms are *Streptococcus pneumoniae*, *Haemophilus influenzae*, and *Moraxella catarrhalis* (Pelton, 2005).

Conditions such as enlarged adenoids or edema from allergic rhinitis can also obstruct the eustachian tube and lead to otitis media. Pacifier use raises the soft palate and thus alters dynamics in the eustacian tube, providing for entry of microorganisms from the nasopharynx (Neto, Hemb, & Silva, 2006). Ethnicity appears to play a role in the incidence of otitis media. Recurrent otitis media has an increased frequency in children of parents who smoke (Brook & Gober, 2005). Children with multiple siblings and those who attend childcare centers have increased rates of recurrent acute otitis media (Harrison, 2005).

Clinical Manifestations

Otitis media is the general term for inflammation of the middle ear. *Acute otitis media* (AOM) is diagnosed when the child has acute onset of ear pain, marked redness of the tympanic membrane upon otoscopy, and middle ear effusion (Figure 19–7 ➤). Recurrent acute otitis media indicates repeated bouts of AOM, such as three in 6 months, or four in 12 months. *Otitis media with effusion* (OME) is evidence of fluid in the middle ear without inflammation (Figure 19–8 ➤). OME sometimes becomes chronic in nature (continuing more than 3 months) and is more commonly associated with hearing loss.

Infants and young children have characteristic behaviors that can indicate otitis media may be present. Pulling at the ear is a sign of ear pain (Figure 19–9 ➤). Diarrhea, vomiting, and fever are typical of otitis media. Irritability and "acting out" may be signs of a related hearing impairment. The child with otitis media often has night awakenings with crying due to increased ear pressure when prone or supine. See Clinical Manifestations of Acute Otitis Media and Otitis Media with Effusion for further details.

◼ COLLABORATIVE CARE

Diagnostic Tests

Diagnosis of otitis media is based on otoscopic examination. Acute otitis media is diagnosed with certainty when there is a history of acute onset, presence of middle ear effusion (bulging or decreased mobility of the tympanic membrane, air fluid behind the membrane or otorrhea or discharge), and signs and symptoms of inflammation (erythema of tympanic membrane or discomfort that makes sleep and other activities difficult for the child) (American Academy of Pediatrics, 2004). Otoscopic examination includes visualization and pneumatic otoscopy. The trained clinician can perform pneumatic otoscopy in which positive air pressure in the external canal is used to measure the movement of the tympanic membrane. A puff of air is blown into the ear canal with a pneumatic otoscope while the practitioner observes tympanic membrane movement (see Chapter 5 ∞ for a further description of this technique).

Special gradient acoustic reflectometry (SGAR) measures the condition of the middle ear by introducing a sound and measuring the tympanic membrane response (Windmill & Windmill, 2006). A flat tympanogram, indicating absence of normal movement for the tympanic membrane, is also suggestive of otitis media. (The tympanogram is described later in this chapter in the section on hearing impairment.)

Occasionally, the middle ear fluid is cultured so that the causative organism can be identified. If the tympanic membrane is not intact, the culture is easy to obtain; in cases with repeated antibiotic treatment failures, a tympanocentesis may be done to aspirate some fluid from the middle ear through the tympanic membrane.

Since otitis media with effusion may only involve fluid in the middle ear, it is best diagnosed by pneumatic otoscopy and tympanometry. Since this type of otitis media is most commonly associated with hearing loss, audiological testing should be performed in the pediatric healthcare home (medical home) if the effusion persists for 3 months or longer. A referral to an audiologist should be made for children who fail testing in the office or are less than 4 years of age (Otitis Media with Effusion, 2004).

Clinical Therapy

Concern has developed about the increasing appearance of drug-resistant microbials as causative agents in otitis media. Based on current knowledge, the American Academy of Pediatrics and the American Academy of Family Physicians joined to establish recommendations in 2004 (American Academy of Pediatrics, 2004). Acute otitis media is now treated with antibiotic therapy for 10 days in children under 6 years, and 5–7 days for children 6 years and over. Consistent with current guidelines, acute otitis media treatment is delayed for 48–72 hours after diagnosis in children 6 months to 2 years with nonsevere illness at presentation AND uncertain diagnosis, or in children 2 years and older without severe symptoms OR with uncertain diagnosis.

When prescribed, the choice of antibiotic depends on the probable organism, ease of administration, cost, previous effectiveness, and any history of allergies. First-line

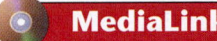

MediaLink

Otitis Media Animation

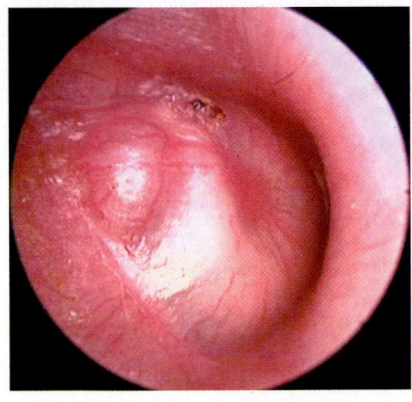

Figure 19–7 ➤ Acute otitis media is characterized by abrupt onset, pain, middle ear effusion, and inflammation. Note the injected vessels and altered shape of the cone of light. See Chapter 5 ∞ for a normal tympanic membrane.
Courtesy of Kevin Kavanagh, MD, FACS.

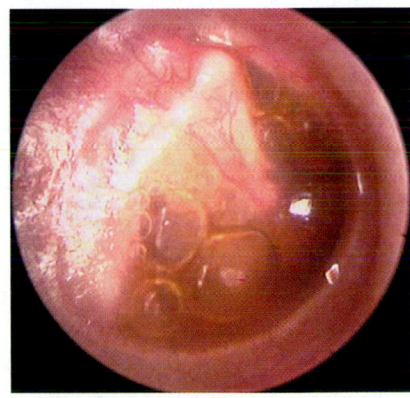

Figure 19–8 ➤ Otitis media with effusion is noted on otoscopy by fluid line or air bubbles. Pneumatic otoscopy or tympanometry shows a nonmobile tympanic membrane. Note that the light reflex is not in the expected position due to a change in tympanic membrane shape from air bubbles. Where would you expect to see the cone of light? See Chapter 5 ∞ for a description of normal findings.
Courtesy of Kevin Kavanagh, MD, FACS.

CLINICAL MANIFESTATIONS | ACUTE OTITIS MEDIA AND OTITIS MEDIA WITH EFFUSION

Etiology	Clinical Manifestations	Clinical Therapy
Acute otitis media—bacterial infection in the middle ear from pathogens transferred from the nasopharynx; most common infectious agents are *S. pneumoniae, H. influenzae, M. catarrhalis*	*Behavioral*—ear pain, pulling at ear, rapid onset, irritability, malaise, poor feeding *Examination*—bulging tympanic membrane, air or fluid bubbles present behind tympanic membrane; immobile or poorly mobile tympanic membrane, red (or other color change such as white, gray, or yellow as long as bulging is present) tympanic membrane, reduced visibility of tympanic membrane landmarks with displaced light reflex	Treat ear pain with local anesthetic, local herbal pain products, or systemic acetaminophen or ibuprofen Observe child's condition for 48–72 hours and if not improved, treat with course of antibiotics
Otitis media with effusion—collection of fluid in the middle ear behind the tympanic membrane, which is not infected with bacteria	*Behavioral*—difficulty hearing or responding as expected to sounds *Examination*—signs of acute inflammation are NOT present; tympanic membrane is retracted or neutral; immobile or partly mobile tympanic membrane; yellow or gray tympanic membrane; opaque or thickened tympanic membrane with visibility of landmarks reduced	Symptomatic treatment or pain Careful observation of hearing acuity over several months Speech assessment if loss of hearing acuity occurs Developmental assessment

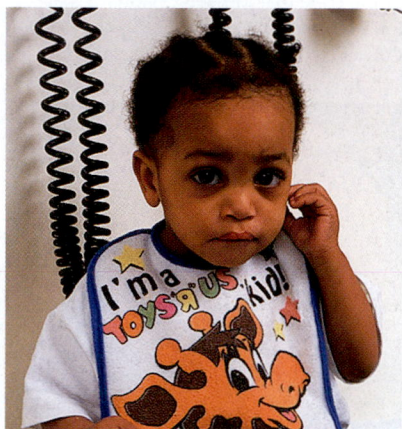

Figure 19–9 ▶ This young child is pulling at the ear and acting fussy, two important signs of otitis media. Ask the parents about the presence of fever and night awakenings, additional signs that are often observed in children with this condition.

therapy is amoxicillin at a dose of 80–90 mg/kg/day. Amoxicillin with clavulanate or cefuroxime are second-line drugs. If an intramuscular drug is preferred, cefdinir at 14 mg/kg/day, cefpodoxime at 10 mg/kg/day, or cefuroxime at 30 mg/kg/day can be prescribed (Zacharyczuk, 2004). See Medications Used to Treat Acute Otitis Media for more details about common medications used.

When antibiotic therapy is not prescribed initially, the child can be given ibuprofen or acetaminophen for pain relief and should return for further treatment if symptoms continue. When the tympanic membrane is intact, topical anesthetic eardrops are sometimes prescribed for several days to provide pain relief.

OME is not treated with antibiotics but is evaluated periodically to be sure there is not an additional AOM that needs treatment. Children with OME generally improve within 3 months. Since this type of otitis is more commonly associated with hearing loss and cochlear damage, follow-up with audiology is essential. If hearing is abnormal, speech testing should be performed (Otitis Media with Effusion, 2004).

Neither decongestants nor antihistamines have been shown to be effective in the treatment of otitis media with or without effusion. Steroids also do not appear to have any long-term beneficial effect. If infection recurs despite antibiotic treatment for acute otitis media or if OME continues 4 months or more with persistent hearing loss

COMPLEMENTARY THERAPY

Naturopathic Extract for Ear Pain in Otitis Media

Because many children with otitis media experience ear pain that can disrupt their sleep, as well as that of family members, anesthetic eardrops have been used for their analgesic effect on the tympanic membrane. Since some families might prefer use of natural remedies for ear pain, a study comparing Naturopathic Herbal Extract Ear Drops (a naturopathic herbal extract of *Allium sativum, Verbascum thapsus, Calendula flores,* and *Hypericum peroforatum, lavender and vitamin E*) with a local anesthetic of ametocaine and phenazone was conducted. About 1/2 of the total of 171 children received each of the pain treatments and parents rated the children after training with a pain tool. Both treatments were effective in decreasing ear pain over the 3 days of the study. There was no significant difference in success rates of local anesthetic and naturopathic agent; in fact, the naturopathic agent was as effective or more effective than anesthetic at each measurement period. It was concluded that herbal pain control may be very beneficial for treatment of ear pain, and can help to decrease the need for antibiotic treatment for every case of otitis media (Sarrell, Cohen, & Kahan, 2003). However, in a collective analysis of several studies, it was concluded that there is as yet insufficient evidence to describe whether or not naturopathic treatment is effective for treatment of ear pain in children (Foxlee, Johansson, Wejfalk, Dawkins, Dooley, & Del Mar, 2006).

MEDICATIONS USED TO TREAT *Acute Otitis Media*		
Medication	**Action/Indication**	**Nursing Implications**
Amoxicillin	Broad-spectrum antibiotic that inhibits mucoprotein synthesis in cell wall of bacteria; used to treat some gram-positive and gram-negative infections.	• Assess for previous allergy to drug, penicillins, cephalosporins. • Take as instructed for entire period prescribed. • If oral suspension is given, refrigerate and shake well before administration. • Teach parents how to administer drug to the child. • Have family report side effects such as rash and diarrhea.
Amoxicillin and clavulanate potassium	Action and use are similar to amoxicillin. However, clavulanate is a β-lactamase inhibitor that enhances effect of amoxicillin.	See amoxicillin
Cefuroxime	A second generation cephalosporin that binds to one or more of the penicillin-binding proteins in cell walls of bacteria; useful in treatment of most gram-negative and some gram-positive infections.	• Assess for previous allergy to drug penicillins, cephalosporins. • Take as instructed for entire period prescribed. • If oral suspension is given, refrigerate and shake well before administration. • Teach parents how to administer drug to the child. • Have family report side effects such as rash and diarrhea.

present, **myringotomy** (surgical incision of the tympanic membrane) may be performed and **tympanostomy tubes** (pressure-equalizing tubes) may be inserted to drain fluid from the middle ear.

NURSING MANAGEMENT

Nursing Assessment and Diagnosis

The tympanic membrane is assessed at each health promotion visit and during examinations for illness. Examine the color, transparency, mobility, presence of landmarks, and light reflex. Ask the parents if the child has had a fever, been fussy, or been pulling at the ears. Observe for signs of impaired hearing, observing for the child's ability to hear whispered or soft sounds.

Several nursing diagnoses that may apply to the child with otitis media are included in the accompanying Nursing Care Plan. Additional nursing diagnoses may include the following:

- Risk for Imbalanced Body Temperature: Hyperthermia related to infectious process
- Fatigue (Child and Parent) related to sleep deprivation
- Disturbed Sensory Perception (Auditory) related to chronic ear infections and altered hearing reception

Planning and Implementation

Preventive measures should be emphasized. Exposure to secondhand smoke in the home increases the incidence of otitis media in children; therefore, parents who smoke should be encouraged to avoid smoking near the child or in the home. Woodburning stoves should also be avoided when possible. If young children are in childcare with fewer than 10 children, incidence decreases. Breast-feeding provides some protection from the disease. Placing babies to sleep with a pacifier may increase incidence and should be avoided in the infant with prior infections (Pelton, 2005).

Most children with otitis media are not hospitalized; therefore, nursing management centers on care of the child in the home. The accompanying nursing care plan summarizes nursing care for the child with otitis media. Parents may not understand why the child with a possible infection is not given antibiotics. Explain to them the problem of developing resistant strains of bacteria. New research indicates that most

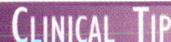
CLINICAL TIP

The *Haemophilus influenzae* type B (Hib) vaccine, which is routinely given to children beginning at 2 months of age, has been influential in reducing the incidence of diseases such as otitis media that are caused by *H. influenzae* type B. Another, more recently recommended immunization for pneumococcal disease has also decreased cases of otitis media from that pathogen. Be sure to check the immunization status of each child to be sure it is up-to-date for Hib and pneumococcal vaccine. (See Chapter 18 ∞ for the recommended immunization schedule.)

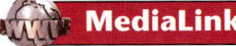
MediaLink

Case Study: Otitis Media

NURSING CARE PLAN | The Child with Otitis Media

GOAL	INTERVENTION	RATIONALE	EXPECTED OUTCOME
1. Acute Pain related to inflammation and pressure on tympanic membrane			
	NIC Priority Intervention: **Pain Management:** *Alleviation or reduction in pain to a level of comfort acceptable to patient and family.*		*NOC Suggested Outcome:* **Pain Level:** *Amount of reported or demonstrated pain.*
The child or parent will indicate absence of pain.	• Give analgesic such as acetaminophen. Use analgesic eardrops. • Have the child sit up, raise head on pillows, or lie on unaffected ear. • Apply heating pad or warm hot water bottle. • Have the child chew gum or blow on balloon to relieve pressure in ear.	• Analgesics after perception or response to pain. • Elevation decreases pressure from fluid. • Heat increases blood supply and reduces discomfort. • Attempts to open the eustachian tube may help aerate the middle ear.	Verbal child states that pain is relieved. Nonverbal child has improved disposition and comfort.
2. Infection related to presence of pathogens			
	NIC Priority Intervention: **Infection Control:** *Minimizing the acquisition and transmission of infectious agents.*		*NOC Suggested Outcome:* **Risk Control:** *Actions to eliminate or reduce health threats.*
The child will be free of infection.	• Encourage breast-feeding of infants. • Instruct the parents to administer analgesics and antibiotics exactly as directed and to complete prescribed course of antibiotic. • Telephone the parents 2–3 days after initial examination. • Examine ear 3–4 days after completion of antibiotic treatment.	• Breast-feeding affords natural immunity to infectious agents. • Taking antibiotics as prescribed minimizes chance for overgrowth of pathogens. Analgesics provide pain relief. • If symptoms have not improved in 48-72 hours, treatment should be evaluated. • Check-up determines if treatment is effective.	The child's temperature is normal, symptoms have disappeared, and tympanic membrane shows no signs of infection.
3. Risk for Caregiver Role Strain related to chronic condition			
	NIC Priority Intervention: **Caregiver Support:** *Provision of necessary support, information, and advocacy to facilitate care by parents.*		*NOC Suggested Outcome:* **Caregiver Performance:** *Provision by family care provider of health care for child.*
The parents will manage the child's condition with minimal stress.	• Determine the parents' ability to manage condition. Provide frequent information and feedback. • Encourage parental input in managing care. • Listen carefully to parental expressions of frustration and fatigue and try to understand parents' feelings.	• Many parents can treat children at home. Knowledge of condition allows parents to make informed decisions and to manage condition effectively. • Active participation increases confidence and ability to manage condition. • Reacting empathically encourages parents to communicate.	The parents express confidence about treating the child and state that stress is reduced.

NURSING CARE PLAN The Child with Otitis Media (continued)

GOAL	INTERVENTION	RATIONALE	EXPECTED OUTCOME
4. Risk for Infection related to knowledge deficit about infection in children			
	NIC Priority Intervention: **Infection Control:** *Minimizing the acquisition and transmission of infectious agents.*		*NOC Suggested Outcome:* **Knowledge:** *Extent of understanding conveyed about infectious disease prevention.*
The parents will state understanding of preventive measures.	• Teach family members to cover mouths and noses when sneezing or coughing and to wash hands frequently. Have parents isolate sick children. • Encourage optimal nutrition, rest, and exercise. • Position bottle-fed infants upright when feeding. Do not prop bottles. • Eliminate allergens and upper respiratory irritants such as tobacco, smoke, and dust.	• Good hygiene prevents spread of pathogens. • Physical well-being helps the body fight disease. • Elevated position prevents passage of milk and pathogens into the eustachian tube. • Fewer irritants and allergens may decrease susceptibility to respiratory infections. Secondhand smoke contributes to higher incidence of otitis media.	Parents express understanding of measures to lead to fewer infections.
5. Risk for Delayed Growth and Development related to hearing loss			
	NIC Priority Intervention: **Developmental Enhancement:** *Facilitating optimal growth and development of the child.*		*NOC Suggested Outcome:* **Growth and Development:** *Milestones of developmental progression.*
The child will have normal hearing. The child will have normal motor and language development.	• Access hearing ability frequently. • Assess motor and language development at each healthcare visit.	• Monitoring detects hearing loss early. • Early detection of developmental delays can lead to appropriate intervention.	The child's general health and hearing improve, and incidence of condition decreases. The child has language and motor development within norms for age group.

children improve after 48 to 72 hours even without antibiotics and that overuse contributes to drug resistance. Encourage parents to bring the child back for care if the condition worsens or has not improved in the recommended time.

Likewise, parents of children with OME need explanations about why there is a waiting period of about 3 months with no medications or other medical care. Explain that antibiotics, steroids, and antihistamines/decongestants have not been effective and that most children improve in 3 months. Assure parents that if the effusion continues beyond that time, the child will be tested for hearing acuity, and, if indicated, for speech development.

The chronic nature of otitis media in some children can create many problems for the family. The child's waking at night with ear pain results in lack of sleep and parental fatigue. Parents often become frustrated and disillusioned because of the inability of the healthcare system to cure the child and may fear a permanent hearing impairment. Reassure parents that as the child grows older, the recurrent infections eventually cease. Provide pain relief techniques such as teaching correct administration of eardrops, oral administration of acetaminophen, and positioning the baby with the head slightly elevated, which often decreases pressure and pain. Provide hearing and language examinations at regular intervals, inform parents of results, and refer to an audiology specialist if hearing problems are identified. For the child with some hearing loss due to otitis media with effusion, a home environment that fosters math, reading, and verbal skills can overcome the effects of lowered hearing during the time of infection. Nurses should focus interventions on helping parents to read and talk with children frequently who have otitis media with effusion.

The child who is having tympanostomy tubes inserted is generally treated in a day surgery setting. Parents and the child will need preparation about what to expect and instructions for safe care upon discharge. (See Families Want to Know: Care of the Child with Tympanostomy Tubes.)

Evaluation

Expected outcomes of nursing care for the child with otitis media include:

- The child will return to normal sleep and feeding patterns.
- The child will maintain normal hearing and speech development.
- Effective pain and temperature management will be achieved for the child.
- The parents will indicate adequate understanding of treatment regimen.

Otitis Externa

Otitis externa is an inflammation of the skin and surrounding soft tissue of the ear canal. It is sometimes called "swimmer's ear" because it is common in children who swim frequently, especially during hot and muggy weather. The ear canal can also be injured by use of cotton-tipped applicators, foreign objects, or sprays used near the face. If the tympanic membrane is not intact because of tympanostomy tubes or breakage of the membrane, there may be drainage visible in the canal; this drainage may irritate the canal and lead to otitis externa. Any irritation of the canal can become infected with bacteria, virus, or fungi; sometimes it represents an allergic reaction. The child usually complains of pain and itching, and may have intense pain when the examiner presses on the tragus, or skin tab in front of the ear. Sometimes the ear appears swollen and redness or drainage of the canal may be seen upon otoscopic examination.

Treatment of otitis externa requires removing the dried and flaking epithelium and cerumen. Burow's solutions or normal saline are used to irrigate and clean the canal. Steroid eardrops are used to decrease inflammation and antibiotic drops are also used if a bacterial infection is suspected. If the child has tympanostomy tubes or a perforated tympanic membrane, non-ototoxic ear antibiotic such as quinolone antibiotic eardrops are used (Rosenfeld et al., 2006). Ibuprofen or acetaminophen is commonly used for pain control. The child should be seen by the healthcare provider if the condition has not improved by 48 to 72 hours. The child should not return to swimming for about 5 days. The ear canal should then be kept dry by using ear plugs or a swim cap for swimming and gently blow drying the canal after bathing. Cotton-tipped applicators or other objects should not be placed in the ear canal so that the skin in the canal can heal. If hair sprays or other solutions are irritating, they should not be used by the child or adolescent.

Nurses should be aware of the signs of otitis externa such as a painful ear, drainage, and irritated canal. Verify that the tympanic membrane is intact during otoscopic examination. Teach families to avoid the irritants identified such as cotton-tipped applicators, sprays, and frequent swimming. Demonstrate proper instillation of drops

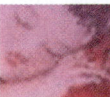

FAMILIES WANT TO KNOW

Care of the Child with Tympanostomy Tubes

After Surgery

- Encourage the child to drink generous amounts of fluids.
- Reestablish a regular diet as tolerated.
- Give pain medication (acetaminophen) as ordered for discomfort and at bedtime.
- Place drops in the child's ears, if instructed.
- Restrict the child to quiet activities.

Following Postoperative Period

- Follow the physician's instructions regarding swimming and water (some caution against swimming and other activities that might get water in ears; others do not).
- Ear plugs can be used to prevent water from getting into the ears.
- Be alert for tubes becoming dislodged and falling out and alert physician (they usually fall out within 1 year).
- Report purulent discharge from the ear, which may indicate a new ear infection. Contact the care provider.

(see *Clinical Skills Manual*) and give instructions for use of acetaminophen for pain relief in the acute period.

Hearing Impairment

Approximately 1 million children in the United States have some form of hearing impairment. Hearing loss is present in 2 out of every 1000 births (Yaeger, McCallum, Lewis, Soslow, Shah, Potsic, Stolle, & Krantz, 2006; Moore, 2006). These hearing impairments are expressed in terms of **decibels** (dB), which are units of loudness, and rated according to severity (Table 19–6). Children who have only a mild hearing loss (35 to 40 dB) may miss 50% of everyday conversation and are considered at high risk for difficulty in school. Children with a hearing loss of more than 90 dB are considered legally deaf. Between 2 and 6 children per 1000 have a hearing loss.

Etiology and Pathophysiology

About 50% of hearing loss is genetically caused, usually with a recessive inheritance pattern with GJB2 gene abnormalities (Yaeger et al., 2006). Another 25% is due to environmental causes around the time of birth; the remainder is due to unknown causes. Although many infants with hearing loss have no known risk factors, identified risks include:

- A family history of congenital hearing loss*
- Positive titer for TORCH infections (toxoplasmosis, rubella, cytomegalovirus, syphilis, herpes)
- Craniofacial abnormalities
- Very low birth weight (<1500 g)*
- Bilirubin >16 mg/dL
- Aminoglycoside medication administration >5 days
- Low Apgar score at 1 or 5 minutes*
- Bacterial meningitis
- Mechanical ventilation >5 days
- Presence of syndromes associated with hearing loss (Down Syndrome, Pierre Robin Syndrome, Arnold-Chiari Malformation)*

*Primary risk factors (Chu, Elimian, Barbera et al., 2003).

Common causes of conductive hearing loss include impacted cerumen, the most frequent reason for conductive loss; otitis externa ("swimmer's ear"); trauma; or a foreign body. Conductive loss also occurs if the tympanic membrane does not fully vibrate, as in otitis media. In these cases, loss may be restored after the infection clears. Chronic and untreated ear infections may lead to ear structural changes and permanent hearing impairment. The loss of acuity may be gradual or rapid and results in diminished hearing in all ranges.

Conditions leading to sensorineural hearing loss may be congenital (maternal rubella), genetic (Tay-Sachs disease), or acquired (such as from ototoxic drugs, bacterial meningitis, or loud noise). In sensorineural hearing loss, high-frequency sounds

SKILL 8–8
Administering an Otic Medication

Table 19–6	SEVERITY OF HEARING LOSS	
Type of Loss	**Decibel Level (dB)**	**Hearing Ability**
Slight/mild	26–40	Some speech sounds are difficult to perceive, particularly unvoiced consonant sounds
Moderate	41–60	Most normal conversational speech sounds are missed
Severe	61–80	Speech sounds cannot be heard at a normal conversational level
Profound	81–90	No speech sounds can be heard
Deaf	> 90	No sound at all can be heard

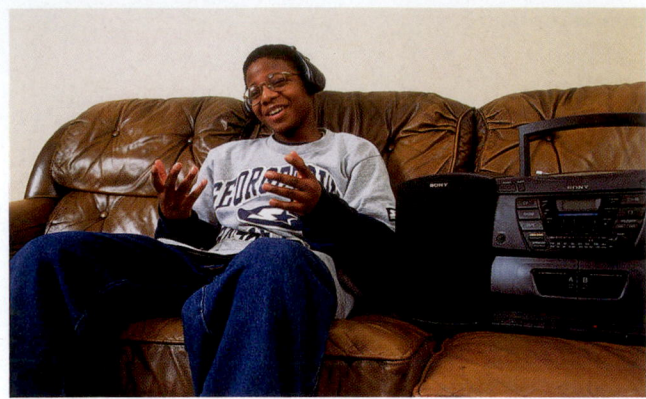

Figure 19–10 ➤ Listening to loud music with headphones or at rock concerts is a frequent cause of hearing loss or tinnitus among teenagers and young adults. This adolescent needs to be informed about the negative outcomes of this activity.

RESEARCH

Noise Exposure

Research has shown that 12% of school-age children may have hearing impairments due to noise exposure, often in ranges not screened during school auditory testing. Hearing loss is even more common among teens, with increasing incidence in the older age groups (Serra, Biassoni, Richter et al., 2005). Preventing these hearing losses is possible, so nurses should identify and find sources of noise in the child's environment. They may include stereos, airplanes, firearms, power tools, machinery, and toys. Encourage use of ear plugs during hazardous activities (Chung, Des Roches, Meunier, & Eavey, 2006). Be aware of the potential harm from iPods or other music since it is in very close contact with the ear and the sound is usually loud and directed into the ear canal with no dissipation into surrounding air. Additionally, the current practice of using headphones for very extended parts of the day increases the risk of injury.

are most affected. Such hearing loss may be preceded by **tinnitus** or ringing in the ears. Teenagers who use earphones at high volumes or attend many rock concerts are at risk for hearing loss (Figure 19–10 ➤). Other noise hazards include firecrackers, guns, and power and farm equipment.

Clinical Manifestations

Hearing is both an innate and a learned behavior. Infants and children who have hearing impairment exhibit a range of behaviors, depending on the child's age and the severity of the deficit (Table 19–7). Infants who hear normally respond to sound in both obvious and subtle ways that do not occur in those with hearing impairment. As children with hearing impairments mature, language skills are affected. Hearing loss is often manifested as a cognitive deficit, a behavioral problem, or both.

Hearing disorders can be classified according to the location of the deficit. **Conductive hearing loss** occurs when conditions in the external auditory canal or tympanic membrane prevent sound from reaching the middle ear. **Sensorineural hearing loss** occurs when the hair cells in the cochlea or along the auditory nerve (cranial nerve VIII) are damaged. This leads to permanent hearing loss. A **mixed hearing loss** indicates a hearing loss having a combination of conductive and sensorineural causes.

■ COLLABORATIVE CARE

Diagnostic Tests

Early identification of hearing loss is a key element in successful treatment. Detection of hearing loss in infants is important to ensure optimal development. Universal screening of all infants is recommended before 1 month of age, with diagnostic audiologic evaluation before 3 months, and beginning of early intervention programs by 6 months of age for those with hearing impairment (Connolly, Carron, & Roark, 2005; Windmill & Windmill, 2006). Many state laws now mandate screening of newborns.

Table 19–7	BEHAVIORS SUGGESTIVE OF HEARING IMPAIRMENT
Age	**Behavior**
Infant	Has a diminished or absent startle reflex to loud sound Does not awaken when environment is very noisy Awakens only to touch Does not turn head to sound at 3–4 months Does not localize sound at 6–10 months Babbles little or not at all
Toddler and preschooler	Speaks unintelligibly, in a monotone, or not at all Communicates needs through gestures Unable to follow directions Appears developmentally delayed, especially in social interactions Appears emotionally immature, yells inappropriately Does not respond to doorbell or telephone Appears more interested in objects than people and prefers to play alone Focuses on facial expressions rather than verbal communications
School-age child and adolescent	Asks to have statements repeated Answers questions inappropriately, except when able to view speaker's face Daydreams and is inattentive Performs poorly at school or is truant Has speech abnormalities or speaks in a monotone Sits close to or turns television or radio up loudly Prefers to play alone

Observations of response to noise in all newborns should be accompanied by more sophisticated testing such as auditory brainstem response or transient evoked otoacoustic emissions, especially in those at high risk of deficits (Figure 19–11 ➤). See Table 19–8 for a description of the common tests used for newborn hearing.

An otoscopic examination with a tympanogram can be performed on an older infant to determine conductive hearing loss. The **tympanogram** is a test that provides a graph of the middle ear's ability to transmit sound. An airtight probe is inserted into the external ear canal and a tone is emitted. The pressure is measured by the probe and plotted on a graph. A flat tympanogram suggests conductive hearing loss (Figures 19–12 A & B ➤). **Audiography** can be used with cooperative children over 3 years of age. Sounds of various frequencies and intensities are presented to the child through earphones, and the child is instructed to raise a hand upon hearing the sound. Although audiography cannot detect hearing loss caused by middle ear effusion, it can indicate sensorineural loss. The hearing of preschool and school-age children is tested by asking them to repeat whispered words. Hearing of school-age children and adolescents is also assessed with the Weber and Rinne tests (see Chapter 5 ∞).

Clinical Therapy

If a hearing loss is uncorrectable, a multidisciplinary team composed of the pediatrician, audiologist, otolaryngologist, speech-language pathologist, nurse, teacher, and social worker should assist the child and family with adaptation to the disability. If the deficit is due to recurrent ear infections, tympanostomy tube insertion may improve hearing.

A hearing aid may be prescribed for a conductive loss. A sensorineural loss is more difficult to treat, but bone conduction hearing aids have been used in some children. Some families choose to have a child treated with a cochlear implant. A cochlear implant is a small electronic device that helps to provide sound for those who are deaf or profoundly hard of hearing. It consists of:

- A microphone to pick up sound that is located outside of the body; it is worn as a headpiece behind the ear
- A speech processor that organizes sound from the microphone; it is worn behind the ear or on a belt
- A transmitter that transfers the sound into electrical impulses; it is part of the headpiece behind the ear
- Electrodes that send the signals to the brain; this receiver is implanted in the skin behind the ear with a wire leading to the cochlear fluid in the middle ear

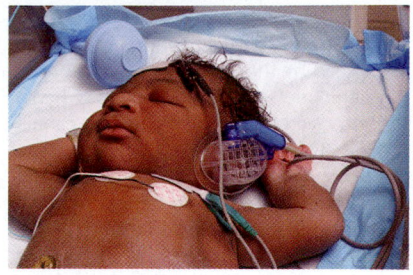

Figure 19–11 ➤ Newborn hearing screening is an effective tool in diagnosing some cases of hearing impairment very early in life.

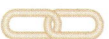

SKILLS 6–20 AND 6–21
Hearing Acuity Screening

Table 19–8	SCREENING TESTS FOR NEWBORN HEARING
Test	**Mechanism of Action**
Otoacoustic Emission (OAE) (either Transient-Evoked [TEOAE] or Distortion-Product [DPOAE])	A measure of low intensity sounds from the cochlear hair cells in response to clicks from a probe placed in the ear canal Sensitive in frequency range above 1500 Hz May show false negative for loss below 1000–1500 Hz Detects inner ear hearing loss by evaluating cochlear and hair cell function Does not detect neural damage to 8th cranial nerve Can be sensitive to outer ear canal obstruction or middle ear effusion, leading to false positive result
Auditory brainstem response (ABR)	Electrical response to auditory stimuli from three surface scalp electrodes Reflects activity of cochlea, cranial nerve 8, and auditory brainstem pathways Detects hearing loss from 1000–8000 Hz May show false negative results for losses in the 500–2000 Hz levels Will give a positive result (indicating hearing loss) if there is damage to cranial nerve 8 or brainstem pathways even if cochlear loss is not present

Figure 19–12 ➤ A, This tympanogram demonstrates normal hearing as evidenced by the curve showing the tympanic membrane's movement when a sound wave is emitted into the ear canal. Mobility is between 0.2 mL and 1.0 mL, the normal range. B, In contrast, note the flat pattern in the second tympanogram, which shows very restricted mobility of the tympanic membrane in response to sound.

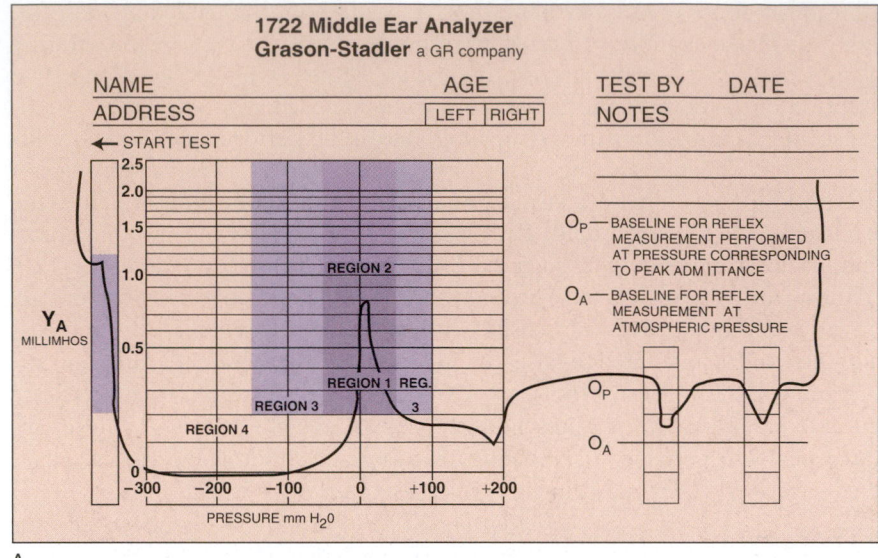

A

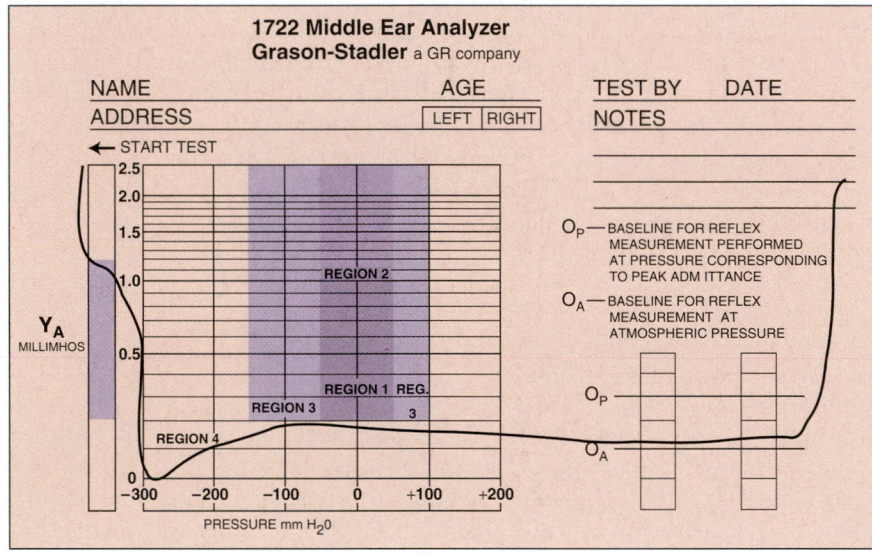

B

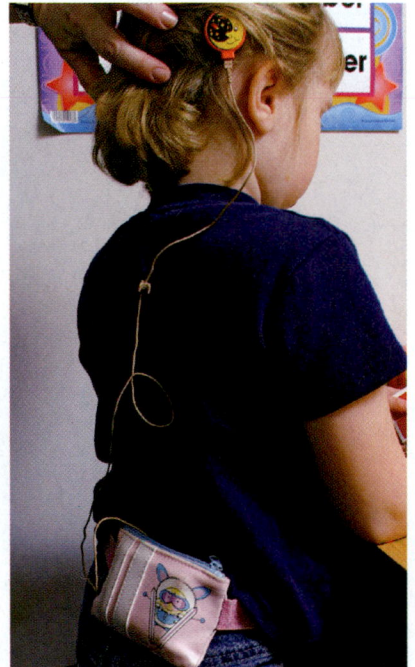

Figure 19–13 ➤ The child with a cochlear implant wears a speech processor, like the one present in this child's waist pack, as well as a microphone to pick up sounds and a transmitter that transfers the sound into electrical impulses. The microphone and transmitter are seen behind the ear. Electrodes that send signals to the brain are implanted in the skin behind the ear with a wire that leads to the middle ear.

Kate, the child introduced in the opening scenario, had a cochlear implant inserted at about 2 years of age (Figure 19–13 ➤). Children with cochlear implants need ongoing speech therapy to teach them the meaning of the new sounds they hear after the implant. There is an elevated risk of bacterial meningitis following implant, so immunization against pneumococcal disease and ongoing monitoring for this potential complication is needed (Wilson-Clark, Squires, & Deeks, 2006).

For children with uncorrectable hearing loss, several approaches are used to enhance communication (Table 19–9). Children with hearing impairment may receive speech therapy and instructions in lip-reading, signing, cuing, and finger-spelling.

NURSING MANAGEMENT
Nursing Assessment and Diagnosis

Nurses conduct newborn hearing tests soon after birth and make observations of the infant's responses to sound. As the child grows, hearing should be assessed at every well-child visit. The best judges of hearing are parents; ask them if they have concerns about their child's hearing. Be alert for parents who believe that their children do not

Table 19-9	COMMUNICATION TECHNIQUES FOR CHILDREN WHO ARE HEARING IMPAIRED

Technique	Description
Cued speech	Supplement to lip-reading; eight hand shapes represent groups of consonant sounds and four positions about the face represent groups of vowel sounds; based on the sounds the letters make, not the letters themselves; child can "see-hear" every spoken syllable a hearing person hears
Oral approach	Uses only spoken language for face-to-face communication; avoids use of formal signs; uses hearing aids and residual hearing
Total communication	Uses speech and sign, finger-spelling, lip-reading, and residual hearing simultaneously; child selects communication technique depending on the situation
Sign language	A separate or foreign language that allows the user to communicate quickly and accurately with others who understand signs. The signs or hand movements represent words or concepts. When a sign is not available, the word can be spelled out using signs. American Sign Language (ASL) is most often used; British Sign Language (BSL) is common in Europe.

have normal hearing since they are often the first to diagnose a hearing impairment. Recall Kate in the opening scenario; her father designed an experiment by clanging pans behind her when he suspected she did not hear. An infant's reaction to rattles, bells, or handclapping 30 cm (12 in.) from the ear is an important observation. Language milestones should be evaluated when the older infant and child are examined. Language development is a major area of focus in deaf children. Deaf infants begin to babble at about 5 to 6 months of age, the same age as hearing infants. However, this babbling ceases several months later in the hearing-impaired child.

School nurses use audiometers to evaluate hearing during screening programs in schools, and refer children who do not pass the screening test. See the *Clinical Skills Manual* for techniques in performing hearing screening. Nurses in offices often use tympanometers to evaluate ear function.

Following are common nursing diagnoses for the child with impaired hearing:

- Disturbed Sensory Perception related to altered sound transmission
- Risk for Impaired Verbal Communication related to hearing loss
- Risk for Delayed Growth and Development related to communication impairment
- Readiness for Enhanced Family Coping related to caring for a child with a hearing impairment

Planning and Implementation
Prevention and Early Identification
Nurses can encourage prevention of hearing loss from exposure to loud noises such as from power and farm equipment and music. Music should be turned down and ear protection should be worn for other activities. Early identification of hearing loss in infants and children is facilitated by newborn screening, developmental assessment, and childhood screening programs. Infants should be tested for hearing loss by 3 months of age; in cases of loss, intervention should begin before 6 months of age (Joint Committee on Infant Hearing, 2000). Be alert for expected language milestones during early childhood. School nurses should be active in hearing conservation education programs in school (Folmer, 2003).

Care in the Community
Most of the care for children with hearing impairment takes place in the community. The nurse integrates special care into the health promotion and health maintenance

LAW & ETHICS

Deafness and Cochlear Implants

Many people who are deaf consider deafness a culture, similar to an ethnic group or group with other common traits and experiences. They believe that they are fully functional, communicate, and socialize with others satisfactorily, and they do not view deafness as a defect. They believe that it is an affront to their culture to consider that someone should try to change from being deaf to hearing. Others note that only a select few can obtain cochlear implants due to their cost and the fact that health insurance may not cover the surgery, instrumentation, or speech therapy. Others are opposed to use of cochlear implants for children because of the surgical risk involved and the fact that children are not old enough to make their own decision about choosing the surgery. However, the earlier the child has the surgery and hears sounds, the more likely speech is to develop. Read about the controversy in resources such as M. Hyde & D. Power (2006). *Cochlear implants in children: Ethics and choices*. Washington DC: Gallaudet University Press. Imagine the difficulty parents have as they try to make the choice about treatment for the child who is hearing impaired. How can nurses support the family as they consider alternatives and then once the treatment decision is made?

SKILLS 6–20 AND 6–21
Hearing Acuity Screening

NURSING ALERT

Although it is recommended that infants with significant hearing loss be identified by 3 months of age and receive treatment by 6 months, most children with hearing deficits are not identified until later in childhood. Early intervention is crucial for maximizing the ability of the child to use any hearing present and to learn communication methods. Development is profoundly impacted by difficulty in communication. Nurses must test all newborns and infants for signs of hearing disorders and refer as needed. Parents often are the first to notice a problem with hearing, so they should be asked their observations of the infant's hearing during each visit (Moore, 2006).

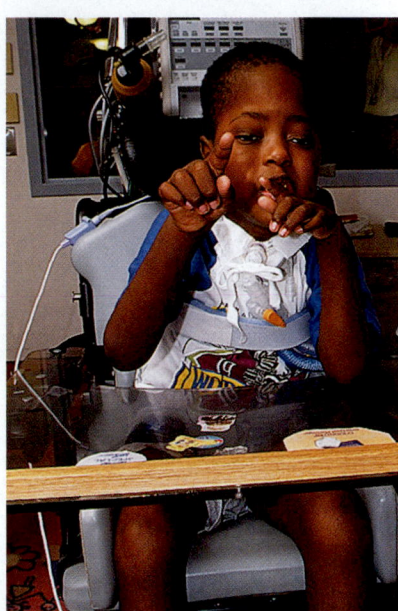

Figure 19–14 ➤ This child with a hearing impairment and tracheostomy is communicating by means of American Sign Language.

MediaLink

Health Promotion and Maintenance Overview: The Child with a Hearing Impairment

visit of children with hearing impairments (Figure 19–14 ➤). Nursing care of the child with a hearing impairment focuses on facilitating the child's ability to receive spoken language and to send information, on helping parents to meet the child's schooling needs, and on providing emotional support to parents. Refer the parents to an early intervention program as soon as the diagnosis of hearing impairment is made, in order to foster the child's development. If a cochlear implant is planned, the child needs surgical care and follow-up to monitor results and integrate sound gradually into the child's life. Parents often need help to decide on the best method for hearing and language enhancement for the child. You may need to interpret information, refer to the Internet and other resources, and help parents connect with parents who have chosen various approaches for their own children.

Children with cochlear implants need regular speech therapy after surgery. Refer parents to appropriate resources. Due to the increased rate of bacterial meningitis in cochlear recipients, particularly that caused by pneumococcus, immunization status is important. The child should be up-to-date for pneumococcal recommendations by 2–3 weeks before implant surgery. Following surgery, recommendations of the Centers for Disease Control and Prevention and cochlear implant should be followed. Parents should be taught the signs and symptoms of meningitis so that they can seek prompt care, if needed.

Facilitate Ability to Receive Spoken Language

Be aware of how the child compensates for hearing loss and use these strategies in communication:

- If hearing loss is mild or temporary or if the child reads lips, first obtain the child's visual attention by lightly touching the child or saying the child's name.
- Position your face 1 to 2 m (3 to 6 ft) from the child's face and make sure that the child's eyes are focused on your face and lips. Make sure the room is well lit, with no backlighting. Speak at a normal rate and tone, and use facial expressions that show caring or concern. If the child does not understand, rephrase the information in shorter, simpler sentences. Use specific, concrete explanations, and give the child time to comprehend. Watch for subtle signs of misinterpretations and give consistent and immediate feedback, since only 30% of the English language is visible on the lips.
- Be familiar with the different types of hearing aids. Hearing aids, which are microphones that amplify all sounds, can be worn in or behind the ear, in the frame of glasses, or on the body with a wire attached to the ear. When talking to a child with a hearing aid, speak slowly and be positioned 15 to 45 cm (6 to 18 in.) from the microphone using a normal conversational tone. Talk to the child even if the child is not looking at you. Make sure the batteries are fresh for the best reception. All sound is amplified, so reduce background noise as much as possible (see Families Want to Know: Care of the Hearing Aid).
- Acoustic feedback, an audible whistling sound that cannot always be heard by the child, is a common problem with hearing aids. To eliminate this sound, readjust the hearing aid to ensure that it is inserted properly and that no hair or ear wax is caught between the ear mold and canal. Turning down the volume may also help.
- A remote microphone system is another type of device designed to improve hearing. This is often used in the classroom situation because it eliminates background noise. The speaker wears a transmitter that picks up the voice and transmits it to a receiver worn by the child.

Facilitate Ability to Send Information

Maintain the child's hearing aid in proper condition. Many children with impaired hearing communicate using speech, which is enhanced through speech therapy. In addition, they are taught to sign, finger spell, or use cued speech (see Figure 19–14). Articulation may be difficult, and understanding what the child is trying to say may be frustrating for both the nurse and the child. Taking time to listen carefully is important.

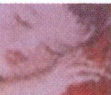

FAMILIES WANT TO KNOW

Care of the Hearing Aid

Families need to know how to maintain the child's hearing aid in proper condition to ensure its function. They can be taught when the child receives the first hearing aid, with at least annual updates to check on knowledge and questions. Items to include in teaching are as follows:

- The three types of hearing aids are those that fit totally in the ear canal, those that fit in the external ear canal, and those that fit behind the ear.

- The hearing aid should be cleaned each day with a damp cloth.
- Change the batteries as needed, usually about once a week. Disconnect the battery when not in use.
- Place the hearing aid in the ear with the volume off, and then slowly turn the volume up to half volume. Adjust as needed.
- Be sure the hearing aid fit is checked yearly, as the child's growth may necessitate a new fitting.

Measures to promote speech and communication development as well as safety are implemented. Ask the parents to explain the child's communication techniques and to help interpret words. Have younger children point to pictures. Use assisted technologies such as a computer or picture board, as well as drawings or gestures, if necessary. This technique is especially helpful for communicating feelings of pain and hunger during hospitalization. If the child signs or finger spells, be sure you understand the signs for important functions. Give older children a paper and pencil to write requests. People other than parents should be able to understand what the child is trying to communicate. Have an interpreter available if the child uses American Sign Language. Learn some common signs to communicate simple words or phrases. Orient the child carefully to new settings such as the hospital room or a new school.

Help Parents to Meet the Child's Educational Needs

Public laws apply to the education of children who are hearing impaired (see Chapter 1 ∞). After diagnosis, the parents and professionals together agree on an Individualized Education Plan (see discussion in Chapter 11 ∞). Childcare and preschool are recommended for children with hearing problems.

- Provide parents with information about adjustments that may have to be made for the hearing-impaired child who attends public school. By sitting at the front of the classroom, the child can hear and see more clearly. The teacher should always face the child when speaking, and background noise should be reduced.
- Tell parents that children who are hearing impaired have the same intelligence quotient (IQ) distribution as children without hearing impairment. However, communication and learning can be difficult, and extra support is needed.
- Children with hearing impairment should reach their intellectual potential, although development in certain areas may take place more slowly than it does in children with no hearing impairment.

Provide Emotional Support

By recognizing the effects of the diagnosis on the family, the nurse can help family members deal with their reactions to the child's hearing loss. Supporting healthy coping is an important intervention to help the parents carry on with their lives.

- Help the parents understand the child's disability and its effect on speech and language development. Provide accurate information about their concerns. Work jointly with other healthcare professionals and social service workers, if necessary.
- Tell the family about the community services available for medical, nursing, psychologic, and financial assistance.

 MediaLink

Resources for the Hearing Impaired

Evaluation

Expected outcomes of nursing care for a child with hearing impairment include:

- The child will demonstrate successful establishment of the communication method.
- The child will manifest growth and developmental milestones to maximum potential.
- An effective Individualized Education Plan will be established and implemented for the child.
- The family will demonstrate positive methods of coping with stress.

Injuries of the Ear

Ear injuries of many types commonly occur in children. Lacerations, infections, and hematomas may occur in the external ear structures, especially the pinna. Children may place foreign objects in the ear, and insects may enter the ear canal.

Rupture of the tympanic membrane may result from head injuries, blows to the ear, or insertion of objects into the ear canal. Serous drainage from the ear can indicate a basilar skull fracture. Be alert for ruptured tympanic membranes in combination with conjunctival and retinal hemorrhage, and other signs of shaken child syndrome (see Chapters 6 and 26 ∞ for further explanation of this syndrome).

See Table 19–10 for information on the emergency treatment of ear injuries. Any injury resulting in earache, decreased hearing, persistent bleeding, or other discharge should be seen by a physician.

DISORDERS OF THE NOSE AND THROAT

Epistaxis

Epistaxis, or nosebleed, is common in school-age children, especially boys. Kiesselbach's plexus, an area of plentiful veins located in the anterior nares, is a usual source of bleed-

> ### NURSING ALERT
>
> Both parents and children should be instructed never to put any object in the child's ear. Some parents believe that the ear canal should be cleaned with a cotton-tipped swab. If the cleaning is too vigorous or the child moves unexpectedly, a ruptured tympanic membrane could result.
>
> If an alkaline button battery (like those found in many toys or watches) is inserted in a child's ear, it can rapidly destroy tissue, causing perforation of the tympanic membrane, destruction of the ossicles, and local tissue ulceration. Removal should be performed with the child under sedation or general anesthesia.

Table 19–10	EMERGENCY TREATMENT OF EAR INJURIES
Injury	**Treatment**
Pinna	
Minor cuts or abrasions	Wash thoroughly with soap and water and rinse well; leave exposed to air if possible or apply adhesive bandage, monitor for infection.
Hematomas	Needle aspiration should be performed and pressure dressing applied; undrained hematomas may become fibrotic; "cauliflower ear" deformity may develop.
Cellulitis or abscesses	Apply moist heat intermittently; make sure that prescribed antibiotic is taken; minor surgery may be performed for an abscess.
Deep lacerations	Apply pressure to stop bleeding; transport to physician's office or emergency department for suturing.
Ear Canal	
Foreign bodies	Have child lie on back and turn head over edge of bed, with affected side down; wiggle earlobe and have child shake head; foreign object may fall out as result of gravity; if object remains in ear, call physician; do not try to remove foreign body with tweezers because this may push the object further into the ear.
Insects	Shine flashlights into ear to try to attract insect; instilling a few drops of mineral oil, olive oil, or alcohol kills insect, and irrigating ear canal gently may remove dead insect (see *Clinical Skills Manual*).
Tympanic Membrane	
Ruptures	Call physician if child has persistent ear pain after blow, blast injury, or insertion of foreign object; cover external ear loosely with piece of sterile cotton or gauze; if tympanic membrane has been ruptured, systemic antibiotics are prescribed.

ing, commonly caused by irritation from nosepicking, foreign bodies, or low humidity. Other causes include forceful coughing, allergies, or infections resulting in congestion of the nasal mucosa. Bleeding from the posterior septum is more serious and may be life threatening. Hospitalization may be necessary. Posterior nosebleeds have a variety of causes, some of which may indicate systemic disease (e.g., bleeding disorder) or injury.

Children with nosebleeds are sometimes brought to the emergency department by a parent who has been unable to stop the flow of blood within a few minutes. Both parent and child may be frightened. Ask the parent briefly about any history of nosebleeds and other contributing factors, including medications. Take the child's pulse and blood pressure to assess for excessive blood loss. Carefully examine the nasal mucosa by asking the child to blow any clots out gently, if possible. Suctioning may be necessary.

Observing the flow may help determine if the blood is coming from an anterior or a posterior location. A nosebleed confined to one side of the nose is almost always anterior, but posterior bleeding can flow on one or both sides. If blood cannot be seen, the child may be swallowing it, resulting in nausea. Suspect posterior bleeding in children who have sustained blunt trauma or in other children at high risk.

The child with anterior bleeding should sit upright quietly. The head should be tilted forward to prevent blood from trickling down the throat, which can lead to vomiting. The nares should be squeezed just below the nasal bone and held for 10 to 15 minutes while the child breathes through the mouth. If the bleeding does not stop, a cotton ball or swab soaked with Neo-Synephrine, epinephrine, thrombin, or lidocaine may be inserted into the affected nostril by the primary care provider to promote topical vasoconstriction or anesthesia. Once the bleeding has stopped, the nostril may have to be cauterized with silver nitrate or electrocautery. If the bleeding cannot be stopped, absorbable packing may be used.

Posterior bleeding must also be stopped by packing, and the child must be monitored carefully. Arterial ligation is occasionally needed. Repeated or severe nosebleeds need further evaluation (Bernius & Perlin, 2006).

Nursing Management

Assess the child's hematocrit or hemoglobin if significant bleeding has occurred. Children with frequent epistaxis should have a complete history taken and physical examination performed to rule out systemic disease.

After the nosebleed has stopped, the child is more vulnerable to recurrent bleeding and should avoid bending over, stooping, strenuous exercise, hot drinks, and hot baths or showers for the next 3 to 4 days. Sleeping with the head elevated on two or three pillows and humidifying the air with a vaporizer may also prevent a recurrence. Provide parents with suggestions for prevention and home management of epistaxis. See Families Want to Know: Prevention and Home Management of Epistaxis.

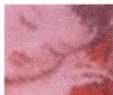

FAMILIES WANT TO KNOW

Prevention and Home Management of Epistaxis

Prevention

- Humidify the child's room, especially during the winter.
- Discourage the child from picking or rubbing the nose or inserting foreign objects into the nose.
- Instruct the child to blow the nose gently and release sneezes through the mouth.

Home Management

- Keep the child calm.
- Sit the child upright with head tilted slightly forward so blood does not run down the nasopharynx.

- Press a roll of cotton under the upper lip to compress the labial artery.
- Apply steady pressure to both nostrils just below the nasal bone with the thumb and forefinger for 15–20 minutes. Time by the clock.
- Apply an ice pack or cold compress to the bridge of the nose or the back of the neck.
- Call the healthcare provider if the bleeding does not stop.
- Avoid vigorous exercise and aspirin or other noncoagulant drugs during the first few days after a nosebleed.

Note: Adapted from Health Care Guide, 2006.

Nasopharyngitis

Nasopharyngitis, also known as the common cold, causes inflammation and infection of the nose and throat and is probably the most common illness of infancy and childhood. More than 200 viruses and numerous bacteria can cause this condition. The most common viruses include rhinovirus and coronavirus, and the most frequently occurring bacterium is group A Streptococcus. See Chapter 20 ∞ for a discussion of respiratory syncytial virus (RSV), a common cause of both upper and lower respiratory illness. The organisms incubate in 1 to 3 days, and the infection is communicable several hours before symptoms develop and for 1 to 2 days after they begin. Symptoms may last 4 to 10 days or longer. The pathogens are believed to spread when the infected person touches the hand of an uninfected person, who then touches his or her mouth or nose, resulting in self-inoculation with infected droplets.

A red nasal mucosa with clear nasal discharge and an infected throat with enlarged tonsils may be apparent in children with nasopharyngitis. Vesicles may be present on the soft palate and in the pharynx. Accompanying symptoms may vary, depending on the child's age (Table 19–11).

Between episodes of nasopharyngitis, the child should be asymptomatic. If a child continues to have upper respiratory infections, the presence of an underlying condition such as allergy, asthma, or polyps should be ruled out.

Nursing Management

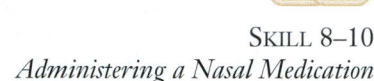

SKILL 8–10
Administering a Nasal Medication

For infants who cannot breathe through the mouth, normal saline nose drops can be administered every 3 to 4 hours, especially before feeding. (Refer to the *Clinical Skills Manual* for instructions on administration of nose drops.) For infants over 9 months of age, nasal stuffiness can be treated with either normal saline nose drops or a decongestant such as phenylephrine (0.125% to 0.25%, depending on the child's age). Older children can use nasal sprays.

Although nose drops and sprays are more effective than systemic decongestants, they should not be used for more than 4 or 5 days or more often than recommended. Antihistamines may be helpful for children with allergic rhinitis or profuse nasal drainage. Long-acting nasal sprays and medications with several ingredients are not recommended.

Room humidification may help prevent drying of nasal secretions. Antipyretics such as acetaminophen reduce fever and make the child more comfortable. Aspirin is not recommended because of its association with Reye's syndrome (refer to Chapter 26 ∞).

Children should avoid strenuous physical activity and engage in quiet play such as reading, listening to music or stories, or watching television or videotapes. Children should not be forced to eat, but the intake of favorite fluids to liquefy secretions should be encouraged. Parents should be told that no medicine or vaccine can prevent the common cold, but eliminating contact with infected persons can reduce the spread of infection. (See Families Want to Know: Teaching About Over-the-Counter Cough and Cold Medications.) Proper hand hygiene and disposal of tissues help to decrease the spread of the infection.

Table 19–11	SYMPTOMS OF NASOPHARYNGITIS	
Infants Younger than 3 Months of Age	**Infants 3 Months of Age or Older**	**Older Children**
• Lethargy • Irritability • Feeding poorly • Fever (may be absent)	• Fever • Vomiting • Diarrhea • Sneezing • Anorexia • Irritability • Restlessness	• Dry, irritated nose and throat • Chills, fever • Generalized muscle aches • Headache • Malaise • Anorexia • Thin nasal discharge, which may later become thick and purulent • Possible sneezing

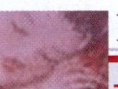

FAMILIES WANT TO KNOW

Teaching About Over-the-Counter Cough and Cold Medications

Parents may try to treat children who have upper respiratory infections with the same medications they are accustomed to taking for a cold. Prepare them during a health promotion visit and help them plan for how to handle medications for the child. Guidelines are as follows:

- Read the label to be sure the medication is recommended for the child's age and condition. Give only the dose recommended for the child's age and weight.
- Be sure you know how to measure the medication. Tablespoon and teaspoon are NOT the same, and using household spoons may lead to incorrect dosing. Use the measuring device that is provided with liquid medications for greatest accuracy.

- Consult the pharmacist, nurse, or doctor if you have questions, if the medication is not recommended for the age of your child, if the child's condition does not improve, or if other symptoms appear.
- Use the child-resistant cap after each opening of the bottle. Store the medication out of reach of all children, preferably in a locked location.
- If you use home remedies or other herbal products to treat colds, be sure to check on their safety for a child with your healthcare provider first.
- Inspect containers and do not buy those that may have tears, imperfections, or tampering.

Adapted from: U.S. Food and Drug Administration. Got a sick kid? Retrieved October 3, 2006, from http:// www.fda.gov/cder/consumerinfo/sickkids.htm

Sinusitis

Sinusitis is an inflammation of one or more of the paranasal sinuses. These sinuses, which have respiratory epithelium and are continuous with the respiratory tract, include the maxillary, ethmoid, frontal, and sphenoid sinuses. The sinuses commonly become infected following a viral upper respiratory infection. It is important to differentiate viral from bacterial sinusitis. In both cases, the child's history reveals a cold for several days, followed by improvement in the cold symptoms, and a decrease in nasal drainage. In bacterial infection, the upper respiratory infection improves but an increase in purulent nasal drainage may be observed, with a fever above 102°F or 39°C. The symptoms persist over 10 days with accompanying facial pain, headache, and fever (Bernius & Perlin, 2006). The most common infectious agents are the same as those for otitis media, namely *Streptococcus pneumoniae*, *Haemophilus influenzae*, and *Moraxella catarrhalis* (Subcommittee on Management of Sinusitis and Committee on Quality Improvement, 2001). Chronic sinusitis may occur in children with uncontrolled allergies and asthma.

Signs and symptoms of sinusitis in children are sometimes nonspecific. A history of recent upper respiratory infection is common, persistent cough from postnasal drip

COMPLEMENTARY THERAPY

Cold Treatments

Many families use home and herbal remedies for treatment of colds. Many of these are harmless and may increase the child's comfort, while others may not help. Echinacea, a product derived from a plant, has been used as an immune stimulant and is commonly used to treat respiratory infections. It is available in capsules, juice, tea, and other preparations. A study funded by the National Center for Complementary and Alternative Medicine did not find echinacea effective in treating upper respiratory tract infections in children from 2 to 11 years of age. While the treatment was generally found to be safe, there was an increased risk of rash in some treated children (Taylor, Weber, Standish et al., 2003).

Some products designed for colds may actually be harmful. Herbal products that contain aristolochic acid, a substance that can cause cancer and kidney disease, can be found on numerous Internet sites, and several are marketed as cold remedies (Gold & Slone, 2003).

Many Hispanic and Asian cultural groups believe in the "hot and cold theory" of disease, in which health problems are viewed as the result of imbalance. For example, Mexican Americans traditionally treat a "cold disease" such as an earache or common cold with "hot" substances. Ask families if they prefer to eat certain foods during an illness. Incorporating such preferences can promote the child's health and increase the family's confidence in healthcare providers.

Nurses should assess what home or herbal remedies families use to treat a child's upper respiratory infection, and evaluate if the treatments are safe. Integrate preferences whenever possible. What questions can you ask to obtain the necessary information? Where will you go to obtain information about safety?

can occur, and nasal discharge or swelling can be apparent. Malodorous breath, fever, mouth breathing, hyponasal speech, and cervical lympadenopathy may be present (Leung & Kellner, 2004). Young children may be anorexic or have difficulty feeding while older children may complain of headache.

A diagnosis of sinusitis is usually based on history and physical examination findings. Percussion and illumination of sinuses are not generally useful in children. Computed tomography (CT), magnetic resonance imaging (MRI), and radiographs may be performed but they can be costly, require sedation of young children, and may be inconclusive. For the child with repeated sinusitis or who appears toxic, aspiration of sinus aspirate may be performed for culture by an otolaryngologist.

Although most primary care providers treat suspected sinusitis with antibiotics, many cases will clear spontaneously without treatment. Amoxicillin is the first choice for therapy; amoxicillin/clavulanate, cephalosporins, azithromycin, and clindamycin are also sometimes used (Bernius & Perlin, 2006; Sinus and Allergy Health Partnership, 2002). Children with recurrent sinusitis should be referred for further care by an otolaryngologist and allergy specialist.

Parents whose child has persistent and purulent nasal drainage should be told to see a healthcare provider, particularly if the drainage is accompanied by facial pain, headache, and fever. Teach parents to correctly administer antibiotics (e.g., to take medications for the full course) if prescribed, and to use saline nose drops if needed for comfort. Infants may need their nose cleared with nose drops and a bulb syringe prior to feedings. (Refer to the *Clinical Skills Manual* for correct use of a bulb syringe.) Antipyretics can be given for fever and to relieve pain.

SKILL 11–20
Performing Nasal/Oral Suctioning

Pharyngitis

Acute pharyngitis is an infection that primarily affects the pharynx, including the tonsils. It is seen most frequently in children 4 to 7 years and is rare in children less than 1 year. Approximately 80% of these infections are caused by viruses (most commonly enteroviruses); the rest are caused by bacteria. Bacterial pharyngitis is commonly known as strep throat, because about 20–40% of bacterial pharyngitis is caused by group A beta-hemolytic *Streptococcus* (GABHS) (Armengol, Hendley, & Schlager, 2006). The major complaint is a sore throat. See the clinical manifestations table below for symptoms of viral pharyngitis and strep throat. Children with symptoms of strep throat who have minimal throat redness and pain, exudate, mild lymphadenopathy, and a low-grade fever, and who have been exposed to someone who has pharyngitis, should have a throat culture. The classic signs of purulent drainage and white patches are not present in all cases of strep throat. A child who finds swallowing difficult or extremely painful, who drools, or who exhibits signs of dehydration or respiratory distress should be seen by a physician immediately. These signs could be indicators

CLINICAL MANIFESTATIONS	VIRAL PHARYNGITIS AND STREP THROAT (GROUP A BETA-HEMOLYTIC STREPTOCOCCUS [GABHS])[a]

Viral Pharyngitis	Strep Throat
Nasal congestion	Abrupt onset
Mild sore throat	Tonsillar exudate[b]
Conjunctivitis	Painful cervical lymphadenopathy[b]
Cough	Anorexia, nausea, vomiting, abdominal pain
Hoarseness	Severe sore throat
Mild pharyngeal redness	Headache, malaise
Minimal tonsillar exudate	Fever > 38.3°C (101°F)
Mildly tender anterior cervical lymphadenopathy	Petechial mottling of soft palate
Fever < 38.3°C (101°F)	

[a]Children 6 months to 3 years of age may have streptococcus with symptoms that resemble those of viral pharyngitis. Children with scarlet fever have the symptoms of strep throat plus a sandpaper-textured erythematous generalized rash and pallor around the lips.
[b]Classic signs of strep throat.

of serious conditions such as epiglottitis (see Chapter 20 ∞) or diphtheria (see Chapter 18 ∞).

Peritonsillar abscess (a tonsil infection that spreads into surrounding tissues and causes cellulites) or retropharyngeal abscess (an infection of the lymph nodes that drain the adenoids, nasopharynx, and paranasal sinuses) are related serious conditions. These conditions may have additional symptoms such as decreased neck movement and respiratory distress (Craig & Schunk, 2003).

The diagnosis of strep throat is made by throat culture, using the rapid or traditional strep tests. Results of the rapid strep test may be available within minutes; those for the traditional test are available in 24 to 48 hours. Early signs of strep throat should be treated with oral penicillin for 10 days or by long-acting penicillin given in one injection immediately, even before the result of the culture is available. If the child is allergic to penicillin, erythromycin is given. Azithromycin and clarithromycin are additional examples of antibiotics used for treatment. Acute symptoms should resolve within 24 hours of therapy, at which time the child is no longer contagious. For pharyngitis that is caused by a virus, symptomatic treatment alone is used.

Nursing Management

Nurses often identify bacterial and viral pharyngitis, take throat cultures as needed, and refer the child for proper treatment. Nursing care focuses on symptomatic relief. Acetaminophen reduces throat pain and generalized fever. Cool, nonacidic fluids and soft foods, ice chips, or frozen juice pops given frequently in small amounts facilitate swallowing and prevent dehydration. Humidification, chewing gum, and gargling with warm salt water (5 g salt to 250 mL water; 1 tsp salt to 8 oz water) soothe an irritated throat. Commercial throat sprays or throat lozenges are not generally more effective than these home remedies. Encourage the child to rest, in order to conserve energy and promote recovery.

Teach parents the importance of completing the entire course of antibiotics if prescribed for bacterial pharyngitis. After about 2 days of the medication, have the parents replace the child's toothbrush with a new one to avoid reinfection by bacteria that can survive on the moist brush. Reinforce to parents the importance of treating streptococcal infections, as untreated infections may lead to rheumatic fever, cervical adenitis, sinusitis, glomerulonephritis, or meningitis.

Tonsillitis and Adenoiditis

Tonsillitis is an infection or inflammation (hypertrophy) of the palatine tonsils. Although most children with pharyngitis may have infected tonsils, they do not necessarily have tonsillitis. The adenoids are lymphatic tissue located on the posterior pharyngeal wall and are sometimes called the pharyngeal tonsils; they can manifest with acute or chronic infection as well (Bahadori & Schwartz, 2006).

Etiology and Pathophysiology

Like pharyngitis, tonsillitis and adenoiditis may be caused by a virus or bacterium. The primary site of infection is the tonsils. The condition tends to recur several times in certain children.

Clinical Manifestations

Symptoms suggestive of tonsillitis include frequent throat infections with breathing and swallowing difficulties; persistent redness of the anterior pillars; and enlargement of the cervical lymph nodes. If children breathe through their mouths continuously, the mucous membranes may become dry and irritated. Adenoiditis is characterized by nasal stuffiness, discharge, and postnasal drip, which results in coughing or excessive clearing of the throat.

■ COLLABORATIVE CARE

Diagnosis is made on the basis of visual inspection and clinical manifestations. Tonsils appear large and inflamed. Enlarged adenoids are diagnosed by radiologic studies.

Symptomatic treatment for tonsillitis is the same as for pharyngitis. Surgical removal of tonsils (tonsillectomy) is often recommended when children have recurrent throat infections (about three per year for 3 years), chronic tonsillitis, obstructive sleep apnea, or malformations causing nasal speech or a facial growth abnormality. If the child is under 3 years of age, the surgery is postponed if possible because it may stimulate growth of other lymphoid tissue in the nasopharynx. If the pharyngeal tonsils (adenoids) are enlarged, as suggested by mouth breathing, snoring, cough, impaired taste and smell, a muffled quality to the voice, and chronic otitis media, then they may be removed at the same time (Bahadori & Schwartz, 2006; Paradise, Bluestone, Colborn et al., 2002).

A technique has been introduced for use with children who have sleep obstruction due to large tonsillar size. Temperature-controlled radiofrequency (TCRF) can reduce the size of tonsils when they are excessively large in children from 4 to 13 years. The target tissue is heated through a submucosal electrode; surgical time and recovery time are lower than in usual tonsillectomy procedures. Children are reported to have increased comfort, decreased snoring and other sleep problems, and a very fast recovery from the procedure (Nelson, 2003).

■ NURSING MANAGEMENT

Nursing Assessment and Diagnosis

Assess the throat carefully during each physical examination. Observe for tonsils that are simply large (a common finding in childhood) and those that are inflamed. Look for the degree of redness and presence of any exudate. Ask if the child has pain or difficulty swallowing. Ask about the history of past tonsillar infections and the length of time of the present discomfort.

If surgery is indicated, take a complete history of the child preoperatively. Monitor vital signs and observe for respiratory distress, hemorrhage, and dehydration postoperatively.

The following nursing diagnoses may apply to the child with tonsillitis:

- Acute Pain related to inflammation of the pharynx
- Risk for Deficient Fluid Volume related to inadequate intake
- Risk for Ineffective Breathing Pattern related to obstruction by enlarged tonsils
- Impaired Swallowing related to inflammation and pain
- Deficient Knowledge (Parents) related to home care following discharge

Planning and Implementation

The nurse provides general supportive care and, if medication is prescribed, encourages completion of the full course of treatment. The nursing management of children with tonsillitis is similar to that of children with pharyngitis (see earlier discussion).

If surgery is indicated, the parents are helped to prepare their child for a short-term surgical procedure with a possible overnight stay in the hospital (see Chapter 13 ∞). Children should be free of sore throat, fever, or upper respiratory infection for at least 1 week before surgery. They should not be given aspirin, ibuprofen, or other medications that alter bleeding time for 2 weeks before surgery, as these medications can increase bleeding. Check if any herbal medications are taken and report them to the physician and anesthesiologist, because some may interfere with anesthetic drugs used in surgery or with normal blood clotting.

Discharge Planning and Home Care Teaching

Discharge planning includes teaching parents about pain management, fluid and nutrition intake, activity restrictions, and possible complications in the postoperative period. Most children have a sore throat for 7 to 10 days after tonsillectomy and adenoidectomy. Advise parents how to relieve the child's throat pain. See Families Want to Know: Care After Tonsillectomy.

Children may experience ear pain, especially when swallowing, between 4 and 8 days after a tonsillectomy. Advise parents that this pain is the result of referred pain from the tonsillar area and does not indicate an ear infection.

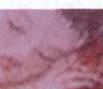

FAMILIES WANT TO KNOW

Care After Tonsillectomy

After a child's tonsillectomy, the parent can institute measures to increase the child's comfort.

- Have the child drink adequate cool fluids or chew gum, as this reduces spasms in the muscles surrounding the throat.
- Give acetaminophen elixir, as ordered.

- Apply an ice collar around the child's neck.
- Have the child gargle with a solution of 2.5 g (0.5 teaspoon) each of baking soda and salt in 8 oz of water.
- Have the child rinse the mouth well with viscous lidocaine and then swallow the solution.

Emphasize to parents the importance of adequate fluid intake. Children should be given any liquid they prefer for the first week, except citrus juices, which may produce a burning sensation in the throat. Red liquids are discouraged initially so that bleeding is not masked by the red fluid. Soft foods such as gelatin, applesauce, frozen juice pops, and mashed potatoes can be added as tolerated.

Children do not need to be confined to bed, but vigorous exercise should be avoided for the first week after surgery. Advise parents that the child may return to school approximately 10 days after a tonsillectomy.

Any surgery carries with it the risk of postoperative complications. Teach parents the normal signs of healing in the postoperative period, as well as signs of complications. See Families Want to Know: Complications of Tonsillectomy and Adenoidectomy.

Evaluation

Expected outcomes of nursing care for the child with tonsillitis include:

- The child will ingest adequate intake of food and fluids.
- Pain and fever will be managed to a level of comfort for the child.
- The child will experience no postoperative complications.
- Complete healing will occur.

DISORDERS OF THE MOUTH

The mouth is an important structure that is directly linked to both the gastrointestinal and respiratory systems. A major type of mouth abnormality is caused by structural problems that occur in the mouth, often in conjunction with other defects. See Chapter 24 ∞ for a description of tracheoesophageal fistula and cleft lip and palate; see Chapter 5 ∞ for a description of examination of the mouth and tongue in infants and children in order to identify abnormalities of the mouth.

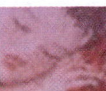

FAMILIES WANT TO KNOW

Complications of Tonsillectomy and Adenoidectomy

Bleeding

- To prevent bleeding, aspirin or ibuprofen should not be given for pain for the first postoperative week. Use acetaminophen instead.
- Bleeding is most likely to occur within the first 24 hours or 7–10 days after the tonsillectomy, when the scar is forming. Report any trickle of bright red blood to the physician immediately.

Pain

- Administer acetaminophen as ordered.
- Offer frequent small amounts of cool liquids. Avoid citrus juice.
- Provide for rest and quiet activities for several days.

Infection

- The back of the throat will look white and have an odor for the first 7–8 days after the surgery. The child may also have a low-grade fever. These are not signs of infection.
- For temperatures over 38.3°C (101°F), acetaminophen may be used.
- Call the physician if the child develops a fever above 38.8°C (102°F).

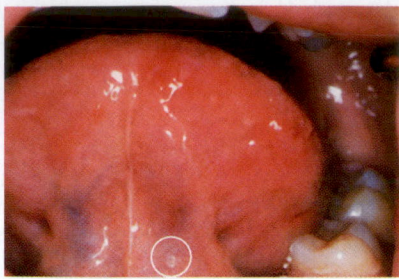

Figure 19–15 ➤ The child with aphthous ulcers in the mouth has discomfort and pain that interfere with ingestion of food and fluids. These ulcers can be caused by infectious organisms and are most common in children with immune suppression. Frequent oral assessment and meticulous oral care are needed by all children at risk of oral ulcers.

A second type of mouth disorder in children is ulceration. Children sometimes have changes in the mucous membranes of the mouth, associated with illnesses, infections, or as a side effect of drug treatments. Mouth ulcers are discussed in the following text.

Trauma is a third cause for mouth disorders in children. Mouth and dental emergencies are discussed in the following text.

Mouth Ulcers

A variety of conditions can cause mouth ulcers in children. They commonly occur in conjunction with certain medications, diseases, or oral trauma (Figure 19–15 ➤). Oral mucosa has a fast rate of growth so that conditions that impair cell synthesis will cause breakdown in the mucosa with lack of new tissue growth. The growth of mucosal tissue requires adequate moisture, so dehydration is a risk factor for development of oral ulcers. See Clinical Manifestations of Mouth Ulcers in Children for the etiology and clinical manifestations for some of the conditions leading to oral ulcers in children.

Collaborative Care

The goals of collaborative care are relief from pain and promotion of ulcer healing. Most mouth ulcers and other oral lesions are diagnosed by history and appearance. Culture of exudate may be helpful in identifying an infective cause. Biopsy may be performed if the cause is not clear or a mouth cancer is possible. Occasionally laboratory blood analysis is done and may show leukocytosis in infectious cases and Stevens-Johnson syndrome.

Most mouth ulcers are treated symptomatically. Since the oral mucosa is fast growing, the cells can rapidly heal. Keeping the mouth clean and administering systemic or topical analgesics can assist with comfort. Foods should be mild and nonirritating. Acyclovir may be administered for treatment of herpes infections. Antibiotics are needed for bacterial infection of oral lesions. Stevens-Johnson syndrome necessitates removing the drug that causes the reaction, and treating the child with oral antihistamines and supportive therapy.

Nursing Management

Nurses assess the oral cavity of all children beginning in the neonatal period. Structural abnormalities are promptly referred for further diagnostic work. Mouth ulcers are examined for size, location, drainage, and pain. For those at risk, such as children on chemotherapy, regular careful examination of the oral mucosa is an important part of care. Some of the appropriate nursing diagnoses for children with oral ulcers include:

- Acute Pain related to injury of oral cavity
- Impaired Oral Mucous Membrane related to chemotherapy or infection
- Imbalanced Nutrition: Less than Body Requirements related to inability to ingest adequate foods

Nurses play an important role in the treatment of oral ulcers. Most ulcers are treated symptomatically and will heal rapidly. Ensure that children have good oral care, including brushing teeth with a soft bristle brush or by use of mouth sponges. Rinse the mouth after all meals and snacks. Teach the family correct administration of oral medications and topical preparations designed to treat infection or provide comfort. When oral mucosa ulcers are predicted, such as with chemotherapy or in AIDS, begin oral protocols before lesions occur to decrease their appearance and severity (Shetty, 2006). Encourage a diet that has only mild foods, and avoid spices and very sweet, sour, and acidic items. Cold foods may be better accepted. Monitor hydration status to ensure adequate fluid intake. Teach parents correct administration of acetaminophen or other analgesic treatment. Use standard precautions to protect the child from infections and prevent their flora from being transferred to other children or family members. Encourage parents to keep children with herpes gingivostomatitis out of contact with other children if active lesions or drooling are present (Blevins, 2003).

Desired outcomes of nursing care for children with oral problems include a decrease in reported oral pain or disruptive effects on dietary intake, structural intactness and normal function of oral mucosal membranes, and ingestion of adequate amounts of fluids and nutrients.

Mouth and Dental Emergencies

Children may experience trauma to the mouth and teeth during falls, sporting activities, and motor vehicle crashes. A predominance of cases occurs in the toddler years as children become more mobile (Bernius & Perlin, 2006). Nurses inform parents of proper treatment for injuries and may provide emergency treatment in schools and other community settings. Injury prevention is encouraged through use of protective gear during sports. See Chapter 23 ∞ for a discussion of oral care during treatment for cancer, and Chapter 6 ∞ for a discussion of protective sporting gear and of body piercing, which may include the oral cavity.

Because the mouth has a profuse blood supply, bleeding may be extensive for even minor injuries. It is best to use clean cloths to absorb the blood and prevent choking on it, and get the child to an emergency facility to have the lesion carefully examined.

Dental injuries may involve fracture of a tooth, luxation (partial extrusion), or avulsion (complete removal). The periodontal ligament holds the tooth in the socket but its attachment is torn during a tooth avulsion (Krause-Parello, 2005). The child should be transported immediately to an emergency facility. If otherwise stable, an emergency dental visit is the best choice. When avulsion has occurred, fast care improves the chance that a permanent tooth can be reimplanted and kept alive. When reimplanted within 30 minutes, the tooth's chances of survival are best (American Association of Endodontics, 2004). Nurses can perform care or teach parents what to do in case of dental emergency. See Families Want to Know: Care of a Tooth Avulsion. Referral to dental resources may be needed. See Chapters 8, 9, and 10 ∞ for specific dental needs for health promotion and health maintenance at each age during childhood and adolescence.

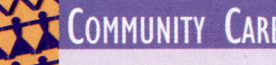

COMMUNITY CARE

Dental Care

For families with financial constraints, dental care is often delayed or not available. Dental caries is the most common cause of chronic disease in childhood. The highest rates of caries occur in Asian and Pacific Islanders, then Hispanics, followed by African Americans and White children (Children's Oral Health, 2003). Ask families about what they do for dental care, and how they would seek care if the child had a dental emergency. Many communities have an association of dentists and dental workers who provide care at clinics and other facilities for children without dental insurance. Nurses can help the families to find resources in their communities to provide regular dental visits and care for dental emergencies.

CLINICAL MANIFESTATIONS | MOUTH ULCERS IN CHILDREN

Disorder	Etiology	Clinical Manifestations
Chemotherapy-related oral mucositis	Many chemotherapy drugs used to treat cancer attack all rapidly growing cells in the body. Lack of intake of sufficient fluids to provide adequate hydration exacerbates the development of mucositis.	The oral mucosa may have painful ulcers that bleed, become infected, or interfere with food intake.
AIDS-related oral mucositis	Some of the drugs used to treat HIV infections and the poor nutritional state of children with AIDS can both promote the development of oral ulcers.	Painful oral ulcers further interfere with adequate food intake.
Stevens-Johnson Syndrome (see Chapter 30 ∞)	*Erythema multiforme* is a rare mucocutaneous disease. *Erythema multiforme major* is also known as Stevens-Johnson syndrome. After a prodromal period with fever, malaise, fatigue, and sore throat, the characteristic lesions of the disease erupt. Stevens-Johnson syndrome may occur with recurrent herpesvirus infection, *Mycoplasma pneumoniae,* or as a reaction to drugs such as nonsteroidal anti-inflammatories, anticonvulsants, and sulfonamides.	Endothelial cells, epithelial cells, and mucosal cells are all affected, causing blisters and erosion of conjunctiva, oral cavity, and genital mucosa. A bullous erythematous rash also is common and a pneumonia can result.
Aphthous ulcers	These lesions are commonly called "canker sores." An allergic or autoimmune cause is suspected, but herpes gingivitis should be ruled out.	They often recur in the same child over time. Ulcers are on the inside of the lips or throughout the mouth; about one to three ulcers occur at a time.
Herpes simplex gingivostomatitis (see Chapter 18 ∞)	Herpesvirus is the causative organism. Herpes simplex infections of the face and nose are referred to as "cold sores."	Multiple ulcers and vesicles of the gingiva, palate, buccal mucosa, lips, and tongue appear. They may be accompanied by skin vesicular lesions characteristic of herpes on the face.
Traumatic ulcers	Trauma to the oral mucosa can lead to ulcers. Children may bite the side of the mouth, may poke a pencil or other object into the mucosa, or can have burns from hot liquids or acidic substances.	One or more ulcerations are visible and may become infected due to the source of trauma.

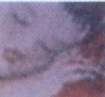

FAMILIES WANT TO KNOW

Care of a Tooth Avulsion

When a tooth is removed during an injury, prompt treatment may influence the chance that it can be reimplanted. If the child's condition is stable, try to reimplant the tooth and then transfer the child to an emergency dental facility.

- Handle the tooth only by the crown (its top) rather than the root in order to avoid further damage.
- Gently rinse the tooth with a stream of sterile saline.
- Insert the tooth into the socket.

- Have the child provide gentle pressure by biting a piece of gauze or a moistened tea bag.

If the child is unstable or has other injuries, enlist emergency medical transportation (call 9-1-1). In this case, the tooth is transported with the child.

- If a dental aid kit is available, it may contain a transport liquid such as Viaspan or Hank's Balanced Salt Solution. If these are not available, alternatives include cold milk, saliva, saline, or water.

Note: Adapted from Krause-Parello, C. A. (2005). Tooth avulsion in the school setting. *Journal of School Nursing, 21,* 279–282.

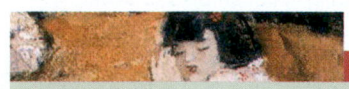

CRITICAL THINKING IN ACTION

Recall Kate, who was described in the opening scenario. She was deaf and had a cochlear implant at 2 years of age. She is now 5 years of age and she hears sounds, is working to integrate sounds with meaning, and attends speech therapy each week. Kate is fortunate that she has two parents who are able to attend speech therapy with her and reinforce learning at home. They are concerned about finding the best kindergarten for her to attend next year.

DISCUSSION

1. Describe the normal speech patterns of a 5-year-old. How are Kate's patterns likely to differ?

2. Refer back to the Denver II Developmental Screening Test described in Chapter 8 . Are there any items for the 5-year-old that might be difficult for Kate? If so, which ones?

3. Which immunization is especially important for Kate to receive in order to prevent a risk of meningitis with her cochlear implant? How will you counsel parents about this and help them find a resource for immunizations?

4. Provide a list of questions that Kate's parents can ask as they visit and evaluate kindergartens. What characteristics will be especially important for them to consider?

Refer to your Prentice Hall Nursing MediaLInk DVD-ROM for answers.

EXPLORE MediaLink 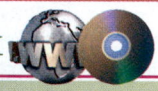 http://www.prenhall.com/ball

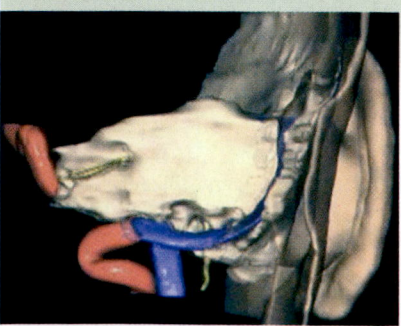

Resources for this chapter can be found on the Prentice Hall Nursing MediaLink DVD-ROM accompanying this textbook, and on the Companion Website at http://www.prenhall.com/ball.

DVD-ROM
Audio Glossary
NCLEX-RN® Review
Animations/Videos
  Deaf Culture
  Ear Abnormalities
  Middle Ear Dynamics
  Otitis Media

COMPANION WEBSITE
Audio Glossary
NCLEX-RN® Review
Care Plan Activity: Retinopathy of Prematurity
Case Study: Otitis Media
MediaLink Application: Early Identification and Intervention for Hearing Loss
WebLinks

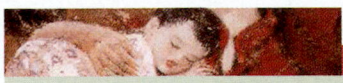

REFERENCES

Abelson, M. B., & Granet, D. (2006). Ocular allergy in pediatric practice. *Current Allergy and Asthma Reports, 6*, 306–311.

Alexander, M. (2003). Ocular allergy: Treatment options for children. *Contemporary Pediatrics* (Supple.), 3–6.

American Academy of Pediatrics. (2001). Sports with high risk of eye injury with appropriate eye protectors. Retrieved July 16, 2004, from http://www.aaporg/policy/01497t2.htm

American Academy of Pediatrics, Committee on Infectious Diseases. (2006). *Red book* (27th ed.). Elk Grove Village, IL: Author.

American Academy of Pediatrics, Committee on Practice and Ambulatory Medicine, Section on Ophthalmology. (2003). Eye examination in infants, children, and young adults by pediatricians. *Pediatrics, 111*, 902–907.

American Academy of Pediatrics, Section on Ophthalmology. (2001). Screening examination of premature infants for retinopathy of prematurity. *Pediatrics, 108*, 809–811.

American Academy of Pediatrics, Subcommittee on Management of Acute Otitis Media. (2004). Diagnosis and management of acute otitis media. *Pediatrics 113*, 1451–1465.

American Association of Endodontics. (2004). Emergency steps for saving a knocked-out tooth. Retrieved May 10, 2006, from http://www.aae.org/patients/avulsed.htm

Armengol, C. E., Hendley, O., & Schlager, T. A. (2006). An office-based guide to diagnosing streptococcal pharyngitis. *Contemporary Pediatrics, 23*(5), 64–78.

Bahadori, R. A., & Schwartz, R. H. (2006). The adenoid in children: Out of sight, out of mind? *Infectious Diseases in Children, 19*(8), 11–12.

Behrman, R. E., Kliegman, R. M., & Jenson, H. B. (2004). *Nelson textbook of pediatrics* (17th ed.). Philadelphia: Saunders.

Bernius, M., & Perlin, D. (2006). Pediatric ear, nose, and throat emergencies. *Pediatric Clinics of North America, 53*, 195–214.

Blevins, J. Y. (2003). Primary herpetic gingivostomatitis in young children. *Pediatric Nursing, 29*, 199–202.

Brook, I., & Gober, A. (2005). Recovery of potential pathogens and interfering bacteria in the nasopharynx of otitis media-prone children and their smoking and non-smoking patients. *Archives of Otolaryngology and Head & Neck Surgery, 131*, 509–512.

Center for Health and Health Care in Schools. (2004). Childhood vision: What the research tells us. Retrieved June 15, 2004, from http://www.healthinschools.org

Centers for Disease Control and Prevention. (2004). Vision impairment. Retrieved August 30, 2006, from http://www.cdc.gov/ncbddd/dd/vision3.htm

Chamley, C. A., Carson, P., Randall, D., & Sandwell, M. (2005). *Developmental anatomy and physiology of children*. St. Louis: Elsevier.

Cheng, K. K., Chang, A. M., & Yuen, M. P. (2004). Prevention of oral mucositis in paedeatric patients treated with chemotherapy: A randomized crossover trial comparing two protocols of oral care. *European Journal of Cancer, 40*, 1208–1216.

Childrens Oral Health National Facts (2003). Washington DC: Childrens Dental Health Project.

Chu, K., Elimian, A., Barbera, J., Ogburn, P., Spitzer, A., & Quirk, J. G. (2003) Antecedents of newborn hearing loss. Obstetrics and Gynecology 101, 584–588.

Chung, J. H., Des Roches, C. M., Meunier, J., & Eavey, R. D. (2006). Evaluation of noise-induced hearing loss in young people using a web-based survey technique. *Pediatrics, 117*, 248–249.

Committee on Sports Medicine and Fitness. (2004). Protective eyewear for young athletes. *Pediatrics, 113*, 619–622.

Connolly, J. L., Carron, J. D., & Roark, S. D. (2005). Universal newborn hearing screening: Are we achieving the Joint Committee on Infant (JCIH) objectives? *Laryngoscope, 115*, 232–236.

Craig, F. W., & Schunk, J. E. (2003). Retropharyngeal abscess in children: Clinical presentation, utility of imaging, and current management. *Pediatrics, 111*, 1394–1398.

Curns, A. T., Holman, R. C., Shay, D. K., Cheek, J. E., Kaufman, S. F., Singleton, R. J., & Anderson, L. J. (2002). Outpatient and hospital visits associated with otitis media among American Indian and Alaska Native children younger than 5 years. *Pediatrics, 109*(3). Retrieved 10/2/06 from http://www.pediatrics.org/cgi/content/full/109/3/e41

Donahue, S. P., Baker, J. D., Scott, W. E., Rychwalski, P., Neely, D. E., Tong, P., Bergsma, D., Lenahan, D., Rush, D., Heinlein, K., Walkenbach, R., & Johnson, T. M. (2006). Lions Clubs International Foundation Core Four Photoscreening: Results from 17 programs and 400,000 preschool children. *Journal of the American Association of Ophthalmology and Strabismus, 10*, 44–48.

Folmer, R. L. (2003). The importance of hearing conservation instruction. *Journal of School Nursing, 19*, 140–148.

Foxlee, R., Johansson, A., Wejfalk, J., Dawkins, J., Dooley, L., & Del Mar, C. (2006). Topical analgesia for acute otitis media. *Cochrane Database Systematic Review, 19*, CD005657.

Gold, L. S., & Slone, T. H. (2003). Aristolochic acid, an herbal carcinogen, sold on the Web after FDA alert. *New England Journal of Medicine, 349*, 1576–1577.

Guttu, M., Engelke, M. K., & Swanson, M. (2004). Does the school nurse-to-student ratio make a difference? *Journal of School Health, 74*, 6–9.

Harrison, C. J. (2005). The microbiology of acute otitis media: Past, present, and future. *Contemporary Pediatrics, 22*(12), 8–16.

Hartmann, E. E., Bradford, G. E., Chaplin, P. K. N., Johnson, T., Kemper, A. R., Kim, S., & Marsh-Tootle, W. (2006). Project universal preschool vision screening: A demonstration project. *Pediatrics, 117*, e226–e237. Retrieved August 30, 2006, from http://pediatrics.aappublications.org/cgi/content/full/117/2/3226

Health Care Guide. (2006). Epistaxis. Retrieved 10/3/06 from http://www.health-care-guide.org/epistaxis.htm

Hyde, M., & Power, D. (2006). Some ethical dimensions of cochlear implantation for deaf children and their families. *Journal of Deaf Students and Deaf Education, 11*, 102–111.

Joint Committee on Infant Hearing. (2000). Joint Committee on Infant Hearing 2000 position statement: Principles and guidelines for early hearing detection and intervention programs. *Pediatrics, 106*, 798–817.

Kimel, L. S. (2006). Lack of follow-up exams after failed school vision screenings: An investigation of contributing factors. *Journal of School Nursing, 22*, 156–162.

Krause-Parello, C. A. (2005). Tooth avulsion in the school setting. *Journal of School Nursing, 21*, 279–282.

Leman, R., Clausen, M. M., Bates, J., Stark, L., Arnold, K. K., & Arnold, R. W. (2006). A comparison of patched HOTV visual acuity and photoscreening. *Journal of School Nursing, 22*, 237–243.

Leung, A. K. C., & Kellner, J. D. (2004). Acute sinusitis in children: Diagnosis and management. *Journal of Pediatric Health Care, 18*, 72–76.

Mah, F. (2006). Bacterial conjunctivitis. *Pediatric Clinics of North America, 53*(Suppl. 1), 7–10.

MMWR. (2005). Visual impairment and use of eye-care services and protective eyewear among children—United States 2002. *MMWR, 54*, 425–429.

Moore, J. (2006). Pediatricians need greater awareness of hearing disorders. *Infectious Diseases in Children, 19*(8), 53–54.

Nageswaran, S., Woods, C. R., Benjamin, D. K., & Shetty, L. (2006). Orvital cellulitis in children. *Pediatric Infectious Disease Journal, 25*, 695–699.

Nelson, L. M. (2003). Temperature-controlled radiofrequency tonsil reduction in children. *Archives of Otolaryngology—Head & Neck Surgery, 129*, 533–537.

Neto, J. F., Hemb, L., & Silva, D. B. (2006). Systematic literature review of modifiable risk factors for recurrent acute otitis media in childhood. *Journal of Pediatrics (Rio J), 82*, 87–96.

Otitis Media with Effusion. (2004). Clinical practice guideline. *Pediatrics, 113*, 1412–1429.

Ottar-Pfeifer, W. (2005). When should children have their eyes checked? *Insight: The Journal of the American Society of Ophthalmic Registered Nurses, 30*(2), 17–22.

Paradise, J. L., Bluestone, C. D., Colborn, K., Bernard, B. S., Rockette, H. E., & Kurs-Lasky, M. (2002). Tonsillectomy and adenotonsillectomy for recurrent throat infection in moderately affected children. *Pediatrics, 110*, 7–15.

Pelton, S. I. (2005). Otitis media: Re-evaluation of diagnosis and treatment in the era of antimicrobial resistance, pneumococcal conjugate vaccine, and evolving morbidity. *Pediatric Clinics of North America, 52*, 711–728.

Phelps, D. L., & Watts, J. L. (2003). Early light reduction for preventing retinopathy of prematurity in very low birth weight infants. *Cochrane Library, 2,* 1–15.

Quinn, G. E. (2005). The "ideal" management of retinopathy of prematurity. *Eye, 19,* 1044–1049.

Rosenfeld, R. M., Brown, L., Cannon, C. R., Dolor, R. J., Ganiats, T. G., Hannley, M., Kokemueller, P., Marcy, S. M., Roland, P. S., Shiffman, R. N., Stinnett, S. S., Witsell, D. L., & American Academy of Otolaryngology—Head and Neck Surgery Foundation. (2006). Clinical practice guideline: Acute otitis externa. *Otolaryngology—Head & Neck Surgery, 134*(4Suppl), S4–23.

Sarrell, E. M., Cohen, H. A., & Kahan, E. (2003). Naturopathic treatment for ear pain in children. *Pediatrics, 111,* e574–579.

Serra, M. R., Biassoni, E. C., Richter, U., Minoldo, G., Franco, G., Abraham, S., Carignani, J. A., Joekes. S., & Yacci, M. R. (2005). Recreational noise exposure and its effects on the hearing of adolescents: Part I: An interdisciplinary long-term study. *International Journal of Audiology, 44,* 65–73.

Scheiner, A. P. (1996). Vision problems: Impairment to blindness. In A. M. Rudolph, J. I. E. Hoffman, & C. D. Rudolph (Eds.), *Rudolph's pediatrics* (20th ed., p. 167). Stamford, CT: Appleton & Lange.

Shetty, K. (2006). Oral lesions commonly associated with pediatric HIV infection—presentation, management, and review of the literature. *General Dentistry, 54,* 284–287.

Sinus and Allergy Health Partnership. (2002). Sinus symptoms. Retrieved on August 30, 2006, from http://www.sahp.org/pnt_symptoms.html#child

Stephenson, M. (2003). Mucopurulent discharge is good sign conjunctivitis is bacterial. *Infectious Diseases in Children, 3,* 32–33.

Subcommittee on Management of Acute Otitis Media, American Academy of Pediatrics. (2004). Diagnosis and management of acute otitis media. *Pediatrics, 113,* 1451–1465.

Subcommittee on Management of Sinusitis and Committee on Quality Improvement, American Academy of Pediatrics. (2001). Clinical practice guideline: Management of sinusitis. *Pediatrics, 108,* 798–808.

Swanson, W. H., & Cohen, J. M. (2003). Color vision. *Ophthalmology Clinics of North America, 16,* 179–203.

Tasman, W., Patz, A., McNamara, J. A., Kaiser, R. S., Trese, M. T., & Smith, B. T. (2006). Retinopathy of prematurity: The life of a lifetime disease. *American Journal of Ophthalmology, 141,* 167–174.

Taylor, J. A., Weber, W., Standish, L., Quinn, H., Goesling, J., McGann, J., & Calabrese, C. (2003). Efficacy and safety of *Echinacea* in treating upper respiratory tract infections in children: A randomized controlled trial. *Journal of the American Medical Association, 290,* 2824–2830.

Teoh, D. L., & Reynolds, S. (2003). Diagnosis and management of pediatric conjunctivitis. *Pediatric Emergency Care, 19,* 48–55.

U.S. Department of Health and Human Services. (2000). *Healthy People 2010.* Washington DC: U.S. Government Printing Office.

U.S. Food and Drug Administration. (2006). Got a sick kid? Retrieved October 3, 2006 from http://www.fda.gov/cder/consumerinfo/sickkids.htm

U.S. Preventive Services Task Force. (2004). Screening for visual impairment in children younger than age 5 years. Retrieved June 1, 2004, from http://www.ahrq.gov/clinic/3rduspstf.visionscr/sicshrs.htm

U.S. Preventive Services Task Force. (2005). Screening for visual impairment in children younger than five years: Recommendation statement. *American Family Physician, 71,* 333–336.

Wheatley, C. M., Dickinson, J. L., Mackey, D. A., Craig, J. E., & Sale, M. M. (2002). Retinopathy of prematurity: Recent advances in our understanding. *Archives of Disease in Childhood, 87,* F78–82.

Wilson-Clark, S. D., Squires, S., & Deeks, S. (2006). Bacterial meningitis among cochlear implant recipients—Canada, 2002. *MMWR, 55*(Sup01), 20–24.

Windmill, S., & Windmill, I. M. (2006). The status of diagnostic testing following referral from universal newborn hearing screening. *Journal of the American Academy of Audiology, 17,* 367–378.

Yaeger, D., McCallum, J., Lewis, K., Soslow, L., Shah, U., Potsic, W., Stolle, C., & Krantz, I. D. (2006). Outcomes of clinical examination and genetic testing of 500 individuals with hearing loss evaluated through a genetics of hearing loss clinic. *American Journal of Medical Genetics, 140,* 827–836.

Zacharyczuk, C. (2004). New guidelines outline AOM management options. *Infectious Diseases in Children,* (April), 24.

ALTERATIONS IN RESPIRATORY FUNCTION

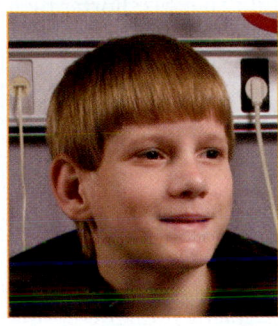

SHAUN, a 13-year-old with cystic fibrosis, has a challenging time with disease management. He lives with his mother and a sister who does not have cystic fibrosis in a town about 50 miles from the cystic fibrosis center at the university medical center. He is in the seventh grade and enjoys riding his bicycle. He usually spends a few days in the hospital each year for intensive therapy sessions to clear his lungs.

Management of cystic fibrosis takes a lot of time each day, whether at home or in the hospital. All of Shaun's care must be scheduled around school and recreation. In most cases, the treatments cut into his recreational time. Shaun has learned to manage many aspects of his care, relieving his mother of some duties. Shaun sets up his nebulizer treatment and correctly measures the amount of DNase to use. After the nebulizer treatment, he uses an oscillating vest for chest physiotherapy for about 20 minutes per treatment. Coughing up the sputum during and after the treatment is very tiring.

Shaun needs many extra calories to grow as well as to meet metabolic demands. His mother works hard to prepare and provide the extra calories he needs throughout the day, and he takes pancreatic enzymes to help him digest food. Because Shaun sometimes has difficulty getting enough calories, he has a gastrostomy tube for night-time feedings. This has made it possible to get enough calories to help support his adolescent growth spurt.

KEY TERMS

adventitious sounds
680
airway remodeling
713
airway resistance
678
apnea 688
compliance 678
cor pulmonale 690
croup 694
dysphagia 698
dysphonia 683
dyspnea 683
grunting 685
hypercapnia 685
hypoxemia 685
hypoxia 685
laryngospasms 696

paradoxical
breathing 680
perfusion 686
periodic breathing
688
pneumothorax 735
polysomnography
690
respiratory effort
680
retractions 680
stridor 684
tachypnea 680
trigger 713
tripod
position 680
ventilation 678

MediaLink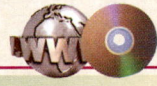

http://www.prenhall.com/ball
See the Prentice Hall Nursing MediaLink DVD-ROM and Companion Website for chapter-specific resources.

LEARNING OUTCOMES

After reading this chapter, you will be able to do the following:

1. Describe unique characteristics of the pediatric respiratory system anatomy and physiology.

2. Describe the development of the child's respiratory system.

3. List the respiratory conditions and injuries that can cause respiratory distress in infants and children.

4. Assess the child's respiratory signs and symptoms to distinguish between mild, moderate, and severe respiratory distress and describe the appropriate nursing care for each level of respiratory distress severity.

5. Differentiate between the signs and symptoms of a child with an upper airway and a lower airway respiratory condition.

6. Develop a nursing care plan for a child with a common acute respiratory condition.

7. Develop a nursing care plan for the child with a chronic respiratory condition.

FOCUS ON
The Respiratory System

ANATOMY AND PHYSIOLOGY

The respiratory system is composed of both the upper and lower airways. The upper airway, containing the nasopharynx and oropharynx, serves as the pathway for gases exchanged during **ventilation**, the movement of oxygen into the lungs and carbon dioxide out of the lungs. The larynx divides the upper and lower airways. The lower airways (trachea, bronchi, and bronchioles) serve as the pathway of gases to the alveoli in the lungs. The left lung is divided into two lobes and the right lung is divided into three lobes. Alveolar sacs surrounded by capillaries are located at the end of the airways and are the site of gas exchange, where oxygen diffuses across the alveolocapillary membrane. Surfactant secreted by alveolar cells coats the inner surface of the alveolus to allow expansion during inspiration. The lung tissue surrounding the airways keeps them from collapsing as the oxygen moves in and carbon dioxide moves out during ventilation. The lungs are positioned in the thoracic cavity, where the ribs and muscles protect the lungs from injury.

The intercostal muscles work with the diaphragm to perform the work of breathing. The diaphragm is a muscle that separates the abdominal and thoracic cavity contents. When the diaphragm contracts, it creates negative pressure that increases the thoracic cavity's volume cavity and pulls air into the lungs. The lungs and chest wall have the ability to expand during inspiration (**compliance**) and then to recoil or return to the resting state with expiration. The work of breathing is tied to the muscular effort required for ventilation, which can be increased in cases of disorders that increase the stiffness of the lungs or obstruct the airways.

The respiratory center in the brain controls respiration, sending impulses to the respiratory muscles to contract and relax. Breathing is usually involuntary as the nervous system automatically adjusts the ventilatory rate and volume to maintain normal gas exchange (Brashers, 2006b). Receptors in the lungs respond to irritants, and increased size or volume of the lungs and increased pulmonary capillary pressure alert the respiratory center to alter the ventilatory rate. Chemoreceptors monitor the pH, $PaCO_2$, and PaO_2 in the arterial blood and send signals to the respiratory center to increase ventilation in cases of arterial hypoxemia. Effective gas exchange requires a near even distribution of ventilation and perfusion of blood in all portions of the lungs. As oxygen diffuses across the alveolocapillary membrane, it dissolves in the plasma and the resulting pressure (PaO_2) helps bind the oxygen to the hemoglobin molecules where it is then transported to the cells for metabolism. Carbon dioxide produced by cellular metabolism is dissolved in the plasma (PCO_2) and/or as bicarbonate and travels back to the lungs where it diffuses across the alveolocapillary membrane (Brashers, 2006b).

PEDIATRIC DIFFERENCES

The child's respiratory tract constantly grows and changes until about 12 years of age. The young child's neck is shorter than an adult's, resulting in airway structures that are closer together.

Upper Airway Differences

The child's airway is shorter and narrower than an adult's. These differences create a greater potential for obstruction (Figure 20–1 ➤). The infant's airway is approximately 4 mm in diameter, about the width of a drinking straw, in contrast to the adult's airway diameter of 20 mm. The child's little finger is a good estimate for the child's tracheal diameter and can be used for a quick assessment of airway size. The trachea primarily increases in length rather than diameter during the first 5 years of life. The tracheal division of the right and left bronchi is higher in a child's airway and at a different angle than the adult's (Figure 20–2 ➤). The cartilage that supports the trachea is more flexible and has the potential to compress the airway if the head and neck are not appropriately positioned. The child's narrower airway causes a greater increase in **airway resistance**, the effort or force needed to move oxygen through the trachea to the lungs, in any condition causing edema of the airway or accumulation of secretions (Figure 20–3 ➤).

Infants, children, and adults can breathe through either the nose or the mouth. Until 4 weeks of age, newborns are obligatory nose breathers. The coordination of mouth breathing is controlled by maturing neurologic pathways; thus, infants up to 2 to 3 months of age do not automatically open the mouth to breathe when the nose is obstructed. The only time a newborn breathes through the mouth is when he or she is crying. Nasal patency in newborns is therefore essential for such activities as breathing and eating.

Lower Airway Differences

At birth the lung tissue contains only 25 million alveoli, which are not fully developed, and the distal bronchioles that extend to the alveoli are narrow and fewer in number than in an adult. After 8 years of age the alveoli begin increasing in size and complexity. The number of alveoli increases to 300 million by adulthood (Brashers, 2006b).

The bronchi and bronchioles are lined with smooth muscle. The newborn does not have enough smooth muscle

AS CHILDREN GROW

Airway Development

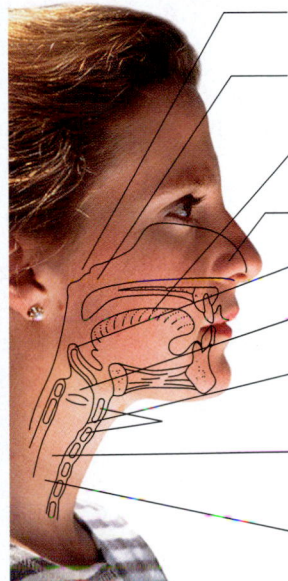

- Smaller nasopharynx, easily occluded during infection.
- Lymph tissue (tonsils, adenoids) grows rapidly in early childhood; atrophies after age 12.
- Small oral cavity and large tongue increase risk of obstruction.
- Smaller nares, easily occluded.
- Long, floppy epiglottis vulnerable to swelling with resulting obstruction.
- Larynx and glottis are higher in neck, increasing risk of aspiration.
- Because thyroid, cricoid, and tracheal cartilages are immature, they may easily collapse when neck is flexed.
- Because fewer muscles are functional in airway, it is less able to compensate for edema, spasm, and trauma.
- The large amounts of soft tissue and loosely anchored mucous membranes lining the airway increase risk of edema and obstruction.

Figure 20–1 ➤ It is easy to see that a child's airway is smaller and less developed than an adult's airway, but why is this important? An upper respiratory tract infection, allergic reaction, positioning of the head and neck during sleep, and the small objects children play with can have serious consequences in the child.

AS CHILDREN GROW

Trachea Position

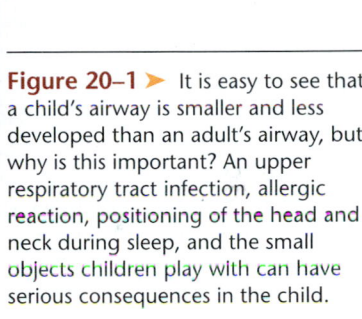

- Bifurcation of trachea in children is at T3 level.
- Right mainstem bronchus in children has a steeper slope than in adults.
- Bifurcation in adults is at T6 level.

Figure 20–2 ➤ In children, the trachea is shorter and the angle of the right bronchus at bifurcation is more acute than in the adult. When you are resuscitating or suctioning, you must allow for the differences. Do you think that this difference is significant in respiratory infection? Why?

bundles to help trap airway invaders. By 5 months of age, however, an infant has enough muscles to react to irritants by bronchospasm and muscle contraction.

Children under 6 years of age use the diaphragm to breathe as the intercostal muscles are immature. By 6 years of age the child uses the intercostal muscles more effectively. The ribs are primarily cartilage and very flexible, and in cases of respiratory distress, the negative pressure caused by the diaphragm movement causes the chest wall to be drawn inward, causing retractions (Figure 20–4 ➤).

Oxygen consumption is higher in children than adults because of their greater metabolic rate. This rate of oxygen consumption increases when the child is in respiratory distress. The child also has fewer muscle glycogen reserves, leading to more rapid muscle fatigue when accessory muscles must be used for breathing (Froh, 2006).

Use the guidelines on the next page to perform a nursing assessment of the respiratory system. Examples of diagnostic and laboratory tests used to evaluate respiratory conditions are provided in the table on pages 681–682.

PATHOPHYSIOLOGY ILLUSTRATED

Airway Diameter

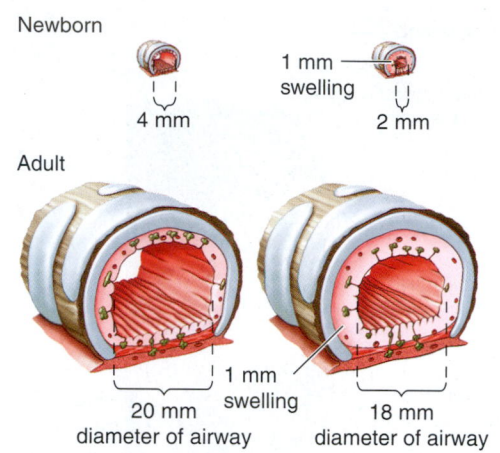

Newborn

1 mm swelling

4 mm

2 mm

Adult

1 mm swelling

20 mm diameter of airway

18 mm diameter of airway

Figure 20–3 ▶ The diameter of an infant's airway is approximately 4 mm, in contrast to an adult's airway diameter of 20 mm. An inflammatory process in the airway causes swelling that narrows the airway, and airway resistance increases. Note that swelling of 1 mm reduces the infant's airway diameter to 2 mm, but the adult's airway diameter is only narrowed to 18 mm. Air must move more quickly in the infant's narrowed airway to get the same amount of air to the lungs. The friction of the quickly moving air against the side of the airway increases airway resistance. The infant must use more effort to breathe and breathe faster to get adequate oxygen.

ASSESSMENT GUIDELINES FOR THE CHILD WITH A RESPIRATORY CONDITION[a]

Assessment Focus	Assessment Guidelines
Position of comfort	• Is the child comfortable lying down? • Does the child prefer to sit up or be in the **tripod position** (sitting forward with arms on knees for support and extending the neck)?
Vital signs	• Assess the rate, depth, and ease of respirations. See Table 5–10 for expected respiratory rate ranges by age. • Assess the pulse for rate and strength. See Table 5–12 for expected heart rate ranges by age.
Lung auscultation	• Are breath sounds bilateral, diminished, or absent? • Are **adventitious sounds** (wheezes, crackles, or rhonchi) present?
Respiratory effort (work of breathing)	• Are there audible inspiratory and expiratory breath sounds or stridor? Is there grunting with expiration? • Is breathing labored? • Are **retractions** (visible appearance of the chest being drawn on inspiration) present or are accessory muscles used to breathe? • Is nasal flaring present? • Is **tachypnea** (abnormally rapid rate of respirations) present? • Can the child say a full sentence or is a breath needed every few words? Is the cry strong or weak? • Do the chest and abdomen rise simultaneously with inspiration or is **paradoxical breathing** present in which the chest and abdomen do not simultaneously rise?
Color	• What is the color of the mucous membranes (pink, pale, mottled, cyanotic)? • Does crying improve or worsen the color?
Cough	• Is the cough dry (nonproductive), wet (productive, mucousy), brassy (noisy, musical), or croupy (barking, seal-like)? • Is the coughing effort forceful or weak?
Behavior change	• Note any sudden behavior changes such as irritability, restlessness, or change in level of responsiveness.
Family history	• Is there a family history of asthma or cystic fibrosis?

[a]Refer to Chapter 5 ∞ for the actual assessment techniques mentioned in this table.

PATHOPHYSIOLOGY ILLUSTRATED

Retraction Sites

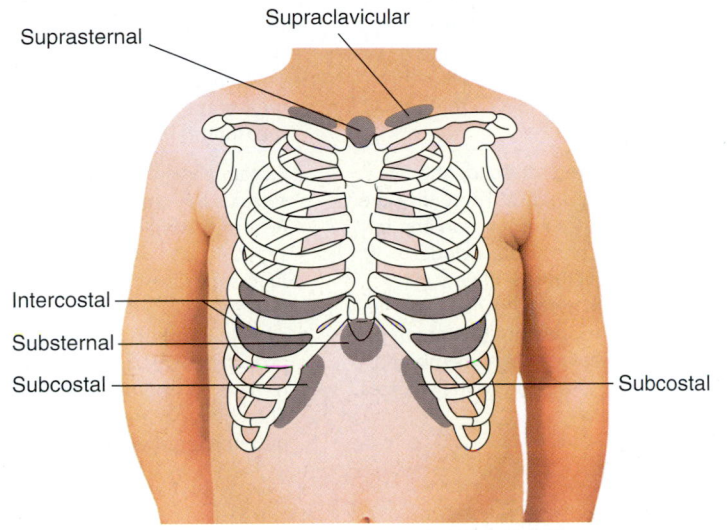

Figure 20–4 ➤ Retractions may occur in the very young infant in the suprasternal area. In the older infant and child, retractions occur when the airway is severely obstructed, as in croup. The depth and location of retractions is associated with the severity of respiratory distress. Isolated intercostal retractions indicate mild distress. Subcostal, suprasternal, and supraclavicular retractions indicate moderate distress. These retractions accompanied by use of accessory muscles indicate severe distress.

DIAGNOSTIC AND LABORATORY PROCEDURES/TESTS FOR THE RESPIRATORY SYSTEM

Diagnostic Procedure/Test	Purpose	Nursing Implications
Bronchoscopy	A flexible, fiberoptic bronchoscope is used to visualize the trachea and bronchi to identify and extract foreign objects in the airway.	• Maintain NPO status pre-procedure. • The child will be sedated for the procedure. Monitor the child according to agency guidelines. • Postoperatively monitor vital signs per protocol. Resume oral feedings as prescribed.
Chest radiograph (x-ray)	Radiographs are commonly used to: • Identify bone structure of the thorax and lung tissue. • Detect abnormalities of the pulmonary system such as air trapping in the alveoli (hyperinflation) or consolidation of lung tissue (pneumonia). • A forced expiratory film may be used in cases of foreign body aspiration to detect local hyperinflation (air trapping) and a mediastinal shift away from the affected side. • Fluoroscopy may be used to detect a foreign body aspiration.	• Explain the procedure to the parents and child. Inform them that the radiograph test usually takes 10 to 15 minutes, and that there may be several taken from different angles. Explain that modern equipment decreases radiation exposure. • Tell the child about the need to hold still for the procedure. Have the child practice holding still and holding a breath in preparation for the test.
Polysomnography (sleep study)	A sleep study that simultaneously records the brain activity, eye movement, and apnea episodes; oxygen desaturation and sleep disturbances are used to identify apnea during sleep and to determine the cause of sleep disorders. Testing for sleep disorders is performed at a sleep laboratory over an 8-hour period.	• Instruct the family to keep a sleep log 1 to 2 weeks prior to sleep studies, including notes about snoring and sleepiness during the day. Review the sleep log. • Instruct the patient/family to avoid caffeine products, sedatives, and naps 1 to 2 days prior to testing. • Obtain a history related to medications, head injury, headache, and seizures. • Explain the procedure to the parents and child.

(continued)

DIAGNOSTIC AND LABORATORY PROCEDURES/TESTS FOR THE RESPIRATORY SYSTEM (continued)

Diagnostic Procedure/Test	Purpose	Nursing Implications
Pulse oximetry	Pulse oximetry provides an estimate of the hemoglobin saturated by oxygen, measured percutaneously (SpO_2). It serves as an alternate to the direct measurement of PO_2 (SaO_2) through arterial blood gas analysis.	• Explain that the sensor needs to be over a nailbed or a central location. • The sensor may stay in place for a constant measurement or be used for periodic measurements.
Spirometry (pulmonary function tests)	Pulmonary function tests are used to identify the severity of obstructive lung disease. These tests are used to establish baselines for comparison and to detect pulmonary dysfunction. Tests include: • Spirometry—measures volume and flow of forced expiration as well as forced vital capacity. • Diffusion capacity test to measure the rate of gas diffusion across the alveolocapillary membrane. • Exercise studies are used to detect early changes in the pulmonary system. • Bronchial provocation studies. • Slow vital-capacity tests. • Flow-volume loop.	• Obtain a list of any oral bronchodilator and steroids the child is taking. • Record the child's age, height, weight, and vital signs. • Assess for signs and symptoms of respiratory distress. • Explain the purpose of tests and procedures; provide teaching as needed to enable the child to have an optimal performance. • The child may need to practice breathing patterns required for the test.
Sweat chloride test	The test is considered the gold standard for diagnosis of cystic fibrosis. Gel pads containing pilocarpine are placed on the child's arms. A small generator attached to the pads stimulates sweating until enough sweat is collected. The arms are covered with plastic. Sweat is analyzed for the concentration of chloride and osmolality.	• Explain the purpose of the test and the need for the child to keep the plastic covering the hands intact for the duration of the test (about 30 minutes).

Laboratory Procedure/Test	Purpose	Nursing Implications
Arterial blood gas analysis	Used to monitor the adequacy of ventilation and oxygenation, the oxygen-carrying capacity of the blood, and acid-base levels. Enables a direct measurement of the blood pH, PO_2, and PCO_2.	• Arterial puncture can be performed on the radial, brachial, and femoral arteries. • Use anesthetizing agent to reduce pain associated with the arterial puncture. • Following the arterial puncture, put pressure over the puncture site for 5 to 10 minutes to prevent hematoma formation.
Cultures	Cultures are taken to isolate microorganisms causing body tissue or body fluid infection. The culture specimen is taken to the laboratory immediately after collection, where it will take 24 to 36 hours to grow the organisms. • Sputum • Nasal wash for respiratory syncytial virus • Gastric wash for tuberculosis	• Hold antibiotics or sulfonamides until after specimen collection, as they may cause false results. If these drugs have been given, list on laboratory slip. • Deliver all specimens immediately to the laboratory, or refrigerate the specimen. • Handle the specimen using strict aseptic technique. • Keep lids on sterile specimen containers. Sputum cups should not be uncovered at the bedside.
Neonatal screening for cystic fibrosis	Blood is collected to test for multiple metabolic disorders and cystic fibrosis (in some states). A positive immunoreactive trypsinogen test leads to more diagnostic tests such as a sweat chloride test.	• A heel capillary puncture is used for blood collection. • All circles on the test card must be completely filled. • Explain the purpose of the test to the parents and let them know that they will be notified if the test is positive.
Protein-purified derivative (PPD), the Mantoux test	Skin test to detect exposure and infection with tuberculosis.	• Solution is injected intradermally and injection site is evaluated within 48 to 72 hours for redness and induration.

Data from: Corbett, J. V. (2004). *Laboratory tests and diagnostic procedures with nursing diagnoses* (6th ed.). Upper Saddle River, NJ: Prentice Hall.

This chapter explores several factors in the child's respiratory system that create ongoing threats to respiratory function and overall health. Most respiratory problems in children produce mild symptoms, last a short time, and can be managed at home. Other respiratory problems are chronic and potentially life threatening. Respiratory conditions are the most common cause of illness requiring hospitalization in children between 1 and 9 years of age, and a leading cause of hospitalization in children between 10 and 15 years of age (Fingerhut, 2005).

Pediatric respiratory conditions may occur as a primary problem or as a complication of nonrespiratory conditions. Respiratory problems may result from structural problems, functional problems, or a combination of both. Structural problems involve alterations in the size and shape of parts of the respiratory tract. Functional problems involve alterations in gas exchange and threats to the process of ventilation due to irritants (such as large particles and chemicals) or invaders (such as viruses or bacteria). Alterations in other organ systems, especially the immune and neurologic systems, may also threaten respiratory function. When reading this chapter, keep the distinction between structural and functional problems in mind to help distinguish between what is normal and what is abnormal about the child's maturing respiratory system. See Chapter 19 ∞ for upper respiratory conditions such as otitis media, sinusitis, and pharyngitis.

RESPIRATORY DISTRESS AND RESPIRATORY FAILURE

Many respiratory conditions associated with difficulty breathing can progress to respiratory distress. If the condition is not managed effectively it can progress to respiratory failure. Foreign body aspiration is a common cause of airway obstruction and respiratory distress, and it is used to illustrate the care of the child in respiratory distress.

Foreign-Body Aspiration

Foreign-body aspiration is the inhalation of any object (solid or liquid, food or nonfood) into the respiratory tract. Aspiration occurs most often during feeding and reaching activities, while crawling, or during playtime in children ages 6 months to 4 years. These young children have a tendency to put small objects in the mouth. However, aspiration may occur in a child of any age.

Etiology and Pathophysiology

In infants over 6 months of age and young children, any number of small objects that make their way into the child's mouth can cause aspiration. Partial or complete airway obstruction can occur. The severity of the obstruction depends on the size and composition of the object or substance and its location within the respiratory tract.

Most aspirated foreign bodies (AFBs) usually cause bronchial, not tracheal, obstruction. An object lodged high in the airway above the vocal cords is frequently expelled by coughing. The right lung is the most common site of lower airway obstruction because of the sloped angle of its bronchus (see Figure 20–2 on page 679). Objects may migrate from higher to lower airway locations. An object may also move back up to the trachea, creating extreme respiratory difficulty. If oxygen is depleted for an extended time, brain damage may occur.

Clinical Manifestations

Children are usually brought to the hospital after a sudden episode of coughing or gagging. The child may have signs of increased respiratory effort such as **dyspnea** (difficulty breathing), tachypnea, nasal flaring, and retractions. As respiratory distress progresses, the child may have a concentrated focus on breathing, have an anxious expression, and sit in a forward position with the neck extended. As the child becomes increasingly hypoxic, behavior changes such as irritability and decreased responsiveness are seen.

Coughing, choking, gagging, **dysphonia** (muffled, hoarse, or absent voice sounds), and wheezing may be brief or may persist for several hours if the object drops below the trachea into one of the mainstem bronchi. In some cases the child may become asymptomatic after coughing for 15 to 30 minutes. If the foreign body drops into

---

CLINICAL TIP

Common items associated with foreign body aspiration and airway obstruction include the following:

- Foods such as nuts, popcorn, or small pieces of raw vegetables or hot dog
- Small, loose toy parts such as small wheels and bells or small magnets
- Household objects and substances such as beads, safety pins, coins, buttons, latex balloon pieces, and colorful liquids (mouthwash, perfume) in enticing packages (screw-top bottles)

NURSING ALERT

If the child cannot say the "P" in words like *puppy* or *Peter Pan,* the child has noticeably diminished expiratory effort.

CLINICAL TIP

These signs and symptoms signal the body's response to increased metabolic demands for oxygenation as a result of airway obstruction, stress, or impending illness:

- Increasing restlessness, irritability, unexplained sudden confusion
- Rapid heart rate accompanied by rapid respiratory rate

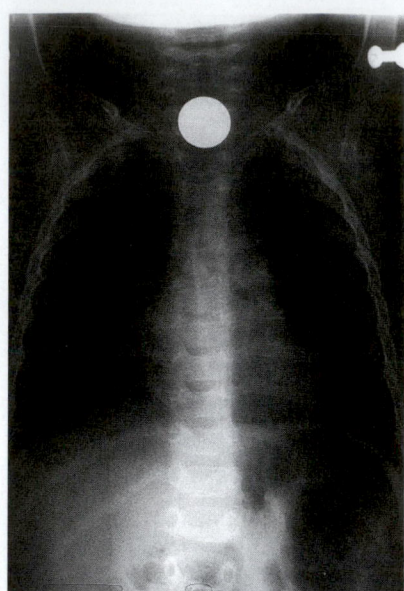

Figure 20–5 ➤ An aspirated foreign body (coin) is clearly visible in the child's trachea on this chest radiograph. Courtesy of Rockwood Clinic, Spokane, WA.

the lower airway and is not removed, the child may present with a chronic cough, persistent or recurrent pneumonia, or a lung abscess weeks later.

COLLABORATIVE CARE

Initial clinical therapy is focused on identifying and treating a potentially life-threatening airway obstruction. If the airway is patent, a careful history is obtained to determine whether aspiration has indeed occurred. Coughing, gagging, or choking associated with feeding or crawling on the floor is usually a confirming event for aspiration. The physical examination often reveals decreased breath sounds, **stridor** (a high-pitched, musical sound that is created by inspiration through a narrowed airway), and respiratory distress in the child without a witnessed aspiration. A forced expiratory radiograph may be ordered to detect local hyperinflation (air trapping) and a mediastinal shift away from the affected side. Sometimes, when the AFB is radiopaque, it can be seen on a radiograph film (Figure 20–5 ➤).

Chest thrusts and back blows or the abdominal thrust is used to remove an object from an obstructed airway. An object lodged in the trachea is a life-threatening situation. Once in the hospital or other emergency facility, fluoroscopy and fiberoptic bronchoscopy may be used to identify, locate, and extract the AFB. See the section on pneumonia, page 705, for care of the child with complications of aspiration.

NURSING MANAGEMENT
Nursing Assessment and Diagnosis

Nursing assessment should initially focus on the physiologic condition to make sure the child has an airway and is breathing. Once the child has a stable airway, the nursing assessment can focus on psychosocial and developmental concerns.

Physiologic Assessment

The child will be in respiratory distress, so constant monitoring is essential. Perform the respiratory assessment following the guidelines on page 680. If the object remains lodged, observe the child for increasing signs of respiratory distress, especially vital signs, audible wheezing on auscultation, and retractions. Note changes in breath sounds, from noisy to decreasing to absent, on the affected side. This can indicate that the object is moving and blocking a mainstem bronchus. Attach the child to a cardiorespiratory monitor and pulse oximeter to assess the child for subtle signs of increasing hypoxia.

SKILLS 11–2 AND 11–3
Using a Cardiorespiratory Monitor and Pulse Oximeter

Psychosocial Assessment

The unexpected and acute nature of the event creates anxiety for both parents and child. The child will be fearful because of difficulty breathing. Assess their coping ability and level of stress.

Developmental Assessment

As the child's condition stabilizes, observe how well the child's abilities match the parents' understanding of age-appropriate behaviors. See Chapters 8 and 9 ∞.

Common nursing diagnoses for a child with an AFB include:

- Ineffective Airway Clearance related to obstruction by foreign body
- Impaired Spontaneous Ventilations related to respiratory muscle fatigue
- Anxiety (Child) related to difficulty breathing, unfamiliar surroundings and procedures
- Risk for Injury related to small objects in environment

SKILL 11–19
Removing a Foreign Body Airway Obstruction

Planning and Implementation

When the airway is totally obstructed administer chest thrusts and back slaps to an infant or abdominal thrusts to a child in an effort to remove the AFB.

If the infant or child has a partially obstructed airway, the period right after aspiration until the AFB is removed is critical. Promptly document and report any subtle changes in the child's respiratory status. The nurse must remain with the child who has a significant obstruction, and have resuscitation equipment at the bedside. Permit the child to stay in a position of comfort. Avoid performing procedures that increase the child's anxiety as sudden movements and increased respiratory efforts may cause the obstruction to move and completely obstruct the airway. Be prepared to perform back blows and chest thrusts for an infant or abdominal thrusts for the child should complete obstruction occur.

After the AFB is removed the child is stabilized and observed for a few hours in a short-stay unit.

Discharge Planning and Home Care Teaching
Discharge planning centers on anticipatory guidance about childproofing the home (see Chapters 8 and 9 ∞). Encourage the parents to learn CPR, and back blows, chest thrusts, or abdominal thrusts.

Evaluation
Expected outcomes of nursing care include:

- The child regains the ability to ventilate spontaneously after removal of the foreign body.
- Parents complete a safety check of the home to prevent future aspiration incidents.

Respiratory Failure

Respiratory failure occurs when the body can no longer maintain effective gas exchange, and often results from a serious acute or chronic respiratory or neuromuscular condition. The physiologic process that ends in respiratory failure begins with hypoventilation of the alveoli. Hypoventilation occurs when the body's need for oxygen exceeds actual oxygen intake, the airway is partially occluded, lung injury has occurred, or the exchange of oxygen and carbon dioxide in the alveoli is disrupted. This disruption may occur for the following reasons:

- A malfunction of respiratory center stimulation (the alveoli do not receive the message to diffuse, such as may occur with narcotic overdose)
- The muscles of ventilation do not work effectively (the child is fatigued from the work of breathing, such as may occur with status asthmaticus or muscular dystrophy)
- Disorders at the alveolar level (the relationship between ventilation and blood flow to the alveoli is impaired) (see Figure 20–6 ➤)

Poor ventilation of the alveoli results in **hypoxemia** (lower-than-normal blood oxygen level) and **hypercapnia** (an excess of carbon dioxide in the blood). See Appendix C ∞ for expected laboratory values by age. When the blood levels of oxygen and carbon dioxide reach abnormal levels, **hypoxia** (lower-than-normal oxygen in the tissues) occurs and respiratory failure begins.

Signs of impending respiratory failure include irritability, lethargy, mottled color or cyanosis, and increased respiratory effort such as dyspnea, tachypnea, nasal flaring, and intercostal retractions. **Grunting** (a moaning or crying-like sound that is produced by forceful expiration against closed vocal cords in an effort to prevent alveolar collapse) helps maintain lung volume and alveolar pressures. This is a sign of severe disease in the newborn (Stoll & Kliegman, 2004).

Arterial blood gases help to identify hypoxemia or hypercapnia. Clinical therapy is directed at improving gas exchange. If hypercapnia exists due to inadequate alveolar ventilation, the child needs assisted ventilation. If hypoxemia exists, the child needs supplemental oxygen. See Figure 20–7 ➤. Some children need both interventions.

> **NURSING ALERT**
>
> Arterial blood gas levels indicative of respiratory failure are a PaO_2 level less than or equal to 50 mmHg, a $PaCO_2$ level greater than or equal to 50 mmHg, and a pH of less than or equal to 7.25 in a patient breathing room air (Brashers, 2006a). Hypoxemia that persists when supplemental oxygen is given is a sign of respiratory failure.

 MediaLink

Ventilation-Perfusion Mismatch Animation

PATHOPHYSIOLOGY ILLUSTRATED

Ventilation-Perfusion Ratio

Airway

From pulmonary artery

Alveolocapillary membrane

Alveolus

To pulmonary vein

A **Normal**

Impaired ventilation

Hypoxemia

B **Low ventilation-perfusion ratio**

Blocked ventilation

Collapsed alveolus

Hypoxemia

C **Shunt**

Figure 20–6 ➤ A ventilation-perfusion mismatch can occur when an infant or child has an abnormal distribution of ventilation or **perfusion** (blood flow in the pulmonary circulation). A, Children with normal lung function and circulation have a ventilation-perfusion ratio of 0.8 to 0.9 because perfusion is greater than ventilation (air exchange) in the lung bases. B, When ventilation is inadequate in areas of the lungs that are adequately perfused, the ventilation-perfusion ratio is low or mismatched, resulting in shunting. Blood passing through the pulmonary capillaries gets less oxygen exchange than normal and hypoxemia occurs. This is the case in asthma due to bronchoconstriction and in pneumonia because alveoli are filled with fluid. C, In the case of neonatal hyaline membrane disease the alveoli are collapsed so ventilation is impaired. Blood flow is adequate through the alveolar capillaries, but no oxygenation occurs by the collapsed alveoli. The ventilation-perfusion ratio is very low with significant shunting that does not respond to oxygen therapy because the capillary bed never gets exposed to the supplemental oxygen. Significant hypoxemia occurs.

Brashers, V. L. (2006a). Alterations in pulmonary function. In K. L. McCance & S. E. Huether, *Pathophysiology: The biologic basis for disease in adults and children,* (5th ed., pp. 1205–1248). St. Louis: Elsevier Mosby.

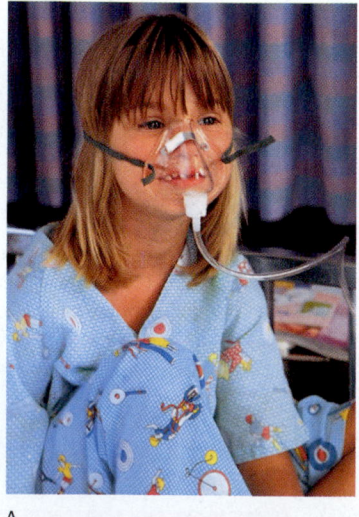

A

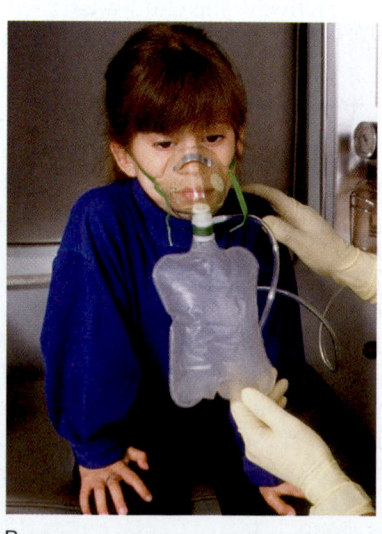

B

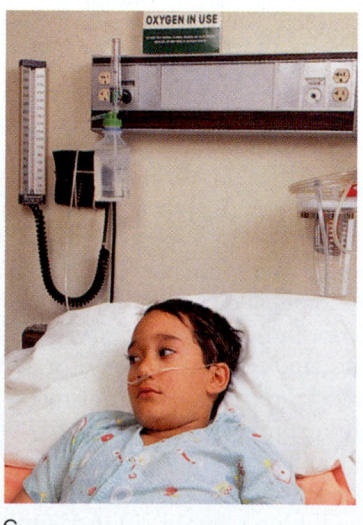

C

Figure 20–7 ➤ Various oxygen delivery devices are used to give supplemental oxygen to children. Oxygen delivery devices are selected to match the concentration of oxygen needed by the child. In respiratory failure, a higher concentration of oxygen is needed to reverse the hypoxemia. Which oxygen delivery device should be used? Are there any contraindications to oxygen use in a child who is hypoxic?

Respiratory problems that do not respond to oxygen therapy, medications, or position changes require the insertion of an artificial airway. As the child's level of responsiveness deteriorates, the ability to keep the airway open decreases. Endotracheal intubation is a short-term, emergency measure to stabilize the airway by placing a tube in the trachea. The tube must be protected and stabilized to prevent its displacement. A tracheostomy is the creation of a surgical opening into the trachea through the anterior neck at the cricoid cartilage. Surgeons prefer to perform this procedure in the operating room; however, a tracheostomy may also be performed in an emergency department or other setting when immediate intervention is needed.

Mechanical ventilation is often needed in addition to a secured airway to provide respiratory support. When respiratory failure cannot be managed, it results in cardiopulmonary arrest. See the clinical manifestations table below.

Nursing Management

Early recognition of impending respiratory failure is the most important aspect of care for a child with any signs of respiratory compromise. Signs and symptoms can progress rapidly, and detection of subtle early signs so that intervention can begin is important to prevent progress to cardiopulmonary arrest. When the child has a chronic respiratory condition, development of respiratory failure may be gradual. Be particularly alert to behavior changes in addition to respiratory signs. Serial blood gases may be needed to monitor the child.

Place a child who has respiratory distress in an upright position (by elevating the head of the bed). Assess respiratory quality and rate, followed by apical pulse rate and temperature. Monitor oxygen saturation with pulse oximetry. Administer oxygen as ordered and keep respiratory emergency equipment at the child's bedside. Monitor the child for changes in vital signs, respiratory status, and level of responsiveness. Be prepared to assist ventilations if respiratory status deteriorates.

Care of the Child with an Artificial Airway

The child with an endotracheal tube or new tracheostomy usually requires admission to the intensive care unit (ICU) for monitoring and ventilatory support. Airway secretions are suctioned as needed and tracheostomy care is provided, if present.

Because endotracheal and tracheostomy tubes prevent vocal cord vibration, intubated children cannot cry or talk. Infants and young children often express initial

NURSING ALERT

When the child in respiratory distress has had increased respiratory effort over a prolonged time period, a decreasing respiratory rate is a critical sign of impending pulmonary arrest. The ventilatory muscles are so fatigued that the child will soon stop breathing.

CLINICAL TIP

Excessive crying and anxiety deplete metabolic reserves and increase oxygen demand. Comfort the child and avoid invasive procedures that will increase distress. Assisted ventilation and vigorous crying may both cause the stomach to become distended and impede diaphragm function. A nasogastric tube may be inserted to prevent stomach distention.

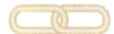

SKILLS 11–13 AND 11–14
Assisted Ventilation

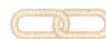

SKILL 11–12
Endotracheal Tube Care

CLINICAL MANIFESTATIONS	RESPIRATORY FAILURE AND IMMINENT RESPIRATORY ARREST
Physiologic Cause	**Clinical Manifestations**
Respiratory Failure These signs occur because the child is trying to compensate for oxygen deficit and airway blockage. Oxygen supply is inadequate; behavior and vital signs reflect compensation and beginning hypoxia.	**Initial Signs** Restlessness Tachypnea Tachycardia Diaphoresis
The child tries to use accessory muscles to assist oxygen intake; hypoxia persists and efforts now waste more oxygen than is obtained.	**Early Decompensation** Nasal flaring Retractions Grunting Wheezing Anxiety and irritability Mood changes Headache Hypertension Confusion
Imminent Respiratory Arrest These signs occur because oxygen deficit is overwhelming and beyond spontaneous recovery. Cerebral oxygenation is dramatically affected; central nervous system changes are ominous.	**Severe Hypoxia** Dyspnea Bradycardia Cyanosis Stupor and coma

frustration when they realize they cannot communicate verbally. When the child is alert, give suggestions for ways to make noise and gain attention, such as striking the mattress. A communication board can be used with older children.

Many children are discharged from the hospital and cared for at home for an extended period with a tracheostomy tube in place. It is essential to teach parents how to maintain the airway, clean the tracheostomy site, and change the tube. A home health-care nurse can provide follow-up care and support for the child and family.

SKILL 11–11
Tracheostomy Care

APNEA

Periodic breathing, an irregular rhythm with pauses of *up to* 20 seconds between breaths, occurs commonly in newborns. This breathing pattern is not apnea. **Apnea** is the cessation of respiration lasting longer than 20 seconds, or any pause in respiration associated with cyanosis, marked pallor, hypotonia, or bradycardia. Apnea may be the first major sign of respiratory dysfunction in the neonate. Apnea of infancy refers to infants with gestational age of 37 weeks or more at the onset of apnea while apnea in infants under that gestational age is described in the following text.

Apnea of Prematurity

Apnea of prematurity is defined as apnea in an infant younger than 37 weeks' gestation and is often associated with immature respiratory control. It may also be a sign of a developing medical condition such as sepsis or infection or a persistent patent ductus arteriosus (Stokowksi, 2005). Apneic episodes often occur during periods of active sleep. Infants are treated with methylxanthines (caffeine and theophylline) and doxapram. Most episodes decrease at approximately 43 weeks' postconceptional age (American Academy of Pediatrics, Committee on Fetus and Newborn, 2003).

Infants are often cared for in the neonatal intensive care unit (NICU) and monitored carefully for apneic episodes. Infants may be discharged with home apnea monitoring if apneic episodes have not stopped by the time of discharge.

Apparent Life-Threatening Event (ALTE)

An ALTE is defined as an episode of apnea accompanied by a color change (cyanosis, pallor, or occasionally ruddiness), limp muscle tone, choking, or gagging in a near-term or term infant who is greater than 37 weeks' gestation. The majority of these events occur in infants under 4 months of age, with a peak incidence between 1 week and 2 months (Davies & Gupta, 2002). These episodes may occur during sleep, wakefulness, or feeding. Some children have multiple episodes. Do not confuse ALTE with Sudden Infant Death Syndrome (SIDS); see page 691.

A variety of identifiable diseases and conditions can potentially cause ALTE, such as gastroesophageal reflux, acute respiratory infection (e.g., pertussis or respiratory syncytial virus), seizures, aspiration while feeding, congenital heart defects, metabolic conditions, and child abuse (Munchausen syndrome by proxy) (Kiechl-Kohlendorfer, Hof, Peglow, et al., 2004; McGovern & Smith, 2004). In some cases, no cause is identified. Nonetheless, ALTE can frighten the parent or observer, who often fears the infant has died. Emergency resuscitation is usually required.

Clinical therapy is focused on identifying the cause of ALTE and then providing effective treatment. The infant is usually admitted to the hospital for evaluation and cardiorespiratory monitoring. Blood is often collected to rule out hematology, electrolyte, infectious, and metabolic conditions. Urine is often collected for urinalysis, culture, and toxicology. Other studies to detect infection include cerebrospinal fluid analysis and culture, and tests for respiratory pathogens. Studies for gastroesophageal reflux may be performed. An electroencephalogram may be performed to investigate seizures as a cause. An electrocardiogram and other cardiac testing may be perfomed to identify any cardiac defects or arrythmias. Radiographic imaging of the chest and brain may be performed. The diagnostic testing selected will be initially focused on the most likely cause identified by history and physical examination. No minimum set of diagnostic tests have been identified to evaluate individual children (Brand, Altman, Purtill et al., 2005). Some children will be sent home on apnea monitors to detect future events.

COMPLEMENTARY THERAPY

Vanilla

The introduction of a pleasant odor (vanillin) into the incubator of a preterm infant with apnea of prematurity was associated with a decrease in episodes of apnea greater than 20 seconds without bradycardia. The 14 infants exposed to the pleasant odor had been unresponsive to traditional treatment for apnea of prematurity with caffeine or doxapram. No side effects to the therapy were noted (Marlier, Gaugler, & Messer, 2005).

NURSING MANAGEMENT

Nursing care includes collecting a detailed history of the event, observing and monitoring cardiorespiratory status, providing supportive care to the infant and family, and anticipating the need for emergency resuscitation and for the diagnostic process.

Monitor Cardiorespiratory Status

Cardiorespiratory monitoring records heart rate and respiratory rate while the infant is awake and asleep. Pulse oximetry provides a noninvasive continuous evaluation of the infant's oxygenation status. An pulse oximetry reading (SpO_2) less than 95% indicates hypoxemia.

Provide Emotional Support

Establishing rapport and open communication with the parents is essential for creating a sense of trust. To obtain further information about the episode, use open-ended questions and active listening skills. Parents are naturally fearful and anxious about the infant's prognosis. Explanations of tests and treatment help to decrease their anxiety and increase their understanding of the situation.

During hospitalization the infant should be held and cuddled to provide a sense of security and well-being. Encouraging parents' participation in the infant's care helps to meet these needs and promotes family bonding. Often parents are hesitant to touch the infant because they are afraid of disconnecting the monitoring cable. Wrapping the cable inside the infant's blanket helps secure the wires, increasing parents' feelings of confidence in handling the infant.

Support the mother to continue breast-feeding and maintain a supply of breast milk by pumping, if necessary. Assure that the mother gets adequate fluids and nutrition. Provide privacy for breast pumping, and store breast milk for future feedings.

Anticipate Emergency Resuscitation

Because the infant who has had ALTE continues to be at risk for cardiopulmonary arrest, keep emergency resuscitation equipment and drugs readily accessible at all times.

Discharge Planning and Home Care Teaching

Identify and address home care needs well in advance of discharge. Teach parents how to operate an apnea monitor and identify when it should be used. Parents who use the monitor during the first week at home are more likely to continue using the monitor in subsequent weeks (Silvestri, Lister, Corwin et al., 2005). See Families Want to Know: Home Care Instructions for the Infant Requiring Apnea Monitoring. Parents also need to learn what to do when the infant has an apneic episode, and how to perform cardiopulmonary resuscitation (CPR) and choking-prevention techniques.

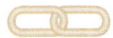

SKILLS 11–18 AND 11–19
Performing Cardiopulmonary Resuscitation

Removing a Foreign Body Airway Obstruction

Obstructive Sleep Apnea

Obstructive sleep apnea syndrome (OSA) is defined as recurrent episodes of partial and complete obstruction of the upper airway during sleep that disrupts normal ventilation and sleep patterns (Bandla, Brooks, Trimarchi et al., 2005). This results in labored breathing and snoring when the child tries to move air past the obstruction. Its incidence peaks between 2 and 6 years of age when tonsils and adenoids are at their largest in contrast to the airway's size. Other contributing factors are obesity and craniofacial abnormalities.

Epidemiology and Pathophysiology

The upper airway contains about 30 muscles that permit the pharynx to collapse, enabling the child to talk and swallow, but also maintain airway patency. When the child is awake, muscle tone is maintained and the airway remains patent even when obstructions such as enlarged adenoids and tonsils, craniofacial anomalies, or obesity are present. During sleep, the airway muscles relax and the pharynx becomes obstructed. When the airway muscles are relaxed, the airway resistance is increased. Reduced upper airway tone and obstruction then results in apnea episodes that lead to hypoventilation, hypoxia, hypercapnia, and an elevated blood pressure. Without treatment,

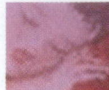

FAMILIES WANT TO KNOW

Home Care Instructions for the Infant Requiring Apnea Monitoring

Apnea Equipment

- Understand monitor type, lead wires, placement of skin electrodes or chest belt, battery power, manual for troubleshooting.

Emergency Preparation

- Notify telephone company, electric company, local rescue squad, and local emergency department (establishes priority status).
- Post phone numbers of rescue squad, physician, equipment company, power company, emergency number, cardiopulmonary resuscitation (CPR) guidelines, and other important numbers (neighbor, parents' work numbers) in at least two places in the home; have at least one added extension phone.
- Keep the apnea monitor battery fully charged.

Safety Precautions

- Place the monitor on a firm surface; keep it away from other appliances (television, microwave oven) and water.
- Ensure that alarms are audible from all locations.
- Double-check that the monitor is on before going to bed.
- Thread cable and wires through the lower end of the infant's clothes.
- Ensure integrity of leads, monitor cable, and power cord (replace if frayed).

Routine Care

- Understand reasons for apnea monitor and frequency of use.
- Be able to attach and detach infant chest leads and belt.

- Evaluate skin for irritation or breakdown from electrode placement and give skin care (no oils or lotion; move patches correctly).

Emergency Care

- Develop plan for respiratory failure and power failure.
- Demonstrate CPR, back blows, and chest thrusts for airway obstruction.
- Understand how to respond to alarms for apnea, bradycardia, or loose lead.

Apnea Alarm

- First observe the infant's respiratory movement to determine if the alarm is for a real event or not.
- If respiration is absent or infant is lethargic, stimulate by calling name and gently touching, proceeding to vigorous touch if needed.
- If no response, proceed with CPR.

Bradycardia Alarm

- Stimulate infant; infant should respond quickly.

Loose Lead

- Check electrode patch. Is it loose? Dirty? Belt loose?
- Check wires from electrode or monitor cable.
- Check power supply. Is battery low? Power failure? Monitor malfunctioning?

---

complications develop that can include failure to thrive, pulmonary hypertension, **cor pulmonale** (obstruction of pulmonary blood flow that leads to right ventricular hypertrophy and heart failure), systemic hypertension, and cognitive impairment. Learning problems and behavior problems may develop.

Clinical Manifestations

Children with OSA snore and have signs of labored breathing during sleep such as retractions and paradoxical breathing. After pauses in snoring or lack of airflow, the child may be noted to snort, gasp, choke, move, or arouse to take a breath. Sleep is restless and the child may sleep in unusual positions to hyperextend the neck and airway. Daytime sleepiness and other symptoms of sleep deprivation (poor attention, increased activity, aggression, acting out behavior, poor school performance) may be noted. Enuresis may occur.

■ COLLABORATIVE CARE

Diagnosis is made by **polysomnography**, a sleep study that simultaneously records the brain activity, eye movement, apnea episodes, oxygen desaturation, and sleep disturbances. Adenotonsillectomy is the most common treatment for OSA and resolution of the condition occurs in the majority of children. Weight loss strategies may be implemented for obese children. Continuous positive airway pressure (CPAP) is used for children with surgical contraindications or those with persistent OSA. Tracheostomy may be necessary in children with craniofacial anomalies or in patients for whom other treatment is not effective.

NURSING MANAGEMENT

In the community setting, all children should be screened for snoring as part of their routine health care. Assess the child for signs of nasal obstruction, mouth breathing, and enlarged tonsils. Determine if the child has symptoms of sleep deprivation or a condition is present that places the child at high risk for OSA. When snoring is present, encourage the parents to keep a sleep diary. Coordinate referral to a sleep center for polysomnogram evaluation and explain the purpose of the test. Discuss how to prepare the child for the strange setting and wires that will be attached during the sleep study. Most pediatric centers will allow the parent to stay with the child during the study.

Following adenoidectomy and tonsillectomy, the hospital nurse monitors the child for bleeding and respiratory distress, such as obstructive sleep apnea and pulmonary edema. Continuous pulse oximetry is used to detect oxygen desaturation. These children are at increased risk for respiratory distress after surgery due to complications of obstructive sleep apnea. They should be carefully monitored postoperatively, particularly 2 to 3 days after surgery when obstructive apnea may occur. Pain is often managed by nonopioid analgesics (acetaminophen) and complementary therapies to avoid additional respiratory depression (Bandla, Brooks, Trimarchi, et al., 2005). See Chapter 19 ∞ for care of the child having an adenoidectomy and tonsillectomy.

Sleep center nurses provide education and support to families of children who need to use CPAP to treat the OSA. The nurse helps identify the best-fitting mask or nasal prong system for CPAP delivery. Parents may need guidance about helping children to go to sleep wearing the mask until they become accustomed to it.

The child may also be referred to an obesity control program to promote weight loss if the excess weight may be contributing to the sleep apnea.

Sudden Infant Death Syndrome

Sudden Infant Death Syndrome (SIDS) is defined as the sudden unexpected death of an infant under 1 year of age. Onset of the fatal episode occurs during sleep and remains unexplained after a thorough investigation, including an autopsy, a review of the circumstances of death, and the clinical history. Various categories of SIDS have been developed to help with future definitions and research (Krous, Beckwith, Byard et al., 2004). It remains a leading cause of death in infants after 1 month of age (American Academy of Pediatrics, Task Force on Sudden Infant Death Syndrome, 2005). SIDS rarely occurs in infants younger than 2 weeks. It is currently unpredictable and in some cases unpreventable.

SIDS is referred to as a "syndrome" because of the many and varied autopsy and clinical findings that characterize most infants who die of the disorder. The autopsy typically does not identify a disease process that caused the death. Current evidence suggests a possible genetic susceptibility to SIDS (American Academy of Pediatrics, Committee on Fetus and Newborn, 2003). A defect in or hypoplasia of the arcuate nucleus, a brain structure that plays a role in regulating breathing, heart beat, body temperature and arousal, may have a role in SIDS (Kato, Franco, Groswasser et al., 2003; Matturri, Ottaviani, & Lavezzi, 2005). Covert homicide may be associated with 6–10% of suspected SIDS deaths (American Academy of Pediatrics, Task Force on Sudden Infant Death Syndrome, 2005). Other proposed causes include respiratory illnesses (potentially as a stress factor on a vulnerable infant) and long QT syndrome, a cardiac dysrhythmia (Daley, 2004). SIDS has not been found to be associated with newborn apnea or immunizations (American Academy of Pediatrics, Task Force on Sudden Infant Death Syndrome, 2005). See Box 20–1 for infant and maternal factors that place infants at risk for SIDS.

The first symptom is a cardiac arrest. Clinical findings include evidence of a struggle or change in position during sleep and the presence of frothy, blood-tinged secretions from the mouth and nares. Typically parents find the infant dead in the crib in the morning or after a nap and report having heard no cries or disturbances during the night.

BOX 20–1
RISK FACTORS FOR SUDDEN INFANT DEATH SYNDROME (SIDS)

Infant Risk Factors

- Race (in decreasing order of frequency): Most common in Native American infants, followed by African American, Hispanic, White, and Asian infants
- Gender: More common in males than females
- Premature or low birth weight
- Age: Most common in infants between 1 and 4 months of age
- Time of year: More prevalent in winter months
- Exposure to passive smoke
- Unsafe sleeping arrangement: Prone or side-lying position, bedsharing, soft bedding or the use of pillows, quilts, or soft toys with bedding
- Overheating due to excessive blankets, clothing on infant, room temperature

Maternal Risk Factors

- Maternal age less than 20 years at first pregnancy, short interval between pregnancies, high parity
- Prenatal and postnatal smoking
- Single parenthood
- Poor prenatal care, intrauterine growth restriction
- Lower socioeconomic status and fewer years of education

Data from: Daley, K. C. (2004). Update on Sudden Infant Death Syndrome. *Current Opinion in Pediatrics, 16*, 227–232; Farrell, P. A., Weiner, G. M., & Lemons, J. A. (2002). SIDS, ALTE, apnea, and the use of home monitors. *Pediatrics in Review, 23*(1), 3–8.

CLINICAL TIP

Guidelines for the support of families experiencing SIDS should include baptism services, religious support, grief counseling, assistance with funeral arrangements, counseling on cessation of breastfeeding, and sibling reactions.

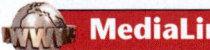
MediaLink

SIDS Support and Resources

■ NURSING MANAGEMENT

The sudden, unexpected nature of the infant's death is often addressed in the emergency department. The nurse's role is to be empathetic and provide support during one of the greatest crises a family must face. Table 20–1 provides guidance for supporting the family during the initial grieving period.

Reassure the parents that they are not responsible for the infant's death and help them contact other family members and mobilize support. Older children may need reassurance that SIDS will not happen to them. Siblings may also believe that bad thoughts or wishes about their baby brother or sister caused the death. Support groups can help parents, siblings, and other family members express these fears and work through their feelings about the infant's death. The First Candle/SIDS Alliance and SHARE are organizations that can help families locate a support group in their area.

Prevention of SIDS

Nurses can play an important role in educating the parents and caregivers about the link between SIDS and infant positioning during sleep. (See Evidence-Based Practice: Infant Sleep Positioning.) All neonates and infants should be placed on the back for sleep every night and for all naps. Prone and side-lying positions both place the infant at risk for SIDS because the side-lying position is unstable. The risk of SIDS is exceptionally high for infants placed in the side-lying position and found in the prone position (American Academy of Pediatrics, Task Force on Sudden Infant Death Syndrome, 2005). Parents should also use a firm mattress and avoid the use of loose bedding, toys, and pillows in the crib. Bed sharing with the parent should be discouraged as it creates an increased risk of SIDS. Use of a sleeper rather than a blanket can help keep the infant warm, but not cause overheating. Infants should be encouraged to have supervised tummy time when awake to promote motor development and to reduce infant skull flattening. See Chapter 26 ∞ for issues related to infant skull flattening (positional plagiocephaly) from sleeping on the back.

| Table 20–1 | SUPPORTIVE CARE FOR THE FAMILY OF AN INFANT WITH SUDDEN INFANT DEATH SYNDROME (SIDS) |

Supportive Care	Rationale
Provide parents with a private area and a support person who reinforces that the infant's death was not their fault.	Parents need to be able to express their grief in their own way and hear that they are not being blamed for the infant's death. Even if a suspicion of abuse exists, parents need to be supported as they express their grief. Comments about blame may be omitted.
Describe how the infant will look and feel. You can say "Paul's [use the infant's name] skin will feel cool. He will be very still and his eyes will be closed." Explain that pooling of blood on the dependent areas will look like bruises.	A gentle explanation prepares the family for the viewing of the infant and demonstrates empathy.
Allow parents to hold, touch, and rock the infant, if desired. Before bringing the infant to parents, wrap in a clean blanket, comb the hair, wash the face, swab the mouth clean, and apply Vaseline to the lips.	Viewing and holding the infant allows parents a chance to say good-bye.
An autopsy is required for all unexplained deaths. You can say to parents, "It is the only way we can be sure of what caused your baby's death."	This step reinforces the physician's explanation about the need for an autopsy.
Answer parents' questions and provide them with sources for further information. Provide literature and the name of a local contact for a SIDS support group, as well as for the national foundation.	Parents may not be able to take in all of your answers. Many hospitals have a social worker who provides ongoing contact with the family. Provide names of resource people and phone numbers for SIDS support groups.
Advise parents that surviving siblings may benefit from psychologic support. Social workers can help the family obtain counseling and support for all members.	Siblings often require emotional support in the weeks and months after the death.
Provide parents with a lock of hair, footprints, and handprints, if they desire. Keep items if the parents don't want them at the time, as they may want them later.	Personal items can be placed in a memory book. This reaffirms the child's existence for many parents.

EVIDENCE-BASED PRACTICE

Infant Sleep Positioning

Problem

In spite of evidence that the supine position for newborns and infants reduces the risk for SIDS, this position is not consistently used by nurses in hospitals.

Evidence

A survey in 58 Missouri hospitals was conducted to examine nurses' knowledge, attitude, and practice in positioning healthy newborns for sleep in the hospital. While nurses no longer used prone positioning for newborns, 75% of 528 responding nurses used side-lying or a mixture of side-lying and supine positioning. However, almost all nurses (96%) reported awareness of guidelines for newborns to sleep on their backs. Reasons nurses gave for using the other sleep position included fear of aspiration, increasing the infant's comfort, and improving the infant's sleep. The majority of nurses reported having encountered an infant in the supine position that was in distress at some time (Bullock, Mickey, Green et al., 2004). Another survey was conducted in eight California hospitals with respondents including 96 newborn nursery staff (predominantly nurses) and 579 mothers. The majority of nurses (68.4%) reported placing infants on their side and 65.3% of nurses advised mothers to use either the side or back positioning for sleep. Aspiration was the primary reason given for the side-lying position. Most nursery staff (72%) reported awareness of guidelines for infant positioning for sleep. The majority of mothers (72%) reported seeing their newborn placed in a nonsupine position by nursery staff, and 44% of mothers were not given recommendations for a sleep position for their newborn. Mothers receiving a recommendation for newborn sleep position were told to use the side or back (Stastny, Ichinose, Thayer et al., 2004).

Implications

The Back to Sleep campaign has been very successful in increasing awareness of the importance of placing infants to sleep in the supine position. Nurses may feel that the side-lying position is safer and prevents aspiration, but not be aware that this position increases the infant's risk for SIDS, especially if the infant rolls to the prone position. Up to 80% of mothers were more likely to use supine positioning for their infant when nurses gave that advice and modeled the position in the hospital (Stastny et al., 2004). Nurses have an important opportunity to model appropriate sleep positioning for newborns and to educate parents about reducing the risk for SIDS.

Critical Thinking

Identify methods to increase the use of supine positioning for newborns and infants who are hospitalized and to promote safe sleep for newborns and infants in the home.

RESEARCH

Pacifier Use

A review of several studies on the association of pacifier use when placing the infant down for sleep, either at night or for naps, has revealed a protective effect against SIDS. Potential mechanisms for the protective effect include increased arousal responsiveness with pacifier use and forward positioning of the tongue that reduces the risk for airway obstruction by the tongue (Hauck, Omojokun, & Siadaty, 2005). The American Academy of Pediatrics now recommends pacifier use for bedtime and naptime, but the pacifier should not be reinserted once the infant falls asleep. Pacifier use should be delayed in breast-fed infants until breast-feeding is well established (American Academy of Pediatrics, Task Force on Sudden Infant Death Syndrome, 2005).

Pregnant women who smoke cigarettes should be educated that exposing the fetus to tobacco places their infant at an increased risk for SIDS (Anderson, Johnson, & Batal, 2005). Referral to a smoking cessation program should be encouraged.

CROUP SYNDROMES

Croup is a term applied to a broad classification of upper airway illnesses that result from swelling of the epiglottis and larynx. The swelling usually extends into the trachea and bronchi. Included under the classification of croup syndromes are viral syndromes, such as spasmodic laryngitis (spasmodic croup), laryngotracheitis, and laryngotracheobronchitis (LTB), as well as bacterial syndromes, such as bacterial tracheitis and epiglottitis (Figure 20–8 ➤).

Epiglottitis, LTB, and bacterial tracheitis are referred to as the "big three" of pediatric respiratory illness because they affect the greatest number of children across all age groups in both sexes. The initial symptoms of all three conditions include inspiratory stridor, a "seal-like" barking cough, and hoarseness. Although LTB is the most common disorder, epiglottitis and bacterial tracheitis are more serious.

Laryngotracheobronchitis

Although the term *croup* is applied to several viral and bacterial syndromes, it is most often used to refer to LTB, a viral invasion of the upper airway that extends throughout the larynx, trachea, and bronchi. Table 20–2 compares LTB and other croup syndromes.

PATHOPHYSIOLOGY ILLUSTRATED

Airway Changes with Croup

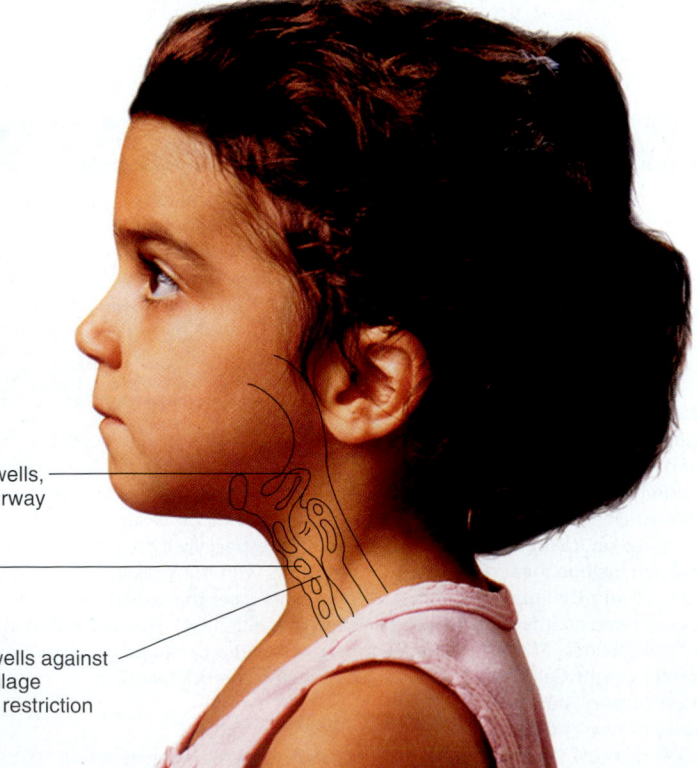

Epiglottis swells, occluding airway

Cricoid cartilage

Trachea swells against cricoid cartilage resulting in restriction

Figure 20–8 ➤ There are two important changes in the upper airway in croup: The epiglottis swells, thereby occluding the airway, and the trachea swells against the cricoid cartilage, causing restriction and narrowing the airway.

| Table 20–2 | OVERVIEW OF VIRAL AND BACTERIAL CROUP SYNDROMES |

| | **Viral Syndromes** | | | **Bacterial Syndromes** | |
	Acute Spasmodic Laryngitis (Spasmodic Croup)	**Laryngotracheobronchitis**	**Laryngotracheitis**	**Bacterial Tracheitis**	**Epiglottitis (Supraglottitis)**
Severity	Least serious	Most common[a]	Most serious; progresses if untreated	Guarded; requires close observation	Most life threatening (medical emergency)[a]
Age affected	3 months to 3 years	3 months to 8 years	3 months to 8 years	1 month to 13 years[a]	2 years to 8 years
Onset	Abrupt onset; peaks at night, resolves by morning (recurs)[a]	Gradual onset; starts as URI, progresses to moderate respiratory difficulty	Gradual onset; starts as URI, progresses to symptoms of respiratory distress	Progressive from URI (1–2 days)	Progresses rapidly (hours)[a]
Clinical manifestations	Afebrile; mild respiratory distress; barking-seal cough	*Early:* mild fever [<39°C (102.2°F)]; hoarseness; barking-seal, brassy, croupy cough; rhinorrhea; sore throat; stridor (inspiratory); apprehension *Progressing to* labored respirations	*Early:* mild fever [<39°C (102.2°F)]; barking-seal, brassy, croupy cough; rhinorrhea; sore throat; stridor (inspiratory); apprehension; restless/irritable *Progressing to* retractions (progressive); increasing stridor; cyanosis	High fever [>39°C (102.2°F)]; URI appears as viral croupy cough; croup initially; stridor (tracheal); purulent secretions	High fever [>39°C (102.2°F)]; URI; intense sore throat; dysphagia[a]; drooling[a]; increased pulse and respiratory rate; prefers upright position (tripod position with chin thrust)[a]
Etiology	Unknown; suspect viral with allergic/emotional influences	Parainfluenza, types I and II, respiratory syncytial virus, influenza A and B viruses, adenovirus, or rubeola virus	Parainfluenza, types I and II, RSV, or influenza	*Staphylococcus*	*Haemophilus influenzae,* streptococcus and staphylococcus

[a]Classic parameter or key point (distinguishes condition).

Etiology and Pathophysiology

Acute viral LTB is most common in children 3 months to 4 years of age but can occur in children up to 8 years of age. Boys are affected more often than girls, and LTB is of greatest concern in infants and children under the age of 6 years, because of potential airway obstruction. The causative organism is usually parainfluenza virus type I, II, or III that appears during winter months. Other viruses causing LTB include influenza A and B, adenovirus, respiratory syncytial virus, and measles (Anonymous, 2005).

Airway tissues respond to the invading virus with inflammation and edema. Copious, tenacious secretions further increase the child's respiratory distress. The laryngeal inflammation causes the airway diameter to narrow in the subglottic area, the airway's narrowest part. Even small amounts of mucus or edema can quickly obstruct the airway. Both the large and small airways can be affected.

Clinical Manifestations

Most children brought to the emergency department with LTB have been ill for a couple of days with upper respiratory symptoms. These symptoms progress to a cough and hoarseness. Fever may or may not be present. Common presenting signs are tachypnea, inspiratory stridor, and a seal-like barking cough. See Table 20–2 for other characteristics of LTB.

■ COLLABORATIVE CARE

Diagnostic Testing

Diagnosis is often made by clinical signs. A stridor assessment score is often used to provide an objective and quantifiable measure of respiratory difficulty that can be compared with future scores. See Table 20–3. Pulse oximetry is used to detect hypoxemia. If the diagnosis of LTB is in question, anteroposterior (AP) and lateral radiographs of the upper airway are taken; these may show the airway narrowing 5 to 10 mm below the vocal cords, called a "steeple sign." Throat cultures and visual inspection of the inner mouth and throat are contraindicated in children with LTB and epiglottitis. These procedures can cause **laryngospasms** (spasmodic vibrations that close the larynx) as a result of the child's anxiety or of probing this reactive and already compromised area.

Clinical Therapy

Clinical therapy consists of maintaining and improving respiratory effort with medications, humidification, and supplemental oxygen when the saturated oxygen level is less than 92% (see Medications Used to Treat Symptomatic Laryngotracheobronchitis). Mist tents are rarely used for laryngotracheobronchitis.

Children with a good response to medications are often sent home from the emergency department after an observation period. Children with moderate to severe symptoms after repeated nebulizer medications are admitted for further observation and treatment. Airway obstruction is a potential complication of LTB. Therefore, the child may require intubation and transfer to the ICU to maintain airway patency if obstruction is imminent. Most children, however, respond positively to the medications and oxygen therapy and are discharged within 48 to 72 hours.

■ NURSING MANAGEMENT

Nursing Assessment and Diagnosis

The initial and ongoing physical assessment of the child with LTB focuses on adequacy of respiratory functioning. Use a stridor assessment scale every 2–4 hours, or more frequently if distress increases. The child should be in an area where continuous visual monitoring is possible to identify changes in airway patency. Pay particular attention to the child's respiratory effort, breath sounds, and responsiveness. Note any change in

Table 20–3	CLINICAL SCORING SYSTEM FOR ASSESSING CHILDREN WITH STRIDOR			
	Criteria for Scoring			
Signs	**0**	**1**	**2**	**3**
Stridor	None	With agitation	Mild at rest	Severe at rest
Retractions	None	Mild	Moderate	Severe
Air entry	Normal	Normal	Decreased	Severe decrease
Color	Normal	Normal	Cyanotic with agitation	Cyanotic at rest
Level of consciousness	Normal	Restless if disturbed	Restless if undisturbed	Lethargic

Scoring: To quantify the severity of stridor, add the individual scores for each of the sign categories. A score between 0 and 15 is possible. The rating of severity is based on total score with < 6 = mild, 7–8 = moderate, and > 8 = severe.

Note: From Perkin, R. M., & Swift, J. D. (2002). Infectious causes of upper airway obstruction in children. *Pediatric Emergency Medicine Reports, 7*(11), 120.

MEDICATIONS USED TO TREAT
Symptomatic Laryngotracheobronchitis

Medication	Action/Indication	Nursing Implications
Beta-agonists and beta-adrenergics (e.g., albuterol, racemic epinephrine): aerosolized through face mask	Rapid-acting bronchodilator, decreases bronchial and tracheal secretions and mucosal edema, used to decrease symptoms of moderate to severe respiratory distress; and constriction of subglottic mucosa and submucosal capillaries. Used until dexamethasone begins working.	Provides only temporary relief; improvement in 30 minutes that lasts about 2 hours, it gives time for the steroid to work; the child may experience tachycardia (160–200 beats/min) and hypertension; dizziness, headache, and nausea; may necessitate stopping medication; reduces the need for artificial airway.
Corticosteroids (e.g., dexamethasone): IM, PO, nebulized budesonide	Anti-inflammatory, used to decrease edema; has a long half-life of 36–54 hours.	The child may experience cardiovascular symptoms (hypertension): requires close observation for individual response; children less frequently need emergency airways; stridor resolves faster.

behavior such as agitation or irritability. Physical exhaustion can diminish the intensity of retractions and stridor. As the child uses the remaining energy reserve to maintain ventilation, breath sounds may actually diminish. Noisy breathing (audible airway congestion, coarse breath sounds) in this situation verifies adequate energy stores. Responsiveness decreases as hypoxemia increases.

A means of communication (sign language or simple word cues) must be established so the older child can alert nursing staff to respiratory difficulty.

The following nursing diagnoses might be appropriate for the child with acute LTB:

- Ineffective Breathing Pattern related to tracheobronchial obstruction, decreased energy, and fatigue
- Risk for Deficient Fluid Volume related to inadequate fluid intake prior to admission
- Readiness for Enhanced Knowledge (Home Management of Croup) related to information about the risk for the child to have future episodes

Planning and Implementation
Maintain Airway Patency
Supplemental oxygen with humidity may be needed for hypoxemia. Cool mist is presumed to moisten airway secretions and soothe the inflamed mucosa, but research has not documented its benefit (Perkin & Swift, 2002). Allow the child to assume a comfortable position with the head elevated, or sitting upright if desired. Be immediately available to attend to the child's respiratory needs, and keep resuscitation equipment at the bedside.

Meet Fluid and Nutritional Needs
The respiratory distress may have interfered with the child's ability and desire to drink fluids and therefore compromised the child's fluid status. Recognizing fluid deficit and monitoring the child's hydration and nutritional status are essential tasks. Fluids promote liquification of secretions and provide calories for energy and metabolism.

Children with LTB usually prefer cool, noncarbonated, nonacidic drinks such as oral rehydration fluids. The parents can be encouraged to give the child oral fluids. An intravenous infusion may be necessary to rehydrate the child, maintain fluid balance, or provide emergency access. Observe the child closely for difficulty in swallowing, which may be an early sign of epiglottitis or bacterial tracheitis.

Discharge Planning and Home Care Teaching

During the child's observation period, take every opportunity to assess the parents' knowledge of symptoms of LTB and discuss actions to take if symptoms recur. For example, instruct parents to call the child's physician if:

- Mild symptoms do not improve after 1 hour of humidity and cool air treatment.
- The child's breathing is rapid and labored.
- The child does not drink adequate fluids and the urine output is reduced.

Evaluation

Expected outcomes of nursing care include:

- The child responds to medications with decreased respiratory distress.
- The child has adequate fluid intake for age.

Epiglottitis (Supraglottitis)

Epiglottitis (also known as supraglottitis) is an inflammation of the epiglottis, the long narrow structure that closes off the glottis during swallowing. Because edema in this area can rapidly (within minutes or hours) obstruct the airway by occluding the trachea, epiglottitis is considered a potentially life-threatening condition. (Table 20–2 compares epiglottitis and other croup syndromes.)

Epiglottitis is caused by bacterial invasion of the soft tissue of the larynx by Streptococcus and Staphylococcus, and by *Haemophilus influenzae* type B (Hib) in unimmunized children. The resulting inflammation and edema in the tissues and surrounding the epiglottis lead to airway obstruction. Since the widespread use of the Hib vaccination, a 10-fold decrease in the incidence of epiglottitis has occurred (Isaacson & Isaacson, 2003).

Characteristically, a previously healthy child suddenly becomes very ill. The child initially develops a high fever (greater than 39°C [102.2°F]), with a sore throat, dysphonia (muffled, hoarse, or absent voice sounds), and **dysphagia** (difficulty in swallowing). As the larynx becomes obstructed, inspiratory stridor and respiratory distress develop. The intense throat pain keeps the child from swallowing, resulting in drooling. To fully open the airway and improve air intake, the child sits up and leans forward with the jaw thrust forward in the classic "sniffing" or tripod posture and refuses to lie down. The child's anxiety increases as it becomes more difficult to breathe.

Diagnosis is often based on physical signs and a lateral neck radiograph (Figure 20–9 ➤), which reveals a narrowed airway and an enlarged, rounded epiglottis, seen as a mass at the base of the tongue. Laryngospasm and airway obstruction can occur as a result of the severe irritation and hypersensitivity of the airway muscles. For this reason, *visual inspection of the mouth and throat is contraindicated in children with suspected epiglottitis.*

Immediate clinical therapy usually involves insertion of an endotracheal tube (often in the operating room) to maintain the airway. The child is then admitted to the pediatric intensive care unit. At the same time a culture of the epiglottis is obtained. If the child develops an airway obstruction, assisted ventilation is performed until the endotracheal tube can be inserted. Antibiotics effective for gram-positive organisms and *H. influenzae* are given until culture sensitivities are available. Antipyretics (acetaminophen, ibuprofen) may be useful in managing fever and sore throat pain.

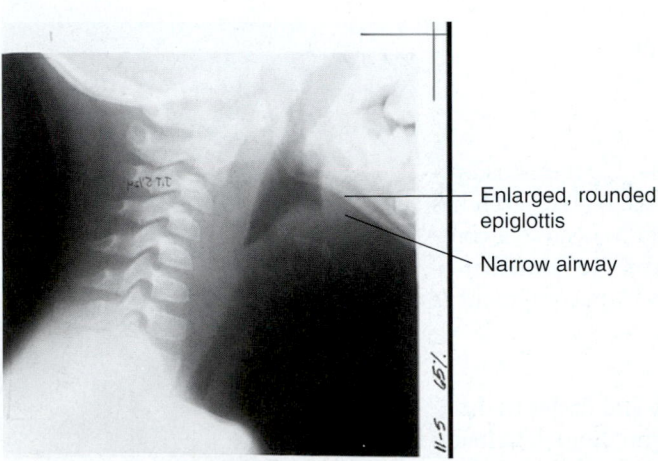

Enlarged, rounded epiglottis

Narrow airway

Figure 20–9 ➤ The phrase "thumb sign" has been used to describe this enlargement of the epiglottis. Recall the trachea's usual "little finger" size. Do you see the stiff, enlarged "thumb" above it in this lateral neck radiograph?

Nursing Management

Nursing management consists of airway management, drug therapy, hydration, and emotional and psychosocial support of the child and parents.

Until the child is intubated, the child is usually sedated and needs to be positioned to maintain the airway and breathe more easily. Observe the child's respiratory and airway status closely and often. Note any change in level of consciousness. Anxiety-provoking procedures are postponed until the airway is stabilized. Crying stimulates the airway, increases oxygen consumption, and can precipitate laryngospasm. Supplemental humidified oxygen may be used initially to reverse hypoxemia.

Until the endotracheal tube is removed, the child is usually managed in the ICU to ensure continual observation. Administer antibiotics to treat bacterial infection and antiviral medications for viral cause. Give IV fluids to provide hydration. Because the child was febrile with a sore throat before admission, fluid intake may have been compromised.

The loss of voice, or even the inability to create sounds, can be frightening to a child. The unfamiliar hospital environment and strange equipment can also create stress for the child and parent alike. Reassure the parents that the child's voice loss is temporary and explain the need for the various pieces of equipment.

Most children show rapid improvement once oxygen, antibiotics, and fluid therapy are started. The endotracheal tube can usually be removed within 1 to 2 days, and home care may involve completing the course of antibiotics. Parents need instructions on proper administration and potential problems of drug therapy.

Bacterial Tracheitis

Bacterial tracheitis is a secondary infection of the upper trachea after viral laryngotracheitis that is most often caused by *Staphylococcus aureus*, *group A streptococcus*, *Moraxella catarrhalis*, or *Haemophilus influenzae*. Airway edema and copious purulent secretions can cause obstruction or the development of a tracheal pseudomembrane (Froh, 2006).

The disorder starts with croupy cough and stridor but progresses with the development of a high fever (greater than 39°C [102.2°F]), respiratory distress, a toxic appearance, and purulent secretions that can obstruct the airway and become life threatening (Froh, 2006). Table 20–2 compares bacterial tracheitis and other croup syndromes.

Because of the similarity of symptoms, bacterial tracheitis is often misdiagnosed initially as LTB. Instead of improving with therapy, however, the child's condition becomes worse. Children generally prefer lying flat to sitting up. This seems to be a position of comfort that allows the child to conserve energy. Diagnosis is often made by blood cultures after the child is found unresponsive to usual LTB management. The subglottis is edematous with ulceration, and thick mucopurulent exudate may obstruct the airway. Intravenous antibiotics are given initially and changed to oral as the child's condition improves over the 10- to 14-day course. Most children need a secured artificial airway for 3 to 11 days and ventilatory support.

Nursing Management

The child with bacterial tracheitis is frequently cared for in the PICU after endotracheal intubation. Mechanical suctioning of the thick tracheal secretions that pool high in the upper airway helps maintain a patent airway. Provide humidified air or oxygen. Antibiotics are administered as ordered. The earlier section on epiglottitis discusses other nursing care interventions that may also be appropriate for the child with bacterial tracheitis.

LOWER AIRWAY DISORDERS

The lower airway, or bronchial tree, lies below the trachea and includes the bronchi, bronchioles, and alveoli. Lower airway disorders occur because a structural or functional problem interferes with the lungs' ability to complete the respiratory cycle. Lower airway disorders include bronchitis, bronchiolitis, bronchopulmonary dysplasia, pneumonia, and tuberculosis.

NURSING ALERT

Observe the child continuously for inability to swallow, absence of voice sounds, increasing degree of respiratory distress, and acute onset of drooling (an ominous sign of supraglottic obstruction). If any of these signs occur, get medical assistance immediately. The quieter the child, the greater the cause for concern.

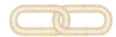

SKILL 11–12
Endotracheal Tube Care

Bronchitis

Acute bronchitis, inflammation of the trachea and bronchi, rarely occurs in childhood as an isolated problem. The bronchi can be affected simultaneously with adjacent respiratory structures during a respiratory illness. Bronchitis is caused most often by a virus but may also result from invasion of bacteria or in response to an allergen or irritant.

The classic symptom of bronchitis is a coarse, hacking cough, which increases in severity at night. Children with bronchitis appear tired. The chest and ribs may be sore because of the deep and frequent coughing. There is often a deep, rattling quality to breathing. Some children have audible wheezing that can be heard without a stethoscope. Treatment is palliative unless a secondary bacterial infection occurs requiring antibiotic therapy.

Nursing Management

Nursing management includes supporting respiratory function through rest, humidification, hydration, and symptomatic treatment. Refer to the sections on asthma and pneumonia for detailed information on treatment measures.

Home care should emphasize the self-limiting nature of the disorder. Advise parents who smoke that quitting or refraining from smoking in the child's presence may benefit the child.

Bronchiolitis

Bronchiolitis is a lower respiratory tract illness that occurs when an infecting agent (virus or bacterium) causes inflammation and obstruction of the small airways, the bronchioles. The peak age for bronchiolitis is 2 to 6 months (Cooper, Banasiak, & Allen, 2003). Infection is most severe in infants under 6 months of age and in children with heart and lung disease. Bronchiolitis is responsible for 90,000 hospital admissions and 4500 deaths per year (Agency for Healthcare Research and Quality, 2003).

Etiology and Pathophysiology

Infection with *respiratory syncytial virus* (RSV) is the most common cause, but other viral (human metapneumovirus and parainfluenza viruses), bacterial, and mycoplasmal organisms may also be responsible. RSV occurs in annual epidemics during the winter and early spring (American Academy of Pediatrics, 2006, p. 561). It is transmitted through direct contact of the contaminated secretions and potentially through inhalation of droplets. Nearly all children have been infected with RSV by 2 years of age, and reinfection is common as infection does not confer immunity (Chavéz-Bueno, Mejías, Jafri et al., 2005).

Viruses, acting as parasites, are able to invade the mucosal cells that line the small bronchi and bronchioles. The invaded cells die when the virus bursts from inside the cell to invade adjacent cells. The membranes of the infected cells fuse with adjacent cells, creating large masses of cells or "syncytia." The resulting cell debris clogs and obstructs the bronchioles and irritates the airway. In response, the airway lining swells and produces excessive mucus. Despite this protective effort by the bronchioles, the actual effect is partial airway obstruction and bronchospasms.

The cycle is repeated throughout both lungs as the airway cells are invaded by the virus. The partially obstructed airways allow air in, but the mucus and airway swelling block expulsion of the air. This creates the wheezing and crackles in the airways. Air trapped below the obstruction also interferes with normal gas exchange, leading to hypoxemia. The child with severe RSV infection is therefore at risk for respiratory failure as the oxygen level decreases and the carbon dioxide level increases. Apnea and pulmonary edema may occur.

Clinical Manifestations

The infant or child with bronchiolitis may have been ill with upper respiratory symptoms such as nasal stuffiness, cough (not usually noted in infants), and fever (less than 39°C [102.2°F]) for a few days. As the illness progresses and the lower respiratory tract

---

CLINICAL TIP

To reduce the exposure of infants at risk for RSV, childcare and healthcare workers should follow principles of good hand hygiene and sanitation of surfaces. The virus can survive on nonporous surfaces for several hours, and on hands for a half hour or more (Chavéz-Bueno, Mejías, Jafri et al., 2005).

becomes involved, symptoms increase and include inspiratory and expiratory wheezing; a deeper, more frequent cough; tachypnea; retractions; and more labored breathing. If severe respiratory distress develops, marked retractions, crackles, cyanosis, and diminished breath sounds are noted. Noisy breath sounds indicate that the child is still able to move air in and out of the lungs.

Parents report that the infant or child is acting more ill—he or she appears sicker, is less playful, and is less interested in eating. Infants, especially, may refuse to feed or may spit up what they do eat along with thick, clear mucus. Dehydration may also be present.

COLLABORATIVE CARE

Diagnostic Testing

The history and physical examination provide the data needed to diagnose bronchiolitis. Chest radiographs show nonspecific findings of inflammation. Enzyme-linked immunoabsorbent assay (ELISA) or direct fluorescent assay performed on a nasal wash specimen are laboratory tests used to identify the virus causing bronchiolitis.

Clinical Therapy

Children who test positive for RSV are isolated, roomed together, or placed on the same ward to minimize the spread of the virus to other hospitalized children. Supportive care is provided, especially when the causative agent is unknown and the condition is mild to moderate in severity. See Table 20–4 for clinical therapies. The child may be intubated and ventilated for apnea or respiratory failure. Aerosolized ribavirin is the only antiviral drug available for treatment. Studies have not confirmed its effectiveness, so it is not used routinely, but it may be used in infants with compromised immune status (Chavéz-Bueno, Mejías, Jafri, et al., 2005).

Table 20–4	CLINICAL THERAPY FOR BRONCHIOLITIS	
Clinical Therapy	**Rationale**
Cardiorespiratory monitor and pulse oximetry	Enable provider to follow course and assess need for specific therapies.
Humidified oxygen therapy via hood or face tent, tent, or nasal cannula	Delivery method determined by desired concentration of oxygen, degree of moisture, and child's response.
Intubation and assisted ventilation (positive end expiratory pressure [PEEP]/continuous positive airway pressure [CPAP])	Used when the child becomes too fatigued to breathe effectively. CPAP helps keep the airway open during inspiration. PEEP increases the mean airway pressure by maintaining the end-expiratory resting lung volume (Frankel, 2004).
Hydration via intravenous or oral fluids	Provider must consider insensible fluid loss, decreased intake, the child's current electrolyte and hydration status, and risk for pulmonary edema.
Systemic medications	Bronchodilators, steroids, and beta-antagonists act directly on inflamed and obstructed airways; bronchodilators help prevent apnea episodes in premature infants; nebulized epinephrine and corticosteroids are occasionally used.
Postural drainage and chest physiotherapy	Helps to further loosen and mobilize trapped mucus.
Suctioning	Removes excessive secretions that child cannot manage to cough or swallow.
High-Risk Infant or Child under 24 Months of age[a]	
Palivizumab (Synargis) IM	Give for 5 consecutive months during RSV season to high-risk children. May prevent RSV bronchiolitis or reduce severity of disease.

[a]Defined as a child with significant congenital heart disease, chronic lung disease associated with prematurity, or an infant who is premature or severely ill and less than 6 months old.

High-risk infants with the following conditions are recommended to receive five monthly intramuscular injections of palivizumab beginning in early November to prevent RSV infection (American Academy of Pediatrics, 2006):

- Infants born before 32 weeks of gestation, particularly if less than 6 months of age at the start of the RSV season. Infants born at 28 weeks and earlier should receive the injections if less than 12 months of age at the start of RSV season.
- Infants and children under 24 months with chronic lung disease associated with prematurity who have required supplemental oxygen, bronchodilator, diuretic, or corticosteroid therapy within 6 months before RSV season.
- Infants and children under 24 months of age with complicated congenital heart disease, particularly those on medication to control congestive heart failure, with cyanosis, and with moderate to severe pulmonary hypertension.
- Immunocompromised infants and children.

Intravenous RSV immune globulin is no longer marketed in the United States.

NURSING MANAGEMENT
Nursing Assessment and Diagnosis

The nursing assessment focuses on airway and respiratory function as the infant may tire with the extra work of breathing and the development of respiratory failure.

Physiologic Assessment

Assess airway and respiratory function carefully. Good observation skills are important to ensure timely interventions for worsening respiratory symptoms and prevention of respiratory distress (see assessment guidelines on page 680 and the Clinical Manifestations of Respiratory Failure on page 687). An oxygen saturation level below 90% is the best indicator of the disease's severity. See the Nursing Care Plan: The Child with Bronchiolitis.

Psychosocial Assessment

Observe children and their parents for signs of fear and anxiety. The unfamiliar hospital environment and procedures can increase stress and have an impact on respiratory status. Observe the young child's reactions to strangers and to the absence of parents. Identify if parents appear anxious, are asking appropriate questions, and observe for nonverbal cues of anxiety. Parents could have financial worries (lost work and wages and cost of hospital stay) and personal concerns (siblings at home) that they may not readily share with nurses.

Common nursing diagnoses for the child with bronchiolitis are included in the nursing care plan.

Planning and Implementation

Nursing management focuses on maintaining respiratory function, supporting overall physiologic function and hydration, reducing the child's and family's anxiety, and preparing the family for home care.

Maintain Respiratory Function

Close monitoring is essential to evaluate the child's improvement or to spot early signs of deterioration. Administer oxygen and pulmonary care therapies. Supplemental oxygen may be provided via nasal cannula, hood, or tent. Use pulse oximetry to evaluate oxygenation.

Patent nares are important to promote oxygen intake. A bulb syringe and saline nose drops can be used to quickly clear the nasal passages. Elevate the head of the bed to ease the work of breathing and drain mucus from the upper airways. Suctioning may be necessary to clear the airway. Chest physiotherapy is often administered by a respiratory therapist.

SKILL 11–20
Performing Nasal Suctioning

NURSING CARE PLAN   The Child with Bronchiolitis

GOAL	INTERVENTION	RATIONALE	EXPECTED OUTCOME
1. Ineffective Breathing Pattern related to increased work of breathing and decreased energy (fatigue)			
	NIC Priority Intervention: **Respiratory Monitoring:** *Collection and analysis of patient data to ensure airway patency and adequate gas exchange.*		*NOC Suggested Outcome:* **Vital Signs Status:** *Temperature, pulse, respiration, and blood pressure within expected range for the child's age.*
The child will return to respiratory baseline.	• Assess respiratory status (Table 20–2) when child is calm and not crying for a minimum of every 2–4 hours, or more often as indicated for an increasing or decreasing respiratory rate and episodes of apnea. Attach cardiorespiratory monitor and pulse oximeter with alarms set. Record and report changes promptly to physician.	• Changes in breathing pattern may occur quickly as the child's energy reserves are depleted. Assessment and monitoring baseline reveal rate and quality of air exchange. Frequent assessment and monitoring provide objective evidence of changes in the quality of respiratory effort, enabling prompt and effective intervention.	The child returns to respiratory baseline within 48–72 hours.
The child's oxygenation status will return to baseline.	• Administer humidified oxygen via mask, nasal cannula, hood, or tent.	• Humidified oxygen loosens secretions and helps maintain oxygenation status and ease respiratory distress.	The child's respiratory effort eases. Pulse oximetry reading remains ≥ 95% oxygen saturation during treatment.
	• Assess pulse oximetry on room air and compare to reading when child is on oxygen.	• Comparison of pulse oximetry readings provides information about improvement status.	
	• Note child's response to ordered medications.	• Medications act systemically to improve oxygenation and decrease inflammation.	The child tolerates therapeutic measures with no adverse effects.
	• Position head of bed up or place child in position of comfort on parent's lap, if crying or struggling in crib or bed.	• Position facilitates improved aeration and promotes decrease in anxiety (especially in toddlers) and energy expenditure.	The child rests quietly in position of comfort.
	• Assess tolerance to feeding and activities.	• Provides an assessment of condition improvement.	
2. Risk for Imbalanced Fluid Volume related to inability to meet body requirements and increased metabolic demand			
	NIC Priority Intervention: **Fluid Management:** *Promotion of fluid balance and prevention of complications resulting from abnormal or undesired fluid levels.*		*NOC Suggested Outcome:* **Hydration:** *Amount of water in intracellular and extracellular compartments of body.*
Child's immediate fluid deficit is corrected.	• Evaluate need for intravenous fluids. Maintain IV, if ordered.	• Previous fluid loss may require immediate replacement.	Child's hydration status is maintained during acute phase of illness as demonstrated by appropriate urine output and moist mucous membranes.
Child will be adequately hydrated, be able to tolerate oral fluids, and progress to normal diet.	• Calculate maintenance fluid requirements and give oral and/or IV fluids.	• Assessment ensures child receives appropriate fluids to maintain hydration while transitioning to oral fluids.	Child takes adequate oral fluids after 24–48 hours to maintain hydration.
	• Maintain strict intake and output monitoring and evaluate specific gravity at least every 8 hours.	• Monitoring proves objective evidence of fluid loss and ongoing hydration status.	

(continued)

NURSING CARE PLAN   The Child with Bronchiolitis (continued)

GOAL	INTERVENTION	RATIONALE	EXPECTED OUTCOME
2. Risk for Imbalanced Fluid Volume related to inability to meet body requirements and increased metabolic demand (continued)			
	• Perform daily weight measurement on the same scale at the same time of day. Evaluate skin turgor.	• Further evidence of improvement of hydration status.	Child's weight stabilizes after 24–48 hours; skin turgor is supple.
	• Assess mucous membranes and presence of tears. Report changes promptly to physician.	• Moist mucous membranes and tears provide observable evidence of hydration.	Child shows evidence of improved hydration.
	• Offer clear fluids and incorporate parent in care. Offer fluid choice when tolerated.	• Choice of fluid offered by parent gains the child's cooperation.	The child accepts beverage of choice from parent or nursing staff.
3. Anxiety (Child and Parent) related to acute illness, hospitalization, uncertain course of illness and treatment, and home care needs			
	NIC Priority Intervention: **Anxiety Reduction:** *Minimizing apprehension, dread, foreboding, or uneasiness related to an unidentified source of anticipated danger.*		*NOC Suggested Outcome:* **Anxiety Control:** *Ability to eliminate or reduce feelings of apprehension and tension from an unidentifiable source.*
Child and parents will demonstrate behaviors that indicate decrease in anxiety.	• Encourage parents to express fears and ask questions; provide direct answers and discuss care, procedures, and condition changes.	• Provides opportunity to vent feelings and receive timely, relevant information. Helps reduce parents' anxiety and increase trust in nursing staff.	Parents and child show decreasing anxiety and decreasing fear as symptoms improve and as child and parents feel more secure in hospital environment. *Parent* freely asks questions and participates in the child's care. The *child* cries less and allows staff to hold and/or touch him or her.
	• Incorporate parents in the child's care. Encourage parents to bring familiar objects from home. Ask about and incorporate in care plan the home routines for feeding and sleeping.	• Familiar people, routines, and objects decrease the child's anxiety and increase parents' sense of control over unexpected, uncertain situation.	
Parents will verbalize knowledge of bronchiolitis symptoms and use of home care methods before the child's discharge from the hospital.	• Explain symptoms, treatment, and home care of bronchiolitis.	• Anticipate potential for recurrence. Assist family to be prepared should respiratory symptoms recur after discharge.	Parent accurately describes respiratory symptoms and initial home care actions.
	• Provide written instructions for follow-up care arrangements, as needed.	• Written, as well as oral, instructions reinforce knowledge. Parents may not "hear" and remember the particulars of home care if only presented orally.	

Support Physiologic Function

Grouping nursing tasks promotes the child's physiologic function by decreasing stress and promoting rest. Medications may be administered to control temperature and promote comfort as needed. An IV infusion may be ordered to rehydrate and maintain fluid balance until the child is capable of taking sufficient oral fluids. Small frequent feedings will help conserve energy in infants who are formula or breast-fed. Thickened formula may improve swallowing and prevent aspiration in infants with RSV bronchiolitis (Gadomski, 2002).

Reduce Anxiety

The need for hospitalization and assistive therapies creates anxiety and fear in the child and parents. An important part of nursing care is anticipating, recognizing, and acting to decrease the child's and parents' anxiety. The parents may be frightened and stressed by the child's continued respiratory difficulty and the assistive equipment at the bedside. Provide parents with thorough explanations and daily updates, and encourage their participation in the child's care. Reassure them that holding or touching the child will not dislodge wires or tubing, and that their presence will calm and support the child.

If the child has been ill for a few days before admission, the parents are likely to be tired. Acknowledging parents' physical and emotional needs creates a spirit of caring and enhances communication between staff and family. Encourage the parents to take turns at the child's bedside and to take breaks for meals and rest.

Discharge Planning and Home Care Teaching

Children are discharged once they show sufficient stability in maintaining adequate oxygenation (as evidenced by easing of respiratory effort, decreased mucus production, and absence of coughing). In most children, symptoms decrease within 24 to 72 hours; however, it may take weeks before all symptoms disappear. The same supportive therapies implemented in the hospital may be needed at home. See Families Want to Know: Discharge Instructions for Bronchiolitis.

Teach the parents proper administration of medications. Acetaminophen may be prescribed for persistent low-grade fevers and general discomfort. Advise parents that RSV infection can recur; therefore, they need to know how to recognize symptoms and when to call the physician.

Evaluation

Expected outcomes of nursing care for the child with bronchiolitis include:

- The child returns to respiratory baseline within 48 to 72 hours.
- The child's hydration status is maintained during the acute phase of the illness.
- Parents and child show decreasing anxiety and decreasing fear as symptoms improve and as child and parents feel more secure in the hospital environment.

Pneumonia

Pneumonia is an inflammation or infection of the bronchioles and alveolar spaces of the lungs. It occurs most often in infants and young children. Pneumonia in children often resolves much sooner than in adults. The key is early recognition, enabling the child to be managed at home rather than in the hospital.

Pneumonia may be viral, mycoplasmal, or bacterial in origin. In children under 5 years of age, pneumonia is most often caused by viruses such as RSV, influenza, parainfluenza virus, adenovirus, rhinovirus, and enterovirus. In children over 5 years,

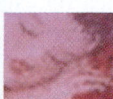

FAMILIES WANT TO KNOW

Discharge Teaching for Bronchiolitis

General care instructions:

- Use a bulb syringe to keep the nares of an infant clear.
- Give fluids to help keep secretions thin and provide calories for energy.
- Encourage active toddlers to rest and take naps during recovery, even though toddlers usually recognize their own activity limits and rest.

Advise parents to call the physician if:

- Breathing is rapid or difficult, or respiratory symptoms interfere with sleep or eating.
- Symptoms persist in a child who is less than 1 year old, has heart or lung disease, or was premature and had lung disease after birth.
- The child acts sicker—appears tired, less playful, and less interested in food (parents just "feel" the child is not improving).

pneumonia is caused by bacteria, such as *Streptococcus pneumoniae*. Children with a condition such as cystic fibrosis or immunosuppression are susceptible to many other bacterial, parasitic, or fungal infections.

Bacterial and viral invaders act differently within the lungs.

- Bacterial invaders circulate through the bloodstream to the lungs, where they damage cells. Cellular debris and mucus cause airway obstruction. Bacteria tend to be distributed evenly throughout one or more lobes of a single lung, a pattern termed *unilateral lobar pneumonia*.
- Viruses frequently enter from the upper respiratory tract, infiltrating the alveoli nearest the bronchi of one or both lungs. There they invade the cells, replicate, and burst out forcefully, killing the cells and sending out cell debris. They rapidly invade adjacent areas, distributing themselves in a scattered, patchy pattern referred to as bronchopneumonia.
- Aspiration of food, emesis, gastric reflux, or hydrocarbons causes a chemical injury and an inflammatory response. Materials with a lower pH cause more inflammation, which sets the stage for bacterial invasion.

Regardless of the causative agent, symptoms include fever, tachypnea, rhonchi, crackles, wheezes, cough, dyspnea, nasal flaring, restlessness, chest pain, and malaise. Decreased breath sounds may be present if consolidation exists. The child also may have poor oral intake, nausea, vomiting, and abdominal pain.

Diagnosis is made by chest radiograph, which shows an abnormal density of tissue, such as a lobar consolidation or patchy consolidation associated with bronchopneumonia. In children over 12 months of age having clinical manifestations associated with pneumonia, a respiratory rate greater than 50 per minute and an oxygen saturation of 96% or less are more likely to be associated with a positive chest radiograph. In children under 12 months of age, nasal flaring is an important finding that is more likely associated with a positive chest radiograph (Mahabee-Gittens, Grupp-Phelan, Brody et al., 2005). The older child may have dullness to chest percussion, increased fremitus, and egophony. There is no clinical way to differentiate bacterial and viral cause because it is difficult to get a sputum culture from children. Blood cultures may be taken. The child's age, severity of symptoms, and presence of an underlying lung, cardiac, or immunodeficiency disease can create varying responses.

Clinical management for all types of pneumonia includes symptomatic therapy (pain and fever control) and supportive care through airway management, fluids, and rest. Mycoplasma and other bacterial pneumonias are treated with organism-sensitive antibiotics; viral pneumonias usually improve without antibiotics. Some children with significant pneumonia are hospitalized for careful monitoring and to receive oxygen and IV fluids to maintain hydration.

Nursing Management

Most children with pneumonia are cared for at home. Nursing care incorporates supportive measures and medical therapies as appropriate. Nursing measures used to manage the child with bronchiolitis are generally applicable to the child with pneumonia.

In addition to ongoing respiratory assessment and supportive therapies (chest physiotherapy, antibiotics, hydration), the child may need relief from pain when coughing and deep breathing. Teach the child and parent how to splint the chest by hugging a small pillow, teddy bear, or doll to make coughing less painful. Pain medication (acetaminophen or ibuprofen) can provide the added benefits of temperature control and may aid in sleep.

The goal of nursing care is to restore optimal respiratory function. Medications, especially antibiotics, must be taken at prescribed intervals and for the full course. Teach parents the proper administration of drugs and any side effects. Follow-up may include a chest radiograph to see if the lungs are clear. Symptoms of pneumonia usually disappear long before the lungs are completely healed. Some children continue to have worsening reactive airway problems or abnormal results on pulmonary function tests. Most children, however, recover uneventfully.

Full immunization of infants is one preventive measure against pneumonia. The pneumococcal conjugate vaccine (PCV7) administered during infancy has significantly reduced the incidence of invasive pneumococcal illness, including pneumonia (Poehling, Talbot, Griffin et al., 2006). A 23-valent pneumococcal vaccine (PPV23) is recommended for children over 2 years of age who are immunosuppressed or have chronic diseases (see Chapter 18 ∞).

Tuberculosis

Tuberculosis (TB) is caused by the organism *Mycobacterium tuberculosis*, which is transmitted through the air in infectious particles called droplet nuclei. The overall incidence of TB in the United States in 2004 was 4.9 cases per 100,000 people (Goldrick, 2005). More than 50% of new U.S. cases of TB occur in individuals who are foreign born (Centers for Disease Control and Prevention, 2004). The number of TB cases in children was 1.5 cases per 100,000 population in 2001 compared to 2.9 cases per 100,000 population in 1993. Children under 5 years of age, racial and ethnic minorities, and foreign-born children were more likely to develop TB than older children (Nelson, Schneider, Wells et al., 2004). More children have latent TB infection (the organism has replicated in the lungs, but no signs of disease are present) than active TB. In young children, the disease develops as an immediate complication of the primary infection.

Epidemiology and Pathophysiology

Children usually acquire a TB infection from infected adults who cough, sneeze, speak, or sing, and send out tiny droplets containing the bacillus. When the child inhales these droplets, the bacillus is small enough to travel directly to the alveoli and cause infection. Frequently, however, the organism is trapped in the upper airway, preventing infection.

Once the organism reaches the alveoli, an immune response is initiated and macrophages surround and wall off the bacillus in small hard capsules, called tubercles. There the bacillus can remain dormant (inactive) indefinitely or can progress to active TB. The tubercle bacillus grows slowly, dividing within the macrophage. When the organisms number 1000 to 10,000 after 2 to 12 weeks, cellular immune response to TB can be elicited with the TB skin test. Up to 40% of untreated infants with latent TB infection develop active TB within 2 to 12 months after initial infection (Reznick & Ozuah, 2005). Infection may progress to active TB even before the TB skin test becomes reactive in infants and children because of their immature immune system (Reznick & Ozuah, 2005).

The tubercle bacilli may spread by the lymphatic system to the hilar lymph nodes and then to the bloodstream and other sites, resulting in TB meningitis or miliary (disseminated) TB. This systemic form of TB (meningeal or miliary tuberculosis) may lead to serious illness or death. Miliary tuberculosis is not, however, transmissible; only active pulmonary TB is communicable.

Clinical Manifestations

Infants, children, and adolescents with latent TB infection will have no symptoms. Clinical manifestations of active TB in infants include a persistent cough, weight loss or failure to gain weight, and low-grade fever. Wheezing and decreased breath sounds may be present. Children with active TB may have fatigue, cough, anorexia, weight loss or growth delay, night sweats, chills, a low-grade fever, and enlarged lymph nodes.

■ COLLABORATIVE CARE

Diagnostic Testing

Screening questions (Box 20–2) should be used to identify infants and children at risk for latent TB infection during health visits every 6 months until 2 years of age and then annually (American Academy of Pediatrics, 2006, p. 682). Only children who have one or more risk factors should have an intradermal tuberculin skin test with purified protein derivative (PPD, the Mantoux test) applied. Children should not be routinely

BOX 20–2
SCREENING QUESTIONS TO IDENTIFY RISK FOR LATENT TB INFECTION

- Was the child born outside the United States?
- Has the child traveled outside the United States?
- Has the child been exposed to anyone with TB disease?
- Does the child have close contact with a person who has a positive TB skin test?
- Does the child spend time with anyone who has been in prison, has been in a shelter, uses illegal drugs, or has HIV infection?
- Has the child drunk raw milk or eaten unpasturized cheese?
- Was any member of the child's household born outside the United States?
- Has a member of the child's household traveled outside the United States?

From: Reznik, M., & Ozuah, P. O. (2005). A prudent approach to screening for and treating tuberculosis. *Contemporary Pediatrics, 22*(11), 73–88.

tested for TB for entry to childcare, camp, or school (Taylor, Nolan, & Blumberg, 2005). Children with a positive PPD then have further diagnostic testing to determine if active TB is present. See Table 20–5 for tests to confirm the diagnosis of active TB. Children who are immunocompromised (e.g., HIV infection, organ transplantation, and malignancies) are at greater risk for rapid progression from latent TB infection to active TB (Taylor, 2005).

Clinical Therapy

Medical management focuses on the diagnosis and treatment of active TB with antitubercular drugs, including isoniazid (INH), rifampicin, pyrazinamide, ethambutol, and streptomycin. Therapy usually involves a 6-month regimen of two or more of these drugs (daily for 2 months and twice weekly for 4 months). Children with latent TB receive either a single daily dose or two to three times weekly dose of isoniazid for 9 months. Daily rifampin may be used if the organism is INH-resistant. Challenges to treatment have occurred with the development of multidrug-resistant TB organisms and failure of infected persons to complete therapy.

Tuberculosis is a major public health problem and must be promptly reported to local health departments. In suspected cases of tuberculosis, the child, immediate family, and supposed carrier should be skin tested for TB.

Table 20–5	DIAGNOSTIC TESTS FOR TUBERCULOSIS
Test	**Indication**
Mantoux test (intradermal injection of 5 tuberculin units of purified protein derivative [PPD])	A positive test confirms latent TB infection and production of antibodies (3–12 weeks after exposure). A repeat PPD should be done in 8 weeks if the first test is negative in a child with risk factors.
Chest radiograph (anteroposterior and lateral views); computed tomography may be used if chest radiograph is not diagnostic	Confirms presence of pulmonary TB (enlargement of hilar, mediastinal, and subcarinal lymph nodes; atelectasis; alveolar consolidation; pleural effusion; focal mass).
Blood cultures for *Mycobacterium tuberculosis*	Confirms TB; defines specific drug sensitivity.
QuantiFERON-g (QFT-g) whole blood assay	Can be used in place of PPD. A negative test should be repeated in 8 to 10 weeks (Taylor, 2005).
Gastric washings (early morning after overnight fast; 3 consecutive days)	Confirms pulmonary TB when positive, but may be negative even with active TB. Used in children under 12 years of age because they do not produce sputum.
Sputum cultures (expectorated or from bronchoscopic examination)	Confirms active pulmonary TB when positive. Used in older children who can produce sputum.
Pleural biopsy for culture and tissue examination	Taken when pleural effusion is present.
Lumbar puncture	Confirms meningeal TB.

NURSING MANAGEMENT

Nursing Assessment and Diagnosis

Nurses have an important role in identifying children with one or more risk factors for TB infection, such as foreign-born children and children residing in states with a higher incidence of TB (California, Texas, New York, Illinois, Georgia, and Florida) (Reznik & Ozuah, 2005). Children at risk should have a PPD applied and read within 48 to 72 hours using the guidelines for interpretation in Box 20–3.

Children who are hospitalized with active TB have their respiratory status assessed as well as energy level, nutritional intake, and weight.

The following nursing diagnoses may be appropriate for the child with TB:

- Effective Therapeutic Regimen Management related to directly observed medication administration
- Risk for Infection (Active TB) related to exposure to infected contact
- Imbalanced Nutrition: Less than Body Requirements related to anorexia and infection

Planning and Implementation

Nursing care centers on administering medications and providing supportive care. Teach parents about the disease process, medications, possible side effects, and the importance of long-term therapy (e.g., that drug therapy may last for 6 to 12 months). Emphasize the importance of taking medications as prescribed on an empty stomach.

Encourage proper nutrition and rest to promote normal growth and development. The child can return to school or childcare when effective therapy has been instituted, adherence to therapy has been documented, and clinical symptoms have diminished substantially (American Academy of Pediatrics, 2006, p. 696). Most children recovering from TB can lead essentially normal lives. The sections on pneumonia earlier in this chapter and on tubercular meningitis in Chapter 26 ∞ discuss other nursing measures appropriate for the child with TB.

> **CLINICAL TIP**
>
> Children with active tuberculosis should receive "directly observed drug therapy" administered by a nurse or other healthcare provider to ensure the drug is being taken. Direct observation should occur at least twice a week for the duration of treatment (Reznik & Ozuah, 2005). Children with latent TB should also receive "directly observed drug therapy" twice a week (American Academy of Pediatrics, 2006, p. 686).

BOX 20–3

INTERPRETING TUBERCULIN SKIN TEST RESULTS IN INFANTS, CHILDREN, AND ADOLESCENTS*

Induration >5 mm
- Children in close contact with known or suspected contagious cases of tuberculosis disease
- Children suspected to have tuberculosis disease: with findings on chest radiograph consistent with active or previously active tuberculosis or clinical evidence of potential tuberculosis disease (i.e., meningitis)
- Children receiving immunosuppressive doses of corticosteroids or having immunosuppressive conditions, including HIV infection

Induration >10 mm
- Children at increased risk of disseminated disease: younger than 4 years of age; with other medical conditions, including Hodgkin's disease, lymphoma, diabetes mellitus, chronic renal failure, or malnutrition
- Children with increased exposure to tuberculosis disease: born in (or parents born in) high-prevalence regions of the world; frequently exposed to adults who are HIV infected, homeless, users of illicit drugs, residents of nursing homes, incarcerated or institutionalized, or migrant farm workers; or travel to high-prevalence regions of the world

Induration >15 mm
- Children 4 years of age or older without any risk factors

* These definitions apply regardless of previous bacille Calmette-Guérin (BCG) immunization.
From: American Academy of Pediatrics. (2006). *Red book: 2006 Report of the Committee on Infectious Diseases* (27th ed., p. 680). Elk Grove Village, IL: Author.

Tuberculosis is a reportable disease. Public health nurses need to evaluate contacts of the child to identify the primary case of TB and other potentially infected family members.

Evaluation

Expected outcomes of nursing care include:

- The child with latent TB infection completes therapy and does not develop active TB.
- The child's contacts are evaluated for TB and those infected are treated.

CHRONIC LUNG DISEASES

Bronchopulmonary Dysplasia

Bronchopulmonary dysplasia (BPD) is the persistance of lung disease following premature birth and respiratory support provided in the neonatal period. It is the most serious chronic respiratory disorder that begins during infancy. BPD usually develops in neonates who are being treated with oxygen and positive-pressure ventilation for respiratory failure or respiratory distress syndrome (Ehrenkranz, Walsh, Vohr et al., 2005). Ventilation on the day of birth is a highly significant predictor of developing BPD. Other contributing factors for development of BPD include chorioamnionitis, postnatal sepsis, and patent ductus arteriosis (Froh, 2006). Bronchopulmonary dysplasia is a major cause of mortality and long-term morbidity in infants.

A changing clinical picture for BPD is emerging as most infants who currently develop BPD are born at 30 weeks of gestation or less and weigh less than 1000 grams. Antenatal steroids and surfactant replacement therapy has reduced the risk for BPD in more mature preterm infants (Ehrenkranz et al., 2005). It is thought that the assisted ventilation (in which tidal volume and inspiratory pressure are not monitored) and provision of oxygen provided at birth may damage the immature lungs. Alveolar sacs begin evolving within the terminal respiratory unit at 26 to 28 weeks' gestation. As a consequence of injury with ventilation on the day of birth, fewer and larger alveoli with less functional surface area occur along with reduced capillary ingrowth to the alveolar region. Other lung changes noted include ventilation-perfusion mismatch, pulmonary hypertension, increased lung fluid, interstitial fibrosis, and smooth muscle hypertrophy. All these injuries lead to increased respiratory effort, higher oxygen requirements, and in severe cases right-sided heart failure (Froh, 2006). Other disorders that contribute to the development of BPD include neonatal pneumonia, meconium aspiration syndrome, fluid overload, and lung hypoplasia (Capper-Michel, 2004).

The infant with BPD has persistent signs of increased respiratory effort, including tachypnea, irritability, nasal flaring, grunting, and retractions. Feeding can create increased oxygen demands the infant cannot meet, leading to failure to thrive. The infant may have wheezing, crackles, and pulmonary edema. The infant has intermittent bronchospasms, mucous plugging, and air trapping. Infants may have episodes of sudden respiratory deterioration with tracheobronchial narrowing and associated expiratory airflow limitations that may be caused by a sudden increase in pulmonary vascular resistance. Cyanosis may be seen in severe cases.

The diagnosis of lung injury is evident by the dependence on oxygen and other clinical manifestations. A chest radiograph often shows hyperexpansion, atelectasis, and interstitial thickening (Capper-Michel, 2004). The air trapping persists and in time causes the chest to assume a barrel shape (Figure 20–10 ➤). Medical management focuses on minimizing the duration of mechanical ventilation and maintaining adequate oxygenation without the use of high inspired oxygen concentrations (Bancalari, Wilson-Costello, & Iben, 2005). Symptomatic treatment that supports respiratory function and good nutrition helps to accelerate lung maturity. A tracheostomy may be performed for long-term airway management to prevent narrowing of the trachea. Chest physiotherapy and medications (diuretics, bronchodilators, anti-inflammatories, and inhaled corticosteroids) are also used (see the medications table on the next page). Frequent

CLINICAL TIP

Severity of BPD is categorized by the need for oxygen to maintain adequate oxygen saturation.

- Mild is the need for 21% oxygen for at least 28 days, but is breathing room air at 36 weeks' postmenstrual age; however, residual lung disease may be present.
- Moderate is the need for less than 30% supplemental oxygen at 36 weeks' postmenstrual age.
- Severe is the need for greater than or equal to 30% supplemental oxygen at 36 weeks' postmenstrual age or positive pressure ventilation or nasal continuous positive airway pressure (CPAP).

PATHOPHYSIOLOGY ILLUSTRATED

Barrel Chest

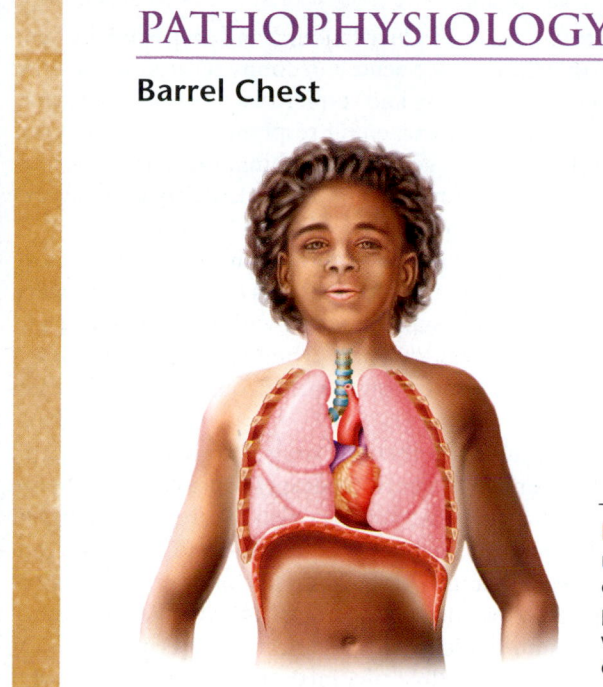

Figure 20–10 ➤ A barrel chest may result from chronic respiratory conditions such as bronchopulmonary dysplasia or asthma, in which air trapping or hyperinflation of the alveoli occur.

rehospitalization is common. With improvement and adequate weight gain, the child is weaned off of oxygen, diuretics, and bronchodilators. However, infants may die due to respiratory failure or infection. Potential long-term outcomes of BPD include developmental delays, growth retardation, impaired cognitive function, and pulmonary dysfunction in adolescents (Belcastro, 2004).

MEDICATIONS USED TO TREAT *Bronchopulmonary Dysplasia*	
Medication	**Action/Indication**
Bronchodilators (beta₂-adrenergics, anticholinergics, theophylline, albuterol nebulizer)	Decreases airway resistance; increases expiratory flow in small airways; stimulates mucous clearance; different drugs work together for best response
Anti-inflammatory agents (corticosteroids, inhaled cromolyn, bechlomethasone)	Reduces pulmonary edema and inflammation in small airways; enhances effect of bronchodilators; helps decrease the need for other drugs and oxygen; for moderate disease only
Diuretics (furosemide, chlorothiazide, spironolactone)	Helps remove excess fluid from lungs; decreases pulmonary resistance and increases pulmonary compliance; may cause electrolyte imbalances
Potassium chloride	Prevents electrolyte imbalances associated with diuretics
Antibiotics	Low-dose prophylactic therapy to prevent severe illness; specific treatment for identified organisms
Palivizumab	Prevents respiratory syncytial virus

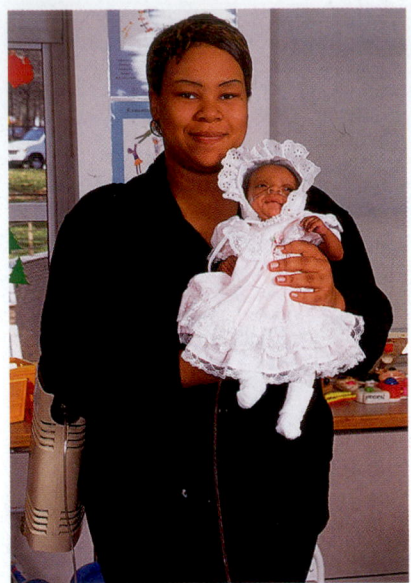

Figure 20–11 ➤ Many children with BPD are cared for at home, with the support of a home care program to monitor the family's ability to provide airway management, oxygen, and ventilator support. This premature infant girl, who is now 4 months old but weighs only about 5 pounds, requires respiratory support, which is provided by a portable oxygen tank.

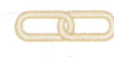

SKILLS 11–2 AND 11–3
Using a Cardiorespiratory Monitor and Pulse Oximeter

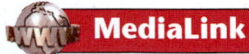

MediaLink

National Asthma Statistics

Nursing Management

Nursing management focuses on promoting respiratory function and preparing the family for home care needs. During hospitalization for acute infections, a cardiorespiratory monitor and pulse oximeter are used. Assess airway and respiratory function, vital signs, color, and behavior changes to identify signs of worsening respiratory symptoms, even when oxygen is provided. Position the infant to facilitate breathing. Observe for airway obstruction when the infant has a tracheostomy and suction as needed. Provide daily tracheostomy care. Organize care to reduce unnecessary physical stimulation.

Administer medications as ordered. Provide fluids and nutrition to meet energy needs; however, fluid management is important to prevent excess fluids and pulmonary edema. Monitor intake and output. A formula supplemented with carbohydrates and medium chain triglycerides (MCT oil) adds calories that promote weight gain. Some children need nasogastric or gastrostomy tube feedings to get adequate nutrition when cyanosis is noted with feeding.

Once home, many infants need ventilation therapy, oxygen, tracheostomy care, multiple medications, fluid restrictions, and high caloric feedings (Figure 20–11 ➤). Some families need home nursing assistance to manage the complex plan of care. Carefully plan and coordinate referrals for needed respiratory supplies, medications, and follow-up care well in advance of the infant's discharge. Infants with BPD do not have the same respiratory reserve as healthy infants, and they may become acutely ill at any time. Teach parents to identify the early signs of respiratory compromise indicating a need for medical intervention and when to seek emergency care. Refer the infant to an early intervention program, as these infants are at increased risk for neuromotor and cognitive development problems (Vaucher, 2002). Suggest ways to provide for the infant's normal development through rest, nutrition, stimulation, and family support. During regular follow-up visits, ensure that the infant receives RSV prophylaxis as described on page 702.

Asthma

Asthma (also called bronchial asthma) is a chronic inflammatory disorder of the airway with airway obstruction that can be partially or completely reversed, and increased airway responsiveness to stimuli (Kieckhefer & Ratcliffe, 2004). It is one of the most common chronic disorders, affecting 11.8% of children between 3 and 17 years of age (Akinbami, Rhodes, & Lara, 2005). Affected children also experience about 2.5 more days of school absence than children without asthma (Wang, Zhong, & Wheeler, 2005). Nearly 9.2 million children under 18 years have been diagnosed with asthma (National Asthma Education and Prevention Program, 2003). Non-Hispanic Black children have a prevalence of asthma that is nearly twice that of non-Hispanic White children (Akinbami, Rhodes, & Lara, 2005). Most children with asthma experience their first symptoms before the age of 5 years.

Asthma is a chronic condition with acute exacerbations or persistent symptoms. Children require continuous coordinated care to control sudden symptoms and minimize long-term airway changes. Although unusual in the past, severe persistent asthma is more common now. Hospitalizations for asthma as well as mortality from asthma in children have significantly increased (Akinbami & Schoendorf, 2002).

Etiology and Pathophysiology

Asthma is a chronic inflammatory disease of the lungs that is caused by multiple factors, including environmental exposures, viral illnesses, allergens, and a genetic predisposition. Several chromosomes are thought to be factors in asthma susceptibility, including chromosomes 5q, 6p, 11q, 12q, and 13q (Foley, 2002). Exposure to environmental factors early in life or in utero is thought to stimulate the onset of asthma. Passive smoke exposure (secondhand smoke), contaminants in indoor air (pet dander, dust mites, cockroach feces, fungal contamination, chemical gases, and pollutants in outdoor air) all contribute significantly to the development of asthma and respiratory problems in children (Solomon, Humphreys, & Miller, 2004).

Inflammation causes the normal protective mechanisms of the lungs (mucous formation, mucosal swelling, and airway muscle contraction) to react excessively in response to a stimulus and cause airway obstruction. The stimulus, or **trigger**, that initiates an asthmatic episode can be inflammatory or noninflammatory. Triggers increase the frequency and severity of smooth muscle contraction, and airway responsiveness is enhanced through inflammatory mechanisms. Asthmatic triggers include exercise, viral or bacterial agents, allergens (mold, dust, pollen, furry pets, birds), fragrances, food additives, pollutants, weather changes (humidity and temperature), stressful events, and emotions. Exercise triggers a bronchospasm by the rapid breathing of cooler and dryer air than the air in the respiratory tract (Baker, Friedman, & Schmitt, 2002).

The reactive airway responses to stimuli are present before the trigger initiates the asthmatic episode. During the acute allergic reaction, an antigen binds to the specific immunoglobulin E surface on the mucosal mast cells, and histamine is released along with intercellular chemical mediators (leukotrienes, prostaglandins, platelet-activating factor, and certain cytokines) resulting in bronchospasm, mucosal edema, and mucous secretion. The late allergic response starts 6 to 9 hours later when inflammatory cells respond and another wave of mediator release occurs. This stimulates more airway inflammation and bronchospasm (Kieckhefer & Ratcliffe, 2004).

Bronchial constriction, airway swelling, and production of copious amounts of mucus causes airway narrowing. Mucus clogs small airways and traps air (Figure 20–12 ➤). The airways swell, creating muscle spasms that may become uncontrolled in the large airways. Decreased perfusion of the alveolar capillaries results from hyperinflation of the alveoli. Hypoxemia leads to an increased respiratory rate, but less air breathed per minute because of airway resistance. Progressive chronic inflammatory changes result in **airway remodeling**, an irreversible thickening and fibrosis of the basement membrane, airway smooth muscle hypertrophy, and mucous gland hypertrophy (Froh, 2006).

Moderate anxiety occurs as the asthma episode begins, and increases as the episode intensifies. Severe anxiety, in turn, intensifies physical responses and symptoms, and a vicious cycle is established. Recognizing and addressing the child's fear and panic are essential for reestablishing normal respirations.

Clinical Manifestations

The sudden appearance of breathing difficulty (cough, wheeze, or shortness of breath) is often referred to as an asthma episode or "asthma attack." The infant or child who has had episodes of frequent coughing or frequent respiratory infections (especially pneumonia or bronchitis) should also be evaluated for asthma. Frequent coughing, especially at night, is the warning signal that the child's airway is very sensitive to stimuli; it may be the only sign in "silent" asthma.

During an acute episode, respirations are rapid and labored and the child often appears tired because of the ongoing exertion of breathing. Nasal flaring and intercostal retractions may be visible. The child exhibits a productive cough and expiratory wheezing, use of accessory muscles, decreased air movement, and respiratory fatigue. In cases of severe obstruction, wheezing may not be heard because of the lack of airflow. The resulting hypoxia, as well as the cumulative effect of previously administered medications, contributes to behaviors ranging from wide-eyed agitation to lethargic irritability. In children who have repeated acute episodes, a barrel chest and the use of accessory muscles of respiration are common findings.

MediaLink

Asthma Animation

■ COLLABORATIVE CARE

Diagnostic Testing

The diagnosis of asthma has four key elements: symptoms of episodic airflow obstruction; partial reversibility of bronchospasm with bronchodilator treatment; exclusion of alternate diagnosis; and confirmation by spirometry of measurement of forced expiratory flow variability. A spirometer measures the volume of air a child can expel from the lungs after a maximum inspiration. Three readings of the forced vital capacity and forced expiratory volume are taken and compared to predicted normal values to assess the severity of airway obstruction. Because the test requires children to cooperate and follow instructions, it is usually administered to children over 4 or 5 years of age. Skin testing may be used to identify allergens that serve as asthma triggers.

PATHOPHYSIOLOGY ILLUSTRATED

Asthma

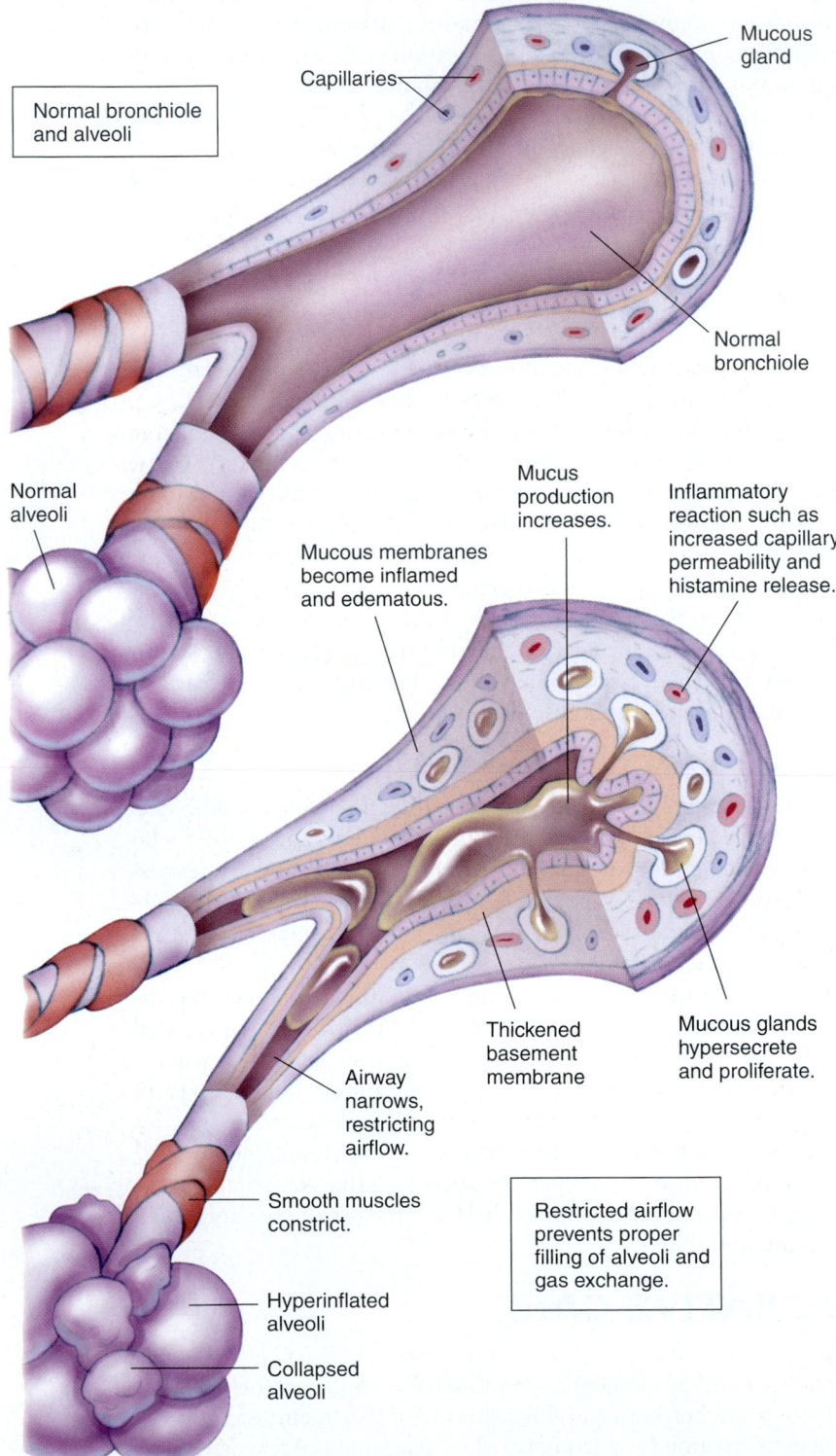

Normal bronchiole and alveoli

Capillaries

Mucous gland

Normal bronchiole

Normal alveoli

Mucous membranes become inflamed and edematous.

Mucus production increases.

Inflammatory reaction such as increased capillary permeability and histamine release.

Thickened basement membrane

Mucous glands hypersecrete and proliferate.

Airway narrows, restricting airflow.

Smooth muscles constrict.

Hyperinflated alveoli

Collapsed alveoli

Restricted airflow prevents proper filling of alveoli and gas exchange.

Figure 20–12 ➤ Some asthma triggers are exercise, infection, and allergies. The figure shows how asthma obstructs airflow through constriction and narrowing of the airway, along with increased production of mucus.

Clinical Therapy

Medical management includes medications, support of parents and child, and education. See the Medications Used to Treat Asthma on pages 717–718 for information about rescue and controller medications used. Pharmacologic treatment is matched to the severity of asthma for long-term control and for management of acute episodes. Tables 20–6 and Table 20–7 show the nationally recommended guidelines for the treatment of children under 5 years of age and children over 5 years of age with acute and chronic asthma, respectively. Control of asthma symptoms is the goal,

Table 20–6	ASTHMA SEVERITY CLASSIFICATION AND PREFERRED CLINICAL THERAPY FOR CHILDREN YOUNGER THAN 5 YEARS OF AGE

Classification (Steps)	Description	Medications for Long-Term Control
Step 1: Mild intermittent	Brief exacerbations with symptoms no more often than twice a week. Night-time symptoms no more than twice a week.	No daily medications needed
Step 2: Mild persistent	Exacerbations more than twice a week, but less than once a day. Night-time symptoms more than twice a month.	Preferred treatment • Low-dose inhaled corticosteroid (with nebulizer or metered-dose inhaler [MDI] with holding chamber with or without face mask or dry powder inhaler [DPI]) Alternate treatment • Cromolyn (nebulizer is preferred or MDI with holding chamber) • OR leukotriene receptor antagonist
Step 3: Moderate persistent	Daily symptoms of coughing and wheezing. Night-time symptoms more than once per week.	Preferred treatment • Low-dose inhaled corticosteroids and long-acting B_2-agonists OR • Medium-dose inhaled corticosteroids Alternate treatment • Low-dose inhaled corticosteroids and either leukotriene receptor antagonist or theophylline If needed (particularly in children and adolescents with recurring severe exacerbations) Preferred treatment • Medium-dose inhaled corticosteroids and long-acting inhaled B_2-agonists Alternative treatment • Medium-dose inhaled corticosteroids and either leukotriene receptor antagonist or theophylline
Step 4: Severe persistent	Continuous daytime symptoms, limited physical activity. Frequent night-time symptoms.	Preferred treatment • High-dose inhaled corticosteroids Plus • Long-acting inhaled B_2-agonists. And if needed, • Oral corticosteroids at 2 mg/kg/day (not to exceed 60 mg per day); repeated efforts should be made to reduce systemic corticosteroids and maintain control with high-dose inhaled corticosteroids.
Quick relief	Bronchodilator as needed for symptoms. Intensity of treatment will depend upon severity of exacerbation. • Preferred treatment: Short-acting inhaled B_2-agonists by nebulizer, face mask, and space/holding chamber • Alternative treatment: oral B_2-agonist With viral respiratory infection • Bronchodilator every 4 to 6 hours up to 24 hours (longer with physician counsel); in general, repeat no more than once every 6 weeks • Consider systemic corticosteroids if exacerbation is severe or patient has a history of previous severe exacerbations Use of short-acting B_2-agonists greater than two times a week in intermittent asthma (daily, or increasing use in persistent asthma) may indicate the need to initiate (increase) long-term control therapy.	

Adapted from: National Asthma Education and Prevention Program. (2002). *Expert Panel Report II: Guidelines for the diagnosis and management of asthma. Update on selected topics 2002* (NIH Publication No 02-5075). Bethesda, MD: National Heart, Lung, and Blood Institute, National Institutes of Health.

Table 20–7	ASTHMA SEVERITY CLASSIFICATION AND PREFERRED CLINICAL THERAPY FOR CHILDREN OLDER THAN 5 YEARS OF AGE	

Classification (Steps)	Description	Medications for Long-Term Control
Step 1: Mild intermittent	Brief exacerbations with symptoms no more often than twice a week. Night-time symptoms no more than twice a week. Asymptomatic and normal PEFR between exacerbations. No emergent visits and no asthma-related absences from school. PEFR greater than or equal to 80% of predicted, with variability less than 20%.	No daily medications needed. Severe exacerbation may occur, separated by long periods of normal lung function and no symptoms; a course of systemic corticosteroids is recommended
Step 2: Mild persistent	Exacerbations more than twice a week, but less than once a day. Night-time symptoms more than twice a month. Exacerbations may affect activity and cause absences from school. PEFR greater than or equal to 80% of predicted with variability of 20–30%.	Preferred treatment • Low-dose inhaled steroid. Alternate treatment • Cromolyn, leukotriene modifier, or nedocromil • OR sustained release theophylline to serum concentration of 5–15 mcg/mL
Step 3: Moderate persistent	Daily symptoms of coughing and wheezing. Exacerbations at least twice a week that may last for days. Night-time symptoms more than once per week. Exacerbations affect activity and several school absences occur. PEF or FEV1 greater than 60% but less than 80% of predicted with variability greater than 30%.	Preferred treatment • Low- to medium-dose inhaled corticosteroid Plus • Long-acting B$_2$-agonists. Alternate treatment • Increase inhaled corticosteroids to within medium-dose range Or • Low-dose inhaled steroid and either leukotriene modifier or theophylline. If needed (particularly in children and adolescents with recurring severe exacerbations) Preferred treatment • Increase inhaled corticosteroids within medium-dose range and add long-acting inhaled B$_2$-agonists Alternative treatment • Increase inhaled corticosteroids within medium-dose range and add either leukotriene modifier or theophylline
Step 4: Severe persistent	Continuous daytime symptoms, limited physical activity. Frequent exacerbations. Frequent night-time symptoms. Limited physical activity. Hospitalizations are frequent with PICU admissions for severe exacerbations. PEF or FEV1 less than or equal to 60% of predicted, with variability greater than 30%.	Preferred treatment • High-dose inhaled corticosteroids Plus • Long-acting inhaled B$_2$-agonists. And if needed, • Oral corticosteroids at 2 mg/kg/day (not to exceed 60 mg per day); repeated efforts should be made to reduce systemic corticosteroids and maintain control with high-dose inhaled corticosteroids.
Quick relief	Bronchodilator as needed for symptoms. Intensity of treatment will depend upon severity of exacerbation. • Preferred treatment: Short-acting inhaled B$_2$-agonists by nebulizer, face mask, and space/holding chamber • Alternative treatment: oral B$_2$-agonist With viral respiratory infection: • Bronchodilator every 4 to 6 hours up to 24 hours (longer with physician counsel); in general, repeat no more than once every 6 weeks • Consider systemic corticosteroids if exacerbation is severe or patient has a history of previous severe exacerbations • Use of short-acting B$_2$-agonists greater than two times a week in intermittent asthma (daily, or increasing use in persistent asthma) may indicate the need to initiate (increase) long-term control therapy.	

Adapted from: National Asthma Education and Prevention Program. (2002). *Expert Panel Report II: Guidelines for the diagnosis and management of asthma. Update on selected topics 2002* (NIH Publication No. 02-5075). Bethesda, MD: National Heart, Lung, and Blood Institute, National Institutes of Health.

MEDICATIONS USED TO TREAT *Asthma*

Rescue Medication	Action/Indication	Nursing Implications
Beta$_2$-agonists (short-acting) Albuterol, metaproterenal, terbutaline, Levalbuterol: inhalation, PO	Relax smooth muscle in airway, increase water content in bronchial mucus to promote muciliary clearance resulting in rapid bronchodilation within 5–10 minutes. Drug of choice for acute therapy (MDI or nebulizer).	• Use this rescue medication before inhaled steroid, wait 1–2 minutes between puffs, wait 15 minutes to give inhaled steroid. Child should hold breath 10 seconds after inspiring. Then rinse mouth and avoid swallowing medication. Use spacer. • Some side effects (tachycardia, nervousness, nausea and vomiting, headaches), but these are usually dose-related. • Repetitive or excessive use can mask increasing airway inflammation and hyperresponsiveness and increase need for higher dosage to get same effect. • Use of more than one canister a month indicates inadequate control.
Corticosteroids Methylprednisolone: IV Prednisone Prednisolone: PO	Diminish airway inflammation and obstruction, enhance bronchodilating effect of Beta$_2$-agonists. Used for moderate to severe acute exacerbations when single Beta$_2$-agonist dose given in emergency department does not resolve symptoms.	• Not used as primary treatment. • Onset of action is 4–6 hours. • Short-term therapy for 3–10 days until symptoms resolve or child achieves 80% peak expiratory flow personal best. • Give with food. • Give daily oral dose in early morning to mimic normal peak corticosteroid blood level. • Assess for potential adverse effects of long-term therapy: decreased growth, unstable blood sugar, immunosuppression
Anticholinergic Ipratropium: inhalation	Inhibits bronchoconstriction and decreases mucus production. Provides additive effects to short-acting Beta$_2$-agonists during acute exacerbation.	• Not for primary treatment. • Side effects include increased wheezing, cough, nervousness, dry mouth, tachycardia, dizziness, headache, palpitations. • Avoid eye contact.

Controller Medication	Action/Indication	Nursing Implications
Beta$_2$-agonists (long-acting) Salmeterol Formoterol: inhalation	Relax smooth muscle in airway, used for nocturnal symptoms and prevention of exercise-induced bronchospasm.	• Should not be used for acute asthma attack. • Should not be used in place of inhaled corticosteroids. • Caution against overdosage as side effects such as tachycardia, tremor, irritability, and insomnia will last 8 to 12 hours. • Report use of more than four puffs a day as this may indicate need for stepped-up therapy.
Methylxanthines Theophylline: PO Aminophylline: IV	Relax muscle bundles that constrict airways; dilate airway; provide continuous airway relaxation; sustained release for prevention of nocturnal symptoms. Aminophylline may be used for emergency adjunct therapy in ICU, but use is controversial.	• Tablet should not be crushed or chewed. • Used for long-term control, so continuous administration needed; works best when a specific amount is maintained in the bloodstream (therapeutic serum level, 10–20 mcg/L). • Requires serum level checks and dose adjustment. • Side effects include tachycardia, dysrhythmias, restlessness, tremors, seizures, insomnia, hypotension, severe headaches, vomiting, and diarrhea.

(continued)

MEDICATIONS USED TO TREAT *Asthma (continued)*

Controller Medication	Action/Indication	Nursing Implications
Mast Cell Inhibitors Cromolyn sodium Nedocromil: aerosol	Anti-inflammatory, inhibit early and late phase asthma response to allergens and exercise-induced bronchospasm; may be used for unavoidable allergen exposure.	• Not used at time of symptom development or acute exacerbation. • Must be used up to four times a day to be effective. • Therapeutic response seen in 2 weeks, maximum benefit may not be seen for 4 to 6 weeks. • Adverse reactions include wheezing, bronchospasm, throat irritation, nasal congestion, anaphylaxis.
Corticosteroids Beclomethasone Budesonide Fluticasone Triamcinolone: aerosol	Anti-inflammatory, controls seasonal, allergic, and exercise-induced asthma; effectively reduces mucosal edema in airways; usually combined with other asthma medications for control. First-line therapy in asthma management.	• Administer with spacer or holding chamber. • Rinse mouth following treatment to reduce chance of thrush and dysphonia. • Monitor growth. • Monitor for headache, gastrointestinal upset, dizziness, infection. • Use exactly as prescribed.
Leukotriene Modifiers Montelukast: PO Zafirlukast: PO	Reduces inflammation cascade responsible for airway inflammation. Improves lung function and diminishes symptoms and need for rescue medications. Adjunct to inhaled corticosteroids in moderate to severe asthma or substitute for inhaled corticosteroids in mild asthma.	• Administer montelukast in evening; may be given with or without food. • Administer zafirlukast 1 hour before or 2 hours after meal. • Family needs to report fever, acute asthma attacks, flu-like symptoms, severe headaches, or lethargy. • Take as prescribed, do not withdraw abruptly.
Other Hyposensitization (allergy shots), subcutaneous	Series of injections that can reduce sensitivity to unavoidable allergens (e.g., environmental organisms–mold, pollen); gradual dose increase over time (called a "build-up") increases the child's tolerance to allergic substances; has been of help in some children.	• Use is controversial; some question about actual effect.

Data from: Baker, V. O., Friedman, J., & Schmitt, R. (2002). Asthma management, part II: Pharmacologic management. *Journal of School Nursing, 18*(5), 257–269; Baren, J. M., & Puchalski, A. (2002). Current concepts in the ED treatment of pediatric asthma. *Pediatric Emergency Medicine, 7*(10), 105–115. Belcher, D. (2002, November). Breathing easier with pediatric asthma: Pharmacologic management. *Advance for Nurse Practitioners*, 37–38, 79;

and if control is not achieved with the prescribed regimen, then the regimen should be changed to correspond to the next step in asthma severity. Once control of asthma symptoms is achieved, the treatment plan can be reviewed in 1 to 6 months to determine if a change to a less aggressive level of asthma treatment is appropriate (Hogan & Wilson, 2003).

Some healthcare providers encourage children to use a peak expiratory flow meter to identify when an obstruction is occurring. This device measures the child's ability to push air forcefully out of the lungs, similar to a spirometer. Medication administration can be based on peak expiratory flow rate (PEFR) readings and the effectiveness of treatment confirmed by improved PEFR numbers.

Most children with acute exacerbations respond to rescue medications provided at home or to aggressive management in the emergency department. Children who do not respond or who are already being managed at home on corticosteroids have a greater chance of being admitted. Some children need mechanical ventilation.

SKILL 11–5
Using a Peak Expiratory Flow Rate (PEFR) Meter

NURSING MANAGEMENT

Nursing Assessment and Diagnosis

The nurse usually encounters the child and family in the emergency department or nursing unit. In these settings, acute care has become necessary because the child's level of respiratory compromise cannot be managed at home.

Physiologic Assessment

Identify the child's current respiratory status first by assessing the ABCs—airway, breathing, and circulation—to make sure the child's condition is not life threatening. If the child is moving air or talking, assess the quality of breathing. Assess the respiratory rate. Inspect the chest for retractions to assess the severity of respiratory distress. Auscultate the lungs for the quality of breath sounds and for the presence or absence of wheezing. Observe the child's color and assess the heart rate. Note whether a cough or stridor is present. Obtain oxygen saturation via pulse oximeter. Determine the severity of symptoms from the criteria provided in Table 20–8 below.

Assess skin turgor, intake and output, and specific gravity. Because asthma can be a symptom of another illness, perform a head-to-toe assessment to identify other associated problems.

Psychosocial Assessment

Assess the child's anxiety. In an older child whose asthma was previously diagnosed, assess whether the child thinks this episode could have been avoided if medication had been taken. Look for clues to hidden stress and self-blaming.

> ### CLINICAL TIP
> A child has good asthma control when the following indications are present:
> - Minimal or no chronic symptoms day or night,
> - Minimal or no exacerbations
> - No limitations on activities, no school missed, parents don't miss work
> - Minimal use of short acting B_2-agonists (less than one time a day or less than one canister a month)
> - Minimal or no adverse effects from medications.
>
> From: National Asthma Education and Prevention Program. (2002). *NAEPP Expert Panel Report: Guidelines for the diagnosis and management of asthma— Update on selected topics 2002* (NIH Publication No. 02-5075). Bethesda, MD: NHLBI, National Institutes of Health.

Table 20–8 | ASTHMA ASSESSMENT CRITERIA BY SEVERITY OF ACUTE EPISODE

Assessment Criteria	Mild	Moderate	Severe
Peak expiratory flow rate (PEFR)[a]	70–90% of predicted or personal best	50–70% of predicted or personal best	Less than 50% of predicted or personal best
Respiratory rate, resting or sleeping	Normal to 30% increase above the mean	30–50% increase above mean	Increase over 50% above mean
Alertness	Normal	Normal	May be decreased
Dyspnea[b]	Absent or mild; speaks in complete sentences	Moderate; speaks in phrases or partial sentences; infant's cry softer and shorter; has difficulty sucking and feeding	Severe; speaks only in single words or short phrases; infant's cry softer and shorter; stops sucking and feeding
Pulsus paradoxus[c]	Less than 10 mmHg	10–20 mmHg	20–40 mmHg
Accessory muscle use	No intercostal to mild retractions	Moderate intercostal retractions with tracheosternal retractions; use of sternocleidomastoid muscles; chest hyperinflation	Severe intercostal retractions, tracheosternal retractions with nasal flaring during inspiration; chest hyperinflation
Color	Good	Pale	Possibly cyanotic
Auscultation	End-expiratory wheeze only	Wheeze during entire expiration and inspiration	Breath sounds becoming inaudible
Oxygen saturation	Greater than 95%	90–95%	Less than 90%
PCO_2	Less than 35	Less than 40	Less than 40

Note: Within each category, the presence of several parameters, but not necessarily all, indicates the general classification of the exacerbation.
[a]For children 5 years of age or older.
[b]Parents' or physicians' impression of degree of children's breathlessness.
[c]Pulsus paradoxus does not correlate with phase of respiration in small children.
From National Asthma Education and Prevention Program. (1994). *Acute exacerbations of asthma: Care in a hospital-based emergency department* (p. 13). Bethesda, MD: National Heart, Lung, and Blood Institute, National Institutes of Health.

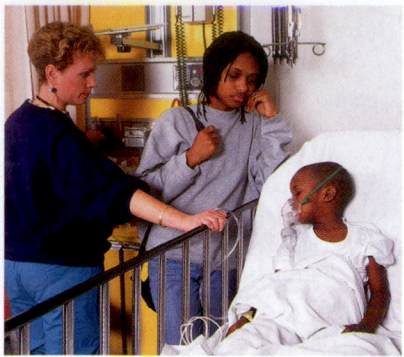

Figure 20–13 ➤ Acute exacerbations of asthma may require management in the emergency department. The child is placed in a semisitting position to facilitate respiratory effort. Providing support to both the child and parent is an important part of nursing care during these acute episodes. This mother is exhausted after a sleepless night of caring for her son.

SKILL 11–1
Using Oxygen Delivery Systems

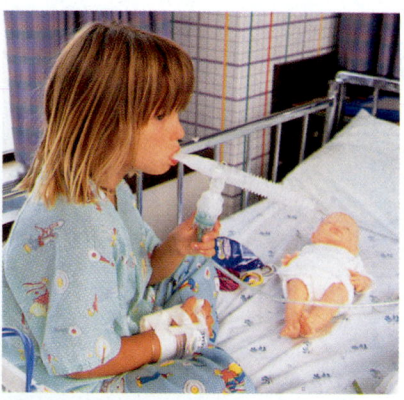

Figure 20–14 ➤ Medications given by aerosol therapy are effective because they reach the bloodstream rapidly, and they allow children more freedom to play and entertain themselves.

Common nursing diagnoses for the child experiencing an acute asthmatic episode include the following:

- Ineffective Airway Clearance related to airway compromise, copious mucous secretions, and coughing
- Impaired Gas Exchange related to airway obstruction, possible additional respiratory illness, and poor response to medication
- Risk for Deficient Fluid Volume related to difficulty in taking adequate fluids with respiratory distress
- Anxiety/Fear (Child or Parents) related to difficulty breathing
- Ineffective Therapeutic Regimen Management (Family) related to lack of understanding about and need for daily management of a chronic disease

Planning and Implementation

Pharmacologic and supportive therapies are used to reverse the airway obstruction and promote respiratory function. Nursing interventions center on maintaining airway patency, meeting fluid needs, promoting rest and stress reduction for the child and parents, supporting the family's participation in care, and educating the family to more effectively manage the child's disease.

Maintain Airway Patency

If the child is exhibiting breathing difficulty, give supplemental oxygen by nasal cannula or face mask. Humidified oxygen should be used to prevent drying and thickening of mucous secretions. Place the child in a sitting (semi-Fowler's) or upright position to promote and ease respiratory effort. Evaluate the effectiveness of positioning and oxygen administration by pulse oximeter and by observing for improved respiratory status.

The respiratory distress and need for supplemental oxygen can be stressful for parents and the child alike (Figure 20–13 ➤). Encouraging the parents' presence can be reassuring for the child. Keep the parents informed of procedures and results, and get their input when developing the treatment plan.

Many medications are given by the aerosol route (Figure 20–14 ➤). See Box 20–4 on page 721 for the different aerosol delivery devices used for children. The advantages of aerosol are that the medication acts quickly, enabling the pulmonary blood vessels to absorb the inhaled medication; systemic effects are minimized; and the inhaled droplets provide the added benefit of moisture. Continuous aerosol treatments may be used for some children with severe exacerbations. Monitor the child for side effects. The frequency of vital sign assessment is related to the severity of symptoms.

Meet Fluid Needs

Fluid therapy is often necessary to restore and maintain adequate fluid balance. Adequate hydration is essential to thin and break up trapped mucous plugs in the narrowed airways. If an adequate oral intake is not possible because of the child's compromised respiratory status, an intravenous infusion may be needed. Additional medications and glucose may also be provided through the IV. Monitor the child's intake and output to avoid overhydration and to prevent pulmonary edema in severe asthma attacks.

As respiratory difficulty diminishes, slowly offer oral fluids. It is safest to offer the asthmatic child room temperature or slightly cooled fluids because iced fluids may precipitate a bronchospasm in some children. Determine the child's fluid preferences and give choices where possible. Monitor intake and output and assess specific gravity frequently to evaluate the child's hydration status. Involving parents in feeding can help gain the child's cooperation in taking oral fluids.

Promote Rest and Stress Reduction

The child who has had an acute asthmatic episode is usually very tired when admitted to the nursing unit. Labored breathing and low oxygen status have left the child exhausted. Put the child in a quiet, private room if possible, but accessible for frequent monitoring, to promote relaxation and rest. Group nursing tasks to avoid repeatedly disturbing the child.

BOX 20–4
MEDICATION ADMINISTRATION—GROWTH AND DEVELOPMENT CONSIDERATIONS

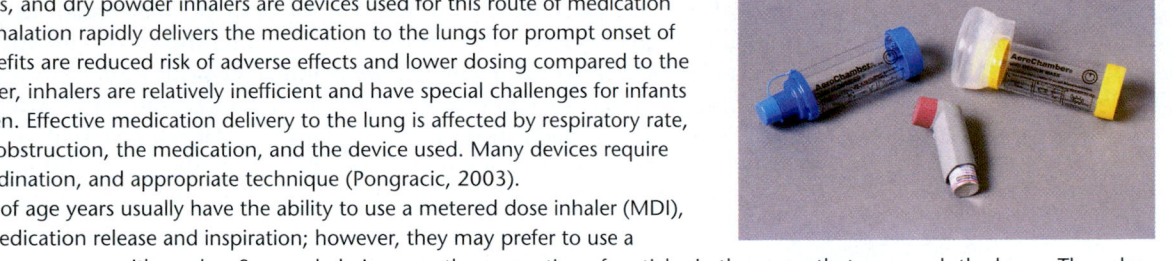

Inhalation is the preferred method of asthma medication administration. Metered-dose inhalers, nebulizers, and dry powder inhalers are devices used for this route of medication administration. Inhalation rapidly delivers the medication to the lungs for prompt onset of action. Other benefits are reduced risk of adverse effects and lower dosing compared to the oral route. However, inhalers are relatively inefficient and have special challenges for infants and young children. Effective medication delivery to the lung is affected by respiratory rate, degree of airflow obstruction, the medication, and the device used. Many devices require cooperation, coordination, and appropriate technique (Pongracic, 2003).

- Children over 5 of age years usually have the ability to use a metered dose inhaler (MDI), coordinating medication release and inspiration; however, they may prefer to use a holding chamber or spacer with a valve. Spacers help increase the proportion of particles in the range that can reach the lungs. They also trap larger particles, preventing them from reaching the mouth and being swallowed, which can cause local and systemic side effects. Valves prevent the escape of medication during use. With proper technique 12–15% of the dose may reach the lower airways. The plastic spacer should be washed with a household detergent and permitted to air dry. This action reduces the electrostatic charge and frees more of the drug for delivery (Meadows-Oliver & Banasiak, 2005). When teaching the child to use an MDI without a spacer, let the child learn to breathe in slowly with straws.
- Spacers have a mouthpiece or mask attachment. When selecting a spacer for infants and young children 4 years and younger, choose one with a mask because they tend to be nasal breathers. Choose a mask size that fits the child's face and that has a flexible seal to prevent an air leak around the facial features. When the young child is uncooperative, it may still be difficult to maintain a seal. Work with young children to improve cooperation for medication delivery with play and distraction. Crying leads to prolonged exhalation and short inspiratory efforts, which reduce lung deposition.
- Some inhaler and spacer brands have a whistle on inhalation that indicates that a breath is too fast or too shallow, but in others it indicates an adequate breath has been taken. When teaching the child and family about inhaler use, make sure you know what the whistle indicates.
- Nebulizers are a device that changes liquid medication to aerosol particles. No coordination of breathing is required, making them easier for young children to use. An added benefit is the humidification provided during treatment. A mask or mouthpiece is used. While nebulizers are not more effective than MDIs with a spacer, they may lead to better outcomes because the child only needs to breathe in and out normally. Nebulizers should not be used with the mouthpiece held away from the mouth, because lung deposition of the medication is significantly reduced and it increases the risk of depositing some medication in the eyes (Meadows-Oliver & Banasiak, 2005). Nebulizers are expensive, need a power source, and take 8 to 10 minutes for the treatment. Infants and young children may have difficulty cooperating for the duration of the nebulizer treatment. Crying and a face mask that is too large for the child's face can further decrease the delivery of the medication to the lower airways.
- Dry powder inhalers (DPI) are activated when the patient takes a breath, so puffs do not need to be coordinated with inhalation. No spacer is required and no propellant is used. They can be used by children 5 years and older. Delivery to the lower airway varies between 15–30%, depending upon the type of inhaler. Children with severe asthma may not be able to produce enough airflow to get an adequate dose of medication.

Data from: Dolovich, M. B., Ahrens, T. C., Hess, D. R., et al. (2005). Device selection and outcomes of aerosol therapy: Evidence-based guidelines. *Chest, 127*, 335–371. Marshik, P. L. (2004). Pharmacologic treatment of pediatric asthma. *Advance for Nurse Practitioners, 12*(3), 35–36, 41–46; Meadows-Oliver, M., & Banasiak, N. C. (2005). Asthma medication delivery devices. *Journal of Pediatric Health Care, 19*(2), 121–123; Pongracic, J. A. (2003). Asthma delivery devices: Age-appropriate use. *Pediatric Annals, 32*(1), 50–54;

Support Family Participation

The parents may stay with the child, but may be exhausted after hours of their child's respiratory distress. Give parents the option of assisting with the child's treatments, rather than expecting them to do it in addition to comforting the child. Provide frequent updates about the child's condition and encourage the parents to take breaks as needed.

Length of hospitalization depends on the child's response to therapy. Any underlying or accompanying health problem, such as preexisting lung disease or pneumonia, can complicate and extend the child's hospital stay. Communicate with the family of the hospitalized child at least once a day about the status of the child's condition.

Discharge Planning and Home Care Teaching

Parents need a thorough understanding of asthma—how to prevent attacks, maintain the child's health, and avoid unnecessary hospitalization. When possible, educate parents when they are rested, and also refer the child to a healthcare provider for more extensive education. Support of parents and the child should focus on helping them to understand and cope with the diagnosis and the need for daily management to promote near normal respiratory function.

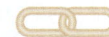

SKILL 8–12

Using a Metered-Dose Inhaler (MDI)

CULTURE

Asthma Management

Asthma occurs in all racial and ethnic groups, but these groups are different in the use of preventive medications for asthma. A recent study investigated these disparities and found a difference in preventive medications used for asthma. Findings revealed that differences in health beliefs, fear of steroids, or communication issues rather than financial barriers may play a role in the use of preventive asthma medications (Lieu, Lozano, Finkelstein et al., 2002). Learn about the family's cultural beliefs and practices. Parents of children from different cultures may have concerns about daily medication regimens. Individualize care through education based on "an assessment of the child's and family's resources, healthcare beliefs, access to healthcare services, and management styles" (Swartz, Cantey-Banasiak, & Meadows-Oliver, 2005).

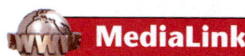

MediaLink

Asthma Symptom Diary

Discharge planning for the asthmatic child focuses on increasing the family's knowledge about the disease, medication therapy, and the need for follow-up care according to guidelines of the National Asthma Education and Prevention Program. The required lifestyle changes may be difficult for the child and parents. The need to modify the home by removing a loved pet, for example, may create stress. When a family will not give up a pet, discuss the need to bathe the pet frequently to reduce animal dander. The nurse can facilitate discussion and clarification of ways to prevent asthma episodes. Teach the family how to measure and interpret peak expiratory flow readings. Discuss rescue medications to manage asthma episodes, as well as controller medications for daily management. Reassure the family that most children with asthma can lead a normal life with some modifications.

Nursing Care in the Community

Nurses provide care to children with asthma in pediatricians' offices, specialty asthma clinics, schools, and summer camps. Once the stress of the acute episode has passed, the community setting is ideal for ongoing coordinated education about asthma management. Help the parents and child to understand the diagnosis and the need for daily management to promote near-normal respiratory function while the child continues to grow and develop normally. See Evidence-Based Practice: Improving Asthma Management.

Key points to cover in asthma education include (Hayes, Djaferis, Gattasso et al., 2004):

- Asthma is a chronic and progressive condition, but parents should expect that it can be controlled.
- The prescribed medication schedule needs to be followed. Discuss strategies to remember daily medications (specific time of day or daily event).
- Discuss possible adverse drug effects.
- Demonstrate proper use of metered dose inhaler, spacer, and peak flow meter.
- Exercise is important for health; asthma induced by exercise can be managed with medication.
- Suggest keeping an asthma symptom diary.

EVIDENCE-BASED PRACTICE

Improving Asthma Management

Problem/Clinical Question

Many children with asthma have less-than-optimal medication management to control symptoms and have increased asthma episodes. What information about the family's knowledge and perceptions about managing the child with asthma could help nurses collaborate more effectively with families to improve asthma management?

Evidence

Recent research on parental beliefs, knowledge, experience of living with a child who has asthma, and attitudes about controller medication was conducted through interviews with 18 mothers of children and adolescents with asthma. Parents indicated that they learned to manage the child's asthma through "trial and error." Even though they learned about medications at one time, they still had gaps in knowledge about medication actions. Parents also wished to have health professionals listen to them regarding their child's healthcare needs. The parents reported that daily medication management was the most difficult aspect of asthma care, but they saw a good response in the child when used (Peterson-Sweeney, McMullen, Yoos et al., 2003). Another study involving the parents of 109 children with asthma explored their attitudes and understanding of asthma. Only 27 of the 78 children with persistent asthma had an appropriate medication regimen, and 17 parents reported using no anti-inflammatory medication even when the child had moderate to severe asthma. Some parents believed inhaled steroids should be a last resort therapy or if steroids were used for a while they would not work when needed. These parents also anticipated that their children would have activity limitations and episodic emergency department visits (Yoos, Kitzman, & McMullen, 2003).

Implications

Demonstrating respect for the parent's knowledge of the child's health status and response to asthma management is an essential step in developing an effective partnership with the parent. It is also important to talk with parents about their beliefs about daily medications for asthma management, use of inhaled steroids, and their expectations of how asthma will affect their child. Gaining an understanding of the family's beliefs can help guide nursing education and collaborative development of a plan to manage the child's asthma.

Critical Thinking

Consider the possible perceptions and beliefs of parents and children with asthma in your practice setting. Develop an education program that integrates these beliefs and perceptions to help improve families' understanding of medication actions, the differences between inhaled and oral corticosteroids, and collaboration with health professionals to improve the control of their child's asthma.

See the Families Want to Know: Home Care Instructions for the Child with Asthma for more information.

If the child has severe asthma and uses high doses of aerosol or oral glucocorticoids to control asthma attacks, monitor the child's growth every 6 months as the disease and medications may affect overall growth. Review the family's daily plan for monitoring the child's respiratory status and the parent's ability to identify the timing and type of stepped-up care needed to manage worsening symptoms. Review and reinforce the child's technique for use of the metered dose inhaler. The goal is to bring asthma attacks under control with stepped-up care before a significant episode occurs (refer to Tables 20–6 and 20–7).

Make sure the child has a supply of medications at school or childcare as well as at home. Help the child learn the signs of early respiratory distress and how to request medications when at school before signs get more serious. Help the parents communicate with school personnel regarding the child's condition, and have an Individual Health Plan (IHP) developed so that medications are given as needed, even in preparation for exercise. An Asthma Action Plan that provides very specific guidelines for the child's care in the event of an asthma episode may be part of the IHP (Borgmeyer, Jamerson, Gyr et al., 2005). For a young school-age child, make sure the child's teacher can help recognize respiratory distress and reduce the child's fear of going to the nurse for rescue medications. See the Nursing Care Plan for more information on care of the child with asthma in the community.

Environmental control is an important part of asthma management. When possible, pets should not be kept in the home (and never in the child's bedroom). Active dust mite control should be attempted, but it is challenging as mites live in carpets, bedding, upholstered furniture, and clothes. To help control dust mites in the child's bedroom, encase the pillow and mattress in plastic covers. Initiate cockroach control. Smoke from cigarettes, woodstoves, and fireplaces all have the potential to trigger an asthma attack.

COMPLEMENTARY THERAPY

Asthma

A study of 310 parents of Hispanic and African American children with asthma revealed that 89% of them had used complementary therapy in the past year to treat their child's asthma episode. Prayer, rubs, and massage were the most common complementary therapies used, and these were sometimes believed to be as effective as medications (Braganza, Ozuah, & Sharif, 2003).

Although exercise is a frequent trigger of asthma symptoms in the majority of patients, the benefits of routine exercise on asthma symptoms have been documented in both children and adults (Chiang, 2005; van Veldhoven, Vermeer, Bogaard et al., 2001). There is no real benefit of one type of exercise over another, although swimming is often recommended. The improvement in cardiovascular fitness along with self-esteem are added benefits that come from routine exercise.

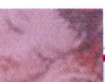

FAMILIES WANT TO KNOW

Home Care Instructions for the Child with Asthma

Identify parents' knowledge about the condition:

1. Review why asthma occurs and assess parents' understanding of the physiologic process. Ask:
   - What happens in your child's lungs during an asthma attack?
   - What are the early warning signs of an asthma episode in your child?
   - What are your child's symptoms and how does he or she respond to them? Does your child use the peak expiratory flow meter to evaluate symptoms? Is a diary maintained of the child's symptoms?
2. Identify asthma triggers and assess parents' understanding of how to prevent, avoid, or minimize their effect in a timely manner. Ask:
   - Do you know your child's personal asthma triggers? Where do most episodes begin? (Suggest that the parents and child keep a notebook to track episodes so they can learn more about these triggers.)
   - What steps can you or have you taken to minimize or eliminate your child's exposure to indoor pollutants (quitting smoking, environmental control, etc.)?

Set up a schedule for parents and children to learn asthma management:

- Discuss when and where to seek emergency medical help.
- Discuss the child's asthma action plan, identifying actions parents can take before seeking medical care.

Review parents' understanding of medication therapy:

- Provide information about medications: name, type of drug, dose, method of administration, expected effect, and possible side effects. Make sure they understand when controller and rescue medications should be used.
- Evaluate the child's technique for the type of inhaler used as the techniques vary. Review the technique for use of the peak flow meter and determination of the child's personal best measurement.

Address associated issues:

- Storage and proper transport of medications.
- Financial considerations of medication cost and lifestyle changes.
- Notification of child's school or teacher; arrangements for the child's use of medications at school.
- Medical identification bracelet or medallion to facilitate assistance when the child is away from home.

NURSING CARE PLAN   The Child With Asthma In The Community Setting

GOAL	INTERVENTION	RATIONALE	EXPECTED OUTCOME
1. Readiness for Enhanced Family Coping related to increased control of asthma with daily therapeutic care			
	NIC Priority Intervention: **Family Support:** *Promotion of family interests and goals.*		*NOC Suggested Outcome:* **Family Normalization:** *Ability of family to develop and maintain routines and management strategies that contribute to optimal functioning when a member has a chronic illness or disability.*
The child and parents will work in partnership with the nurse to improve the child's asthma management.	• Listen to the family's concerns about asthma management and respond with information to correct any misconceptions.	• The parents' concerns may not be the same as the nurse's. If the parents' concerns are not addressed, the parents may not comply with recommended care.	The parents express greater confidence in averting and managing their child's asthma attacks.
	• Teach the family skills (assessment, use of equipment, and giving medications) for managing the child's asthma.	• Proper use of equipment and appropriate medication dosage will help alleviate asthma symptoms.	Parents appropriately call to ask questions about initiating home management or going to the emergency department for an asthma episode.
	• Provide telephone consultation to the parents during management of the first few asthma attacks.	• Support and reinforcement of learning during an asthma attack will increase the parents' confidence in managing future attacks.	
	• Educate the parents about when to call for future medical advice or to seek emergency treatment.	• Parents need guidelines for judging the severity of asthma attacks.	
2. Ineffective Family Management of Therapeutic Regimen related to knowledge deficit			
	NIC Priority Intervention: **Family Involvement Promotion:** *Facilitating family participation in the emotional and physical care of the patient.*		*NOC Suggested Outcome:* **Family Functioning:** *Ability of the family to meet the needs of its members through developmental transitions.*
The child and parents will recognize early signs of an asthma episode and begin appropriate treatment.	• Teach the child and parents to use a peak flow meter.	• The peak flow meter helps quantify changes in respiratory status before symptoms are detected.	The number of asthma attacks requiring medical intervention is reduced.
	• Help the child recognize his or her personal best peak flow and range indicating development of asthma symptoms.	• Identifying a personal best peak flow helps establish the ranges to be used for future symptom identification.	
	• Teach the family and child to give medications when the peak flow falls to the yellow range.	• Giving medications before an asthma attack becomes established may help avert the actual attack.	
	• Teach the child and family to monitor the child's response to medications with the peak flow meter.	• Monitoring the response gives the family information to determine when home care is inadequate and medical intervention is needed.	
3. Ineffective Health Maintenance related to lack of school asthma management plan			
	NIC Priority Intervention: **Health System Guidance:** *Facilitating a patient's location and use of appropriate health services.*		*NOC Suggested Outcome:* **Health Promoting Behavior:** *Actions to sustain or promote optimal wellness, recovery, and rehabilitation.*

NURSING CARE PLAN   The Child With Asthma In The Community Setting (continued)

GOAL	INTERVENTION	RATIONALE	EXPECTED OUTCOME
3. Ineffective Health Maintenance related to lack of school asthma management plan (continued)			
An Individual Health Plan (IHP) will be developed to help control and manage the child's asthma symptoms.	• Provide the family with educational materials to give to the school nurse and school administrators.	• School personnel need the latest information about effective asthma management in school settings.	Implementation of the individual health plan reduces the number of school absences for asthma attacks that occur during school hours and increases participation in school activities.
	• Advocate for all children to have an asthma management plan developed.	• Establishing a school policy will help all children with asthma receive appropriate care.	
	• Support the family to have a school health plan that includes the healthcare provider's written orders customized for the child.	• The child with asthma needs a personalized care plan to be most successful in controlling asthma attacks.	
	• Include in the IHP participation in regular school/class activities such as field trips and physical education, and what to do if asthma symptoms occur at school.	• Participation, even with modification or premedication, prior to activities promotes self-esteem and peer relationships.	
	• Help the family to obtain extra equipment and medications that can be provided to the school.	• Schools will provide care, but the families must provide all supplies, equipment, and medications.	
	• Work with the parents and school nurse to teach the specific asthma interventions to a designated person in the school nurse's absence.	• School nurses often travel between several schools. The school administrator or secretary often serves as the backup care provider.	
4. Risk for Situational Low Self-Esteem (child) related to need to seek special care during school hours			
	NIC Priority Intervention: **Self-Esteem Enhancement:** *Assisting a patient to increase his or her personal judgment of self-worth.*		*NOC Suggested Outcome:* **Self-Esteem:** *Personal judgment of self-worth.*
The child's improved control over asthma will increase his or her self-esteem and peer relationships.	• Assess the child's peer relationships and opportunities for age-appropriate interactions.	• Assessment is important to identify the best strategies to support the child and family.	The child establishes friendships and engages in activities with peers.
	• Motivate the child and family to gain increased control of asthma so the child can participate in normal childhood activities.	• Motivation may increase compliance with recommended daily asthma control interventions.	
	• Identify types of conflict and teasing the child experiences with peers, and teach the child defense tactics to deal with them.	• If the child is able to gain some control over these situations, his or her self-esteem will be improved.	

Evaluation

Expected outcomes of nursing care include:

- The child recognizes early asthma symptoms and uses rescue medications, hydration, and relaxation breathing before severe respiratory distress occurs.
- The child and family implement a daily treatment plan for asthma and reduce the child's number of asthma episodes.
- The child with a serious asthma attack responds to oxygen, fluids, and medication therapy, avoiding hospital admission.

Status Asthmaticus

Status asthmaticus is unrelenting, severe respiratory distress and bronchospasm in an asthmatic child, which persists despite pharmacologic and supportive interventions. Without immediate intervention the child with status asthmaticus may progress to respiratory failure and die. The child is placed in an ICU and may require endotracheal intubation with assisted ventilation. The section on respiratory failure earlier in the chapter gives additional information on the nurse's role in providing emergency respiratory care.

Cystic Fibrosis

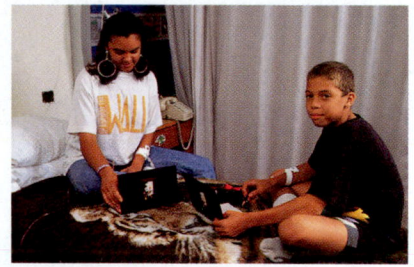

Figure 20–15 ➤ Cystic fibrosis is an inherited autosomal recessive disorder of the exocrine glands, so it is not uncommon to see siblings with it such as this brother and sister.

Cystic fibrosis (CF) is a common inherited autosomal recessive disorder of the exocrine glands that results in physiologic alterations in the respiratory, gastrointestinal, integumentary, musculoskeletal, and reproductive systems. The incidence of CF varies by race—1:3300 in Whites, 1:17,000 in Blacks, 1:8000 in Hispanics, and 1:32,000 in Asian Americans (McMullen & Bryson, 2004). There are nearly 1000 mutations of the CF Transmembrane conductance regulator (CFTR) gene that can cause CF (Orenstein, Winnie, & Altman, 2002). Approximately 20,000 children and 10,000 adults have CF in the United States (Cystic Fibrosis Foundation, 2004) (Figure 20–15 ➤). The median life span for individuals with cystic fibrosis is 35 years (Cystic Fibrosis Foundation, 2005).

Etiology and Pathophysiology

A gene isolated on the long arm of chromosome 7 directs the function of the CFTR. With a defective CFTR, the exocrine and epithelial cells have defective chloride-ion transport and decreased water flows across cell membranes. This results in an abnormal accumulation of viscous, dehydrated mucus that affects the respiratory, gastrointestinal, and genitourinary systems. Inflammation and lung changes are present as early as 4 weeks of age. Ultimately, all body organs with mucous ducts become obstructed and damaged (McMullen & Bryson, 2004).

Because of the blocked pancreatic ducts and resulting pancreatic damage, the natural enzymes necessary to digest fats and proteins are not secreted, and malabsorption results in the majority of children by 1 year of age. As the pancreas becomes increasingly damaged, some children and adolescents develop insulin deficiency and a distinct form of diabetes with features of both type 1 and type 2 diabetes. Cystic fibrosis-related diabetes is found more commonly in females, and in individuals who are older, have pancreatic insufficiency, have more pulmonary problems, and are a specific homozygous genotype (δ F508) (Marshall, Butler, Stoddard et al., 2005).

The lungs are always filled with mucus, which the respiratory cilia cannot clear. This causes air to become trapped in the small airways, resulting in atelectasis (pulmonary collapse). Secondary respiratory infections occur because secretions provide an environment conducive to bacterial growth. Respiratory failure is the leading cause of mortality.

Nearly all males who have CF are sterile because of blockage or absence of the vas deferens. Females have difficulty conceiving because of chronic illness and increased mucous secretions in the reproductive tract, which interfere with the passage of sperm (McMullen & Bryson, 2004).

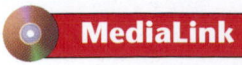

MediaLink

Cystic Fibrosis Animation

Metabolic function is altered as a result of the imbalances created by excessive electrolyte loss through perspiration, saliva, and mucous secretion. The children are at risk for dehydration secondary to electrolyte imbalance. The "salty taste" of the skin is the result of sodium chloride that makes its way through skin pores to the skin's surface.

Clinical Manifestations

The primary symptom of CF is the production of thick, sticky mucus. One of the earliest signs is meconium ileus, a small bowel obstruction in the newborn's first 48 hours of life. Stools of the child with cystic fibrosis characteristically are frothy (bulky and large quantity), smell foul, contain fat (are greasy), and float. Constipation is common and intestinal obstruction may occur in older children. Rectal prolapse, resulting from the large, bulky, difficult-to-pass stools, may occur.

Other signs and symptoms include a chronic moist, productive cough and frequent respiratory infections. Frontal headaches, facial tenderness, and purulent nasal discharge are signs of a chronic sinus infection. Nasal polyps are found in 10% of children with CF (McMullen & Bryson, 2004). Most children have difficulty maintaining and gaining weight despite a voracious appetite because of malabsorption and frequent infections. Infants and children may have a delayed bone age, short stature, and delayed onset of puberty. Clubbing of the tips of the fingers and toes occurs as the disease progresses (Figure 20–16 ➤).

Some adolescents and young adults in later stages of CF often report chronic pain. Chest pain is most commonly reported and may be musculoskeletal in origin, related to regular use of accessory muscles for breathing. Headaches may be related to hypoxia, hypercarbia, or sinusitis (Hubbard, Broome, & Antia, 2005).

■ COLLABORATIVE CARE

Diagnostic Testing

Cystic fibrosis is usually diagnosed in infancy or early childhood with one of three major presentations: newborn meconium ileus, malabsorption or failure to thrive, or chronic recurrent respiratory infections. Some children with a milder form of the disease, however, may reach the teen or young adult years before symptoms appear.

Recent advances in localization of the CF gene have led to successful techniques for prenatal diagnosis and carrier testing. Genetic testing to identify the majority of CF gene alterations is available to adults with a positive family history, partners of people with CF, couples planning a pregnancy in a high-risk population, and couples seeking prenatal testing. Rare CF gene alterations are not always detected by genetic testing (Cystic Fibrosis Foundation, 2004).

Newborn screening using dried blood samples for immunoreactive trypsinogen is mandated in some states, and genetic testing of the child's DNA is performed to confirm a positive test (Parad & Comeau, 2003). A sweat chloride test by pilocarpine iontophoresis is used to test children with classic symptoms or a positive family history (McMullen & Bryson, 2004). A sweat chloride concentration of 50 to 60 mEq/L is suspicious. If the chloride concentration is greater than 60 mEq/L, it is diagnostic with other signs. The positive sweat chloride test is repeated to confirm the diagnosis (Figure 20–17 ➤). A spirometer is used on children older than 6 years to monitor pulmonary function. Sputum cultures are obtained to identify infectious organisms and antibiotic sensitivities.

Clinical Therapy

Clinical therapy focuses on maintaining respiratory function, managing infection, promoting optimal nutrition and exercise, and preventing gastrointestinal blockage (Table 20–9). See Medications Used to Treat CF on page 729. Newly diagnosed newborns will have no or minimal symptoms and near-normal lung function if aggressively treated. Chronic infection and the inflammatory response ultimately lead to permanent lung damage.

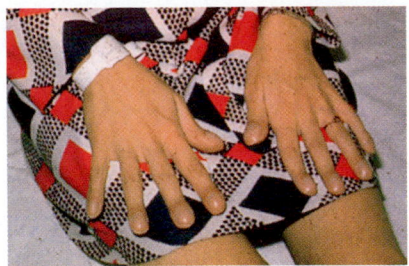

Figure 20–16 ➤ Digital clubbing.

RESEARCH

Cystic Fibrosis Survival Outcomes

A recently published study reported survival outcomes for children who had cystic fibrosis diagnosed either by prenatal or newborn screening or due to symptoms occurring beyond 1 month of age (not meconium ileus). Children diagnosed because of meconium ileus at birth had the worst survival outcomes compared to all other groups despite early treatment. Children diagnosed within 1 month of age because of non-meconium ileus symptoms or prenatal or newborn screening had significantly better survival than children diagnosed with symptoms after 1 month of age up to 10 years of age (Lai, Cheng, & Farrell, 2005). Early diagnosis enabled aggressive treatment to promote nutrition, leading to improved growth and cognitive outcomes (Farrell, Lai, Li et al., 2005).

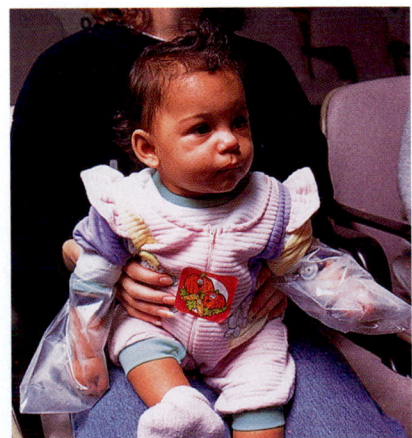

Figure 20–17 ➤ This 6-month-old girl is being evaluated for cystic fibrosis using the sweat test.

Table 20–9	CLINICAL THERAPY FOR CYSTIC FIBROSIS	

Clinical Therapy	Rationale
Respiratory Therapy	
Exercise and physical fitness	Promotes maintenance of lung function.
Chest physiotherapy twice a day for all lung segments (percussion or vibration, patient is positioned to promote sputum drainage)	In association with coughing and breathing techniques, secretions move to bronchi from lung areas; this is often preceded by aerosol medication to increase moistness of mucus.
Immunizations	Prevention of viral and some bacterial infections.
Chest tube drainage of air leaks	Resolves pneumothorax.
Thoracostomy to sew over ruptured alveoli	Repairs area of recurrent pneumothorax and prevents future episode in same location.
Lung transplantation	Reversal of respiratory failure.
Gastrointestinal Tract Therapy	
Acid suppression preparation	Gastroesophageal reflux worsens lung function, enteric coating of enzyme supplements is affected by high acid content in duodenum.
Hyperosmolar enemas, isotonic fluid lavage of the intestines (oral or NG tube)	Enema relieves meconium ileus in most infants, fluid lavage reduces distal intestinal obstruction.
Nutritional Needs	
Pancreatic enzyme supplements	Assists in digestion of nutrients and decreasing fat and bulk.
Well-balanced diet with 120–150% of RDA recommended calories, 200% of RDA recommended protein, and moderate fat	Promotes essential nutrients for health, growth, and weight maintenance; nutritional counseling to support high caloric intake, and cultural-socioeconomic issues.

Collaborative care with physicians, nurses, respiratory therapists, and nutritionists have led to improvements in medical management and optimal nutrition that have prolonged the lives of children with CF. However, new complications such as CF-related diabetes must be carefully coordinated along with the progression of the disease. Lung transplantation is occasionally performed, and approximately 50% of cases survive for the first 5 years (McMullen & Bryson, 2004). Cystic fibrosis is ultimately terminal, however, because of the progressive multisystem changes and the difficulty of long-term infection management.

NURSING MANAGEMENT

Care of the child with previously diagnosed CF is the focus of the following discussion.

Nursing Assessment and Diagnosis
Physiologic Assessment

Physical assessment of the child focuses on adequacy of respiratory function. The child with CF usually is admitted with symptoms of an upper respiratory infection. Obtain a set of baseline vital signs. Assess the child's respiratory status. Auscultate the chest for breath sounds, crackles, and wheezes. Inquire about the frequency and character of the child's cough and characteristics of sputum as changes may be related to a new infection. Note any cyanosis or clubbing of the extremities.

Evaluate the child's growth, plotting the weight and height on a growth curve. Determine whether the child is maintaining an appropriate growth pattern or is malnourished. Inquire about the child's appetite and dietary intake. How are nutritional supplements, pancreatic enzymes, and vitamins used?

Assess the child's stooling pattern. Identify whether the child has problems with abdominal pain or bloating, and whether these problems can be related to eating,

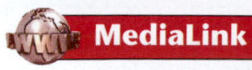

MediaLink

Care Plan Activity: The Child with Cystic Fibrosis

MEDICATIONS USED TO TREAT *Cystic Fibrosis*

Medications	Actions
Aerosol bronchodilators	Opens large and small airways; use before chest physiotherapy, and with symptoms; few studies exist to demonstrate their effectiveness.
Aerosol Dornase Alfa	Loosens, liquefies, and thins pulmonary secretions; decreases risk of developing pulmonary infections requiring parenteral treatment in some patients (McMullen & Bryson, 2004).
Corticosteroids and high-dose ibuprofen on alternate days	Anti-inflammatory agents: Reduces inflammatory response to infection; alternate day use to decrease side effects of steroids; decreases progression of lung damage in preadolescents with mild disease; may be used for a limited time.
Antibiotics (oral, IV, and inhalation)	Treats infections; higher doses than normal and prolonged courses may be needed; antibiotic selection should be based upon culture sensitivities; intermittent administration of tobramycin by inhalation improves pulmonary function.
Pancreatic enzyme supplements (Cotazym-S, Pancrease, Viokase)	Assists in digestion of nutrients decreasing fat and bulk; given prior to food ingestion, taken with meals and snacks.
Multivitamins and vitamin E in water-soluble form, vitamins A, D, and K given when deficient, iron supplementation	Cystic fibrosis interferes with vitamin production; supplements are required in water-soluble form for better absorption (vitamins A, D, E, and K are naturally fat soluble); iron deficiency results from malabsorption syndrome.
Ursodeoxycholate	May slow progression of hepatic lesion in CF; given when patient has elevated liver enzymes or evidence of portal hypertension.
Lactulose	May abort early distal intestinal obstruction syndrome and prevent recurrences.
Montelukast	Leukotriene receptor antagonist that may help reduce airway inflammation.

stooling, or other activities. Palpate the abdomen for liver size, fecal masses, and evidence of pain.

Psychosocial Assessment

The emotional stress of this chronic disease may not be readily apparent on admission, particularly if the child's symptoms are mild and not imminently life threatening. Ongoing observation of the child's and parents' behavior helps direct nursing interventions throughout hospitalization. Parents may feel guilt as carriers of the disease. Siblings may also show signs of difficulty in dealing with the illness. School-age children and adolescents often are embarrassed at being viewed as different from playmates and peers. Ask how the child and adolescent feel about the need for a special diet, medications, and limitations.

Ask parents how the child's illness has affected day-to-day functioning, any potential conflicts with family activities, and how they have adapted to the child's plan of care.

Investigate the need of and options for respite. The nurse should ask what parents have told the child and siblings about the disease. What kinds of questions have the child and siblings asked about CF, and how have parents answered them? Has the child ever asked about his or her life expectancy? If not, what would parents say if asked?

Developmental Assessment

Observe the adolescent for the appearance of secondary sex characteristics, which are often delayed. Adolescent concerns regarding body image and desire to be like peers should be explored. Investigate challenges in adhering to the treatment regimen.

Common nursing diagnoses for the child with cystic fibrosis include the following:

- Ineffective Airway Clearance related to thick mucus in lungs
- Risk for Infection related to the presence of mucous secretions and airway obstruction
- Imbalanced Nutrition: Less than Body Requirements related to the need for increased calories to meet metabolic needs
- Parental Role Conflict related to interruptions in family life due to the home care regimen and child's frequent exacerbations

Planning and Implementation

Nursing management involves supporting the child and family initially, when the diagnosis is made; during subsequent hospitalizations; and during visits to specialty and primary healthcare providers. The nurse's role begins with implementing specific medical therapies and providing nursing care to meet the child's physiologic and psychosocial needs. Respiratory therapy, medications, and diet must be coordinated to promote optimal body function. Psychosocial support and reinforcement of the child's daily care needs are important in preparation for home care.

Children with cystic fibrosis require periodic hospitalization when a severe infection occurs or for a pulmonary and nutritional assessment. The child is usually placed in a single room to reduce the spread of infectious organisms with standard precautions. Children with CF are not co-roomed to reduce the risk for transfer of the infectious organisms Pseudomonas and *Burkholderia cepacia*. Respect the parents' experiences as the child's primary care provider and include them in the child's routine care as much as possible. However, parents may view the hospital stay as a break from the rigorous daily pulmonary routine at home and need support in taking advantage of some "down" time. While the family is often proficient at providing physical care to the child, the nurse should take the opportunity to review basic and new information about respiratory care, medications, and nutrition, especially as the child matures and begins to assume some responsibility for self-care.

Provide Respiratory Therapy

Chest physiotherapy is usually performed one to three times per day before meals to clear secretions from the lungs, as coughing may stimulate vomiting (Figure 20–18 ➤). Parents and other family members can learn to help with these necessary treatments. Pulmonary care may involve aerosol treatments and antibiotics when indicated (see the medications table on the previous page).

Administer Medications and Meet Nutritional Needs

Antibiotics for acute exacerbation are provided by oral, inhalation, and intravenous routes. Because children with CF have an increased clearance of most antibiotics, they need higher doses and long treatment courses. Renal function needs to be monitored and serum antibiotic levels may be taken to ensure therapeutic dosing.

Digestive problems can be eased with pancreatic enzymes and dietary modification. Pancreatic enzyme supplements come in powder sprinkles and capsule form and, are taken orally with all meals and large snacks. The amount needed is individualized, based on the child's nutritional needs and digestive response to these supplements. Families need to learn which foods if any to avoid that contribute to a child's gastrointestinal problems. The goal is to achieve near-normal, well-formed stools and adequate weight gain.

COMMUNITY CARE

Cystic Fibrosis and B. cepacia

Individuals with cystic fibrosis who are infected with *Burkholderia cepacia* are no longer permitted to attend events or camps sponsored by the Cystic Fibrosis Foundation. This policy was developed to reduce the health risk in individuals with cystic fibrosis that are not yet infected with this organism. *B. cepacia* can cause a serious respiratory illness and may lead to a rapid decline in lung function (Cystic Fibrosis Foundation, 2006).

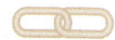

SKILL 11–25
Performing Chest Physiotherapy/Postural Drainage

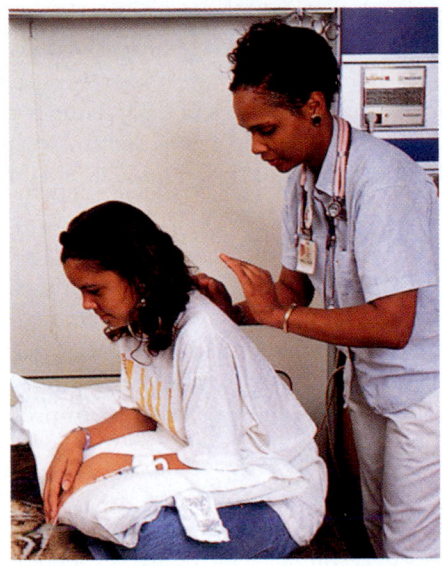 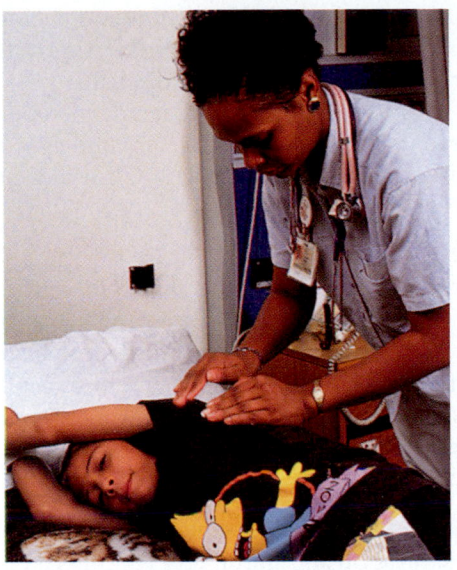 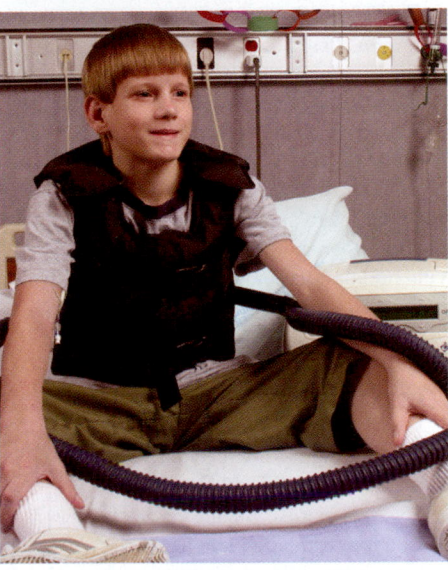

A   B   C

Figure 20–18 ➤ Postural drainage can be achieved by clapping with a cupped hand on the chest wall over the segment to be drained to create vibrations that are transmitted to the bronchi to dislodge secretions. A, If the obstruction is in the posterior apical segment of the lung, the nurse can do this with the child sitting up. B, If the obstruction is in the left posterior segment, the child should be lying on the right side. Several other positions can be used depending on the location of the obstruction. C, A high-frequency chest wall oscillation vest is another option for chest physiotherapy that the child can independently manage.

Fat-soluble vitamins (A, D, E, and K) are not completely absorbed from food; therefore, they must be taken in water-soluble form. Multivitamins taken twice daily usually are sufficient to prevent deficiency. The diet should be well-balanced, with an emphasis on high caloric value. Fats and salt are both necessary in the diet. Balanced with pancreatic enzyme supplements, moderate fat intake adds an important source of extra fuel. Respiratory complications cause additional energy expenditure, and some children require supplemental nasogastric or gastrostomy feedings to gain and maintain weight.

Provide Psychosocial Support

Help the parents and child learn what they must do to maintain health after discharge. Emotional support is essential because the diagnosis of this disorder creates anxiety and fear in both the parents and the child. They need assistance with emotional and psychosocial issues relating to discipline, body image (stooling and odor), frequent rehospitalization, the potential fatal nature of the illness, the child's feeling of being different from friends, and overall financial, social, and family concerns. Because the disorder is inherited, families may have more than one child with cystic fibrosis. Parents may have unspoken feelings of anger and guilt, blaming themselves for their children's condition. Link the family (parents, siblings, and affected child) to support groups.

Discharge Planning and Home Care Teaching

Review the family's potential need for financial assistance due to the out-of-pocket costs for medications, supplies, equipment, and medical follow-up. Home care of the child with CF is expensive and can be draining on the family's finances. If the family requires financial assistance, refer them to the appropriate social services.

Review chest physiotherapy techniques with the parents, which should be performed as often as two or three times a day. An alternate bronchial hygiene therapy for children over age 4 years involves a vest that has an air pulse generator that rapidly inflates and deflates the vest. Deep breathing and coughing help move the loosened secretions. Encourage the child to exercise and participate in physical activities as this helps improve lung function, endurance, and airway clearance.

Managing the child's nutritional needs is important and takes time and energy. Parents need to learn how to prepare high-calorie foods, provide needed enzymes

CLINICAL TIP

Parents often have a difficult time getting the child with CF to eat the extra calories needed for optimal nutrition, setting the stage for a potential mealtime battleground. To be successful, parents need guidance about managing mealtime behaviors in addition to guidelines for preparing nutritional calorie-dense foods. Increase calorie intake by adding fats and high-calorie snacks between meals and before bed. Extra intervention, such as a gastrostomy tube for night-time feedings, may be needed when the child's weight is 85–90% of ideal weight for height. Children with adequate nutrition have a longer life expectancy.

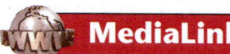

MediaLink

Cystic Fibrosis Family Support

before meals, give daily vitamins and decide what foods should be avoided or eliminated because of the child's digestive problems. Make a referral to a nutritionist either before or at the time of discharge.

Cystic fibrosis affects all family members and disrupts activities of daily living for everyone. It is important to refer families to family counseling and group therapy with families of other children with CF if indicated. The Cystic Fibrosis Foundation is a source for family information.

Care in the Community

Nurses may encounter the child with cystic fibrosis in any of the following settings: clinics specializing in the disease, pediatricians' offices, and schools. The primary goal is to slow the progression of the disease by promoting optimal nutrition and assisting the family to reduce the incidence of infection. Nurses may also provide home care to the child with cystic fibrosis following hospitalization for an acute exacerbation or provide hospice care.

Assessment

Perform the physical assessment as described for the hospitalized child. Obtain oxygen saturation and spirometry readings if changes in respiratory status are suspected. Observe the child's physical appearance, noting overall body proportions and any changes characteristic of long-term CF. The antibiotic tobramycin is associated with hearing loss, so assess hearing acuity on a regular basis.

Inquire about the family's and child's emotional and psychosocial responses to managing the illness. These issues are very important when the child is going through major developmental stages.

Management

Review the child's use of bronchodilators and airway clearance techniques. To prevent a change in pulmonary status from progressing, short-term additional therapies may be recommended. These may include intravenous and aerosol medications and antibiotics, an increase in the number of times chest physiotherapy is performed each day, and changes in dietary management. Assist the family to select the best time to fit the additional treatment into their schedule.

Malnutrition is a major problem for children with CF. Parents often need to plan meals and snacks for the young child to ensure that adequate calories are consumed. Arrange for a consultation with a nutritionist if the family would benefit from new strategies to help meet the child's nutritional needs.

Children with CF lose more than normal amounts of salt in their sweat. This loss can become intensified during hot weather, strenuous exercise, and fever. Parents should allow the child to add extra salt to food and should permit some salty snacks (pretzels with salt, pickles, carbonated soda). During periods of increased sweating, the child should be encouraged to drink more fluids and increase salt intake. Teach parents to recognize early symptoms of salt depletion, including fatigue, weakness, abdominal pain, and vomiting, and to contact the child's healthcare provider if these symptoms occur.

Adolescents with CF need special assistance in coping with their disorder, especially as survival into adulthood is common. Help them identify normal adolescent changes versus those related to CF. Adolescents must learn how to cope with the difference they know exists between themselves and peers. Provide information about potential infertility along with guidelines for safe sexual practices to reduce the risk for sexually transmitted infections. Females with CF may be able to conceive and should be offered contraception.

Gradual assumption of responsibility for daily disease management is necessary. Adherence with the daily disease management may be a problem during adolescence. Individualized planning to achieve adolescents' daily care regimen while enabling them to interact with peers and participate in school activities may be most helpful. Link adolescents to services to assist with planning appropriate educational and occupational goals for their future. Palliative care planning should be initiated as the disease progresses to respiratory failure.

Evaluation

Expected outcomes of nursing care include:

- The child and family develop proficiency in providing the daily pulmonary care and reducing the incidence of respiratory infections.
- The child and family develop a schedule and routine for daily pulmonary care that fits into family and school activities.
- The child consumes adequate calories and pancreatic enzymes to support growth and to stay within desirable weight ranges.

INJURIES OF THE RESPIRATORY SYSTEM

Airway compromise after an unintentional injury can cause death if not managed quickly and effectively. Children are vulnerable to changes in respiratory function after injury because the child's small airway can become easily obstructed. The airway may be obstructed by the tongue, small amounts of blood, mucus, or foreign debris, as well as swelling in the respiratory tract or adjacent neck tissue. If the child's neck is flexed or hyperextended, the soft laryngeal cartilage may also compress and obstruct the airway.

Smoke-Inhalation Injury

Exposure to fire conditions causes dramatic responses in a child's respiratory tract. Inhalation injury increases the child's risk for mortality, prolongs hospitalization, and increases risks for complications related to burns (Perry, 2003).

The severity of the smoke-inhalation injury is influenced by the type of material burned and whether the child was found in an open or closed space. The composition of materials determines how easily they ignite, how fast they burn, and how much heat they release. These factors influence the production of smoke and toxic gases. Smoke, a product of the burning process that is composed of gases and particles, is generated in varying volumes and density and consumes oxygen from the air. The type and concentration of toxic gases, which are usually invisible, affect the severity of pulmonary damage. The duration of exposure to the smoke produced and any toxic gases contribute significantly to the child's prognosis.

Exposure to extreme heat, common in house fires, leads to surface injury and upper airway damage. The upper airway normally removes heat from inhaled gases, sparing the lower airway from thermal damage. However, this action results in marked edema, placing the small child at particular risk for airway obstruction. Edema develops rapidly over a few hours and may lead to acute respiratory distress syndrome.

Carbon monoxide (CO) is a clear, colorless, odorless gas present in all fire conditions as the fire consumes oxygen. The CO molecule binds more firmly to hemoglobin than does oxygen. As a result, CO replaces oxygen in the blood cells and hypoxia results. The longer the exposure to CO, the greater the hypoxia. The brain receives inadequate oxygen, resulting in confusion. This accounts for the inability of fire victims to escape as confusion progresses to loss of consciousness. The process can be rapidly reversed, however, if supplemental oxygen or hyperbaric oxygen treatment is provided before hypoxia becomes too severe (Kao & Nañagas, 2004).

Damage to the lower airway most often results from chemicals or toxic gas inhalation. Soot is carried deep into the lungs, where it combines with water in the lungs to deposit acid-producing chemicals on the lung tissue. These acids burn the tissue, causing loss of cilia, loss of surfactant, and edema. Tissue destruction, pulmonary edema, and disruption of gas exchange produce the initial insult to the lungs and potential airway obstruction. Days later, the damaged tissue sloughs off, obstructing the airways. Because the cilia that normally help remove debris have been destroyed, the lungs become a breeding ground for microorganisms. Pneumonia becomes a major health concern. The damaged alveoli heal with scarring that can greatly reduce future lung function.

Burns of the face and neck, singed nasal hairs, soot around the mouth or nose, and hoarseness with stridor or voice change all indicate inhalation injury, even when the child initially has no respiratory distress. Edema develops rapidly over a few hours and may lead to airway obstruction with signs such as tachypnea, stridor, coughing, and wheezing. Respiratory distress develops and can lead to respiratory failure.

Nursing Management

Most children who survive smoke-inhalation injury are admitted for close observation, airway management, and ventilatory support, if indicated. Initial treatment is 100% humidified oxygen administered through a nonrebreather mask. Respiratory assessment and pulmonary therapy are usually required to reestablish adequate oxygenation and respiratory function. If respiratory distress develops, aggressive airway management with an endotracheal tube, mechanical ventilation, and monitoring are usually provided in an intensive care unit. Care is provided as described for the child with respiratory failure.

Blunt Chest Trauma

Blunt chest trauma with thoracic injury is second only to brain injury as the leading cause of injury death in children. A thoracic injury is an indicator of a severe injury in the child (Pitetti & Walker, 2005). Chest injuries may not be obvious and can be extremely difficult to evaluate.

Most children who die after sustaining severe blunt trauma were hypoxic because of poor airway and ventilatory control. A child's elastic, pliable chest wall and thin abdominal muscles provide minimal protection to underlying organs. This elasticity of the ribs often prevents rib fractures, but the energy from blunt trauma is transferred directly to the internal organs, often causing a pulmonary contusion or pneumothorax. A rib fracture in children under 12 years old indicates trauma of significant force. Children also have a more mobile mediastinum permitting structures in the chest to shift, such as occurs with a tension pneumothorax.

Pulmonary Contusion

A pulmonary contusion is the most common thoracic injury, defined as bruising damage to the tissues of the lung. This causes bleeding into the alveoli, which may lead to capillary rupture in the air sacs. Pulmonary edema develops in the lower airways as blood and fluid from damaged tissues accumulate. The lower airway becomes obstructed, leading to a ventilation-perfusion mismatch, poor compliance, hypoxemia, and hypoventilation (Pitetti & Walker, 2005).

Initially the child may appear asymptomatic. Respiratory distress, along with fever, wheezing, hemoptysis, and crackles, often develops over several hours. Careful observation is required during the first 12 hours after the injury to detect decreased perfusion related to ventilatory impairment.

Chest radiographs or computed tomography are used to diagnose a pulmonary contusion, but it may take several hours for evidence to appear on radiographic images. Children with severe injury to the lungs will require mechanical ventilation with low airway pressures. Other therapy includes fluid restriction, supplemental oxygen, pain control, incentive spirometry, and avoiding prolonged immobilization. Pneumonia is a potential complication that may progress to respiratory failure (Pitetti & Walker, 2005).

Nursing Management

Nursing care centers on providing necessary physiologic support, such as oxygen therapy, positioning, positive pressure ventilation, fluid management, and comfort measures. Observe for hemoptysis (fresh blood in the emesis), dyspnea, decreased breath sounds, wheezes, crackles, and a transient temperature elevation.

Inspect the thorax for symmetric chest wall movement and equal presence of breath sounds in both lungs. The child may initially appear well but requires careful and thorough monitoring to detect signs of deterioration. Children with significant injuries are cared for in the ICU with ventilator support.

Intake and output should be carefully monitored to reduce the severity of pulmonary edema. Incentive spirometry should be performed while assisting the child to reduce discomfort associated with coughing.

NURSING ALERT

When monitoring the status of a child who has a pulmonary contusion, do not rely on the child's color as an indicator of adequate oxygenation. Cyanosis in children is often a late indicator of respiratory distress.

CLINICAL TIP

The child's level of consciousness is an excellent indicator of respiratory function. Agitation and lethargy can signal increasing hypoxia.

Support the parents who are anxious about the potential life-threatening nature of the child's injury. See Chapter 14 ∞ for suggested support for families and siblings.

Pneumothorax

A **pneumothorax** occurs when air enters the pleural space because of tears in the tracheobronchial tree, the esophagus, or the chest wall. If blood collects in the pleural space, it is called a *hemothorax*, and if blood and air collect, it is called a *pneumohemothorax*. A pneumothorax is one of the more common thoracic injuries in pediatric trauma patients.

There are three types of pneumothorax: open, closed, and tension. An open pneumothorax, sometimes referred to as a sucking chest wound, results from any penetrating injury that exposes the pleural space to atmospheric pressure, thereby collapsing the lung. A sucking sound may be heard as the air moves through the opening on the chest wall. A mediastinal shift is often seen.

A closed pneumothorax is sometimes caused by blunt chest trauma with no evidence of rib fracture (Figure 20–19 ➤). The chest may be compressed against a closed glottis (such as may occur with breath holding), causing a sudden increase in pressure within the thoracic cavity. The pressure increase is transferred to the alveoli, causing them to burst. A single burst alveolus may be able to seal itself off, but with the destruction of many alveoli the lung collapses. Breath sounds are decreased or absent on the injured side, and the child is in respiratory distress. A chest radiograph often reveals air in the chest. Treatment usually involves a thoracostomy so a chest tube can be inserted. A closed drainage system is attached to help remove the air and any blood while reinflation of the lung occurs by reestablishing negative pressure.

A tension pneumothorax is a life-threatening emergency that results when the air leaks into the chest during inspiration but cannot escape during expiration. Internal pressure continues to build, compressing the chest contents and collapsing the lung. Venous return to the heart is impaired as the trachea, heart, vena cava, and esophagus

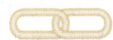

SKILLS 11–15 THROUGH 11–17
Chest Tubes

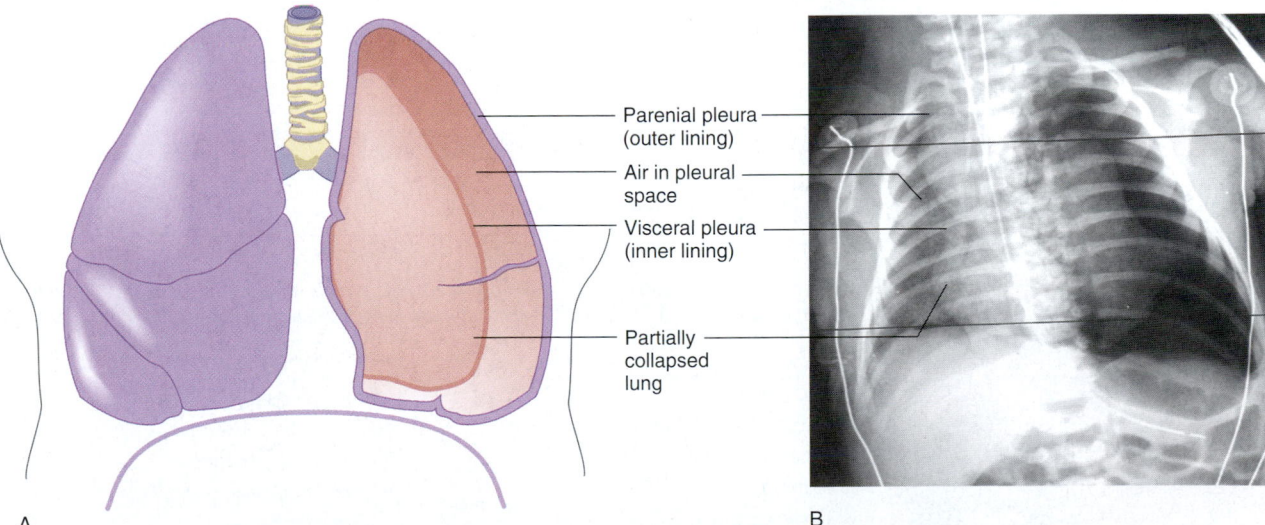

PATHOPHYSIOLOGY ILLUSTRATED

Pneumothorax

A

- Parenial pleura (outer lining)
- Air in pleural space
- Visceral pleura (inner lining)
- Partially collapsed lung

B

Figure 20–19 ➤ A, A pneumothorax is air in the pleural space that causes a lung to collapse. Whether the air results from an open injury or from bursting of alveoli due to a blunt injury, it is important to focus on airway management and maintain lung inflation. B, Tension pneumothorax, note the collapsed lung on the patient's right side and the deviation of the child's heart and trachea to the right side of the chest.
Note: B, Courtesy of Dorothy I. Bulas, M.D., Professor of Radiology and Pediatrics, Children's National Medical Center, Washington, DC.

are compressed toward the unaffected lung when the mediastinum shifts, leading to decreased cardiac output. Signs of tension pneumothorax include increasing tracheal deviation, respiratory distress, decreased or absent breath sounds on one side, decreased chest wall movement, and paradoxical breathing. A needle or tube thoracostomy is immediately required to relieve the pressure in the chest. This is usually performed before a chest radiograph is taken. Complications include hemothorax (if the thoracostomy and chest tube are improperly placed), lung tissue injury, and scarring from poor tube placement (especially if the tube is placed too near the breast in girls).

Nursing Management

Nursing management focuses on airway management and maintaining lung inflation. The child arrives on the nursing unit with a chest tube and drainage system in place. In this case, continued close observation for respiratory distress is essential. Carefully monitor vital signs and respiratory function. If a hemothorax occurs, monitor blood draining into the chest tube drainage system and the child's physiologic status for hypovolemic shock. See Chapter 21∞ for management of the child in hypovolemic shock.

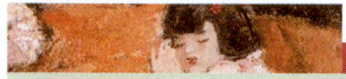

CRITICAL THINKING IN ACTION

Recall Shaun, the 13-year-old from the opening scenario. He is in the hospital for infection management and aggressive physical therapy. Because he has cystic fibrosis and infectious organisms in his lungs, he is in a single room and cannot interact with the other children on his unit. Shaun needs to use a mask when he leaves the nursing unit. He is not feeling ill and welcomes company and distractions. His mother and sister are only able to visit after work. This is an optimal time to continue teaching Shaun to manage his condition.

1. What is Shaun's developmental stage, and what information and self-care skills should be included in a teaching plan for Shaun to correspond to that stage?

2. What information should be reviewed with Shaun about his condition and the treatments needed to keep it from progressing?

3. What signs should Shaun learn to recognize that might indicate a new infection?

4. What approaches might be taken to help Shaun schedule his treatments around school and recreational activities that might increase adherence to the schedule?

 Refer to your Prentice Hall Nursing MediaLink DVD-ROM for answers.

EXPLORE MediaLink

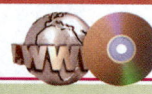 http://www.prenhall.com/ball

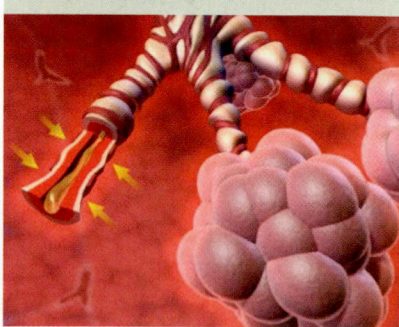

Resources for this chapter can be found on the Prentice Hall Nursing MediaLink DVD-ROM accompanying this textbook, and on the Companion Website at http://www.prenhall.com/ball.

DVD-ROM
Audio Glossary
NCLEX-RN® Review
Animations/Videos
  Asthma
  Cystic Fibrosis
  Gas Exchange in the Lungs
  Foreign Body Airway Obstruction
  Pnuemonia
  Respiratory Trauma
  SIDS
  Ventilation-Perfusion Mismatch

COMPANION WEBSITE
Audio Glossary
NCLEX-RN® Review
Care Plan Activities
  Bronchopulmonary Dysplasia
  Cystic Fibrosis
MediaLink Application: Using a Metered-Dose Inhaler
WebLinks

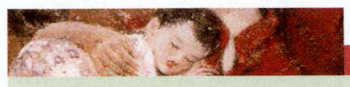

REFERENCES

Agency for Healthcare Research and Quality. (2003). Management of bronchiolitis in infants and children, summary (Evidence Report/Technology Assessment: Number 69, AHRQ Publication Number 03-E009). Rockville, MD: Author. Accessed March 29, 2004, from http://www.ahrq.gov/clinic/epcsums/broncsom.htm.

Akinbami, L. J., Rhodes, J. C., & Lara, M. (2005). Racial and ethnic differences in asthma diagnosis among children who wheeze. *Pediatrics, 115*(5), 1254–1260.

Akinbami, L. J., & Schoendorf, K. C. (2002). Trends in childhood asthma: Prevalence, health care utilization, and mortality. *Pediatrics, 110*(2), 315–322.

American Academy of Pediatrics. (2006). *Red book: 2006 Report of the Committee on Infectious Diseases* (27th ed.). Elk Grove Village, IL: Author.

American Academy of Pediatrics, Committee on Fetus and Newborn. (2003). Apnea, Sudden Infant Death Syndrome, and home monitoring. *Pediatrics, 111*(4), 914–917.

American Academy of Pediatrics, Committee on Infectious Diseases and Committee on Fetus and Newborn. (2003). Revised indications for the use of palivizumab and respiratory syncytial virus immune globulin intravenous for the prevention of respiratory syncytial virus infections. *Pediatrics, 112*(6), 1442–1446.

American Academy of Pediatrics, Task Force on Sudden Infant Death Syndrome. (2005). The changing concept of Sudden Infant Death Syndrome: Diagnostic coding shifts, controversies regarding the sleeping environment, and new variables to consider in reducing risk. *Pediatrics, 116* (5), 1245–1255.

Anderson, M. E., Johnson, D. C., & Batal, H. A. (2005). Sudden Infant Death Syndrome and prenatal maternal smoking: Rising attributed risk in the Back to Sleep era. *BMC Medicine, 3*, 4, Accessed January 10, 2006 from http://www.biomedcentral.com/1741-7015/3/4

Anonymous. (2005). Laryngotracheobronchitis (croup). *Clinician Reviews, 15*(3), 47.

Baker, V. O., Friedman, J., & Schmitt, R. (2002). Asthma management, part I: An overview of the problem and current trends. *Journal of School Nursing, 18*(3), 128–137.

Baker, V. O., Friedman, J., & Schmitt, R. (2002). Asthma management, part II: Pharmacologic management. *Journal of School Nursing, 18*(5), 257–269.

Bancalari, E., Wilson-Costello, D., & Iben, S. C. (2005). Management of infants with bronchopulmonary dysplasia in North America. *81*(2), 171–179.

Bandla, P., Brooks, L. J., Trimarchi, T., & Helfaer, M. (2005). Obstructive sleep apnea syndrome in children. *Anesthesiology Clinics in North America, 23*, 535–549.

Baren, J. M., & Puchalski, A. (2002). Current concepts in the ED treatment of pediatric asthma. *Pediatric Emergency Medicine Reports, 7*(10), 105–115.

Belcastro, M. R. (2004). Bronchopulmonary dysplasia: A new look at an old problem. *Newborn and Infant Nursing Reviews, 4*(2), 121–125.

Belcher, D. (2002, November). Breathing easier with pediatric asthma: Pharmacologic management. *Advance for Nurse Practitioners*, 37–38, 79.

Borgmeyer, A., Jamerson, P., Gyr, P., Westhus, N., & Glynn, E. (2005). The school nurse role in asthma management: Can the action plan help? *Journal of School Nursing, 21*(1), 23–30.

Braganza, S., Ozuah, P. O., & Sharif, I. (2003). The use of complementary therapies in inner-city asthmatic children. *Journal of Asthma, 40*(7), 823–827.

Brand, D. A., Altman, R. L., Purtill, K., & Edwards, K. S. (2005). Yield of diagnostic testing in infants who have had an apparent life-threatening event. *Pediatrics, 115*(4), 885–893.

Brashers, V. L. (2006a). Alterations in pulmonary function. In K. L. McCance & S. E. Huether, *Pathophysiology: The biologic basis for disease in adults and children* (5th ed., pp. 1205–1248). St. Louis: Elsevier Mosby.

Brashers, V. L. (2006b). Structure and function of the pulmonary system. In K. L. McCance & S. E. Huether, *Pathophysiology: The biologic basis for disease in adults and children*. (5th ed., pp. 1181–1204). St. Louis: Elsevier Mosby.

Bullock, L. F. C., Mickey, K., Green, J., & Heine, A. (2004). Are nurses acting as role models for the prevention of SIDS? *Maternal Child Nursing, 29*(3), 172–177.

Capper-Michel, B. (2004). Bronchopulmonary dysplasia. In P. J., Allen, & J. A. Vessey, *Primary care of the child with a chronic condition* (4th ed., pp. 282–298). St. Louis: Mosby.

Centers for Disease Control and Prevention. (2004). Trends in tuberculosis—United States, 1998–2003. *Morbidity and Mortality Weekly Report, 53*(10), 209–214.

Chávez-Bueno, S., Mejías, A., Jafri, H. S., & Ramilo, O. (2005). Respiratory syncytial virus: Old challenges and new approaches. *Pediatric Annals, 34*(1), 62–68.

Chiang, L. (2005). Exploring the health related quality of life among children with moderate asthma. *Journal of Nursing Research, 13* (1), 31–39.

Cooper, A. C., Banasiak, N. C., & Allen, P. J. (2003). Management and prevention strategies for respiratory syncytial virus (RSV) bronchiolitis in infants and young children: A review of evidence-based practice interventions. *Pediatric Nursing, 29*(6), 452–456.

Corbett, J. V. (2004). *Laboratory tests and diagnostic procedures with nursing diagnoses* (6th ed.). Upper Saddle River, NJ: Prentice Hall.

Cystic Fibrosis Foundation. (2004). Genetic carrier testing for CF. Accessed March 10, 2004, from http://www.cff.org

Cystic Fibrosis Foundation. (2005). Median age of survival for people with CF increased to 35 years in 2004. Accessed July 8, 2005, from http://www.cff.org

Cystic Fibrosis Foundation. (2006). B. cepacia policy. Retrieved February 28, 2006, from http://www.cff.org/Uploaded files/living_with_cf/Files/b%20B_cepacia%20_policy.pdf

Daley, K. C. (2004). Update on Sudden Infant Death Syndrome. *Current Opinion in Pediatrics, 16*, 227–232

Davies, F., & Gupta, R. (2002). Apparent life threatening events in infants presenting to an emergency department. *Emergency Medicine Journal, 19*, 11–16.

Dolovich, M. B., Ahrens, T. C., Hess, D. R., et al. (2005). Device selection and outcomes of aerosol therapy: Evidence-based guidelines. *Chest, 127*, 335–371.

Ehrenkranz, R. A., Walsh, M. C., Vohr, B. R., Jobe, A. H., Wright, L. L., Fanaroff, A. A., et al. (2005). Validation of the National Institutes of Health consensus definition of bronchopulmonary dysplasia. *Pediatrics, 116*(6), 1353–1360.

Farrell, P. A., Weiner, G. M., & Lemons, J. A. (2002). SIDS, ALTE, apnea, and the use of home monitors. *Pediatrics in Review, 23*(1), 3–8.

Farrell, P. M., Lai, H. J., Li, Z., Kosorok, M. R., Laxova, A., Green, C. G., et al. (2005). Evidence of improved outcomes with early diagnosis of cystic fibrosis through neonatal screening: Enough is enough! *Journal of Pediatrics, 147*(3), S30–S36.

Fingerhut, L. (2005). Hospital discharges, ages 1 to 21 years, 2003. *National Hospital Discharge Survey*, unpublished data.

Foley, S. M. (2002). Infant asthma: Genetic predisposition and environmental influences. *Newborn and Infant Nursing Reviews, 2*(4), 200–206.

Frankel, L. R. (2004). Mechanical ventilation. In R. E. Behrman, R. M. Kliegman, & H. B. Jenson, *Nelson textbook of pediatrics* (17th ed., pp. 303–306), Philadelphia: Saunders.

Froh, D. L. (2006). Alterations in pulmonary function in children. In K. L. McCance & S. E. Huether (Eds.), *Pathophysiology: The biologic basis for disease in adults and children* (5th ed., pp. 1249–1278). St. Louis: Elsevier Mosby.

Gadomski, A. (2002). Bronchiolitis dilemma: A happy wheezer and his unhappy parent. *Contemporary Pediatrics, 19*(11), 40–59.

Goldrick, B. A. (2005). Update: Tuberculosis in the United States. *American Journal of Nursing, 105*(7), 85–86.

Hauck, F. R., Omojokun, O. O., & Siadaty, M. S. (2005). Do pacifiers reduce the risk for Sudden Infant Death Syndrome: A meta-analysis. *Pediatrics, 116*(5), e716–e723.

Hayes, E., Djaferis, M., Gattasso, S., Hosmer, T., & Williamson, K. (2004). Documenting to improve pediatric asthma outcomes. *Advance for Nurse Practitioners, 12*(9), 51–56.

Hogan, M. B., & Wilson, N. W. (2003). Asthma in the school-aged child. *Pediatric Annals, 32*(1), 20–25.

Hubbard, P. A., Broome, M. E., & Antia, L. A. (2005). Pain, coping, and disability in adolescents and young adults with cystic fibrosis: A web-based study. *Pediatric Nursing, 31*(2), 82–86.

Isaacson, G., & Isaacson, D. M. (2003). Pediatric epiglottitis caused by group G beta-hemolytic streptococcus. *Pediatric Infectious Disease Journal, 22*(9), 846–847.

Kao, L. W., & Nañagas, K. A. (2004). Carbon monoxide poisoning. *Emergency Medical Clinics of North America, 22*(4), 985–1018.

Kato, I., Franco, P., Groswasser, J., Scaillet, S., Kelmanson, I., & Kahn, A. (2003). Incomplete arousal processes in infants who were victims of sudden death. *American Journal of Respiratory and Critical Care Medicine, 168*(1), 1298–1303.

Kiechl-Kohlendorfer, U., Hof, D., Peglow, U. P., Traweger-Ravanelli, B., & Kiechl, S. (2004). Epidemiology of apparent life-threatening events. *Archives of Diseases in Childhood, 90*, 297–300.

Kieckhefer, G., & Ratcliffe, M. (2004). Asthma. In P. L. Jackson & J. A. Vessey (Eds.), *Primary care of the child with a chronic condition* (4th ed., pp. 174–197). St. Louis: Mosby.

Krous, H. F., Beckwith, J. B., Byard, R. W., Rognum, T. O., Bajanowski, T., Corey, T., et al. (2004). Sudden Infant Death Syndrome and unclassified sudden infant deaths: A definitional and diagnostic approach. *Pediatrics, 114*(1), 234–238.

Lai, H. J., Cheng, Y., & Farrell, P. M. (2005). The survival advantage of patients with cystic fibrosis diagnosed through neonatal screening: Evidence from the United States Cystic Fibrosis Foundation registry data. *Journal of Pediatrics, 147*(3), S57-S63.

Lieu, T. A., Lozano, P., Finkelstein, J. A., Chi, F. W., Jensvold, N. G., and others. (2002). Racial/ethnic variations in asthma status and management practices among children in managed Medicaid. *Pediatrics, 109*(5), 857–865.

Mahabee-Gittens, E. M., Grupp-Phelan, J., Brody, A. S., Donnelly, L. F., Bracey, S. E. A., Duma, E. M., et al. (2005). Identifying children with pneumonia in the emergency department. *Clinical Pediatrics, 44*, 427–435.

Marlier, L., Gaugler, C., & Messer, J. (2005). Olfactory stimulation prevents apnea in premature newborns. *Pediatrics, 115*(1), 83–88.

Marshall, B. C., Butler, S. M., Stoddard, M., Moran, A. M., Liou, T. G., & Morgan, W. J. (2005). Epidemiology of cystic fibrosis-related diabetes. *Journal of Pediatrics, 146*, 681–687.

Marshik, P. L. (2004). Pharmacologic treatment of pediatric asthma. *Advance for Nurse Practitioners, 12*(3), 35–36, 41–46.

Matturri, L., Ottaviani, G., & Lavezzi, A. M. (2005). Techniques and criteria in pathologic and forensic-medical diagnostics in sudden unexplained infant and perinatal death. *American Journal of Clinical Pathology, 124*(2), 259–268.

McGovern, M. C., & Smith, M. B. H. (2004). Causes of apparent life threatening events in infants: A systematic review. *Archives of Diseases in Childhood, 89*, 1043–1048.

McMullen, A. H., & Bryson, E. A. (2004). Cystic fibrosis. In P. J. Allen & J. A. Vessey, *Primary care of the child with a chronic condition* (4th ed., pp. 404–425). St. Louis, Mosby.

Meadows-Oliver, M., & Banasiak, N. C. (2005). Asthma medication delivery devices. *Journal of Pediatric Health Care, 19*(2), 121–123.

National Asthma Education and Prevention Program. (1994). *Acute exacerbations of asthma: Care in a hospital-based emergency department* (p. 13). Bethesda, MD: National Heart, Lung, and Blood Institute, National Institute of Health.

National Asthma Education and Prevention Program. (2002). *Expert Panel Report II: Guidelines for the diagnosis and management of asthma. Update on selected topics 2002* (NIH Publication No. 02-5075). Bethesda, MD: National Heart, Lung, and Blood Institute, National Institutes of Health.

National Asthma Education and Prevention Program. (2003). *Managing asthma: A guide for schools* (NIH Publication No. 02-2650). Bethesda, MD: National Institutes of Health, National Heart, Lung, and Blood Institute.

National Center for Health Statistics. (2004). Summary health statistics for U.S. children: *National Health Interview Survey, 2002, 10*(221), 87(PHS)–1549. Available at http://www.cdcc.gov/nchs

Nelson, L. J., Schneider, E., Wells, C. D., & Moore, M. (2004). Epidemiology of childhood tuberculosis in the United States, 1993–2001: The need for continued vigilance. *Pediatrics, 114*(2), 333–341,

Orenstein, D. M., Winnie, G. B., & Altman, H. (2002). Cystic fibrosis: A 2002 update. *Journal of Pediatrics, 140*(2), 156–164.

Parad, R. B. & Comeau, A. M. (2003). Newborn screening for cystic fibrosis. *Pediatric Annals, 32*(8), 528–535.

Perkin, R. M., & Swift, J. D. (2002). Infectious causes of upper airway obstruction in children. *Pediatric Emergency Medicine Reports, 7*(11), 117–128.

Perry, C. M. (2003). Thermal injuries. In P. A. Moloney-Harmon & S. J. Czerwinski, *Nursing care of the pediatric trauma patient* (pp. 277–294). Philadelphia: Saunders.

Peterson-Sweeney, K., McMullen, A., Yoos, H. L., & Kitzman, H. (2003). Parental perceptions of their child's asthma: Management and medication use. *Journal of Pediatric Nursing, 17*(3), 118–125.

Pitetti, R. D., & Walker, S. (2005). Life-threatening chest injuries in children. *Clinical Pediatric Emergency Medicine, 6*, 16–22.

Poehling, K. A., Talbot, T. R., Griffin, M. R., Craig, A. S., Whitney, C. G., et al. (2006). Invasive pneumococcal disease among infants before and after introduction of pneumococcal conjugate vaccine, *Journal of the American Medical Association, 295*(14), 1668–1674.

Pongracic, J. A. (2003). Asthma delivery devices: Age-appropriate use. *Pediatric Annals, 32*(1), 50–54

Reznik, M., & Ozuah, P. O. (2005). A prudent approach to screening for and treating tuberculosis. *Contemporary Pediatrics, 22*(11), 73–88.

Silvestri, J. M., Lister, G., Corwin, M. J., Smok-Pearsall, S. M., Baird, T. M., et al. (2005). Factors that influence use of a home cardiorespiratory monitor for infants. *Archives of Pediatrics and Adolescent Medicine, 159*(1), 18–24.

Solomon, G., Humphreys, E. H., & Miller, M. D (2004). Asthma and the environment: *Connecting the dots. Contemporary Pediatrics, 21*(8), 73–81.

Stastny, P. F., Ichinose, T. Y., Thayer, S. D., Olson, R. J., & Keens, T. G. (2004). Infant sleep positioning by nursery staff and mothers in newborn hospital nurseries. *Nursing Research, 53*(2), 122–129.

Stokowski, L. A. (2005). A primer on apnea of prematurity. *Advances in Neonatal Care, 5*(3), 155–170.

Stoll, B. J., & Kliegman, R. M. (2004). The newborn infant. In R. E. Behrman, R. M. Kliegman, & H. B. Jenson, *Nelson textbook of pediatrics* (17th ed, pp. 523–527). Philadelphia: Saunders.

Swartz, M., Cantey-Banasiak, N., & Meadows-Oliver, N. (2005). Barriers to effective pediatric asthma care. *Journal of Pediatric Health Care, 19*, (2): 71–79.

Taylor, Z. (2005). Guidelines for the investigation of contacts of persons with infectious tuberculosis. *Morbidity and Mortality Weekly Report, 54*(RR15), 1–37.

Taylor, Z., Nolan, C. M., & Blumberg, H. M. (2005). Controlling tuberculosis in the United States: Recommendations from the American Thoracic Society, CDC, and Infectious Diseases Society of America. *Morbidity and Mortality Weekly Report, 54*(RR12), 1–81.

van Veldhoven, N. H., Vermeer, A., Bogaard, J. M., Hessels, M. G., Wijnroks, L., Colland, V. T., et al. (2001, August). Children with asthma and physical exercise: Effects of an exercise programme. *Clinical Rehabilitation, 15*(4), 360–370.

Vaucher, Y. E. (2002). Bronchopulmonary dysplasia: An enduring challenge. *Pediatrics in Review, 23*(10), 349–357.

Wang, L. Y., Zhong, Y., & Wheeler, L. (2005). Direct and indirect costs of asthma in school-age children. *Preventing Chronic Disease, 2*(1), 1–10. Accessed August 25, 2005, from http://www.cdc.gov/pcd/issues/2005/jan/04_0053.htm

Yoos, H. L., Kitzman, H., & McMullen, A. (2003). Barriers to anti-inflammatory medication use in childhood asthma. *Ambulatory Pediatrics, 3*(July), 181–190.

ALTERATIONS IN CARDIOVASCULAR FUNCTION

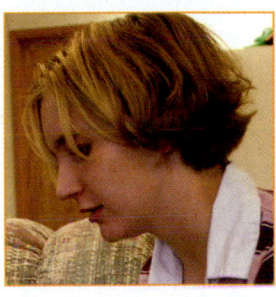

TINA, who is 16 years old, was diagnosed with transposition of the great arteries at birth. She had a Senning procedure, also called venous switch palliative surgery, as a newborn. Her parents were very concerned when she was born and throughout her early childhood because of her heart defect and the possible disabilities that she might have. However, other than the usual childhood illnesses, Tina grew and developed as expected. Her parents were careful to make sure she had regular health promotion care and always received antibiotic prophylaxis for infective endocarditis before dental care. Her parents tried to follow the pediatrician's advice to treat her as a normal child.

One year ago, Tina felt dizzy and tired more quickly with exercise and activity, indicating the potential development of a rhythm disturbance or right ventricular failure. Following a comprehensive cardiac evaluation, Tina was found to have an episodic slow ventricular heart rate, and received a pacemaker. Tina's current exercise limitations are no strenuous activities or competitive sports. She is now seen every 6 months in the pediatric cardiac clinic to monitor for further changes in her condition.

Tina, a junior in high school, is trying to figure out what she would like to do when she graduates. She has average grades in school and likes computers. She has a boyfriend and hopes to have a family some day. She has no idea if her heart condition will be a problem for her as she begins to think about future jobs. In the past, her parents have always made the decisions about her visits and treatment. What kinds of jobs can she do? Will she need any special treatment if she gets pregnant? What other information does she need as she prepares for her future?

KEY TERMS

arrythmias **783**
cardiac output **741**
cardiomegaly **768**
compliance **741**
desaturated
  blood **741**
digitalization **769**
dyslipidemia **785**
endocardium **780**
hemodynamics
  740
holosystolic **752**
hypercyanotic
  episode **757**
hypoxemia **741**
inotropic
  medicines **769**
palliative
  procedure **747**
polycythemia **742**
preload **758**
radiofrequency
  ablation **783**
shock **787**
shunt **746**
stenosis **758**
stroke volume **741**
syncope **746**
systemic vascular
  resistance **741**

MediaLink

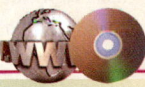

http://www.prenhall.com/ball

See the Prentice Hall Nursing MediaLink DVD-ROM and Companion Website for chapter-specific resources.

LEARNING OUTCOMES

After reading this chapter, you will be able to do the following:

1. Describe the anatomy and physiology of the cardiovascular system, focusing on the flow of blood and action of the heart valves.

2. Identify at least three differences in cardiac functioning between infants and adults.

3. Recognize the signs of congestive heart failure in an infant and child.

4. Develop a nursing care plan for a child with congestive heart failure.

5. Describe the pathophysiology associated with congenital heart defects with increased pulmonary circulation, decreased pulmonary circulation, and obstructed systemic blood flow.

(continued)

Learning Outcomes, continued

6. Develop a nursing care plan for the infant with a congenital heart defect cared for at home prior to corrective surgery.

7. Develop a nursing care plan for the child undergoing open heart surgery.

8. Identify heart diseases acquired during childhood and how they differ from congenital defects.

9. Describe the pathophysiology of hypovolemic shock, distributive shock, and cardiogenic shock.

FOCUS ON
The Cardiovascular System

ANATOMY AND PHYSIOLOGY OVERVIEW

The heart is divided into four chambers, two atria and two ventricles. Atrioventricular valves (tricuspid and mitral) separate the atria from the ventricles. They open and close to control the flow of blood to the ventricles. The semilunar valves (pulmonary and aortic) open when the ventricles pump blood and close to prevent the backflow of blood to the ventricles. The great arteries (aorta and pulmonary artery) carry blood away from the heart to either the body or the lungs. Pulmonary veins and the superior and inferior vena cava return blood to the heart. See Figure 21–1 ➤ for the anatomy of the heart.

The heart is the pump that circulates the blood through the systemic and pulmonary systems. Blood flows to the lungs for oxygen and carbon dioxide exchange. The oxygen-saturated blood then returns to the heart to be pumped out to the systemic circulation to oxygenate the tissues. The oxygen saturation of blood in each heart chamber and pressures generated by each chamber are also illustrated on Figure 21–1. See Table 21–1 for **hemodynamics** (passage of blood through the heart and pulmonary system and pressures generated by the blood) of the normal heart. The heart's electrical conduction system controls the rhythmic pumping (Figure 21–2➤).

Transition from Fetal to Pulmonary Circulation

Blood flows from the placenta to the fetus through the umbilical vein to the ductus venosus (the fetal vascular channel between the umbilical vein and the inferior vena cava) and into the right atrium of the heart. The foramen ovale, an

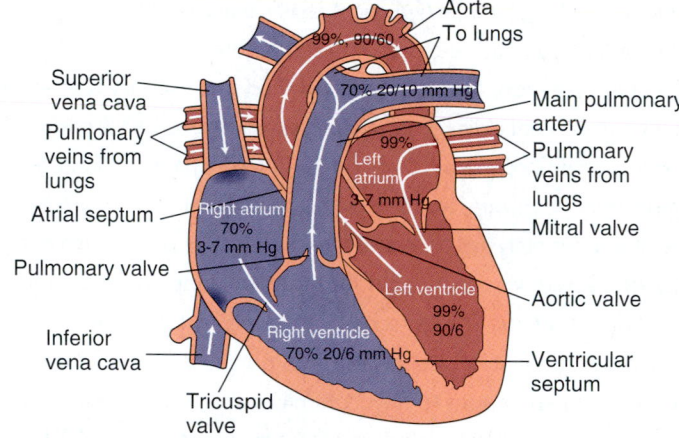

Figure 21–1 ➤ Normal pressure gradients and oxygen saturation levels in the heart chambers and great arteries. The ventricle on the right side of the heart has a lower pressure during systole than the left ventricle because less pressure is needed to pump blood to the lungs through the rest of the body.

opening between the atria of the fetal heart, allows blood to flow from the right atrium to the left atrium and then into the left ventricle. Blood is then pumped into the aorta and systemic circulation. Some blood returns from the head and upper extremities to the superior vena cava and right atrium. Some blood travels to the right ventricle where it is pumped into the pulmonary artery. The majority of this blood passes through the ductus arteriosus, the vascular channel between the pulmonary artery and the aorta, and into the systemic circulation. A small amount of the blood from the pulmonary artery goes to the lungs. Blood eventually returns to the placenta by way of the umbilical arteries.

Table 21–1	HEMODYNAMICS OF THE NORMAL HEART	
Action	**Right Side of Heart**	**Left Side of Heart**
Blood return to heart	Systemic circulation by way of the superior and inferior vena cavae.	Lungs by way of the left and right pulmonary veins.
Diastolic phase	Pulmonary valve closes and tricuspid valve opens. Blood flows from the vena cavae through the right atrium and tricuspid valve into the right ventricle.	Aortic valve closes and mitral valve opens. Blood flows from the pulmonary veins through the left atrium and mitral valve into the left ventricle.
Systolic phase	Tricuspid valve closes and pulmonary valve opens. Blood is pumped from the right ventricle into the pulmonary artery and passes into the right and left pulmonary arteries and lungs.	Mitral valve closes and aortic valve opens. Blood is pumped from the left ventricle into the aorta where it enters the systemic circulation.

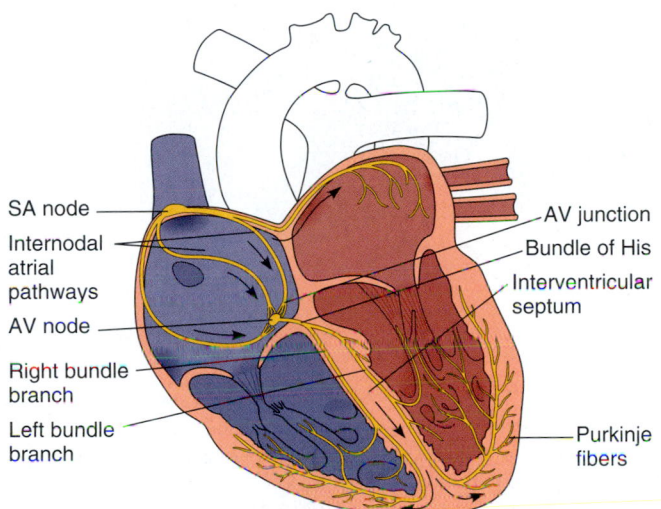

SA node
Internodal atrial pathways
AV node
Right bundle branch
Left bundle branch

AV junction
Bundle of His
Interventricular septum
Purkinje fibers

Figure 21–2 ➤ Electrical conduction system of the heart. Depolarization normally follows a sequence that begins in the sinoatrial (SA) node and travels through the atrial muscle to the atrioventricular (AV) junction, and then through the AV node to the ventricular muscles. The pathway in the ventricles begins in the bundle of His and divides into the right and left bundle branches. The pathway terminates in the Purkinje system so that the impulse spreads across the myocardium.

After the umbilical cord has been cut, the newborn must quickly adapt to receiving oxygen from the lungs. The transition from fetal to pulmonary circulation occurs in just a few hours. The first breath expands the lungs and blood that previously flowed through the ductus arteriosus to the aorta begins flowing to the lungs. Increased pulmonary blood flow and decreased pulmonary vascular resistance results. Pressure in the left atrium increases as increased blood flow is returned from the lungs through the pulmonary veins.

Systemic vascular resistance (the force or resistance of the blood in the body's blood vessels that helps return blood to the heart) increases and right atrial pressure falls after the umbilical cord is cut. Increased pressure in the left atrium stimulates closure of the foramen ovale. The flaps of the foramen ovale close and fibrin deposits permanently seal the opening unless there is excess pressure on the right side of the heart. The ductus arteriosus, responding to higher oxygen saturation, normally constricts and closes within 10 to 15 hours after birth. Permanent closure occurs by 10 to 21 days after birth, unless

oxygen saturation remains low. Fetal tissues are accustomed to low oxygen saturation. This may explain why newborns with cyanotic heart disease appear relatively comfortable even when the arterial partial pressure of oxygen (PaO_2) is 20–25 mmHg, in contrast to healthy newborns who have a PaO_2 of 83–108 mmHg. Older children and adults would rapidly develop acidosis and cerebral anoxia with such a low PaO_2. Figure 21–3 ➤ compares fetal and postnatal circulation through the heart.

Pediatric Differences

Cardiac Functioning

Infants have a greater risk of heart failure than older children because the immature heart is more sensitive to volume or pressure overload. During infancy the heart's muscle fibers are less developed and less organized, resulting in limited functional capacity. Less **compliance** (amount of distention or expansion the ventricles can achieve to increase stroke volume) of the heart muscle means that the **stroke volume** (amount of blood ejected with each contraction) cannot increase substantially until the heart muscle is fully developed at 5 years of age. The heart muscle fibers develop during early childhood; by 9 years of age, the weight of the heart has increased by six times (Connor, 2006). As the child's heart grows and develops, the systolic blood pressure rises, reaching adult levels by puberty.

The infant's metabolic rate and oxygen requirements double at birth, so the heart rate is high to maintain a high **cardiac output** (volume of blood ejected from the left ventricle each minute) and adequate oxygen transport. During stress, exercise, fever, or respiratory distress, infants and children have tachycardia, which increases their cardiac output. The infant has little cardiac output reserve capacity until oxygen requirements begin to decrease.

Oxygenation

Oxygen bound to hemoglobin is transported to the tissues by the systemic circulation. Hematocrit and hemoglobin concentrations appropriate for the child's age are necessary for adequate oxygen transport (see Chapter 20 ∞). The oxygen arterial saturation is the amount of oxygen that can potentially be delivered to the tissues. **Desaturated blood** results when oxygenated and unoxygenated blood mix because of a congenital heart defect. Cyanosis, which indicates **hypoxemia** (lower-than-normal amounts of oxygen in

AS CHILDREN GROW

Transition of Fetal Circulation to Pulmonary Circulation

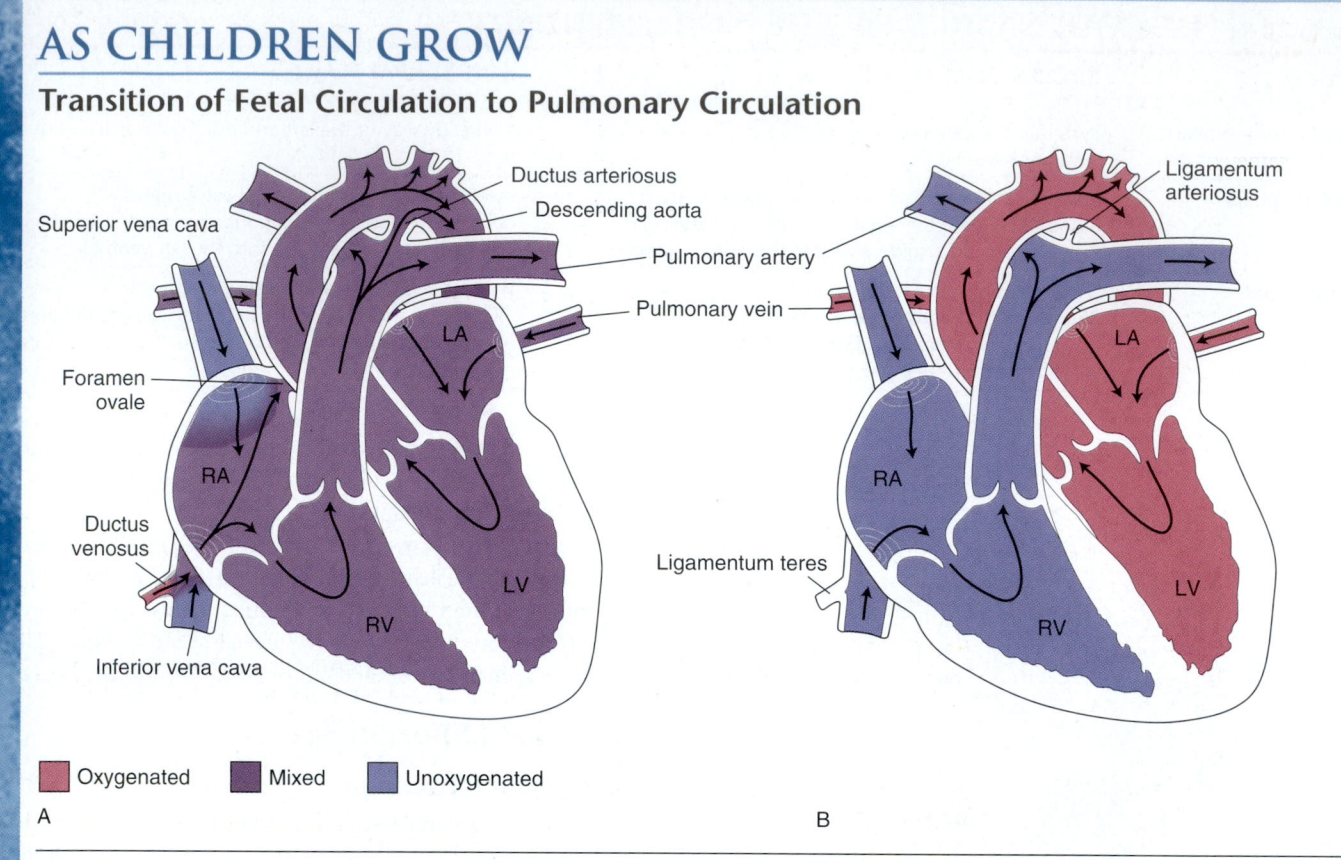

Figure 21–3 ➤ The arrows indicate the flow of blood through the heart while the color indicates level of oxygen saturation in the blood. A, Fetal circulation. B, Pulmonary circulation. LA, left atrium; LV, left ventricle; RA, right atrium; RV, right ventricle.

CLINICAL TIP

A pulse oximeter provides a noninvasive measurement of the arterial oxygen saturation level (SpO₂). A reading of 95–98% is normal in children. A value of less than 85% for more than 30 seconds is a major hypoxic event (Popovich, Richiuso, & Danek, 2004).

NURSING ALERT

Extreme polycythemia, a hemoglobin concentration greater than 20 g/dL and a hematocrit greater than 55–60%, is dangerous. Blood viscosity is increased, and the child is at risk for a thromboembolism (Park, 2002).

---

the blood), results from a concentration of 5 or more grams of deoxygenated hemoglobin per 100 mL of blood or from arterial saturations less than 85%.

The child's bone marrow responds to chronic hypoxemia by producing more red blood cells to increase the amount of hemoglobin available for oxygenation. This increase is known as **polycythemia**. A hematocrit value of 50% or higher is common in children with cyanotic heart defects.

Children respond to severe hypoxemia with bradycardia. Cardiac arrest in children generally results from prolonged hypoxemia related to respiratory failure or shock rather than from a primary cardiac insult as in adults. Bradycardia is therefore a significant warning sign of cardiac arrest. Appropriate management of hypoxemia often reverses bradycardia and prevents cardiac arrest.

Numerous diagnostic procedures and laboratory tests are used for the diagnosis of cardiac conditions. See the accompanying table on the following pages.

Performing a nursing assessment of the child with a potential or actual cardiac condition involves a careful review of the signs and symptoms in many body systems and analysis of their relationship to cardiac functioning. Use the guidelines on page 745 to perform a comprehensive nursing assessment of the cardiovascular system.

Alterations in cardiovascular function may be the result of a congenital defect, acquired infection, or injury. Congenital heart disease is the leading cause of death, excluding prematurity, during the first year of life. It is estimated that about one-third of children born with congenital heart disease die as a result of their cardiac disease, and about one-third of those deaths occur in the first year of life (Connor, 2006). Rapid advances in the treatment of congenital heart defects allow children to have surgery at younger ages. As a result, the nursing care required to identify and manage responses of infants and children with heart disease has become more challenging.

DIAGNOSTIC PROCEDURES AND LABORATORY TESTS USED TO EVALUATE CARDIAC CONDITIONS

Diagnostic Procedure	Purpose	Nursing Implications
Cardiac catheterization	An invasive procedure that passes a radiopaque catheter through a large vein or artery in an arm or leg to the heart. The catheter is threaded to the heart chambers or coronary arteries, or both, guided by fluoroscopy, which enables precise measurement of oxygen saturation within the heart's chambers and great arteries and pressure gradients in the pulmonary vessels or heart chambers. This helps identify: • Congenital heart defects • Cardiac valvular disease • Coronary artery disease In some cases a biopsy of the heart muscle may also be obtained to evaluate muscle function problems, inflammation, or heart transplant rejection. Also, cardiac catheterization can aid in evaluation of artificial valves and rhythm disturbances.	• No food or fluid 6 to 8 hours prior to test. • Obtain history of hypersensitivity to iodine, seafood, or contrast dye. Antihistamines and/or steroids may be ordered prior to the procedure if allergy exists. Assess for an allergic reaction during the procedure. • Oral anticoagulant therapy is discontinued. • An IV may be started for administering sedation or emergency drugs, as needed. • Vital signs and heart rhythm are monitored during the procedure. • Once the catheter and guidewires are removed, apply direct pressure on the catheterization site for 15 minutes and then apply a pressure dressing for 6 hours. • Monitor the site for bleeding and assess the distal extremity for pulse, capillary refill, and temperature according to agency guidelines. • Maintain bed rest for 6 hours after the procedure and then limit activities for 24 hours. • Monitor intake and output as the contrast dye causes diuresis.
Chest radiograph study	As the most common form of imaging, radiographs use irradiation to obtain images and capture them on film for diagnostic and screening purposes. They reveal the size and contour of the heart and characteristics of pulmonary vascular markings.	• Explain the procedure to parents and child. Inform them that several images may be taken from different angles. • Explain that modern equipment decreases radiation exposure. • Have the child practice holding still and holding a breath in preparation for the test.
Echocardiogram	This is a noninvasive ultrasound study of the heart. An ultrasound probe (transducer) is held over the chest to produce an ultrasound beam to the tissues. The reflected sound waves or tissues are then transformed into scans, graphs, or sounds (Doppler). It identifies the heart size, structure, pattern of movement, hemodynamics, blood flow, and blood flow disturbances.	• Explain the procedure to parents and child. Inform the child of the need to hold still for the procedure. • Inform the child that a gel will be applied to the skin and a transducer will move over the area, but that the test causes no pain.
Electrocardiogram (ECG)	This records the electrical impulses of the heart via electrodes and a galvanometer (ECG machine). Electrodes with electropaste or pads are strapped to the four extremities, and chest electrodes are applied. The lead selector is turned to read the 12 standard leads. Purposes of this procedure include: • Detection of cardiac dysrhythmias • Identification of electrolyte imbalances • Monitoring ECG changes during the stress test	• Obtain a list of current medications, and when last taken. • When applying the chest and extremity leads, explain to the child that the procedure is not painful. • Tell the child about the need to hold still for a very short time. A pacifier or bottle may help the infant hold still. • Teach methods to relieve anxiety and remain relaxed.
Exercise testing	A test performed with a treadmill or stationary exercise bicycle will evaluate exercise tolerance. ECG leads, a blood pressure cuff, and sometimes an oxygen consumption monitor are attached and the adolescent begins the exercise. Acceleration and pitch of the treadmill or bicycle are increased at intervals until the adolescent is fatigued or a predetermined endpoint is reached. This enables ECG recording with controlled increase in activity to identify significant cardiac compensation or inadequate cardiac output.	• Inform the adolescent about the test, what to expect, and that the test can be stopped at any time. • Instruct the adolescent to report vertigo, extreme shortness of breath, chest pain, and excessive fatigue. • Ensure that the adolescent understands that the test is of greater value when the exercise continues to the predetermined stopping level. • Take baseline vital sign measurements prior to the exercise.

(continued)

DIAGNOSTIC PROCEDURES AND LABORATORY TESTS USED TO EVALUATE CARDIAC CONDITIONS

Diagnostic Procedure	Purpose	Nursing Implications
Holter monitor (ambulatory electrocardiography)	ECG leads are attached and a portable recorder is used to enable continuous 24- to 48-hour recording of the ECG on magnetic tape. It is used to detect rhythm disturbances, changes in heart rate with activity or during sleep, as well as responses to antiarrhythmic medications.	• The child may not swim or bathe in a tub or shower until the electrodes are removed. • The child can engage in other usual activities. • A diary of any events or emotional stress that cause symptoms should be kept. A daily schedule of sleep, eating, exercise, and other activities may be requested.
Hyperoxitest	Arterial blood is collected before and at least 10 minutes after giving the child 100% oxygen. It measures differences in arterial blood gas level when an infant has central cyanosis to help distinguish between cardiac disease, pulmonary disease, or central nervous system depression (Park, 2002).	• Follow guidelines for arterial blood collection from the upper right side of the body, as described later. • Adminster oxygen through a plastic hood for at least 10 minutes to replace all alveolar air with oxygen.
Magnetic resonance imaging	MRI produces results similar to those of a CT scan, but it does not use ionizing radiation. The MRI scanner is a large, doughnut-shaped cylinder. The child lies on a table and is guided into the cylinder until the body part to be imaged is within the magnetic field. It provides images of the heart's myocardium, structure, valve function, blood vessels, and other soft tissues.	• Prepare the child for sounds, size of equipment, and tunnel. • Ensure that the child has no metallic implants, and is not connected to metal equipment (e.g., oxygen tank). • Use sedation, if needed, to keep the infant or child still. • Monitor the child according to agency guidelines.

Laboratory Test	Purpose	Nursing Implications
Arterial blood gases	Blood is collected from an artery to monitor the adequacy of ventilation and oxygenation, the oxygen-carrying capacity of the blood and acid-base levels. It enables a direct measurement of the arterial blood pH, partial pressures of oxygen and carbon dioxide, and bicarbonate.	• Perform arterial puncture on the radial, brachial, and femoral arteries, if desired. • Use anesthetizing agent to reduce pain associated with the arterial puncture. • Following blood collection, put pressure over the puncture site for 5 to 10 minutes to prevent hematoma formation.
Complete blood count	Blood is collected from a vein or capillary puncture. The hematocrit and hemoglobin levels are assessed to identify polycythemia or anemia. The white blood cell count provides evidence of infection.	• Inform the child about what to expect and how to cooperate. • Use the approved skin preparation and wipe the skin dry with gauze. • Warm the skin prior to blood collection to improve blood flow. • Apply pressure briefly and cover with a bandage.
Serum digoxin level	Blood is collected from a vein to assess the drug level for therapeutic range or toxicity.	• Collect 1 mL of blood. • Record the dosage, route, and time since last digoxin dose on the requisition.
Anti-streptolysin-O antibody titer	This provides documentation of a recent group A beta-hemolytic streptococcal infection.	• Follow guidelines for venous blood collection.
Erythrocyte sedimentation rate (ESR)	ESR measures the speed with which red blood cells settle in a tube of anticoagulated blood. It provides evidence of inflammation or infection but does not reveal location. Changes in the ESR help evaluate the condition's acuteness.	• Collect 5 mL of uncoagulated blood. • Follow guidelines for venous blood collection.
C-reactive protein	This nonspecific test provides evidence of inflammation but does not reveal the location. It is used to monitor rheumatic fever.	• Collect 3 mL of venous blood. • Follow guidelines for venous blood collection.
Serum lipid panel	This detects dyslipidemias.	• Fasting is not needed for total cholesterol screening. • Fasting for 12 hours is needed for a total lipid panel.

Data from: Corbett, J. V. (2004). *Laboratory tests and diagnostic procedures with nursing diagnoses* (6th ed.). Upper Saddle River, NJ: Prentice Hall; and Park, M. (2002). *Pediatric cardiology for practitioners* (4th ed., pp. 374–375). St. Louis: Mosby.

ASSESSMENT GUIDELINES FOR THE CHILD WITH A CARDIAC CONDITION*

Assessment Focus	Assessment Guidelines
Respirations	• Inspect the rate, depth, and respiratory effort. • Is a cough present? • Identify the signs of increased respiratory effort: *tachypnea* (abnormally rapid rate of respirations), dyspnea, retractions, nasal flaring, and expiratory grunting. • Auscultate breath sounds for adventitious sounds (wheezes, crackles).
Pulses	• Assess the pulse rate, rhythm, and quality. • Compare the apical, brachial, and radial pulse rates. • Compare the brachial and femoral pulses for strength.
Blood pressure	• Compare the blood pressure to expected value for age, sex, and height percentiles (see Table 5–14). • Compare blood pressure values between upper and lower extremities.
Color	• Observe overall color: note pallor, dusky color, or cyanosis. • Contrast color in peripheral and central locations (e.g., nailbeds to mucous membranes). Note whether crying improves or worsens color.
Heart	• Inspect the anterior chest for bulging or *heaving* (lifting of the chest wall during contraction). • Palpate the chest wall for pulsations, heaves, or vibrations. • Locate the point of maximum intensity. • Auscultate the heart for the heart sounds and their quality (loud versus weak, distinct versus muffled). Muffled or indistinct sounds are associated with congestive heart failure or a heart defect. • Are extra heart sounds or murmurs present? Describe murmurs by intensity, location, radiation, timing, and quality. • Auscultate the heart with the child in sitting and reclining positions to detect differences in heart sounds.
Fluid status	• Observe for signs of periorbital, facial, or peripheral edema. • Observe for abdominal distention. • Palpate the liver to detect hepatomegaly. • Observe for signs of dehydration with acute illnesses.
Activity and behavior	• Is exercise intolerance present? • Does the child tire with feeding? • Identify changes in activity level or behavior.
General	• Assess growth. • Note presence of diaphoresis and when it occurs.

*See Chapter 5 ∞ for actual techniques of assessment.

CONGENITAL HEART DISEASE

Congenital heart disease refers to a defect in the heart or great vessels, or persistence of a fetal structure after birth. Congenital heart defects occur in an estimated 1% of all pregnancies and one in every 170 live births (Neilson & Robin, 2002). More than 35 types of heart defects have been documented. Deaths from heart defects have declined dramatically over the past 50 years, and now approximately 85% of newborns with congenital heart disease are expected to survive to adulthood (Green, 2004). This is attributed to diagnostic advances, surgical technique refinements, and intensive care.

Etiology and Pathophysiology

Most congenital heart defects develop during the first 8 weeks of gestation. They are usually the result of a combined or interactive effect of genetic and environmental factors, such as:

- Fetal exposure to drugs such as phenytoin, lithium, warfarin, and alcohol.
- Maternal viral infections such as rubella or coxsackie B5.
- Maternal metabolic disorders such as phenylketonuria, diabetes mellitus, and hypercalcemia.
- Maternal complications of pregnancy such as increased age and antepartal bleeding.
- Genetic factors (family recurrence patterns); transmission is higher when the mother is the affected parent (Park, 2002).
- Chromosomal abnormalities such as Turner syndrome, Noonan syndrome, Marfan syndrome, DiGeorge syndrome, cri du chat syndrome, Down

MediaLink

Congenital Heart Defects Animation

syndrome, and trisomy syndromes 13, 15, 18, and 21. The prevalence of heart defects in children with Down syndrome is about 50% and in children with trisomy 13 and 18 the incidence increases to 90% or more (Park, 2002).

Deletion of chromosome 22q11 is associated with development of several cardiovascular defects such as interrupted aortic arch, truncus arteriosus, tetralogy of Fallot, and ventricular septal defects (Goldmuntz, 2004). Knowledge about other chromosome deletions or mutations associated with cardiovascular defects is emerging. Because of this genetic component, the incidence of congenital heart defects is expected to slowly rise as people with some of these defects survive and have children of their own. Depending on the type of defect, signs and symptoms may be present at birth or develop later.

Congenital heart defects previously were categorized as to whether the child had or did not have cyanosis (cyanotic or acyanotic). Defects are now categorized by pathophysiology and hemodynamics. These categories include the following:

- Increased pulmonary blood flow (see page 749)
- Decreased pulmonary blood flow (see page 757)
- Obstructed systemic blood flow (see page 765)
- Mixed defects in which infant survival is dependent upon mixing of systemic and pulmonary blood (see page 757)

Clinical Manifestations

The presence of a heart murmur is often the first indication of a congenital heart defect. A loud murmur indicates blood is flowing with higher pressure than normal to get through a narrowed valve or vessel, or through a **shunt** (movement of blood between the systemic and pulmonary circulation through an abnormal anatomic opening, such as through the right and left ventricles). Other clinical manifestations and the timing of their appearance vary by the pathophysiology and severity of the defect. See the clinical manifestations table below. Some infants and children may be asymptomatic except for a heart murmur, such as with a small atrial septal defect. Older children with the diagnosis of congenital heart disease may have additional symptoms such as exercise intolerance, chest pain, arrhythmias, and **syncope** (transient loss of consciousness

CLINICAL MANIFESTATIONS	HEART DEFECTS BY PATHOPHYSIOLOGY	
Pathophysiology	**Clinical Manifestations**	**Types of Defects**
Increased pulmonary blood flow	Tachypnea, tachycardia, murmur, congestive heart failure, poor weight gain, diaphoresis, periorbital edema, frequent respiratory infections	Patent ductus arteriosus, atrial septal defect, ventricular septal defect, atrioventricular canal defect (endocardial cushion defect), truncus arteriosus, total anomalous pulmonary venous return
Decreased pulmonary blood flow	Cyanosis, hypercyanotic episodes, poor weight gain, polycythemia	Pulmonic stenosis, tetralogy of Fallot, pulmonary atresia, tricuspid atresia, transposition of the great arteries
Obstructed systemic blood flow	Diminished pulses, poor color, delayed capillary refill time, decreased urine output, congestive heart failure with pulmonary edema	Coarctation of aorta, aortic stenosis, hypoplastic left heart syndrome, mitral stenosis, interrupted aortic arch
Mixed defects— postnatal survival is dependent upon mixing of systemic and pulmonary blood	Cyanosis, poor weight gain, pulmonary congestion, or congestive heart failure may occur with increased shunting	Transposition of great arteries, total anomalous pulmonary venous connection, truncus arteriosus, double outlet right ventricle

and muscle tone after exercise or activity). Clinical manifestations for specific heart defects will be found in later sections with their focus on conditions associated with increased pulmonary blood flow, decreased pulmonary blood flow, obstruction to systemic blood flow, and mixed defects.

COLLABORATIVE CARE

Diagnostic Tests

The history and physical examination findings may lead to a suspicion of a congenital heart defect. See pages 743–744 for multiple tests and procedures used to diagnose cardiac defects.

Clinical Therapy

One-third of infants born with congenital heart defects develop life-threatening symptoms in the first few days of life. Treatment for congenital heart defects depends on the severity of symptoms and whether the condition is imminently life threatening. Interventional catheterization or surgical correction is the treatment of choice for many defects. Many heart defects can be completely repaired with restoration of normal hemodynamics and physiology. For complex heart defects, treatment may only be a **palliative procedure**, a surgical or interventional cardiac catheterization procedure that does not create normal anatomic or hemodynamic results. A palliative procedure may be used for children with a potentially fatal or lethal condition or as an initial procedure while the infant is small before definitive corrective surgery can be performed. Table 21–2 lists the types of interventions during cardiac catheterization and surgical procedures performed on children with congenital heart defects.

NURSING MANAGEMENT OF THE CHILD UNDERGOING A CARDIAC CATHETERIZATION

Cardiac catheterization is a diagnostic and an interventional procedure, often performed on an outpatient basis. However, some children will be admitted for observation after the procedure to monitor for complications or for surgery scheduled to follow the catheterization. The child is given nothing by mouth (NPO) for several hours, except for medications, and arrives at the catheterization laboratory 1 to 2 hours before the procedure. In preparation for the procedure, the child is asked to void and is given an oral sedative.

Assessment and Diagnosis

Before the procedure, assess the child using the guidelines on page 745. Pay particular attention to the child's vital signs, hematocrit and hemoglobin concentrations, and capillary refill time. In addition, collect baseline data on skin temperature, color, and strength of pedal and popliteal pulses for comparison with postcatheterization assessments.

For several hours after the procedure, monitor the child for potential complications such as arrhythmia, bleeding, hematoma development, thrombus formation, and infection. No bleeding should occur at the catheterization site. Assess vital signs, perfusion of the lower extremities (pulses, temperature, color, capillary refill time, and sensation), and the pressure dressing over the catheterization site every 15 minutes for 1 hour and then every 30 minutes for 1 hour. Be sure to check under the buttocks to make sure blood does not ooze out and run under the child. The child's vital signs should remain stable. Monitor intake and output because the contrast medium may cause diuresis.

The following nursing diagnoses may apply to the child who undergoes cardiac catheterization:

- Fear related to separation from support system in a stressful situation
- Risk for Imbalanced Fluid Volume related to inadequate fluid intake due to NPO status and diuretic effect of contrast medium

| Table 21–2 | **CLINICAL INTERVENTIONS FOR CONGENITAL HEART DEFECTS** |

Cardiac Catheterization Procedure	Intervention	Therapeutic Use, Defect Treated
Angioplasty	Dilatation of coarctation of aorta or a stenotic vessel during cardiac catheterization	Palliative or corrective for COA
Balloon valvuloplasty	A deflated balloon is inserted into the opening of a narrowed valve and inflated to stretch the valve open during cardiac catheterization	Corrective or palliative for PS, AS
Patent ductus arteriosus closure	Closure of ductus arteriosus by an umbrella or coil device during cardiac catheterization	Corrective for PDA
Rashkind–Balloon atrial septostomy	Creation of larger defect (at the foramen ovale) between atria to increase blood mixing, performed during cardiac catheterization	Palliative for TGA
Transcatheter closure	Closure of a septal defect by a device such as aseptal occluder during cardiac catheterization	Corrective for ASD, VSD

Surgical Procedure	Intervention	Therapeutic Use, Defect Treated
Aorta end-to-end anastomosis	Resection of the narrowed section of the aorta and connection of the proximal and distal sections	Corrective for COA
Blalock-Taussig shunt, modified	Creation of aorto-pulmonary conduit (from the subclavian artery to pulmonary artery) to increase pulmonary blood flow	Palliative for TOF, other defects of decreased pulmonary blood flow
Brock	Blind incision of pulmonary valve	Corrective for PS
Damus-Kaye-Stansel	Pulmonary artery is cut in two with the proximal section attached to the ascending aorta and the distal section to the right ventricle	Corrective for TGA, complex single-ventricle defects
Fontan	Creation of conduit between inferior vena cava and pulmonary artery to increase pulmonary blood flow—total right heart by-pass. This permits the right ventricle to assume the responsibility for the systemic circulation and eject blood into the aorta.	Palliative for HLHS, single-ventricle defects
Glenn	Superior vena cava connected to right pulmonary artery along with closure of aorto-pulmonary shunt; systemic venous blood from the head sent to the lungs directly without ventricular pumping	Palliative for HLHS, single-ventricle defects
Jatene (arterial switch)	Aorta and pulmonary arteries transected and re-anastomosed to opposite stumps; coronary arteries moved to the new aorta area	Corrective for TGA
Mustard or Senning (venous switch or intra-atrial baffle)	Baffling blood in atria to reestablish a proper blood flow in transposition of great arteries	Palliative for TGA
Norwood	Atrial septectomy, anastomosis of the main pulmonary artery to the aorta, and an arterial-pulmonary shunt	Palliative for HLHS
Norwood with Sano modification	Creation of a right ventricle to pulmonary artery conduit so that both the direct pulmonary and aorta blood flow originate in the right ventricle	Palliative for HLHS
Patch aortoplasty	Insertion of a Dacron patch to expand the lumen of the aorta	Corrective for COA
Pulmonary artery banding	Placement of constricting band around pulmonary artery to reduce pulmonary blood flow	Palliative for VSD, AV canal, single-ventricle defects
Rastelli	Creation of a conduit between the right ventricle to pulmonary artery with closure of the ventricular septal defect; in the case of truncus arteriosus, the pulmonary arteries are removed from the truncus	Corrective for TGA with pulmonic stenosis, TOF, tricuspid atresia, truncus arteriosus
Ross	The diseased aortic valve replaced with the patient's pulmonic valve (pulmonary autograft), and a homograft (valve from a human donor) replaces the pulmonic valve	Corrective for AS
Subclavian flap aortoplasty	Division of the distal subclavian artery and insertion of a flap into the aorta through the coarcted segment	Corrective for COA
Transplant	Replacement of diseased heart with donor heart	Corrective for HLHS, complex defects, cardiomyopathies

AS—aortic stenosis, ASD—atrial septal defect, AV—atrioventricular, COA—coarctation of aorta, HLHS—hypoplastic left heart syndrome, PDA—patent ductus arteriosus, PS—pulmonic stenosis, TGA—transposition of great arteries, TOF—tetralogy of Fallot, VSD—ventricular septal defect

- Impaired Tissue Perfusion (Cardiopulmonary) related to mechanical reduction of arterial and venous blood flow
- Decreased Cardiac Output related to ventricular restriction (obstruction by balloon catheter)

Planning and Implementation

Prepare the child for cardiac catheterization with age-appropriate information. A tour of the catheterization laboratory may reduce the child's fears about the large equipment. Because the child will be sedated but arousable for the procedure, explain the sensations that he or she will experience.

Nursing care during a cardiac catheterization focuses on monitoring the child's vital signs, reassuring the child, and providing emergency care if necessary. After the catheters and guidewires are removed at the end of the procedure, direct pressure must be applied for 15 minutes. A pressure dressing is then placed over the site for 6 hours.

The child is kept on bed rest for 6 hours with an effort to keep the leg straight for several hours. Avoid elevating the head of the bed as flexion of the hips is not permitted during this period. Activity is then limited for 24 hours. Provide quiet diversional activities to keep the child occupied.

Encourage the child to drink small amounts of clear liquids initially, and then progress to other fluids and food as the child tolerates them. Infants and children treated with diuretics have a greater potential for dehydration. The child's intake and output should be balanced, so provide adequate fluids to maintain hydration status.

Discharge Planning and Home Care Teaching

Children are routinely discharged several hours after the cardiac catheterization. Teach the parents to watch the child for signs of complications and make sure they know when to notify the physician. See Families Want to Know: Home Care After Cardiac Catheterization.

Children whose heart defect is corrected by cardiac catheterization have the same risks for infective endocarditis as children with surgical correction. Use the information in the medication table on the next page to teach parents about infective endocarditis prophylaxis.

Evaluation

Expected outcomes of nursing care include:

- Any potential complications (thrombosis or hemorrhage) following cardiac catheterization are rapidly identified and cared for.
- The child maintains fluid balance.

Congenital Heart Defects That Increase Pulmonary Blood Flow

Etiology and Pathophysiology

The most common congenital heart defects result from a connection between the left and right side of the heart (septal defect) or between the great arteries (patent ductus

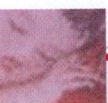

FAMILIES WANT TO KNOW

Home Care After Cardiac Catheterization

- Encourage fluids to help flush the dye out of the body and to prevent dehydration.
- Allow no active or rough play for the first 24 hours. Permit quiet play such as games, puzzles, and videos for the first 24 hours after the procedure.
- Check for signs of complications several times in the first 24 hours after catheterization:

- Fever
- Bleeding or a bruise increasing in size at the catheterization site
- Foot on side of catheterization site is cooler than other foot
- Loss of feeling in foot on side of catheterization
- Notify the healthcare provider immediately if any of these signs are noted within the first 24 hours after the catheterization.

MEDICATIONS USED FOR *Infective Endocarditis Prophylaxis in Children*

Procedure	Antibiotic Recommendations	Nursing Considerations
For dental, oral, or upper respiratory tract procedures	Amoxicillin **For Children Allergic to Penicillin:** Clindamycin, cephalexin, cefadroxil, azithromycin, clarithromycin	• One large dose is given 1 hour before the procedures. • In high-risk patients, a smaller dose may be given 6 hours after the procedure.
For genitourinary and gastrointestinal procedures	Ampicillin, gentamicin, amoxicillin **For Children Allergic to Penicillin:** Vancomycin, gentamicin	• Teach parents and the child to keep at least one dose in the home to take before dental visits or for dental emergencies. • Dentists and physicians can write a prescription.

Note: Modified from Dajani, A. S., Taubert, K. A., Wilson, W., Bolger, A. F., Bayer, A., et al. (1997). Prevention of bacterial endocarditis: Recommendations of the American Heart Association. *Journal of the American Medical Association, 277*(22), 1794–1801.

arteriosus) that allows blood to flow between the left and right side of the heart. The pressures on the left side of the heart are higher than on the right side, so blood shunts from the left side of the heart to the right side and increases the amount of blood pumped to the lungs. The size of the connection and how much blood passes through it determine how quickly the child develops signs of congestive heart failure (CHF). The increased blood flow to the lungs causes increased pulmonary vascular resistance (constriction of the pulmonary vascular bed) in an effort to reduce the blood flow, as well as pulmonary artery hypertension (see page 777). Right ventricular hypertrophy (RVH) develops to overcome the increasing pulmonary vascular resistance and deliver the blood to the lungs.

Clinical Manifestations

The infant's heart rate, respiratory rate, and metabolic rate are increased due to the high pulmonary blood flow. Sucking breast milk or formula takes energy, and diaphoresis often occurs with feeding. The infant may be unable to take in enough calories to support the metabolic rate and growth, so poor weight gain is noted. If CHF develops, signs include dyspnea, tachypnea, intercostal retractions, and periorbital edema (see page 767). Frequent respiratory infections occur as the wet environment in the lungs supports bacterial growth. See Table 21–3 for the pathophysiology, clinical manifestations, and clinical therapy for specific congenital heart defects with increased pulmonary blood flow.

COLLABORATIVE CARE

Diagnostic Tests

See the table on pages 743-744 for tests used to diagnose the condition. Coagulation studies, platelet counts, and serum electrolytes are often obtained for children in preparation for open-heart surgery, in addition to a chest radiograph, complete blood count, and urinalysis.

Clinical Therapy

Surgery to correct or manage defects that cause significant increased pulmonary blood flow is performed early in infancy to prevent irreversible pulmonary artery hypertension, the major complication of these defects. Unless complications develop before surgery,

Table 21–3	PATHOPHYSIOLOGY, CLINICAL MANIFESTATIONS, AND CLINICAL THERAPY FOR HEART DEFECTS THAT INCREASE PULMONARY BLOOD FLOW

Pathophysiology, Clinical Manifestations, and Clinical Therapy	**Anatomy**

PATENT DUCTUS ARTERIOSUS (PDA)

A common congenital defect caused by persistent fetal circulation that accounts for 10% of all congenital heart defects (Rome & Kreutzer, 2004). When pulmonary circulation is established and systemic vascular resistance increases at birth, pressures in the aorta become greater than in the pulmonary arteries. Blood is then shunted from the aorta to the pulmonary arteries, increasing circulation to the pulmonary system. It is a common problem of preterm infants, and is present in nearly all preterm infants less than 27 weeks' gestation (Tran, 2002). The ductus arteriosus in the preterm newborn is not as responsive to the increased oxygen content with the conversion to pulmonary circulation, and it is less likely to close.

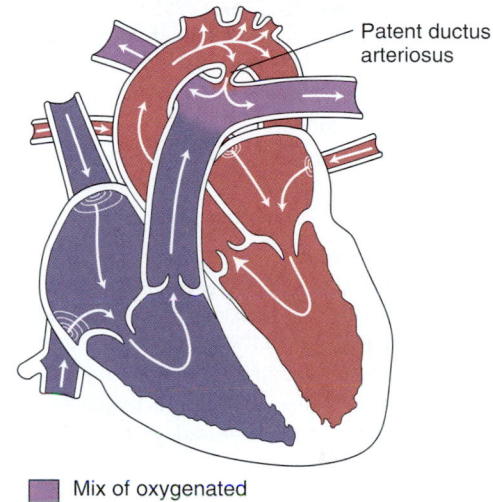

Patent ductus arteriosus

Mix of oxygenated and unoxygenated blood

Clinical Manifestations

Dyspnea; tachypnea; tachycardia; full, bounding pulses; widened pulse pressure; hypotension may be noted when cardiac output is low.

CHF, intercostal retractions, hepatomegaly, and growth failure when a large PDA exists.

A continuous "machinery" murmur during systole and diastole, and a thrill in the pulmonic area.

High risk for frequent respiratory infections, pneumonia, and infective endocarditis.

Diagnostic Procedures

The chest radiograph and ECG show left ventricular hypertrophy.

The PDA can be visualized, and left-to-right shunt can be measured on echocardiogram.

Clinical Therapy

Surgical ligation of PDA is the treatment of choice.

Intravenous indomethacin often stimulates closure of the ductus arteriosus in premature infants.

Transcatheter closure by obstructive device is sometimes attempted in children over 18 months of age. Prophylaxis for infective endocarditis is required until the PDA is closed.

Prognosis: No long-term sequelae occur if treated before pulmonary vascular disease develops. If PDA is not treated, the child's life span is shortened because pulmonary hypertension and pulmonary vascular obstructive disease develop.

ATRIAL SEPTAL DEFECT (ASD)

This opening in the atrial septum permits left-to-right shunting of blood. Three types of ASDs occur: ostium secundum; ostium primum, which is an endocardial cushion defect with anomalies of one or both of the tricuspid and mitral valves; and sinus venosus, which is associated with partial anomalous pulmonary venous connection. The opening may be small, as when the foramen ovale fails to close, or large, as when the septum may be completely absent. Of children with congenital heart defects, 10% have an ASD (Rome & Kreutzer, 2004).

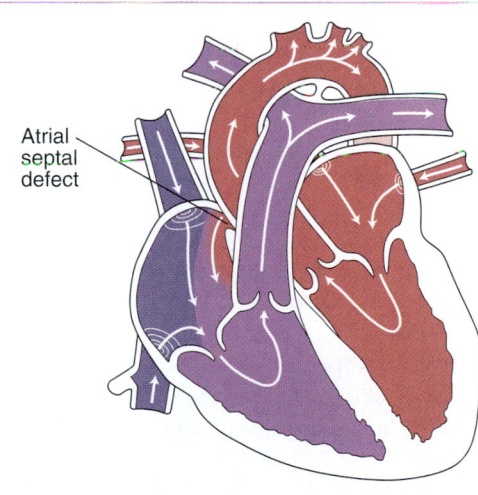

Atrial septal defect

Clinical Manifestations

Infants and young children usually have no symptoms. Small and moderate-size ASDs may not be diagnosed until preschool years or later.

CHF, easy tiring, and poor growth occur with a large ASD.

A soft systolic ejection murmur occurs in the pulmonic area with wide splitting of S2. The split second sound is fixed through all phases of respiration.

Diagnostic Procedures

Echocardiogram identifies a dilated right ventricle due to blood overload and the shunt size.

The chest radiograph and ECG reveal little information unless the ASD is large, has excessive shunting, and right ventricular hypertrophy is present.

Clinical Therapy

Spontaneous closure of some ASDs occurs within the first 4 years of life. No activity limitations are needed.

Surgery to close or patch the ASD is performed when significant increased pulmonary blood flow causes CHF, or when spontaneous closure has not occurred by 4 years of age.

Secundum ASDs may be closed by a transcatheter device (septal occluder) during cardiac catheterization.

Prognosis: Many persons with uncorrected small- and moderate-sized ASDs have lived to middle age without symptoms, but CHF and pulmonary hypertension may develop in untreated adults. Atrial arrhythmias may also occur in adults.

(continued)

Table 21–3	PATHOPHYSIOLOGY, CLINICAL MANIFESTATIONS, AND CLINICAL THERAPY FOR HEART DEFECTS THAT INCREASE PULMONARY BLOOD FLOW (continued)

Pathophysiology, Clinical Manifestations, and Clinical Therapy	Anatomy

VENTRICULAR SEPTAL DEFECT (VSD)

An opening in the ventricular septum causes increased pulmonary blood flow. Blood is shunted from the left ventricle directly across the open septum into the pulmonary artery. This is the most common congenital heart defect, accounting for 40% of all defects (Rome & Kreutzer, 2004).

Clinical Manifestations

Only 15% of VSDs are large enough to cause CHF, an increased number of pulmonary infections, and pulmonary hypertension.

A systolic murmur is auscultated at the third or fourth left intercostal space at the sternal border.

Diagnostic Procedures

A chest radiograph and ECG reveal little when VSDs are small. An enlarged heart and pulmonary vascular markings on chest radiograph may be seen when a large VSD causes shunting. Right and left ventricular hypertrophy may be seen on ECG.

Echocardiogram establishes the diagnosis if shunting is present.

Cardiac catheterization is used only in preparation for surgery. Findings reveal increased oxygen in the right ventricle and increased systolic pressure in the right ventricle and pulmonary artery.

Clinical Therapy

Most small VSDs close spontaneously within the first 6 months of life. Treatment is conservative when no signs of CHF or pulmonary artery hypertension are present.

Surgical patching of VSD during infancy is performed when poor growth is evident.

Closure of VSD by transcatheter device (i.e., Rashkind device) during cardiac catheterization may be attempted for some defects.

Prophylaxis for infective endocarditis is required.

Prognosis: Highest risk associated with surgical repair is in the first few months of life. Children respond well to surgery and experience substantial catch-up growth. Tachyarrhythmias and right bundle branch block are possible complications.

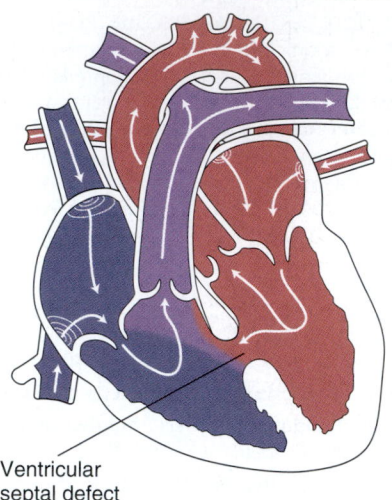

Ventricular
septal defect

ATRIOVENTRICULAR (AV) CANAL (ENDOCARDIAL CUSHION DEFECT)

AV canal refers to a combination of defects in the atrial and ventricular septa and portions of tricuspid and mitral valves. Approximately 2% of children with congenital heart defects have a total AV canal (Park, 2002). This defect is associated with Down syndrome. Endocardial cushions are fetal growth centers for mitral and tricuspid valves and AV septum. The most complex AV canal defect results in one AV valve and large septal defects between both atria and ventricles.

Clinical Manifestations

Severity of symptoms depends on the amount of mitral regurgitation and the left-to-right shunting of blood across the septum.

Infants have CHF, tachypnea, tachycardia, poor growth, recurrent respiratory infections, and repeated respiratory failure.

A **holosystolic** (heard the entire phase of systole) murmur is loudest at the left lower sternal border, and the intensity reflects the amount of mitral regurgitation. S1 is accentuated and S2 is split.

Diagnostic Procedures

On chest radiograph, cardiomegaly and pulmonary vascular markings are present.

On ECG, atrial enlargement, right ventricular hypertrophy, and an incomplete right bundle branch block are noted.

Echocardiogram reveals dilation of the ventricles, septal defects, and details of valve malformation.

Cardiac catheterization reveals increased oxygen in the right atrium, and increased right ventricle and/or pulmonary artery pressure.

Clinical Therapy

Surgery is performed during infancy to prevent pulmonary vascular disease.

Palliative pulmonary artery banding may be used to reduce blood flow to the lungs and CHF so the infant can grow before corrective surgery.

Oxygen may be required until surgery, but it may increase pulmonary blood flow and worsen CHF.

Patches are placed over septal defects, and valve tissue is used to form functioning valves. The mitral valve may be replaced.

Prophylaxis for infective endocarditis is required.

Prognosis: Information on long-term survival following successful surgery is lacking. Arrhythmias and mitral valve insufficiency occur postoperatively. There is no difference in short-term survival rates between infants with and without Down syndrome.

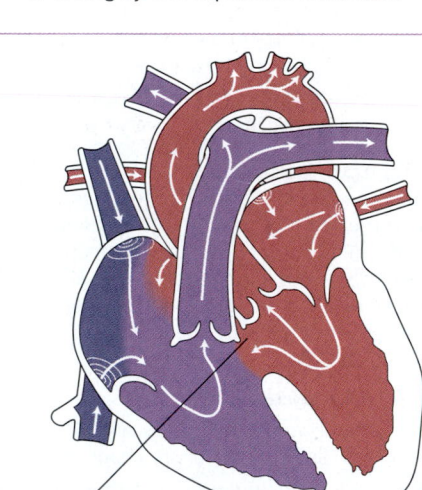

Atrioventricular
canal defect

the child should make a complete recovery without limitations. See Figure 21–4 ➤.

Conservative treatment, such as waiting until the child is symptomatic or older, may be selected for some children with these defects. For example, a small ventricular septal defect may close spontaneously, or repair of an atrial septal defect may be postponed until preschool or early school-age years. Indomethacin may be given to preterm infants with a patent ductus arteriosis when immediate closure of the ductus is needed. Interventional cardiac catheterization may be performed for defects. See Table 21–3.

Postpericardiotomy syndrome is a potential surgical complication when surgery involves an incision through the pericardium, leading to pericardial and pleural inflammation. The cause is unknown, but it may result from a viral infection, an autoimmune response, or a reaction to blood in the pericardium. The syndrome generally develops within a few weeks to a few months after surgery, more often in children over 2 years than in infants. It is characterized by a high fever up to 40°C (104°F) and severe chest pain that worsens with deep inspiration and in supine position. The median duration of the condition is 2 to 3 weeks. Mild cases are treated with bed rest and nonsteroidal anti-inflammatories (NSAIDs). Severe cases may need hospitalization and more aggressive treatment with pericardiocentesis, diuretics, and corticosteroids (Park, 2002).

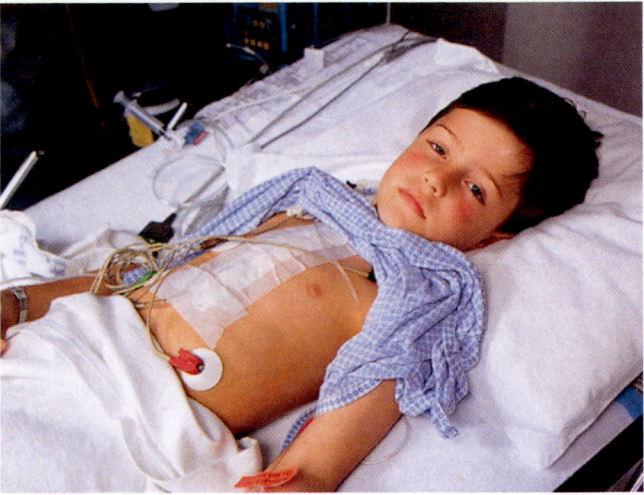

Figure 21–4 ➤ A child with atrial septal defect repair. Surgery is performed with this type of defect to prevent pulmonary artery hypertension.

NURSING MANAGEMENT PRIOR TO SURGERY

Nursing Assessment and Diagnosis

Physiologic Assessment

Prior to surgery, the infant or child is seen regularly to assess growth and to detect signs of worsening CHF. Many infants with a small defect will have no problems with growth. Failure to gain weight is an indication of an increased metabolic rate and inability to consume adequate calories for both metabolic function and growth. Assessment of length and head circumference helps to determine the full impact of the condition on growth.

Psychosocial Assessment

Assess the parents' ability to cope with the infant's diagnosis. Parents may initially be in shock and feel guilty or anxious. Parents need an opportunity to express their feelings and learn to cope with the child's illness. The initial period of diagnosis, hospitalization, and early care of the infant at home are very stressful. Parents need special support if their infant has a life-threatening heart defect.

Examples of nursing diagnoses associated with heart defects having increased pulmonary blood flow and their complications include:

- Excess Fluid Volume related to heart failure and pulmonary vasculature overload
- Ineffective Infant Feeding Pattern related to shortness of breath and fatigue
- Risk for Infection related to pulmonary vascular congestion and chronic illness
- Interrupted Family Processes related to crisis of child's serious illness

CLINICAL TIP

Resources for parents of a child with a congenital heart defect include:

- *If Your Child Has a Congenital Heart Defect* by the American Heart Association.
- *The Parent's Guide to Children's Congenital Heart Defects* by Gerri Freid Kramer and Shari Maurer, Three Rivers Press.
- *King of Hearts: The True Story of the Maverick Who Pioneered Open Heart Surgery* by G. Wayne Miller.

Planning and Implementation
Family Education

Participate with members of the cardiology team to provide information and educate the family about the child's condition. Information may include the following:

- General information about the congenital heart disease, including a description of the heart's anatomy and physiology and the defect.
- Information about genetic and environmental influences associated with congenital heart disease.
- Overview of the child's prognosis and timing of medical and surgical interventions.
- Interventions for congestive heart failure if they develop (see page 771 for care guidelines).

Psychosocial Support

Parents often need support for anxiety about an uncertain surgical outcome. Determine if parents have a support system as they learn about the infant's diagnosis and make difficult decisions about the child's surgery. If the parents do not have adequate support systems, identify some resources for support, such as social services, pastoral services, or a parent of a child with a similar heart defect. Some parents may be concerned that signing consent for surgery places the child in even more danger of illness or even death.

Parents should be offered genetic counseling if planning a future pregnancy.

Home Care

Children are often managed at home until surgery. Parents should encourage feeding to promote growth, but allow the infant to feed for up to 30 minutes. Breast-feeding is encouraged because of its beneficial effects for the infant. A high caloric formula may be used if the infant does not gain enough weight. Feedings through a nasogastric or gastrostomy tube may also be given at night or 24 hours a day to ensure that adequate calories are ingested. Even when nasogastric or gastrostomy feedings are used, encourage the infant to take some formula orally to provide positive oral stimulation. See feeding suggestions for the infant with CHF on page 773.

Efforts should be made to reduce the infant's exposure to infectious diseases. Wash hands frequently. Respiratory infections make hypoxemia worse in children with cyanosis. Fever increases the metabolic rates and oxygen demands. Vomiting and diarrhea may cause an electrolyte disturbance and digoxin toxicity (Cook & Higgins, 2004). The physician should be notified about fever, poor feeding, vomiting, and diarrhea.

Health promotion visits are important. Provide all immunizations according to the recommended schedule. Monthly prophylaxis for respiratory syncytial virus (RSV) with palivizumab should be provided during the peak season. See Chapter 20 ∞.

Preparation for Surgery

When the child is preschool age or older, prepare the child for the settings, equipment, and experiences to expect before and after surgery. Follow guidelines for preoperative treatment described in Chapter 13 ∞. If an infant or toddler is having surgery, provide parents with information about how the child will look, equipment that will be used, and what care will be provided in the immediate postoperative period.

Evaluation

- Nutritional intake is adequate with oral feeding and supplemental nasogastric supplementation as necessary.
- The child maintains a growth pattern that follows the established growth curve percentile.
- The child receives all immunizations and RSV prophylaxis to reduce the potential for acute illnesses.

NURSING MANAGEMENT AT THE TIME OF SURGERY

The goals of nursing management are to perform assessments, provide supportive care to the family, and meet the child's nursing care needs before and after surgery.

Nursing Assessment and Diagnosis

At the time of surgery, the child needs a careful history and physical examination to detect any acute illnesses. Assess the child's behavioral patterns, heart function, respiratory function, weight, and fluid status. Refer to Table 21–3.

In the immediate postoperative period the child will be cared for in the intensive care unit. When the child returns to the general nursing unit, assessment focuses on signs of surgical complications such as infection, arrhythmias, and impaired tissue perfusion. Pain assessment is also important.

Monitor the vital signs, including blood pressure. The child may not be on a cardiac monitor, so auscultate the apical pulse to detect an irregular heart rate or bradycardia, which are both signs of reduced cardiac output that require immediate intervention. Assess the respiratory system for breath sounds, respiratory effort, and signs of distress that may indicate pneumonia or fluid in the pleural space. Check pulse oximetry, capillary refill, extremity warmth, pedal pulses, level of consciousness, and urine output to assess impaired tissue perfusion. Reduced urine output is another sign of decreased cardiac output.

Monitor the child's temperature and inspect the surgical incision site. Fever, excessive incisional pain, spreading erythema around the incision, and wound drainage beginning 3 to 4 days postoperatively may be early signs of infection.

Examples of nursing diagnoses following cardiac surgery include the following:

- Ineffective Breathing Pattern related to respiratory muscle fatigue
- Acute Pain related to surgical incision and expansion of chest with coughing and deep breathing exercises
- Risk for Imbalanced Fluid Volume related to impact of surgery on heart's pumping action
- Risk for Infection related to surgery and chronic disease status

Planning and Implementation

Pain Management

Pain management with 24-hour intravenous opioids should be provided for several days postoperatively until the child is taking fluids. Once the child is taking oral fluids and foods, oral analgesics may be given around the clock. Follow the guidelines for pain management provided in Chapter 15 ∞. Teach parents and caregivers to lift and move the child carefully and avoid stress on the incision to reduce potential pain.

Promote Respiratory Function

Encourage the child to take deep breaths and cough or to perform spirometry exercises regularly to promote full lung expansion. Chest physiotherapy may be performed in children under 3 years of age.

Manage Fluids and Nutrition

Encourage the infant or child to begin oral fluids and nutrition when permitted. Although oral fluids are rarely limited, intake and output should be carefully assessed. Parents may be encouraged to bring in favorite foods for the child when they can be tolerated. Administer antibiotics as ordered. If intravenous antibiotics are continued after the child's oral intake is normal, the line can be converted to a heparin or saline lock.

Activity

Encourage the child to increase activity gradually with longer periods out of bed every day, but ensure adequate rest periods to promote healing. Provide diversional activities and opportunities for therapeutic play so the child can better manage the stresses associated with pain and frightening procedures.

CLINICAL TIP
Use a pillow or stuffed animal held against the chest to reduce the pain from coughing and deep breathing.

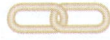

SKILL 9–3
Infusing Medication: Medication Lock in Place
SKILL 11–25
Performing Chest Physiotherapy
SKILL 11–26
Using the Incentive Spirometer

RESEARCH

PTSD and Heart Surgery

Children between 5 and 12 years of age were evaluated for symptoms of posttraumatic stress disorder (PTSD) 1 to 3 days before and 4 to 8 weeks after undergoing heart surgery. No children had PTSD at the preoperative assessment, even though 18 (42%) had had prior cardiac surgery. Results indicated that the number of PTSD symptoms increased in children who spent 48 hours or more in the intensive care unit. No significant relationship was found in PTSD scores for children with prior cardiac surgery or chronological age. These findings are similar to findings of other studies of PTSD in children after hospitalization for other serious medical illnesses and injuries such as cancer and liver transplantation (Connolly, McClowry, Hayman et al., 2004). See Chapter 27 ∞ for more information about PTSD.

Discharge Planning and Home Care Teaching

Infants and children may be discharged from the hospital within a few days of surgery. Parents need information spread over several days to prepare for care of the child at home. Encourage a nutritious diet and snacks so the infant or child has an opportunity to catchup for previous growth deficits. Acetaminophen or ibuprofen may be used for pain management after discharge. See Families Want to Know: Care of the Child After Cardiac Surgery.

Prepare parents for potential behavior problems of young children that may result from the stress of hospitalization, such as nightmares, separation anxiety, and overdependence on parents. Encourage parents to reassure children about their security, and to promote play and other means to deal with their feelings. If the child's symptoms continue for several weeks, a referral for psychological evaluation and care may be needed.

Reassure parents of children with a complete correction of the cardiac defect that there should be no further cardiovascular problems. Provide parents with full information about the child's defect and the surgery performed to share with the child's current and future healthcare providers. Encourage parents to allow the child to live a normal and active life.

Children are at risk for infective endocarditis, especially within the first 6 months after surgery. See the medication table on page 750 for prophylactic antibiotics needed for invasive procedures. Any unexplained fever or malaise seen in the 2 months following surgical repair or after dental work may be a sign of infection. The child should be examined for petechiae and splenomegaly and evaluated for infective endocarditis. (See page 780.)

Evaluation

Examples of expected outcomes of nursing care include the following:

- The child's pain is effectively managed.
- Full lung expansion is maintained with incentive spirometry exercises or chest physiotherapy.
- The child's incision heals without infection.
- Catch-up growth occurs over the next few months to years.

FAMILIES WANT TO KNOW

Care of the Child After Cardiac Surgery

- Place infants and children in car safety seats for travel home from the hospital. Place a small blanket over the incision to prevent the straps from rubbing.
- Sponge bathe the infant or use a tub bath with a low water level. Avoid soaking the incision until sutures are out, the steristrips are off, and the incision is healed. Clean the incision daily with gentle baby or pH-balanced soap. Do not use oils, creams, lotions, or ointments on the incision. Cover the incision with a clean shirt or bib to keep it clean and dry.
- Pick up infants and young children by placing one hand under the head and the other hand under the hips. Avoid picking the child up under the arms.
- Allow the child to increase activity gradually as tolerated, starting with quiet play for the first week at home. Report increased

fatigue or decreased activity tolerance to the physician. Postpone rough play, bike riding, and strenous activities for 6 weeks until the sternum incision has healed completely. Allow the child to return to school in about 3 weeks.
- Report any signs of wound infection, fever, flulike symptoms, chest pain, increased respiratory rate or respiratory distress, appetite change, or irritability to the physician.
- Acetaminophen or ibuprofen can be given for pain control. Use the recommended dose for the child's weight.
- Antibiotics should be given for dental and surgical procedures as directed (some children need them for several months and some for the rest of their lives). Report any unexplained fever or illness during the first 2 months following surgery as the child is at higher risk for infective endocarditis during that time.

Defects Causing Decreased Pulmonary Blood Flow and Mixed Defects

Information about these defect categories is combined because the clinical therapy and nursing interventions are similar. Distinguishing features are described by etiology, pathophysiology, and clinical manifestations.

Etiology and Pathophysiology

DEFECTS CAUSING DECREASED PULMONARY BLOOD FLOW Defects that obstruct the pulmonary blood flow result in little or no blood reaching the lungs to get oxygenated. If an atrial or ventricular septal opening exists between the left and right side of the heart, right-sided pressures exceed those on the left, resulting in right-to-left shunting. In this case, cyanosis often results.

The bone marrow is stimulated to produce more red blood cells to increase the hemoglobin available to carry oxygen. Polycythemia may result and place the child at risk for thromboembolism. Over time platelet survival is reduced and clotting factors are impaired, increasing the infant's risk of bleeding with surgery. Brain abscesses are also more common in children with cyanotic heart defects.

When infants and children with cyanosis rise in the morning, they may experience an abrupt decrease in systemic resistance and pulmonary blood flow. This physiologic change can trigger a **hypercyanotic** (hypoxic or "tet") **episode** when combined with a sudden increase in cardiac output and venous return associated with crying, feeding, exercise, a warm bath, and straining with defecation. The partial pressure of oxygen (PO_2) is lowered, and the partial pressure of carbon dioxide (PCO_2) rises. Hypoxemia becomes progressively worse as the respiratory center in the brain overreacts, increasing the respiratory effort. The extra respiratory effort further increases the cardiac output and contributes to a life-threatening decline unless rapid intervention is successful.

MIXED DEFECTS Many complex congenital heart defects involve a combination of defects that make the newborn dependent upon mixing pulmonary and systemic circulations for survival during the postnatal period. This mixing of oxygen-saturated and desaturated blood results in a general desaturated systemic blood flow and cyanosis. Pulmonary congestion occurs because of increased pulmonary blood flow and obstruction of systemic flow.

Clinical Manifestations

DEFECTS CAUSING DECREASED PULMONARY BLOOD FLOW Clinical manifestations in infants initially include cyanosis shortly after birth, dyspnea, and a loud murmur. The skin may initially be ruddy or mottled before cyanosis is observed. Cyanosis that does not respond as expected to oxygen is a classic sign. Signs and symptoms of chronic hypoxemia include fatigue, clubbing of the fingers and toes, exertional dyspnea, and delayed developmental milestones. See Figure 21–5 ➤. The infants may need to stop sucking periodically during feedings to breathe, and diaphoresis may be seen with the increased work of feeding. These infants have a higher metabolic rate, and inadequate calories may be consumed, resulting in poor weight gain. See Table 21–4 for the pathophysiology, clinical manifestations, and clinical therapy for these defects.

When the infant or child has severe obstruction to pulmonary blood flow, hypercyanotic episodes can occur suddenly. Toddlers with uncorrected cyanotic heart disease often squat to relieve dyspnea (Figure 21–6 ➤). The knee–chest position reduces the cardiac output by decreasing the venous return from the lower extremities and by increasing the systemic vascular resistance. Hypercyanotic episodes usually appear between 2 months and 2 years of age. Signs include increased rate and depth of respirations; increased heart rate; increased cyanosis, pallor, and poor tissue perfusion; diaphoresis; irritability and crying; and seizures and loss of consciousness.

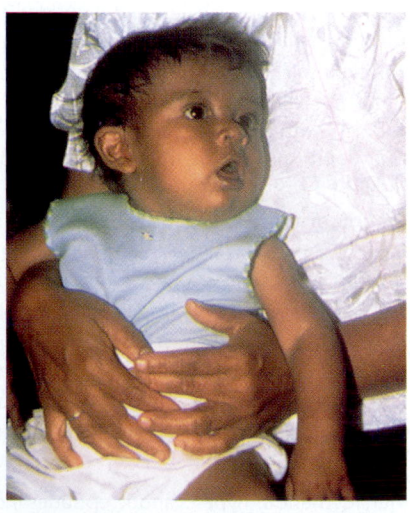

Figure 21–5 ➤ This infant is cyanotic due to a heart defect that reduces pulmonary blood flow.

Table 21–4	PATHOPHYSIOLOGY, CLINICAL MANIFESTATIONS, AND CLINICAL THERAPY FOR DEFECTS WITH DECREASED PULMONARY BLOOD FLOW

Defect Pathophysiology, Clinical Manifestations, and Clinical Therapy   **Anatomy**

PULMONIC STENOSIS (PS)

Stenosis (narrowing of the valve, valve area, or great artery above the valve) can be above valve, below valve, or at valve. Stenosis obstructs blood flow into the pulmonary artery, which increases **preload** (the volume of blood in the ventricle at the end of diastole that stretches the heart muscle before contraction) and results in right ventricular hypertrophy. This is the second most common congenital heart defect, accounting for 8–12% of all cases (Park, 2002). Stenosis may progress in the subvalvular area as the heart muscle grows and develops.

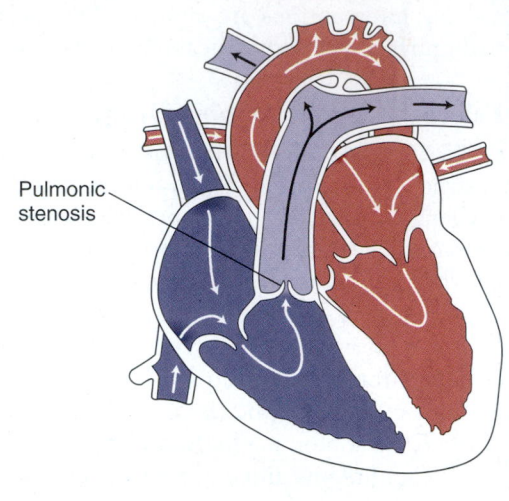

Pulmonic stenosis

Clinical Manifestation

Children with mild stenosis may have no symptoms and grow normally.

In moderate stenosis, dyspnea and fatigue occur on exertion. Signs of CHF and hepatosplenomegaly are rare but may result from chronic pressure overload. Heart failure and chest pain on exertion occur in severe cases.

A loud systolic ejection murmur with a widely split S2 and thrill may be found in the pulmonic listening area.

Diagnostic Procedures

The chest radiograph may show an enlarged pulmonary artery with normal heart size and normal pulmonary vascularity.

The ECG may show right atrial enlargement and right ventricular hypertrophy.

An echocardiogram provides information about the pressure gradient across the valve and size of valve ring.

▢ Decreased unoxygenated blood flow

Cardiac catheterization findings include increased right ventricular pressure and a normal or slightly lowered pulmonary artery pressure.

Clinical Therapy

Dilation by balloon valvuloplasty, performed during cardiac catheterization, treats simple pulmonic stenosis.

Surgical valvotomy may be used when other defects such as VSD are present.

Surgical resection may be needed for narrowing above the valve area. Pulmonary regurgitation may result, but is not a significant problem.

Prognosis: Pulmonic stenosis does not typically increase in severity. Lifelong infective endocarditis prophylaxis is necessary.

TETRALOGY OF FALLOT (TOF)

Four defects—pulmonic stenosis, right ventricular hypertrophy, ventricular septal defect (VSD), and overriding of aorta—make up the condition. Some children have a fifth defect, an open foramen ovale or atrial septal defect (ASD). About 10% of children with congenital heart defects have TOF (Park, 2002). Elevated pressures in the right side of the heart cause a right-to-left shunt.

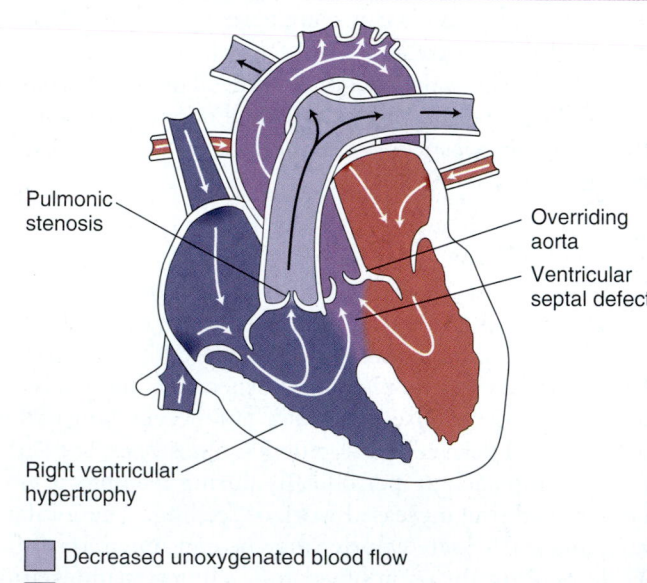

Pulmonic stenosis

Overriding aorta

Ventricular septal defect

Right ventricular hypertrophy

Clinical Manifestations

The infant becomes hypoxic and cyanotic as the ductus arteriosus closes. The degree of pulmonary stenosis determines the severity of symptoms.

A systolic murmur is heard in the pulmonic area and transmitted to the suprasternal notch. A thrill may be palpated in the pulmonic area.

Polycythemia, hypoxic episodes, metabolic acidosis, poor growth, clubbing, and exercise intolerance may develop.

Toddlers with uncorrected defects instinctively squat (assume a knee–chest position) to decrease the return of systemic venous blood to the heart. See Figure 21–6 ➤ .

▢ Decreased unoxygenated blood flow

▢ Mixed oxygenated and unoxygenated blood

Diagnostic Procedures

A chest radiograph shows the boot-shaped heart due to the large right ventricle, decreased pulmonary vascular markings, and a prominent aorta.

The ECG shows right ventricular hypertrophy.

The echocardiogram shows the VSD, obstruction of pulmonary outflow, an overriding aorta, and the size of the pulmonary arteries.

Cardiac catheterization provides details about the anatomic defects.

Blood tests reveal an elevated hematocrit and hemoglobin and an increased clotting time.

Clinical Therapy

Management of hypercyanotic episodes includes placing the infant in the knee–chest position, calming the child, giving oxygen, and administering morphine and propranolol intravenously. Monitoring the child for metabolic acidosis or prolonged unconsciousness is critical.

A total repair is often performed before 6 months of age when the infant has a hypercyanotic episode. Palliative shunt procedure (e.g., Blalock-Taussig) may be performed to allow the child to grow and improve outcomes with corrective surgery.

Prognosis: Not all children are cured by surgery, but most have improved quality of life and improved longevity. Arrhythmias may be residual problems (Park, 2002). Lifelong infective endocarditis prophylaxis is required.

Table 21–4	PATHOPHYSIOLOGY, CLINICAL MANIFESTATIONS, AND CLINICAL THERAPY FOR DEFECTS WITH DECREASED PULMONARY BLOOD FLOW (continued)

Defect Pathophysiology, Clinical Manifestations, and Clinical Therapy	Anatomy

PULMONARY OR TRICUSPID ATRESIA

Pulmonary atresia is the absence of communication between the right ventricle and the pulmonary artery, either at the site of the pulmonary valve or in the main pulmonary artery. It occurs in fewer than 1% of children with congenital heart defects. In tricuspid atresia, the tricuspid valve is absent. It occurs in 1–3% of congenital heart defects (Park, 2002). Blood flows to the left side of the heart through the foramen ovale. The PDA provides the only flow of blood to the pulmonary arteries. A ventricular septal defect (VSD) or transposition of the great arteries (TGA) is also often present.

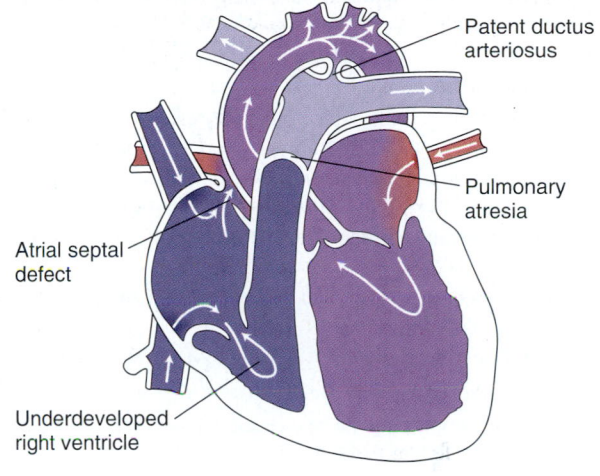

Clinical Manifestations

Cyanosis is present at birth.

Tachypnea, CHF, pulmonary edema, hepatomegaly, acidosis, hypoxic episodes, clubbing, polycythemia, and growth delays occur.

A continuous murmur from the PDA is heard in the pulmonic area. A single S2 is heard in the aortic area, and a harsh systolic murmur may be heard in the tricuspid area.

Diagnostic Procedures

The chest radiograph may reveal a normal size or slightly enlarged sized heart.

The ECG may reveal right atrial hypertrophy.

The echocardiogram shows a small hypoplastic right ventricular cavity and tricuspid valve, an absent right ventricular outflow tract, a dilated right atrium, and right-to-left shunting across the atrial septum.

Clinical Therapy

Prostaglandin E1 is given immediately to maintain a patent ductus arteriosus. Digoxin and diuretics are also used.

The Rastelli balloon atrial septostomy is performed to increase the atrial opening.

A Rastelli or modified Fontan procedure results in improved survival.

Prognosis: Outcome depends upon the size of the pulmonary outflow tract developed by surgery and the fibrosis in the right ventricle. The child has increased risk for arrhythmia and right ventricular dysfunction.

Older children may have additional symptoms such as exercise-induced dizziness and syncope, which are serious signs indicating a need for medical evaluation.

MIXED DEFECTS   These complex congenital heart defects cause varying degrees of cyanosis and CHF. When the pulmonary vascular resistance is lower than the systemic resistance, pulmonary congestion develops, followed by CHF. When the pulmonary blood flow is decreased, the infant will have more severe cyanosis and polycythemia (Suddaby, 2001). See Table 21–5 for the pathophysiology, clinical manifestations, and clinical therapy for these complex mixed defects.

COLLABORATIVE CARE

Diagnostic Tests

See Tables 21–4 and 21–5 for diagnostic tests and clinical therapy for these individual defects.

Clinical Therapy

Early management of these defects is important to prevent secondary damage to the heart, lungs, and brain, including the adverse effects of hypoxemia on the child's cognitive and psychomotor development. Corrective surgery is often performed in infancy. A palliative procedure may be performed first to preserve life in children with potentially lethal heart defects and complications (see Table 21–4). With some defects, corrective surgery can be postponed with a palliative procedure, giving the infant an

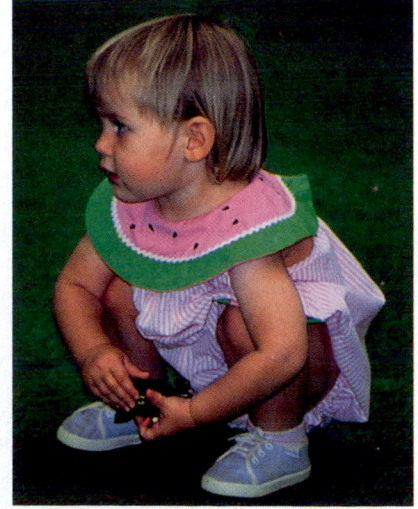

Figure 21–6 ➤ A young child with an uncorrected or partially corrected defect that reduces pulmonary blood flow may squat (assumes a knee–chest position) to reduce systemic blood flow return to the heart.

Table 21–5

PATHOPHYSIOLOGY, CLINICAL MANIFESTATIONS, AND CLINICAL THERAPY FOR MIXED DEFECTS

Defect Pathophysiology, Clinical Manifestations, and Clinical Therapy   **Anatomy**

TRANSPOSITION OF THE GREAT ARTERIES (TGA)

The pulmonary artery is the outflow tract for the left ventricle, and the aorta is the outflow tract for the right ventricle, creating parallel circulations. The condition is life threatening at birth, and survival initially depends on an open ductus arteriosus and foramen ovale. This condition occurs in about 5% of children with congenital heart disease (Park, 2002). An ASD or VSD may also be present with TGA.

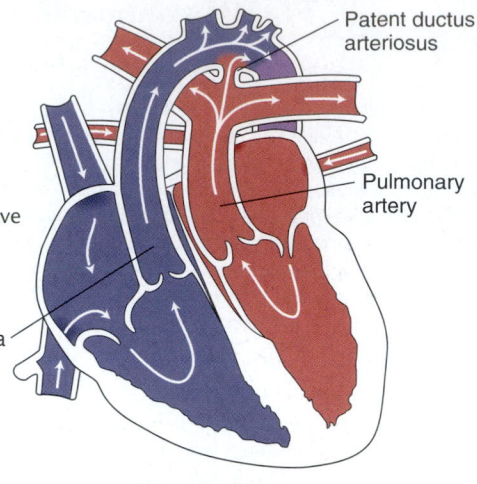

Clinical Manifestations

Cyanosis, apparent soon after birth, progresses to hypoxia and acidosis. Cyanosis does not improve with oxygen administration. Cyanosis may be less apparent when a large VSD is present.

CHF may develop immediately or over days or weeks. Tachypnea (60 breaths per minute) is often present without retractions or other signs of dyspnea.

A systolic murmur is present if a VSD is present; no other murmur is generally heard. S2 is loud.

Infants take a long time to feed and need frequent rest periods because of rapid respiratory rate and fatigue.

Growth failure may be evident as early as 2 weeks of age if corrective surgery is not performed.

Diagnostic Procedures

A chest radiograph may reveal a classic egg-shaped heart on a string (narrow superior mediastinum) with enlarged ventricles and increased pulmonary vascular markings.

The ECG reveals right ventricular hypertrophy.

The echocardiogram often shows the abnormal position of the great arteries rising from ventricles.

A hyperoxitest confirms a cyanotic congenital heart defect.

Cardiac catheterization shows increased right ventricular pressure, and the catheter can enter the aorta through the right ventricle.

Blood tests reveal an increased hematocrit and hemoglobin or polycythemia.

Clinical Therapy

Prostaglandin E1 is ordered to maintain a patent ductus arteriosus until a palliative procedure can be performed. Oxygen is administered for severe hypoxemia.

Balloon atrial septostomy may be performed during cardiac catheterization in newborns as a first stage. This may also be corrected surgically. Other defects may be repaired in stages as the infant grows.

Corrective surgery (arterial switch) is usually performed before 1 week of age.

Prognosis: Survival without surgery is impossible. The 5-year survival following an arterial switch is greater than 80% (Park, 2002). Arrhythmias, decreased right ventricular function, pulmonary vascular disease, and sudden death are long-term complications after the Mustard and Senning procedures, so follow-up every 6 to 12 months is needed (Park, 2002). Other complications of surgical repair include pulmonary artery or aortic stenosis, coronary artery obstruction, and mitral regurgitation. Infective endocarditis prophylaxis may be necessary.

TRUNCUS ARTERIOSUS

A single large vessel empties both ventricles and provides circulation for the pulmonary, systemic, and coronary circulations. A VSD is usually present. This occurs in less than 1% of congenital heart defects (Park, 2002).

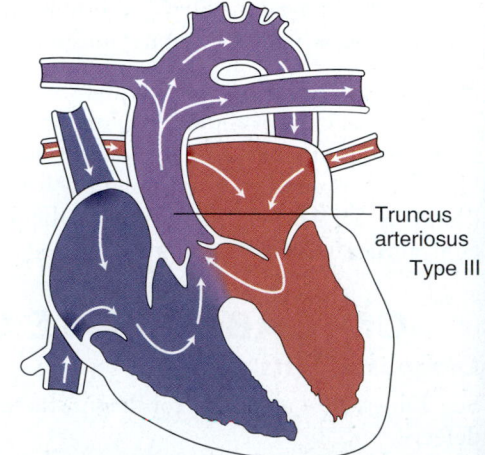

Clinical Manifestations

Cyanosis develops soon after birth; however, this is also a condition of increased pulmonary blood flow. Severe CHF, dyspnea, retractions, fatigue, poor feeding, poor growth, polycythemia, clubbing, increased pulse pressure, bounding peripheral pulses, a widened pulse pressure, frequent respiratory infections, and cardiomegaly occur.

The VSD produces a harsh systolic murmur in the lower sternal border. A systolic click may be heard in the apex and pulmonic area.

Diagnostic Procedures

The chest radiograph shows cardiomegaly, a large aorta, and increased pulmonary vascular markings.

The ECG reveals right and left ventricular hypertrophy.

The echocardiogram shows the absence of two semilunar valves.

Cardiac catheterization documents a left-to-right shunt at the level of the ventricle, equal pressure in the ventricles, the truncus, and pulmonary arteries.

Clinical Therapy

A Rastelli procedure is performed to close the VSD and create a passage to pulmonary arteries. Repeated surgery is necessary to enlarge the pulmonary artery conduit.

Digoxin and diuretics are given.

Prognosis: Survival is improved, but truncal valve stenosis and regurgitation result. The long-term prognosis is unknown. The child should not participate in competitive sports.

Table 21–5	PATHOPHYSIOLOGY, CLINICAL MANIFESTATIONS, AND CLINICAL THERAPY FOR MIXED DEFECTS (continued)

Defect Pathophysiology, Clinical Manifestations, and Clinical Therapy   **Anatomy**

TOTAL ANOMALOUS PULMONARY VENOUS RETURN

The pulmonary veins empty into the right atrium or veins leading to the right atrium rather than into the left atrium. The foramen ovale must remain patent for mixed blood from the right atrium to pass to the systemic circulation. Any obstruction of the pulmonary veins increases the condition's severity. It occurs in about 1% of children with a congenital heart defect (Park, 2002).

Clinical Manifestations

Mild cyanosis and frequent respiratory infections occur. Increased cyanosis may occur with feedings as the filled esophagus compresses the common pulmonary vein.

If the pulmonary veins are obstructed in any way, cyanosis will be increased. Increased pulmonary blood flow will result in signs of CHF.

A precordial bulge may be palpated. The S2 has a wide, fixed split when there is no pulmonary vein obstruction. An ejection murmur and gallop rhythm may be heard in the pulmonic area.

Diagnostic Procedures

The chest radiograph shows cardiac enlargement, a large pulmonary artery, and increased pulmonary blood flow.

The ECG reveals hypertrophy of the right atrium and ventricle.

The echocardiogram shows enlargement of the right atrium, a patent foramen ovale, and lack of connection between the pulmonary veins and left atrium.

Cardiac catheterization shows a higher oxygen level in the right atrium and the abnormal circulation.

Clinical Therapy

Prostaglandin E1 is given to maintain patent ductus arteriosus.

Hypoxemia and CHF are treated.

Balloon atrial septostomy may be performed to promote better mixing of blood so surgery can be delayed until the infant is stabilized.

Surgery to reconnect or baffle the pulmonary veins to the left atrium is performed.

Prognosis: Survivors have lived more than 20 years after correction.

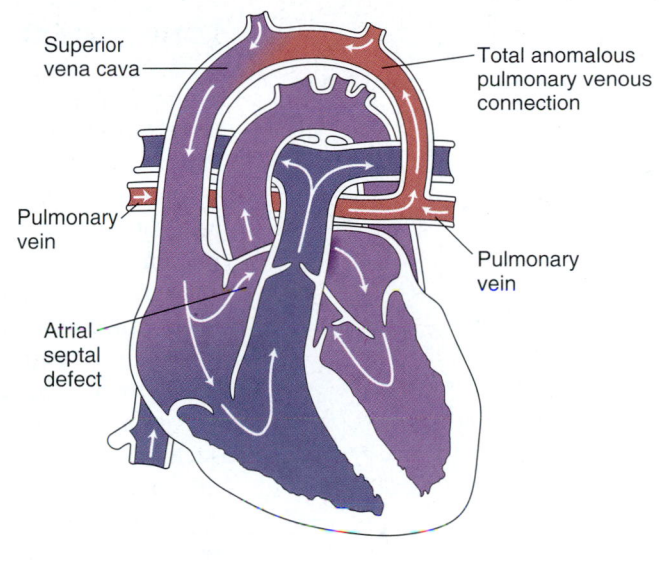

opportunity to grow and improve the success of corrective surgery. See Figure 21–7 ➤ for various palliative shunts (surgically created channels for blood flow) that may be performed. See Tables 21–4 and 21–5 for clinical therapy for specific congenital heart defects. Antibiotic prophylaxis for infective endocarditis is needed before and after surgical correction for many of these defects.

If closure of the ductus arteriosus causes life-threatening cyanosis in newborns, prostaglandin E1 (PGE1) is given to reopen the ductus arteriosus and to improve pulmonary or systemic blood flow. Treatment with PGE1 provides time to transfer the newborn to a cardiac center for diagnostic evaluation and medical or surgical intervention. The child's hemoglobin and hematocrit values are monitored for polycythemia or anemia. If the blood viscosity becomes too high, red cell pheresis may be performed. These infants also do not tolerate anemia well as they have less oxygen-carrying hemoglobin.

Hypercyanotic episodes are aggressively treated. To decrease the pulmonary vascular resistance, the initial treatment involves calming the child, giving oxygen, and administering morphine and propranolol intravenously. Packed red blood cells may be administered to improve oxygen delivery to the

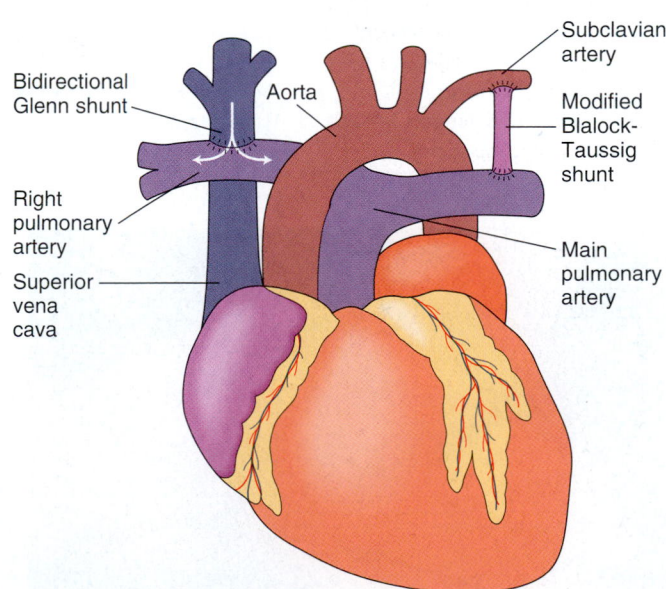

Figure 21–7 ➤ Anatomic location of the modified Blalock-Taussig and Glenn shunts for palliative procedures.

tissues when the child is anemic. Postpone all unpleasant procedures. To increase the systemic vascular resistance, the infant is placed in knee–chest position and given intravenous fluids to expand circulatory volume. Dopamine or phenylephrine (Neosynephrine) is also given. Once a hypercyanotic episode has occurred, immediate palliative or corrective surgery is often scheduled.

LONG-TERM CLINICAL THERAPY   Children with complex congenital heart defects require long-term care following palliative or corrective heart surgery. Some need multiple stages of surgery, revisions of previous surgeries, valve replacements, or interventional cardiac catheterization to reopen valves or vessels that have become stenotic. Some children need an implanted pacemaker for arrhythmias that may be associated with anomalies of the conduction system or unavoidable surgical incisions in areas of the sinoatrial node or sinoventricular node, such as occurred with Tina in the opening scenario. The Mustard, Senning, and Fontan procedures, as well as tetralogy of Fallot (TOF) repairs, are associated with increased risk of arrhythmias. A pacemaker or an implantable cardioverter-defibrillator may be used in older children with life-threatening ventricular arrhythmias, as described for Tina in the opening scenario (Gregoratos, Abrams, Epstein et al., 2002).

Infants with complex congenital heart defects, in conjunction with conditions such as congestive heart failure, prolonged hypoxemia, profound acidosis, or low cardiac output, increase the infant's risk for long-term neurologic sequelae. Inadequate nutrition during the first year of life may affect brain development during the period of most rapid brain growth. Cardiopulmonary bypass and deep hypothermic circulatory arrest used in most surgery may cause insult to the neurologic system, such as intraventricular hemorrhage. Seizures have been noted in the immediate postoperative period (Connor, Arons, Figueroa et al., 2004).

Most preschool and school-age survivors of congenital heart disease have average intelligence abilities. Some children with complex defects such as transposition of the great arteries (TGA) and single ventricles have an increased risk for neurodevelopmental problems (Forbess, Visconti, Hancock-Friesen, et al., 2002). Visuospatial, visual-motor, and speech deficits may be present even when IQ scores are within normal ranges.

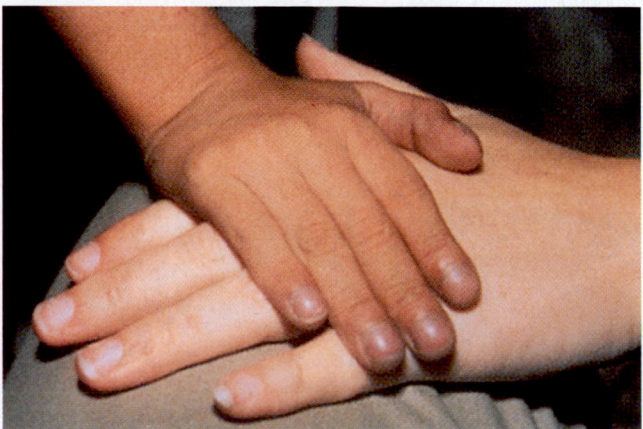

Figure 21–8 ➤ Clubbing of the fingers in an older child is one manifestation of a heart defect that reduces pulmonary blood flow.

> **NURSING ALERT**
>
> Common side effects of PGE₁ therapy include cutaneous vasodilation, bradycardia, tachycardia, hypotension, seizure activity, fever, and apnea.

NURSING MANAGEMENT

Nursing management of the hospitalized child focuses on monitoring PGE1 therapy for newborns, treating hypercyanotic episodes, supporting families to care for the child at home, and providing postsurgical care.

Nursing Assessment and Diagnosis
Physiologic Assessment Before Surgery

Newborns receiving PGE1 therapy are cared for in an intensive care nursery where their cardiovascular status can be closely monitored until palliative procedures are performed.

Prior to or between stages of surgery, the infant or child is seen regularly to assess growth, and for signs of deterioration in cardiac status. These children are at risk for growth problems that affect height and weight, and potentially the head circumference, so measurements need to be plotted on the same growth curve to monitor the significance of the growth problems.

The child needs careful observation for signs of increased cyanosis in the morning or at other high-risk times. Observe for neurologic signs of thromboembolism due to polycythemia such as headache, dizziness, excessive irritability, and paralysis. Older children with cyanotic defects may have clubbing of the fingers and toes (Figure 21–8 ➤).

Assessment Following Surgery

Children are admitted to the intensive care unit following surgery. Refer to the section on post-surgery nursing assessment of the child with increased pulmonary blood flow on page 755 for nursing care guidelines. Once the child returns to the general nursing unit, monitor the child's heart functioning. Assess vital signs, pulse oximetry, skin color, and skin perfusion by capillary refill and distal pulses. Monitoring fluid intake and output following surgery is critical. A sudden sustained increase in pulse and respirations and a decrease in peripheral perfusion may be early signs of hemorrhage. Signs of respiratory distress may indicate the development of a pneumothorax or CHF.

Psychosocial Assessment

Assess the parents' need for information and emotional support. In many cases, the infant's condition is first identified at birth; however, a defect could have been identified prenatally by sonogram. The parents will be grieving the loss of a perfect newborn and be extremely anxious about the infant's condition and prognosis. See Evidence-Based Practice: Parental Stress Associated with Having a Child with a Congenital Heart Defect.

Examples of nursing diagnoses that may apply to a child with decreased pulmonary blood flow include:

- Decreased Cardiac Output related to ventricular restriction and an obstructed outflow tract
- Risk for Infection related to unfiltered bacteria in the blood and sites of blood shunting that promote bacterial growth
- Caregiver Role Strain related to care of a child with chronic illness
- Activity Intolerance related to cyanosis and dyspnea on exertion
- Delayed Growth and Development related to congenital anomaly and hypoxemia

Planning and Implementation
Home Care of the Child Before Surgery

Infants with tetralogy of Fallot and other serious defects are often managed at home to grow and potentially improve surgical outcome. Parents are usually anxious during the wait for surgery. They may fear that the infant will not survive until surgery or that they will be unable to manage any problems the infant may have. Provide information and teach parents how to care for the infant at home. Arrange for home healthcare nursing and other community services that may be required. Many of these children require supplemental nutrition. Oxygen is available only for emergencies as it has no effect on improving the child's usual oxygen saturation level.

Promoting Development

Cyanosis with or without congestive heart failure often results in delayed gross motor skills. Make referrals to community-based early-intervention programs to help parents learn about realistic developmental goals and to promote the child's development. Encourage parents to treat the infant as normally as possible. Children with mild cyanotic lesions do not need to adjust activity. The child with moderate to severe disease should be able to tolerate crying for a few minutes without difficulty.

Caring for a Hypercyanotic Episode

Teach parents to observe for signs of worsening cyanosis, particularly in the morning, that could signal the beginning of a hypercyanotic episode. Provide guidelines for the initial care of the hypercyanotic episode. The parents should call for an ambulance and try to calm and reassure the infant. The infant should be placed in knee–chest position by holding the infant facing the chest, placing one arm under the knees, and folding the legs upward toward the infant's chest. Use the other arm to support the infant's back. If oxygen is available, provide it in a manner that does not further upset the infant. If none is available in the home it will be administered in the ambulance during transport to the emergency department.

An emergency plan should be developed for the infant in anticipation of acute problems such as a hypercyanotic episode or respiratory distress, and parents should

> ### CLINICAL TIP
> Crying may improve cyanosis caused by lung disease or disorders of the central nervous system. In children with cyanotic heart disease, crying usually makes the cyanosis worse. Prolonged crying should not be permitted because it causes fatigue and further hypoxia.

> ### NURSING ALERT
> Hypercyanotic episodes become life threatening if not treated immediately. The child who becomes progressively more hypoxic and limp, and loses consciousness, may have a seizure or cerebrovascular accident and die. If they occur when the infant is at home, parents should begin recommended treatment and call 9-1-1 or their emergency number.

EVIDENCE-BASED PRACTICE

Parental Stress Associated with Having a Child with a Congenital Heart Defect

Clinical Question

Do parents of a child with a congenital heart defect have any more or less stress than parents with children having other chronic conditions?

Evidence

Prior studies identified that parents of infants with congenital heart defects reported higher stress than parents of children with cystic fibrosis or cleft lip and/or cleft palate (Goldberg, Morris, Simmons et al., 1990; Pelchat, Ricard, Bouchard et al., 1999). A 36-item self-report Parenting Stress Index (PSI) was used recently to measure the amount of stress experienced by parents of young children with congenital heart defects. The PSI has three subscales to help interpret findings: parental distress, parent-child dysfunctional interaction, and difficult child. The 80 parents of children with congenital heart disease reported significantly greater stress than the parent population in whom the PSI had been normalized; and 17.5% reported a total stress score at or above the 90th percentile. The parents also had significantly higher stress scores for the Difficult Child subscale. Parenting stress was not related to the severity of the child's heart disease (Uzark & Jones, 2003). A second study compared the parents of 26 children with a complex heart defect requiring multiple surgeries and 32 children with a simple defect (ventricular septal defect) requiring a single surgery. No significant differences were found in parental stress (even when scores of mothers and fathers were analyzed separately) by the type of their child's congenital heart defect (Mörelius, Lundh, & Nelson, 2002). These findings were consistent with those of a study that included children with 11 different types of congenital heart defects (Davis, Brown, Bakeman, & Campbell, 1998).

Implications

The heart is known to be an organ essential for survival, so it is appropriate for parents to be fearful of their child's survival. However, these studies reveal that most parents of children with congenital heart defects do have significant stress, and the stress is not related to the severity of the heart defect. It is therefore an important nursing role to identify factors that could contribute to the parent's stress and help them find coping mechanisms. Families need information about the child's condition that is reinforced in future visits, especially when the child has a simple heart defect. Allow the parents to tell their stories of living with the child to help understand their stresses and strengths. A family assessment may help identify social supports, strengths, and resources available (see Chapter 2 ∞). Encourage the parents to raise the child as close to normal as possible. Help them by providing age-appropriate expectations about development and activity and discussing strategies for discipline.

Critical Thinking

Refer back to Tina's story in the opening scenario. What stresses do you believe Tina's parents experienced at the time of her birth? What stresses and concerns did they experience when Tina developed a complication of her congenital heart disease? Identify two nursing interventions to help this family cope with Tina's current health status, and to help a family with an infant having a serious congenital heart defect.

---

learn cardiopulmonary resuscitation. The local rescue squad should be informed about the presence of a child with special needs in the community. Provide the parents with a card or brief history form with information about the child's condition, medications, necessary emergency care, and the physician's name so emergency care providers have vital information for medical care.

Preventing Serious Illnesses

Teach parents to report signs of illness to the physician. Vomiting and diarrhea may lead to dehydration, which is a particular risk in children with polycythemia because the blood can become even more viscous. Fever increases the metabolic rate and causes further stress on the heart. Aggressive management with antipyretic medication and fluid volume replacement is sometimes necessary. Signs of infective endocarditis (low-grade fever, fatigue, and malaise) occurring within 2 months of surgery or a high-risk procedure should be reported. Parents should be taught about the need to request antibiotic prophylaxis for the child.

Although parents may travel with cyanotic children, they should talk with the physician before taking them to areas of high altitude. Supplemental oxygen when traveling on an airplane may be necessary.

Hospital-Based Care of the Infant and Child

If a hypercyanotic episode occurs in an infant or toddler prior to surgery, immediately place the child in the knee–chest position and administer oxygen. Administer morphine as ordered. Immediately notify the physician for further orders if these procedures are ineffective and the episode continues. Avoid any unpleasant or anxiety-provoking procedures.

Following surgery, the child is initially cared for in the intensive care unit until heart function has stabilized. Once the child returns to the general nursing unit, nursing care is the same as described for the child having surgery for increased pulmonary blood flow. See page 755.

Evaluation

Examples of expected nursing care outcomes include the following:

- The parents recognize a hypercyanotic episode and initiate appropriate emergency treatment.
- The parents manage fever and medical illnesses to prevent dehydration and thromboembolism.
- The child becomes stable following surgery and has no complications.
- The child attains expected development following surgical repair of the congenital heart defect.

Defects Obstructing Systemic Blood Flow

Etiology and Pathophysiology

An anatomic stenosis of the aorta causes obstruction to blood flow and results in a pressure load on the left ventricle and decreased cardiac output. The greater the narrowing, the more obstructed blood flow is to the circulation. This results in higher pressure in the ventricle and decreased cardiac output. Neonates with severe left outflow obstruction or left ventricular dysfunction may develop decreased cardiac output and shock.

Clinical Manifestations

Low cardiac output is responsible for the following clinical manifestations: diminished pulses, poor color, delayed capillary refill time, and decreased urinary output. The blood cannot move past the obstruction, so it backs up into the left atrium and then the lungs, causing congestive heart failure and pulmonary edema. In children with mild obstruction, the child may have leg cramps, cooler feet than hands, and stronger pulses and higher blood pressure in the upper extremities than the lower extremities. Decreased blood supply to the gastrointestinal tract may lead to necrotizing enterocolitis. See Chapter 24 ∞. See Table 21–6 for the pathophysiology, clinical manifestations, and clinical therapy for the congenital heart defects that obstruct systemic blood flow.

Collaborative Care

See Table 21–6 for diagnostic tests and clinical therapy for these individual defects.

PGE1 and inotropic medications may be required to support the newborn's systemic circulation until the obstruction is relieved or ventricular function improves.

Children with hypoplastic left heart syndrome who have survived because of palliative surgery or heart transplant often have seizures, decreased IQ scores, or cerebral palsy. They may also have renal failure, complete heart block, respiratory failure, and sepsis (Connor, Arons, Figueroa et al., 2004).

Nursing Management

Children with aortic stenosis and coarctation of the aorta should have nursing care as described in the nursing management of defects that increase pulmonary blood flow on page 753. Infants with hypoplastic left heart syndrome (HLHS) should have nursing care as described in the nursing management of defects that decrease pulmonary blood flow and mixed defects on page 762.

Parents of children with life-threatening defects such as HLHS must make decisions very quickly about the best treatment for their child. There is no cure, and a decision must be made that is best for their individual situation (palliative care, Norwood procedure, or heart transplant). Parents are faced with the potential death of the newborn before having an opportunity to grieve the loss of a normal infant. Parents do not have much time to carefully weigh the information about the various treatment options. However, it is important to try to support parents through this difficult decision-making period. Share the following information with parents so they are fully informed for decision making: information about each of the treatment options and their associated mortality, the intense care that the surviving child will require, potential cognitive and developmental outcomes, and unknown long-term survival. If parents choose comfort or palliative care,

MediaLink

Health Promotion and Maintenance Overview: The Adolescent with Congenital Heart Disease

CLINICAL TIP

The blood pressure is usually 10 to 15 mmHg higher in the legs than in the arms.

COMPLEMENTARY THERAPY

Congenital Heart Defects

Caution parents of children with congenital heart defects to avoid using complementary therapies such as herbal products that may interfere with the medications prescribed to manage the child's heart condition. Products containing ginkgo are known to interact with warfarin, which is of particular concern for any child on anticoagulant therapy. Full research on many of these herbal remedies has not been conducted, so the potential side effects and interactions with prescribed medications are not known (Cook & Higgins, 2004).

Table 21–6	PATHOPHYSIOLOGY, CLINICAL MANIFESTATIONS, AND CLINICAL THERAPY FOR DEFECTS THAT OBSTRUCT THE SYSTEMIC BLOOD FLOW

Defect Pathophysiology, Clinical Manifestations, and Clinical Therapy   **Anatomy**

AORTIC STENOSIS (AS)

Narrowing of the aortic valve obstructs blood flow to systemic circulation. The valve is often bicuspid rather than tricuspid. The pressure gradient across the valve usually increases as the child grows and cardiac output increases. Aortic stenosis accounts for 3–6% of all cases of congenital heart defects (Park, 2002).

Clinical Manifestations

Most infants and children are asymptomatic with normal growth and development. Life-threatening aortic stenosis is detected in some newborns. CHF develops in infants with significant stenosis.

The blood pressure is normal, but a narrow pulse pressure may be noted. Peripheral pulses may be weak. The child may complain of chest pain after exercise, but exercise intolerance is uncommon. Syncope and dizziness are serious signs that require intervention.

A systolic heart murmur and thrill occur in the aortic or pulmonic areas with transmission to the neck. An ejection click may be heard. Splitting of the S2 may be noted with severe aortic stenosis.

Diagnostic Procedures

The chest radiograph is usually normal, but may reveal a slight prominence of the left ventricle and aorta with increased severity.

The ECG is usually normal in mild cases, but may show mild left ventricular hypertrophy and inverted T waves with increased severity.

An echocardiogram reveals the number of the valve cusps, pressure gradient across valve, and size of aorta.

Stress testing may be used in asymptomatic children to determine the amount of obstruction present with exercise.

Clinical Therapy

Newborns with life-threatening aortic stenosis need PGE1 to maintain a patent ductus arteriosus until the aortic valve can be dilated.

The aortic valve may be successfully dilated by balloon valvuloplasty during cardiac catheterization. Surgical valvuloplasty may also be performed. Surgical treatment is palliative rather than curative.

Aortic valve replacement is performed when stenosis is severe or if significant regurgitation results from other interventions.

Prognosis: Chest pain, syncope, and sudden death can occur in symptomatic children, particularly during vigorous exercise. Stenosis is usually progressive during childhood as the valve calcifies. Valve replacement may be necessary once the child reaches adulthood, requiring lifelong anticoagulant therapy. Lifelong infective endocarditis prophylaxis is required.

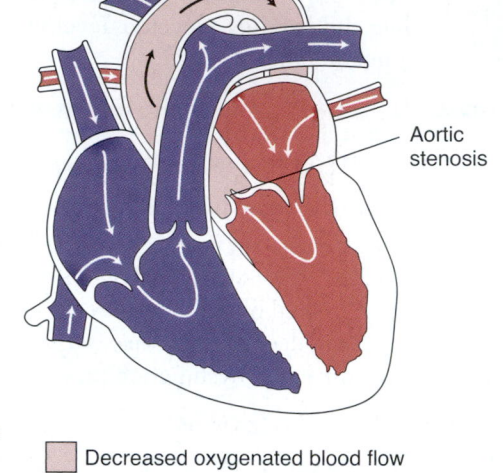

Aortic stenosis

☐ Decreased oxygenated blood flow

☐ Mixed oxygenated and unoxygenated blood

COARCTATION OF THE AORTA (COA)

Narrowing or constriction in the descending aorta, often near the ductus arteriosus or left subclavian artery, obstructs the systemic blood outflow. This defect is common, occurring in 5% of all children with congenital heart disease (Rome & Kreutzer, 2004). Up to 30% of girls with Turner syndrome have COA (Park, 2002).

Coarctation of aorta

Clinical Manifestations

Many children are asymptomatic and grow normally, but constriction is progressive. Up to 30% of infants develop CHF by 3 months of age.

Blood pressure in legs is lower than in the arms. Brachial and radial pulses are typically bounding, but femoral pulses are weak or absent. Older children may complain of weakness and pain in the legs after exercise.

S2 is loud and single on auscultation. A systolic ejection murmur may be heard at the upper right and middle or lower left sternal border. A thrill may be palpated in the suprasternal notch.

Diagnostic Procedures

The chest radiograph may reveal cardiomegaly, pulmonary venous congestion, and indentation of the descending aorta. Rib notching is rarely seen before 10 years of age. MRI shows the site of coarctation.

ECG shows left ventricular hypertrophy; right ventricular hypertrophy may be seen in severe cases.

Echocardiogram shows the size of the aorta, the actual coarctation, and the function of the aortic valve and left ventricle.

Clinical Therapy

Balloon dilation occurs during cardiac catheterization for initial relief and re-coarctation. Balloon dilation on infants under 3 months of age may be performed through the umbilical artery to avoid injury to the femoral artery (Rao, Jureidini, Balfour et al., 2003).

Surgical resection with end-to-end anastomosis or with patching using the subclavian artery may be performed. Repair in the first year of life is preferred to decrease exposure to hypertension.

Prognosis: If coarctation recurs, balloon valvuloplasty is usually performed. Persistent hypertension in adulthood is common. Infective endocarditis prophylaxis is needed.

Table 21–6	PATHOPHYSIOLOGY, CLINICAL MANIFESTATIONS, AND CLINICAL THERAPY FOR DEFECTS THAT OBSTRUCT THE SYSTEMIC BLOOD FLOW (continued)

Defect Pathophysiology, Clinical Manifestations, and Clinical Therapy	Anatomy

HYPOPLASTIC LEFT HEART SYNDROME (HLHS)

This is one of the most severe defects with absence or stenosis of mitral and aortic valves, an abnormally small left ventricle, a small aorta, and aortic or mitral stenosis or atresia. It occurs in 1% of congenital heart defects (Park, 2002).

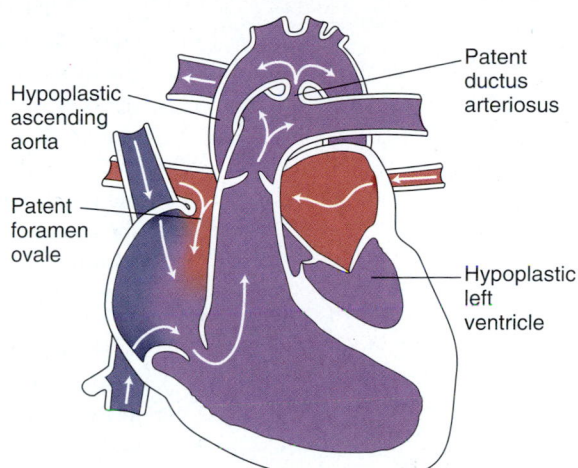

Clinical Manifestations

With closure of the ductus arteriosus the newborn has progressive cyanosis, tachycardia, tachypnea, dyspnea, retractions, and decreased peripheral pulses.

A systolic murmur may be present or absent.

Poor peripheral perfusion, pulmonary edema, and CHF lead to shock, acidosis, and death.

Diagnostic Procedures

The chest radiograph shows cardiomegaly and increased pulmonary vascularity.

The echocardiogram shows the small left ventricle. This condition may be diagnosed prenatally.

Cardiac catheterization may be performed in preparation of surgical intervention or to perform an atrial septostomy to promote blood mixing.

Clinical Therapy

Prostaglandin E1 is given to maintain a patent ductus arteriosus.

Supplemental oxygen is avoided.

Three treatment options include comfort or palliative care, the Norwood procedure, and heart transplantation.

Many infants waiting for a heart transplant die because of the scarcity of donor hearts.

The Norwood procedure has become a more common intervention as outcomes have improved. Surgery is performed in three stages. The Norwood procedure is performed in the first week of life, followed by the Glenn procedure at about 3 to 8 months of age, and the Fontan procedure at between 18 months and 3 years of age.

Prognosis: Without surgery, the median survival time is 3 days. HLHS is the largest contributor of infant deaths due to congenital heart disease. Mortality rates in infants having a first stage Norwood procedure are approximately 10–20% in the first year of life (Cook & Higgins, 2004). Some large centers have achieved a 70% 5-year survival rate with the Norwood procedure (Chang, Chen, & Klitzner, 2002). The child will have some limitations in physical activity because of a single ventricle. Many children have significant neurocognitive and neurodevelopmental impairment whether treated with transplantation or staged Fontan procedure (Mahle, Visconti, Freier et al., 2006; Shillingford & Wernovsky, 2004; Ikle, Hale, Fashaw et al., 2003). Failure of the single ventricle occurs over time, and these children may require a heart transplant during adolescence or adulthood.

interventions such as PGE1 are discontinued and the infant is given appropriate pain medication and comfort. Seek the support of clergy, social workers, or other supportive individuals in the family's life to assist them through this period. Reassure parents that they are good parents, no matter what decision they make. See Chapter 14 ∞.

CONGESTIVE HEART FAILURE

Congestive heart failure (CHF) is a disorder of circulation in which cardiac output is inadequate to support the body's circulatory and metabolic needs. It may result from a congenital heart defect that causes increased blood flow to the lungs or obstructed blood flow to the systemic circulation, from problems with heart contractility, or from pathologic conditions that require high cardiac output, such as severe anemia, acidosis, or respiratory disease. In addition, CHF results from acquired heart disease such as cardiomyopathy or Kawasaki disease.

Etiology and Pathophysiology

Blood volume overloads associated with congenital heart defects are the most common cause of congestive heart failure in infants. Up to 90% of infants who develop CHF do so within the first 6 to 12 months of life (Connor, 2006). Some defects allow blood to flow from the left side of the heart to the right so that extra blood must be pumped to the pulmonary system rather than through the aorta when the left ventricle contracts.

This overloads the pulmonary system, and if prolonged can lead to pulmonary artery hypertension, an often irreversible condition leading to life-threatening pulmonary vascular resistance (pulmonary artery hypertension is discussed on page 777). Obstructive congenital defects (i.e., abnormally small pulmonary vessels) restrict the flow of blood so the heart muscle hypertrophies to work harder and force blood through these structures.

When cardiac output remains insufficient, the body's organs and tissues do not receive adequate oxygen. The muscle tone in the veins increases to improve blood return to the heart. Blood flow to the kidneys, skin, spleen, and extremities is reduced by the sympathetic nervous system. The kidneys respond to the lowered circulating volume by activating the renin-angiotensin mechanism to retain salt and water. A sympathetic response increases the heart rate, heart muscle contractility, and peripheral vascular resistance to maintain blood flow to the heart, brain, and lungs (Connor, 2006). Without intervention, the compensatory mechanisms increase their intensity, demanding more effort from the compromised heart. This results in progressive systemic edema and pulmonary congestion. Initially one side of the heart may fail, but eventually failure is bilateral.

Clinical Manifestations

Congestive heart failure often develops subtly, and symptoms may not be recognized at first. The infant tires easily, especially during feeding. Weight loss or lack of normal weight gain, diaphoresis, irritability, and frequent infections may be evident. Older children may have exercise intolerance, dyspnea, abdominal pain or distention, and peripheral edema. See the clinical manifestations table below.

As the disease progresses, symptoms such as tachypnea, tachycardia, pallor or cyanosis, nasal flaring, grunting, retractions, cough, or crackles may occur. Generalized fluid volume overload is seen more commonly in toddlers and older children. Periorbital and facial edema and hepatomegaly are signs of fluid volume excess. Jugular vein distention is seen in older children.

Cardiomegaly, enlargement of the heart by hypertrophy of its walls, occurs as the heart attempts to maintain cardiac output. Cyanosis, weak peripheral pulses, cool extremities, hypotension, and heart murmur are precursors of cardiogenic shock, which can occur if congestive heart failure is not adequately treated. (Cardiogenic shock is discussed on page 793.)

■ COLLABORATIVE CARE

Diagnostic Tests

Diagnosis is based primarily on clinical manifestations such as tachycardia, respiratory distress, and crackles. A chest radiograph study reveals cardiac enlargement and venous congestion or signs of pulmonary edema. Echocardiography may be performed to diagnose specific cardiac defects or dysfunction. An electrocardiogram may show tachycardia, bradycardia, or ventricular hypertrophy.

Clinical Therapy

The goals of medical management are to make the heart work more efficiently and to remove excess fluid. This decreases the heart's work and improves systemic circulation

CLINICAL MANIFESTATIONS	CONGESTIVE HEART FAILURE
Cause	**Clinical Manifestation**
Pulmonary venous congestion	Tachypnea, wheezing, crackles, retractions, cough, grunting, nasal flaring, feeding difficulties, irritability, tiring with play
Systemic venous congestion	Hepatomegaly, ascites, peripheral edema
Impaired cardiac output	Tachycardia, diminished pulses, hypotension, capillary refill time greater than 2 seconds, pallor, cool extremities, oliguria
High metabolic rate	Failure to thrive or slow weight gain

without flooding the pulmonary system. Diuretics, such as furosemide, chlorothiazide, and spironolactone, are given to promote fluid excretion. Because most diuretics (except for spironolactone) cause potassium loss, serum potassium levels are monitored and potassium supplements may be ordered.

Inotropic medicines (agents that improve the velocity of contractility of the heart) and afterload-reducing agents (angiotensin-converting enzyme inhibitors) are sometimes used to lessen the heart's workload and help it to work more efficiently.

Digoxin is the drug most commonly used to improve the heart's ability to contract and therefore increase its output. Occasionally a higher-than-normal dose is given initially, followed by a lower maintenance dose. This process, called **digitalization**, helps the child achieve therapeutic blood levels more quickly. Beta-blockers such as propanolol and carvediol may be used to treat chronic heart failure (Azeka, Ramires, Valler et al., 2002). See Medications Used to Treat CHF below.

Surgery or interventional cardiac catheterization to correct a congenital heart defect may become the treatment of choice. Cardiac transplantation may be performed for children with end-stage cardiomyopathy or complex congenital heart defects such as hypoplastic left heart syndrome.

Other medical therapy is supportive. Airway management, ventilatory support, rest, and fluid and dietary management are also part of the treatment plan. Oxygen may be ordered (Figure 21–9 ➤). Most children improve rapidly after medication is administered.

> **NURSING ALERT**
>
> Digoxin and digitoxin are both digitalis preparations but are not the same drug. Digoxin is the drug of choice in pediatrics. Digitoxin is 10 times more powerful than digoxin, and is rarely used in children. Read labels carefully and double-check doses to ensure that you give the child the right dose of the right drug.

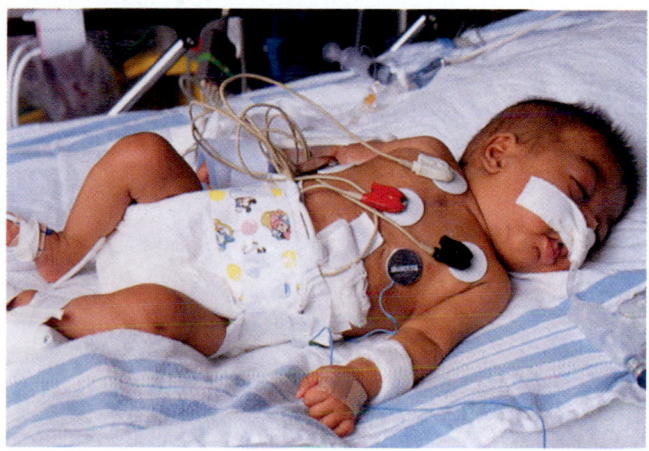

Figure 21–9 ➤ Jooti is receiving intravenous fluids and oxygen. Her condition is being continuously monitored for congestive heart failure.

■ # NURSING MANAGEMENT

Nursing Assessment and Diagnosis

As diagnosis of CHF depends primarily on physical symptoms, nursing observations are important. Psychosocial assessment is important in learning how the family is coping with the demands and stresses of the child's condition.

MEDICATIONS USED TO TREAT *Congestive Heart Failure*

Drug	Action
Digoxin	Increases myocardial contractility by improving systemic circulation
Furosemide	Rapid diuresis

Thiazides
    Chlorothiazide (suspension)
    Hydrochlorthiazide (tablets)
	Maintenance diuresis, decreases absorption of sodium, water, potassium, chloride, and bicarbonate in renal tubules

Spironolactone	Maintenance diuresis (potassium-sparing)
ACE (angiotensin-converting enzyme) inhibitor	Promotes vascular relaxation and reduced peripheral vascular resistance
Propranolol	Increases contractility
Carvedilol	Improves left ventricular function, promotes vasodilation of systemic circulation for chronic heart failure and dilated cardiomyopathy

Physiologic Assessment

Assess the child's vital signs, behavioral patterns (e.g., playfulness, irritability), cardiac function, respiratory function, and fluid status using the guidelines on page 745. Use the age-specific heart and respiratory rates in Chapter 5 ∞ to identify tachycardia and tachypnea. Obtain a detailed history of the onset of symptoms from the parents, as CHF often develops slowly.

Psychosocial Assessment

Take a history of the child's previous hospitalizations and assess the family's knowledge about the child's condition. Families of children with CHF are anxious and fear the potentially serious outcome of the problem and the need to provide ongoing care. Assess the family's anxiety level and coping strategies. Evaluate the family's economic status. Medication is crucial to treatment, and a family's inability to afford or obtain the necessary medications jeopardizes the child's survival.

Developmental Assessment

Since fatigue limits the activities of the child with CHF, the child does not have the opportunity to practice the skills needed to attain normal developmental milestones. Assess development with a tool such as the Denver II (see Chapter 7 ∞). In addition, parents can provide information about the attainment of expected developmental milestones such as sitting, manipulating objects, standing, or walking. When CHF is well controlled, the child's energy level increases and developmental skills often improve. In infants and toddlers, assessments every 2 to 3 months are useful to observe development and evaluate disease management.

Parents may limit the child's contact with other children because of frequent infections and exercise intolerance. Ask parents about contact and play with other children and a typical day's activity schedule.

Several nursing diagnoses that may apply to the child with congestive heart failure can be found in the accompanying Nursing Care Plan. The primary nursing diagnosis is decreased cardiac output related to cardiac anomaly.

Planning and Implementation

Nursing care for the child with congestive heart failure focuses on administering and monitoring effects of medications, maintaining adequate oxygenation and myocardial function, promoting rest, fostering development, providing adequate nutrition, and providing emotional support to the child and family. The Nursing Care Plan that follows summarizes the nursing care for the child who is hospitalized with CHF.

Administer and Monitor Prescribed Medications

Children with CHF usually receive digoxin and furosemide. These medications are potent and must be correctly administered. Observe the child carefully for digoxin toxicity. Early signs include cardiac arrhythmias in children. Early indicators in adults (nausea, vomiting, anorexia, diarrhea, visual disturbance) are rarely the initial signs of toxicity in children. Serum digoxin levels are taken 6 to 8 hours after a dose. A therapeutic serum level ranges from 0.8 to 2 ng/mL; levels over 2 ng/mL are toxic (Bindler, Howry, Wilson et al., 2005). Monitor serum digoxin levels closely during antibiotic therapy as altered intestinal flora may precipitate digoxin toxicity.

Measure intake and output carefully. Weigh the infant's diapers before and after changing to measure urine output (1 g = 1 mL urine). Observe for changes in peripheral edema and circulation. Weigh the child daily at the same time. If ascites is present, take serial abdominal measurements to monitor changes. Turn the child frequently, and provide skin care when edema is present (see Figure 16–11 ∞).

Maintain Oxygenation and Myocardial Function

Oxygen therapy may be ordered. Make sure that tubing is patent, the oxygen flow rate is correct, the oxygen delivery device is working properly, and humidification is provided. Keep the child calm and quiet. Position the child in a semi-Fowler's or 45-degree angle position to promote maximum oxygenation.

SKILLS 6–1 THROUGH 6–7
Growth Measurements
SKILL 6–22
Output Measurement

> ### NURSING ALERT
>
> Before giving the digitalizing dose of digoxin, establish baseline vital signs, the quality of peripheral pulses, and clinical symptoms, and also obtain an ECG. Check serum electrolytes, and hepatic and renal function. Assess hydration status, and hydrate if hypovolemic.
>
> Before giving any dose of digoxin, take the apical pulse for 1 minute. If bradycardia is detected (less than 60 to 100 beats/min in children, dependent upon age, less than 60 beats/min in adolescents, or below a guideline noted in the physician's order) or changes in heart rhythm or quality are noted, withhold the medication and call for a physician's advice before administering the drug (Bindler, Howry, Wilson et al., 2005).

NURSING CARE PLAN The Child Hospitalized with Congestive Heart Failure

GOAL	INTERVENTION	RATIONALE	EXPECTED OUTCOME
1. Decreased Cardiac Output related to cardiac anomaly (VSD)			
	NIC Priority Intervention: **Hemodynamic Regulation:** *Optimization of heart rate, preload, afterload, and contractility.*		*NOC Suggested Outcome:* **Cardiac Pump Effectiveness:** *Extent to which blood is ejected from the left ventricle per minute to support systemic perfusion pressure.*
The child's cardiac output will be sufficient to meet the body's metabolic demands.	• Administer digoxin as ordered.	• Digoxin increases contractility of the heart and force of contraction.	The child's cardiac output is sufficient as indicated by increased energy, adequate feeding intake, and decreased edema.
	• Take apical pulse and listen to heart sounds regularly, especially before each dose of digoxin. Record apical pulse with each recorded dose of digoxin.	• Digoxin may cause bradycardia. Pulse and heart sounds provide information about heart functioning.	
	• Use cardiac monitor if ordered.	• Monitor tachycardia and arrhythmias.	
	• Prevent injury by monitoring for digoxin side effects and serum potassium level.	• Digoxin is a potent drug with serious side effects. Hypokalemia increases the risk of digoxin toxicity.	The child maintains normal serum levels of potassium and therapeutic levels of digoxin.
	• Provide for rest periods each hour.	• Rest decreases the need for high cardiac output.	The child rests hourly and has adequate energy to eat and play.
	• Place child in semi-Fowler's position.	• Position facilitates lung expansion.	
The child will manifest adequate oxygenation.	• Evaluate respiratory rate and sounds. Take pulse oximetry readings to determine oxygen saturation.	• Absence of tachypnea and adventitious sounds and oxygen saturation above 95% indicate ease of respiration.	The child has normal respiratory rate for age with no evidence of adventitious sounds or diaphoresis.
	• Provide oxygen and humidification, if ordered. Observe for diaphoresis, a sign of increased respiratory effort.	• Supplemental oxygen decreases tachypnea, and humidification moistens secretions to keep the airway clear.	
2. Excess Fluid Volume related to heart failure			
	NIC Priority Intervention: **Fluid Management:** *Promotion of fluid balance and prevention of complications resulting from abnormal or undesired fluid levels.*		*NOC Suggested Outcome:* **Fluid Balance:** *Balance of water in the intracellular and extracellular compartments of the body.*
The child's peripheral and central edema will decrease. Intake and output will be balanced once excess fluid is excreted.	• Administer diuretics as ordered.	• Diuretics mobilize fluids and facilitate excretion.	The child's intake and output are proportional, and electrolyte levels remain within normal ranges.
	• Weigh daily. Measure abdominal girth daily. Observe for peripheral edema.	• Evaluations demonstrate effectiveness of treatment.	
	• Measure intake and output carefully. Weigh diapers to obtain output of young child.	• Adequate output is a good indicator of renal perfusion.	
	• Maintain fluid-restricted diet if ordered.	• Fluid restriction is sometimes used to decrease cardiac load.	
	• Monitor electrolytes.	• Electrolyte imbalance is common when fluids are restricted and diuretics are given.	

(continued)

NURSING CARE PLAN The Child Hospitalized with Congestive Heart Failure (continued)

GOAL	INTERVENTION	RATIONALE	EXPECTED OUTCOME
3. Risk for Impaired Skin Integrity related to altered fluid status			
	NIC Priority Intervention: **Pressure Management:** *Minimizing pressure to body parts.*		*NOC Suggested Outcome:* **Tissue Integrity: Skin and Mucous Membranes:** *Structural intactness and normal physiologic function of skin and mucous membranes.*
The child's peripheral and central edema will decrease.	• Provide skin care for edematous body parts and elevate extremities.	• Edematous skin injures easily. Elevation promotes return of fluid from extremities.	The child has no skin breakdown after edema resolves.
	• Change child's position frequently.	• Position change promotes circulation to skin over pressure points.	
	• Inspect skin frequently for redness and skin breakdown over pressure points.	• Inspection identifies earliest stages of skin breakdown.	
4. Imbalanced Nutrition: Less than Body Requirements related to high metabolic needs and rapid tiring while feeding			
	NIC Priority Intervention: **Nutrition Management:** *Assistance with or provision of a balanced dietary intake of food and fluids.*		*NOC Suggested Outcome:* **Nutrition Status:** *Extent to which nutrients are available to meet metabolic needs.*
The infant or child will demonstrate normal weight gain for age.	• Hold infant at 45-degree angle for feeding.	• Position facilitates breathing while eating.	The infant or child gains recommended weight according to growth grids. All dietary requirements are met, and mealtimes are pleasant.
	• Record intake carefully.	• Evaluation of intake indicates whether caloric and other nutritional needs are met.	
	• Weigh child daily.	• Weight indicates growth (in absence of edematous symptoms of congestive heart failure).	
	• Give frequent small meals with rest periods in between.	• Digesting small meals requires less energy.	
	• Use high-calorie formula or give high-calorie snacks.	• High-calorie formulas and snacks provide calories efficiently.	
	• Use soothing approaches such as holding infants for feeding and having parents eat with older child.	• Restful approach facilitates intake with minimum cardiac work.	
	• Transition to supplemental nasogastric feeding if the infant is not able to gain weight.	• Nasogastric feeds provide added calories but do not force the infant to use energy to eat.	

NURSING CARE PLAN The Child Hospitalized with Congestive Heart Failure (continued)

GOAL	INTERVENTION	RATIONALE	EXPECTED OUTCOME
5. Compromised Family Coping related to situational crisis with child's disease			
	NIC Priority Intervention: **Caregiver Support:** *Provision of necessary information, advocacy, and support to facilitate primary patient care by someone other than healthcare professional.*		*NOC Suggested Outcome:* **Family Coping:** *Family actions to manage stressors that tax family resources.*
Parents will express lessened anxiety as hospitalization proceeds.	• Encourage parents to room-in or stay with child. Explain procedures and treatment. Involve parents in care as much as possible. Have parents plan child's play periods.	• Involvement in child's care lessens parental anxiety and fear of unknown.	Parents participate in developing and implementing the treatment plan and providing care to the child.
	• At discharge, provide clear instructions and information about what to do in an emergency, and whom and where to call with questions.	• Having resources available provides feelings of security.	
	• Allow parents to verbalize questions, concerns, and feelings. Refer parents to support groups or other resources as needed	• Emotional support is needed to lessen anxiety.	

Promote Rest

Group assessments and interventions together to ensure that the child has some uninterrupted rest each hour. Feedings should last no more than 20 to 30 minutes. Frequent small feedings generally work best, with burping after every half ounce of intake to minimize vomiting. Rocking is restful for infants. Encourage older children to engage in quiet activities such as playing board games or watching television.

Foster Development

Encourage parents to play with the child, using toys to stimulate eye–hand coordination and fine motor movements. Such toys include rattles, blocks, and stuffed animals for infants and books, paper and pencil, and dolls for older children. Encourage sitting, standing, or walking for short periods with adequate rest afterward to promote the development of large muscles. Singing, talking, and playing music facilitate cognitive and language skills.

Provide Adequate Nutrition

Teach parents about feeding techniques. Encourage the mother who chooses to breast-feed the infant, as the antibodies in breast milk reduce infections, and the milk is naturally low in sodium. However, the sucking involved in breast- or bottle-feeding may cause dyspnea that forces the infant to rest frequently during feeding.

Infants should be burped frequently to permit rest and prevent vomiting. In addition, they may need small frequent feedings and longer feeding periods. Make sure parents understand that changes in feeding habits (decreased intake, vomiting, sleeping through feedings, increased perspiration with feedings) may indicate deteriorating cardiac status.

The infant needs adequate nutrition to support growth. Some infants need a higher caloric formula (24 to 30 calories per ounce) to obtain adequate nutrition. It is not unusual for infants with heart problems to develop failure to thrive as the result of feeding difficulties (see Chapter 4 ∞). When infants have significant dyspnea with

CLINICAL TIP

Positioning the baby in an infant seat at a 45-degree angle decreases venous return to the heart and decreases its metabolic demand. This is a favorable position for feeding and interacting with the infant to promote development (Cook & Higgins, 2004).

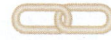

SKILL 12–3
Administering a Gavage/Tube Feeding

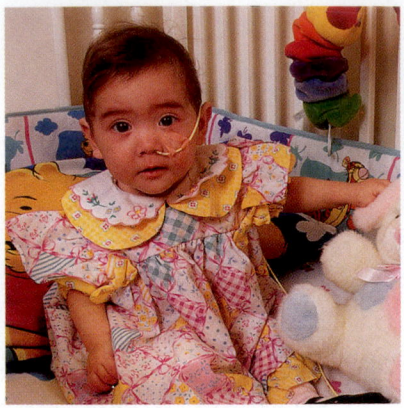

Figure 21–10 ➤ Infants with cardiac conditions often require supplemental feedings to provide sufficient nutrients for growth and development. The parents of this infant girl have been taught how to give her nasogastric feedings at home.

feeding, special feeding techniques are needed such as nutritional supplementation by nasogastric or gastrostomy tube (Figure 21–10 ➤). Parents are often advised to give the infant a chance to feed normally for a specific period. The remainder of the formula is then given by nasogastric or gastrostomy tube.

Provide Emotional Support

When a child is hospitalized with CHF, the family is often anxious about his or her condition. Give parents a chance to express their concerns. Explain the child's treatment regimen, and make sure family members understand the child's need for nutrition and rest. Answering questions about the child's prognosis and the ultimate outcome can be reassuring to some families. Refer parents to the appropriate support groups as talking with parents of children with cardiac conditions may be a source of emotional support.

Discharge Planning and Home Care Teaching

Identify and address home care needs well in advance of discharge. While the child is hospitalized, teach the family about the administration of medications and signs of a worsening condition.

Demonstrate administration of drugs, and then supervise while the parents measure and administer medications. Teach parents about the toxic effects of digoxin and other drugs. Advise them to notify the physician immediately if any of these side effects occur. (See Families Want to Know: Administering Digoxin below.)

Show parents how to feed the child to maximize nutritional intake. Tell them to watch for symptoms such as increased feeding difficulty, irritability, lethargy, breathing difficulty, and puffiness around the eyes or extremities, which indicate that CHF is worsening. Parents are frequently taught to take the child's pulse and to report any significant change to the physician. An increase in pulse rate can signal CHF, and a decrease can indicate digoxin toxicity.

Teach parents to identify signs of dehydration when the child is managed on diuretics. An acute illness could lead to dehydration more quickly when the child takes these medications.

Care in the Community

Parents play a critical role in the care of the child with heart disease by facilitating normal development and limiting the incidence of congestive heart failure. The nursing care plan on the next page summarizes the home care for a child with CHF.

The family is often overprotective and reluctant to leave the child with other caregivers. Find out if a knowledgeable person is available for respite care who can safely administer medications and watch the child. Show the family how to assess the child's energy level, and how to observe for feeding problems and edema. Observe medication administration and correct any errors. Watch the child as he or she feeds and make suggestions as necessary.

FAMILIES WANT TO KNOW

Administering Digoxin

- Take the child's pulse prior to giving digoxin. Report to the physician when the pulse rate falls below or rises above guidelines provided.
- Administer the medication exactly as prescribed at the same time each day. The parents should decide if the medication will be given with food or without food, and be consistent in giving it the same way each day.
- Do not repeat the digoxin dose if the child vomits unless directed to do so by the physician.
- Do not give the child over-the-counter medications for colds, coughs, allergies, GI upset, or obesity without approval.

- Do not give the child on digoxin herbal preparations such as ginseng, ma huang, or ephedra. They interact with digoxin and may cause digoxin toxicity or arrhythmias.
- Keep the medication locked and out of reach of children. In case of accidental ingestion, immediate medical care is needed. Be sure to keep the Poison Control Center number on all phones.
- Remind the child's healthcare providers about the potential interaction between digoxin and certain antibiotics (e.g., tetracycline, erythromycin, clarithromycin, and beta-lactams) so that safe antibiotics can be prescribed when needed (Bindler, Howry, Wilson et al., 2005).

NURSING CARE PLAN   The Child with Congestive Heart Failure Being Cared for at Home

GOAL	INTERVENTION	RATIONALE	EXPECTED OUTCOME
1. Delayed Growth and Development related to effects of physical disability			
	NIC Priority Intervention: **Developmental Enhancement:** *Teaching parents to facilitate optimal gross motor, fine motor, language, cognitive, social, and emotional growth of preschool children.*		*NOC Suggested Outcome:* **Child Development (2 years):** *Milestones of physical, cognitive, and psychosocial progression by 2 years of age.*
The child will meet developmental milestones for age group.	• Perform baseline developmental assessment.	• Assessment provides comparison for later assessments and basis for planning specific games, toys, and activities.	The child displays normal language, fine motor, and gross motor activity.
	• Plan for short play periods after rest.	• Short play periods maintain energy and facilitate play.	
	• Introduce age-appropriate toys and activities such as rattles for infants and blocks for toddlers.	• Play activities facilitate learning and mastery of developmental tasks.	
	• Plan for interactions with healthy children.	• Social skills are learned through contact with others.	
2. Ineffective Therapeutic Regimen Management related to complexity of therapeutic regimen			
	NIC Priority Intervention: **Mutual Goal Setting:** *Collaborating with the family to identify and prioritize care goals, then developing a plan for achieving those goals.*		*NOC Suggested Outcome:* **Compliance Behavior:** *Actions taken on the basis of professional advice to promote wellness, recovery, and rehabilitation.*
Parents will demonstrate correct administration of medications.	• Have parents prepare the medication dosages and administer the digoxin, diuretics, and other medications to the child under the supervision of the home health nurse.	• Demonstration techniques used to administer medications provide opportunities to identify dosage errors and to suggest methods to help assure the child gets all needed medications.	Parents report that the child continues to demonstrate improvement and adequate cardiac output with absence of congestive heart failure. Medications are given as prescribed.
Parents will state side effects of medications and symptoms of congestive heart failure.	• Describe side effects of medications. Give parents handouts with telephone number to call to ask questions or report side effects.	• If side effects are understood, serious complications can be avoided.	
	• Describe subtle onset of congestive heart failure and its symptoms (increasing weakness, exhaustion, irritability, difficulty feeding, cough or difficult respirations, edema).	• Parents can evaluate child regularly and note subtle changes requiring medical management.	
3. Imbalanced Nutrition: Less than Body Requirements related to chronic illness and tiring while feeding			
	NIC Priority Intervention: **Weight Gain Assistance:** *Facilitation of body weight gain.*		*NOC Suggested Outcome:* **Nutritional Status: Food and Fluid Intake:** *Amount of food and fluid taken into the body over a 24-hour period.*
The infant or child will demonstrate normal weight gain for age.	• Teach parents methods to promote food intake related to positioning, size of feedings, and food choices.	• Positioning, frequency of feedings, size of feedings, and use of high-caloric foods can enhance nutritional intake.	The infant or child shows normal weight gain.
	• Observe feeding during home visit.	• Feedback can assist parents in integrating positive feeding techniques.	Parents report and demonstrate successful feedings of child.

(continued)

NURSING CARE PLAN   The Child with Congestive Heart Failure Being Cared for at Home

GOAL	INTERVENTION	RATIONALE	EXPECTED OUTCOME
4. Activity Intolerance (Child) related to poor cardiac output			
	NIC Priority Intervention: **Energy Management:** *Regulating energy use to treat or prevent fatigue and optimize function.*		*NOC Suggested Outcome:* **Energy Conservation:** *Extent of active management of energy to initiate or sustain activity.*
The child will perform all necessary activities of daily living without undue tiring.	• Help parents alternate activities and rest throughout the child's day.	• Activities to promote development must be alternated with rest due to decreased cardiac output.	The child performs necessary activities and rests frequently each day.
	• Have parents limit child's exposure to persons with contagious disease.	• When the child is ill and tired, the immune system can be compromised.	
	• Help family plan quiet surroundings to provide for child's rest.	• Home setting may need to be altered to promote rest.	
5. Caregiver Role Strain (Parent) related to 24-hour responsibility for child's care			
	NIC Priority Intervention: **Caregiver Support:** *Provision of the necessary information, advocacy, and support to facilitate primary patient care by someone other than a healthcare professional.*		*NOC Suggested Outcome:* **Caregiver Endurance Potential:** *Factors that promote family care provider continuance over an extended period of time.*
Parents will express ability to meet own needs.	• Assess family and community supports. Provide information related to respite care.	• Variable family and community supports are available.	Parents report some time away from the child and report renewal in caring for the child.
	• Encourage parents to seek activities to meet personal needs.	• Parents need time to meet own personal needs in order to successfully care for child.	

Evaluation

Expected outcomes of nursing care can be found in the Nursing Care Plans on pages 771–773 and 775–776.

CARDIOMYOPATHY

Cardiomyopathy is a serious disorder of the heart's muscle that occurs most often during infancy and adolescence.

Hypertrophic cardiomyopathy (HCM) occurs due to autosomal dominant transmission and is caused by mutations in any one of 10 genes (Maron, 2004). It is often unrecognized until sudden death occurs. Approximately 36% of young athletes who die suddenly have HCM (American Heart Association, 2003). Treatment used to prevent sudden death when HCM is diagnosed often includes an implantable cardioverter-defibrillator or antiarrhythmic medications (Maron, 2004). Children with hypertrophic cardiomyopathy and other genetic cardiovascular diseases should avoid exercise such as sprinting, body building, ice hockey, basketball, racquetball, soccer, tennis, and scuba diving due to the risk for sudden cardiac death (Maron, Chaitman, Ackerman et al., 2004).

Conditions leading to dilated cardiomyopathy include neuromuscular disorders such as muscular dystrophy and viral myocarditis (Lipshultz, Sleeper, Towbin et al., 2003). Immunosuppression with cyclosporine and prednisone has improved the long-term survival of children with dilated cardiomyopathy (Gagliardi, Bevilacqua, Bassano et al., 2004). Almost 40% of children with symptoms of cardiomyopathy die of the condition within 2 years or receive a heart transplant (Strauss & Lock, 2003).

Nursing Management

Nursing management for dilated cardiomyopathy is the same as for children with CHF unless or until a heart transplant is performed. Nursing management for hypertrophic cardiomyopathy involves frequent visits to assess the child's condition and to review progress with antiarrhythmic medications (see page 784).

HEART TRANSPLANTATION

Approximately 260 heart transplants are performed in children each year (Gabrys, 2005). Indications for heart transplantation include end-stage cardiomyopathy and congenital heart disease with ventricular failure such as hypoplastic left heart syndrome (Blume, 2003). With improved immunosuppressive protocols and surgical techniques, survival rates are increasing (85% at 1 year, 75% at 5 years, and 65% at 10 years) (Gabrys, 2005). The use of ventricular assist devices and extracorporeal membranous oxygenation (ECMO) prior to and following transplant has been found to improve the child's recovery from end-organ failure and enhance transplantation outcome (Blume, Naftel, Bastardi et al., 2006).

Rejection is a major cause of mortality and morbidity. The immunosuppression regimen usually includes calcineurin inhibitors (cyclosporin or tacrolimus), cell toxins (azathioprine), and corticosteroids. Rejection is not always associated with symptoms, so an endomyocardial biopsy is performed during cardiac catheterization frequently during the first year after transplant to detect rejection, and then annually if no rejection occurs.

Infection is another cause of mortality and morbidity. Bacterial, fungal, and viral (i.e., cytomegalovirus) infections cause the most problems; however, some common childhood illnesses (acute otitis, colds) may be well tolerated. Certain antibiotics (macrolide category) should be avoided because they cause a significant elevation of cyclosporine and tacrolimus levels that could potentially lead to renal failure (Gabrys, 2005).

> **NURSING ALERT**
>
> Signs of acute rejection of a transplanted heart include the following: low-grade fever, increasing resting heart rate, fatigue, abdominal pain, nausea, vomiting, and decreasing exercise tolerance. Chronic rejection involves rapidly progressive coronary artery narrowing. However, because the transplanted heart does not have the usual nerve connections, the child or adolescent does not usually experience chest pain (Gabrys, 2005).

Nursing Management

Depending upon the age at time of transplant, the child may not have had all immunizations (see Chapter 18 ∞). Live virus vaccines are contraindicated in children with heart transplants. Help parents arrange for school and childcare center administrators to immediately alert the family if any cases of measles, mumps, rubella, and chickenpox occur. Preventive treatment for the child can be provided as necessary. Handwashing and other methods to reduce the spread of infection should be encouraged both at home and at school.

After recovery from surgery, children may have near-normal exercise capabilities, normal heart function, and return to school and other activities. Immunosuppressive medications will be continued long term and can cause a variety of physical side effects such as hair growth, gum hyperplasia, weight gain, moon face, acne, rashes, and osteoporosis (Josephson, 2005). Children and adolescents may need support to develop positive self-esteem. Children often develop hypertension and may be treated with calcium channel blockers. Hypercholesterolemia and graft coronary artery disease can become causes of late transplant failure.

Organ rejection is a major concern of families. Provide education for the parents and child to recognize the signs and to seek treatment promptly. Adolescents need special attention to promote adherence to the immunosuppression protocol.

PULMONARY ARTERY HYPERTENSION

Pulmonary artery hypertension is a complication of many congenital heart defects (particularly those with systemic to pulmonary shunting such as a large ventricular septal defect), as well as pulmonary conditions and congenital diaphragmatic hernia. Excessive pulmonary blood flow over time leads to pulmonary vascular vasoconstriction to decrease the blood flow. The smooth muscle in the small pulmonary arteries increases to sustain vasoconstriction if the excess pulmonary blood flow is not controlled.

The pulmonary artery pressure must increase to push blood across the vascular bed. Inflammation, hypertrophy of pulmonary vessels, and fibrosis develop. The increased pressure leads to a right-to-left shunt and right heart function is impaired. The condition may become life threatening (Granton & Rabinovitch, 2002).

Hypoxemia results from pulmonary hypertension and helps maintain the vasoconstriction. The infant displays tachypnea, cyanosis, retractions, and fatigue. Feeding is difficult, and weight loss with fluid and electrolyte imbalance is likely. Older children have exertional dyspnea, chest pain, and syncope.

Clinical therapy involves surgery to correct an obstructive lesion or close a defect. Therapy for pulmonary artery hypertension related to noncardiac conditions involves bronchodilators, antibiotics, corticosteroids, and low-flow oxygen. No cure is available, but these measures can prolong life. A heart transplant or heart-lung transplant may be performed (Granton & Rabinovitch, 2002).

Nursing care focuses on promoting rest for oxygen conservation, monitoring fluid intake and output carefully, and administering medications and oxygen. Airplane travel may be possible with supplemental oxygen. Exercise should be tailored to avoid dyspnea. Give parents needed support and information about their child.

ACQUIRED HEART DISEASES

Rheumatic Fever

Rheumatic fever is an inflammatory disorder of connective tissue that follows an initial infection by some strains of group A beta-hemolytic streptococci. This disorder causes changes in the heart, joints, brain, and skin tissues. Although not common, the disorder has occurred more frequently in the intermountain west region of the United States since the 1980s and into the 21st century (Tani, Veasy, Minich et al., 2003).

The exact cause of the disorder is unknown. Probable causes include an immune response to the M proteins in the streptococcal organisms that affect the normal tissues of the heart, joints, central nervous system, and skin in a genetically predisposed child (Connor, 2006). From 1 to 3 weeks after an untreated streptococcal infection, the hallmark signs of rheumatic fever may occur. Aschoff bodies (hemorrhagic bullous lesions) develop in the heart's connective tissue. Endocarditis may lead to permanent mitral or aortic heart valve damage. The child's joints become inflamed and painful (migratory polyarthritis), although this condition improves in several weeks. Subcutaneous nodules may be palpable near joints. A skin rash called erythema marginatum, with pink macules and blanching in the middle of the lesions, is frequently seen on the trunk and proximal extremities. Spiking fever often occurs. A condition known as Sydenham chorea (St. Vitus dance), which is characterized by aimless movements of the extremities and facial grimacing, may be seen if the central nervous system is involved.

Diagnosis is based on clinical signs (Jones criteria; see Table 21–7) and laboratory testing for antistreptolysin-O (ASLO). An ASLO titer of 333 Todd units in children indicates a recent streptococcal infection (Connor, 2006).

Clinical therapy includes antibiotics (penicillin, sulfadiazine, or erythromycin) to eradicate the streptococcal infection. Aspirin is used to treat carditis if present (for 3 to 4 weeks or longer), and to control joint inflammation and reduce fever. Children should be monitored carefully by echocardiogram for potential heart involvement. Steroids may be used for severe carditis with CHF. Most children recover fully. Long-term antibiotic prophylaxis to reduce the risk of recurrent attacks are given well into adulthood. Children with residual valve damage need antibiotic prophylaxis to prevent infectious endocarditis.

Nursing Management

The nurse's most important role is prevention of rheumatic fever. Nurses in clinics, offices, and schools need to ensure that all children with possible streptococcal infections have a throat culture taken. Even if the sore throat is mild, a culture is needed if family members or other contacts have had a streptococcal infection. Emphasize to the family the importance of giving the child all doses of the antibiotic as prescribed when a culture is positive.

Table 21–7	GUIDELINES FOR DIAGNOSIS OF INITIAL ATTACK OF RHEUMATIC FEVER (JONES CRITERIA, UPDATED 1992 AND CONFIRMED IN 2002)*

Major Manifestations	Minor Manifestations
Clinical Findings	**Clinical Findings**
Carditis	Arthralgia
Polyarthritis	Fever
Chorea	**Laboratory Findings**
Erythema marginatum	Elevated acute-phase reactants
Subcutaneous nodules	Erythrocyte sedimentation rate
	C-reactive protein
	Prolonged PR interval

Supporting evidence of antecedent group A streptococcal infection: (1) positive throat culture or rapid streptococcal antigen test; (2) elevated or rising streptococcal antibody titer.

*If supported by evidence of preceding group A streptococcal infection, the presence of two major manifestations or one major and two minor manifestations indicates a high probability of acute rheumatic fever.

Note: Data from Special Writing Group of the Committee on Rheumatic Fever, Endocarditis, and Kawasaki Disease of the Council on Cardiovascular Disease in the Young of the American Heart Association. (1992). Guidelines for the diagnosis of rheumatic fever. Jones Criteria, 1992 update. *Journal of the American Medical Association, 268*(15), 2069–2073; Ferrieri, P. (2002). Proceedings of the Jones Criteria workshop. *Circulation, 106,* 2521–2523.

In a case of severe rheumatic fever, the child is hospitalized for a period of time. Nursing care focuses on assessing the child's condition, promoting recovery, and ensuring adherence with the treatment regimen.

During the acute inflammatory phase, take the child's temperature at least every 4 hours and monitor vital signs. The child is on bed rest while monitoring for the onset of carditis, and for 4 weeks if carditis develops. Auscultate the child's heart and note any unusual sounds. Observe the child for changes in skin, joints, or behavior. Be sure family members have throat cultures done to identify possible asymptomatic streptococcal carriers.

Administer antibiotics and aspirin as ordered. The child is usually lethargic and often has joint pain. Aspirin often relieves pain dramatically after a few doses. Position and handle the child's joints carefully. Provide quiet activities, as the child is often confined to bed. Encourage visits or telephone calls from family members and friends. Provide emotional support to the child with *chorea* (purposeless involuntary movements) that can last for 5 to 15 weeks and be disturbing. Encourage the family to participate in the child's hospital care.

During the recovery phase, the child is generally cared for at home. Activities may be limited, especially if heart damage is suspected. Help parents plan quiet activities, such as playing board games, working with computers, or reading, and arrange rest periods after the child returns to school. Reassure the child and parents that the effects of chorea will eventually subside.

On discharge, a daily oral low-dose antibiotic is prescribed or a monthly long-acting antibiotic injection is given. Make sure the child and parents understand the importance of taking prescribed medications until adulthood to prevent future infection and possible heart damage from recurrent rheumatic fever. Stress the importance of telling future healthcare providers, including dentists and surgeons, about the child's rheumatic fever history so prophylactic antibiotics can be given to prevent infective endocarditis during invasive procedures.

Make sure the parents understand that the child's future sore throats may be streptococcal and that a throat culture should be taken even when the child is taking daily antibiotics. The child may need additional antibiotics for the infection. Emphasize the importance of follow-up care to prevent new infections and to monitor heart function.

Infective Endocarditis

Infective endocarditis is an inflammation of the lining, valves, and arterial vessels of the heart caused by bacterial, enterococci, and fungal infections. Children who have a congenital heart defect, rheumatic heart disease, an artificial valve, a central venous catheter, or who have had heart surgery are at risk for infective endocarditis (Ferrieri, Gewitz, Gerber et al., 2002). In children with heart defects, a high velocity or turbulent blood flow can injure the **endocardium**, the tissue lining of the heart chambers. Indwelling catheters positioned in the right side of the heart also damage the endocardium or valve endothelium. Infections may occur after the causal organism enters the bloodstream during dental work or surgery and lodges on damaged or abnormal endocardial tissue. Common infectious organisms include gram positive cocci, such as alpha-hemolytic streptococci, staphylococci, and enterococci (Ferrieri et al., 2002). Children at risk may also develop endocarditis following body piercing of the nose and tongue (Goldrick, 2003).

Symptoms can be mild and develop slowly, or they can be severe and develop rapidly. Common symptoms are fever (often with elevations in the afternoon), fatigue, weakness, joint and muscle aches, weight loss, and diaphoresis. Signs may include a new or changing murmur, CHF, dyspnea, hematuria, petechia, and conjunctival hemorrhages (Ferrieri et al., 2002). Children with indwelling catheters may initially have pulmonary signs related to septic pulmonary embolism.

Infective endocarditis is diagnosed primarily by blood culture; however, urine and cerebrospinal fluid also may be cultured. Elevated erythrocyte sedimentation rate, anemia, elevated C-reactive protein level, increased white blood cell count, alterations in the electrocardiogram, and changes in heart sounds and murmurs are indicators of the condition. Two-dimensional echocardiography is used to identify vegetation or infective lesions in the heart, the extent of valve damage, and cardiac function.

Clinical therapy consists of administering antibiotics such as penicillin G or ampicillin, ceptriaxone, gentamicin, vancomycin, and nafcillin, dependent upon the sensitivity of the cultured organism. Intravenous administration is preferred, with therapy continuing for 2 to 8 weeks until the infective organism is eradicated. Serum levels of antibiotics are monitored to maintain a therapeutic range. Surgery may be necessary to replace a heart valve or because of risk of embolism. If CHF occurs, bed rest and medications such as digoxin and furosemide are prescribed.

Nursing Management

Nursing care focuses on assessing the child's respiratory and cardiovascular status, administering medications, and teaching the parents about the child's care. Take the child's vital signs and assess oxygen saturation and level of consciousness as CHF and embolism may occur.

Administer medications as ordered and monitor serum antibiotic levels. Monitor for side effects of antibiotics and for infiltration or extravasation at the infusion site. Keep invasive procedures to a minimum. Use careful aseptic technique in performing venipunctures, urinary catheterizations, and other procedures.

The child is often lethargic and on bed rest. Encourage parents to assist with the child's care and plan quiet age-appropriate activities. At discharge, arrange home healthcare nursing. Home infusion therapy may also be ordered. Instruct parents about care needed for the child's recuperation. Reinforce the need for follow-up visits. In addition, home schooling will be needed during the recovery period.

Nursing care also focuses on prevention of endocarditis. Children at risk should be encouraged to have the best possible dental health to reduce the potential sources of many causative organisms that originate in the oral cavity (Ferrieri et al., 2002). Children at high risk for endocarditis should be discouraged from body piercing and tattoos as endocarditis may occur even with prophylaxis. Explain the importance of telling physicians and dentists about the child's risk for endocarditis so that they will take care to prevent infection before invasive procedures.

Kawasaki Disease

Kawasaki disease is an acute systemic inflammatory illness. It is the leading cause of acquired heart disease in children in North America and most developed countries. The annual incidence is 18.5 cases per 100,000 children, but the incidence is 47.7 cases per 100,000 in Hawaiian children. Children under 5 years of age account for 75% of cases, and nearly half of those cases occur in children under 2 years. Although this disorder is most common in Asian children, it is seen in all races (Chang, 2002).

Etiology and Pathophysiology

The etiology of Kawasaki disease is unknown, but the primary cause is thought to be infectious in genetically predisposed children. It does not appear to be spread by person-to-person contact, but there is often a preceding upper respiratory tract infection. A multisystem inflammatory disease involves the small and medium-sized arteries, including the coronary arteries. Coronary artery damage can lead to aneurysms, ischemic heart disease, and potentially infarcts.

Clinical Manifestations

There are three stages of the disease: acute, subacute, and convalescent. The acute stage is characterized by fever, irritability, conjunctival hyperemia, red throat, swollen hands and feet, rash on the trunk, enlargement of the cervical lymph nodes, diarrhea, and hepatic dysfunction (Figure 21–11 ➤). The subacute stage is characterized by cracking lips and fissures, desquamation of the skin on the tips of the fingers and toes starting at 10 days after the fever begins, joint pain, cardiac disease, and thrombocytosis. In the convalescent stage, 6 to 8 weeks after disease onset, the child appears normal but may have lingering signs of inflammation. Other clinical signs may include abdominal pain, paralytic ileus, diarrhea, vomiting, dysuria, aseptic meningitis, and arthritis.

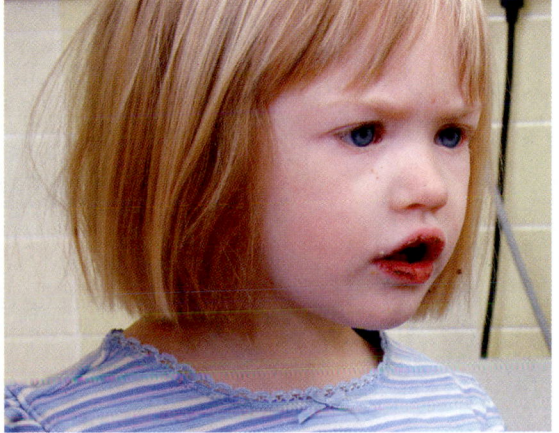

Figure 21–11 ➤ This child has returned for one of her frequent follow-up visits to assess her cardiac status after treatment for Kawasaki syndrome. Notice the lips that show inflammation and cracking.

■ COLLABORATIVE CARE

Diagnostic Tests

Diagnosis is based on clinical signs using the criteria given in Box 21–1. Blood studies show some abnormalities such as elevated erythrocyte sedimentation rate, elevated white blood cell count, mild anemia, thrombocytosis, elevated platelet count, and elevated C-reactive protein level. A two-dimensional echocardiogram is used to reveal

---

BOX 21–1

DIAGNOSTIC CRITERIA FOR KAWASAKI DISEASE

Kawasaki disease is diagnosed when a high spiking fever over 39°C (102.2°F) for 5 days or longer is present along with four of the following five principal features:

- Changes in the extremities: acute changes include erythema of palms, soles and edema of feet, sometimes painful induration of hands and feet; subacute changes include periungual peeling of fingers and toes in weeks 2 and 3
- Changes in the lips and oral cavity: dry, peeling, cracking lips, strawberry tongue, diffuse erythema of the buccal and pharyngeal mucosae
- Bilateral bulbar conjunctival redness without exudate, usually painless
- Polymorphous exantham (erythematous maculopapular rash) on trunk and extremities may involve perineal region
- Cervical lymphadenopathy, greater than 1.5 cm in diameter, usually unilateral and in anterior cervical triangle

Adapted from: Newberger, J.W., Takahasi, M., Gerber, M. A., et al. (2004). Diagnosis, treatment, and long-term management of Kawasaki disease: A statement for health professionals from the Committee on Rheumatic Fever, Endocarditis, and Kawasaki Disease, Council on Cardiovascular Disease in the Young, American Heart Association. *Circulation, 110* (October 26), 2747–2771.

specific vascular changes in the heart and coronary arteries, including assessment of the internal coronary vessel diameters.

Clinical Therapy

Kawasaki disease is treated with intravenous immunoglobulin (2 g/kg given in a single infusion) and aspirin. High doses of aspirin (80 to 100 mg/kg/day in four divided doses) are given while the fever is high. The dose is decreased to 3 to 5 mg/kg/day or less once the fever has dropped for its antiplatelet activity. High doses of immune globulin given before the 10th day of fever reduce the incidence of coronary artery lesions and aneurysms, as well as decrease fever and inflammatory signs (Newberger et al., 2004).

Children are usually hospitalized for 3 or more days, depending upon the presence of cardiac lesions and how long the fever persists. Most children recover fully. Careful monitoring for cardiac disease continues for several weeks or months. Coronary aneurysms and coronary artery stenosis with risk of thrombosis are the most serious complications. Children without cardiac complications during the first month of Kawasaki disease generally have no long-term cardiac impairment (Newberger et al., 2004).

■ NURSING MANAGEMENT

Nursing care focuses on promoting comfort, monitoring for early signs of complications or disease progression, and supporting the family.

Nursing Assessment and Diagnosis

Assessment is important in identifying signs of Kawasaki disease, as the acute phase of this disorder is commonly confused with other diseases. The nurse in the community must be alert to early signs and symptoms.

When the child is hospitalized, take the temperature every 4 hours and before each dose of aspirin. Carefully assess the extremities for edema, redness, and desquamation every 8 hours. Examine the eyes for conjunctivitis and the mucous membranes for inflammation. Monitor the child's dietary and fluid intake and weigh the child daily. Carefully assess heart sounds and rhythm.

Several nursing diagnoses may apply to the child with Kawasaki disease. They include:

- Risk for Imbalanced Body Temperature related to inflammatory process
- Impaired Oral Mucous Membranes related to inflammation and decreased fluid intake
- Impaired Skin Integrity due to edema, diaphoresis, and skin desquamation
- Interrupted Family Processes due to child's acute and potentially life-threatening illness

Planning and Implementation

Administer aspirin and immune globulin as ordered. Monitor for side effects of aspirin such as bleeding and gastrointestinal upset. Administer intravenous immune globulin as a blood product, carefully regulating the infusion rate to run slowly according to the physician's orders, and watching for any reactions to the infusion. The infusion rate should not be over 1 mL/min. If symptoms of reaction occur, stop the infusion immediately (see Chapter 17 ∞).

Promote the child's comfort. Keep the child's skin clean and dry, and lubricate the lips. Use cool compresses to make the feverish child more comfortable. Change the child's clothes and bed linens frequently. Give the child frequent small feedings of soft foods and liquids that are neither too hot nor too cold.

Use passive range of motion exercises to facilitate joint movement. Because the child with Kawasaki disease is often lethargic and irritable, plan rest periods and quiet age-appropriate activities. Encourage the parents to participate in their child's care. This comforts and reassures the child. Give the parents information about the disease and the child's treatment.

Before the child is discharged, teach the parents to administer aspirin as ordered and to watch for side effects. Advise the parents that the child may need to avoid contact sports or other activities that could cause bleeding. Have them take the child's temperature daily and report any fever above 37.8°C (100°F) to the physician. Emphasize the need for follow-up care to monitor for cardiac complications.

Evaluation

Examples of expected nursing care outcomes include:

- The child's skin care promotes healing and protects from further damage and infection.
- The parents are educated to monitor the child for complications and to provide ongoing care to the child.

CARDIAC ARRHYTHMIAS

Cardiac **arrhythmias** (abnormal rhythms or dysrhythmias) occur frequently in children, but less often than in adults. These include tachyarrhythmias (sinus tachycardia) and bradyarrhythmias (sinus bradycardia) that occur with acute conditions such as hypoxia, acidosis, increased intracranial pressure, hypothermia, and hypoglycemia. Most of these arrhythmias resolve once the condition is treated. Less common arrhythmias are often associated with congenital heart disease, including atrial fibrillation, atrial flutter, ventricular fibrillation, and heart block. Arrhythmias must be recognized because they cause decreased cardiac output and CHF, or an even more serious arrhythmia may develop that could result in sudden death.

Supraventricular Tachycardia

Supraventricular tachycardia (SVT), the most common pediatric pathologic arrhythmia, is the abrupt onset of a rapid, regular heart rate, often too fast to count (Green, Kitchen, & Ray, 2005). Neonates and young children may be predisposed to the condition because of a congenital heart defect or Wolff-Parkinson-White syndrome. Short periods of arrhythmia (several seconds), which may be caused by paroxysmal atrial tachycardia, are rarely dangerous. However, prolonged episodes of continuous SVT for more than 24 hours may lead to CHF. Cardiac output is affected because diastolic filling cannot occur with such a rapid heart rate. Prolonged episodes of SVT are life threatening and can progress to CHF or cardiogenic shock if untreated (Green, Kitchen, & Ray, 2005).

Early signs in infants include poor feeding, irritability, diaphoresis, and pallor. Older children may have episodes of altered consciousness (dizziness or syncope). The presenting heart rate in infants with supraventricular tachycardia (SVT) may be 220 beats/min or higher. In older children, a heart rate higher than 180 beats/min may be seen (Doniger & Sharieff, 2006).

Electrocardiography, including a 24-hour rhythm recording after the acute episode, confirms the diagnosis. Vagal stimulation such as applying ice or iced saline solution to the face of an infant may reduce the heart rate. An older child can perform Valsalva's maneuver (holding the breath and straining, or blowing forcefully on the thumb) to increase intrathoracic and venous pressures and thus slow the heart rate. Adenosine given intravenously is the recommended emergency medication for chemical cardioversion when vagal stimulation does not work. Synchronized cardioversion may be used for life-threatening episodes of shock if other treatments are not effective. Sedation and analgesia may be given prior to cardioversion.

Recurrent attacks are common, and digoxin and propranolol may be given to reduce the frequency of episodes (Green, Kitchen, & Ray, 2005). **Radiofrequency ablation** uses energy to destroy a very small section of the myocardium through which an accessory conduction pathway passes that triggers tachycardia (Pappone, Manguso, Santinelli et al., 2004). The procedure is performed in a cardiac catheterization laboratory; when successful, medications taken to control SVT can be discontinued.

NURSING ALERT

Inform the parents of a child with Kawasaki disease to postpone any scheduled immunizations for 11 months after immune globulin administration, as immune response to the vaccine may not be fully effective. Influenza vaccine should be administered because of the risk for Reye's syndrome with long-term aspirin therapy (American Academy of Pediatrics, 2006, p. 415).

GROWTH & DEVELOPMENT

Criteria for Bradycardia

The criteria for bradycardia by age group is as follows (Hanish, 2001):

- Infants to 3 years less than 100 beats per minute
- Children 3 to 9 years less than 60 beats per minute
- Children 9 to 16 years less than 50 beats per minute
- Adolescents over 16 years less than 40 beats per minute

NURSING ALERT

When applying ice or iced saline to the face of an infant, take care to avoid pressure on the eyes as retinal damage could occur. Also ensure that the child's airway is unobstructed by the ice packs.

Nursing Management

During the acute episode, the nurse monitors the child's level of consciousness, rhythm strips, and pulse oximetry on a constant basis. A change in the child's level of consciousness may indicate the beginning of cardiopulmonary compromise (Green, Kitchen, & Ray, 2005). The nurse also assesses the impact of the acute episode on the parents and their ability to be supportive to the child.

Nurses support other healthcare providers during the process of cardioversion. The nurse assists with Valsalva's maneuvers, administers intravenous medications, and monitors the child's condition. Nurses also have a role in providing support to families during the acute crisis (see Chapter 14 ∞). Educate parents to help them prevent and recognize future episodes, as certain other medications can trigger another episode and should be avoided. The child with SVT should not use cardiac stimulant drugs such as decongestants. Teach parents how to perform Valsalva's maneuvers for home management and when to call the healthcare provider.

Long QT Syndrome

Long QT Syndrome is a rhythm disturbance of autosomal dominant and autosomal recessive inheritance that puts children at risk for ventricular fibrillation and sudden death. It may also result from electrolyte abnormalities (hypokalemia, hypocalcemia, and hypomagnesemia) and medications (Doniger & Sharieff, 2006). It is thought to be associated with some cases of Sudden Infant Death Syndrome.

The arrhythmia commonly occurs without warning and often results in death. Depending upon the type of Long QT Syndrome, it may be triggered by demanding physical exercise, extreme emotional stress, or a loud noise. It may also occur during sleep (Balaji, 2004). Early signs include a fast heart rate (too fast to count), irritability, lethargy, poor feeding, poor perfusion (cool pale skin, increased capillary refill time), decreased responsiveness, decreased blood pressure, and sudden death.

If the child is resuscitated or evaluated because of early signs, the arrhythmia is commonly detected by electrocardiogram. Treatment of the acute episode includes cardiac pacing, correcting electrolyte abnormalities, administering lidocaine infusion, and withdrawing drugs that prolong the QT interval. Beta-blockers (e.g., propanalol) and class 1B antiarrhythmic agents (mexiletene and phenytoin) are often effective in treating the condition (Balaji, 2004). A pacemaker is often recommended for children with type 3 Long QT Syndrome. Children with the condition should not engage in competitive sports. In addition, swimming should be supervised.

Nursing Management

Nursing care of children with Long QT Syndrome focuses on assessing the child's condition, administering medications, and providing emotional support to the child and parents. Children are treated in the emergency department or intensive care unit. The child is placed on a cardiac monitor, and frequent assessment is critical. Report continued abnormal rates or rhythms to the physician. Carefully observe and record changes in level of consciousness, color, weakness, irritability, and feeding pattern. Administer medications as ordered. Have emergency drugs and resuscitation equipment available at the bedside. Provide for rest and adequate nutrition.

Episodes of arrhythmia are frightening for both the child and parents. Carefully explain the treatment plan and home care. Teach parents to take the child's apical pulse. Make sure parents are trained in cardiopulmonary resuscitation. Provide telephone numbers of emergency medical facilities and help parents plan how to seek emergency care. Emphasize that prescribed medications help prevent or reduce the frequency of the episodes. The child with Long QT syndrome should avoid any medications that prolong the QT interval, such as macrolide antibiotics, some antiarrhythmics, tricyclic antidepressants, and antihistamines (Balaji, 2004). Discuss safety measures with the family to reduce or manage a future episode.

NURSING ALERT

When the child is diagnosed with Long QT Syndrome, ensure that all family members get tested for the condition as it is transmitted in an autosomal dominant or autosomal recessive pattern. Identifying previously undiagnosed family members with the condition and providing treatment may prevent their sudden death.

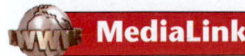

MediaLink

Long QT Syndrome

DYSLIPIDEMIA

Dyslipidemia is a condition in which one or more lipids (total cholesterol, low-density lipoproteins, triglycerides, high-density lipoproteins) have an abnormal level in the blood. It is important to identify children who have a genetic history or lifestyle that makes them more susceptible to future coronary heart disease and to implement preventive health measures to reduce the child's risk of disease and premature death as an adult. The factors that increase risk for coronary artery calcium are obesity and increased body mass index, elevated blood pressure in childhood, and dyslipidemia (Kavey, Daniels, Lauer et al., 2003).

Some children have primary dyslipidemia due to familial hypercholesterolemia, and may have cholesterol levels as high as 600 to 1000 mg/dL and lipid deposits in their corneas and tendons. As the excessive fat circulates, it causes changes in blood vessels. Children may also have secondary dyslipidemia resulting from a diet rich in saturated fat, too little exercise, diseases such as diabetes, and use of drugs such as anabolic steroids (Kingsbury, 2003). More often, children have milder lipid abnormalities that arise from a combination of heredity and lifestyle factors. The fatty streaks that appear in childhood become fibrous plaques in adolescence. These atherosclerotic plaques continue to grow in adulthood and may cause hemorrhage, thrombi, and occlusion of vessels.

A blood test identifies hyperlipidemia. Cholesterol, including total cholesterol (TC) and high-density lipoprotein cholesterol (HDL-C), and triglycerides are measured. See Table 21–8. The low-density lipoprotein cholesterol (LDL-C) level is calculated using an equation based on the triglyceride, HDL, and total cholesterol levels. All children over 2 years of age with the following risk factors should be screened with a fasting lipid panel: a family history of cardiovascular disease before age 55 years (parents or grandparents) or who have a parent with elevated total serum cholesterol (240 mg/dL); blood pressure greater than 90th percentile for age, sex, and height; body mass index greater than 85th percentile; and diabetes (Kavey, Daniels, Lauer, et al., 2003). If the child's total serum cholesterol is greater than or equal to 200 mg/dL, a fasting lipid profile should be performed.

The primary management of dyslipidemia in most children includes dietary modifications, exercise, and other changes in lifestyle. The child's diet is carefully analyzed and changes are made to satisfy the dietary guidelines given in Table 21–9. It is hoped that careful monitoring and management of lipid levels in childhood will decrease the incidence of cardiovascular disease.

If the child continues to have high serum lipid levels, a lipid specialist should be consulted. Cholestyramine or colestipol, which bind bile acid in the intestine, and niacin are sometimes prescribed in children over 10 years. Lovastatin may be prescribed for adolescents for treatment of familial hypercholesterolemia, and soon may be prescribed for younger children. A recent study of statin therapy in children 8 to 18 years with familial hypercholesterolemia revealed that carotid atherosclerosis regressed without an

Table 21–8	LABORATORY VALUES FOR ASSESSMENT OF DYSLIPIDEMIA IN CHILDREN BETWEEN 2 AND 19 YEARS OLD	
Test	**Recommended Level**	**Levels of Higher Risk**
Total cholesterol	< 170 mg/dL	Borderline: ≥170–199 mg/dL Abnormal: ≥200 mg/dL
LDL-C	< 100 mg/dL	Borderline: 100–129 mg/dL Abnormal: ≥ 130 mg/dL
Triglyceride	< 200 mg/dL	Abnormal: ≥ 200 mg/dL
HDL-C	≥ 40 mg/dL	Abnormal: < 40 mg/dL

Adapted from: Giddings, S., Dennison, B. A., Birch, L. L., et al. (2005). Dietary guidelines for children and adolescents: A guide for practitioners. Consensus statement from the American Heart Association. *Circulation, 112,* 2061–2075.

Table 21–9	RECOMMENDED NUTRIENT INTAKE IN CHILDREN AND ADOLESCENTS WITH HYPERLIPIDEMIA
Nutrient	**Recommended Intake**
Saturated fatty acid	Less than 7% of calories
Total fat	Less than 30% of calories
Cholesterol	Less than 200 mg/day

Data from: Giddings, S., Dennison, B. A., Birch, L. L., et al. (2005). Dietary guidelines for children and adolescents: A guide for practitioners. Consensus statement from the American Heart Association. *Circulation, 112,* 2061–2075.

adverse effect on growth, maturation, hormone levels, or liver or muscle tissue (Wiegman, Hutten, de Groot et al., 2004).

Nursing Management

Nursing care focuses on identifying children at risk for dyslipidemia, providing education about diet and exercise, and monitoring eating patterns. Identification and management of dyslipidemia takes place in many community settings. Office and clinic nurses identify children who need to have serum lipid measured. Nurses in schools provide education on ways to reduce risk factors. The child's history of exercise patterns, weight percentile, and dietary intake provides important information. Obtain information on familial heart disease, hypertension, diabetes, and smoking to determine risk factors. Although a screening for total cholesterol level does not require fasting, the child needs to fast for 12 hours before blood is drawn for a complete lipid evaluation.

Work with nutritionists to provide dietary teaching and monitor family eating patterns. Emphasize the importance of teaching and modeling food choices that help lower lipid levels. Help the child select an enjoyable moderate-to-intense activity such as running, biking, swimming, soccer, hiking, fast walking, aerobic dancing, and rollerblading to participate in every day for 30 minutes at least three to four times a week. Discourage smoking by the child or the parents as it increases the risk for coronary heart disease.

Include the entire family in the treatment plan, as changing eating and exercise patterns is difficult for a single family member. The family of a child with dyslipidemia requires continual teaching and reinforcement. Periodically perform nutrition assessments and evaluation of family diet.

HYPERTENSION

Hypertension is present in 350,000 (1–5%) children and adolescents (Peters & Flack, 2003). Trends since 1988 have demonstrated a substantially increased systolic and diastolic blood pressure among children and adolescents in the United States. Increasing body mass index accounts for some of the increased blood pressure trends (Muntner, He, Cutler et al., 2004). Secondary hypertension in infants and prepubescent children is often associated with underlying conditions such as kidney disease or heart defects. Primary or essential hypertension may be associated with a genetic or familial predisposition and obesity. Hypertension is defined as a systolic blood pressure and/or diastolic blood pressure that is greater than or equal to the 95th percentile for gender, age, and height, averaged over three readings (National High Blood Pressure Education Program Working Group on High Blood Pressure in Children and Adolescents, 2004).

The child with documented hypertension should have blood chemistry (BUN, creatinine, and electrolytes), complete blood count with platelets, urinalysis, and urine culture tests done to detect secondary causes of hypertension. Renal ultrasonography may also be performed. Serum lipid studies and a fasting glucose should be performed to identify dyslipidemia or diabetes. Polysomnography may be performed to identify a

RESEARCH

Coronary Heart Disease and Family History

A recent study of 113 children with parents who developed coronary heart disease before 50 years of age examined their lifestyle and physical activity in particular. Children reported a wide range of activities. Even though 81% reported that peers participated on sports teams and were physically active, peer influence had only a slight influence on the child's activity. However, when the father was active, the child was more likely to be active (Gilmer, Harrell, Miles et al., 2003). Encouraging the entire family to be active will be better than encouraging the child to individually increase activity.

CULTURE

Blood Pressure

A recent study contrasted the blood pressure of 13- and 14-year-old children in the eighth grade in three states. The sample of 1740 children had the following racial and ethnic heritage: White (14.3%), Black (22%), Hispanic (50%), Native American (2%), and mixed heritage (11.7%). No significant differences in blood pressure were found to be related to racial or ethnic origin; however, a larger number of children than expected (23.9%) had high blood pressure. High blood pressure was most often attributable to body mass index (BMI) (Jago, Harrell, McMurray et al., 2006).

sleep disorder. A drug screen may be appropriate to identify substances that could cause hypertension (National High Blood Pressure Education Program Working Group on High Blood Pressure in Children and Adolescents, 2004).

Nonpharmacologic measures for reduction of blood pressure include weight reduction dietary counseling for obesity, reduced sedentary activities (television, videos, computer time), increased physical activity, increased fruits and vegetables, and reduced sodium. Medications (ACE inhibitors, angiotensin-receptor blockers, beta-blockers, calcium channel blockers, and diuretics) are used for children with secondary hypertension and poor response to lifestyle modifications.

Nursing Management

A complete history is taken to evaluate the child's persistent high blood pressure, identifying potential risk factors such as a family history for hypertension, smoking, or a systemic disease. Is the child obese? How many servings of fruits does the child eat daily? What is the daily number of dairy product servings? What is the child's daily salt intake? What are the child's daily exercise routines? Take the child's blood pressure regularly to monitor changes. Consistently use the right arm for the reading, and compare the blood pressure in the leg to that in the arm. Compare readings to the expected blood pressure reading for gender, age, and height percentile (see Table 5–14 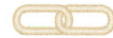). Monitor the child's blood pressure every 3 to 6 months. Assure that the correct-sized blood pressure cuff and appropriate technique is used to assess the blood pressure.

SKILL 6–10
Measuring Blood Pressure

Teach both the child and the parents how to improve the diet and develop exercise routines. Provide suggestions about substitute seasonings for salt and a list of salty foods to avoid. Emphasize the importance of avoiding smoking. Teaching that involves the entire family is usually the most effective. Instruct the family on correct administration of prescribed medications when used.

INJURIES OF THE CARDIOVASCULAR SYSTEM

Shock

Shock is an acute, complex state of circulatory dysfunction resulting in failure to deliver sufficient oxygen and other nutrients to meet cell and tissue demands. It can be caused by a variety of conditions such as hemorrhage, dehydration, sepsis, obstruction of blood flow, and cardiac pump failure.

COMPLEMENTARY THERAPY

Transcendental Meditation for Stress Management and Blood Pressure Control

The relationship between stress and cardiovascular reactivity and subsequent development of primary hypertension in adults has been documented. African American adolescents have been found to exhibit greater blood pressure reactivity to stress than Caucasian adolescents. A randomized clinical trial with 35 adolescents 15 to 18 years of age with high normal resting blood pressure (between 85th and 95th percentiles) compared the impact of a 2-month transcendental meditation program with a control group that received lifestyle education sessions. Each group had similar numbers of males and females, but 34 of the participants were African American and 1 was Caucasian. Participants in the transcendental meditation group practiced two 15-minute sessions while sitting comfortably with eyes closed to obtain a deeply restful state of wakefulness. Participants in the control group attended seven weekly 1-hour health education sessions. The study was conducted in collaboration with the public school system. Anthropometric measurements, heart rate, blood pressure, cardiac output, and total peripheral resistance were evaluated at the beginning of the study and during exposure to stressful experiences (a car driving simulation and a social situation interview). Study results revealed that the transcendental meditation group had greater decreases in resting systolic blood pressure and a trend toward greater decreases in diastolic blood pressure than the control group, particularly with the car driving simulation. Transcendental meditation shows promise as a potential complementary therapy to help control blood pressure in adolescents. Further study is needed to determine if the blood pressure reductions are sustained long term with this intervention (Barnes, Treiber, & Davis, 2001).

Hypovolemic Shock

Hypovolemic shock is a clinical state of inadequate tissue and organ perfusion resulting from the movement of blood or plasma out of the intravascular compartment leading to inadequate intravascular volume (Figure 21–12 ➤). The blood or plasma in the vascular space may be decreased because of hemorrhage or fluid movement into the interstitial spaces.

ETIOLOGY AND PATHOPHYSIOLOGY

Major causes of decreased intravascular blood volume include:

- Hemorrhage from significant injury
- Plasma loss from burns, nephrotic syndrome, and sepsis
- Fluid and electrolyte loss associated with dehydration, diabetic ketoacidosis, and diabetes insipidus

Shock results in inadequate delivery of oxygen and nutrients to cells and accumulation of toxic wastes in the capillaries. The reduction in circulating blood volume

PATHOPHYSIOLOGY ILLUSTRATED

Hypovolemic Shock

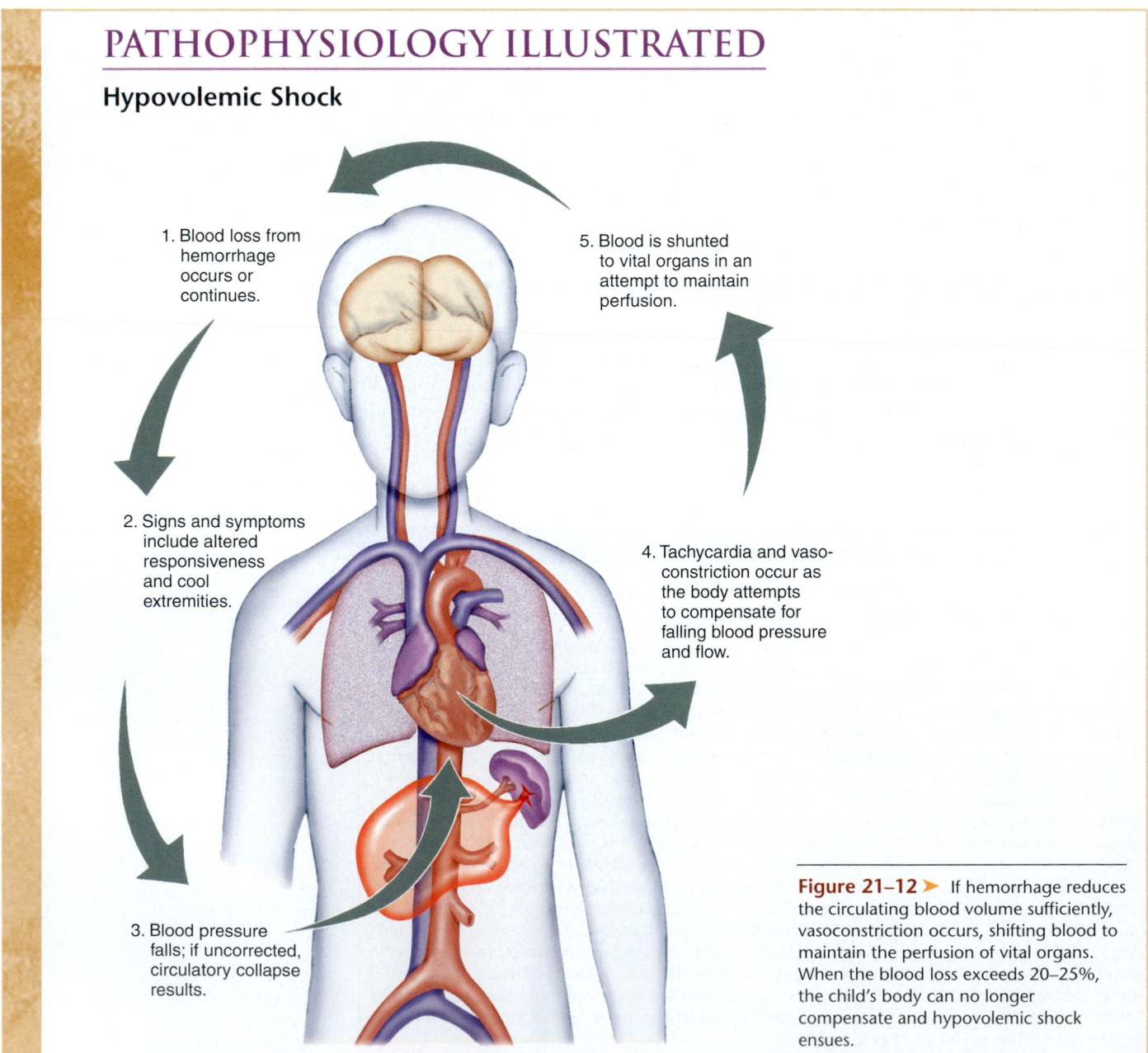

1. Blood loss from hemorrhage occurs or continues.

2. Signs and symptoms include altered responsiveness and cool extremities.

3. Blood pressure falls; if uncorrected, circulatory collapse results.

4. Tachycardia and vasoconstriction occur as the body attempts to compensate for falling blood pressure and flow.

5. Blood is shunted to vital organs in an attempt to maintain perfusion.

Figure 21–12 ➤ If hemorrhage reduces the circulating blood volume sufficiently, vasoconstriction occurs, shifting blood to maintain the perfusion of vital organs. When the blood loss exceeds 20–25%, the child's body can no longer compensate and hypovolemic shock ensues.

causes a decrease in cardiac output and mean arterial pressure. Cellular hypoxia and acidosis develop simultaneously. The accumulation of toxins and inadequate tissue oxygenation cause cellular damage.

The child's body attempts to compensate by the following measures:

- The renin-angiotensin-aldosterone system is stimulated to retain sodium and water when perfusion of the kidneys is decreased.
- The antidiuretic hormone is secreted when the atria have reduced blood volume leading to water retention.
- The heart rate and myocardial contractility increase to improve cardiac output.
- The respiratory rate increases to improve oxygenation and decrease waste accumulation in the cells.
- The hydrostatic pressure falls, permitting fluid to shift into the vascular space and increasing the circulating blood volume.
- The peripheral vasculature constricts to maintain the systemic vascular resistance and to increase perfusion to the vital organs as long as possible.

The child can compensate until 20–25% of volume loss occurs, and then life-threatening hypotension results.

CLINICAL MANIFESTATIONS   Signs of early hypovolemic shock in children are nonspecific but need to be recognized before hypotension occurs. Signs that the child is compensating for a decreased blood volume are tachycardia, usually sustained at a rate greater than 130 beats per minute; increased respiratory effort; delayed capillary refill (greater than 2 seconds); weak peripheral pulses; pallor; and cold extremities (signs of decreased perfusion). Urine output decreases (less than 0.5–1 mL/kg/hour in infants and young children) when renal blood flow drops. In cases of dehydration, dry mucous membranes and poor skin turgor are also present.

If treatment is not begun in the early stages of hypovolemic shock, the condition progresses until the child can no longer compensate. At that time the systolic blood pressure drops and the pulse pressure narrows. Reduced cerebral blood flow ultimately results in a decreased level of consciousness. If shock is not reversed, the condition progresses to cardiopulmonary failure. Clinical Manifestations of Hypovolemic Shock below compares the signs associated with early, uncompensated, and profound shock.

CLINICAL MANIFESTATIONS | HYPOVOLEMIC SHOCK

System	Early Shock	Uncompensated Shock	Profound Shock
Cardiac and respiratory	Tachycardia, weak distal pulses, full central pulses; normal systolic blood pressure; tachypnea	Tachycardia, absent distal pulses, weak central pulses, decreasing systolic blood pressure; tachypnea	Frank hypotension; bradycardia; weak or absent central pulses; bradypnea
Neurologic	Normal, anxious, irritable, or combative behavior	Confusion, lethargy, decreased pain response	Coma
Skin	Mottled appearance; capillary refill time greater than 2 seconds; cool, clammy extremities	Cyanosis; capillary refill time greater than 3 seconds; dusky, cold extremities	Pale, cold skin
Renal	Decreased urine output, increased specific gravity	Markedly decreased urine output; increased specific gravity	No urine output

Data from: Markenson D. S., (2002). *Pediatric prehospital care* (pp. 174–175). Upper Saddle River, NJ: Brady, Prentice Hall; Waisman, H., & Eichelberger, M. R. (1993). Hypovolemic shock. In M. R. Eichelberger (Ed.), *Pediatric trauma: Prevention, acute care, rehabilitation* (p. 182). St. Louis, MO: Mosby-Yearbook.

CLINICAL TIP

Signs that a child with hypovolemic shock is responding to fluid resuscitation include slowing of the heart rate to less than 100 beats per minute, improved color, improved responsiveness, increased warmth of extremities, and a faster capillary refill time. The systolic blood pressure should be greater than 80 mmHg (Stafford, Blinman, & Nance, 2002).

GROWTH & DEVELOPMENT

Blood Volume

The child's total blood volume varies by weight. The child has approximately 80 mL of blood for every kilogram of body weight.
- Newborn: 3 kg × 80 mL = 240 mL (1 cup)
- 5-year-old child: 25 kg × 80 mL = 2000 mL (2 quarts)
- 13-year-old child: 50 kg × 80 mL = 4000 mL (1 gallon)

CLINICAL THERAPY No laboratory tests can be used to evaluate the volume deficit rapidly enough to diagnose hypovolemic shock. The child is examined for characteristic signs to confirm the diagnosis. Laboratory tests commonly performed after hypovolemic shock is diagnosed include hematocrit and hemoglobin, arterial blood gases, serum electrolytes, glucose, osmolality, blood urea nitrogen, and urinalysis.

Emergency care focuses on improving tissue perfusion. An open airway is established, oxygen is administered, and ventilation is assisted if necessary. Bleeding is controlled, and an intravenous or intraosseous line is started to provide large volumes of crystalloid fluids.

Ringer's lactate solution is the preferred fluid for initial resuscitation. A fluid volume of 20 mL/kg is administered rapidly over 5 minutes. The same amount of fluid is given in 5 minutes if the child's physiologic condition does not improve after fluid is first administered. If no improvement is seen after the second fluid bolus, blood or albumin is usually ordered.

Once the child's physiologic condition is stabilized, the cause of the hypovolemic shock becomes the focus of examination and treatment. If no external bleeding is evident, determine whether an injury may be causing internal bleeding. For example, the liver and spleen are highly vascular organs that have little protection from direct blunt forces. Significant bleeding from injury to one of these organs can cause hypovolemic shock without evidence of bleeding. An acute illness such as gastroenteritis with prolonged vomiting and diarrhea can also result in dehydration and hypovolemic shock.

NURSING MANAGEMENT

Nursing Assessment and Diagnosis

Ask the parent (or child, if appropriate) about possible injuries or the duration and severity of acute illnesses. If external bleeding is apparent, determine the amount of blood lost. Although children lose the same amount of blood from a laceration as adults, the total volume of blood lost is proportional to their weight.

Frequently assess the child's heart rate, respiratory rate, blood pressure, capillary refill time, level of consciousness with the Glasgow Coma Scale (see Chapter 26 ∞), color, and skin temperature to identify any changes that indicate improvement or deterioration in the child's condition. Monitor urine output and specific gravity hourly, as it is a good indicator of adequate fluid volume.

Assess the parents' response and coping mechanisms to the child's potential life-threatening injury. Families are unprepared for the abrupt change in the child's condition because of the unpredictability of the injury. See Chapter 14 ∞.

Several nursing diagnoses may apply to the child with hypovolemic shock. They include:

- Decreased Cardiac Output related to hypovolemia
- Deficient Fluid Volume related to active fluid volume loss due to vomiting and diarrhea
- Ineffective Tissue Perfusion (Cardiopulmonary, Renal, and Cerebral) related to hemorrhage and inadequate hemoglobin to transport of oxygen across alveolar and capillary membrane
- Ineffective Airway Clearance related to altered level of consciousness
- Compromised Family Coping related to life-threatening condition of the child

Planning and Implementation

Nurses in the emergency department and intensive care unit participate in the resuscitation of the child in hypovolemic shock. Assist with the child's assessment and the establishment of intravenous access. Calculate and prepare the amount of intravenous fluid needed for administration according to the child's weight (20 mL/kg). Ensure rapid administration of warmed fluids by intravenous push or pressure bag. Warmed intravenous fluids are used for resuscitation because hypothermia may interfere with the child's response to treatment. Monitor the child's physiologic response to the fluid bolus within 5 minutes. Prepare a second and third fluid bolus. Keep the child covered or use heat lamps to reduce body-heat loss.

When packed red blood cells are administered, verify that the correct blood has been obtained for the child. Change the intravenous fluid to normal saline solution to prevent clotting during blood administration. Assess the child carefully for a transfusion reaction (see Chapter 22 ∞). Monitor the child's physiologic circulatory responses for improvement or deterioration in status. Notify the physician of any deterioration.

Provide support to the child and family during the acute phase of treatment. Parents and children with hypovolemic shock resulting from injury are usually apprehensive. The child may be fearful because of the sudden hospitalization or agitated because of an altered level of consciousness. Determine the causes of the child's anxiety. The parents often fear for the child's life in cases of severe injury. Update the parents about the child's condition frequently. Explain the care being provided and how it helps the child. Listen to their concerns and correct any misconceptions. When hospital policy permits, support the parents who desire to be present during resuscitation of the child.

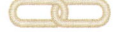

SKILL 9–6
Administering Blood or Blood Products

Evaluation

Examples of expected nursing care outcomes include:

- The child receives adequate fluid resuscitation to prevent progression to uncompensated shock.
- The family copes with the stress of the child's injury.

Maldistributive Shock

Maldistributive shock is an abnormal distribution of blood volume, usually resulting from a decrease in systemic vascular resistance. Causes of maldistributive shock include anaphylaxis, sepsis, and spinal cord injury.

Immunodeficient children are at high risk for septic shock. Septic shock begins as an infection and progresses to sepsis with a bacterial toxin. Once the toxin enters the circulatory system, the body's inflammatory processes go out of control. White blood cells multiply throughout the body and macrophages produce cytokines, which dilate the blood vessels and increase permeability. The blood accumulates in the extremities because of loss of vascular muscle tone causing vasodilation, increased venous capacity, and increased capillary permeability. Less blood is returned to the heart, so preload drops and cardiac output falls. Congestion occurs in some tissue beds, causing edema. This reduces the delivery of oxygen and nutrients to the cells. Bacteria may then be trapped and multiply unchecked (Figure 21–13 ➤). As the metabolism is altered, and less blood is delivered to vital organs, cardiac and other vital organ dysfunction occurs. Toxic shock syndrome is one form of septic shock that may rapidly progress and cause death.

Septic shock has three phases: compensated, uncompensated, and refractory.

- The compensated phase is characterized by fever, tachycardia, tachypnea, warm extremities, bounding pulses, and brisk capillary refill. Urine output may be normal. Responsiveness may be decreased. Perfusion appears adequate; however, because of infection and fever, oxygen demand in the tissues is much higher and perfusion is really inadequate. Cardiac output is high but systemic vascular resistance is low, leading to an uneven flow and pooling in the extremities. Blood moves sluggishly, and anaerobic metabolism and lactic acidosis occur in tissue beds where oxygen no longer circulates. Microvascular thrombi may cause further blood flow obstruction.
- In the uncompensated phase, hypotension and inadeqate oxygen and nutrient delivery to the tissues occurs. Cellular damage from the infection may become so significant that the metabolic processes cannot be supported even when adquate fluids have been given to maintain intravascular volume. Poor tissue perfusion of the vital organs occurs and multiple organ failure begins.

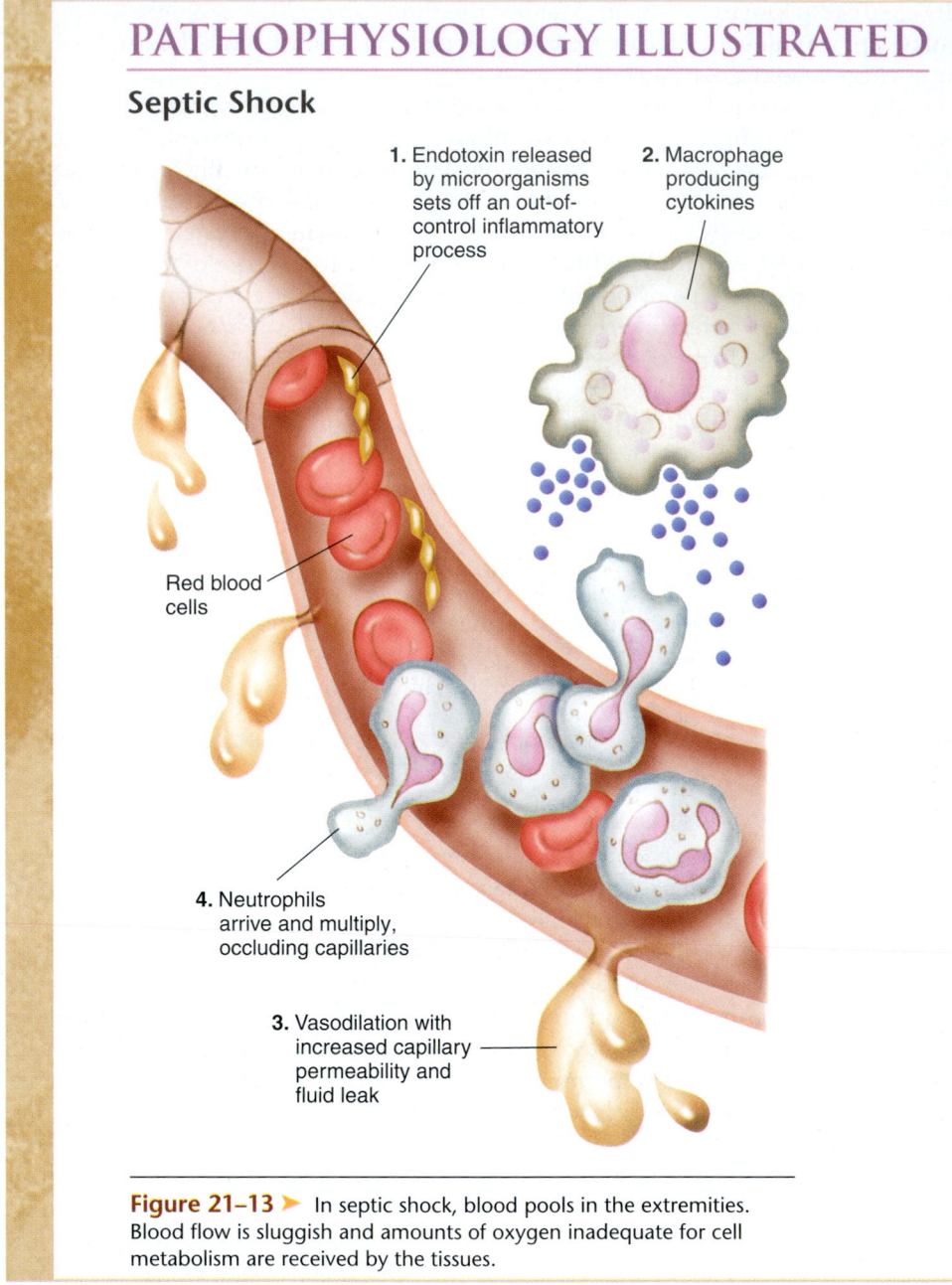

PATHOPHYSIOLOGY ILLUSTRATED

Septic Shock

1. Endotoxin released by microorganisms sets off an out-of-control inflammatory process

2. Macrophage producing cytokines

Red blood cells

4. Neutrophils arrive and multiply, occluding capillaries

3. Vasodilation with increased capillary permeability and fluid leak

Figure 21–13 ➤ In septic shock, blood pools in the extremities. Blood flow is sluggish and amounts of oxygen inadequate for cell metabolism are received by the tissues.

- In the refractory phase, the shock becomes irreversible. Cardiac output falls as the myocardium becomes unresponsive.

Treatment for septic shock is begun even before the diagnosis is confirmed with appropriate antibiotics effective for the suspected organism. Fluid resuscitation is used to stabilize the circulation and ensure adequate tissue perfusion. Vasopressors are given during the hypodynamic phase. Metabolic acidosis is treated. Nutrition with enteral or parenteral support may be initiated early. Morbidity and mortality are high even when treatment is initiated early. Complications include disseminated intravascular coagulation and adult respiratory distress syndrome.

NURSING MANAGEMENT   The child is cared for in the intensive care unit. Nursing care is focused on careful assessment and monitoring of the child for signs that the condition is progressing. The nurse supports other healthcare professionals in promoting the child's oxygenation, physiologic, and hemodynamic status with oxygen, IV fluids, and medication administration. Parents are supported as described in Chapter 14 ∞.

Obstructive Shock

Obstructive shock occurs when a blockage of the main bloodstream interferes with tissue perfusion (Figure 21–14 ➤). Causes in children include compression of the vena cava, pericardial tamponade, pulmonary embolism, tension pneumothorax, pleural effusion, and congenital heart defects with outflow obstruction (e.g., coarctation of the aorta). Management is focused on treatment of the underlying condition.

Cardiogenic Shock

Cardiogenic shock is an abnormality of myocardial function in which the heart fails to maintain adequate cardiac output and tissue perfusion (Figure 21–15 ➤). Causes of cardiogenic shock in children may include CHF, cardiovascular surgery, severe obstructive congenital heart disease such as hypoplastic left heart syndrome, cardiomyopathy, and arrhythmias such as bradycardia and supraventricular tachycardia. Cardiogenic shock may also be an end stage for other acute and chronic conditions such as sepsis, prolonged shock, asphyxia, hypoglycemia, and muscular dystrophy.

Clinically, cardiogenic shock resembles hypovolemic shock with low cardiac output. Tachycardia, tachypnea, decreased oxygen saturation, hypotension, diminished peripheral pulses, and cool, pale extremities are common signs. The child becomes disoriented and restless as the compensatory mechanisms fail. Increased systemic vascular resistance puts more stress on the failing heart. Each contraction causes more blood to accumulate in the heart and pulmonary vessels, eventually leading to CHF, metabolic acidosis, and circulatory collapse. Signs of respiratory distress are seen as CHF develops.

The goals of medical treatment are rapid restoration of myocardial function with adequate ventilation, resolution of the initial metabolic insult, correction of arrhythmias, management of fluids, and administration of diuretics and inotropic drugs.

PATHOPHYSIOLOGY ILLUSTRATED

Mediastinal Shift in Obstructive Shock

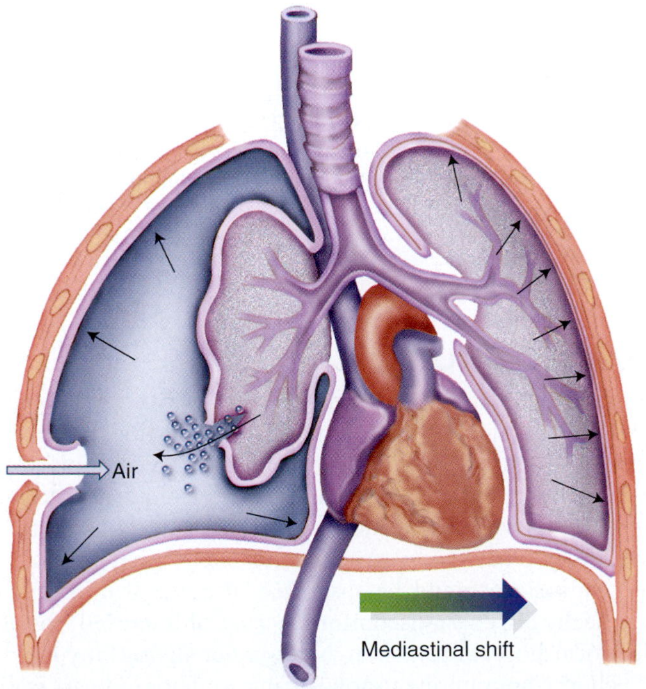

Air

Mediastinal shift

Figure 21–14 ➤ Compression of the great arteries can occur when a tension pneumothorax causes a mediastinal shift of the heart and great arteries and obstructs blood flow to and from the heart.

PATHOPHYSIOLOGY ILLUSTRATED

Cardiogenic Shock

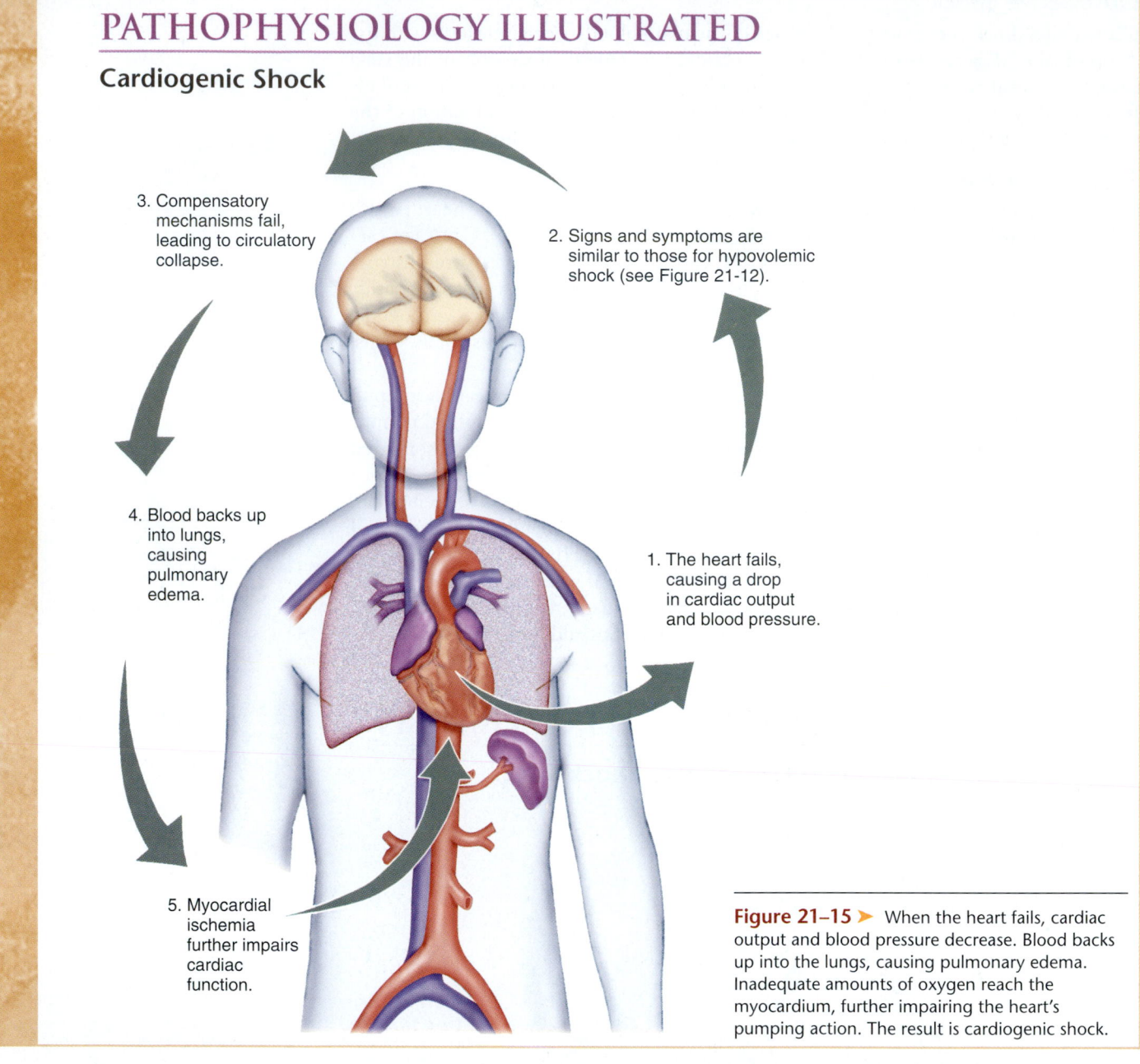

3. Compensatory mechanisms fail, leading to circulatory collapse.

2. Signs and symptoms are similar to those for hypovolemic shock (see Figure 21-12).

4. Blood backs up into lungs, causing pulmonary edema.

1. The heart fails, causing a drop in cardiac output and blood pressure.

5. Myocardial ischemia further impairs cardiac function.

Figure 21–15 ➤ When the heart fails, cardiac output and blood pressure decrease. Blood backs up into the lungs, causing pulmonary edema. Inadequate amounts of oxygen reach the myocardium, further impairing the heart's pumping action. The result is cardiogenic shock.

MYOCARDIAL CONTUSION

Myocardial contusion, a rare injury in children, results from a strong, blunt force against the chest wall that injures the heart muscle. Blood flow to areas of the heart muscle is disrupted, or myocardial cells are directly destroyed. This potentially life-threatening condition is often associated with a motor vehicle–related injury. It most often occurs in adolescents who have struck the steering wheel of a motor vehicle during a crash or children who have been struck in the chest with a baseball.

A myocardial contusion should be suspected in cases of injury to the anterior chest. The child typically has chest discomfort because of fractured ribs or a chest wall contusion. An electrocardiogram reveals arrhythmias or signs of myocardial infarct. A two-dimensional echocardiogram may show an abnormality in heart wall movement. Cardiac treponin I levels and cardiac isoenzyme concentrations may be monitored for elevation. Because of the risk of sudden arrhythmias, the child is admitted to the intensive care unit for cardiac monitoring. Long-term problems could potentially include aneurysm, myocardial rupture, and post-contusion pericarditis.

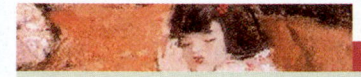

CRITICAL THINKING IN ACTION

ADOLESCENT WITH A CONGENITAL HEART DEFECT

Recall Tina, the 16-year-old in the opening scenario who was born with transposition of the great arteries. She recently had a pacemaker placed to help manage the episodic slow ventricular heart rate. Up until this time, Tina's parents made all of her healthcare decisions. Now Tina must become much more involved in her health care.

1. What is the potential explanation for the development of an arrhythmia so many years after the original heart surgery?

2. What emotional and behavioral responses should be expected from Tina when learning about her new physical limitations?

3. Develop a teaching plan to educate Tina about her congenital heart condition and self-management to maintain her health status.

4. Develop a transition plan for Tina to begin taking responsibility for all aspects of her health care.

 Refer to your Prentice Hall Nursing MediaLink DVD-ROM for answers.

EXPLORE MediaLink   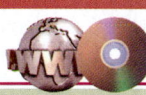 http://www.prenhall.com/ball

Resources for this chapter can be found on the Prentice Hall Nursing MediaLink DVD-ROM accompanying this textbook, and on the Companion Website at http://www.prenhall.com/ball.

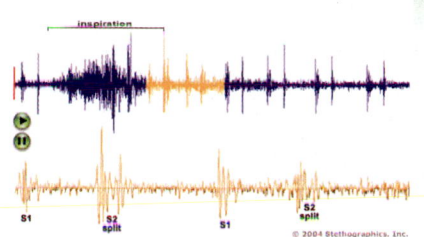

DVD-ROM
Audio Glossary
NCLEX-RN® Review
Animations
  Congenital Heart Defects
  Heart Sounds

COMPANION WEBSITE
Audio Glossary
NCLEX-RN® Review
Care Plan Activity: Pediatric Heart Transplant
Case Study: A Child with Congestive Heart Failure
MediaLink Application: Teaching Plan: Healthy Heart Curricula
WebLinks

REFERENCES

American Academy of Pediatrics, Committee on Infectious Disease. (2006). *Red book: Report of the Committee on Infectious Disease* (27th ed., p. 415). Elk Grove Village, IL: Author.

American Heart Association. (2003). Youth and cardiovascular diseases—Statistics. Accessed August 4, 2003, from http://www. americanheart.org

Azeka, E., Ramires, J. A. F., Valler, C., & Bocchi, E. A. (2002). Delisting infants and children from the heart transplantation waiting list after carvedilol treatment. *Journal of the American College of Cardiology, 40*(11), 2034–2038.

Balaji, S. (2004). Medical therapy for sudden death. *Pediatric Clinics of North America, 51*, 1379–1387.

Barnes, V. A., Treiber, F. A., & Davis, H. (2001). Impact of transcendental meditation on cardiovascular function at rest and during acute stress in adolescents with high normal blood pressure. *Journal of Psychosomatic Research, 51*, 597–605.

Bindler, R. M., Howry, L. B., Wilson, B. A., Shannon, M. T., & Stang, C. L. (2005). *Pediatric drug guide.* Upper Saddle River, NJ: Prentice Hall.

Blume, E. D. (2003). Current status of heart transplantation in children: Update 2003. *Pediatric Clinics of North America, 50,* 1375–1391.

Blume, E. D., Naftel, D. C., Bastardi, H. J., Duncan, B. W., Kirklin, J. K., et al. (2006). Outcomes of children bridged to heart transplantation with ventricular assist devices: A multi-institutional study. *Circulation, 113,* 2313–2319.

Canobbio, M. M. (2001). Health care issues facing adolescents with congenital heart disease. *Journal of Pediatric Nursing, 16*(5), 363–370.

Chang, R. K. (2002). Hospitalizations for Kawasaki disease among children in the United States, 1988–1997. *Pediatrics, 109*(6), e87–e93.

Chang, R. R., Chen, A.Y., & Klitzner, T. S. (2002). Clinical management of infants with hypoplastic left heart syndrome in the United States, 1988–1997. *Pediatrics, 110*(2), 292–298.

Connolly, C., McClowry, S., Hayman, L., Mahony, L., & Artman, M. (2004). Posttraumatic stress disorder in children after cardiac surgery. *Journal of Pediatrics, 144*(4), 480–484.

Connor, J. A. (2006). Alterations in cardiovascular function in children. In K. L. McCance & S. E. Huether (Eds.), *Pathophysiology:*

The biologic basis for disease in adults and children. (5th ed., pp. 1147–1180). St. Louis: Mosby.

Connor, J. A., Arons, R. R., Figueroa, M., & Gebbie, K. M. (2004). Clinical outcomes and secondary diagnoses for infants born with hypoplastic left heart syndrome. *Pediatrics, 114*(2), e160–e165.

Cook, E. H., & Higgins, S. S. (2004). Congenital heart disease. In P. J. Allen & J. A. Vessey, *Primary care of the child with a chronic condition* (4th ed., pp 382–403). St. Louis: Mosby.

Corbett, J. V. (2004). Laboratory tests and diagnostic procedures with nursing diagnoses (6th ed.). Upper Saddle River, NJ: Prentice Hall.

Dajani, A. S., Taubert, K. A., Wilson, W., Bolger, A. F., Bayer, A., Ferrieri, P., et. al. (1997). Prevention of bacterial endocarditis: Recommendations of the American Heart Association. *Journal of the American Medical Association, 277*(22), 1794–1801.

Davis, C. C., Brown, R. T., Bakeman, R., & Campbell, R. (1998). Psychological adaptation and adjustment of mothers of children with congenital heart disease: Stress, coping, and family functioning. *Journal of Pediatric Psychology, 23*(4), 219–228.

Doniger, S., & Sharieff, G. Q. (2006). Pediatric dysrhythmias. *Pediatric Clinics in North America, 53,* 85–105.

Fernandes, S. M., & Landzberg, M. J. (2004). Transitioning the young adult with congenital heart disease for life-long medical care. *Pediatric Clinics of North America, 51,* 1739–1748.

Ferrieri, P. (2002). Proceedings of the Jones Criteria workshop. *Circulation, 106,* 2521–2523.

Ferrieri, P., Gewitz, M. H., Gerber, M. A., Newburger, J. W., Dajani, A. S., et al. (2002). Unique features of infective endocarditis in childhood. *Pediatrics, 109*(5), 931–943.

Forbess, J. M., Visconti, K. J., Hancock-Friesen, C., Howe, R. C., Bellinger, D. C., & Jonas, R. A. (2002). Neurodevelopmental outcome after congenital heart surgery: Results from an institutional registry. *Circulation, 106*(Suppl I), I95–I102.

Gabrys, C. A. (2005). Pediatric cardiac transplants: A clinical update. *Journal of Pediatric Nursing, 20*(2), 139–143.

Gagliardi, M. G., Bevilacqua, M., Bassano, C., Leonardi, B., Boldrini, R., et al. (2004). Long term follow up of children with myocarditis treated by immunosuppression and of children with dilated cardiomyopathy. *Heart, 90,* 1167–1171.

Giddings, S., Dennison, B. A., Birch, L. L., Daniels, S. R., Gilman, M. W., et al. (2005). Dietary guidelines for children and adolescents: A guide for practitioners. Consensus statement from the American Heart Association. *Circulation, 112,* 2061–2075.

Gilmer, M. J., Harrell, J. S., Miles, M. S., & Hepworth, J.T. (2003). Youth characteristics and contextual variables influencing physical activity in young adolescents of parents with premature coronary heart disease. *Journal of Pediatric Nursing, 18,* 159–168.

Goldberg, S., Morris, P., Simmons, R. J., Fowler, R. S., & Levinson, H. (1990). Chronic illness in infancy and parenting stress: A comparison of three groups of parents. *Journal of Pediatric Psychology, 15,* 347–358.

Goldmuntz, E. (2004). The genetic contribution to congenital heart disease. *Pediatric Clinics of North America, 51,* 1721–1737.

Goldrick, B. A. (2003). Endocarditis associated with body piercing. *American Journal of Nursing, 103*(1), 26–27.

Granton, J. T., & Rabinovitch, M. (2002). Pulmonary artery hypertension in congenital heart disease. *Cardiology Clinics, 20,* 441–457.

Green, A. (2004). Outcomes of congenital heart disease: A review. *Pediatric Nursing, 30*(4), 280–284.

Green, A., Kitchen, B., & Ray, T. (2005). Supraventricular tachycardia in children: Symptoms distinguish from sinus tachycardia. *Journal of Emergency Nursing, 31*(1), 105–108.

Gregoratos, G., Abrams, J., Epstein, A. E., Freedman, R. A., Hayes, D. L., et al. (2002). ACC/AHA.NASPE 2002 guideline update for implantation of cardiac pacemakers and antiarrhythmia devices: A report of the American College of Cardiology, American Heart Association Task Force on Practice Guidelines. Accessed May 4, 2004, from http://www.acc.org/clinical/guidelines/pacemaker/pacemaker.pdf

Hanish, D. (2001). Pediatric arrhythmias. *Journal of Pediatric Nursing, 16*(5), 351–362.

Higgins, S. S., & Tong, E. (2003). Transitioning adolescents with congenital heart disease to adult health care. *Progressive Cardiovascular Nursing, 18*(2), 93–98.

Ikle, L., Hale, K., Fashaw, L., Boucek, M., & Rosenberg, A. A. (2003). Developmental outcome of patients with hypoplastic left heart syndrome treated with heart transplantation. *Journal of Pediatrics, 142*(1), 20–25.

Jago, R., Harrell, J. S., McMurray, R. G., Edelstein, S., El Ghormli, L., & Bassin, S. (2006). Prevalence of abnormal lipid and blood pressure values among ethnically diverse population of eighth-grade adolescents and screening implications. *Pediatrics, 117*(6), 2065–2073.

Josephson, M. A. (2005). Improving medication adherence in transplant recipients: Managing the physical side effects of immunosuppression. *Medscape Transplantation, 6*(2). Accessed August 22, 2005, from http://www.medscape.com/viewartical/508880.htm

Kavey, R. E. W., Daniels, S. R., Lauer, R. M., Atkins, D. L., Hayman, L. L., & Taubert, K. (2003). American Heart Association guidelines for primary prevention of atherosclerotic cardiovascular disease beginning in childhood. *Journal of Pediatrics, 142*(4), 368–372.

Kingsbury, K. J. (2003). Understanding the essentials of blood lipid metabolism. *Progressive Cardiovascular Nursing, 18*(1), 13–18.

Lipshultz, S. E., Sleeper, L. A., Towbin, J. A., Lowe, A. M., Orav, E. J., Cox, G. F., et al. (2003). The incidence of pediatric cardiomyopathy in two regions of the United States. *New England Journal of Medicine, 348* (April 24), 1647–1655.

Mahle, W. T., Visconti, K. J., Freier, M. C., Kanne, S. M., Hamilton, W. G., et al. (2006). Relationship of surgical approach to neurodevelopmental outcomes in hypoplastic left heart syndrome. *Pediatrics, 117*(1), e90–e97.

Mahle, W. T., & Wernovsky, G. (2001). Long-term developmental outcome of children with complex congenital heart disease. *Clinics in Perinatology, 28*(1), 235–247.

Maron, B. J. (2004). Hypertrophic cardiomyopathy in childhood. *Pediatric Clinics of North America, 51,* 1305–1346.

Maron, B. J., Chaitman, B. R., Ackerman, M. J., Bayés de Luna, A., Corrado, D., et al. (June 8, 2004). Recommendations for physical activity and recreational sports participation for young patients with genetic cardiovascular diseases. *Circulation, 109,* 2807–2816.

Mörelius, E., Lundh, U., & Nelson, N. (2002). Parental stress in relation to the severity of congenital heart disease in the offspring. *Pediatric Nursing, 28*(1), 28–32.

Muntner, P., He, J., Cutler, J. A., Wildman, R. P., & Whelton, P. K. (2004). Trends in blood pressure among children and adolescents. *Journal of the American Medical Association, 291*(17), 2107–2113.

National High Blood Pressure Education Program Working Group on High Blood Pressure in Children and Adolescents. (2004). The fourth report on the diagnosis, evaluation, and treatment of high blood pressure in children and adolescents. *Pediatrics, 114*(2), 555–576.

Neilson, D. E., & Robin, N. H. (2002). Advances in the genetics of pediatric heart disease. *Contemporary Pediatrics, 19*(1), 85–100.

Newberger, J. W., Takahasi, M., Gerber, M. A., (2004). Diagnosis, treatment, and long-term management of Kawasaki disease: A statement for health professionals from the Committee on Rheumatic Fever, Endocarditis, and Kawasaki Disease, Council on Cardiovascular Disease in the Young, American Heart Association, *Circulation, 110* (October 26), 2747–2771.

Pappone, C., Manguso, F., Santinelli, R., et al. (2004). Radiofrequency ablation in children with asymptomatic Wolff-Parkinson-White syndrome. *New England Journal of Medicine, 351*(12), 1197–1205.

Park, M. K. (2002). *Pediatric cardiology for practitioners* (4th ed.). St. Louis: Mosby.

Pelchat, D., Ricard, N., Bouchard, J. M., Perreault, M., Saucier, J. F., Berrthiaume, M., et al. (1999). Adaptation of parents in relation to their 6-month-old infant's type of disability. *Child: Care, Health and Development, 25,* 377–397.

Peters, R. M., & Flack, J. M. (2003). Diagnosis and treatment of hypertension in children and adolescents. *Journal of the American Academy of Nurse Practitioners, 15*(2), 56–63.

Popovich, D.M., Richiuso, N., & Danck, G. (2004). Pediatric health care providers' knowledge of pulse oximetry. *Pediatric Nursing, 30*(1), 14–20.

Rao, P. S., Jureidini, S. B., Balfour, I. C., Singh, G. K., & Chen, S. (2003). Severe aortic coarctation in infants less than three months: Successful palliation by balloon angioplasty. *Journal of Invasive Cardiology, 15*(4), 202–208.

Rome, J. J., & Kreutzer, J. (2004). Pediatric interventional catheterization: Reasonable expectations and outcomes. *Pediatric Clinics of North America, 51,* 1589–1610.

Shillingford, A. J., & Wernovsky, G. (2004). Academic performance and behavioral difficulties after neonatal and infant heart surgery. *Pediatric Clinics of North America, 51,* 1625–1639.

Special Writing Group of the Committee on Rheumatic Fever, Endocarditis, and Kawasaki Disease of the Council on Cardiovascular Disease in the Young of the American Heart Association. (1992). Guidelines for the diagnosis of rheumatic fever. Jones Criteria, 1992 update. *Journal of the American Medical Association, 268*(15), 2069–2073.

Stafford, P. W., Blinman, T. A., & Nance, M. L. (2002). Practical points in evaluation and resuscitation of the injured child. *Surgical Clinics of North America, 82,* 273–301.

Stephens, P., & Paridon, S. M. (2004). Exercise testing in pediatrics. *Pediatric Clinics of North America, 51,* 1569–1587.

Strauss, A., & Lock, J. E. (2003). Pediatric cardiomyopathy—A long way to go. *New England Journal of Medicine, 348* (April 24), 1703–1705.

Suddaby, E. C. (2001). Contemporary thinking for congenital heart disease. *Pediatric Nursing, 27*(3), 233–238, 270.

Tani, L. Y., Veasy, G., Minich, L. L., & Shaddy, R. E. (2003). Rheumatic fever in children younger than 5 years: Is the presentation different? *Pediatrics, 112*(5), 1065–1068.

Tran, J. T. (2002). Current treatment strategies of symptomatic patent ductus arteriosis. *Journal of Pediatric Health Care, 16*(6), 306–310.

Uzark, K., & Jones, K. (2003). Parenting stress and children with heart disease. *Journal of Pediatric Health Care, 17*(4), 163–168.

Wiegman, A., Hutten, B. A., de Groot, E., Rodenburg, J., Baccker, H. D., et al. (2004). Efficacy and safety of statin therapy in children with familial hypercholesterolemia. *Journal of the American Medical Association, 292*(3), 331–337.

ALTERATIONS IN HEMATOLOGIC FUNCTION

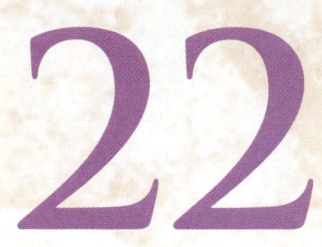

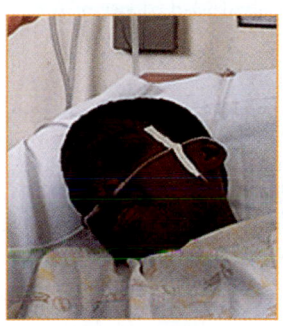

MICHAEL, a 12-year-old boy, is admitted to the hospital with severe abdominal pain. He was diagnosed with sickle cell anemia at 1 year of age and has been in fairly good health. He has, however, been hospitalized on two previous occasions with complications of the disease. Recently, Michael has had several viral illnesses, leading his physician to suspect that his spleen is filled with abnormal cells, which are impairing his immune function.

Michael is small for his age and has several bruises on his lower legs. His respirations are rapid and he appears anxious. Michael's parents are knowledgeable about sickle cell anemia, as his uncle also has the disease. They know that Michael is experiencing an episode of sickle cell crisis.

An intravenous infusion is started, and Michael is medicated for pain. The nurse attempts to perform multiple tests and procedures together to allow Michael time to rest in-between. Michael is receiving oxygen by nasal cannula to increase his oxygen saturation to normal levels.

What immediate and long-term care does Michael require? What do Michael and his parents need to know about this crisis? How could you help them manage the challenges of this condition? This chapter will assist you in planning care for children like Michael who have disorders of the hematologic system.

KEY TERMS

allogeneic transplantation 833
anemia 799
autologous transplantation 833
ecchymosis 824
erythropoiesis 798
hemarthrosis 824
hematopoiesis 820
hemochromatosis 819
hemoglobinopathy 806
hemosiderin 819

hemosiderosis 812
isogeneic transplantation 833
leukopenia 799
menorrhagia 803
neutropenia 822
pancytopenia 822
petechiae 822
polycythemia 799
priapism 807
purpura 822
thrombocytopenia 799
vaso-occlusion 807

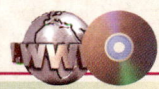

MediaLink

LEARNING OUTCOMES

After reading this chapter, you will be able to do the following:

1. Describe the function of red blood cells, white blood cells, and platelets.

2. Discuss the pathophysiology and clinical manifestations of the major disorders of red blood cells affecting the pediatric population.

3. Discuss the pathophysiology and clinical manifestations of the major disorders of white blood cells affecting the pediatric population.

4. Discuss the pathophysiology and clinical manifestations of the major disorders of platelets affecting the pediatric population.

5. Describe the nursing management and collaborative care of a child with a hematologic disorder.

6. Discuss nursing implications for a child receiving hematopoietic stem cell transplantation (HSCT).

FOCUS ON
The Hematologic System

ANATOMY AND PHYSIOLOGY

Blood has two components: a fluid portion called plasma and a cellular portion known as the formed elements of the blood. The cellular elements are red blood cells or RBCs (erythrocytes), white blood cells or WBCs (leukocytes), and platelets (thrombocytes) (Figure 22–1 ➤). Table 22–1 gives normal values for these blood components in children.

Red Blood Cells

Red blood cells, or erythrocytes, are the most abundant of the cellular elements of blood. They are formed through a process called **erythropoiesis**. The primary function of red blood cells is to transport oxygen from the lungs to the tissues. These cells also help to carry carbon dioxide back to the lungs. Hemoglobin, a red pigment composed of protein and

Figure 22–1 ➤ Types of blood cells.

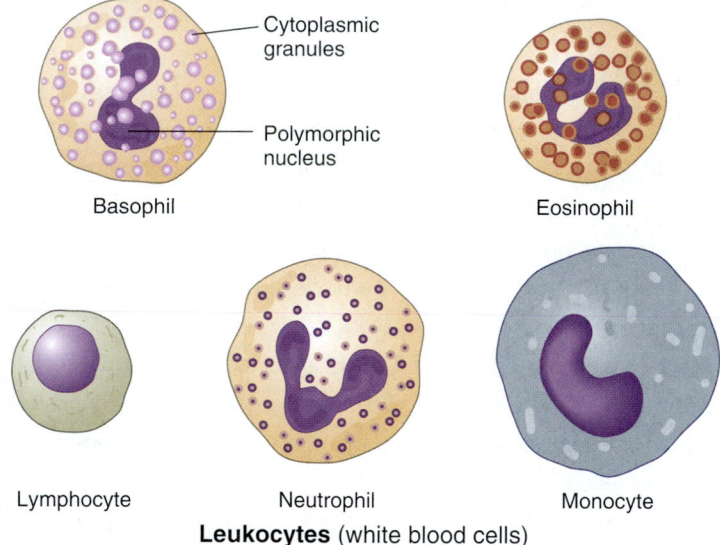

Cytoplasmic granules

Polymorphic nucleus

Basophil

Eosinophil

Lymphocyte

Neutrophil

Monocyte

Leukocytes (white blood cells)

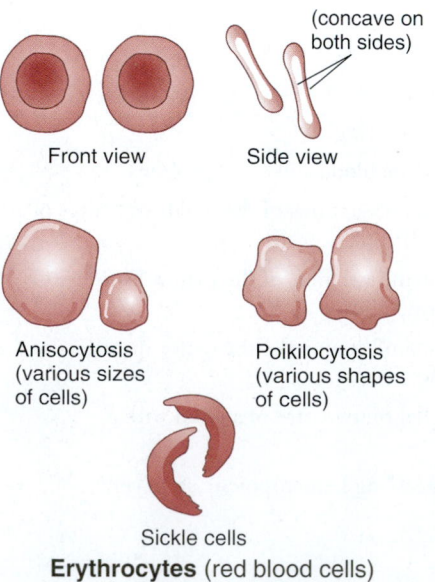

(concave on both sides)

Front view

Side view

Anisocytosis (various sizes of cells)

Poikilocytosis (various shapes of cells)

Sickle cells

Erythrocytes (red blood cells)

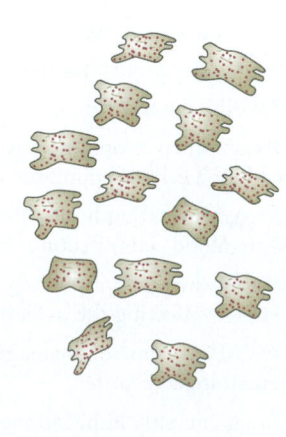

Thrombocytes (Platelets)

Table 22–1	NORMAL BLOOD VALUES IN CHILDREN			
	Newborn	**2 Years**	**12 Years**	**18 Years**
Red blood cells (RBCs) (values $\times 10^6$/microL)	3.4–5.5	4.0–4.9	4.0–5.3	3.8–5.4
Hematocrit (Hct) (%)	37.4–56.1	31.7–37.7	34.0–43.9	33.0–46.2
Hemoglobin (Hgb) (g/dL)	12.7–18.6	10.5–12.7	11.2–14.8	10.7–15.7
White blood cells (WBCs) (values $\times 10^3$/microL)	6.8–14.3	5.3–11.5	4.5–10.1	4.4–10.2
Platelets (values $\times 10^3$/microL)	164–351	204–405	165–335	143–326

Note: Modified from Soldin, S. J., Brugnara, C., & Hicks, J. M. (2003). *Pediatric reference ranges* (4th ed.). Washington, DC: AACC Press.

iron which is contained in the RBC, is essential to this function. The normal life span of a red blood cell is about 120 days. See Chapter 21 ∞ for a discussion of fetal hemoglobin and its unique characteristics, as well as its effect on hemoglobin levels in the newborn period.

Polycythemia is an above-average increase in the number of red cells in the blood. Any condition that causes the quantity of oxygen transported to the tissues to decrease ordinarily increases the rate of red blood cell production. When a child becomes anemic secondary to hemorrhage, for instance, the bone marrow immediately begins to produce large quantities of red cells. **Anemia** is a reduction in the number of red blood cells; the various types of anemia will be discussed in this chapter.

White Blood Cells

White blood cells, or leukocytes, are the mobile units of the body's protective system. They are formed in bone marrow and lymph tissue. There are five types of white blood cells, each with a distinct function (Table 22–2). A differential blood count indicates the percentages of the different types of white cells present in the blood and is sometimes useful in identifying the cause of an illness. For example, infections cause an increase in neutrophils, and allergies are related to an increase in eosinophils. The role of lymphocytes is discussed with acquired immunodeficiency syndrome in Chapter 17 ∞. A decrease in the number of white blood cells is called **leukopenia**, and can be caused by immune or bone marrow disorders.

Table 22–2	WHITE BLOOD CELLS AND THEIR FUNCTIONS	
Type	**Function**	**Value (% of total)**
Neutrophils	Phagocytosis	32.3–72.9%
Eosinophils	Allergic reactions	2.4–4.8 %
Basophils	Inflammatory reactions	1%
Monocytes (macrophages)	Phagocytosis, antigen processing	3.5–13.4%
Lymphocytes	Humoral immunity (B cell), cellular immunity (T cell)	13.5–52.8%

Platelets

Platelets, or thrombocytes, are cell fragments that can form hemostatic plugs to stop bleeding. They are synthesized from components in the red bone marrow and are stored in the spleen. A deficiency of platelets can lead to a bleeding disorder and is termed **thrombocytopenia.**

PEDIATRIC DIFFERENCES

Production of *red blood cells* occurs in the fetus by the second week of gestation, with white blood cell and platelet production beginning at 8 weeks. Most of this early production occurs first in the embryonic yolk sac and then in the liver; however, by 20 to 24 weeks' gestation, liver production decreases as bone marrow production begins to predominate (Chamley, Carson, Randall, & Sandwell, 2005; Ohls & Christensen, 2004). At birth, hematopoiesis, or blood cell production, occurs in the marrow of almost every bone. The flat bones, such as the sternum, ribs, pelvic and shoulder girdles, vertebrae, and hips, retain most of their hematopoietic activity throughout life.

Fetal RBCs contain fetal hemoglobin, which has a high level of affinity for oxygen. The fetus must extract oxygen from the maternal circulation, which has lower oxygen saturation than the atmosphere. Therefore, the developing fetus needs this enhanced ability. Fetal hemoglobin is present in decreasing amounts after birth, with normal hemoglobin gradually increasing.

Blood volume of the newborn infant is 80 mL/kg of body weight (London et al., 2007). At birth, the newborn has a naturally occurring elevation in red blood cells (RBCs) and hemoglobin due to a high level of erythropoietin, which stimulates red cell production (see Table 22–1). Additional contributors to these higher levels are the transfusion of blood from the placenta at birth and low extracellular fluid volume from low oral intake after birth. Once the newborn begins breathing air and the oxygen level in the blood increases, this production slows (Polin, Fox, & Abman, 2004). Levels of RBCs and hemoglobin fall until about 2 to 3 months of age (to about 9–11 g/dL), and then begin increasing. Adult levels are reached during adolescence. Teenage males have red blood cell levels slightly higher than teenage females (see Appendix C ∞).

The *white blood cell* count is highest at birth, although levels vary greatly among infants. By 1 week of age, white blood cell values stabilize. Throughout childhood, there is a very slow decrease in white blood cell count (Boxer, 2004).

Platelet levels in newborns are lower than in older children and adults. Levels of many clotting factors, particularly those requiring vitamin K for activation (factors II, VII, IX, X, and anticoagulant factors — proteins C and S), are also lower in infants. For this reason, all newborns receive a prophylactic injection of vitamin K at birth. Values of platelets and other coagulation products soon reach normal childhood levels (Montgomery & Scott, 2004).

Examples of diagnostic and laboratory tests used to evaluate the hematologic system are provided in the accompanying table. Use the guidelines on page 802 to perform a nursing assessment of this system.

DIAGNOSTIC PROCEDURES AND LABORATORY TESTS FOR THE HEMATOLOGIC SYSTEM

Laboratory Test	Purpose	Nursing Implications
Complete blood count (CBC)	The CBC measures all cell types in the serum, including red blood cells and white blood cells.	• Collect the blood sample in tubes according to agency laboratory protocol. • Collect blood samples from children in a treatment room or laboratory rather than in a hospital room or outpatient examination room. • Arrange for transport to the laboratory in the required manner.
Clotting indices	Several studies assist in diagnosis and management of clotting disorders: • Platelet count = numbers of platelets in mm^3 • Mean platelet volume (MPV) = volume of platelets in serum, measured in cubic micrometers (microm^3) • Bleeding time = time before clotting occurs to stop bleeding from a small puncture, measured in minutes • Prothrombin time (PT) = a measure of clotting factor II, plasma protein in sec • Partial thromboplastin time (PTT) = demonstrates lack of various clotting factors, measured in sec • Thrombin time = the time it takes blood to clot when thrombin is added, measured in sec • Activated clotting time (ACT) = often used to monitor heparin effects, measured in sec • Factors VIII and IX = measures the two clotting factors most commonly abnormal in hemophilia, measured in % • Fibrinogen = factor I, a plasma protein measured in mg/dL	• Collect the blood sample in tubes according to agency laboratory protocol. • Collect blood samples from children in a treatment room or laboratory rather than in a hospital room or outpatient examination room. • Arrange for transport to the laboratory in the required manner.
Iron indices	Several indices indicate the function of iron in serum and are thus helpful in diagnosis of iron deficiency anemia: • Serum iron = microgram/deciliter (mcg/dL) • Serum ferritin = measure of ferritin, the iron storage protein in ng/mL • Total iron-binding capacity (TIBC) = measure of transferrin, a plasma protein that transports iron in micrograms/deciliter (mcg/dL) • Transferrin saturation = calculation derived from serum iron and TIBC, measured in % • Free erythrocyte protoporphyrin (FEP) = protoporphyrin is used in synthesis of heme but will not be used if adequate iron is not available, causing a rise in levels of FEP, measured in microgram/deciliter (mcg/dL) • Reticulocyte count = measure of amount of reticulocytes, which are immature RBCs, in % • Erythrocyte sedimentation rate (ESR or sed rate) = speed with which RBCs settle in a tube, measured in mm/hr • Erythropoietin assay = a kidney hormone that regulates RBC production, measured in m/units/mL	• Collect the blood sample in tubes according to agency laboratory protocol. • Collect blood samples from children in a treatment room or laboratory rather than in a hospital room or outpatient examination room. • Arrange for transport to the laboratory in required manner.

DIAGNOSTIC AND LABORATORY TESTS FOR THE HEMATOLOGIC SYSTEM (continued)

Laboratory Test	Purpose	Nursing Implications
Red blood cell indices	A variety of tests are used to provide information about red blood cell (erythrocyte) amount and quality: • RBC count = number of RBCs/mm^3 of blood • Hematocrit = packed red cell volume, obtained when serum is centrifuged; amount in % of packed red cells that collect at the bottom of the sample • Hemoglobin = grams/100 mL of hemoglobin (the protein-iron compound in RBCs that carries oxygen); approximately one-third of the hematocrit • Hemoglobin electrophoresis can be used to identify the specific types of hemoglobin that are abnormal • Sickledex or sickle-turbidity test mixes blood with a special solution in which sickled hemoglobin is not soluble; it is a quick screening test for sickle cell disease and sickle cell trait; positive results must be followed by hemoglobin electrophoresis • Mean corpuscular volume (MCV) = average size of RBCs in cubic micrometers (microm^3) or femtoliters (fl) • Mean corpuscular hemoglobin concentration (MCHC) = amount of hemoglobin in one RBC in picograms (pg) • RBC cell distribution width (RDW) = % range of RBC cell size; wide distribution indicates many new cells are present	• Collect the blood sample in tubes according to agency laboratory protocol. • Collect blood samples from children in a treatment room or laboratory rather than in the hospital room or outpatient examination room. • Arrange for transport to the laboratory in the required manner.
White blood cell indices	A variety of tests are used to measure the amount of WBCs and their comparative amounts in the serum: • WBC count = total number of WBCs in blood in mm^3 • Differential—proportion of each of the types of WBCs (bands or young neutrophils, neutrophils or "segs," eosinophils, basophils, lymphocytes, monocytes)	• Collect the blood sample in tubes according to agency laboratory protocol. • Collect blood samples from children in a treatment room or laboratory rather than in the hospital room or outpatient examination room. • Arrange for transport to the laboratory in the required manner.
Additional blood tests	Various additional tests may assist in diagnosis of hematologic disorders: • Serum folic acid = indicates a potential cause of anemia, measured in ng/mL • Vitamin B$_{12}$ = indicates a potential cause of anemia, measured in pg/mL • Glucose-6-Phosphate-Dehydrogenase (G-6-PD) = this test measures an enzyme normally present in RBCs; a deficiency may indicate a genetic cause of anemia, measured in units/g	• Collect the blood sample in tubes according to agency laboratory protocol. • Collect blood samples from children in a treatment room or laboratory rather than in the hospital room or outpatient examination room. • Arrange for transport to the laboratory in the required manner.

Data from: Corbett, J. V. (2004). *Laboratory tests and diagnostic procedures with nursing diagnoses* (6th ed.). Upper Saddle River, NJ: Prentice Hall Health; Kee, J. L. (2005). *Handbook of laboratory & diagnostic tests with nursing implications* (5th ed.). Upper Saddle River, NJ: Prentice Hall Health.

ASSESSMENT GUIDELINES FOR THE CHILD WITH A HEMATOLOGIC SYSTEM ALTERATION

Assessment Focus	Assessment Guidelines
Family history	• Does a family member have sickle cell anemia/trait or other inherited anemia? • Does a family member have hemophilia or another inherited clotting alteration?
Growth and development	• Growth should be regular and in the same growth curve percentiles on growth charts. Nutritional intake should meet recommendations for age and weight. Developmental milestones should emerge at expected times. The child should display usual energy levels and regular sleep patterns. Delayed growth and development and lethargy can indicate anemia or other disorders.
Skin	• Assess for pallor, flushing, rashes, ecchymosis. • Observe for bleeding/clotting time.
Joints	• Observe for edema, pain, inflammation, and range of motion.
Additional assessments	• Assessments of pain in various body parts, frequent infection, and other factors may suggest diseases such as sickle cell anemia or other hematologic disorders.

The hematologic system is one of the few body systems that regulate, directly or indirectly, all other body functions. Because blood is involved in the function of all tissues and organs, changes in the blood may result in altered functioning of many body organs and structures. A tendency toward easy bruising is a characteristic sign of many bleeding disorders. Other signs include nosebleeds, pallor, frequent infections, and lethargy. This chapter discusses the most common disorders of the blood and blood-forming organs in children. (See Chapter 23 ∞ for a discussion of leukemia.)

ANEMIAS

Anemia is defined as a reduction in the number of red blood cells, the quantity of hemoglobin, and the volume of packed red cells to below-normal levels. This condition can be caused by loss or destruction of existing red blood cells or by an impaired or decreased rate of red cell production. Anemia also can be a clinical manifestation of an underlying disorder, such as lead poisoning or hypersplenism (a syndrome characterized by splenomegaly and blood cell deficiencies). Common childhood anemias are discussed in this section.

Iron Deficiency Anemia

Iron deficiency anemia is the most common type of anemia and the most common nutritional deficiency in children. It affects 3% of children younger than 2 years of age, 6–18% of toddlers, 9–11% of adolescent females, and less than 1% of adolescent males (Carley, 2003; White, 2005).

Etiology and Pathophysiology

The body requires iron for the production of hemoglobin. Insufficient quantities of iron limit hemoglobin production, in turn affecting the production of red blood cells. RBCs are needed to carry oxygen throughout the body, so anemia results in less oxygen reaching cells and tissues.

Iron deficiency anemia can occur secondary to blood loss, malabsorption, or poor nutritional intake. See Chapter 4 ∞ for a discussion of iron deficiency anemia due to deficits in nutritional intake. Increased internal demands (such as rapid growth periods) can also lead to anemia. Rapidly growing adolescents whose diets are high in fat and low in vitamins and minerals are particularly susceptible to iron deficiency anemia. Infants who do not take in adequate solid foods after 6 months of age and are fed only breast milk or formula that is not fortified with iron are also at risk because neonatal iron stores have been depleted by this time and their iron needs are not being met. Similarly, among mothers whose nutritional status during pregnancy was inadequate, and infants who were born prematurely or are products of multiple births, insufficient iron may have been stored in the latter part of pregnancy, placing the infant at higher risk for anemia in the first months of life.

Chronic blood loss is always a potential cause of iron deficiency anemia. The infant who has had bleeding in the neonatal period, the child who loses blood as a result of conditions such as hemophilia or parasitic gastrointestinal illness, and the adolescent girl who has **menorrhagia** (heavy menstrual bleeding) may all be at risk of anemia.

Clinical Manifestations

Clinical manifestations and severity of symptoms are directly related to the amount of iron deficiency. Pallor, fatigue, and irritability are characteristic findings. With prolonged anemia, nailbed deformities, growth retardation, developmental delay, tachycardia, and systolic heart murmur can occur. Pica, or consumption of non-food items, is also associated with iron deficiency anemia. Lead poisoning is associated with anemia and may worsen since lead absorption increases in the anemic state.

COLLABORATIVE CARE

Diagnostic Tests

Diagnosis is made on the basis of laboratory studies; findings include low hemoglobin level, mean corpuscular volume, serum iron, RBC count, reticulocytes (immature or newly released red blood cells), iron-binding capacity, and serum ferritin <15 ng/mL. Microscopic analysis (Figure 22–2 ➤) reveals red blood cells are microcytic (small) in size and hypochromic (pale) in appearance (Carley, 2003). A diet history and analysis can provide information related to food intake; see Chapter 4 ∞ for guidelines about diet history.

Clinical Therapy

Treatment of iron deficiency anemia involves correction of the iron deficiency with oral elemental iron preparations and a diet high in iron. Ferrous sulfate at a dose of 3 to 6 mg/kg/day for about 4 weeks is a common treatment, followed by evaluation for its effectiveness. If the anemia is improving, treatment usually continues for about 2 months (Carley, 2003; American Academy of Pediatrics, 2004). Because oral iron preparations cause several side effects such as constipation and gastrointestinal discomfort, the child may receive iron supplements (to restore blood levels of iron) while the iron content of the diet is increased above the recommended dietary allowances (RDAs). Oral supplements can then be tapered off once the child's food intake can supply the needed iron; the child is evaluated in about 6 months for recurring anemia.

If the anemia is not improved by iron intake, further diagnostic studies are needed. If it is a result of bleeding, the cause is identified and treated to prevent future excess blood loss. Other causes such as myelosuppression or genetic diseases are treated as appropriate. If lead poisoning has occurred, removal from the source and treatment to facilitate lead excretion are needed (see Chapter 6 ∞).

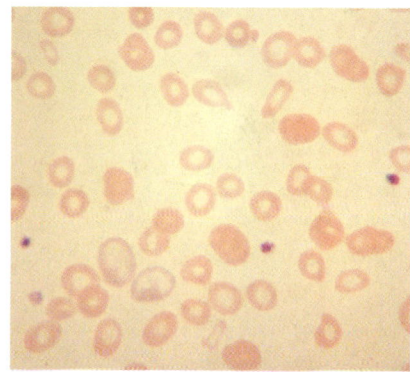

Figure 22–2 ➤ In iron deficiency anemia, red blood cells appear hypochromic as a result of decreased hemoglobin synthesis.
Courtesy of Dr. Ed Wong, Laboratory Medicine, Children's National Medical Center, Washington, DC.

NURSING MANAGEMENT

Nursing Assessment and Diagnosis

Children with iron deficiency anemia are usually identified and treated in the community unless they have another serious illness. Nursing care focuses on screening for the disorder and educating the parents and children about the causes of iron deficiency anemia, dietary management, and the importance of complying with the medication regimen.

Screening for anemia is recommended at 9–12 months of age, at 15–18 months of age, and again at adolescence. Premature infants are generally screened at 4 months

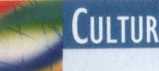

CULTURE

Chi

According to traditional Chinese beliefs, a person who does not feel well is lacking in chi (inner energy) and blood. Chinese Americans who follow traditional practices may be hesitant to have blood drawn for laboratory studies for fear of causing bodily weakness.

(Committee on Nutrition, 2004). A hematocrit or hemoglobin level is obtained for screening. More detailed tests, such as those identified previously in the collaborative care section, are performed if the blood test is abnormal. Children at high risk for nutritional deficiencies, such as those in low-income groups and Women, Infants, and Children (WIC) programs, may require additional tests. Most children in Head Start are screened annually by nurses. In addition, children showing signs of anemia should be screened. Height and weight measurements should be obtained at each healthcare visit, plotted on growth charts, and compared with percentiles obtained at previous visits. Slow downward trends in percentiles are of concern and require further nutritional analysis. A diet history and analysis provide information related to food intake (see Chapter 4 ∞ for guidelines about diet analysis). Developmental screening tests should be performed to assess for developmental delays (see Chapter 7 ∞).

Nursing diagnoses that may apply to the child with iron deficiency anemia include:

- Imbalanced Nutrition: Less than Body Requirements related to dietary intake
- Ineffective Tissue Perfusion related to lack of oxygen
- Activity Intolerance related to decreased oxygen-carrying capacity
- Risk for Delayed Growth and Development related to decreased tissue perfusion

Planning and Implementation

Dietary management is the preferred long-term treatment for iron deficiency anemia. Teach the family and child about foods that are rich in iron. Include teaching about foods with vitamin C as well since this vitamin enhances absorption of iron (Table 22–3). The infant over 6 months of age should have a diet that includes breast milk or iron-fortified formula and baby cereals with iron fortification. Avoid cow's milk in the first year of life since it can cause bleeding from the gastrointestinal tract, contributing to anemia. If the older infant or toddler consumes large quantities of milk and refuses to eat solid food, restriction on milk intake may be required. Older infants and toddlers can be provided with finger foods such as thinly sliced meats. Adolescents can be encouraged to eat foods with a high iron content, such as hamburgers and dried fruits. Protein is needed for blood cell production, and folic acid helps to convert iron from ferritin to hemoglobin; encourage adequate amounts of these nutrients in the diet.

Oral iron preparations, usually ferrous sulfate, are given to correct anemia (see Medications Used to Treat Iron Deficiency Anemia on the next page). Teach the child and family that the liquid iron preparation should be taken through a straw because it stains the teeth. Instruct about side effects such as black, green, or "tarry" stools; constipation; and a foul aftertaste. Emphasize the importance of drinking fluids and eating foods high in dietary fiber to minimize these side effects.

Iron overdose can occur if the treated child or others in the family ingest excessive amounts of the drug. Abdominal pain, vomiting, bloody diarrhea, shortness of breath, and shock can occur. Teach safe storage of the medication to avoid poisoning.

Table 22–3	FOOD SOURCES OF IRON AND VITAMIN C
Iron-Rich Foods	**Vitamin C-Rich Foods**
Meats, fish, poultry	Orange juice
Vegetables	Citrus fruits
Dried fruits	Strawberries
Legumes	Tomatoes
Enriched grain products	Broccoli
Whole-grain cereals	Green leafy vegetables
Iron-fortified dry cereals	Potatoes
	Some dry cereals

MEDICATIONS USED TO TREAT *Iron Deficiency Anemia*

Medication	Action/Indication	Nursing Implications
Ferrous sulfate	Corrects anemia caused by iron deficiency	Common side effects include gastrointestinal symptoms such as nausea, anorexia, constipation, abdominal distress, black stools.
	A variety of doses and preparations are available, such as tablets, capsules, syrup, elixir, and drops	Give on empty stomach if possible; if gastric distress occurs, give with or immediately after meals; if gastric distress continues, report to prescriber as formulation may need to be changed to ferrous gluconate.
		Monitor bowel movements and suggest increased fluid and fiber.
		Monitor development, sleep, and activity/fatigue patterns.
		Monitor hemoglobin and reticulocytes to measure effectiveness of therapy.
		Dilute liquid preparations well in water (avoid milk and fruit juice unless manufacturer states those fluids are acceptable for mixing) and give through a straw or place on the back of the tongue to prevent teeth staining and to mask taste; rinse the mouth with clear water immediately after ingestion.
		Instruct families to keep this drug locked and out of reach of children; poisoning is a serious risk.

Evaluation

Expected outcomes of nursing care include:

- The child's laboratory results manifest a normal red blood cell level.
- The family verbalizes understanding of treatment regimen.
- The child consumes recommended dietary intake.
- The child is free of side effects of oral iron therapy.
- The child is active and achieves appropriate growth and development milestones.

Normocytic Anemia

In normocytic anemia, the red blood cells, although decreased in number, are of normal size with a pale center. This type of anemia may occur as a result of hemorrhage, disease-induced inflammation, disseminated intravascular coagulation (DIC; see the discussion later in this chapter), Glucose-6-Phosphate-Dehydrogenase (G-6-PD) deficiency, hemolytic-uremic syndrome (see Chapter 25 ∞), or several other conditions. When one of these conditions exists in a child diagnosed with anemia, the infectious or inflammatory condition should be suspected as the cause of the identified anemia and treated first. Some of the infectious and inflammatory causes of anemia are listed in Table 22–4.

The etiology of normocytic anemia associated with chronic inflammation or infection is related to increased red blood cell destruction, decreased iron release from

Table 22–4	INFECTIOUS AND INFLAMMATORY CAUSES OF ANEMIA	
Infections		**Inflammations**
Haemophilus influenzae type b		Arthritis
HIV/AIDS		Cancers
Orbital cellulitis		Chronic heart or liver disease
Meningitis		
Septic arthritis		

storage sites, and ineffective bone marrow response. In hemorrhage, anemia is a direct result of loss of blood.

Clinical manifestations are similar to those seen in iron deficiency anemia, with the possible occurrence of hepatomegaly and splenomegaly, as well. Microscopic examination of red blood cells confirms diagnosis. Treatment of normocytic anemia depends on the underlying cause. When the anemia is associated with inflammation or infection, the underlying condition is treated. For anemia caused by renal failure, recombinant human erythropoietin is administered. When hemorrhage is the underlying cause, the source of the bleeding is identified and treated. In acute emergencies, blood products are infused to make up for some of the losses.

Nursing management of normocytic anemia depends on the cause of the decreased red blood cells. Children with inflammatory or infectious diseases require careful assessment and management of medication and other treatment regimens. Administer blood products and other intravenous fluids as ordered to restore blood volume. Follow-up and home visits are used to assess hematocrit, hemoglobin, and dietary intake. (Refer to the discussion later in this chapter for management of DIC; to Chapter 24 for management of intestinal infections; and to Chapter 25 ∞ for management of hemolytic-uremic syndrome.)

 MediaLink

Sickle Cell Anemia Animation

Sickle Cell Disease

Sickle cell disease is a hereditary **hemoglobinopathy**, characterized by the partial or complete replacement of normal hemoglobin with abnormal hemoglobin S (Hgb S) in red blood cells. This causes occlusion of small blood vessels, ischemia, and damage to affected organs. Sickle cell anemia is the most common type of sickle cell disease (Table 22–5). Sickle cell trait (carrying one gene for the disease) affects 1 in 8 African Americans and sickle cell disease occurs in about 1 of 400 Black infants born in the United States; about 2000 infants affected by the disease are born annually in the United States (Kral, Brown, Connelly et al., 2006; Wilson, Krishnamurti, & Kamat, 2003). The disorder is found primarily in Blacks, although occasionally it affects people of Mediterranean descent.

Table 22–5	SICKLE CELL DISORDERS
Sickle Cell Trait (Hgb SA)	Most common form of sickle cell disease in the United States
	Heterozygous condition (child has one sickle cell hemoglobin gene and one normal hemoglobin gene)
	Child is carrier of sickle cell anemia and rarely has symptoms of the disease
Sickle Cell Anemia (Hgb SS)	Homozygous condition (child has two sickle hemoglobin genes)
	Child is subject to sickle cell crises
Sickle Cell Syndromes	*Sickle cell–Hgb C disease (Hgb SC)*
	Second most frequent form of sickle cell disease in Blacks
	Different from sickle cell anemia only in that the sickle cell assumes a C shape instead of an S shape
Rare Combination of Conditions	Combination of sickle cell trait and thalassemia trait most often seen in people of Mediterranean descent
	Sickle Cell–β-Thalassemia Disease (Hgb SB)

Etiology and Pathophysiology

Sickle cell anemia is an autosomal recessive disorder. If both parents have the trait, with each pregnancy the risk of having a child with the disease is 25%. (See Chapter 3 ∞ for a discussion of recessive gene transmission.)

In sickle cell anemia, the hemoglobin in the red blood cell acquires an elongated crescent or sickle shape (Figure 22–3 ➤). This is caused by a genetic mutation in which the amino acid valine replaces the amino acid glutamic acid. The sickled cells are rigid and obstruct capillary blood flow. Microscopic obstructions lead to engorgement and tissue ischemia. This local tissue hypoxia causes further sickling and ultimately large infarctions.

Damaged tissues in organs throughout the body become scarred, resulting in impaired function. For example, children with sickle cell anemia can suffer from splenic sequestration when blood is trapped in the spleen, a life-threatening complication. Many children must undergo splenectomy in early childhood, leading to severely compromised immunity. Infection rate is subsequently high due to impaired immunity, and bacterial infections are the leading cause of death in young children with sickle cell disease.

Stroke is a significant risk to children with sickle cell anemia and can lead to developmental delay, mental retardation, and other neurologic outcomes (National Heart, Lung, and Blood Institute, 2002). Other complications of sickle cell disease can include acute chest syndrome with pulmonary hypertension, pulmonary infiltrate and infection; aplastic crisis or temporary cessation of bone marrow blood cell production; **priapism** or sustained and painful penile erection; and gallstone formation (Wilson, Krishnamurti, & Kamat, 2003).

Sickling may be triggered by fever and emotional or physical stress. Precipitating factors for sickle cell crisis include increased blood viscosity (such as from a low fluid intake or fever) and hypoxia or low oxygen tension. Potential causes of hypoxia or low oxygen tension include high altitudes, poorly pressurized airplanes, hypoventilation, vasoconstriction when cold, or an emotionally stressful event. Any condition that increases the body's need for oxygen or alters the transport of oxygen (such as infection, trauma, or dehydration) may result in sickle cell crisis.

Sickled cells can resume a normal shape when rehydrated and reoxygenated. The membrane of these cells becomes more fragile, however, and cell life is shortened to 10 to 20 days rather than the usual 120 days. In response, bone marrow spaces enlarge to produce more red blood cells. Continuous formation and destruction of the child's red blood cells contributes to the severe hemolytic anemia that is characteristic of sickle cell anemia (Tanyi, 2003). See Figure 22–4 ➤ for further information.

Clinical Manifestations

The manifestations of sickle cell disease range over nearly all of the organ systems. Pathologic changes occur in most body systems and result in multiple signs and symptoms (Figure 22–5 ➤). Affected children are usually asymptomatic until 4 to 6 months of age because sickling is inhibited by high levels of fetal hemoglobin. Clinical manifestations are directly related to the shortened life span of blood cells (hemolytic anemia) and tissue destruction resulting from **vaso-occlusion** (blockage of a blood vessel). Illness results from recurrent vaso-occlusive events that involve painful crises and chronic organ damage. Sickle cell crises are acute exacerbations of the disease that vary markedly in severity and frequency. Table 22–6 outlines the most common types of crises affecting children with sickle cell disease, and Box 22–1 lists some of the common precipitating factors. Notice that infections, impaired respirations, neurologic symptoms, pain, and skin changes are common manifestations of the disease. Crises in these systems may occur individually or in combination. Michael, the boy described at the beginning of this chapter, was in sickle cell crisis. Both his lungs and spleen are affected by the present crisis.

The most common reason for hospitalization of the child with sickle cell anemia is acute painful episodes (Beyer & Simmons, 2004). The sickled RBCs cause vaso-occlusion, microinfarction, and ischemia. Pain results from avascular necrosis

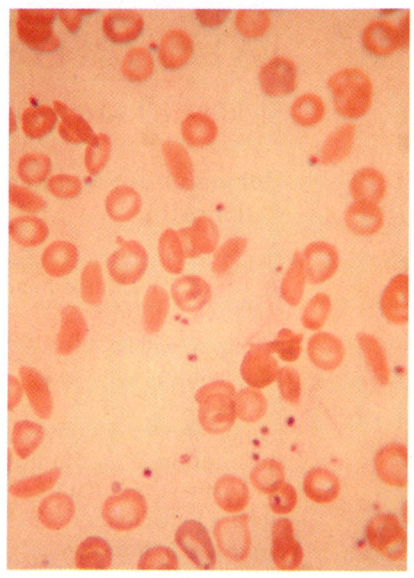

Figure 22–3 ➤ Many of these red blood cells show an elongated crescent shape characteristic of sickle cell anemia. Courtesy of Dr. Ed Wong, Laboratory Medicine, Children's National Medical Center, Washington, DC.

BOX 22–1

PRECIPITATING FACTORS CONTRIBUTING TO SICKLE CELL CRISIS

- Fever
- Dehydration
- Altitude
- Extremes in temperature
- Vomiting
- Emotional distress
- Fatigue
- Alcohol consumption
- Pregnancy
- Elevated hemoglobin levels
- Elevated reticulocyte counts
- Excessive exercise or physical activity
- Acidosis

PATHOPHYSIOLOGY ILLUSTRATED

Sickle Cell Anemia

Hemoglobin S and Red Blood Cell Sickling

Sickle cell anemia is caused by an inherited autosomal recessive defect in Hb synthesis. Sickle cell hemoglobin (HbS) differs from normal hemoglobin only in the substitution of the amino acid valine for glutamine in both beta chains of the hemoglobin molecule.

When HbS is oxygenated, it has the same globular shape as normal hemoglobin. However, when HbS loses its oxygen, it becomes insoluble in intracellular fluid and crystallizes into rodlike structures. Clusters of rods form polymers (long chains) that bend the erythrocyte into the characteristic crescent shape of the sickle cell.

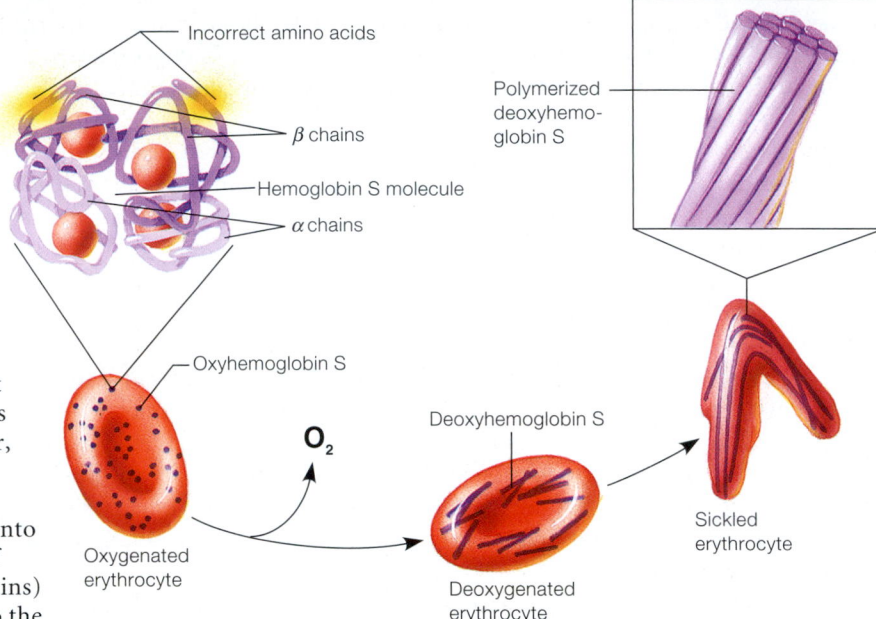

Incorrect amino acids

β chains

Hemoglobin S molecule

α chains

Polymerized deoxyhemoglobin S

Oxyhemoglobin S

Oxygenated erythrocyte

O₂

Deoxyhemoglobin S

Deoxygenated erythrocyte

Sickled erythrocyte

The Sickle Cell Disease Process

Sickle cell disease is characterized by episodes of acute painful crises. Sickling crises are triggered by conditions causing high tissue oxygen demands or that affect cellular pH. As the crisis begins, sickled erythrocytes adhere to capillary walls and to each other, obstructing blood flow and causing cellular hypoxia. The crisis accelerates as tissue hypoxia and acidic metabolic waste products cause further sickling and cell damage.

Sickle cell crises cause microinfarcts in joints and organs, and repeated crises slowly destroy organs and tissues. The spleen and kidneys are especially prone to sickling damage.

Microinfarct

Necrotic tissue

Damaged tissue

Inflamed tissue

Hypoxic cells

Mass of sickled cells obstructing capillary lumen

Capillary

Figure 22–4 ▶ The etiology, pathophysiology, and disease process of sickle cell anemia.

PATHOPHYSIOLOGY ILLUSTRATED

Clinical Manifestations of Sickle Cell Anemia

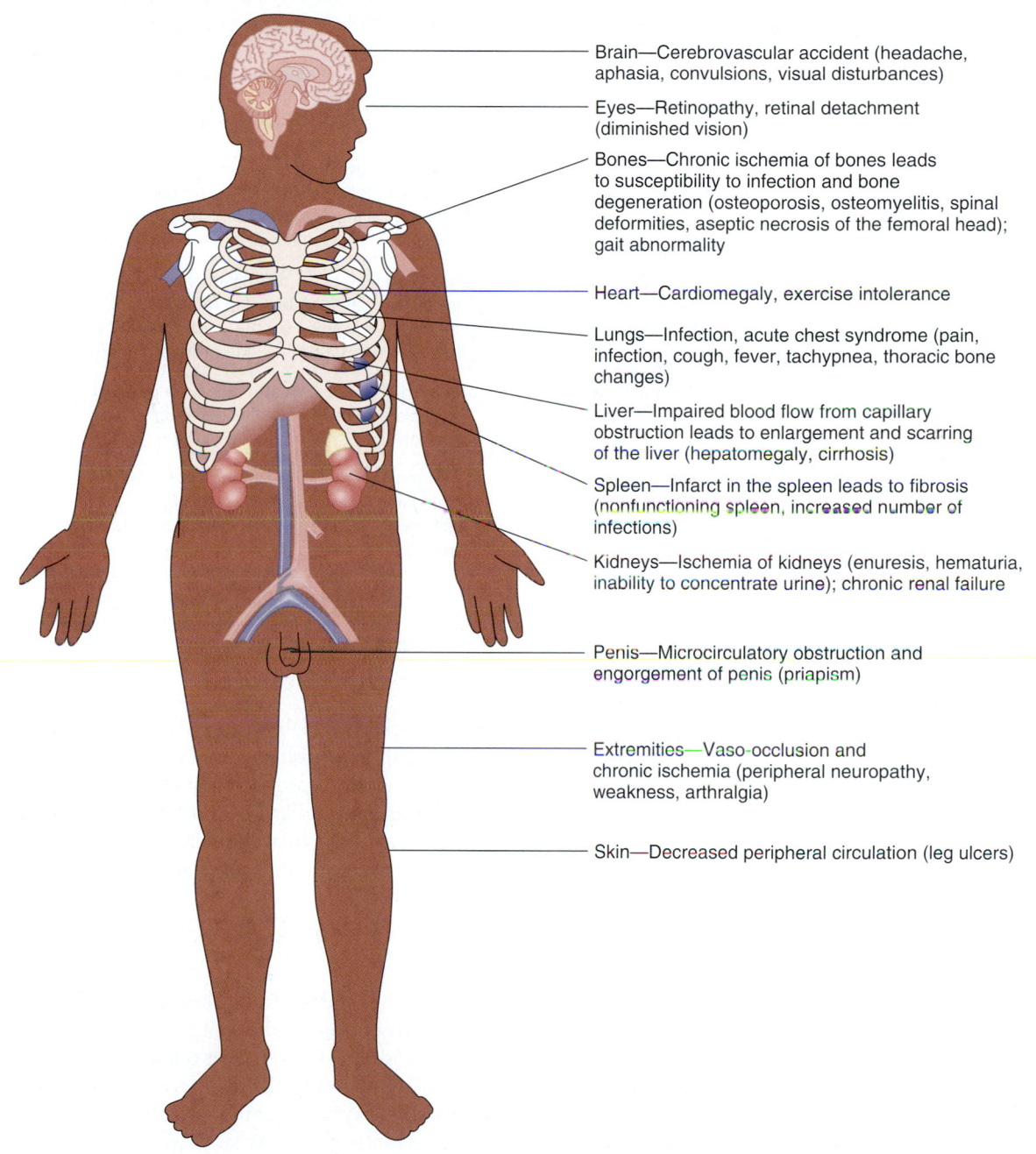

Brain—Cerebrovascular accident (headache, aphasia, convulsions, visual disturbances)

Eyes—Retinopathy, retinal detachment (diminished vision)

Bones—Chronic ischemia of bones leads to susceptibility to infection and bone degeneration (osteoporosis, osteomyelitis, spinal deformities, aseptic necrosis of the femoral head); gait abnormality

Heart—Cardiomegaly, exercise intolerance

Lungs—Infection, acute chest syndrome (pain, infection, cough, fever, tachypnea, thoracic bone changes)

Liver—Impaired blood flow from capillary obstruction leads to enlargement and scarring of the liver (hepatomegaly, cirrhosis)

Spleen—Infarct in the spleen leads to fibrosis (nonfunctioning spleen, increased number of infections)

Kidneys—Ischemia of kidneys (enuresis, hematuria, inability to concentrate urine); chronic renal failure

Penis—Microcirculatory obstruction and engorgement of penis (priapism)

Extremities—Vaso-occlusion and chronic ischemia (peripheral neuropathy, weakness, arthralgia)

Skin—Decreased peripheral circulation (leg ulcers)

Figure 22–5 ➤ The clinical manifestations of sickle cell anemia result from pathologic changes to structures and systems throughout the body.

of the bone marrow, and is typically experienced in the back, abdomen, chest, and joints. Children with sickle cell anemia can also experience chest tightness and shortness of breath, which are diagnostic for acute chest syndrome and medical crisis.

Pain intensity and duration vary depending on the individual and the location. Pain may be transient in a localized area, such as the wrist, to severe, generalized pain that lasts for several days or weeks and may require hospitalization. The pain is often severe enough to require opioid analgesics and the use of a patient-controlled analgesic

Table 22–6	TYPES OF SICKLE CELL CRISES

Type of Crisis	Clinical Manifestations
Vaso-Occlusive Crises (Thrombotic)	Most common type of crisis; may last for days or weeks
	Precipitated by dehydration, exposure to cold, acidosis, or localized hypoxemia
	Caused by stasis of blood with clumping of cells in the microcirculation, ischemia, and infarction
	Thrombosis and infarction of local tissue may occur if the crisis is not reversed
	Cerebral occlusion can result in stroke, manifested by paralysis and/or other central nervous system complications
	Extremely painful; symptoms include fever, tissue engorgement, painful swelling of joints in hands and feet, priapism, and severe abdominal pain
Splenic Sequestration	Life-threatening crisis; death can occur within hours
	Caused by pooling of blood in the spleen; since the spleen can hold much of the body's blood supply, cardiovascular collapse can result
	Clinical manifestations include profound anemia, hypovolemia, and shock
Aplastic Crises	Diminished production and increased destruction of red blood cells
	Triggered by viral infection or depletion of folic acid
	Signs include profound anemia, pallor, fatigue
Acute Chest Syndrome	Common cause of hospitalization for sickle cell disease
	Most common from 2–4 years of age
	Pulmonary infiltrate of abnormal blood cells leads to lower respiratory tract symptoms
	Clinical manifestations include fever, cough, chest and back pain, dyspnea, hypoxemia
	Pulmonary infection, infarct, and fat embolism may occur and can lead to pulmonary failure and death

Data from: Bryant, 2005; Wilson, Krishnamurti, & Kamat, 2003.

(PCA) pump. Children with sickle cell trait rarely have sickle cell crises. However, because they have some abnormal hemoglobin, they may develop symptoms of the disease under conditions of abnormally low oxygen such as flying in an unpressurized airplane over 7000 feet or during anesthesia. The most common symptoms experienced by those with sickle cell trait are splenic infarction and hematuria. However, most persons who carry the trait never have symptoms, even with low oxygen concentrations.

■ COLLABORATIVE CARE

Diagnostic Tests

The initial diagnosis of sickle cell anemia in newborns is often made by testing cord blood using hemoglobin electrophoresis. The sickle-turbidity test (Sickledex) may be used for quick screening purposes in children over 6 months of age, once the fetal hemoglobin levels have fallen. Hemoglobin electrophoresis is performed to verify positive Sickledex test results. Newborn screening of infants for hemoglobinopathies occurs in most states. It is recommended that all newborns be screened, as sickle cell disease can occur in several groups in addition to African Americans, such as those of Mediterranean, South American, Arabian, and East Indian descent (Kral et al., 2006). A child's heritage cannot be predicted from appearance or name alone.

Serum analysis of blood reveals the degree of anemia, with hemoglobin of 6–10 g/dL characteristic of severe syndromes (Segal, Hirsh, & Feig, 2002). Reticulocyte values are elevated, demonstrating the marrow activity that attempts to replace destroyed and nonfunctional red cells. These values are monitored regularly to measure the response of the bone marrow and state of the anemia.

Clinical Therapy

No cure for sickle cell anemia exists. Management focuses on pain control, hydration, oxygenation, prevention of infection, and prevention/treatment of associated compli-

COMPLEMENTARY THERAPY

Sickle Cell Disease and Pain

Management of pain for children with sickle cell disease is a major challenge, both for healthcare providers and families. A nursing study that determined effectiveness of pain control and types of comfort measures used by families provides information that can be applied in caring for children with sickle cell disease in the hospital and at home. The mothers in this study described a combination of traditional medicine and complementary approaches. They emphasized the importance of keeping the child healthy, in order to avoid crisis, by avoiding overheating or chilling. Regular medical checkups, adequate hydration, and immunizations were considered important. Being alert to early signs of pain was also important. Families could begin pharmacological treatment as well as complementary therapies such as applying heat by baths and hot towels to decrease pain and increase relaxation; touching, holding, and massaging the extremities or chest and back; praying together; and using distraction and diversionary activities such as playing games and taking drives. Nurses can learn from and apply these approaches with families. Ask them what they do to identify pain early and alleviate it. Add to the list of interventions the family can try and then partner with them to evaluate results. Continue to emphasize medical care while integrating the other comfort measures the family and child find helpful into nursing care plans (Beyer, J. E., & Simmons, L. E. (2004). Home treatment of pain for children and adolescents with sickle cell disease. *Pain Management Nursing, 5,* 126–135).

cations. Treatment of crises involves hydration, oxygen, pain management, and bed rest to reduce energy expenditure. Neonatal screening, early intervention, prophylactic antibiotics, and parent education have allowed children with sickle cell disease to live into adulthood. Prognosis depends on the severity of the child's disease; children with more frequent exacerbations and hospitalization have poorer prognosis.

PAIN CONTROL, HYDRATION, AND OXYGENATION Parenteral analgesics, such as morphine, are generally administered around the clock or via patient-controlled analgesia. Pain medications should not be ordered on an "as needed" basis, as this increases the child's anxiety and delays medication administration. Oral and intravenous fluid replacement also promotes pain relief since dehydration is often a cause of crisis. Fluids reduce the viscosity of the blood, so adequate hydration is essential. Oxygen is usually administered to provide comfort and decrease incidence of pulmonary complications.

PREVENTION AND TREATMENT OF INFECTION Children who are functionally asplenic or have had a splenectomy have a resultant decreased capability to fight infection. For this reason, infection is a serious condition requiring immediate attention. Daily prophylactic penicillin VK 125 mg twice daily is recommended for children from 2 months to 3 years. From 3 to 5 years of age, the recommended dosage is doubled to 250 mg twice daily. Amoxicillin or injections of Bicillin every 3 weeks can be substituted. If the child is allergic to penicillin, erythromycin ethyl succinate (20 mg/kg divided into two doses) can be used for prophylaxis (Wilson, Krishnamurti, & Kamat, 2003).

When an infection is suspected, cultures (blood, urine, and throat) are obtained to identify the source of infection and the offending organism. Aggressive antibiotic therapy is implemented immediately.

It is recommended that the pneumococcal vaccine [PCV 7 for infants and toddlers or 23-valent for children over 2 years of age] be administered to all infants and children with sickle cell disease (National Institutes of Health, 2002). The *Haemophilus influenzae* type b (Hib) vaccine series should be started at 2 months of age and continued at recommended ages to prevent infection with Hib, which was once the most common cause of epiglottitis, a life-threatening disorder. Other vaccines such as the influenza and meningococcal vaccines may also be administered.

TRANSFUSION OF RED BLOOD CELLS Another therapeutic measure is transfusion of red blood cells. The benefits of transfusions include improved blood and tissue oxygenation, a reduction in sickling, and a temporary suppression of the production of RBCs containing HbS (Ogedegbe, 2002). Several types of blood transfusion are used.

RESEARCH

Chronic Blood Transfusion

A cerebrovascular event or stroke is a common occurrence in children with sickle cell disease since 11% of children from 2 to 10 years of age experience this complication. After a child manifests a stroke, a blood transfusion is given every 3 weeks on an ongoing basis in order to reduce hemoglobin S from 90% to less than 30–50%. Several transfusion techniques are used:

- Simple blood transfusion supplies whole blood to the child.
- Manual partial exchange transfusion separates abnormal RBCs from the affected child and replaces them with transfused healthy cells.
- Erythrocytopheresis is an automated RBC procedure that removes RBCs with hemoglobin S by machine and simultaneously replaces them with normal packed RBCs.

Nurses commonly start peripheral intravenous lines to administer transfusions, and maintain central lines when they are used. They are uniquely positioned to perform research on the types of transfusions used, their complication rates, and family satisfaction with the approach. Insurance reimbursement, family time and travel to clinics for the transfusions, and protection from strokes all need to be explored (Lindsey et al., 2005).

A complication associated with frequent transfusions is an overload of iron in the body. The iron is stored in tissues and organs (**hemosiderosis**), because the body has no way of excreting it. For this reason, an iron-chelating drug such as deferoxamine may be given with vitamin C to promote iron excretion. Another complication of multiple transfusions is the development of alloimmunization to red cell and platelet antigens (Ogedegbe, 2002). Alloimmunization occurs when the child's immune system reacts against antigens on the donated tissues (for example, blood and stem cells).

Additionally, chronic transfusions have proven to be an effective treatment of stroke complications related to sickle cell disease. In children who have had strokes from the disease, periodic transfusions (about every 3 to 4 weeks) can reduce the incidence of future strokes (National Heart, Lung, and Blood Institute, 2002). If administered early in the crisis, blood transfusions may relieve the ischemia caused by vaso-occlusion in major organs and body parts such as the spleen, lung, kidney, brain, and penis. Exchange transfusion is preferred in order to reduce the potential of fluid volume excess.

OTHER THERAPIES   Treatment with hydroxyurea has been helpful in adults, and is now being used more frequently in children. This cytotoxic medication decreases production of abnormal blood cells and leads to a lesser amount of pain being experienced. Additionally, hydroxyurea increases fetal hemoglobin production and red cell mean corpuscular volume (Ogedegbe, 2002). Side effects of hydroxyurea include bone marrow suppression, headaches, dizziness, nausea, and vomiting.

Hematopoietic stem cell transplantation (HSCT) may be considered; however, a recurrence of the disease is demonstrated in approximately 10% of recipients. Refer to the discussion regarding HSCT later in this chapter.

LAW & ETHICS

Genetic Testing and Confidentiality

Information about genetic testing is confidential and must not be shared with persons other than those tested. In the 1970s, when genetic testing for sickle cell disease and trait first became available, discrimination in jobs and insurance occurred against Blacks who had the trait for sickle cell disease.

NURSING MANAGEMENT

Nursing Assessment and Diagnosis

The nurse with a specialty in genetics may be involved in sickle cell gene testing and counseling to identify and inform carriers and children who have the disease. Once a child is diagnosed with the disease, a comprehensive physical assessment is essential because sickle cell anemia can affect any body system.

Physiologic Assessment

In children who are known to have sickle cell anemia, obtain a detailed history from the parents or child about past crises, precipitating events, medical treatment, and home management. Measure the child's height and weight accurately and compare them with past measurements, since failure to thrive is common. Ask about chronic or acute pain that the child is experiencing. Pain may occur in nearly any body part, but most commonly manifests as headache, extremity pain, or abdominal discomfort. Use a pain scale and identify pain perception in each body part where pain exists (see Chapter 15 ∞). Assess the pain management protocols the family has used and what has been most successful.

The ill child with sickle cell disease should receive a careful multisystem assessment. Fever, neurological changes such as decreased alertness or behavioral changes, and respiratory symptoms are emergency conditions that necessitate prompt treatment. When the child is in crisis, assess pain and note the presence of any signs of inflammation or infection. Carefully monitor the child for signs of shock (see Chapter 21 ∞).

Psychosocial Assessment

The child with sickle cell disease experiences a chronic illness that interferes with activities of daily living. Disturbed self-concept and body image, guilt about disturbing the family routines, depression, and isolation can occur. Carry out an assessment of the child's developmental status with a concentration on friends, family support, and self-concept.

The family of a child with sickle cell disease requires a thorough psychosocial assessment. If the child is newly diagnosed with the disorder, the family will need assistance to deal with feelings related to the disease's serious, life-threatening nature. Assess parents' understanding of the disease transmission and ask whether genetic counseling has been obtained. Determine whether the family has adequate healthcare coverage to pay for the child's medical expenses. Ask older children about their knowledge of the disease, and explore their feelings related to the management of a chronic condition. When siblings or other family members are carriers, counseling is needed periodically during the life span so that implications for dating, marriage, and having children can be understood.

Several nursing diagnoses that may apply to the child with sickle cell anemia are presented in the accompanying Nursing Care Plan. Other nursing diagnoses may include the following:

- Risk for Impaired Tissue Perfusion (Cerebral) related to interrupted blood flow
- Caregiver Role Strain related to child's chronic illness
- Risk for Interrupted Family Processes related to having a child with a chronic illness
- Delayed Growth and Development related to effects of physical disability
- Impaired Physical Mobility related to pain

Planning and Implementation

The accompanying Nursing Care Plan summarizes nursing care for the child with sickle cell anemia. Nursing management for the child in crisis focuses on increasing tissue perfusion, promoting hydration, controlling pain, preventing infection, ensuring adequate nutrition, preventing complications, and providing emotional support to the child and family. Refer back to Michael in the opening scenario to determine how many of the following interventions will apply in that situation.

Promote Increased Tissue Perfusion

Administer blood transfusions and oxygen as ordered. The child frequently travels to a clinic to receive the treatment every 3 weeks and nurses commonly start and maintain the lines and infusions used. To prevent hemolysis, the intravenous fluid used before and after a blood transfusion must be saline rather than D_5W. In small children, the blood is usually infused without saline because the child cannot manage the extra volume. Monitor for transfusion reactions. (See Clinical Manifestations of Blood Transfusion Reactions on page 816.) Encourage the child to rest. Work with the child and family to avoid emotional stress and plan with the family for the trips to the healthcare facility. Any activities that increase cellular metabolism also result in tissue hypoxia, so the family needs assistance to plan the child's daily activities. Schedule caregiving activities and play during hospitalizations and clinic visits to allow for optimal rest.

> ### LAW & ETHICS
>
> #### Blood Transfusions and Religious Beliefs
>
> Jehovah's Witnesses and some other religious groups are opposed to the transfusion of blood products. Ethical issues arise when blood transfusion is the treatment of choice for a childhood disease, since parents may choose not to consent to treatment. The courts have generally accepted that the child's life is of the greatest importance and temporarily make the child a ward of the court in order to allow medical personnel to administer the needed blood product. Recent advances in synthetic clotting factor production and research into blood volume expanders that can successfully treat some conditions have decreased the incidence of disagreement between religious and medical interventions. However, nurses may care for children and families when court-ordered therapy is being carried out. Sensitivity to the family's beliefs, a caring approach to the child, and provision of information about care are needed (Woolley, 2006).

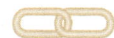

SKILL 9–6
Administering Blood or Blood Products

> ### NURSING ALERT
>
> Nurses should consider the following principles when administering blood and blood products:
> - Become familiar with the transfusion policies and procedures where you work.
> - Verify the blood type, patient number, donor number, and Rh factor with another RN.
> - Check the blood for sediment or any nonuniform or unusual characteristics.
> - Never infuse cold blood because it may increase sickling; use a blood-warming coil to bring blood to room temperature.
> - Assess the child's history for previous transfusion reactions.
> - Blood reactions can occur as soon as the blood transfusion begins. Administer the first 20 mL of blood slowly and observe the child carefully for a reaction. Repeatedly assess the child according to hospital policy.
> - Assess the child's vital signs before transfusion and every 15–30 minutes throughout transfusion.
> - Remain with the child during the first 20 minutes of the transfusion to monitor for any undesirable reactions.
> - If transfusion reaction occurs, immediately discontinue the transfusion, change the IV to normal saline, and notify the primary healthcare provider. (Refer to the *Clinical Skills Manual* for the procedure for administering blood or blood products.)

NURSING CARE PLAN The Child with Sickle Cell Anemia

GOAL	INTERVENTION	RATIONALE	EXPECTED OUTCOME
1. Ineffective Tissue Perfusion (All Systems) related to affinity of hemoglobin for oxygen			
	NIC Priority Intervention: **Circulatory Care:** *Promotion of arterial and venous circulation.*		*NOC Outcome:* **Tissue Perfusion:** *Extent to which blood flows through the vessels of the body vasculature and maintains tissue function.*
The child will show few signs and symptoms of tissue hypoxia.	• Instruct child to avoid physical exertion, emotional stress, low oxygen environments (e.g., airplanes, high altitudes), and known sources of infection.	• Decreased activity and exposure reduce body's need for oxygen.	The child has no shortness of breath and shows no signs of hypoxia.
	• Administer blood transfusions as ordered.	• Packed cells increase number of red blood cells available to carry oxygen to tissue cells. Transfusions promote circulation.	
	• Perform several caregiving activities together when possible.	• Grouping activities allows for optimum rest.	
	• Give oxygen as ordered.	• High concentration of oxygen in alveoli increases diffusion of gas across membranes.	
Repeated cerebrovascular accidents will be avoided.	• Administer and teach the family to administer prophylactic transfusions for the child who has had a cerebrovascular accident.	• Lowers potential for a future cerebrovascular accident.	The child does not suffer a cerebrovascular accident.
2. Risk for Deficient Fluid Volume related to inadequate fluid intake and dehydration			
	NIC Priority Intervention: **Fluid Management:** *Promotion of electrolyte balance and prevention of complications resulting from abnormal or undesired fluid levels.*		*NOC Suggested Outcome:* **Hydration:** *Amount of water in the intracellular and extracellular compartments of the body.*
The child will maintain or be restored to adequate hydration.	• Calculate the child's daily fluid requirements. Monitor the child's usual fluid consumption and make necessary adjustments. Encourage the child to take fluids. Observe for signs of dehydration.	• Optimizing fluid intake ensures that the child gets needed fluid. Dehydration exacerbates crises.	The child shows signs of adequate hydration.
	• Record intake and output.	• Recording enables you to monitor daily fluid intake and spacing throughout the day.	
	• Instruct family to report fever, vomiting, diarrhea, or other signs of fluid imbalance immediately.	• Early intervention can be effective in minimizing complications from dehydration. Child may need oral or intravenous rehydration therapy.	

NURSING CARE PLAN   The Child with Sickle Cell Anemia (continued)

GOAL	INTERVENTION	RATIONALE	EXPECTED OUTCOME
3. Chronic Pain related to chronic physical disability and clustering of sickled cells			
	NIC Priority Intervention: **Pain Management:** *Alleviation of pain or a reduction in pain to a level of comfort acceptable to the patient.*		*NOC Suggested Outcome:* **Comfort Level:** *Feelings of physical and psychologic ease.*
The child will verbalize that pain is controlled.	• Administer analgesics, such as morphine or hydromorphine (Dilaudid), as ordered. Continuous intravenous infusion is used for the duration of a painful crisis.	• Pain of sickle cell crises is excruciating.	The child is pain free, or pain control is significantly improved.
	• Position carefully.	• Joints and extremities can be extremely painful.	
	• Ask family what pain relief measures are helpful and integrate them into care for the child.	• Complementary therapy such as holding the child, massage, warmth, distraction, and other measures may be instrumental in managing the child's pain.	
4. Risk for Infection related to chronic disease and splenic malfunction			
	NIC Priority Intervention: **Infection Control:** *Minimizing the acquisition and transmission of infectious agents.*		*NOC Suggested Outcome:* **Risk Control:** *Actions to eliminate or reduce actual, personal, and modifiable health threats.*
The child will not develop infection.	• Ensure adequate nutrition by providing high-calorie high-protein diet. Ensure that the child's immunizations are up-to-date. Report any signs of infection to physician immediately.	• Chronically ill children are at greater risk of infection.	The child is free of infection.
	• Isolate the child from possible sources of infection. Instruct parents about signs of infection and encourage them to seek prompt health care.	• Restriction of persons with infection decreases the child's contact with infectious agents. Prompt care for infection reduces the chance of sickle cell crisis.	
5. Deficient Knowledge (child and parents) related to lack of exposure about cause and treatment of sickle cell anemia			
	NIC Priority Intervention: **Teaching Disease Process:** *Assisting the patient to understand information related to a specific disease process.*		*NOC Suggested Outcome:* **Knowledge:** *Extent of understanding conveyed about sickle cell disease.*
The child and family will verbalize understanding of risk factors for sickle cell crises and how to minimize them.	• Review basics of sickle cell disease. Teach the child and family about signs and symptoms of crises.	• Knowledge of disease helps ensure compliance with treatment regimen and adherence to preventive measures.	The child and parent can verbalize precipitating events of crises.
	• Arrange for genetic counseling and testing for sickle cell trait for family members if desired.	• Questions and concerns regarding future pregnancies can be allayed through knowledge of disease and transmission.	

CLINICAL MANIFESTATIONS | BLOOD TRANSFUSION REACTIONS

Type of Reaction	Clinical Manifestation	Etiology	Clinical Therapy
Allergic reaction	Urticaria, itching, respiratory distress	Immune response to protein in the blood	Stop the transfusion; call physician; administer antihistamines as ordered; monitor vital signs; maintain intravenous infusion of normal saline; keep intravenous line open; check urine for hematuria.
Hemolytic reaction	Fever, chills, hematuria, headache, chest pain; can progress to shock	Mismatched blood, history of multiple transfusions, or infusion with a solution containing dextrose or other additives	
Febrile or septic	Chills, fever, headache, decreased blood pressure, nausea and/or vomiting, and leg and back pain	Usually a result of contamination of blood; may also be caused by idiopathic conditions	Inform primary healthcare provider.
Circulatory overload	Labored breathing, chest or lower back pain, productive cough with crackles heard on auscultation, and distended neck veins; central venous pressure may increase	Results from infusion of excessive amounts of fluid or too rapid administration	Diuretics may be ordered.

GROWTH & DEVELOPMENT

Encouraging Fluid Intake

To encourage fluid intake in a small child:

- Use a favorite cup or glass.
- Use straws.
- Take advantage of times the child is thirsty, such as on awakening or after play.
- Leave a cup within easy reach of the child.
- Offer frozen juice pops, crushed ice drinks, and flavored ice chips.

NURSING ALERT

Neither hot nor cold compresses should be used for pain management in the child who has sickle cell anemia. Ischemic tissue is fragile and has reduced sensation, increasing the risk of burn injury. Cold compresses promote sickling.

Promote Hydration

The child with sickle cell anemia is adversely affected by dehydration. Calculate the child's fluid maintenance requirements (minimum daily fluid intake) (see Chapter 16 ∞) and monitor the child's oral fluid intake. Administer intravenous fluids as ordered. Adjust oral intake as necessary to keep the child well hydrated.

Pain Management

Administer prescribed analgesics around the clock during crises. If patient-controlled analgesia is used, be sure that the constant infusions run as ordered and that the parent or child understands the use of bolus infusions, when needed (see Chapter 15 ∞). Reposition the infant and young child carefully, supporting joints and extremities on pillows or special mattresses. Assist the child to assume a comfortable position. Avoid putting stress on painful joints or other body parts. See Evidence-Based Practice: Sickle Cell Anemia and Pain Management.

Prevent Infection

Infection makes the child more susceptible to a crisis, and the crisis, in turn, increases susceptibility to infection. Teach the parents how to administer antibiotics for prophylaxis or treatment of infection. Be sure they have the finances and other resources to obtain and give daily antibiotics. Because infections can be particularly virulent and can cause death in these children, parents should be instructed to obtain immediate care when the child is ill. Encourage the use of the pneumococcal vaccine for all infants and children with the disease. The *Haemophilus influenzae* type b (Hib) vaccine series should be started at 2 months of age and continued at recommended ages to prevent another common source of infection. See Chapter 18 ∞ for further information about recommended immunizations.

Ensure Adequate Nutrition

Emphasize the importance of adequate nutrition to promote growth. Encourage the child to eat a high-protein, high-calorie diet. Emphasize the importance of folic acid and vitamin C supplements as prescribed. Perform regular growth measurements and, if slow growth is apparent, perform 24-hour diet recalls and other nutritional assessments.

Prevent Complications of Crises

Observe the child for signs of increasing anemia and shock (mental status change, pallor, vital sign changes). Maintain ongoing monitoring of the child's neurologic status for evidence of altered cerebral function. Assess for an enlarged spleen by gentle palpation. Administer blood transfusions and watch the child for any adverse reaction. Assess growth and developmental milestones.

EVIDENCE-BASED PRACTICE

Sickle Cell Anemia and Pain Management

Problem

Severe episodes of sickle cell crisis require hospitalization for pain management. Pain relief is the primary goal for healthcare providers and is most significant to the child experiencing pain. However, different pain management regimens may be used during each hospitalization and effective regimens are not well documented. Studies are needed to identify effective pain management strategies for children with sickle cell disease. In addition, parents use a variety of pain relief measures at home, but these may not be integrated into care when the child becomes hospitalized, leading to poor pain management.

Evidence

Nurse researchers conducted a descriptive longitudinal study with 27 children to evaluate the pain management strategies used in sickle cell disease when they experienced pain during a vaso-occlusive episode. The children ranged in age from 5 to 19 years; there were 40 hospital admissions during the 9-month study. The researchers noted several surprising findings from the study. First, they found that children on average self-administered only 35% of the pain medication that was prescribed. Second, they found that the children did not report significant pain relief. It is assumed that adequate pain relief was not achieved during hospitalization because the dose of analgesics administered was too low. Another study of 21 female caretakers of children with sickle cell disease found a variety of techniques were used to manage pain at home. Oral medications, massage, warmth to painful body parts, and other techniques were considered helpful.

Implications

Hospitalized children who self-administered their medication consistently undermedicated themselves and failed to achieve pain relief.

Children may not be taught how to use the PCA device properly and may interpret that they should use it as little as possible. Thus, healthcare provider practices influence the child's pain management. In addition, children and families have developed many effective pain relief measures at home that may not be included in hospital care. More information is needed about methods of integrating these techniques.

Recommendations include the need to evaluate whether increasing analgesic use to the amount prescribed would increase the amount of pain relief. Additional research is needed to determine the effectiveness of different PCA regimens and to evaluate the effectiveness of pain management algorithms. Evaluation tools are needed to measure effectiveness of the child's self-medication by PCA. Tools for evaluating home care pain management are needed. Nurses must be willing to integrate the family's measures into care while the child is hospitalized.

Critical Thinking

How will you determine if the child in sickle cell crisis is obtaining adequate pain relief. (Consult Chapter 15 ∞ for ideas.) What personal beliefs of healthcare providers may influence effective pain management? How can these beliefs be addressed? If the primary healthcare provider has prescribed a subtherapeutic dosage of pain medication for a child in sickle cell crisis, what action could you take?

References

Beyer, J. E., & Simmons, L. E. (2004). Home treatment of pain for children and adolescents with sickle cell disease. *Pain Management Nursing, 5,* 126–135.

Jacob, E., Miaskowski, C., Savedra, M., Beyer, J. E., Treadwell, M., & Styles, L. (2003). Management of vaso-occlusive pain in children with sickle cell disease. *Journal of Pediatric Hematology/Oncology, 25,* 307–311.

Provide Emotional Support

Sickle cell anemia is a chronic disease that is accompanied by life-threatening episodic crises. Family members often need support to help them deal with their feelings about the diagnosis and its implications. Explore resources in the home and community to see if parents will be able to administer medications and fluids and to provide adequate nutrition. Assess their knowledge of signs of infection and of sickle cell crisis and when to seek medical care for the child. Refer the parents for genetic counseling, particularly if they plan to have more children. Encourage adolescents and young adults in the family to receive genetic counseling and testing, as well. Referrals to support groups and contact with others with the disease can be helpful.

Collaborate with family members and provide them with ongoing support to deal with the stress of having a child with a chronic condition. (See Families Want to Know: Home Care Considerations for the Child with Sickle Cell Anemia.) Provide resources, respite care for parents, and information as needed for siblings. Sickle cell disease and some other hematologic disorders of childhood require that parents provide ongoing monitoring and care for their children with these chronic conditions. Refer to Chapter 12 ∞ for a discussion of chronic disorders in children. Refer parents to support groups such as the National Association of Sickle Cell Disease for further information.

Discharge Planning and Home Care Teaching

Home care needs should be identified and addressed well in advance of discharge. Provide parents with information about sickle cell disease and the child's treatment. Even parents of a child previously diagnosed with the disorder may benefit from information about the disease process and its management. Explain the basic effect of tissue hypoxia and the effects of sickling on circulation.

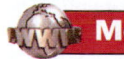

MediaLink

Sickle Cell Anemia Resources

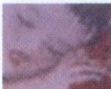

FAMILIES WANT TO KNOW

Home Care Considerations for the Child with Sickle Cell Anemia

- Follow recommended schedules for well-child care visits.
- Be sure the child is up-to-date with immunizations, including hepatitis B, annual influenza, pneumococcal vaccine, and tuberculosis skin test.
- Special testing, such as heart and eye examinations, may be needed periodically to check for any sequelae of the disease.
- Special medications, such as antibiotics, may be needed; pain relief medicine and blood transfusions may be administered.
- Dehydration is dangerous. Be sure the child gets extra fluids in hot weather, when ill, during physical activity, and during travel.

- As the child develops, provide information about the disease and encourage self-care. Be sure the school personnel understand the child's diagnosis and any care required during school hours.
- Contact your healthcare provider if the child has a high fever, a common illness that lasts more than a day, seizures, change in behavior, severe pain, abnormal skin color or breathing pattern, or any other symptoms of concern.

COMMUNITY CARE

Sickle Cell Crisis and School

Children who have episodes of sickle cell crisis miss school for prolonged and repeated periods. In addition, if they have experienced strokes as a disease complication, they often have learning difficulties and neurological changes. Teachers may have difficulty understanding why children with a blood disease are frequently absent and why they may have trouble with concepts in the classroom that they previously understood. School and other community-based nurses are ideally situated to provide information to teachers about sickle cell disease so that they understand the challenges faced by children with the disease. While teachers commonly have some knowledge about the disease, they are often not fully cognizant of the neurological sequelae and the importance of the Individualized Education Plan and its frequent evaluation and revision (King, Tang, Ferguson, & DeBaun, 2005). Outline the topics that you would address to inform teachers about the effect of sickle cell anemia on a child's ability to learn.

Teach parents to look for signs of dehydration, such as dry mucous membranes, weight loss, and sunken fontanels in infants. Give specific instructions about how many ounces of liquid the child needs to drink each day. Emphasize that increased fluid intake is needed to replace the fluids lost from overheating or exposure to hot weather. Make sure both the child and family understand the triggers and precipitating factors for sickle cell crises. Encourage them to avoid situations that cause crises. Instruct the child and parents about signs and symptoms of crises that should be reported to their healthcare provider.

Provide the family with careful instructions about infusion therapy. When regular blood infusions are used, the resulting iron overload is damaging to body organs. Children treated with transfusions need infusion of deferoxamine (Desferal) for iron overload. The medication is usually given by subcutaneous or intravenous routes over 8 to 10 hours. Prompt recognition of side effects and careful management of the lengthy infusion process are important. The child needs to be monitored for skin reactions and allergic responses. Have parents demonstrate the infusion technique and state what to do in case of reactions. Pain management is needed during infusion as the site may be tender and uncomfortable.

Instruct parents that it is important to inform all treating physicians and dentists of the child's medical condition. Special precautions are necessary when the child undergoes surgery of any kind, as hypoxia resulting from anesthesia is a major surgical risk. The child should also wear a medical identification tag or bracelet.

Family members need ongoing support to deal with the stress of having a child with a chronic condition. Provide resources, respite care for parents, and information as needed for siblings.

Encourage older children with sickle cell anemia to participate in activities with other children between crises, but to avoid strenuous physical exertion and contact sports. Play and social interactions that promote learning and development are important.

Care in the Community

The child may receive home care nursing for transfusion therapy or may need to travel frequently for infusions at a medical center. The nurse partners with the child and family to establish a plan of care. An Individualized School Health Plan will need to be established. The nurse can assist the family and school with establishing this plan.

School personnel must be aware of the child's disease, since prompt care is essential if the child exhibits any sign of sickle cell crisis. The nurse can identify key staff members in the school and partner with them to ensure essential management actions are understood by all staff members. Members of the school staff should be instructed in management of emergencies and contact numbers for parents should be readily available. Assist the family and school to plan an appropriate schedule of activities without overprotecting the child. Children with sickle cell disease should not engage in activities, such as running and heavy exercise, that may increase oxygen demand, resulting in sickling.

Evaluation

Expected outcomes of nursing care for the child with sickle cell anemia include the following:

- The child expresses that pain is successfully managed to a state of comfort.
- The child demonstrates adequate hydration to prevent cell sickling.
- The child displays no side effects of disease in the respiratory system, central nervous system, and body organs.
- The child has normal immune status and freedom from infection.
- Family and healthcare personnel promptly recognize and treat complications of the disease.
- The child meets normal growth and developmental milestones.
- Parents and other family members are referred for and receive information to manage and understand the disease.
- The family demonstrates adequate knowledge of the disease and treatment regimens.

Thalassemias

The thalassemias are a group of inherited blood disorders of hemoglobin synthesis characterized by anemia that can be mild to severe. They affect one of the two pairs of polypeptide chains (alpha and beta polypeptides) in the hemoglobin chain. There are three types of Beta-thalassemia (β-thalassemia). β-thalassemia major, also known as Cooley's anemia, is the most common type. Alpha-thalassemia (α-thalassemia) varies from the trait to the fatal Alpha-thalassemia major, in which all four alpha-forming genes are defective.

The thalassemias occur most often in people of Mediterranean descent but are also found among Middle Eastern, Asian, and African populations. Over 5% of populations at risk are affected by the disease (Catlin, 2003). β-thalassemia is an autosomal recessive disorder, so if both parents carry the abnormal gene, with each pregnancy there is a 25% chance of passing the disorder on to the child.

Etiology and Pathophysiology

In β-thalassemia, defective hemoglobin is synthesized as a result of impaired production of the beta chain of hemoglobin A (HbA). To compensate for decreased HbA, production of HbF (fetal hemoglobin) increases. The RBCs are fragile and are easily destroyed, shortening their life span (Figure 22–6 ➤). As hemolysis increases, **hemosiderin** (iron-containing pigment accumulated from hemoglobin as the red blood cells are destroyed) is deposited in the skin, causing a bronze appearance. Chronic anemia leads to hyperplasia of the bone marrow cavity and thinning of the bone marrow cortex as the bone marrow attempts to compensate for the anemia. Pathologic fractures and skeletal deformities may occur as a result of these bone marrow changes. Splenomegaly results from hyperactivity of the spleen and from pooling of cells.

The three types of β-thalassemia are

- Thalassemia minor, or thalassemia trait (produces mild anemia)
- Thalassemia intermedia (produces moderate anemia)
- Thalassemia major (produces anemia requiring transfusion)

Long-term complications related to **hemochromatosis** (excessive absorption and accumulation of iron in the body) include gallbladder disease, liver enlargement and cirrhosis, growth retardation, endocrine complications, jaundice, and cardiac complications including heart failure. Skeletal changes include pathological fractures, skeletal deformities such as an enlarged head, and thickened cranial bones. Death is generally the result of heart failure resulting from severe anemia or iron overload. Other causes of death include liver disease and infection. However, with improvement in treatment, survival is now possible through the second and third decades of life.

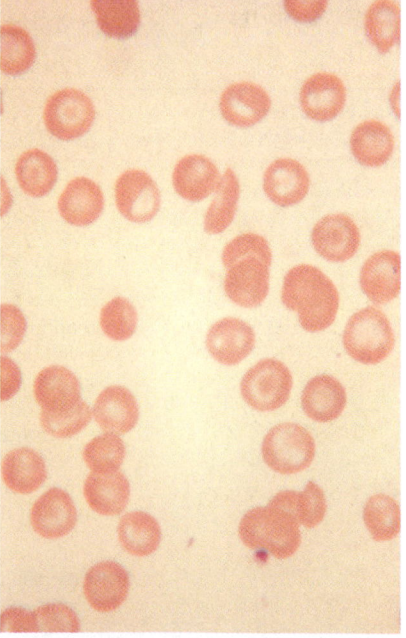

Figure 22–6 ➤ Red blood cell appearance in β-thalassemia. What characteristic abnormalities can be seen on this microscopic view?
Courtesy of Dr. Ed Wong, Laboratory Medicine, Children's National Medical Center, Washington, DC.

In á-thalassemia, the defect occurs on the alpha chain of adult hemoglobin. As with β-thalassemia, the severity of the disorder is dependent upon the number of genes that are defective.

The four types of á-thalassemia are:

- Alpha trait. Defect in a single alpha chain-forming gene.
- Alpha-thalassemia minor. Defect in two genes.
- Hemoglobin H disease. Defect in three genes.
- Alpha-thalassemia major. Defect in all four alpha-forming genes.

Clinical Manifestations

Clinical manifestations of β-thalassemia are caused by the defective synthesis of hemoglobin, structurally impaired red blood cells, and the shortened life span of the RBCs. The infant with β-thalassemia manifests pallor, failure to thrive, hepatosplenomegaly, and severe anemia (hemoglobin < 6 g/dL) that leads to chronic hypoxia. (See Clinical Manifestations of β-Thalassemia below.) Hemochromatosis may result as the body conserves iron from the destroyed red cells as well as from the transfused cells. Manifestations of chronic hypoxia include lethargy, exercise intolerance, anorexia, headache, and bone pain. The liver enlarges as a result of hemosiderosis, and the spleen enlarges as a result of extramedullary **hematopoiesis** and increased hemolysis of red blood cells.

The child with alpha trait is generally symptom free. Clinical manifestations of á-thalassemia minor are similar to those of β-thalassemia minor. Manifestations of hemoglobin H disease are similar, though they tend to be milder, to those of β-thalassemia major. á-thalassemia major results in hydrops fetalis, intrauterine congestive heart failure (the oxygen is unable to be related to the tissues due to defective alpha chains), cardiomegaly, and hepatomegaly.

■ COLLABORATIVE CARE

Diagnostic Tests

Diagnosis is made by hemoglobin electrophoresis, which reveals a decreased production of one of the globin chains in hemoglobin and an elevated F and A hemoglobin.

CLINICAL MANIFESTATIONS	β-THALASSEMIA	
Body Organs	**Clinical Manifestations**	**Clinical Therapy**
Red blood cells (anemia)	Hypochromic and microcytic changes Folic acid deficiency Frequent epistaxis	Hypertransfusion program Administer folic acid and increase dietary consumption of folic acid and vitamin C
Skeletal changes	Osteoporosis Delayed growth Susceptibility to pathologic fractures Facial deformities: enlarged head, prominent forehead due to frontal and parietal bossing, prominent cheek bones, broadened and depressed bridge of nose, enlarged maxilla with protruding front teeth, eyes with mongolian slant and epicanthal fold	Assess growth and plot on chart—monitor for delays in growth Teach safety precautions to avoid fractures
Heart	Chronic congestive heart failure Myocardial fibrosis Murmurs	Monitor for signs of congestive heart failure EKG and echocardiogram may be conducted to assess heart function
Liver/gallbladder	Hepatomegaly Hepatic insufficiency	MRI or CT scans may be conducted to evaluate liver and gallbladder Liver biopsy may be performed
Spleen	Splenomegaly	MRI or CT scans may be conducted to evaluate spleen
Endocrine system	Delayed sexual maturation Fibrotic pancreas, resulting in diabetes mellitus	Assess sexual maturation using the Tanner staging
Skin	Darkening of skin	Assess for skin changes

A complete blood count (CBC) reveals a decreased hemoglobin, hematocrit, and reticulocyte count. Thalassemia can be detected early in infancy as characteristic erythrocyte cell changes often can be recognized in infants by 6 weeks of age. Prenatal testing using chorionic villus sampling (CVS) or amniocentesis can detect or rule out thalassemia in the fetus.

A chest radiograph may be performed to evaluate heart size. MRI and CT scans may be performed to evaluate the liver. A liver biopsy may be performed to evaluate the degree of hemachromatosis.

Clinical Therapy

Treatment for thalassemia is supportive. The goal of medical management is to maintain normal hemoglobin levels. Blood transfusion every 2 to 4 weeks is the conventional therapy used to treat children with severe disease (thalassemia major). Since iron overload is a side effect of this treatment, children may need to receive an iron-chelating drug such as deferoxamine, which binds excess iron so it can be excreted by the kidneys. Deferoxamine 30–40 mg/kg/day is infused over 8–12 hours during the child's sleep for 5 days each week by a mechanical pump. The medication may be administered subcutaneously or intravenously. A port provides ease of intravenous access and reduced irritation for the child. Pain, induration, and erythema are common side effects with subcutaneous infusions. A newer oral chelator, deferasirox (Exjade), is under investigation and may provide similar efficacy to deferoxamine infusion (Piga, Galanello, Forni et al., 2006). Exjade could potentially simplify treatment by use of daily oral administration.

Other potential complications of long-term transfusion therapy are transfusion reactions and alloimmunization (antibody formation). Hematopoietic stem cell transplantation (HSCT) from a matched sibling may be offered as an alternative therapy for children with the disorder.

Diet is normal for age and should include folic acid and ascorbic acid (vitamin C). Iron should not be administered and foods rich in iron should be avoided.

■ NURSING MANAGEMENT

Nursing Assessment and Diagnosis

Assess for the classic manifestations of pallor, failure to thrive, severe anemia, skin discoloration, and hepatosplenomegaly. Assess heart sounds, breath sounds, and respiratory effort. Assess for signs of infection. Assessment also includes monitoring for signs of iron overload, including abdominal pain, vomiting, and bloody diarrhea, leading to shortness of breath and shock. As previously mentioned, immediate emergency treatment is required as death may result from iron overdose.

Nursing diagnoses for the child with thalassemia may include:

- Risk for Infection related to splenectomy
- Deficient Knowledge related to disease process and management
- Activity Intolerance related to anemia
- Disturbed Body Image related to discoloration of skin
- Ineffective Tissue Perfusion (All Systems) related to anemia

Planning and Implementation

Care for the child with thalassemia is generally managed at home unless the child has a coexisting complication. Transfusions of packed cells are often given. Partner with the family to teach parents the technique for subcutaneous infusion of deferoxamine (to prevent iron overload) if that route is to be used for therapy at home.

Home care nurses may provide care to the child receiving intravenous infusions. Needles and tubing should be discarded after use and should not be reused. The subcutaneous injection sites most often chosen are the areas with the most subcutaneous fat, such as the abdomen, upper arms, thighs, or buttocks. Rotate injection sites for each treatment.

Chronic toxicity may result from usually high doses of deferoxamine, and resulting complications include hearing loss and renal calcium loss. Blurred vision, decreased visual acuity, and night blindness may occur. Blurred vision should be immediately reported. Periodic ophthalmologic examinations are recommended. Inform parents and the child that deferoxamine discolors urine to a reddish color.

If the child has undergone a splenectomy, the risk for infection is increased. Teach the parents and child infection control measures, including proper handwashing and aseptic technique for infusion. Long-term prophylactic antibiotics are generally prescribed.

Provide parents information about thalassemia and its treatment, and encourage them to obtain genetic counseling. The nurse provides emotional support to the child and parents and implements measures to assist them in coping with a chronic life-threatening illness.

Encourage parents to take an active role in the child's treatment regimen. Partner with the parents and child to provide opportunities for physical activities, such as swimming, that do not increase the risk of fractures. Collaborate with the family and school to establish an emergency treatment plan. Discuss potential body image changes with the child and provide an opportunity for them to express their concerns. The child may require referral for counseling to help to cope with the body image changes.

Compliance with transfusion therapy often becomes an issue as children reach adolescence. Offering the adolescent a choice regarding treatment options, such as when to undergo transfusion, can help to improve compliance. Adolescents with β-thalassemia and parents of newly diagnosed children can be referred to the Thalassemia Action Group, a national organization for patients, or to the Cooley's Anemia Foundation.

MediaLink

β-thalassemia Resources

Evaluation

Expected outcomes of nursing care for the child with thalassemia include:

- The child remains free from infection.
- The child and family demonstrate understanding of treatment regimen and signs of potential complications.
- The child engages in age-appropriate, safe activities.
- The child develops a positive body image.
- The child demonstrates effective tissue perfusion throughout the body.

Aplastic Anemia

Aplastic anemia is a deficiency of the blood cells that results from failure of the bone marrow to produce adequate numbers of circulating blood cells. The condition may be congenital or acquired. Aplastic anemia is more common between the ages of 15–25 years and in the Asian population. Most aplastic anemia is immune-mediated and results from a combination of environmental exposure with an individual's genetically determined response to the environmental agent (Corbeel, 2005; Young, Calado, & Scheinberg, 2006; Young & Maciejewski, 2004).

Congenital aplastic anemia (Fanconi anemia) is a rare autosomal recessive syndrome consisting of multiple congenital anomalies. Symptoms can include **purpura** (bleeding into the tissues) (Figure 22–7 ➤), **petechiae** (pinpoint lesions), bleeding, fatigue, and pallor. Laboratory findings include **neutropenia** (decreased number of neutrophils) or anemia, and thrombocytopenia (low platelet count) that progresses to **pancytopenia** (decreased number of blood cell components).

Children with congenital aplastic anemia are at risk for developing malignancies such as acute nonlymphocytic leukemia. The treatment of choice is bone marrow transplantation; however, the prognosis is poor, and death usually results from overwhelming infection, hemorrhage, or malignancy.

Acquired aplastic anemia in children is either idiopathic or occurs from a drug reaction. It can develop after exposure to ionizing radiation or insecticides or after ingestion of drugs such as sulfonamides, chloramphenicol, quinacrine, benzene solvents

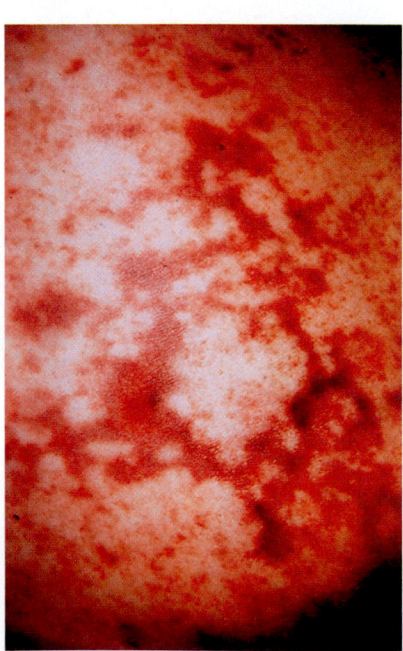

Figure 22–7 ➤ Nonpalpable purpura with bleeding into the tissues below the skin.
Courtesy of the Department of Hematology/Oncology, Children's National Medical Center, Washington, DC.

in model airplane glue, or lead. This type of anemia can also be a result of an infectious process such as viral hepatitis or mononucleosis.

Clinical manifestations are related to the degree of bone marrow failure and can include petechiae, purpura, bleeding, pallor, weakness, tachycardia, and fatigue. Diagnosis is made by blood studies, which reveal leukopenia (low white blood cell count) with marked neutropenia, thrombocytopenia, and pancytopenia; and by bone marrow aspiration, which reveals yellow, fatty bone marrow instead of red bone marrow.

After identification of the disorder, the child is removed from any causal agents and the underlying disorder is treated. Therapy involves preventing complications associated with neutropenia, thrombocytopenia, and anemia. Supportive treatment includes transfusions of packed cells and/or platelets. Immunosuppressive drug therapy is effective for many children because it is believed the child's immune system is reacting against the bone marrow. Immunosuppressive agents include antithymocyte globulin (ATG) and cyclosporine. Cyclosporine may be given in combination with androgens to stimulate blood cell production (Aplastic Anemia and MDS International Foundation, 2003). Antibiotics are administered if infection is confirmed. The treatment of choice is hematopoietic stem cell transplantation from a compatible sibling or family member donor. The family and child require psychosocial support during this life-threatening illness.

NURSING MANAGEMENT

Nursing care is similar to care provided for the child with leukemia (see Chapter 23 ∞). Nursing actions focus on preventing bleeding, administering and monitoring blood transfusions, preventing infection, encouraging mobility as tolerated, educating the parents and child about the disorder, and providing emotional support.

The nurse partners with the child and family to assist the child with activities of daily living and cluster patient care to conserve energy since fatigue, poor tissue oxygenation, and weakness may be experienced. Observe for complications associated with administration of blood products, including transfusion reaction and fluid overload. For the child receiving hematopoietic stem cell transplantation, refer to the section discussing HSCT later in this chapter.

Families require support in dealing with a child who has a life-threatening disease. A collaborative approach with the use of social service, spiritual care, and other support services offers comfort and education to families with these special needs. Assistance with both personal and social resources can help families to cope with these challenging circumstances (Pelchat & Lefebvre, 2004). Expected outcomes of nursing care include maintenance of normal levels of white and red blood cells and platelets to support body functions.

CLOTTING DISORDERS

The body depends on a complex mechanism to ensure proper clotting of blood. Platelets and several clotting factors are required. Platelets can be decreased (the condition known as thrombocytopenia) for several reasons:

- The bone marrow is injured or unable to produce platelets (see aplastic anemia discussion in this chapter)
- Loss or excessive dilution of blood
- Pooling of blood in the spleen (see description of sickle cell disease earlier in this chapter)
- A variety of medical conditions such as disseminated intravascular coagulation (see following section), hemolytic-uremic syndrome (see Chapter 25 ∞), or infection
- Immune response (idiopathic thromcytopenic purpura (see description later in this chapter) (Buchanan, 2005).

Clotting factors are most often deficient due to genetic causes; see the discussions of hemophilia and von Willebrand's disease that follow.

Hemophilia

Hemophilia refers to a group of hereditary bleeding disorders that result from a deficiency in specific clotting factors. Hemophilia A, or classic hemophilia, is caused by a deficiency of factor VIII in the blood and accounts for 80% of persons with hemophilia. About 1 in 5000 male births result in hemophilia A. Hemophilia B, known as Christmas disease, is caused by a deficiency of factor IX. Of persons with hemophilia, 15% have hemophilia B. The severity of the disease may range from mild to severe bleeding tendencies. Hemophilia C (a deficiency in factor XI) is an autosomal recessive disease, occurring equally in males and females. The bleeding in factor XI deficiency is generally less severe than in factor VIII and IX deficiencies (Curry, 2004; Robertson & Shilkofski, 2005).

Etiology and Pathophysiology

Genes for clotting factors VIII and IX are located near the terminal long arm of the X chromosome (Montgomery & Scott, 2004). Hemophilia A and B are X-linked recessive traits, which manifest almost exclusively as affected males and carrier females. A daughter who inherits the trait from her father has a 50% chance at each pregnancy of transmitting it to her sons (refer to Chapter 3 ∞ for a description of genetic transmission). As many as one-third of the children affected by hemophilia do not have a family member with a history of a clotting disorder. In these cases, the disorder is caused by a new mutation (Montgomery & Scott, 2004).

The degree of bleeding is related to the amount of clotting factor, which is dependent upon the phase of coagulation affected, and the severity of the injury. Potential complications of hemophilia include internal hemorrhaging, transfusion reactions, shock, and death.

Clinical Manifestations

Hemophilia is manifested in different children by bleeding tendencies that range from mild to moderate or severe. Children with hemophilia often do not manifest symptoms until after 6 months of age as they become more mobile and incur injuries and bleeding from falls or from tooth eruption. Spontaneous bleeding, **hemarthrosis** (bleeding into a joint space), and deep tissue hemorrhage occur. Affected children frequently experience bleeding into the joint spaces of the knees, ankles, and elbows. Bleeding into joint spaces or bursae causes the child to have limited motion because of pain, tenderness, and swelling. Bone changes, contractures, and disabling deformities can result from immobility and from the effects of blood in the joint structures.

Male children may have bleeding after circumcision. Other signs and symptoms include easy bruising **(ecchymosis)**, nosebleeds, hematuria, and bleeding after tooth extraction; minor trauma; or minor surgical procedures. Large subcutaneous and intramuscular hemorrhages sometimes occur. Bleeding into the tissues of the neck, mouth, or chest is particularly serious because of the potential for airway obstruction. Retroperitoneal and intracranial bleeding may also occur and can be life threatening.

Females who carry the trait for hemophilia do not usually manifest symptoms of the disease. However, they may have prolonged bleeding during dental work, surgery, or trauma.

■ COLLABORATIVE CARE

Diagnosis of affected individuals and carriers can be done before birth through chorionic villus sampling or amniocentesis. Genetic testing of family members is increasingly being used to identify carriers. Diagnosis can also be made on the basis of the history, physical examination, and laboratory data. Laboratory tests will show low levels of factor VIII or IX, and prolonged activated partial prothrombin time (APPT). Prothrombin time (PT), thrombin time (TT), fibrinogen, and platelet count are normal. See Table 22–7.

The goal of medical management is to control bleeding by replacing the missing clotting factor. A synthetic drug that is effective against mild hemophilia is desmopressin acetate (DDAVP). An analog of vasopressin, DDAVP is administered intravenously and causes a two- to fourfold increase in factor VIII activity.

| Table 22–7 | DIAGNOSTIC TESTS FOR CLOTTING DISORDERS | |

TEST	NORMAL VALUE	
Bleeding time	2–9 minutes	
Fibrinogen	200–500 mg/dL (5.9–14.7 μmol/L)	
Partial thromboplastin time (PTT)	42–54 seconds	
Platelet count (3 10³/μl)	Males	Females
Newborns	164–351	234–346
1–2 months	275–567	295–615
2–6 months	275–566	288–598
6 months–2 years	219–452	229–465
2–6 years	204–405	204–402
6–12 years	194–364	183–369
12–18 years	165–332	185–335
> 18 years	143–320	171–326
Prothrombin time (PT)	11–15 seconds	
Thrombin time (π)	12–16 seconds	

Adapted from Soldin, S. J., Brugnara, C., & Wong, E. C. (2003). *Pediatric Reference Ranges* (4th ed.) Washington, DC: AACC Press.

Replacement therapy with the needed factor is indicated when the child experiences a mild or major hemorrhage or faces a life-threatening situation. Prompt and adequate treatment is needed to prevent serious bleeding episodes and their sequelae.

The outlook for children with hemophilia has been greatly improved by the availability of transfusion therapy. Transfusions started at home and early interventions prevent many disease complications. In the past, many children with factor VIII deficiency died in the first 5 years of life. Today, children with moderate or mild hemophilia can lead normal lives. See Table 22–8 for types of blood products available for infusion in hemophilia and other disorders.

RESEARCH

Gene Therapy

Gene therapy is being explored for treatment of hemophilia. One approach is to infuse carrier organisms into the body where they would act on target cells to promote manufacture of deficient clotting factor. Efforts in animal models such as dogs are underway. These research approaches offer the promise of new treatment options in the future (Warrington & Herzog, 2006).

■ NURSING MANAGEMENT

Nursing management for the child with hemophilia involves thorough assessments of the child at each healthcare visit, and implementation with interventions that are designed to manage pain, ensure physical mobility, and enhance developmental progression.

| Table 22–8 | TYPES OF BLOOD AND BLOOD PRODUCTS FOR ADMINISTRATION |

Type of Blood or Blood Product	Indication for Use
Whole blood	To replace blood volume Generally given in hemorrhagic emergencies and shock
Packed red blood cells	To increase oxygen-carrying capacity in anemia and some leukemias
Fresh frozen plasma	To expand blood volume
Cryoprecipitate	To replace factor VIII, factor XIII, von Willebrand's factor, and fibrinogen
Clotting factors	
Factor VIII	To treat factor VIII deficiency (Hemophilia A) and von Willebrand's disease
Factor IX	To treat factor IX deficiency (Hemophilia B)
Albumin	To expand blood volume in shock and trauma

Nursing Assessment and Diagnosis

Physiologic Assessment

Be aware of the history of bleeding disorder in the family of any infant or young child. Observe for prolonged bleeding or oozing of blood. At times, children with mild disorders are diagnosed after incidents such as prolonged nosebleeds or seeping after a venipuncture or intravenous start.

Once the disorder is diagnosed, obtain a complete medical history from the parents or child. In particular, ask about previous episodes of bleeding and the occurrence of hemophilia or any other bleeding disorders in family members. The history of bleeding will vary, and provides clues to the severity of the disease.

Assess the child for any joint pain, swelling, or permanent deformity, particularly around the knees, elbows, ankles, and shoulders. Evaluate range of motion for all joints and level of physical activity. Assess for pain in any body part. Note the presence of hematuria and mild flank pain. Assess the skin for evidence of ecchymosis or petechia. A neurologic assessment should be conducted, as the risk for intracranial hemorrhage and bleeding can lead to peripheral neuropathies.

Psychologic Assessment

It is difficult for families to manage care of the hemophiliac child, especially if the disease is severe. Assess the family's coping mechanisms and support systems. Determine the ability of the family's resources to manage procedures and treatment; the factor concentrates and infusion equipment are costly. Inquire if the parents have respite care that enables them to take time for themselves while knowing that the child is cared for safely. Assess older children's understanding of the disease, limitations, and their adaptation to it.

Developmental Assessment

Because the child with hemophilia may have physical activity restrictions, physical skills may be delayed. Perform frequent developmental assessments, being particularly attentive to fine and gross motor skills.

The most important nursing diagnosis for the child with hemophilia is Risk for Injury related to bleeding disorder. Following are other nursing diagnoses that may apply:

- Acute Pain related to bleeding episodes
- Risk for Injury related to excessive bleeding
- Impaired Physical Mobility related to joint stiffness or contractures
- Deficient Knowledge Deficit related to lack of exposure to illness
- Interrupted Family Processes related to family role shift required to care for a child with a chronic illness
- Delayed Growth and Development related to effects of physical disability

Planning and Implementation

Nursing care focuses on preventing and controlling bleeding episodes, limiting joint involvement and managing pain, and providing emotional support. Both short-term interventions and long-term management are necessary.

Prevent and Control Bleeding Episodes

Bleeding problems are rare in infants with hemophilia. As children learn to walk and develop other motor skills, however, they often fall and suffer cuts and bruises. The risk of injury can be reduced by emphasizing to parents the need for close supervision and a safe environment. Parents should encourage children to play with toys that are safe and age-appropriate. When the child is learning to walk, a helmet is recommended to protect the head from injury during falls. The home environment should be adapted to promote safety, such as by removing rugs that cause tripping and padding furniture with sharp edges.

If dental surgery or tooth extraction is necessary, it is performed in a controlled environment by experienced staff. Use of a dental irrigation device is often recommended if the child has excess bleeding from gums. Advise adolescents to shave only with an electric razor.

Control any superficial bleeding by applying pressure to the area for at least 15 minutes. Immobilize and elevate the affected area, and apply ice packs to promote vasoconstriction. Follow prescriptions for administration of factor replacement. Carefully monitor the child's condition for any side effects when factor replacement therapy is administered. If the child sustains a head, abdominal, or other major injury, immediate medical attention is required.

When the child is hospitalized, use nursing approaches to minimize the chance of bleeding. Ensure that the hospital environment is safe by orienting the child to the room and keeping the floor and room clear of hazards as much as possible.

Limit Joint Involvement and Manage Pain

During bleeding episodes, hemarthrosis is managed by elevating and immobilizing the joint and applying ice packs. Administer analgesics as ordered. Once bleeding has been controlled, range-of-motion exercises are performed to strengthen muscles and joints and to prevent flexion contractures. Physical therapy may be required. Because excessive weight can place an added stress on joints, encourage the child to maintain an appropriate weight. Note that oral opioids may be required for pain relief.

Provide Emotional Support

The needs of families with hemophiliac children are best met through a comprehensive team approach. Refer the parents for genetic counseling as soon as possible after diagnosis. It is important to identify family members who carry the trait, as they may suffer excessive bleeding during surgery.

Encourage the parents to verbalize their feelings. Be understanding and sensitive to their needs. Mothers may feel guilty about having transferred the disease to the child and may benefit from assistance in dealing with these feelings. Refer to counseling as appropriate. Partner with the family to explain the disorder and how it affects both the child and other family members. Refer the parents and child to organizations such as the National Hemophilia Foundation for further information.

Discharge Planning and Home Care Teaching

The child may be hospitalized briefly during the first manifestation of bleeding or diagnosis and management. Most care will subsequently take place in the home. Home care needs should be identified and addressed well in advance of discharge. Advise parents to have the child wear a medical identification tag. Dentists and other healthcare providers should be aware of the diagnosis.

Explain the cause of bleeding so both the child and parents understand the disease process. Teach the child and family how to identify internal bleeding. Signs and symptoms such as joint pain, abdominal pain, and obvious bleeding are indicators for immediate factor infusion. Make sure the child and parents know what situations could cause bleeding to occur. Teach parents to give acetaminophen instead of aspirin or other drugs that prolong bleeding time to relieve pain.

Instruct the parents and the child, when appropriate, in the preparation and administration of factor concentrate. If infusion of the missing factor is scheduled on a regular basis, bleeding episodes can be controlled or avoided. Have the parents demonstrate the procedure and make sure they can properly administer the product. The parents need to be familiar with properties of the factor concentrate to correctly prepare the mixture. As the child advances in age, he or she can assume some of the management responsibilities of care.

The child will need an Individual School Health Plan (see Chapter 11 ∞). Members of the school staff should be instructed in management of emergencies, and infusion equipment should be readily available. The nurse can identify key staff members in the school and teach them the actions that need to be taken.

Help the family and school to plan an appropriate schedule of activities without overprotecting the child. Children with hemophilia should not engage in contact sports such as football and soccer, which may result in injury and trauma. Instead, sports such as swimming, hiking, and bicycling should be encouraged.

CLINICAL TIP

Take the following precautions when caring for children with bleeding disorders:

- Avoid taking temperatures rectally or giving suppositories.
- Check blood pressure by cuff as infrequently as possible.
- Avoid intramuscular or subcutaneous injections.
- Use only paper or silk tape for dressings.
- When indicated, perform mouth care every 3 hours with a glycerin swab.
- Except for factor replacement therapy, avoid all venipunctures.
- Use a peripheral fingerstick to obtain blood samples.
- Insert a saline lock, if needed, to provide access for blood when repeat venous draws are needed. Heparin flush must *not* be used in the lock.
- Do not give aspirin or other drugs that alter bleeding time.

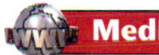

MediaLink

Hemophilia Resources

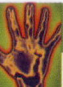

GROWTH & DEVELOPMENT

The Child with Hemophilia

The needs of children with hemophilia differ at various ages. Young toddlers may need helmets or knee pads to protect them from bleeding as they become ambulatory. Preschoolers and school-age children benefit from planning for activities that encourage activity without creating large risk of physical impact and subsequent bleeding. Encourage adolescents with hemophilia to participate in leisure activities that are important to their peers such as computer games, reading clubs, and crafts. Physical activity is very important for the health and maintenance of a healthy weight, so help the teen to find activities such as swimming, biking, and others that do not generally create physical impact. Knee pads, elbow pads, and helmets should be used when participating in any physical sports. Coaches, teachers, and others should be well informed about how to treat bleeding episodes and the importance of prompt treatment. The child can carry a cell phone to contact the family members who can bring supplies to start an infusion, if needed.

Explain how the parents can coordinate their child's care with a number of health professionals. Provide ongoing case management, assisting the family to take on this task, if able.

Hemophilia is not only a debilitating disorder for the child, but can also be financially draining for the family. Frequent outpatient visits, emergency department visits, hospital admissions, and the cost of factor concentrate can exhaust a family's resources. If indicated, referral should be made to appropriate social services (e.g., the state's maternal and child health program for children with special healthcare needs) and organizations such as the National Hemophilia Foundation. Sharing experiences with other families of children with hemophilia can provide support. Investigate the availability of summer camps for children and teens with hemophilia and refer these resources to families.

Evaluation

Expected outcomes of nursing care include the following:

- The child will be free from injury that could cause bleeding.
- Normal joint mobility will be maintained.
- Pain will be successfully managed to a level of comfort for the child.
- Safe and timely infusions will be provided as needed to treat the disease and prevent complications.
- The child will demonstrate normal growth and developmental progression.
- The child and family will demonstrate adequate knowledge of disease management, including recognition of bleeding and prompt initiation of infusions.
- Family members will verbalize that they have adequate support to provide care for the child with a chronic illness of hemophilia and to deal with genetic implications of the disease.

Von Willebrand's Disease

Like hemophilia, von Willebrand's disease is a hereditary bleeding disorder. There are about 20 different disorders involving a deficiency of von Willebrand's factor (vWF), which is a plasma protein and the carrier for clotting factor VIII, thereby playing a necessary role in platelet adhesion. The most common form of the disorder is transmitted as an autosomal dominant trait, and it can occur in both males and females. The gene for the disease is located on chromosome 12.

Normally, vWF concentration increases in the area of an injury and binds to platelets to facilitate their binding to the damaged vessel wall. With von Willebrand's disease, the vWF is not sufficient in quantity or is dysfunctional; therefore, clot forming and bleeding control is impaired.

The three types of von Willebrand's disease and their characteristics are:

- Type I   Decreased amount of normal vWF, autosomal dominant, most common form
- Type II   Presence of abnormal vWF, autosomal dominant
- Type III Near complete absence of vWF, autosomal recessive (Curry, 2004)

The characteristic manifestations are easy bruising and epistaxis. Children with von Willebrand's disease also frequently have gingival bleeding and increased bleeding with lacerations or during surgery or dental work. The disease may not be diagnosed until a surgical or dental procedure leads to bleeding. Affected teenage girls may have menorrhagia (increased menstrual bleeding). Gastrointestinal bleeding can occur, although hemarthrosis is uncommon.

Diagnosis of von Willebrand's disease is made after laboratory studies reveal decreased von Willebrand's factor levels, von Willebrand's factor antigen levels, and factor VIII activity; reduced platelet agglutination; prolonged bleeding time; and prolonged or normal activated partial thromboplastin time (APPT).

Treatment is similar to that for the child with hemophilia and involves infusion of von Willebrand's protein concentrate. Desmopressin (DDAVP) is administered to promote release of stored vWF and to prevent bleeding associated with dental or surgical procedures. Locally administered medications such as aminocaproic acid are sometimes used to manage bleeding in the mucous membranes.

Nursing Management

Nursing care is the same as for a child with hemophilia, which is described in the previous section. Teach parents about the disorder and instruct them not to give the child any aspirin or other drugs that can cause bleeding or inhibit platelet function. Teach management of bleeding episodes and intravenous infusion techniques, as for hemophilia. The prognosis is good, and children with von Willebrand's disease usually have a normal life expectancy. Expected outcomes of nursing care include prompt management of bleeding and prevention of disease complications.

Disseminated Intravascular Coagulation

Disseminated intravascular coagulation (DIC) is a life-threatening, acquired pathologic process in which the clotting system is abnormally activated, resulting in widespread clot formation in the small vessels throughout the body. It is a complication of other serious illnesses in infants and children, such as infection, sepsis, hypoxia, shock, trauma, burns, liver disease, necrotizing enterocolitis, cancer, and viruses.

The disorder results from increased protease activity that is caused by unregulated release of thrombin. Excess thrombin is generated, followed by deposition of fibrin strands in body tissues. These changes slow the circulating blood and cause tissue hypoxia, resulting in eventual tissue necrosis. The circulating fibrin fragments later begin to interfere with platelet aggregation and other aspects of the clotting mechanism, resulting in bleeding or hemorrhage. The disease process commonly interferes with function in the respiratory, cardiovascular, hepatic, renal, neurologic, and gastrointestinal systems (Oren, Cingoz, & Duman, et al., 2005).

The sequence of events for DIC is as follows (LeMone & Burke, 2004):

1. Widespread formation of tiny blood clots occurs within the microcirculation of all body organs.
2. The fibrinolytic pathway is activated, promoting the dissolution of the clots that have been formed.
3. The amount of thrombin that enters the systemic circulation greatly exceeds that of clotting inhibitors to regulate it.
4. The deposit of thrombin decreases blood flow to organs, which may eventually cause tissue ischemia, infarction, and necrosis.
5. The excessive amounts of thrombin also activate platelet aggregation — causing thrombocytopenia with an increased risk of bleeding — and the fibrinolytic pathway (causing bleeding).
6. Plasma begins to break down fibrin before a stable clot is formed.
7. Fibrin degradation products, which are potent anticoagulants, are released and further increase bleeding.
8. Clotting factors are depleted, the ability to form clots is lost, and hemorrhage occurs.

Symptoms can include diffuse bleeding manifested by hematuria, petechiae, or purpura; an injection site that continues to ooze; circulatory collapse; and major vessel thrombosis. See Clinical Manifestations of Disseminated Intravascular Coagulation on the next page for further signs and symptoms.

Collaborative Care

The prothrombin time and partial thromboplastin time are prolonged, platelet count and fibrinogen levels are increased, and levels of fibrin-fibrinogen split products are high.

Clinical therapy is supportive and includes identification and treatment of the underlying disorder; replacement of depleted coagulation factors, fibrinogen, and

CLINICAL MANIFESTATIONS | DISSEMINATED INTRAVASCULAR COAGULATION

Etiology	Clinical Manifestations	Clinical Therapy
Cardiovascular System Tachycardia Hypotension Circulatory collapse Major vessel thrombosis	Decreased perfusion, shock Inappropriate clotting	Administer fluids as ordered; monitor intake and output Monitor vital signs
Respiratory System Tachypnea Decreased breath sounds	Impaired gas exchange due to microclots in the pulmonary vasculature	Monitor respiratory status Maintain ventilatory support if required
Central Nervous System Confusion Coma Seizures	Impaired cerebral perfusion	Conduct neurologic assessment every 2 hours during critical period, then every 4 hours until stabilized
Urinary System Oliguria Anuria Renal failure Hematuria	Impaired renal perfusion Impaired clotting mechanisms lead to bleeding	Monitor urine output hourly Maintain patent urinary catheter Monitor urine for blood
Gastrointestinal System Gastrointestinal bleeding Abdominal distention Bleeding from mucous membranes Occult blood in stool or emesis	Impaired clotting mechanisms lead to bleeding	Monitor for occult blood in stools and emesis Monitor for overt signs of bleeding from gums Measure abdominal girth every 4 hours
Integumentary System Petechiae Purpura Ecchymosis Bleeding or oozing from wounds or intravenous access site Pallor Cool extremities Cyanosis of extremities Gangrene	Impaired clotting mechanism leads to bleeding Impaired tissue perfusion	Monitor skin for evidence of bleeding Protect from injury Monitor distal pulses, temperature, and capillary refill
General: weakness, malaise Oozing from body orifices	Shock, decreased perfusion Impaired clotting mechanism leads to bleeding	Cluster care to allow for rest periods Maintain bed rest

platelets; and anticoagulant therapy (heparin). Oxygen is administered, and perfusion is measured. The clinical manifestations table lists further steps in clinical therapy.

Nursing Management

DIC is a complex disorder that is managed by a critical care team. Nursing care focuses on assessing the bleeding, preventing further injury, and administering prescribed therapies.

Because all body systems can be involved, careful assessment of all systems is needed on a continual basis. Observe for petechiae, ecchymoses, and oozing every 1 to 2 hours. Check dependent areas, as blood will pool there. Intravenous sites are particularly prone to oozing and should be assessed every 15 minutes. Examine stool for the presence of blood, and measure blood loss as accurately as possible. Assess extremities for capillary refill, warmth, and pulses. Frequently assess vital signs and level of consciousness. Measure intake and output. Monitor urine for the presence of blood. BUN and creatinine are monitored to assess renal function.

Institute bleeding control precautions, monitor prescribed therapy (transfusion, anticoagulant therapy), and report any signs of complications. Monitor oxygen saturation and arterial blood gases. The child may require mechanical ventilation. Maintain patency of the airway and ensure correct endotracheal tube position.

Implement measures to maintain skin integrity, such as gentle repositioning. Implement a nutritional plan of tube feedings or total parenteral nutrition. Identify the family's coping strategies and support system to facilitate their ability to manage this life-threatening crisis.

Expected outcomes of nursing care are management of bleeding and adequate functioning of all body systems, as well as effective family coping.

Idiopathic Thrombocytopenic Purpura

Idiopathic thrombocytopenic purpura (ITP), also known as autoimmune thrombocytopenic purpura, is a disorder characterized by increased destruction of platelets, even though platelet production in the bone marrow is generally normal. When the rate of platelet destruction exceeds the rate of platelet production, the number of circulating platelets decreases and blood clotting slows, causing bleeding, often into the mucosa and cutaneous tissues. The condition can be acute when it improves within 6 months, or chronic if it continues for a longer time.

Etiology and Pathophysiology

ITP is the most common bleeding disorder in children. It occurs annually in 2.5 to 5 children per 100,000, with a peak age of 5.5 years. The acute condition occurs most frequently in children 1 to 10 years of age and the chronic condition is most common in children over 9 years (Panepinto & Brousseau, 2005).

The cause of ITP is unknown but it usually follows a viral infection such as Epstein-Barr virus, varicella, or human immunodeficiency virus. It is also seen in a small number (1 in 25,000) of children after measles-mumps-rubella vaccination (Buchanan, 2005). An antibody that acts against platelets binds to the platelet surface, reacts with membrane glycoproteins, and causes platelet destruction in the liver and spleen (Buchanan, 2005; Panepinto & Brousseau, 2005).

Clinical Manifestations

Symptoms include multiple ecchymoses and petechiae. Mucosal bleeding such as in the mouth or nose are common presentations. The child has typically been well, has a history of recent viral illness, and then develops onset of bruising and bleeding that concerns parents. A rare complication is intracranial hemorrhage, which occurs most commonly in severe thrombocytopenia.

◼ COLLABORATIVE CARE

Diagnosis is made by history and through physical and laboratory findings, which show a decreased platelet count and antiplatelet antibodies in the peripheral blood. Platelet count is less than $20 \times 10^3/microL$. The child has normal hemoglobin and white blood cell counts. Direct and indirect Coombs' tests may be performed to detect the presence of antibodies (Kuhne, Buchanan, & Zimmerman et al., 2003).

If the child has minor thrombocytopenia and minimal bleeding, some clinicians do not treat ITP but observe the child closely. Families need instructions to identify bleeding, especially intracranial, and to seek care immediately. Children must avoid contact sports until platelet counts return to normal. As is common in many autoimmune conditions, most children improve without treatment within 6 months. However, most children are treated with a variety of medications. Corticosteroids (prednisone or methylprednisolone) are commonly given as treatment, usually for several days up to 3 weeks (Beck et al., 2005). Within 3–10 days, the platelet count shows improvement. Alternatively, intravenous immunoglobulin is sometimes administered, as is anti-D immunoglobulin. These infusions improve platelet count within 24–48 hours but require intravenous infusion, often in an outpatient facility (Panepinto & Brousseau, 2005). Children who relapse are treated similarly in subsequent eruptions of the disease.

A few children, most often those with extremely low platelet counts, develop life-threatening complications such as intracranial hemorrhage, gastrointestinal bleeding, or other serious bleeding. They receive critical care which includes hospitalization on a critical care unit, high dose corticosteroids, intravenous immune globulins, and splenectomy.

NURSING MANAGEMENT

Nursing care focuses on controlling and reducing the number of bleeding episodes. Assess vital signs and level of consciousness. Assess for evidence of bleeding, including petechiae and purpura. The abdomen is assessed for hepatosplenomegaly. Monitor for nosebleeds, oozing at intravenous sites, gastrointestinal bleeding, and indications of intracranial bleeding. Signs of intracranial bleeding include vomiting and seizures.

Preventive measures are similar to those for the child with hemophilia. Teach parents to use acetaminophen, rather than aspirin or other drugs that influence bleeding time, to control pain. The child should avoid contact sports and other activities that may increase the risk of injury. Be sure the family and child are aware of the signs and symptoms indicating bleeding, including signs of intracranial bleeding. Provide emotional support for the child and family who are often concerned about the sudden and unexpected nature of the disease.

Expected outcomes of nursing care are prevention of bleeding and restoration of normal coagulation patterns with no serious sequelae.

Meningococcemia

Meningococcemia is the most severe disease process that follows infection with *Neisseria meningitidis* or, occasionally, other microorganisms such as *H. influenzae* or *Streptococcus pneumoniae*. The disorder is thought to be an immune response to the endotoxins of the organism.

Onset is sudden: A respiratory infection is followed by high fever, petechial rash, massive skin and mucosal hemorrhage, hypotension, disseminated intravascular coagulation, and shock. The child, usually under 2 years of age, is critically ill and demonstrates multisystem disease. Symptoms can progress to a critical level within 12 to 48 hours of onset. Commonly the skin turns pink and then black as the tissues are damaged from reduced oxygen delivery. Limbs may need to be amputated as a result of impaired circulation.

Treatment consists of antibiotics, removal from sources of infection, and multisystem shock management. (See Chapter 21 for a description of distributive shock and Chapter 26 ∞ for a discussion of meningitis.) Prompt administration of antibiotics to the child who manifests fever with purpura can decrease the severity of outcome. Depending on the child's condition, total parenteral nutrition, sedation and pain relief, dialysis, or amputation may be required. Close contacts of the child should receive prophylactic antibiotics.

Nursing Management

Nursing care of the child with meningococcemia is complex. Treatment must begin quickly and the child generally has a lengthy hospitalization in a pediatric intensive care unit. Thorough assessments of all body systems are performed. Intravenous infusions must be administered when ordered to ensure correct and timely administration of antibiotics and other therapies. Urinary output is measured to evaluate kidney function. Meticulous skin care is necessary to preserve the integrity of tissues. Care is taken to prevent further infections. Nutritional support in the form of total parenteral nutrition is common. The family needs support to deal with the changing critical nature of the child's illness and the possibility that death or permanent, severe deformities will result. When the child improves, continuing comprehensive care in the hospital and then in the community is needed to manage complex issues related to growth, development, nutrition, amputations, and prosthetics. Expected outcomes of nursing care include prevention of further infection, maintenance of body systems during the acute phase of illness, positive adjustment to amputations and deformities resulting from the disease, and end-of-life care when the child does not survive the disease.

HEMATOPOIETIC STEM CELL TRANSPLANTATION (HSCT)

Hematopoietic stem cell transplantation is a treatment used for diseases such as severe combined immunodeficiency disease, severe and unresponsive aplastic anemia, and leukemia (refer to Chapters 17 and 23 ∞). Sources of stem cells include bone marrow, peripheral blood, and cord blood. Hematopoietic stem cells exist primarily in the bone marrow but also circulate in the peripheral blood. These cells can grow into new body cells and so have become useful to treat immune and hematologic diseases when restoration of normal cells is needed. Stem cells can be obtained from bone marrow, cord blood, or peripheral blood and frozen for later use (Trigg, 2004).

■ COLLABORATIVE CARE

There are three types of hematopoietic stem cell transplants: autologous, isogeneic (or syngeneic), and allogeneic. In **autologous transplantation**, the child's own marrow is taken, treated, stored, and reinfused after the child has received chemotherapy. In **isogeneic transplantation**, the marrow is taken from a genetically identical twin. In **allogeneic transplantation**, the donor, usually a sibling, has a compatible human leukocyte antigen (HLA). Human leukocyte antigens are proteins found on the surface of nearly all nucleated cells within the body, and they are responsible for regulating the immune response. When no relative is found to match the child, a histocompatible donor may be sought from the National Bone Marrow Registry. With the development of the National Bone Marrow Registry, bone marrow transplantation from HLA-matched unrelated donors has become possible for some children.

Clinical Therapy

PRE-TRANSPLANT PHASE   After a thorough evaluation of the child, including HLA typing, evaluation of organ functions, and laboratory studies, the child receives high doses of chemotherapy and, sometimes, total body irradiation directed at destroying circulating blood cells and the diseased bone marrow in the ill child. Common chemotherapeutic agents used include cyclophosphamide, busulfan, cytarabine, carmustine, and lomustine (Ryan, Kristovich, Haugen, Coyne, & Hubbell, 2002). The chemotherapy program for destruction of bone marrow ranges from 4 to 12 days. During this time, the child is cared for in strict isolation in a special unit that provides a negative pressure environment (Figure 22–8 ➤). Measures are implemented to prevent transmission of infection, such as irradiating food and sterilizing utensils and other items used in the room.

TRANSPLANT PHASE   Following the immunosuppression procedure, the child receives an intravenous transfusion with the donor stem cells. This procedure is similar to administration of a blood product. The healthy stem cells migrate to the bone marrow. Healthy bone marrow, capable of making blood cells, is the anticipated result. If the transplantation is successful, the donor cells implant in the child's marrow and begin to produce blood cells within approximately 2 to 4 weeks.

POST-TRANSPLANT PHASE   Pancytopenia (marked decrease in RBCs, WBCs, and platelets) lasts for several weeks following the transplantation. The major risks during this period are infection, anemia, and bleeding. Transfusion of red blood cells and platelets may be required. The child's illness and the side effects related to the chemotherapy may alter nutritional status. Total parenteral nutrition (TPN) may be implemented in order to meet the child's nutritional needs during this period.

Except for children receiving syngeneic transplants, immunosuppressive agents are administered to prevent graft-versus-host disease. Once the bone marrow begins to produce new cells, graft-versus-host disease (rejection) is the major threat. Refer to Chapter 17 ∞ for a discussion of this disease.

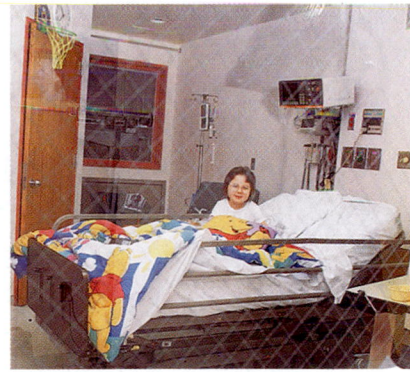

Figure 22–8 ➤   The child undergoing bone marrow transplantation is hospitalized in a special sterile unit while receiving chemotherapy before the transfusion. The child remains in the unit for several weeks afterward until the new marrow produces enough cells to maintain health.

GROWTH & DEVELOPMENT

Hospitalization

Hospitalizations of children undergoing bone marrow and other stem cell transplantation are usually lengthy. Evaluate the child's age and developmental stage and establish developmental goals to be met during the hospitalization. Implement nursing plans to meet the child's developmental needs and encourage further growth. Evaluate the child's developmental status on follow-up visits and inquire about the family's observations of developmental milestones.

MediaLink

Health Promotion and Maintenance Overview: The Child with Hematopoietic Stem Cell Transplantation

NURSING MANAGEMENT

Monitor the child undergoing HSCT by assessing the skin, mucous membranes, gastrointestinal function, respiratory function, cardiac function, and hydration status. Multisystem assessment is needed. Because graft-versus-host disease may occur at any time, even after the child returns home, frequent thorough assessments are necessary after discharge.

Supportive care after the transplantation procedure focuses on preventing infection, controlling bleeding, maintaining adequate nutrition and hydration, monitoring for signs of rejection, and providing psychosocial support. The treatment is lengthy, the child is often critically ill, and parents may have traveled to a medical center many miles from home for the procedure. Ask parents about other family members and how they are managing. Provide information about inexpensive housing available near the medical center, such as in a Ronald McDonald house. Encourage parents to discuss their feelings with other parents of children receiving bone marrow transplantation. Organizations such as the Bone Marrow Transplant Family Support Network can serve as resources for families.

When the child is ready for discharge, be sure the family is prepared to administer medications, recognize signs of graft-versus-host disease, provide adequate nutrition for the child, and perform other necessary care. Arrange for follow-up visits and provide the names of local healthcare contact persons who can offer support and provide information. The child may need tutors or other educational assistance to promote integration back into the school setting.

The major expected outcome of nursing care is the proper activity of bone marrow in the child with resulting normal levels and function of blood cells. Other outcomes are provision of family support, ongoing care and education for the child, adequate nutrition, and prevention of infection.

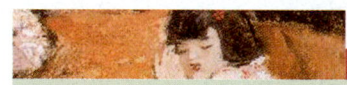

CRITICAL THINKING IN ACTION

Recall Michael, the child in the opening scenario who is admitted with sickle cell crisis. Michael is receiving intravenous and oral fluids, oxygen, and opioids via a patient-controlled analgesia (PCA) pump. His hemoglobin on admission was 7.7 g/dL, hematocrit was 22%. Michael's father has returned to work and he visits in the evenings. Michael's mother remains at the hospital with her son.

DISCUSSION

1. Considering Michael's age and developmental stage, what communication techniques will the nurse implement when teaching Michael about his disease and treatment?

2. Refer to Chapter 15 ∞ to plan the pain assessment and management techniques that can be used with Michael.

3. What are the expected levels of hemoglobin and hematocrit at Michael's age? Why are his levels abnormal? Describe how sickle cell disease influences blood values.

4. What are the most immediate care needs while Michael is hospitalized? What additional immediate care will he require at home?

 Refer to your Prentice Hall Nursing MediaLink DVD-ROM for answers.

EXPLORE MediaLink

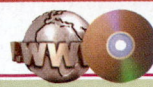

http://www.prenhall.com/ball

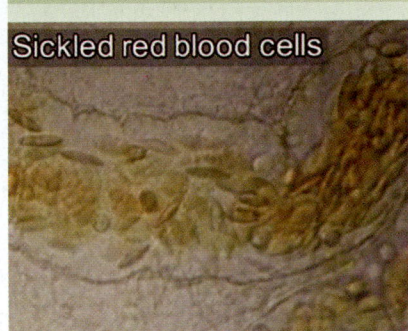

Sickled red blood cells

Resources for this chapter can be found on the Prentice Hall Nursing MediaLink DVD-ROM accompanying this textbook, and on the Companion Website at http://www.prenhall.com/ball.

DVD-ROM

Audio Glossary
NCLEX-RN® Review
Animations/Videos
  Blood Cells
  Sickle Cell Anemia

COMPANION WEBSITE

Audio Glossary
NCLEX-RN® Review
Care Plan Activity: A School-age Child with Hemophilia
Case Study: An Adolescent in Sickle Cell Crisis
MediaLink Applications
  Carrier Testing of Hemophilia
  Sickle Cell Anemia
WebLinks

REFERENCES

American Academy of Pediatrics Committee on Nutrition. (2004). *Pediatric nutrition handbook* (5th ed.). Elk Grove Village, IL: American Academy of Pediatrics.

Aplastic Anemia and MDS International Foundation. (2003). Retrieved June 1, 2004, from http://www.aplastic.org/pdfs/ACQUIRED-APLASTIC-ANEMIA-BASIC-EXPLANATIONS.pdf

Beck, C. E., Nathan, P. C., Parkin, P. C., Blanchette, V. S., & Macarthur, C. (2005). Corticosteroids versus intravenous immune globulin for the treatment of acute immune thrombocytopenic purpura in children: A systematic review and meta-analysis of randomized controlled trials. *Journal of Pediatrics, 147*, 521–527.

Beyer, J. E., & Simmons, L. E. (2004). Home treatment of pain for children and adolescents with sickle cell disease. *Pain Management Nursing, 5*, 126–135.

Boxer, L. A. (2004). Leukopenia. In R. E Behrman, R. M. Kliegman, & H. B. Jenson (Eds.), *Nelson textbook of pediatrics* (17th ed., pp. 717–723). Philadelphia: W. B. Saunders.

Bryant, R. (2005). Asthma in the pediatric sickle cell patient with acute chest syndrome. *Journal of Pediatric Health Care, 19*, 157–162.

Buchanan, G. R. (2005). Thrombocytopenia during childhood: What the pediatrician needs to know. *Pediatrics in Review, 26*, 401–409.

Carley, A. (2003). Anemia: When is it iron deficiency? *Pediatric Nursing, 29*, 128–133.

Catlin, A. J. (2003). Thalassemia: The facts and the controversies. *Pediatric Nursing, 29*, 447–451.

Chamley, C., Carson, P., Randall, D., & Sandwell, W. (2005). *Developmental anatomy and physiology of children*. St. Louis: Elsevier.

Corbeel, L. (2005). Immune-mediated aplastic anemia. *European Journal of Pediatrics, 164*, 698–699.

Corbett, J. V. (2004). *Laboratory tests and diagnostic procedures with nursing diagnosis* (6th ed.). Upper Saddle River NJ: Prentice Hall Health.

Curry, H. (2004). Bleeding disorder basics. *Pediatric Nursing, 30*, 402–429.

Jacob, E., Miaskowski, C., Savedra, M., Beyer, J., Treadwell, M., & Styles, L. (2003). Management of vaso-occlusive pain in children with sickle cell disease. *Journal of Pediatric Hematology/Oncology, 25*, 307–311.

King, A. A., Tang, S., Ferguson, K. L., & DeBaun, M. R. (2005). An education program to increase teacher knowledge about sickle cell disease. *Journal of School Health, 74*, 11–14.

Kral, M. C., Brown, R. T., Connelly, M., Cure, J. K., Besenski, N., Jackson, S. M., & Abboud, M. R. (2006). Radiographic predictors of neurocognitive functioning in pediatric sickle cell disease. *Journal of Child Neurology, 21*, 37–44.

Kuhne T., Buchanan, G. R., Zimmerman, S., Michaels, L. A., Kohan, R., Berchtold, W., & Imback, P. (2003). A prospective comparative study of 2540 infants and children with newly diagnosed idiopathic thrombocytopenic purpura (ITP) from the intercontinental childhood ITP study group. *Journal of Pediatrics, 143*, 605–608.

LeMone, P., & Burke, K. M. (2004). *Medical surgical nursing: Critical thinking in client care* (2nd ed.). Upper Saddle River, NJ: Prentice Hall.

Lindsey, T., Watts-Tate, N., Southwood, E., Routhieaux, J., Beatty, J., Calamaras, D., Phillips, M., Lea, G., Brown, E., & DeBaun, M. R. (2005). Chronic blood transfusion therapy practices to treat strokes in children with sickle cell disease. *Journal of the American Academy of Nurse Practitioners, 17*, 277–282.

London, M. L., Ladewig, P. W., Ball, J. W., & Bindler, R. C. (2007). *Maternal & child nursing care* (2nd ed.). Upper Saddle River, NJ: Prentice Hall Health.

Montgomery, R. R., & Scott, J. P. (2004). Hemorrhagic and thrombotic diseases. In R. E Behrman, R. M. Kliegman, & H. B. Jenson (Eds.), *Nelson textbook of pediatrics* (17th ed., pp. 1651–1674). Philadelphia: W.B. Saunders.

National Heart, Lung, and Blood Institute. (2002). The management of sickle cell disease. Retrieved June 1, 2004, from http://www.nhilbi.nih.gov/health/prof/blood/sickle/sc_mngt.pdf

National Institutes of Health. (2002). The management of sickle cell disease. Retrieved October 4, 2006 from http://www.nhlbi.nih.gov/health/prof/blood/sickle/sc_mngt.pdf

Ogedegbe, H. O. (2002). Sickle cell disease: An overview. *Laboratory Medicine, 7*, 515–543.

Ohls, R. K., & Christensen, R. D. (2004). The hematopoietic system. In R. E. Behrman, R. M. Kliegman, & H. B. Jenson (Eds.), *Nelson textbook of pediatrics* (17th ed., pp. 1599–1604). Philadelphia: W.B. Saunders.

Oren, H., Cingoz, I., Duman, M., Yilmaz, S., & Irken, G. (2005). Disseminated intravascular coagulation in pediatric patients. *Pediatric Hematology and Oncology, 22*, 679–688.

Panepinto, J. A., & Brousseau, D. C. (2005). Acute idiopathic thrombocytopenic purpura of childhood—diagnosis and therapy. *Pediatric Emergency Care, 21*, 691–695.

Pelchat, D., & Lefebvre, H. (2004). A holistic intervention programme for families with a child with a disability. *Journal of Advanced Nursing, 48*, 124–131.

Piga, A., Galanello, R., Forni, G. L., Cappellini, M. D., Origa, R., Zappu, A., Donato, G., Bordone, E., Lavagetto, A., Zanaboni, L., Sechaud, R., Hewson, N., Ford, J. M., Opitz, H., & Alberti, D. (2006). Randomized phase II trial of deferasirox (Exjade, ICL670), a once-daily, orally-administered iron chelator, in comparison to deferoxamine in thalassemia patients with transfusional iron overload. *Haematologica, 91*, 873–880.

Polin, R. A., Fox, W. W., & Abman, S. H. (2004). *Fetal and neonatal physiology* (3rd ed.). Philadelphia: Saunders.

Robertson, J., & Shilkofski, N. (Eds.). (2005). *The Harriet Lane handbook* (17th ed., pp. 353–357). Philadelphia: Elsevier Mosby.

Ryan, L. G., Kristovich, K. M., Haugen, M. S., Coyne, K. D., & Hubbell, M. M. (2002). Hematopoietic stem cell transplantation. In

C. R. Baggott, K.P. Kelly, D. Fochtman, & G. V. Foley, *Nursing care of children and adolescents with cancer* (3rd ed., pp. 212–255). Philadelphia: Saunders.

Segal, G. B., Hirsh, M. G., & Feig, S. A. (2002). Managing anemia in pediatric office practice: Part 1. *Pediatrics in Review, 23,* 75–83.

Soldin, S. J., Brugnara, C., & Wong, E. C. (2003). *Pediatric Reference Ranges* (4th ed.). Washington DC: AACC Press.

Tanyi, R. A. (2003). Sickle cell disease: Health promotion and maintenance and the role of primary care nurse practitioners. *Journal of the American Academy of Nursing Practitioners, 15,* 389–397.

Trigg, M. E. (2004). Hematopoietic stem cells. *Pediatrics, 113,* 1051–1057.

Warrington, K. H., & Herzog, R. W. (2006). Treatment of human disease by adeno-associated viral gene transfer. *Human Genetics, 119,* 571–603.

White K. E. (2005). Anemia is a poor predictor of iron deficiency among toddlers in the United States: For heme the bell tolls. *Pediations, 115,* 315–320.

Wilson, R. E., Krishnamurti, L., & Kamat, D. (2003). Management of sickle cell disease in primary care. *Clinical Pediatrics, 42,* 753–761.

Woolley, S. (2006). Children of Jehovah's Witnesses and adolescent Jehovah's Witnesses: What are their rights? *Archives of Disease in Children, 90,* 715–719.

Young, N. S., Calado, R. T., & Scheinberg, P. l. (2006). Current concepts in pathophysiology and treatment of aplastic anemia. *Blood, 108,* 2509–2519.

Young, N. S., & Maciejewski, J. P. (2004). The pathophysiology of acquired aplastic anemia. *New England Journal of Medicine, 336,* 1365–1372.

ALTERATIONS IN CELLULAR GROWTH

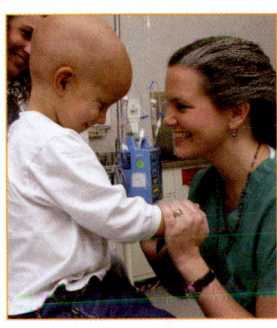

Sam, a 4-year-old, had several bruises on his legs that puzzled his parents since he had not been engaged in any activities that would have caused them. He also appeared to be lethargic compared to his usual energetic self. Suspecting an influenza after he also began to manifest a respiratory infection, Sam's parents brought him to the pediatric office. The physician's assessment showed hepatosplenomegaly, so a complete blood count was obtained. Low amounts of red blood cells and platelets were seen with high levels of white blood cells. The physician suspected leukemia and referred Sam to the oncology center that afternoon. Sam's mother was devastated; she had never suspected this diagnosis.

The next few days were a blur of making phones calls, arranging care for two older children, and then staying with Sam during his lumbar puncture, bone marrow aspiration, several body scans, and placement of a central line. Sam remained in the hospital for induction therapy and then went home. He is now returning for his next series of consolidation therapy treatments at the oncology clinic. The nurse who planned care in the immediate diagnostic period prepared him appropriately for every procedure, and now sees Sam at each visit. Although Sam has remained well, the nurse provided information for his parents about common side effects of chemotherapy drugs and the treatment regimen. She offered information about nutritional intake and answered the mother's questions at each visit. The two older siblings were able to attend a recent clinic visit, which allows them to understand Sam's condition and feel that they are part of his care. The family has many resources and adequate psychosocial support. The nurse identified the family's greatest need as knowledge, since they have many questions at each visit.

KEY TERMS

apoptosis 839	neutropenia 867
benign 838	oncogenes 844
biotherapy 851	pancytopenia 879
cachexia 845	phantom pain 885
carcinogens 843	polypharmacy 867
chemotherapy 848	protocol 849
complementary	protooncogenes
therapies 853	844
debulk 847	radiation 851
extravasation 866	secondary cancers
leukocytosis 879	857
leukopenia 879	staging 847
malignant 838	thrombocytopenia
metastasis 838	855
myelosuppression	tumor suppressor
867	genes 845
neoplasms 838	

MediaLink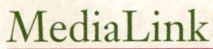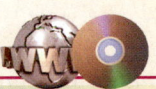

http://www.prenhall.com/ball

See the Prentice Hall Nursing MediaLink DVD-ROM and Companion Website for chapter-specific resources.

LEARNING OUTCOMES

After reading this chapter, you will be able to do the following:

1. Describe the incidence, known etiologies, and common clinical manifestations of cancer.

2. Synthesize information about diagnostic tests and clinical therapy for cancer to plan comprehensive care for children undergoing these procedures.

3. Integrate information about oncologic emergencies into plans for monitoring all children with cancer.

(continued)

Learning Outcomes, continued

4. Recognize the most common solid tumors in children, describe their treatment, and plan comprehensive nursing care.

5. Plan care for children and adolescents of all ages who have a diagnosis of leukemia.

6. Recognize the most common soft-tissue tumors in children, describe their treatment, and plan comprehensive care.

7. Describe the impact of cancer survival on children and use this information to plan for ongoing physiological and psychosocial care.

FOCUS ON
Cellular Growth

ANATOMY AND PHYSIOLOGY

Abnormal cellular growth can occur in any area of the body. Why are some growths called cancer and others are not? Changes in cellular growth within the body are called **neoplasms** (meaning new growth). A neoplasm is further classified as benign or malignant. **Benign** means that a growth does not endanger life or health; it tends not to recur after treatment. **Malignant** means that progressive growth of the tumor will, if not checked by treatment, result in spread to other sites in the body (**metastasis**), resulting in death. The common term for this type of cellular growth is *cancer*.

PEDIATRIC DIFFERENCES

Cancers in children often have different etiology than those in adults. Most adult cancers are epithelial in origin, while in children the nonepithelial or embryonal cell types predominate. They more often occur in deep body tissues and therefore may not be visible or palpable until quite large (Baggott, Kelly, Fochtman, & Foley, 2002). While many adult cancers are slow-growing and result from exposure to carcinogens over time, most childhood cancers are fast-growing, with a child who appears healthy becoming ill within several weeks or months (Thompson, 2003). Different types of cancers predominate at various ages in childhood, demonstrating the multiple causes and their relationship to age and development (Figure 23–1 ➤). Occasionally, an environmental exposure is linked to the incidence of cancer in children.

Although not common, some neonates have cancer that is diagnosed soon after birth. The types of cancers most common in this age group include brain tumors, neuroblastoma, leukemia, retinoblastoma, and teratomas (arising from primary germ layers). While treatments are usually as effective in neonates as in older children, the rapid growth of this age makes side effects of therapy more serious.

A major physiologic difference between adults and children that affects cellular growth involves the immune system and how well it functions in the body's defense. The rate of cell growth in children can also play a role in the rapidity with which some childhood cancers progress. The continuing presence of fetal cells in small children is related to some cancers.

The immune system defends the body against foreign organisms and substances through two responses: nonspecific and specific. In a nonspecific response, the components of the immune system attack a variety of targets. Nonspecific components include phagocytic (cell destroying) cells such as mononuclear leukocytes, polymorphonuclear (PMN) leukocytes, natural killer (NK) cells, and complements (noncellular proteins) that work together to destroy invading cells and substances. During the first month of a child's life, the nonspecific response is immature, so phagocytic cells have little ability to move toward cancer cells and fulfill their function. The nonspecific response is also impaired in premature and small-for-gestational-age (SGA) infants.

In a specific response, T lymphocytes and immunoglobulin (Ig) attack only one type of invader. The specific response capability also is immature in infants. B-cell production of various proteins called immunoglobins (IgM, IgG, and IgA) is below adult levels, so that the infant is vulnerable to bacterial and viral infections. (For a discussion of immune function, see Chapter 17 ∞.)

AS CHILDREN GROW

Types of Cancer by Age Group

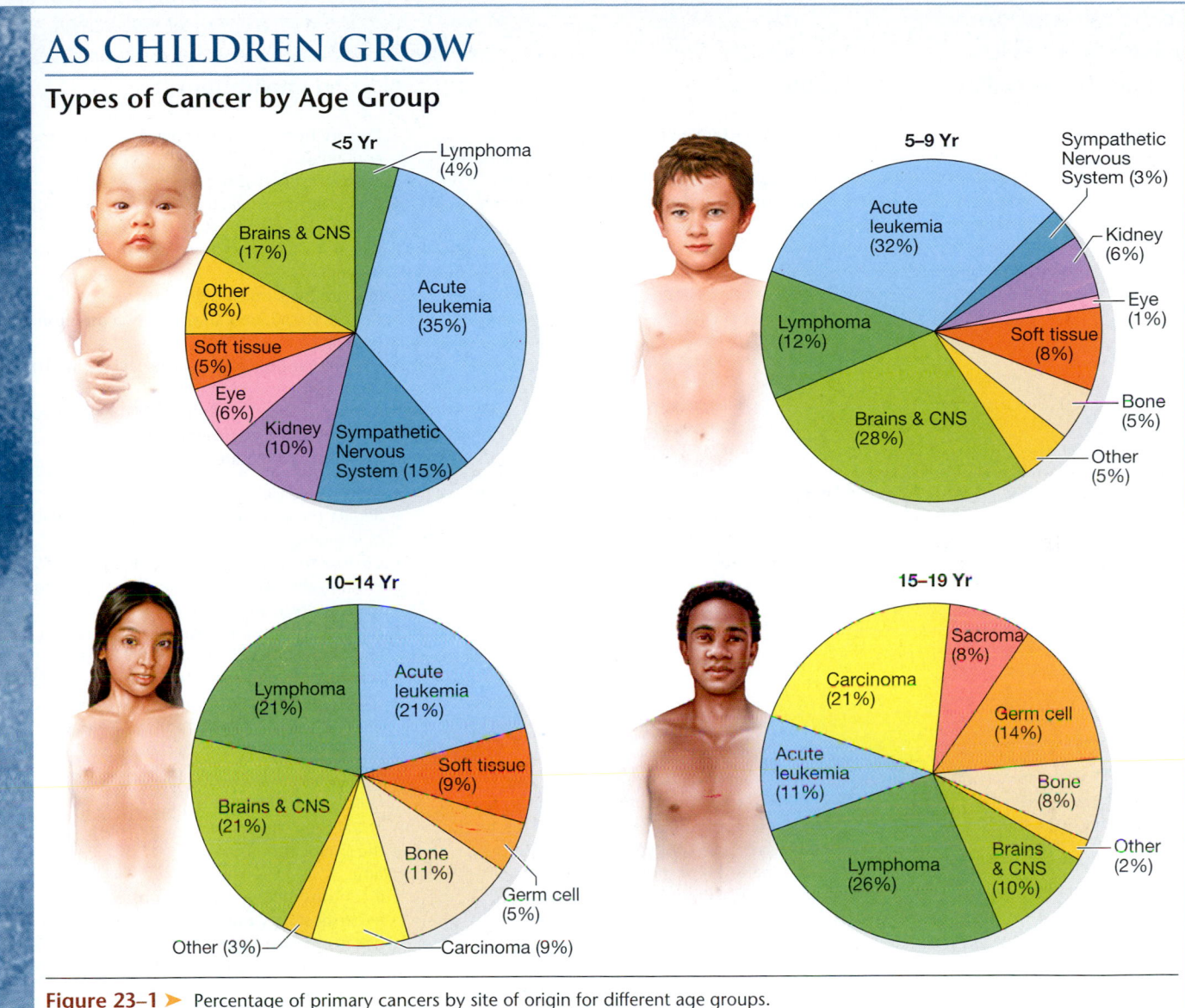

Figure 23–1 ➤ Percentage of primary cancers by site of origin for different age groups.
Data from Gurney, J. G. & Bondy, M. L. (2004). *Epidemiology of childhood and adolescent center.* In R. E. Behrman, R. M. Kliegman & H. B. Jensen. *Nelson Textbook of Pediatrics,* 17th ed. Philadelphia: Saunders, pg. 1679–1681.

In children, many cells are growing quickly; this fast growth can lead to the proliferation of both cancerous and normal cells. Cell division that is out of control may normally trigger a mechanism called **apoptosis**, whereby the cell "realizes" something is wrong and destroys itself. The process of apoptosis or physiologic cell death limits the growth of cancerous cells. However, this recognition of abnormality and subsequent destruction of cells may not be well developed in young children (Wuchter, Richter, Oltersdorf et al., 2004).

Examples of diagnostic and laboratory tests used for cancer are provided in the accompanying table. Use the assessment guidelines on page 842 to identify and monitor alterations in cellular growth.

DIAGNOSTIC PROCEDURES/LABORATORY TESTS FOR ALTERATIONS IN CELLULAR GROWTH

Diagnostic Procedure	Purpose	Nursing Implications
Biopsy	Removal and examination of tissue from the body; commonly used in solid tumor diagnosis. Pathologic results are used to diagnose the tumor type and plan the treatment regimen.	• Prepare necessary instruments and specimen containers. • Teach the child about the procedure. • Label specimens accurately and arrange for transport as recommended for specimen. • Monitor vital signs during and following the procedure. • Prepare the surgical site. • Adhere to sedation and analgesia monitoring guidelines. • Ensure that the child remains still during the procedure. • Apply dressing to the site after the procedure. • Teach the family to monitor the site for infection and to care for the wound.
Bone marrow aspiration	Marrow is removed from the pelvic or iliac crest bones through a needle with a syringe used for aspiration. The test is definitive for leukemia and many types of solid tumors.	• Teach the child about the procedure. • Sedate the child; adhere to sedation monitoring guidelines. • Cleanse the site according to agency protocol. • Position the child appropriately—side-lying for the iliac crest, supine for the sternum. • After the procedure, maintain the child on bed rest for at least 1 hour. Assess vital signs according to agency protocol and the child's condition. Monitor for signs of bleeding such as tachycardia and hypotension. Provide pain relief.
Computed tomography (CT) or computerized axial tomography (CAT)	A narrow beam of radiation examines body sections from different angles, producing a two-dimensional cross-section of the structures. A contrast media (or dye) can be ingested for abdominal scans or given intravenously for scans of the brain to enhance visualization.	• Depending on the body system evaluated, the child may be NPO or require bowel evacuation. • Teach the child about the procedure, including the size of equipment, noises, and length of time. • If contrast medium is used, obtain history of hypersensitivity to iodine, seafood, or contrast dye from other radiographic procedures. Report to the healthcare provider and staff in the CT scan area. • Use sedation, if needed, for young children to ensure that they remain still. Monitor children with sedation according to guidelines.
Lumbar puncture	A lumbar puncture is performed at L3-4 or L4-5 to remove cerebral spinal fluid. The fluid is analyzed for WBCs, RBCs, glucose, and proteins.	• Prepare the child for the procedure. • Sedate the children; monitor the child according to sedation guidelines. • Prepare the surgical site. • Position and hold the child in the care provider's preferred position. • Apply dressing to the site. • Monitor the site for bleeding, and the child for changes in vital signs. The child will be kept on bed rest for at least 1 hour.
Magnetic resonance imaging (MRI)	A large magnet is used to deliver radio waves to the body part to be imaged. The energy field produced can be transferred as a visual image to the computer. Soft-tissue abnormalities can be visualized by MRI.	• Prepare the child for the procedure, including the size of equipment, sounds, time, and tunnel. • Ensure that the child has no metallic objects or implants and is not connected to metal equipment. • Use sedation for young children, if needed, to ensure that they are still for the procedure; monitor the child with sedation according to guidelines.

DIAGNOSTIC PROCEDURES/LABORATORY TESTS FOR ALTERATIONS IN CELLULAR GROWTH (continued)

Diagnostic Procedure	Purpose	Nursing Implications
Positron-emission tomography (PET) scan and single photon emission computed tomography (SPECT)	Normal body substances such as glucose or oxygen are made radioactive with fluorine 18 and administered intravenously. PET then measures areas of positron-emitting isotope concentration. Organ activity, such as of the brain, can be measured. SPECT is similar but uses conventional radioisotopes such as technetium 99m and iodine 123.	• Prepare the child for the procedure. • Monitor vital signs. • Start IVs as needed—generally one for injection of contrast and the other to draw blood gases. • Since contrast medium is used, obtain a history of hypersensitivity to iodine, seafood, or contrast dye from other radiographic procedures. Report to the healthcare provider and staff in the CT scan area.
Radiograph (X-ray)	Radiographs use irradiation to obtain images and capture them on film for diagnosis and screening. They are used to visualize organs and body structure. Chest, abdominal, and skeletal radiographs are commonly performed to evaluate the presence of tumors.	• Explain the procedure to the child. • Tell the child about the need to hold still for the procedure. Have the child practice holding a breath while being still. • Note that radiopaque materials for tests such as GI studies and aivp administered within 3 days of the radiograph may distort images.
Scans	A variety of nuclear medicine scans that use radioactive isotopes can assist in imaging specific body parts. Bone scans that use technetium 99m compounds, gallium scans, thallium-201, and 1-metaiodobenzylguanidine (MIBG) are common examples.	• Prepare the child for the test. • If contrast medium is used, obtain a history of hypersensitivity to iodine, seafood, or contrast dye from other radiographic procedures. Report to the healthcare provider and staff in the CT scan area. • Start an IV for injection of contrast material. • Sedate young children, if needed, to ensure that they are still; monitor according to sedation guidelines.
Ultrasound	An ultrasound probe (transducer) is held over the skin above the body part to produce an ultrasound beam aimed at the tissues. The reflected sound waves are then transformed into graphs or pictures of the tissues. It may produce initial information about a body mass.	• Prepare the child for the procedure. • Maintain NPO status as ordered. • Confirm that the child has not received any tests that interfere with results, such as GI series.

Laboratory Tests	Purpose	Nursing Implications
Complete blood count (CBC)	The CBC measures types of all cells in the serum. It includes leukocytes (white blood cells or WBCs), WBC differential, erythrocytes (red blood cells or RBCs), and thrombocytes (platelets). Findings can assist in diagnosis of several types of cancers and their treatments.	• Prepare the child. • Perform the test in a treatment room rather than the child's hospital room or clinic examination room. • Label and transport specimens according to policy.
Red blood cell indices	A variety of RBC indices provide information about the number and quality of red blood cells. They include hematocrit, hemoglobin, mean corpuscular volume, mean corpuscular hemoglobin concentration, and mean corpuscular hemoglobin.	• Prepare the child. • Perform the test in a treatment room rather than the child's hospital room or clinic examination room. • Label and transport specimens according to policy.
Serum chemistry panel	Serum electrolytes, minerals (iron, copper), renal function studies such as BUN and creatinine, liver function studies such as bilirubin, ALT, and AST may all be helpful in diagnosing particular types and locations of tumors.	• Prepare the child. • Perform the test in a treatment room rather than the child's hospital room or clinic examination room. • Label and transport specimens according to policy.

DIAGNOSTIC PROCEDURES/LABORATORY TESTS FOR ALTERATIONS IN CELLULAR GROWTH (continued)

Laboratory Tests	Purpose	Nursing Implications
Tumor markers	Markers are parts of cells or metabolites associated with certain cancers. Serum and urine analysis of substances such as α-fetoprotein, homovanillic acid, vanillylmandelic acid, and catecholamine are often performed to assist with diagnosis of specific tumors.	• Prepare the child. • Perform the blood test in a treatment room rather than the child's hospital room or clinic examination room. If the examination is of urine, instruct the child about collecting the specimen if old enough to understand. For the young child, apply a urine bag. • Label and transport specimens according to agency policy.
Urinalysis	Analysis of urine for RBCs, WBCs, tumor markers, and abnormal cells assists in diagnosis of certain tumors and infections.	• Instruct the child about collecting the specimen if old enough to understand. For the young child, apply a urine bag. • Label and transport specimens according to agency policy.

Data from: Corbett, J. V. (2004). *Laboratory tests and diagnostic procedures with nursing diagnoses* (6th ed.). Upper Saddle River, NJ: Prentice Hall Health; Kee, J. L. (2005). *Handbook of laboratory & diagnostic tests with nursing implications* (5th ed.). Upper Saddle River, NJ: Prentice Hall Health; Baggott, C. R., Kelly, K. P., Fochtman, D., & Foley, G.V. (2002). *Nursing care of children and adolescents with cancer* (3rd ed.). Philadelphia: W.B. Saunders.

ASSESSMENT GUIDELINES FOR THE CHILD WITH AN ALTERATION IN CELLULAR GROWTH

Assessment Focus	Assessment Guidelines
Growth and development parameters	• Assess the child's weight and height and plot on growth grids; be alert for weight loss. • Inquire about nutritional intake and any recent changes in appetite. • Perform developmental assessment and be alert for slow progress or regression. • Ask about school performance for children enrolled in school; include this data in every assessment of children who were treated for cancer in the past.
Pain	• Pain is abnormal if there is no known acute injury or chronic condition; assess any pain for length, duration, and type. • Be alert for limping, headache, decreased activity level, or other symptoms indicative of pain.
Skin	• Evaluate skin for bruising and other signs of bleeding. • Be alert for pallor and other signs of anemia. • Describe skin lesions.
EENT and sensory	• Inspect the symmetry and general condition of the eyes, ears, mouth, throat, head, and neck. • Inspect eye movements, corneal light reflex, and red reflex. • Evaluate hearing and vision and note any recent changes.
Chest, heart, and respiratory system	• Inspect the shape of the chest, respiratory rate, and ease of respirations. • Auscultate heart and lungs. • Ask about endurance and activity levels.
Abdomen	• Be alert for abdominal masses. Stop palpation immediately if any are noted and inform the physician. • Repeated vomiting, anorexia, and weight loss are important for diagnosis and to monitor for side effects of treatment.
Urinary and gastrointestinal systems	• Evaluate frequency of urination and feces. • Assess for intake and evidence of vomiting or food intolerance. • Ask about blood or other discoloration in urine or stool. • Be alert for urinary tract infections.
Musculoskeletal system	• Observe for expected developmental tasks. • Be alert for asymmetry of bone or muscle. • Observe for limping and other abnormalities.

CHILDHOOD CANCER

The care of children who have cancer is a challenging specialty in pediatric nursing. For several years, the child undergoes aggressive treatments that may be life threatening and cause serious illness. Often the prognosis is quite hopeful; at other times, a terminal result may be expected. Frequently the child is cared for at home with outpatient visits for treatments and occasional hospitalizations when needed for conditions such as fever and neutropenia. The periods of hospitalization are times of intense physical vulnerability for the child and intense emotional vulnerability for both the child and the family. For some cancers, multiple hospitalizations are needed to carry out therapy. To monitor the child closely, nurses need a sound knowledge of physiologic and psychologic responses, medical interventions, and nursing care. Effective communication skills are also necessary to support the child and family and promote realistic hope.

During 2006, in the United States, cancer was diagnosed in approximately 9500 children from birth to 14 years of age, while about 12,500 children under 20 years were diagnosed with cancer. In children under 15 years of age, cancer is the leading cause of disease-related death, and the second leading cause of death following accidents. In 2006, about 1560 U.S. children died of cancer. One-third of the deaths were from leukemia (American Cancer Society, 2006a; Thompson, 2003). However, mortality rates have declined by about 48% since 1975, and the rates continue to improve. The overall survival rate is 80% for childhood cancer (Baggott, Kelly, Fochtman, & Foley, 2002). Children treated in the 1980s, 1990s, and 2000s had significantly lower mortality rates than those treated in the 1960s and 1970s due to multimodal therapies including multiagent chemotherapy, surgery, and radiation therapy. Survival rates vary for different types of cancer, ranging from 66% for neuroblastoma to 95% for Hodgkin's disease. Mortality rates are higher for females than males, for those diagnosed before 5 years of age, and for children with a central nervous system tumor or leukemia (American Cancer Society, 2006a).

Etiology and Pathophysiology

Alterations in cellular growth occur in response to external and internal stimuli. Neoplasms are caused by one or a combination of three factors: (1) external stimuli that cause genetic mutations, (2) immune system and gene abnormalities, and (3) chromosomal abnormalities.

External Stimuli

External stimuli may affect the child's general health and cause mutations in body cells. **Carcinogens** are chemicals or industrial processes that, when combined with genetic traits and in interaction with one another, result in cancer. Several carcinogens cause cancers that are diagnosed during childhood. Others cause cancers that begin in childhood but are not identified until adulthood. Some chemicals suspected of causing childhood cancer include diethylstilbestrol or DES (maternal use of therapeutic estrogen hormones), anabolic androgenic steroids, alkylating chemotherapy agents, and immunosuppressants used for organ transplantation. Radiation exposure has been known to cause cancers such as leukemia and thyroid tumors in children exposed to nuclear fallout from atomic bombs, other nuclear accidents, and other excessive radiation sources.

External stimuli may also lead to secondary cancers in children, or those occurring after treatment for a primary cancer, and of a different cellular type than the primary cancer. Secondary cancers can result when the child is treated for a primary cancer with high doses of radiation. Excessive exposure to ultraviolet radiation from the sun predisposes children to development of skin cancer in adulthood. See Families Want to Know: Cancer Prevention.

Immune System and Gene Abnormalities

One critical function of a normal immune system is immune surveillance, in which phagocytic cells circulate throughout the body, detecting and destroying abnormal and

MediaLink

Cancer

FAMILIES WANT TO KNOW

Cancer Prevention

Many parents ask what they can do to decrease the incidence of cancer in children as they grow into adulthood. Four major teaching areas to address are as follows:

1. Have children increase their intake of fruits, vegetables, and whole grains. Aim for five or more servings of fruits and vegetables daily. Most children do not eat enough of these foods, and higher intake throughout life is associated with lower rates of several cancers in adulthood. Additionally, higher vitamin C and potassium intake in the first 2 years of life is associated with lower rates of childhood leukemia (Kwan, Block, Selvin, Month, & Buffler, 2004).

2. Protect skin with sunscreen. Early excessive exposure to sun and severe sunburns causing blistering have an increased chance of skin cancers in adulthood.

3. Discourage smoking among children and be sure children are not exposed to environmental tobacco smoke. This will decrease future chances of developing lung cancer.

4. Have homes tested for radon. Be alert for exposure to any potential hazardous substances in the home or on parents' clothing if they work in industries with chemicals or other harmful substances.

cancerous cells. Children with congenital immune deficiencies, such as Wiskott-Aldrich syndrome, in which immune surveillance may fail are at high risk for cancer. A form of non-Hodgkin's lymphoma develops in some children treated with drugs that suppress the immune system. Children with acquired immunodeficiency syndrome (AIDS) may be at higher risk of certain types of cancer, such as Hodgkin's disease, non-Hodgkin's lymphoma, leiomyosarcoma, and Kaposi's sarcoma.

Viruses and other substances may act in the body to alter the immune system, thereby allowing cancer to occur (Figure 23–2 ➤). Their action is based on changing certain genes that normally regulate cellular growth and development (called **protooncogenes**) to related genes that allow unregulated cell division and cancerous growth (called **oncogenes**). Among cancers thought to be linked to virus action and the change of protooncogenes to oncogenes are certain leukemias, rhabdomyosarcoma, Burkitt's lymphoma, and some forms of Hodgkin's disease. Genetic changes (mutations) can include autosomal dominant, autosomal recessive, and X-linked transfer. In these cases, the resulting cancers often occur relatively early in life. Cancers of these types are typ-

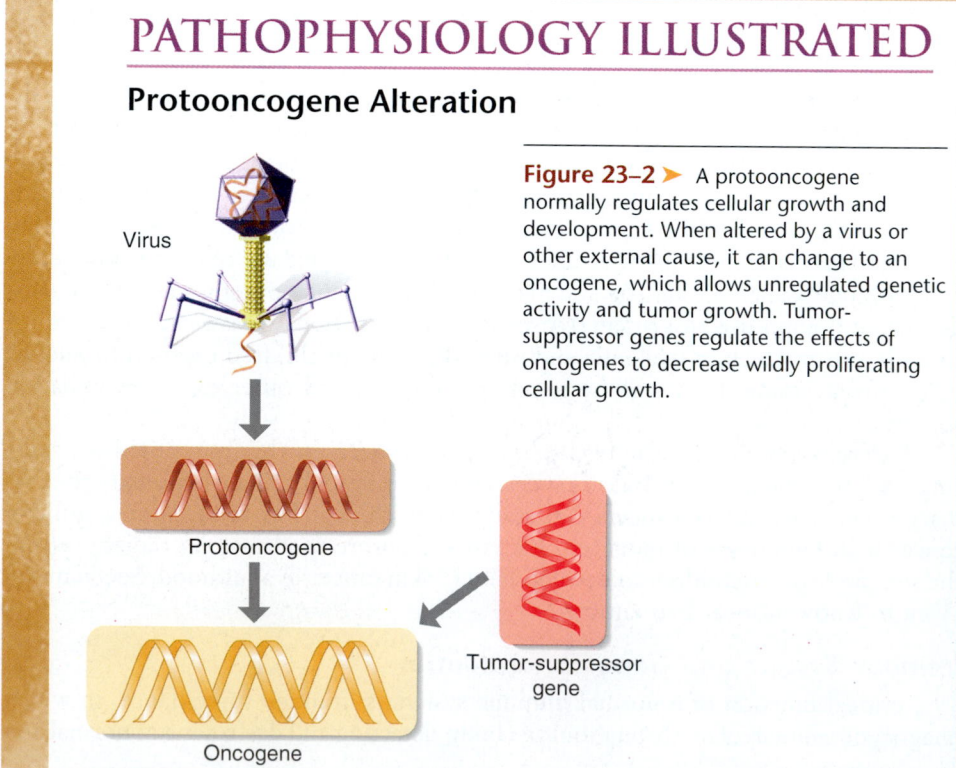

PATHOPHYSIOLOGY ILLUSTRATED

Protooncogene Alteration

Virus

Protooncogene

Oncogene

Tumor-suppressor gene

Figure 23–2 ➤ A protooncogene normally regulates cellular growth and development. When altered by a virus or other external cause, it can change to an oncogene, which allows unregulated genetic activity and tumor growth. Tumor-suppressor genes regulate the effects of oncogenes to decrease wildly proliferating cellular growth.

ically aggressive since the child has inherited the abnormal gene, so it is within each cell, rather than a single mutation of one gene in a specific cell. Due to progress that is being made in the Human Genome Project (see Chapter 3 ∞), there is increasing ability to perform genetic testing for certain familial cancers. Examples of cancers that are sometimes caused by genetic abnormalities within families include retinoblastoma (described later in this chapter), Wilms' tumor (described in this chapter), multiple endocrine neoplasia, type 2 (thyroid cancer), and familial adenomatous polyposis (invasive colon cancer). Not all cases of these cancers are familial, but their incidence suggests the need for careful history taking to identify any other cases in the family.

Tumor suppressor genes counteract the effect of oncogenes, keeping cellular growth within normal limits. When tumor suppressor genes are missing, unstemmed cellular growth can occur. These genes are commonly missing in children with retinoblastoma and Wilms' tumor.

Chromosomal Abnormalities

Normal chromosomes undergo change as a part of the genetic process. Although most of the changes are not harmful, some changes do result in chromosomal abnormalities such as hyperploidy (a greater-than-normal number of chromosomes), deletion, translocation, and breakage.

Some of these chromosomal abnormalities have been linked to an increased incidence of cancer. Children with Down syndrome have a relative risk over 30 times higher for developing leukemia than nonaffected children (Agha et al., 2005). Children who are missing a band of genetic material on chromosome 13 often have retinoblastoma. Similarly, a Wilms' tumor often develops in children missing part of the genetic material from chromosome 11. Regardless of the location of abnormal cellular growth, the pathophysiologic process is similar. The altered cell begins to multiply as directed by the altered genetic structure of its DNA and the absence or inactivation of tumor suppressor genes. Each new cell transmits the new or altered pattern to the next generation. As the abnormal cells replicate, they form a growing neoplastic mass. Normal cells usually die as the increased metabolic rate of the neoplastic cells depletes available nutrition. The altered DNA in the tumor cells may also cause the abnormal cells to invade adjoining tissue. Through continued growth, the mass invades, disrupting a major vessel or a vital organ.

Clinical Manifestations

Each type of childhood cancer signals its presence differently. Because many of the presenting signs and symptoms of cancer are typical of common childhood illnesses, a delay in diagnosis can occur. In some cases, no symptoms are noted until the cancer is advanced. Children commonly present with presence of cancer in a site other than its origin at the time of diagnosis due to this difficulty in recognition of the disease. Some of the common presenting symptoms of cancer follow:

- *Pain* may be the result of a neoplasm either directly or indirectly affecting nerve receptors through obstruction, inflammation, tissue damage, stretching of visceral tissue, or invasion of susceptible tissue. The pain may be in any body part, such as abdominal pain, bone and joint discomfort, or headache.
- **Cachexia** is a syndrome characterized by anorexia, weight loss, anemia, asthenia (weakness), and early satiety (feeling of being full).
- *Anemia* may be experienced during times of chronic bleeding or iron deficiency. In chronic illness the body uses iron poorly. Anemia is also present in cancers of the bone marrow when the number of red blood cells (RBCs) is reduced, in part because of the presence of large numbers of other bone marrow products. Treatment of cancer often promotes further anemia.
- *Infection* is usually a result of an altered or immature immune system. In addition, infection occurs when bone marrow cancers inhibit maturation of normal immune system cells. Infection may also occur in children who are treated with corticosteroids. Because their immune response is altered, the normal signs of infection may not appear.

- *Bruising* or ecchymosis can occur if the bone marrow cannot produce enough platelets. Prolonged bleeding also occurs after minor trauma.
- *Neurologic symptoms* may result from impingement on the brain or nervous system. Signs of increased intracranial pressure, decreased or altered consciousness, eye abnormalities, or other neurologic or behaviorial changes may be evident.
- *Palpable mass* may be present for certain cancers. This is most commonly abdominal but may be mediastinal, or in the neck or other sites.

A variety of other symptoms can occur depending on the location of the cancer. Subcutaneous nodules may appear if leukocytosis is present, superior vena cava syndrome (obstruction of the superior vena cava by a mass and leading to increased venous pressure and involvement of the lungs and other mediastinal structures) or respiratory difficulty can occur with mediastinal tumors (such as neuroblastoma), and enlarged lymph nodes are common with lymphomas (Bleyer, 2004; Hon, Leung, Chik et al., 2005).

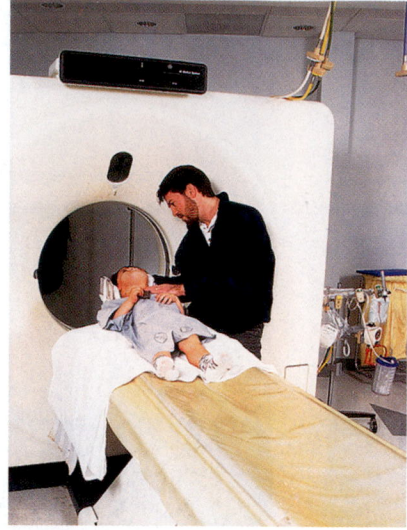

Figure 23–3 ➤ Computed tomography (CT) can be a frightening procedure for children. This 2-year-old boy is comforted by his father before the procedure.

NURSING ALERT

Any child who has an implanted metallic object in the body should not undergo MRI scanning because of the strong magnetic field generated. Metallic objects include orthodontic braces, metal dental bridgework, surgical clips or plates, and orthopedic rods. Remove all jewelry and clothes with metal snaps from the child before the test.

COLLABORATIVE CARE

Diagnostic Tests

The most common diagnostic tests performed on children with cancer are complete blood count with differential, bone marrow aspiration, lumbar puncture, radiographic examination, magnetic resonance imaging (MRI), computed tomography (CT), ultrasound, and biopsy of tumors (Figure 23–3 ➤). See Table 23–1 for normal laboratory values and abnormalities common in cancer.

Additional tests of serum may be helpful in diagnosis. Studies that are informative for certain cancers are nuclear medicine scans with radioactive isotopes such as gallium or iodine, bone scan with technetium 99m, or positron emission tomography (PET) and single photon emission computed tomography (SPECT) that combine nuclear medicine with CT (Yang, Kim, & Inoue, 2006). Specific tests such as pulmonary function tests and echocardiograms may be used to determine if the lungs or heart may be affected by the cancer.

The blood work is very detailed and includes:

- RBC, WBC, platelets (CBC with differential).
- Hemoglobin and hematocrit.
- RBC indices such as mean corpuscular volume (MCV), mean corpuscular hemoglobin concentration (MCHC), and mean corpuscular hemoglobin (MCH).

Table 23–1	SELECTED DIAGNOSTIC TEST RESULTS FOR CHILDHOOD CANCER		
Test	**Purpose**	**Normal Laboratory Values**	**Diagnostic Values**
Bone marrow aspiration	Examines bone marrow	<5% blast cells (immature)	>25% blast cells in acute lymphoblastic leukemia, most with hypercellular marrow
Lumbar puncture	Examines cerebrospinal fluid	Cell count (µL) Polymorphonuclear leukocytes 0 Monocytes 0–5 RBCs 0–5	Presence of malignant cells indicates central nervous system involvement
Complete blood count and differential	Examines cellular components of blood	WBC <10,000/µL Platelets 150,000–400,000/µL Hemoglobin 12–16 g/dL	WBC <10,000/µL Platelets 20,000–100,000/µL Hemoglobin 7–10 g/dL
Absolute neutrophil count (ANC)	Blood component ratio: % of segmental neutrophils plus % of bands (immature neutrophils) times WBC count	ANC > 1000	ANC < 500 risk of infection

- WBC indices (manual differential) which include the percent of all five types (basophils, eosinophils, monocytes, lymphocytes, neutrophils; neutrophils are further divided into segmented and banded).
- Absolute neutrophil count (ANC), which uses both the segmented (mature) and bands (immature neutrophils) as a measure of the body's infection fighting capability; calculated by adding percentage of segmented neutrophils to percentage of bands, and then multiplying this percentage by the WBC count.
- Serum chemistry, which includes electrolytes, including sodium, potassium, chloride, calcium, magnesium, phosphorus, and carbon dioxide.
- Additional studies that provide important diagnostic clues in some cases; for example, renal function studies such as blood urea nitrogen (BUN) and creatinine; liver studies such as total bilirubin, alanine aminotransferase (ALT), aspirate aminotransferase (AST), lactic dehydrogenase (LDH), and blood urea nitrogen (BUN); alkaline phosphatase may be elevated; uric acid is commonly elevated in leukemia.
- Certain substances, or markers, that are elevated with some specific tumors; for example, α-fetoprotein may be elevated in liver tumors, vanillylmandelic acid (VMA) and homovanillic acid (HVA) may be elevated in adrenal tumors, and elevated catecholamines are found in neuroblastoma.

Urinalysis is performed, as the presence of abnormal cells such as RBCs (hematuria) may assist in diagnosis of some kidney tumors. Histological or laboratory analysis of tumor cells is often critical in diagnosis. A needle biopsy or endoscopic procedures of some tumors can be performed to obtain tumor cells. If the tumor is removed during surgery, the entire tumor is available for study. The borders are examined to be certain it has been totally removed, and lymph nodes may also be removed to analyze possible spread via the lymph system.

The tests are aimed at identifying the source of the cancer and any metastases to additional sites. This enables the physician to stage the cancer. **Staging** refers to the process of labeling the type, severity, and spread of cancer cells, which will determine the recommended treatment. Stage number 1 indicates less severe cancer without spread to other parts of the body, while higher numbers indicate both greater severity and spread to other sites.

Clinical Therapy

Clinical therapy for cancer is extremely complex and is managed by a specialist in pediatric oncology. The cancer itself is treated, its effects on the body must be addressed, and the side effects of treatment also require management. All children and adolescents suspected of having cancer should be referred to a pediatric cancer center and have their care coordinated by that center (American Cancer Society, 2003a).

Cancer is treated with one or a combination of therapies: surgery, chemotherapy, radiation, biotherapy, and bone marrow or hematopoietic stem cell transplantation. Many families also choose some type of complementary therapy, in addition to traditional medical approaches. The treatment plan is determined by the type of cancer, site of primary tumor, and the degree and sites of metastasis (spread to other sites in the body).

The goal of treatment may be curative, supportive, or palliative. Curative treatment rids the child's body of the cancer. Supportive treatment includes transfusions, pain management, antibiotics, and other interventions to assist the body's defenses and increase the child's comfort. Palliative treatment is designed to make the child as comfortable as possible when no curative treatment is possible (see Chapter 14 ∞ for a detailed discussion of palliative care for children). Whatever combination of treatment is used, families have many questions and need resources for information.

SURGERY   Surgery is used to remove or **debulk** (reduce the size of) a solid tumor. An example of a cancer that is commonly treated with surgery is a Wilms' tumor. Surgery is also used to determine the stage and type of cancer since the tumor cells can be examined microscopically once removed, and various body organs can be inspected for signs of cancer during the surgery.

CHEMOTHERAPY **Chemotherapy** is the administration of specific drugs that kill both normal and cancerous cells. The administration of various chemotherapeutic drugs is timed to achieve the greatest cellular destruction. The schedule is determined by the cell's cycle of replication (Figure 23–4 ➤). Several chemotherapeutic drugs are administered simultaneously to maximize their lethal impact on cells at all stages of activity. Table 23–2 provides examples of common chemotherapy drug

PATHOPHYSIOLOGY ILLUSTRATED

Chemotherapy Drug Action

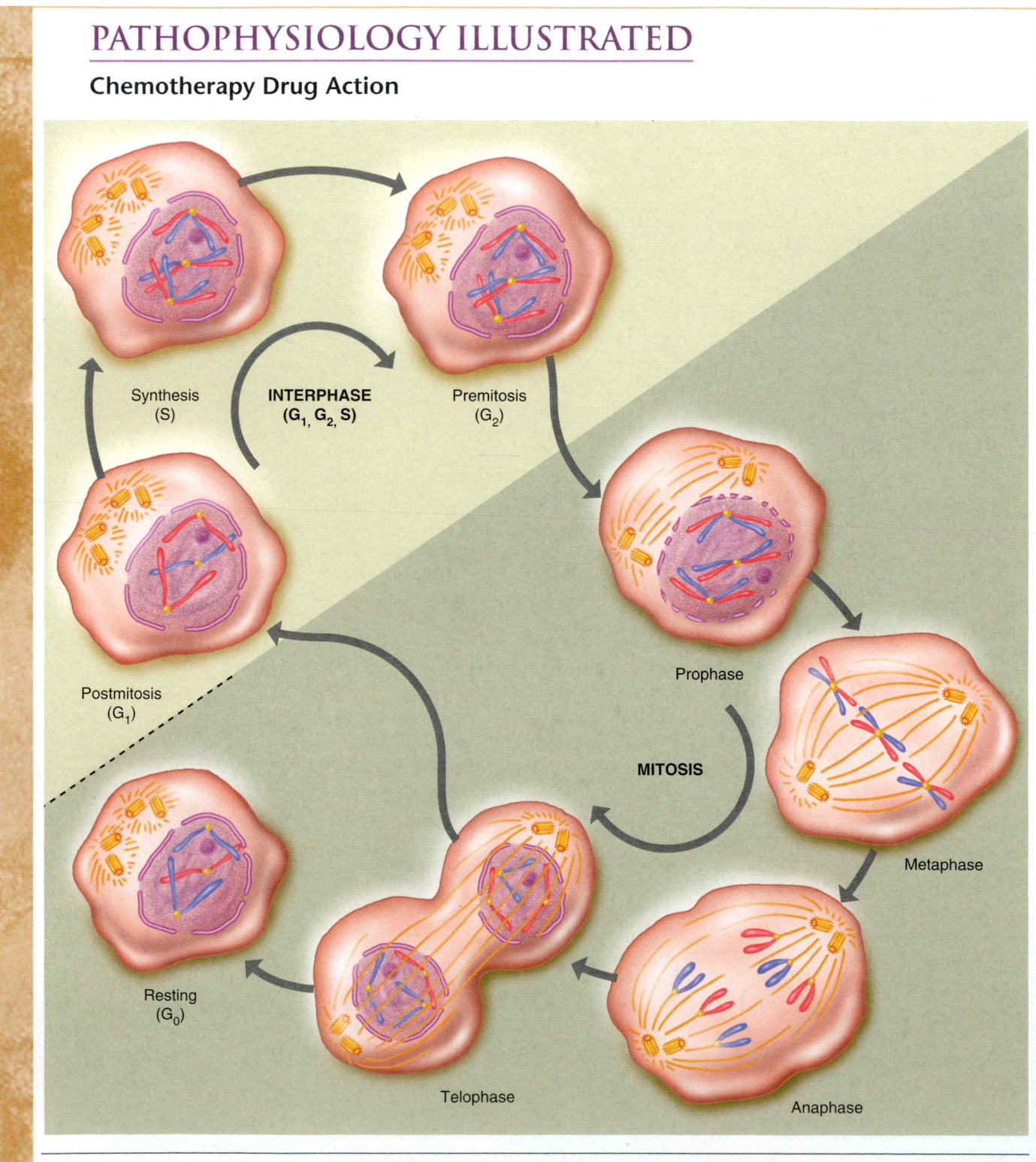

Synthesis (S)

INTERPHASE (G₁, G₂, S)

Premitosis (G₂)

Postmitosis (G₁)

Prophase

MITOSIS

Metaphase

Resting (G₀)

Telophase

Anaphase

Figure 23–4 ➤ Chemotherapy drugs either act at specific parts of the cell cycle or are nonspecific for action (act throughout all cell phases).

Table 23–2	COMMONLY USED CHEMOTHERAPY DRUG COMBINATIONS

Acronym	Drug Combination
A-COPP	Adriamycin (doxorubicin) + cyclophosphamide + vincristine (Oncovin) + procarbazine + prednisone
ABVD	Adriamycin (doxorubicin) + bleomycin + vinblastine + dacarbazine
ABVE	Adriamycin (doxorubicin) + bleomycin + vincristine + etoposide
ABVE-PC	Adriamycin (doxorubicin) + bleomycin + vincristine + etoposide + prednisone + cyclophosphamide
ACE	Adriamycin (doxorubicin) + cyclophosphamide + etoposide
AOPE	Adriamycin (doxorubicin) + Oncovin (vincristine) + prednisone + etoposide
APE	Adriamycin (doxorubicin) + procarbazine + etoposide
BEACOPP	bleomycin + etoposide + Adriamycin (doxorubicin) + cyclophosphamide + vincristine + procarbazine + prednisone
CAF	cyclophosphamide + doxorubicin + fluorouracil
CAMP	cyclophosphamide + doxorubicin + methotrexate + procarbazine
CAVe	lomustine + doxorubicin + vinblastine
CAVE or ECHO or CAPO or EVAC or VOCA	etoposide + cyclophosphamide + doxorubicin + vincristine
CHOP	cyclophosphamide + doxorubicin + vincristine + prednisone
CHOR	cyclophosphamide + doxorubicin + vincristine
CISCA	cisplatin + cyclophosphamide
CMF	cyclophosphamide + methotrexate + fluorouracil
COPP	cyclophosphamide + vincristine + procarbazine + prednisone
CY-VA-DIC	cyclophosphamide + vincristine + doxorubicin + dacarbazine
EBVP	etoposide + bleomycin + vinblastine + prednisone
FAC	fluorouracil + doxorubicin + cyclophosphamide
MACC	methotrexate + doxorubicin + cyclophosphamide + lomustine
MOPP	mechlorethamine + vincristine + procarbazine + prednisone
MTX + MP + CTX	methotrexate + mercaptopurine + cyclophosphamide
OEPA	vincristine + etoposide + prednisone + Adriamycin (doxorubicin)
OPPA	vincristine + prednisone + procarbazine + Adriamycin (doxorubicin)
PVB or VBP	vinblastine + bleomycin + cisplatin
T-2	dactinomycin + doxorubicin + vincristine + cyclophosphamide
VAMP	vinblastine + Adriamycin (doxorubicin) + methotrexate + prednisone
VAP	vincristine + dactinomycin + cyclophosphamide
VEPA	vinblastine + etoposide + prednisone + Adriamycin (doxorubicin)
VP-L-asparaginase	vincristine + prednisone + L-asparaginase

Note: From Bindler, R., & Howry, L. (2005). *Pediatric drug guide.* Upper Saddle River, NJ: Prentice Hall Health.

combinations. See Medications Used to Treat Cancer through Chemotherapy on pages 850–851.

Whereas DNA in a normal cell can repair itself after chemotherapy, the DNA in a neoplastic cell cannot. The particular chemotherapy treatment protocol used is based on research into different types of cancer cells. A **protocol** is a plan of action for chemotherapy that is based on the type of cancer, its stage, and the particular cell type (Figure 23–5 ➤).

Other drugs used in the treatment of children with cancer include colony-stimulating factors, antiemetics, and nutritional supplements. Colony-stimulating factors are hormonelike glycoproteins that enhance blood cell production and counteract the myelosuppressive effects of chemotherapy drugs (see Medications Used to Treat Cancer: Colony-Stimulating Factors on page 852). For example, erythropoietin is

MEDICATIONS USED TO TREAT *Cancer through Chemotherapy*

Medication	Action/Indication	Nursing Implications
Cell Cycle Specific Agents **Antimetabolites** • 5-Azacytidine • 5-Fluorouracil • 6-Mercaptopurine • 6-Thioguanine • Cytosine arabinoside (cytarabine) • Hydroxyurea • Methotrexate	The antimetabolites work at synthesis phase of cell division; interface with function of nucleic acid; inhibit DNA or RNA synthesis	• Most common side effects are nausea and vomiting, myelosuppression, stomatitis. Specific agents such as methotrexate and cytarabine can cause neurologic toxicity with high doses. • Consult drug books and package inserts for detailed list of side effects. • Obtain baseline CBC, liver function, renal function. • Monitor I&O and body weight. Ensure hydration and output levels ordered by oncologist. • Monitor VS and cardiovascular and respiratory function. • Watch for bleeding and signs of infection. • Monitor carefully during administration for signs of anaphylaxis.
Vinca alkaloids • Etoposide • Teniposide • Irinotecan • Paclitaxel • Vinblastine • Vincristine	Act during mitosis; bind with cell proteins to inhibit nucleic acid and protein synthesis	• Common side effects include nausea and vomiting, abdominal cramping and diarrhea, constipation, paralytic ileus, hair loss, hypotension or hypertension, peripheral neuropathy and neurological toxicity (latter especially with vinblastine and vincristine). • Obtain baseline blood work. • Consult specific drug information for period of maximum myelosuppressive effect. • Be alert for bruising, infection, and other signs of myelosuppression. • Monitor carefully during administration for signs of anaphylaxis.
Miscellaneous—G_1 phase activity • L-asparaginase	Causes depletion of asparagine, needed by cancer cells; makes cell in G_1 phase vulnerable to other agents; interferes with prosynthesis. Used in combination with other agents in leukemia and other cancers.	• Administered intravenously. • Major side effects are severe nausea and vomiting, hypersensitivity, renal failure, myelosuppression, acid–base imbalance. • CBC, serum amylase, glucose, coagulation factors, bone marrow function, liver function tests performed before therapy and twice weekly. • Monitor I&O, neurologic status, gastrointestinal symptoms, abdominal pain.
Miscellaneous—G_2 phase activity • Etoposide	Works at G_2 phase; binds cellular proteins to cause metaphase arrest; also acts on S phase of DNA synthesis. Used with other agents, particularly in recurrent disease.	• Administered orally and intravenously. • Common side effects are nausea and vomiting, myelosuppression, hair loss, diarrhea. Can cause anaphylaxis; hypotension and IV site pain with rapid infusion. • Perform baseline CBC, liver and renal function tests. • Check IV site frequently since extravasation can cause necrosis. • Monitor VS during infusion and stop drug if hypotension occurs.
Cell Cycle Nonspecific Agents **Alkylating agents** • Cyclophosphamide • Carboplatin • Cisplatin • Busulfan • Chlorambucil • Ifosfamide • Thiotepa • Mechlorethamine • Melphalan • Procarbazine • Dacarbazine	Substitute an alkyl group for a hydrogen atom, leading to blockage of DNA replication. Used for treatment of many cancers, either alone or in conjunction with other agents.	• Most are administered orally and/or intravenously. Array of side effects depending on specific drug. Some common side effects are nausea and vomiting, diarrhea, myelosuppression, hair loss, neuropathies, pulmonary toxicity, renal damage; secondary tumors later in life associated with some agents. • Obtain CBC and full blood work before and during treatment. • Monitor for side effects of the specific agents administered. Ensure generous hydration and monitor I&O. Teach family the importance of long-term monitoring for secondary tumors.
Antibiotics • Doxorubicin • Mitomycin-C • Dactinomycin • Bleomycin • Daunorubicin • Idarubicin • Mitoxantrone	Interfere with nucleic acid, inhibiting DNA or RNA synthesis. Used in combination with other agents to treat leukemia and other childhood cancers.	• Most are administered intravenously. • Common side effects include nausea and vomiting, myelosuppression, oral ulcers, skin and pulmonary toxicity. Several have cumulative dose toxicity, such as cardiac abnormalities (doxorubicin) and skin/pulmonary (bleomycin); total dose the child has received must be monitored. • Obtain baseline CBC and other blood studies and monitor throughout therapy. • Monitor VS, lung function, cardiac function, neurologic status throughout and following therapy. Be alert for signs of myelosuppression and mucosal ulcers.

MEDICATIONS USED TO TREAT *Cancer through Chemotherapy (continued)*

Medication	Action/Indication	Nursing Implications
Cell Cycle Nonspecific Agents (continued)		
Nitrosoureas • Carmustine • Lomustine	Cross breakage in DNA strands so that DNA and RNA replication cannot occur. Used in lymphomas and other childhood cancers. Can cross blood-brain barrier.	• Administered orally (lomustine) or intravenously (carmustine). Major side effect is myelosuppression. • Others include pulmonary fibrosis, eye infarction, skin changes, hair loss, nausea, and vomiting. • Obtain baseline and periodic CBC and other studies. • Monitor pulmonary function, skin, and signs of infection or bleeding.
Hormones • Prednisone • Prednisolone • Dexamethasone	Analog of hydrocortisone; anti-inflammatory; delayed and depressed immune response. Used in conjunction with other agents for many types of childhood cancer.	• Often administered orally. • Numerous side effects including edema, moon face, mood lability, increased appetite, disturbed sleep, immunosuppression, disturbed glucose control, osteoporosis. • Teach child and family the effects of the drug. Minimize exposure to persons with infection. Monitor for infections in all systems. • Monitor weight regularly. Take VS. Teach to take as directed. Drug must be tapered slowly at end of therapy.
Topoisomerase I inhibitor • Irinotecan • Mitoxantrone • Topotecan	Inhibit the enzyme topoisomerase I in the cell nucleus, relaxing DNA and preventing its duplication. Used in conjunction with other agents to treat ALL and other childhood cancers.	• Administered intravenously: topotecan can be given intrathecally. • Common side effects include nausea and vomiting, diarrhea, fever, dehydration, myelosuppression. Can alter liver function and cause skin changes. • Obtain baseline and periodic CBC and other studies, including liver function. • Monitor for signs of myelosuppression, gastrointestinal distress, change in liver function.

produced in the kidney, and a recombinant form (epoetin) is available which can be used to treat anemia of cancer, thereby decreasing the number of transfusions needed. Filgrastim (Neupogen) increases production of neutrophils by the bone marrow. Antiemetics, such as ondansetron (Zofran), are used to treat the nausea and vomiting that are common side effects of therapy. Nutritional supplements can be given to maintain nutritional status. Some children need periodic treatment with antibiotics or antiviral drugs to treat infections that occur as a result of decreased immune response.

RADIATION   **Radiation** therapy involves the use of unstable isotopes that release varying levels of energy to cause breaks in the DNA molecule and thereby destroy cells. Radiation has been used as a treatment method since shortly after its discovery in the early 1900s. It is often used for the local and regional control of cancer, and in combination with surgery and chemotherapy.

The area to be irradiated (treatment field) includes the tumor site and sometimes other involved areas, such as lymph glands. The goal is to irradiate the tumor but not irradiate healthy adjacent tissue. The total dose of radiation is divided (or fractionated) and given over several weeks. A common course of radiation treatment might be once daily 4 or 5 days per week for a period of 2 to 7 weeks. Examples of cancers treated with radiation include Hodgkin's disease, Wilms' tumor, retinoblastoma, rhabdomyosarcoma, and CNS disease in leukemia.

BIOTHERAPY   **Biotherapy** is the use of biologic retooling and molecular intervention to produce targeted cancer therapy. Biologic retooling uses parts of the human body that are programmed to destroy cells, and applies them to the cancer cells. An example of this technique includes development of antibodies that are tumor-specific to certain cancers, and produced by the body in response to antigens of cancer cells (Henderson, Mossman, Nairn, & Cheever, 2005). These antibodies promote apoptosis or death of the cancerous cells. Another example is the group of drugs that stimulate the body's own immune

Protocol = Map or plan of action

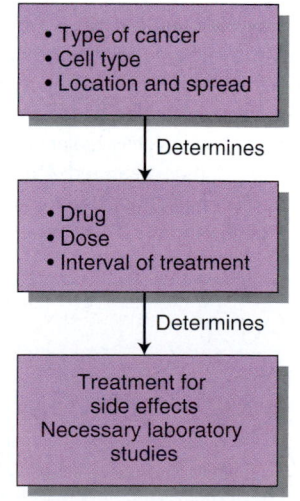

Figure 23–5 ➤ Chemotherapy protocol. A protocol is a map or plan of action that directs therapy by identifying the drug and its accompanying treatment.

MEDICATIONS USED TO TREAT *Cancer: Colony-Stimulating Factors*

Medication	Action/Indication	Nursing Implications
Epoetin alfa (human recombinant erythropoietin)	This glycoprotein stimulates the bone marrow in RBC formation; useful when numbers of RBCs are low due to chemotherapy effects	• Give subcutaneously or intravenously. • Do not shake and do not use if discolored or particles are present. Single-dose vials only so discard any solution that is not used. • Obtain blood tests before therapy and periodically after; improvement in hematocrit should be seen in 7–14 days. • Monitor blood pressure before and during therapy as hypertension can result. • Monitor for change in neurologic response and headache; both seizures and strokes are possible side effects.
Filgrastim (Neupogen) and pegfilgrastim (Neulasta)	This human granulocyte colony-stimulating factor (G-CSF) increases production of neutrophils by the bone marrow	• Administered subcutaneously and intravenously; prepare as directed for IV infusion to prevent its absorption by IV tubing. • Single-dose vials only so discard any solution that is not used. • Incompatible with many medications; check package insert; do not give within 24 hours before or after chemotherapy drugs or their effect may be decreased. • Obtain baseline and twice weekly CBC. • Monitor for side effects such as bone pain and heart arrhythmias; report fevers and be alert for other signs of infection when neutrophil count is low.
Oprelvekin (Neumega)	A hematopoietc growth factor, interleukin-11, that increases platelet count; useful in low platelet count due to chemotherapy effects on bone marrow	• Administered subcutaneously. • Single-dose vials only so discard any solution that is not used. • Obtain baseline CBC and platelet count; monitor platelets throughout treatment. • Monitor for side effects such as edema, fever, CNS changes, tachycardia, respiratory problems, and skin rash. • Take daily weights and monitors for fluids retention.

► NURSING ALERT

Nurses who care for a child receiving implant radiation or who work in a radiation department must wear a dosimeter film badge at all times. The cumulative radiation exposure is thus measured. The nurse must avoid radiation exposure for a period of time if recommended levels are exceeded.

response. Cancer vaccines are under development that may work to help the body fight cancers. The actions of many of these agents are not completely understood, and some agents have more than one effect. For example, interferon has both antiviral and antiproliferative effects on some malignant cells. Interferon and tumor necrosis factor (TNF) are undergoing clinical trials to study their effectiveness and to develop protocols for their safe use against selected cancers.

Molecular targeting involves interference with metabolic pathways (for example, through enzyme disruption) in the tumor cells. It may also disturb the cell's growth and development and thereby depress proliferation. For example, the signaling system in cancer cells that leads to proliferation is triggered by kinases, a specific type of enzyme that leads to transfer of phosphates among molecules. Drug therapy can interfere with the action of specific kinases, leading to cancer cell proliferation arrest (Faivre, Djelloul, & Raymond, 2006). Astrocytoma (discussed later in the section on brain tumors), for example, is a cancer in which research on therapy to interfere with metabolic pathways that is proving useful (Butowski, Sneed, & Chang, 2006).

An additional type of biological therapy is gene therapy, which is an attempt to replace a faulty gene with a normal one. Genetic technology is rapidly growing and shows promise for treatment of cancer and some other childhood diseases in the future. This complex field includes research to identify genes that lead to disease, recombinant techniques to enable genetic engineering, and studies of enzymes active in DNA and RNA formation. Nurses will need to have increased knowledge of this important work in the future as increased technologies are used in cancer treatment (Loescher & Merkle, 2005).

BONE MARROW AND HEMATOPOIETIC STEM CELL TRANSPLANTATION

Bone marrow and hematopoietic stem cell transplantation are used to treat leukemia, neuroblastoma, and some noncancerous conditions such as aplastic anemia. The goal of therapy is to administer a lethal dose of chemotherapy and radiation that will kill the cancer, and then to resupply the body with bone marrow stem cells either from the child's own marrow that was previously removed and stored (autologous transplant) or from a compatible donor (allogeneic transplant). Umbilical cord blood is another source of stem cells used for transplant. Peripheral blood stem cells are increasingly being used for transplant. The donor, whether autologous or allogeneic, can be given growth factors prior to donation to stimulate production of stem cells. An advantage of peripheral stem cells is that they can be collected easily rather than by the painful and invasive procedure of a bone marrow aspiration (Elfenbein, 2005).

Transplantation has become the treatment of choice for some cancers in the event a relapse occurs while the child is receiving another form of cancer therapy. First, a histocompatible donor must be located. The child then receives intensive chemotherapy, often followed by total body irradiation. Beginning 7 to 10 days before the transplant, this treatment kills all circulating blood cells and bone marrow contents. Supportive care is needed to treat the effects of nausea, diarrhea, and pain. Following this treatment, the child is intravenously transfused with the transplant stem cells. New blood cells usually form within 2 to 8 weeks (Alcoser & Rodgers, 2003). (See Chapter 17 ∞ for a complete description of care for the child undergoing transplantation.)

COMPLEMENTARY THERAPIES   Many families use **complementary therapies** to treat a child's cancer. These approaches to care are also referred to as alternative or unconventional, and may involve nutritional supplements, herbal ingestion, touch therapy, and mind-body interventions. Little research has been done on complementary therapies, although up to 80% of children have used at least one such therapeutic approach (Post-White & Hawks, 2005).

Mind-body therapies and touch are the most frequently used approaches. Some people use nutrition and herbal therapies with foods such as carrots, garlic, green tea, cabbage, citrus fruits, ginger root, and willow bark, which are thought to be effective in the prevention and treatment of cancer (Post-White & Hawks, 2005). Healthcare providers should be aware of these practices, inquire in a nonjudgmental manner about what therapies are used, and attempt to learn about specific therapies and practices. Although some herbs and nutritional products such as St. John's Wort may decrease serum concentration of chemotherapeutic agents, and others may act as hormones in the body, most are not known to negatively impact contemporary medical treatment. The families should be assisted in seeking information and supported in use of their chosen therapies. Intake of fruits and vegetables is associated with lower cancer incidence in adults, and some foods such as garlic and oranges may slow cancer growth or enhance medical chemotherapy. Some individuals use herbal supplements to treat cancer; these supplements include cat's claw (bark of a tree root), mistletoe, and shark cartilage. The Food and Drug Administration has allowed testing of the efficacy of some herbal treatments for cancer. Several cancer drugs such as vincristine and paclitaxel are obtained from plant products. Some herbs are useful in the treatment of nausea and vomiting, and others can boost the immune system's function.

PALLIATIVE CARE   Despite modern medicine practices and complementary therapies, some children do not survive childhood cancer. In these cases, the focus of health care is to provide comfort and emotional support for the child and family. Too often, healthcare providers feel uncomfortable when a child is expected to die and may withdraw from close contact with the child or family, fail to provide adequate comfort measures, and leave the family without access to needed resources. When delay in the recognition of prognosis occurs, children experience greater suffering and less integration of palliative care. Some of the symptoms for which children are commonly undertreated include pain, dyspnea, nutrition, elimination, and fatigue. Additionally, care may be required by a wide array of specialists that can lead to fragmentation of care and lack of integrated palliative approaches (Himmelstein, Hilden, Boldt, & Weissman, 2004).

The presence of a palliative care team and an integrated plan of care; collaboration between families, the primary care provider, and other practitioners; and focus on the child's developmental level and the needs of the family can enhance the care provided for the dying child (Himmelstein et al., 2004; Rushton, 2005). Parents state that an advanced care directive that outlines the medical care plans for the child is helpful in preserving the child's quality of life and increases the child's comfort (Hammes, Klevan, Kempf, & Williams, 2005). See Chapter 14 ∞ for a detailed description of palliative care for children with terminal disease.

Special Issues in Childhood Cancer

ONCOLOGIC EMERGENCIES Oncologic emergencies may result from the cancer itself or as a side effect of treatment. They can be organized into three groups: metabolic, hematologic, and those involving space-occupying lesions.

Metabolic Emergencies Several types of emergencies can arise from metabolic changes in the body. The first of these metabolic emergencies results from the lysis (dissolving or decomposing) of tumor cells and rapid release of their contents into the blood, a process called *tumor lysis syndrome*. This cell destruction releases high levels of uric acid, potassium, phosphates, and calcium into the blood and can lower serum sodium levels, possibly resulting in cardiac arrhythmias and renal failure. This syndrome is seen most commonly in children with non-Hodgkin's lymphoma and acute lymphocytic leukemia (Alavi, Arzanian, Abbasian, & Ashena, 2006; Cantril & Haylock, 2004; Spinazze & Schrijvers, 2006). See the Clinical Manifestations of Tumor Lysis Syndrome table for more details on manifestations and management of tumor lysis syndrome.

A second type of metabolic emergency is septic shock. During periods of immune suppression the child is vulnerable to overwhelming infection, resulting in circulatory failure, hypothermia or hyperthermia, tachypnea, mental changes, inadequate tissue perfusion, and hypotension. Septic shock can be fatal (see Chapter 21 ∞ for a description of septic shock), but early and aggressive therapy improves outcomes (Haut, 2005). Factors contributing to massive infection include inadequate neutrophil production, abnormal granulocytes (not able to be actively phagocytic), erosions through normal barriers such as blood vessels and mucous membranes, and altered bone marrow production caused by chemotherapy and some forms of radiation. Such infections must be vigorously treated with antimicrobial therapy and hydration management.

A third type of metabolic emergency occurs when large amounts of bone are destroyed by treatment and decreased renal tubular excretion, resulting in hypercalcemia

CLINICAL MANIFESTATIONS TUMOR LYSIS SYNDROME

Etiology	Clinical Manifestations	Clinical Therapy	Nursing Implications
Breakdown of malignant cells releases intracellular components into blood	Hyperuricemia Hyperkalemia Hyperphosphatemia Hypocalcemia	• Vigorous hydration with 2–4 times maintenance fluid • Correction of electrolyte imbalances • Administration of allopurinol or urate oxidase (Rasburicase) to reduce conversion of metabolic by-products to uric acid	• Administration of fluids, beginning before therapy • Careful intake and output measures • Daily weight • Urine specific gravity (should remain < 1.010) • Monitoring for desired and side effects of drug therapy
Electroyte imbalance causes metabolic acidosis and serious abnormalities	Cardiac arrhythmias Impaired renal function Tetany, neurological and mental status changes	• ECG monitoring • Medications such as furosemide to facilitate potassium excretion • Dialysis may be needed	• Administration of electrolytes and medications • Urine pH (should remain 7.0 to 7.5) • Perform Trousseau's and Chvostek's signs for tetany monitoring and assess neurological function • Perform mental status examination • Obtain laboratory specimens as needed

(elevated calcium in the serum). Hypercalcemia is most common in children with acute lymphocytic leukemia and rhabdomyosarcoma. Treatment includes hydration, bisphosphonates, glucocorticoids, and adequate intake of phosphate by oral supplement (Spinazze & Schrijvers, 2006).

Some children develop syndrome of inappropriate antidiuretic hormone (SIADH) and have excessive release of ADH. The resulting decreased urinary output leads to water intoxication. See Chapter 29 ∞ for a detailed description of SIADH.

Hematologic Emergencies   Hematologic emergencies result from bone marrow suppression or infiltration of brain and respiratory tissue with high numbers of leukemic blast cells (hyperleukocytosis). Bone marrow suppression results in anemia and **thrombocytopenia** (decreased platelets) with resultant hemorrhage. Disseminated intravascular coagulation (DIC) occurs in some children and is a life-threatening complication. (See Chapter 22 ∞ for a thorough description of this condition.) Gastrointestinal and central nervous system bleeding (strokes) are common. Disruption of normal WBC production and resulting hyperleukocytosis can lead to obstruction of small blood vessels throughout the body.

Treatment involves infusion of packed red blood cells for anemia; and platelet transfusion, vitamin K, and fresh frozen plasma for thrombocytopenia and hemorrhage. Hyperleukocytosis is treated by hydration, diuresis, respiratory support, and plasmaphoresis, if needed (Haut, 2005).

Space-Occupying Lesions   Extensive tumor growth may result in spinal cord compression, increased intracranial pressure, brain herniation, seizures, massive hepatomegaly, and superior vena cava syndrome (obstruction of the superior vena cava by tumor). These emergencies are often caused by neuroblastoma, medulloblastoma, astrocytoma, Hodgkin's disease, or lymphoma. After biopsy of the mass, treatment involves radiation therapy, chemotherapy, and corticosteroids.

PSYCHOSOCIAL NEEDS   The diagnosis of cancer is devastating for families. They cannot believe that their vibrant young child or adolescent has a potentially life-threatening disease. Families are in a state of crisis when the diagnosis is made; their first response is typically shock. Despite this, parents must gather resources to support the child, make treatment decisions, and adjust family life to integrate the needs of the child with cancer. Some families need to travel a great distance for the child's treatments and others may have financial constraints that make healthcare costs a major concern. For nearly everyone, parental work schedules, as well as arrangements for other children, must be adjusted. Most cancer treatment will last for a minimum of several months up to several years, necessitating nearly constant adaptation. See Families Want to Know: Cancer Therapy.

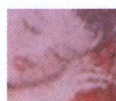

FAMILIES WANT TO KNOW

Cancer Therapy

Most parents are not aware of the effects of cancer treatment and how they can help children through this experience. Depending on the stage and type of treatment, there are several ways to help:

- Children in radiation and chemotherapy are fatigued. Provide extra rest periods with shorter activity periods between them.
- Have essential items packed in case the child develops a complication and needs to be taken to stay in the hospital for a few days. Several hospital stays of a few days are normal during treatment.
- When concerned about a symptom in the child, ask the care provider. Parents are often key in identifying problems early.
- Parents are usually concerned about central line care, but feel more comfortable after a few days of caring for the line.

- Children may not feel hungry, so nutritional intake is needed when they are ready to eat.
- Remember that the child is still at the normal developmental age. Treat children based on their ages, not as if they are older or younger.
- Try to maintain contact with the child's peer group and family members.
- Seek information from other parents and resources on cancer care.
- Remind parents to get time away and relax so that parental energy remains high and they are better able to deal with the child's therapy.

The child reacts to the diagnosis based on age and developmental stage. Infants and toddlers are unaware of the severity of the disease, while preschoolers are beginning to understand the illness. However, they may think they caused their illness, and are confused about why the parent cannot make the illness go away. School-age children can understand a diagnosis of cancer and benefit from opportunities to talk about the experience. Adolescents find contact with others who have gone through their experience reassuring and supportive. A comprehensive review of studies on communicating with children and adolescents about their cancer found a lack of clear guidance for effective interventions. However, some benefit from structured youth groups and camping activities designed to lower anxiety and improve knowledge, coping, and well-being (Scott, Entwistle, Sowden, & Watt, 2003). Group therapy sessions, computer programs about cancer and treatment, and school reintegration all show potential for assisting youth who are adjusting to cancer.

CANCER SURVIVAL   Children with cancer have a variety of common psychologic and physiologic challenges, regardless of their specific types of cancer. They and their families are dealing with a complex illness that influences their lives for years. The impact of this experience extends into all areas of function. Over the past 20 to 30 years, treatment for childhood cancers has been increasingly successful. About 1 in 1000 young adults is a survivor of childhood cancer, and by 2010 it is expected that 1 in 250 adults will be a cancer survivor (Florin & Hinkle, 2005). The success of new modalities and treatment combinations has, however, created special healthcare needs for many survivors (Figure 23–6 ➤).

Surgery can have many results. Body organs may be removed and manipulated, leading to adhesions, intestinal obstruction, visual impairment, neurologic disruption, and sterility. Removal of the spleen can lead to serious infections. Amputation necessitates the need for prosthetic devices and physical rehabilitation.

Radiation has several long-term effects. It can impair the growth of bones, teeth, and eyes, leading to conditions such as scoliosis, leg length discrepancy, low bone mineral density, cataracts, or poor dental health. Hypothyroidism can be observed in those who have had head and neck radiation (Skinner, Hamish, Wallace, & Levitt, 2006).

Figure 23–6 ➤ Survivors of childhood cancer. A, Nicole, 11 years old, is undergoing chemotherapy for Ewing's sarcoma. Her mother emphasizes, "It's our faith that has gotten us through this. The hardest part is how busy you are coming to treatments all the time. Nicole's younger brother sometimes feels neglected." B, According to Jesse, who is 10 years old and waiting for a bone marrow transplant, "The thing that has helped me the most [in dealing with acute lymphoblastic leukemia] is all the mail I got from my friends." His mother adds, "We're just really positive and think that everything will turn out all right." C, Cassie, 19 months old, has been diagnosed with neuroblastoma. At this age, it is hard for her to understand what is happening. Her mother has stayed with her each time she has come to the hospital, which has helped Cassie adjust to therapy. Her caregivers are confident that she will respond well to her treatment.

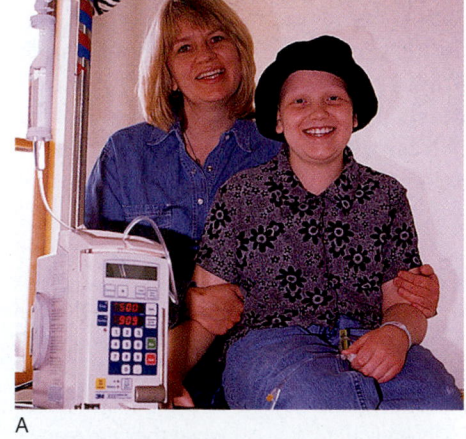

A

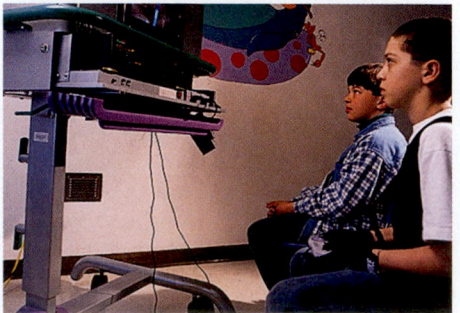

B

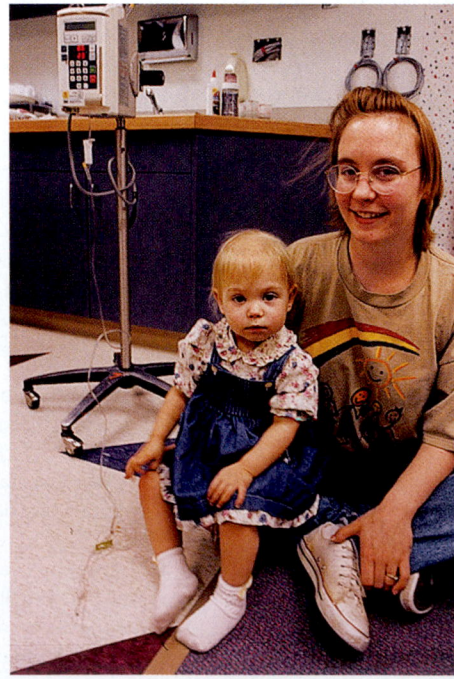

C

Cardiotoxicity and pulmonary toxicity can result from mediastinal radiation, while delayed puberty and sterility can result from radiation effects to the cranium and spinal regions. Impaired neurocognitive performance may occur as long-term effects of treatment, especially with higher doses of radiation. Some studies have found lower behavioral and social competence in treated children, and higher rates of post-traumatic stress syndrome (Rourke, Hobbie, Schwartz, & Kazak, 2006).

Secondary cancers, most commonly solid tumors, occur in some survivors. **Secondary cancers** are also called second malignant neoplasm (SMN) and are those that occur subsequent to the primary cancer and treatment but are of a different histologic type. Cancers of the thyroid, CNS, breast, and skin are examples of described secondary neoplasms. Most of these cancers can be effectively treated, emphasizing the need for thorough and frequent monitoring of the treated cancer patient (Haddy, Mosher, Dinndorf, & Reaman, 2004).

Chemotherapy can cause a wide variety of effects, both during its administration and for years afterward. See Clinical Manifestations of Common Side Effects of Chemotherapy on page 868. Cardiomyopathy can occur with some drugs, especially the anthracyclines. Temporary and/or permanent pulmonary toxicity and renal complications can develop. Neurologic effects of some drugs can lead to hearing loss (e.g., cisplatin and ifosfamide), cataracts, and paraplegia (e.g., intrathecal methotrexate for leukemia). Learning disabilities and change in intelligence quotient (IQ) occur in some children. Infertility may also result (Nelson & Meeske, 2005). Although radiation is responsible for most secondary tumors, some chemotherapy drugs have also been implicated.

The diagnosis and stress of treatment, along with the risk of recurrence, are significant stressors for the child with cancer. Families may find it difficult to obtain full insurance coverage for the child who has had a prior cancer. Employment can be a potential problem for cancer survivors if employers have concerns about the earlier cancer diagnosis. Most people with cancer report fear of recurrence of the disease, which is another stressor. Depression, suicidal thoughts, and concerns about appearance have been found by some researchers to be more common in survivors of childhood cancer (Recklitis, O'Leary, & Diller, 2003), while other researchers have found rates of depression to be similar among those treated for cancer and those in the population at large (Zebrack et al., 2006).

Conversely, hopefulness and the sense of having an added purpose in life can be positive outcomes for many cancer survivors. Some meet with others who have recently been diagnosed or work on fundraising events that support cancer research. The highest risk for long-term psychological distress in adult survivors of childhood cancer occurs in those with poor health status, low income, low education, and unemployment. Thus, encouraging children with cancer to meet educational goals will maximize their chances of psychological adaptation (Zebrack et al., 2006).

A recent consensus group of experts identified barriers to optimal care for cancer survivors, including:

- Lack of knowledge about survivorship by healthcare professionals
- Lack of knowledge about risks and care recommendations by the cancer survivor
- Lack of awareness about cancer survivorship by the general public
- Paucity of research on survivorship

Therefore, additional education of healthcare professionals and the public, as well as research into survivor issues, are recommended (Houldin, Curtiss, & Haylock, 2006).

NURSING MANAGEMENT
Nursing Assessment and Diagnosis

Children who have cancer have all of the usual health promotion and health maintenance requirements; in addition, they require astute assessments to identify any of the possible outcomes of cancer and its treatment.

History

During any child's health promotion visit, nurses should determine if there is a history of cancer in the family. In particular, if more than one person has had cancer, and if young children in the extended family have been affected, complete a genogram to isolate cases in the family (see Chapter 3 ∞). A history of exposure to known carcinogens is also important. Does a parent work in an industry with chemicals or asbestos that might remain on clothing worn home? Was the child treated with radiation or chemotherapy for a previous cancer? Does the child have an identified condition such as Down syndrome? Does the child have any recognized congenital anomalies? A number of conditions are more commonly associated with certain types of cancer.

Physiologic Assessment

When performing any physiologic assessment on children, the nurse considers the possible signs and symptoms of cancer. These include anemia, frequent infections, bleeding disorders, loss of weight, fatigue, pain, and changes in mental health and neurological status. Assessment of children with the most significant types of childhood cancers is presented in separate sections throughout this chapter.

Once cancer has been diagnosed, a thorough physical assessment of all systems is needed to help identify the presence and extent of cancer (see Chapter 5 ∞). Systems needing particularly thorough assessments are neurologic, respiratory, cardiac, and gastrointestinal. Assess hydration status and the tumor site if it is visible. These assessments will be completed regularly at each treatment and monitoring visit. Height and weight should be carefully measured, and compared with prior findings for the child. Nutritional intake histories may be pertinent as well. Observe immunization status, developmental milestones, gait and coordination, as well as any changes in mental status. Evaluate pain, fatigue, infections, bruising, shortness of breath, and elimination problems, and perform periodic laboratory studies.

Psychosocial Assessment

Assessment of stress and coping abilities, as well as knowledge of the condition and cognitive level, support systems, developmental level, and body image, provides data that help determine the appropriate nursing interventions for the child with cancer and his or her family.

Stress and Coping

The diagnosis of cancer is a major stressor for both the child and his or her family. Although each child's prognosis and each family's coping mechanisms are unique, most families deal with the diagnosis in a manner similar to that of other families who have a child with a life-threatening illness (see Chapter 14 ∞). Assess the family (and child, if old enough) for their understanding and acceptance of the diagnosis. Evaluate if the family has told the child about the diagnosis and whether the family needs assistance in deciding how to do this. Ask what the parents have told siblings; if they need suggestions, help and support them to decide how much and when to share information with the child's siblings (Packman, Greenhalgh, Chesterman et al., 2005).

Assess the level of anxiety during healthcare visits and scheduled treatments. Evaluate the family's methods of coping, such as the ability to integrate relaxing and meaningful activities into family life, the use of support systems in the extended family and the community, and the ability to alter expectations to take into account the child's health status (Figure 23–7 ➤). Concurrent stressors increase the family's difficulty in coping with childhood cancer. Evaluate the family for stressors such as illness or death of another family member, occupational changes, financial problems, relocation, and change in vacation plans. Evaluate the family's knowledge of the U.S. Family Leave Act, which provides for parental use of sick time to treat an ill family member.

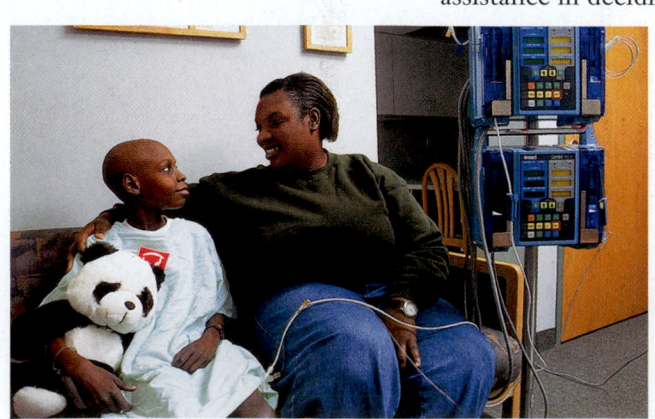

Figure 23–7 ➤ The child with cancer depends on parents and family members to provide support. Nurses can assist families to draw upon their strengths to help the child.

Knowledge

People who are anxious tend to narrow their scope of attention and may read unintended messages into the behaviors of healthcare personnel. Anxiety also limits a person's ability to retain information.

The child's knowledge of cancer and its treatment should be assessed throughout the treatment period. As the child matures cognitively, new evaluations of knowledge are needed. Cancer and its treatment are complex topics and parents are exposed to information in various forms, including written material, news reports, and Internet web sites and resources. Evaluate their knowledge and information sources, providing them with opportunities to ask questions. Evaluate the learning styles of the child and family in order to adapt approaches to meet their needs.

Support Systems

Cancer treatment generally occurs over a long period of time. The extended family is crucial in providing necessary support to the child, parents, and siblings. Identify key persons in the family. They may be the parents, grandparents, or aunts and uncles. Thoroughly assess the coping strategies used by the family to meet the various challenges posed by the child's illness. This information helps to predict the success of interventions, such as home care with intravenous medications, and to decide when referrals for other supportive therapies are needed.

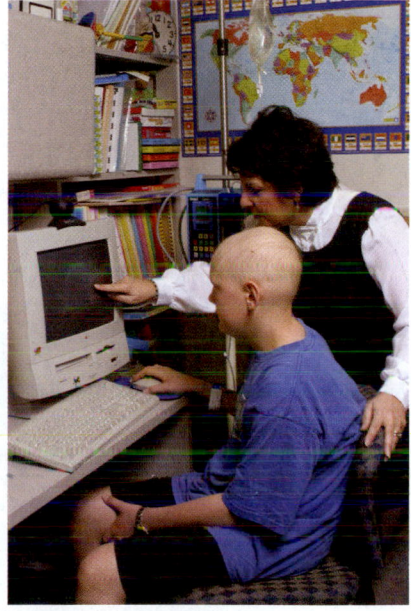

Assess family resources to identify support systems available to help the family during crises and if a child is expected to die. Extended supports include friends, jobs, insurance coverage, faith-based affiliations, cultural support systems, the healthcare system, and the school system (Figure 23–8 ➤). Inquire if the insurance carrier provides for a case manager in complex health needs such as cancer. Parents commonly lose contact with close friends following the diagnosis of cancer in a child. This is an additional stressor for the family. Jobs are often a source of support because coworkers may have gone through the same experience. It may also be comforting for parents to return to a job where they can feel a sense of security in tangible accomplishments. However, jobs can also be a source of stress if employers are unsympathetic to the demands of the child's hospitalization and clinic or office visits.

Faith-based affiliations can be an important source of support. Evaluate whether such affiliations are meaningful for the family and, if so, plan for visits from the appropriate clergy. In some cultures, spiritual leaders are an important part of the family's support. Enable a healer to visit the child and conduct a healing ceremony if that will be supportive to the family and child.

Figure 23–8 ➤ This teacher is able to come to the pediatric oncology center to work with students while their chemotherapy is administered. What are the benefits of having her work with students in this setting?

The child's return to school may pose difficulties for the child with cancer, or, alternatively, it may be a source of support to be connected again to peers. The child is encouraged to go to school, even if only for half a day per week, to stay connected to

---

🖐 GROWTH & DEVELOPMENT

Adolescents Diagnosed with Cancer

During much of childhood, parents are told first about the child's diagnosis, and then assisted in their planning of what the child can understand and how the information is best relayed. However, the adolescent is more independent in decision making and establishing support systems. Therefore, joint discussions between the healthcare providers and parents and teens are generally helpful, followed by individual sessions when the adolescent can meet individually with the healthcare team and have questions answered. The teen needs information about the diagnosis and treatment regimens, as well as an atmosphere where feelings can be discussed and assistance is offered in locating other teens with cancer for further discussion and support (Bradlyn, Kato, Beale, & Cole, 2004). Adolescence is a distinct developmental stage that overlaps both childhood and adulthood. Asking for adolescents' perspectives may be the best way of understanding the experience of cancer and offering the support they need. Two questions are suggested: "During treatment there are good days and there are bad days. What makes a good day for you? How has being sick been for you?" (Hinds, 2004). The nurse can ask these questions and examine the answers for clues to the protective factors or support the teen experiences, as well as the areas that need assistance.

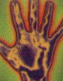 **GROWTH & DEVELOPMENT**

Cancer and Age Considerations

Children of different ages experience differing threats to body image as a result of cancer treatment. A preschool girl may be most upset at hair loss, since she will look like a boy. A school-age child has the most difficult time with changes that interfere with the developmental task of industry. Amputation, which decreases the child's ability to participate in activities such as sports, dancing, and school work, can be a major challenge during the school-age years. Teenagers are often most worried about such changes as hair loss and cushingoid features, which cause them to look different from peers.

peers. Evaluate the school's ability to accept a medically vulnerable child into the classroom. Nurses who work in the oncology department of the hospital or clinic can ask if the family will give consent to visit the school, meet with the school nurse, and plan together to meet the child's educational needs. Assess whether the other children and teachers have been prepared for the appearance and needs of the child with cancer. Arrangements can be made for tutors to help the child keep up with school work if he or she cannot attend school. An Individualized Education Plan is needed (see a description of the IEP in Chapter 12 ∞). Parents need information about the legal right to this plan since the child is newly ill and they will likely not have been exposed to this in the past.

Developmental Assessment

Developmental assessment of children should be performed regularly during treatment for cancer. This assessment should be done at times when the child feels well so that results are accurate. Children under 6 years of age who have cancer should receive regular developmental assessment with a standardized tool such as the Denver II Developmental Screening Test (see Chapter 7 ∞). A home healthcare nurse, or a nurse in the pediatric healthcare home (medical home) who sees the child for a general health supervision visit, can perform such testing. Assessment of the child's physical and neurologic development helps in determining the progress made during treatment and provides a baseline for evaluating the long-term effects of treatment. Recommend referral to a neuropsychologist for testing early in treatment and determine if changes in developmental performance are noted. Observe developmental milestones at each contact with the child and refer for further assessment if regression has occurred. Performance in school and social activities with friends also provides important information about expected developmental milestones in older children.

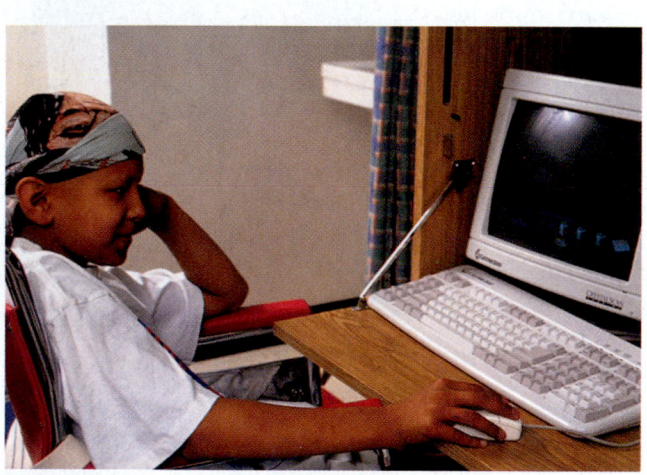

Figure 23–9 ➤ One of the most common threats to a child's body image at any age is hair loss induced by chemotherapy. Use of hats can improve self-concept.

Body Image

Body image disturbances occur when a child cannot integrate changes and continues to cling to old images despite their inconsistency with reality. Common means for assessing body image are drawings, colored pictures cut out by the child to form a collage, discussion, and observation. Drawing is an especially powerful tool that assists children in handling the stress of the disease and enhances communication with healthcare providers (Rollins, 2005). See Chapter 13 ∞ for further discussion of these and other assessment techniques that can be used with children.

Hair loss, surgical scars, and cushingoid changes are three common treatment-induced threats to body image. Most children being treated for cancer experience hair loss (Figure 23–9 ➤). Children who have cranial surgery lose hair as part of the surgical preparation. Chemotherapy also frequently results in some degree of hair loss. The speed of hair loss is unique to the child and can be as rapid as overnight or slower, evidenced by hair left on the pillow and in the hairbrush. Assess for hair loss and assist the child to deal with it in the method he or she chooses.

A second challenge to the child's body image is surgery. The scars of cranial and neck surgery are obvious, as are amputation and limb salvaging. Abdominal surgery for lymphoma is more easily concealed but is still a threat to the child's body image.

A third source of altered body image is the cushingoid features such as round and flushed face, prominent cheeks, double chin, and generalized obesity that result from the use of corticosteroids (Figure 23–10 ➤). As the child's weight increases, stretch marks similar to those women experience in pregnancy may occur. These stretch marks often remain after the corticosteroids are decreased.

Assessment for Impact of Cancer Survival

Nurses are involved with families when a diagnosis of cancer is made, during the therapy process, and in the years that follow. The family needs support as treatment concludes and the child is integrated back into his or her usual home and community roles

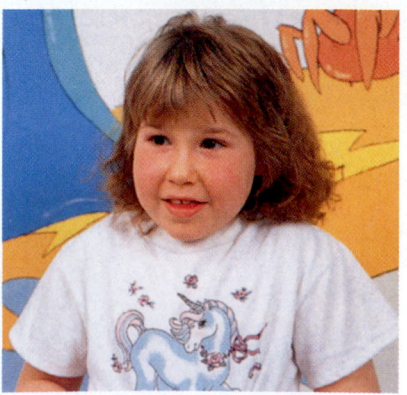

Figure 23–10 ➤ The child with cushingoid changes frequently has a rounded face and prominent cheeks.

(Labay, Mayans, & Harris, 2004). For a child who survives cancer, ongoing care is essential (Hudson & Findlay, 2006; Landier, Bhatia, Eshelman et al., 2004). Evaluate the child regularly with thorough physical, psychosocial, developmental, and cognitive assessments. Carefully monitor all body systems (e.g., cardiovascular; respiratory; musculoskeletal; eye, ear, nose, and throat; genitourinary). Record height, weight, and general growth patterns. Ask about the child's interactions with peers and performance at school. Children who have received cranial radiation and intrathecal chemotherapy need regular scholastic evaluations. Be alert for signs and symptoms that could indicate a secondary tumor.

Assess the need for physical rehabilitation, support related to visual impairment, or treatment for cardiac or musculoskeletal abnormalities. Facilitate periodic evaluations in a healthcare agency so that serious outcomes of treatment can be identified early. Ask the parents about insurance coverage and other financial difficulties with ongoing care.

The accompanying Nursing Care Plans include several diagnoses that may be appropriate for the child with cancer who is receiving care in the hospital or at home. Among the many other diagnoses that may be appropriate for a child with cancer are the following:

- Diarrhea related to radiation therapy and chemotherapy
- Impaired Urinary Elimination related to chemotherapy
- Impaired Oral Mucous Membrane related to chemotherapy and radiation therapy
- Impaired Skin Integrity related to altered nutritional state, effects of medication, radiation, and immobilization
- Ineffective Individual Coping related to situational crises of chronic and acute illness
- Disturbed Sleep Pattern related to biochemical agents, anxiety, and unfamiliar surroundings
- Deficient Diversional Activity related to frequent lengthy treatments
- Disturbed Body Image related to chronic illness and treatments
- Deficient Knowledge (Child or Parents) related to lack of exposure to disease or treatments
- Anticipatory Grieving related to actual or potential loss of significant other

Planning and Implementation

The nursing care of children newly diagnosed with cancer and their families includes immediate physiologic and psychologic support, along with anticipatory guidance about imminent and future medical interventions. The family should be assisted and supported in making decisions about types of treatment that are appropriate for their child.

Nursing care of the hospitalized child with cancer and the child receiving ongoing therapy at home is summarized in the accompanying nursing care plans. These care plans are designed for the child who is beyond the cancer diagnosis phase and is receiving chemotherapy.

Physiologic care of the hospitalized child focuses on providing support during treatment. This includes ensuring optimal nutritional intake, administering medications, managing the multiple side effects of chemotherapy and radiation, ensuring adequate hydration, preventing infection, and managing pain.

Ensure Optimal Nutritional Intake

The high metabolic rate of cancer growth depletes the child's nutritional stores. In addition, is the catabolic effect of chemotherapy and radiation on normal cells, necessitates additional cellular replacement. The child needs increased nutritional intake at a time when nausea and vomiting are occurring as drug side effects, when taste and smell have been altered, and when decreased activity, fatigue, pain, and general health status result in diminished appetite. This often leads to extreme concern on the part of parents, who may focus excessive attention on the child's intake. See Families Want to Know: Nutrition and the Child with Cancer on page 866.

COMMUNITY CARE

Hair Loss

For many parents, especially those with daughters, the loss of the child's hair can be devastating. Ask the parents and the child what this issue is like for them. Prepare them for the fact that it can be rapid or slow. Find out how they will plan to cope. Some children want their hair cut very short so its loss will not be as traumatic. Offer resources for wigs, hats, or other ideas. Put them in touch with children who have lost hair and with those who have regrown it.

NURSING CARE PLAN — Hospital Care of the Child with Cancer

GOAL	INTERVENTION	RATIONALE	EXPECTED OUTCOME
1. Chronic Pain related to tissue injury			
	NIC Priority Intervention: **Pain Management:** *Alleviation or reduction in pain to a level of comfort acceptable to patient.*		*NOC Suggested Outcome:* **Comfort Level:** *Feelings of physical and psychologic ease.*
The child will report reduced pain that is manageable.	• Give analgesics as ordered.	• Adequate medications can reduce pain.	• The child experiences pain reduced to the level that allows child to interact appropriately and gain rest.
	• Teach relaxation techniques, deep breathing and distraction.	• Nonpharmacologic methods work with the medication to reduce pain.	
2. Disturbed Sleep Pattern related to lack of sleep privacy/control			
	NIC Priority Intervention: **Sleep Enhancement:** *Facilitation of regular sleep/wake cycles.*		*NOC Suggested Outcome:* **Rest:** *Extent and pattern of diminished activity for mental and physical rejuvenation.*
The child will sleep for hours appropriate to age. The child will report feeling rested.	• Alter the environment to allow designated rest periods.	• A quiet environment encourages relaxation needed for resting.	The child rests and sleeps for an age-appropriate amount of time per day.
	• Plan care to reduce frequency of interruptions during normal rest and sleep times.	• Reduced interruptions allow continuous sleep and rest.	
3. Imbalanced Nutrition: Less than Body Requirements related to inability to ingest or digest food or absorb nutrients			
	NIC Priority Intervention: **Nutrition Management:** *Assistance with and provision of a balanced dietary intake.*		*NOC Suggested Outcome:* **Nutritional Status:** *Extent to which nutrients are available to meet metabolic needs.*
The child will maintain adequate nutritional intake.	• Offer small feedings. Encourage favorite foods. Refer to dietitian for special meals. Weigh daily.	• Measures can increase caloric intake. Taste changes and mouth sores alter desire for food.	The child maintains admission weight.
The child will experience reduced effects of chemotherapy (i.e., nausea and vomiting)	• Teach the child distraction and relaxation techniques. Give antiemetics according to orders.	• Pharmacologic and non-pharmacologic methods are effective in helping to reduce nausea.	The child has minimal side effects of nausea and vomiting.
4. Risk for Constipation related to change in usual foods and eating patterns			
	NIC Priority Intervention: **Constipation Management:** *Prevention and alleviation of constipation.*		*NOC Suggested Outcome:* **Bowel Elimination:** *The ability of the gastrointestinal tract to form and evacuate stool effectively.*
The child will reestablish normal bowel pattern.	• Record all output by size and description. Administer stool softeners. Test stool for guaiac. Report changes in stool to physician. Encourage adequate fluid intake.	• Chemotherapy or tumor may create constipation, diarrhea, or blood in stool.	The child has normal bowel pattern.
5. Fluid Volume Excess or Deficient related to medications			
	NIC Priority Intervention: **Fluid Management:** *Promotion of fluid balance and prevention of complications resulting from abnormal fluid levels.*		*NOC Suggested Outcome:* **Fluid Balance:** *Balance of water in the intracellular and extracellular compartments of the body.*
The child will be adequately hydrated.	• Record all intake. Monitor intravenous rate and solution as appropriate.	• Some drugs (e.g., cyclophosphamide) necessitate a high level of fluid intake to prevent complications.	The child demonstrates adequate hydration. Mucous membranes are hydrated.

NURSING CARE PLAN	Hospital Care of the Child with Cancer (continued)		
GOAL	**INTERVENTION**	**RATIONALE**	**EXPECTED OUTCOME**
5. Fluid Volume Excess or Deficient related to medications (continued)			
	• Test specific gravity of urine daily.	• Renal function may be affected by chemotherapy.	• Specific gravity remains within normal range.
6. Risk for Infection related to immunosuppression, invasive procedures, malnutrition, or pharmaceutical agents			
	NIC Priority Intervention: **Infection Protection:** *Prevention and early detection of infection in patient at risk.*		*NOC Suggested Outcome:* **Risk Control:** *Actions to eliminate or reduce health threats.*
The child will remain free of infection.	• Wash hands often. Maintain in isolation if needed.	• Handwashing is effective to reduce organisms. Transmission-based precautions may be needed to safeguard child.	The child remains infection free.
	• Monitor temperature. Report elevation to physician.	• Elevated temperature is a sign of infection.	
	• Administer intravenous antibiotics as ordered. Monitor temperature. Use cooling mattress as ordered. Report elevations over 38°C (101°F) to physician.	• Multiple antibiotics are needed to deal with bacterial and lung infections during neutropenia. Blood cultures may be taken to identify organism.	The child with an infection is effectively treated.
7. Ineffective Individual Coping related to situational crisis			
	NIC Priority Intervention: **Coping Enhancement:** *Assisting a patient to adapt to stressors that interfere with meeting life demands and roles.*		*NOC Suggested Outcome:* **Coping:** *Actions to manage stressors that tax an individual's resources.*
The child will demonstrate normal adaptive coping methods.	• Encourage drawings and other therapeutic play for expression of feelings. Allow for expression of angry feelings, such as hitting dolls and throwing sponge balls. Discuss how to behave during treatments.	• Expression of feelings helps identify avoidance coping for further intervention. Play is a normal way for child to express self and ideas. Misinterpretations can be corrected. Knowledge of appropriate and helpful behaviors supports self-esteem.	The child continues to use usual coping strategies expected for developmental stage.
8. Ineffective Health Maintenance related to complex treatment, and lack of resources			
	NIC Priority Intervention: **Health System Guidance:** *Facilitating use of health services.*		*NOC Suggested Outcome:* **Knowledge:** *Health Behaviors: Extent of understanding conveyed about promotion and protection of health.*
The child will state understanding of treatments and procedures.	• Use age-appropriate teaching methods. Content areas include child's cancer, medications (actions and side effects), how to deal with body changes, and how to deal with response of others to those changes. Correct misinterpretations. Anticipate upcoming events and teach the child and family about them.	• Education helps by increasing understanding, removing fantasy, and clarifying fears. Education promotes the use of new learning in all areas of life.	The child demonstrates age-appropriate knowledge of the cancer, its treatments, and medications. The child has age-appropriate understanding of how to deal with changes in the body.

NURSING CARE PLAN Home Care of the Child with Cancer

GOAL	INTERVENTION	RATIONALE	EXPECTED OUTCOME
1. Risk for Infection related to immunosuppression, chemotherapy, and presence of invasive lines			
	NIC Priority Intervention: **Infection Protection:** *Prevention and early detection of infection in child at risk.*		*NOC Suggested Outcome:* **Risk Control:** *Actions to eliminate or reduce health risks.*
The child will remain infection free.	• Educate the child and parents about meaning of blood counts.	• Knowledgeable parents and child can protect themselves.	The child remains infection free.
	• Encourage parents/family members to use masks when they are ill.	• Masks help decrease airborne infection if used properly.	
	• Encourage good handwriting at all times.	• Handwashing is best prevention.	
	• Advise the child's teacher to tell parents if the child is exposed to communicable illness at school.	• Exposure can be reported to physician for possible use of antibiotic, antiviral drug, or admission for treatment.	All exposures are reported to physician immediately.
	• Clean vascular access site and provide care per protocol. Observe for signs of infection. Report infection to physician.	• Care helps to prevent infection and maintain an open line.	
2. Imbalanced Nutrition: Less than Body Requirements related to inability to ingest or digest adequate quantities of food or absorb adequate nutrients			
	NIC Priority Intervention: **Nutrition Management:** *Assistance with and provision of a balanced dietary intake.*		*NOC Suggested Outcome:* **Nutritional Status:** *Extent to which nutrients are available to meet metabolic needs.*
The child will maintain adequate nutritional intake.	• Encourage small and frequent high-calorie meals. Encourage small bites of a variety of foods.	• Measures to increase caloric intake. Taste changes and favorite foods may no longer be preferred.	The child maintains normal weight for height.
	• Promote good oral hygiene and use of nonalcohol mouthwashes.	• Mouth ulcers cause discomfort when eating, alcohol is painful on open ulcers.	
	• Teach home enteral and parenteral nutrition, if ordered.	• Enternal or parenteral nutritional support may be used to enhance intake.	
3. Ineffective Management of Therapeutic Regimen related to complex therapy			
	NIC Priority Intervention: **Family Involvement:** *Facilitating family participation in the emotional and physical care of the child.*		*NOC Suggested Outcome:* **Care Management:** *Family ability to manage complex therapy.*
The child will comply with oral medication regimen.	• Educate parents and child about the importance of taking medication as prescribed.	• Understanding can assist parents and child in placing importance on medication intake.	The child takes all medications according to prescription.
	• Set up calendar with dates, times, and medications clearly labeled.	• Visual reminders can help them recall instructions.	
	• Reward the child for taking medications.	• Reinforcing desired behaviors through rewards is effective with children.	

NURSING CARE PLAN Home Care of the Child with Cancer (continued)

GOAL	INTERVENTION	RATIONALE	EXPECTED OUTCOME
4. Delayed Growth and Development related to serious illness			
	NIC Priority Intervention: **Developmental Enhancement:** *Facilitating parents/caregivers to promote optimal/growth and development of child.*		*NOC Suggested Outcome:* **Child Growth and Development:** *Normal increase in body size and developmental skills.*
The child will demonstrate normal physical, emotional, and cognitive development.	• Encourage play appropriate to age.	• Normal activities support self-esteem and self-knowledge.	The child continues to develop physically, emotionally, and cognitively at a normal pace.
	• Encourage the child to attend school.	• School is the work of the child and promotes cognitive and social growth.	
	• Encourage communicating with peers when unable to attend school.	• Peer contacts help the child in normal developmental tasks.	
	• Work with teachers to support reentry to school. Use puppets, videotape, and discussion with classmates.	• Classmates need to understand what has happened to their friend without asking the child directly.	
5. Fatigue related to disease state			
	NIC Priority Intervention: **Energy Management:** *Regulating energy use to prevent fatigue and optimize function.*		*NOC Suggested Outcome:* **Energy Conservation:** *Extent of management of energy to initiate and sustain activity.*
The child will maintain energy levels necessary for normal activities.	• Problem solve ways to save energy for play and school.	• The child and parents are assisted to see school and play as important.	The child plans use of time effectively to maintain energy for school and play.
	• Plan with child for quiet activities during low-energy times.	• Child is empowered to select and plan own activities.	The child conserves energy during times of increased fatigue.
6. Interrupted Family Processes related to situational crisis			
	NIC Priority Intervention: **Family Process Maintenance:** *Minimization of family process disruption events.*		*NOC Suggested Outcome:* **Family Process:** *Extent of maintenance of family support system.*
The child and family will demonstrate healthy adaptation.	• Encourage open communication.	• Open discussion allows problem solving and ego support.	Parents report better communication between themselves and the children.
	• Suggest that all family members develop support networks.	• Network expands support systems.	Family members report an increase in friends with whom they can share feelings.
	• Parents should be proactive with siblings about their feelings and needs.	• Siblings feel valued and problems are confronted early.	
	• Encourage attendance of all family members at oncology camps.	• Oncology camps promote open discussion between peers for further support and fun.	Family reports attending oncology camp and describe benefit of sharing with other families in same situation.

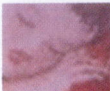

FAMILIES WANT TO KNOW

Nutrition and the Child with Cancer

Because of the effects of cancer and chemotherapy or other treatment, the child often has a poor appetite. Mucosal sores lead to difficulty chewing and swallowing. Parents can enhance the child's nutritional intake in the following ways.

- Provide frequent small feedings rather than three meals daily.
- Integrate the child's favorite foods into daily menus.
- Have nutritious snacks available for times when the child feels like eating.
- Sprinkle dried milk on top of cereals and other foods.
- Serve smooth, soft foods. Milkshakes with added peanut butter, puddings, and soft casseroles may be well tolerated and preferred. Try a variety of liquid protein-calorie supplements to find those the child likes.
- Avoid making food an area for disagreement. Do not force foods, but make them readily available.

- If the child is vomiting due to therapy, do not encourage food at that time. Food aversions may develop to foods that are vomited.
- Administer antiemetics as ordered during therapy because they can prevent nausea and vomiting.
- Report weight loss and increased fatigue.
- Bring the child in for scheduled health visits so growth, development, and effects of therapy can be monitored.
- Request a temporary feeding tube to ensure adequate nutrition. Feedings at night can often increase intake and promote health. Occasionally a central line is inserted to provide total parenteral nutrition.
- Recognize that supplements and tube feedings will usually be covered by insurance if the provider writes an order for them.

CLINICAL TIP

Several precautions must be taken during administration of chemotherapy drugs. Usually the child receiving intravenous medications has a central line or implantable port. The line is maintained carefully; if any drugs are given through a peripheral line, extreme caution and frequent monitoring is used to prevent extravasation, which can seriously injure tissues. Likewise, healthcare providers must avoid inadvertent contact with these potent drugs. The Occupational Safety and Health Administration (OSHA) publishes an instruction manual entitled *Controlling Occupational Exposure to Hazardous Drugs* that outlines general guidelines, protective equipment, and procedures.

MediaLink

OSHA

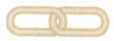

Administration of Medication: Calculation

The goals of nutrition therapy during treatment for cancer are to prevent or reverse any nutritional deficiencies, preserve the child's lean body mass, minimize any side effects that influence nutritional state, allow for the child's growth needs, and improve overall quality of life (Eldridge, 2004). Administer antiemetic drugs to lessen nausea from chemotherapy. Offer frequent, small meals. It may be helpful to offer the child's favorite foods at times when nausea and vomiting are decreased. Ask the family what treatments they use to decrease the child's nausea and vomiting. Perform 24-hour dietary recalls to assess the child's intake, and evaluate height and weight regularly. Special nutritional products may be given orally, nasogastric or nasoduodenal tube feedings may be given, or total parenteral nutrition may be necessary. When the child's nutritional status is deteriorating or parenteral nutrition is used, perform weekly studies of serum electrolytes, liver chemistry, glucose, and triglycerides. Partner with both the oncologist and the dietitian to plan interventions appropriate for meeting the needs of individual children.

Palliative care is administered when a child is not expected to be cured. Nutritional support becomes especially important during this time to improve quality of life, enhance comfort, and support the immune system. Children should be offered foods that they like and which are easy to eat. Soft, non-spicy foods like puddings, eggs, and purées offer qualities like high energy density as well as ease in consumption and digestion. Ensure adequate fluids and supplement fluids with powdered milk or energy supplements.

Administer Medications

One important intervention of the oncology nurse is administering medications safely. Most chemotherapeutic drugs are prescribed and calculated as dose per meter squared (dose/m^2), with m^2 calculated from the child's height and weight. (Refer to the section on administering medications in the *Clinical Skills Manual*.)

Several chemotherapeutic drugs are often used in combinations (see Table 23–2). These drugs are prepared with special techniques under laminar flow devices to minimize potential toxic effects on healthcare providers. Gloves and other hazardous drug protocols are used. Care must be taken to avoid **extravasation** of intravenous drugs (leakage into the soft tissue around the infusion site), as this can cause permanent tissue damage.

Special techniques such as generous hydration and accompanying medications help to decrease side effects. In addition to chemotherapy drugs, the nurse administers other medications, such as antiemetics to control nausea, vitamin supplements, and antibiotics. Antiemetics such as oldansetron are given prophylactically when a cancer agent is administered that has known emetic effects. Parents are asked about complementary therapy and medications they are obtaining from other sources and using at home. All medications must be safely administered and the child should be monitored for side effects. **Polypharmacy** (the use of several drugs at one time to treat multiple health conditions) can lead to multiple side effects and can challenge the body's ability to metabolize and excrete drugs.

Parents and children must become well informed about the drugs to be administered and the side effects that may occur. Telephone numbers, web sites and other resources are needed for provision of information when questions arise. Inform the family about the phases of drug trials if the child is asked to participate. The phases of clinical drug trials are:

Phase 1—This is the first clinical trial to involve people; it seeks to answer the question: "Is the treatment safe?" It is the phase with the greatest risk since the drug has not previously been tested in people.

Phase 2—Once a drug is found to be reasonably safe, phase 2 trials seek to establish its effectiveness.

Phase 3—If a drug is found to be generally safe and effective, in phase 3 it is compared to other standard treatments. It seeks to ask if it is better than what is already available. After this phase, the Food and Drug Administration deliberates and decides if the drug should be approved.

Phase 4—The approved drug is still tested in phase 4 to determine if there are better ways to prescribe it, regarding dosage, length of treatment, and other factors (American Cancer Society, 2004).

Manage Treatment Side Effects

All cancer treatments affect some normal body cells as well as cancer cells, causing a wide variety of side effects. A frequent occurrence is **myelosuppression**, or suppression of blood cell production in the bone marrow. Be alert for signs of a decreased white blood cell count, such as infections. **Neutropenia** is present when the absolute neutrophil count (ANC) is < 500 cells/mm^3 or if between 500–1000 cells/mm^3 when chemotherapy is being given and falling levels are anticipated. At these levels, children will be given a broad-spectrum antibiotic; granulocyte colony-stimulating factor (G-CSF) may also be given (see Table 23–2 and the medications table on page 852) (Bryant, 2003). Take the child's temperature, isolate the child from others with infections, and perform serum laboratory studies as ordered. See Clinical Manifestations of Common Side Effects of Chemotherapy.

Protect the child from bruises and be alert for signs of bleeding such as petechiae, nosebleeds, dark colored or bloody stools, and presence of blood in vomit and urine. These are all effects of decreased platelets. When thrombocytopenia occurs, minimize needlesticks and other intrusive procedures. Be ready to deal with nosebleeds and watch for bleeding gums. Report any bleeding episodes to the physician. Be sure parents know that the child should avoid contact sports or other rough activities and that any health-care provider, such as a dentist, should be informed of the child's treatment and condition (Bryant, 2003). Infusions to increase platelets are sometimes administered.

Inadequate red blood cell production can result in anemia. Encourage the child to eat iron-rich foods and administer nutritional supplements, as needed. Blood transfusions are sometimes required to treat severe anemia.

Chemotherapy affects all rapidly growing cells in the body, but especially those of the mucous membranes. Evaluate the effects of hair loss on the child. Provide good oral hygiene with a soft toothbrush, foam wand, or water irrigation device. Report oral breakdown promptly. (See Families Want to Know: Oral Care.) Be alert for blood in vomitus and stool, which can be indicators of bleeding in the gastrointestinal tract.

Radiation can cause burns to the skin. Examine the skin daily during hospitalization or weekly when making home visits. Leave the marks on the skin that outline the radiation target area. Avoid use of lotions, powders, and soaps on the target skin area. Some children may need to be anesthetized to ensure correct positioning for radiation; postanesthesia care will then be needed.

NURSING ALERT

A treatment known as *leucovorin rescue* is used in conjunction with high-dose methotrexate chemotherapy. Leucovorin (citrovorum factor) is a form of folic acid that helps to protect normal cells from the destructive action of methotrexate. It is started within 24 hours of methotrexate administration and is given along with hydration therapy. Usual administration is every 6 hours X 72 hours or until serum methotrexate is at the desired level.

LAW & ETHICS

Clinical Trials

When unapproved investigational drugs are given in a clinical trial, consent by parents is mandatory. They should know the potential benefits and harm to the child. Children who are cognitively able should also give assent verbally or in writing. This assent can usually be obtained from children by the age of 7–9 years, depending on the child's level of understanding. Conferences that are held with the families, including children, to discuss the disease and potential treatments, identify risks and benefits of treatment, and ensure that the choices are voluntarily made are an important part of oncology practice (Chappuy, Doz, Blanche et al., 2006). Even when the family has given consent for a clinical trial, they may have additional questions. Nurses can clarify information and refer the family to the research investigator for further explanations.

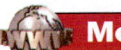
MediaLink

Care Plan Activity: The Child Undergoing Chemotherapy

CLINICAL MANIFESTATIONS | COMMON SIDE EFFECTS OF CHEMOTHERAPY

Side Effect	Manifestations	Clinical Therapy
Bone marrow suppression	Evidence of suppression usually appears 7–10 days after administration of chemotherapy recovery is usually complete within 3–4 weeks	Blood transfusions are administered when anemia is severe (Hgb, 7 g/dL) or platelets are very low Some institutions use a low microbial to decrease the possibility that infections organisms will colonize the intestine Septra is used for pneumocystis carinii pneumonia prophylaxis; nystatin and oral vancomycin for antifungal and antibacterial prophylaxis Instruct the family and child about the importance of protecting the body from bruising during periods of mild to moderate thrombocytopenia (platelet count, < 5,000/mm^3) Careful handwashing is essential Encourage use of masks if family or staff have nasopharyngeal infections
Nausea and vomiting	Symptoms may occur immediately or 5–6 hours after administration of chemotherapy and may last 48 hours	Antiemetics, such as antaneutron, Kytril, Raglan, and Benadryl are used to treat this side effect Teach relaxation techniques, hypnosis, and systematic desensitization (a hypnotic process that progressively reduces reactions to objects that cause strong emotional or physical responses) to help to decrease the child's symptoms Encourage mild exercise and change of diet (eating only easily digestible foods) 12 hours before chemotherapy
Anorexia and weight loss	May occur at any time	Hyperalimentation is necessary if dietary changes are unsuccessful in halting the child's weight loss Pay careful attention to changes in taste that affect food preferences Referral to a dietician may be helpful to achieve successful modification of the child's diet
Mouth sores	The oral mucositis resulting from chemotherapy usually occurs within 3–4 days and is often a contributing factor in anorexia	Antifungal agents, such as nystatin or clotrimazole, lessen the possibility of candidal infection Promote good oral hygiene, use soft foam wand or water irrigation to clean teeth; commercial mouthwashes are not recommended because they contain alcohol and increase drying of the oral cavity
Constipation	Can occur at any time in treatment but becomes more common as therapy progresses and dietary intake and physical activity decrease	Stool softeners and laxatives are used to treat this side effect Advise parents to increase fluids and fibrous foods in the child's diet
Pain	Pain can occur at any time and is best understood by subjective explanations of the child.	Acetaminophen, morphine, steroids, nonsteroidal anti-inflammatory drugs, and antidepressants may be used to manage pain Careful pain assessment is important; the location of the pain may provide a clue to its cause, for example, metastasis to the skull, infiltration of joints, or damage to soft tissue; pain associated with chemotherapy may also be related to oral mucositis, myalgia, or tumor embolization; painful polyneuropathy can follow treatment with vincristine or cisplatin Acetaminophen for pain can mask the presence of fever, which signals infection; careful and complete physical assessment is needed to identify infection Pharmacologic, nonhypnotic (deep breathing, self-control), and hypnotic methods often prove helpful to children with pain from multiple etiologies.

Ensure Adequate Hydration

Hydration management can be a challenge as the child may not be thirsty but is excreting large numbers of cell fragments and other substances as a result of treatment. Offer frequent small amounts of fluid. Include frozen ice pops or other fluid-containing foods such as Jell-O. Measure intake and output. To ensure adequate excretion, a number of chemotherapy drugs are given with intravenous fluids. It is important to administer fluids as ordered, monitor intravenous lines carefully, and ensure that the recommended urinary output excretion rate is maintained after drug administration.

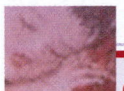

FAMILIES WANT TO KNOW

Oral Care

Since cancer treatment and poor nutritional status can adversely affect the oral status of children, families need help to plan and carry out prophylactic and treatment measures. Children continue to lose teeth, have new teeth erupt, and require nutrients to help in building teeth not yet erupted, even during cancer treatment. Some suggestions are:

- Provide a visit to the dentist early in treatment for assessment, treatment of dental disease, and to establish a prevention plan.
- Floss and brush teeth twice daily with a soft bristle brush and rinse with water. Use mouthwash as prescribed (normal saline or chlorhexidine are most common).
- Toothpaste can be used unless it causes discomfort.

- Avoid hot, spicy foods and choose mild flavors and soft textures.
- When granulocyte counts fall below 500/mm^3 or platelets fall below 40,000/mm^3, toothettes or gauze can be used to clean the teeth. Avoiding brushes will help to prevent bleeding and infection.
- Medications may be used to prevent infection. They may include antibacterial mouthwash, antibacterial lozenges and suspension to treat mucositis. Continue oral fluoride if it is not present in the drinking water.
- If bleeding, infection, or other oral care needs emerge, consult with the dentist and pediatric oncologist to develop a treatment plan.

Adapted from Wohlschlaeger, 2004.

Prevent and Treat Infection

Children with cancer have an altered immune system, both from the disease and from the effects of immunosuppressant drugs, and must be kept away from persons with known infections. Teach parents to avoid taking the child to places that attract large gatherings of people, such as department stores, once the child returns home. Emphasize the need to report any exposure to contagious diseases, especially chickenpox. Signs of infection may be masked by some drugs, so be alert for any signs of mild infection. Fever, malaise, and mild respiratory infection must be reported promptly. Follow recommendations for the immunization of children with cancer as published by the Centers for Disease Control and Prevention and the American Academy of Pediatrics. Usually no immunizations are given to the child until 6 months after receiving chemotherapy. Immunity may be lost from some prior immunizations, requiring titer levels and repeat immunization later.

Teach administration of any drugs being used to prevent infection such as pentamadine or sulfa preparations for pneumocystis pneumonia prophylaxis. Management of infections is critical. Children are often hospitalized, and central lines are used for antibiotic administration. Blood cultures and cultures of infected body parts help to establish the causative organisms. Due to lowered immune status, unusual organisms are sometimes identified. Administer medication treatment on time and as ordered. Ensure standard precautions and transmission-based precautions are followed. Temperature, vital signs, and assessment of all body systems are performed at admission and at least every 4 hours. (See Families Want to Know: Reportable Events for Children Receiving Chemotherapy.)

RESEARCH

Cancer and Immunizations
Children being treated for cancer are known to have low immune response to many immunizations. Special schedules that may include titer levels to determine immune status are recommended. Researchers studied immune response in 44 children with various types of cancer after immunization with the annual influenza vaccine. Protective titer rates were reached for 72% of the children. The vaccine was considered safe and protective. Children on chemotherapy and low white blood cell count had the lowest response rates (Matsuzaki, Suminoe, Koga et al., 2005). Nurses should consult the Centers for Disease Control and Prevention (CDC) to read the current recommendations each year for the administration of immunizations for children with cancer.

FAMILIES WANT TO KNOW

Reportable Events for Children Receiving Chemotherapy

Report the following events to your child's oncologist if they occur while the child is receiving chemotherapy:

- Temperature above 38°C (101°F)
- Any bleeding, such as nosebleeds, blood in stool or urine, petechiae, bruising
- Pain or discomfort with urination or defecation
- Sores in the mouth
- Vomiting or diarrhea
- Persistent pain anywhere, including headache

- Signs of infection, such as cough, fever, runny nose, tugging at ears
- Signs of infection in central lines, such as redness, drainage, or tenderness
- Exposure to communicable diseases, especially varicella (chickenpox)

Inform dentists and other healthcare providers that the child is receiving chemotherapy prior to procedures. Prophylactic antibiotics should be given before and after dental care.

Note: Adapted from Bindler, R. M., & Howry, L. B. (2005). *Pediatric drug guide.* Upper Saddle River, NJ: Prentice Hall.

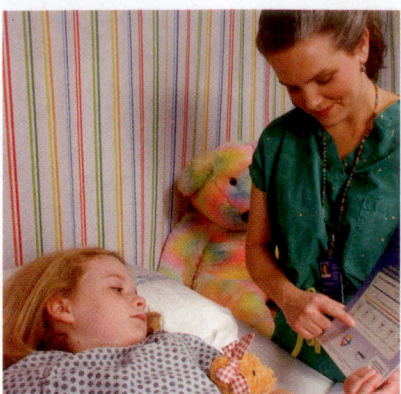

Figure 23–11 ➤ The nurse is having the child rate her pain by pointing to the face that most closely matches the way she feels. Note her stuffed animals that provide comfort.

COMPLEMENTARY THERAPY

Pain Management

Children have many painful and invasive procedures during cancer treatment. In addition to use of medication, they will be helped by a variety of other pain management techniques. These include:

- Parent's presence during procedures as a support person.
- Use of distraction and relaxation. Either a parent or healthcare provider can work with the child and integrate techniques, such as singing, counting, telling stories, and blowing bubbles. Children and teens can be taught to visualize positive scenes, use rhythmic breathing, or listen to music (Tsao & Zeltzer, 2005).
- Hypnosis has been used successfully to manage both pain and nausea/vomiting during cancer treatment with children from 5–18 years (Richardson, Smith, McCall, & Pilkington, 2006).

Manage Pain

The child with cancer may experience pain from the disease itself and from the medical interventions, such as lumbar puncture, bone marrow aspiration, and frequent intravenous infusions and blood draws. Use all possible pain management techniques to keep the child comfortable, as this will assist with comfort and encourage cooperation throughout the long treatment period. (See Chapter 15 ∞ for suggestions on methods of pain management.) Nurses must examine research on effective pain management for children and integrate findings into practice (Figure 23–11 ➤).

Sedation (see Chapter 15 ∞) may be used for some procedures. Administer sedation as ordered for young children who are undergoing lumbar punctures, radiation, and other procedures. Coordinate painful or intrusive tests so they can be done together while the child is sedated. Topical anesthetics such as EMLA cream may be used to numb the skin before a blood draw or an intravenous start.

When possible, include the parents in comforting the child during and after painful procedures. Find what techniques work at home to relieve pain and insert them into care of the child in the health facility.

Provide Psychosocial Support

A diagnosis of cancer generates many emotions within the family. Initially parents experience shock and anger. They need basic information about the disease and the purpose of the tests that will be performed. Instructions often need to be repeated as parents may not process information the first time it is presented due to their increased stress levels. Assist the parents to plan how and when to tell the child the diagnosis. What the child needs to know is based on his or her developmental level and understanding.

After progressing from the initial state of shock about the diagnosis, the family needs to learn more about the disease, including the pathophysiology, treatment, and expected outcome or the prognosis. Clarify the family's understanding of these areas and be ready to answer questions. Provide verbal explanations and written material. Parents may talk with friends, purchase books, or search the Internet for information. Find out where they are getting information and provide additional resources when appropriate. Correct misconceptions and misinformation.

The family needs many strategies to deal with the challenge of long-term treatment for cancer. As the child experiences remissions and exacerbations or complications, the family feels alternately hopeful and discouraged. (See Evidence-Based Practice: Cancer and Stress.) Help the family to identify support systems and intervene as needed to enhance these systems. Facilitate contact with extended family members who might be of help, faith-based or spiritual connections, social service agencies, and other resources such as the Internet and parent support groups. Assist parents who are

CLINICAL TIP

EMLA cream, or eutectic mixture of local anesthetics, is a combination of lidocaine 2.5% and prilocaine 2.5% in an emulsion. Apply a thick layer of the cream to intact skin and cover with an occlusive dressing. Leave in place 1 hour for minor procedures and 2 hours for major procedures. Do not use EMLA on infants who are a gestational age of less than 37 weeks, under 20 kg, or in those under 12 months receiving treatment with methemoglobin-inducing agents. For all infants, be certain that parents realize the importance of limiting the area and duration as ordered and to keep the cream in a safe place in the home to avoid ingestion by any children.

Another measure that can be effective for local anesthetic delivery is iontophoresis. A low-voltage electrical current is applied to intact skin in the area needing anesthesia. The current forces drug molecules (commonly lidocaine hydrochloride and epinephrine) across the stratum corneum. The local anesthetic is effective in approximately 10–15 minutes and has been tested for safety in children as young as 5 years of age (Pasero, 2006).

Some fast-acting sprays are available for even more minor anesthesia. Intradermal injection of anesthesia with lidocaine is generally used for more painful and invasive procedures such as central line insertion. They may be combined with sedation to assist the child to relax. Sedation monitoring protocols need to be followed.

concerned about job obligations and financial concerns. In addition, consider the impact on siblings when a child is being treated for cancer. They may alternately resent and feel guilty for the sibling's illness. They may not understand the treatments or disease. School progress may be slowed and teachers may not be aware of the sibling's stress.

The child undergoing treatment for cancer needs support appropriate to his or her developmental stage and cognitive level (Figure 23–12 ➤). (See Chapters 3 and 13 ∞ for developmental levels and effective support strategies for children of different ages.) Younger children primarily need support during painful procedures and separation from parents. They need to learn about procedures and feel comfortable touching the equipment that is used in their care. Older children also need intervention strategies to assist in working through feelings related to treatments (Figure 23–13 ➤). A major developmental task of adolescence is to attain independence and control, but cancer often interferes with adolescents' ability to achieve this task. Therefore, plan nursing strategies that empower adolescents as much as possible.

Talk with the child's teachers before he or she returns to school after treatment to explain the child's condition. Arrange for tutors if necessary to assist the child with school work during hospitalization and home care. Explore the option of summer camp for children with cancer. The Make-a-Wish Foundation strives to make dreams come true for ill children by sponsoring them for a desired activity or outing. Refer the child to this foundation, if appropriate.

The siblings of a child who has cancer can be stressed by the changes in the family. They may grieve over the ill brother or sister and may feel sad and depressed. They also can experience anger, guilt, or resentment and may have a lack of knowledge about the disease and treatment. Inquire about siblings and ask what they know about the child's condition. Find out who is caring for siblings and whether their teachers have been informed about the family situation. Include siblings in the child's care when possible. Invite them to visit and to participate both during hospitalization and at home care visits. They can be involved in play therapy sessions and recreational activities with the ill child. Ask the parents if the siblings are demonstrating symptoms such as depression, behavioral changes, or decrease in school performance and suggest interventions as appropriate.

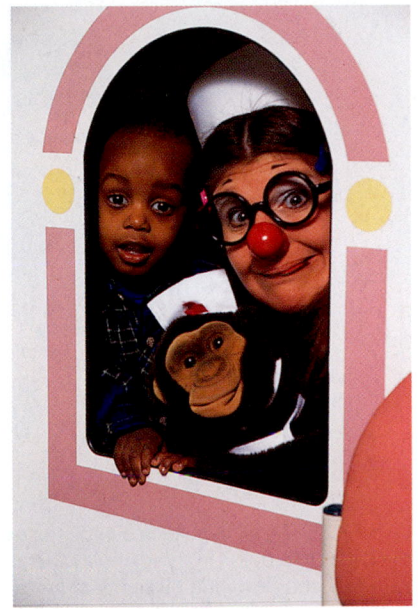

Figure 23–12 ➤ Clowns from the Big Apple Clown Care Unit can help to ease the stress of hospitalization for seriously ill children and their families. Here, a clown doctor and her puppet distract a toddler who is waiting for his clinic appointment.

EVIDENCE-BASED PRACTICE

Cancer and Stress

Problem

The family of a child with cancer experiences profound stress, and each member of the family needs time and support to adjust to the new roles they must take on in the family. However, the needs of family members are often overlooked as the ill child becomes the center of treatment and attention. Family members often provide care for the child, which can be emotionally and physically draining, and can also deplete family financial resources.

Evidence

Major changes in the family were identified by a research study that interviewed family members when a child was diagnosed with leukemia (McGrath, Paton, & Huff, 2005). They included:
- Relocation to be closer to the treatment center
- Interruption of normal activities of daily life for family members
- Placing life "on hold" and deferring usual activities, such as classes and vacations
- Readjustment to home when the child improves and the family resumes usual living patterns
- Concerns related to school and employment for family members
- Financial difficulties

In another study, parents in 86 families that had a child with cancer focused on the needs of the 159 well siblings in those families. About 50% of the parents stated that they anticipated that the well siblings would manifest some problems because of the diagnosis of cancer. Parents frequently observed depression or withdrawal among the siblings, and believed that they had received inadequate information about how to support and help the siblings. Difficulty in scheduling times for the sibling to come to the treatment center and learn more about the cancer treatment was noted. A weekend intervention program for siblings was instituted to offer activities and counseling designed to support siblings. The peer support of meeting with others was helpful to the children (Ballard, 2004).

Implications

Being a family member when a child has cancer is a stressful event. Both parents and siblings express a need for information about the ill child's condition and treatment. Nurses should provide information at each health encounter and frequently ask what questions the family members have. Ask about siblings and include them in visits, whenever possible. Plan peer support group sessions for the siblings so they can discuss their experiences and feelings with other siblings. In addition to information, support is vital. Ask who the parents and siblings have told about the ill child. Who can they turn to when they want to talk? Who can the parents call upon for help at home? Who can the siblings invite to school performances and other events if the parents are unable to attend?

Critical Thinking

Consider the opening scenario that describes Sam, who has leukemia, and his family. What information do his parents need? How can you best support his older siblings?

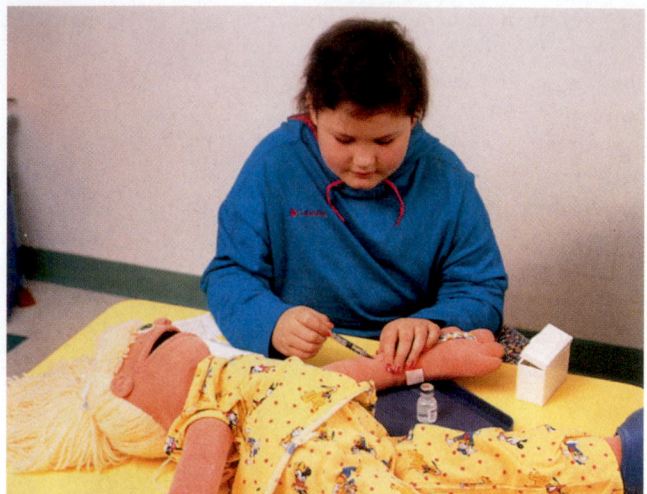

Figure 23–13 ➤ A child in a pediatric oncology clinic is giving injections to a doll. This type of play therapy helps the child deal with fear, thus lowering his or her stress level.

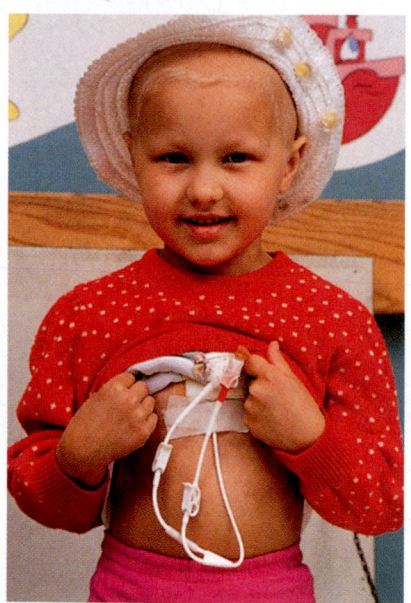

Figure 23–14 ➤ A vascular access device allows chemotherapeutic agents to be administered without the need for repeated "sticks" to the child.

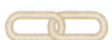

SKILL 9–8:
Caring for a Central Venous Catheter Site

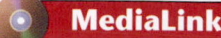

MediaLink

Health Promotion and Maintenance: The Child with Cancer

They may benefit from speaking with a school counselor or can be referred to a support group for siblings of children with cancer. Some cancer summer camps welcome siblings as well as children with cancer.

The family of a child with cancer is faced with a life-threatening illness. Refer to Chapter 14 ∞ for strategies to assist the family in coping with this stress. For some types of cancer, the child may experience a remission with treatment, but then a recurrence of disease later as cancer cells grow again. In this case, the family may become angry or depressed about the relapse. Repeated treatments challenge the family's support systems. Waiting for the outcome of diagnostic tests can be an especially challenging time, so provide information as soon as possible. If the child's illness progresses, refer the family to hospice to assist them in caring for the terminally ill child and in working through the grieving process. Explore support groups and information related to cancer in order to share this information with families as well.

Care in the Community

Preparation for home care centers on creating a normal environment while supporting the child's physiologic and psychosocial responses to the cancer and treatments. Education is the primary focus of discharge planning. Teach the parents how to ensure adequate nutritional intake, to be alert for signs of infection, to protect the child from exposure to communicable diseases during times of neutropenia, to administer medications at home, and to handle vomiting and pain. Assist the parents and child to deal with any obstacles to normal development and functioning. Teach the parents and family about symptoms that need to be treated immediately.

Home management of a vascular access device or central line, such as a Broviac catheter (refer to the *Clinical Skills Manual*), is an initial challenge for parents (Figure 23–14 ➤). Alternatively, an implanted port may be used and allows the child freedom to swim and engage in other activities. Parents will need information about whatever device the child has received. Details about cleaning the site, keeping the line open, and other needed care are demonstrated and reviewed. After teaching the parents, observe them performing the procedure before the child is discharged.

Emphasize the need for the child and family to have usual family activities, including recreational activities. Play distracts the child and is essential in reducing fears. Children, parents, and siblings often benefit from participation in cancer support groups and cancer summer camps. These activities create additional support systems, build the child's self-esteem, and enhance coping skills through role modeling.

Make home visits to evaluate the family's strengths and needs. Be sure that the family has adequate support from a hospice and other end-of-life services when the child's condition is terminal. The presence of a palliative care team; an integrated plan of care; collaboration between families, the primary care provider, and other practitioners; and focus on the child's developmental level and the needs of the family can enhance the care provided for the dying child.

Health Promotion and Health Maintenance

Treatment for cancer is generally a long process; most children are treated for a period of 2–3 years. Since normal developmental stages progress during this time, health promotion and health maintenance visits should still occur. Some usual care may have to be altered, but many of the same developmental concerns of all children should be addressed. Help parents to view the child as a "normal" child who is ill for a period of time, but still needs to have limits set on behavior, develop healthy lifestyles, and have environmental stimulation to learn to talk, read, or perform motor and cognitive tasks.

After the treatment is complete, the child should be closely monitored for any sequelae of cancer survivorship (see the section earlier in the chapter about issues of survivorship). The possibility of treatment-related physical and psychological side effects necessitates clear instructions to the family, with increasing information provided to the child as cognitive development proceeds. Periodic laboratory and diagnostic tests may be needed, in addition to thorough physical and psychological examinations. Guidelines for healthcare professionals and survivors have been developed by the Children's Oncology Group, and vary according to the type of cancer and the therapies received (Children's Oncology Group, 2004). When the child transfers to the care of a healthcare professional that serves adults, provide a clear and complete summary of the cancer and treatment so that appropriate follow-up can be maintained (Florin & Hinkle, 2005).

Evaluation

The following expected outcomes of nursing care for the child with cancer relate to the specific disease, treatments, and responses:

- The child has adequate nutritional intake to promote normal growth.
- Hydration is adequate to support body processes and ensure drug and cancer cell product elimination.
- Side effects of the cancer and therapies are promptly identified and treated.
- Pain is managed to a level of comfort satisfactory to the child and family.
- The family uses resources to provide necessary support during hospitalizations and treatments.
- The child and family demonstrate knowledge of management needed for treatment regimens.
- All family members accept the prognosis in order to support the child.

Brain Tumors

Central nervous system or brain tumors are the most commonly occurring solid tumors in children and the second most common malignancy, after leukemia. Each year approximately 3200 children and adolescents in the United States are diagnosed with tumors of the brain and central nervous system, accounting for one in five childhood cancers (American Cancer Society, 2005; Ryan-Murray & Petriccione, 2002).

Etiology and Pathophysiology

While a few cases are associated with other diseases, the cause of most brain tumors is unknown. An association may exist between parents who work in the aircraft or agricultural industry, or among paints, solvents, radiation, and electromagnetic fields, and the higher incidence of brain tumors in children (Ryan-Murray & Petriccione, 2002).

Brain tumors in children usually occur below the roof of the cerebellum and involve the cerebellum, midbrain, and brainstem (Figure 23–15 ➤). In contrast, brain tumors in adults are usually located above the areas between the cerebrum and cerebellum.

The most common brain tumors in children are medulloblastoma, cerebral and cerebellar astrocytoma, ependymoma (from the ependymal cells lining the brain ventricles and spinal canal), and gliomas of the cerebrum or brainstem. Less common are supratentorial embryonal tumors and craniopharyngioma.

Clinical Manifestations

Brain tumors in children can be manifested by behavioral and nervous system changes that occur either rapidly or more slowly and subtly. Some common symptoms include headache (most common manifestation), nausea, vomiting, dizziness, change in vision or hearing, fatigue, and mental status changes, such as educational or behavioral problems (Wilne, Ferris, Nathwani, & Kennedy, 2006). See the clinical manifestations table for common manifestations of certain types of tumors. Brainstem tumors can present with weight deficits, and may be mistakenly diagnosed as an eating disorder of infancy and childhood (failure to thrive). This may delay proper treatment. See Clinical Manifestations of Brain Tumors on the next page.

Medulloblastomas, brain tumors in the external layer of the cerebellum, account for 20% of childhood brain tumors, and commonly occur in children ages 5 to 6 years.

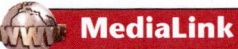
MediaLink

Cancer Guidelines

CLINICAL TIP

Some children with brain tumors have nonspecific signs. They may have a slight behavior change, perform poorly at school, or show some incoordination. Be alert to such signs and to the parents' statement that they notice a change in the child. Report such findings so appropriate assessments can be made.

PATHOPHYSIOLOGY ILLUSTRATED

Sites of Brain Tumors in Children

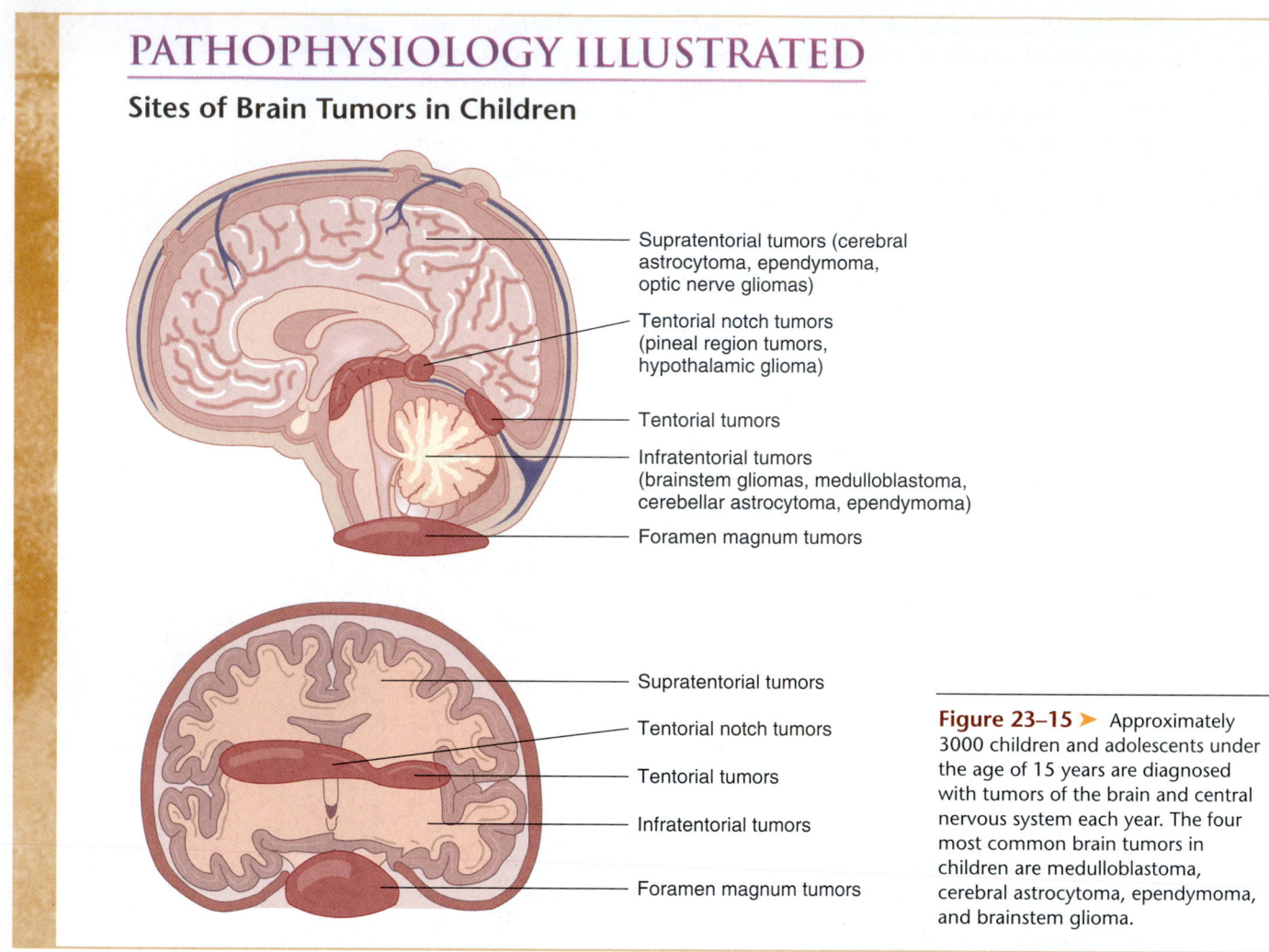

Supratentorial tumors (cerebral astrocytoma, ependymoma, optic nerve gliomas)

Tentorial notch tumors (pineal region tumors, hypothalamic glioma)

Tentorial tumors

Infratentorial tumors (brainstem gliomas, medulloblastoma, cerebellar astrocytoma, ependymoma)

Foramen magnum tumors

Supratentorial tumors

Tentorial notch tumors

Tentorial tumors

Infratentorial tumors

Foramen magnum tumors

Figure 23–15 ➤ Approximately 3000 children and adolescents under the age of 15 years are diagnosed with tumors of the brain and central nervous system each year. The four most common brain tumors in children are medulloblastoma, cerebral astrocytoma, ependymoma, and brainstem glioma.

They are fast growing and therefore often present with sudden onset of symptoms such as increased intracranial pressure, manifested by increased head circumference in infants, vomiting, headache, ataxia, and vision changes. Astrocytomas arise from glial cells and can be either above or below the area between the cerebrum and cerebellum. They comprise 40% of childhood brain tumors, and vary from low-grade cerebellar to low-grade cerebral or high-grade tumors. The presenting symptoms vary depending on the location of the tumor. Endocrine, vision, and behavioral changes are all possible, as well as increased intracranial pressure and seizures. Ependymomas commonly

CLINICAL MANIFESTATIONS | BRAIN TUMORS

Tumor	Etiology	Clinical Manifestations	Clinical Therapy
Medulloblastoma	External layer of cerebellum	Headache, vomiting, ataxia	Surgery; chemotherapy with lomustine, vincristine, prednisone, cisplatin, radiation
Astrocytomas	Glial cells, supratentorial or infratentorial	Seizures, visual disturbances, increased intracranial pressure, vomiting	Surgery; chemotherapy with vincristine, dactinomycin; radiation
Ependymoma	Fourth ventricle, posterior fossa	Hydrocephalus	Surgery, radiation
Brainstem gliomas	Pons	Cranial nerve (VI and VII) tract signs, nystagmus, ataxia, motor symptoms	Surgery, radiation

occur in the fourth ventricle of the posterior fossa and comprise 10% of childhood brain tumors. Impaired growth, hydrocephalus, seizures, and cranial nerve impairments are the most common manifestations. Brainstem gliomas are located in the pons and typically spread into the surrounding tissue. Gliomas, which can occur in the brainstem or as supratentorial lesions, account for 6.5% of all brain tumors in children (Tamber & Rutka, 2003). Cranial nerve impairments, mental status changes, seizures, and motor symptoms occur.

COLLABORATIVE CARE

Diagnostic Tests

The first step in diagnosing brain tumors is a detailed health history and physical examination. Onset of symptoms, severity, and presentation of neurological symptoms is recorded. Brain tumors are then definitively diagnosed by means of computed tomography (CT; Figure 23–16A ➤), magnetic resonance imaging (MRI; Figure 23–16B ➤), positron emission tomography (PET), single-photon emission computed tomography (SPECT), myelography, and angiography. These tests are used to assess sensory pathway integrity and disease- or drug-related sensory dysfunction. Other tests that may be performed are use of tumor markers such as α-fetoprotein and human chorionic gonadotropin. Analysis of DNA is also useful in some types of cancer when a genetic basis is related to the cancer type. Lumbar puncture is used to identify abnormal cells in the cerebrospinal fluid. Bone marrow aspiration identifies any extracranial primary neoplastic growth, as cancers in other sites can metastasize to the brain.

Clinical Therapy

Treatment depends on the type of brain tumor. Surgery is a common treatment, and may be performed to obtain a biopsy specimen, to debulk (reduce the tumor size by partial removal) or excise the tumor, or to treat any hydrocephalus that may be present. During surgery, radiology images allow the neurosurgeon to see computerized images of the brain while at the same time stimulating nerves to determine their functioning. These techniques provide rapid feedback to the neurosurgeon. Laser surgery, which has delicate precise control and accuracy, is used when tumors are close to sensitive neural or vascular structures.

Radiation is commonly used in the treatment of brain tumors. A combination of radiation and chemotherapy following surgery has improved the survival chances of children with medulloblastoma and ependymoma. Intrathecal administration of chemotherapy is useful in some cases. However, the blood-brain barrier is a factor in the effectiveness of chemotherapy for children with brain tumors. For example,

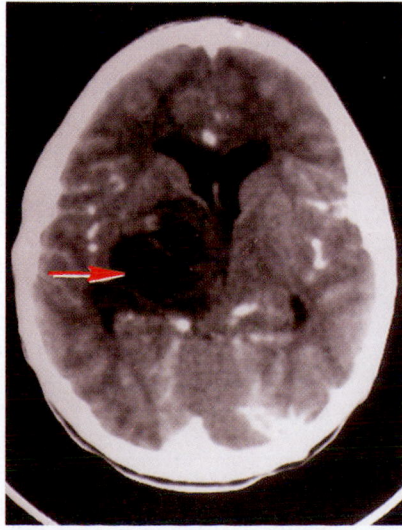
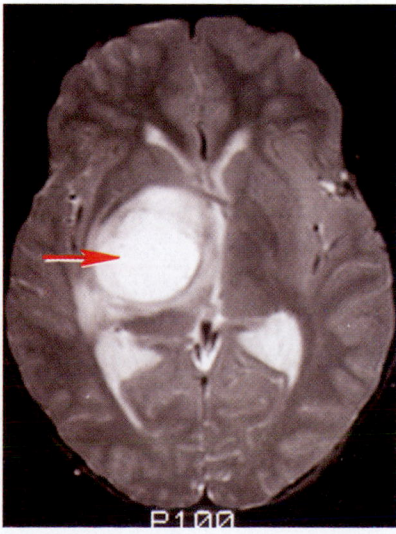

A   B

Figure 23–16 ➤ Radiologic imaging of a child with a brain tumor. A, CT scan. B, MRI.
Courtesy of Carlos Sivit, MD, Children's National Medical Center, Washington, DC.

when methotrexate is administered intrathecally (in the spinal canal), only a small amount crosses normal brain capillaries. Bone marrow and stem cell transplantation is an increasingly used treatment option.

Many new approaches are being investigated and some are expected to emerge as viable treatments in the years ahead. New combinations of chemotherapeutic agents, delivery of medications and radiation directly to the tumor, gene therapy, and cytokine-producing therapy to activate the immune system are examples of emerging treatments (Tamber & Rutka, 2003).

Complications of treatment for children with brain tumors are significant. They include severe infections (associated with high-dose chemotherapy), seizure activity, sensorimotor defects, hydrocephalus, and growth problems. Care is taken to treat infections early and aggressively. If a cerebrospinal shunt is used, infection or blockage can occur (see Chapter 26 ∞ for further discussion of cerebrospinal shunts in children). Anticonvulsants are commonly given prophylactically following surgery. Endocrine problems, such as growth hormone changes, hypothyroidism, and panhypopituitarism, may occur when the tumor is in the hypothalamic-pituitary area. Treatment may also lead to impaired cognitive function and emotional or behavioral problems in some children. Memory deficits and selective attention deficits are the most common problems.

Diabetes insipidus is a special consideration in children with midline brain tumors, such as those that compress the hypothalamus, pituitary stalk, or posterior pituitary gland. Manifestations of diabetes insipidus include voiding of large amounts of dilute urine with a specific gravity of less than 1.005 to 1.010 (see Chapter 29 ∞).

NURSING MANAGEMENT
Nursing Assessment and Diagnosis

The focus of physiologic assessment of the child with a brain tumor is determined by its presentation (Table 23–3). Presenting signs can be categorized as follows:

- Nonspecific signs related to increasing intracranial pressure
- Secondary signs related to displacement of intracranial structures
- Focal signs suggesting direct involvement of the brain and cranial nerves

Thorough neurologic examination before surgery is essential to provide a record of baseline functioning and allow the evaluation of the child's changing physiologic status before surgery. Ask if the child has manifested slow changes over time or has had quickly developing symptoms. Measurement of head circumference and assessment of the anterior fontanel are necessary in children under the age of 18 months.

Perform developmental screening on young children using the Denver II or other developmental test (see Chapter 7 ∞). Ask about the child's social interactions, school performance, and any behavior changes that have occurred.

Table 23–3	PHYSIOLOGIC ASSESSMENT OF BRAIN TUMORS	
Clinical Manifestations	**Assessment**
Nonspecific signs: headache, morning vomiting, somnolence, irritability	Level of consciousness, pupil response, pupil shape and size
Secondary signs: disturbances of cranial nerves; other signs depend on site of tumor	All cranial nerves
Focal signs: truncal ataxia (midline brain tumors), general nystagmus, head tilting	Motor ability, head positions when watching television or looking at people (double vision, sixth cranial nerve involvement)

The following nursing diagnoses can be identified for the child with a brain tumor, depending on the type and location of the tumor:

- Imbalanced Nutrition: Less than Body Requirements related to loss of appetite
- Impaired Physical Mobility related to tumor pressure on coordination centers
- Delayed Growth and Development related to effects of disability
- Impaired Memory related to neurologic disturbance
- Acute Pain related to tumor, diagnostic tests, and treatment

Planning and Implementation

The child with a brain tumor requires multidisciplinary care by a neurologist, neurosurgeon, pediatrician, dietitian, social worker, and other specialists. The nurse can act as a case manager to coordinate the complex care needed by the child and help the family to understand treatment.

For the nursing care of children immediately following surgery, refer to Chapter 13 ∞. In addition, close monitoring of neurologic status is needed postoperatively (refer to Chapter 26 ∞). Subtle alterations such as visual differences, behavior or alertness variations, and gait changes can herald serious problems from the tumor or pressure in the brain. Many children return from surgery with a ventricular-peritoneal shunt. Be especially alert for signs of increased intracranial pressure and infection. Observe for seizure activity. Administer drugs such as antibiotics and anticonvulsants as ordered.

Signs and symptoms of diabetes insipidus may occur following brain surgery (see Chapter 29 ∞ for a description of diabetes insipidus). Nursing care includes hourly measurement of intake and output, measurement of serum sodium levels every 4 to 6 hours, accurate fluid replacement, and frequent assessment of neurologic status. An indwelling urinary catheter is useful for accurate measurement of urinary output.

Discharge Planning and Home Care Teaching

Teach the parents to watch for an increase in voiding of dilute urine. Be sure they can recognize the signs of infection and changes in the child's neurologic status. Once the child is ready for discharge, chemotherapy or radiation may begin; inform parents of the reason and potential side effects of these treatments. Assist the family in obtaining any special equipment they may need to care for the child at home, such as a wheelchair, bed rails, or dressings. The American Cancer Society is a potential resource for assistance with these needs.

Children with brain tumors, especially those who have received radiation, often have some permanent sequelae. They may have slowed development, incoordination, learning disabilities, or other effects. These sequelae are most common in children who are 3 years of age or younger at the time of radiation therapy. Perform accurate height and weight measurements at each healthcare visit. Assess developmental milestones. Ask about progress in school and any special services that might be needed. Perform thorough neurologic assessments. Support the family as they learn to deal with unknown or changed expectations for the child's performance (Freeman, O'Dell, & Meola, 2003).

Evaluation

Expected outcomes of nursing care for the child with a brain tumor depend on the site of the tumor, clinical therapy, and medical outcome. Possible outcomes include the following:

- Nutritional intake will be adequate to support growth and prevent malnutrition.
- A safe environment will be maintained for the child.
- Physical mobility to maximum level allowed by developmental level and alterations of disease will be attained.
- An environment will be provided to meet normal developmental milestones within the child's capability.
- Pain will be successfully managed to reach a comfort level.
- Parents display understanding of the diagnosis and treatment plan.

RESEARCH

Concerns of Children with Brain Tumors and Their Siblings

In a study of 87 families, children with a brain tumor and their siblings were asked to identify their concerns. The main concerns of children with a tumor included:

- Keeping up with school work and special needs at school
- Changes in physical activity level
- Changes in appearance
- Mood variations
- Getting together with friends

Concerns of siblings included:

- Worry about what might happen to the ill sibling
- Keeping up with school work
- Information about cause of the tumor
- Help in dealing with the ill sibling regarding activity, mood, appearance, pain

For both groups, information by healthcare providers and support by family, friends, and clergy were identified as the most helpful factors (Freeman, O'Dell, & Meola, 2003). Nurses can ask both affected children and their siblings what their concerns are throughout the treatment. Provide information that they desire and facilitate supportive contact with friends and clergy.

Neuroblastoma

Neuroblastoma is the solid tumor most commonly occurring outside the cranium of children. It is responsible for 8–10% of childhood cancers and 15% of cancer deaths in children. The average age at onset is 22 months; it is the most common tumor in infants during the first year of life. Prognosis varies, depending on the staging of the tumor (Table 23–4) and the age of the child, with more favorable outcomes in infants under 1 year of age, and in presenting sites in the pelvis or thorax. Less favorable outcomes are associated with the presence of N-myc oncogen amplification. Survival rates are 98% for stages 1 and 2, but drop to 22% for stage 4 (Kim & Chung, 2006).

Neuroblastoma is commonly a smooth, hard, nontender mass that can occur anywhere along the sympathetic nervous system chain. A frequent location is the abdomen, although other sites are the adrenal, thoracic, and cervical areas. It is nearly unheard of after 10 years of age, and is usually diagnosed in children under 5 years of age, while the median age at diagnosis is 2 years (McManus & Gilchrist, 2004).

Etiology and Pathophysiology

Neuroblastoma originates in primitive neurocrest cells that form the adrenal medulla, paraganglia, and sympathetic nervous system of the cervical sympathetic chain and the thoracic chain. Fifty percent of neuroblastomas develop in the adrenal medulla, 20% develop in the thorax, and the remaining 30% are elsewhere along the sympathetic chain (McManus & Gilchrist, 2004). Lymph node metastasis is common.

The cause of neuroblastoma is unknown. Theories that have been proposed center on the possible effects of environmental factors such as prenatal drug exposure from the mother and disturbed cellular nerve growth factors. Canada has recently noted a drop in neuroblastoma rates commensurate with fortification of flour with folate (French, Grant, Weitzman, Ray, Vermeulen, Sung, Greenberg, & Koren, 2003). A genetic defect found in many cases of neuroblastoma is a deletion of the short arm of chromosome 1 (1p del). Oncogenes are present in neuroblastoma cells in a DNA sequence known as N-myc, located on chromosome 2. High levels of the N-myc oncogene are associated with rapid disease progression and a poorer prognosis (Kim & Chung, 2006).

Clinical Manifestations

The location of the mass determines the symptoms. Altered bowel and bladder function occur when the mass is retroperitoneal; characteristic signs are weight loss, abdominal fullness, irritability, fatigue, and fever. Dyspnea or infection may occur when

Table 23–4	INTERNATIONAL NEUROBLASTOMA STAGING SYSTEM
Stage	**Description**
1	Localized tumor confined to the area of origin; complete gross excision, with or without microscopic residual disease; identifiable ipsilateral and contralateral lymph nodes negative microscopically
2A	Unilateral tumor with incomplete gross excision; identifiable ipsilateral and contralateral lymph nodes negative microscopically
2B	Unilateral tumor with complete or incomplete gross excision; with positive ipsilateral regional lymph nodes; identifiable contralateral lymph nodes negative microscopically
3	Tumor infiltrating across the midline with or without regional lymph node involvement; or unilateral tumor with contralateral regional lymph node involvement; or midline tumor with bilateral regional lymph node involvement
4	Dissemination of tumor to distant lymph nodes, bone, bone marrow, liver, and/or other organs (except as defined in stage 4S)
4S	Localized primary tumor as defined for stage 1 or 2 with dissemination limited to liver, skin, and/or bone marrow

Note: Adapted from Castleberry, R.P. (1997). Biology and treatment of neuroblastoma. *Pediatric Clinics of North America, 44,* 919–938.

the tumor is mediastinal. Neck and facial edema may result from vena cava syndrome if the tumor is mediastinal and large. Intracranial lesions may be present with periorbital ecchymosis. Malaise, fever, and a limp can occur if there has been metastasis to the bone. Bone marrow disease can manifest as **pancytopenia** (abnormal depression of all cellular blood components) with neutropenia (causing infections) and anemia (causing fatigue). Metastatic spread can result in an array of symptoms affecting multiple organs.

COLLABORATIVE CARE

The International Neuroblastoma Staging System (INSS) recommends different diagnostic and laboratory evaluations for diagnosis of the primary disease and of metastases (Table 23–5).

Routine blood cell counts are needed, including CBC with differential. The test may reveal anemia and thrombocytopenia. There is no classic WBC response, although thrombocytopenia may occur in association with disseminated intravascular coagulation. **Leukocytosis** (higher than normal leukocyte count) and **leukopenia** (lower than normal leukocyte count) have been observed with bone marrow involvement. Serum electrolytes, liver function studies, LDH, coagulation studies, and urinalysis are performed. Baseline cardiac function is evaluated if doxorubicin will be used in treatment.

Tumor markers include VMA, HVA, dopamine, ferritin, NSE, LDH, and a ganglioside GD2. Vanillylmandelic acid (VMA) and homovanillic acid (HVA) are byproducts of adrenal hormones and their levels are usually elevated in the urine and blood (see Appendix C ∞ for normal values). Urinary catecholamines are increased. Elevations in dopamine, ferritin, NSE (an enzyme in neural tissue), LDH, and GD2 (a sugar and lipid molecule on the surface of neural cells) are seen. All of these laboratory findings are used initially to diagnose the disease and later to follow its progress. A biopsy or surgical removal of the tumor will be followed by analysis of its type and genetic abnormalities. Areas of necrosis and calcification in major organs are readily identifiable with radiologic tests and MRIs. These tests also help in the staging of the disease by identifying metastases.

Clinical Therapy

The stage of the tumor (see Table 23–4) determines the treatment protocol. Surgical excision of the mass is performed and may be the only treatment in low risk stages. With higher risk, surgery is followed by chemotherapy consisting of a combination of drugs. Several courses of chemotherapy may be needed prior to surgery when the mass is large or wrapped around major blood vessels. Chemotherapy may include:

- Cyclophosphamide
- Ifosfamide
- Doxorubicin
- Cisplatin
- Carboplatin
- Teniposide
- Etoposide

Table 23–5	DIAGNOSTIC TESTS FOR NEUROBLASTOMA
Tests for Initial Diagnosis	**Tests for Metastases**
Tumor tissue diagnosis by light microscopy, or Biopsy of tumor cells plus laboratory evaluation showing increased urine or serum catecholamines (two separate measures each more than 3 standard deviations above the norm for age)	Bone marrow aspirate and biopsy Radiolabeled scanning with metaiodobenzylguanidine (MIBG) Bone scan Skeletal radiograph CT or MRI of abdomen, liver, brain, eye orbits MRI of spine Chest radiograph, with added CT or MRI if radiograph shows lesions

Radiation is often used, especially in disseminated disease. HSCT may be performed for advanced disease, sometimes followed by the biological modifier *cis*-retinoic acid and fenretinide (to promote apoptosis). Studies are being conducted involving GD2, natural killer cells, and other treatments, as well as gene therapy to interrupt growth of abnormal cells. Neuroblastoma is most responsive to treatment in children under 1 year of age.

■ NURSING MANAGEMENT
Nursing Assessment and Diagnosis

The presenting site of the tumor, such as the neck or abdomen, is assessed by observation and inspection. Palpation is contraindicated. Carefully document related functioning, such as bowel and bladder function. Take vital signs to watch for elevated temperature and vital sign changes caused by a thoracic mass. Observe gait and coordination. Take weight and height measurements and compare them with earlier percentiles for the child. Specific assessments during treatment will depend on the treatment methods used (refer to the earlier discussions of chemotherapy and radiation treatment). Psychosocial and emotional assessment of the family are needed.

The following nursing diagnoses may be appropriate for the child with neuroblastoma, depending on the location and extent of the presenting disease:

- Impaired Gas Exchange related to ventilation-perfusion imbalance
- Impaired Physical Mobility related to neuromuscular impairment
- Disturbed Sensory Perception Alteration (Visual) related to altered sensory perception
- Chronic Pain related to tumor pressure and injury to tissues
- Anticipatory Grieving (Family) related to potential loss of significant person

Planning and Implementation

The nursing management of the child with neuroblastoma can encompass the three phases of medical treatment: chemotherapy, surgery, and radiation. Specific postsurgical care depends on the size and site of the tumor. Normal postoperative care includes providing fluid support and respiratory care and preventing infection.

Nursing care during the chemotherapy phase includes minimizing side effects, preventing infection, teaching parents about the medications their child is receiving, and monitoring the young child's physical and emotional growth and development. When radiation is part of the treatment, use common nursing measures described earlier in the chapter. Topics for parent and family teaching and discharge planning are presented in Families Want to Know: The Child with Neuroblastoma. Ongoing support and connection to resources to assist in management of the child's treatment at home will be needed. When the prognosis is poor, parents may appreciate referrals to hospice, to other parents who have experienced similar child illnesses, and to other community resources. See Chapter 14 ∞ for additional nursing care for end of life.

Evaluation

Expected outcomes of nursing care for the child with neuroblastoma include the following:

- The child's respiratory exchange is adequate to support daily activities.
- Physical mobility is achieved to maximum level possible considering developmental age.
- Sensory/perceptual alterations are successfully managed to provide for safety and sensory input.
- Pain is successfully managed to level of comfort.
- Family members display acceptance and integration of diagnosis.

CLINICAL TIP

Many oncology centers provide notebooks with information on chemotherapy and other relevant treatment approaches to families shortly after diagnosis. Information that is pertinent to the child is highlighted during the teaching sessions. Blank pages are included to encourage parents to use the notebook for recording information, tests and results, personal thoughts, and questions.

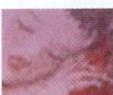

FAMILIES WANT TO KNOW

The Child with Neuroblastoma

Surgery phase

- Teach the parents to observe for signs of infection at the wound site and to take the child's temperature, if necessary.
- Assist the family to provide pain management including medication administration and various comfort measures.
- Teach the parents the importance of keeping accurate records of urine output and bowel movements and to notify physician if child does not have a bowel movement at least every 3 days.
- Continue with progression to a regular diet.

Chemotherapy phase

- The child frequently has a central line placed early in the chemotherapy phase. The central line greatly reduces the emotional trauma associated with chemotherapy and blood tests.
  - Teach the child how to help the parents with cleaning of the central line.

- Teach the child how to protect the central line.
- Teach the parents how to clean and dress the site of the central line.
- Have the parents practice central line care with a model and then on the child before discharge to increase the parents' confidence.
- Give the parents written and illustrated information about care of a central line.
- Arrange for home care dressing supplies before discharge.
- Give the parents detailed chemotherapy information.
- Teach administration of any medications that the parent will perform via central line or other routes.
- Refer the family to the American Cancer Society for coloring books and other resources for children receiving chemotherapy.

Wilms' Tumor (Nephroblastoma)

Nephroblastoma, sometimes called Wilms' tumor, is a common intrarenal abdominal tumor of childhood. It accounts for 6–7% of all childhood tumors (Jaffe & Huff, 2004). The incidence is approximately 8.1 cases per million children annually. Wilms' tumor occurs most frequently between 2 and 5 years of age, but may also occur in adolescents and adults (Kim & Chung, 2006).

Etiology and Pathophysiology

Wilms' tumor is associated with several congenital anomalies: aniridia (absence of the iris), hemihypertrophy (abnormal growth of half of the body or a body structure), genitourinary anomalies, nevi, and hamartomas (benign, nodulelike growths). This connection suggests a genetic link; chromosome deletions at 11p13 and 11p15 (locations for WT1 and WT2 genes) have been associated with Wilms' tumor. There is a high incidence of tumors in Beckwith-Wiedemann syndrome, which is characterized by macroglossia and hypoglycemia (Kline & Sevier, 2003). However, most children with Wilms' tumor have no other abnormalities. A tumor suppressor gene has been identified that acts to promote normal kidney development. This gene and others may be missing in children with Wilms' tumor. Wilms' tumor grows very quickly, doubling its size in 11 to 13 days. Such fast growth generally contributes to a large tumor by the time of diagnosis. However, chemotherapy drugs have significantly increased survival rates for children Wilms' tumor, with even stage III and IV groups having a 10-year survival rate, or 75% and 55%, respectively (Kutluk, Varan, Buyukpamukcu et al., 2006). Tissue type is associated with outcome, with anaplastic tumors having a less favorable prognosis.

Clinical Manifestations

Wilms' tumor is usually an asymptomatic, firm, lobulated mass located to one side of the midline in the abdomen. Often a parent discovers the mass during the child's bath. Hypertension caused by increased renin activity related to renal damage is reported in 25% of cases. Hematuria is sometimes present. Bilateral Wilms' tumors occur in 5–10% of cases (Jaffe & Huff, 2004).

■ COLLABORATIVE CARE

The diagnosis of Wilms' tumor is based on an ultrasound study of the abdomen and an intravenous pyelogram. CT scanning or MRI of the lungs, liver, spleen, and brain may be performed to identify any metastasis. This information is used in staging the tumor (Table 23–6). A complete blood count is obtained, as well as BUN and creatinine

Table 23–6	NATIONAL WILMS' TUMOR STUDY STAGING SYSTEM
Stage	**Description**
I	The tumor is limited to the kidney and completely excised. The surface of the renal capsule is intact. The tumor is not ruptured before or during removal. No residual tumor is apparent beyond the margins of the excision.
II	The tumor extends beyond the kidney but is completely excised. Regional extension of the tumor is present, i.e., penetration through the outer surface of the renal capsule into the perirenal soft tissues. Vessels outside the kidney substance are infiltrated or contain tumor thrombus. Biopsy may have been performed on the tumor, or local spillage of tumor confined to the flank has occurred. No residual tumor is apparent at or beyond the margin of excision.
III	Residual nonhematogenous tumor is confined to the abdomen. Any of the following may occur: Lymph nodes on biopsy are found to be involved in the hilus, the periaortic chains, or beyond. Diffuse peritoneal contamination by the tumor has occurred, such as by spillage of tumor beyond the flank before or during surgery, or by tumor growth that has penetrated through the peritoneal surface. Implants are found on peritoneal surfaces. The tumor extends beyond the surgical margins either microscopically or grossly. The tumor is not completely resectable because of local infiltration into vital structures.
IV	Hematogenous metastasis: deposits are present beyond stage III, e.g., lung, liver, bone, and/or brain.
V	Bilateral renal involvement is present at diagnosis. An attempt should be made to stage each side according to the above criteria on the basis of extent of disease before biopsy.

Note: Adapted from Green, D. M., Grigoriev, Y. A., Nan, B., Takashima, J. R., Norkool, P. A., D'Angio, G. J., & Breslow, N. E. (2001). Congestive heart failure after treatment for Wilms' tumor: A report from the National Wilms' Tumor study group. *Journal of Clinical Oncology, 19,* 1926–1934.

levels, and liver function tests are performed. Histologic examination is performed for tissue typing once the tumor is removed.

Treatment is multifaceted and increasingly successful. About 90% of early stages and 70% of metastatic cases have long-term survivial (Kutluk et al., 2006; Pritchard-Jones, 2002). Surgery is performed to remove the affected kidney, to examine the opposite kidney, and to look for other sites of metastasis. Chemotherapy or radiation therapy, alone or in combination, is sometimes used before surgery to reduce the size of the tumor. Children with stage III and IV disease often receive vincristine, dactinomycin, and doxorubicin; cyclophosphamide is sometimes added as well. Radiation may also follow surgery, especially in disseminated disease. Children whose tumors are almost completely excised and who have a favorable prognosis do not require irradiation of the tumor bed.

Long-term complications of treatment include liver damage, portal hypertension, and mild cirrhosis, which may occur in children treated for right-sided Wilms' tumor. Radiation damage (such as thinning or weakening) of the skeleton, pelvis, and thorax has been reported. Kyphosis and scoliosis may occur from irradiation of vertebral bodies and the pelvis. Glomerular damage to the remaining kidney may also occur. Second malignancies in the original radiation field have occurred with orthovoltage radiation, but recent changes in radiation therapy have reduced this risk.

NURSING MANAGEMENT
Nursing Assessment and Diagnosis

Perform a thorough baseline assessment of the child. Do not palpate the abdomen, as this may potentially spread the cancerous cells. Monitor the child's blood pressure carefully as hypertension is a common finding that may require treatment.

NURSING ALERT

If a mass is felt during palpation of a child's abdomen, stop palpating immediately and report the finding to the physician. Never palpate the liver or abdomen of a child with Wilms' tumor as this could cause a piece of the tumor to dislodge. Place a sign on the child's bed and in the chart alerting health providers not to palpate the child's abdomen.

Nursing diagnoses for a child with Wilms' tumor will differ depending on the phase of treatment. Common nursing diagnoses may include the following:

- Risk for Infection related to inadequate defenses
- Impaired Urinary Elimination related to anatomic obstruction
- Ineffective Cardiopulmonary Tissue Perfusion related to hypertension caused by mechanical reduction of blood flow
- Risk for Caregiver Role Strain related to child's illness severity
- Risk for Impaired Home Maintenance related to child's disease

Planning and Implementation

Nursing management can be divided into two phases: the postrenal surgery phase and the chemotherapy phase. (See Chapter 13 ∞ for general care of the child after surgery.) Drawings and special teaching dolls with removable kidneys can be used to teach young children about the surgery. Although chemotherapy may occur at two different times, before and after surgery, nursing management considerations remain the same.

Nursing care during the postrenal surgery phase focuses on pain management and close monitoring of fluid levels. A large incision is necessary to remove the kidney, and the resultant postoperative shift of organs and fluid in the abdominal cavity may create discomfort for the child. Frequently reposition the child and use noninvasive and pharmacologic pain interventions to improve the child's comfort. Gentle handling is important. Monitor fluids closely following surgery to prevent hypovolemia and to assess the shift of fluids out of the third space and out of the body. Assess daily weight, intake and output (I&O), and urine specific gravity. Monitor the function of the remaining kidney. Take blood pressure measurements frequently to watch for signs of shock and to assess the functioning of the remaining kidney.

During the chemotherapy phase, monitor the child for side effects of drugs, the potential for infection from the central line site, and the function of the remaining kidney. Advise parents about home care needs, administration of medications, and monitoring for drug side effects and ongoing needs for health monitoring. Ensure that care is well coordinated among all the healthcare providers.

Evaluation

Desired outcomes for nursing care of the child with nephroblastoma include balanced intake and output, normal vital signs, recovery from surgery, and successful family management of postsurgical care and ongoing treatments.

Bone Tumors

Osteosarcoma

Osteosarcoma is the most common tumor affecting the skeleton of children, with an incidence of 5.6 cases per million children. Its peak incidence is during the rapid growth years, at 13 years for girls and 14 years for boys (Hartford, Wodowski, Rao et al., 2006). The tumor is usually located at the metaphysis of the distal femur, proximal tibia, or proximal humerus.

ETIOLOGY AND PATHOPHYSIOLOGY   Bone tissue produced by osteosarcoma never matures into compact bone. Although the cause of osteosarcoma is unknown, radiation exposure (either environmental or treatment related) is associated with its development. Survivors of retinoblastoma have a greatly increased incidence of osteosarcoma. An abnormality of gene p53 has been noted in some cases of this cancer, leading to oncogene malformations and possibly to an absence of tumor suppressor genes (Wunder, Gokgoz, Parkes et al., 2005).

CLINICAL MANIFESTATIONS   The common initial symptoms of osteosarcoma are pain and swelling. The pain can be referred to the hip or back, which can delay diagnosis. Pulmonary metastasis occurs in 20% of cases. Other metastatic sites include kidney, adrenals, brain, and pericardium. When lung metastasis is the only site, lung resection may be successful for treatment. Disseminated metastases and bone lesions have poorer prognosis.

COLLABORATIVE CARE

Diagnosis of osteosarcoma is made through radiographic tests of the affected area and bone scan. CT or MRI scans of involved bone and other potential cancer sites are performed. A complete blood count, liver studies, and renal studies are performed for clues to potential metastases. A blood test for serum alkaline phosphatase (level may be elevated) and tumor biopsy can confirm the diagnosis. Arteriography may be performed if limb-salvage surgery is contemplated. Cardiac assessments are performed to establish baseline function prior to treatment with doxorubicin.

Treatment involves both surgery and chemotherapy. The surgery is either a limb-salvage procedure or limb amputation. In limb-salvage procedures, the tumor is removed and an internal prosthesis is inserted. A limb-salvage procedure is possible if bone growth has taken place and a neurobundle (area where several nerves converge) is not involved in the tumor. If these two criteria are not met, limb amputation is necessary. Physical rehabilitation will be needed after either amputation or limb-salvage procedure. At the time of diagnosis, most children have metastases (even though they may not be identifiable), so chemotherapy is needed. Chemotherapy may be started before surgery, especially in cases where limb-salvage surgery is performed. It is also given postoperatively to treat and prevent metastasis. Aggressive chemotherapy following surgery has improved the survival rate. Drugs commonly used for osteosarcoma include:

- Doxorubicin
- Cisplatin
- Ifosfamide with mesna
- Methotrexate with leucovorin rescue

Radiation is generally not effective in treating osteosarcoma, although it may be used with chemotherapy for recurrence at other sites.

Ewing's Sarcoma

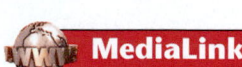

MediaLink

Case Study: A Teen with Ewing's Sarcoma

Ewing's sarcoma is a malignant, small, round cell tumor usually involving the diaphyseal (shaft) portion of the long bones. The most common sites are the femur, pelvis, tibia, fibula, ribs, humerus, scapula, and clavicle, but any bone may be involved. Ewing's sarcoma occurs in two children per million, is most common in Whites and Hispanics, and is rare in Black and Asian children. The incidence is highest in children between the ages of 5 and 20 years, with a median of 14 years (Khoury, 2005).

Translocations on chromosomes 11 and 22 have been identified in children with Ewing's sarcoma; these are t(11;22)(q24;q12). In addition, these tumors express a protooncogene, c-myc.

The symptoms are similar to those of osteosarcoma and may include pain, swelling, fever, an elevated WBC count, elevated erythrocyte sedimentation rate, and elevated C-reactive protein. Some children present with a fracture of the affected bone. A tumor biopsy is necessary for diagnosis. Diagnostic tests are the same as those for osteosarcoma.

Initial treatment for Ewing's sarcoma is chemotherapy to reduce the tumor, followed by surgical removal of the entire bone or intensive high-dose irradiation of the entire bone. Limb-salvage procedures are now commonly performed rather than amputation. Surgery is preferred because of the possibility of a secondary cancer from radiation. Chemotherapy is always used following initial treatment, as undetectable metastases are nearly always present. Medications used to treat Ewing's sarcoma include:

- Vincristine
- Doxorubicin
- Cyclophosphamide
- Dactinomycin
- Etoposide
- Ifosfamide

NURSING MANAGEMENT

Nursing Assessment and Diagnosis

Physiologic assessment of the child with a bone tumor includes assessment of the site before surgery. Assess the child's pain or discomfort, mobility, and gait. Take careful vital signs, especially noting temperature and respirations. Psychologic assessment of the child and family are needed, especially if amputation is planned. Body image disturbances occur when a limb is lost, particularly with school-age children and adolescents. Assess the child's understanding of the treatment and of care after surgery. Inquire about support systems that are available for assistance.

Observe the wound postoperatively for infection and hemorrhage. Assess circulation above and below the operative site. If edema is found, elevate the limb. If a limb-salvage procedure is performed, the child's extremity will be intact but it will not function as before, because muscle insertion sites and mass have been removed with the tumor during surgery. Detailed charting of the condition of the surgical site and limb function is important.

If the limb has been amputated, assess the child for the following signs indicating a disturbed body image:

- Refusal to look at or touch the altered or missing body part
- Preoccupation with loss or change
- Feelings of shame or embarrassment, either verbalized or demonstrated
- Distorted perception of normal body (easily seen in the child's drawings of the body)
- Fears of rejection or unwanted attention from others
- Overexposure or hiding of the affected body part
- Actual or perceived change in the structure and function of the body or body parts

Psychosocial assessment of the child and family is discussed in more detail earlier in this chapter in the Childhood Cancer section (see pages 858–860).

Appropriate nursing diagnoses for the child with a bone tumor are based on the treatment and needs of each child:

- Risk for Infection related to amputation
- Impaired Skin Integrity related to mechanical forces of prosthesis
- Impaired Physical Mobility related to musculoskeletal impairment
- Impaired Adjustment related to disability and lifestyle change
- Disturbed Body Image related to treatment and injury
- Chronic Pain related to physical injury of tissues

Planning and Implementation

Care of the child after surgery involves general postoperative care (see Chapter 13 ∞). The child who has had an amputation has special needs regarding skin care and rehabilitation. Inspect the tissue at the surgical site, using sterile technique, and turn the child at least every 2 hours. The site needs to heal completely before chemotherapy can begin and a prosthesis can be made. Pain management is a major nursing care need. When amputation has occurred, the adolescent will often experience **phantom pain**. This pain, which feels as if it is in the amputated extremity, is caused by trauma to the nerves in the area of the amputation. Acknowledge the pain as real since the nerve endings are intact and the patient is perceiving real discomfort. Medicate adequately and use additional pain control measures such as repositioning the limb using gentle movement, supporting the limb, and using distraction or deep breathing (Siddle, 2004).

Discuss insurance and other financial arrangements with the parents, as prosthetics can be expensive. Physical rehabilitation will be needed as well. Referral to a Shriners Hospital is an option for some families.

Implement plans to help the child deal with body image disturbance. Plan for a visit from another child who is well adjusted to a prosthesis. Help the child to gradually learn how to care for the stump. Slow progress may be made as the child first looks briefly, then for longer periods, and finally is willing to touch the stump. Show the child how it is possible to continue with sports such as baseball, skiing, or biking with a prosthesis. A discussion group with others can be very useful for adolescents. Plan with the child how to tell friends about the surgery and what issues he or she may face upon return to school. Make plans for elevator access if needed and emergency evacuation procedures. Some children or adolescents may need referral for counseling to assist in dealing with body image disturbance.

The child will be receiving physical rehabilitation while hospitalized and after discharge. When the child is discharged, explain to the family the importance of bringing the child for outpatient chemotherapy and physical rehabilitation visits. Special arrangements may be needed at the child's school to facilitate a wheelchair, crutches, or ambulation with a new prosthesis. Call or visit the school to evaluate the presence of buttons to open doors, wide doorways to facilitate passage, and any limitations of the building. Contact school personnel to plan for the child's return. The child will need careful management of a schedule that permits both healing of the surgical site with rehabilitation and then the demands of chemotherapy.

Follow-up care is needed to monitor for progress and to be alert for signs of metastases. See the discussion of cancer survivorship earlier in this chapter. Fracture may be a sign of recurrent tumor. All body systems such as the lungs, heart, kidneys, and liver are monitored for signs of recurrence. Consider carefully the drugs the child received and the long-term side effects, such as cardiac change with doxorubicin.

Evaluation

The following expected outcomes of nursing care for the child with a bone tumor focus on the treatments required and adaptation to changes in lifestyle:

- The surgical site heals with no signs of infection.
- The child adapts to changes in mobility status.
- The child manifests successful adjustment to changes required in school settings.
- Healthy, intact skin is maintained at the surgical site.
- The child shows evidence of positive body image.
- Pain is managed to a comfort level.
- The child and family successfully integrate continuing medical therapy into family life.

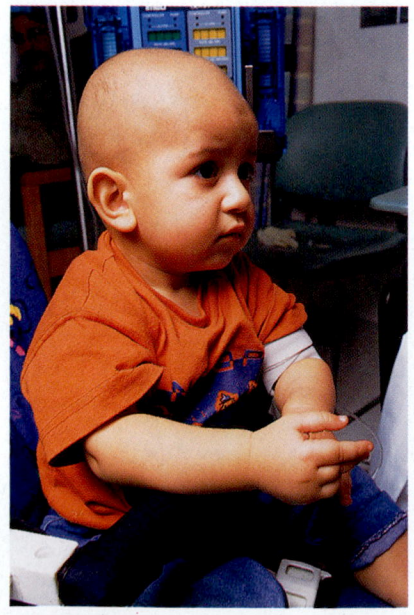

Figure 23–17 ➤ Acute lymphoblastic leukemia is the most common type of leukemia in children and the most common cancer affecting children under 5 years of age.

Leukemia

Leukemia is among the most commonly diagnosed pediatric malignancies in children under 14 years of age. A cancer of the blood-forming organs, leukemia is characterized by a proliferation of abnormal white blood cells in the body. Several types of leukemia are differentiated, depending on the blood cells affected. The main types are acute lymphoblastic leukemia (ALL), acute nonlymphocytic leukemia (acute myelogenous leukemia), and the rare chronic leukemias of childhood.

The most common type of childhood leukemia is acute lymphoblastic leukemia (ALL), which accounts for 25% of all childhood cancer and 78% of leukemias in children. Sam, described in the opening scenario, has ALL. The peak age at onset is 2 to 3 years. ALL is more common in Whites and in boys (Figure 23–17 ➤) (American Cancer Society, 2006b). Subtypes of ALL are based on the French-American-British (FAB) system of classification, and the three subtypes are L1, L2, and L3.

Acute nonlymphocytic leukemia (ANLL) refers to all leukemias from myeloid cells. About 17% of childhood leukemias are ANLL. ANLL is most common in children younger than 2 years of age and in adolescents. It is more common in males than females, and in Asians/Pacific Islanders, Hispanics, and Whites than in Blacks (Brown, 2006). There are several subtypes of ANLL in the FAB classification (Bennett & Konrokji, 2005):

- M0 = acute nonlymphocytic leukemia without maturation
- M1 = acute nonlymphocytic leukemia with poor maturation
- M2 = acute nonlymphocytic leukemia with maturation
- M3 = acute promyelocytic leukemia
- M4 = acute myelomonocytic leukemia
- M5 = acute monocytic leukemia
- M6 = erythroleukemia
- M7 = acute megakaryocytic leukemia

Because chronic leukemias such as chronic myelocytic, chronic myelomonocytic, and chronic lymphocytic leukemia are rare in children, the following discussion will focus on ALL and ANLL.

Etiology and Pathophysiology

The causes of leukemia are not well understood. Some investigators theorize that exposure to infectious agents can predispose children to leukemia. Genetic factors are also believed to play a role in some types of the disease. For instance, children with chromosomal defects such as Down syndrome, neurofibromatosis type I, Bloom syndrome, and Shwachman syndrome have an increased incidence of ALL, and chromosomal abnormalities are present in most children with ALL (Bennett & Konrokji, 2005). Children with immune deficiency states, such as ataxia-telangiectasia, congenital hypogammaglobulinemia, and Wiskott-Aldrich syndrome, have an increased risk of ALL. Certain racial and ethnic groups have poorer outcomes from leukemia.

Ionizing radiation when in utero, and chemical agents such as treatment of an earlier cancer with chemotherapy (alkylating agents and topoisomerase II inhibitors), are thought to play some role in the development of ANLL. There are several chromosomal and genetic abnormalities associated with ANLL. For example, trisomy 8 is associated with all subtypes of the disease (Jaff, Chelghoum, Elhamri et al., 2006). Leukemia occurs when the stem cells in the bone marrow produce immature WBCs that cannot function normally. These cells proliferate rapidly by cloning instead of through normal mitosis, causing the bone marrow to fill with abnormal WBCs. The abnormal cells then spill out into the circulatory system where they steadily replace the normally functioning WBCs. As this occurs, the protective lymphocytic functions such as cellular and humeral immunity are reduced, leaving the body vulnerable to infections.

The malignant WBCs rapidly fill the bone marrow, replacing stem cells that produce erythrocytes (red blood cells) and other blood products such as platelets, thereby decreasing the amount of these products in circulation. The stem cells are replaced by leukemic clones, eventually resulting in anemia. Children with leukemia commonly experience abnormal bleeding because of the reduced platelet amounts.

Clinical Manifestations

Children with ALL and ANLL usually have fever, pallor, overt signs of bleeding, lethargy, malaise, anorexia, and large joint or bone pain. Petechiae, frank bleeding, and joint pain are cardinal signs of bone marrow failure. Enlargement of the liver and spleen (hepatosplenomegaly) and changes in the lymph nodes (lymphadenopathy) are common. If the leukemia has infiltrated the central nervous system (entered it by means of the circulatory or lymphoid system), the child may exhibit signs such as headache, vomiting, papilledema, and sixth cranial nerve palsy (inability to move the eye laterally). These findings are caused by the leukemic cells massing and putting pressure on nerves. The testicles, spinal cord, and bone marrow are common sites for infiltration. The leukemic cells in the testicle become a mass that causes the testicle to enlarge, often painlessly.

MediaLink

Leukemia

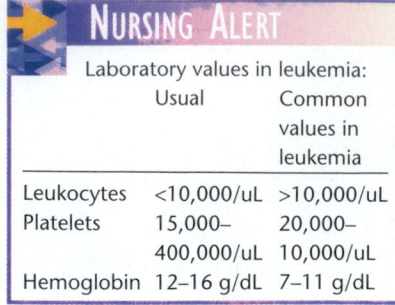

COLLABORATIVE CARE

Diagnostic Tests

Diagnosis is based initially on blood counts and bone marrow aspiration. Blood counts reveal anemia, thrombocytopenia, and neutropenia. Bone marrow aspiration, the definitive test, reveals immature and abnormal lymphoblasts and hypercellular marrow. Percent of blast cells in marrow is measured; 25% lymphoblasts is definitive for the disease (Brown, 2006). Neutropenia, thrombocytopenia, and anemia are commonly noted. Other abnormal laboratory findings include elevated serum uric acid and elevated calcium, potassium, and phosphorus levels. New laboratory studies such as rapid flow cytometric assay are making the presence of even very small numbers of leukemic cells possible, so that treatment can be used to improve prognosis in children with minimal residual disease. Leukemic cells are examined and classified by FAB type, and DNA analysis may provide clues about genetic changes; all of these considerations are used to establish the protocol for treatment. Cells of children with ALL are either B cell or T cell; these classifications are also used to establish treatment protocols.

Clinical Therapy

Treatment of ALL involves radiation and chemotherapy. Radiation is used for central nervous system disease, in T-cell leukemia, and for testicular involvement. Chemotherapy is organized into four phases:

1. Induction
   - Prednisone
   - Vincristine
   - L-asparaginase
   - Daunorubicin
2. Consolidation
   - L-asparaginase
   - Doxorubicin
3. Delayed intensification
   - Vincristine
   - ARA-C
   - Cyclophosphamide
4. Maintenance of remission
   - 6-mercaptopurine
   - 6-thioguanine
   - Methotrexate

Additional drugs used for treatment of central nervous system disease or prophylaxis include intrathecal methotrexate.

Maintenance therapy may continue for 2 to 3 years, causing decreased resistance to infection for this prolonged period of time.

Treatment of ANLL involves use of a wide variety of drugs during the induction and consolidation phases. They include:

1. Induction phase
   - Daunorubicin
   - Coxorubicin
   - Mitoxantrone
   - Cytarabin
2. Consolidation phase
   - Etoposide
   - Teniposide

Maximum cell death occurs during the *induction phase*. The cells that remain after this period are more resistant to treatment. After 3 to 4 weeks, when a remission has occurred, central nervous system prophylaxis begins. Drugs are used in combination with cranial irradiation. During the *consolidation phase*, chemotherapy with L-asparaginase and doxorubicin is administered. *Delayed intensification* uses additional drugs to target the leukemic cells that have survived. Treatment during the *maintenance phase* is aimed at destroying the remaining leukemic cells. Combinations of active drugs are used to prevent resistance. Many complications can occur with such high doses and combinations of drugs; therefore, much of the clinical therapy is aimed at managing these effects. In addition, long-term complications such as central nervous system toxicity; damage to the pituitary, liver, kidneys, gastrointestinal tract, heart, lungs, gonads, blood, and immune system; and secondary malignancies can occur.

The prognosis for children with leukemia is much improved with current therapy. However, several risk factors affect the long-term outcome. The most favorable findings are as follows:

- Age at onset between 2 and 10 years
- Initial hemoglobin level less than 10 g/dL
- Low initial WBC count
- Lack of B- or T-cell antigens
- Absence of extramedullary (outside bone marrow or spinal cord) involvement
- Rapid response to chemotherapy

The most important factor is the initial leukocyte count. The higher the leukocyte count (over 50,000/mm^3) at diagnosis, the worse the prognosis. For children in the low-risk group, the probability of prolonged survival is as high as 90%. Infants under 12 months of age have a poor prognosis. Treatment methods and duration are adjusted for each child, depending on that child's risk factors. More aggressive treatment is undertaken for those in the higher risk groups.

Approximately 10% of children have a relapse within a year after completing treatment (Carroll, 2003). Treatment for relapse consists of additional chemotherapy drugs. The prognosis is best if the relapse occurs late after the initial diagnosis and after the initial treatment is completed. Bone marrow transplantation is a treatment option for the child who has a relapse with ALL who then achieves a second remission; the transplant is given when the child is in remission. Transplant is also used for children with ANLL; they do not need to be in remission for the transplant to be performed. Chemotherapy itself can create numerous complications, affecting all body organs. Secondary malignancies sometimes occur later in life. Overall, 80% of children with leukemia are cured (Carroll, 2003).

NURSING MANAGEMENT

Nursing Assessment and Diagnosis

A thorough physical assessment is important to ensure prompt identification of problems without injuring the child who has deficient coagulation and immune function. Perform assessments every 8 hours or more often depending on the chemotherapy regimen. Observe carefully for bruising and other new sites of bleeding, and for fever or other signs of infection. Once chemotherapy has begun, closely monitor renal functioning through specific gravity, intake and output (I&O), and daily weight measurement. Monitor dietary intake, nausea, vomiting, and constipation. Observe for mucosal sores in the mouth. A central line is usually in place for intravenous infusion of medications, so careful assessment of the line for proper functioning and for signs of infection is needed. Ask the parents about any behavioral changes. Central nervous system infiltration can affect the child's level of consciousness, causing irritability, vomiting, and lethargy. However, these nonspecific signs can also be induced by chemotherapeutic drugs and antiemetics. Frequent venipunctures, bone marrow aspirations, and lumbar punctures require pain assessment and an evaluation of the level of knowledge and coping skills of the child and family.

Leukemia causes many changes in the body, and confirmation of the disease is difficult for families to face. Among the many nursing diagnoses that might be appropriate for the child with leukemia are the following:

- Imbalanced Nutrition: Less than Body Requirements related to inability to ingest food
- Risk for Infection related to altered immune system functioning
- Risk for Injury related to bleeding
- Activity Intolerance related to generalized weakness
- Chronic Pain related to chemotherapy and disease process
- Disturbed Sleep Pattern related to chemotherapy drugs and disease process
- Anxiety (Child and Parent) related to change in health status

Planning and Implementation

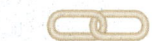

CHAPTER 1
Transmission-based Precautions

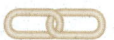

SKILL 9–6:
Administering Blood or Blood Products

Bone marrow suppression necessitates transmission-based precautions (refer to the *Clinical Skills Manual*). Instruct parents in the prevention of infection and use nursing care measures to prevent infection as well. Perform careful handwashing; take temperature frequently; give mouth care with antibacterial mouth washes; and inspect the skin, mouth, rectal area, and central line site for any signs of infection. Care of mouth ulcers and other side effects of chemotherapy are presented in the Nursing Care Plan for Hospital Care of the Child with Cancer, earlier in this chapter.

Special attention to renal function is needed when the child receives cyclophosphamide. Gross hematuria is a side effect of this drug. Hydration with intravenous fluids to attain a specific gravity of less than 1.010 prevents or reduces the severity of hematuria. It also prepares the kidneys to manage products of tumor cell breakdown. To achieve this desired specific gravity, the child receives intravenous fluids at 1.5 times maintenance volume for at least 6 to 8 hours before and at least 1.5 hours after administration of the drug. Other chemotherapy drugs have different infusion times, while some do not require hydration prior to infusion. Check drug references carefully for recommendations with each drug. Evaluate the infusion site before and frequently during infusion. Although extravasation is not as common with central lines used in cancer treatment as in peripheral lines, it still can occur. Many chemotherapy agents are extremely toxic to tissues. In addition, lysis of the cancer cells can produce toxic side effects (see oncologic emergencies described earlier in the chapter). Careful monitoring of I&O is required to record the intravenous fluids, assess kidney functioning, and monitor excretion of by-products from destroyed tumor cells. Monitor specific gravity every 8 hours, as well as before and during administration of the drug, and when the intravenous fluids are reduced to maintenance volume levels. Daily weight measurements are important to assist in planning adequate hydration during chemotherapy, as well as to measure nutritional status.

Drug side effects may necessitate infusion of platelets or packed red blood cells. See the *Clinical Skills Manual* for techniques to be used in these situations.

Many children are treated in an oncology clinic, staying in the hospital only on the day of intravenous drug administration, and receive oral medications at home. The time at the hospital is used to assess how the family is managing issues such as nutrition, sleep, medication administration, and obtaining psychosocial support. Careful teaching for the family is needed to ensure safe drug administration and identification of issues requiring further care.

Nurses play a key role in the long-term multidisciplinary treatment of children with leukemia. The impact of a diagnosis of leukemia and the long-term nature of treatment can severely stress the coping abilities of both the child and the family. Consider the shock to the family when Sam, described in the chapter opener, was diagnosed with leukemia, a possibility they had never considered. Ongoing psychosocial assessment and emotional support are essential (see the general discussion of psychosocial assessment in the Childhood Cancer section, pages 858–860). Referral to support groups and social services may be beneficial. Assist the family in exploration of alternative therapies such as relaxation, imagery, and nutritional support that may aid the child. Be alert for any interactions that could occur between alternative therapies and the medical regimen. (See Families Want to Know: Chemotherapy for Leukemia.)

Evaluation

Following are expected outcomes for nursing care of the child with leukemia.

- The child is adequately hydrated to allow for elimination of drugs and cell components.
- The child maintains normal urinary output.
- The child remains free from infection.
- Blood values are maintained within normal limits.
- The family successfully adapts to parenting a child with a chronic illness.
- The parents demonstrate adequate knowledge related to the disease process and treatment regimens.

Soft-Tissue Tumors

Hodgkin's Disease

Hodgkin's disease, a disorder of the lymphoid system, usually arises in a single lymph node or an anatomic group of lymph nodes (Figure 23–18 ➤). There are approximately three cases per 100,000 people, with the peak occurrence in adolescent boys. Hodgkin's disease has a childhood form but is rare in those under 14 years, and almost never seen in those under 5 years. Most cases involve a young adult form that affects those between 15 and 40, and an older adult form, usually seen in persons over 55 years (American Cancer Society, 2003b).

ETIOLOGY AND PATHOPHYSIOLOGY   Hodgkin's disease occurs in clusters and has been reported in families. This suggests a possible genetic link as well as an infectious agent or environmental hazard.

CLINICAL MANIFESTATIONS   The main symptom of Hodgkin's disease is nontender, firm lymphadenopathy, usually in the supraclavicular and cervical nodes but occasionally in the mediastinal area. A mediastinal growth can cause respiratory difficulty because of pressure on the trachea or bronchi. Fever, night sweats, and weight loss occur in one-third of children with Hodgkin's disease; these symptoms and elevated sedimentation rate are associated with a more aggressive form of the disease (Schwartz, 2003). The leukocyte count and erythrocyte sedimentation rate (ESR) may be elevated.

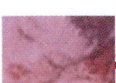

FAMILIES WANT TO KNOW

Chemotherapy for Leukemia

Physical Care

- Have rest periods each day.
- Avoid areas of exposure to people with illnesses.
- Drink generous amounts of water.
- Eat a healthy diet, using frequent, small, and nutritious meals to obtain enough nutrients.
- Take medicines prescribed to decrease nausea.
- Maintain good oral hygiene with soft toothbrush and water pik.
- Avoid sun exposure and check skin each day for any signs of bruises, pressure areas, cuts, or scratches.
- Allow time and eat foods to promote bowel elimination.
- Report any signs of infection, changes in condition, or other concerns.

Emotional Care

- Be prepared for loss of hair with plans for hats, wigs, or other alternatives.
- Continue contact with friends via phone, internet, and in person when possible.
- Try relaxation techniques to aid in sleep and management of treatments.
- Talk with clergy, teachers, parents, counselors, friends, or other supportive people about the experience of having leukemia.

PATHOPHYSIOLOGY ILLUSTRATED

Hodgkin's Disease

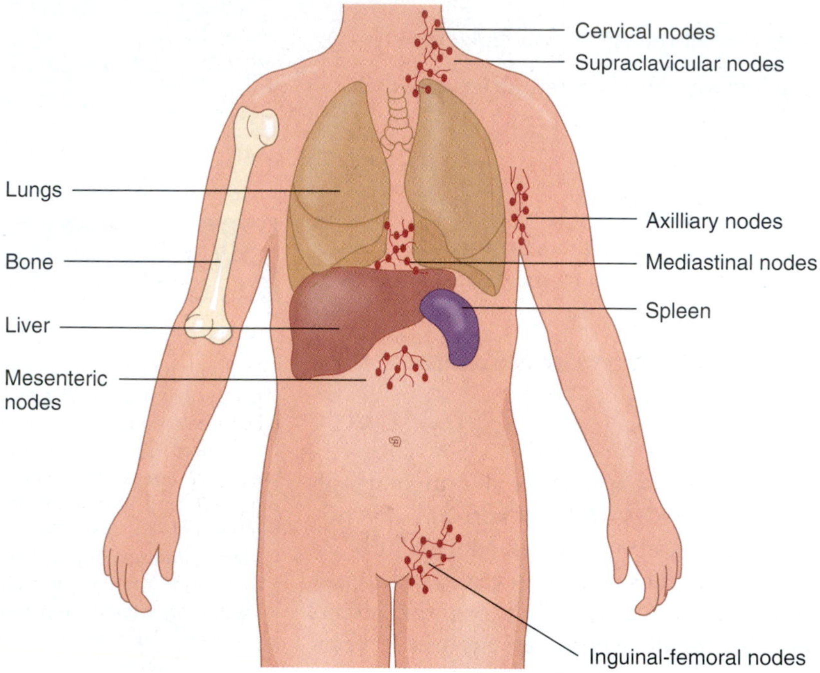

Figure 23–18 ➤ Lymph nodes and organs affected in Hodgkin's disease in children.

COLLABORATIVE CARE

CLINICAL TIP

An oral contrast medium is often given to children having CT scanning of the abdomen and pelvis. Mixing this contrast medium with fruit juice or punch makes it more palatable. Mix it in a small amount so the child can easily drink it all.

Diagnosis is based on lymph node biopsy; Reed-Sternberg cells (large cells with two nucleoli) are present. A staging classification is used to determine disease severity (Table 23–7). The basis for staging is data obtained from the history, physical examination, chest radiograph study (for metastasis), chest CT scan, CT or MRI scans of the retroperitoneal nodes, lymphangiogram if there is retroperitoneal involvement, laboratory studies (complete blood count, erythrocyte sedimentation rate, serum copper level, liver function tests), and a radionuclide scan with gallium. Bone marrow biopsy, bone scan, or a staging laparotomy may be performed in certain situations when advanced disease is suspected. Minimally invasive surgery can be used to

Table 23–7 STAGING SYSTEM FOR HODGKIN'S DISEASE

Stage	Description
I	Disease within a single lymph node region
IE	Disease within a single extralymphatic organ
II	Disease within two or more lymph node regions on the same side of the diaphragm
IIE	Disease within extralymphatic organ, and of one or more lymph node regions on the same side of the diaphragm
III	Disease of lymph node regions on both sides of the diaphragm
IIIE	Disease of lymph node regions on both sides of the diaphragm with involvement of extralymphatic organ
IIIS	As in III, plus disease within spleen
IIISE	As in III, plus disease in extralymphatic organs and spleen
IV	Disseminated disease within one or more lymphatic organs with or without lymph node involvement

biopsy or remove the spleen for diagnosis, avoiding the potential complications of major surgery.

Treatment is commonly performed in outpatient settings unless complications develop that require hospitalization. A four-drug chemotherapy combination has been found to be the most effective drug treatment. Drugs commonly used include:

- Adriamycin
- Bleomycin
- Vinblastine
- Dacarbazine
- Etoposide
- Prednisone
- Cyclophosphamide
- Procarbazine
- Methotrexate
- Mechlorethamine

Common drug combinations (see Table 23–2) are:

- ABVD
- ABVE
- ABVE-PC
- ASCT
- BEACOPP
- COPP
- EBVP
- MOPP
- OEPA
- OPPA
- VAMP
- VEPA

Radiation is commonly added, with low doses for children who are still growing, and larger doses for those who are physically mature or whose disease is more advanced at diagnosis. The 5-year survival rate is approximately 80–90%, depending on the stage of the disease at diagnosis (American Cancer Society, 2003b). Bone marrow transplantation or HSCT is a treatment option in children with advanced disease or relapse.

Non-Hodgkin's Lymphoma

About 12% of pediatric cancers are lymphoma; of these, 40–45% are Hodgkin's and 55–60% are non-Hodgkin's. There are three types of pediatric non-Hodgkin's lymphoma: (1) lymphoblastic lymphoma (30–40%), (2) small noncleaved cell (Burkitt's) lymphoma (40–50%), and (3) large cell lymphoma (15%) (Mann, Attarbaschi, Steiner et al., 2006). Lymphomas of all types are the third most common group of malignancies in children, following leukemia and brain tumors. Non-Hodgkin's lymphomas are malignant tumors of lymphoreticular (internal framework of the lymph system) origin. The peak incidence for lymphomas occurs between the ages of 7 and 11 years, and they are three times more common in boys than in girls. The cure rate is 80% (Mann, Attarbaschi, Steiner et al., 2006).

Lymphoblastic non-Hodgkin's lymphomas are caused by T-cell abnormalities. These abnormal T cells are diffuse, highly malignant, and very aggressive and do not mature. T-cell lymphomas produced by these cells often occur in children with congenital or acquired immunodeficiency states, chronic immune stimulation, or autoimmune disease. Some lymphomas have B-cell abnormalities, most specifically Burkitt's lymphoma; 8q24 chromosomal translocation may be found in these cases, and it is sometimes associated with Epstein-Barr virus infection. Large cell lymphomas are variable in cell type affected and may also manifest chromosomal translocations (Mann, Attarbaschi, Steiner et al., 2006).

Children with non-Hodgkin's lymphoma frequently present with fever and weight loss. The lymph glands are usually enlarged or nodular, with the most frequent sites being the cervical, axillary, inguinal, and femoral nodes. However, the disease may be diffuse, without nodular glands. The anterior mediastinum is the primary site for T-cell lymphomas. Tumors that occur in this area may compress the airway (causing breathing difficulty) or superior vena cava (leading to swelling of the face, neck, or arms), and can cause pain. Jaw involvement is common in Burkitt's lymphoma. An abdominal mass may cause pain, nausea, and vomiting.

The symptoms of lymphoma are often nonspecific and treatments may already have been tried with antibiotics or other medication if a mass is thought to be an infection. A careful history will help determine the progression and possible location of disease. CBC is performed; additional blood tests include renal and liver function, electrolytes, uric acid, and LDH. Bone marrow aspiration and lumbar puncture are performed. Chest radiograph, bone scan, gallium scan, CT, and MRI can help to isolate affected body organs. Diagnosis is confirmed by tissue biopsy.

A staging system is used to describe the tumor mass and extension to other body areas (Table 23–8). Treatment is tailored to the type of cancer and its stage. Stages I and II may be treated with drugs such as vincristine, cyclophosphamide, prednisone, and methotrexate for several months. Intrathecal medication is added if head and neck cancers are present. Stages III and IV are treated with additional drugs (up to 9 total) for longer periods of time (1–2 years). Radiation is uncommonly used and may be helpful to treat a tumor that is impinging on a body part. Surgery is used to biopsy the tumor mass and treat any complications caused by the cancer. Bone marrow transplantation or HSCT is used for children with recurrent disease.

Rhabdomyosarcoma

Rhabdomyosarcoma is the most common soft-tissue sarcoma diagnosed in children, and is especially common in children under 5 years of age. The 5-year survival rate is 64% (Punyko, Gurney, Baker et al., 2006). It occurs most often in the muscles around the eyes (extraorbital), in the neck, and less commonly in the abdomen, genitourinary tract, and the extremities. Genitourinary, bladder, and prostate cancers are more common in children under 5 years, while paratesticular and extremity cancer is more common among adolescents. Rhabdomyosarcoma occurs more often in Whites than in Blacks or Asians. It is uncommon in newborns; if it is present in this age group, abdominal or pelvic sites are the most common locations.

The cause of rhabdomyosarcoma is unknown. However, it is more common in children with neurofibromatosis and Li-Fraumeni syndrome. Mutations in a tumor suppressor gene p53 is sometimes seen. The abnormal cells arise from mesenchyme, which normally grows into muscle, fat, and bone.

Table 23–8	ST. JUDE CHILDREN'S RESEARCH HOSPITAL STAGING CLASSIFICATION FOR NON-HODGKIN'S LYMPHOMA	
Stage	**Description**	
I	Single tumor or node area involved; no tumor in abdomen or mediastinum	
II	Single tumor with lymph node involvement; or two node areas or tumor on same side of diaphragm; or GI tumor in one site	
III	Two tumors or node areas on different sides of the diaphragm; or a primary mediastinal, intraabdominal, or epidural tumor	
IV	Any involvement with CNS or bone marrow metastases	

Adapted from: Hussong, M. R. (2002). In C. R. Baggott, K. P. Kelly, D. Fochtman, & G. V. Foley, *Nursing care of children and adolescent with cancer* (3rd ed., p. 539). Philadelphia: Saunders.

Tumors occurring close to the eye produce swelling, ptosis, visual disturbances, and eye movement abnormalities (Figure 23–19 ➤). When the tumor occurs in the genitourinary tract, the result can be obstruction, hematuria, dysuria, vaginal discharge, and a protruding vaginal mass. Rhabdomyosarcoma occurring in the abdomen may be asymptomatic. There is rapid metastasis to the lungs, bones, bone marrow, and distant lymph nodes.

Diagnosis is confirmed by CT, MRI, PET, bone marrow aspiration, and biopsy. CBC, renal and liver studies, and urinalysis are performed. Lumbar puncture may be used in head and neck tumors. A useful biologic marker, Desmin, allows differentiation of rhabdomyosarcoma from other round cell tumors. A significant number of children have metastatic disease at the time of diagnosis, so chest and lung CT scans are performed; regional lymph node biopsies also help to establish the extent of disease (Rodeberg & Paidas, 2006).

Treatment includes surgical removal of the tumor when possible. However, if the tumor involves other structures, removal may not be possible. Many children have metastasis at the time of diagnosis, so the primary tumor is removed. Surgery is followed by wide-field radiation and chemotherapy with a combination of drugs. Some commonly used drugs include:

- Vincristine
- Actinomycin
- Cyclophosphamide (VAC therapy)

Prognosis depends on the site, staging (Table 23–9), and histologic findings, with about 70% of children now surviving (Rodeberg & Paidas, 2006).

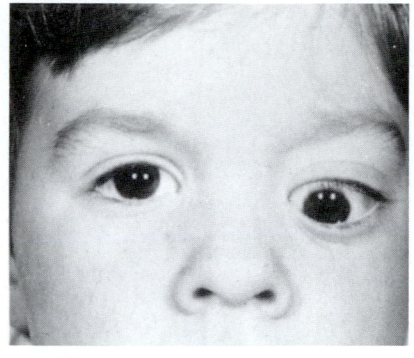

Figure 23–19 ➤ Rhabdomyosarcoma is characterized by ptosis and swelling. From Vaughn, D., Asbury, T., & Riordan-Eva, P. (1995). *General ophthamology* (14th ed.). Norwalk, CT: Appleton & Lange.

Retinoblastoma

Retinoblastoma is an intraocular malignancy of the retina. It may be bilateral (20–30%) or unilateral. In 40% of children, the disease is inherited by an autosomal dominant gene. The RB gene undergoes a mutation that predisposes the child to retinoblastoma (de Andrade, da Hora Barbosa, Vargas et al., 2006). Family history is therefore important to collect, although many cases occur after a recent mutation. In this case, there is no family history of the cancer.

The first sign of retinoblastoma is a white pupil, termed leukokoria or cat's-eye reflex (Figure 23–20 ➤). The red reflex is absent, asymmetrical, or of a differing color in the affected eye. Other symptoms may include a fixed strabismus (a constant deviation of one eye from the other), orbital inflammation, glaucoma, and heterochromia (irises of different colors).

Retinoblastoma is usually diagnosed when the child is between 1 and 2 years of age. A family history should alert healthcare providers so that regular ophthalmologic examinations can be performed frequently on infants and young children in the family. The appearance of a unilateral tumor demands regular examinations of the healthy eye since bilateral disease can develop. In some children a pineal gland tumor can also develop, causing central nervous system symptoms. The overall tumor-free survival rate is 90%, 5 to 10 years after diagnosis (Kids Data, 2006).

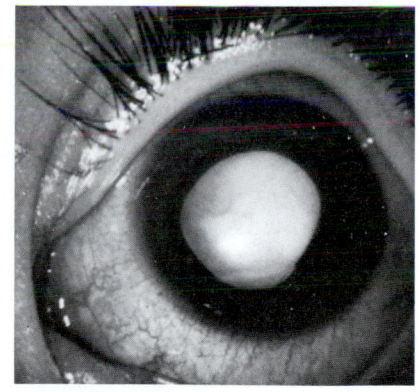

Figure 23–20 ➤ Retinoblastoma is characterized by leukokoria, a white reflection in the pupil. From Hathaway, W. E., Hay, W. W., Jr., Groothuis, J. R., & Paisley, J. W. (1993). *Current pediatric diagnosis and treatment* (11th ed.). Norwalk, CT: Appleton & Lange.

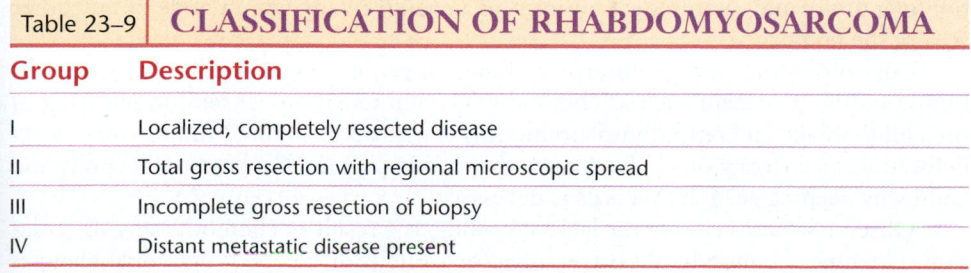

Table 23–9	CLASSIFICATION OF RHABDOMYOSARCOMA
Group	**Description**
I	Localized, completely resected disease
II	Total gross resection with regional microscopic spread
III	Incomplete gross resection of biopsy
IV	Distant metastatic disease present

Note: From Wexler, L. H., & Helman, L. J. (2005). Rhabdomyosarcoma and the undifferentiated sarcomas. In P. A. Pizzo & D. G. Poplack (Eds.), *Principles and practices of pediatric oncology* (5th ed.). Philadelphia: Lippincott Williams Wilkins.

Children at risk for retinoblastoma due to family history can be tested for the RB1 gene. Diagnostic tests include full ocular examination and CT or MRI scans of the eye orbit. All children with a history of retinoblastoma in the family should be examined by an ophthalmologist after birth, at 6 weeks, every 2–3 months until 2 years, every 4 months until 3 years, and then annually (de Andrade, da Hora Barbosa, Vargas et al., 2006) to aid in early diagnosis. Tumors are classified according to a staging system, from a very small localized tumor (group I) to tumors involving more than half the retina and with seeding into the vitreous (group V).

Treatment for retinoblastoma may include removal of the eye (enucleation) when there is permanent retinal damage or failure to respond to other treatment. Other surgical treatments involve cryotherapy or photocoagulation (argon laser therapy). Radiation is nearly always used, either as the sole treatment or before surgery to shrink the tumor. Chemotherapy is occasionally used but is generally ineffective as the drugs often fail to penetrate sufficiently into the eye. Chemotherapy drugs include carboplatin, etoposide, vincristine, and cyclosporine. Multiple therapies are more commonly used in children with bilateral retinoblastoma. Children with retinoblastoma are at increased risk of developing a secondary tumor, including another retinoblastoma or a sarcoma, most commonly osteogenic sarcoma. However, most young children who have been treated for the disease have good health and normal mental abilities several years after treatment. Over 90% of children with small unilateral tumors survive. Increased size and invasion by a tumor decrease success of treatment. The most common sequela of retinoblastoma is a decrease in visual acuity.

NURSING MANAGEMENT

Nursing management of retinoblastoma begins with astute assessments that may identify the condition, extends through the treatment process in support for the child and family, and includes ongoing care to ensure the child's normal developmental progression.

Nursing Assessment and Diagnosis
Physiologic Assessment

Careful family histories can sometimes identify children at risk who need frequent physical examinations. For example, if a family history of retinoblastoma is present, the child should receive frequent eye examinations. Physiologic assessment of the child with a soft-tissue tumor, such as Hodgkin's disease, non-Hodgkin's lymphoma, rhabdomyosarcoma, and other lymphomas, focuses on the child's general condition. Accurate height and weight measurements are essential to provide a baseline against which to measure the child's growth during treatment, as well as for calculation of chemotherapeutic drug dosages.

Observe the area of the tumor, such as the face, neck, and abdomen, and describe any changes. Monitor respiratory status if the tumor is on the face or neck. Report any changes in respiratory pattern to the physician. Avoid palpation of any tumor site or enlarged area, as metastasis can be influenced by injudicious palpation and manipulation of a tumor site. Notify the physician of a change in any lymph node or any other area of the body.

Gastrointestinal and genitourinary function can be altered by the presence of a tumor and by treatment such as chemotherapy and radiation. Careful monitoring of the child's intake and output measurement is essential. Abdominal tumors may affect defecation, so charting of all bowel movements is important. Explain to the family and child why keeping accurate records is necessary.

Observe wounds closely for lack of healing as a result of chemotherapy or radiation. Examine the mouth and extremities for wounds or ulcers. Nutritional changes caused by treatment will affect the body's ability to support healthy cells and heal wounds.

A thorough eye examination is warranted for any child who has a family history of retinoblastoma or has undergone treatment for a prior tumor. Assess the color and position of the iris, eye movements, cover-uncover test, and other eye tests described in Chapter 5 ∞. Ask whether the child has been evaluated by an ophthalmologist.

Psychosocial Assessment

Assessment of the family's psychosocial status and coping mechanisms is an essential component of nursing care. Refer to the general discussion of psychosocial assessment in the Childhood Cancer section earlier in this chapter. Assessment of body image is needed when the child has a soft-tissue tumor affecting the appearance of the head and neck. Even after treatment is successfully completed, lasting mental health changes can be apparent. Survivors of childhood lymphoma more commonly report depression and somatic distress (symptoms such as pains in the heart or chest, dizziness, weakness) than other individuals (Zebrack et al., 2006). Ask about symptoms of depression such as loneliness, lack of interest, anxiety, and suicidal thoughts. Survivors of rhabdomyosarcoma are less likely to complete high school than their siblings, and report higher incidences of pain (Punyko et al., 2006).

The location and type of soft-tissue tumor determine the specific nursing diagnoses for a particular child. Common nursing diagnoses may include the following:

- Altered Tissue Perfusion (Peripheral) related to interruption of blood flow
- Ineffective Breathing Pattern related to effect of tumor deformity on neck or chest wall
- Impaired Swallowing related to acquired anatomic defect
- Delayed Growth and Development related to effects of treatment
- Disturbed Body Image related to illness and treatment
- Disturbed Sensory Perception (Visual) related to illness

Planning and Implementation

Nursing management of children with soft-tissue tumors varies depending on the specific tumor. (See Families Want to Know: The Child with a Soft-Tissue Tumor.) Children with lymphoma affecting the mediastinum may need respiratory support. Position the child so that the head is elevated. Administer chemotherapy drugs as ordered, maintaining adequate fluids to facilitate excretion of the resultant breakdown products. Monitor the central line used for chemotherapy administration, and teach parents care of the central line when the child is at home.

For the child with a rhabdomyosarcoma involving the bladder, monitor urinary output carefully. Report hematuria and painful urination. Monitor the changes that occur during therapy. For example, in children with eye tumors, observe for a decrease in ptosis, which may indicate successful treatment. Administer pain medications as needed and use distraction and other techniques to decrease the child's discomfort. Emphasize to parents the need for follow-up CT and MRI scans after completion of treatment.

When the child with retinoblastoma undergoes removal of the eye, the parents and child will need detailed instructions on postsurgical care. Demonstrate to the

FAMILIES WANT TO KNOW

The Child with a Soft-Tissue Tumor

- Teach the family about the chemotherapy drugs and their side effects.
- Teach about the care of surgically placed venous access devices.
- Provide written and illustrated information about the chemotherapy protocol(s).

- Provide radiation and surgery education specific to the tumor treatment.
- Refer the family to nutrition resources such as dietitians to improve the child's nutritional status.

parents care of the socket and use of a conformer to maintain the eye socket's shape. When healing is complete and the child receives a prosthetic eye, instruct parents about its insertion and care. The child can gradually be taught to take over this care when old enough. Encourage periodic healthcare visits to monitor for signs of a tumor in the other eye. Interventions to encourage normal developmental milestones are adapted if sensory alteration has resulted.

Attention is directed at the body changes of the cancer and its treatment. Children and adolescents may need suggestions to deal with hair loss, disfigurement, and issues related to living with a serious illness. Referral to other children and teens with similar concerns may be helpful. Parents of all children need help to encourage normal development in the child with cancer.

The child with a soft-tissue tumor often receives chemotherapy or radiation, or sometimes both modalities. Nursing management during chemotherapy and radiation was discussed earlier in this chapter in the general sections on these treatment measures (see pages 847–855) and in the Nursing Care Plan for Hospital Care of the Child with Cancer. Generally, the family will need help to adjust to the diagnosis of a life-threatening disease and to the care of the ill child. Refer to Chapter 13 ∞ for a description of postsurgical care. Consult Chapter 19 ∞ for strategies to assist the child and family if the child has a visual impairment resulting from a retinoblastoma. Topics for parent and family teaching and discharge planning are similar to those previously presented. Referral resources to support the families of children with these types of cancer can be found at our Companion Website.

Care in the Community

Reinforce with families the importance of long-term follow-up after treatment for a soft-tissue tumor. Increased risk for secondary cancers is possible for 2–3 decades, and early identification can help with prompt diagnosis (Hudson & Findlay, 2006). Partner with other healthcare providers to supply instructions to families as the child transitions from oncology treatment back to the pediatrician so they understand the importance of telling all care providers about the cancer and treatment. Establish oncology clinics to track and examine survivors. As children grow into the teen and young adult years, help them to take over this important task in their care. Some recommended annual examinations include:

- CBC
- Physical examination with special attention to skin, abdomen, and thyroid
- Monitoring for signs of hypo- and hyperthyroidism
- Neurological and developmental examinations; monitoring of school performance
- First mammogram at 25 years in those with chest radiation
- Pap and pelvic exams for teen and young adult women
- Mental status assessment (Smith, 2002)

Evaluation

The following expected outcomes of nursing care for the child with a soft-tissue tumor are examples that illustrate the varied tumor presentations:

- Treatment side effects are successfully managed.
- The surgical site heals with no signs of infection.
- The child successfully adapts to sensory loss.
- The child achieves growth and development to maximum potential.
- The parents and family achieve anticipatory grieving in cases of terminal disease.

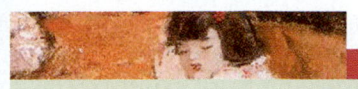

CRITICAL THINKING IN ACTION

Recall 4-year-old Sam, who was described in the opening scenario. He was recently diagnosed with acute lymphocytic leukemia (ALL) and has begun treatment. Both his mother and father are strong supports, and his older siblings, Jeffrey (6 years) and Blake (8 years), are worried about and protective of their younger brother. On a recent clinic visit, Sam's hemoglobin was found to be 6 g/dL.

1. Sam has had several procedures already that are painful and have required sedation. Plan to prepare him for a lumbar puncture for which he will be sedated. Consider his age as you plan how far ahead to tell him, how to explain the room he will be in, and how you will include his parents in the procedure.

2. Lack of all blood cellular components is a side effect of leukemia treatment. Explain why Sam's hemoglobin is low. What is the expected level?

What colony-stimulating factor might be used in his treatment to increase RBCs? What dietary teaching can you do to enhance hemoglobin levels?

3. Infection is a frequent complication of treatment for leukemia. During Sam's clinic visit, what assessments will you make to monitor for infection?

4. Jeffrey and Blake are attending one of Sam's clinic visits when he receives chemotherapy. What questions and activities will you plan for them during the visit? What can you do to increase their knowledge and help them feel like they are part of Sam's care? Could their concern for Sam influence their own school performance? What should their teachers know about the fact that they have a sibling who has leukemia?

 Refer to your Prentice Hall Nursing MediaLink DVD-ROM for answers.

EXPLORE MediaLink 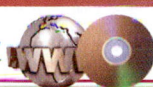 http://www.prenhall.com/ball

Resources for this chapter can be found on the Prentice Hall Nursing MediaLink DVD-ROM accompanying this textbook, and on the Companion Website at http://www.prenhall.com/ball

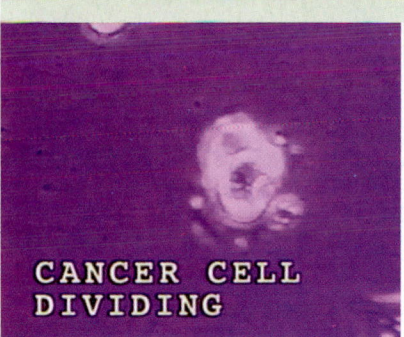

CANCER CELL DIVIDING

DVD-ROM
Audio Glossary
NCLEX-RN® Review
Animations/Videos
  Cancer
  Leukemia

COMPANION WEBSITE
Audio Glossary
NCLEX-RN® Review
Care Plan Activity: Child Undergoing Chemotherapy
Case Study: Ewing's Sarcoma
MediaLink Application: Childhood Cancer
WebLinks

REFERENCES

Agha, M. M., Williams, J. I., Marrett. L., To, T., Zipursky, A., & Dodds, L. (2006). Congenital abnormalities and childhood cancer. *Cancer, 106,* 1418–1419.

Alavi, S., Arzanian, M. T., Abbasian, M. R., & Ashena, Z. (2006). Tumor lysis syndrome in children with non-Hodgkin lymphoma. *Pediatric Hematology and Oncology, 23,* 65–70.

Alcoser, P. W., & Rodgers, C. (2003). Treatment strategies in childhood cancer. *Journal of Pediatric Nursing, 18,* 103–112.

American Cancer Society. (2003a). National Action Plan for Childhood Cancer. Retrieved February 16, 2004, from http://www.cancer.org

American Cancer Society. (2003b). What are the key statistics about Hodgkin disease in children? Retrieved June 14, 2006, from http://www.cancer.org/docroot/CRI/content/CRI_2_4_1x_What_Are_the_Key_Statistics_about_Hodgkin_Disease_in_Children.asp?sitearea=

American Cancer Society. (2004). Clinical trials: What you need to know. Retrieved June 12, 2006, from http://www.cancer.org/docroot/ETO/content/ETO_6_3_Clinical _Trials

American Cancer Society. (2005). What are the key statistics about brain and spinal cord cancers? Retrieved September 7, 2006, from http://www.cancer.org/docroot/CRI

American Cancer Society. (2006a). Cancer facts and figures. Retrieved June 7, 2006, from http://www.cancer.org/docroot/STT/stt_o.asp

American Cancer Society. (2006b). What are the key statistics about childhood leukemia? Retrieved September 7, 2006, from http://www.cancer/docroot/CRI/content/

Baggott, C. R., Kelly, K. P., Fochtman, D., & Foley, G. V. (2002). Nursing care of children and adolescents with cancer (3rd ed.). Philadelphia: Saunders.

Ballard, K. L. (2004). Meeting the needs of siblings of children with cancer. *Pediatric Nursing, 30*, 394–402.

Bennett, J. M., & Konrokji, R. S. (2005). The myelodysplastic syndromes: Diagnosis, molecular biology and risk assessment. *Hematology, 10*, (Suppl 1), 258–269.

Bindler, R. M., & Howry, L. B. (2005). *Pediatric drug guide*. Upper Saddle River, NJ: Prentice Hall.

Bleyer, A. (2004). Principles of diagnosis; Principles of Treatment. In R. E. Behrman, R. M. Kliegman, & H. B. Jenson (eds). *Nelson Textbook of Pediatrics* (17th ed.). Philadelphia: Saunders.

Bradlyn, A. S., Kato, P. M., Beale, I. L., & Cole, S. (2004). Pediatric oncology professionals' perceptions of information needs of adolescent patients with cancer. *Journal of Pediatric Oncology Nursing, 21*, 335–342.

Brown, P. (2006). Answers to key questions about childhood leukemias. *Contemporary Pediatrics, 23*(3), 81–84, 87, 90.

Bryant, R. (2003). Managing side effects of childhood cancer treatment. *Journal of Pediatric Nursing, 18*, 113–125.

Butowski, N. A., Sneed, P. K., & Chang, S. M. (2006). Diagnosis and treatment of recurrent high-grade astrocytoma. *Journal of Clinical Oncology, 10*, 1273–1280.

Cantril, C. A., & Haylock, P. J. (2004). Tumor lysis syndrome. *American Journal of Nursing, 104*(4), 49–52.

Carroll, W. L. (2003). Race and outcome in childhood acute lymphoblastic leukemia. *Journal of the American Medical Association, 290*, 2061–2062.

Castleberry, R. P. (1997). Biology and treatment of neuroblastoma. *Pediatric Clinics of North America, 44*, 919–938.

Chappuy, H., Doz, F., Blanche, S., Gentet, J.C., Pons, G. & Treluyer, J. M. (2006). Parental consent in paediatric clinical research. *Archives of Disease in Childhood, 91*, 112–116.

Children's Oncology Group. (2004). Long-term follow-up guidelines for survivors of childhood, adolescent, and young adult cancers. Retrieved June 7, 2006, from http://www.survivorshipguidelines.org

De Andrade, A. F., da Hora Barbosa, R., Vargas, F. R., Ferman, S., Eisenberg, A. L., Fernandes, L., & Bonvicino, C. R. (2006). *Cancer Genetics and Cytogenetics 167*, 43–46.

Eldridge, B. (2004). Medical nutritional therapy for cancer prevention, treatment and recovery. In L. K. Mahan & S. Excott-Stump, *Krause's food, nutrition and diet therapy* (11th ed.). Philadelphia: W.B. Saunders.

Elfenbein, G. J. (2005). Granulocyte-colony stimulating factor primed bone marrow and granulocyte-colony stimulating factor mobilized peripheral blood stem cells are equivalent for engraftment: Which to choose? Pediatric Transplantation, 9(Suppl 7), 37–47.

Faivre, S., Djelloul, S., & Raymond, E. (2006). New paradigms in anticancer therapy: Targeting multiple signaling pathways with kinase inhibitors. *Seminars in Oncology, 33*, 407–420.

Florin, T. A., & Hinkle, A. S. (2005). A guide to caring for cancer survivors. *Contemporary Pediatrics, 22*(8), 31–48.

Freeman, K., O'Dell, C., & Meola, C. (2003). Childhood brain tumors: Children's and siblings' concerns regarding the diagnosis and phase of illness. *Journal of Pediatric Oncology Nursing, 20*, 133–140.

French, A. E., Grant, R., Weitzman, S., Ray, J. G., Vermeulen, M. J., Sung, L., Greenberg, M., & Koren, G. (2003). Folic acid food fortification is associated with a decline in neuroblastoma. *Clinical Pharmacology Therapy, 74*, 288–294.

Green, D. M., Grigoriev, Y. A., Nan, B., Takashima, J. R., Norkool, P. A., D'Angio, G. J., & Breslow, N. E. (2001). Congestive heart failure after treatment for Wilms' tumor: A report from the National Wilms' Tumor study group. *Journal of Clinical Oncology, 19*, 1926–1934.

Gurney, J. G. & Bondy, M. L. (2004). Epidemiology of Childhood and Adolescent Cancer. In R. E. Behrman, R. M. Kliegman & H. B. Jensen. Nelson Textbook of Pediatrics, 17th ed. Philadelphia: Saunders, 1679–1681.

Haddy, T. B. K., Mosher, R. B., Dinndorf, P. A., & Reaman, G. H. (2004). Second neoplasms in survivors of childhood and adolescent cancer are often treatable. *Journal of Adolescent Health, 34*, 324–329.

Hammes, B. J., Klevan, J., Kempf, M., & Williams, M. S. (2005). Pediatric advance care planning. *Journal of Palliative Medicine, 8*, 766–773.

Hartford, C. M., Wodowski, K. S., Rao, B. N., Khoury, J. D., Neel, M. D., & Daw, N. C. (2006). Osteosarcoma among children age 5 years or younger. *Journal of Pediatric Hematology and Oncology, 28*, 43–47.

Haut, C. (2005). Oncological emergencies in the pediatric intensive care unit. *AACN Clinical Issues, 16*, 232–245.

Hawks, R. (2006). Complementary and alternative medicine research initiative in the children's oncology group and the role of the pediatric oncology nurse. *Journal of Pediatric Oncology Nursing, 23*, 261–264.

Henderson, R. A., Mossman, S., Nairn, N., & Cheever, M. A. (2005). Cancer vaccines and immunotherapies: Emerging perspectives. *Vaccine, 23*, 2359–2362.

Himmelstein, B. P., Hilden, J. M., Boldt, A. M., & Weissman, D. (2004). Pediatric palliative care. *New England Journal of Medicine, 350*, 1752–1762.

Hinds, P. S. (2004). Adolescent-focused oncology nursing research. *Oncology Nursing Forum, 31*, 281–287.

Hon, K. L., Leung, A., Chik, K.W., Chu, C.W., Cheung, K. L., & Fok, T. F. (2005). Critical airway obstruction, superior vena cava syndrome, and spontaneous cardiac arrest in a child with acute leukemia. *Pediatric Emergency Care, 21*, 844–846.

Houldin, A., Curtiss, C. P., & Haylock, P. J. (2006). Executive summary: The state of the science on nursing approaches to managing late and long-term sequelae of cancer and cancer treatment. *American Journal of Nursing, 106*(3), 54–59.

Hudson, M. M., & Findlay, S. (2006). Health-risk behaviors and health promotion in adolescent and young adult cancer survivors. *Cancer 107*, (7 Suppl), 1695–1701.

Hussong, M. R. (2002) *Non-Hodgkin's Lymphoma*. In C. R. Baggott, K. P. Kelly, D. Fochtman, & G.V. Foley, *Nursing care of children and adolescents with cancer* (3rd ed., pp. 536–544). Philadelphia: Saunders.

Jaff, N., Chelghoum, Y., Elhamri, M., Tigaud, I., Michallet, M., & Thomas, X. (2006). Trisomy 8 as sole anomaly or with other clonal aberrations in acute myeloid leukemia: Impact on clinical presentation and outcome. *Leukemia Research 31*, 67–73.

Jaffe, N. & Huff, V. (2004). Neoplasms of the kidney. In R. E. Behrman, R. M. Kliegman, & H. B. Jensen (eds). *Nelson textbook of pediatrics* (17th ed). Philadelphia: Saunders.

James, K., Keegan-Wells, D., Hinds, P. S., Kelly, K. P., Bond, D., Hall, B., Mahan, R., Moore, I. M., Roll, L., & Speckhart, B. (2002). The care of my child with cancer: Parents' perceptions of caregiving demands. *Journal of Pediatric Oncology Nursing, 19*, 218–228.

Khoury, J. D. (2005). Ewing sarcoma family of tumors. *Advances in Anatomy and Pathology, 12*, 212–220.

Kids Data. (2006). Net five-year cancer survival rates. Retrieved September 7, 2006, from http://www.kidsdata.org

Kim, S., & Chung, D. H. (2006). Pediatric solid malignancies: Neuroblastoma and Wilms' tumor. *Surgical Clinics of North America, 86*, 469–487.

Kline, N. E., & Sevier, N. (2003). Solid tumors in children. *Journal of Pediatric Nursing, 18*, 96–102.

Kutluk, T., Varan, A., Buyukpamukcu, N., Atahan, L., Caglar, M., Akyuz, C., & Buyukpamukcu, M. (2006). Improved survival of children with Wilms' tumor. *Journal of Pediatric Hematology and Oncology, 28*, 423–426.

Kwan, M. L., Block, G., Selvin, S., Month, S., & Buffler, P. A. (2004). Food consumption by children and the risk of childhood abuse leukemia. *American Journal of Epidemiology, 160*, 1098–1107.

Labay, L. E., Mayans, S., & Harris, M. B. (2004). Integrating the child into home and community following the completion of cancer treatment. *Journal of Pediatric Oncology Nursing, 21*, 165–169.

Landier, W., Bhatia, S., Eshelman, D. A., Forte, K. J., Sweeney, T., Hester, A. L., Darling, J., Armstrong, F. D., Blatt, J., Constine, L. S., Freeman, C. R., Friedman, D. L., Green, D. M., Marina, N., Meadows, A. T., Negla, J. P., Oeffinger, K. C., Robison, L. L., Ruccione, K. S., Sklar, C. A., & Hudson, M. M. (2004). Development of risk-based guidelines for pediatric cancer survivors: The Children's Oncology Group Long-Term Follow-Up Guidelines from the Children's Oncology Group Late Effects Committee and Nursing Discipline. *Journal of Clinical Oncology, 1522*, 4979–4990.

Loescher, L. J., & Merkle, C. J. (2005). The interface of genomic technologies and nursing. *Journal of Nursing Scholarship, 37*, 111–119.

Mann, G., Attarbaschi, A., Steiner, M., Simonitsch, I., Strobl, H., Urban, C., Meister,

B., Haas, O., Dworzak, M., & Gadner, H. (2006). Early and reliable diagnosis of non-Hodgkin lymphoma in childhood and adolescence. *Pediatric Hematology and Oncology, 23*, 167–176.

Martel, D., Bussieres, J. F., Theoret, Y., Lebel, D., Kish, S., Moghrabi, A., & Laurier, C. (2005). Use of alternative and complementary therapies in children with cancer. *Pediatric Blood and Cancer, 44*, 660–668.

Matsuzaki, A., Suminoe, A., Koga, Y., Kinukawa, N., Kusuhara, K., & Hara, T. (2005). Immune response after influenza vaccination in children with cancer. *Pediatric Blood and Cancer, 45*, 831–837.

McGrath, P., Paton, M. A., & Huff, N. (2005). Beginning treatment for pediatric acute myeloid leukemian: The family connection. *Issues in Comprehensive Pediatric Nursing, 28*, 97–114.

McMancus, J. & Gilchrist, G. S. (2004). Neuroblastoma. In. R. E. Behrman, R. M. Kliegman, & H. B. Jensen (eds.). *Nelson Textbook of Pediatrics (17th ed.).* Philadelphia: WB Saunders.

Nelson, M. B., & Meeske, K. (2005). Recognizing health risks in childhood cancer survivors. *Journal of the American Academy of Nurse Practitioners, 17*(3), 96–103.

Packman, W., Greenhalgh, J., Chesterman, B., Shaffer, T., Fine, J., Van Zutphen, K., Golan, R., & Amylon, M. D. (2005). Siblings of pediatric cancer patients: The quantitative and qualitative nature of quality of life. *Journal of Psychosocial Oncology, 23*, 87–108.

Pasero, C. (2006). Lidocaine iontophoresis for dermal procedure analgesia. *Journal of PeriAnesthesia Nursing, 21*, 48–52.

Post-White, J., & Hawks, R. G. (2005). Complementary and alternative medicine in pediatric oncology. *Seminars in Oncology Nursing, 21*, 107–114.

Pritchard-Jones, K. (2002). Controversies and advances in the management of Wilms' tumor. *Archives of Disease in Childhood, 87*, 241–244.

Punyko, J. A., Gurney, J. G., Baker, K. S., Hayashi, R. J., Hudson, M. M., Liu, Y., Robison, L. L., & Mertens, A. C. (2006). Physical impairment and social adaptation in adult survivors of childhood and adolescent rhabdomyosarcoma: A report from the Childhood Cancer Survivors Study. *Psycho-Oncology 16*, 26–37

Recklitis, C., O'Leary, T., & Diller, L. (2003). Utility of routine psychological screening in the childhood cancer survivor clinic. *Journal of Clinical Oncology, 231*, 787–792.

Richardson, J., Smith, J. E., McCall, G., & Pilkington, K. (2006). Hypnosis for procedure-related pain and distress in pediatric cancer patients: A systematic review of effectiveness and methodology related to hypnosis interventions. *Journal of Pain and Symptom Management, 31*, 70–84.

Rodeberg, D., & Paidas, C. (2006). Childhood rhabdomyosarcoma. *Seminars in Pediatric Surgery, 15*, 57–62.

Rollins, J. A. (2005). Tell me about it: Drawing as a communication tool for children with cancer. *Journal of Pediatric Oncology Nursing, 22*, 203–211.

Rourke, M. T., Hobbie, W. L., Schwartz, L., & Kazak, A. D. (2006). Posttraumatic stress disorder (PTSD) in young adult survivors of childhood cancer. *Pediatric Blood Cancer.*

Rushton, C. H. (2005). A framework for integrated pediatric palliative care: Being with dying. *Journal of Pediatric Nursing, 20*, 311–325.

Ryan-Murray, J., & Petriccione, M. M. (2002). Central nervous system tumors. In C. R. Baggott, K. P. Kelly, D. Fochtman, & G. V. Foley, *Nursing care of children and adolescents with cancer* (3rd ed., pp. 503–523). Philadelphia: Saunders.

Schwartz, C. L. (2003). The management of Hodgkin disease in the young child. *Current Opinions in Pediatrics, 15*, 10–16.

Scott, J. T., Entwistle, V. A., Sowden, A. J. & Watt, I. (2003). Communicating with children and adolescents about their cancer. *Cochrane Library Issue, 2*, Oxford: Update software.

Siddle, L. (2004). The challenge and management of phantom limb pain after amputation. *British Journal of Nursing, 13*, 664–667.

Skinner, R., Hamish, W., Wallace, B., & Levitt, G. A. (2006). Long-term follow-up of people who have survived cancer during childhood. *Lancet, 7*, 489–498.

Smith, P. C. K. (2002). The role of the primary care advanced practice nurse in evaluating and monitoring childhood cancer survivors for a second malignant neoplasm. *Journal of Pediatric Oncology Nursing, 19*, 84–96.

Spinazze, S., & Schrijvers, D. (2006). Metabolic emergencies. *Critical Reviews in Oncology/Hematology, 58*, 79–89.

Tamber, M. S., & Rutka, J. T. (2003). Pediatric supratentorial high-grade gliomas. *Neurosurgery Focus, 14*(2), 1–8.

Thompson, S. W. (2003). When kids get cancer. *RN, 55*(7), 29–33.

Tsao, J. C., & Zeltzer, L. K. (2005). Complementary and alternative medicine approaches for pediatric pain: A review of the state-of-the-science. *Evidence Based Complementary and Alternative Medicine, 2*, 149–159.

U.S. Department of Labor. (2003). OSHA Technical Manual. Retrieved February 19, 2004, from http://www.osha.gov

Wexler, L. H. & Helman, L. J. (2005). Rhabdomyosarcoma and the undifferentiated sarcomas. In P. A. Pizzo & D. G. Poplack (eds.) *Principles and practices of pediatric oncology* (5th ed.). Philadelphia: Lippincott Williams Wilkins.

Wilne, S. H., Ferris, R. C., Nathwani, A., & Kennedy, C. R. (2006). The presenting features of brain tumors: A review of 200 cases. *Archive of Diseases in Children, 91*, 502–506.

Wohlschlaeger, A. (2004) Prevention and treatment of mucositis: A guide for nurses. *Journal of Pediatric Oncology Nursing, 21*, 281–287.

Wuchter, C., Richter, S., Oltersdorf, D., Karawajew, L., Ludwig, W. D., & Tamm, I. (2004). Differences in the expression pattern of apoptosis-related molecules between childhood and adult de novo acute myeloid leukemia. *Haematologica, 89*, 363–364.

Wunder, J. S., Gokgoz, N., Parkes, R., Bull, S. B., Eskandarian, S., Davis, A. M., Beauchamp, C. P., Conrad, E. U., Grimer, R. J., Healey, J. H., Malkin, D., Mangham, D. C., Rock, M. J., Bell, R. S., & Andrulis, I. L. (2005). TP53 mutations and outcome in osteosarcoma: A prospective, multicenter study. *Journal of Clinical Oncology, 23*, 1483–1490.

Yang, D. J., Kim, E. E., & Inoue, T. (2006). Targeted molecular imaging in oncology. *Annals of Nuclear Medicine, 20*, 1–11.

Zebrack, B. J., Zevon, M. A., Turk, N., Nagarajan, R., Whitton, J., Robison, L. L., & Zeltzer, L. K. (2006). Psychological distress in long-term survivors of solid tumors diagnosed in childhood: A report from the Childhood Cancer Survivor Study. *Pediatric Blood Cancer.*

24 ALTERATIONS IN GASTROINTESTINAL FUNCTION

KEY TERMS

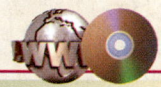

MediaLink

http://www.prenhall.com/ball

See the Prentice Hall Nursing MediaLink DVD-ROM and Companion Website for chapter-specific resources.

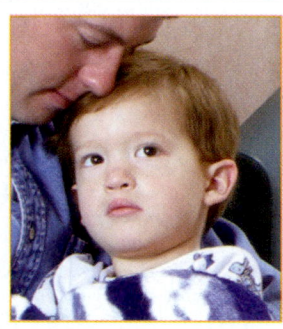

JASON is a 3-year-old who has just been admitted to the pediatric unit following surgery for a ruptured appendix. He had complained of his stomach hurting last night, but this morning his condition appeared worse and he had a temperature of 102°F. Worried that this was not just a virus, his mother took him to the pediatrician. On the way to the doctor's office Jason told his mother that his pain "just went away." While at the pediatrician's office he complained of feeling bad all over. On examination his abdomen was rigid and no bowel sounds were heard. A complete blood count revealed a white blood count (WBC) of 22,000 mm³. The pediatrician diagnosed that Jason had appendicitis and most likely had a ruptured appendix. He referred Jason to the emergency department for assessment and surgical consultation. A CT scan confirmed a diagnosis of appendicitis. During surgery the appendix was found to have ruptured.

Jason had an appendectomy and his wound was left open and packed with saline-soaked gauze. The gauze was covered with a dry dressing. Montgomery straps have been placed on Jason's abdomen to decrease the skin irritation related to dressing changes that must be performed three times a day. Jason now has a peripheral line for intravenous fluids, pain medication, and intravenous antibiotics. He also has a nasogastric tube to suction and a Foley catheter.

Jason's parents are at the bedside and are very anxious about the surgery and the open wound. They feel guilty that the appendix was ruptured and wonder if they could have done something to prevent it. This is Jason's first hospitalization. They are worried that he will have a lot of pain and wonder how he will cope with the hospitalization.

LEARNING OUTCOMES

After reading this chapter, you will be able to do the following:

1. Describe the anatomic and physiologic characteristics of the developing gastrointestinal system.

2. Discuss the pathophysiological processes associated with specific gastrointestinal disorders in the pediatric population.

3. Identify signs and symptoms that may indicate a disorder of the gastrointestinal system.

4. Describe nursing management and plan care for disorders of the gastrointestinal system.

5. Analyze developmentally appropriate approaches for nursing management of gastrointestinal disorders in the pediatric population.

6. Discuss nursing management of the child with an injury to the gastrointestinal system.

FOCUS ON
The Gastrointestinal System

ANATOMY AND PHYSIOLOGY REVIEW

The gastrointestinal tract includes the esophagus, stomach, pancreas, small intestine, and large intestine. Through the gastrointestinal (GI) tract, a child ingests and absorbs the foods and fluids necessary to sustain life and promote growth. Elimination of waste products is another role of the GI tract (Doughty, 2004). The organs of the GI tract are located in the abdomen. Other organs located in the abdominal region include the gallbladder, liver, and spleen. The abdomen is generally divided into four quadrants for purposes of assessment. See Figure 24–1 ➤ for the abdominal organs and structures in each quadrant.

Esophagus and Stomach

The esophagus is a continuous tube that allows food to pass to the stomach (Rudolph, 2003). Food enters the esophagus through the mouth, where it is chewed. Initial enzyme secretion then occurs to begin food digestion. (See Chapter 19 ∞ for more information related to the mouth and pharynx.) The stomach is located in the left upper quadrant (LUQ) of the abdomen. The role of the stomach is to store food and to secrete enzymes and digestive juices that aid in the digestion of the food (Table 24–1). Hydrochloric acid stimulates the stomach's pepsinogens to become pepsins which break down proteins and are active in acidic levels (pH of 3 or less). The stomach propels food that is partially digested into the duodenum (a part of the small intestine) (Simone, 2003).

Pancreas

The pancreas is located behind the stomach and has several functions. The pancreas secretes enzymes, electrolytes, and

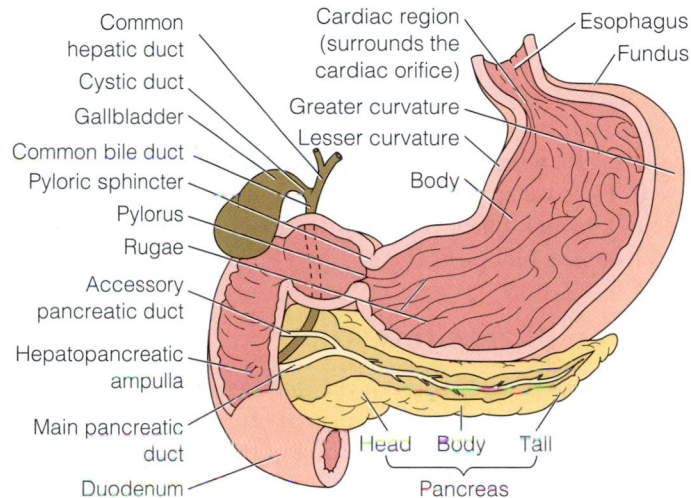

Figure 24–1 ➤ The internal anatomic structures of the stomach, including the pancreatic cystic and hepatic ducts; the pancreas; and the gallbladder.

bicarbonate that aid in the digestion and absorption of fats, proteins, and carbohydrates. Another key function of the pancreas is to regulate blood glucose metabolism through production of insulin, glucagon, and gastrin (Simone, 2003).

Liver and Gallbladder

The liver, the largest organ in the abdomen, is located in the right upper quadrant (RUQ). Its primary functions include production of blood clotting factors, fibrinogen and prothrombin; secretion of bile and **bilirubin** (yellow pigment produced from the breakdown of red blood cells); metabolism of fat, protein, and carbohydrates; detoxification of hormones,

Table 24–1	ENZYMES USED IN DIGESTION	
Enzyme	**Source**	**Function**
Amylase	Secreted by salivary glands	Converts starches to disaccharides
Hydrochloric Acid	Secreted by stomach	Stops action of amylase; converts pepsinogen to pepsin that is instrumental in converting proteins to polypeptides
Amylase	Secreted by pancreas	Converts starches to disaccharides
Enterokinase	In small intestine	Converts chymotrypsinogen & trypsinogen to trypsin
Chymotrypsin and trypsin	In small intestine	Converts polypeptides to di- and tri-peptides and then to amino acids
Bile salts	From bile and secreted to small intestine	Emulsifies fats
Lipase	From pancreas and small intestine	Converts fats to fatty acids and glycerol

Adapted from: Chamley, C. A., Carson, P., Randall, F., & Sandwell, M. (2004). *Developmental anatomy and physiology of children.* St. Louis: Elsevier.

drugs, and other substances; and storage of vitamins A, D, E, and K and glycogen (Simone, 2003). The gallbladder is a small organ located behind the liver. The gallbladder stores and concentrates the bile that is produced in the liver. It then releases stored bile as needed into the duodenum. Bile includes a variety of substances such as water, salts, bilirubin, and cholesterol. A major role of bile is to emulsify fats so that fatty acids become soluble and absorbable.

Spleen

The spleen is located in the LUQ of the abdomen and is a very vascular organ. The spleen contains about 30% of the circulating platelets and is a site for red blood cell production as well. Defense against infection is another key role of the spleen. Through phagocytosis, infectious organisms are filtered from the blood (Pearson, 2003; Simone, 2003).

Small and Large Intestine

The small intestine consists of the duodenum, the jejunum, and the ileum. Each part of the small intestine plays a vital role in the digestion and absorption of carbohydrates, amino acids, fats, and vitamins. About 90% of absorption takes place in the small intestine (Chamley, Carson, Randall, & Sandwell, 2004). The intestinal wall is covered with small villi, the brush border, through which absorption occurs. Ab-

sorption occurs both through diffusion (commonly monosaccharides, amino acids, fatty acids, and glycerol) and active transport (commonly disaccharides, dipeptides, and tripeptides). A complex system of innervation and secretions maintains a basic pH that facilitates metabolism and absorption. The large intestine includes the cecum, the appendix, the colon (consisting of ascending, transverse, descending, and sigmoid portions), and the rectum which passes to the exterior through the anus. The primary function of the large intestine is reabsorption of fluid and electrolytes from the GI tract and excretion of wastes (Rudolph, 2003; Simone, 2003). Large intestine bacteria synthesize vitamin K and facilitate some vitamin B absorption.

PEDIATRIC DIFFERENCES

Although the fetus makes sucking and swallowing movements in utero and ingests amniotic fluid, the GI system is immature at birth. The processes of absorption and excretion do not begin until after birth because the placenta provides nutrients and removes waste. Sucking is a primitive reflex that occurs whenever the lips or cheeks are stroked. The infant does not have voluntary control over swallowing until about 6 weeks of age.

The stomach capacity of the newborn is quite small, and intestinal motility (**peristalsis**) is greater than in older children (Figure 24–2 ➤). These characteristics explain the

AS CHILDREN GROW

Stomach Capacity Increases Throughout Childhood

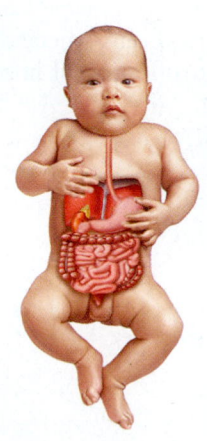

Stomach capacity throughout early childhood	
Age	Capacity (mL)
Newborn	10 to 20
1 week	30 to 90
2 to 3 weeks	75 to 100
1 month	90 to 150
3 months	150 to 200
1 year	210 to 360
2 years	500

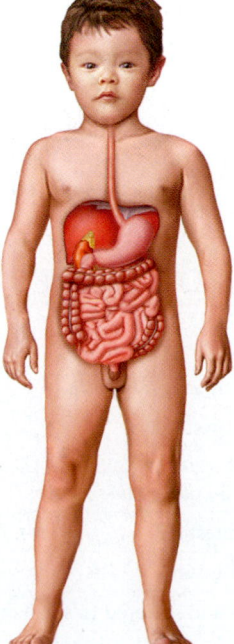

Figure 24–2 ➤ Parents should be reminded that the young infant has a small stomach as compared to the older child or adolescent. Amounts per feeding should be determined accordingly using the guidelines seen here.
From: Chamley, C. A., Carson, P., Randall, D., & Sandwell, M. (2004). *Developmental anatomy and physiology of children* (p. 217). St. Louis: Elsevier.

newborn's need for small, frequent feedings and the increased frequency and liquid consistency of bowel movements. Because of the relaxed cardiac sphincter, infants frequently regurgitate small amounts of feedings.

Digestion takes place in the duodenum. Infants have a deficiency of several enzymes: amylase (which digests carbohydrates), lipase (which enhances fat absorption), and trypsin (which catabolizes protein into polypeptides and some amino acids). Enzymes are usually not present in sufficient quantities to aid digestion until 4 to 6 months of age. Thus, abdominal distention from gas is common.

Liver function is also immature. After the first few weeks of life the liver is able to conjugate bilirubin and ex-crete bile. The processes of **gluconeogenesis** (formation of glycogen from noncarbohydrates), plasma protein and ketone formation, vitamin storage, and **deamination** (removal of amino group from amino compound) remain immature during the first year of life.

By the second year of life, digestive processes are fairly complete. Stomach capacity increases to accommodate a three-meals-per-day feeding schedule. At about the same time, myelination of the spinal cord becomes complete and voluntary control over excretory functions can be achieved. See the accompanying tables for laboratory and diagnostic tests and guidelines for assessment of the gastrointestinal system.

DIAGNOSTIC PROCEDURES/LABORATORY TESTS FOR THE GASTROINTESTINAL SYSTEM

Diagnostic Procedure	Purpose	Nursing Implications
Abdominal ultrasound	Ultrasound is a noninvasive procedure used to detect tissue abnormalities by visualizing body tissue structure or wave-form analysis of Doppler studies. Can be useful in diagnosis of tumors. Helps determine size, structure, and position of the spleen, liver, and pancreas. An ultrasound probe (transducer) is held over the abdominal area to produce an ultrasound beam to the tissues. The reflected sound waves or tissues are then transformed into scans, graphs, or sounds (Doppler).	• Administer sedation if prescribed and monitor child according to agency guidelines. • Maintain NPO status pre-procedure if ordered. • Explain procedure to parents and child. Inform them that the procedure is painless, and there is no exposure to radiation. • Confirm the child has not received any tests that will interfere with results, (e.g., upper GI series). • Explain to the child that a gel will be placed on the abdomen. • Instruct the child to remain still during the procedure.
Barium enema	Barium or barium and air is administered via a tube through the rectum to the colon. The large intestine is visualized to detect any abnormalities. Fluoroscopy is used to monitor the process and radiographs are taken.	• If procedure is planned ahead of time, give parents any special instructions regarding diet, laxatives, and/or enemas.
Computer tomography (CT) of the abdomen	Narrow radiograph beam is used to examine the structures of the abdomen. CT with or without iodine contrast (dye) may be performed. Dye enhances visualization of structures. Useful in diagnosis of tumors, obstruction, bleeding, and perforation of the liver, spleen, or pancreas.	• Assess for iodine allergy if contrast is to be used. • Will need intravenous access if contrast is used. • NPO for at least 4 hours for CT with contrast. • Administer sedation as ordered and monitor according to agency guidelines.
Endoscopy	A flexible, fiberoptic endoscope is used to visualize the internal structures of the esophagus, stomach, and duodenum. This procedure is also used to collect cytologic specimens, and confirm GI pathology.	• Maintain NPO status pre-procedure. • The child will be sedated for the procedure. Monitor the child according to agency guidelines. • Inform child that some pressure will be felt upon endoscope insertion. • Resume oral feedings as prescribed.
GI series	Upper GI and small bowel series are fluoroscopic and radiographic examinations of the esophagus, stomach, and small intestine. Oral barium or water-soluble contrast agent is swallowed. The barium or contrast is observed as it passes through the digestive tract and films are taken. This series identifies: • Esophageal, gastric, or duodenal ulcers • Polyps, tumors, or hiatal hernias in the GI tract • Pyloric stenosis • Foreign bodies, varices, or strictures	• Maintain NPO status pre-procedure. A low-residue diet may be ordered before the test. • Withhold medications as ordered. • Record vital signs; note epigastric pain or discomfort. • Inform child that all of the liquid must be swallowed, but that the test will not cause pain or discomfort.

DIAGNOSTIC PROCEDURES/LABORATORY TESTS FOR THE GASTROINTESTINAL SYSTEM (continued)

Diagnostic Procedure	Purpose	Nursing Implications
Intraesophageal pH probe monitoring	Considered the gold standard test for diagnosing gastroesophageal reflux disease and for evaluating atypical symptoms such as apnea, stridor, or cough. Probe is placed in the distal esophagus to detect pH changes below 4.0. pH is measured and recorded every 4 to 8 seconds.	• Ensure pH probe is secured. • Prevent infant or child from inadvertent removal of probe. May need to mitten infant and young child's hands using soft bandaging. • Probe is left in place to measure pH for 24 hours. • Monitor and record pH measurements per protocol. • Instruct parents to keep diary of child's activities while probe is in place, (e.g., feeding, sleeping, etc.).
Radiograph (X-ray) - Flat plate of the abdomen	Radiographs use irradiation to obtain images and capture them on film for diagnostic and screening purposes. Useful in detecting abdominal masses, obstruction, trauma, and fluid in the abdomen.	• Infants and young children may need to be immobilized. • Explain to the child that the procedure will not hurt. • Ask child to hold still. • Have adolescent females wear a protective lead apron.

Laboratory Test	Purpose	Nursing Implications
Bilirubin (Serum)	To monitor bilirubin levels associated with jaundice of the newborn and liver disease in children.	• Explain the reason for the tests. • Obtain specimen via protocol. • Support child during procedure. • Monitor child for signs of jaundice that would indicate need for bilirubin testing.
Stool for ova and parasites	Stool is collected for laboratory analysis for ova and parasites.	• Assist in collection of specimen. • Use precautions when handling stool to avoid spread of infection to self and others.
Stool for occult blood	Stool is examined for blood that is present in minute quantities and can be seen only on microscopic examination or through chemical testing.	• Assist in collection of specimen. • Send the specimen to the laboratory or examine on the unit with special testing kit per instructions. • For adolescent females, make sure the specimen does not contain menstrual discharge.

Data from: Corbett, J. V. (2004). *Laboratory tests and diagnostic procedures with nursing diagnoses* (6th ed.). Upper Saddle River, NJ: Prentice Hall Health; Kee, J. L. (2005a). *Handbook of laboratory & diagnostic tests with nursing implications* (5th ed.). Upper Saddle River, NJ: Prentice Hall Health; Kee, J. L. (2005). *Laboratory and diagnostic tests with nursing implications* (7th ed.). Upper Saddle River, NJ: Prentice Hall Health.

GUIDELINES FOR ASSESSMENT OF A CHILD WITH A GASTROINTESTINAL CONDITION*

Assessment Focus	Assessment Guidelines
Abdomen	• Observe the shape of the abdomen. • Note any abdominal distention. • Observe for peristaltic waves (visible rhythmic contractions of the intestinal wall smooth muscle). • Palpate the abdomen and note if it is soft or firm. • Does the child complain of pain or tenderness during palpation? Does the infant cry? • Describe any masses palpated by location, shape, size, and consistency. • Palpate the liver for size and tenderness. • Palpate the spleen for size and tenderness.
Esophagus	• Note the presence of increased oral secretions, tolerance of feedings, spitting up, emesis, and recurrent respiratory infections. Observe amount, color, and frequency of emesis. • Note if emesis is associated with feeding and whether or not it is projectile.
Stomach umbilicus	• Note amount of intake, frequency of feedings, and growth. • Observe the umbilicus for protrusion. Palpate the size of the umbilical ring.
Bowel sounds	• Auscultate for bowel sounds in all four quadrants prior to palpation.
Stool	• Observe color, consistency, and size of stool. Note any changes in stool patterns.

*See Chapter 5 ∞ for actual techniques and order of abdominal assessment.

STRUCTURAL DEFECTS

Structural defects can involve one or more areas of the GI tract. These defects occur when growth and development of fetal structures are interrupted during the first trimester. This can leave the structure incomplete, resulting in **atresia** (absence or closure of a normal body orifice), malposition, nonclosure, or other abnormalities.

Cleft Lip and Cleft Palate

Cleft lip and cleft palate are two distinct facial defects (Figure 24–3 ➤). Incomplete fusion of the lip occurs in approximately 1 in 700 births (Cleft Palate Foundation, 2005). It is more common in Native Americans and Asians than in Whites, and less common in Blacks. Incomplete fusion of the palate occurs in approximately 1 in 2000 births. Cleft lip and cleft palate are the fourth most common birth defects in the United States (Merritt, 2005a).

Etiology and Pathophysiology

Cleft lip with or without cleft palate results when the maxillary processes fail to fuse with the elevations on the frontal prominence during the sixth week of gestation. Normally union of the upper lip is complete by the seventh week. Fusion of the secondary palate occurs between 5 and 12 weeks of gestation. Failure of the tongue to move downward at the correct time prevents the palatine processes from fusing.

The intrauterine development of the hard and soft palates is completed in the first trimester. It is during this time that other major organ systems develop. Ten percent of children with cleft lip and palate will have an associated syndrome. When cleft lip or cleft palate occurs alone, the incidence of an associated syndrome increases to 30–50%, respectively (Merritt, 2005a). These children have an increased incidence of dental deformity, otitis media, hearing loss, and speech problems (Johansson & Ringsberg, 2004). There is an increased incidence in families with a prior history of cleft lip or palate. The cause is believed to be multifactorial, involving a combination of environmental and genetic influences. When fortification of cereals and breads with folate began in the United States in 1996 as a measure to decrease neural tube defects, the incidence of orofacial clefts also decreased. Folic acid supplementation prior to conception may decrease the incidence of cleft lip and/or palate (van Rooij et al., 2003).

Clinical Manifestations

A cleft that involves the lip is apparent at birth. It may be a simple dimple in the vermilion border of the lip or a complete separation extending to the floor of the nose. The defect may be unilateral or bilateral and may occur alone or in combination with a cleft palate defect. Varying degrees of nasal deformity may also be present.

Cleft palate defects are less obvious when they occur without a cleft lip and may not be detected at birth. Clefts of the hard palate form a continuous opening between the mouth and nasal cavity and may be unilateral or bilateral, involving just the soft palate or both the soft and hard palate.

■ COLLABORATIVE CARE

Medical management of cleft lip and palate requires the combined efforts of a multidisciplinary team. Because speech, hearing, and dentition may be affected, coordinated care by specialists in plastic surgery, hearing, speech, and dentistry is necessary.

Successful imaging of the face via ultrasound can be performed at 15 weeks' gestation; however, the optimal timing for prenatal diagnosis of cleft lip is at 20–22 weeks' gestation (Johnson & Sandy, 2003). The cleft lip is usually repaired by about 2 to 3 months of age (Figure 24–4 ➤). Some institutions have reported successful repair in the neonatal period (Sandberg, Magee, & Denk, 2002). The lip is sutured together using either a diagonal incision or a staggered suture line (z-plasty) (Merritt, 2005b). If the defect is severe, the child may need more than one operation to achieve total repair. After surgery, soft elbow immobilizers are used to prevent flexion of the arms. The child should receive distraction and pain medication as needed to prevent crying, as prolonged crying may disrupt the suture line.

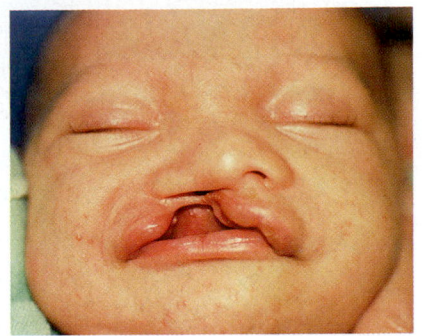

A

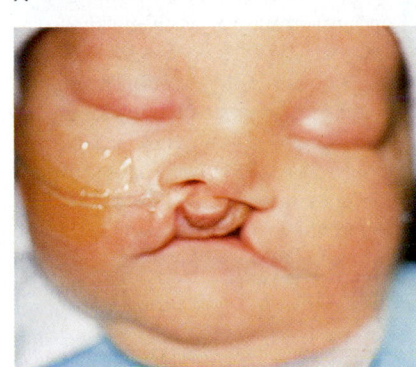

B

Figure 24–3 ➤ A, Unilateral cleft lip.
B, Bilateral cleft lip.
Courtesy of Dr. Elizabeth Peterson, Spokane, WA.

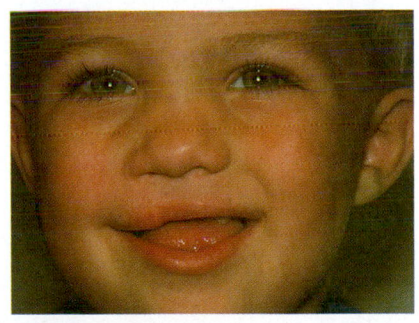

A

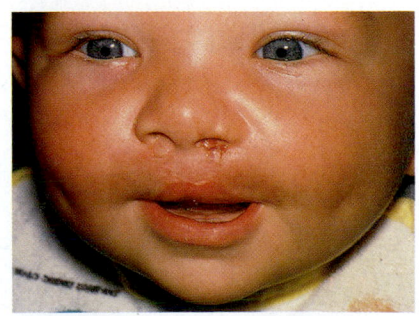

B

Figure 24–4 ➤ A, Repaired unilateral cleft lip. B, Repaired bilateral cleft lip.
Courtesy of Dr. Elizabeth Peterson, Spokane, WA.

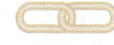

SKILL 4–6
Applying Elbow Immobilizers

CULTURE

Cleft Lip and Cleft Palate

In many developing countries, infants do not have access to surgery for correction of cleft lip and palate. They may grow into childhood and adulthood with these abnormalities. Medical teams from the United States, Canada, and other countries sometimes travel to developing nations for short medical missions, performing surgery on the children and teaching local doctors surgical techniques. Are their medical mission teams from your area that perform these surgeries? What is the planning required for such trips to perform surgery safely and care for the children? What is the impact on the communities served?

MediaLink

Case Study: The Child with Cleft Palate

Early closure of the lip enables the infant to form a better seal around the nipple for feeding. The sucking motion strengthens the muscles necessary for speech. Special feeding devices such as longer nipples with enlarged holes are available to help meet the infant's nutritional needs before surgical correction.

Timing of the cleft palate repair varies among surgeons and depends on the size and severity of the cleft. Most surgeons perform closure operations before the child reaches 18 months of age (Merritt, 2005b). This protects the formation of tooth buds and allows the infant to develop more normal speech patterns.

Infants with cleft lip and cleft palate are prone to recurrent otitis media, which can lead to tympanic membrane scarring and hearing loss. Antibiotics are prescribed to treat any infections that might lead to an ear infection. Because infants with chronic otitis media often have difficulty hearing, speech patterns may be altered. These infants require early, continuous intervention to prevent complications. (Refer to Chapter 19 ∞ for care of the child with chronic otitis media.) The child who has had cleft palate repair requires orthodontic care. Early visits permit assessment of tooth eruption and the need for future orthodontic work.

NURSING MANAGEMENT

Nursing care involves facilitating feeding, providing emotional support, performing preoperative and postoperative care, assisting parents to coordinate care and maintain a healthy home environment, and making appropriate referrals.

Nursing Assessment and Diagnosis

Physiologic Assessment

A cleft lip defect is observable at birth. A cleft palate defect is usually noted during the newborn assessment by palpation of the hard and soft palate with the finger (Merritt, 2005b). A description of the location and extent of the defect helps the nurse determine the correct method of feeding. Thorough and complete physical assessment is needed since additional defects are sometimes present.

Psychosocial Assessment

Assessment of the family's reactions is an integral part of the overall nursing assessment. Physical deformities, especially of the face, can be devastating to parents. A poorly corrected defect can lead to low self-esteem in the older child. Assess the child's developmental level and social interactions with peers.

The accompanying Nursing Care Plan lists common nursing diagnoses for the infant with a cleft lip and/or palate. Other diagnoses that might be appropriate include:

- Anxiety (Parent) related to situational crisis and threat to self-concept
- Ineffective Infant Feeding Pattern related to anatomic abnormality
- Risk for Caregiver Role strain related to complexity of caregiving tasks
- Risk for Impaired Home Maintenance Management related to infant's defect(s) and inadequate family support

Planning and Implementation

Nursing care involves providing emotional support, performing postoperative care, helping parents coordinate care and maintain a healthy home environment, and making appropriate referrals. See Nursing Care Plan: The Infant with a Cleft Lip and/or Palate for a summary of nursing care.

Facilitate Feeding

Feeding problems for the infant with cleft lip or cleft palate depend on the severity of the anatomic defect. Infants with cleft lip and/or cleft palate are generally able to breast- or bottle-feed with the assistance of lactation consultants and education related to positioning and feeding techniques (Reid, 2004). If breast-feeding is not possible, the mother can be assisted to pump her breasts in order for the milk to be fed by a special nurser.

NURSING CARE PLAN The Infant with a Cleft Lip and/or Palate

GOAL	INTERVENTION	RATIONALE	EXPECTED OUTCOME
Preoperative Care			
1. Compromised Family Coping related to birth of a child with a defect			
	NIC Priority Intervention: **Family Involvement:** *Facilitating family participation in the emotional and physical care of the child.*		*NOC Suggested Outcome:* **Positive Coping:** *Extent of coping mechanisms and ability to perform child's physical and emotional care.*
Parents will begin bonding process with the infant.	• Help parents to hold the infant and facilitate feeding process.	• Contact is essential for bonding.	Parents hold, comfort, and show concern for the infant.
	• Point out positive attributes of infant (e.g., hair, eyes, alertness).	• Helps parents see the child as a whole, rather than concentrating on the defect.	
	• Explain surgical procedure and expected outcome. Show pictures of other children's cleft lip repair.	• Eliminating unknown factors helps to decrease anxiety.	
The family's coping ability will be maximized. Parents will verbalize the nature and sequelae of the defect.	• Assess parents' knowledge of the defect, their degree of anxiety and level of discomfort, and the interpersonal relationships among family members.	• Helps to determine the appropriate timing and amount of information to be given regarding the child's defect.	The family demonstrates improved coping ability before discharge.
	• Explore the reactions of extended family members.	• Extended family is an important source of support for most parents of a newborn. Family members can often help promote acceptance and compliance with the treatment plan.	Parents receive necessary support to care for their infant.
	• Support open visitation.	• Allows parents to continue the bonding process.	
	• Encourage parents to participate in caretaking activities (holding, diapering, feeding).	• Participation in infant care decreases anxiety and provides parents with a sense of purpose.	
	• Provide information about the etiology of cleft lip and palate defects and the special needs of these infants. Encourage questions.	• Concrete information allows parents time to understand the defect and reduces guilt.	
	• Refer to parent support groups.	• Support groups allow parents to express their feelings and concerns, to find people with concerns similar to their own, and to seek additional information.	
2. Imbalanced Nutrition: Less than Body Requirements related to the infant's inability to ingest nutrients			
	NIC Priority Intervention: **Nutrition Management:** *Provision of a balanced dietary intake of foods and fluids.*		*NOC Suggested Outcome:* **Nutrition Status:** *Amount of food and fluid taken into the body over a 24-hour period.*
The infant will gain weight steadily.	• Assess fluid and calorie intake daily. Assess weight daily (same scale, same time, with infant completely undressed). Teach parents signs of adequate fluid intake such as frequent wet diapers.	• Provides an objective measurement of whether the infant is receiving sufficient caloric intake to promote growth. Using the same scale and procedure when weighing the infant provides for comparability between daily weights.	The infant maintains adequate nutritional intake and gains weight appropriately.

(continued)

GOAL	INTERVENTION	RATIONALE	EXPECTED OUTCOME
2. Imbalanced Nutrition: Less than Body Requirements related to the infant's inability to ingest nutrients (continued)			
	• Observe for any respiratory impairment.	• Any symptoms of respiratory compromise will interfere with the infant's ability to suck. Feedings should be initiated only if there are no signs of respiratory distress.	
	• Provide weight and appropriate calories and fluid amounts. If the infant needs an increased number of calories to grow, referral to a nutritionist should be made. Formulas with higher calorie concentrations per ounce are available without increasing total fluids.	• Provides optimal calories and fluids for growth and hydration.	
	• Facilitate breast-feeding.	• Breast milk is recommended as the best food for an infant. The process of breast-feeding helps to promote bonding between mother and infant.	Successful breast-feeding is achieved if desired.
	• Hold the infant in a semisitting position.	• Makes swallowing easier and reduces the amount of fluid return from the nose.	
	• Give the mother information on breast-feeding the infant with a cleft lip and/or palate such as plugging the cleft lip and eliciting a letdown reflex before nursing.	• Information and specific suggestions may encourage the mother to persist with breast-feeding.	
	• Contact the La Leche League for the name of a support person.	• The La Leche League promotes breast-feeding for all infants. It can provide support people with experience who will aid the mother.	
	• If the mother is unable to breast-feed (or prefers not to), initiate bottle-feeding: Hold infant in an upright or semisitting position for feeding.	• Facilitates swallowing and minimizes the amount of fluid return from the nose.	Feeding provides necessary nutrients and is a positive experience for parents and infant.
	• Place nipple against the inside cheek toward the back of the tongue. May need to use a premature nipple (slightly longer and softer than regular nipple with a larger opening) or a Brecht feeder (an oval bottle with a long, soft nipple). Special commercial feeders are also available.	• Use of longer, softer nipples makes it easier for the infant to suck. A Brecht feeder decreases the amount of pressure in the bottle and makes the formula flow more easily.	
	• Feed small amounts slowly.	• Small amounts and slow feeding do not tire the infant as quickly as do larger amounts given at a faster rate. They also decrease the calories used during feeding.	

GOAL	INTERVENTION	RATIONALE	EXPECTED OUTCOME
2. Imbalanced Nutrition: Less than Body Requirements related to the infant's inability to ingest nutrients (continued)			
	• Burp frequently, after 15–30 mL of formula has been given.	• Frequent burping prevents the accumulation of air in the stomach, which can cause regurgitation or vomiting.	
	• Initiate nasogastric feedings if the infant is unable to ingest sufficient calories by mouth.	• Adequate nutrition must be maintained. Use of a feeding tube allows the infant who has difficulty with oral feeding to receive adequate nutrition for growth.	
3. Risk for Aspiration (Breast Milk, Formula, or Mucus) related to anatomic defect			
	NIC Priority Intervention: **Aspiration Precautions:** *Prevention or minimization of risk factors in the patient at risk of aspiration.*		*NOC Suggested Outcome:* **Airway Maintenance:** *Toleration of enteral feedings without aspiration.*
The infant will have no episodes of gagging or aspiration.	• Assess respiratory status and monitor vital signs at least every 2 hours.	• Allows for early identification of problems.	The infant exhibits no signs of respiratory distress.
	• Hold upright for 30 minutes after feeding.	• Prevents aspiration of feedings.	
	• Keep head of bed elevated.		
	• Feed slowly and use adaptive equipment as needed.	• Facilitates intake while minimizing risk of aspiration.	
	• Burp frequently (after every 15–30 mL of fluid).	• Helps to prevent regurgitation and aspiration.	
	• Position upright for feedings.	• Minimizes passage of feedings through cleft.	
	• Keep suction equipment and bulb syringe at bedside.	• Suctioning may be necessary to remove milk or mucus.	
4. Deficient Knowledge (Parent) related to lack of exposure and unfamiliarity with resources			
	NIC Priority Intervention: **Teaching, Disease Process:** *Assisting the patient to understand information related to cleft lip/palate.*		*NOC Suggested Outcome:* **Knowledge:** *Extent of understanding conveyed about cleft lip/palate treatment.*
Before discharge, parents will verbalize home care methods for care of the infant with cleft lip and palate defect.	• Explain care and treatment (both short-term and long-term). Discuss potential complications.	• Assists the family to deal with the physical and psychosocial aspects of a child with a congenital defect.	Parents accurately describe and demonstrate feeding techniques to facilitate optimal growth of the infant; describe interventions if respiratory distress occurs; and take the written instructions home with them on discharge.
	• Demonstrate feeding techniques and alternatives. Allow parents to demonstrate before discharge.	• Provides visual instructions. Redemonstration confirms learning.	
	• Provide written instructions for follow-up care arrangements.	• Written instructions reinforce verbal instruction and provide a reference after discharge.	
	• Introduce the parents (if possible) to a primary care provider in the setting where the infant will receive follow-up care after discharge.	• Continuity of care is important. Since the infant will require long-term follow-up, a contact with the new provider is helpful.	

(continued)

NURSING CARE PLAN The Infant with a Cleft Lip and/or Palate (continued)

GOAL	INTERVENTION	RATIONALE	EXPECTED OUTCOME
Postoperative Care			
1. Imbalanced Nutrition: Less than Body Requirements related to inability to ingest nutrients			
	NIC Priority Intervention: **Nutrition Management:** *Promotion of a balanced dietary intake of foods and fluids.*		*NOC Suggested Outcome:* **Nutritional status:** *Extent to which nutrients are available to meet metabolic needs.*
The infant will receive adequate nutritional intake.	• Maintain intravenous infusion as ordered.	• Provides fluid when NPO.	The infant receives adequate nutritional intake. Infant resumes usual feeding patterns and gains weight appropriately.
	• Begin with clear liquids, then give half-strength formula or breast milk as ordered.	• Ensures adequate fluids and nutrients.	
	• Use Asepto syringe or dropper in side of mouth.	• Avoids suture line and resultant accumulation of formula in that area.	
	• Do not allow pacifiers.	• Sucking can disrupt suture line.	
	• Give high-calorie soft foods after cleft palate repair.	• Rough foods, utensils, and straws could disrupt the surgical site.	
2. Risk for Infection related to location of surgical procedure			
	NIC Priority Intervention: **Infection Control:** *Minimizing the acquisition and transmission of infectious agents.*		*NOC Suggested Outcome:* **Risk Control:** *Actions to eliminate or reduce actual, personal, or modifiable health risks.*
The infant's mucosal tissue will heal without infection.	• Assess vital signs every 4 hours.	• Elevated temperature may indicate infection.	The infant remains free of infection in the oral cavity. Tissues remain intact and pink.
	• Assess oral cavity every 2 hours or as needed for tenderness, reddened areas, lesions, or presence of secretions.	• Aids in identifying infection.	
	• Cleanse suture line with normal saline or sterile water, if ordered.	• Helps decrease the presence of bacteria.	Healing process progresses without adverse events in postoperative period.
	• Cleanse the cleft areas by giving 5–15 mL of water after each feeding.	• Prevents accumulation of carbohydrates, which encourage bacterial growth.	
	• If a crust has formed, use a cotton swab to apply a half-strength peroxide solution.	• Helps loosen the crust, aiding in removal.	
	• Apply antibiotic ointment to suture line as ordered.	• Counteracts the growth of bacteria.	
	• Use careful handwashing and sterile technique when working with suture line.	• Prevents the spread of microorganisms from other sources.	

NURSING CARE PLAN The Infant with a Cleft Lip and/or Palate (continued)

GOAL	INTERVENTION	RATIONALE	EXPECTED OUTCOME
3. Ineffective Breathing Pattern related to surgical correction of defect			
	NIC Priority Intervention: **Airway Management:** *Facilitation of patency of air passages.*		*NOC Suggested Outcome:* **Vital Signs Status:** *Temperature, pulse, respiration, and blood pressure within expected range for the infant/child.*
The infant will maintain an effective breathing pattern.	• Assess respiratory status and monitor vital signs at least every 4 hours.	• Allows for early identification of problems.	The infant shows no signs of respiratory infection or compromise.
	• Apply a cardiorespiratory monitor and pulse oximeter.	• Enables early detection of abnormal respirations and oxygenation facilitating prompt intervention.	
	• Keep suction equipment and bulb syringe at bedside. Gently suction oropharynx and nasopharynx as needed.	• Gentle suctioning will keep the airway clear. Suctioning that is too vigorous can irritate the mucosa.	
	• Provide cool mist for first 24 hours postoperatively if ordered.	• Moisturizes secretions to reduce pooling in lungs. Moisturizes oral cavity.	
	• Reposition every 2 hours.	• Ensures expansion of all lung fields.	
4. Impaired Tissue Integrity related to mechanical factors			
	NIC Priority Intervention: **Wound Care:** *Prevention of wound complications and promotion of wound healing.*		*NOC Suggested Outcome:* **Wound Healing:** *The extent to which cells and tissues have regenerated following intentional closure.*
Lip and/or palate will heal with minimal scarring or disruption.	• Position the infant with cleft lip repair on back.	• Prone position could cause rubbing on suture line.	Lip/palate heals without complications.
	• Use soft elbow immobilizers. Remove every 2 hours and replace. Do not leave the infant unattended when immobilizers are removed.	• Prevents the infant's hands from rubbing surgical site. Regular removal allows for skin and neurovascular checks.	
	• Maintain suture line or Steri-Strips placed over cleft lip repair.	• Maintaining suture line will minimize scarring.	
	• Avoid metal utensils or straws after cleft palate repair.	• These devices may disrupt suture line.	
	• Keep the infant well medicated for pain in initial postoperative period. Have parents hold and comfort the infant.	• Good pain management minimizes crying, which can cause stress on suture line. Increases bonding and soothes the child to decrease crying.	
	• Provide developmentally appropriate activities (i.e., mobiles, music).	• Soothes and keeps the infant calm.	

For infants requiring assistance to feed, several wide-based nipples, squeezable bottles, and other special bottles are available (Figure 24–5 ➤). Some infants may require a device placed in the mouth to enable them to establish suction. Several companies provide special nursers that may be helpful for children with cleft lip or palate. See Families Want to Know: Feeding the Infant with Cleft Lip or Cleft Palate on page 914.

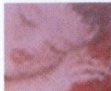

FAMILIES WANT TO KNOW

Feeding the Infant with Cleft Lip or Cleft Palate

The nurse assists the family to maintain feeding methods to promote the infant's growth and development. Inform the parents of the following:

- The infant with a cleft may require additional time to feed, which may produce fatigue. Allow the child additional time to eat and provide opportunities for rest after feeding.
- Feed the infant with the head and chest elevated since gravity helps to prevent milk from coming through the baby's nose.
- Breast-feeding is encouraged if possible; special techniques can help you to achieve success.

- Burp the baby frequently since infants with cleft palate tend to swallow air during feedings.
- A feeding specialist is available to assist, and can suggest specially designed bottles and other feeding techniques to facilitate feeding your baby.
- Maintain follow-up appointments so that infant is weighed and evaluated for growth and development.
- Inform your primary care provider if the infant has difficulty feeding or develops a problem such as vomiting or respiratory difficulty.

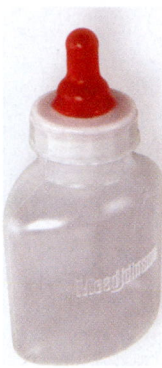
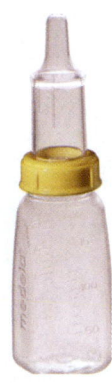

Figure 24–5 ▶ Special bottles and nipples for the child with cleft lip and/or cleft palate. The cleft palate nurser (A) and the SpecialNeeds® Feeder (B) both have longer, softer nipples and make it easier for the child to feed from a bottle. A, photo courtesy of Mead Johnson & Company; B, courtesy of Medela AG, Switzerland.

MediaLink

Cleft Palate Resources

CLINICAL TIP

Nurses can provide compassionate care to the family of the child born with cleft lip or cleft palate by pointing out the infant's positive aspects rather than focusing on the cleft. Examples include "Congratulations on the birth of your new son. He has beautiful hair and long eyelashes. The cleft lip/palate is correctable. We will refer you to a team of professionals who will work together to correct the opening."

Provide Emotional Support

Parent-infant bonding is jeopardized when a child is born with a cleft lip with or without an accompanying cleft palate (Coy, Speltz, & Jones, 2002). Parents may need assistance to view their infant as a whole person, rather than focusing solely on the physical defect. Promote parent-infant bonding by explaining the nature of the structural defect and the procedure for correction. Interact and speak to the infant in the parents' presence and point out positive attributes such as alertness, soft skin, or active movements. Self-blame is common among parents. Parents can also be referred to the Cleft Palate Foundation for information about the disorder. Pictures of children who have had repair are available at this web site. Seeing pictures of children who have had a successful repair offers reassurance to parents.

Parental anxiety is a typical response when children undergo surgery, and it is heightened when the surgery involves an infant. To minimize anxiety, give clear, concise explanations to parents. Allow sufficient time for parents to ask questions. Encourage parents to hold and cuddle the infant before surgery.

Provide Postoperative Care

Provide general postoperative care for the infant. (See Nursing Care Plan: The Infant with a Cleft Lip and/or Palate in this chapter and Nursing Care Plan: The Child Undergoing Surgery in Chapter 13 ∞.) Assess vital signs frequently and maintain the infant's airway. Measure intake and output. When oral fluids with clear liquids are started, they may be given through a dropper, syringe, or special feeder. Position the infant in a sitting position for the feedings to avoid aspiration. The infant then progresses to half-strength formula or breast milk. After each feeding, clean the suture line with water or normal saline to avoid accumulation of feedings.

It is important to maintain the suture line to ensure healing. Position the infant in a supine position to avoid rubbing the suture line on the bedding. Keep elbows in soft immoblizers. Maintain the suture line or Steri-Strips placed over the incision. Place antibiotic ointment on the incision site as ordered. Medicate the infant regularly to control pain and to minimize crying and stress on the suture line. After cleft palate surgery, avoid the use of metal utensils or straws, which may disrupt the surgical site.

Care in the Community

Pre- and postoperative management involves many different healthcare professionals. In addition to hospital, clinic, and home health nurses, members of the healthcare team often include specialists such as the plastic surgeon, orthodontist, speech pathologist, and pediatrician (Johansson & Ringsberg, 2004). The parents are the best coordinators of the child's care. Encourage them to keep a diary listing the professionals with whom they talk and the content of the discussions.

Identify and address home care needs well in advance of discharge. Discuss all aspects of the infant's care with the parents throughout hospitalization and after surgery. Involve parents in the infant's care to increase their comfort level before discharge and to promote bonding. Teach them feeding techniques, how to recognize signs of infection, how to position the infant, and how to care for the suture line.

Discuss with the parents the financial implications of long-term care. Private insurance does not always cover all the costs of care necessary for the child. Refer parents to social services familiar with programs and financial aid for which the parents and child may be eligible. Relief of financial worries enables parents to concentrate on caring for the child.

Teach parents how to care for the child after discharge. If the child has siblings, emphasize that they will need preparation to accept the child. Sibling rivalry can be heightened when one child receives more attention at the home. Remind parents of the importance of setting limits and of spending time with each child. Determine whether additional family supports are necessary. Provide parents with information on support groups, physicians, social workers, Internet resources, and local services that can help maintain family continuity.

Discuss ways to prevent the infant from touching the suture line. Teach parents how to bundle an infant in a blanket with arms tucked inside the blanket. A front-sling baby carrier may also be used to immobilize the arms. Front-sling carriers provide the additional benefits of comforting the infant through contact with the parent and of holding the infant upright, which aids in optimal positioning after feedings.

After surgical repair, parents need to be taught how to feed the infant and identify signs of complications (fever, vomiting, respiratory distress). Referral to a home healthcare agency for support may be helpful. Encourage follow-up visits with healthcare professionals. The child may need further evaluation of speech development, presence of ear infections, or a recommendation for plastic surgery.

Evaluation

Expected outcomes of nursing care in the preoperative period include:

- The child does not experience respiratory distress and maintenance of normal respirations.
- Positive parent-infant bonding is established.
- The parents express a feeling of support and comfort by family and community.
- The child achieves and maintains a normal weight.
- The parent has knowledge of the defect, its correction, and the child's needs.

Expected outcomes of postoperative nursing care include:

- The child will be free of infection.
- The surgical site will heal without complications.
- The child will not experience respiratory distress.
- The child will have effective pain management.
- The child will have fluid and electrolyte balance and adequate weight gain.
- The parents will verbalize appropriate home care after surgery.

Esophageal Atresia and Tracheoesophageal Fistula

Esophageal atresia is a malformation that results from failure of the esophagus to develop as a continuous tube during the fourth and fifth weeks of gestation. Esophageal atresia occurs in approximatley 1 in 4000 births, with 90% of those affected also having a tracheoesophageal fistula (Orenstein, Peters, Khan, Youssef, & Hussain, 2004).

In esophageal atresia, the foregut fails to lengthen, separate, and fuse into two parallel tubes (the esophagus and trachea) during fetal development. Instead, the esophagus may end in a blind pouch or develop as a pouch connected to the trachea by a fistula (tracheoesophageal fistula) (Figure 24–6 ➤). Esophageal atresia is often associated with a maternal history of polyhydramnios. Associated anomalies may occur, including congenital heart defects, gastrointestinal or urinary tract anomalies, and musculoskeletal abnormalities (Orenstein et al., 2004).

GROWTH & DEVELOPMENT

Cleft Lip Healing

An infant who has had a cleft lip repair needs stimulation to provide distraction. This approach will minimize crying, which can damage the suture line. Soft, colorful toys, mobiles, and other visual objects are helpful. Music also can be used to soothe the infant. Parental presence is comforting and reassuring.

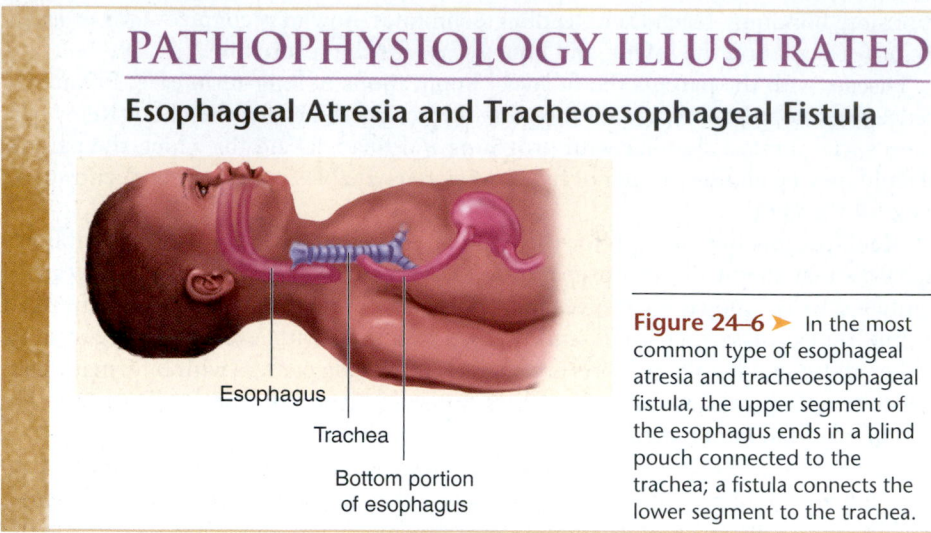

PATHOPHYSIOLOGY ILLUSTRATED

Esophageal Atresia and Tracheoesophageal Fistula

Esophagus

Trachea

Bottom portion
of esophagus

Figure 24–6 ➤ In the most
common type of esophageal
atresia and tracheoesophageal
fistula, the upper segment of
the esophagus ends in a blind
pouch connected to the
trachea; a fistula connects the
lower segment to the trachea.

Symptoms in the newborn include excessive salivation and drooling, often accompanied by cyanosis, choking, coughing, and sneezing. During feeding, the infant returns fluid through the nose and mouth. Aspiration places the infant at risk for pneumonia. Depending on the type of defect, the abdomen may become distended because of air trapping.

Collaborative Care

Diagnosis is usually confirmed by attempting to pass a 5 or 8 French nasogastric tube into the stomach. In most cases, the tube meets resistance and can be advanced only minimally. Specific defects and associated anomalies are determined by radio examination. Echocardiogram and abdominal ultrasound are performed. Careful examination of the lungs is needed. A delay in diagnosis can be fatal because ingested fluid or secretions may enter the lungs.

A tube is inserted to suction the upper pouch. Intravenous antibiotics and fluids are begun. Surgery is performed as soon as possible. Surgical correction may be accomplished in several stages. The first stage usually involves ligation of the fistula and insertion of a gastrostomy tube. In the second stage, the two ends of the esophagus are reconnected, if possible. When surgical closure (anastomosis) is not possible, a gastrostomy tube must remain in place for use in feeding. Potential postoperative complications include gastroesophageal reflux, aspiration, and stricture formation. The prognosis is usually good with surgery.

Nursing Management

The nurse may recognize the signs and symptoms in the immediate newborn period. Assess for difficulty feeding and excessive drooling. Assess for the classic signs of choking, coughing, and cyanosis. Assess for respiratory distress and assess the lung sounds carefully. Esophageal atresia is a surgical emergency. Preoperatively the infant requires close observation and intervention to maintain a patent airway. Suction should be readily available to remove any secretions that accumulate in the nasopharyngeal airway. Place the infant with the head of the bed slightly lowered to minimize aspiration of secretions into the trachea. Use continuous or low intermittent suction to remove secretions from the blind pouch. Withhold oral fluids, and provide maintenance intravenous fluids.

After surgery, measure gastrostomy drainage, and administer intravenous fluids and antibiotics. Total parenteral nutrition may be needed until gastrostomy or oral feedings are tolerated.

The parents require emotional support throughout the infant's hospitalization. Clearly explain all procedures. Encourage parents to bond with the infant by stroking and talking to the infant. Eliciting questions and allowing parents to participate in the infant's care, especially feeding (when permitted), can facilitate bonding and help to prepare parents for care of the infant after discharge.

Once enteral feedings have been established, the infant may be discharged from the hospital with a gastrostomy tube in place (Figure 24–7 ➤). Teach the parents about gastrostomy tube care and feeding, signs of infection, and how to prevent postoperative complications. (See Families Want to Know: Teaching the Family About Gastrostomy Tube Feedings.)

The outcomes of nursing care will depend on the extent of the defect and correction. Examples include:

- Adequate intake of fluids to promote hydration and growth
- Absence of respiratory distress
- Positive parent-infant bonding
- Absence of infection
- Parental use of support and information resources regarding the condition

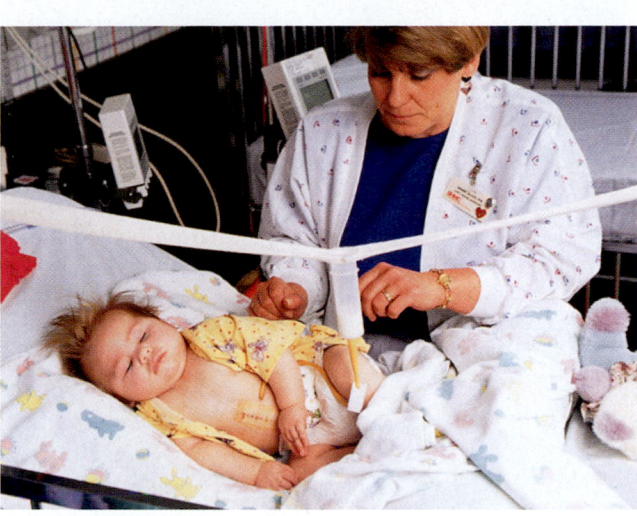

Figure 24–7 ➤ A gastrostomy tube is used to feed the child with a gastrointestinal disorder such as esophageal atresia.

Pyloric Stenosis

Pyloric stenosis is a hypertrophic obstruction of the circular muscle of the pyloric canal. The disorder is common and occurs in approximately 1–3 cases per 1000 live births (Gasseling, 2004). There is an increased incidence in first born males (Morash, 2002).

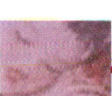

FAMILIES WANT TO KNOW

Teaching the Family About Gastrostomy Tube Feedings

The infant or child who has difficulty swallowing, consuming oral feedings, or gaining weight may be a candidate for gastrostomy tube placement. Feedings via gastrostomy tube are generally preferred instead of nasogastric feedings if the child will need enteral feedings but will not be needed more than 1–3 months (Burd & Burd, 2003). Children with chronic conditions such as failure to thrive, cystic fibrosis, neurological impairment, or gastrointestinal anomalies may need to have a gastrostomy tube placed for long-term enteral feedings (Borkowski, 2005). Parents of children who have or will receive a gastrostomy tube need clear instructions to maximize the benefit of the device to the child. See Chapter 13 ∞ for general guidelines related to teaching plans.

General Principles

Preoperatively

- Assess what the family knows about gastrostomy tube placement.
- Assess the parents and extended family members' willingness to learn about care of the gastrostomy tube and enteral feedings.
- Show the family pictures or dolls with gastrostomy tubes and explain what the child's abdomen will look like in the immediate postoperative period.
- Provide the family with a booklet about gastrostomy tubes and enteral feedings.

Postoperatively

- Show the family the child's gastrostomy tube.
- Reassess the family's understanding of the tube.
- When feedings are ordered, demonstrate the first feeding to the parents while explaining each step.
- Actively involve a family member in the second feeding. With subsequent feedings have a family member feed the child with the nurse watching.
- Teach the family how to administer medications.
- Teach the family daily care of the tube and the site surrounding the tube.
- Teach the family how to troubleshoot common complications.
- Provide family with phone numbers to call if needed.
- All family members that are involved in care of the child should practice feeding the child and administering medications to the child prior to discharge. This allows the nurse to assess for understanding of the procedure and gives the family confidence in their ability to care for the child. Some children will need bolus feedings, others may have continuous feedings via a feeding pump, and others may have bolus feedings during the day and continuous feedings at night.

Data from: Borkowski, S. (2005, May). Irritation, redness, and drainage at the site of a pediatric gastrostomy. *The Clinical Advisor*, 90–91; Burd, A., & Burd, R. S. (2003). The who, what, why and how-to guide for gastrostomy tube placement in infants. *Advances in Neonatal Care, 3,* 197–205; Gracey, K., Burd, A., & Burd, R. (2003). Guide for home gastrostomy tube care. *Advances in Neonatal Care, 3,* 206–207; and Holmes, S. (2004). Enteral feeding and percutaneous endoscopic gastrosotomy. *Nursing Standard, 18*(20), 41–43.

Etiology and Pathophysiology

The exact cause of pyloric stenosis is unknown, although frequently there is a family history of the disorder. Hypertrophy of the circular pylorus muscle results in stenosis of the passage between the stomach and the duodenum, partially obstructing the lumen of the stomach (Figure 24–8 ➤). The lumen becomes inflamed and edematous, which narrows the opening until the obstruction becomes complete. At this time vomiting becomes more forceful. As the obstruction progresses, the infant becomes dehydrated and electrolytes are depleted, resulting in metabolic imbalances.

Clinical Manifestations

Symptoms usually become evident 2 to 8 weeks after birth, although onset may vary. Initially the infant appears well or regurgitates slightly after feedings. The parents may describe the infant as a "good eater" who vomits occasionally. The symptoms in the early stages may be attributed erroneously to overfeeding, milk allergy, feeding intolerance, or gastroesophageal reflux (Morash, 2002). As the obstruction progresses, the vomiting becomes projectile. In **projectile vomiting**, the contents of the stomach may be ejected up to 3 feet from the infant. The vomitus is nonbilious and may become blood tinged because of repeated irritation to the esophagus. The infant is always hungry, appears irritable, fails to gain weight, and has fewer and smaller stools. The infant may become dehydrated and may develop metabolic alkalosis.

■ COLLABORATIVE CARE

On physical examination, visible peristaltic waves across the abdomen and an olive-sized mass in the right upper quadrant are often found. An abdominal ultrasound, to determine the diameter and length of the pyloric muscle, is usually performed to confirm the diagnosis. A thickened pylorus of >4 mm in diameter and length of >18 mm for the pyloric channel are diagnostic of pyloric stenosis (Blumer, Zucconi, Cohen, Scriven, & Lee, 2004). An upper gastrointestinal (UGI) study may also be performed, and reveals a narrowing of the pyloric channel, preventing the passage of the contrast

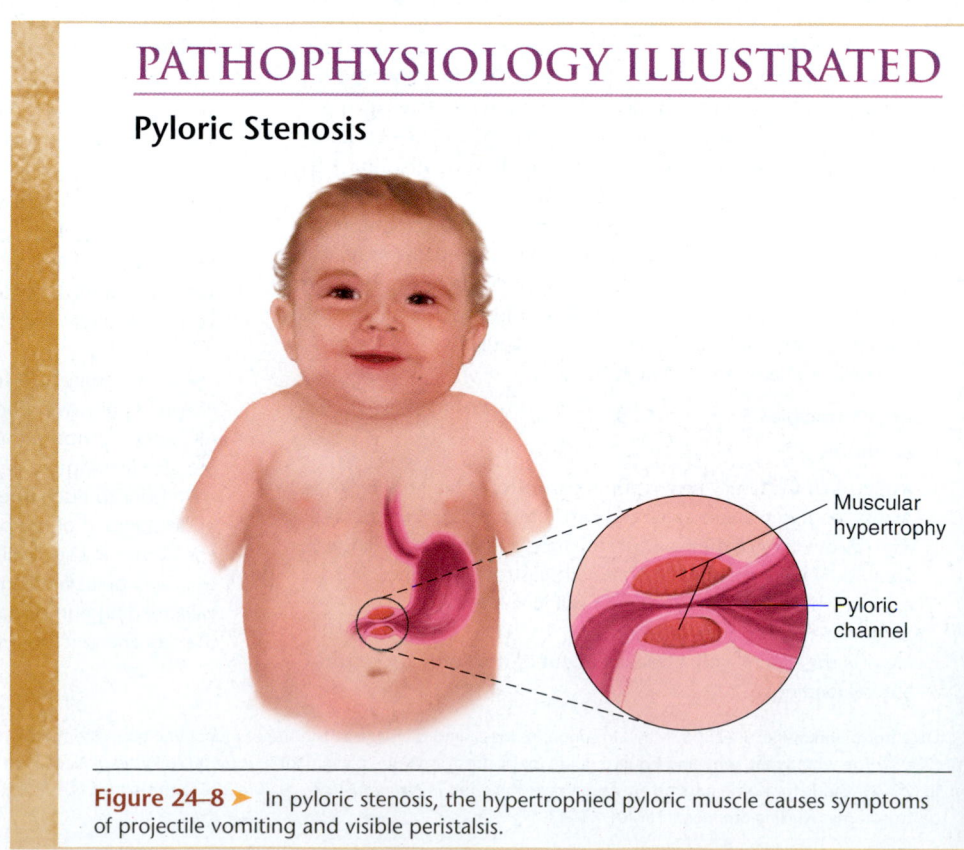

PATHOPHYSIOLOGY ILLUSTRATED

Pyloric Stenosis

Muscular hypertrophy

Pyloric channel

Figure 24–8 ➤ In pyloric stenosis, the hypertrophied pyloric muscle causes symptoms of projectile vomiting and visible peristalsis.

medium. Blood tests determine the degree of dehydration, electrolyte imbalance, and anemia (see Chapter 16 ∞); common findings are hypochloremia and metabolic alkalosis. Early diagnosis will decrease the frequency with which infants present with an alteration in electrolytes (Colletti, 2004).

Surgical correction is the treatment of choice. Preoperatively the infant's condition is stabilized with intravenous fluids and electrolytes. A nasogastric tube is inserted to decompress the stomach. Surgery is performed as soon as possible after the infant's condition is stabilized. Open pyloromyotomy is performed though a periumbilical incision or through a small, transverse upper abdominal incision. Laparoscopic pyloromyotomy is currently used in many cases, and patients undergoing this surgical method reach full feeding sooner, have less emesis, and average a shorter hospital stay than those having an open procedure (Zitsman, 2003). With both procedures, the circular muscle fibers are released to allow the passage of food and fluid.

The prognosis is good. The infant is usually taking fluids within a few hours following surgery and discharged on full strength formula within 24 hours after surgery.

NURSING MANAGEMENT

Nursing Assessment and Diagnosis

Observe the infant's abdomen for the presence of peristaltic waves. Bowel sounds are hyperactive on auscultation. Auscultate before palpating the abdomen since palpation can cause a change in bowel patterns. Palpation reveals an olive-shaped mass in the right upper quadrant of the abdomen.

Assess skin turgor, fontanels, urinary output, and mucous membranes to determine whether hydration is adequate. Measure vomitus and describe vomiting episodes. Be alert for signs of an electrolyte imbalance, particularly low levels of serum chloride, sodium, and potassium, and an elevated pH. (See Chapter 16 ∞ for a discussion of these electrolyte imbalances.)

Assess the parents' level of anxiety related to the child's condition.

Among the nursing diagnoses that might be appropriate for the child with pyloric stenosis are:

- Deficient Fluid Volume related to active fluid volume loss
- Imbalanced Nutrition: Less than Body Requirements related to vomiting and inability to ingest nutrients
- Disturbed Sleep Pattern related to discomfort and hunger
- Altered Family Processes related to health status of family member

Planning and Implementation

Nursing care centers on meeting the infant's fluid and electrolyte needs, minimizing weight loss, promoting rest and comfort, preventing infection, and providing supportive care for parents.

Meet Fluid and Electrolyte Needs

Because projectile vomiting will continue until the obstruction is relieved surgically, withhold oral feedings. Administer intravenous fluid therapy to correct fluid and electrolyte imbalances and to maintain adequate hydration. Because gastric fluid is high in potassium, hypokalemia can result. (See Chapter 16 ∞ for a discussion of this electrolyte imbalance and the signs of its occurrence.) Monitor intake and output (including vomitus) and urine specific gravity. Inform parents that all diapers will be weighed to measure the infant's output of urine and stool.

Minimize Weight Loss

The infant loses weight because of frequent vomiting. Monitor weight daily both preoperatively and postoperatively. Begin small, frequent feedings of clear liquids within 4 to 6 hours postoperatively. If clear liquids are tolerated, advance the infant to formula or breast milk feedings.

Promote Rest and Comfort

During the preoperative period the infant is hungry and cries often. Swaddle the infant to maintain warmth and provide comfort. Encourage the parents to hold and cuddle the infant. Provide a pacifier to meet the infant's need to suck.

Postoperatively the infant is uncomfortable because of the surgical incision. Instruct parents to avoid pressure on the incision. When diapering the infant, slide the diaper gently under the buttocks rather than lifting the legs. Swaddling, rocking, and use of a pacifier help to relax the infant. Analgesics can be administered to relieve discomfort as ordered. (See Chapter 15 ∞ for a discussion of pain management.)

Prevent Infection

Postoperatively the incision is covered with collodion or Steri-Strips and should be kept clean and dry. Check the incision site for redness, swelling, or discharge. Monitor the infant's temperature every 4 hours. Auscultate lungs for clear respiratory sounds.

Provide Supportive Care

The need for hospitalization and surgery creates anxiety for parents. Encourage them to participate in the infant's care and to discuss their fears and concerns. Provide simple and clear explanations about the infant's condition and care. Advise parents that occasional vomiting after surgery may occur.

Discharge Planning and Home Care Teaching

Instruct parents to observe the incision for redness, swelling, or discharge and to notify the physician immediately if these occur or if the infant's temperature is higher than 38.5°C (101°F). To reduce the possibility of infection, advise parents to fold the infant's diaper so that it does not touch the incision. Provide instructions about feeding to ensure the infant's intake. See Evidence-Based Practice: Postoperative Feeding Methods Following Pyloromyotomy in Infants, and Families Want to Know: Home Care Instructions Following Pyloromyotomy.

Evaluation

Expected outcomes of care include pain control, intake of recommended fluid and food with absence of vomiting, and manifestation of normal growth patterns.

Gastroesophageal Reflux

Gastroesophageal reflux (GER), the return of gastric contents into the esophagus, is the result of relaxation of the lower esophageal sphincter. Gastroesophageal reflux is one of the most common gastrointestinal disorders in children, affecting approximately

---

EVIDENCE-BASED PRACTICE

Postoperative Feeding Methods Following Pyloromyotomy in Infants

Clinical Question

How long should the infant be NPO following pyloromyotomy?

Evidence

Nurse researchers, in collaboration with a pediatric surgeon, conducted a 6-month retrospective study of 36 hypertrophic pyloric stenosis patients to compare conventional regimen feeds to ad lib feeds according to surgeon preference. The study revealed that the interval from the operating room to toleration of full feedings was less than with the ad lib group as compared to the conventional regimen group. Significant decrease in length of stay was also noted. These findings led to practice changes at the hospital where the study was conducted.

Implications

Postoperative feeding methods for infants following surgical correction (pyloromyotomy) of pyloric stenosis have remained unchanged for several decades. Conventional feeding methods include a prolonged NPO period following pyloromyotomy, with slow, incremental increases in volume and strength of feedings once feeding has resumed. Recent evidence indicates that a more liberal feeding method may prove beneficial, rather than harmful, to the infant.

Critical Thinking

How is feeding tolerance determined in the post-pyloromyotomy infant? If a surgeon prescribes conventional regimen feeding for post-pyloromyotomy infants, what collaborative approach could the nurse take to improve feeding approach?

Reference

Morash, D. (2002). An interdisciplinary project that changed practice in feeding methods after pyloromyotomy. *Pediatric Nursing, 28*(2), 113–117.

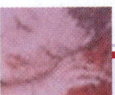

FAMILIES WANT TO KNOW

Home Care Instructions Following Pyloromyotomy

The infant is generally discharged home the day following surgery. Partner with the family to provide home feeding and care instructions. The following information is provided:

- The infant may be bottle- or breast-fed.
- An infant will sometimes vomit after some feedings following surgery—this does not mean the surgical correction was unsuccessful.
- If the infant vomits, offer a bottle or breast as soon as he or she is interested in feeding again
- The infant should be burped after every 1 to 2 ounces during feeding. If breast-feeding, burp the infant every 5 to 10 minutes.
- After feeding, place the baby in an upright position, holding for approximately 30 minutes, or position the infant on the right side with the head and upper body slightly elevated.
- The infant should not play or be rocked for 30 minutes following feedings.

- Administer analgesics as prescribed. Inform the healthcare provider if you believe your infant is not obtaining adequate pain relief.
- Keep the surgical wound area clean and dry. The bandage or strips may fall off, and this is normal. If not, they will be removed at the follow-up visit.
- The infant should be sponge bathed only. Tub baths are not allowed until the wound has healed or as instructed by the healthcare provider.
- Notify the healthcare provider if the infant demonstrates any of the following:
  - Redness, drainage, bleeding, or swelling at the surgical site.
  - The infant has a fever of 100.5°F or higher.
  - The infant is inconsolable.
  - The infant vomits the majority of 2 feedings in a row.

40–65% of infants ages 1–4 months. GER resolves by 1 year of age in most children with only 1% of those affected continuing to exhibit symptoms (Henry, 2004). There is a higher incidence in premature infants, and males are affected three times more often than females. Children with neurological impairments, such as cerebral palsy, more commonly experience gastroesophageal reflux. Some "spitting up" after feedings is considered normal in newborn infants, because of the weak cardiac sphincter of the stomach. However, regurgitation that continues and increases in frequency may be caused by GER and requires further investigation.

Gastroesophageal reflux disease (GERD) is a more serious manifestation of GER; it is a pathological condition in infants manifested by poor weight gain, esophagitis, neurobehavioral changes, and persistent respiratory symptoms or complications (Arguin & Swartz, 2004). Gastroesophageal reflux disease is diagnosed in approximately one in every 300 infants (Henry, 2004). Those children most at risk include those with neurologic disorders, syndromes, trisomy 21, bronchopulmonary dysplasia, and tracheoesophageal fistula (Henry, 2004).

Regurgitation after feeding is the most common sign of gastroesophageal reflux in infants. The infant may spit a small amount or may have episodes of forceful vomiting (Sondheimer, 2003). Children with gastroesophageal reflux are frequently hungry and irritable. They eat often but still lose weight. They have a history of vomiting and frequent upper respiratory infections and are at risk for aspiration and apneic episodes.

Collaborative Care

Diagnosis is confirmed by a thorough history of the child's feeding patterns and by diagnostic evaluation using contrast upper GI series, pH probe monitoring (insertion of a small catheter into the esophagus through the nose that is left in place for 18 to 24 hours to measure pH and thus determine number of reflux episodes), or nuclear medicine scintiscan (gastric emptying study) (Henry, 2004). The child should be tested for cow's milk protein allergy since there is an association between gastroesophageal reflux and cow's milk allergy (Arguin & Swartz, 2004).

Treatment depends on the severity of the condition. Uncomplicated GER may require only lifestyle changes that include small frequent feedings and adding rice cereal to formula in the infant's bottle to thicken feedings (Arguin & Swartz, 2004). Commercial thickened formulas that are nutritionally balanced are available. Breast milk does not thicken with rice cereal addition, but the breast-feeding mother should be encouraged to continue and feed small amounts at a time with frequent burping. The infant should be held in an upright position for 20–30 minutes after feeding (Arguin & Swartz, 2004). Fatty foods and citrus juices are avoided. Medications (proton pump inhibitors, antacids, and histamine antagonists) may be prescribed to reduce the amount of stomach acid and lessen the child's discomfort. See Medications Used to Treat GER/GERD on page 923.

Surgery may be indicated for those children with GER who do not respond to medications, especially if the child has potentially life-threatening complications such as respiratory symptoms (Gremse, 2004). Surgery involves the creation of a valve mechanism by wrapping the greater curvature of the stomach (fundus) around the distal esophagus (Nissen fundoplication). A gastrostomy tube is generally placed during the surgery to provide a means for venting the stomach. This will decrease the incidence and discomfort of gas that frequently accumulates after the Nissen fundoplication (Henry, 2004).

Nursing Management

Nursing management focuses on obtaining a thorough history of the child's feeding patterns. Observe vomiting episodes and document amount, color, and consistency of emesis.

Monitor the infant's weight daily and plot on a growth chart to note progress. Observe for any signs of respiratory distress, and keep the infant's nose and mouth clear of vomitus.

Adequate nutrition must be maintained. Infants receiving oral feedings should be given small, frequent feedings. Elevate the head of the crib to prevent aspiration if vomiting should occur. Prone positioning is no longer recommended in infants due to the risk of sudden infant death syndrome (SIDS). The infant is placed or held in the supine position. The child may be placed in a harness to maintain the desired position. Parents are encouraged to hold their infant in an upright position for 20 to 30 minutes following feedings. Minimize seated positioning such as in an infant seat since this increases intra-abdominal pressure and promotes reflux (Henry, 2004).

If the child has a gastrostomy tube, it is important to maintain skin integrity around the stoma site. Secure the tube so the infant cannot dislodge or pull on it, and check daily to be sure the length is the same, indicating correct placement.

Discharge planning focuses on instructing parents in how to feed and position the infant, as well as how to provide comfort and emotional support. Encourage parents to hold and cuddle the infant during all feedings. Providing the infant with a pacifier helps to meet nonnutritive sucking needs. Teach parents how to suction the nose and mouth if vomiting occurs.

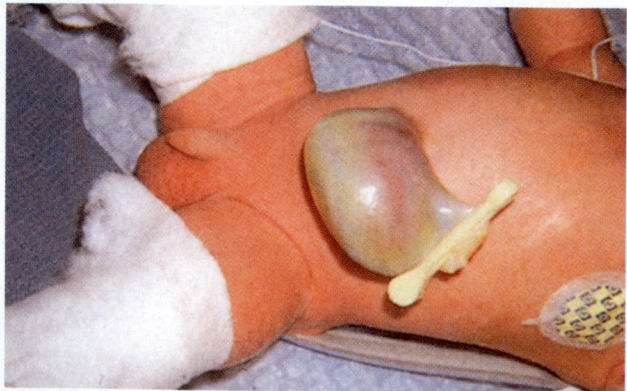

Figure 24–9 ▶ In omphalocele, the size of the sac depends on the extent of the protrusion of abdominal contents through the umbilical cord.
From Rudolph, A.M., Hoffman, J.I.E., & Rudolph, C.D. (Eds). (1991). Rudolph's pediatrics (19th ed., p. 1040). Stamford, CT: Appleton & Lange.

Omphalocele and Gastroschisis

Omphaloceles are congenital malformations in which intra-abdominal contents herniate through the umbilical cord (Figure 24–9 ▶). They result when the abdominal contents, such as intestines and liver, fail to return to the abdomen when the abdominal wall begins to close by the tenth week of gestation. The protrusion is covered by a translucent sac (peritoneum) into which the umbilical cord inserts. Omphalocele has a prevalence of 2.5 in 10,000 births (Weir, 2003). Omphalocele is often associated with other congenital anomalies such as cardiac defects; genitourinary anomalies; trisomy 13, 15, 18, or 21; craniofacial abnormalities; and diaphragmatic abnormalities (Azizkhan & Frykman, 2003).

The size of the sac varies depending on the extent of the protrusion. Rupture of the sac results in evisceration of the abdominal contents. Treatment involves protecting the sac from injury,

MEDICATIONS USED TO TREAT *Gastroesophageal Reflux*

Medication	Action/Indication	Nursing Implications
Histamine H-2 receptor antagonists Zantac (Ranitidine) Pepcid (Famotidine) Tagament (Cimetidine)	Inhibition of the histamine-2 receptor on the gastric parietal cell, thus blocking gastric acid secretion	May be administered with or without food If antacids are prescribed, administer 2 hours before or after H-2 antagonists Teach parents to avoid OTC medications without checking with healthcare provider Monitor for side effects: Bradycardia Constipation Nausea Fatigue Confusion Dizziness Headache Irritability Rash Thrombocytopenia
Proton Pump Inhibitors Prevacid (Lanzoprazole) Prilosec (Omeprazole)	These powerful inhibitors of acid secretion alleviate symptoms and help to heal esophagitis Blocks the final common pathway of acid production by inhibiting activated proton pumps in the gastric parietal cell canaliculus	Administer in the morning on an empty stomach Monitor for side effects: Abdominal pain Diarrhea Dizziness Fatigue Headache Hematuria Nausea Proteinuria Rash Teach family to inform primary healthcare provider if severe diarrhea occurs Teach family to inform primary healthcare provider if changes in urinary elimination, such as pain or discomfort associated with urination, occur
Prokinetic Agents Reglan (Metoclopramide)	Promotes gastric emptying Improves gut motility	Monitor for side effects: Mild sedation Fatigue Restlessness Nausea Rash Headache Insomnia Diarrhea Constipation Teach the family

Data from: Bindler, R., & Howry, L. (2005). *Pediatric drug guide.* Upper Saddle River, NJ: Prentice Hall Health.
Gremse, D. A. (2002). Gastroesophageal reflux: Life-threatening disease or laundry problem? *Clinical Pediatrics, 41*(6), 369–372.
Henry, S. M. (2004). Discerning differences: Gastroesophageal reflux and gastroesophageal reflux disease infants. *Advances in Neonatal Care, 4,* 235–247.
Wall, G. C., & Jacoby, H. I. (2002). Gastroesophageal reflux disease. *American Journal of Pharmaceutical Education, 66*(2), 148–152.

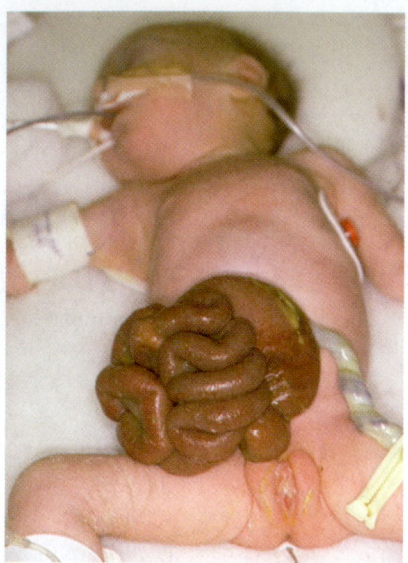

Figure 24–10 ➤ The newborn with gastroschisis has abdominal contents located outside the abdominal wall. Used with permission of the authors and the University of Iowa's Virtual Hospital®, http://www.vh.org

providing fluids and warmth, and surgical repair to replace the abdominal contents and close the abdominal wall. For smaller defects, primary closure is accomplished with one surgery. If the defect is severe, surgical correction may be performed in several steps. If an omphalocele occurs without associated defects, the child usually recovers from the surgery without incident and leads a normal life.

A related condition is **gastroschisis**, a congenital defect of the ventral abdominal wall, characterized by herniation of abdominal viscera outside the abdominal cavity through a defect in the abdominal wall to the side (most often to the right) of the umbilicus (Figure 24–10 ➤). The most common abdominal organs involved are the small intestine and ascending colon. Unlike the omphalocele, no membrane covers the organs. Gastroschisis occurs in approximately 1 in 10,000 births and has a survival rate of 92% (Weir, 2003). Gastroschisis has a much lower incidence of associated anomalies than omphalocele (Williams, Butler, & Sundem, 2003).

Collaborative Care

Elevated maternal serum alpha-fetoprotein (MSAFP) levels are seen in both gastroschisis and omphalocele. Routine prenatal determination of MSAFP and ultrasonography lead to early diagnosis and coordination of the team of specialists needed to manage these congenital anomalies, including geneticists, neonatologists, and pediatric surgeons (Weir, 2003). Intensive care is needed to manage fluid status, temperature regulation, infection control, and vital signs. Surgical care is instituted as soon as possible. Current trends are to suture a prosthetic silo around a gastroschisis defect, allowing for return of the intestines to the abdominal cavity (Weir, 2003).

Nursing Management

Be alert for signs of associated congenital anomalies. (Refer to the discussions of tracheoesophageal fistula earlier in this chapter; to genitourinary anomalies in Chapter 25; and to congenital heart defects in Chapter 21 ∞.)

Immediately after birth, follow physician protocol for maintaining the omphalocele sac or for the exposed abdominal contents in gastroschisis, such as with sterile gauze soaked in warm normal saline solution covered with sterile plastic. Monitor vital signs at least hourly, paying close attention to temperature, as the infant can lose heat through the sac. The child should be in a warmer or isolette for maintenance of temperature control. Inspect the area for signs of infection.

Because the infant is NPO preoperatively, maintain fluid and electrolyte balance with intravenous fluids. Postoperative care includes measures to control pain, prevent infection, maintain fluid and electrolyte balance, and ensure adequate nutritional intake. Attainment of bowel motility and function varies and is often delayed for weeks after surgery; parenteral nutrition for the infant is used during this period (Ashburn, Pranikoff, & Turner, 2002).

Throughout the infant's hospitalization, parents need clear, accurate explanations about the infant's condition. To help the parents deal with the crisis of an acutely ill newborn, provide emotional support and encourage parents to express their feelings. When the child has multiple anomalies, parents need ongoing support for the lengthy treatment, numerous hospitalizations, and management of nutritional intake.

Expected outcomes of nursing care depend on the severity of defect and its correction. Some examples include maintenance of normal vital signs, prompt identification of additional problems, healing of surgical site without signs of infection, pain control, proper intake of fluids, and establishment of an intake to support growth patterns.

INTUSSUSCEPTION

Intussusception occurs when one portion of the intestine prolapses and then invaginates or telescopes into another (Figure 24–11 ➤). It is one of the most frequent causes of intestinal obstruction during infancy, with an incidence of 1 to 4 in 1000 births. Most cases occur in boys between the ages of 3 months and 6 years (Wyllie, 2004). The etiology of intussusception is multifactorial and direct causes cannot always be identified.

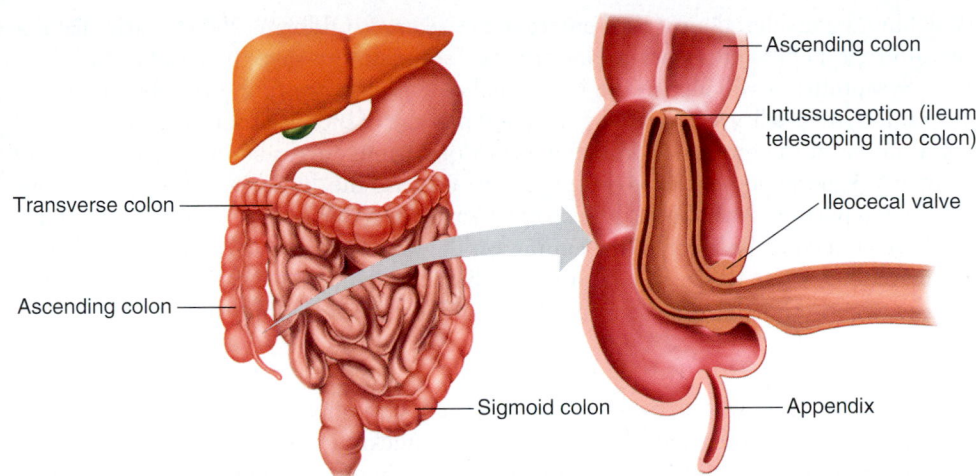

Figure 24–11 ➤ In infants, intussusception is commonly associated with viral illnesses and gastroenteritis.

Labels in figure: Ascending colon · Intussusception (ileum telescoping into colon) · Ileocecal valve · Transverse colon · Ascending colon · Sigmoid colon · Appendix

Viral infection, use of medications that influence gut motility, and the body's inflammatory mediators such as cytokine, nitric oxide, and prostaglandins are all associated with increased rates of intussception.

The most common site of intussusception is the ileocecal valve. Telescoping of the intestine obstructs the passage of stool. The walls of the intestine rub together, causing inflammation, edema, and decreased blood flow. This can lead to necrosis, perforation, hemorrhage, and peritonitis.

The onset is usually abrupt. A previously healthy infant or child suddenly experiences acute abdominal pain with vomiting and passage of brown stool. There may be periods of comfort between acute episodes of pain. As the condition worsens, painful episodes increase. The stools become red and resemble currant jelly because of the mix of blood and mucus. A palpable mass may be present in the upper right quadrant or mid-upper abdomen.

Diagnosis is made on the basis of the history and confirmed by radiographs and ultrasound of the abdomen. A contrast enema using barium, air, or water-soluble contrast can be both diagnostic and therapeutic. In some cases the hydrostatic pressure from the contrast moves the bowel back into place (Nelson & Hostetler, 2002). If the intussusception is not resolved during this procedure, surgical intervention to reduce the invaginated bowel and remove any necrotic tissue is necessary. Surgery usually corrects the problem.

Nursing management focuses on maintaining or restoring fluid and electrolyte balance. Intravenous fluids are started immediately. Serum electrolyte monitoring is essential to correct imbalances.

Postoperative care focuses on monitoring for early signs of infection, managing the child's pain, and maintaining nasogastric tube patency. Assess vital signs, check for abdominal distention, and listen for bowel sounds every 4 hours. After normal bowel function returns, begin clear liquid feedings. Feedings are advanced to half-strength formula or milk and other foods as the infant or child tolerates it.

Discharge usually occurs shortly after the infant or child begins taking full feedings. Instruct parents to watch for infection and to call the physician if symptoms recur, a fever develops, or appetite decreases.

Volvulus

During the 7–12th week of gestation the small intestine undergoes rapid growth. In normal development the intestine rotates counterclockwise as it settles into its permanent position inside the abdominal cavity. Malrotation of the intestine occurs in 1 out of 6000 live births and can lead to complications in the infant (Aiken & Oldham, 2005). If the bowel does not rotate normally during this process the child is at risk for **volvulus**, a twisting of the intestine (Doughty, 2004). Volvulus disrupts blood flow in the intestines and can lead to necrosis of the bowel, short bowel syndrome, and death.

> **NURSING ALERT**
>
> The passage of a normal brown stool may indicate that an intussusception has been reduced. Report this finding to the primary care provider immediately since the course of treatment may be altered, especially in the case of a planned surgical reduction.

Volvulus is considered a surgical emergency (Aiken & Oldham, 2005). Early diagnosis and treatment is necessary to preserve the bowel and to save the child's life.

Symptoms of volvulus in the infant include bilious vomiting, firm abdomen with distention, irritability secondary to pain, and passage of bloody stools. Confirmation of malrotation of the intestine through contrast or barium enema supports a diagnosis of volvulus. Emergency exploratory surgery to untwist the bowel is essential (Meyers, 2003). If a portion of the bowel is necrotic, that portion of the bowel is removed. An ostomy may need to be created, depending on the amount of bowel removed (Aiken & Oldham, 2005). See the section on ostomies beginning on page 930. The child is at risk for developing short bowel syndrome if a significant amount of bowel is removed.

Nursing Management

The infant or child who presents to the emergency room with bilious vomiting and a firm and distended abdomen should be assessed quickly to determine the cause of the symptoms. Once volvulus has been diagnosed, nursing management focuses on keeping the child NPO, administering intravenous fluids, assessing vital signs, and reporting symptoms of a worsening condition. The child who has had surgery to correct uncomplicated volvulus will need care similar to that described for the child with intussusception. If the child had necrotic bowel removed he or she may have an ostomy for a period of time.

Hirschsprung Disease

Hirschsprung disease, also known as congenital aganglionic megacolon, is a congenital anomaly in which inadequate motility causes mechanical obstruction of the intestine. Genetics plays a role in the development of most cases of Hirschsprung disease (Milla, 2003). The disease occurs in approximately one in every 5000 live births, and the incidence of transmitting this disease to offspring is approximately 3% (Swenson, 2002). Males are affected more commonly than females (Milla, 2003). Hirschsprung disease can occur as a single anomaly or in combination with congenital heart defects and chromosomal abnormalities such as Down syndrome.

The absence of autonomic parasympathetic ganglion cells in the colon prevents peristalsis at that portion of the intestine, resulting in the accumulation of intestinal contents and abdominal distention. In most cases the area lacking ganglion cells is limited to the rectum and sigmoid (Milla, 2003). In contrast, disorders that affect bowel motility but are not related to the absence of ganglionic cells are referred to as pseudo-Hirschsprung disease (Milla, 2003).

Clinical manifestations of Hirschsprung disease vary depending on the child's age at onset. In newborns, symptoms include failure to pass meconium in the first 48 hours after birth, abdominal distention, and emesis (Swenson, 2002). If Hirschsprung disease is not treated, the condition can lead to fever, bloody diarrhea, abdominal distention, and enterocolitis (Biggs & Dery, 2006).

The older infant or child may have a history of failure to gain weight and severe **constipation** (difficult and infrequent defecation with passage of hard, dry stool). On examination the rectum may be empty. Abdominal distention is generally present (Swenson, 2002). The child may have a history of passage of pencil thin stools (Biggs & Dery, 2006).

Collaborative Care

Diagnosis is made on the basis of the history, bowel patterns, anorectal manometry (reaction of the anal sphincter to distention of the rectum), radiographic contrast studies, and rectal biopsy for presence or absence of ganglion cells. Rectal biopsy has proven to be the most reliable test for confirmation of the diagnosis (Swenson, 2002).

Treatment in infancy involves surgical removal of the aganglionic bowel. In severe cases or in ill infants, a temporary colostomy is created. Timing of closure of the colostomy and reanastomosis varies among surgeons with the procedure being performed sometime between 2–4 months of age (Black, 2005) in some infants and much later in others.

The return of normal bowel function depends on the amount of bowel involved. Some fecal incontinence and constipation may persist following surgery. A serious complication is enterocolitis (inflammation of the intestines), which is manifested by symptoms such as GI bleeding and **diarrhea**, frequent, watery stools. Enterocolitis can occur before or after surgery, resulting in ischemia and ulceration of the bowel wall. Treatment includes intravenous fluids, antibiotics, and placement of a nasogastric tube for decompression of the abdomen (Milla, 2003).

Nursing Management

Nursing assessment in the newborn period includes careful observation for the passage of meconium. Because newborns are often discharged within 24 hours of birth, tell parents to notify the physician if no stool is passed within 48 hours of birth or if the abdomen becomes distended. When the disease is diagnosed later in infancy or in childhood, take a thorough history of weight gain, nutritional intake, and bowel habits.

Nursing management consists of carefully monitoring fluid and electrolyte balance and maintaining nutrition. Teach parents how to ensure regular bowel movements. Daily rectal irrigations with normal saline solution are necessary to promote adequate elimination and prevent obstruction.

If surgical correction is necessary, nursing care includes monitoring for infection, managing pain, maintaining hydration, measuring abdominal circumference to detect any distention, and providing support to the child and family. Parents need instruction in ostomy care if the child has a colostomy (refer to the discussion later in this chapter). Provide appropriate referrals to an ostomy support group and enterostomal nurse specialist when indicated. Teach parents to be alert for and immediately report signs of complications. These include diarrhea and pelvic abscess from leakage of intestinal contents at the surgical site (characterized by fever and pain). Children occasionally develop constipation, and parents may need guidance to adapt the diet and fluid intake to manage this complication. Because some children develop malabsorption, be alert for signs of poor growth or malnutrition (see Chapter 4 ∞).

Expected outcomes of nursing care include prompt identification of obstruction, maintenance of normal bowel patterns, adequate hydration, and maintenance of clear skin.

CLINICAL TIP

Teach parents to prevent skin breakdown in the rectal area by changing diapers frequently, cleansing the area carefully, and applying protective ointment at each diaper change.

Anorectal Malformations

Malformations of the anus and rectum are common congenital anomalies. Minor anomalies occur in 1 in 4000 to 5000 births. They are often associated with anomalies of the genitourinary tract, musculoskeletal system, and neurological system (Gereige & Frias, 2002). Chromosomal abnormalities such as trisomy 13, 18, or 21 may coexist, and some babies have VACTERL conditions. VACTERL refers to the presence of three or more of the following anomalies: anal atresia, vertebral anomalies, congenital heart disease, tracheoesophageal fistula, radial limb defects, and reno-urinary anomalies (Davies, Creighton, & Wilcox, 2004).

Types of defects include *anal stenosis* (a thickened and constricted anal wall) and *anal atresia* (absence of anal opening) (Figure 24–12 ➤). Diagnosis is usually made at birth or during the newborn assessment of anorectal structures and rectal patency. Failure to pass meconium may indicate a malformation high in the colon. Stool in the urine indicates a fistula between the colon and urinary tract. Ribbonlike stools may occur with some malformations. Ultrasound and lower GI radiographic studies confirm the diagnosis and demonstrate the extent of the anomaly. Higher defects are often less apparent at birth and involve more complicated treatment.

Medical management depends on the extent of the malformation. Some stenosed anal openings can be treated with dilation alone. An imperforate anal membrane is excised surgically, followed by daily manual dilations. More severe defects

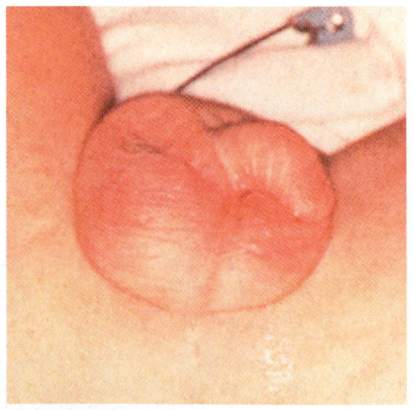

Figure 24–12 ➤ Anorectal malformations, which are often obvious at birth, can range from mild stenosis to a complex syndrome that includes associated congenital anomalies.

require reconstructive surgery. A temporary colostomy is performed to rest the bowel after reconstruction and allow for healing of a new anal opening. The colostomy is generally closed in a few months.

Nursing Management

During the initial newborn assessment, inspect the perineal area for a poorly developed anal dimple or sacral anomalies. Observation and recording of passage of meconium are essential.

Once the diagnosis has been made, intravenous fluids are initiated and a nasogastric tube is inserted to decompress the stomach. Monitor the child's intake and output and cardiorespiratory functioning. Provide emotional support to the parents and give them information about the upcoming surgery.

Postoperative care centers on preventing infection and respiratory complications from surgery, as well as maintaining hydration. Observe the incision for signs of infection, and provide careful wound care. Avoid taking rectal temperatures in children who have had anorectal surgery. Assess vital signs at least every 4 hours. Once the child's condition is stable, clear fluid oral intake is allowed, advancing to half- and full-strength formula or breast milk as tolerated. The infant will have a colostomy after surgery, and careful skin care around the stoma is essential to prevent breakdown of the fragile area. See page 931 for stoma care.

The child with associated abnormalities may need several surgeries and interventions to treat all of the conditions present. Partnering with families and the group of healthcare providers will assist in case management that facilitates the child's health and development. Health promotion and health maintenance that include support of family members, ensuring immunizations, and monitoring developmental status is important.

CARE IN THE COMMUNITY Infants are increasingly discharged shortly after birth, so parents need clear instructions about normal newborn stools and what abnormalities to report.

After surgery, teach parents how to take the infant's temperature using the axillary route. Have them demonstrate the proper technique before discharge. Explain the signs and symptoms of infection. Discuss feeding regimens and bowel habits necessary to maintain adequate nutrition for growth and development. Advise parents that children with anorectal malformations may have difficulty achieving bowel control. Patience in toilet training is important. When the child reaches an age appropriate for toilet training, encourage the family to speak with a healthcare provider to discuss the child's progress.

If a colostomy is performed, teach parents how to care for the ostomy site (see discussion of ostomies later in this chapter). Reassure parents that the colostomy will be closed in the future, and help them plan for that hospitalization. Refer them to ostomy support groups in the community or online. Discuss follow-up care and long-term management. Arrange follow-up visits and home care visits to evaluate the child's ostomy site and monitor growth.

Expected outcomes of nursing care include adequate fluid intake, normal bowel patterns, parental knowledge of ostomy or other treatment protocols, and eventual success with toilet training.

Hernias

A **hernia** is the protrusion or projection of an organ or a part of an organ through the muscle wall of the cavity that normally contains it. This protrusion may result from the failure of normal openings to close during fetal development or from weakness in the supporting musculature. When intra-abdominal pressure increases (as when the infant cries or strains to pass stool), the weakened area separates, causing a protrusion of underlying organs. Inguinal hernias are the most common type of hernia occurring in children (see Chapter 25 ∞). Other hernias that occur frequently in children are diaphragmatic and umbilical.

Diaphragmatic Hernia

In a diaphragmatic hernia, abdominal contents protrude into the thoracic cavity through an opening in the diaphragm. Sites of herniation include the substernal space, posterolateral region, and the esophageal hiatus. The posterolateral site (foramen of Bochdalek) is the most common location. The cause is a delay or failure in closure of the pleuroperitoneal musculature. The overall incidence of diaphragmatic hernia is 1 in 2000 to 3000 live births (Walsh & Adzick, 2003). Associated anomalies, particularly cardiac defects, occur in some infants.

A diaphragmatic hernia is a life-threatening condition with an overall mortality rate of 50% (Walsh and Adzick, 2003). Severe respiratory distress occurs shortly after birth. As the infant cries, abdominal organs extend into the thorax, decreasing the size of the thoracic cavity. The infant becomes dyspneic and cyanotic. Characteristic findings include a barrel-shaped chest and sunken abdomen.

Some cases of congenital diaphragmatic hernia are diagnosed in utero by ultrasound. If not identified prenatally the condition is first identified postnatally by physical signs and symptoms; confirmation is made by chest radiologic examination. MRI is helpful in confirming the diagnosis and in determining the position of organs in the chest and abdomen (Hedrick et al., 2004). Immediate respiratory support is essential. Extracorporeal membrane oxygenation (ECMO) may be used to provide cardiopulmonary bypass to rest the lungs. Alternatively, inhaled nitric oxide (iNO) and high-frequency oxygen ventilation (HFVO) preoperatively may improve survival outcomes and decrease morbidity associated with congenital diaphragmatic hernia (Bagolan et al., 2004).

The infant is positioned with the head and thorax higher than the abdomen to facilitate downward movement of abdominal organs. A nasogastric tube is inserted to decompress the stomach. Ventilator support is necessary to manage respiratory compromise. Intravenous fluids are administered through an umbilical artery catheter.

Once the infant's condition is stabilized, the defect is corrected surgically. The prognosis is poor. Even after surgery the infant may do well initially and then manifest severe respiratory decompensation.

■ NURSING MANAGEMENT

The infant with a diaphragmatic hernia is admitted to the neonatal intensive care unit (NICU) and requires continuous monitoring for respiratory distress. Preoperative management centers on providing supportive care to the infant and parents. Place the child on a cardiorespiratory monitor and note the infant's vital signs every 30 minutes. Observe for worsening of respiratory compromise. Maintain intravenous fluid administration. Promote decreased stimulation to keep the infant calm and thus maintain low abdominal pressure. Keep parents informed about the infant's condition, and provide emotional support both before and after surgery.

Postoperative care includes positioning the infant on the affected side to facilitate expansion of the lung on the unaffected side, observing closely for signs of infection, maintaining respiratory support, and carefully monitoring fluid and electrolyte balance. Before discharge, instruct parents in wound care, prevention of infection, and feeding techniques.

Due to the high rate of infant mortality associated with this condition, palliative care may need to be discussed with the parents if the child's condition is deteriorating and unresponsive to treatment. Comfort measures for the infant may become the focus of care. Refer to Chapter 14 ∞ for this discussion.

Umbilical Hernia

An umbilical hernia results from a weak or imperfectly closed umbilical ring (Figure 24–13 ➤). The condition is often associated with diastasis recti (lateral separation of the abdominal muscles). Umbilical hernia is a common condition in childhood and occurs more frequently in African American children than White children (Stoll & Kleigman, 2004).

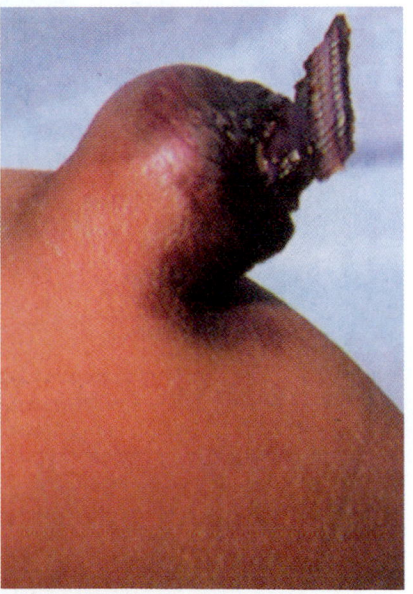

Figure 24–13 ➤ The umbilical hernia of the newborn usually closes as the muscles strengthen in later infancy and childhood. *Note:* From Zitelli, B., & Davis, H. (Eds.). (2002). *Atlas of pediatric physical diagnosis* (4th ed., p. 43). Philadelphia: Mosby.

The hernia appears as a soft swelling covered by skin. The herniated area protrudes with coughing, crying, or straining during a bowel movement. It is easily reduced by pushing the bowel back through the fibrous ring. The size of the defect may vary among individuals. Contents of the hernia include omentum or portions of the small intestine.

Most defects resolve spontaneously by 3 to 4 years of age. Surgery is indicated in cases of **strangulation**, closure of the umbilical ring around a portion of the bowel, preventing it from moving back into the abdomen. Surgery is also recommended if the defect does not resolve by 3 to 4 years of age (Marinkovic & Bukanica, 2003).

Nursing management is generally supportive. Instruct parents not to apply tape, straps, or coins to reduce the hernia. This can cause strangulation of the hernia, necessitating immediate surgery. If surgery is required, it is usually performed in an outpatient surgery unit. Postoperatively, teach parents how to care for the surgical site, to watch for bleeding, and to recognize signs of infection. Reinforce the importance of returning for follow-up evaluation.

OSTOMIES

An intestinal **ostomy** is an opening, or **stoma**, on the abdominal surface allowing the small or large intestine to divert fecal matter. It provides an outlet when a distal surgical anastomosis, obstruction, or nonfunctioning structure prevents normal elimination (Figure 24–14 ➤). Depending on the integrity and function of anatomic structures, the ostomy may be temporary or permanent. Infants and small children with necrotizing enterocolitis, Hirschsprung disease, volvulus, or intussusception may require a temporary colostomy or ileostomy. Ostomies may also be indicated for children with inflammatory bowel disease, intestinal tumors, or abdominal trauma.

An ostomy may be elective or a surgical emergency. In all cases it affects a child's lifestyle, alters body image, causes anxiety, and increases the risk for alterations in physiologic processes (electrolyte imbalance, increased nutritional requirements). For adolescents, it may also result in dependence at a time when autonomy is a major developmental need (Figure 24–15 ➤).

In assessing the family and child approaching ostomy surgery, it is important to determine their ability to understand and accept the physical changes that will occur. Parents may feel guilt and anger about the ostomy surgery when the child has a genetically transmitted disease, is injured, or has developed an obstruction from necrosis of the bowel. Encourage the parents and child to express their feelings, and correct any misunderstandings. Parents and older children may be referred for counseling and to support groups to help them deal with their feelings. Adolescents often benefit from a visit with an adolescent ostomate (someone who has an ostomy) who can answer questions about living with an ostomy.

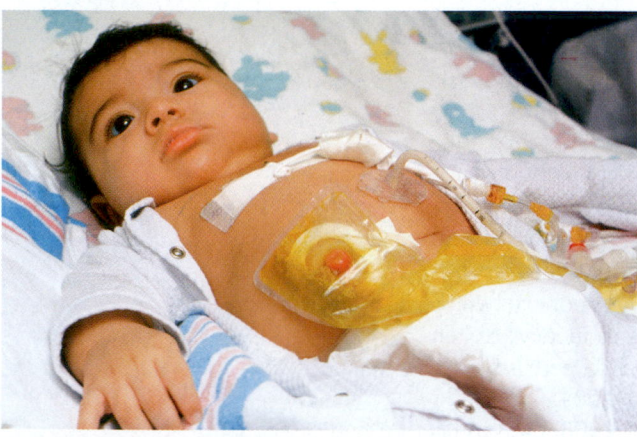

Figure 24–14 ➤ This infant has several gastrointestinal problems and requires ostomies both for gastric feedings and for drainage of fecal material. Note the appearance of the healthy stoma.

Figure 24–15 ➤ Nursing strategies to address altered perceptions of body image and increased feelings of dependence are important when working with adolescents who have ostomies. Support groups or a visit from another teenager who has had an ostomy can facilitate positive coping, as demonstrated by this teenage girl.

◼ NURSING MANAGEMENT
Preoperative Care

Preoperative education focuses on educating the child and family and preparing them for postoperative management. Discuss how the appliance will look, and explain the purpose of the pouch in developmentally appropriate terms. Encourage the parents and child to touch and manipulate all equipment. A younger child can be shown how to place a pouch on a doll. Older children can practice placing a pouch on their skin. These measures help relieve anxiety by providing information and increasing familiarity with the appliance.

In addition to discussion of the appliance, preoperative education should include discussion of pain control and measures that will be used to prevent postoperative complications (turning, coughing, and breathing deeply). Gear the instructions to the child's developmental level. Encourage parental participation to promote compliance.

Postoperative Care

Postoperative care of a child with an ostomy is similar to that for any child who undergoes abdominal surgery. (See the discussion of nursing management for appendicitis and Nursing Care Plan: The Child Undergoing Surgery in Chapter 13 .) Management of the stoma may be done by an "ostomy nurse" or other nurses. Major interventions involve ensuring proper function of the stoma, identifying complications, and instituting daily stoma care. Assess the stoma, quality and amount of fecal matter, skin condition, and adherence of the pouch. Evaluate for the most common complications, which are prolapse, retraction, stenosis, and skin breakdown around the stoma. Evaluate the family's understanding and their ability to care for the ostomy.

Care in the Community

Identify and address home care needs well in advance of discharge. Instructions include skin care, care of the stoma, appliance removal and application, and frequency of appliance changes. Begin teaching immediately after surgery with responsibility for care transferred gradually to the parents and child as they are ready. Discuss diet, activity level, hygiene, clothing, equipment, and financial considerations. Arrange for periodic home visits to see how the family is managing.

Parents and children can be referred to the United Ostomy Association or a local ostomy group for information and support. Make referrals to social services, counseling, and a home health agency, if appropriate.

Expected outcomes of nursing care include successful adjustment to the ostomy, thorough evacuation of the bowel, absence of infection and other complications, intact skin, and formation of a positive self-image in the child.

INFLAMMATORY DISORDERS

Inflammatory disorders are reactions of specific tissues of the GI tract to trauma caused by injuries, foreign bodies, chemicals, microorganisms, or surgery. These disorders may be acute or chronic and may involve various segments of the GI tract.

Appendicitis

Appendicitis is an inflammation of the vermiform appendix, the small sac near the end of the cecum. The condition occurs most often in adolescent boys (10 to 19 years of age). Appendicitis is the most common cause for emergency abdominal surgery in children and adolescents in the United States (Kosloske, Love, Rohrer, Goldthorn, & Lacey, 2004). Children account for 1/4 to 1/3 of the appendectomies performed every year in more than 250,000 Americans (Ziegler, 2004). The incidence of ruptured appendix is much higher in children less than 4 years of age as compared to older children and adolescents. Infants and young children are unable to verbalize the presence of symptoms such as pain and nausea. They may also have symptoms that are not specific to appendicitis (Kwok, Kim, & Gorelick, 2004). These factors may lead to a delayed diagnosis of appendicitis, increasing the risk of perforation.

Etiology and Pathophysiology

Appendicitis almost always results from an obstruction in the appendiceal lumen. It can be caused by a fecalith (hard fecal mass), parasitic infestations, stenosis, hyperplasia of lymphoid tissue, or a tumor. Continued secretion of mucus following acute obstruction of the lumen increases pressure, causing ischemia, cellular death, and ulceration.

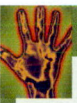

SKILLS 13–3 AND 13–4
Ostomy Care

MediaLink

Ostomy Resources

GROWTH & DEVELOPMENT

Ostomy Maintenance

The preschooler has some manual dexterity and can help with some parts of the procedure for changing an ostomy appliance and cleaning the stoma. Teach the child using a doll or stuffed animal. Many school-age children are able to care for their ostomy independently. Teach them how to avoid leakage around the bag, which could be embarrassing. Adolescents are generally totally independent in their self-care of ostomies. However, they may need support to deal with the fact that they are different from their peers.

CLINICAL TIP

Avoid adhesive enhancers on the skin of newborns and premature infants. Their skin layers are so thin that removal of the appliance can strip off the skin. Remember also that adhesive contains latex and its constant use is not advised due to risk of latex allergy development (see Chapter 17). Latex-free alternatives are available.

The appendix may perforate or rupture, resulting in fecal and bacterial contamination of the peritoneum. Peritonitis spreads quickly and if untreated can result in small bowel obstruction, electrolyte imbalances, septicemia, and hypovolemic shock. Early diagnosis and treatment of appendicitis is essential to minimize complications related to rupture (Kwok et al., 2004).

Clinical Manifestations

At onset, symptoms include periumbilical cramps, abdominal tenderness, and fever. In adolescent and young adult females, symptoms must be differentiated from those associated with ovulation (mittelschmerz), ruptured ectopic pregnancy, and pelvic inflammatory disease. As the inflammation progresses, pain in the right lower abdomen becomes constant. Pain is often most intense at McBurney's Point, halfway between the anterior superior iliac crest and the umbilicus (Figure 24–16 ➤). The location of the appendix varies in some children so the pain may occur elsewhere (Jaffe & Berger, 2005). Symptoms progress to include guarding, rigidity, and rebound tenderness following palpation over the right lower quadrant. Vomiting, diarrhea, or constipation may be present. As appendicitis progresses, the child remains motionless, usually in a side-lying position with knees flexed. If the appendix ruptures, there is usually fever, sudden relief from abdominal pain, guarding and distention of the abdomen, rapid breathing, pallor, chills, and irritability.

PATHOPHYSIOLOGY ILLUSTRATED

Appendicitis Pain

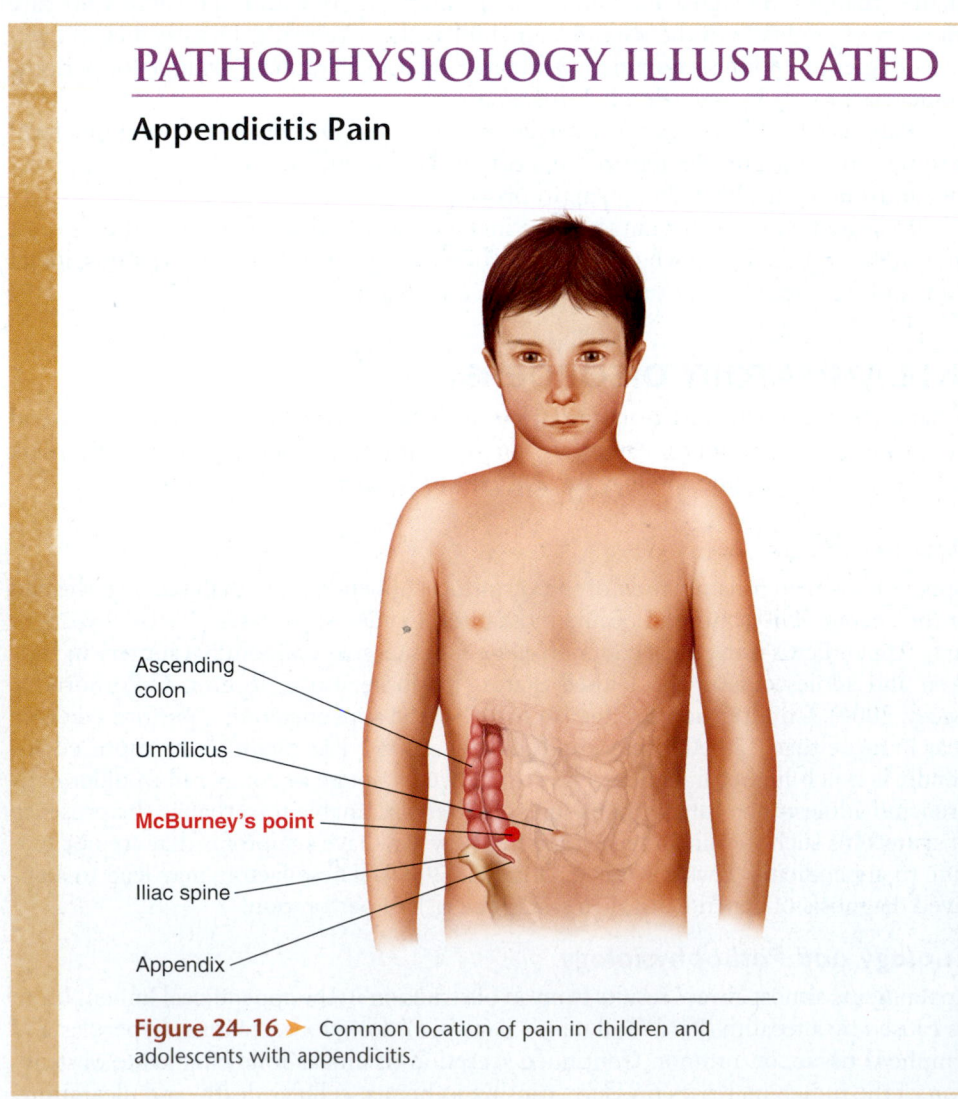

Figure 24–16 ➤ Common location of pain in children and adolescents with appendicitis.

COLLABORATIVE CARE

Diagnostic Tests

Diagnosis of appendicitis in young children can be difficult because their pain may be less localized and their symptoms more diffuse than in the older child. Continuing evaluations over several hours are often needed to establish the diagnosis.

An elevated white blood cell count (above 15,000/mm^3) may occur. In the opening scenario, Jason had a WBC of 22,000/mm^3 which was clearly indicative of infection. In addition to an elevated WBC, a history of abdominal pain, presence of a fecalith in the right lower abdomen on radiograph, and an elevated C-reactive protein help establish the diagnosis. While an abdominal ultrasound can be helpful in the diagnosis of appendicitis, computed tomography (CT) is preferred and has been found to be most reliable (Jaffe & Berger, 2005; Kwok, Kim, & Gorelick, 2004).

Clinical Therapy

Treatment involves immediate surgical removal (appendectomy), either through laparoscopic or open method (Vegunta, Ali, Wallace, Switzer, & Pearl, 2004). Preoperatively the child is kept NPO. Intravenous fluids, electrolytes, and antibiotics are administered. Postoperatively the child has an abdominal incision, and intravenous antibiotics may be administered to prevent infection. The child with uncomplicated appendicitis will generally be discharged the next day.

With ruptured appendix, some surgeons prefer to close the wound, while others will leave the wound open, with or without placement of drains (Emil et al., 2003). If the wound is left open, it is packed with sterile saline-soaked gauze. The child will have a nasogastric tube to decompress the abdomen and will remain NPO until signs of bowel function are present such as the presence of bowel sounds or passage of flatus or stool. The child will also have an intravenous line for administration of intravenous fluids and medications. After surgery for a ruptured appendix the child will receive antibiotics for several days. A combination of Ampicillin, Gentamicin, and Clindamycin is used by some surgeons. Ampicillin is omitted from the regimen in the presence of penicillin allergy. Flaygl is substituted for Clindamycin in some cases (Emil et al., 2003). The exact regimen varies among surgeons. Morphine is generally given for pain. Recovery is usually complete following uncomplicated removal of the appendix.

NURSING MANAGEMENT

Nursing management includes collaborative identification of the child with appendicitis, preoperative and postoperative care, and preventing complications.

Nursing Assessment and Diagnosis

Physiologic Assessment

Preoperatively, a detailed assessment of the child's pain is necessary to differentiate appendicitis from other illnesses (see Chapter 15 ∞). Ask the child to point to the painful area and to describe the pain. Recognize that localizing the pain may be difficult for young children. Note onset, location, and intensity of pain; precipitating factors; and relief measures tried. During abdominal assessment, palpate last to avoid causing additional pain. Assess vital signs to determine baseline values, and monitor every 4 hours thereafter.

Postoperatively, assess fluid volume status every 2 hours. Assess skin turgor, eyes, and mucous membranes for signs of dehydration. Monitor intake and output. Assess for signs of return of bowel function as previously listed. Assess for pain using the appropriate scale. (See Chapter 15 for pain assessment and pain management.) Careful attention should also be paid to the wound site for signs of infection such as increased redness or drainage. Vital signs should be monitored at least every 4 hours. Changes in vital signs, especially temperature, may be indicative of infection.

Psychosocial Assessment

Because appendicitis usually occurs in school-age children and adolescents, assessment of the child's coping skills is important. Adolescents, because of their preoccupation with body image, may be concerned about the surgical scar. Assess the parents' and child's anxiety about the sudden hospitalization and need for emergency surgery.

Among the nursing diagnoses that might be appropriate for the child with appendicitis are:

- Acute Pain related to inflammation and surgery
- Risk for Deficient Fluid Volume Deficit related to fluid volume loss and inadequate fluid volume intake
- Anxiety/Fear related to surgery
- Risk for Infection related to surgical procedure
- Risk for Ineffective Airway Clearance related to decreased mobility and refusal to cough

Planning and Implementation

Nursing management focuses on promoting comfort, maintaining hydration, providing emotional support, supporting respiratory function, providing care of the surgical site, and monitoring for symptoms of infection.

Promote Comfort

Preoperatively administer analgesics as ordered and note relief from pain. Manage postoperative pain in a similar manner. The child should be placed in a semi-Fowler or side-lying position on the right side. If the appendix has ruptured, lying on the right side helps the peritoneal cavity drain and facilitates comfort. Postoperatively the child with a ruptured appendix will require intravenous pain medication frequently and prior to scheduled dressing changes if the wound was left opened. The child who has an appendectomy for uncomplicated appendicitis will need oral or intravenous pain management for postoperative pain control.

Maintain Hydration

An intravenous infusion is initiated preoperatively and continued until bowel function returns after surgery. Once bowel sounds return and after the nasogastric tube has been removed, offer water in small amounts and then other clear fluids. The child should be monitored closely to make sure he or she does not become nauseated after he or she begins taking oral fluids. If the child had a ruptured appendix and has a nasogastric tube for awhile after surgery, accurate assessment of the amount of output from the nasogastric tube is essential. The child may have orders to replace the amount of fluid lost from the nasogastric tube with additional intravenous fluids. The nurse should be alert to an increase in nasogastric drainage postoperatively, as this drainage should decrease over time. Any concerns should be reported promptly to the physician.

Provide Emotional Support

For many children, this may be their first hospitalization and their first experience with healthcare personnel beyond their usual provider. The nurse must elicit a history, perform a physical examination, coordinate diagnostic tests, and prepare the child for surgery in a short period of time. Emotional support is essential for both child and parents. Good preoperative education can reduce anxiety. Answer any questions the child or parents may have.

Support Respiratory Function

General anesthesia during surgery compromises respiratory function. It is important for the child to turn, cough, and breathe deeply to prevent atelectasis. While the child with uncomplicated appendicitis is usually willing to get out of bed and walk soon after surgery, the child with a ruptured appendix is generally hesitant to move, and may need to be repositioned by family or staff. The child will need to get out of bed as soon

---

NURSING ALERT

Be alert to the child who does not complain of pain postoperatively following surgery for a ruptured appendix. This child still needs pain medication. While the child may not verbally complain of pain, he or she will cry when approached and will resist or refuse to move in the bed. Proper pain management will facilitate the child's recovery and will help prevent respiratory complications related to immobilization.

CLINICAL TIP

When a child has a nasogastric tube in place, the nurse must keep an accurate measurement of the amount of output from the tube so that adequate fluid replacement can be given. Loss of large amounts of stomach contents without fluid replacement may lead to metabolic alkalosis. Infants are especially at risk for acid/base imbalances.

as his or her condition allows and walk 2–3 times a day to decrease the risk of pulmonary complications and decrease recovery time. Encourage the child to splint the incision area with a pillow during coughing to decrease pain. Incentive spirometry is frequently ordered for the child. Young children may be resistant to this procedure or may be too young to understand the procedure. An effective alternative approach is to give the child bubbles to blow. Praise and rewards such as stickers each time the child completes the task will likely increase compliance with the procedure and decrease the likelihood of complications. Consider Jason in the opening scenario. What activities would be appropriate to prevent respiratory complications?

Recognize Symptoms of Infection

Assess vital signs and observe the abdominal incision every 4 hours for redness, edema, or drainage. If a drain is present, assess drainage for color, consistency, and amount. The amount of drainage from the wound should decrease gradually as the wound heals. Administer antibiotics as prescribed. The child with an open wound will require wet to dry dressing changes 2–3 times a day, depending on physician orders.

Discharge Planning and Home Care Teaching

For non-rupture the child is discharged once bowel function returns and he or she has a bowel movement. Give parents instructions on reestablishing a nutritious diet slowly and as tolerated. Teach parents to recognize the signs and symptoms of infection and to seek early treatment. If the appendix was ruptured, the child will be hospitalized for several days for intravenous antibiotics. If the wound was left open, it is generally closed after a few days and prior to discharge. Prepare the child and family for this procedure. Sedation or anesthesia is used to decrease the child's anxiety and discomfort.

Normal activities can be resumed fairly quickly, but the child should avoid strenuous activities and contact sports in the immediate postoperative period. Parents should check with the child's physician before allowing the child to resume sports activities. Home tutoring may be needed for a short time so the child can keep up with school work.

Evaluation

Expected outcomes of nursing care include:

- The child's pain is effectively managed.
- The child will not develop a secondary infection.
- The child and parent verbalize understanding of the condition and treatment.
- Effective airway clearance is maintained.
- Adequate hydration is achieved and maintained.
- Restoration of normal nutritional intake will occur.
- The child experiences decreased fear and anxiety associated with the hospitalization and procedures.

Necrotizing Enterocolitis

Necrotizing enterocolitis (NEC) is a potentially life-threatening inflammatory disease of the intestinal tract that occurs primarily in premature infants. It affects from 4–13% of very low birth weight infants (Bell, 2005), and has an overall mortality rate of 25–30% (Tudehope, 2004). NEC is considered the most common emergency condition of the gastrointestinal tract in infants in the neonatal intensive care unit (NICU) (Parker, Moniaci, & Fike, 2003). It can be caused by several factors including intestinal ischemia, bacterial or viral infection, and immaturity of the gut.

The disease occurs most often in the distal ileum and proximal colon (McCollough & Sharieff, 2006).

The infant may initially show signs of feeding intolerance (increased gastric residuals, vomiting, irritability, and abdominal distention). These signs are caused by inflammation and dilation of the bowel and accumulation of gas in the intestine. Bloody diarrhea may be present because of the hemorrhagic bowel. Signs of sepsis usually follow, and the infant's condition rapidly deteriorates (Parker et al., 2003).

> **NURSING ALERT**
>
> Signs of sepsis include:
> - Hypothermia or hyperthermia
> - Abdominal distention
> - Jaundice
> - Anorexia
> - Respiratory distress
> - Vomiting
> - Hepatomegaly
> - Lethargy

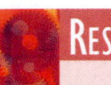

NURSING ALERT

Cholestasis is a disruption of bile flow. This is the most common problem in survivors of necrotizing enterocolitis. It is a complication of total parenteral nutrition (TPN) and commonly occurs 2 weeks after TPN therapy has been initiated. It is characterized by an elevated bilirubin (greater than 2 mg/dL), hepatomegaly, and elevated serum transaminase.

RESEARCH

Necrotizing Enterocolitis Treatment

New treatments for necrotizing enterocolitis are being attempted with probiotics, live and beneficial microorganisms that promote normal gut flora. *Lastobacillus acidophilus* and *Bifidobacterium infantis* are examples of organisms that can be administered by special formula (Kliegman & Willoughby, 2005).

Diagnosis is made on the basis of characteristic clinical findings and the presence of free peritoneal gas, dilated bowel loops, bowel distention, and bowel wall thickening on abdominal radiographs. Stools and emesis are monitored for occult blood. Laboratory data reveals anemia, leukopenia, leukocytosis, thrombocytopenia, electrolyte imbalance, and metabolic or respiratory acidosis. Blood cultures may be positive for the organism present.

Necrotizing enterocolitis requires prompt intervention. All enteral feedings are discontinued, an orogastric tube is inserted to prevent gastric distention, and intravenous fluids are started. Total parenteral nutrition may be initiated. Antibiotics are administered prophylactically or to treat sepsis. Radiographs of the abdomen should be performed every 6–8 hours to see if intestinal perforation has occurred (Parker et al., 2003). Perforation or necrosis of the bowel necessitates surgical resection of the bowel. An ileostomy or colostomy may be performed.

All cases of necrotizing enterocolitis are treated with strict enteric precautions to prevent the spread of infection to other premature infants on the unit. Early aggressive enteral formula feedings of premature infants is avoided because of the increased incidence of the disease in these cases. Human milk has been shown to protect against the disease; thus, breast-feeding or feeding the mother's expressed milk is the feeding method of choice for premature infants.

Long-term complications of necrotizing enterocolitis include short bowel syndrome, strictures, **cholestasis** (disruption of bile flow), impaired nutrition and growth, and delayed developmental performance.

Nursing Management

Nursing care centers on prevention and early detection of necrotizing enterocolitis to minimize bowel loss, and providing postoperative care. Feedings should be progressed very slowly with frequent assessment of feeding tolerance and abdominal girth. Even minimal changes in circumference can indicate necrotizing enterocolitis; report them to the physician. Maintaining fluid and electrolyte balance is essential. Careful assessment for infection and maintenance of skin integrity is also important. Gradually reestablish feedings once bowel function returns.

Because the symptoms of necrotizing enterocolitis do not appear until approximately 5 to 7 days after feedings are begun, parents may not be prepared for the infant's decline. Recovery is slow and can be complicated. Give clear explanations and encourage parents to ask questions and express their fears and concerns. If the infant's condition worsens, offer support for the parents of a child with life-threatening illness (see Chapter 14 ∞).

Once the child is discharged, frequent follow-up is needed. Parents need specific education related to feedings, medications, and any other treatments prescribed. The infant requires regular and thorough physical assessments to check weight gain, assess development, and identify signs of complications.

Expected outcomes of nursing care for the child with necrotizing enterocolitis include successful treatment of infection, absence of signs of sepsis, management of fluid and electrolyte status, and provision of adequate nutrition. If surgery is performed, complete healing without infection or other complication is desired. If the infant is not successfully treated, support and comfort for the parents is a necessary outcome (see Chapter 14 ∞). When the child survives, long-term outcomes include normal developmental progression and nutrition to support growth.

Meckel's Diverticulum

Meckel's diverticulum results when the omphalomesenteric duct, which connects the midgut to the yolk sac during embryonic development, fails to atrophy. Instead, an outpouching of the ileum remains, usually located near the ileocecal valve. The pouch contains gastric or pancreatic tissue, which secretes acid, causing irritation and ulceration.

Meckel's diverticulum is the most common GI malformation and cause of lower GI bleeding in children; it occurs in 2% of the population, although many people are asymptomatic and do not know they have the disorder (Brown & Stevenson, 2003).

Clinical manifestations usually appear by 2 years of age. The most common sign is painless dark or bright red rectal bleeding, which results from the obstruction or ulceration. Often blood is passed without stool. Abdominal pain is uncommon, but when it occurs, it may resemble the pain of appendicitis. The child may have symptoms of intussusception, incarcerated hernia, volvulus, or intestinal obstruction. If untreated, diverticulitis may progress to perforation and peritonitis.

Diagnosis is based on the history. Contrast studies are usually not helpful because the diverticulum is often too small to visualize and may not fill with barium. Radionuclide imaging and scanning can usually detect the gastric tissue, confirming the diagnosis.

Treatment is surgical excision of the diverticulum and removal of any involved bowel. The prognosis is good following surgical excision.

Nursing Management

Preoperatively an intravenous infusion is initiated to correct fluid and electrolyte imbalances. Monitor intake and output. Observe for rectal bleeding, and test stools for occult blood. Keep the child on bed rest. Assess vital signs every 2 hours, and monitor for signs of shock. Postoperative care is similar to that for an infant or child undergoing abdominal surgery. (See the earlier discussion of postsurgical nursing management of appendicitis and Nursing Care Plan: The Child Undergoing Surgery in Chapter 13 ∞).

At discharge, parents need instructions on caring for the surgical site, preventing infection, providing an adequate diet, and administering prescribed medications.

Inflammatory Bowel Disease
Crohn's Disease and Ulcerative Colitis

Inflammatory bowel disease (IBD) encompasses two distinct chronic disorders, Crohn's disease and ulcerative colitis, that have similar symptoms and treatment (see the clinical manifestations table below). Genetics and environmental factors are involved in the development of IBD. Onset of both of these disorders is most common in adolescence and young adulthood, but either disease can begin in early childhood (Hyams, 2004). Inflammatory bowel disease differs from irritable bowel syndrome, which is discussed in the section on feeding and elimination disorders in Chapter 4 ∞.

Crohn's disease is a chronic, inflammatory process. It can occur randomly throughout the GI tract, with the ileum, colon, and rectum the most common sites. A distinct feature of Crohn's disease is the development of enteric fistulas between loops

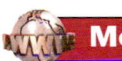

MediaLink

Crohn's and Colitis Foundation of America

CLINICAL MANIFESTATIONS	ULCERATIVE COLITIS AND CROHN'S DISEASE	
	Ulcerative Colitis	**Crohn's Disease**
Type of lesions	Continuous, superficial involvement	Segmental, transmural (through the wall) involvement
Clinical manifestations		
Anal or perianal lesions	Rare	Common
Anorexia	Mild to moderate	Can be severe
Diarrhea	Often severe	Moderate
Growth retardation	Mild	Significant
Pain	Present	Common
Rectal bleeding	Present	Absent
Weight loss	Moderate	Severe
Risk of cancer	Slightly increased	Greatly increased

of bowel or nearby organs. Mucosal ulcers begin in small locations, and then grow in size and depth into the mucosal wall. Submucosal inflammation can be severe. The etiology is unknown. There is strong evidence to support a genetic association. Crohn's disease is more common in Whites and 3 to 6 times more prevalent in individuals of Jewish descent. It most often develops in adolescents and young adults and has an incidence of 10 out of 100,000 children younger than age 18 years (Baron, 2002).

The onset of Crohn's disease is subtle. Crampy abdominal pain is usually reported first, followed by diarrhea. Other symptoms include fever, anorexia, growth failure or weight loss, general malaise, and joint pain. Diagnosis is based on laboratory evaluation (anemia is common; an elevated erythrocyte sedimentation rate, hypoalbuminemia, and thrombocytosis are other possible findings), diffuse abdominal tenderness, and radiologic and biopsy examinations.

Ulcerative colitis is a chronic recurrent disease of the colon and rectal mucosa of unknown etiology. Inflammation is limited to the mucosa and can involve the entire length of the bowel with varying degrees of inflammation, ulceration, hemorrhage, and edema. Emotional and other psychosocial factors may influence the presentation and course of the disease. It is more prevalent among persons of Jewish heritage. The disease develops before 20 years of age with peak onset at about 12 years.

The first symptom of ulcerative colitis is usually diarrhea. Lower abdominal pain and cramping are present before and during a bowel movement and are relieved by the passage of stool and flatus. The stool is often mixed with blood and mucus. Weight loss or delayed growth, nutritional deficiencies, and arthralgias often occur as effects of the disease.

■ COLLABORTIVE CARE

Collaborative care focuses on promoting remission of the disease, promoting optimal nutritional intake, and promoting optimal growth and development.

Diagnostic Tests

Diagnosis centers on evaluating the cause and identifying the extent of involved bowel and differentiating an infectious process (organisms such as *Shigella* and *Salmonella*) from ulcerative colitis. Endoscopy with biopsy is helpful to determine the extent and severity of the inflammatory process. Laboratory and bone age studies help to identify related nutritional, growth, and blood abnormalities. Common serum findings include elevated erythrocyte sedimentation rate, elevated C-reactive protein, hypoalbuminemia, thrombocytosis, and antineutrophil cytoplasmic antibodies (ANCA).

Clinical Therapy

Crohn's disease and ulcerative colitis have periods of remission and exacerbation (Tanaka & Kazuma, 2005). Treatment for both diseases includes pharmacologic interventions (antibiotic, anti-inflammatory, immunosuppressive, and antidiarrheal medications), nutrition therapy, and, in severe cases, surgery. Corticosteroids are given orally and as enemas to children with more severe disease. For children with milder disease, sulfasalazine decreases the number of relapses. (See the Medication Administration table on the next page.)

A nutritionist is part of the team treating the child. The goal of nutrition therapy is to provide adequate caloric intake and nutrients necessary for growth. Vitamin, iron, zinc, and folic acid supplementation is frequently required. Total parenteral nutrition (TPN) is often given to treat nutritional deficiencies and malnutrition, which accompany inflammatory bowel disease. A high-protein, high-carbohydrate, low-fiber diet with normal amounts of fat is recommended.

If other treatment measures fail to reduce inflammation, surgery is generally indicated. A temporary colostomy or ileostomy is performed to allow the bowel to rest. In Crohn's disease, however, ulcerations tend to recur elsewhere in the GI tract. Biologic therapies such as Infliximab (Remicade) have been effective in patients with persistent disease despite treatment (Baron, 2002). In ulcerative colitis, removal of the diseased bowel provides a permanent cure.

SKILL 12–3
Administering a Gavage/Tube Feeding

MEDICATIONS USED TO TREAT *Inflammatory Bowel Disease*

Medication	Indication	Nursing Implications
Aminosalicylates • Sulfasalazine • Mesalamine	Used for anti-inflammatory effect Inhibition of prostaglandins known to cause diarrhea and affect mucosal transport	Administer after meals Do not crush or chew sustained released tablets Teach patient or parents to supplement daily intake of iron Monitor for side effects: • Nausea • Vomiting • Bloody diarrhea • Anorexia • Rash • Headache
Corticosteroids • Prednisone • Prednisolone • Hydrocortisone enema	Used for anti-inflammatory effect	Administer oral medications with meals to reduce gastric irritation Teach family to avoid abrupt discontinuation of medication Teach family to report delayed wound healing Monitor for side effects: • Nausea • Vomiting • Cushingoid appearance • Immunosuppression • Growth suppression • Hypertension • Acne • Altered moods
Immunosuppressants • 6-Mercaptopurine (6-MP) • Azathioprine • Cyclosporine • Methotrexate	Used for immunosuppressive effect	Monitor for side effects: • Nausea • Vomiting • Anorexia • Diarrhea • Bone marrow suppression • Infection • Mucositis Teach family to avoid exposing child to persons with infection Teach family the importance of good hygiene for child to avoid infection
Biologic therapies • Tumor necrosis factor-α • Infliximab (Remicade) • Interleukin-10 • Thalidomide	Prevents TNF-alpha from binding to its receptors (TNF-alpha have been found in stools of patients with Crohn's disease)	Reconstitute IV preparation according to manufacturer directions and administer according to agency protocol Monitor for side effects: Infusion reactions—fever, chills, chest pain, hypotension, dyspnea, urticaria Discontinue IV infusion if infusion reaction is evident
Antibiotics • Metronidazole • Ciprofloxacil	Antibacterial against anaerobic bacteria and some gram-negative bacteria	Extended release form should not be chewed or crushed Administer with food or milk to reduce gastrointestinal distress Monitor for side effects: • Fever • Headache • Diarrhea • Nausea • Vomiting • Fungal overgrowth

Data from: Baron, M. L. (2002). Crohn disease in children. *American Journal of Nursing, 102* (10), 26–34; Bindler, R., & Howry, L. (2005). *Pediatric drug guide.* Upper Saddle River, NJ: Prentice Hall Health; Hyams, J. (2005). Inflammatory bowel disease. *Pediatrics in Review, 26* (9), 314–320; Plante, M. L. (2004). Crohn's disease. *Advance for Nurse Practitioners* (May 2004), 28–35.

NURSING MANAGEMENT

Nursing management occurs mainly in the community and home and focuses on helping the child and family adjust to the emotional impact of a chronic disease, administering medications and diet therapy, monitoring nutritional status, monitoring growth status, and providing appropriate referrals.

Assessment and Diagnosis

Assess for abdominal distention, tenderness, and pain. Monitor bowel sounds and stool pattern; measure abdominal girth.

Nursing diagnoses that apply to the child with inflammatory bowel disease may include:

- Diarrhea related to disease process
- Imbalanced Nutrition: Less than Body Requirements related to bowel inflammation and poor nutritional intake
- Pain (Acute or Chronic) related to inflammatory disease process
- Risk for Deficient Fluid Volume related to loss of fluids through diarrhea
- Disturbed Body Image related to disease process, presence of stoma, and medication side effects

Planning and Implementation

Provide emotional support and counseling to help the child adjust to feeling "different" from peers. Inability to compete with peers and frequent absences from school can affect the child's self-esteem. Collaborate care with parents and assist them in contacting the school district to arrange for tutoring in case extended absences from school become necessary. Encourage the child who is not attending school regularly to maintain contact with friends through telephone calls, cards, and visits.

Body image is a major concern for children and adolescents with inflammatory bowel disease. Corticosteroid therapy causes growth retardation and delayed sexual maturation. Encourage the child to discuss feelings about these side effects. If a permanent colostomy or ileostomy is required, the nurse can assist the child and family to understand the need for surgical treatment. (See the discussion of ostomies earlier in this chapter.) Introduce the child and family to other children who have stomas.

Providing adequate stress reduction may be helpful in the control of inflammatory bowel disease. Collaborate with the parents to teach young children relaxation techniques, such as deep breathing, progressive tensing and relaxing of muscles, and visualization of favorite places. Encourage busy school-age children and teens to have quiet and restful times each day, in addition to physical activity periods.

Teach parents about medication administration and diet therapy. Reinforce to both the parents and child the importance of adhering to a strict medication regimen. Emphasize that medications should be continued even when the child is asymptomatic. Discuss the side effects of the drugs and what to do if any of these symptoms occur. (See Families Want To Know: Dietary Instructions for Inflammatory Bowel Disease.)

GROWTH & DEVELOPMENT

Stress Reduction for IBD

Providing adequate stress reduction may be helpful in control of inflammatory bowel disease. Teach young children relaxation techniques, such as deep breathing, progressive tensing and relaxing of muscles, and visualization of favorite places. Encourage busy school-age children and teens to have quiet and restful times each day, in addition to physical activity periods.

FAMILIES WANT TO KNOW

Diet Instructions for Inflammatory Bowel Disease

- Several small feedings are usually better tolerated than three meals daily.
- Limiting fiber intake can help to decrease intestine motility and inflammation. Peel fruits and avoid large quantities of whole grains and nuts.
- If the child is not eating well, offer high-calorie meals. If lactose intolerance is not a problem for the particular child, cream soups, milkshakes, puddings, and custards can be offered.

- Liquid dietary supplements may be helpful to ensure protein and caloric requirements are met.
- Watch for foods that cause intestinal problems for the individual child, and avoid them in the future.
- Avoid having mealtime become a reason for family strife. Seek help of nurses and dietitians if needed.

Since immune status may be altered by steroid use, have families avoid contact with infectious diseases when the child is taking steroids. Instruct them to report any diseases and fevers the child experiences, and to report the use of steroids to all healthcare providers. Immunization schedules may need to be altered.

Parents also will require instructions for TPN if it is used, as well as information about care of a central venous catheter, including dressing changes, sterile and nonsterile techniques, signs of infection, how to handle infusion pumps and tubing, and how to measure the child's intake and output. Assist parents in obtaining equipment and supplies necessary for the child's care. Have parents demonstrate their mastery of care for the central venous catheter and their understanding of TPN techniques during home visits and appointments for health care.

Refer parents to social services, the visiting nurse association, and home healthcare agencies if they are not receiving any of these services. For information about inflammatory bowel disease, refer families to the Crohn Colitis Foundation.

Evaluation

Expected outcomes of nursing care for the child with inflammatory bowel disease include the following:

- Normal growth and development milestones are achieved.
- The child demonstrates absence of gastrointestinal distress.
- The child and family demonstrate successful management of medications without demonstration of side effects.
- The child remains free from infection due to central line.
- A positive body image is achieved.
- The child demonstrates integration of stress-lowering practices into daily life.

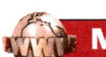

MediaLink

Inflammatory Bowel Disease Resources and Support

Peptic Ulcer

A peptic ulcer is an erosion of the mucosal tissue in the lower end of the esophagus, in the stomach (usually along the lesser curvature), or in the duodenum (*gastric ulcer* is the term sometimes used when the stomach mucosa is affected). Boys are more likely to have peptic ulcers than girls. Peptic ulcers are much less common in children than in adults. African American and Hispanic children are at greater risk for peptic ulcers (Simpson & Ivey, 2003).

Ulcers are classified as primary or secondary, depending on their etiology. Primary peptic ulcers occur in healthy children. Secondary (stress) ulcers occur in children with a preexisting illness or injury (often a burn) and in children receiving medications such as salicylates, corticosteroids, and nonsteroidal anti-inflammatory drugs. Diet usually is not a major factor in the development of peptic ulcers in children, although caffeine and alcohol consumption in adolescents may exacerbate the disease. It is now known that ulcers in both adults and children are often caused by *Helicobacter pylori*, a gram-negative rod (Vaira et al., 2005). This organism is transmitted by the fecal-oral or oral-oral routes. Infections often occur in several members of a family, especially when the family's water supply is contaminated.

Clinical manifestations vary according to the age of the child and location of the ulcer. The most common symptom is abdominal pain (burning) associated with an empty stomach, which may awaken the child at night. Vomiting and pain after meals, anemia, occult blood in stools, and abdominal distention may also be present.

Diagnosis is based on the history and radiologic studies. *H. pylori* can be diagnosed by culture of the organism taken via gastroscopy, and by measuring urea in the urine and on the breath, since the organism hydrolyzes urea. The goals of medical management are to relieve discomfort and promote healing. When *H. pylori* is the causative agent, antimicrobial agents such as bismuth salts, tetracycline, and metronidazole combination are given. Other drug combinations, such as a combination of antacids in liquid form (Maalox, Mylanta) and histamine antagonists (ranitidine, cimetidine, and famotidine), are also used. Antibody titers are measured several times over

6 months to evaluate the effectiveness of therapy. The prognosis is usually good with early intervention.

Nursing Management

Nurses may identify children with peptic ulcer disease by looking for the symptoms and noting family history of *H. pylori* infection. Nursing care centers on interventions to promote adequate nutritional intake, promote healing, and prevent recurrences. Provide a nutritionally sound, age-appropriate diet. Omit foods only if they exacerbate the disorder.

Antibiotics must be given as scheduled. Emphasize the importance of continuing drug therapy. The family needs encouragement to continue the medications as ordered and to return for follow-up visits. Children who attend school may prefer to take antacids in the form of tablets, which are easier to carry than liquid preparations. A permission form to take medications at school needs to be filled out by the prescriber. Parents should check with the child's physician before giving any additional medication. Caution parents to avoid aspirin products, which irritate the gastric mucosa. If an antipyretic or pain medication is needed, acetaminophen should be given. Advise parents to read medication labels if they are unsure of product contents.

Because psychologic stress can contribute to peptic ulcer disease, help the parents and child identify sources of stress in the child's life. Assess coping mechanisms and provide referral for psychologic counseling, if appropriate. Teach relaxation techniques and recommend community classes on yoga or other stress reduction.

DISORDERS OF MOTILITY

Fluids are produced in large quantities as part of normal GI functioning. As food passes through the intestines, fluids are reabsorbed and moderately soft stool is formed and evacuated. In disorders such as diarrhea and constipation, fluid production is altered, causing either more or less fluid to be reabsorbed. This can severely alter the characteristics of the stool. Reabsorption of too little water produces diarrhea and can lead to fluid and electrolyte alterations. Reabsorption of too much fluid can cause constipation, which if untreated can lead to bowel obstruction.

Gastroenteritis (Acute Diarrhea)

Gastroenteritis is an inflammation of the stomach and intestines that may be accompanied by vomiting and diarrhea. It can affect any part of the GI tract. Diarrhea is a common problem in children, accounting for 13% of hospitalizations in children less than 5 years of age (Van Niel, Feudtner, Garrison, & Christakis, 2002). It may be an acute problem, caused by viral, bacterial, or parasitic infections, or a chronic problem. Rotavirus is the leading cause of gastroenteritis in children (Hsu et al., 2005). Acute gastroenteritis affects approximately 30 million children per year in the United States (Reeves, Shannon, & Fleisher, 2002). Children under age 5 years average approximately two episodes of gastroenteritis each year. Infants and small children with gastroenteritis or diarrhea can quickly become dehydrated and are at risk for hypovolemic shock if fluid and electrolyte losses are not replaced (see Chapter 16 ∞).

Etiology and Pathophysiology

Diarrhea in children can have many different causes (Table 24–2). The specific etiology is not always identified. The common mechanism is a decrease in the absorptive capacity of the bowel through inflammation, decrease in surface area for absorption, or alteration of parasympathetic innervation. Children in childcare centers and those living in substandard housing with improper sanitation are at increased risk.

Clinical Manifestations

Diarrhea may be mild, moderate, or severe. In mild diarrhea, stools are slightly increased in number and have a more liquid consistency. In moderate diarrhea the child has several loose or watery stools. Other symptoms include irritability, anorexia, nau-

Table 24–2	CAUSES OF DIARRHEA IN CHILDREN
Etiology	**Bowel Manifestations**
Emotional stress (anxiety, fatigue)	Increased motility
Intestinal infection (bacteria [*E. coli, Salmonella, Shigella*], viral [human rotavirus, enteric adenovirus], fungal overgrowth)	Inflammation of mucosa; increased mucus secretion in colon
Food sensitivity (gluten, cow's milk)	Decreased digestion of food
Food intolerance (lactose, introduction of new foods, overfeeding)	Increased motility; increased mucus secretion in colon
Medications (iron, antibiotics)	Irritation and suprainfection
Colon disease (colitis, necrotizing enterocolitis, enterocolitis)	Inflammation and ulceration of intestinal walls; reduced absorption of fluid; increased intestinal motility
Surgical alterations (short bowel syndrome)	Reduced size of colon; decreased absorption surface

sea, and vomiting. Moderate diarrhea is usually self-limiting, resolving without treatment within 1 or 2 days. In severe diarrhea, watery stools are continuous. The child exhibits symptoms of fluid and electrolyte imbalance (see Chapter 16 ∞), has cramping, and is extremely irritable and difficult to console.

COLLABORATIVE CARE

Diagnosis is based on the history, physical examination, and laboratory findings. A thorough history may help identify the cause. Ask parents about recent exposure to illnesses, use of antibiotics, travel, food and formula preparation, food sensitivities or allergies, and whether the child attends childcare. Physical examination provides a guide to the severity of dehydration (see Chapter 16 ∞). The stool can be examined for the presence of ova, parasites, infectious organisms, viruses, fat, and undigested sugars. Laboratory evaluation of serum and urine helps identify electrolyte imbalances and other deficiencies.

Medical management depends on the severity of the diarrhea and fluid and electrolyte imbalances. The goal of treatment is to correct the fluid and electrolyte imbalances. For mild dehydration the child is rehydrated with oral rehydration therapy (see Chapter 16). This may be accomplished at home or in the short-stay observation unit in a hospital with oral rehydration solutions such as Pedialyte, Infalyte, and Rehydralyte. Carbonated and very sugary beverages should not be given. Fermentation of sugar in the GI tract causes increased gas, abdominal distention, and an increased frequency of diarrhea. For moderate and severe dehydration, rehydration is accomplished by intravenous infusion with a solution chosen to correct the specific imbalances. (see Chapter 16 ∞ for information about solutions to correct dehydration).

If the diarrhea is caused by bacteria or parasites, antimicrobial therapy may be prescribed. Antiemetics and antidiarrheals are generally not used in young children since they can mask the signs and symptoms of more serious illness (Thielman & Guerrant, 2004).

NURSING MANAGEMENT
Nursing Assessment and Diagnosis

The nurse may encounter the child and family in the emergency department, urgent care center, clinic, or office. The child may be cared for over several hours at a clinic or urgent care center so that dehydration is treated with intravenous infusion and/or oral rehydration, and then sent home with instructions for parents to care for the child. If the child is hospitalized, it is important to assess onset, frequency, color, amount, and consistency of stools. If the child is also vomiting, monitor the amount and type of vomitus. Initial and ongoing physical assessment of the child focuses on observing for signs and symptoms of dehydration, which reflect underlying fluid and electrolyte status. Evaluate urinary output and specific gravity. An accurate weight must be obtained on admission and daily thereafter. Monitor vital signs every 2 to 4 hours. A febrile child has increased water loss, contributing to the dehydration. Assess skin integrity, especially in the perineal and rectal areas, and note any breakdown or rashes.

The accompanying Nursing Care Plan lists common nursing diagnoses. Other diagnoses that might also be appropriate include:

- Anxiety (Child and Parent) related to change in health status
- Disturbed Sleep Pattern related to pain
- Imbalanced Nutrition: Less than Body Requirements related to inability to ingest sufficient nutrients

Planning and Implementation

Nursing care focuses on providing emotional support, promoting rest and comfort, and ensuring adequate nutrition and hydration. See Nursing Care Plan: The Child with Gastroenteritis for a summary of nursing care.

Provide Emotional Support

The child may have been ill for several days or become suddenly ill a short time before seeking health care. The child and parents are usually anxious, so it is important to allow them to talk and ask questions. The child may require blood tests to help direct rehydration therapy. Most children are cared for at home, although care in a 24-hour monitoring unit may occur. For hospitalized children, use therapeutic play techniques, such as allowing the child to manipulate equipment, to help reduce anxiety (see Chapter 13 ∞). To promote trust, be honest if a procedure will hurt. Encourage the child to express anger, fear, and pain.

Promote Rest and Comfort

Most children with gastroenteritis are quite ill and awaken frequently with periods of vomiting and diarrhea. Provide a quiet, restful environment. Darken the room and keep interruptions to a minimum. To reduce the child's anxiety, encourage parents to room in. Place the child's favorite toys and comfort objects within reach. Keep the child's mouth moistened with a glycerine swab, a wet washcloth, or an occasional ice chip. Provide skin care after each episode of diarrhea. Avoid using commercial baby wipes that contain alcohol as these irritate the skin and cause discomfort for the child.

Ensure Adequate Nutrition and Hydration

Offer liquids throughout the illness, even if an intravenous infusion is in place. Follow guidelines for oral rehydration therapy in Chapter 16 ∞. Find out what fluids the family uses at home. Small amounts of normal diet for age are provided. Infants are breast-fed or given formula. Avoid cow's milk-based formula or regular milk until the diarrhea resolves. The child's diet progresses based on tolerance for feedings. Apple juice and other fruit juices should be avoided since they contain high amounts of carbohydrates which pull circulating fluids into the gut and can prolong the presence of diarrhea.

Discharge Planning and Care in the Community

Discharge teaching should begin on arrival at the healthcare facility. Teach family members that handwashing is the most important measure that can be taken to prevent the spread of gastroenteritis. Tell parents what to expect as the child's GI system returns to normal. Teach the parents about the symptoms of dehydration and what to do if diarrhea recurs. Be sure that parents understand the recommended diet progression. Emphasize the necessity of good hygiene practices to prevent the spread of microorganisms that can cause gastroenteritis. If the child attends childcare, have the parent inform the care center about the infection so the staff can be alerted to watch for other cases and can take steps to prevent the spread of infection.

> **NURSING ALERT**
>
> Handwashing is the most important health maintenance measure that can be taken to prevent the spread of gastroenteritis. Wash your hands often, and particularly before and after care of each child. Instruct parents in the importance of handwashing, especially when caring for the child with gastroenteritis. Teach children in childcare centers and schools how to wash their hands effectively to prevent the spread of infectious diseases.

NURSING CARE PLAN | The Child with Gastroenteritis

GOAL	INTERVENTION	RATIONALE	EXPECTED OUTCOME
1. Diarrhea related to infectious process			
	NIC Priority Intervention: **Diarrhea Management:** *Prevention and alleviation of diarrhea.*		*NOC Suggested Outcome:* **Fluid and Electrolyte Balance:** *Balance of water and electrolytes in the intracellular and extracellular compartments of the body.*
The child's bowel function will be restored to normal.	• Obtain baseline vital signs and monitor every 2–4 hours.	• Fluid and electrolyte imbalances can alter vital body functions.	The child's bowel function returns to normal.
	• Observe stools for amount, color, consistency, odor, and frequency.	• Aids in the diagnosis and in monitoring the child's status.	
	• Test stools for occult blood.	• Frequent defecation and some infectious organisms can cause bleeding.	
	• Monitor results of stool culture and sample for ova and parasites.	• Rapid notification of the physician will facilitate treatment.	
	• Wash hands well before and after contact with the child.	• Helps prevent transmission of microorganisms.	
	• Isolate the child until the cause of the diarrhea is determined.	• Prevents exposure of other patients and staff.	
	• Assist the child with toileting and hygiene.	• The child may be weak, incontinent, physically impaired, or anxious and require assistance to use the bathroom.	
	• Administer prescribed oral rehydration and intravenous solutions.	• Provides necessary fluids and nutrients.	
	• Notify the physician if diarrhea persists, stool characteristics change, or other symptoms of dehydration electrolyte imbalance occur.	• Ensures early intervention.	
2. Deficient Fluid Volume related to active fluid volume loss			
	NIC Priority Intervention: **Fluid Monitoring:** *Collection and analysis of patient data to regulate fluid balance.*		*NOC Suggested Outcome:* **Fluid and Electrolyte Balance:** *Balance of water and electrolytes in the intracellular and extracellular compartments of the body.*
The child will remain hydrated and will begin to drink fluids within 24 hours of admission.	• Monitor intake and output. Be sure to document time of each voiding.	• Will determine if output exceeds input. Long periods of time without urine output can be an early indicator of poor renal function. A child should produce 1–2 mL of urine/kg/hr.	The child has normal fluid and electrolyte balance as indicated by laboratory evaluation and physical examination.
	• Compare admission weight to preadmission weight. Assess weight daily.	• The degree of dehydration can be determined by the percentage of weight loss. Daily weights aid in determining progress toward rehydration.	
	• Assess level of consciousness, skin turgor, mucous membranes, skin color and temperature, capillary refill, eyes, and fontanels every 4 hours.	• Will determine degree of hydration and adequacy of interventions.	

(continued)

NURSING CARE PLAN **The Child with Gastroenteritis** (continued)

GOAL	INTERVENTION	RATIONALE	EXPECTED OUTCOME
2. Deficient Fluid Volume related to active fluid volume loss (continued)			
	• Assess for vomiting.	• Vomiting frequently accompanies diarrhea and contributes to the child's fluid loss.	
	• Provide oral fluid and electrolyte replacement solution if able to tolerate.	• Less invasive than IV fluids. Provides for replacement of essential fluids and electrolytes.	
	• Provide and maintain IV replacement therapy, as ordered.	• Use of IV replacement is based on the degree of dehydration, ongoing losses, insensible water losses, and electrolyte results.	
3. Risk for Impaired Skin Integrity related to altered fluid status			
	NIC Priority Intervention: **Skin Surveillance:** *Collection and analysis of patient data to maintain skin integrity.*		*NOC Suggested Outcome:* **Tissue Integrity:** *Structural intactness and normal physiologic function of skin.*
The child will remain free of skin breakdown and rashes.	• Assess skin of perineum and rectum for signs of skin breakdown or irritation.	• Early assessment and intervention can prevent worsening of the condition.	The child's perianal and rectal tissue remains pink and intact.
	• Provide prevention or restorative care for infants as follows:		
Preventive care:			
	• Change diapers every 2 hours or as needed.	• Minimizes skin contact with chemical irritants from stool and urine.	
	• Use cloth diapers rather than disposable.	• Minimizes the mechanical and chemical irritation from disposables.	
	• Wash diaper area after each soiling.	• Removes traces of stool if present.	
	• Apply A & D ointment, Aquaphor, or another barrier ointment with each diaper change.	• Provides a barrier and protects intact or reddened skin from becoming excoriated.	
Restorative care:			
	• Place the infant prone and leave the buttocks open to air.	• Promotes air circulation to the area.	
	• Notify the physician if the skin is severely broken or peeling or if a rash is present.	• Additional measures may be needed to ensure skin healing.	
	• For toddlers and older children: Tub bathe at least daily (if condition allows) in tepid water. Pat the area dry.	• Helps loosen any fecal matter without scrubbing, which can cause additional irritation to the skin.	
	• Discourage the wearing of underwear if possible.	• Allows air to circulate and prevents accumulation of moisture.	
	• Apply A & D ointment or Aquaphor at least four times daily.	• Provides a barrier and protects intact or reddened skin from becoming excoriated.	

Evaluation

Expected outcomes of nursing care for the child with gastroenteritis include:

- Fluid and electrolyte balance is restored.
- The child achieves adequate nutritional intake to support growth and development.
- The child achieves adequate rest and sleep.
- Normal bowel function for the child is restored.
- The family describes signs of dehydration and appropriate interventions.
- The family acknowledges the importance of handwashing in decreasing transmission of infectious agents.

Constipation

Constipation is a common complaint in the pediatric population and accounts for approximately 25% of referrals made to pediatric gastroenterologists (Coughlin, 2003). Constipation is characterized by a decrease in the frequency or passage of stools; the formation of hard, dry stools; or the oozing of liquid stool past a collection of hard, dry stool. Because stooling patterns vary among children, identification of an abnormal pattern is sometimes difficult. Infants usually have several bowel movements a day. For a young child, one bowel movement a day may be normal. As the child grows, however, three to four bowel movements a week may be a normal pattern. Constipation is characterized by "pebble-like, hard stools for a majority of bowel movements for at least 2 weeks, firm stools ≤2 times per week for at least 2 weeks, and no evidence of structural, endocrine, or metabolic disease" (Lembo & Camilleri, 2003).

Breast-fed infants may have bowel movements as frequently as with every feeding or just one bowel movement every several days. Because of differences in fat digestion and absorption, bottle-fed infants are more prone to hard stools (Coughlin, 2003).

Because stool patterns vary among children, identification of an abnormal pattern is sometimes difficult. For a young child, one bowel movement a day may be normal. As the child grows, however, three to four bowel movements in a week may be a normal pattern.

Etiology and Pathophysiology

Constipation may be caused by an underlying disease, diet, or psychologic factor (Table 24–3.) It may result from defects in filling, or more commonly emptying, of the rectum. Pathologic causes of defective filling include ineffective colonic propulsive activity, caused by hypothyroidism or use of medication, and obstruction, caused by a structural anomaly (stricture or stenosis) or by an aganglionic segment (Hirschsprung disease). If the rectum fails to fill, stasis leads to excessive drying of the stools. Emptying of the rectum depends on the defecation reflex. Lesions of the spinal cord, weakness of the abdominal muscles, and local lesions blocking sphincter relaxation all may impede attempts to defecate.

Table 24–3	INFLUENTIAL FACTORS IN CHILDHOOD CONSTIPATION	
Physical Factors in Infancy	**Physical Factors in Children**	**Psychological Factors in Children**
Familial stool patterns	Hypertrophied rectum	Embarrassment/shame related to soiling
High milk and low fiber intake	Residual stool blockage (fecalith)	related to early or coercive toilet training,
Cow's milk allergy	Overflow fecal soiling around a solid stool	or to lack of privacy
Hard stools	Poor rectal sensation	Fear of pain from hard stool
Dehydration	Diseases that influence gastrointestinal or	Being too busy to use the bathroom
Perianal group A streptococcal infection	neurologic systems such as celiac disease,	Parental blame/anger related to soiling and
Medications such as diuretics, and analgesia	cerebral palsy	toiling refusal
Intestinal or anal conditions such as		Teasing and bullying related to incontinence
Hirschsprung disease, cystic fibrosis,		Decreased mobility/activity
anorectal malformations		

Adapted from: Clayden, G., & Keshtgar, A. S. (2003). Management of childhood constipation. *Postgraduate Medical Journal, 79*, 616–621.

Constipation during infancy is rare and is most often caused by mismanagement of diet. The transition from formula to cow's milk may cause a transient constipation because the bowel must adjust to the increased protein content of cow's milk.

Constipation occurs most frequently in the toddler and preschool-age groups. This increased incidence is often associated with learning to control body functions. Many children do not like the sensations of a bowel movement and may begin withholding stool, which accumulates in and dilates the rectum until the next urge to defecate. The increasingly hard and painful bowel movement reinforces the child's behavior, and a pattern develops (Clayden & Keshtgar, 2003). See discussion in this chapter on encopresis.

Constipation in the school-age child and adolescent usually results in overflow fecal incontinence. Some children with constipation are discovered during their school years after being evaluated for recurrent urinary tract infections or enuresis (Clayden & Keshtgar, 2003).

■ COLLABORATIVE CARE

Collaborative care focuses on determining the underlying pathologic cause of constipation, correcting any structural defect, obstruction, or eliminating contributing factors, and assisting the child to establish routine bowel elimination habits.

Diagnostic Tests

Diagnosis is based on a thorough history and physical examination. When constipation occurs along with growth failure, vomiting, or abdominal pain, further investigation is necessary to rule out other disorders.

Clinical Therapy

Dietary management is the treatment of choice for constipation that has no underlying pathologic cause. Constipation in young infants can usually be corrected by increasing the amount of fluids or adding 2 ounces of pear or apple juice to daily intake. Increasing physical activity and fluid intake may be effective for some children.

Removing constipating foods (e.g., bananas, rice, and cheese) from the child's diet often decreases the constipation. Increasing the child's intake of high-fiber foods (whole grain breads, raw fruits and vegetables) and fluids also promotes bowel elimination. A single glycerin suppository or enema may be needed to remove hard stool, followed by dietary and fluid management.

In the school-age child, constipation may occur due to limited time for toileting. Busy school-age children may delay toileting. Children may also be hesitant to use an unfamiliar bathroom. Encouragement from parents and relaxation of bathroom privileges at school promote regularity and return of bowel patterns within a short time. Children may need to get up earlier to have breakfast and time for toileting before going to school.

Constipation may follow surgery, especially in children who are immobilized, such as by traction or a body cast. Stool softeners and a diet high in fiber and fluids are given to prevent and treat constipation.

Pharmacologic management of severe constipation usually occurs in two stages. The first stage involves softening the stool with medications such as lactulose, and the second stage involves evacuation of stool with a laxative. The evacuation phase is the most difficult for the child and those who are managing the child's constipation (Clayden & Keshtgar, 2003).

Once a stool softener is administered, the most effective means to evacuate the stool while causing the least amount of stress and anxiety to the child is considered. Suppositories and enemas can cause fear in children. Polyethylene glycol electrolyte solution (Golytely) can be administered orally or instilled via a nasogastric tube to promote stool evacuation (Biggs & Dery, 2006). More recently electrolyte-free polyethylene glycol (Miralx) has been used effectively (Kinservik & Friedhoff, 2004). Once the stool has been evacuated, a routine stimulant laxative is given to prevent reaccumulation of stool in the bowel. Senokot or Bisacodyl is usually the stimulant laxative of choice (Biggs & Dery, 2006).

RESEARCH

Bowel Elimination and STR

A recent study was conducted to determine whether constipation and painful bowel elimination occur as a result of stool toileting refusal (STR) or occur before STR. In this prospective longitudinal study of toilet training, 380 children between the ages of 17 and 19 months were followed (Blum, Taubman, & Nemeth, 2004). Researchers found that when hard or painful bowel movements or painful bowel elimination were associated with STR, the first episode of constipation occurs generally before the STR (Blum et al., 2004). This suggests that constipation is a chronic problem for many children, and it is not being treated effectively. Painful bowel elimination associated with hard bowel movements are thus factors that contribute to STR and not solely the result of STR (Blum et al., 2004).

Behavior Management

Behavior modification may prove beneficial to managing constipation. For younger children, providing rewards for overcoming the fear of toilets or for toileting at routinely scheduled times are effective. Older children also respond to rewards (Clayden & Keshtgar, 2003). Rewards can be simple items such as an afternoon spent with the parent playing a game. For children with psychological issues, child and family psychotherapy may be necessary. In these cases, the family is referred to a child and family counselor.

■ NURSING MANAGEMENT

Nursing care focuses on teaching parents what constitutes normal bowel patterns in children and the importance of diet in maintaining such patterns.

Nursing Assessment and Diagnosis

Assess the child's diet history and obtain a description of bowel patterns and habits from parents. When was the child toilet trained and have those patterns changed? Has there been incontinence in the toilet-trained child? Ask what the family does to treat constipation. Ask about frequency, consistency, and the presence of blood in the stools. Ask the child or parents about pain upon passing of stool. Assessment of the child's food likes and dislikes may provide a clue to the cause of constipation. Assess fluid intake and level of activity. Assess for previous history of gastrointestinal complications or surgery, as well as present medications. Ask parents when the newborn passed meconium.

Physical Assessment

Palpate the abdomen and assess the child's abdomen for firmness or tenderness, and the presence of palpable mass (retained stool). Assess for bowel sounds. If a digital rectal examination is performed, assess for presence of stool in rectum. Assess for hemorrhoids, anal fissures, or other abnormalities of the abdomen or perineum.

Nursing diagnoses that may apply to the child with constipation include:

- Constipation related to dietary, nutritional, and/or elimination habits
- Bowel Incontinence related to leakage around formed stool

Planning and Implementation

Regular bowel habits are encouraged by placing the child on the toilet 30 minutes after a meal or around the time bowel elimination usually occurs. Providing positive reinforcement during toilet training helps to prevent a withholding pattern.

Partner with the family and teach parents dietary measures to promote regularity of bowel movements. Children can be given a high-fiber diet that includes fruits and vegetables. Cut fresh fruits, dried fruits, and fruit juice can be offered as snacks. A glycerin suppository can be used periodically if needed. This is a natural stimulant and lubricant of the bowel.

Caution parents to avoid frequent use of laxatives, stool softeners, and enemas, since overuse can cause bowel dependency. Herbal stimulant laxatives are discouraged for children less than 12 years, although other intestinal motility aids are not generally harmful. Ask the family about any herbs they may commonly use.

Evaluation

Expected outcomes of nursing care for the child with constipation include:

- The child establishes a routine bowel elimination pattern.
- The child is free from constipation.

Encopresis

Encopresis is an abnormal elimination pattern characterized by the recurrent soiling or passage of stool at inappropriate times by a child who should have achieved bowel continence. Encopresis is reported to occur in 55% of boys and 35% of girls with

---

COMPLEMENTARY THERAPY

Herbal Laxatives

Herbal laxatives are used by some cultures as complementary therapies. The safety and effectiveness of many of these laxatives have not been established in children. Psyllium, for example, has been approved for use as an ingredient in bulk laxatives but no studies have evaluated its safety or effectiveness in treating constipation in children. Cascara sagrada and senna are stimulant laxatives that have been approved by the FDA for use in children older than 2 years of age to treat constipation. Stimulant laxatives should be used with caution in children, however, as they can lead to dependency as well as abdominal pain. Senna has also been associated with skin problems in children, including diaper rash and blistering (Gardiner & Kemper, 2005).

constipation (Biggs & Dery, 2006). Children with primary encopresis have never achieved bowel control. Children with secondary encopresis have been continent of stool for several months.

Encopresis is usually associated with voluntary or involuntary retention of stool in the lower bowel and rectum, leading to constipation, dilation of the lower bowel, and incompetence of the inner sphincter. The retention of stool is usually a result of being "too busy"; the child puts off going to the bathroom because there are activities occurring and it would be an inconvenience to leave. The retention of stool leads to constipation that is untreated and chronic. Loose stool leaks around the hard feces, and the child becomes unaware of a need to eliminate. Soiling may occur during the day or night. Bowel movements are irregular, painful, small, and hard. The child may be ridiculed by peers because of his or her offensive body odor. This rejection leads to withdrawal and behavioral problems, often resulting in altered school performance and attendance. The child continues to hold stool because the passage has become painful. Parents commonly seek health care, believing that the child has diarrhea or constipation.

The underlying constipation that leads to encopresis may be caused by the stress of environmental changes (e.g., birth of a sibling, moving to a new house, attending a new school), issues of anger and control related to bowel training, diet, a full schedule of activities, or a genetic predisposition.

A thorough history, physical examination, and diagnostic studies (possibly including barium enema) are necessary to rule out organic causes and anatomic abnormalities. Examination of mental health and cognitive functioning may be indicated. Information about the child's toilet-training habits and parents' attitudes concerning those habits is obtained. A dietary history, including eating habits and types of foods eaten, is often helpful. Physical examination sometimes reveals a nontender mass in the lower abdomen.

Treatment may include behavior modification techniques, dietary changes, use of lubricants to clear the bowel of impacted stool and encourage normal defecation, and psychotherapy. Behavior modification programs that reward and reinforce appropriate toileting habits can be successful. Dietary changes include incorporating high-fiber foods such as fruits, vegetables, and whole grain cereals into the diet. Limiting intake of refined and highly processed foods and dairy products also may be helpful. Drugs such as mineral oil, bulk-forming laxatives, and stool softeners are used temporarily to empty the bowel. The child should sit on the toilet for several minutes after morning and evening meals. It takes several months for the bowel to be retrained to respond to sphincter stimulation. Psychotherapy involving the child and family may be indicated in instances of dysfunctional parent-child relationships.

Nursing Management

Prevention of encopresis is the nursing goal. Partner with parents to teach toilet-training techniques, emphasizing the child's developmental readiness (see Chapter 3 ∞). Parents are encouraged to praise the child for successes and avoid punishment and power struggles. Encourage high-fiber diets and regular times for elimination.

Nursing care centers on educating the child and parents about the disorder and its treatment and providing emotional support. Explain the treatment plan, including dietary changes and use of laxatives or stool softeners. Reassure the child that he or she has a healthy body and, with treatment, will achieve normal functioning. The child is monitored by the nurse for at least 6 months to be certain new patterns have been established.

INTESTINAL PARASITIC DISORDERS

Intestinal parasitic disorders occur most frequently in tropical regions. Outbreaks take place where water is not treated, food is incorrectly prepared, or people live in crowded conditions with poor sanitation. In the United States, outbreaks of diseases caused by protozoa or helminths (worms) are increasing. A common cause of infection in the United States is camping and ingesting untreated water. Young children, especially those in childcare, are most at risk of infection. Young children often lack good hygiene practices and are likely to put objects and their hands into their mouths. See Clinical Manifestations: Common Intestinal Parasitic Disorders on the next page.

CLINICAL MANIFESTATIONS	COMMON INTESTINAL PARASITIC DISORDERS			
Parasitic Infection	**Transmission, Life Cycle, Pathogenesis**	**Clinical Manifestations**	**Clinical Therapy**	**Comments**
Giardiasis Organism: protozoan *Giardia lamblia* 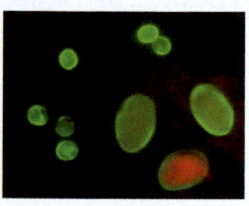	Transmission is through person-to-person contact, unfiltered water, improperly prepared infected food, and contact with animals. Cysts are ingested and passed into the duodenum and proximal jejunum, where they begin actively feeding. They are excreted in the stool.	May be asymptomatic. *Infants:* diarrhea, vomiting, anorexia, failure to thrive. *Older children:* abdominal cramps; intermittent loose, foul-smelling, watery, pale, and greasy stools.	Available medications include furazolidone and quinacrine. Furazolidone has fewer side effects than quinacrine but is more expensive. Metronidazole is also effective but is not licensed in the United States for treatment of giardiasis.	Most common intestinal parasitic organism in the United States. Infection may resolve spontaneously in 4–6 weeks without treatment. Parents or caregivers should wear gloves when handling diapers or stool of parasite-infected infant or child.
Enterobiasis (Pinworm) Organism: nematode *Enterobius vermicularis* 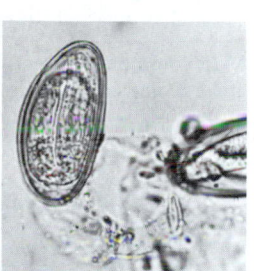	Transmission is from discharged eggs inhaled or carried from hand to mouth. Eggs hatch in the upper intestine and mature in 15–28 days. Larvae then migrate to the cecum. After mating, the female migrates out of the anus and lays up to 17,000 eggs. Movement of worms causes intense itching. Scratching deposits eggs on the hands and under the nails.	Intense perianal itching, irritability, restlessness, and short attention span; in females, can migrate to the vagina and urethra to cause infection. Itching intensifies at night when the female comes to the anal opening to lay eggs.	Available medications include mebendazole, pyrantel pamoate, and piperazine citrate. The child and all household members should be treated at the same time. Treatment may be repeated in 2–3 weeks.	Most common helminthic infection in the United States. Transmission is increased in crowded conditions such as housing developments, schools, and day care centers.
Ascariasis (Type of Roundworm) Organism: nematode *Ascaris lumbricoides* 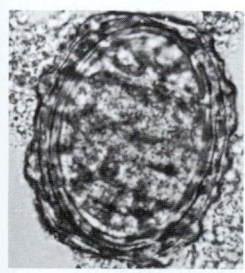	Transmission is from discharged eggs carried from hand to mouth. Adult lays eggs in small intestine. Eggs are excreted in stool, where they incubate for 2–3 weeks. Swallowed eggs hatch in the small intestine. Larvae may penetrate intestinal villi, entering the portal vein and liver, then moving to the lung. Larvae that ascend to upper respiratory tract are swallowed and proceed to the small intestine, where they repeat the cycle.	Mild infection may be asymptomatic. Severe infection may result in intestinal obstruction, peritonitis, obstructive jaundice, and lung involvement.	Available anthelmintic medications include mebendazole, pyrantel pamoate, or piperazine citrate. Stools should be examined 2 weeks after treatment and monthly for 3 months. Family members and contacts of the child should be treated if indicated. If the child has intestinal obstruction, treatment may include administering piperazine through a nasogastric tube and duodenal suction. Obstructing worms sometimes have to be surgically removed.	Most common in warm climates. Primarily affects children 1–4 years of age.

(continued)

CLINICAL MANIFESTATIONS | COMMON INTESTINAL PARASITIC DISORDERS (continued)

Parasitic Infection	Transmission, Life Cycle, Pathogenesis	Clinical Manifestations	Clinical Therapy	Comments
Hookworm disease Organism: nematode *Necator americanus* 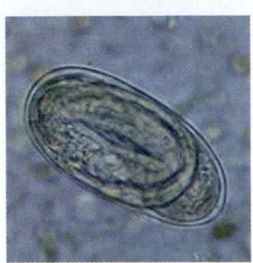	Transmission is through direct contact with infected soil containing larvae. Worms live in the small intestine and feed on villi, causing bleeding. Eggs are deposited in the bowel and excreted in feces. Eggs hatch in damp shaded soil. Larvae attach to and penetrate the skin then enter the bloodstream, migrating to the lungs. Larvae then migrate to the upper respiratory passages and are swallowed.	In healthy individuals mild infection seldom causes problems. More severe infection may result in anemia and malnutrition. Presence of larvae on the skin may cause burning and itching, followed by redness and papular eruption.	Available medications include mebendazole and pyrantel pamoate. Stools should be examined 2 weeks after treatment and monthly for 3 months. Family members and contacts of the child should be treated if indicated.	Children should wear shoes when outdoors, although other unprotected areas of the skin may still come in contact with larvae.
Strongyloidiasis (Type of Roundworm) Organism: nematode *Strongyloides stercoralis*	Transmission is from the ingestion of discharged larvae in the soil. Life cycle is similar to that of the hookwarm, except the threadworm does not attach to the intestinal mucosa and feeding larvae (rather than eggs) may be deposited in the soil.	Mild infection may be asymptomatic. Severe infection may result in abdominal pain and distention, nausea, vomiting, and diarrhea. Stools may be large and pale, with mucus. Severe infection may lead to a nutritional deficiency.	Available medications include thiabendazole or mebendazole. Treatment may need to be repeated if symptoms recur after treatment. Family members and contacts of the child should be examined and treated if indicated.	Most common in older children and adolescents.

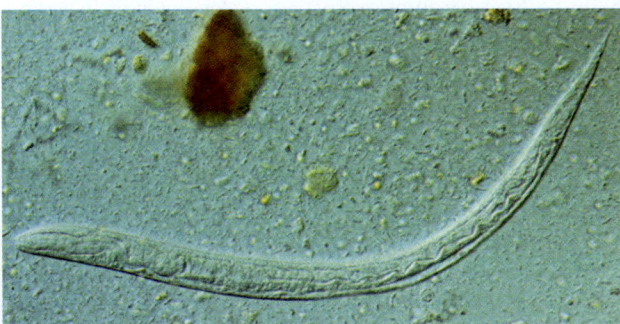

Parasitic Infection	Transmission, Life Cycle, Pathogenesis	Clinical Manifestations	Clinical Therapy	Comments
Visceral larva migrans (toxocariasis) Organism: nematode *Toxocara canis* or *T. catis,* commonly found in dogs and cats 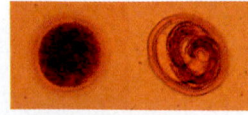	Transmission is through the ingestion of eggs in the soil. Ingested eggs hatch in the intestine. Mobile larvae then migrate to the liver and eventually to all major organs (including the brain). Once migration is complete, they encapsulate in dense fibrous tissue.	Most cases are asymptomatic. Affected children may have a low-grade fever and recurrent upper airway diseases. Severe symptoms include hepatomegaly, pulmonary infiltration, and neurologic disturbances. In all cases there is a hypereosinophilia of the blood.	There is no specific treatment. Corticosteroids have been used in severe cases. Thiabendazole has been recommended but efficacy is not established (infection usually resolves spontaneously).	Most common in toddlers. Deworm household pets monthly if indicated. Keep children away from areas contaminated with animal droppings.

Giardia lamblia, Strongyloidiasis, Hookworm, and Toxocariasis courtesy of the Centers for Disease Control and Prevention, Atlanta, GA. Ascariasis and Enterobiasis from: Murray, D. L. (2003). Infectious diseases. In C. D. Rudolph & A. M. Rudolph (Eds.), *Rudolph's pediatrics* (21st ed., pp. 1102, 1106). New York: McGraw Hill.

MEDICATIONS USED TO TREAT *Intestinal Parasitic Infections*

Diloxanide furoate	Piperazine citrate
Furazolidone	Pyrantel pamoate
Iodoquinol	Tetracycline
Mebendazole	Thiabendazole
Metronidazole	Trimethoprim/sulfamethoxazole
Paromomycin	

Data from: Bindler, R. M., & Howry, L. B. (2005). *Pediatric drugs and nursing implications* (3rd ed.). Upper Saddle River, NJ: Prentice Hall Health.

Another common cause of parasitic infection in the young child is related to exposure to pets and wildlife. Pets should be checked for parasites and treated for worms regularly. Sandboxes should be kept covered when not in use and children should be taught good handwashing after exposure to their pets (CDC, 2006b).

Laboratory examination of stool specimens identifies the causative organism (protozoa, worms, larvae, or ova). Treatment usually involves an anthelmintic. See the Medication Administration box above. Nursing care centers on preventive teaching. Emphasize the importance of good hygiene practices, especially careful handwashing, after toileting and when handling food. Instruct parents to give prescribed medications as directed even if the child's condition seems to be improved.

FEEDING DISORDERS

Feeding problems that interfere with a child's ability to ingest or tolerate formulas and foods usually become apparent during the first year of life. To prevent complications of poor nutrition, feeding methods or diet may need to be altered. The following discussion focuses on the common disorders of colic and rumination. See Chapter 4 for a discussion of food allergy and sensitivity and of feeding disorder of infancy and childhood (failure to thrive). See Chapter 4 ∞ for a discussion of the eating disorders anorexia nervosa and bulimia.

Colic

Colic is a feeding disorder characterized by paroxysmal abdominal pain of intestinal origin and severe crying. Approximately 5–28% percent of infants have colic during the first few months of life. Episodes of colic usually begin when the infant is between 2 and 6 weeks of age. Symptoms generally subside by 3 months of age (Miller, 2003). The etiology of colic is unknown. Proposed causes include feeding too rapidly and swallowing large amounts of air.

Characteristically the infant with colic cries loudly and continuously, often for several hours. The infant's face may become flushed. The abdomen is distended and tense. Often the infant draws up the legs and clenches the hands. Episodes occur at the same time each day, usually in the late afternoon or early evening. Crying may stop only when the child is completely exhausted or after passage of flatus or stool. Carrying the child in the upright position is often helpful.

The symptoms initially may resemble intestinal obstruction or peritoneal infection. These conditions must be ruled out along with sensitivity to formula. Treatment is supportive. Usually by 3 months of age the severity and frequency of symptoms decrease.

Nursing Management

Nursing care requires a thorough history of the infant's diet and daily schedule and the events surrounding episodes of colicky behavior. Assess the infant's feeding patterns and diet including type, frequency, and amount of feeding (if breast-feeding, maternal

---

NURSING ALERT

Vomiting and feeding disorders can occur throughout childhood as well as in infancy. In older children, a pattern of **chronic vomiting** (low-grade nearly daily emesis) or **cyclic vomiting** (repeated severe vomiting of an sepisodic nature) can occur. These patterns differ from vomiting seen in colic or gastroesophageal reflux. Chronic vomiting is often associated with upper gastrointestinal tract diseases such as gastritis and esophagitis while cyclic vomiting is indicative of a syndrome known as abdominal migraine (Bullard & Page, 2005). Continuous vomiting of any nature should be evaluated.

COMPLEMENTARY THERAPY

Chamomile

A warm towel soaked in chamomile tea and wrapped around the infant's abdomen may relieve symptoms associated with colic. In addition, chamomile tea may be given orally to relieve pain related to teething and stomach ache (Duke, 2004).

diet history), as well as frequency of burping. Assess episodes of colic for onset, duration, and characteristics of cry. What measures are used to relieve crying? How effective are they? When possible, observe the feeding method. Parents of infants with colic are often tired and frustrated. They require frequent reassurance that they are not to blame for the infant's condition. Suggest ways of alleviating some of the infant's symptoms and discomfort. See Families Want to Know: Suggestions for Alleviating Colic.

Rumination

Rumination is a rare and serious form of chronic regurgitation of recently ingested food into the mouth, followed by rechewing and reswallowing or expelling the material (Chial, Camilleri, Williams, Litzinger, & Perrault, 2003). Chewing movements and mouthing of fingers often precede or accompany regurgitation. Close observation may reveal the infant actively initiating gagging with the tongue and fingers. The condition may lead to malnutrition and growth failure in infancy.

Rumination is most often associated with poor maternal-infant bonding. This kind of behavior is seen in infants deprived of tactile, visual, or auditory stimuli for long periods. The infant substitutes repetitive self-stimulation for the lack of appropriate external stimulation. (See the discussion of eating disorders of infancy and childhood in Chapter 4 ∞.)

Diagnostic evaluation focuses on ruling out an organic cause and determining the degree and type of nutritional deficiencies. Treatment involves correcting the nutritional deficits and developing normal feeding patterns. An interdisciplinary approach with medical and nursing staff and social services is often involved in helping parents meet the infant's nutritional and psychologic needs (see Chapter 4).

Nursing Management

Nursing care focuses on establishing a warm, caring relationship with the infant and the parents. Making eye contact with the infant, providing food regularly, and stimulating the infant through all the senses are ways to break the pattern of rumination.

Parents need to be included in the infant's care. Discuss proper nutrition and demonstrate feeding techniques and interactions that promote development. Determine the parents' support needs and make a referral to social service agencies as appropriate. A parent preoccupied with financial or other problems is less likely to attend to an infant's needs, resulting in continuation or recurrence of the pattern of rumination.

DISORDERS OF MALABSORPTION

Malabsorption occurs when a child cannot digest or absorb nutrients in the diet. Disorders of malabsorption include celiac disease, lactose intolerance, and short

FAMILIES WANT TO KNOW

Suggestions for Alleviating Colic

Provide Rhythmic Movement—Front-carrying sling carriers
Infant swing (battery-operated swing provides continuous motion)
   Car ride

Alternate Positions—Swaddle infant in a soft, stretchy blanket with knees flexed up against abdomen or with legs straight
   Place infant prone on parent's arm, supporting the body with one hand under the abdomen and cradling the head in the crook of the other arm

Reduce Environmental Stimuli—Respond to crying
   Provide quiet, soothing music

Prevent sudden loud noises
Avoid smoking

Provide Various Tactile Stimuli—Offer a pacifier
   Provide a warm bath
   Massage abdomen

Alter Intake—Feed smaller amount and burp frequently
   Use a bottle with a collapsible bag to prevent sucking air
   Breast-feeding mothers: eliminate milk products and spicy or gas-producing foods
   Hold upright for 1/2 hour after feeding

bowel syndrome. Cystic fibrosis, a common cause of malabsorption, is discussed in Chapter 14 ∞.

Celiac Disease

Celiac disease, or gluten-sensitive enteropathy, is a chronic malabsorption syndrome (Nehring, 2004). While it was previously thought to be more prevalent in European countries, recent data show that the prevalence of celiac disease in the general population of the United States is 1 in 133 people, similar to that of those countries in Europe (Hill & Hill, 2005). It is also more common among members of the same family, so a genetic factor may play a role in etiology. It is estimated that 4–17% of children with Down syndrome have celiac disease (Nehring, 2004). Current research is directed at locating the potential genetic abnormalities that occur in celiac disease, and using knowledge of genetics to carry out antibody titer level diagnostic testing (Hoffenberg et al., 2004). Celiac disease is an immunological disorder (Zelnik, Pacht, Obeid, & Lerner, 2004) characterized by an intolerance for gluten, a protein found in wheat, barley, rye, and oats. Inability to digest glutenin and gliadin (protein fractions) results in the accumulation of the amino acid glutamine, which is toxic to mucosal cells in the intestine. Damage to the villi ultimately impairs the absorptive process in the small intestine.

In the early stages, celiac disease affects fat absorption, resulting in excretion of large quantities of fat in the stools (steatorrhea). Stools are greasy, foul smelling, frothy, and excessive. As changes in the villi continue, the absorption of protein, carbohydrates, calcium, iron, folate, and vitamins A, D, E, K, and B_{12} becomes impaired.

Symptoms usually occur when solid foods containing gluten are introduced to the child's diet (in the first 2 years of life), although celiac disease is sometimes first diagnosed in adulthood. The child exhibits chronic diarrhea, vomiting, irritability, malabsorption, abdominal pain, and failure to thrive (Zelnik, Pacht, Obeid, & Lerner, 2004). (Figure 24–17 ➤). If diagnosis is delayed, the child begins to show evidence of protein deficiency (wasted musculature, abdominal distention), delayed dentition, and changes in bone density due to hypocalcemia.

Diagnosis is confirmed through measurement of fecal fat content, jejunal biopsy, and improvement with removal of gluten products from the diet. Serum antigliadin antibody (AGA) and reticulin antibody levels are elevated. IgA antiendomuysial antibodies and IgA antitussue transglutaminase antibodies are commonly used in diagnosis (Murdock & Johnston, 2005).

Symptoms usually improve within a few days to weeks after dietary intervention. The intestinal villi return to normal in about 6 months. Growth should improve steadily, and height and weight should reach normal range within 1 year. Vitamin supplementation may be needed for a time if the child has become malnourished.

Nursing Management

Nursing care focuses on supporting the parents in maintaining a gluten-free diet for the child. Thoroughly explain the disease process to the parents. Emphasize the necessity of following a gluten-free diet (Allen, 2004; Thorn, 2005). Help parents understand that celiac disease requires lifelong dietary modifications that should not be discontinued when the child is symptom free. Discontinuation of the diet places the child at risk for growth retardation and the development of GI cancers in adulthood. All children with celiac disease should be seen by a dietitian several times during childhood. Nutritional assessment and continued teaching to maintain a gluten-free diet take place at these visits. Dietary management is made difficult by hidden gluten in many prepared foods, such as chocolate candy, prepared meats, ice cream, soups, condiments, and food starch.

An infant or toddler's diet is easily monitored at home. When the child enters school, however, ensuring adherence to dietary restrictions becomes more difficult. In addition to easily identified gluten-based foods, such as bread, cake, doughnuts, cookies, and crackers, the child must also avoid processed foods that contain gluten as a

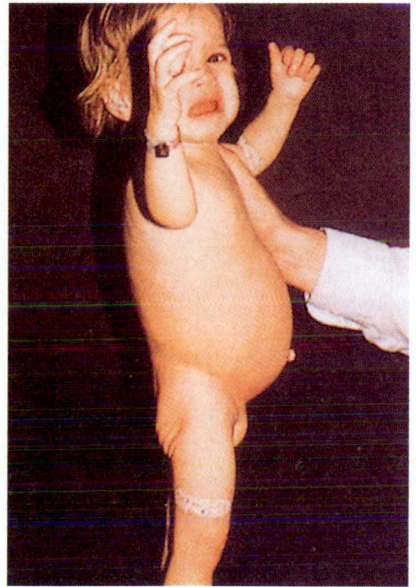

Figure 24–17 ➤ The child with celiac disease commonly shows failure to grow and wasting of extremities. The abdomen can appear large due to intestinal bloating and malnutrition.
Note: From Zitelli, B. J., & Davis, H. W. (Eds.). (2002). *Atlas of pediatric physical diagnosis,* (4th ed., p. 345). St. Louis: Mosby.

filler. School-age children and adolescents are often tempted to eat these foods, especially when among peers. Emphasize the need for compliance while meeting the child's developmental needs.

The child's special dietary needs can place a financial burden on the family. Parents need to purchase prepared rice or corn flour products or make their own bread and bakery products. Advise parents that getting a dietary prescription enables them to deduct the cost of these ingredients and commercially prepared products as a medical expense.

Because the entire family must adapt to the diet, parents and siblings need support and management skills. For information and support, refer parents and children to several organizations, including the American Celiac Society, the Celiac Sprue Association/United States of America, and the Gluten Intolerance Group. Written materials are also available from Children's Memorial Hospital in Chicago.

Expected outcomes of nursing care include:

- Maintenance of normal dietary patterns
- Adequate absorption of essential nutrients as demonstrated by normal growth patterns and absence of deficiency symptoms
- Child and family knowledge of sources of dietary gluten

MediaLink

Celiac Disease Support and Resources

Lactose Intolerance

Lactose intolerance is the inability to digest lactose, a disaccharide found in milk and other dairy products. It results from a congenital or acquired deficiency of the enzyme lactase. Congenital lactase deficiency of infancy is rare. See Chapter 4 ∞ for a general discussion of food intolerance. Abdominal pain, flatulence, and diarrhea occur shortly after birth when the infant is unable to hydrolyze lactose. Lactose intolerance occurs in approximately 70% of African Americans and Native Americans and >90% of Asian Americans (Barnard, 2003). Diarrhea develops rapidly after the child ingests milk and milk products. Some children can tolerate small ingestions of lactose but have symptoms when larger amounts are consumed. Incidence of lactose intolerance increases with advancing age throughout childhood.

Diagnosis is based on a thorough history and a hydrogen breath test, which measures the amount of hydrogen left after fermentation of unabsorbed carbohydrates. A lactose-free diet may eliminate the symptoms, confirming the diagnosis. Treatment for infants includes switching to a soy-based formula. For older children, eliminating lactose-containing foods is recommended. Enzyme tablets such as LactAid can be added to milk or sprinkled on foods to aid digestion.

Nursing Management

Nursing care is primarily supportive. Carefully explain dietary modifications to parents and discuss alternate sources of calcium (see Chapter 4 ∞). Discuss the need for supplementation of calcium and vitamin D to prevent deficiencies. Teach families how to read food labels to find hidden sources of lactose. For example, milk solids may be found in breads, cakes, candies, salad dressings, margarine, and processed food. Suggest lactase tablets for children who want to eat some dairy products.

Short Bowel Syndrome

Short bowel syndrome is a decreased ability to digest and absorb a regular diet because of a shortened intestine. Loss of intestine may result from extensive bowel resection for treatment of necrotizing enterocolitis or inflammatory disorders or from a congenital bowel anomaly such as intestinal malrotation, gastroschisis, or atresia.

The extent and location of the involved bowel determine the severity of the disorder. Because specific types of absorption occur primarily in certain parts of the bowel, the section lost determines which vitamins and other nutrients are inadequate. During the first 3 months after bowel resection, watery diarrhea is common. In the transition period, the remaining bowel usually increases its absorptive surface area and partially compensates for the absent intestine. At first, the infant or young child requires nutritional support to provide sufficient nutrients for growth and development. In the initial period, the child only receives TPN. Once the bowel begins to recover, in addition to TPN, feedings by mouth or by tube may be started in small amounts. Feedings by this method stimulate the bowel and prevent atrophy of the mucosa (Baron & Blaber 2005). It is essential that the child receive the appropriate nutritional components regardless of the method in which nutrition is delivered.

Nursing Management

Nursing care focuses on meeting the child's nutritional and fluid needs and teaching parents how to care for the child at home. Establishing an adequate nutritional intake and bowel pattern is a lengthy process. TPN is provided initially until a feeding regimen can be established. Oral and enteral feedings are instituted gradually to allow the bowel time to compensate. Provide support to the family and child throughout this period. Teach parents how to prepare and administer total parenteral feedings and care for the central line Once enteral or tube feedings are begun, teach management of the feeding pump and care of the feeding tube. Ensure regular bowel function and maintain skin integrity. Arrange home visits to monitor the child's growth and development, care of the central line and tube feeding site, and any side effects such as fluid and electrolyte imbalance and diarrhea.

HEPATIC DISORDERS

The liver is one of the most vital organs in the body. Thus, any inflammatory, obstructive, or degenerative disorder that affects liver function can be life threatening. The following discussion focuses on four common liver disorders in children: hyperbilirubinemia, biliary atresia, viral hepatitis, and cirrhosis.

Hyperbilirubinemia

Newborns have more RBCs per kilogram of weight than adults, and because the lifespan of the RBC is shorter in newborns than adults, they are at risk for producing more bilirubin than their livers are capable of metabolizing (Shaw, 2003). Thus, bilirubin levels are normally high at this age, causing physiologic jaundice. **Hyperbilirubinemia**, an abnormally elevated serum bilirubin level, requires timely assessment and appropriate intervention to prevent central nervous system injury (AAP, 2004).

Etiology and Pathophysiology

Physiologic jaundice occurs in up to 60% of full-term infants and 80% of preterm infants (Askin & Diehl-Jones, 2003). Jaundice is usually visible 2–4 days after birth and lasts until day 6. Peak bilirubin concentration reaches 6–7 mg/dL; however, near-term newborns of 37 weeks' gestation may reach or exceed levels of 13 mg/dL. Preterm infants are more susceptible to the abnormal bilirubin levels of hyperbilirubinemia, with 63% reaching bilirubin levels of 10–19 mg/dL (Shaw, 2003).

Clinical Manifestations

Jaundice in the infant is first evident on the face, and then progresses to the trunk and finally to the extremities. Jaundice may be difficult to see in babies with dark skin color. Symptoms of hyperbilirubinemia include (AAP, 2004):

- Visible jaundice head to toe, including the sclera
- Lethargy or irritability
- Poor breast-feeding or bottle-feeding

> **NURSING ALERT**
>
> The section of the intestine that is resected will determine the vitamin and nutrient deficiencies of the child with short bowel syndrome. When the ileum is resected, bile salts, fluids, and electrolyte absorption decrease so diarrhea can result. Loss of ileum also leads to steatorrhea and fat-soluble vitamins. When the colon is resected, fluid and electrolyte management is impaired. Resection of the jejunum is compensated for effectively by adaptation of the remaining bowel (Jackson & Buchman, 2004).

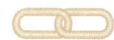

SKILL 12–3
Administering a Gavage/ Tube Feeding

CLINICAL TIP

If phototherapy is already in progress, total serum bilirubin (TSB) should be drawn with the phototherapy lights turned off because phototherapy lights can alter TSB results (Shaw, 2003).

COLLABORATIVE CARE

Diagnostic Tests

A blood test, performed by heelstick or venipuncture, measures total serum bilirubin (TSB) in the newborn. A transcutaneous bilirubin (TcB) measurement device is a noninvasive method for estimating serum bilirubin in infants. This method for measuring bilirubin is generally within 2–3 mg/dL of the total serum bilirubin (TSB) and can be performed instead of the TSB in many cases, especially those infants in which the TSB is less than 15 mg/dL (AAP, 2004).

Clinical Therapy

Phototherapy most effectively reduces serum bilirubin in newborns with physiologic jaundice. The point at which phototherapy is implemented depends on whether or not the infant is full or preterm and how many hours old the infant is at the time the bilirubin rises. The goal of phototherapy is to keep the TSB below the exchange transfusion level (AAP, 2004). The American Academy of Pediatrics provides specific guidelines that clinicians can follow in determining the appropriate treatment (AAP, 2004).

Phototherapy is thought to reduce the amount of indirect, or unconjugated, bilirubin in the baby's bloodstream by promoting excretion via the intestines and kidneys. Phototherapy exposes the infant's skin to blue light at certain wavelengths, which changes bilirubin into water-soluble forms that can be excreted. Phototherapy also facilitates excretion of unconjugated bilirubin through the liver and speeds passage through the bowel (Shaw, 2003). Phototherapy causes bleaching of the skin; therefore, visual assessment and transcutaneous assessment of jaundice are not reliable once treatment has been initiated (AAP, 2004).

Sick term infants and premature, or low-birth-weight, infants should receive phototherapy in an open warmer or incubator to ensure temperature stability (Shaw, 2003). However, a large term infant can be placed nude in an open bassinet during phototherapy (AAP, 2004). The infant receives adequate phototherapy when the fluorescent tubes are placed within approximately 10 cm of the infant's body. However, halogen spotlights cannot be used in this manner due to risk of burns, and manufacturer's recommendations must be followed (AAP, 2004). In most cases, the newborn's diaper can stay in place, which makes it easier to manage increased urine output and loose stools. However, if bilirubin levels are at dangerous levels the diaper should be removed to expose more of the infant's skin surface to the effects of the phototherapy light (AAP, 2004) (Figure 24–18 ➤). The infant will need total serum bilirubin levels

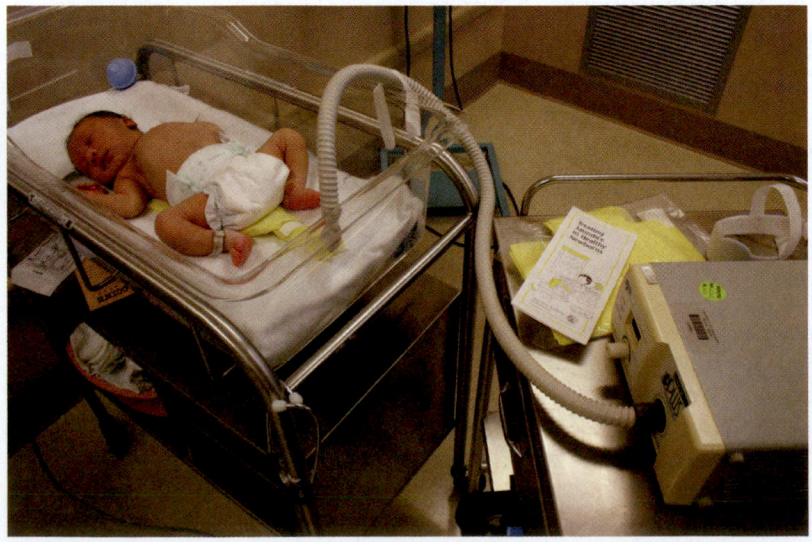
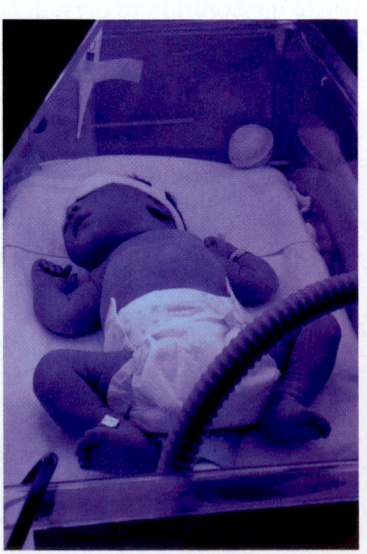

Figure 24–18 ➤ A, Infant receiving phototherapy on a phototherapy blanket. B, Infant receiving phototherapy in an incubator with overhead phototherapy lights. The infant is wearing eye shields.

checked periodically during treatment to evaluate response to treatment and possibly 24 hours after discharge to see if the bilirubin increases after treatment is discontinued (AAP, 2004).

Many newborns with hyperbilirubinemia are also mildly dehydrated. When breast-fed, supplemental fluid intake in the form of milk-based formula may be used to improve hydration and inhibit the enterohepatic circulation of bilirubin. Without evidence of dehydration, intravenous fluid or supplementation with dextrose water is not recommended for term or near-term infants receiving phototherapy (AAP, 2004).

CLINICAL TIP

The infant's eyes are covered during phototherapy to prevent retinal damage, but eye protection should be removed during feeding and interaction with parents and caregivers (AAP, 2004).

NURSING MANAGEMENT

The nurse in the newborn nursery and in the outpatient setting plays a critical role in identifying the newborn at risk and providing parent education related to hyperbilirubinemia. While the nurse in the newborn nursery may be providing care to an infant for a few days after birth, many infants are discharged home within 24 hours. The infant may be evaluated for jaundice in the outpatient setting and then admitted to the pediatric unit for treatment. Nurses working in acute care settings must familiarize themselves with the care of very young infants who require treatment for hyperbilirubinemia.

Nursing Assessment and Diagnosis

The newborn should be assessed for jaundice at least every 8–12 hours by using digital pressure to blanche the skin. Adequate lighting should be used (Blackwell, 2003). If the nurse suspects the presence of jaundice, the infant's primary care provider should be notified. A TcB (transcutaneous bilirubin) measurement or TSB (total serum bilirubin) level is indicated (Holcomb, 2005).

Feeding Assessment

The mother who is breast-feeding should nurse her infant at least 8–12 times per day for the first several days (Holcomb, 2005). The nurse should be alert to mothers and infants who are having difficulty and require lactation support during the hospital stay and following discharge.

The infant who is breast-fed should have 4–6 very wet diapers and 3–4 stools per day by the fourth day of life. Meconium stool should have transitioned to mushy, mustard-colored yellow stools by day 3 to 4 (AAP, 2004). If these parameters are not met, the infant may be at risk for dehydration due to inadequate intake, thus increasing the risk of hyperbilirubinemia (AAP, 2004). Because many mothers and term newborns are discharged within 24 hours after birth, this is important information to teach parents prior to discharge.

Nursing Diagnoses

Nursing diagnoses that may apply to the newborn with hyperbilirubinemia may include:

- Deficient Fluid Volume related to decreased oral intake and ineffective breast-feeding
- Risk for Impaired Parent/Newborn Attachment related to disruption of parental/newborn interaction due to hospitalization and treatment
- Risk for Imbalanced Body Temperature related to phototherapy
- Risk for Injury related to phototherapy
- Risk for Neurological Impairment related to hyperbilirubinemia

Planning and Implementation

The role of the nurse is to identify the newborn at risk for hyperbilirubinemia, educate parents about newborn jaundice, and care for the newborn and family undergoing treatment for this condition. For the infant undergoing phototherapy, the nurse should monitor the infant frequently, ensuring that the infant is receiving the phototherapy properly. Vital signs should be assessed every 4–8 hours, especially the infant's temperature, which might indicate signs of infection or signs of hypothermia in an infant

NURSING ALERT

In cases of severe and untreated hyperbilirubinemia, bilirubin encephalopathy can cause serious neurological sequelae. The term *acute bilirubin encephalopathy* is used to describe the acute effects of bilirubin toxicity in the first weeks of life. The term *kernicterus* is used when referring to chronic and permanent brain damage related to bilirubin toxicity (Holcomb, 2005).

whose clothing is removed for phototherapy. An accurate measurement of intake and output is essential to make sure the infant is not dehydrated. Assist the family in breast- or bottle-feeding as appropriate.

Care in the Community

Problems with breast-feeding in the first week of life can contribute to low caloric intake, dehydration, and subsequent risk of neonatal hyperbilirubinemia (AAP, 2004). The nurse plays a critical role in assessing adequacy of breast-feeding prior to hospital discharge and coordinating with the newborn's care provider in making appropriate referrals to lactation specialists and support groups in the community when necessary.

For term infants who develop uncomplicated hyperbilirubinemia, home phototherapy may be appropriate (AAP, 2004). Serum bilirubin levels must be monitored regularly at the physician's office, neighborhood laboratory, or by the home healthcare worker. A visiting or home healthcare nurse often visits the family to establish the phototherapy and inform parents about the care needed. The nurse partners with other professionals such as staff from a medical supply company to service equipment, lactation specialist, and pediatrician to coordinate services.

Evaluation

Expected outcomes of nursing interventions include:

- The term or near-term newborn at risk for hyperbilirubinemia is identified prior to discharge and receives appropriate and timely follow-up.
- The infant's parents understand the basics of newborn jaundice and know who and when to call if they suspect development of hyperbilirubinemia.
- The infant receives appropriate and timely intervention if hyperbilirubinemia occurs.
- The infant's nutritional and fluid intake are adequate to meet growth and development requirements.
- The infant does not develop neurological sequelae as a result of hyperbilirubinemia.

Biliary Atresia

Biliary atresia results when the extrahepatic bile ducts fail to develop or are closed (Askin & Diehl-Jones, 2003; Bezerra, 2005). The disorder leads to cholestasis, fibrosis, and cirrhosis (Kelly, 2002). Biliary atresia is the most common cause of pathologic jaundice in infants and is the leading indication for pediatric liver transplantation (Bezerra, 2005).

Initially the newborn is asymptomatic. Jaundice may not be detected until 2 to 3 weeks after birth. At that point bilirubin levels increase, accompanied by abdominal distention and hepatomegaly. As the disease progresses, splenomegaly occurs. The infant experiences easy bruising, prolonged bleeding time, and intense itching. Stools have puttylike consistency and are white or clay colored because of the absence of bile pigments. Excretion of bilirubin and bile salts results in tea-colored urine. Failure to thrive and malnutrition occur as the destructive changes of the disease progress.

The cause of biliary atresia is unknown. Absence or blockage of the extrahepatic bile ducts results in blocked bile flow from the liver to the duodenum. This altered bile flow soon causes inflammation and fibrotic changes in the liver. In addition to blockage, the disease can also be caused by hepatocellular dysfunction. Lack of bile acids also interferes with digestion of fat and absorption of fat-soluble vitamins A, D, E, and K, resulting in steatorrhea and nutritional deficiencies. Without treatment the disease is fatal.

Diagnosis is based on the history, physical examination, and laboratory evaluation. Laboratory findings reveal elevated bilirubin levels, elevated serum aminotransferase and alkaline phosphatase values, prolonged prothrombin time, and increased ammonia levels. Ultrasound rules out other causes, and a liver biopsy is performed. Because liver damage develops rapidly in infants with biliary atresia, early diagnosis is essential.

Treatment involves surgery to attempt correction of the obstruction (hepato-portoenterostomy) and supportive care. In the hepatoportoenterostomy (Kasai procedure), a segment of the intestine is anastomosed to the porta hepatis. In most children this is a palliative treatment to promote bile drainage, maintain as much hepatic function as possible, and prevent the complications of liver failure. Supportive treatment is directed at managing the bleeding tendencies by administering oral vitamin K; preventing rickets through vitamin D supplementation; controlling itching and irritability with cholestyramine and antihistamines; and promoting adequate nutrition. Low dose oral antibiotics are administered to prevent cholangitis (Kelly, 2002). The 5-year survival rate following the Kasai procedure is 35–50% (Askin & Diehl-Jones, 2003).

Although the Kasai procedure improves the prognosis, complications of liver disease continue to develop; liver transplantation is eventually needed. Donor shortage is the major factor limiting the use of liver transplantation (Tran, Nissen, Poordad, & Martin, 2004). Advances in transplantation surgery now make it possible to perform partial liver transplants from living donor resections. This enables transplantation to be performed when the child is in optimal health, rather than waiting until an appropriate-size cadaver liver is available, and allows for donations from close family members who are often good tissue matches. The 1-year survival rate for pediatric liver transplant has improved to 85% (Carroll, Goodman, Superina, Whitington, & Alonso, 2003).

Nursing Management

Nursing care in the initial stages of biliary atresia is the same as that for any healthy newborn. As symptoms develop, the focus of nursing care becomes long-term management and support.

Diagnosis of this potentially fatal disorder can be devastating to parents. Provide emotional support and offer frequent explanations of tests during the initial diagnostic evaluation. As the disease progresses, the infant becomes irritable because of intense itching and the accumulation of toxins. Tepid baths may help to relieve itching and provide comfort. Dry skin by patting rather than rubbing to avoid further skin irritation. Promote rest by grouping nursing activities while the infant is awake. Care following a hepatoportoenterostomy is similar to that for a child undergoing abdominal surgery. (See the earlier discussion of postsurgical nursing management for appendicitis and Nursing Care Plan: The Child Undergoing Surgery in Chapter 13 ∞). Posttransplant care includes immunosuppressant drugs and close monitoring for vascular complications. Refer to Chapter 17 ∞.

Discharge planning focuses on teaching parents how to care for the child's skin, providing for nutritional needs, administering medications, and monitoring for increasing symptoms of liver disease. When the child has received a transplant, teach parents how to identify signs of rejection (nausea, vomiting, fever, and jaundice), as well as the administration and side effects of immunosuppressant medications. Refer parents to support groups, clergy, or social services if indicated. They will need ongoing visits from a home healthcare nurse to help them manage the child's complex care. The main expected outcomes of nursing care are the parent's ability to cope with the child's health status and to provide the necessary care. The child is expected to function at maximum potential considering the extent of disease. Palliative care may need to be discussed with the family if it becomes evident the child will not survive. See Chapter 15 ∞.

Viral Hepatitis

Hepatitis is an inflammation of the liver caused by a viral infection (Figure 24–19 ➤). It may be acute or chronic. Acute hepatitis is rapid in onset and if untreated may

PATHOPHYSIOLOGY ILLUSTRATED

Viral Hepatitis

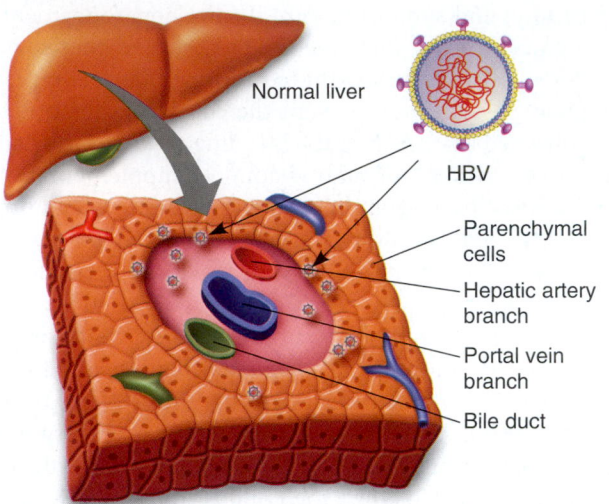

Normal liver

HBV

Parenchymal cells

Hepatic artery branch

Portal vein branch

Bile duct

① Virus invades parenchymal cells, causing local degeneration and necrosis

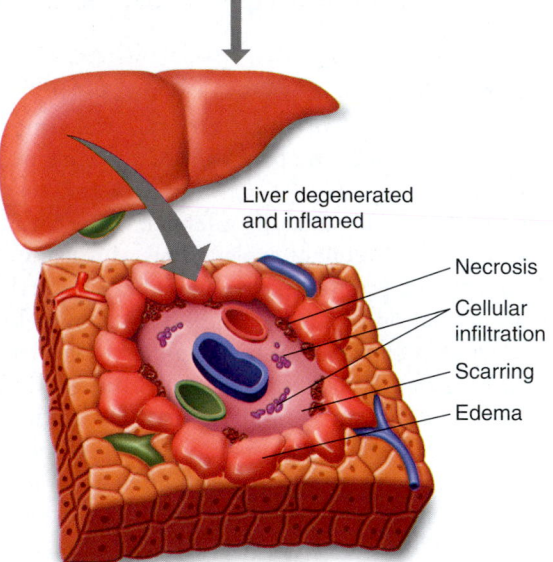

Liver degenerated and inflamed

Necrosis

Cellular infiltration

Scarring

Edema

② Infiltration by lymphocytes, macrophages, and other white blood cells causes inflammation that blocks drainage

③ Structural changes occur in parenchymal cells, resulting in altered liver function:

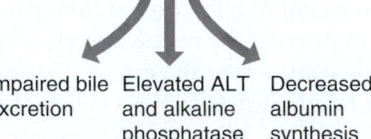

Impaired bile excretion

Elevated ALT and alkaline phosphatase levels

Decreased albumin synthesis

Figure 24–19 ▶ The hepatitis virus causes degeneration and necrosis of the liver, which results in abnormal liver function and illness.

develop into chronic hepatitis. The most frequently diagnosed causative organisms are hepatitis A virus (HAV), hepatitis B virus (HBV), hepatitis C virus (HCV), hepatitis D virus (HDV), and hepatitis E virus (HEV). Other types of non-A, non-B have been identified, such as hepatitis G. An estimated 136,000 cases of hepatitis occur annually in the United States, and one third of these are in children. Most cases are types A and B. See Table 24–4.

Etiology and Pathophysiology

Hepatitis A is the most common form of acute viral hepatitis. It is highly contagious and traditionally has been called infectious hepatitis. Infection occurs primarily through the fecal-oral route. Transmission is by direct person-to-person spread or through ingestion of contaminated water or food (particularly shellfish). Hepatitis A frequently occurs in children in childcare settings where hygiene practices are poor. Food handlers can spread hepatitis A if not aware of their infection; it is a common cause of foodborne illness. The virus can live on surfaces for 1 month. Because the virus is transmitted in the early stages of the disease when individuals are often asymptomatic or only mildly ill, large numbers of people may be exposed before the diagnosis is confirmed (see Table 24–4). Most children recover from hepatitis A; however, in rare instances end-stage liver disease can develop (Snyder & Pickering, 2004).

Hepatitis B, known traditionally as serum hepatitis, is a serious disease. Transmission is usually by the parenteral route through the exchange of blood or any body secretion or fluid. Other common transmission routes include sexual activity and transmission from mother to fetus in utero. Adolescents who use intravenous drugs and have unprotected sexual intercourse are at risk for contracting hepatitis B. Major sources for the spread of HBV are healthy chronic carriers. All body fluids of infected individuals are potentially contaminated with the virus.

The hepatitis C virus is transmitted primarily through blood and blood products, and blood banks now test for this virus. Infected children have commonly had repeated transfusions (as in sickle cell disease or hemophilia). Intravenous drug use, body piercing, and multiple sexual partners are also risk factors. Infected mothers may infect their children during birth (CDC, 2005).

Hepatitis D (delta virus) is a defective virus that can gain entry to a human only in connection with hepatitis B. This virus is suspected when someone diagnosed with hepatitis B has diminishing liver function, increasing jaundice, and deteriorating mental status.

Table 24–4	COMPARISON OF HEPATITIS TYPES			
Type	**Immunization Available**	**Prophylaxis**	**Primary Transmission**	**Incubation Period**
Hepatitis A	Yes	Immune globulin Hepatitis A vaccine	Fecal-oral	1 month
Hepatitis B	Yes	Hepatit's B immune globulin Hepatitis B vaccine	Needlesticks or sharps exposure Intravenous drug use During birth Sexual activity	100–120 days
Hepatitis C	No	None	Needlesticks or sharps exposure Intravenous drug use During birth	7–9 weeks
Hepatitis D	No	Hepatitis B vaccine	Needlesticks or sharps exposure Intravenous drug use During birth Sexual activity	2–4 months
Hepatitis E	No	None	Fecal oral	40 days

Adapted from: http://www.cdc.gov/hepatitis (2005); Snyder, J. D., & Pickering, L. K. (2004). Viral hepatitis. In R. E. Behrman, R. M. Kliegman, & H. B. Jenson (Eds.), *Nelson textbook of pediatrics* (17th ed., pp. 1324–1331). Philadelphia: Saunders.

Hepatitis E infection is primarily transmitted through contaminated water and is most common in developing countries. Outbreaks may occur in flooding and rainy seasons. A related infection transferred primarily through blood transfusion is hepatitis G (Snyder & Pickering, 2004).

The liver's response to injury by the viruses that cause hepatitis is similar (see Pathophysiology Illustrated: Viral Hepatitis). Initially, invasion of the parenchymal cells by the virus results in local degeneration and necrosis. Subsequent infiltration of the parenchyma by lymphocytes, macrophages, plasma cells, eosinophils, and neutrophils causes inflammation that blocks biliary drainage into the intestine. Impaired bile excretion causes a buildup of bile in the blood, urine, and skin (jaundice). Structural changes in the parenchymal cells account for other altered liver functions. Regeneration of parenchymal cells occurs within 3 months, and most children completely recover.

In some children, however, a progressive and total destruction of the hepatic parenchyma known as acute fulminating hepatitis develops. Children with this form of the disease usually die of liver failure within 2 weeks of onset unless they receive a liver transplant. Another complication, chronic active hepatitis, may lead to scarring of the liver and progressive deterioration of liver function. The prognosis depends on the degree of liver involvement. In some people, especially those who develop chronic hepatitis, liver cancers and cirrhosis can develop.

Clinical Manifestations

Acute hepatitis infection is characterized by two phases, the anicteric (absence of jaundice) phase and the icteric (jaundice) phase. The anicteric phase usually lasts 5 to 7 days. Signs and symptoms include nausea, vomiting, anorexia, malaise, fatigue, right upper quadrant pain, hepatosplenomegaly, and fever. The child becomes irritable, looks ill, and requires rest. In the icteric phase, signs and symptoms include darkening of urine, clay-colored stools, and the characteristic yellowing of the skin and sclera. However, many children with hepatitis do not have jaundice, leading to difficulty in disease diagnosis and management. As the jaundice worsens, the child begins to feel better. This phase lasts approximately 4 weeks. Complete recovery with return of normal liver function and laboratory values may take 1 to 3 months.

In some cases, hepatitis becomes chronic. A person with chronic hepatitis carries the virus, can transfer it to others, and may develop serious liver disease after several years.

■ COLLABORATIVE CARE

Diagnosis is often made on the basis of a thorough history and physical examination. A history of exposure to persons with the disease is significant. Physical examination reveals a tender, enlarged liver, abdominal pain, and flulike symptoms. Laboratory evaluation includes serologic testing (to detect the presence of antigens and antibodies to HAV, HBV, HCV, or HDV) and liver function studies.

The three goals of medical management are early detection to prevent complications, support and monitoring during the acute phase of the disease, and prevention of the spread of the disease. Early diagnosis is essential to follow the course of the illness and identify potential complications. Management includes bed rest during the flulike phase. If prothrombin times are increased, vitamin K is administered.

The spread of viral infections can be interrupted by elimination of the virus from the infected population, institution of proper hygiene, and passive or active immunization. To date, no antiviral agent has been developed to combat the hepatitis viruses. Prevention depends on breaking the cycle of infection. Active immunization for hepatitis A, a two-dose series, is recommended for all people at risk of acquiring and transmitting the disease and for children and childcare workers in certain states with endemic disease (see Chapter 18 ∞). People at risk include childcare staff and food handlers. Since childhood vaccination in high-risk areas was recommended, the overall hepatitis A rate has declined steadily, and in 2002, it was the lowest yet recorded (3.1/100,000) (Centers for Disease Control and Prevention (CDC), 2004). The CDC now recommends that all children receive the hepatitis A vaccine at 1 year of age (CDC, 2006a).

Immunization for hepatitis B, a three-dose series, is recommended for all children and at-risk adults. The first dose is given within 12 hours of birth to the infant born of an infected mother (refer to the discussion of immunization in Chapter 18 ∞). A total of 7996 acute hepatitis B cases in the United States were reported in 2002, representing more than a 65% decrease since 1990 (21,102 cases). This decline in hepatitis B rates coincides with the implementation of a national strategy to achieve the elimination of hepatitis B virus (HBV) infection. The rate among children aged ≤18 years, the age group covered by the recommendation for routine childhood immunization, has declined by approximately 90% since 1990 (CDC, 2004).

Passive immunity to HAV can be achieved with standard pooled immune globulin. It must be administered within 2 weeks of exposure. Passive immunity to HBV can be achieved with hepatitis B immune globulin (HBIG). Used for one-time exposure and for infants of infected mothers, it is given within 12 hours of birth.

NURSING MANAGEMENT

Nursing Assessment and Diagnosis

The nurse usually encounters the child and family in an outpatient setting. In addition to observing the child for characteristic signs of hepatitis (jaundiced skin and sclera), assess for abdominal pain, anorexia, nausea and vomiting, malaise, and arthralgia. Also get a history of the child's contacts over the past 45 days for HAV and up to 180 days for HBV. For an infant, the hepatitis history of the mother and other family members is important.

Common nursing diagnoses for the child with acute hepatitis might include:

- Risk for Imbalanced Nutrition: Less than Body Requirements related to anorexia, nausea and vomiting
- Fatigue related to disease state
- Risk for Deficient Diversional Activity related to malaise and forced inactivity
- Risk for Body Image Disturbance (Older Child) related to jaundice
- Anxiety (Parent and Child) related to threat to health status
- Pain related to liver injury

Planning and Implementation

Nursing care involves home and community considerations, as children are seldom admitted to the hospital for hepatitis treatment. The hospitalized child is placed in isolation. Prevention of the disease is integrated into all health care by discussion of immunization and standard precautions. When hepatitis cases have occurred in the family or community, parents need additional detailed information about health precautions and infection-control measures. In addition, teach parents the importance of checking with health professionals before administering any medications (even nonprescription medicines), maintaining adequate nutrition, promoting rest and comfort, and providing diversional activities.

Prevent Spread of Infection

Teach the parents and the child infection-control measures to help prevent transmission of the virus. For parents, reinforce good hygiene practices, such as washing hands before and after toileting and proper disposal of soiled diapers. Siblings of a child with hepatitis B who have not already been immunized with the hepatitis B vaccine should be vaccinated immediately. Contacts of the child with hepatitis A should receive immune serum globulin and the first immunization in the hepatitis A series. Rifampin may be given in some cases. All health providers should receive the hepatitis B immunization series and use standard precautions at all times with everyone in health care.

Maintain Adequate Nutrition

Initially, encourage the child to eat favorite foods. Once the anorexia and nausea have resolved, a high-protein, high-carbohydrate, low-fat diet is recommended. Increased

CLINICAL TIP

Nurses in childcare centers can provide assessment of the center's procedures and teaching to prevent hepatitis A transmission. Help the center to set standards about:

- Handwashing after each diaper change
- Proper disposal of diapers
- Cleaning diaper-changing surfaces after each diaper change
- Never having food handlers perform diaper changes
- Instructing parents to keep children at home for at least 2 weeks after a diagnosis of hepatitis A
- Informing parents of other children when there is a case of hepatitis A and teaching them the symptoms of the condition

protein helps maintain protein stores and prevent muscle wasting. Increased carbohydrates ensure adequate caloric intake and prevent protein depletion. Low-fat foods lessen stomach distention. Offer the child small, frequent feedings.

Promote Rest and Comfort

Bed rest is necessary only if the child has severe fatigue and malaise. However, most children voluntarily limit their activities during the initial phase of the disease. Keep the child quiet and comfortable. Offer comfort items such as favorite toys, blankets, and pillows.

Provide Diversional Activities

Hospitalized children with hepatitis are kept in isolation. Nonhospitalized children with hepatitis do not need to be isolated, but they should be kept at home for 2 weeks following the onset of symptoms. Parents who cannot take time off from work may need to arrange home sitters to stay with the child. Offer suggestions for diversional activities during this period. Young children can be given a new toy or favorite activities. Older children and adolescents can be given board games, puzzles, books or magazines, movies, or video games. Phone calls and short visits from friends help school-age children and adolescents maintain contact with peers.

Evaluation

Expected outcomes of nursing care for hepatitis include the following:

- New cases of hepatitis are prevented.
- The child will have normal liver function.
- Normal growth and development are achieved.
- Effective pain management will be achieved.
- The child will not develop chronic liver disease.

Cirrhosis

Cirrhosis is a degenerative disease process that results in fibrotic changes and fatty infiltration in the liver. It can occur in children of any age as the end stage of several disorders, including biliary atresia (Kelly, 2002). The diffuse destruction and regeneration of the hepatic parenchymal cells result in an increase in fibrous connective tissue and disorganization of the liver structure. The balance between destruction and regeneration determines the specific clinical presentation.

Clinical manifestations of cirrhosis vary. When the disease process results from obstruction, as in biliary atresia, jaundice is an initial sign that intensifies with progression of the disease. In other diseases that cause cirrhosis, jaundice may be a late sign, intermittent, or absent. Anemia can occur as a result of chronic blood loss from the GI tract. Pruritus is common, particularly in children with biliary malformations. Clubbing of the digits and cyanosis are other common findings. Severe end-stage complications signaling hepatic failure can occur at any time and with little warning. Diagnostic evaluation is based on the child's history of infection or disease with liver involvement. Physical examination may reveal jaundice, skin changes, ascites, and hemodynamic changes. Laboratory evaluation reveals abnormal liver function tests. A liver biopsy may help determine the extent of the parenchymal damage.

Medical management focuses on treating the child's symptoms and achieving optimal nutritional status and growth. See the clinical manifestations table on the next page for a summary of treatment. Liver transplantation is the most common treatment for biliary atresia and metabolic disorders and is the only treatment for end-stage liver disease.

Nursing Management

Nursing care focuses on monitoring physiologic and psychosocial changes to identify early signs of end-stage hepatic failure. Monitor vital signs every 2 to 4 hours. Measure weight daily to assess for fluid retention. Close monitoring of electrolytes and liver function test results helps determine the need for fluid replacement therapy.

CLINICAL MANIFESTATIONS	CIRRHOSIS COMPLICATIONS	

Etiology	Clinical Manifestations	Clinical Therapy
Fluid and electrolyte imbalance	Ascites	Restrict sodium, protein, and fluids. Administer diuretics (e.g., furosemide [Lasix]). Administer intravenous albumin.
Liver dysfunction	Hepatic encephalopathy	Restrict protein. Administer lactulose to control increased ammonia levels. Administer antibiotics. Correct any imbalances that can lead to coma (fluid and electrolyte imbalance).
Esophageal varices	Hemorrhage	Administer blood and blood products. Replace fluid and electrolytes. Administer vitamin B complex and vitamin K. Insert Sengstaken-Blakemore tube in cases of severe bleeding.

Careful administration of medications and monitoring for side effects are necessary because drug metabolism is altered in liver disorders. If ascites is present, provide a low-sodium, low-protein diet and restrict fluids. Remove all water pitchers, glasses, and straws to minimize the child's desire to drink.

Parents of a child with cirrhosis are coping with a life-threatening disorder, and their anxiety and stress are high. The child may be awaiting a liver transplantation that represents the only hope for recovery. Support parents and encourage them to talk about their fears and concerns (see Chapter 14 ∞). Encourage parents to participate in the child's care. Referral to a support group or counseling may be beneficial. See Chapter 15 ∞ for discussion on palliative care.

INJURIES TO THE GASTROINTESTINAL SYSTEM
Abdominal Trauma

The majority of abdominal injuries are caused by blunt trauma (85%) with penetrating trauma accounting for the remainder. Approximately 50% of abdominal injury in children is related to blunt trauma from a motor vehicle accident (Simone, 2003). In addition, ATV (all-terrain vehicle) injuries are increasing in the United States as the popularity of these devices increases (Brandenberg, 2004). The child may suffer severe abdominal trauma, including injury to the spleen and liver. Child abuse involving kicking or punching the abdomen is another major cause of blunt abdominal trauma. Penetrating trauma occurs due to impalement on an object, stabbing, or gunshot wounds. Children are more likely to have abdominal injuries because of the smaller amount of subcutaneous tissue surrounding organs, less developed abdominal muscle tone, and proportionately larger solid organs than in adults (Simone, 2003).

The kind of injury determines the extent of organ damage. High-velocity blunt trauma, which may occur in motor vehicle crashes, usually involves multiple organs. Solid organs such as the liver and spleen can be bruised or lacerated. The sudden increase in abdominal pressure that occurs with a lapbelt injury causes hollow organs such as the stomach, intestines, and bladder to burst. Sports-related abdominal trauma is often associated with a direct blow to the abdomen and a single organ is usually injured. Bicycle crashes can result in abdominal injury if the handlebars hit the child in the abdomen (Simone, 2003).

Clinical manifestations of abdominal injury include pain, abdominal distention, muscle guarding, decreased or absent bowel sounds, nausea and vomiting, hypotension, and shock. The external abdomen and back may have penetrating wounds, abrasions, bruising, or markings (e.g., tire tracks or lapbelt marks) that provide a clue to injury beneath the skin surface. Ecchymosis and contusions in the lower abdominal area are classic visible signs of seatbelt trauma (Eckert, 2005). See Chapter 5 ∞ for techniques of abdominal assessment.

The injured child is rapidly assessed for airway, breathing, and circulation, and is stabilized before examination of the abdomen is performed. An IV line is inserted for fluid management. A nasogastric tube is inserted to decompress the stomach and to detect the presence of blood. Plain abdominal radiographs may reveal air in the abdomen. An ultrasound can reveal free fluid in the abdomen. A CT scan assesses multiple organs for injury and for the presence of free fluid in the abdomen. A rectal examination is performed to assess the bowel wall and to detect rectal bleeding. Baseline laboratory studies, including complete blood count, coagulation tests, blood type, and cross-match, are done. In addition, electrolytes and enzyme studies to detect liver, spleen, and pancreas injuries are obtained (Simone, 2003).

Treatment of a liver or spleen injury takes place in the ICU and focuses on monitoring the child's physical status for hypovolemic shock, maintaining adequate fluid volume with IV fluids or blood products, and allowing the solid organ to heal without surgery in most cases. Pain management with opioids is initiated. Serial hematocrit levels are monitored to detect hemorrhage during this period. Parenteral or enteral nutrition may be initiated within 24 to 48 hours after admission to prevent infection and promote wound healing (Simone, 2003).

Exploratory laparotomy is performed to resect hollow organ injuries or to repair liver or spleen lacerations when bleeding is not controlled. The spleen is salvaged whenever possible to help maintain immune function (Potoka & Saladino, 2005). The child is maintained on strict bedrest until bleeding is controlled and the child has not required blood transfusions for at least 2 days. The child is usually kept in the hospital for 5 to 7 days to monitor for symptoms of bleeding (Simone, 2003). No strenuous activity is allowed for 6 to 8 weeks. The prognosis is generally good.

Nursing Management

Nursing care includes initial and ongoing assessments of the child's condition. Monitor vital signs every hour as warranted. Tachycardia and hypotension may indicate hypovolemia or internal bleeding. Strict monitoring of intake and output will give information to the child's fluid status. The child should have a Foley catheter in place for accurate output measurement unless a uretheral injury is suspected (Simone, 2003). Monitor the respiratory status as abdominal injuries may also have thoracic involvement. Abdominal distention, immobility, and pain may all affect the child's ability to take deep breaths (Simone, 2003). Additional nursing care includes maintenance of the nasogastric tube, administration of antibiotics and intravenous fluids, and monitoring of lab studies as appropriate (Simone, 2003). Any concerns should be reported to the physician immediately.

The child and parents are usually fearful and anxious when the child is admitted with a serious injury. If the injury was preventable, parents may have feelings of guilt or anger. Provide emotional support and avoid judgmental comments or statements that assign blame. With a child on strict bedrest, providing diversional activities is essential once the child is feeling better.

When the child's condition is stabilized, the focus of nursing care shifts to preventive teaching. Parents should be taught safety measures to prevent future injuries. Discuss the use of car safety restraint devices for riding in an automobile (see Chapters 8–10 ∞). If the child's injury was the result of a bicycle fall or crash, discuss the importance of the proper bicycle size and safety measures such as use of a helmet and proper use of hand signals.

Refer to Chapter 6 ∞ for information related to injury to the GI system due to poisoning and ingestion of foreign objects.

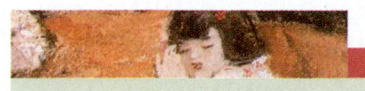

CRITICAL THINKING IN ACTION

POSTOPERATIVE APPENDECTOMY

Recall Jason from the chapter opening scenario, a 3-year-old who has just been admitted to the pediatric unit after surgery for a ruptured appendix. Jason is groggy from the anesthesia, but is scared. He complains of "tummy" pain and wants the tubes "out now." He cries as the nurse approaches to perform an initial assessment.

1. Why was Jason at increased risk for ruptured appendix compared to a school-age child?

2. What are the priorities of postoperative nursing care for Jason?

3. Considering Jason's developmental age, how can the nurse help Jason adapt to the hospitalization experience? (Refer to Chapter 13).

4. What interventions are most appropriate with a 3-year-old to decrease the risk of pulmonary complications associated with surgery?

Refer to your Prentice Hall Nursing MediaLink DVD-ROM for answers.

EXPLORE MediaLink

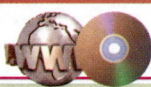   http://www.prenhall.com/ball

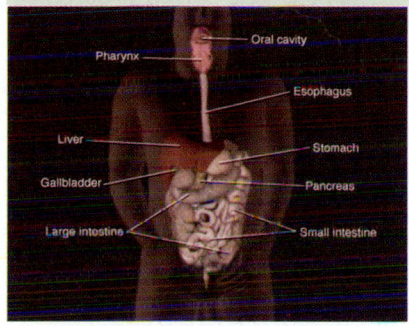

Resources for this chapter can be found on the Prentice Hall Nursing MediaLink DVD-ROM accompanying this textbook, and on the Companion Website at http://www.prenhall.com/ball.

DVD-ROM
NCLEX-RN® Review
Audio Glossary
Animations/Videos
  Appendicitis
  Digestive System

COMPANION WEBSITE
Audio Glossary
NCLEX-RN® Review
Care Plan Activity: Managing Emesis in Pediatric Conditions
Case Study: The Child with a Cleft Palate
MediaLink Application: Teaching Plan for Foreign Travel
WebLinks

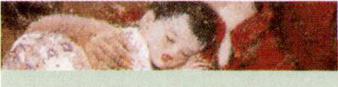

REFERENCES

Aiken, J. J., & Oldham, K. T. (2005). Malrotation. In K. W. Ashcraft, G. W. Holcomb, & J. P. Murphy (Eds.), *Pediatric surgery* (4th ed., pp. 435–447). Philadephia: Saunders.

Allen, P. L. J. (2004). Guidelines for the diagnosis and treatment of celiac disease in children. *Pediatric Nursing, 30*(6), 473–476.

American Academy of Pediatrics. (2004). Management of hyperbilirubinemia in the newborn infant 35 or more weeks of gestation. *Pediatrics, 114*(1), 297–316.

Arguin, A. L., & Swartz, M. K. (2004). Gastroesophageal reflux in infants: A primary care perspective. *Pediatric Nursing, 30,* 45–52.

Ashburn, D. A., Pranikoff, T., & Turner, C. S. (2002). Unusual presentations of gastroschisis. *The American Surgeon, 68,* 724–727.

Askin, D. F., & Diehl-Jones, W. L. (2003). The neonatal liver part III: Pathophysiology of liver dysfunction. *Neonatal Network, 22*(3), 5–15.

Azizkhan, R. G., & Frykman, P. K. (2003). Abdominal wall defects. In C. D. Rudolph, & A. M. Rudolph (Eds), *Rudolph's pediatrics* (21st ed., pp. 1399–1400). New York: McGraw Hill.

Bagolan, P., Casaccia, G., Crescenzi, F., Nahom, A., Trucchi, A., & Giorlandino, C. (2004). Impact of a current treatment protocol on outcome of high-risk congenital diaphragmatic hernia. *Journal of Pediatric Surgery, 39,* 313–318.

Baron, M. L. (2002). Crohn disease in children. *American Journal of Nursing, 102*(10), 26–34.

Baron, M., & Blaber, M. E. (2005). Short-bowel syndrome in children. *American Journal of Nursing, 105*(9), 72C–72H.

Barnard, N. D. (2003). The milk debate goes on and on and on! *Pediatrics, 112,* 448.

Bell, E. F. (2005). Preventing necrotizing enterocolitis: What works and how safe? *Pediatrics, 115,* 173–175.

Bezerra, J. A. (2005). Potential etiologies of biliary atresia. *Pediatric Transplantation, 9,* 646–651.

Biggs, W. S & Dery W. H, (2006). Evaluation and treatment of constipation in infants and children. *American Family Physician, 73*(3), 469–477.

Bindler, R. M., & Howry, L. B. (2005). *Pedirtic drugs & nursing implications* (3rd ed.). Upper Saddle River, NJ: Prentice Hall Health.

Black, T. L. (2005). Congenital megacolon. In M. R., Dambro & J. A., Griffith (Eds.), *Griffith's 5-minute clinical consult* (13th ed., p. 260). Philadelphia: Lippincott, Williams, & Wilkins.

Blackwell, J. T. (2003). Management of hyperbilirubinemia in the healthy term newborn. *Journal of the American Academy of Nurse Practitioners, 15*(5), 194–198.

Blum, J., Taubman, B., & Nemeth, N. (2004). During toilet training, constipation occurs before stool toileting refusal. *Pediatrics, 113,* 1791–1792.

Blumer, S. L., Zucconi, W. B., Cohen, H. L., Scriven, R. J., & Lee, T. K. (2004). The vomiting neonate: A review of the ACR appropriateness criteria and ultrasound's role in the workup of such patients. *Ultrasound Quarterly, 20*(3), 79–89.

Borkowski, S. (2005,). Clinical challenge. Case 1. Irritation, redness, and drainage at the site of a pediatric gastrostomy. *The Clinical Advisor for Nurse Practitioners, 8*(5).

Brandenberg, M. A. (2004). All-terrain vehicle injuries: A growing epidemic. *Annals of Emergency Medicine, 43*(4), 536–537.

Brown R. L., & Stevenson, R. J. (2003). Congenital anomalies of the stomach and intestine. In C. D. Rudolph, & A. M. Rudolph (Eds.), *Rudolph's pediatrics* (21st ed., pp. 1405–1407). New York: McGraw Hill.

Bullard, J., & Page, N. E. (2005). Cyclic vomiting syndrome: A disease in disguise. *Journal of Pediatric Nursing, 31*, 27–29.

Burd, A., & Burd, R. S. (2003). The who, what, why and how-to guide for gastrostomy tube placement in infants. *Advances in Neonatal Care, 3*, 197–205.

Carroll, C. L., Goodman, D. M., Superina, R. A., Whitington, P. F., & Alonso, E. M. (2003). Timed pediatric risk of mortality scores predict outcomes in pediatric liver transplant recipients. *Pediatric Transplantation, 7*, 289–295.

Centers for Disease Control and Prevention. (2004). Summary of notifiable diseases, 2002. *MMWR, 51*, 1–84. http://www.cdc.gov.mmwr/preview/mmwrhtml/mm5153a1.htm

Centers for Disease Control and Prevention. (2005). Hepatitis C fact sheet. Retrieved October 16, 2005, from http://www.cdc.gov/hepatitis

Centers for Disease Control and Prevention. (2006a). Prevention of hepatitis A through active or passive immunization. *MMWR, 55*, 1–23.

Centers for Disease Control and Prevention. (2006b). What every pet owner should know about roundworms & hookworms. http://www.cdc.gov/healthypets/

Chamley, C. A., Carson, P., Randall, F., & Sandwell, M. (2004). *Developmental anatomy and physiology of children*. St. Louis: Elsevier.

Chial, H. J., Camilleri, M., Williams, D. E., Litzinger, K., & Perrault, J. (2003). Rumination syndrome in children and adolescents: Diagnosis, treatment, and prognosis. *Pediatrics, 111*, 158–162.

Clayden, G., & Keshtgar, A. S. (2003). Management of childhood constipation. *Postgraduate Medical Journal, 79*, 616–621.

Cleft Palate Foundation. (2005). Retrieved Sept. 18, 2005, from http://www.cleftline.org/aboutclp/

Colletti, J. E. (2004). Pyloric stenosis. *Canadian Journal of Emergency Medicine, 6*, 444–445.

Corbett, J. V. (2004). *Laboratory tests and diagnostic procedures with nursing diagnoses* (6th ed.). Upper Saddle River, NJ: Prentice Hall Health.

Coughlin, E. C. (2003). Assessment and management of pediatric constipation in primary care. *Pediatric Nursing, 29*, 296–302.

Coy, K., Speltz, M. L., & Jones, K. (2002). Facial appearance and attachment in infants with orofacial clefts: A replication. *The Cleft Palate-Craniofacial Journal, 39*, 66–72.

Davies, M. C., Creighton, S. M., & Wilcox, D. T. (2004). Long-term outcomes of anorectal malformations. *Pediatric Surgery International, 20*, 567–572.

Doughty, D. (2004). Structure and function of the gastrointestinal tract in infants and children. *Journal of Wound, Ostomy and Continence Nursing, 31*, 207–212.

Duke, J. (2004, Spring/Summer). Chamomile: Use in pregnancy and pediatrics. *Journal of the American Herbalists Guild*, 57–58.

Eckert, K. (2005). Penetrating and blunt abdominal trauma. *Critical Care Nursing Quarterly, 28*, 41–59.

Emil, S., Laberge, J., Mikhail, P., Baican, L., Glageole, H., Nguyen, L., et al. (2003). Appendicitis in children: A ten year update of therapeutic recommendations. *Journal of Pediatric Surgery, 38*, 236–242.

Gardiner, P., & Kemper, K. J. (2005). Which herbs and supplements spell relief? *Contemporary Pediatrics, 22*(8), 50–55.

Gasseling, J. (2004). Hypertrophic pyloric stenosis. *Radiologic Technology, 75*, 314–316.

Gereige, R. S., & Frias, J. L. (2002). Is it more than just constipation? *Pediatrics, 109*, 961–965.

Gracey, K., Burd, A., & Burd, R. (2003). Guide for home gastrostomy tube care. *Advances in Neonatal Care, 3*, 206–207.

Gremse, D. A. (2002). Gastroesophageal reflux: Life-threatening disease or laundry problem? *Clinical Pediatrics, 41*(6), 369–372.

Gremse, D. A. (2004). GERD in the pediatric patient: Management considerations. *Medscape General Medicine, 6*(2).

Hedrick, H. L, Crombleholme, T. M., Flake, A. W., Nance, M. L., von Allmen, D., Howell, L. J., Johnson, M. P., Wilson, R. D., & Adzick, N. S. (2004). Right congenital diaphragmatic hernia: Prenatal assessment and outcome. *Journal of Pediatric Surgery, 39*, 319–323.

Henry, S. M. (2004). Discerning differences: Gastroesophageal reflux and gastroesophageal reflux disease infants. *Advances in Neonatal Care, 4*, 235–247.

Hill, K. D., & Hill, I. D. (2005). Celiac disease: Fundamentals for pediatricians. *Contemporary Pediatrics, 22*(10), 65–77.

Hoffenberg, E. J., Emery, L. M., Barriga, K. J., Bao, F., Taylor, J., Eisenbarth, G. S., et al. (2004). Clinical features of children with screening-identified evidence of celiac disease. *Pediatrics, 113*, 1254–1259.

Holcomb, S. S. (2005). Managing jaundice in full-term infants. *The Nurse Practitioner, 30*(1), 6–7, 11–12.

Holmes, S. (2004). Enteral feeding and percutaneous endoscopic gastrosotomy. *Nursing Standard, 18*(20), 41–43.

Hsu, V. P., Staat, M. A., Roberts, N., Thieman, C., Bernstein, D. L., Bresee, J., et al. (2005). Use of active surveillance to validate international classification of disease code estimates of rotavirus hospitalizations in children. *Pediatrics, 115*, 78–82.

Hyams, J. (2004). Inflammatory bowel disease. In R. E. Behrman, R. M. Kliegman, H. B. Jenson (Eds.) *Nelson textbook of pediatrics* (17th ed., pp. 1248–1249). Philadelphia: Saunders.

Hyams, J. (2005). Inflammatory bowel disease. *Pediatrics in Review, 26*(9), 314–320.

Jackson, C. S., & Buchman, A. L. (2004). The nutritional management of short bowel syndrome. *Nutritional Clinical Care, 7*, 114–121.

Jaffe, B. M., & Berger, D. H. (2005). The appendix. In F. Charles Brunicardi, Dana K. Andersen, Timothy R. Billiar, David L. Dunn, John G. Hunter, Jeffrey B. Matthews, Raphael E. Pollock & Seymour I. Schwartz (Eds.), *Schwartz's principles of surgery* (8th ed., pp. 1119–1137). New York: McGraw-Hill.

Johansson, B., & Ringsberg, K. C. (2004). Parents' experience of having a child with cleft lip and palate. *Journal of Advanced Nursing, 47*, 165–173.

Johnson, N., & Sandy, J. R. (2003). Prenatal diagnosis of cleft lip and palate. *The Cleft Palate-Craniofacial Journal, 40*, 186–189.

Kee, J. L. (2005a). *Handbook of laboratory & diagnostic tests with nursing implications* (5th ed.). Upper Saddle River, NJ: Prentice Hall Health.

Kee, J. L. (2005b). *Laboratory and diagnostic tests with nursing implications* (7th ed.). Upper Saddle River, NJ: Prentice Hall Health.

Kelly, D. A. (2002). Managing liver failure. *Postgraduate Medical Journal, 78*, 660–667.

Kliegman, R. M., & Willoughby, R. E. (2005). Prevention of necrotizing enterocolitis with probiotics. *Pediatrics, 115*, 171–172.

Kinservik, M. A., & Friedhoff, M. M. (2004). The efficacy and safety of Polyethylene Glycol 3350 in the treatment of constipation in children. *Pediatric Nursing, 30*(3), 232–237.

Kosloske, A. M., Love, C. L., Rohrer, J. E., Goldthorn, J. F., & Lacey, S. R. (2004). The diagnosis of appendicitis in children: Outcomes of a strategy based on pediatric surgical evaluation. *Pediatrics, 113*, 29–34.

Kwok, M. Y., Kim, M. K., & Gorelick, M. H. (2004). Evidence-based approach to the diagnosis of appendicitis in children. *Pediatric Emergency Care, 20*, 690–698.

Lembo, A., & Camilleri, M. (2003). Chronic constipation. *The New England Journal of Medicine, 349*, 1360.

Marinkovic, S., & Bukanica, S. (2003). Umbilical hernia in children. *Medicinski Pregled, 56* (5–6), 291–294.

McCollough, M., & Sharieff, G. Q. (2006). Abdominal pain in children. *Pediatric Clinics of North America, 53*, 107–137.

Merritt, L. (2005a). Part 1. Understanding the embryology and genetics of cleft lip and palate. *Advances in Neonatal Care, 5*(2), 64–71.

Merritt, L. (2005b). Part 2. Physical assessment of the infant with cleft lip and/or palate. *Advances in Neonatal Care, 5*(3), 125–134.

Meyers, R. L. (2003). Neonatal emergencies. In C. D. Rudolph & A. M. Rudolph (Eds.), *Rudolph's pediatrics* (21st ed., pp. 202–207). New York: McGraw Hill.

Milla, P. J. (2003). Hirschsprung disease and other neuropathies. In C. D. Rudolph & A. M. Rudolph (Eds.), *Rudolph's pediatrics* (21st ed., pp. 1461–1463). New York: McGraw Hill.

Miller, K. E. (2003). Colic: Prevalence, risk factors, and potential sequelae. *American Family Physician, 67*, 2005–2006.

Morash, D. (2002). An interdisciplinary project that changed practice in feeding methods after pyloromyotomy. *Pediatric Nursing, 28*, 113–117.

Murdock, A. M., & Johnston, S. D. (2005). Diagnostic criteria for celiac disease: Time for change? *European Journal of Gastroenterology and Hepatology 17*, 41–43.

Murray, D. L. (2003). Infectious diseases. In C. D. Rudolph & A. M. Rudolph (Eds.), *Rudolph's pediatrics* (21st ed., pp. 1102, 1106). New York: McGraw Hill.

Nehring, W. M. (2004). Down syndrome. In P. L. Allen & J. A. Vessey, *Primary care of the child with a chronic condition* (pp. 445–468). St. Louis: Mosby.

Nelson, K. S., & Hostetler, M. A. (2002). A listless infant with vomiting. *Hospital Physician, 38*(2), 40–46.

Orenstein, S., Peters, J., Khan, S., Youssef, N., & Hussain, S. (2004). Congenital anomalies: Esophageal atresia and tracheoesophageal fistula. In R. E. Behrman, R. M. Kliegman, & H. B. Jenson (Eds.), *Nelson textbook of pediatrics* (17th ed., p. 1219). Philadelphia: Saunders.

Parker, L. A., Moniaci, V. K., & Fike, D. L. (2003). Surgical intervention for the treatment of necrotizing enterocolitis. *Newborn and Infant Nursing Reviews, 3*(2), 64–70.

Pearson, H. A. (2003). The spleen. In C. D. Rudolph & A. M. Rudolph (Eds.), *Rudolph's pediatrics* (21st ed., pp. 1560–1562). New York: McGraw Hill.

Plante, M. L. (2004). Crohn's disease. *Advance for Nurse Practitioners,* (May, 2004), 28–35.

Potoka, D. A., & Saladino, R. A. (2005). Blunt abdominal trauma in the pediatric patient. *Clinical Pediatric Emergency Medicine, 6,* 23–31.

Reeves, J. J., Shannon, M. W., & Fleisher, G. R. (2002). Ondansetron decreases vomiting associated with acute gastroenteritis. *Pediatrics, 109*(4), e62.

Reid, J. (2004). A review of feeding interventions for infants with cleft palate. *The Cleft Palate-Craniofacial Journal, 41,* 268–278.

Rudolph, C. (2003). Structures and development of the gastrointestinal tract. In C. D. Rudolph & A. M. Rudolph (Eds.), *Rudolph's pediatrics* (21st ed., pp. 1305–1313). New York: McGraw Hill.

Sandberg, D. J., Magee, W. P., & Denk, M. J. (2002). *AORN Journal, 75,* 490–499.

Shaw, N. M. (2003). Assessment and management of the hematologic system. In C. Kenner & J. W. Lott (Eds.) *Comprehensive neonatal nursing: A physiologic perspective,* (3rd ed., pp. 586–602). St. Louis, MO: Saunders.

Simone, S. (2003). *Abdominal/genitourinary injuries.* In P. A. Moloney-Harmon & S. J. Czerwinski (Eds.), *Nursing care of the pediatric trauma patient* (pp. 227–247). Philadelphia: Saunders.

Simpson, T., & Ivey, J. (2003). Pediatric management problems. *Pediatric Nursing, 29,* 310.

Snyder, J. D., & Pickering, L. K. (2004). Viral hepatitis. In R. E. Behrman, R. M. Kliegman, & H. B. Jenson (Eds.), *Nelson textbook of pediatrics* (17th ed. pp. 1324–1331). Philadelphia: Saunders.

Sondheimer, J. (2003). Gastroesophageal reflux. In W. Hay, A. Hayward, M. Levin, & J. Sondheimer (Eds.), *Current pediatric diagnosis and treatment* (16th ed., pp. 614–615). New York: Lange Medical Books/McGraw-Hill.

Stoll, B. J., & R. M. Kleigman (2004). The umbilicus. In R. E. Behrman, R. M. Kliegman, & H. B. Jenson (Eds.), *Nelson textbook of pediatrics* (17th ed., pp. 608–609). Philadelphia: Saunders.

Swenson, O. (2002). Hirschsprung's disease. *Pediatrics, 109,* 914—918.

Tanaka, M., & Kazuma, K. (2005). Ulcerative colitis: Factors affecting difficulties of life and psychological well-being of patients in remission. *Journal of Clinical Nursing, 14,* 65–73.

Thielman, N. M., & Guerrant, R. L. (2004). Acute infectious diarrhea. *The New England Journal of Medicine, 350,* 38.

Thorn, M. (2005). Celiac disease. *Advance for Nurses, 7*(2), 21–23.

Tran, T. T., Nissen, N., Poordad, F. F., & Martin, P. (2004). Advances in liver transplantation: New strategies and current care expand access, enhance survival. *Postgraduate Medicine, 115*(5), 73–85.

Tudehope, D. I. (2004). The epidemiology and pathogenesis of neonatal necrotizing enterocolitis. *Journal of Paediatric Child Health, 41,* 167–168.

Vaira, D., Gatta, L., Ricci, C., Tampieri, A., Cavina, M., Bernabucci V. (2005). Symposium on peptic acid disease. Peptic ulcer and *Helicobacter pylori*: Update on testing and treatment. *Postgraduate Medicine, 117*(6), 17–22, 46.

Van Niel, C. W., Feudtner, C., Garrison, M. M., & Christakis, D. A. (2002). Lactobacillus therapy for acute infectious diarrhea in children: A meta-analysis. *Pediatrics, 109,* 678–684.

Van Rooij, I. A., Vermeij-Keers, C., Kluijtmans, J., Ocke, M. C., et al. (2003). *Does the interaction between maternal folate intake and the methylenetetrahydrofolate reductase polymorphisms affect the risk of cleft lip with or without cleft palate? Journal of Epidemiology, 157,* 583.

Vegunta, R. K., Ali, A., Wallace, L. J., Switzer, D. M., & Pearl R. H. (2004). Laparoscopic appendectomy in children: Technically feasible and safe in all stages of acute appendicitis. *The American Surgeon, 70,* 198–202.

Wall, G. C., & Jacoby, H. I. (2002). Gastroesophageal reflux disease. *American Journal of Pharmaceutical Education, 66*(2), 148–152.

Walsh, D. S., & Adzick, N. S. (2003). Fetal disorders and their prenatal management. In C. D. Rudolph & A. M. Rudolph (Eds.), *Rudolph's pediatrics* (21st ed., pp. 77–79). New York: McGraw Hill.

Weir, E. (2003). Congenital abdominal wall defects. *Canadian Medical Association Journal, 169,* 809.

Williams, T., Butler, R., & Sundem, T. (2003). Management of the infant with gastroschisis: A comprehensive review of the literature. *Newborn and Infant Nursing Reviews, 3*(2), 55–63.

Wyllie, R. (2004). Stomach and intestines: Ileus, adhesions, intussusception, and closed loop obstructions. In R. E. Behrman, R. M. Kliegman, & H. B. Jenson, (Eds.), *Nelson textbook of pediatrics* (17th ed., pp. 1228–1232; 1241–1243). Philadelphia: Saunders.

Zelnik, N., Pacht, A., Obeid, R., & Lerner, A. (2004). Range of neurological disorders in patients with celiac disease. *Pediatrics, 113,* 1672–1677.

Ziegler, M. M. (2004). The diagnosis of appendicitis: An evolving paradigm. *Pediatrics, 113,* 130–132.

Zitelli, B., & Davis, H. (Eds.). (2002). *Atlas of pediatric physical diagnosis* (4th ed.). Philadelphia: Mosby.

Zitsman, J. L. (2003). Current concepts in minimal access surgery for children. *Pediatrics, 111,* 1239–1245.

25

ALTERATIONS IN GENITOURINARY FUNCTION

KEY TERMS

azotemia **994**

balanitis **1017**

chordee **984**

circumcision **1017**

cryptorchidism **1018**

cystitis **978**

dialysate **1006**

disequilibrium

   syndrome **1007**

dysfunctional

   voiding **987**

end-stage renal

   disease (ESRD)

   1000

enuresis **987**

hydronephrosis **979**

incarceration **1019**

nephron **973**

neurogenic

   bladder **978**

oliguria **994**

osteodystrophy **996**

phimosis **1017**

pyelonephritis **978**

pyeloplasty **982**

renal insufficiency

   999

stent **984**

uremia **994**

uremic frost **1001**

vesicoureteral

   reflux **978**

MediaLink

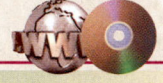

http://www.prenhall.com/ball

See the Prentice Hall Nursing MediaLink DVD-ROM and Companion Website for chapter-specific resources.

TERRELL, who is now 7 years old, was born with posterior urethral valves, which caused damage to his kidneys. Despite undergoing surgery to correct the defect at 2 years of age, his kidney function continued to deteriorate. End-stage renal disease was diagnosed 2 years ago, and dialysis treatment was initiated. Terrell requires a kidney transplant; however, no family member is able or willing to donate a kidney. As a result, Terrell has been placed on the transplant list for a cadaver kidney.

Terrell was initially treated with peritoneal dialysis, but after experiencing several peritoneal infections in the first year, he started hemodialysis. Terrell visits the dialysis center three afternoons a week for treatments lasting approximately 3 to 4 hours.

What are the special concerns of the nurse in monitoring a child who is receiving hemodialysis treatment? Is Terrell at any higher risk for infection than other children? Does he require a special diet? What are the potential complications for Terrell's growth and development? What are the psychological effects of renal disease on the child and family? How is his education managed to provide time for learning and peer interaction? The answers to these questions and information about numerous other genitourinary conditions are presented in this chapter.

LEARNING OUTCOMES

After reading this chapter, you will be able to do the following:

1. Describe the pathophysiologic processes associated with genitourinary disorders in the pediatric population.

2. Discuss the nursing management of a child with a structural defect of the genitourinary system.

3. Develop a nursing care plan for the child with a urinary tract infection.

4. Describe the growth and developmental issues for the child with chronic renal failure.

5. Outline a plan to meet the fluid and dietary restrictions of a child with a renal disorder.

6. Describe psychosocial issues for the child requiring surgery on the genitourinary tract.

7. Develop a nursing care plan for the child with acute and chronic renal failure on dialysis.

8. Describe the nursing education for the adolescent with a sexually transmitted infection.

FOCUS ON
The Genitourinary System

ANATOMY AND PHYSIOLOGY

The genitourinary system is made up of the urinary and reproductive organs. The urinary system—composed of the kidneys, ureters, bladder, and urethra—has an important function in excreting wastes and maintaining the acid-base and fluid and electrolyte balance (Figure 25–1 ➤) Normal renal function requires the following: unimpaired renal blood flow, adequate glomerular ultrafiltration, normal tubular function, and unobstructed urine flow.

The functional unit of the kidney, the **nephron**, contributes to the formation of urine. The nephron is a tubular structure containing the renal corpuscle, proximal convoluted tubule, loop of Henle, distal convoluted tubule, and collecting duct. The renal corpuscle is composed of the glomerulus (a small group of capillaries) that loops into the Bowman's capsule (Figure 25–2 ➤). The glomerular capillaries serve as the filtration membrane where metabolic wastes and fluids are separated from the blood cells and plasma

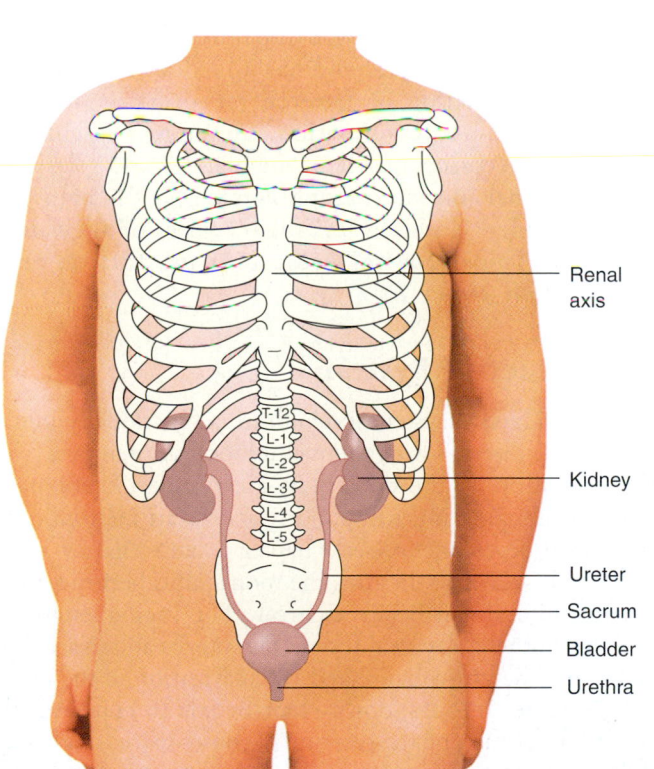

Figure 25–1 ➤ The kidneys are located between the twelfth thoracic (T12) and third lumbar (L3) vertebrae.

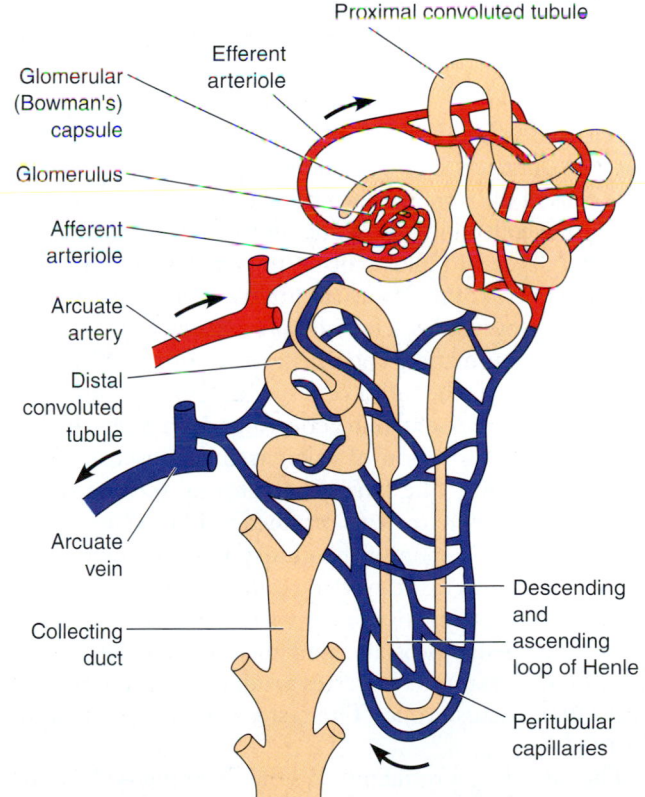

Figure 25–2 ➤ The nephron is the structural and functional unit of the kidneys. A nephron holds 6 glomeruli, Bowman's capsule, proximal tubule, loop of Henle, distal tubule, and the collecting duct.

proteins to form the urine. The kidney maintains the rate of blood flow to keep the glomerular filtration rate fairly constant. The urine flows through the proximal convoluted tubule, the loop of Henle, and into the distal convoluted tubule and collecting duct. Water, electrolytes, and other substances are reabsorbed or secreted in the tubules, including the following (Huether, 2006):

- *Proximal tubule* Sodium chloride, glucose, potassium, amino acids, bicarbonate, urea, and water are reabsorbed.
- *Loop of Henle* Water and sodium are reabsorbed, leading to urine concentration and secretion of urea.
- *Distal tubule* Sodium chloride, bicarbonate, and water are reabsorbed; potassium, urea, hydrogen ions, and ammonia ions are secreted.
- *Collecting tubule* Water is reabsorbed; sodium, potassium, hydrogen ions, and ammonia ions may be reabsorbed or secreted.

The presence of antidiuretic hormone (ADH) secreted by the posterior pituitary gland causes more water reabsorption, leading to urine concentration. Absence of ADH leads to dilute urine. See Chapter 16 ∞ for more information about fluid and electrolyte physiology.

Urine from the nephron flows into the calyces in the renal pelvis and is funneled into the ureters. The lower end of the ureters connects into the bladder's posterior aspect. The muscle cells of the ureters move urine to the bladder by peristalsis. Urine collects in the bladder until the internal urethral sphincter relaxes and allows urine to pass into the urethra. Voluntary control of the external urethral sphincter is gained as the child's nervous system matures. Contraction of the bladder during urination compresses the lower end of the ureter and prevents the reflux of urine back into the ureter.

The kidney is essential in activating vitamin D, which is needed for the absorption of calcium and phosporus from the small intestine. The kidney secretes erythropoietin to stimulate the bone marrow to produce red blood cells. The renin-angiotensin system of the kidney is a hormonal regulator that can increase the systemic blood pressure.

The male reproductive system is composed of the testes and scrotum, penis, prostate, and the vas deferens, which drains into the urethra. The testes produce the primary male sex hormone, testosterone. The testes produce sperm after puberty.

The female reproductive system is composed of the ovaries, fallopian tubes, uterus, and vagina. The ovaries produce the primary female sex hormone, estrogen. Beginning between 8 and 12 years of age, the ovaries produce increasing amounts of sex hormones to initiate puberty and sexual maturation. After puberty, the ovaries produce the ovum that may be fertilized by the sperm during its passage through the fallopian tube into the uterus. Complex hormonal factors are involved in puberty, the menstrual cycle, and pregnancy.

PEDIATRIC DIFFERENCES

Urinary System

All of the nephrons that will make up the mature kidney are present at birth. The kidneys grow and the tubular system matures gradually during childhood, reaching full size by adolescence. Most renal growth occurs during the first 5 years of life. This increase in size is due primarily to enlargement of the nephrons. The kidney's efficiency also increases with age. During the first 2 years of life, the kidneys are less efficient at regulating electrolyte and acid-base balance (see Chapter 16 ∞) and eliminating some drugs from the body. After the age of 2 years, the kidneys' efficiency markedly increases. Urinary output per kilogram of body weight decreases as the child ages because the kidney becomes more efficient at concentrating urine. The expected output is as follows:

- Infants—2 mL/kg/hr
- Children—0.5 to 1 mL/kg/hr
- Adolescents—40 to 80 mL per hour

Bladder capacity increases with age from 20 to 50 mL at birth to 700 mL in adulthood. A child's bladder capacity (in ounces) can be estimated by adding 2 to the child's age (e.g., a 4-year-old has a bladder capacity of 6 ounces). Stimulation of "stretch receptors" within the bladder wall initiates urination. Simultaneous contraction of the detrusor muscle of the bladder and relaxation of the internal and external sphincters result in emptying of the bladder. Children less than 2 years of age cannot maintain bladder control because of insufficient nerve development (Figure 25–3 ➤).

Reproductive System

The reproductive system in children is functionally immature until puberty. Throughout childhood the genitalia (with the exception of the clitoris in girls) enlarge gradually. The hormonal changes of puberty accelerate anatomic and functional development (see Chapter 5 and Figures 5–40, 5–41, and 5–42 ∞). In girls, the mons pubis becomes more prominent and hair begins to grow. The vagina lengthens, and the epithelial layers thicken. The uterus and ovaries enlarge, and the musculature and vascularization of the uterus also increase. In boys, downy hair begins to appear at the base of the penis, and the scrotum becomes increasingly pendulous as the testes enlarge. The penis grows longer and wider.

See Figure 25–4 ➤ for a description of a color wheel, used to describe and standardize urine color. Examples of diagnostic and laboratory tests used to evaluate genitourinary system function are provided in the accompanying table. Use the guidelines on page 978 to perform a nursing assessment of the genitourinary system.

AS CHILDREN GROW

Development of the Genitourinary System

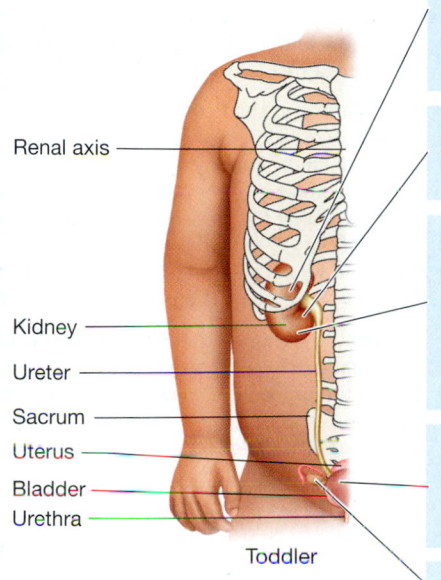

All nephrons are present at birth, the ureters are short, and tubules have smaller surface area resulting in diminished water reabsorption. Nephrons grow in size, and the kidneys and the tubule system gradually develop during childhood to reach adult size during adolescence.

Glomerular filtration rate is at 30% to 50% of adult levels throughout first year of life. Glomerular filtration rate increasess during childhood.

Kidneys are less efficient at regulating electrolyte and acid-base balance, and less able to concentrate urine. Diarrhea, infection, improper feeding may lead to severe acidosis and fluid imbalance. Efficiency of the kidneys in regulating electrolytes and acid-base balance increases after 2 years of age.

Average daily urine output is up to 15 to 50 mL at birth to 400 mL at 2 months of age. Average daily urine output increases during childhood and reaches 700 to 1500 mL during adolescence.

Reproductive system immature.

Reproductive system matures after puberty.

Renal axis

Kidney

Ureter

Sacrum

Uterus

Bladder

Urethra

Toddler

Adolescent

Figure 25–3 ➤ Development of the genitourinary system (Toddler versus the Adolescent).
Data from: Huether, S. E. (2006). Alterations of renal and urinary tract function in children. In K. L. McCance & S. E. Huether, *Pathophysiology: The biologic basis for disease in adults and children* (5th ed., pp. 1337–1352). St. Louis: Elsevier Mosby.

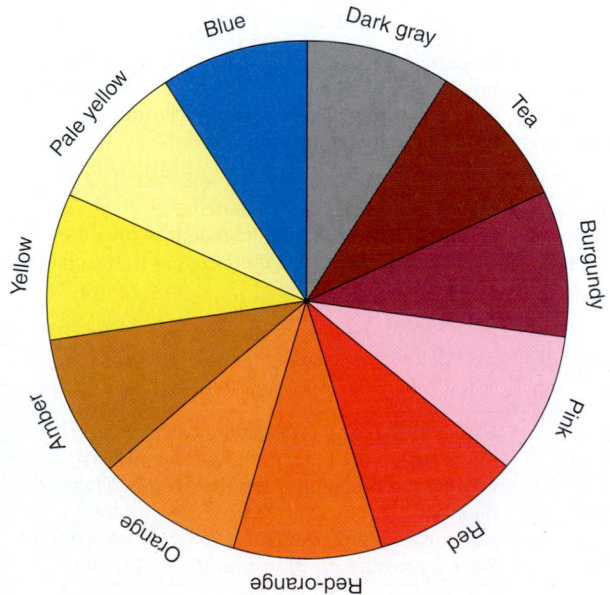

Figure 25–4 ➤ A color wheel, such as the one shown here, can be used as a guide in standardizing descriptions of urine color. Normal urine is *pale yellow*. Changes in urine color can indicate the following alterations: *yellow*—concentrated urine; *amber*—bile in urine; *orange*—alkaline or concentrated urine; *red-orange*—acid pH, medications; *red*—blood; menses; *pink*—dilute blood; *burgundy*— laxatives; *tea*—melanin, hematuria; *dark gray*—medications, dyes; *blues*—dyes, medications.
Note: From Cooper, C. (1993). What color is that urine specimen? *American Journal of Nursing, 93,* 37. Copyright © 1993 Connie Cooper, RN, MSN; graphics by Mike O'Grady, RN, MSN

DIAGNOSTIC PROCEDURES/LABORATORY TESTS FOR GENITOURINARY SYSTEM CONDITIONS

Diagnostic Procedure	Purpose	Nursing Implications
CT (computed tomography)	Provides detailed visualization of structures of the urinary tract and major renal blood vessels using a radiograph beam and computers to create cross-sectional and three-dimensional images.	• Infant or child may be NPO and require bowel evacuation prior to study. • Prepare child for size of equipment and the need to stay still on the table. • Assess for allergies if contrast medium is used. • Provide sedation, if needed. • Encourage fluids after the procedure to flush out the contrast media.
Cystoscopy	A flexible fiber optic scope is inserted through the urethra into the bladder. Shows interior urethra and bladder. May be done simultaneously with voiding cystourethrogram (see page 977)	• Note infants and children are NPO prior to the study. • Administer sedation. • Provide antibiotic prophylaxis to children with cardiac anomalies • Force fluids after the procedure to detect problems with voiding. • Note that dysuria and frequency may be experienced for a short time after the procedure.
Diuretic renogram	An IV administration of a radioactive medication is given as sequential images are taken of the kidneys, ureters, and bladder. Imaging continues when furosemide is administered IV. The test evaluates renal function and enables comparison of the right and left sides. This test helps distinguish between obstructive and nonobstructive lesions, or the presence of a dilated ureter.	• Hydrate the child before the test. IV fluids are used for hydration during the test. • Explain the procedures to be performed and how the child can cooperate. • Catheterize the child is to drain urine during the procedure.
Intravenous pyelogram (intravenous urography)	A contrast medium excreted by the urinary system is administered IV. Radiographs are initially taken every minute for 5 minutes to visualize the kidney cortex. More radiographs are taken 15 minutes later as the dye collects in the kidney pelvis, enters the ureters, and passes to the bladder. A post-void radiograph is taken to see how well the bladder empties. Images identify structural defects, tumors, and show the kidney's collecting system, distal ureters, and bladder.	• Assess for allergies as contrast medium is used. Premedication with an antihistamine or corticosteroid may be given to minimize allergic risk in these children. Monitor children carefully as a reaction may still occur. • Obtain a serum creatinine and BUN, if needed, to assess renal function prior to giving the contrast medium. • Infants and children may be NPO or allowed clear liquids prior to the study. An IV is started for injection of contrast. • Encourage fluids after the procedure to flush out the contrast media.
MRI (magnetic resonance imaging)	Uses a large magnet and radio waves delivered to the body part to be imaged. The energy field produced can be transferred as a visual image to the computer. The test provides detailed visualization of structures of the urinary system.	• Prepare child for sounds, size of equipment, and tunnel, as well as need to stay still on the table. • Ensure that the child has no metallic implants. • Provide sedation if needed.
Radionucleotide renal scan with dimercaptosuccinic acid (DMSA)	A radioactive element is tagged to DMSA and administered IV. A series of CT scans are taken over 20 minutes to 4 hours to assess the kidney perfusion and function. The test detects renal parenchymal lesions, renal atrophy, or scars. It differentiates between hydronephrosis caused by obstructive lesions, reflux, or a cyst.	• Ensure the child is well hydrated. • Perform catheterization, if needed, to measure urine output. Explain catheterization to the child.
Renal biopsy	Removal and examination of tissue from the kidney. The needle insertion is monitored by fluoroscopy or scanning. Pathologic results are used to diagnose the presence and/or extent of renal involvement in specific disorders or to determine a tumor type.	• Ensure infants and children are NPO for several hours before the biopsy, if physician orders. • Provide site preparation and bowel evacuation, if needed. • Administer pre-procedural sedation as prescribed. Place a pressure dressing over the biopsy site.

DIAGNOSTIC PROCEDURES/LABORATORY TESTS FOR GENITOURINARY SYSTEM CONDITIONS

Diagnostic Procedure	Purpose	Nursing Implications
Renal or bladder ultrasound	Ultrasound waves are sent into the body with a small transducer held against the skin. The transducer then receives returning sound waves bouncing off of underlying structures. The test may identify large renal scars, renal anomalies, obstruction, abscesses, masses, and hydronephrosis.	• Explain the procedure to the child. Keep the parent present to promote the young child's cooperation. • Administer fluids as prescribed.
Voiding cystourethrogram or radionuclide cystography	A cystoscope is passed into the urethra and bladder to examine the interior of the bladder. Ureteral catheters may also be passed to obtain urine samples from each kidney pelvis. A contrast medium may be used to examine structures. Bladder structure and function, urethral anatomy, and bladder masses are examined. The test may detect vesicoureteral reflux.	• Explain catheterization to child and that the bladder will be filled. • Provide coaching strategies for parents accompanying the child to help the child cope. • Assess for allergies (iodine, shellfish, or contrast media) as contrast media is used. • Encourage fluids after the procedure to flush out the contrast media.

Laboratory Tests	Purpose	Nursing Implications
Bladder capacity	Collection of urine when the child has urgency to void. It provides information on the amount of urine the bladder will hold.	• Force fluids and measure the amount of urine voided when the child has the urgency to void.
Blood urea nitrogen	Blood test of the urea nitrogen level that reflects the glomerular filtration rate and glomerular functioning.	• Prepare the child for a venipuncture. • Be sure the child is adequately hydrated.
Creatinine clearance	Urine is collected for 2, 12, or 24 hours to measure creatinine excreted. A serum blood sample is collected during the urine collection interval to measure the serum creatinine level. A rate of creatinine clearance is calculated from urine and blood levels to provide a measure of glomerular function.	• Explain the urine collection process. The first specimen is discarded and the time is recorded. All subsequent urine is collected, including the last void at the end of the collection period. • Note that no preservatives are needed for the urine.
Urinalysis	Collection of urine to measure the specific gravity and pH, and to detect the presence of glucose, ketones, protein, blood cells, casts, crystals, and microorganisms. Dipstick and reagent strips can be used to assess for glucose, protein, and bacteria in the urine.	• Use a urine collection bag for infants and children who are not toilet trained. • Give fluids if unable to void.
Urine culture	Collection of a clean-catch or catheterization urine specimen to detect the presence of an infection in the urinary system.	• Explain the process for cleaning the perineum and collecting the urine midstream in a sterile cup. • Clean the perineum and collect a catheter specimen midstream in a sterile container.
Urine protein-to-creatinine ratio	Collection of urine (either 24 hour or first voided morning specimen) to assess urine protein excretion.	• Use the first voided morning specimen due to difficulty in obtaining 24-hour urine specimen in young children.
Vaginal and urethral cultures	A culture swab is inserted into the endocervical section of the vagina in adolescent girls. A swab is used to collect exudate from the urethra in adolescent boys. The presence of sexually transmitted infections can be detected.	• Explain the culture collection process to the adolescent. • Use standard precautions for collection of the specimen. • Follow agency guidelines for handling the culture and transfer to the laboratory.

Data from: Kraus, S. J. (2001). Genitourinary imaging in children. *Pediatric Clinics of North America, 48*(6), 1381–1423; Hanson, K. A. (2003). Diagnostic tests and tools in the evaluation of urologic disease, Part II. *Urologic Nursing, 23*(6), 405–415; and Corbett, J. V. (2004). Laboratory tests and diagnostic procedures with nursing diagnoses (6th ed.). Upper Saddle River, NJ: Prentice Hall Health.

ASSESSMENT GUIDELINES FOR THE CHILD WITH A GENITOURINARY CONDITION

Assessment Focus	Assessment Guidelines
Urine characteristics	• Does the urine have a strong odor, a dark or unusual color, or appear cloudy? See Figure 25–4.
Pain or discomfort	• Is there pain or burning with urination? • Is there flank or abdominal pain? • Is there scrotal or testicular pain?
Edema	• Is there generalized edema?
Appearance of genitalia	• What is the location of the urethra on the glans penis? • Is the scrotum large or underdeveloped? Are rugue present? Are testes palpable in the scrotum? • Do the genitalia have characteristic male or female appearance, or are the genitalia ambiguous? • Is there vaginal or urethral discharge? • Are there lesions on the genitalia?
Sexual development	• What is the stage of pubertal development? See Figures 5–40 , 5–41 , and 5–42 ∞ .

M any infections, structural disorders, and disease processes alter genitourinary function. Because the kidneys and other urinary system organs perform several essential body functions, including removing waste products and maintaining fluid and electrolyte balance, disorders that affect these organs pose a significant threat to the health of children.

Although the reproductive system is functionally immature until puberty, uncorrected structural defects and sexually transmitted diseases can have both psychologic and physiologic implications for the developing child.

URINARY TRACT INFECTION

A urinary tract infection (UTI) which may be bacterial, viral, or fungal occurs in the urinary tract. **Cystitis** is a lower UTI that involves the urethra or bladder. **Pyelonephritis** is an upper UTI that involves the ureters, renal pelvis, and renal parenchyma. UTIs can be acute or chronic (the latter is either recurrent or persistent).

UTIs are the second most common infections in children. An estimated 3% of females and 1% of males will have a UTI by age 11 years (National Kidney and Urological Diseases Information Clearinghouse, 2003).

Etiology and Pathophysiology

The urinary tract is normally sterile. The most common mechanism is with an organism entering the genitourinary tract and ascending from the urethra to the bladder and up toward the kidney. Many first UTIs are caused by *Escherichia coli*, a common gram-negative enteric bacterium. Other causative organisms include *Staphylococcus*, *Klebsiella*, *Proteus*, *Pseudomonas*, *Enterobacter*, and *Enterococcus*.

Urinary stasis enhances the risk of UTI. Stasis may be caused by abnormal anatomic structures or abnormal function (e.g., a **neurogenic bladder** in which an interrupted nerve supply from meningomyelocele or spinal cord trauma impairs bladder voiding function and leads to incomplete bladder emptying). Children normally void five to six times a day. Infrequent voiding, common in school-age children, results in incomplete emptying of the bladder and urinary stasis. Other factors associated with increased risk of UTI include an irritated perineum, uncircumcised male in first 6 months of life, constipation, masturbation, sexual abuse, and sexual activity in adolescent females (Dulczak & Kirk, 2005).

Another cause of UTI is **vesicoureteral reflux**, the backflow of urine from the bladder into the ureters during voiding. Bacteria in the urine may be swept up to the kidneys leading to pyelonephritis. The vesicoureteral reflex also prevents complete emptying of the bladder; because urine returns to the bladder, it creates a reservoir for bacterial growth (Huether, 2006). Vesicoureteral reflux can also result from a structural anomaly in which the ureters insert into the bladder in an abnormal position.

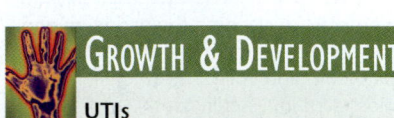

GROWTH & DEVELOPMENT

UTIs

Most urinary tract infections among newborns and young infants occur in boys, as obstructive structural defects predisposing an infant to infection have a higher incidence in males. The incidence of UTIs in older infants and children is higher in girls because the shorter female urethra (2 cm [1 in.] in young girls) has closer proximity to the anus and vagina, increasing the risk of contamination by fecal bacteria.

Renal scarring can result from **hydronephrosis** (accumulation of urine in the renal pelvis as a result of obstructed outflow) or pyelonephritis due to the inflammatory and ischemic effects of the infection. Scars have been associated with hypertension, proteinuria, and kidney failure. The risk of kidney damage increases in the following instances:

- UTI in an infant less than 1 year of age
- Delay in diagnosis and effective antibacterial treatment for an upper UTI
- Anatomic obstruction or nerve supply interruption
- Recurrent episodes of upper UTIs

Clinical Manifestations

Symptoms depend on the infection's location as well as the child's age. Symptoms in the newborn period tend to be nonspecific—unexplained fever, failure to thrive, poor feeding, vomiting and diarrhea, strong-smelling urine, and irritability. Any child under 2 years of age with a fever of unknown origin should be tested for a UTI. The more "classic" symptoms of lower UTI are not seen until the toddler years, as listed in the clinical manifestations table below. About 40% of UTIs are asymptomatic.

COLLABORATIVE CARE

Diagnostic Tests

A urine specimen is examined for the presence of bacteria. Dipsticks can be used to screen for urinary tract infection. A dipstick positive leukocyte esterase test identifies white blood cells and pyuria, and a positive nitrite dipstick detects gram-negative bacteria (Raszka & Khan, 2005). The UTI is diagnosed when a midstream clean-catch urine culture yields greater than 100,000 colony-forming units (cfu) of a single bacteria, or greater than 50,000 cfu of a single bacteria are cultured from a sterile catheter specimen (Dulczak & Kirk, 2005). Urine cultures do not distinguish between upper and lower UTIs (Raszka & Khan, 2005). Antibiotic sensitivity for the specific organisms cultured is then determined.

Radiologic studies may be performed to detect structural abnormalities and renal scarring. The most common tests performed are a renal and bladder ultrasound soon after the diagnosis and a voiding cystourethrogram (VCUG) obtained to test for vesicoureteral reflux (Dulczak & Kirk, 2005). Renal and bladder ultrasound and DMSA scanning are used to detect pyelonephritis and renal scarring (Dulczak & Kirk, 2005).

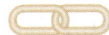

SKILLS 7–7 THROUGH 7–12
Collecting Urine Samples

CLINICAL TIP

Urine obtained from infants using urine collection bags may be used for urinalysis and to screen for UTI, but the specimen collection procedure is not sterile. Confirmation of a UTI must be made with urine collected by a clean-catch or catheterization procedure (Raszka & Khan, 2005).

NURSING ALERT

Urine specimens collected for culture must be delivered to the laboratory within 1 hour or the specimen must be refrigerated to prevent the growth of organisms that occur with prolonged room temperature exposure.

CLINICAL MANIFESTATIONS	URINARY TRACT INFECTIONS	
Type of UTI	**Clinical Manifestations**	**Clinical Therapy**
Lower UTI—cystitis	Frequency, dysuria, urgency, enuresis, strong-smelling urine, cloudy urine, hematuria, abdominal or suprapubic pain.	5- to 7-day course of trimethoprim or sulfamethoxazole or antibiotic matching organism sensitivity, encourage oral fluids, analgesic such as acetaminophen or pyridium.
Upper UTI—pyelonephritis	High fever, chills, abdominal pain, flank pain, costovertebral angle tenderness, persistent vomiting, moderate to severe dehydration. Infants may have nonspecific signs such as poor appetite, failure to thrive, lethargy, irritability. Older children may have signs of cystitis.	Rehydration, antipyretics, IV antibiotics initially, then transitioned to oral antibiotics matching organism sensitivity for a total of 7 to 10 days.

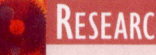

RESEARCH

VUR and Prophylactic Antibiotics

A randomized control trial of 218 children, ages 3 months to 18 years, diagnosed with pyelonephritis and mild or moderate vesicoureteral reflux (VUR) evaluated the effect of prophylactic antibiotics on outcomes. Half the children received antibiotics and the remainder did not. Children were seen every 3 months for the year of the study, and each had a urine culture at each visit. Results indicated that the presence of mild or moderate VUR did not increase the incidence of UTI, pyelonephritis, or renal scarring following an acute episode of pyelonephritis. The children who did not receive prophylactic antibiotics had no more infections or renal scarring than the children who did receive antibiotics (Garin, Olavarria, Nieto et al., 2006).

Clinical Therapy

Antibiotic therapy is begun as soon as urine samples have been collected. Antibiotics are selected based upon the age of the child, sensitivity of the cultured organism, and the child's signs and symptoms. The antibiotic is changed if necessary after culture sensitivity is determined. Follow-up cultures may be obtained 48 to 72 hours after drug therapy has started if the child is still febrile (Raszka & Khan, 2005). Children with pyelonephritis should be maintained on antibiotic prophylaxis until radiologic tests are performed to detect any structural defects.

Children who appear ill and cannot tolerate oral antibiotics are often hospitalized because they need rehydration and parenteral antibiotic treatment until afebrile for 24 hours. Infants may develop permanent kidney damage or generalized sepsis if the UTI is not treated aggressively. If a structural defect is identified, surgical correction may be necessary to prevent recurrent infections that could lead to renal damage.

Follow-up urine cultures should then be obtained according to the frequency specified by agency guidelines. Children with pyelonephritis may have repeat urine cultures monthly for 3 months, every 3 months for 6 months, and then annually. Most reinfections occur within a year, and subsequent infections may be asymptomatic. For children with vesicoureteral reflux or recurrent infections, a long-term, suppressive dose of an antibiotic may be ordered in an attempt to keep the urine sterile and to prevent subsequent pyelonephritis and renal scarring, but there is limited evidence that this is effective (Raszka & Khan, 2005). Children with renal scarring should have their blood pressure monitored.

■ NURSING MANAGEMENT

Nursing Assessment and Diagnosis

Nursing assessment for the child with a suspected UTI involves assessing the infant or child for signs of acute or chronic illness, examining the genitourinary system, and collecting a urine specimen for culture.

Physiologic Assessment

Take a history of urinary symptoms. Assess the infant for toxic (very ill) appearance, fever, and oral fluid intake. Evaluate the child's oral fluid intake. Assess for quality, quantity, and frequency of voiding. Measure the child's height and weight and plot the data on a growth curve to identify any change in growth pattern associated with a chronic illness. Take the infant's or child's blood pressure. Palpate the abdomen and suprapubic and costovertebral areas for masses, tenderness, and distention.

Observe the urinary stream if possible and perform a urinalysis, including specific gravity. Proper collection of the urine specimen is essential. Get a clean-catch urine specimen if the child is able to cooperate. If not, get a catheterized sample. An early morning urine specimen is preferred because the urine is more concentrated.

Psychosocial Assessment

Sexually active adolescents may deny having symptoms because they fear disclosing their sexual activity to their parents. Careful questioning may be necessary to elicit a response despite these concerns. Be open and approachable, and give the patient and family the chance to address their concerns.

Common nursing diagnoses for the child with a UTI include:

- Impaired Urinary Elimination related to recurrent urinary tract infections
- Risk for Disproportionate Growth related to chronic infection and renal damage
- Urinary Retention related to infrequent voiding habits or vesicoureteral reflux
- Ineffective Therapeutic Regimen Management related to lack of knowledge of preventive measures (adequate fluid intake, proper hygiene, signs of infection and prophylactic antibiotics)
- Risk for Deficient Fluid Volume related to fever and inadequate intake

Planning and Implementation

Nursing care for the hospitalized child with a complicated UTI centers on administering prescribed medications, promoting rehydration, assessing renal function, and teaching parents and older children how to minimize the risk of future infection.

Administer antibiotics and antipyretics as prescribed to maintain therapeutic drug levels and reduce fever. Encourage fluid intake to dilute the urine and flush the bladder. Frequent voiding minimizes urinary stasis. Document intake and output. Assess renal function by comparing the child's output to the expected measure of 1 mL/kg/hr and weigh the child daily.

Because bladder training is such an important milestone for young children, any disorder that affects voiding may have developmental implications. A toddler who has been toilet trained may regress and require diapers temporarily due to incontinence related to the UTI. An older child may develop enuresis after a prolonged period of being dry at night. A preschooler may perceive the infection as punishment for an imagined wrong such as masturbation. Reassure parents that this is normal and emphasize that they should offer the child support rather than disapproval.

Care in the Community

Children with UTIs are usually cared for at home. Teach parents that antibiotics must be taken for the full course and that they may be continued even after the symptoms disappear to prevent a recurrence. Teach prevention through proper hygiene and avoidance of risk behaviors. See Families Want to Know: Prevention of Urinary Tract Infections.

Give parents specific guidelines for oral fluid intake. Make sure the amount of fluids recommended for a 24-hour period equals the maintenance fluids needed plus additional fluids required because of fever and diuresis to flush out pathogens (see Chapter 16 ∞). Suggest that the parents avoid giving the child caffeinated and carbonated beverages as these may potentially irritate the bladder mucosa.

Encourage the child to void more frequently even after the infection has cleared. A wristwatch with an alarm may be a helpful reminder. The child with a neurogenic bladder needs to have clean intermittent catheterization performed several times a day to reduce urinary stasis and the potential for UTI.

Teach parents the signs and symptoms of recurrent infection so they can seek care promptly.

Evaluation

Expected outcomes of nursing care include:

- The child increases fluid intake and number of times voiding each day.
- Future UTIs are prevented.

FAMILIES WANT TO KNOW

Prevention of Urinary Tract Infections

- Teach proper perineal hygiene. Girls should always wipe the perineum from front to back after voiding.
- Encourage the child to drink plenty of fluids and avoid long periods of "holding urine."
- Caution against tight underwear; children should wear cotton rather than nylon underwear.
- Encourage the child to void more frequently and to fully empty the bladder.
- Discourage bubble baths, bath oils, and hot tubs, which can irritate the urethra.
- Instruct sexually active adolescent girls to void before and after sexual intercourse to prevent urinary stasis and flush out bacteria introduced during intercourse.

STRUCTURAL DEFECTS OF THE URINARY SYSTEM
Obstructive Uropathy

Obstructive uropathy refers to structural or functional abnormalities of the urinary system that interfere with urine flow. The pressure caused by urine backup compromises kidney function and often causes hydronephrosis. Physiologic changes that may occur as a result of hydronephrosis include:

- Cessation of glomerular filtration when the pressure in the kidney pelvis equals the filtration pressure in the glomerular capillaries. To compensate, the blood pressure increases to increase the glomerular filtration pressure. However, increasing pressure on the glomeruli leads to cell death.
- Metabolic acidosis results when the distal nephrons' ability to secrete hydrogen ions is impaired.
- Impairment of the kidney's ability to concentrate urine results in polydipsia and polyuria.
- Obstruction results in urinary stasis, promoting bacterial growth.
- Restriction of urinary outflow causes progressive renal damage and chronic renal failure if untreated.

Obstructive uropathy may be caused by several congenital lesions such as ureteropelvic junction obstruction, posterior urethral valves, and stenosis or hypoplasia of the ureterovesicular junction (Figure 25–5 ➤).

- The ureteropelvic junction (UPJ), the tapered point where the renal pelvis transitions to the ureter, is the most common site of obstruction of the upper urinary tract in infants and children.
- Posterior urethral valves (PUV), abnormal folds of mucosa in the male urethra, are the most common cause of anatomic bladder outlet obstruction, occurring in approximately 1 in 5000 to 8000 live male births (Vogt, 2002).
- Stenosis of the distal ureter at the ureterovesicular junction leads to dilation of the entire ureter, renal pelvis, and kidney (Huether, 2006).
- Other conditions that can lead to hydronephrosis include prune-belly syndrome, myelomeningocele and neoplasms. See Box 25–1 for information on prune-belly syndrome.

See the clinical manifestations table on the next page for the differing signs and symptoms of obstructive uropathy by location.

Early diagnosis and treatment is needed to prevent kidney damage and deterioration of renal function. Prenatal ultrasound may detect hydronephrosis and PUV. A diuretic enhanced radionuclide scan and voiding cystourethrogram are performed when UPJ or ureterovesicular obstruction is suspected. See page 976–977 for diagnostic tests commonly used to identify urinary tract conditions.

The goals of surgical correction or diversion are to lower the pressure within the collecting system, which reduces renal damage, and to prevent stasis, which decreases the risk of infection. Surgical correction may necessitate **pyeloplasty** (removal of an obstructed segment of the ureter and reimplantation into the renal pelvis) or valve repair or reconstruction, depending on the cause of the obstruction. Urinary incontinence resulting from sphincter weakness is a common problem after surgery. Urinary diversion may be performed in conditions such as meningomyelocele and prune-belly syndrome.

Nursing Management

Preoperative nursing care focuses on preparing the parents and child for the diagnostic testing and the surgical procedure, as well as addressing parents' concerns about the postsurgical outcome. Give parents a chance to discuss concerns about how the disorder will affect the child's long-term renal functioning.

Postoperative care involves monitoring vital signs and intake and output and observing for signs of urine retention, such as decreased output and bladder distention. Many children are discharged with stents or catheters. Teach parents how to change

---

BOX 25–1
PRUNE-BELLY SYNDROME

Prune-belly syndrome, also known as Eagle–Barrett syndrome, is another cause of hydronephrosis. In this congenital defect, the abdominal musculature fails to develop. The skin covering the abdominal wall is thin and resembles a wrinkled prune. Urinary tract anomalies include a large bladder without muscle tone, vesicoureteral reflux, and renal dysplasia. Because of the lack of muscular development, ureters become dilated and hydronephrosis develops, making the infant at high risk for recurrent urinary tract infection (Palmer, 2003). Prune-belly syndrome occurs predominantly in males (95%), with an incidence of 1 in 35,000 to 50,000 births (Vogt, 2002).

PATHOPHYSIOLOGY ILLUSTRATED

Obstruction Sites

Stenosis of the ureteropelvic valve

Stenosis of the ureterovesicular junction

Stenosis of the posterior urethral valve

Kidney

Ureter

Bladder

Urethra

Figure 25–5 ➤ The common sites of obstruction in the upper and lower urinary tract. Why would damage from posterior urethral valves potentially be worse than other obstructions? Upper urinary tract infections are often unilateral. Renal failure is most likely to occur when both kidneys are affected by hydronephrosis.

dressings, double diaper, care for catheters, assess pain and give analgesics, and recognize signs of possible obstruction or infection. Parents should encourage the child to participate in age-appropriate activities. However, children should avoid contact sports because of their potential to injure the bladder.

Hypospadias and Epispadias

Hypospadias and epispadias are congenital anomalies involving the abnormal location of the urethral meatus in males (Figure 25–6 ➤). Both defects result when the urethral

CLINICAL MANIFESTATIONS	OBSTRUCTIVE LESIONS OF THE URINARY SYSTEM
Obstructive Lesion	**Clinical Manifestations**
Ureteropelvic junction obstruction	In infants: abdominal mass (enlarged kidney), hypertension, urinary tract infection In children: hematuria, pain, intermittent nausea and vomiting
Posterior urethral valves	In infants: abdominal mass (enlarged kidney), distended bladder, poor urinary stream, urinary tract infection, sepsis, low specific gravity, polyuria, increased creatinine level, failure to thrive In children: urinary frequency and incontinence
Ureterovesicular junction obstruction	Urinary tract infection (recurrent or chronic), hematuria, pain, abdominal mass (enlarged kidney), enuresis

Figure 25–6 ➤ Hypospadias and epispadias. A, In hypospadias, the urethral canal is open on the ventral surface of the penis. B, In epispadias, the canal is open on the dorsal surface.

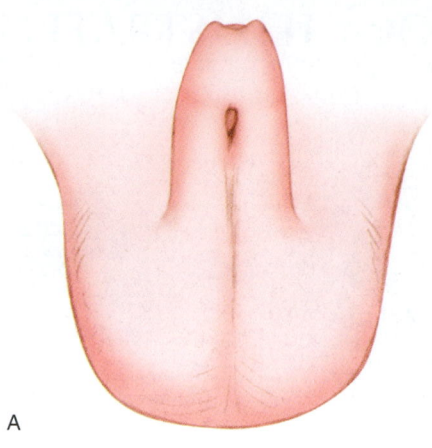
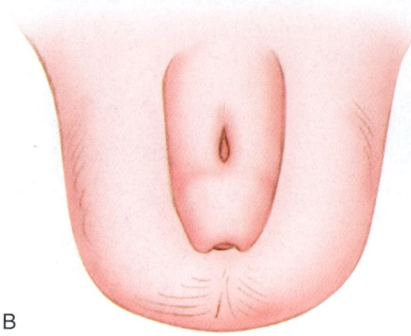

A   B

folds fail to fuse completely over the urethral groove. The reported incidence of hypospadias is 1 in every 125 live male births (Stokowski, 2004). The incidence of epispadias is 1 in 40,000 to 118,000 live births (Huether, 2006).

With hypospadias, the urethral meatus can be located anywhere along the course of the urethra on the ventral or undersurface of the penile shaft, from the perineum to the tip of the glans. Most cases are mild, with the meatus slightly off center from the tip of the penis; in severe cases, the meatus is located on the scrotum. Hypospadias often occurs in conjunction with congenital **chordee**, a shortage of skin on the ventral side of the penis that causes the penis to bow. Associated defects may include undescended testes and partial absence of the foreskin (Huether, 2006).

In epispadias, the meatal opening is located on the dorsal surface of the penile shaft. The opening may be small or a fissure may extend the entire length of the penis. Epispadias and exstrophy of the bladder are the same condition, but epispadias is the milder expression of the condition (Huether, 2006). See section on exstrophy of the bladder on the next page.

Diagnosis is made by prenatal ultrasound or by examination at birth. The infant should not be circumcised because the dorsal foreskin tissue may be used for surgical repair.

The defects are corrected surgically, usually during the first year of life, to minimize psychologic effects when the child is older. Surgery is usually performed in a single operation, often as an outpatient procedure. The goals of surgical repair are:

- Placement of the urethral meatus at the end of the glans penis with satisfactory caliber and configuration for a urinary stream (enabling the child to void in a standing position)
- Release of chordee to straighten the penis (enabling future sexual function).

A caudal nerve block is often used for postoperative pain relief. Anticholinergic medications may be prescribed to relieve bladder spasms.

Nursing Management

It is important to address parents' concerns at the time of birth. Preoperative teaching can relieve some of their anxiety about the future appearance and functioning of the penis.

Postoperative care focuses on protecting the surgical site from injury. The infant or child returns from surgery with the penis wrapped in a simple dressing, and sometimes a urethral **stent** (a device used to maintain patency of the urethral canal) is placed to keep the new urethral canal open. Fresh blood may be seen on the dressing and in the stent during the immediate postoperative period, but the urine should become less bloody over a few hours. Plan care to ensure that the stent does not get removed. Refer to the hospital's policy for the appropriate use of immobilizers in this situation.

SKILL 4–6
Applying Elbow Immobilizers

Encourage fluid intake to maintain adequate urinary output and patency of the stent. Begin with clear liquids or breast milk. Other infants may start with half strength formula and progress to full strength formula as tolerated. Hourly documentation of intake and output is essential. Notify the physician if there is no urine drainage for 1 hour as this may indicate obstruction.

Pain may be associated with bladder spasms. Anticholinergic medications such as oxybutynin or hyoscyamine may be prescribed. Ibuprofen or acetaminophen may also be given for pain. Antibiotics are often prescribed until the urinary stent falls out.

Patients are often discharged the day of surgery. Discharge teaching should include instructions for parents about care of the reconstructed area, double diapering to protect the stent, fluid intake, medication administration, and signs and symptoms of infection (Figure 25–7 ➤). Tell parents when the child needs to see the physician for dressing removal. See Families Want to Know: Caring for the Child After Hypospadias and Epispadias Repair.

Bladder Exstrophy

Bladder exstrophy is a rare defect in which the posterior bladder wall extrudes through the lower abdominal wall (Figure 25–8 ➤). Failure of the abdominal wall to close during fetal development results in eversion and protuberance of the bladder wall and a wide separation of the rectus muscles and the symphysis pubis. The upper urinary tract is usually normal. The defect occurs in approximately 1 in every 400,000 live births and is five times more common in boys than girls (Huether, 2006).

The bladder mucosa appears as a mass of bright red tissue, and urine continually leaks from the ureters onto the skin. Females have a bifid (split) clitoris. Males have a short, stubby penis, and the glans is flattened with dorsal chordee and a ventral prepuce. Epispadias and undescended testes (see page 1018) occur with this disorder in males. Inguinal hernias may develop in both males and females (Leung, Robson, & Wong, 2005).

FAMILIES WANT TO KNOW

Caring for the Child After Hypospadias and Epispadias Repair

- A double diapering technique protects the urinary stent after surgery for hypospadias or epispadias repair. The inner diaper collects stool; the outer diaper, urine (Figure 25–7). Make sure the penis is flat against the abdomen when putting on the diaper, and wrap the diaper tightly. Make sure the catheter or stent is not kinked.

- Restrict the infant or toddler from activities (e.g., playing on riding toys) that put pressure on the surgical site. Do not hold the infant or child straddled on the hip. Limit the child's activity for 2 weeks.
- Sponge bathe the child until the catheter has been removed.
- Note that the urine will be blood tinged for several days.
- Provide pain medication (ibuprofen or acetaminophen) with food or milk as prescribed.
- Encourage the infant or toddler to drink fluids to ensure adequate hydration. Provide fluids in a pleasant environment or using a special cup. Offer fruit juice, fruit-flavored ice pops, fruit-flavored juices, flavored ice cubes, and gelatin.
- Be sure to give the complete course of prescribed antibiotics to avoid infection.
- Call the physician for any of the following concerns:
  - A swollen or discolored penis
  - Redness, swelling, or drainage around the incision
  - A large amount of bright red bleeding
  - Urine coming from any place except the end of the catheter
  - Fever that does not go down when the child is given acetaminophen

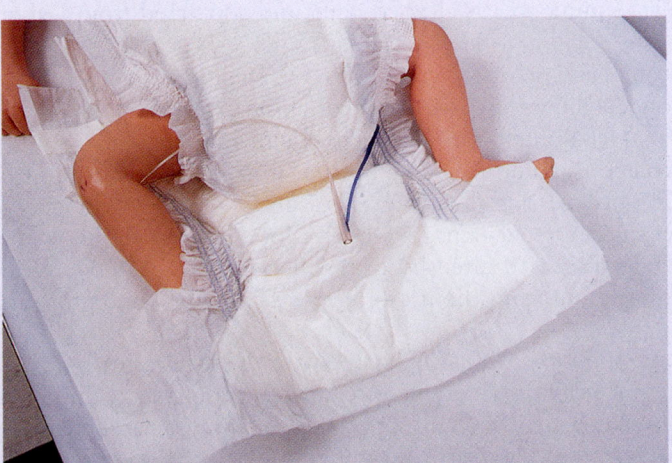

Figure 25–7 ➤ In double diapering, the inner diaper collects stool and the outer diaper collects urine from the draining stent.

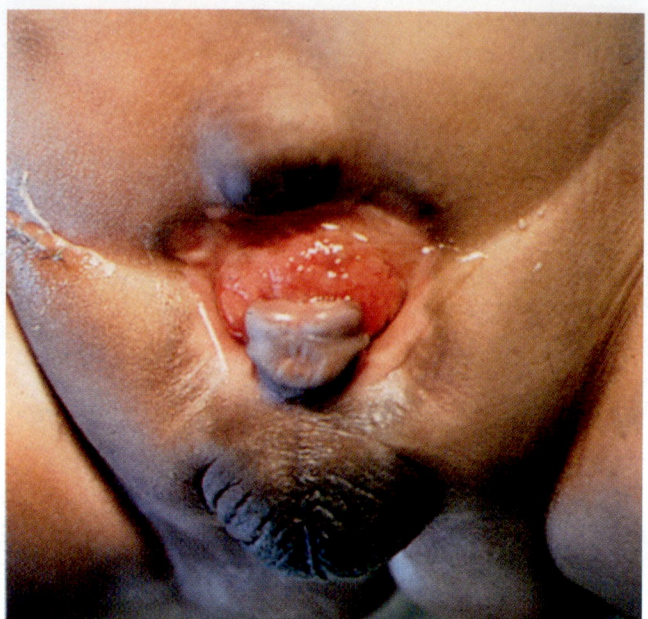

Figure 25–8 ▶ This child has bladder exstrophy, noted by extrusion of the posterior bladder wall through the lower abdominal wall.

Prenatal diagnosis may be made with ultrasound. Diagnosis is also made at the time of birth based on physical appearance. A renal ultrasound is used to identify hydronephrosis or other renal abnormalities.

The exposed bladder tissue is covered with plastic wrap until surgery is performed to reduce the exposure to air and infectious organisms. Surgical reconstruction is performed in several stages. Primary closure of the bladder and abdominal wall is usually completed within 24 to 48 hours after birth. The wound and pelvis are immobilized to promote healing. An osteotomy (see Chapter 28 ∞) to rotate the innominate bones of the pelvis to approximate the symphysis pubis reduces tension on the closed bladder and abdominal wall to promote healing. Epispadias repair is often performed at age 1 to 2 years or at the same time as a surgical procedure to improve continence. Surgery to reconstruct the bladder neck and reimplant the ureters is performed when the bladder has achieved capacity of at least 60 mL (Leung, Robson, & Wong, 2005). The goals of surgical reconstruction include:

- Closure of the bladder and abdominal wall
- Urinary continence, with preservation of renal function
- Creation of functional and normal-appearing genitalia
- Improvement of sexual functioning

Some children require permanent urinary diversion because a functional bladder cannot be reconstructed.

Following surgical reconstruction, a voiding cystourethrogram is used to evaluate for vesicoureteral reflux. Regular urinalysis should be performed to detect urinary tract infections. Because the bladder epithelium is abnormal, it is prone to neoplasms. Periodic examination and cystoscopy after the age of 20 years is recommended to detect malignancies.

Nursing Management

The newborn with exposed bladder tissue on the abdomen is assessed for other obvious defects such as epispadias or ambiguous genitalia. The skin surface around the exposed bladder is assessed for excoriation due to leaking urine and covered with plastic wrap for protection from the diaper. The parents are assessed for their response to the infant with a congenital defect and their need for psychosocial support.

Preoperative nursing care centers on preventing infection and trauma to the exposed bladder. The bladder mucosa is covered in sterile plastic wrap to prevent trauma and irritation, and the surrounding area is cleaned daily and protected from leaking urine with a skin sealant.

Postoperatively the wound and pelvis are immobilized to facilitate healing. Internal and external immobilization techniques are used for pelvic closure (see Chapter 28 ∞). Avoid abduction of the infant's legs. Nursing care includes maintaining proper alignment, monitoring peripheral circulation, and providing meticulous wound and skin care.

Monitor renal function by assessing the adequacy of urine output and blood and urine chemistries to detect signs of renal damage. Observe for any signs of obstruction in the drainage tubes such as increased intensity of bladder spasms, decreased urine output, or urine or blood draining from the urethral meatus. Promote comfort and give antibiotics as ordered.

Parents need emotional support to help them cope with the disfiguring nature of the infant's defect and the uncertainty of complete repair. To promote parent–infant bonding, encourage parents to participate in all aspects of the infant's care, including bathing, feeding, and wound care. Discharge teaching should include instructions about dressing changes and diapering, and the need to immediately report any signs of infection or change in renal function. Emphasize the need for routine follow-up visits after surgery to assess urinary function and to ensure that the next stages of surgery for continence control are performed at the appropriate time in the child's development. However, these children do not always achieve continence. Parents need help to promote the child's self-esteem and self-confidence with sexual identity and function. Psychologic counseling may help the child during adolescence.

ENURESIS

Enuresis is repeated involuntary voiding by a child old enough that bladder control is expected, usually about 5 to 6 years of age. (See Table 25–1 for bladder control milestones.) Enuresis can occur either at night (nocturnal), during the day (diurnal), or both night and day. Nocturnal enuresis accounts for approximately 50% of cases and occurs more often in boys than in girls, with 3.5:1 ratio, whereas diurnal enuresis is more common in girls. Enuresis can be primary, intermittent, or secondary. In primary enuresis the child has never had a dry night. It is thought to be due to a maturational delay and small functional bladder, not stress or a psychologic cause. In intermittent enuresis the child has occasional nights or periods of dryness. With secondary enuresis a child who has been reliably dry for 6 to 12 months begins bed-wetting. It is associated with stress, infections, and sleep disorders. Between 5 to 7 million children older than 5 years (or 5% of school-aged children) have primary nocturnal enuresis (Mercer, 2003; Nield, & Kamat, 2004). Approximately 10% of children with enuresis experience both day and night wetting (Nield, & Kamat, 2004)

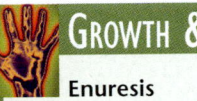

GROWTH & DEVELOPMENT

Enuresis

An estimated 15–20% of children who are partially toilet trained will continue to have wetting episodes after 5 years of age. An estimated 45% of 7- to 10-year-olds and 2.8% of 11- to 12-year-olds continue to have nocturnal enuresis more than once a week (Nield & Kamat, 2004).

Epidemiology and Pathophysiology

Enuresis may result from neurologic or congenital structural disorders, illness, or stress. Nocturnal enuresis occurs frequently in children whose parents, siblings, and other relatives have a history of bedwetting (Huether, 2006). In most children with primary enuresis, the bladder has a smaller functional capacity, and neuromuscular maturation of the inhibitory fibers is delayed. Often children with nocturnal enuresis are harder to arouse and may fail to respond to full bladder signals. Some children may produce more urine and exceed the functional bladder capacity due to a lack of circadian rhythm of vasopressin that helps concentrate the urine during sleep (Nield & Kamat, 2004). Some children with daytime enuresis may have **dysfunctional voiding**, an abnormality in the storage or emptying phase of urination (Berry, 2005). Minor abnormalities of the bladder neck and urethra are also associated with enuresis. Some children are believed to have mild developmental delays. Children with obstructive sleep apnea have a higher rate of enuresis (Brooks & Topol, 2003). The majority of cases are not associated with structural or neurologic pathology.

Table 25–1	MILESTONES IN THE DEVELOPMENT OF BLADDER CONTROL

Age	Developmental Milestone
1 1/2 years	Child passes urine at regular intervals.
2 years	Child announces when he or she is voiding.
2 1/2 years	Child makes known need to void; can hold urine.
3 years	Child goes to the bathroom by himself or herself; holds urge if preoccupied with play.
2 1/2–3 1/2 years	Child achieves nighttime bladder and bowel control.
4 years	Child shows great interest in going to bathrooms when away from home (shopping centers, movies).
5 years	Child voids approximately seven times a day; prefers privacy; is able to initiate emptying of bladder at any degree of fullness.

Clinical Manifestations

Children with diurnal enuresis may have frequency, urgency, constant dribbling, and involuntary loss of control after voiding. Children with nocturnal enuresis have bedwetting.

■ COLLABORATIVE CARE

Diagnostic Tests

Urinalysis on the first voided specimen is performed. The specific gravity provides information about the child's ability to concentrate the urine. Screening for a UTI with dipsticks is performed. Diabetes mellitus, diabetes insipidus, or renal insufficiency should be ruled out in children with both enuresis and polyuria or oliguria. The child's functional bladder capacity may be measured. Bladder sonography to measure residual urine after voiding and uroflow (the rate of urine flow) measurement are sometimes performed, but are not considered essential (Nield & Kamat, 2004).

A thorough history can help identify potential causes of enuresis (Box 25–2). Enuretic children often have a history of constipation. Rectal pressure on the posterior bladder wall stimulates the bladder to empty.

The child's lower spine is examined for fistulas, sacral dimples, or tufts of hair that could be signs of occult spina bifida. Prolonged hospitalization, family stressors, and preoccupation with school concerns also have been associated with secondary enuresis.

Clinical Therapy

A multitreatment approach is usually most effective. Fluid restriction, bladder training, and enuresis alarms are common approaches (Table 25–2). A spontaneous cure happens in 15% of children each year, regardless of intervention or lack of intervention.

BOX 25–2
QUESTIONS TO ASK WHEN TAKING AN ENURESIS HISTORY

Family History

Is there a family history of renal or urinary structural abnormalities?
Is there a family history of bedwetting?

Family Management

How serious is the problem for the family?
What happens when the child wets? (Who gets up and changes sheets?)
How is the child treated? Is the child punished or blamed for wetting?
What remedies have been tried?

Toilet Training

Did the child have a difficult time with toilet training?
What method of toilet training did you use? When was toilet training initiated?
What are the child's current voiding and stooling patterns?
How long is the child's longest dry period, and when does it occur?
Does the child have a history of constipation or encopresis?

Stressors

How is the child doing in school? How are relationships with peers?
Are there any changes in the home, such as a new sibling or death in the family?
Are any new or chronic stressors present in the child's life?
How does the problem interfere with play and other activities?

Risk Factors

Diabetes
- Does the child void often or have urgency?
- Is the child frequently thirsty?

Urinary Tract Infection
- Does the child experience burning on urination?
- Has the child had a urinary tract infection before?

Table 25–2	TREATMENT APPROACHES FOR ENURESIS
Approach	**Description**
Fluid restriction	Fluid intake is limited in the evening and before the child goes to bed.
Bladder exercises	The child drinks a large amount and then holds urine as long as he or she can. The child practices stopping voiding midstream. Exercises should continue for at least 6 months.
Timed voiding	The child with diurnal enuresis is instructed to void every 2 hours and to use a double voiding pattern; this trains the bladder to empty completely and avoid overdistention.
Enuresis alarms	A detector strip is attached to the child's pants. The alarm sounds a buzzer that alerts the child when wetting occurs, so the child can get up and finish voiding in the bathroom. This works best for children over 7 years old, and takes 3 to 4 months for success.
Reward system	Set realistic goals for the child and reinforce dry days or nights with stars and stickers on a chart.
Medications	Imipramine is prescribed nightly for 2 to 4 months and then tapered over several months to reduce the rate of relapse. It is effective in 50–70% of children. Desmopressin is prescribed to children with nocturnal enuresis for special events such as camp or sleepovers. Oxybutynin is used for diurnal enuresis to relieve urgency and frequency from bladder irritability.

Some children with nocturnal enuresis are treated with medications.

- Imipramine, a tricyclic antidepressant, is often used but requires close monitoring because of its effects on mood and sleep-arousal patterns and the associated danger of overdoses.
- Desmopressin, given as a nasal spray or oral tablet, has an antidiuretic effect but is not used long term because of its expense. It is usually reserved for times when the child is away from home for a short period (e.g., sleepovers or camp).
- Oxybutinin, an anticholinergic medication, is used for children with urgency or an overactive detrusor muscle.

Relapse often occurs when medications are stopped.

NURSING MANAGEMENT
Nursing Assessment and Diagnosis

Nurses assist in the evaluation of the child with enuresis, obtaining much of the history listed in Box 25–2. A review of the child's elimination patterns and developmental milestones and the parents' methods of toilet training are also essential information. Identify how many bathroom breaks are given during the day at school and if the child uses them. If the child does not use the bathroom at school, identify the reasons. Assess for associated conditions by examining the child's lower spine for fistulas, sacral dimples, or tufts of hair that could be signs of occult spina bifida.

Assess the child's and family's feelings and frustrations about the problem of bedwetting and their motivation to implement therapies.

Nursing diagnoses that apply to the child with enuresis may include:

- Impaired Urinary Elimination related to inability to control voiding during the day or at night
- Overflow urinary incontinence related to ignoring urge to void during activities

COMPLEMENTARY THERAPY

Biofeedback and Enuresis

Biofeedback is a complementary therapy that may be used for some cases of enuresis when the child and parents are highly motivated. In the case of bladder sphincter dysfunction, when the pelvic floor muscles contract during voiding, the child may have urgency and frequency associated with daytime or nighttime enuresis. During biofeedback training, the child learns to identify the differences in relaxation and contraction of the bladder muscles, as well as straining. They then learn to sustain and maintain a relaxed pelvic floor and voluntary sphincter opening (Liberti, 2005).

- Risk for Situational Low Self-Esteem related to embarrassment over lack of bladder control
- Readiness for Enhanced Knowledge (enuresis management) related to motivation of the child.

Planning and Implementation

Teach the child and parents about the physiologic development of bladder control and causes and treatment of enuresis. Explore feelings of guilt or blame. Make sure the parents are aware that the child cannot control the wetting. Psychosocial support is an essential part of care since stress is an important cause of secondary enuresis. Provide emotional support to the parents and child, and encourage the child's participation in the treatment plan. Refer the child for counseling or therapy, if appropriate.

Assess the parents' and child's motivation and readiness for interventions. The child needs to be an active participant in the treatment plan for daytime or nighttime wetting. For daytime wetting, the child may need a reminder to go to the bathroom such as a vibrating watch. A discussion with the child's teacher may make it possible for the child to have additional or private bathroom breaks.

Before parents buy an enuresis alarm, suggest that the alarm clock be used in the child's room for several nights to see if the child will arouse. The child may need the parent's help to arouse initially. Find out whether the child shares a room with others who will be disturbed by the alarm. Ask if the child and parents are willing to persist with an enuresis alarm, as it may take months to work.

Encourage children and parents who are frustrated by how long it takes to see progress. Remind the child that it takes practice and hard work to be good at tasks such as sports or learning to ride a bicycle. Involve the child in bedding changes, but do not make it a punishment. Help parents think of ways to reduce the work of bedding changes, such as disposable underpads. The child may want to consider using pull-ups for sleepovers or family vacations, when changing wet bedding is a problem (Bennett, 2005).

Evaluation

Evaluation of nursing care may include

- The child and family choose one or more interventions that prefer and they persist in using them.
- The child has an increased number of dry nights.

RENAL DISORDERS

Nephrotic Syndrome

Nephrotic syndrome does not refer to a specific disease, but rather to a clinical state characterized by edema, massive proteinuria, hypoalbuminemia, hypoproteinemia, hyperlipidemia, and altered immunity. Congenital nephrotic (CNF) syndrome, an autosomal recessive disorder, is extremely rare. The CNF gene is localized on chromosome 19 (Huether, 2006). Primary nephrotic syndrome results from a disease that affects only the kidney, such as glomerulonephritis.

Approximately 90% of children with nephrotic syndrome have a type of primary disease called minimal change nephrotic syndrome (MCNS) that is steroid-responsive (Ruth, Kemper, Leumann et al., 2005). MCNS usually occurs in children between the ages of 2 and 7 years, with an incidence of 2 per 100,000 children, and it is more common in males than females. African American and Hispanic children experience a greater incidence of nephrotic syndrome, and the disorder in these children is more virulent, progresses more rapidly to renal failure, and has a poorer prognosis (Robinson, Nahata, Mahan et al., 2003). MCNS derives its name from the normal or only minimally changed appearance of the glomeruli on light microscopic evaluation. Because MCNS is the most common form of nephrotic syndrome, it is the focus of the following discussion.

Etiology and Pathophysiology

The cause of primary MCNS is unknown, but an immune system role is strongly suspected as an upper respiratory infection often precedes the onset of edema by 2 to 3 days (Robinson et al., 2003). The mechanism of increased glomerular permeability is unknown; however, it may be related to the release of permeability factors from abnormal circulating T cells and the loss of a negative charge in the glomerular capillary wall (Huether, 2006). In MCNS, increased permeability of the glomerular membrane permits large, negatively charged molecules such as albumin to pass through the membrane and be excreted in the urine. Proteinuria results in decreased oncotic pressure and edema, because fluid remains in the interstitial spaces instead of being pulled back into the vascular compartment (Robinson et al., 2003). Immunoglobulins are lost, resulting in altered immunity. Loss of protein in the urine, as well as insufficient albumin production by the liver and a decreased albumin concentration as a result of salt and water retention by the kidney, contribute to hypoalbuminemia. Hypercoagulability occurs because of loss of antithrombin III in the urine and reduced levels of factors IX, XI, and XII. The liver, stimulated perhaps by hypoalbuminemia or decreased osmotic pressure, responds by increasing synthesis of lipoprotein, resulting in hyperlipidemia. Acute renal failure is a rare complication of MCNS, most likely due to changes in glomerular permeability (Walle, Mauel, Raes et al., 2004).

Clinical Manifestations

In most children, edema develops gradually over several weeks. Children may have a history of periorbital edema on waking that resolves during the day as fluid shifts to the abdomen and lower extremities. Other signs include snug fit of clothing and shoes, pallor, hypertension, irritability, anorexia, hematuria, decreased urine output, and nonspecific malaise. The child's urine may be frothy or foamy. Parents often do not seek medical treatment until generalized edema develops on the child's extremities, abdomen, or genitals (Figure 25–9 ▶). Respiratory distress from pleural effusion may occur in some cases.

Massive edema resulting in a dramatic weight gain and abdominal pain, with or without vomiting, may occur, depending on the amount of albumin lost and the amount of sodium ingested. The child becomes malnourished as a result of protein loss in the urine. The skin is pale and shiny with prominent veins, and the hair becomes more brittle. An increased risk of thrombosis is present.

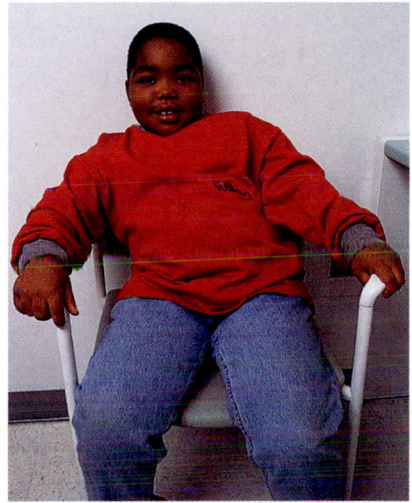

Figure 25–9 ▶ This boy has generalized edema, a characteristic finding in nephrotic syndrome.

COLLABORATIVE CARE

Diagnostic Tests

Diagnosis is based on the history, characteristic symptoms, and laboratory findings. Urinalysis as well as serum albumin, sodium, BUN, cholesterol, and electrolytes are ordered. Hypoalbuminemia of less than 25 g/L and urinary protein excretion of greater than or equal to 40 mg/m^2/hour are the criteria for diagnosing nephrotic syndrome in childhood (Ruth, Kemper, Leumann et al., 2005). Microscopic hematuria may also be present. Renal ultrasound may be performed to detect structural kidney problems.

Diagnostic testing for a relapse is the presence of 2+ proteinuria by dipstick testing for 3 consecutive days (Ruth, Kemper, Leumann et al., 2005).

Clinical Therapy

Children may be hospitalized when severe edema or a major infection is present, but are usually treated as outpatients. Clinical therapy focuses on decreasing proteinuria, relieving edema, managing associated symptoms, improving nutrition, and preventing infection. A corticosteroid (such as prednisone) is prescribed to decrease proteinuria. In most children, urine protein levels fall to trace or negative values within 2 to 3 weeks of the start of therapy. Children who respond successfully to therapy continue to take corticosteroids daily for 6 weeks, and then take 6 weeks of alternate-day treatment. Approximately 90% of children experience complete remission with corticosteroid therapy.

CLINICAL TIP

A protein-to-creatinine (PR/CR) ratio of the first morning void is used to estimate protein excretion in children because of the challenges in obtaining 24-hour urines. Normal PR/CR ratios are less than 0.2 in children over 2 years and less than 0.5 in children 6 months to 24 months of age (Hogg, Furth, Lemley et al., 2003).

Relapses occur in up to 70% of children, and are often associated with a respiratory infection or live virus immunization. Relapses may become less frequent during adolescence; however, long-term studies have revealed that many adults continue to have relapses (Fakhouri, Bocquet, Taupin et al., 2003; Ruth, Kemper, Leumann et al., 2005).

Children who have a relapse after drug therapy is discontinued get repeat therapy. Other medications used include diuretics, antihypertensive agents, and antibiotics. Immunosuppressive or immunomodulator medications, including cyclophosphamide, chlorabucil, cyclosporine, or levamisole, are steroid-sparing agents that may be used when children with nephrotic syndrome frequently relapse (Fakhouri, Bocquet, Taupin et al., 2003). Since diuretics can precipitate hypovolemia, hyponatremia, and hypokalemia, electrolyte levels should be carefully monitored. Intravenous administration of albumin may occasionally be ordered in the child with massive edema who is resistant to diuretics (Robinson et al., 2003). Analgesics may be ordered for pain related to edema or flank pain from a urinary tract infection.

A normal diet for the child's age is recommended. No attempt should be made either to restrict or to increase protein intake. A "no added salt" diet is recommended during corticosteroid treatment as these children have an elevated total body sodium even though serum sodium concentrations are low (Hogg, Portman, Milliner et al., 2000).

NURSING MANAGEMENT
Nursing Assessment and Diagnoses
Physiologic Assessment

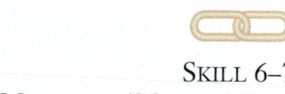
SKILL 6–7
Measuring Abdominal Girth

Careful assessment of the child's hydration status and edema is essential. Carefully monitor intake and output. Weigh the child daily using the same scale, and measure abdominal girth to monitor changes in edema and ascites (see Figure 16–14 ∞ on page 516). Monitor vital signs every 4 hours to watch for signs of respiratory distress, hypertension, or circulatory overload. Test urine for proteinuria and specific gravity at least once each shift. Assess for hypovolemia during periods of diuresis. Assess for skin breakdown.

Psychosocial Assessment

Children and parents are often fearful or anxious on admission. Because edema often develops gradually, parents may feel guilty if they did not seek medical attention immediately. School-age children with generalized edema are often concerned about their appearance. Careful questioning may be necessary to elicit these concerns. The child hospitalized for a recurrence of nephrotic syndrome may be frustrated or depressed. Assess individual and family coping mechanisms, support systems, and level of stress.

Common nursing diagnoses for the child with MCNS include:

- Risk for Infection related to immunosuppressive therapy
- Risk for Impaired Skin Integrity related to edema, lowered resistance to infection and injury, immobility, and malnutrition
- Excess Fluid Volume related to renal dysfunction and sodium retention
- Imbalanced Nutrition: Less than Body Requirements related to loss of appetite and protein loss in urine
- Fatigue related to fluid and electrolyte imbalance, albumin loss, altered nutrition, and renal failure
- Deficient Diversional Activity related to fatigue, immobility, and social isolation

Planning and Implementation

Nursing care is mainly supportive and focuses on administering medications, preventing infection, preventing skin breakdown, meeting nutritional and fluid needs, promoting rest, and providing emotional support to the parents and child.

Administer Medications

It is important to give prescribed medications at the scheduled times. Watch for side effects of corticosteroids such as moon face, increased appetite, increased hair growth, abdominal distention, and mood swings, as well as adverse effects such as hypertension, nausea, and hyperglycemia. An evaluation of fasting blood sugar may be needed during therapy. If the child is receiving albumin intravenously, monitor closely for hypertension or signs of volume overload caused by fluid shifts. If diuretics are used, observe for shock. The child may need to have albumin infused simultaneously with diuretics.

Prevent Infection

Children with MCNS are at risk for infection because of the loss of immunoglobulins in the urine and corticosteroid therapy. Careful hand hygiene is important. Use standard precautions. Strict aseptic technique is essential during invasive procedures. Monitor the child's white blood cell count when cytotoxic drugs are given as bone marrow suppression is a side effect. Monitor vital signs carefully to detect early signs of infection that may be masked by corticosteroid therapy. Decrease the child's social contacts during immunosuppressive treatment, and caution parents and children to avoid exposure to people with respiratory infections and communicable diseases. Emphasize the importance of avoiding shopping malls, sporting arenas, grocery stores, game stores, and other public areas where the risk of exposure to such infections is increased.

Prevent Skin Breakdown

Meticulous skin care is essential to prevent skin breakdown and potential infection. Assess the skin repeatedly, turn the child frequently, and use therapeutic mattresses (e.g., egg crate, airflow) to help prevent skin breakdown. Keep the skin clean and dry.

Meet Nutritional and Fluid Needs

Keep the child's food preferences in mind when planning menus. Encourage the child to eat by presenting attractive meals with small portions. Socialization during meals may improve the child's appetite. Fluids are not usually restricted except during severe edema.

Promote Rest

Provide opportunities for quiet play as tolerated, such as drawing, playing board games, listening to tapes, and watching videos. Adjust the child's daily schedule to allow rest periods after activities. Signs of fatigue may include irritability, mood swings, or withdrawal. Tell the parents and child about the importance of rest. Limiting visitors during the acute phase of the illness may be necessary. Telephone and computer contacts may be encouraged as an alternative to visitors. To provide a sense of control, encourage the child to set his or her own limits on activity.

Provide Emotional Support

Parents and children often need support to cope with this chronic disease. Thoroughly explain the child's disease and treatment regimen to parents. Parental anxiety in combination with the hospitalization may interfere with the child's independence. Help parents promote the child's independence by allowing the child to choose from the menu or to select the daily activity schedule. This gives the child some sense of control.

Children with MCNS may have a distorted body image because of sudden weight gain and edema. They may refuse to look in the mirror, refuse to participate in care, and take less interest in their appearance. Encourage children to express their feelings. Help them maintain a normal appearance by promoting normal grooming routines. Encourage children to wear their own pajamas rather than hospital gowns. Scarves or hats may be used to lessen the child's edematous appearance. Adolescents can be encouraged to write their feelings in a journal as a coping mechanism. These children may have a long-term psychosocial adjustment since they have a chronic condition with concerns about potential relapse (Ruth, Landolt, Neuhaus et al., 2004).

Discharge Planning and Home Care Teaching

Explain the disease process, prognosis, and treatment plan to parents and school-age children. Make sure parents know how to administer medications and can identify potential side effects. Inform parents about restricting fluid intake until the edema resolves.

Instruct parents about the need to monitor urine daily for protein, and have them keep a diary to record the results. Monitoring the child's weight each week may help identify early stages of fluid retention. This helps parents to spot a relapse before edema occurs.

Tutoring may be required for a short period after discharge. However, encourage parents to allow the child to return to normal activities once the acute episode has resolved. Emphasize the importance of avoiding contact with people with infectious diseases, because of the child's reduced immunity. Reinforce to parents that it is important to follow the "no added salt" diet as long as the child is receiving corticosteroid therapy or shows signs of MCNS. Warn them that steroids stimulate appetite, so they need to control the child's food intake and weight gain. No live immunizations should be given to the child who is relapsing or taking corticosteroid therapy. Withhold immunizations until 6 months after the completion of corticosteroid therapy. Although immunizations may trigger a relapse, pneumococcal vaccine and other immunizations are important to protect the child from serious preventable infections.

Most children do well with corticosteroid therapy; however, relapses are common. Even children with frequent relapses can experience a spontaneous resolution of MCNS before 30 years of age. Children should have periodic bone density evaluations because of the repeated steroid therapy (Gulati, Godbole, Singh et al., 2003).

Evaluation

Expected outcomes of nursing care include:

- The child responds to corticosteroid therapy.
- Dietary guidelines of "no added" salt are followed and food intake is controlled during corticosteroid therapy.
- Relapses are identified by parents before generalized edema occurs.
- The child receives the additional recommended immunizations.

A discussion of Wilms' tumor can be found in Chapter 23 ∞.

Renal Failure

Renal failure, which may be acute or chronic, occurs when the kidney is unable to excrete wastes and concentrate urine. Acute renal failure occurs suddenly (over days or weeks) and may be reversible, whereas in chronic renal failure, kidney function diminishes gradually and permanently over months or years.

Both types of renal failure are characterized by **azotemia** (accumulation of nitrogenous wastes in the blood) and sometimes **oliguria** (urine output less than 0.5 to 1 mL/kg/hr), indicating the kidney's inability to excrete metabolic waste products. The degree of renal impairment is estimated by the glomerular filtration rate (Hogg, Furth, Lemley et al., 2003). **Uremia** occurs when there is an excess of urea and other nitrogenous waste products in the blood.

Acute Renal Failure

Acute renal failure (ARF) is a sudden loss of adequate renal function in which the kidneys are unable to clear metabolic wastes and to regulate extracellular fluid volume, sodium balance, and acid-base homeostasis. ARF is seen in 2–3% of children cared for in pediatric intensive care units, and up to 8% of infants cared for in neonatal intensive care units (Vogt & Avner, 2004). Potential causes include hemolytic uremic syndrome, acute glomerulonephritis, sepsis, poisoning, hypovolemia, obstructive uropathy, and complication of cardiac surgery. Hematologic-oncologic complications, bone marrow transplantation, and respiratory failure have become more common causes of ARF in the last few years (Bock, 2005).

ETIOLOGY AND PATHOPHYSIOLOGY ARF may be caused by prerenal or postrenal factors as well as actual kidney damage (Figure 25–10 ➤).

- Prerenal ARF is a result of decreased perfusion to an otherwise normal kidney in association with a systemic condition. Hypovolemia (hemorrhage or

PATHOPHYSIOLOGY ILLUSTRATED

Acute Renal Failure

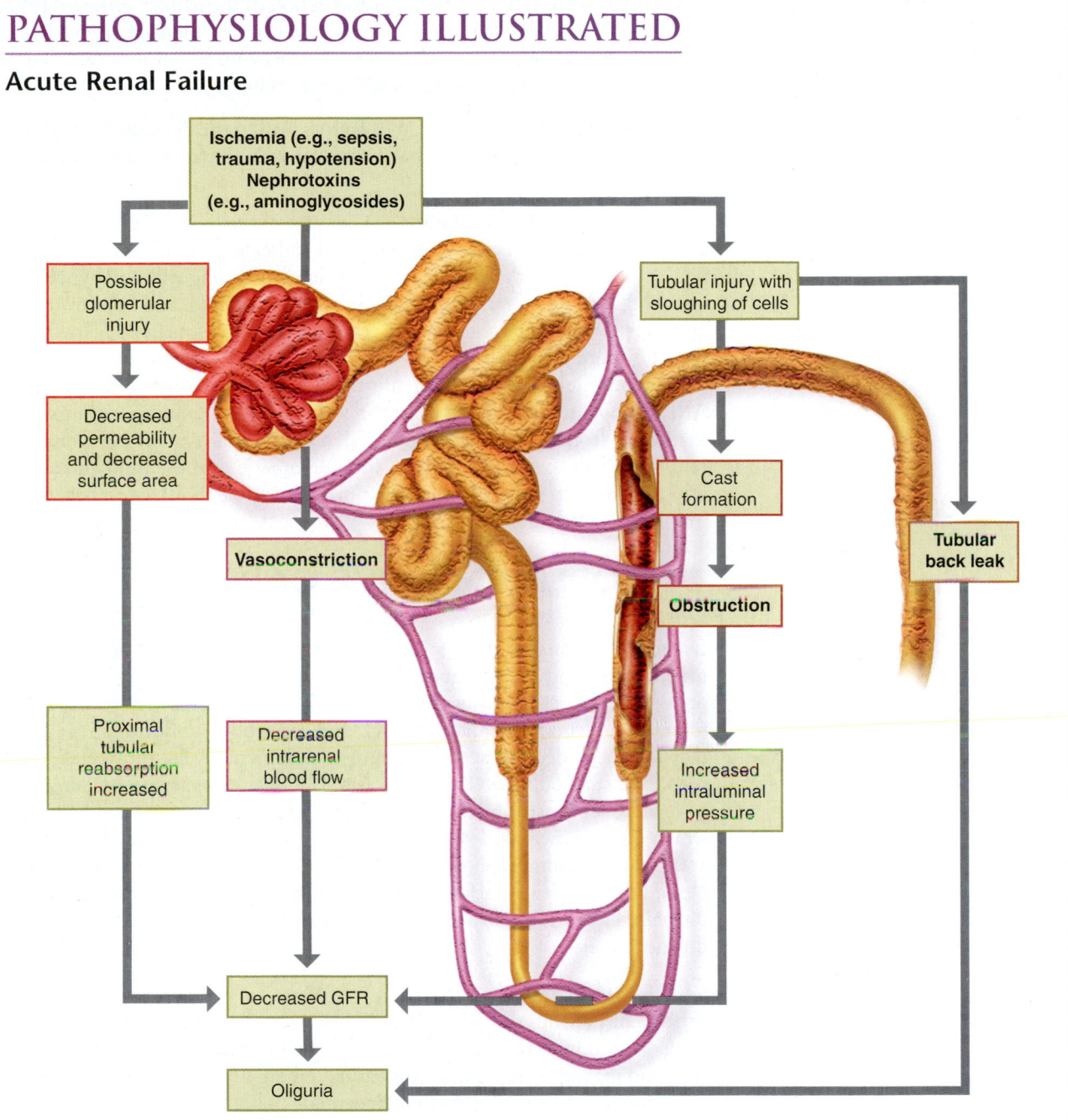

Figure 25–10 ➤ The initial kidney injury is usually associated with an acute condition such as sepsis, trauma, and hypotension, or is the result of treatment for an acute condition with nephrotoxic medication. Injury to the kidney can occur because of glomerular injury, vasoconstriction of capillaries, or tubular injury. All consequences of injury lead to decreased glomerular filtration and oliguria.

dehydration), septic shock, or cardiac failure may precipitate prerenal ARF. This is the most common type of ARF in infants and young children.

- Primary kidney damage (intrinsic factors) may result from infection, diseases such as hemolytic-uremic syndrome or acute glomerulonephritis, cortical necrosis, nephrotoxic drugs, or accidental ingestion of drugs or poisons. The structure most susceptible to damage is the kidney tubule. Injury to the tubule resulting in acute tubular necrosis is the most frequent cause of intrinsic renal failure in children.

- Postrenal ARF is caused by obstruction of the urinary flow from both kidneys, such as occurs in posterior urethral valves or a neurogenic bladder. Children may have oliguria, or normal or increased urine output. Renal failure without oliguria usually indicates a less severe renal injury.

In some cases a combination of factors lead to the development of ARF. Children who recover from ARF may have residual kidney damage and compromised renal function.

CLINICAL MANIFESTATIONS Characteristically, a healthy child suddenly becomes ill with nonspecific symptoms that indicate a significant illness or injury (e.g., nausea, vomiting, lethargy, edema, gross hematuria, oliguria, and hypertension). These symptoms are a result of electrolyte imbalances, uremia, and fluid overload. The child appears pale and lethargic. See the clinical manifestations table below and on the next page for more information.

Hyperkalemia is the most life-threatening electrolyte disorder associated with ARF. Hyponatremia affects central nervous system function, resulting in symptoms that range from fatigue to seizures. Edema occurs as a result of sodium and water retention. (Refer to Chapter 16 ∞ for a discussion of these fluid and electrolyte alterations.) Children with ARF are also more susceptible to infection because of depressed immune functioning.

■ COLLABORATIVE CARE

Diagnostic Tests

Diagnosis of renal failure is based primarily on urinalysis, urine culture, complete blood count, and serum chemistry tests, including BUN, serum creatinine, sodium, potassium, and calcium levels (Table 25–3). These tests may reveal hematuria, proteinuria, infection, anemia, acidosis, and electrolyte abnormalities. Additional tests may include toxicology screens, serum complement levels, antinuclear antibodies, and blood and stool cultures (Boydstun, 2005). The kidneys are normal in size and no signs of renal **osteodystrophy** (a complex bone disease process of chronic kidney disease in which there is increased resorption of bone caused by chronic hyperparathyroidism) are found on radiograph. Various imaging studies to assess kidney structures, renal blood flow, and renal perfusion and function may be performed to determine whether the child has ARF or chronic renal failure. A renal biopsy may be required to examine the glomeruli.

Clinical Therapy

Treatment depends on the underlying cause of the renal failure. The goal is to minimize or prevent permanent renal damage while maintaining fluid and electrolyte balance and managing complications. Initial emergency treatment of children with fluid depletion focuses on rapid fluid replacement at 20 mL/kg of saline or lactated Ringer's solution given over 5 to 10 minutes and repeated as needed to ensure renal perfusion

CLINICAL MANIFESTATIONS	ACUTE VERSUS CHRONIC RENAL FAILURE
Type of Renal Failure	**Clinical Manifestations**
Acute renal failure	Dark urine or gross hematuria, headache, edema, fatigue, crackles, gallop heart rhythm, hypertension, hematuria, lethargy, nausea and vomiting, oliguria. Mass in flank area if a cyst, tumor, or obstructive lesion is present.
Chronic renal failure	Fatigue, malaise, poor appetite, nausea and vomiting, failure to thrive or short stature. Headache, decreased mental alertness or ability to concentrate, secondary enuresis, chronic anemia, hypertension, edema. Fractures with minimal trauma, rickets, valgus bone deformity.

CLINICAL MANIFESTATIONS | ELECTROLYTE IMBALANCES IN ACUTE AND CHRONIC RENAL FAILURE

Electrolyte Imbalance and Cause	Clinical Manifestations
Hyperkalemia Results from inability to adequately excrete potassium derived from diet and catabolized cells. In metabolic acidosis, potassium also moves from intracellular fluid to extracellular fluid.	• Peaked T waves, widening of QRS waves on ECG • Dysrhythmias: ventricular dysrhythmias, heart block, ventricular fibrillation, cardiac arrest • Diarrhea • Muscle weakness
Hyponatremia In the acute oliguric phase, hyponatremia is dilutional, related to the accumulation of fluid in excess of solute.	• Change in level of consciousness • Muscle cramps • Anorexia • Abdominal reflexes, depressed deep tendon reflexes • Cheyne-Stokes respirations • Seizures
Hypocalcemia Phosphate retention (hyperphosphatemia) due to impaired renal function depresses the serum calcium concentration. Calcium is deposited in injured cells. Hyperkalemia and metabolic acidosis may mask the common clinical manifestations of severe hypocalcemia.	• Muscle tingling • Changes in muscle tone • Seizures • Muscle cramps and twitching • Positive Chvostek's sign (contraction of facial muscles after tapping facial nerve just anterior to parotid gland)

and stabilize blood pressure. Albumin may also be administered when blood loss is the cause of circulatory depletion. If oliguria persists after restoration of adequate fluid volume, intrinsic renal damage is suspected.

Children with fluid overload, like those with pulmonary edema, need diuretic therapy, as well as dialysis if they respond poorly to diuretics. Once the child is stabilized, fluid requirements are calculated to maintain *zero water balance* (intake should

Table 25–3 | DIAGNOSTIC TESTS FOR RENAL FAILURE

Test	Normal Values	Findings in Renal Failure
Urinalysis		
pH	4.5–8	Acidic urine
Osmolarity	50–1400 mosm/L	Greater than 500—prerenal ARF
		Less than 350—intrinsic ARF
Specific gravity	1.001–1.030	High: prerenal ARF Low: intrinsic ARF Normal: postrenal ARF
Protein	Negative	Positive
Blood Chemistry		
Potassium	3.5–5.8 mmol/L	Elevated
Sodium	135–148 mmol/L	Normal, low, or high, depends solely on the amount of water in the body
Calcium	2.2–2.7 mmol/L	Low
Phosphorus	1.23–2 mmol/L	High
Urea nitrogen	3.5–7.1 mmol/L	Increased
Creatinine	0.2–0.9 mmol/L	Increased
pH	7.38–7.42	Low acidic

ARF: acute renal failure

equal urine output and insensible fluid loss). Eliminate all potential sources of potassium intake until hyperkalemia is controlled (see Chapter 16 ∞). Remember that catabolic states or extensive tissue injury may raise potassium levels. Other electrolyte imbalances are treated. Nutrition must be maintained with extra carbohydrate intake during the catabolic state. Antibiotics are prescribed for infection. Nephrotoxic antibiotics such as aminoglycosides are avoided. See Medications Used to Treat Complications of Acute Renal Failure below.

Children whose ARF is unresponsive to management require dialysis to correct severe electrolyte imbalances, manage fluid overload, and cleanse the blood of waste products. The clinical situation and age of the child determine whether hemodialysis or peritoneal dialysis is used. Refer to the renal replacement therapy section on page 1005.

Prognosis depends on the cause of ARF. When renal failure results from drug toxicity or dehydration, the prognosis is generally good. However, ARF that results from diseases such as hemolytic-uremic syndrome or acute glomerulonephritis may be associated with residual kidney damage.

MediaLink

Care Plan Activity: A School-age Child with Acute Renal Failure

NURSING MANAGEMENT
Nursing Assessment and Diagnoses

A complete history and physical examination are necessary to identify progression of symptoms and possible causes for renal failure.

Physiologic Assessment

Assess vital signs, level of consciousness, and other neurologic indicators to help identify clinical signs of electrolyte imbalance (see the clinical manifestations table on page 997). Measure the child's weight on admission to provide a baseline for evaluating changes in fluid status. Monitor urinalysis, urine culture, and blood chemistry studies. Inspect urine for color (see Figure 25–4). Cloudy urine may indicate infection; tea-colored urine suggests hematuria. Assess urine specific gravity as well as intake and output.

MEDICATIONS USED TO TREAT *Complications of Acute Renal Failure*

Complication	Medication	Action or Indication	Nursing Implications
Hyperkalemia (greater than 5.8 mmol/L)	Kayexalate Calcium gluconate 10%, IV	Exchanges sodium for potassium Counteracts potassium-induced increased myocardial irritability	May require up to 4 hours to take effect. Monitor for ECG changes. Intravenous infiltration may result in tissue necrosis.
	Albuterol	Beta-agonist effects cause potassium to be shifted into the cells	Give by aerosol.
Metabolic acidosis	Sodium bicarbonate or sodium citrate	Helps correct metabolic acidosis by exchanging hydrogen for potassium	*Do not mix with calcium.* Complications include fluid overload, hypertension, and tetany.
Hypocalcemia (less than 2.2 mmol/L)	Calcium gluconate 10%	Used in presence of tetany; provides ionized calcium to restore nervous tissue function to control serum phosphorus	Administer slowly to prevent bradycardia. Monitor for ECG changes.
Malignant hypertension (blood pressure greater than 95% for age, sex, and height percentile)	Sodium nitroprusside, nitroglycerin	Relaxes smooth muscle in peripheral arterioles	Administer by continuous intravenous infusion; fall in blood pressure is seen within 10–20 minutes.

Psychosocial Assessment

The unexpected and acute nature of the child's hospitalization creates anxiety for both parents and the child. Assess for feelings of anger, guilt, or fear associated with the hospitalization. Such feelings are likely if ARF developed as a result of dehydration, a preventable injury, or poisoning. Assess coping mechanisms, family support systems, and level of stress.

Several nursing diagnoses may apply to the child with ARF, including:

- Ineffective Renal Tissue Perfusion related to hypovolemia, sepsis, or drug toxicity
- Excess Fluid Volume related to renal dysfunction and sodium retention
- Imbalanced Nutrition: Less than Body Requirements related to anorexia, nausea, vomiting, and catabolic state
- Risk for Infection related to invasive procedures and monitoring equipment, and diminished immune functioning
- Compromised Family Coping related to sudden hospitalization and uncertain prognosis of child

Planning and Implementation

Nursing care focuses on preventing complications, maintaining fluid balance, administering medications, meeting nutritional needs, preventing infection, and providing emotional support to the child and parents.

Prevent Complications

Complications are best prevented by ensuring compliance with the treatment plan. Careful monitoring of vital signs, intake and output, serum electrolytes, and level of consciousness can alert the nurse to changes that indicate potential complications.

Maintain Fluid Balance

Estimate the child's fluid status by daily monitoring of weight (on the same scale at the same time of day), intake and output, and blood pressure two or three times a day. Also monitor serum chemistry values, especially for sodium. The aim of maintaining fluid balance is to achieve a stable serum sodium concentration and a decrease in body weight by 0.5–1% a day.

If the child has oliguria, limit fluid intake, including parenteral nutrition, to replacement of insensible fluid loss (what is excreted by the lungs, skin, and gastrointestinal tract), which is about one third the daily maintenance requirements in afebrile children. If the child is febrile, fluid administration is increased by 12% for each centigrade degree of temperature elevation.

Administer Medications

Because the kidney's ability to excrete drugs is impaired in ARF, dosages of all medications should be adjusted. The actual dosage of the drug can be reduced or the time interval between doses may be increased. Check drug levels to monitor for drug toxicity. Know the signs of drug toxicity for each medication the child is receiving.

Meet Nutritional Needs

Children are at risk for malnutrition because of their high metabolic rate during ARF. Parenteral or enteral feeding may be used initially to minimize protein catabolism. The diet is tailored to the individual child's need for calories, carbohydrates, fats, and amino acids or protein hydrolysates. Depending on the degree of renal failure, sodium, potassium, and phosphorus may be restricted. Initiate oral feeding as soon as the child can tolerate it.

Prevent Infection

The child with ARF is extremely susceptible to nosocomial infections because of altered nutritional status, compromised immunity, and numerous invasive procedures. Good hand hygiene and standard precautions are imperative to decrease the risk of infection. Use sterile technique for all invasive procedures and when caring for lines. Drainage from catheter sites should be cultured to check for the presence of infectious organisms. Assess vital signs and lung sounds frequently.

CLINICAL TIP

If the serum sodium concentration rises and weight falls, insufficient fluids are being administered. If the serum sodium level falls and the weight increases, excessive fluids are being administered.

CLINICAL TIP

The child with **renal insufficiency** (decrease in the kidneys' ability to conserve sodium and concentrate the urine) is at greater risk for fluid loss with illness. In cases of acute gastrointestinal illness, these children are at greater risk for dehydration and ARF.

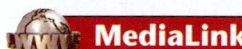

MediaLink

Acute Renal Failure Resources

Provide Emotional Support

The sudden onset of ARF presents parents with an unexpected threat to their child's life. Both the child and the parents experience anxiety because of the unexpected hospitalization and the uncertainty of the prognosis. Parents often feel guilty, regardless of the cause of renal failure. This guilt is intensified when renal failure is a result of dehydration or poisoning. Encourage parents to verbalize their fears and help them work through feelings of guilt. Explain procedures and treatment measures to decrease anxiety. Encouraging parents and older siblings to participate in the child's care can increase their sense of control.

Discharge Planning and Home Care Teaching

Encourage parental involvement early in the child's hospitalization. Be sure parents understand the importance of administering medications correctly. Teach family members proper technique for measuring blood pressure so they can monitor the child's blood pressure for hypertension, if ordered. Make sure the parents can identify signs of progressive renal failure (see chronic renal failure discussion).

Diet counseling is a key component of discharge planning and is usually performed by a renal dietitian. Depending on the degree of renal failure, the child's diet may include restrictions on protein, water, sodium, potassium, and phosphorus. The parents should be given written guidelines listing appropriate food choices to assist in menu planning. Ethnic and cultural preferences should be considered in listing menu options.

Continued monitoring of renal function during follow-up examinations is critical as deterioration may occur over time. Referral to support groups can be helpful for both parents and children. The National Kidney Foundation is a source of numerous publications.

Evaluation

Expected outcomes of nursing care include:

- The child's fluid status is balanced with edema-associated weight loss. Electrolyte and acid-base balance is restored.
- Nutritional needs are met.
- The child acquires no secondary infections.

Chronic Renal Failure

Chronic renal failure (CRF) is a progressive, irreversible reduction in kidney function. The prevalence of CRF is approximately 18 per 1 million children (Vogt & Avner, 2004).

ETIOLOGY AND PATHOPHYSIOLOGY In children, CRF usually results from developmental abnormalities of the kidney or obstructed urine flow and reflux, hereditary diseases such as polycystic kidney disease, infections such as hemolytic-uremic syndrome, and glomerulonephritis. (See discussions on hemolytic-uremic syndrome and glomerulonephritis later in the chapter.)

The gradual, progressive loss of functioning nephrons ultimately results in **end-stage renal disease (ESRD)**. ESRD is characterized by minimal renal function (less than 10% of normal), uremic syndrome, anemia, and abnormal blood values. In ESRD, the kidneys can no longer maintain homeostasis and the child requires dialysis.

The kidneys excrete excess acid in the body and regulate the body's fluid and electrolyte balance. Renal failure disrupts this fluid and electrolyte balance. As renal failure progresses, metabolic acidosis occurs because the kidneys cannot excrete the acids that build up in the body. Retention of excessive sodium and water is a common cause of the elevated blood pressure associated with CRF.

Renal osteodystrophy occurs as the kidneys are unable to produce activated vitamin D and to excrete phosphorus, causing phosphorus levels to rise and serum calcium levels to fall. The parathyroid gland responds by drawing calcium and phosphorus from the bones to maintain the adequate serum calcium and phosphorus levels. Hypocalcemia may occur as the parathyroid glands become less responsive to vitamin

D and lower serum calcium levels (Legg, 2005). Osteodystrophy increases the child's risk for spontaneous fractures and rickets.

Growth retardation is caused by disturbances in the metabolism of calcium, phosphorus, and vitamin D; decreased caloric intake; and metabolic acidosis. The kidneys also produce erythropoietin (the growth factor responsible for the production and maturation of red cells); lack of erythropoietin and progressive renal disease are the underlying causes of the anemia of CRF.

CLINICAL MANIFESTATIONS   Children with CRF frequently have no symptoms initially. Early renal failure with glomerular filtration rate (GFR) of 50–75% of normal has few or no clinical signs. As progression continues, renal insufficiency occurs with polyuria as the kidneys cannot concentrate the urine. Symptoms become more classic as CRF occurs with pallor, headache, nausea, and fatigue. Decreased mental alertness and ability to concentrate may be seen. The child may have anemia leading to tachycardia, tachypnea, and dyspnea on exertion. As the disease progresses, the child loses his or her appetite and has complications of renal impairment, including hypertension, pulmonary edema, growth retardation, osteodystrophy, delayed fine and gross motor development, and delayed sexual maturation. Contrast these signs with those of acute renal failure on the clinical manifestations table on page 996.

In ESRD, the most advanced form of CRF, renal failure adversely affects all body systems. As the severity of the clinical and biochemical disturbances resulting from progressive renal deterioration increases, uremic symptoms develop. Signs and symptoms of uremic syndrome include nausea and vomiting, progressive anemia, anorexia, dyspnea, malaise, **uremic frost** (urea crystals deposited on the skin), unpleasant (uremic) breath odor, headache, progressive confusion, tremors, pulmonary edema, and congestive heart failure.

COLLABORATIVE CARE

Diagnostic Tests

Laboratory evaluation, including serum electrolytes, phosphate, BUN, and creatinine levels and pH, is used to confirm the diagnosis of chronic kidney disease and the stage of CRF. An early morning urine sample is collected for culture, and to calculate the protein-to-creatinine ratio. The child's glomerular filtration rate (GFR) is calculated from prediction equations using the serum creatinine level and the patient's height and gender. An online GFR calculator is available through the National Kidney Foundation.

Imaging studies are performed to identify renal diseases that could be causing the renal failure. A renal biopsy may sometimes be performed.

Clinical Therapy

CRF is irreversible. However, the course of the disease is variable. Some children progress quickly to renal failure, necessitating dialysis. Other children are managed with a combination of medication and diet therapy for some time before significant renal impairment occurs. Frequent modifications in the treatment plan are often necessary to address the child's changing status. The goals of treatment are to slow the progression of renal disease and to prevent complications. See Medications Used to Treat Children with Chronic Renal Failure on page 1002.

Dietary management focuses on maximizing caloric intake for growth while limiting phosphorus, potassium, and sodium intake as needed to keep electrolytes in balance. Adequate calcium needs to be part of the meal plan. Tube feedings or parenteral nutrition may be required to achieve optimal protein intake, especially in children under 1 year of age. When CRF is present, optimal intake of high-quality protein (meat, fish, poultry, and egg whites) for infants is 2 to 2.5 g/kg/day; for older children it is 1.5 to 2 g/kg/day. Complex carbohydrates should be chosen along with vegetables and fruits that are lower in potassium. Vegetable oils, hard candy, sugar, honey, and jelly may be recommended to add calories to the child's diet.

Children who progress to ESRD require renal replacement therapy. The timetable for dialysis or renal transplantation is different from that of adults; transplantation is the

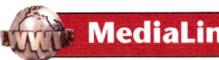

MediaLink

GFR Calculator

MEDICATIONS USED TO TREAT *Children with Chronic Renal Failure*

Medication	Action or Indication	Nursing Considerations
Vitamin and mineral supplement (Nephrocaps)	Add vitamins and minerals missing from heavily restricted diet	Only prescribed vitamins should be used; over-the-counter brands may contain elements that are harmful.
Phosphate-binding agents: Calcium carbonate (Tums), calcium acetate (PhosLo), or sevelamer hydrochloride (Renagel)	Reduce absorption of phosphorus from the intestines	Ensure that phosphate-binding agent is aluminum-free.
Calcitriol (Rocaltrol)	Replace the calcitriol the kidneys are no longer producing to keep calcium balance normal	Monitor serum calcium level. Ensure that calcium supplement is provided.
Epoetin alfa (Epogen, Procrit)	Stimulates bone marrow to produce red blood cells, treats anemia due to CRF	Given by IV or subcutaneous injection. Monitor blood pressure as hypertension is an adverse effect. Monitor hematocrit and serun ferritin level according to facility guidelines.
Iron supplementation	Treat iron deficiency when epoetin alfa is prescribed	May be administered orally or IV during hemodialysis.
Growth hormone (rhGH)	Used to stimulate growth in children with CRF	Record accurate height measurements at regular intervals.
Antihypertensive agents: Angiotensin-converting enzyme (ACE) inhibitor (enalapril, lisinopril) Loop diuretics	Used with proteinuric kidney disease as it slows the progression to ESRD; used when volume overload is present	Monitor renal function and electrolyte balance.

goal so the child has an optimal chance for a more normal childhood. Earlier initiation can prevent some complications of ESRD. In addition to the GFR, nonspecific signs such as uremic syndrome, poorly controlled hypertension, renal osteodystrophy, failure of head circumference measurement to increase normally, developmental delay, and poor growth are used in determining when to initiate therapy. (Refer to "Renal Replacement Therapy" section later in this chapter.) Infection is the most common morbidity in children receiving renal replacement therapy.

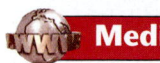

MediaLink

Case Study: A Child with Chronic Renal Failure

NURSING MANAGEMENT
Nursing Assessment and Diagnoses

Nursing assessment focuses on identifying signs and symptoms of renal failure and associated complications, and assessing the psychosocial effects of renal failure on the child and family.

Physiologic Assessment

The initial and ongoing assessment of the child focuses on identifying complications of renal failure. Observe for signs of edema, poor growth and development, osteodystrophy, and anemia. Assess vital signs, particularly the blood pressure. Observe for signs of electrolyte alterations (see page 997).

Psychosocial Assessment

As renal disease progresses, the number of stressors on the child and family increases. Denial and disbelief are commonly the first reactions. A thorough family assessment can help to identify particular needs of the child and family (see Chapter 2 ∞). The development of ESRD is particularly challenging during childhood and adolescence because of differences in appearance and social, psychological, and physical issues. Nonadherence with treatments can endanger the adolescent's life.

Nursing diagnoses for the child with CRF are similar to those previously listed for ARF. Additional diagnoses might include:

- Delayed Growth and Development related to decreased protein and caloric intake and loss of protein in dialysate
- Impaired Social Interaction related to impaired immunity and hemodialysis schedule during school hours
- Activity Intolerance related to anemia and fatigue
- Ineffective Therapeutic Regimen Management related to complexity of care plan and economic difficulties
- Disturbed Body Image related to short stature and visible external catheter for dialysis

Planning and Implementation
Hospital-Based Care

Children with CRF are usually hospitalized for one or more of the following reasons: initial diagnostic evaluation, dialysis treatment initiation, problems with the treatment plan, infection, or another problem. Nursing care for the hospitalized child with CRF focuses on monitoring for side effects of medications, preventing infection, meeting nutritional needs, and providing emotional support and anticipatory teaching.

Monitor for Side Effects of Medications

Watch for signs of electrolyte imbalance such as weakness, muscle cramps, dizziness, headache, and nausea and vomiting in children taking diuretics. Supervise the child's activities closely to prevent falls resulting from dizziness, especially at the beginning of diuretic therapy. If antihypertensive medications such as hydralazine are being administered, monitor the child's weight to detect excessive gain resulting from water and sodium retention.

Prevent Infection

The child with CRF is susceptible to infections. Be alert for signs of infection, such as elevated temperature; cloudy, strong-smelling urine; dysuria; changes in respiratory pattern; or productive cough. Emphasize to the child and family the importance of good hand hygiene.

Meet Nutritional Needs

Maintaining adequate nutritional intake in a child with CRF who has dietary restrictions is challenging. Provide small, frequent feedings and present meals attractively to encourage the child to eat. A renal dietitian works with families of children with chronic renal failure to develop meal plans that fit a restricted diet. See Table 25–4 for foods that children with CRF should avoid.

Provide Emotional Support

Progressive CRF requires a total lifestyle change for the child and family. The parents and child need opportunities to express and work through their feelings related to the disease, prognosis, and treatment restrictions. Help children express their feelings through drawings or therapeutic play.

The need for ongoing dialysis treatments and the wait for a suitable donor kidney are stressful for both parents and the child. Identify effective coping methods and family support systems to promote treatment compliance. The National Kidney Foundation and local support groups for kidney disease can give the family information or additional support.

Discharge Planning and Home Care Teaching

Parents need to understand the necessity of long-term treatments and follow-up care. Help the family develop a schedule for medication administration that fits with their routine. Emphasize the importance of consistency in administration times. Teach parents how to recognize medication side effects and complications.

 MediaLink

Chronic Renal Failure Support

LAW & ETHICS

Kidney Failure and Medicare
In 1972, Congress made children with permanent kidney failure (needing regular dialysis or having a kidney transplant) eligible for Medicare to pay for needed medical care. Medicare coverage can help supplement other health insurance programs that the child is eligible for (National Kidney and Urological Diseases, 2005).

| Table 25–4 | NUTRITIONAL INFORMATION FOR THE CHILD WITH KIDNEY DISEASE |

High Sodium Content Foods	High Potassium Content Foods	High Phosphorus Content Foods
Soups and sauces: e.g., gravy, spaghetti and tomato sauce, barbeque sauce, steak sauce *Processed lunchmeats*: bologna, ham, salami, hot dogs, etc. *Smoked meat and fish*: bacon, chipped beef, corned beef, ham, lox Sauerkraut, pickles, and other pickled foods *Seasonings*: horseradish, soy sauce, Worchestershire sauce, meat tenderizer, and monosodium glutamate (MSG)	*Fruit*: apricots, avocados, bananas, citrus fruits, fresh pears, nectarines, dates, figs, cantaloupe and other melons, prunes, and raisins *Vegetables*: celery, dried beans, lima beans, potatoes, leafy greens, spinach, tomatoes, winters squash *Whole grains*: especially those containing bran Sardines, clams Peanuts *Dairy products*: milk, ice cream, pudding, yogurt Potassium-containing salt substitutes	*Dairy products*: milk, cheese, yogurt, custard, pudding, ice cream Dried beans, peas Nuts, peanut butter Chocolate Dark cola Sausage, hot dogs

Children with kidney disease have restricted diets, generally low in sodium, potassium, and phosphorus. The nurse can help families remember that certain foods must be avoided or eaten in very small quantities by reviewing this table.

MediaLink

Health Promotion and Maintenance Overview: CRF

CLINICAL TIP

Review the child's immunizations on every visit in an effort to have the child fully immunized prior to kidney transplantation. Live virus vaccines cannot be given when the child is immunocompromised following the transplant. Make sure the child also receives the 23-valent pneumococcal and meningococcal vaccines. Some children receive a kidney transplant prior to reaching ESRD (Benfield, 2003).

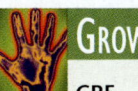

GROWTH & DEVELOPMENT

CRF

School-age children with CRF may not understand the consequences of nonadherence with dietary restrictions and may perceive these restrictions as punishment. Adolescents often resent the dietary restrictions and ongoing dialysis treatments, which pose a threat to their independence and evolving sense of self. Noncooperation, depression, and hostility are common responses.

Appropriate referrals are made to home care nursing agencies as indicated. Home care nurses teach the parents of the child receiving peritoneal dialysis to perform the treatment and to identify complications, as well as provide necessary support and reassurance.

Care in the Community

Children with CRF require frequent outpatient visits to monitor the progression of signs and symptoms, and to evaluate the effectiveness of current treatments. The blood pressure is monitored. Blood and urine tests are performed to monitor renal function. Radiographs of the bones are often taken at 6-month intervals to assess changes caused by osteodystrophy.

When assessing the child, compare height, weight, and head circumference to age-specific norms to identify growth retardation and to plot progress. Assess developmental progress using the Denver II or another screening tool (see Chapter 7 ∞). Assess the adolescent for signs of delayed sexual maturation and, in girls, amenorrhea. Encourage the child to get regular exercise.

Promote good dentition and oral hygiene. Regular dental visits are important to reduce infections. Make sure the family understands the need for antibiotic prophylaxis before certain invasive procedures, including dental care (see the medications table on page 750).

Review any dietary restrictions with parents. Provide sample menus for meal planning to help parents incorporate dietary changes into daily meals. A renal dietitian usually helps the child make food selections and restrict fluids and sodium as necessary, taking into account the child's likes and dislikes and cultural background. Collaborate with the family to help them implement the appropriate meal plan, and check to see if there are any problems with obtaining and preparing the foods the child should eat. High caloric supplements may be needed because of anorexia. Discuss possible behavioral responses to dietary restrictions and limitations imposed by the treatment plan.

Parents should be encouraged to register the young child for the Early Education Program to promote development and interaction with other children. The dialysis schedule for school-age children should enable the child to participate in school, or home tutoring should be provided. Educational progress needs to be assessed in children with ESRD, and additional educational assistance should be provided as needed to promote optimal education attainment.

School-age children and adolescents are often embarrassed about being seen as different from peers. The metabolic abnormalities interfere with the child's height growth and delay pubertal development. Ask the child how he or she feels about the need to follow a special diet, take medications, and undergo dialysis treatments. To minimize the psychologic consequences of coping with a chronic disease, encourage parents to promote the child's participation in age-appropriate activities. Attendance at school and contacts with peers promote normal growth and development. Work to promote the child's self-worth and a healthy self-esteem. Encourage adolescents to participate in a program that helps them transition to adult health services and job skill training.

Begin teaching the child during early adolescence about the health condition, medications taken and their actions, how to access emergency help, and problems caused by nonadherence to treatment. (See Evidence-Based Practice: Living with End-Stage Renal Disease.) As the adolescent ages, have the family begin giving more responsibility for self-care, such as making appointments for health care, obtaining prescription refills, and seeking out adult healthcare professionals and a dialysis program.

Give the parents timely information about the disease process, dialysis treatments, and issues related to renal transplantation, as the child's renal impairment progresses.

Evaluation

Expected outcomes of nursing care include:

- The child is fully immunized with childhood and additional vaccines.
- The child's fluid status is maintained.
- The child eats foods that meet nutritional needs while adhering to dietary restrictions.

Renal Replacement Therapy

Renal replacement therapy is the treatment for renal failure and includes both dialysis and renal transplantation. In 2002, 6982 children between birth and 19 years of age received some form of renal replacement therapy. Hemodialysis has emerged as the dominant form of dialysis when treatment is initiated. Approximately 680 children under

---

COMPLEMENTARY THERAPY

Herbal Supplements and Children with Chronic Renal Failure

Herbal supplements should not be used in children with CRF as they may contain harmful minerals, such as potassium, or they are toxic to the kidneys. The child's body is unable to clear waste products like healthy children. There is also the risk for interaction between the herbs and medications taken that could place the child at risk for rejection of a transplanted kidney (National Kidney Foundation, 2004).

EVIDENCE-BASED PRACTICE

Living with End-Stage Renal Disease

Clinical Question

End-stage renal disease is a serious chronic condition that requires significant adaptations in lifestyle and complex medical treatments that take a toll on the child and family. What is the impact of the condition on adolescents?

Evidence

A study of 35 adolescents, ages 13 to 18 years, was conducted to evaluate their perceptions of themselves and living with end-stage renal disease. Twenty-one of the adolescents provided responses that clustered into one of four groups:
- Normalization, $n=8$ (identified selves as independent and leading as normal a life as possible)
- Illness causes a barrier to normalcy, $n=5$ (the physical effects of the disease such as shortened stature affected how they looked and how they were treated by society), had psychological effects
- Illness management was parent focused, $n=5$ (adolescents wished to be independent but perceived that they were dependent upon parents to help care for them)
- Illness management was self-focused, $n=3$ (perceived that ongoing treatment for renal disease was very hard, and they perceived that they were different from their peers)

The study group of adolescents was 65.7% White and 28.6% African American. They were predominantly from intact families and 68.6% had positive treatment outcomes due to renal transplants (Snethen, Broome, Bartels, & Warady, 2001).

Practice Implications

Children and adolescents who develop end-stage renal disease are expected to develop adaptive functioning skills as well as cope with the consequences of the disease (physical trauma and operative scars, corticosteroid side effects, dietary restrictions, growth failure, and responses of peers). The adolescent experiences delayed development of separation and independence (Benfield, 2003). Parents must modify lifestyles and their hopes and dreams for their children's future. Strategies for managing the disease differ for every family. Normalization is a coping process in which the family views the care of the child with a chronic condition as a "normal" part of life, rather than an inconvenience or something outside of their routine. They choose to focus on the normal aspect of the child's life and the family's life. In cases when normalization cannot be achieved or sustained, the adolescent's condition may have recently changed or another family stressor is present. These families view their life and their child as different from other families because of the child's condition. Nurses can be effective in working with families by listening to the issues and offering suggestions. Often the opportunity to talk through the child's management plan will help the family consider different strategies that may be effective. The nurse may also provide linkages to community resources that may help the family.

Critical Thinking

Initiate a discussion with an adolescent with end-stage renal disease, and listen to the adolescent's description of living with the condition. Develop a nursing care plan to help the child take the next steps in self-management.

19 years begin hemodialysis each year, and there are nearly 1350 children treated by dialysis at any time (Chand, Brier, Strife et al., 2005). Many of the metabolic abnormalities of the chronic renal failure that impact a child's growth and development are improved by kidney transplantation (Benfield, 2003). By the 18th month of ESRD treatment, transplant is the dominant treatment method (United States Renal Data System, 2004).

PERITONEAL DIALYSIS   In peritoneal dialysis, the peritoneum of the abdomen is the membrane through which the body's waste products pass from the blood to the abdominal cavity. A catheter is inserted through the abdominal wall into the peritoneal cavity. The dialysis solution (**dialysate**) that enters the abdomen contains dextrose that pulls body wastes and extra fluid into the abdominal cavity. These wastes and extra fluid leave the body with the drained dialysate. This method of dialysis is beneficial to small children since it allows continuous removal of fluids and waste products, decreasing the toxic effects of waste products on the child's developing body. The child can ambulate and interact with the environment. Dietary and fluid restrictions are less severe. The timing of the treatment can be set to minimize the interruption of school, play, or other social events.

Two types of peritoneal dialysis are commonly used: continuous ambulatory peritoneal dialysis and automated peritoneal dialysis. Graduated cylinders are used to monitor the volume of fluid exchanged.

- Continuous ambulatory peritoneal dialysis (CAPD) uses gravity to instill prefilled bags of dialysate into the peritoneal cavity four or five times a day. The fluid remains in the cavity for 4 to 8 hours. An attached bag is folded under the child's clothes, permitting normal activity. After the allotted time, the dialysate is drained by hanging the bag lower than the pelvis. The repeated connections and disconnections with this method are time consuming for the child and family and increase the risk of infection.
- Automated peritoneal dialysis uses an automatic cycler to instill and drain the dialysate about five times over a 10-hour period, usually overnight. One additional exchange may be needed during the day. With this method the number of connections and disconnections is minimized, which reduces demands on the family as well as the risk of infection. This is the preferred peritoneal dialysis method since a more customized schedule can be developed to allow children to attend school (Verrina, Zacchello, Edefonti et al., 2001).

In children receiving peritoneal dialysis for ARF, a percutaneously placed catheter can be used for a few weeks. In children with CRF, a catheter is placed surgically for long-term use.

The primary complications of peritoneal dialysis are peritonitis and abdominal hernia (Table 25–5). Signs and symptoms of peritonitis associated with peritoneal dialysis include cloudy dialysate, fever, vomiting, diarrhea, abdominal pain, and tenderness. Chronic alterations in the peritoneal membrane transport capacity may result from peritonitis, and may lead to peritoneal membrane failure (Warady, Schaefer, Holloway et al., 2000). Peritonitis is treated with antibiotics infused in the dialysate.

Teach the family to perform peritoneal dialysis and to use sterile technique when performing dialysis and doing catheter care. Peritoneal dialysis is time consuming, and family members must be committed to managing this procedure daily. Help the family develop home routines that minimize disruptions to daily family life. For additional information, refer to Nursing Care Plan: The Child Receiving Home Peritoneal Dialysis.

HEMODIALYSIS   In hemodialysis, the blood flows through a machine with a special filter that removes body wastes and extra fluids. Blood is pumped out of the body and through a dialyzer, where waste products and extra fluids diffuse out across a semipermeable membrane. Dialysate is pumped in the direction opposite blood flow to promote waste extraction. Differences in osmolarity and concentration between the child's

Table 25–5	COMPLICATIONS OF PERITONEAL DIALYSIS
Complication	**Cause**

Peritonitis

Cloudy dialysate, abdominal pain, tenderness, leukocytosis, fever (neonatal hypothermia), constipation	*Staphylococcus aureus, Staphylococcus epidermidis,* fungal infections, gram-negative rods (risk is proportional to duration of dialysis and inversely proportional to age)

Pain

During inflow	Too rapid a rate of infusion, too large a volume of dialysate, encasement of catheter in a false passage, extremes in temperature of dialysate
During outflow at end of emptying	Omentum entering catheter at end of outflow

Leakage

Fluid around catheter, edema of penis or scrotum secondary to leakage into abdominal subcutaneous tissue, fluid leakage to pleural spaces through diaphragm	Overfilling of abdomen; catheter that has migrated from peritoneal cavity

Respiratory Symptoms

Shortness of breath, decreased breath sounds in lower lobes, inadequate chest expansion	Abdominal fullness that compromises diaphragm movement, hole in diaphragm allowing dialysate into chest cavity

blood and the dialysate alter the intravascular electrolyte concentration and reduce the intravascular volume. Hemodialysis is provided to children in the critical care setting and in a special center. Treatment is usually performed three times a week, with each session lasting approximately 3 to 4 hours. Continuous renal replacement therapy (CRRT) is a form of continuous hemodialysis used when the child has acute renal failure, multiple organ failure, and hemodynamic instability.

In emergency hemodialysis and for infants, a double-lumen cannula is inserted into a large vein (e.g., the femoral, jugular, or subclavian vein). Children over 20 kg (44 lb) may have a central venous catheter, or have an artificial blood vessel created, such as an arteriovenous shunt or fistula as the venous access for dialysis. Two needles are inserted into the arteriovenous fistula, one to carry blood to the dialyzer and the other to return cleaned blood to the body.

Hemodialysis is more efficient than peritoneal dialysis but requires close monitoring for symptoms related to hypotension or rapid changes in fluid and electrolyte balance. Uncommonly, a **disequilibrium syndrome** (rapid changes in the body's water and electrolyte balance during treatment) may occur during or soon after the dialysis procedure is initiated. Other complications include access thrombosis and infection. Heparin is used to achieve an active clotting time of 150%, which reduces the risk of thrombosis.

Nursing management focuses on care of the child during dialysis and teaching the child and family about the administration of heparin and the control of bleeding from minor trauma. Carefully monitor fluid balance in the child undergoing hemodialysis. Check vital signs and blood pressure every half hour. Monitor oral intake and urinary output every half hour when the child is on the dialysis equipment. Weigh the child before and after the dialysis to determine any fluid imbalances that must be adjusted in the next hemodialysis session.

Because fluid and dietary limitations (reduced potassium, sodium, and phosphorus-containing foods) are needed more often with hemodialysis than with peritoneal dialysis, make sure the family knows how to plan and provide for the child's daily nutritional needs. Review ways to reduce the risk of infection, including the daily care of the catheter site. Encourage showering rather than tub baths. Activities such as swimming may be discouraged.

RESEARCH

Hemodialysis in Nighttime Home Treatment

Hemodialysis in nighttime home treatment has been used in adults for many years. A recent study was reported about the experience of treating four adolescents with significant renal disease with dialysis nightly in the home. The program was successfully implemented with few technical problems, and the well-being of the adolescents was improved, but there were issues related to the intensity of the workload on families and their anxieties (Geary, Piva, Tyrrell et al., 2005).

NURSING ALERT

Monitor the child receiving hemodialysis for complications that can occur suddenly.
- Hypotension. Sudden nausea and vomiting, abdominal cramping, tachycardia, and dizziness
- Rapid fluid and electrolyte exchange. Muscle cramping, nausea and vomiting, and dizziness
- Disequilibrium syndrome. Restlessness, headache, nausea and vomiting, blurred vision, muscle twitching, and altered level of consciousness

GOAL	INTERVENTION	RATIONALE	EXPECTED OUTCOME
1. Imbalanced Nutrition: Less than Body Requirements related to poor appetite, feeling of fullness after a small amount, and loss of protein in dialysate			
	NIC Priority Intervention: **Nutrition management:** *Assistance with or provision of a balanced dietary intake of foods and fluids*		*NOC Suggested Outcome:* **Nutrition Status: Food and Fluid Intake.** *Amount of food and fluid taken into the body over a 24-hour period.*
The child will obtain adequate nutrients each day.	• With a nutritionist, develop a meal plan to identify the amounts of essential nutrients needed.	• Parents need concrete guidelines for food preparation.	The child's intake is adequate to maintain an expected growth pattern.
	• Provide small, frequent meals of needed nutrients.	• The child will feel full with smaller amounts of food because of the dialysate.	
	• Make mealtimes pleasant and avoid battles over the child's intake.	• The child will be more inclined to eat if there is less stress.	
	• Provide supplements by tube feeding if oral intake is inadequate.	• Adequate nutrition is important for growth and development, and must be supported if oral intake is inadequate.	
2. Risk for infection related to daily invasive procedure			
	NIC Priority Intervention: **Infection Control:** *Minimizing the acquisition and transmission of infectious agents.*		*NOC Suggested Outcome:* **Infection Status:** *Presence and extent of infection.*
The child will not develop peritonitis.	• Wash hands, use sterile gloves, and perform aseptic technique for connection and disconnection of catheters.	• Aseptic technique reduces chance of introducing bacteria into the abdomen.	The child does not develop peritonitis.
	• Perform daily catheter site care.	• Skin around the catheter site will have fewer organisms that could potentially cause infection.	
If peritonitis occurs, it will be treated appropriately.	• Observe for signs of infection (fever, abdominal pain, cloudy dialysate).	• Early identification of infection will reduce complications.	Hospitalization will not be needed for peritonitis due to early identification and prompt treatment.
	• Report signs of infection to physician immediately.	• Rapid intervention may reduce need for hospitalization.	
3. Caregiver role strain related to daily dialysis treatments			
	NIC Priority Intervention: **Caregiver Support:** *Provision of necessary information, advocacy, and support to facilitate primary patient care by someone other than a healthcare professional*		*NOC Suggested Outcome:* **Caregiver Performance: Direct Care:** *Provision by family care provider of appropriate personal and health care for a family member or significant other.*
The family copes with daily demands for the child's dialysis treatments.	• Discuss the importance of daily, consistent dialysis treatments for the child's overall health status.	• If parents understand the need for consistent dialysis treatments, they are more likely to adhere to guidelines.	The family adheres with daily dialysis treatment guidelines.
	• Collaborate with the family to identify strategies that could reduce the impact of dialysis on the family's life.	• When the family participates in planning care, compliance is more likely.	
	• Refer the family to local support groups for emotional support, treatment strategies, and respite care.	• Support groups may help the family develop effective coping strategies.	

NURSING CARE PLAN The Child Receiving Home Peritoneal Dialysis (continued)

GOAL	INTERVENTION	RATIONALE	EXPECTED OUTCOME
4. Disturbed body image related to small size and perception of being and looking different			
	NIC Priority Intervention: **Body Image Enhancement:** *Improving a patient's conscious and unconscious perceptions and attitudes toward his/her body.*		*NOC Suggested Outcome:* **Psychosocial Adjustment: Life Change:** *Psychosocial adaptation of an individual to a life change.*
The child will develop a sense of self-worth and self-esteem.	• Identify and emphasize strengths the child has (e.g., interaction style, skills, or cognitive abilities) despite being smaller than peers.	• Perception of personal strengths should increase self-esteem.	The child effectively interacts with peers and participates in age-appropriate activities.
	• Assist the child and family to identify popular clothing styles that hide the protuberant abdomen, dialysate bag, and catheter.	• Clothing that conforms to current styles will help the child feel less different from peers.	
	• Increase the child's participation in self-care as appropriate for developmental age.	• Ability to perform self-care increases the child's sense of control.	
	• Promote participation in safe activities with peers.	• Social interaction with peers helps reinforce similarities with others.	
	• Encourage the child to participate in support groups with other children receiving dialysis when possible.	• Interactions with other affected children provide a chance to express feelings and frustrations, and to develop successful coping strategies.	
5. Ineffective health maintenance related to chronic condition			
	NIC Priority Intervention: **Health System Guidance:** *Facilitating a patient's location and use of appropriate health services.*		*NOC Suggested Outcome:* **Health-Seeking Behaviors:** *Actions to promote optimal wellness, recovery, and rehabilitation.*
The child's routine health maintenance visits will be integrated with the management of the chronic condition.	• If a renal specialty team is not conveniently located and providing general health care, make sure the child has a primary care provider working in collaboration with the renal team.	• A source of health maintenance and acute minor illness care is important, especially if the family lives a distance from the tertiary care center.	The child is fully immunized at appropriate intervals and the family has a source of regular care in the community.
	• Assess the child regularly for height growth and developmental progress and signs that the chronic condition is being managed effectively.	• Routine assessments will allow potential complications to be identified earlier.	
	• Provide immunizations as recommended for the child with a chronic condition.	• Live virus vaccines must be given prior to kidney transplant. Immunizations may reduce the risk of potentially life-threatening infections in a child at high risk.	
	• Provide anticipatory guidance related to safety, developmental progress, appropriate physical activities, and behavior management.	• Information will help the family support the child's health status and promote development.	

NURSING ALERT

Signs of rejection following a kidney transplant include fever, increased BUN and serum creatinine levels, pain and tenderness over the abdomen, irritability, and weight gain. However, because the size of the kidney transplanted is often large in comparison to the child's size, rejection may be further advanced before symptoms appear, making it more difficult to reverse the rejection process (Benfield, 2003).

KIDNEY TRANSPLANTATION   Kidney transplantation provides the only alternative to long-term dialysis for children with ESRD. It can normalize physiology and may let children grow normally. Because delaying transplantation has adverse effects on growth and development, children are given some priority over adults awaiting transplantation. Blood type compatibility between the donor and recipient is essential for a transplant to be successful. A human leukocyte antigen (HLA) system match also improves survival of the graft. A living relative donor kidney has a higher survival rate than a cadaver kidney. Children and their families are carefully screened prior to transplantation in an effort to identify problems that could lead to rejection of the kidney or infection that could be life threatening if the immune system is suppressed.

After transplantation, the child must take immunosuppressive medications such as corticosteroids, azathioprine, cyclosporine, tacrolimus, and polyclonal antibodies, as well as monoclonal antibodies to suppress rejection. See Chapter 17 ∞. Immunosuppression regimens use various combinations and sequences of these drugs to reduce the incidence of acute and chronic rejection. Chronic rejection is the most important cause of transplanted kidney loss (Benfield, 2003).

Complications of immunosuppression therapy include opportunistic infection, lymphomas and skin cancer, and hypertension. Nonadherence to therapy is the primary cause of transplanted kidney loss (in 10–15% of pediatric kidney transplant recipients). Nonadherence is highest among families with crises or who do not provide adequate support, and in adolescents who are responsible for taking their medications, or have mild cognitive impairment or depression (Feinstein, Keich, Becker-Cohen et al., 2005). Adherence is higher in adolescents when their parents are knowledgeable and supportive, and when they promote the adolescent to become competent in self-care (Pool & Korus, 2002). Some primary kidney diseases, such as glomerulonephritis and hemolytic-uremic syndrome, can also recur in the transplanted kidney.

Nursing management includes teaching parents about the transplantation process before it occurs to help prepare them for the experience. Discuss all aspects of the child's care that will have an impact on the family's life, including follow-up appointments, medications, and general health promotion. Following transplant, monitor adherence to immunosuppression treatment at each visit in an effort to identify issues early. Monitor the child's blood pressure as many of these children will need antihypertensive medications. Teach parents about the signs of acute and chronic rejection and infection, including when and how to notify the child's physician if immediate care is required.

Polycystic Kidney Disease

Polycystic kidney disease (PKD) is a genetic disorder that has autosomal recessive and autosomal dominant forms. Liver abnormalities are associated with both forms of the disease. The incidence of the autosomal recessive form is 1 per 20,000 live births, and is most often detected in fetuses and infants (Guay-Woodford & Desmond, 2003). The autosomal dominant form is the most commonly inherited kidney disease, with a prevalence of 1 per 400 to 500 individuals. The autosomal dominant PKD results from mutations on the PKD1 locus on chromosome 16 and PKD2 on chromosome 4. The autosomal recessive gene (PKHD1) is located on chromosome 6 (National Kidney and Urologic Diseases Information Clearinghouse, 2004).

In PKD, cellular hyperplasia of the collecting ducts causes them to dilate. Fluid secreted into these ducts enables cyst sacs to form. Initially, cysts are usually less than 2 mm in size and do not obstruct urinary flow. As the child grows, however, the cysts become larger and fibrosis occurs. The cysts slowly replace much of the kidney's mass and reduce kidney function. Tubular atrophy may occur in some children, whereas others have minimal changes in renal function. PKD is associated with liver abnormalities that progress to fibrosis, portal hypertension, and biliary infection, which become more severe with age.

Newborns with autosomal recessive PKD may have enlarged kidneys, which are detected at birth. Those with the most severe form of the disease die shortly after birth of pulmonary hypoplasia. Clinical manifestations in infants with autosomal recessive PKD include Potter facies (low-set ears, small jaw, and a flattened nose). Hypertension develops early in infancy and is often severe. Infants may have expected urine output or oliguria. Polyuria and polydipsia develop with progressive renal insufficiency. Respiratory distress and feeding intolerance may develop from the enlarged kidneys. As uremia develops, infants and children develop renal osteodystrophy and progressive developmental delay and growth failure.

Sonogram or renal biopsy confirms the diagnosis. The disease is often diagnosed on prenatal ultrasound. Liver function tests are usually normal initially. A liver biopsy may also be performed. Other family members should be screened for subclinical cases of PKD.

Treatment is supportive. Medications such as diuretics are prescribed for hypertension, and fluid and electrolyte abnormalities are managed. Antibiotics treat urinary tract infection. Growth hormones may be used in some children to promote growth. Renal osteodystrophy is treated to suppress the parathyroid hormone. Many children develop ESRD by 10 years of age. Renal dialysis or a transplant prolong survival; however, liver problems may continue to complicate the child's health, even when the renal condition is well controlled. Up to 20–30% of children die by age 15 years (Davis & Avner, 2004).

Nursing Management

Nursing care is the same as that for the child with renal insufficiency and chronic renal failure. Observe the child for signs of progressive renal impairment. Make sure the family schedules and keeps follow-up appointments to assess growth, developmental progress, and the effectiveness of the treatment plan. Family teaching for home management focuses on medications, a diet adequate in protein and calories to support growth, management of acute gastrointestinal illnesses to prevent dehydration, and care for the child with progressive renal insufficiency and a liver disorder. Since the disease is inherited, the family should be referred for genetic counseling.

Hemolytic-Uremic Syndrome

Hemolytic-uremic syndrome (HUS), an acute renal disease, is the most common cause of acute renal failure. HUS is also an important cause of chronic renal failure. It occurs most often in children under age 4 years with a peak between 1 and 2 years. The syndrome has a classic triad of signs: (1) hemolytic anemia, (2) thrombocytopenia, and (3) ARF.

The development of HUS is often linked to bacterial and viral organisms, such as *Escherichia coli* strain 0157:H7, which is found in undercooked meat and unpasteurized milk. This organism produces a toxin that attaches to the glomeruli, collecting ducts, and distal tubules. The toxin damages the lining of the glomerular arterioles, causing the endothelial cells to swell and become occluded with platelets and fibrin clots. This partial occlusion damages the red blood cells, resulting in hemolytic anemia. Platelets cluster in areas of vascular endothelial damage, causing thrombocytopenia. Glomerular filtration is decreased, resulting in hematuria and proteinuria. Oliguria and ARF develop in nearly 50% of affected children (Huether, 2006). *Streptococcus pneumoniae* is another important organism causing HUS that is not associated with diarrhea or a gastrointestinal site of infection (Constantinescu, Bitzan, Weiss et al., 2004).

An episode of severe gastroenteritis with bloody diarrhea, upper respiratory infection, or UTI precedes the development of HUS by 1 to 2 weeks, followed by 1 to 5 days without symptoms. Signs and symptoms of HUS include hypertension, pallor, bruising, and oliguria. The child may also have fever, anorexia, vomiting and diarrhea, abdominal pain, mild jaundice, and edema or ascites. Neurologic involvement is indicated by irritability, lethargy, and seizures.

The urine is tested for hematuria and proteinuria. Serum chemistries often reveal hyperkalemia and metabolic acidosis as a result of renal failure. A peripheral blood smear with fragments of red blood cells, fibrin fragments, and a decreased platelet count (<150,000/mm^3) confirm the diagnosis. The hematocrit is less than 30%.

Treatment focuses on the complications of ARF and includes fluid restrictions and a high-calorie, high-carbohydrate diet that is low in protein, sodium, potassium, and phosphorus. Enteral nutrition is sometimes needed. The use of antibiotics is controversial; medications may include calcium gluconate or calcium chloride, aluminum hydroxide gel to bind to phosphorus, kayexalate to remove excess potassium, and antihypertensive agents. Transfusions of fresh packed red blood cells may be ordered to treat severe anemia. Platelets are given if the child is bleeding or if surgery is needed. Transfusions should be administered carefully to prevent hypertension caused by hypervolemia. About 40% of children need dialysis, and approximately 3–5% of those affected will die (Trachtman, Cnaan, Christen et al., 2003). Peritoneal dialysis is preferred unless the child has severe colitis and abdominal tenderness. Some children may develop chronic renal failure; however, most regain normal renal function (Huether, 2006).

Nursing Management

Nursing care is the same as that for the child with ARF, described earlier. Careful monitoring of neurologic signs, laboratory values, fluid and electrolyte balance, and bleeding is essential. Monitor daily weights and assess intake and output. Assess the child for abdominal discomfort from diarrhea. Observe the child carefully for signs of progressive renal impairment.

Discharge planning focuses on teaching parents about medications and dietary and fluid restrictions. Follow-up visits are necessary to evaluate the effectiveness of the treatment plan. Teach parents that HUS can be largely prevented by cooking ground beef to 155°F throughout, meaning no rare hamburgers. Teach them to wash hands carefully when handling raw ground meats, and to make sure utensils touching raw meat do not come into contact with cooked meats.

Acute Postinfectious Glomerulonephritis

Glomerulonephritis is an inflammation of the glomeruli of the kidneys. In children, it is most often a response to a nephrogenetic strain of group A beta-hemolytic streptococcal infection of the skin or pharynx. It is also caused by other organisms, including *Staphylococcus, Pneumococcus,* and *Coxsackie* viruses. The incidence of acute postinfectious glomerulonephritis (APIGN) is highest in children who are 2 to 12 years of age, and the disorder is more common in boys than in girls (Lang & Towers, 2001). Early antibiotic therapy for streptococcal infection does not seem to prevent the development of APIGN (Patel & Bissler, 2001). Other causes of glomerulonephritis in children and adolescents include immunologic abnormalities, effects of drugs or toxins, systemic diseases, and viruses (Gray, Huether, & Forshee, 2006). The focus of this discussion is APIGN.

Etiology and Pathophysiology

The child with APIGN usually becomes ill after recovering from a strain of group A beta-hemolytic streptococcal infection of the upper respiratory tract or the skin that attacks the kidney. Signs of APIGN develop after 10 to 21 days.

Glomerular damage occurs as a result of an immune complex reaction that localizes on the glomerular capillary wall. Antibody-antigen complexes become lodged in the glomeruli, leading to inflammation and obstruction. The glomerular membranes are thickened and capillaries in the glomeruli are obstructed by damaged tissue cells, leading to a decreased glomerular filtration rate. Vascular permeability increases, allowing protein, red blood cells, and red cell casts to be excreted. Sodium and water are retained, expanding the intravascular and interstitial compartments and resulting in the characteristic finding of edema (Figure 25–11 ➤).

Clinical Manifestations

Many children are asymptomatic. In other children, the onset is usually abrupt with flank or midabdominal pain, irritability, malaise, and fever. Microscopic hematuria is present in nearly all cases, and gross hematuria, resulting in tea-colored urine, is found in up to 50% of cases and may last for 1 to 2 weeks. Mild periorbital edema occurs early, along with dependent edema of the feet and ankles. Edema may progress in severity to cause a pulmonary effusion (dyspnea, cough, and crackles) or ascites (Gray, Huether, & Forshee, 2006). Acute hypertension may cause an encephalopathy that includes headache, nausea, vomiting, irritability, lethargy, and seizures. Oliguria may or may not be present.

PATHOPHYSIOLOGY ILLUSTRATED

Acute Postinfectious Glomerulonephritis

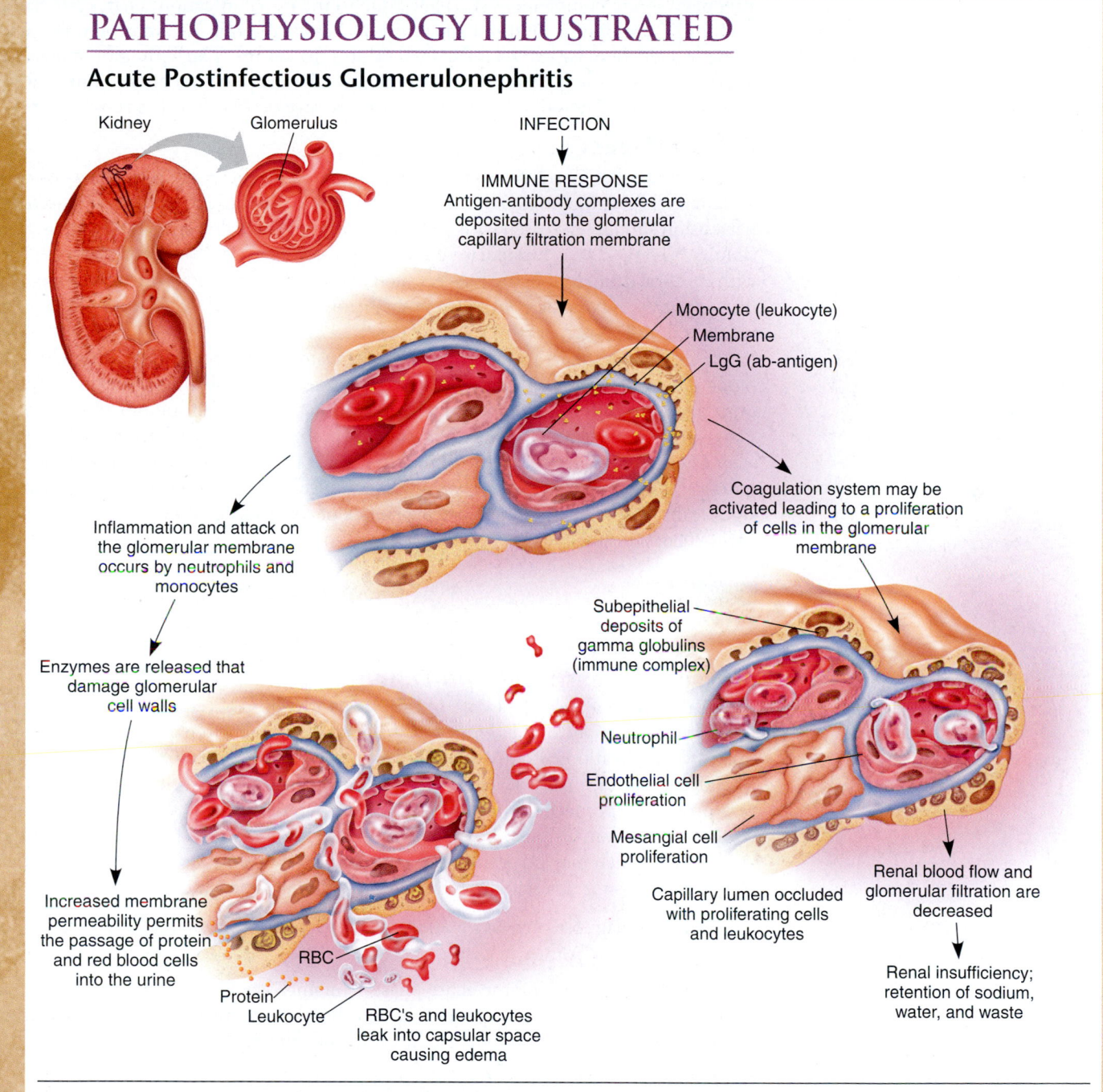

Kidney

Glomerulus

INFECTION

IMMUNE RESPONSE
Antigen-antibody complexes are deposited into the glomerular capillary filtration membrane

Monocyte (leukocyte)
Membrane
LgG (ab-antigen)

Coagulation system may be activated leading to a proliferation of cells in the glomerular membrane

Inflammation and attack on the glomerular membrane occurs by neutrophils and monocytes

Enzymes are released that damage glomerular cell walls

Subepithelial deposits of gamma globulins (immune complex)

Neutrophil

Endothelial cell proliferation

Mesangial cell proliferation

Capillary lumen occluded with proliferating cells and leukocytes

Renal blood flow and glomerular filtration are decreased

Renal insufficiency; retention of sodium, water, and waste

Increased membrane permeability permits the passage of protein and red blood cells into the urine

RBC

Protein
Leukocyte

RBC's and leukocytes leak into capsular space causing edema

Figure 25–11 ➤ Infection from group A beta-hemolytic *Streptococcus* leads to an immune response that causes inflammation and damage to the glomeruli. Protein and red blood cells are allowed to pass through the glomeruli. Blood flow to the glomeruli is reduced due to obstruction with damaged cells and renal insufficiency results, leading to the retention of sodium, water, and waste.

■ COLLABORATIVE CARE

Diagnostic Tests

The serum BUN and creatinine concentrations are elevated. Serum protein is decreased due to mild or moderate proteinuria. The white blood cell count and erythrocyte sedimentation rate may be elevated, and serum lipid levels are increased in about 40% of cases. An elevated antistreptolysin O (ASO) titer reflects the presence of antibodies from a recent pharyngeal streptococcal respiratory infection, but the ASO level associated with a recent skin infection is low. The anti-DNase B titer is helpful for detecting antibodies associated with recent skin infections. Up to 90% of children have a reduced serum complement (C3) level due to the initial infection. Urinalysis reveals hematuria, proteinuria, and red and white cell casts. Anemia is common in the acute phase, usually because extracellular fluid dilutes the serum. The hemoglobin level and hematocrit value may decrease during the late phase as a result of hematuria. Renal biopsy is rarely required unless there is a progressive deterioration in renal function.

Clinical Therapy

Treatment focuses on relief of symptoms and supportive therapy. Bed rest is a key component of the treatment plan during the acute phase. Edema and mild to moderate hypertension should be treated with sodium restriction and a diuretic such as furosemide (Lau & Wyatt, 2005). Immediate emergency care is needed for severe hypertension with cerebral dysfunction; medication such as diazoxide or hydralazine is administered intravenously. A course of antibiotics may be given to ensure eradication of the original infectious agent.

Fluid requirements are determined by careful monitoring of urinary output, weight, blood pressure, and serum electrolytes. Initially, only insensible fluid losses are replaced until the status of renal function is known. Dietary restriction of sodium and potassium intake may be necessary; with severe azotemia, protein intake may have to be limited.

The prognosis for over 90% of children with APIGN is good. Clinical signs, proteinuria, and hematuria resolve within several weeks. Most children recover without significant loss of renal function or recurrence of the disorder (Gray, Huether, & Forshee, 2006).

■ NURSING MANAGEMENT

Nursing Assessment and Diagnoses

As with other renal disorders, care of the child with APIGN requires careful monitoring of vital signs and fluid-electrolyte balance to evaluate renal functioning and to identify complications. Frequently monitor the blood pressure, which can rise as high as 200/120 mmHg. With severe hypertension, assess for signs of central nervous system problems (headache, blurred vision, vomiting, decreased level of consciousness, confusion, and convulsions). Monitor urine for proteinuria, hematuria, and output. Assess edema, which may be periorbital or dependent and shifts as the child's position is changed. Assess for a pulmonary effusion (crackles, dyspnea, and cough).

Nursing diagnoses are provided in the accompanying Nursing Care Plan.

Planning and Implementation

Bed rest is required during the acute phase. Nursing care focuses on monitoring fluid status, preventing infection, preventing skin breakdown, meeting nutritional needs, and providing emotional support to the child and family.

Monitor Fluid Status

Monitor vital signs, fluid and electrolyte status, and intake and output. Hypovolemia can occur as a result of fluid shifting from vascular to interstitial spaces despite the outward clinical signs of excess fluid retention. Monitor the degree of ascites by measuring abdominal girth. Document urine specific gravity. Make sure parents and visitors understand the need to limit fluids to prevent excessive intake.

Prevent Infection

Impaired renal function puts the child at risk for infection. Monitor for signs of infection, including fever, increased malaise, and an elevated white blood cell count. Instruct the family in good hand hygiene. Limit visitors, and screen for upper respiratory infections. Screen family members for the presence of streptococcal infection and refer for treatment, if necessary.

Prevent Skin Breakdown

Dependent areas or areas prone to pressure are vulnerable to skin breakdown. Turn the child frequently. Pad bony prominences or susceptible areas with sheepskin, or protect

NURSING CARE PLAN The Child with Acute Postinfectious Glomerulonephritis

GOAL	INTERVENTION	RATIONALE	EXPECTED OUTCOME
1. Excess Fluid Volume related to decreased glomerular filtration and increased sodium retention			
	NIC Priority Intervention: **Fluid Management:** *Promotion of fluid balance and prevention of complications resulting from abnormal and undesired fluid levels.*		*NOC Suggested Outcome:* **Fluid Balance:** *Balance of water in the intracellular and extracellular compartments of the body.*
The child will regain normal fluid balance.	• Assess for edema (periorbital or dependent areas).	• Sodium and water retention leads to edema.	The child maintains urine output that is balanced to intake. The child receives the appropriate amount of fluid each day.
	• Calculate fluid intake and plan amounts to offer throughout the day.	• An intake/output ratio of 1:1 reflects normal hydration and kidney function.	
	• Limit foods with moderate to high sodium content.	• Further reduction in sodium intake will help balance fluid and sodium retention.	
	• Document intake and output.	• Prevents excessive fluid intake.	
	• Perform daily weight measurement on same scale at the same time of day.	• Changes in weight can indicate fluid retention or improvement in condition.	
	• Administer prescribed medications (diuretics and antihypertensives).	• Diuretics cause excretion of excess fluid by preventing reabsorption of water and sodium. Antihypertensives increase excretion of water and sodium and cause vasodilation.	
2. Risk for Infection related to renal impairment and corticosteroid therapy			
	NIC Priority Intervention: **Infection Protection:** *Prevention and early detection of infection in a patient at risk.*		*NOC Suggested Outcome:* **Risk Detection:** *Actions to identify personal health threats.*
The child will develop no secondary infection.	• Assess temperature every 4 hours. Observe for signs of infection.	• The child is at risk for secondary infection.	The child's temperature remains within normal limits and the child is free of secondary infection.
	• Obtain throat culture and other cultures as ordered.	• Cultures can identify causative microorganisms in secondary infections or presence of residual streptococcal infection.	
3. Risk for Impaired Skin Integrity related to tissue edema			
	NIC Priority Intervention: **Bed Rest Care:** *Promotion of comfort and safety and prevention of complications for a patient unable to get out of bed.*		*NOC Suggested Outcome:* **Tissue Integrity: Skin and Mucous Membranes:** *Structural intactness and normal physiological function of skin and mucous membranes.*
The child's skin integrity will remain intact.	• Assess skin for redness, abrasions, and breakdown secondary to edema, bed rest, and skin rubbing against sheets.	• Ensures early identification and implementation of preventive measures.	The child develops no areas of redness, abrasions, or skin breakdown over pressure points.
	• Encourage position changes every 1–2 hours. Provide skin care. Use a therapeutic mattress.	• Prolonged pressure leads to decreased circulation and skin breakdown.	

(continued)

NURSING CARE PLAN The Child with Acute Postinfectious Glomerulonephritis (continued)

GOAL	INTERVENTION	RATIONALE	EXPECTED OUTCOME
4. Imbalanced Nutrition: Less than Body Requirements related to loss of appetite			
	NIC Priority Intervention: **Nutrition Management:** *Assistance with or provision of balanced dietary intake of foods and fluids.*		*NOC Suggested Outcome:* **Nutritional Status: Nutrient Intake:** *Adequacy of nutrients taken into the body.*
The child will maintain adequate caloric intake.	• Maintain meal schedule similar to that at home. Serve food in age-appropriate serving sizes.	• Normal routines and small frequent serving sizes help child feel less overwhelmed by calories needed.	The child maintains pre-illness body weight and tolerates the daily food intake that meets nutritional requirements.
	• Assess for food likes and dislikes. Provide favorite foods if allowed.	• Favorite foods may encourage child to eat.	
5. Activity Intolerance related to fluid and electrolyte imbalance, infectious process, and altered nutrition			
	NIC Priority Intervention: **Energy Management:** *Regulating energy use to treat and prevent fatigue and optimize function.*		*NOC Suggested Outcome:* **Energy Conservation:** *Extent of active management of energy to initiate and sustain activity.*
The child will progress in activity tolerance without excessive fatigue as the disease process improves.	• Maintain bed rest during acute stage. Encourage gradual activity increase as the condition improves.	• Rest decreases the production of waste materials, which place increased stress on the kidneys.	The child avoids fatigue and exhibits the ability to tolerate activity for a longer period each day.
	• Provide quiet play for the developmental stage of the child (e.g., coloring books, music, videos, television).	• Quiet activities minimize energy expenditure and stress on the kidneys.	
6. Effective Therapeutic Regimen Management related to parent's ability to manage child's medication schedule and treatment regimen at home			
	NIC Priority Intervention: **Anticipatory Guidance:** *Preparation of patient for an anticipated developmental and/or situational crisis.*		*NOC Suggested Outcome:* **Compliance Behavior:** *Actions taken on the basis of professional advice to promote wellness, recovery, and rehabilitation.*
The parents will state knowledge of the child's treatment regimen after discharge.	• Assess parents' understanding of the need for adherence to medication schedule, fluid limits, and dietary restrictions.	• Diuretics, antihypertensives, fluid limits, and dietary restrictions in sodium and potassium are central to the treatment plan.	The parents administer medications as prescribed. The child's sodium and potassium levels reflect adherence to dietary restrictions.
	• Collaborate on development of best schedule for giving medications to match child's and family's routines.	• Partnering with the family improves adherence.	
	• Inform parents about potential side effects of prescribed medication and signs of complications.	• Allows for early intervention in case of problems to prevent complications.	

skin with a transparent dressing. Make sure the child's bed is free of crumbs or sharp toys. Keep sheets tight and free of wrinkles.

Meet Nutritional Needs

A team approach (including the nurse, renal dietitian, parents, and child) is often needed to meet the child's nutritional needs. In most cases, the child follows a "no added salt" and low-protein diet. Anorexia presents the greatest challenge to meeting daily nutritional requirements during the acute phase of the disease. To increase the child's appetite, encourage parents to bring the child's favorite foods from home, serve foods in age-appropriate quantities, and allow the child to eat with other children or with family members.

Provide Emotional Support

Parents of a child with APIGN often feel guilty. Parents may blame themselves for not responding more quickly to the child's initial symptoms or may believe they could have prevented the development of glomerular damage. Discuss the etiology of the disease and the child's treatment, and correct any misconceptions. Emphasize that it is not possible to predict which of the few children with streptococcal infection will develop APIGN.

Discharge Planning and Home Care Teaching

Children are hospitalized for a few days, but it may take 3 weeks for hypertension and gross hematuria to resolve and longer for the disorder to resolve completely. Discharge planning focuses on teaching parents about the child's medication regimen, potential side effects of medications, dietary restrictions, and signs and symptoms of complications. Teach parents how to take the child's blood pressure and how to test urine for albumin, if ordered. Emphasize that it is important to avoid exposing the child to people with upper respiratory tract infections. Advise parents to allow the child to gradually return to his or her normal routine and activities after discharge, with periods allowed for rest.

Evaluation

Expected outcomes of nursing care are the following:

- The child receives appropriate fluid volume each day and maintains or regains normal urine output of 0.5–1 mL/kg/hr.
- The child develops no areas of redness, abrasions, or skin breakdown over pressure points.
- The child's temperature remains within normal limits and child is free of secondary infection.
- Child maintains pre-illness weight and tolerates daily intake that meets nutritional requirements.
- The parents administer medications as prescribed. The child's sodium and potassium levels reflect adherence to dietary restrictions.

STRUCTURAL DEFECTS OF THE REPRODUCTIVE SYSTEM

Phimosis

In **phimosis**, the foreskin over the glans penis cannot be retracted. As a result of natural adhesion, phimosis is a normal finding in uncircumcised infants and young males. Generally the foreskin separates from the glans during childhood, and intermittent erections lead to physiologic foreskin retraction. Obstructions to urine flow may occur when there is narrowing of the preputial opening, causing a dribbling stream. **Balanitis** (inflammation or infection of the glans penis) may occur as a result of the obstructed urine flow.

Paraphimosis, the most serious complication of phimosis, occurs when the foreskin cannot be returned to its normal position over the glans. Blood flow to the penis becomes obstructed with swelling of the glans. Ischemic injury to the glans penis occurs if the constriction is not relieved. Paraphimosis is a medical emergency and requires immediate intervention to preserve the glans penis.

Circumcision, surgical removal of the foreskin, has long been a common practice performed in some countries and cultures during the newborn period to prevent phimosis, for ease of proper male hygiene, and to prevent urinary tract infections and penile cancer. The procedure removes the skin covering the end of the penis. Circumcision is considered comparatively safe; however, complications such as damage to the urethra and disfigurement to the penis may occur.

CULTURE

Circumcision

The Jewish and Islamic faiths practice circumcision for religious and cultural reasons. Circumcision is an uncommon practice in Asia, Central America, South America, and most of Europe. Rates of circumcision in North America may be as high as 64% (Singh-Grewal, Macdessi, & Craig, 2005).

NURSING ALERT

Circumcision is contraindicated in neonates with blood dyscrasias, family history of bleeding disorder, and those that are premature. Anomalies such as hypospadias, epispadias, and chordee are other contraindications since the foreskin may be needed for later reconstruction (Lerman & Liao, 2001).

Analgesia is provided for neonatal circumcision to prevent pain and physiologic stress on the neonate. Sucrose pacifiers, EMLA cream, dorsal penile nerve block, and subcutaneous ring block are methods used (Lerman & Liao, 2001). See Chapter 15 ∞ for more information on pain management.

Betamethasone cream (0.05%) or betamethasone ointment (0.1%) applied twice daily for 4 to 8 weeks to the outer prepuce is an effective alternative to surgery with few side effects. Often the child is able to achieve foreskin retraction without surgery (Ashfield, Nickel, Siemens et al., 2003).

Nursing Management

Nursing initially focuses on educating the parents about cleansing the foreskin and penis of the uncircumcised newborn male. Educate the parents to avoid forcibly retracting the foreskin and prevent complications such as scarring or paraphimosis. Frequent diaper changes help to prevent diaper rash and irritation. When the child is older and the foreskin separates from the penis and easily retracts, teach the parents and the child to pull back the foreskin for cleaning and then to return it to its normal position.

The family requires adequate information when making an informed decision for routine circumcision of their newborn, including the risks and benefits of circumcision, potential complications, and pain relief for the infant during and following circumcision. The American Academy of Pediatrics does not recommend routine circumcision as there is no scientific evidence of the potential medical benefits of the surgery (American Academy of Pediatrics, 1999).

If circumcision is requested by parents of the newborn or it is the method of treatment for phimosis, nursing care focuses on preoperative preparation of the infant, including the advocacy for and assistance in giving the newborn local anesthesia. Postoperatively, the nurse assesses the infant's vital signs and the operative site. Educate the parents to provide proper care for the surgical site, as newborns are discharged within 24 hours of surgery. See Families Want to Know: Care Following Circumcision.

If topical steroids are prescribed as treatment, the nurse educates the family to ensure the proper application of the medication along with methods of good hygiene.

Cryptorchidism

Cryptorchidism (undescended testes) occurs when one or both testes fail to descend through the inguinal canal into the scrotum. Normally, the testes descend during the seventh to ninth month of gestation.

Cryptorchidism may be the result of a testosterone deficiency, an absent or defective testis, or a structural problem such as a narrow inguinal canal, short spermatic cord, or adhesions. The disorder occurs in 3–6% of term male infants and in 20–30% of preterm infants (Morgan & McCance, 2006). The higher temperature in the abdomen than in the scrotum results in morphologic change to the testis that are apparent by 1 year of age. Complications of cryptorchidism include infertility and malignancy.

FAMILIES WANT TO KNOW

Care Following Circumcision

Instruct the family to wash hands well before and after each diaper change and to follow these instructions for care following circumcision:

- Cover the head of the penis with a generous amount of petroleum jelly with each diaper change until the redness goes away.

- A pale yellow crust around the incision site and on the glans is normal for several days after surgery.
- Use cotton balls moistened with tap water to gently clean the head of the penis.
- Contact the healthcare provider if there is increased redness, bleeding, or swelling of the head of the penis.

Adapted from: Kaufman, M. W., Clark, J. Y., & Castro, C. L. (2001). Neonatal circumcision: Benefits, risks, and family teaching. *Maternal Child Nursing, 26*(1), 200.

Cryptorchidism is usually detected during the newborn examination when palpation of the scrotum fails to reveal one or both testes. It is not unusual for boys with cryptorchidism to have an inguinal hernia as well. In a majority of cases, the testes descend spontaneously by 3 months of age. An undescended testis may be located in the inguinal canal, abdomen, perineum, or even the thigh. Ultrasound, CT scan, and MRI may be used to identify the location of the testes. A diagnostic laparoscope may also be needed to locate the testis. When neither testis can be located, hormonal or chromosomal evaluation may be performed to detect an intersex disorder.

An orchiopexy is performed at 1 year of age before further damage to the testes occurs. An incision is made at the location of the testis, either in the abdomen or in the inguinal area. Blood vessels are disentangled to allow the testis to reach into the lower scrotum. A second incision is made in the scrotum at the point where the testis is stitched to the inside wall to keep it in place. A protective sealant is often put over the incision that peels off in 3 to 5 days. If the testis is defective or undeveloped, it may be removed surgically to decrease the risk of later malignancies and a prosthesis may be placed in the scrotum. The goals of surgery are repair of any hernia, enhanced fertility, and psychologic benefit. The orchiopexy also makes it easier to examine the testis for tumors. The risk of testicular cancer is 35 to 50 times greater in men with a history of cryptorchidism (Morgan & McCance, 2006).

Nursing Management

Preoperative nursing care includes preparing the parents and child for the procedure and addressing parents' concerns about the postsurgical outcome. Orchiopexy is often performed as an outpatient procedure. If the child is hospitalized, postoperative nursing care focuses on maintaining comfort and preventing infection. Encourage bed rest, and monitor voiding. Apply ice to the surgical area, and administer prescribed analgesics to relieve pain.

Discharge instructions should include demonstration of proper incision care. The diaper area should be cleaned well with each diaper change to decrease the chance of infection. Sponge bathe the child for 2 days after surgery, after which a tub bath or shower may be taken. No medicine or ointment should be placed over the incision. Teach parents to identify signs of infection such as redness, warmth, swelling, and discharge and to notify the physician if they are discovered. Ibuprofen or acetaminophen may be given for pain. Inform parents to avoid straddling the infant across the hip and to permit no strenuous activity or straddle toy riding for 2 weeks after surgery to promote healing and to prevent injury.

Inguinal Hernia and Hydrocele

An inguinal hernia is a painless inguinal or scrotal swelling of variable size that occurs when abdominal tissue such as bowel extends into the inguinal canal. A hydrocele is a fluid-filled mass in the scrotum. A hernia is found in 1–5% of term infants and up to 11% of preterm infants, more commonly in boys than girls (Burd & Burd, 2002).

During fetal development, a peritoneal sac precedes the testicle's descent to the scrotum. The lower sac enfolds the testis to become the tunica vaginalis, and the upper sac atrophies before birth. Fluid may become trapped in the tunica vaginalis and cause the hydrocele. When the tunica vaginalis does not atrophy, an abdominal structure may move into it. In males, the bowel is the most frequent tissue protruding into the groin, and in females an ovary or fallopian tube is a common finding (Katz, 2001).

Diagnosis is made by physical examination at birth or in early infancy. Palpation of the scrotum reveals a round, smooth, nontender mass. Transillumination helps determine whether the mass is a hernia or hydrocele (see Chapter 5 ∞). Parents may report an intermittent bulge in the groin or swelling in the scrotum. Swelling associated with a hernia may become more apparent with straining. Some hernias reduce in size during sleep.

Outpatient surgery is performed at an early age (usually after 3 months of age to reduce anesthesia risks) to avoid **incarceration** (hernia cannot be reduced and circulation to trapped tissue is impaired), which is a medical emergency. A nerve block may

> **NURSING ALERT**
>
> Inguinal hernias can become incarcerated when a bit of bowel becomes trapped in the inguinal opening and the blood supply is constricted. The child has an acute onset of pain, abdominal distention, vomiting, and an irreducible mass. Other findings may include an edematous scrotum, poor feeding, and bloody stools (Burd & Burd, 2002). Efforts are made to reduce the hernia before surgery by sedating the child and applying firm manual pressure on the affected side. If the hernia is reduced, surgery is often performed several days later. If the hernia cannot be reduced, emergency surgery is performed (Coppola, 2005).

be given in the operating room to reduce postoperative pain. The prognosis is generally excellent. Most hydroceles without inguinal hernia resolve spontaneously as the fluid reabsorbs by the time an infant is 1 to 2 years of age.

Nursing Management

Nursing care for hydrocele and inguinal hernia includes explaining the disorder and its treatment and providing preoperative and postoperative teaching and care. Inform parents that the scrotum may be edematous and may appear bruised after surgery. Incision care involves careful cleaning of the diaper area. The incision is covered with a protective sealant rather than a dressing. Acetaminophen is provided for pain.

Testicular Torsion

Testicular torsion is an emergency condition in which the testis suddenly rotates on its spermatic cord, cutting off its blood supply. The arteries and veins in the spermatic cord become twisted and interrupt the blood supply, leading to vascular engorgement and ischemia. Testicular torsion occurs in approximately 1 in 4000 males before 25 years of age, with the highest incidence at puberty (Sessions, Rabinowitz, Hulbert et al., 2003; McAndrew, Pemberton, Kikiros et al., 2002). Often the testicles are positioned horizontally in the scrotum, a congenital anomaly known as a bell clapper deformity, which predisposes the boy to this condition.

Manifestations include severe pain and erythema in the scrotum, nausea and vomiting, abdominal pain, and scrotal swelling that is not relieved by rest or scrotal support. The testes are tender on palpation and become edematous. The cremasteric reflex is absent. Symptoms generally start when the child is sleeping or inactive, but they can occur after trauma, sexual activity, or exercise. The testis is positioned higher in the scrotum than the unaffected testis because of the shortened vascular pedicle. A testicular scan or Doppler flow sonogram may be performed if immediately available; however, a risk for delay in treatment and misdiagnosis with these procedures is possible (McAndrew et al., 2002).

Torsion must be reduced within 4 to 6 hours to save the testis. Manual reduction with an analgesic is sometimes attempted, but emergency surgery is more common. During surgery (orchipexy), the testis is untwisted and stitched to the side of the scrotum in the correct position. The procedure is usually performed bilaterally to prevent future torsion in the other testis.

Nursing Management

Nursing management involves psychologic support for the child and family related to the need for emergency surgery and concern about the child's future fertility. Reassure parents that as only one testis is usually involved, fertility should not be affected. The child often goes home within a few hours of surgery; thus, the child and family need to be taught about proper care of the incision and pain management. Explain to parents that the child should not lift heavy objects for 4 weeks or participate in strenuous activity for 2 weeks after surgery to promote healing. Teach the adolescent testicular self-examination.

SEXUALLY TRANSMITTED INFECTIONS

Sexually transmitted infections (STIs) are a major national public health concern and they pose a significant health risk to children and adolescents. Numerous organisms of bacterial, parasitic, and viral origin, including the human immunodeficiency virus (HIV), have been identified as causative agents of sexually transmitted infections. Children and adolescents can become infected with sexually transmitted organisms through sexual experimentation, sexual play, molestation, and sexual abuse. Some diseases, such as chlamydia, syphilis, and gonorrhea, acquired after the neonatal period are almost always indicative of sexual contact (CDC, 2002).

Of the 15 million new STI cases each year, approximately 25% occur in adolescents. Female adolescents have the highest reported rates of STIs, and they also have

NURSING ALERT

When a child younger than 10 years is found to have gonorrhea or other sexually transmitted infection, consider the possibility of sexual abuse. When anorectal symptoms are found, suspect molestation (see Chapter 6 ∞).

the potential for more complications, such as pelvic inflammatory disease (Shafii & Burstein, 2004). Results from the Centers for Disease Control National Youth Risk Behavioral Surveillance (2004) demonstrated that 46.7% of high school students had engaged in sexual intercourse and 37% of sexually active adolescents had not used a condom during their last sexual intercourse. Adolescents are considered an at-risk population related to their inexperience and lack of knowledge about STIs. Recent studies have determined that adolescents possess minimal knowledge about non-HIV sexually transmitted diseases, their treatments, and their curability (Clark, Jackson, & Allen-Taylor, 2002).

Factors contributing to the risk to the child and adolescent include the avoidance of protective barriers, multiple sexual partners, frequent sexual activity, and failure to seek medical treatment until symptoms are well advanced. The adolescent who acquires an STI has a 40% chance of acquiring another STI within a year, especially if gonorrhea is the first infection (Stamm & McGregor, 2001). The rates of chlamydia and gonorrhea are highest in the female age group of 15–19 years (Centers for Disease Control and Prevention, 2002).

Frequently diagnosed STIs are chlamydia, genital herpes (herpes simplex type 2), gonorrhea, genital warts (Human papillomavirus), trichomoniasis, and syphilis. Refer to the table on the next page for information about clinical manifestations and clinical therapy for the most common STIs.

State and local health departments are responsible for controlling the spread of STIs through health promotion programs, staff training, reporting systems, diagnosis, treatment, patient counseling, and the notification of sex partners. To reduce all sexually transmitted infections, the CDC recommends abstinence from sexual contact, or a long-term mutually monogamous relationship with a partner who has been tested for STIs and is known to be uninfected (CDC, 2002). A new vaccine has been approved for adolescents to prevent human papillomavirus. See Chapter 18 ∞.

Human immunodeficiency virus is discussed in Chapter 17, and Hepatitis B, another infection that can be transmitted sexually, is discussed in Chapter 24 ∞.

NURSING MANAGEMENT
Nursing Assessment and Diagnosis

Nursing assessment focuses on identifying signs and symptoms indicative of sexually transmitted infections, assessing for the potential for asymptomatic sexually transmitted infections, and assessing the psychosocial impact on the child or adolescent with a sexually transmitted infection.

The nurse usually encounters the child or adolescent and family in the emergency department, outpatient clinic, or nursing unit. Since adolescents are often afraid of the consequences of reporting symptoms, good assessment and communication skills are important considerations for the nurse, particularly when asking questions about sexual activity, partners, and the possibility of abuse. Essential to communication is maintaining a warm, encouraging, nonjudgmental approach and conveying acceptance when discussing sexual health issues with the child or adolescent. In order to achieve the adolescent's cooperation, confidentiality must be assured. Offer support to the adolescent and encourage the seeking of parental guidance and involvement.

Assess the child or adolescent for manifestations as described in the clinical manifestations table on the next page. When a child or adolescent is diagnosed with one STI, it is essential to screen for the presence of other STIs, as these diseases may coexist. Adolescents who are symptomatic may postpone care due to feeling uncomfortable about genital examinations. Given that many adolescents have subclinical cases or are asymptomatic, routine screening of sexually active adolescents is recommended.

CLINICAL TIP

Questions that may be useful in collecting a sexual history include:

- Do you hang out with boys, girls, or mixed groups?
- Are some of your friends involved in a romantic relationship? How about you?
- Have any of your friends had a pregnancy scare or an STI? Has that happened to you?
- Are you currently involved in a romantic relationship? Is sex a part of this relationship?
- Has anyone ever touched you in a way that you did not like? Forced you to have sex?
- In your opinion, what is the best way for a teen to protect herself or himself from getting an STI? Any other ways? Do you protect yourself? How?

Adapted from: McEvoy, M., & Coupey, S. M. (2002). Sexually transmitted infection: A challenge for nurses working with adolescents. *Nursing Clinics of North America, 37*(3), 461–474.

CLINICAL MANIFESTATIONS | SEXUALLY TRANSMITTED INFECTIONS

Disease and Organism	Clinical Manifestations and Complications	Clinical Therapy and Patient Education
Chlamydia *Chlamydia trachomatis*	The clinical manifestations in adolescent females include yellow mucopurulent endocervical discharge, dysuria, pelvic pain, mild abdominal pain, vaginal spotting, cervicitis, salpingitis, and pelvic inflammatory disease (PID). Cases are frequently asymptomatic. Manifestations in adolescent males include urethritis, mucoid gray or clear discharge, dysuria, proctitis, epididymitis. Complications associated with chlamydia in females include pelvic inflammatory disease (PID) and infertility. Chlamydia is a leading cause of early infant pneumonia and conjunctivitis (pink eye) in newborns.	Diagnosis by culture or a nucleic acid-amplified test on the urine. Recommended medication therapy includes doxycycline, or erythromycin for 7 days, or single-dose azithromycin. HIV-positive persons with chlamydia receive the same treatment as those who are HIV negative. All sex partners should be evaluated, tested, and treated. Encourage abstinence from sexual intercourse until they and their sex partners have completed treatment, to prevent reinfection. Encourage use of condoms. All sexually active female adolescents should be screened at least annually for chlamydia.
Genital Herpes *Herpes simplex virus* 1 (HSV-1) or 2 (HSV-2).	Most infected with HSV-2 are not aware of their infection. Presentation can be variable and ranges from no symptoms to systematic involvement. Common symptoms include dull pain, itching, and small lesions or pimples on genitalia, buttocks, or thighs. Two types of lesions develop, either fluid-filled blisters on an erythematous base or, more commonly, painful papules and ulcers. Ulcers can appear between vaginal folds, in the posterior cervix, on the glans penis, or on the shaft of the penis, in the rectum, or in the anus. Ulcers heal within 2–4 weeks. Lymph nodes closest to lesions are frequently enlarged. The disease frequently recurs 4–5 times a year with episodes lasting 5–10 days. Triggers include stress, menses, or trauma.	Diagnosis is confirmed by virology and type-specific serologic tests. There is no permanent cure. Recommended drug therapy is acyclovir given for 7–10 days. Antiviral medications can shorten and prevent outbreaks during the period of time the person takes the medication. Daily suppressive therapy for symptomatic herpes can reduce transmission to partners. A cesarean delivery is usually performed for infected pregnant women. Discourage oral sex if ulcers are present in the mouth, on the lips, in the vagina, or on the penis. Discourage anal sex when lesions are active. Encourage use of condoms, although they may not prevent transmission. Emphasize that the patient remains contagious, even after lesions are healed.
Gonorrhea *Neisseria gonorrhoeae*	Symptoms and severity vary from mild to severe and are different for males and females. In females, areas that can be infected include urethra, cervix, fallopian tubes, and Bartholin and Skene glands. In males, areas include urethra, prostate, seminal vesicles, epididymis, and Littre and Cowper glands. Of females, 51% are asymptomatic (Burstein & Murray, 2003). The classic sign is discharge from the vagina and urethra; however, infections involving the conjunctiva, pharynx, and anus area are also seen. Prepubescent girls: heavy, thick green or creamy vaginal discharge, vulvovaginitis. Adolescent girls: purulent vaginal discharge, cervicitis; fallopian tube; and pelvic inflammatory disease involvement can lead to sterility. Prepubescent and adolescent boys: yellow pus-like urethral discharge, erythematous meatus, frequency, dysuria, and painful or swollen testicles. Although many men with gonorrhea may have no symptoms at all, some men have some signs or symptoms that appear 2 to 5 days after infection; symptoms can take as long as 30 days to appear. Symptoms and signs of rectal infection in both genders include discharge, anal itching, soreness, bleeding, or painful bowel movements. However, they may be asymptomatic. Infections in the throat may cause a sore throat, but they are usually asymptomatic. Transmission to neonate during vaginal delivery can cause blindness, joint infection, or sepsis. Gonorrhea is a common cause of pelvic inflammatory disease (PID).	Diagnosis by culture of vaginal or urethral discharge or nucleic acid-amplified test on the urine. Recommended drug therapy includes a single dose of ceftriaxone IM, or a single oral dose of cefixime, ciprofloxacin, ofloxacin, or levofloxacin plus treatment for chlamydia if chlamydia infection is not ruled out (Workowski &Berman, 2006). Sexual partners should be treated if adolescent has had sexual contact within 60 days of onset of symptoms. Encourage use of condomsor abstinence. Emphasize the importance of taking all of the medication prescribed to cure gonorrhea. The individual and all sex partners must avoid sex until they have completed their treatment for gonorrhea.

CLINICAL MANIFESTATIONS	SEXUALLY TRANSMITTED INFECTIONS (continued)

Disease and Organism	Clinical Manifestations and Complications	Clinical Therapy and Patient Education
Human Papillomavirus (HPV)	HPV the most common STD in adolescents, has been found in 40% of sexually active females (American Academy of Pediatrics, 2003). Warts are small, flat, and fleshy-colored with a cauliflower appearance. Adolescent females: warts clustered or alone on the vulva, perineal area, vagina, or cervix; itching, bleeding, burning, irritation. A subclinical infection may be detected through a Pap smear. Specific types of HPV cause 90% of cervical cancers (American Academy of Pediatrics, 2003). Adolescent males: warts on the penis, near base of penis on scrotal skin, or near anus.	Diagnosis is based upon physical findings or biopsy. The PAP test may be abnormal. No cure exists. Treatment includes cryotherapy, topical podophyllin, laser ablation, or chemical cautery with trichloracetic acid. Encourage abstinence or condom use, although condoms are not sufficient to prevent contact transmission. The disorder is transmissible even after treatment.
Trichomoniasis, *Trichomonas vaginalis*	Adolescent females: pale yellow to gray-green discharge that may be frothy or have a fishy odor, dysuria, vulvar pruritis, occasional abdominal pain; symptoms worsen during menses. Adolescent males: most common site is the urethra; mucoid or purulent urethral discharge, pruritis, dysuria; however, males are usually asymptomatic.	Diagnosis by culture. Metronidazole orally as a single dose or for 7 days. Both partners should be treated at the same time to eliminate the parasite. Avoid drinking alcohol during and for several days after treatment if a single dose is used. Sexual contact should be avoided until both partners are cured. No follow-up test is needed if symptoms resolve after treatment.
Syphilis, *Treponema pallidum*	Appearance of classic signs and symptoms of syphilis depends on the stage of disease. *Primary state* manifests an ulcer on the labia, within vagina, on penis, in anus, or on lips or tongue that appears at invasion site approximately 2 weeks to 3 months after infection. Ulcer has an indurated border and smooth base (chancre), and it is painless. Lymphadenopathy is usually present. Ulcer spontaneously heals within 5 weeks. *Second stage* appears up to 10 weeks after initial infection with fever, malaise, lymphadenopathy, patchy alopecia, and diffuse rash. Rash can be macular, papular, papulosquamous, or bullous, and appearance on the palms and soles is classic. Flat mucous patches called condylomata lata appear on genitals. *Latent stage* is asymptomatic and follows the second stage by about 6 weeks. It can last for several years or be lifelong. *Tertiary stage* occurs more than 2 years after onset and manifests as neurosyphilis, cardiovascular disease, ophthalmic, or congenital syphilis.	Diagnosis by serologic tests or direct fluorescent antibody tests of lesion exudate. Due to the risk of fetal death, every pregnant woman should have a blood test for syphilis. Syphilis is easy to cure in its early stages. Recommended drug therapy includes single IM injection of benzathine penicillin G. For children allergic to penicillin, erythromycin is given by mouth for 15 days. Saline compresses and a topical antibiotic are often used to treat lesions on the skin. Treat all sexual contacts within 90 days to 1 year of diagnosis, depending upon the stage when diagnosed. During syphilis treatment, abstain from sexual contact with new partners until the syphilis sores are completely healed. Encourage abstinence or the use of condoms plus spermicidal foams, cream, or jelly to prevent infection.

Data From: Centers for Disease Control and Prevention. (2002). Sexually transmitted diseases treatment guidelines, 2002. *Morbidity and Mortality Weekly Report, 51*(RR-6), 1–82; Burstein, G. R., & Murray, P. J. (2003). Diagnosis and management of sexually transmitted disease pathogens among adolescents. *Pediatrics in Review, 24*(3), 75–81.

Nursing diagnoses that may apply to the child or adolescent with a sexually transmitted infection include:

- Anxiety related to presence of sexually transmitted infection
- Pain related to genital irritation
- Deficient Knowledge (Sexually Transmitted Infections) related to cause, transmission, treatments, and prevention
- Disturbed Body Image related to genital lesions, presence of genital infection

Planning and Implementation

The nurse focuses on identifying adolescents at risk for STIs, providing appropriate education, and preventing transmission and complications.

When counseling the adolescent, reinforce the importance of treating all sexual partners and modifying high-risk sexual behaviors. Notification of all sexual partners is essential to treat infected partners and to reduce the risk of reinfection (Fortenberry,

Brizendine, Katz, & Orr, 2002). Encourage sexually active adolescents to receive hepatitis B immunization if not already obtained.

Care in the Community

Education includes promoting abstinence, which means avoiding *any* type of sexual contact with a partner. (See Families Want to Know: Preventing STIs and Their Consequences.) The nurse, in partnership with schools and community organizations, is active in sexual health promotion through schools, health clinics, community services, and groups or organizations.

Work with sexually active adolescents to identify methods of reducing the risk of contracting STIs. Suggestions include the use of latex condoms (though the possibility of STI transmission still exists even with the use of latex condoms), voiding immediately after sexual intercourse, and appropriate genital hygiene with soap and water. Assist adolescents to avoid sexual partners who are at higher risk for STIs, such as intravenous drug users and those who have multiple sexual partners. Emphasize to the adolescent that even with applying these measures, there is no guaranteed protection against STIs except when using abstinence. Explain to the adolescent that some STIs, such as chlamydia, are asymptomatic.

Additional teaching includes dispelling myths of how STIs are spread. Instruct the child or adolescent that STIs are not contracted from sharing bath towels, clothing, and drinking glasses, or from sitting on toilet seats. Inform the female taking contraceptives that birth control offers no protection against STIs.

Evaluation

Expected outcomes for the child or adolescent with a sexually transmitted infection are:

- The child or adolescent remains free from pain.
- An understanding of the transmission, prevention, and treatment of sexually transmitted infections is demonstrated by the adolescent.
- The adolescent has a positive body image.
- Reduced anxiety is displayed by the child or adolescent.

Pelvic Inflammatory Disease (PID)

Pelvic inflammatory disease (PID) is an infection of the upper genital tract caused by the ascending spread of organisms in the cervix and vagina. The majority of cases of PID are caused by *chlamydia trachomatis* or *Neisseria gonorrhea*. It is estimated that between 10–40% of untreated gonorrhea and chlamydia infections result in PID (Bortot, Risser, & Cromwell, 2004).

The infection ascends into the uterus and fallopian tubes during the menses when the cervix mucosal plug is open and retrograde menstrual blood can flow into the fallopian tubes. A significant complication is Fitz-Hugh-Curtis syndrome, in which the anterior surface of the liver and adjacent parietal peritoneum become infected (Bortot, Risser, & Cromwell, 2004).

FAMILIES WANT TO KNOW

Preventing STIs and Their Consequences

Collaborate with the child and family to promote the following recommendations in preventing STIs and their consequences:

- Abstinence is the best method to prevent STIs.
- Limit the number of sexual contacts; practice mutual monogamy.
- Always use condoms and spermicidal gels or foams for vaginal and anal intercourse.

- Refrain from oral sex if partner has active sores in the mouth, vagina, anus, or penis.
- Reduce high-risk sexual behaviors. Use of recreational drugs and alcohol can increase sexual risk taking.
- Seek care as soon as symptoms are noticed and make sure your partner gets treatment.
- Seek annual screening for STIs.

Signs and symptoms of PID may include fever, mild or dull bilateral lower abdominal pain, dysmenorrheal pain that is worse or longer lasting than usual, dysuria, vaginal discharge, pain with sexual activity, prolonged or increased menstrual bleeding, nausea, and vomiting. Most cases are mild. Some females complain of right upper quadrant pain when Fitz-Hugh-Curtis syndrome is present.

No specific laboratory test exists for PID. During a pelvic examination, uterine or adnexal tenderness or tenderness with cervical motion is present. Other criteria that help support the diagnosis of PID include an elevated erythrocyte sedimentation rate, elevated C-reactive protein level, white blood cells seen on microscopic examination of vaginal secretions, and documented cervical infection with gonorrhea or chlamydia (Centers for Disease Control and Prevention, 2002). A transvaginal sonogram may reveal thickened and fluid-filled fallopian tubes with or without free pelvic fluid. A pregnancy test, HIV test, and cultures for STIs should be performed.

Parenteral antibiotic therapy is often used for the first 24 hours before converting to oral antibiotics for the remaining 14 days of treatment. Common intravenous antibiotics used include cefotetan or cefoxitin plus doxycycline or clindamycin plus gentamycin. Oral antibiotics may include ofloxacin, levofloxacin, and ceftriaxone or cefoxitin plus doxycycline. Follow-up physical examination is performed in 72 hours to monitor treatment adherence and to detect improvement in symptoms and reduced pelvic tenderness. Hospitalization and IV antibiotics are initiated if no improvement is noted.

Nursing Management

A sexual history should be obtained from all adolescent females to identify the risk for sexually transmitted infection and PID. Adolescents at greater risk for PID include those who have multiple sexual partners, a history of a previous sexually transmitted infection, use sex for survival, lack consistent condom use, and use douching (Eissa & Cromwell, 2003). Less than 10% of adolescents with PID have signs of a severe infection. Encourage adolescents who are sexually active to have a pelvic examination to detect signs of a sexually transmitted infection and PID.

Administer medications intravenously for the first 24 hours, making arrangements for the adolescent to return for a second dose 12 hours after the first. Provide education for the ongoing treatment with oral antibiotics, ensuring that the adolescent understands the importance of taking all medications on schedule for the full 14 days. Provide signs of adverse effects and actions to take if they occur.

Determine if the adolescent's parents have been informed about the illness, and assist the adolescent to discuss the health problem with the parents. If parents are unaware of the health problem, discuss the importance of telling the parents so that they can help identify any problems that develop during treatment.

Provide counseling about methods to reduce the risk for reinfection with a sexually transmitted infection. Provide information about the potential consequences of infertility, ectopic pregnancy, and chronic abdominal pain for this infection and the increased risk for these consequences with subsequent infections. Encourage regular health visits with screening for sexually transmitted infections, as future chlamydia and gonorrhea infections may be asymptomatic.

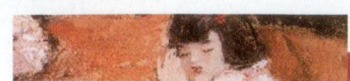

CRITICAL THINKING IN ACTION

Recall Terrell, the child in the opening scenario with ESRD secondary to posterior ureteral valves. Terrell receives hemodialysis three times a week since peritonitis resulted after peritoneal dialysis. Terrell is on the transplant list for a cadaver kidney as no one in the family is able to donate a kidney.

Terrell has been gaining weight and is edematous. Upon evaluation, his primary nurse at the dialysis center discovers that Terrell has been drinking cokes and eating "junk food" at school. Terrell asks the nurse not to tell his mother because she will be mad, but that he just can't help eating and drinking what he isn't supposed to.

DISCUSSION

1. What approach does the nurse take in discussing this nutritional issue with Terrell and his family?

2. How does Terrell's growth and development level affect his adherence to the treatment regimen?

3. Terrell's family receives a call that a donor kidney is available and Terrell is immediately taken to the medical center for a transplant. What discussions should have occurred with Terrell's family prior to the transplant? Following the transplant, what are the most important elements of teaching for Terrell and the family?

4. Establish three priority nursing diagnoses for Terrell's long-term post-transplant care. What interventions will be implemented? How will they be evaluated?

 Refer to your Prentice Hall Nursing MediaLink DVD-ROM for answers.

EXPLORE MediaLink 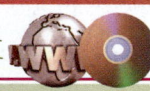 http://www.prenhall.com/ball

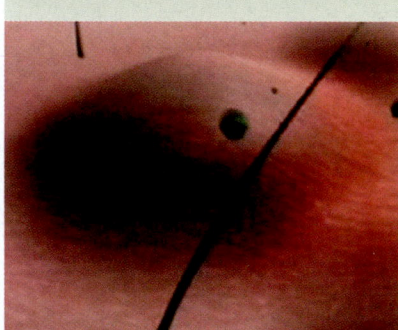

Resources for this chapter can be found on the Prentice Hall Nursing MediaLink DVD-ROM accompanying this textbook, and on the Companion Website at http://www.prenhall.com/ball.

DVD-ROM
Audio Glossary
NCLEX-RN® Review
Animations/Videos
   Renal Function
   Sexually Transmitted Infections

COMPANION WEBSITE
Audio Glossary
NCLEX-RN® Review
Care Plan Activity: A School-age Child with Acute Renal Failure
Case Study: A Child with Chronic Kidney Failure
MediaLink Application: Child Having Nocturnal Enuresis
WebLinks

REFERENCES

American Academy of Pediatrics. (1999). Circumcision policy statement. *Pediatrics, 103*(3), 686–693. Retrieved April 1, 2006, from http://aappolicy.aappublications.org/cgi/content/abstract/pediatrics;103/3/686

American Academy of Pediatrics. (2003). *Red book: Report of the Committee on Infectious Disease* (26th ed.). Chicago, IL: Author.

Ashfield, J. E., Nickel, K. R., Siemens, D. R., MacNeily, A. E., & Nickel, J. C. (2003). Treating phimosis with topical steroids in 194 children. *Journal of Urology, 169*(3), 1106–1108.

Benfield, M. R. (2003). Current status of kidney transplant: Update 2003. *Pediatric Clinics of North America, 50,* 1301–1334.

Bennett, H. J. (2005). Clinical tips for helping patients overcome bedwetting. *Contemporary Pediatrics, 22*(9) 92–96.

Berry, A. (2005). Helping children with dysfunctional voiding. *Urologic Nursing, 25*(3), 193–200.

Bock, K. R. (2005). Renal replacement therapy in pediatric critical care medicine. *Current Opinion in Pediatrics, 17,* 368–371.

Bortot, A. T., Risser, W. L., & Cromwell, P. F. (2004). Coping with pelvic inflammatory disease in the adolescent. *Contemporary Pediatrics, 21*(4), 33–48.

Boydstun, I. I. (2005). Acute renal failure. *Adolescent Medicine Clinics, 16*(1), 1–9.

Brooks, L. J., & Topol, H. I. (2003). Enuresis in children with sleep apnea. *The Journal of Pediatrics, 142*(5), 515–518.

Burd, A. J., & Burd, R. S. (2002). Inguinal hernia in the premature infant: Management of a common problem. *Neonatal Network, 21*(7), 39–47.

Burstein, G. R., & Murray, P. J. (2003). Diagnosis and management of sexually transmitted disease pathogens among adolescents. *Pediatrics in Review, 24*(3), 75–81.

Centers for Disease Control and Prevention. (2002). Sexually transmitted diseases treatment guidelines, 2002. *Morbidity and Mortality Weekly Report, 51,* (RR-6), 1–82.

Centers for Disease Control and Prevention. (2004). Youth Risk Behavioral Surveillance—United States 2003. *Morbidity and Mortality Weekly Report, 53*(SS-2).

Chand, D. H., Brier, M., Strife, F., and the Medical Review Board of the Renal Network,

Inc. (2005). Comparison of vascular access type in pediatric hemodialysis patients with respect to urea clearance, anemia management, and serum albumin concentration. *American Journal of Kidney Disease, 45*(2), 303–308.

Chesney, R. W., & Wyatt, R. J. (2003). Racial disparities in renal transplant in children. *Pediatrics, 112*(2), 409–410.

Clark, L. R., Jackson, M., & Allen-Taylor, L. (2002). Adolescent knowledge about sexually transmitted diseases. *Sexually Transmitted Diseases, 29*(8), 436–443.

Constantinescu, A. R., Bitzan, M., Weiss, L. S., Christen, E., Kaplan, B. S., Cnaan, A., & Trachtman, H. (2004). Non-enteropathic hemolytic uremic syndrome: Causes and short-term course. *American Journal of Kidney Diseases, 43*(6), 976–982.

Coppola, C. P. (2005). A surgeon in your corner. *Pediatric Annals, 34*(11), 903–908.

Corbett, J. V. (2004). Laboratory tests and diagnostic procedures with nursing diagnoses (6th ed.). Upper Saddle River, NJ: Prentice Hall Health.

Davis, I. D., & Avner, E. D. (2004). Anatomic abnormalities associated with hematuria. In R. E. Behrman, R. M. Kliegman, & H. B. Jenson, *Nelson textbook of pediatrics* (17th ed, pp. 1749–1750). Philadelphia: Saunders.

Dulczak, S., & Kirk, J. (2005). Overview of the evaluation, diagnosis, and management of urinary tract infections in infants and children. *Urologic Nursing, 25*(3), 185–191.

Eissa, M. A. H., & Cromwell, P. F. (2003). Diagnosis and management of pelvic inflammatory disease in adolescents. *Journal of Pediatric Health Care, 17*(3), 145–147.

Fakhouri, F., Bocquet, N., Taupin, P., Presne, C., Gagnadoux, M. F., Landais, P., et al. (2003). Steroid sensitive nephrotic syndrome: From childhood to adulthood. *American Journal of Kidney Diseases, 41*(3), 550–557.

Feinstein, S., Keich, R., Becker-Cohen, R., Rinat, C., Schwartz, S. B., & Frishberg, Y. (2005). Is noncompliance among adolescent renal transplant recipients inevitable? *Pediatrics, 115*(4), 969–973.

Fortenberry, J. D., Brizendine, E. J., Katz, B. P., & Orr, D. P. (2002). The role of self-efficacy and relationship quality in partner notification by adolescents with sexually transmitted infections. *Archives of Pediatric and Adolescent Medicine, 156*(11), 1133–1137.

Garin, E. H., Olavarria, F., Nieto, V. G., Valenciano, B., Campos, A., & Young, L. (2006). Clinical significance of primary vesicoureteral reflux and urinary antibiotic prophylaxis after acute pyelonephritis: A multicenter, randomized controlled study. *Pediatrics, 117*(3), 626–632.

Geary, D. F., Piva, E., Tyrrell, J., Gajaria, M. J., Picone, G., Keating, L. E., & Harvey, E. A. (2005). Home nocturnal hemodialysis in children. *Journal of Pediatrics, 147*(3), 383–387.

Gray, M., Huether, S. E., & Forshee, B. A. (2006). Alterations of renal and urinary tract function. In K. L. McCance & S. E. Huether, *Pathophysiology: The biologic basis for disease in adults and children* (5th ed., pp. 1301–1335). St. Louis: Elsevier Mosby.

Guay-Woodford, L. M., & Desmond, R. A. (2003). Autosomal recessive polycystic kidney disease: The clinical experience in North America. *Pediatrics, 111*(5), 1072–1080.

Gulati, S., Godbole, M., Singh, U., Gulati, K., & Srivastava, A. (2003). Are children with idiopathic nephrotic syndrome at risk for metabolic bone disease? *American Journal of Kidney Diseases, 41*(6), 1163–1169.

Hanson, K. A. (2003). Diagnostic tests and tools in the evaluation of urologic disease, Part II. *Urologic Nursing, 23*(6), 405–415.

Hogg, R. J., Furth, S., Lemley, K. V., Portman, R., Schwartz, G. J., et al., (2003). National Kidney Foundation's kidney disease outcomes quality initiative clinical practice guidelines for chronic kidney disease in children and adolescents: Evaluation, classification, and stratification. *Pediatrics, 111*(6), 1416–1421.

Hogg, R. J., Portman, R. J., Milliner, D., Lemley, K. V., Eddy, A., & Ingelfinger, J. (2000). Evaluation and management of proteinuria and nephrotic syndrome in children: Recommendation from a pediatric nephrology panel established at the National Kidney Foundation Conference on Proteinuria, Albuminuria, Risk, Assessment, Detection, and Elimination (PARADE). *Pediatrics, 105*(6), 1242–1249.

Huether, S. E. (2006). Alterations of renal and urinary tract function in children. In K. L. McCance & S. E. Huether, *Pathophysiology: The biologic basis for disease in adults and children* (5th ed., pp. 1337–1352). St. Louis: Elsevier Mosby.

Katz, D. A. (2001). Evaluation and management of inguinal and umbilical hernias. *Pediatric Annals, 30*(12), 729–735.

Kaufman, M. W., Clark, J. Y., & Castro, C. L. (2001). Neonatal circumcision: Benefits, risks, and family teaching. *Maternal Child Nursing, 26*(1), 200.

Kraus, S. J. (2001). Genitourinary imaging in children. *Pediatric Clinics of North America, 48*(6), 1381–1423.

Lang, M. M., & Towers, C. (2001). Identifying poststreptoccal glomerulonephritis. *The Nurse Practitioner, 26*(8), 34–49.

Lau, K. K., & Wyatt, R. J. (2005). Glomerulonephritis. *Adolescent Medicine Clinics, 16*(1), 67–85.

Legg, V. (2005). Complications of chronic kidney disease. *American Journal of Nursing, 105*(6), 40–49.

Lerman, S. E., & Liao, J. C. (2001). Neonatal circumcision. *Pediatric Clinics of North America, 48*(6), 1539–1557.

Leung, A. K. C., Robson, W. L. M., & Wong, A. L. (2005, February). What's your diagnosis? Bladder exstrophy. *Consultant for Pediatricians, 4*, 77–80.

Liberti, J. (2005). Biofeedback therapy in pediatric urology. *Urologic Nursing, 25*(3), 206–210.

McAndrew, H. F., Pemberton, R., Kikiros, C. S., & Gollow, I. (2002). The incidence and investigation of acute scrotal problems in children. *Pediatric Surgery International, 18*, 435–437.

McEvoy, M., & Coupey, S. M. (2002). Sexually transmitted infection: A challenge for nurses working with adolescents. *Nursing Clinics of North America, 37*(3), 461–474.

Mercer, R. (2003). Dry at night: Treating nocturnal enuresis. *Advance for Nurse Practitioners, 11*(2), 26–32.

Morgan, K., & McCance, K. L. (2006). Alterations of the reproductive systems. In K. L.

McCance & S. E. Huether, *Pathophysiology: The biologic basis for disease in adults and children* (5th ed., pp. 771–861). St. Louis: Elsevier Mosby.

Myers, P. S. (2002). Transitioning an adolescent dialysis patient to adult health care. *Nephrology Nursing Journal, 29*(4), 375–376.

National Kidney and Urological Diseases. (2005). Financial help for treatment of kidney failure. NIH Publication 05-476F. Retrieved July 31, 2006, from http://www.kidney.niddk.nih.gov/kudiseases/pubs/financialhealth/index.htm#assistance

National Kidney and Urological Diseases Information Clearinghouse, (2003). Urinary tract infections in children. NIH Publication No. 04-4246. Retrieved December 13, 2004 from, http://www.kidney.niddk.nih.gov/kudiseases/pubs/uitchildren/index.htm

National Kidney and Urological Diseases Information Clearinghouse, (2004). Polycystic kidney disease. NIH Publication No. 05-4008. Retrieved December 19, 2004, from http://www.kidney.niddk.nih.gov/kudiseases/pubs/polycystic/index.htm

National Kidney Foundation. (2004). Use of herbal supplements in chronic kidney disease. Retrieved December 23, 2004, from http://www.kidney.org/atoz/atozPrint.cfm?id=123

Nield, L. S., & Kamat, D. (2004). Enuresis: How to evaluate and treat. *Clinical Pediatrics, 43*, 409–415.

Palmer, J. S. (2003). Genetic diseases in pediatrics. *Urologic Clinics of North America, 30*, 161–169.

Patel, H. P. & Bissler, J. J. (2001). Hematuria in children. *Pediatric Clinics of North America, 48*(6), 1519–1537.

Pool, R., & Korus, M. (2002). Pediatric kidney transplantation: Growth, development, and nursing implications. *Progress in Transplantation, 12*(2), 129–135.

Raszka, W. V., & Khan, O. (2005). Pyelonephritis. *Pediatrics in Review, 26*(10), 364–369.

Ritz, S. (2002). Pediatric hemodialysis and peritoneal dialysis: Report rewards program. *Journal of Renal Nutrition, 12*(3), 199–204.

Robinson, R. F., Nahata, M. C., Mahan, J. D., & Batisky, D. L. (2003). Management of nephrotic syndrome in children. *Pharmacotherapy, 23*(8), 1021–1036.

Ruth, E. M., Kemper, M. J., Leumann, E. P., Laube, G. F., & Neuhaus, T. J. (2005). Children with steroid-sensitive nephrotic syndrome come of age: Long-term outcome. *Journal of Pediatrics, 147*(2), 202–207.

Ruth, E. M., Landolt, M. A., Neuhaus, T. J., & Kemper, M. J. (2004). Health-related quality of life and psychosocial adjustment in steroid-sensitive nephrotic syndrome. *Journal of Pediatrics, 145*, 778–783.

Sessions, A. E., Rabinowitz, R., Hulbert, W. C., Goldstein, M. M., & Mevorach, R. A. (2003). Testicular torsion: Direction, degree, duration, and disinformation. *Journal of Urology, 169*(2), 663–665.

Shafii, T., & Burstein, G. R. (2004). An overview of sexually transmitted infections among adolescents. *Adolescent Medicine Clinics, 15*(2), 201–214.

Singh-Grewal, D., Macdessi, J., & Craig, J. (2005). Circumcision for prevention of urinary tract infection in boys: A systematic review of randomized trials and observational studies. *Archives of Diseases in Childhood, 90,* 853–858.

Snethen, J. A., Broome, M. E., Bartels, J., & Warady, B. A. (2001). Adolescent's perception of living with end-stage renal disease. *Pediatric Nursing, 27*(2), 159–167.

Stamm, C. A., & McGregor, J. A. (2001). Diagnosing and treating STDs in young women. *Contemporary Pediatrics, 18*(2), 53–67.

Stokowski, L. A. (2004). Hypospadias in the neonate. *Advances in Neonatal Care, 4*(4), 206–215.

Trachtman, H., Cnaan, A., Christen, E., Gibbs, K., Zhao, S., Acheson, D. W., et al. (2003). Effect of an oral Shiga toxin-binding agent on diarrhea-associated hemolytic uremic syndrome in children. *Journal of American Medical Association, 290*(10), 1337–1344.

United States Renal Data System (2004). 2004 annual data report. Retrieved December 13, 2004, from http://www.usrds.org/atlas.htm

Verrina, E., Zacchello, G., Edefonti, A., Sorino, P., Rinaldi, S., et al. (2001). A multicenter survey on automated peritoneal dialysis prescription in children. *Advances in Peritoneal Dialysis, 17,* 264–268.

Vogt, B. A. (2002). A newborn with a urinary tract anomaly: What role for the general pediatrician? *Contemporary Pediatrics, 19*(10), 131–153.

Vogt, B. A., & Avner, E. D. (2004). Renal failure. In R. E. Behrman, R. M. Kliegman, & H. B. Jenson, *Nelson textbook of pediatrics* (17th ed., pp. 1767–1775). Philadelphia: Saunders.

Walle, J. V., Mauel, R., Raes, A., Vanderkerckhove, K., & Donckerwolcke, R. (2004). ARF in children with minimal change nephrotic syndrome may be related to functional changes of the glomerular basement membrane. *American Journal of Kidney Diseases, 43*(3), 399–404.

Warady, B. A., Schaefer, F., Holloway, M., Alexander, S., Kandert, M., et al. (2000). Consensus guidelines for the treatment of peritonitis in pediatric patients receiving peritoneal dialysis. *Peritoneal Dialysis International, 20*(6), 610–624.

Workowski, K. A. & Berman, S. M. (2006). Sexually transmitted diseases treatment guidelines, 2006. Morbidity and Mortality Weekly Report, 55(RR-11), 43–44.

ALTERATIONS IN NEUROLOGIC FUNCTION

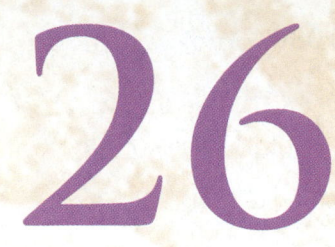

26

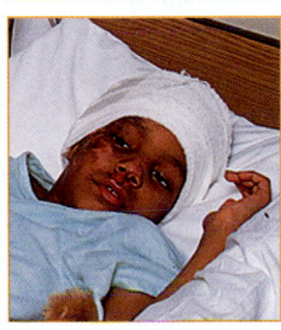

ANTWAN, 7 years old, was injured when he was struck by a car and thrown several feet into the air. He was unconscious upon admission to the emergency department and showed some signs of increased intracranial pressure (dilated and fixed pupils). Antwan was treated for shock, and his neurologic status and vital signs were frequently assessed. The initial evaluation revealed that Antwan had sustained several contusions of the brain, but no skull fracture. He was intubated and medicated to manage the increased intracranial pressure.

Antwan's intracranial pressure has now stabilized, and he has been moved to the general pediatric care unit. However, he still has not totally regained consciousness. He is restless and agitated, and unable to follow directions. His parents stay at his bedside and provide auditory and tactile stimulation, hoping he will eventually respond. Physical therapy has been initiated to prevent contractures and to maintain function. Long-term rehabilitation will be needed to help Antwan and his family achieve the best outcome possible after this injury.

What is the nurse's role in acute care of the child who has a brain injury? What support does the family need to contribute to the child's care? How does the nurse work with other healthcare professionals to plan the long-term care of a child such as Antwan?

LEARNING OUTCOMES

After reading this chapter, you will be able to do the following:

1. Describe the anatomy and physiology of the neurologic system.
2. Describe the nursing assessment process and tools used for infants and children with altered levels of consciousness and other neurologic conditions.
3. Differentiate between the signs of a seizure and status epilepticus in infants and children, and describe appropriate nursing management for each condition.
4. Differentiate between signs of bacterial meningitis, viral meningitis, encephalitis, Reye's syndrome, and Guillain-Barré syndrome in infants and children.
5. Describe the nursing care for the child with myelodysplasia and hydrocephalus.
6. Describe the focus of community-based nursing care for the child with cerebral palsy.
7. Distinguish between the assessment findings of the child with a mild, moderate, and severe traumatic brain injury.
8. Describe initiatives to prevent drowning in children.

KEY TERMS

areflexia **1084**
assistive technology **1081**
aura **1041**
automatisms **1042**
autonomic dysreflexia **1092**
cerebral edema **1049**
cerebral perfusion pressure **1036**
clonic **1041**
coma **1036**
consciousness **1036**
Cushing's triad **1084**
diplegia **1077**
encephalopathy **1056**
febrile seizures **1041**
focal **1040**

fontanels **1032**
herniation **1085**
intracranial pressure **1036**
intractable seizures **1044**
microcephaly **1060**
myelination **1032**
myelodysplasia **1066**
nuchal rigidity **1049**
obtunded **1036**
opisthotonic position **1049**
postictal period **1041**
posturing **1036**
status epilepticus **1043**
stupor **1036**
tonic **1041**

MediaLink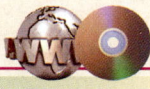

http://www.prenhall.com/ball

See the Prentice Hall Nursing MediaLink DVD-ROM and Companion Website for chapter-specific resources.

FOCUS ON
The Neurologic System

ANATOMY AND PHYSIOLOGY

The brain, spinal cord, and nerves are the major structures of the nervous system (Figure 26–1 ➤). The brain is protected by the skull and covered by three layers of tissue called the meninges—the dura mater, arachnoid, and pia mater. Cerebrospinal fluid circulates within the ventricles of the brain and around the brain and spinal cord.

The brain is a complex organ that controls, regulates, or coordinates many body functions, including cognition, emotions, behaviors, the senses, and motor ability. Stimuli are received from the environment and the brain enables response for adaptation, survival, and maintenance of body functions. See Table 26–1 for the primary functions of the brain's cerebrum, the cerebellum, and the brainstem. The brainstem connects the cerebral hemispheres, the cerebellum, and the spinal cord. The 12 cranial nerves arise from the brainstem and have many important sensory and motor functions (Table 26–2).

The spinal cord, covered by the vertebrae, transmits impulses to and from the brain, conveying sensory information and relaying impulses that stimulate motor responses. Spinal nerves have sensory and motor components that send and receive information to specific body locations. Nerve impulses are transmitted by chemical and electrical conduction that enable the impulse to travel through the synapses with the next neuron. Examples of these chemical substances involved in impulse transmission include norepinephrine, acetylcholine, dopamine, histamine, and serotonin.

The peripheral nerves permit transmission of impulses from the nerve pathways to the cerebral cortex through simple spinal reflex arcs. The upper motor neurons consist of the fibers originating in the anterior horn of the spinal cord that travel to the brainstem and the nerve cells in the cerebral cortex. The lower motor neurons consist of the peripheral nerves and branches that transmit impulses to the anterior horn of the spinal cord.

Figure 26–1 ➤ Transverse section of the brain and spinal cord. Knowledge of the anatomy of the brain is helpful in understanding the symptoms of neurologic dysfunction.

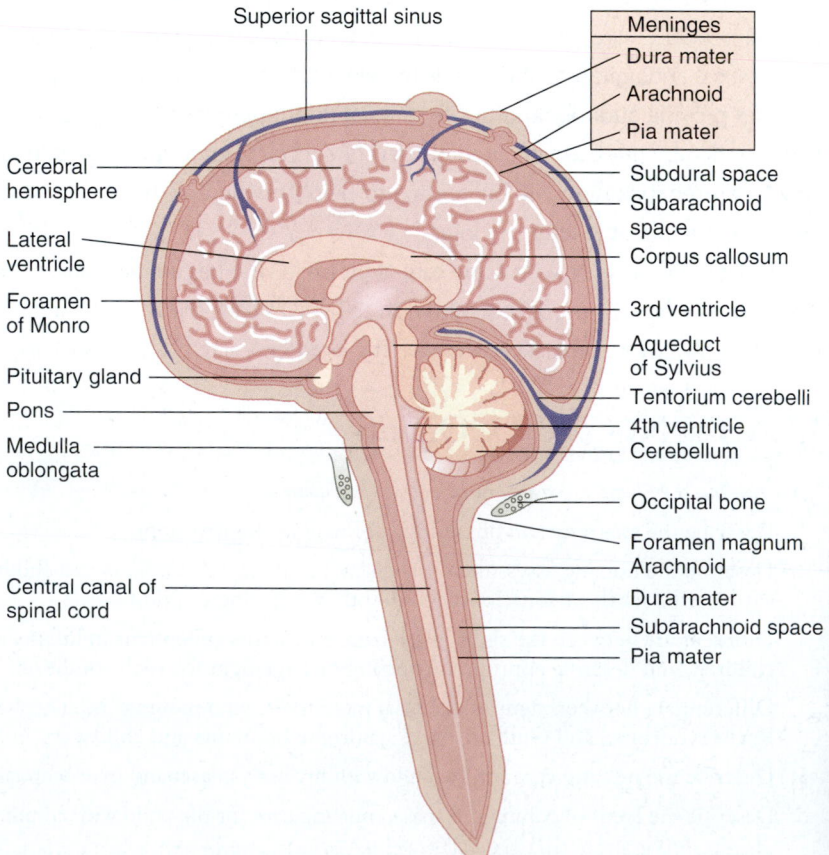

Superior sagittal sinus

Meninges
- Dura mater
- Arachnoid
- Pia mater

Cerebral hemisphere

Lateral ventricle

Foramen of Monro

Pituitary gland

Pons

Medulla oblongata

Central canal of spinal cord

Subdural space
Subarachnoid space
Corpus callosum
3rd ventricle
Aqueduct of Sylvius
Tentorium cerebelli
4th ventricle
Cerebellum
Occipital bone
Foramen magnum
Arachnoid
Dura mater
Subarachnoid space
Pia mater

Table 26–1	THE BRAIN STRUCTURES AND THEIR PRIMARY FUNCTIONS

Brain Structure	Functions and Control
Cerebrum	Higher mental functions, general movement, perception, and integration of all functions in lobes below
Frontal lobe	Voluntary skeletal muscle movement, fine repetitive motion, eye movements, motor aspects of speech
Parietal lobe	Interpretation of sensations (taste, visual, smell, hearing, temperature, pressure, pain, texture, two-point discrimination); recognition of body parts, proprioception
Occipital lobe	Vision center and interpretation of vision
Temporal lobe	Hearing or the perception, reception, and interpretation of sounds, long-term memory
Insula (corpus callosum)	Coordination of activities between the two hemispheres of the cerebrum
Limbic system	Mediates certain primitive behavior responses, visceral emotional responses, feeding behaviors, biologic rhythms, and the sense of smell
Thalamus	Processing center for interpretation of most sensations except smell; relay center for sensory motor information
Hypothalamus	Maintains the internal environment (temperature, autonomic nervous system function, endocrine function, wakefulness), regulates emotional expression
Cerebellum	Provides conscious and reflexive control of muscle tone, maintains balance and posture
Brainstem	Location of the descending and ascending motor and sensory pathways; connects the cerebrum, cerebellum, and spinal cord; location of the origin of the 12 cranial nerves

Table 26–2	THE CRANIAL NERVES AND THEIR FUNCTIONS

Cranial Nerves	Function
Olfactory (I)	Reception and interpretation of smell
Optic (II)	Visual acuity, visual fields
Oculomotor (III)	Many eye movements, raise the eyelids, pupil constriction
Trochlear (IV)	Inward and downward eye movement
Trigeminal (V)	Opening and closing the jaw, chewing; sensation in the eye (cornea, eyelids); sensation of the eyelids, face, mouth and nose mucosa, tongue, and ear
Abducens (VI)	Lateral eye movement
Facial (VII)	Facial expression, eye closure, and speech sounds involving the lips. Taste sensation on anterior two thirds of tongue and sensation in pharynx
Acoustic (VIII)	Sense of hearing and equilibrium
Glossopharyngeal (IX)	Muscles for swallowing and guttural speech; gag reflex; taste sensation of posterior one third of tongue, sensation in nasopharynx
Vagus (X)	Sensation behind ear and for a portion of the external ear canal; involuntary control of the heart and lungs
Spinal accessory (XI)	Shrug the shoulders and turn the head
Hypoglossal (XII)	Tongue movement; swallowing, speech sounds involving the tongue

The autonomic nervous system maintains a steady state of the internal body organs' and glands' involuntary functions. It is divided into the sympathetic nervous system, which mobilizes the body to respond in times of need or stress; and into the parasympathetic nervous system, which works to conserve and restore energy.

PEDIATRIC DIFFERENCES

The brain and spinal cord are formed early in gestation from the neural plate, which evolves into the neural groove and neu-ral folds by the third week of gestation. The neural groove deepens and the neural folds develop laterally and close to form the neural tube, which becomes the central nervous system (CNS). The neural folds close first in the cervical region. Closure then progresses in both the cranial and caudal directions. The brain develops from the cranial end of the neural tube, and the spinal cord develops from the other end (Padgett, 2006).

Any insult (such as inadequate folic acid) or critical event (teratogen, infection, substance abuse, or trauma) during this early gestational period can result in a CNS malformation. Such defects account for approximately one third of all apparent congenital malformations in live infants; 90% of these are neural tube defects. CNS defects are responsible for 40% of infant deaths in the first year of life (Padgett, 2006).

The anatomic and physiologic differences between the nervous systems of children and adults help explain why children and adults have different neurologic problems (Figure 26–2 ➤). For example, the brain and spinal cord are protected by the skeletal structures of the skull and vertebrae. In infants, however, the cranial bones and vertebrae are not completely ossified. The infant's brain and spinal cord are thus at greater risk for injury resulting from trauma. The bones of the skull are separated but held together with bands of connective tissue to allow for normal brain growth. **Fontanels** are spaces of connective tissue covering the brain at the junction of skull bones that gradually close and ossify. The posterior fontanel closes at 3 months of age and the anterior fontanel closes at about 18 to 24 months of age. See Figure 5–9 ∞. The suture lines between skull bones interlock as early as 6 months of age; by 12 years of age the sutures are completely ossified and cannot be separated (Padgett, 2006).

At birth, the nervous system is complete but immature. The infant is born with all of the nerve cells that will exist throughout life, but maturation of these nerve cells continues after birth. The number of glial cells and dendrites, which enable receipt of nerve impulses, continues to increase until approximately 4 years of age. Brain growth results in increasing head circumference in infants and toddlers, and continues until the child is 12 to 15 years of age.

Myelination, the progressive covering of axons with layers of myelin or a lipid protein sheath, is also incomplete at birth. Lack of myelination is associated with the presence of primitive reflexes. As the myelination progresses, the primi-

AS CHILDREN GROW

Anatomic Differences in the Structures of the Nervous System Between Children and Adults

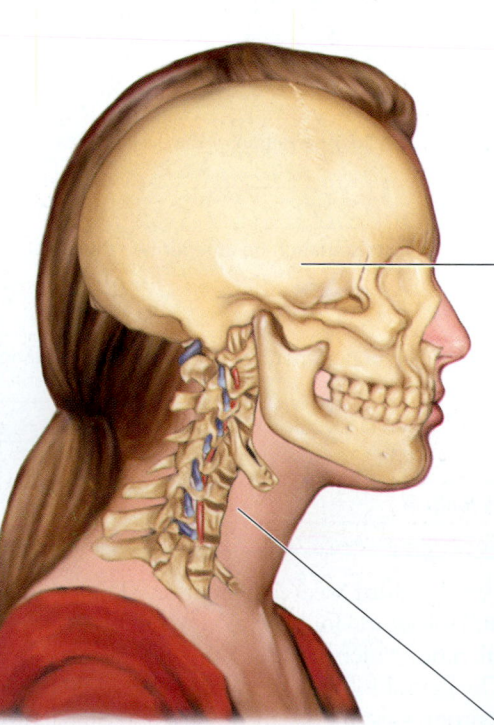
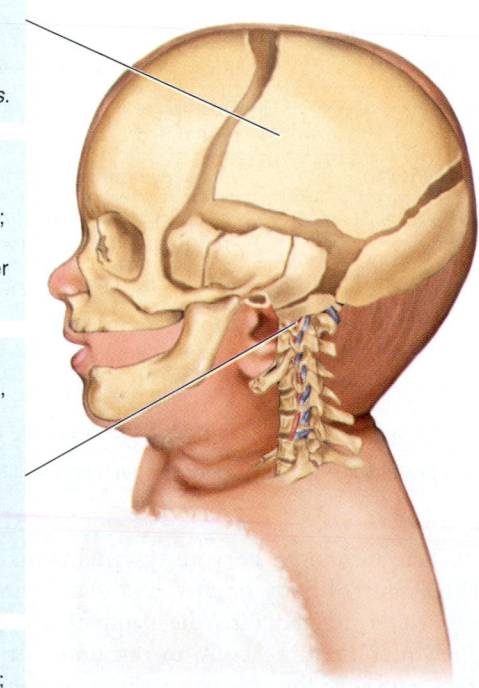

Top heavy, head is large in proportion to body; neck muscles poorly developed; thin cranial bones not well developed; unfused sutures; skull expands until age 2 years. *Prone to brain injury and skull fracture with falls.*

Head size proportional to body; neck muscles well developed, can reduce risk for brain injuries; sutures are ossified by age 12 years; no expansion of skull after 5 years.

Excessive spinal mobility; immature muscles, joint capsule, and ligaments of cervical spine; wedge-shaped, cartilaginous vertebral bodies; incomplete ossification of vertebral bodies. *Greater risk for high cervical spine injury at C1-C2 level or vertebral compression fractures with falls.*

Well developed muscles and ligaments reduce spinal mobility; vertebral bodies completely formed and ossified.

Figure 26–2 ➤ The skull and brain grow and develop rapidly during early childhood.

tive reflexes disappear. See Table 5–21 ∞ for the expected appearance and disappearance of primitive reflexes during early infancy. This process continues throughout childhood, proceeding in a cephalocaudal direction, permitting voluntary movement. The myelination process accounts for the progressive acquisition of fine and gross motor skills and coordination during early childhood, and it is ultimately responsible for the speed and accuracy of nerve impulses.

The brain depends upon a continuous blood flow to meet its high demands for oxygen. Through an autoregulatory process, the cerebral blood vessels dilate to maintain the cerebral blood flow in response to physiologic changes such as fluctuating cerebral perfusion pressure from decreased cardiac output, increased intracranial pressure, or constriction of the neck's blood vessels due to positioning. When blood flow and oxygenation is not maintained, the brain cells become damaged in a very short time. Because the nervous system helps to control and coordinate many body functions, alterations in neurologic function can have widespread effects on the body's metabolism.

Examples of diagnostic and laboratory tests used to evaluate neurologic system function are provided in the accompanying table. Use the guidelines found on page 1035 to perform a comprehensive nursing assessment of the neurologic system. The Glasgow Coma Scale is also used to assess the level of consciousness, and to provide a score for future comparison. See Table 26–3 for assessment criteria to use with children at different ages.

DIAGNOSTIC PROCEDURES/LABORATORY TESTS USED TO EVALUATE NEUROLOGIC CONDITIONS

Diagnostic Procedure	Purpose	Nursing Implications
Computed tomography (CT)	The CT scan produces a narrow radiograph beam that examines the brain or spinal cord from different angles, producing a two-dimensional cross-section of the structures. It can be performed with or without iodine contrast media; it is not invasive unless contrast dye is used. CT of the brain evaluates the density of intracranial tissues and structures to identify congenital anomalies, hemorrhage, tumors, swelling, or infection. CT of the spine is used to identify fractures and injury to spinal ligaments.	• Inquire about allergy to iodine, seafood, or contrast dye used for other radiographic procedures. Antihistamines and/or steroids may be ordered prior to the procedure if an allergic reaction is suspected. Assess for an allergic reaction during procedure. • Prepare child for the procedure by describing the size of equipment, noises, and other sensations that will be experienced, and how the child can help during the procedure. • When sedation is required to help keep an infant or small child still, monitor the child according to agency guidelines.
Electroencephalogram (EEG)	Electrodes are applied to the scalp to record brainwave activity. The electrical activity in various lobes of the brain is used to identify the potential for seizures, to determine brain death, and to detect other abnormalities such as a tumor, abscess, or intracranial hemorrhage.	• Obtain a list of current medications and when last taken to identify any that could alter the EEG result. • EEGs are usually performed with the child lying down or seated in a reclining chair. • Prepare the child for the procedure by describing the placement of electrodes, and equipment to be used. Indicate that the procedure is not painful. • Observe for seizures, and describe seizure activity. • Inform parents to wash the child's hair to remove the electrode gel.
Intracranial pressure (ICP) monitoring	A burr hole is placed through the skull and a ventricular catheter or bolt is inserted to monitor ICP pressure when it reaches dangerous heights.	• Informed consent is needed for the invasive procedure. • Provide pain management and sedation. • Keep parents informed about the child's condition.
Lumbar puncture	A lumbar puncture is performed at the L3–4 or L4–5 level to obtain cerebrospinal fluid (CSF). The CSF pressure is measured, and then fluid is collected in sterile test tubes that are numbered by sequence of collection. CSF is cultured and analyzed for glucose and protein content, and the cells present.	• Hold the infant or child in the knee-chest position and keep the child still during the procedure. Assess the child's breathing during the procedure. • Assess vital signs at specified times and assess for changes in neurological function. • Administer analgesics as ordered for headache.

(continued)

DIAGNOSTIC PROCEDURES/LABORATORY TESTS USED TO EVALUATE NEUROLOGIC CONDITIONS

Diagnostic Procedure	Purpose	Nursing Implications
Magnetic resonance imaging (MRI)	MRI produces results similar to those of CT, but does not use ionizing radiation. The MRI examines specific characteristics of the brain tissue in multiple planes for detailed imaging and to identify the anatomic cause of disorders. MRI may also permit the study of CSF flow dynamics.	• Prepare the child for sounds, size of equipment, and tunnel. • Ensure that the child has no metallic implants, and is not connected to metal equipment (e.g., oxygen tank). • Allow the parent to stay with the child during the procedure. • Sedation may be needed to keep the infant or child still. Monitor the child according to agency guidelines.
Positron emission tomography (PET) scan	PET uses CT to measure emission of positive electrons from radioactive substances injected into the bloodstream or given by inhalation. PET is most effective in measuring cerebral blood flow and metabolic processes in the brain.	• Assess for allergies as contrast medium is used. • Monitor vital signs. • Start two IVs; one for contrast and the other to draw blood gases. • Do not provide sedation; the child must be alert.
Radiograph (X-ray)	Radiographs use irradiation to obtain images and capture them on film for diagnostic and screening purposes. Skull radiographs are used to detect fractures, spreading suture lines, and unexpected characteristics such as bone erosion or degeneration. Spinal radiographs are used to assess the vertebrae for alignment, fractures, unusual separation, or bony defects.	• Explain procedure to parents and child. Inform them that more than one radiograph may be taken from different angles to detect problems. Explain that modern equipment decreases radiation exposure. • Tell the child about the need to hold still for the procedure. Have the child practice holding still and holding a breath in preparation for the test.
Ultrasonography	A noninvasive procedure performed by placing an ultrasound transducer over the brain through the anterior fontanel, producing an ultrasound beam to the tissues. The reflected sound waves are transformed into scan graphs. Ultrasound is used to visualize the anatomic structure of the brain of newborns and young infants with an open anterior fontanel.	• Administer sedation as prescribed. • Explain the procedure to parents and the child. Inform them that the procedure is painless, and there is no radiation exposure. • Instruct the child to remain still during the procedure.

Laboratory Test	Purpose	Nursing Implications
Arterial blood gases	Direct measurement of the blood pH, Po_2, and Pco_2. They are used to monitor the adequacy of ventilation and oxygenation in cases of altered consciousness that is essential for reducing the risk for increased ICP.	• Perform arterial puncture on the radial, brachial, and femoral arteries. • Use anesthetizing agent to reduce the pain associated with the arterial puncture. • Following the arterial puncture, put pressure over the puncture site for 5 to 10 minutes to prevent hematoma formation.
Cultures	Cultures are taken to isolate microorganisms causing body tissue or body fluid infection. Common cultures taken include: • Cerebrospinal fluid • Blood	• Hold antibiotics or sulfonamides until after specimen collection, as they may cause false results. If these drugs have been given, list them on a laboratory slip. • Immediately deliver all specimens to the laboratory, or refrigerate the specimens. • Handle specimens using strict aseptic technique.
Complete blood count	Assesses hematocrit and hemoglobin levels; WBC and differential provides evidence of infection and whether bacterial or viral.	• Explain procedure to child and parents.
Toxicology screening	Screening of blood, urine, meconium, and hair for drugs or other substances that could cause neurologic insult.	• Chain of custody for specimens may be needed.

ASSESSMENT GUIDELINES FOR THE CHILD WITH A NEUROLOGIC CONDITION

Assessment Focus	Assessment Guidelines
Level of consciousness	• Is the infant or child lethargic or hard to arouse? • Is the infant or child irritable or difficult to console? • Note that the Glasgow Coma Scale provides a numerical score for future comparison. See Table 26–3.
Cranial nerves	• Assess the cranial nerves. See Table 5–20 ∞. See also Table 26–5 for methods to indirectly assess cranial nerves in the unconscious child.
Fontanels and sutures	• Palpate fontanels and suture lines on the scalp of the infant.
Cognitive function	• Are the child's verbal skills developmentally appropriate for age? • Does the child follow directions appropriately?
Pupils	• Check the pupils for size and reaction to light and accommodation. See Figure 26–3 ➤.
Vital signs	• Assess heart rate, respiratory rate, and blood pressure. • Monitor for an increased systolic blood pressure, a widened pulse pressure, bradycardia, and irregular respirations (late signs of increased intracranial pressure)
Posture and movement	• Inspect the infant's posture and movement by using the primitive reflexes. See Table 5–21 ∞. • Observe the child's play or other spontaneous activity to assess strength as well as symmetry and smoothness of movements. • Are the child's motor skills developmentally appropriate for age? Were motor skills acquired at the appropriate age? Has the child lost a previously acquired skill? • Evaluate muscle strength and tone, comparing side to side. Is any weakness present? • Test the child's coordination for smoothness and symmetry of response. • Assess deep tendon reflexes for smoothness and symmetry of response. See Table 5–22 ∞.
Neck stiffness	• Assess for neck stiffness (nuchal rigidity).
Pain	• Assess level of pain when present.

Table 26–3	GLASGOW COMA SCALE FOR ASSESSMENT OF COMA IN INFANTS AND CHILDREN

Category	Score	Infant and Young Child Criteria	Older Child and Adult Criteria
Eye opening	4	Spontaneous opening	Spontaneous
	3	To loud noise	To verbal stimuli
	2	To pain	To pain
	1	No response	No response
Verbal response	5	Smiles, coos, cries to appropriate stimuli	Oriented to time, place, and person; uses appropriate words and phrases
	4	Irritable; cries	Confused
	3	Inappropriate crying	Inappropriate words or verbal response
	2	Grunts, moans	Incomprehensible words
	1	No response	No response
Motor response	6	Spontaneous movement	Obeys commands
	5	Withdraws to touch	Localizes pain
	4	Withdraws to pain	Withdraws to pain
	3	Abnormal flexion (decorticate)	Flexion to pain (decorticate)
	2	Abnormal extension (decerebrate)	Extension to pain (decerebrate)
	1	No response	No response

Add the score from each category to get the total. The maximum score is 15, indicating the best level of neurologic functioning. The minimum is 3, indicating total neurologic unresponsiveness.

Note: From Teasdale, G., & Jennett, B. (1974). Assessment of coma and impaired consciousness. *Lancet, 2,* 81–84; and James, H. E. (1986). Neurologic evaluation and support in the child with acute brain insult. *Pediatric Annals, 15*(1), 16–22.

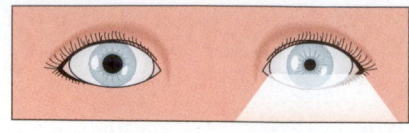

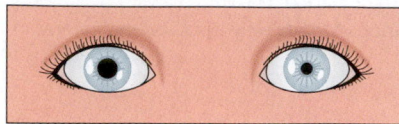

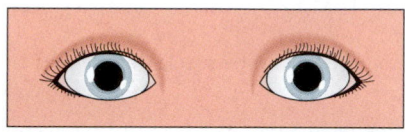

Figure 26–3 ➤ Pupil findings in various neurologic conditions with altered consciousness. A, A unilateral dilated and reactive pupil is associated with an intracranial mass. B, A fixed and dilated pupil may be a sign of impending brainstem herniation. C, Bilateral fixed and dilated pupils are associated with brainstem herniation from increased intracranial pressure.

ALTERED STATES OF CONSCIOUSNESS

Level of consciousness (LOC) is perhaps the most important indicator of neurologic dysfunction. **Consciousness**, the responsiveness of the mind to sensory stimuli, has two components: *alertness*, or the ability to react to stimuli, and *cognitive power*, or the ability to process the data and respond either verbally or physically. *Unconsciousness*, in contrast, is depressed cerebral function, or the brain's inability to respond to stimuli. Altered levels of consciousness can be further categorized as:

- *Confusion.* Disorientation to time, place, or person. The child may seem alert. Answers to simple questions may be correct, but responses to complex ones may be inaccurate.
- *Delirium.* State characterized by confusion, fear, agitation, hyperactivity, or anxiety.
- *Lethargy.* Limited spontaneous movements, sluggish speech, drowsy, falls asleep easily.
- **Obtunded.** Limited response to the environment; the child falls asleep unless given verbal or tactile stimulation.
- **Stupor.** Response to vigorous stimulation only; the child returns to the unresponsive state when the stimulus is removed. For example, the child may react to a needlestick but not respond to a milder stimulus such as touching the skin.
- **Coma.** Severely diminished response or unconsciousness; the child cannot be aroused even by painful stimuli.
- *Persistent vegetative state.* Permanent loss of function of the cerebral cortex with reflexive responses only (eyes following objects, response to pain, hand grasping, facial grimacing, groaning or other sounds).

Etiology and Pathophysiology

Many conditions may alter the level of consciousness, including the following: trauma, hypoxia, infection, poisoning, seizures, endocrine or metabolic disturbances, electrolyte or acid–base imbalance, CNS pathology, and a congenital structural defect. Any of these pathologic processes can also cause increased **intracranial pressure** (force exerted by brain tissue, cerebrospinal fluid, and blood within the cranial vault). Decreased **cerebral perfusion pressure**, the amount of pressure needed to ensure that adequate oxygen and nutrients will be delivered to the brain, often results when the arterial blood flow to the brain is reduced due to increased intracranial pressure. Discovering the cause of the decreased level of consciousness is essential so that immediate treatment can begin, to prevent possible secondary effects of the illness or injury.

Clinical Manifestations

Decline in a child's level of consciousness often follows a sequential pattern of deterioration. A child may first appear awake and alert, and may respond appropriately. Initial changes may be subtle: a slight disorientation to time, place, and person. The child may become restless or fussy, and actions that normally calm or soothe the child only increase irritability. As responsiveness decreases, the child may become drowsy but still respond to loud verbal commands and withdraw from painful stimuli. Keeping the child awake is sometimes difficult. Then response to pain progresses from purposeful to nonpurposeful. The child may exhibit decorticate or decerebrate **posturing**, abnormal positions assumed after injury or damage to the brain (Figure 26–4 ➤). The timing of the decline in function varies by the child as well as the condition causing alteration in consciousness. In some cases, the decline will be rapid and stages may be skipped, such as when the child has a serious brain injury.

Clinical manifestations of increased intracranial pressure are provided in Table 26–4.

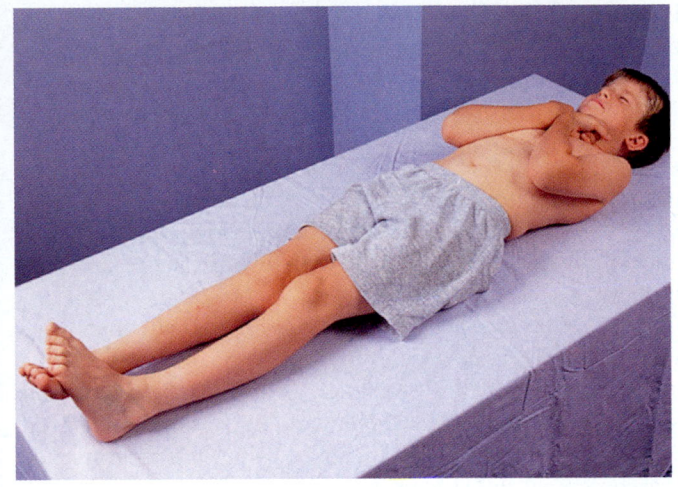

A

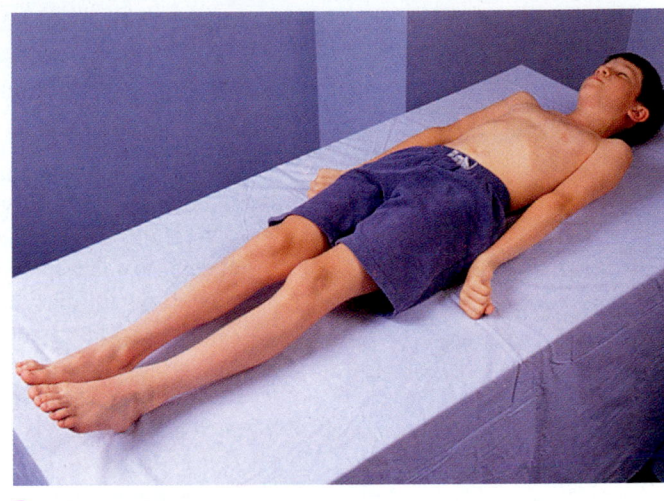

B

Figure 26–4 ➤ A, Decorticate posturing, characterized by rigid flexion, is associated with lesions above the brainstem in the corticospinal tracts. B, Decerebrate posturing, distinguished by rigid extension, is associated with lesions of the brainstem.

Table 26–4	SIGNS OF INCREASED INTRACRANIAL PRESSURE
Timing of Signs	**Signs**
Early signs	Headache Visual disturbances, diplopia Nausea and vomiting Dizziness or vertigo Slight change in vital signs Pupils not as reactive or equal Sunsetting eyes Seizures Slight change in level of consciousness, restlessness
Infant has above signs plus:	Irritability Bulging fontanel Wide sutures, increased head circumference Dilated scalp veins High-pitched, catlike cry
Late signs	Significant decrease in level of consciousness Cushing's triad • Increased systolic blood pressure and widened pulse pressure • Bradycardia • Irregular respirations Fixed and dilated pupils

■ COLLABORATIVE CARE

Diagnostic Tests

The Glasgow Coma Scale is used to quantify the level of consciousness, thus enabling future comparison of improvement or deterioration in the child's condition. Pediatric criteria take into account the child's developmental age for each category of the test (see Table 26–3).

Laboratory tests include a complete blood cell count, blood chemistry, clotting factors, and blood culture; toxicology assessments of both blood and urine; and urinalysis with culture. A lumbar puncture may be performed to assess the cerebrospinal fluid for protein, glucose, or blood cells. An electroencephalogram (EEG) identifies damaged or nonfunctioning areas of the brain. Computed tomography (CT) or magnetic

> ## NURSING ALERT
>
> Assess the child for increased intracranial pressure prior to performing a lumbar puncture to make sure there is not a risk for herniation. In addition to checking for the signs of increased intracranial pressure listed in Table 26–4, make sure that an ophthalmoscopic examination has been performed to determine if papilledema, or pressure on the optic nerve, is present. The lumbar puncture should be postponed if any signs of increased intracranial pressure are present.

> ## GROWTH & DEVELOPMENT
>
> **Glasgow Coma Scale Assessment**
>
> Following are developmentally appropriate cues in the Glasgow Coma Scale Assessment:
>
> - Eye opening. Note whether eye opening is spontaneous or occurs in response to stimuli.
> - Verbal response. Crying in an infant is a positive response. The 2-year-old child who says "no" to each command is also responding in an age-appropriate way.
> - Motor response. Motor score is probably the most critical aspect of this test, since the child cannot control reflexes. A fearful toddler may refuse to open his or her eyes or talk to strangers, but the child's reflexes should automatically respond to appropriate stimuli. Ask the child to reach for a finger puppet or doll rather than your hand. This makes the child feel less threatened, and the toy can be a reward.

resonance imaging (MRI) is used to detect any lesions, structural abnormalities, vascular malformations, or edema. Skull radiographic studies are used to detect fractures or bony malformations.

Clinical Therapy

Clinical therapy focuses on early diagnosis of the cause of an altered level of consciousness and intervention to prevent further insult to the central nervous system. The child is treated with oxygen, and assisted ventilation is provided when gas exchange is inadequate. Any metabolic, acid-base, or electrolyte imbalances are corrected. Antibiotics are initiated for suspected infection.

Efforts are made to maintain the cerebral perfusion pressure so that adequate oxygen and nutrients are supplied to brain tissue. In cases of hypovolemia, intravenous fluids are given. In cases of poor perfusion and fluid overload, a vasopressor medication such as dopamine is administered to increase cardiac output and perfusion of the brain. If the intracranial pressure is markedly increased and is caused by an obstruction leading to the accumulation of cerebrospinal fluid, a ventricular tap can be performed to decrease the pressure, temporarily relieving a life-threatening condition.

■ NURSING MANAGEMENT

Nursing Assessment and Diagnosis

Initially assess the child's physiologic status, focusing on the child's responsiveness to the environment or stimuli, ability to maintain the airway, vital signs, and breathing patterns. A baseline neurologic assessment should be performed, using the guidelines on page 1035. Repeated assessments should be performed and compared with baseline findings. Use the Glasgow Coma Scale (Table 26–3) to assess the child at specified intervals.

Assess the child's cranial nerves (see Table 5–20 ∞). The child's responses may differ significantly when stress and anxiety are reduced, so encourage the parents to take part in the examination to reduce the child's anxiety. In the unconscious child, cranial nerve assessment and interpretation are more challenging (Table 26–5).

Assess the child's airway. The presence of a cough or gag reflex indicates that the child is able to protect the airway from aspiration. Assess the child's respiratory effort and color. Monitor pulse oximetry and arterial blood gas measurements. Adequate air exchange to keep oxygen and carbon dioxide levels within normal ranges and maintaining acid-base balance are critical to reduce the risk of hypoxemia and increased intracranial pressure. If the child cannot maintain an adequate respiratory effort, mechanical ventilation will be necessary.

Table 26–5	ASSESSMENT OF CRANIAL NERVES IN THE UNCONSCIOUS CHILD	
Cranial Nerves	**Reflex**	**Assessment Procedure and Normal Findings[a]**
II, III	Pupillary	Shine a light source in the eye. *Rapid, concentrically constricting pupils indicate intact cranial nerves, II, III.*
II, IV, VI	Oculocephalic	Should be performed with eyes held open (doll's eyes) and head turned from side to side. *Eyes gazing straight up or logging slightly behind head motion indicate intact cranial nerves.* Precaution: Cervical spine injury must be ruled out before this assessment is performed.
III, VIII	Oculovestibular	Place the head in a midline and slightly elevated position. Inject ice water into the ear canal. *Eyes deviating* toward *the irrigated ear indicate intact cranial nerves III, VIII.* Precautions: Cervical spine injury must be ruled out before this assessment is performed. Tympanic membrane must be intact; otherwise, brain may be filled with bacteria-laden fluid. *Note:* This assessment is usually performed by a physician.
V, VII	Corneal	Cornea is gently swabbed with sterile cotton swab. *A blink indicates intact cranial nerves V, VII.*
IX, X	Gag	Pharynx is irritated with tongue depressor or cotton swab. *Gagging response indicates intact cranial nerves IX, X.*

[a]Italic indicates normal findings.

Among the nursing diagnoses that might be appropriate for the child with an altered level of consciousness or increased intracranial pressure are:

- Ineffective Breathing Pattern related to neuromuscular dysfunction associated with increased intracranial pressure
- Risk for Aspiration related to poor control of secretions with decreased level of consciousness
- Imbalanced Nutrition: Less than Body Requirements related to decreased level of consciousness
- Risk for Impaired Skin Integrity related to agitation and skin rubbing against sheets
- Impaired Verbal Communication related to physiologic condition of decreased level of consciousness
- Interrupted Family Processes related to care of a child with an acquired disability

Planning and Implementation
Hospital-Based Care

Nursing care of the child with altered consciousness or increased intracranial pressure focuses on maintaining airway patency, monitoring neurologic status, performing routine care, providing sensory stimulation, and providing emotional support to parents. Nursing care for the child with increased intracranial pressure is described on page 1085.

Ensure that the child's airway is clear at all times. If the child is having difficulty managing secretions or does not have a gag reflex, intubation or a tracheostomy is performed. Frequent suctioning may be required. Keep suction apparatus with catheters, oxygen, resuscitation bag and mask, and extra tracheostomy tubes (if applicable) at the bedside. Perform pulse oximetry or arterial blood gas analysis at regular intervals to ensure that gas exchange is adequate. Mechanical ventilation may be required.

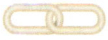

SKILL 11–23
Tracheostomy Tube Suctioning

Perform routine neurologic checks. Evaluate pupil size and reactivity, eye movements, and motor function (see Figure 26–3). Monitor vital signs. Increased systolic blood pressure, a wide pulse pressure, and bradycardia indicate increased intracranial pressure. Observe for the other signs of increased intracranial pressure listed in Table 26–4. Anticipate that seizures may occur. Raise and pad the side rails to protect the child from injury.

Perform routine nursing care. If the corneal reflex is absent, place artificial tears in the eyes and cover them with gauze, taping over so they remain closed. Perform routine mouth care by brushing the teeth and using swabs with water.

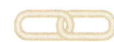

SKILL 12–3
*Administering a Gavage/
Tube Feeding*

Provide adequate nutrition. Nutrients may initially be supplied intravenously, although a nasogastric or gastrostomy tube may be inserted if the child remains unconscious or is not alert enough to take food by mouth.

Prevent complications associated with immobility (muscle atrophy, contractures, and skin breakdown) as described in the nursing practice box. Support physical therapy efforts with extra passive range of motion exercises.

Provide sensory stimulation. Because the child with a severely altered level of consciousness may still be able to hear, talking to him or her may be beneficial. Listening to music or tapes of family members talking or reading can soothe a child who has an altered level of consciousness when family members cannot be present. Explain all procedures and actions to the family and the child, even though the child's state of consciousness is altered.

When the child becomes more alert, gradually and repeatedly orient the child to time, place, and person, depending on his or her age and level of understanding. Encourage parents to bring objects or toys from home to make the environment more familiar and promote a feeling of security.

Provide emotional support to the child and family. Explain the child's condition in simple terms. Encourage parents to take part in the child's care and therapy as much as possible. If the child's usual functioning has been permanently impaired, refer the family to the appropriate psychologic and social services for emotional support.

CLINICAL TIP
Care of the Immobile Child
- Help keep the body in proper alignment with splints or rolls made of towels or blankets.
- Perform passive or gentle range of motion exercises three or four times per day according to physician's orders.
- Maintain skin integrity:
  - Change position every 2 hours.
  - Place child on foam or egg-crate mattress or sheepskin covering.
  - Massage child gently using lotion.
  - Cover skin exposed to rubbing with transparent film.

(See Chapter 14 ∞ for more information about helping families cope with a child's life-threatening illness.) Give family members opportunities to express their feelings.

Discharge Planning and Home Care Teaching

The child's transition from the hospital to home, a long-term care facility, or inpatient rehabilitation center must be well planned. A case manager or social worker should be identified who can help plan the child's long-term care needs, including home health nursing, adaptation of the home, and purchase of special equipment.

Care in the Community

Home care nurses play a vital role in the care of the child with an acquired neurologic dysfunction and prolonged altered consciousness. Teach the family how to care for the child with severe neurologic dysfunction and to perform routine procedures such as maintaining the airway, providing skin care, feeding, positioning, performing exercises, and offering stimulation. Regular follow-up visits are needed to assess the child's progress and to modify the treatment plan.

The child also needs to be linked with community rehabilitation services through an early intervention program or school-based program. The home health nurse or case manager should help the family have an Individual Education Plan developed for the child (see Chapter 12 ∞).

Evaluation

Expected outcomes of nursing care include the following:

- The child's airway is maintained and the brain is adequately oxygenated.
- Complications of immobility are prevented.
- The family provides appropriate care to the child with prolonged altered consciousness to promote minimal long-term disabilities.

SEIZURE DISORDERS

Seizures are periods of abnormal electrical discharges in the brain that cause involuntary movement, as well as behavior and sensory alterations. They are a common neurologic disorder in children. Approximately 2–4% of children have one or more seizures during childhood from a variety of causes, most often during infancy. *Epilepsy* is a chronic disorder characterized by recurrent, unprovoked seizures secondary to a CNS disorder. Infants are susceptible to developing epilepsy in the first year of life, with an incidence of 1 per 1000. The incidence decreases with age. The median age for the development of epilepsy is 5 to 6 years of age. In the United States, approximately 150,000 to 325,000 children between 5 and 14 years of age have epilepsy (Blair & Selekman, 2004).

Etiology and Pathophysiology

Seizures are believed to be the result of abnormal excessive concurrent electrical discharges from the cortical neuronal network of cells on the surface of the brain. Chemical changes within the neurons create an electrical negativity that enables the transfer of information between neurons. When an excessive number of these cells become excited, they discharge abnormally. These cells can be triggered by either environmental or physiologic stimuli such as emotional stress, anxiety, fatigue, infection, or metabolic disturbances. An acute insult such as a CNS infection, hypoxia, and brain trauma are the most common causes in children.

Some seizures are idiopathic, or not provoked by known stimuli. Genetic factors may lower the seizure threshold by making brain cells more vulnerable to abnormal electrical discharges. Acquired seizures may be caused by underlying pathologic conditions such as trauma, infection, hypoglycemia, hypotonic dehydration, electrolyte imbalance, endocrine dysfunction, toxins, tumors, or lesions that may be manifested at any time.

Partial, or **focal**, seizures are caused by abnormal electrical activity in one hemisphere or a specific area of the cerebral cortex, most often the temporal, frontal, or parietal lobes. The seizure may spread regionally and the symptoms are related to the region of the cortex affected.

In contrast, generalized seizures are the result of diffuse electrical activity that often begins in both hemispheres of the brain simultaneously and spreads throughout the cortex into the brainstem. As a result, movements and spasms displayed by the child are bilateral and symmetric.

The length of a seizure, especially of a generalized seizure, is important because the airway may be compromised during the tonic phase. The basal metabolic rate rises during the peak of seizure activity, increasing the body's demand for oxygen and glucose. During a seizure, the child may become pale or cyanotic as a result of hypoxia. The child may also become hypoglycemic if glucose demand is excessive.

Febrile seizures are generalized seizures that usually occur in children as the result of rapid temperature rise above 39°C (102°F) in association with an acute illness. No evidence of intracranial infection or other defined cause is found. They are usually seen between 3 months and 5 years with a peak incidence between 17 to 24 months of age. There is often a family history of febrile seizures. In addition, children who have one febrile seizure have a 30–50% greater chance of having future seizures (Gill & Gieron-Korthals, 2002). The lower convulsive threshold of infants may explain this type of seizure.

Clinical Manifestations

The symptoms of a seizure depend on its type and duration. Seizures are classified into two types: *partial (focal) seizures* and *generalized seizures*. The specific characteristics of the various types of partial and generalized seizures are presented in the clinical manifestations table on the next page. Tonic-clonic seizures are the most common seizure type in children (Weinstein, 2002). The initial manifestations of the **tonic** phase of a generalized seizure are unconsciousness and continuous muscular contraction. The tonic phase is followed by the **clonic** phase, characterized by alternating muscular contraction and relaxation. During the **postictal period** following seizure activity, the level of consciousness is decreased. The length of the postictal period varies among children. An **aura**, an olfactory or visual sensory sensation, may provide an early warning sign of a seizure. When the child recognizes the pattern of an aura, he or she may have time to avoid injury by getting to the floor.

Febrile seizures involve generalized tonic-clonic movements that last less than 15 minutes.

COLLABORATIVE CARE

Diagnostic Tests

After the child's first seizure, it is essential that a thorough history be taken from the parent, primary caretaker, or witnesses to the event. Details such as the description and length of the seizure, presence or absence of an aura, and whether or not the child lost consciousness should be noted. This information helps to identify the type of seizure according to the International Classification of Epileptic Seizures.

Perform a complete physical and neurologic examination. Laboratory tests that may be ordered include a complete blood cell count, blood chemistry, urine culture, and lumbar puncture. If the child is taking any anticonvulsants, the serum drug blood level is monitored regularly. An electroencephalogram (EEG) is often performed at a follow-up visit between seizures. A lead level, toxicology screening, and radiologic tests such as CT scanning or MRI and angiography may be performed to identify a cerebral lesion or metabolic disorder in the brain.

Clinical Therapy

Many seizures are self-limiting and require no emergency intervention. Children with febrile seizures are usually not treated with an anticonvulsant at the time of the seizure because of their side effects. Long-term anticonvulsants are not recommended for simple febrile seizures (Shinnar & O'Dell, 2004). Instead, parents are taught to lower

CLINICAL MANIFESTATIONS FOR VARIOUS TYPES OF SEIZURES

Type of Seizure and Cause	Clinical Manifestations
Partial Seizures *Complex partial seizures* (psychomotor seizures) Lesions, cysts, or tumors Perinatal trauma Focal sclerosis (i.e., scarring of the mediotemporal lobe from prolonged febrile seizures) Vascular anomalies (i.e., arteriovenous malformations) Brain trauma	*Onset:* 3 years of age to adolescence Consciousness is impaired immediately or gradually after a simple partial onset; lasts 30 seconds up to 5 minutes; post-seizure amnesia or confusion May have abnormal motor activity, twitching, loss of tone, sensory changes such as tingling or numbness, may progress to a generalized seizure Aura frequently present, unusual taste or odor Feelings of anxiety, fear, or déjà vu (sensation that event occurred before) Abdominal pain Staring into space, mental confusion Posturing **Automatisms**—lip smacking, lip chewing, sucking
Simple partial seizures (focal seizures) Focal damage (e.g., with cerebral palsy) Tumors or lesions Arteriovenous malformation Brain abscesses	*Onset:* any age No loss of consciousness; lasts less than 30 seconds; no post-seizure confusion No aura Motor responses may involve one extremity, part of extremity, or ipsilateral extremities with eyes and head turning in opposite direction Sensory responses involve paresthesias (decreased sensation or tingling); auditory, olfactory, or visual sensations; autonomic (sweating, papillary dilation) or psychic symptoms Motor and sensory involvement may be combined and progress to generalized seizure Jacksonian march (rare in children): tonic contractions of either fingers of one hand, toes of one foot, or one side of face become clonic or tonic-clonic movements; activity then "marches" up to adjacent muscles of either affected extremity or same side of body (such as face)
Generalized Seizures *Tonic-clonic seizures* (grand mal seizures) Cerebral damage from perinatal trauma, brain trauma, tumors, structural lesions, metabolic and neuromuscular degenerative disorders Genetic link Many are idiopathic	*Onset:* any age, rare before 6 months of age, strong familial incidence Abrupt onset seizure, 1–2 minute loss of consciousness, post-seizure confusion (few minutes to hours) May or may not have aura Body becomes stiff and rigid when all muscles contract (tonic phase), followed by rhythmic jerking motions (clonic phase) Drooling or foaming at mouth as secretions are not swallowed Eyes roll upward or deviate to one side with pupils dilated Abdominal or chest wall rigidity with leg, head, and neck extended, and arms flexed or contracted Cry or grunt as air is forced out when diaphragm and chest muscles contract Urinary or bowel incontinence as muscles become flaccid during clonic phase Characterized by sleepiness, difficulty in arousal; hypertension; diaphoresis; headache, nausea, vomiting; poor coordination, decreased muscle tone; confusion, amnesia; slurred speech; visual disturbances; combativeness
Absence seizures (petit mal, or lapse seizures) Hyperventilation Genetic predisposition	*Onset:* age 3–12 years with remission in adolescence More prevalent in females May go on to develop other generalized seizures Hyperventilation or flashing lights may trigger a seizure Brief loss of consciousness, usually lasts 5–10 seconds, rarely exceeds 30 seconds, no post-seizure confusion, lethargy, or sleepiness Frequent attacks (50–100 per day), may cluster, interfere with learning No aura Child may continue simple movements such as walking or looking, but ceases activities such as reading; slight increase or loss of muscle tone (head may droop, handheld objects may be dropped) Staring; usually a glazed eye appearance, episodes may be confused with daydreaming or inattentiveness Rolling of eyes, eye blinking, ptosis or fluttering of eyelids Amnesia
Myoclonic seizures Progressive or degenerative encephalopathy like Tay-Sachs disease	*Onset:* as early as 2 years, but more prevalent in school-age child or adolescent No loss of consciousness, child recovers in seconds, no postictal period Attacks occur most often upon falling asleep or awakening Quick involuntary muscle jerks, may appear to drop or throw object; sudden flexion and bending of upper torso and head, extremity, or body contractions; may be limited to one body part or whole body

CLINICAL MANIFESTATIONS	FOR VARIOUS TYPES OF SEIZURES (continued)
Type of Seizure and Cause	**Clinical Manifestations**
Infantile spasms (myoclonic epilepsy of infancy, salaam seizures) Prenatal and perinatal encephalopathy Metabolic disorder Tuberous sclerosis Microcephaly Evolve into Lennox-Gaustaut syndrome	*Onset:* begin at age 3 months and resolve by 2 years Positive history of gestational difficulties, developmental delays, or other neurologic abnormalities May occur with altered consciousness as part of a complex partial seizure Occur in clusters, 5 to 150 per day Episodes of abrupt flexor (jackknife seizures), extensor or mixed jerks occurring in flurries when infant is awakening or throughout wakefulness Eye rolling, either upward or downward Crying, pallor, or cyanosis Regression in development and irritability Seizure activity increases in intensity and severity over time
Akinetic or atonic seizures (drop attacks) Gray matter degenerative diseases and subacute seizures Sclerosing panencephalitis Many are idiopathic	*Onset:* first seen at 2 years, disappear by 6 years Momentary loss of consciousness Falls to ground with sudden loss of postural tone; inability to break fall; is limp for a period of time Quickly regains consciousness

fevers by using antipyretics and keeping the child cool with light clothing. They must also protect the child from injury if there is a future seizure. As 30–40% of children experience a second febrile seizure, rectal diazepam or diazepam gel may be prescribed for the parents to have at home for treatment of a future febrile seizure, especially when they live a distance from medical care (Shinnar & O'Dell, 2004).

Any child with a generalized seizure lasting longer than 10 minutes needs to be monitored for electrolytes, glucose, blood gases, increasing fever, and abnormal blood pressure. Anticonvulsants are given intravenously or rectally to control the seizure, as the longer the seizure lasts the harder it is to stop (Wheless, 2004). Monitor for continued motor activity and the potential for **status epilepticus** (a continuous seizure that lasts for more than 30 minutes or a series of seizures during which consciousness is not regained). The postictal period ranges from 30 minutes to 2 hours. Management of the child in status epilepticus is described in Table 26–6.

Table 26–6	MANAGEMENT OF STATUS EPILEPTICUS
Type of Care	**Clinical Therapy**
Emergency assessment and management	• Maintain a patent airway. Muscle rigidity may compromise the airway. • Perform a jaw thrust maneuver if the airway is obstructed. • Keep suction equipment at the bedside in case secretions are excessive. • Give oxygen by mask, as increased metabolic demands deplete oxygen stores. • Monitor vital signs and circulation with pulse oximeter and cardiorespiratory monitor. • Perform neurologic assessment.
Ongoing urgent management	• Establish an intravenous line to administer any necessary fluids or medications. • Administer glucose if the child is hypoglycemic; the physical stress of the seizure may result in declining glucose levels. • Insert a nasogastric tube. • Protect the child from injury. • Manage thermoregulation.
Medications	• Administer benzodiazepines such as diazepam, lorazepam, or midazolam. If there is no response, the dose may be repeated. Phenytoin or phenobarbital may be necessary if seizure activity continues. Cumulative doses of drugs may produce apnea, so be prepared to assist ventilations.

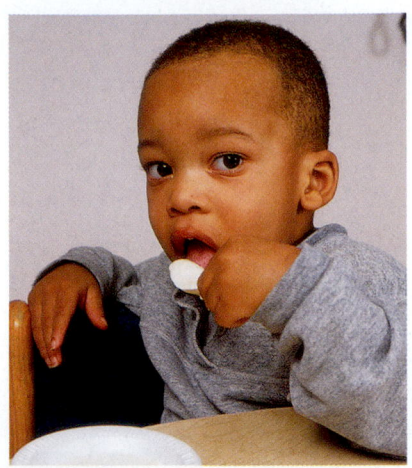

Figure 26–5 ▶ The family must make an effort to make the high-fat diet appealing to the child on a ketogenic diet, despite their personal feelings about eating large amounts of food such as mayonnaise, as this child is doing.

Most seizure disorders are treated with anticonvulsants. A single medication (monotherapy) is preferred for seizure control to minimize the side effects such as sleepiness, decreased attention and memory, difficulty with speech, ataxia, and diplopia. Monotherapy works for 60–70% of children with new onset epilepsy (Blair & Selekman, 2004). See Medications Used to Treat Seizure Disorders below. Other medications are added when necessary to control seizures. Serum drug levels are monitored to achieve therapeutic levels or identify if toxicity is possible. Therapeutic ranges of medications may be exceeded to control seizures when tolerated by the child. Medication dosage adjustments are often needed as the child grows. Approximately 25–30% of children have refractory or **intractable seizures**, seizures that continue to occur even with optimal medical management (Danielpour & Peacock, 2000). These children are often treated with multiple anticonvulsants. Regular blood testing is performed to identify any developing hematologic or liver problems, as well as to determine if therapeutic ranges of medications are maintained.

Surgery may occasionally be performed to remove a tumor, lesion, or portion of the brain that has been identified as causing the seizures, particularly when seizures are not responsive to medication. Cerebral hemispherectomy is sometimes performed for a child with intractable epilepsy (Jonas, Nguyen, Hu et al., 2004). A vagal nerve stimulator is another option for children who are unable to tolerate multiple medications and are not candidates for surgery (Blair & Selekman, 2004).

A ketogenic diet is occasionally used for children under the age of 8 years with myoclonic and absence seizures. This diet involves a high intake of fat (90%), an adequate intake of protein (1 gm/kg), and very low intake of carbohydrates. Caloric intake is calculated at 75% and fluids are restricted to 80% of usual (Freeman, 2003). The ketosis caused by the diet is believed to produce anticonvulsant effects. The diet is customized to the child to maintain the ideal body weight, maximize ketosis, and achieve optimal seizure control. Family motivation must be high to prepare the food and maintain the child on the diet for several years. See Figure 26–5 ▶. The child's urine ketone values are monitored weekly or more frequently. The most common complications are constipation, hyperlipidemia, and kidney stones. Constipation is treated with medium chain triglycerides (MCT oil) and increasing fluids. Kidney stones are treated by increasing fluid intake and alkalinizing the urine. Some children have discontinued the diet after becoming seizure-free and require no antiepileptic medications. Other children have a dramatically reduced incidence of seizures (Kossoff, Pyzik, McGrogan et al. 2002).

A trial of antiepileptic medication withdrawal is often attempted for children who have been seizure-free for 2 years (Goldstein, 2004). Approximately 60–70% of children are successfully weaned from antiepileptic medications and have no seizures (Blair & Selekman, 2004).

MEDICATIONS USED TO TREAT *Seizure Disorders*

Emergency Medications	Partial Seizures	Generalized Seizures	Absence Seizures
Diazepam	Carbamazepine	Phenytoin	Ethosuximide
Lorazepam	Oxcarbazepine	Oxcarbazepine	Valproic acid
Fosphenytoin	Lamotrigine	Topiramate	Lamotrigine
	Topiramate	Valproic acid	
		Carbamazepine	
		Gabapentin	
		Levetiracetam	
		Vigabatrim	
		Phenobarbital	

Data from: Sankar, R. (2004). Initial treatment of epilepsy with antiepileptic drugs. *Neurology, 63*(Suppl. 4), S30–S39.

NURSING MANAGEMENT

Nursing Assessment and Diagnosis

Assess and monitor the child's physiologic status. Observe the specific seizure activity, level of consciousness, vital signs, and signs of hypoxia. During the postictal period, monitor the child's vital signs, perform neurologic checks, and keep the environment safe. Once the child is stable, a more definitive assessment can be made. Level of consciousness is one of the most important indicators of neurologic function. Remember that the child's lack of response may be the result of the postictal state.

Collect and analyze historical information about the seizure activity, clustering, aura, description of motor activity or changes in muscle tone, automatisms, and any changes in development or school performance to help determine the type of seizures the child has. See Box 26–1.

Assess the family's adaptation to the seizure disorder, including how well the family is coping with the uncertainty of when the next seizure will occur.

Common nursing diagnoses for the child with a seizure disorder include:

- Ineffective Breathing Pattern related to neuromuscular dysfunction during the tonic phase of a seizure
- Ineffective Airway Clearance related to inability to control or manage secretions during the seizure
- Risk for Trauma related to fall with onset of seizure activity
- Chronic Low Self-Esteem related to seizures and loss of bowel and bladder control during seizure activity
- Anxiety related to unpredictable nature of seizure disorder
- Ineffective Therapeutic Regimen Management related to poor adherence with medications
- Readiness for Enhanced Family Processes related to care of a child with a chronic disorder

Planning and Implementation

Nursing care focuses on maintaining airway patency, ensuring safety, administering medications, and providing emotional support. Both acute care and long-term management are involved.

Maintain Airway Patency

Place nothing in the child's mouth during a seizure as loose teeth may be knocked out and aspirated. Position the child on his or her side so secretions can drain. Monitor the child to ensure adequate oxygenation: the child's color should be pink, the heart rate

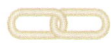

SKILL 11–2
Pulse Oximetry

BOX 26–1

HISTORY QUESTIONS TO ASK ABOUT SEIZURES

- Did the child complain of not feeling well or feeling "funny" just before the seizure?
- Did the child complain of headache, nausea, or muscle pain? Did the child vomit?
- Did the child suffer any trauma before the seizure?
- Did the child get into any medications or poisons before the seizure?
- Was the child sick or feverish before the seizure?
- What movements of the arms and legs were seen? On both sides of the body? On one side of the body or in one extremity only?
- Was the child's vision normal?
- Were the pupils dilated or the eyes deviated to one side?
- Was the child aware of surroundings? Could the child respond to questions?
- Was the child incontinent of urine or stool?
- How long did the episode last? When did the child begin to wake up?
- Was the child lethargic, weak, or uncoordinated upon arousal?
- Was the child injured during the convulsion?
- Did the child's skin color change (pale, red, blue)?

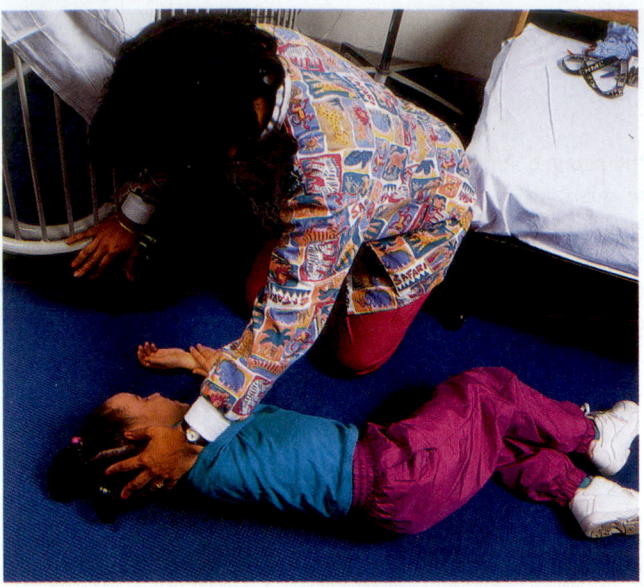

Figure 26–6 ➤ A child who has a seizure when standing should be gently assisted to the floor and placed in a side-lying position. Clear the area of any objects that might cause harm to the child.

should be at a normal or slightly elevated rate for age, and the pulse oximetry reading should be greater than 95%. Oxygen is usually administered when the pulse oximetry reading (SpO_2) falls below 95%.

Ensure Safety

Protect the child from self-harm during violent seizures (Figure 26–6 ➤). If the child is in bed, the side rails should be padded to prevent injury. Children who have frequent, recurrent seizures should wear helmets to protect their heads during falls. All children with seizure disorders should wear some form of medical alert identification.

Administer Medications

Take special precautions when administering intravenous medications (diazepam, lorazepam, or fosphenytoin) for the emergency management of status epilepticus. Give these medications very slowly over several minutes to minimize the risk of respiratory or circulatory collapse.

Medications for the ongoing management of seizures are given orally. Crushing pills and mixing them in a teaspoonful of applesauce, pudding, or other soft food make them more palatable and easier for the child to swallow.

Provide Emotional Support

The loss of control of body movements and possible loss of consciousness make seizures frightening and difficult to accept for the child, parents, and other family members. Parents often feel guilty about the child's seizure disorder and compensate by not disciplining or restricting the child appropriately. Stress the need to treat the child as normally as possible. Refer the child and family to support groups and counseling services, if indicated.

Discharge Planning and Home Care Teaching

Encourage parents to express their fears and anxieties. Answer their questions honestly, and refer them to organizations such as the Epilepsy Foundation of America, where they can get more information about the child's disorder. Be sure parents know how to administer medications and keep the child safe. Discuss with them whom to call with questions and when to return for follow-up.

Care in the Community

Children and adolescents need to have growth, as well as the medication plasma level, monitored carefully in order to maintain the level within therapeutic range—neither too low to be ineffective nor too high to cause toxic effects. Rapid changes in weight may lead to loss of seizure control if medication dosage is not appropriately adjusted (Marin, 2005).

Educate the child and parents about medication regimens. Explain the purpose of each drug, its schedule for administration, and the importance of giving all doses. Explain the use of rectal valium (Diastat) for acute management of a seizure. Teaching the older child to take medications without parental intervention gives the child a feeling of control. Provide information about the side effects of medications ordered, and alert parents to the signs of toxic reactions or undermedication. Regular dental care is also important because of the effect of phenytoin (Dilantin) on the gingiva. Explain the importance of follow-up visits to healthcare providers so that medication blood levels and the effectiveness of the child's medications can be monitored. See Evidence-Based Practice: Supporting Children with Epilepsy.

The parents of children with recurrent febrile seizures should be taught how to properly administer antipyretics. Parents need to know, however, that antipyretics may not prevent a future febrile seizure associated with an acute illness. The potential tox-

CLINICAL TIP

When the child on a ketogenic diet is hospitalized, it is important to limit glucose and dextrose from all sources. Normal saline intravenous fluid should be used. Medications in elixirs or syrups cannot be used because of the sugar content. Alternatively obtain medications in pill form, crush them, and mix with an allowable food approved by the pharmacy.

CLINICAL TIP

When a child is NPO due to illness or on the day of surgery, seizure medications are usually given with a swallow of water. Obtain medication orders in these cases.

MediaLink

Epilepsy and Seizure Resources

CLINICAL TIP

The blood for serum drug levels is ideally obtained just prior to a dose so that it can be representative of the child's lowest serum level.

EVIDENCE-BASED PRACTICE

Supporting Children with Epilepsy

Clinical Question

Children who develop epilepsy during childhood are faced with many issues, such as making an adjustment to living with a chronic condition, managing their condition, and telling friends about the seizures. What information and support do school-age children need to live with epilepsy and manage their lives?

Evidence

A scale developed to measure the psychosocial care needs of children with seizures was tested with a total of 63 children (average age of 10.5 years) at both 3 months and 6 months after the first seizure. Children were most satisfied with explanations they received from healthcare providers about their condition, but they were least satisfied with an opportunity to ask questions 3 months after the first seizure. Children wanted more information about activity restrictions, protection from injury, and handling future seizures. They also wanted to talk with other children their age with seizures and learn how to handle seizures at school (Austin, Dunn, & Huster et al., 1998; McNelis, Musick, Austin et al., 1998). In another study, 8 school-age children who had lived with epilepsy for at least a year were interviewed. They understood the need for medications, knew the medication name, and knew the dosage schedule. However, 6 of the children did not like taking the medication

or the side effects it generated. Most of the children had found a way to educate their peers and to fit in with their peer group. Some of the children had identified warning signs of an impending seizure and took measures to prevent future seizures such as getting plenty of sleep, drinking adequate fluids, performing some exercise, staying out of the sun, and avoiding getting angry (Hightower, Carmon, & Minick, 2002).

Implications

While the sample sizes for these studies are not large, information about living with epilepsy from the child's perspective is important. Learning about the child's understanding and perceptions helps the nurse to determine strategies that may help the child cope more effectively and to enhance development of self-esteem. As the child grows, self-management of the condition becomes increasingly important, along with preventive measures that can become part of the child's daily routine, such as sleep, hydration, nutrition, and avoiding certain types of stimulation.

Critical Thinking

Develop a teaching plan for a child between 10 and 12 years old with generalized seizures who is beginning to assume more responsibility for daily care. Be sure to include safety as well as self-esteem enhancement along with recognizing signs of seizures, nutrition, hydration, and medication administration.

---

icity of an anticonvulsant in a child with febrile seizures is often considered greater than the risk of the seizures, and parents can be reassured that complications from febrile seizures are rare.

Adolescent females need to be educated about the potential teratogenicity of some anticonvulsants, such as valproic acid and carbamazepine that are associated with neural tube defects and heart defects. Contraception should be used when the adolescent is sexually active, until a pregnancy is desired. Anticonvulsants with a lower risk for birth defects may be ordered at that time.

Teach families about safety guidelines for the child. Families of children with severe seizure disorders need to develop an emergency care plan so that emergency personnel know about their needs for care in advance (see Chapter 12). See Families Want to Know: Safety for the Child with a Seizure Disorder.

Assist the family to work with school administrators to develop an Individual Health Plan so the child can receive needed medications and care during school hours. Teachers and school administrators should know what to do if the child has a seizure and what information to report about the seizure. Parents may want to provide a towel and change of clothing for the child to use if incontinence occurs along with the seizures.

Physical activity and exercise are important for all children. Encourage the child's participation in sports when adequate supervision is provided. Activities such as rope climbing, rock or mountain climbing, tree climbing, snow skiing, scuba diving, and sky diving are more dangerous if seizures are not well controlled. Swimming and water sports require one-to-one supervision.

The child may be afraid of having a seizure in front of friends. Reassure the child and family that taking medications regularly should control seizures. Children need to be able to explain to peers what a seizure is and what to do if they are present when one occurs. However, adolescents are often hesitant to reveal a seizure disorder to peers because of embarrassment over being different. A support group may be valuable to help relieve those feelings. Summer camps for children with seizures can be a safe and comfortable place for the child to enjoy outdoor activities. Encourage parents to boost the child's self-image by emphasizing what the child can do, rather than focusing on contraindicated activities. Depending on state laws, most adolescents can drive after they have been seizure-free for at least 2 years.

CLINICAL TIP

Some antiepileptic medications cause a drug interaction with oral contraceptive pills that can lead to contraceptive failure. Effective contraception may require increasing the amount of estrogen in the contraceptive hormones or the use of medroxyprogesterone injections (Marin, 2005).

FAMILIES WANT TO KNOW

Safety for the Child With a Seizure Disorder

Children with epilepsy have more injuries of all sorts, including burns and falls. These children are also at increased risk for death due to drowning. Planning for safety includes the following:

- The child should not be left alone in the bathtub.
- Children who do bathe alone should use the shower.
- A buddy and lifeguard should always be present when the child swims.

- A life vest should always be worn when boating.
- A child with frequent seizures should wear a helmet to protect the head in case of a fall.
- The child should not play or stand around open flames or outdoor grills.
- The child should avoid areas where fall risks are increased.
- A form of medical identification should be worn (e.g., medical alert bracelet).

Evaluation

Expected outcomes of nursing management include the following:

- The child achieves good seizure control with medication, ketogenic diet, or surgical intervention.
- The child's self-esteem is enhanced through participation in well-supervised sports and activities.

INFECTIOUS DISEASES

Bacterial Meningitis

Meningitis, an inflammation of the meninges, can be caused by either bacterial or viral agents. Bacterial meningitis is more virulent than viral meningitis and is sometimes fatal. Newborns and infants are at greatest risk for bacterial meningitis. Infants and children who develop meningitis have the potential for acute complications and long-term morbidity.

Etiology and Pathophysiology

Meningitis may occur secondary to other infections such as otitis media, sinusitis, pharyngitis, cellulitis, pneumonia, tuberculosis, or septic arthritis; brain trauma; or a neurosurgical procedure. Three organisms cause a majority of cases in children between 2 months and 12 years of age: *Haemophilus influenzae* type b, *Neisseria meningitidis*, and *Streptococcus pneumoniae*. Group B Streptococcus and gram-negative enteric bacilli are most likely to cause meningitis in newborns (Chávez-Bueno & McCracken, 2005). See Chapter 18 ∞ for more information about these infectious organisms. Children who are immunosuppressed, or who have a ventriculoperitoneal shunt, cochlear implant, or penetrating head injury, are at greater risk for developing meningitis (Chávez-Bueno & McCracken, 2005).

In many cases, bacteremia spreads the infectious agent to the CNS where it enters the subarachnoid space. An inflammatory response then follows (Figure 26–7 ➤). White blood cells accumulate, covering the surface of the brain with a thick, white, purulent exudate. The brain then becomes hyperemic and edematous. If the infection spreads to the ventricles, they can become obstructed and impede the flow of cerebrospinal fluid, causing increased intracranial pressure and hydrocephalus. The infection may trigger the syndrome of inappropriate antidiuretic hormone (SIADH).

Clinical Manifestations

Symptoms are variable and depend on the child's age, the pathogen, and the length of the illness before diagnosis. Onset may be sudden or the illness may develop over 1 to 2 days. Symptoms in the young infant may include fever, change in feeding pattern, vomiting, or diarrhea. The anterior fontanel may be bulging or flat. The infant may be alert, restless, lethargic, or irritable. However, rocking or cuddling, which normally calms a fussy infant, only irritates the infant with meningitis.

CLINICAL TIP

Haemophilus influenzae type b was the most common cause of bacterial meningitis in children prior to the use of the Hib conjugate vaccine (American Academy of Pediatrics, 2006, p. 311). Immunization of infants with the pneumococcal vaccine is reducing the incidence of meningitis caused by *Streptococcus pneumoniae* (Black, Shinefield, Baxter et al., 2004).

PATHOPHYSIOLOGY ILLUSTRATED

Central Nervous System Infection

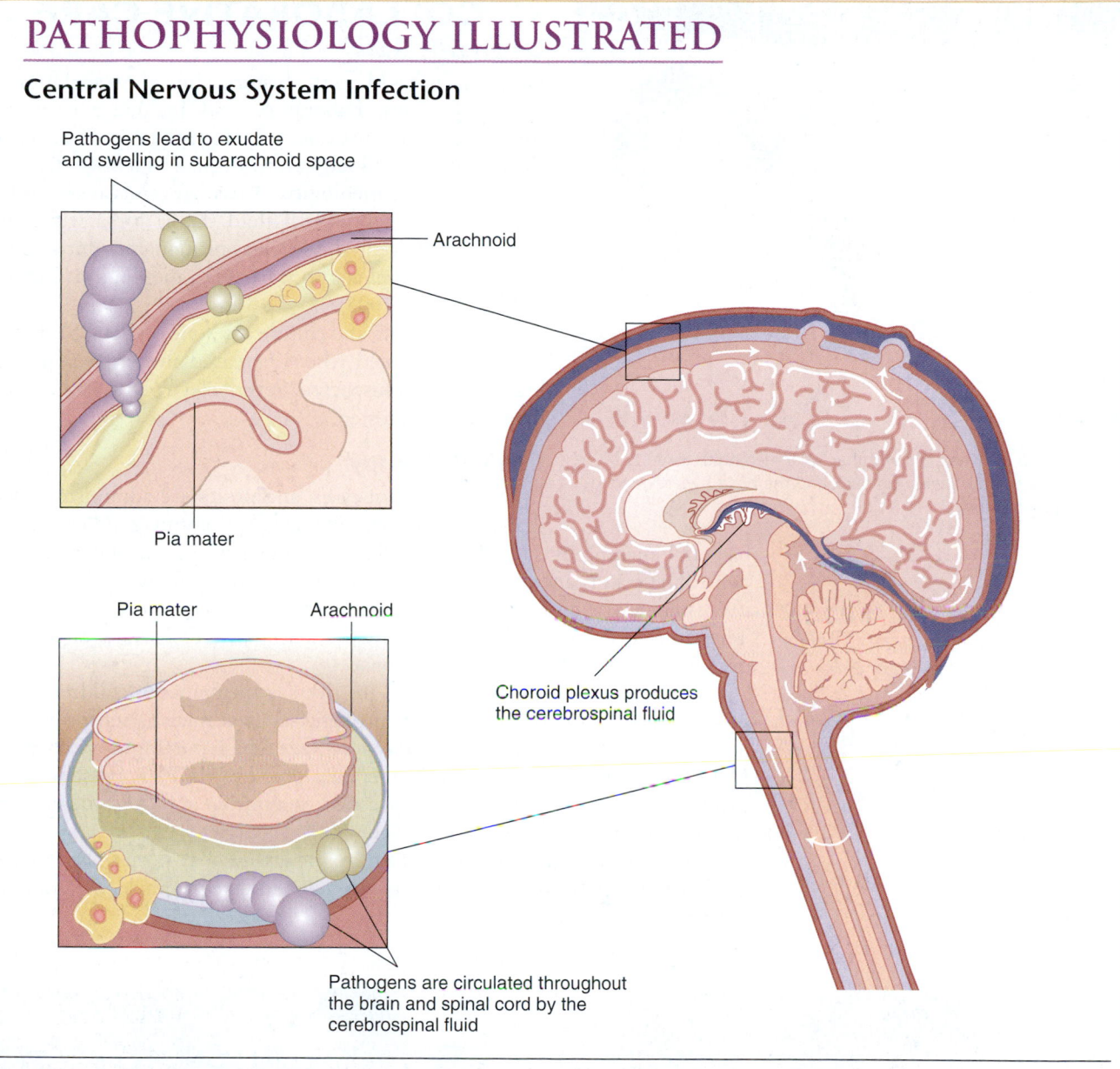

Pathogens lead to exudate and swelling in subarachnoid space

Arachnoid

Pia mater

Pia mater

Arachnoid

Choroid plexus produces the cerebrospinal fluid

Pathogens are circulated throughout the brain and spinal cord by the cerebrospinal fluid

Figure 26–7 ➤ After bacteria reach the central nervous system, the pia mater, the arachnoid, and the cerebrospinal fluid-filled subarachnoid space become infected. The cerebrospinal fluid then circulates the pathogens throughout the brain and spinal cord.

Older children are usually febrile. They can have confusion, delirium, or impaired consciousness; can be irritable, lethargic, or confused; may have vomiting; and may complain of muscle or joint pain. A hemorrhagic rash, first appearing as petechiae and changing to purpura or large necrotic patches, may be seen in meningococcal meningitis (see Chapter 18 ∞). The child also displays other symptoms consistent with meningeal irritation: headache (most often frontal), photophobia, esotropia, and **nuchal rigidity** (resistance to neck flexion). The infant may assume an **opisthotonic position**, in which the head and neck are hyperextended, to relieve discomfort (Figure 26–8 ➤). The child may have a positive Kernig's or Brudzinski sign, or both, on examination (Figure 26–9 ➤).

Symptoms can progress to include seizures, apnea, **cerebral edema** (the increase in intracellular and extracellular fluid in the brain that results from anoxia, vasodilation, or vascular stasis), subdural effusion, hydrocephalus, disseminated intravascular coagulation (DIC), shock, and increased intracranial pressure.

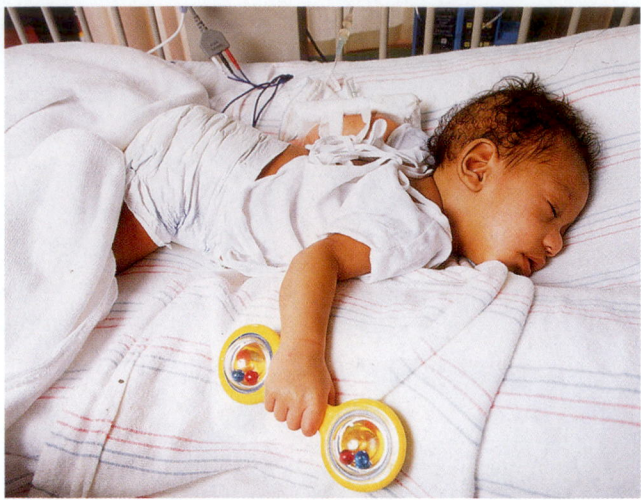

Figure 26–8 ➤ The child with bacterial meningitis assumes an opisthotonic position, with the neck and the head hyperextended, to relieve discomfort.

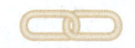

SKILL 4–2
Positioning a Child for a Lumbar Puncture

■ COLLABORATIVE CARE

Diagnostic Tests

Diagnosis is based on the history, clinical presentation, and laboratory findings. Laboratory tests include a complete blood count, blood cultures, serum electrolytes and osmolality, and clotting factors. Blood cultures usually identify the responsible bacteria causing meningitis. A lumbar puncture is performed to evaluate the cerebrospinal fluid (CSF) for a white blood cell count and differential, as well as protein and glucose levels. The CSF glucose level is low in bacterial meningitis (Chávez-Bueno & McCracken, 2005).

A Gram stain and culture are done on the CSF. CT scanning may be performed when increased intracranial pressure or a brain abscess is suspected. Serum electrolytes and blood urea nitrogen are also tested.

Clinical Therapy

In the majority of cases, antibiotics are administered as soon as diagnostic tests are obtained. Antibiotics commonly used to treat bacterial meningitis include ampicillin, aminoglycosides, cefotaxime, ceftriaxone, penicillin G, and vancomycin. Antibiotics are often changed once culture and sensitivity results are known, since many organisms have resistance to certain antibiotics. These medications are administered intravenously for 7 to 21 days, depending on the organism and the child's clinical response.

Corticosteroids (dexamethasone) are given as an adjunct to children over 6 weeks of age to reduce the risk of severe neurologic sequelae such as sensorineural hearing loss, especially in cases of *Haemophilus influenzae* type b meningitis (Chávez-Bueno & McCracken, 2005). If increased intracranial pressure (ICP) is present, medications used to reduce ICP include antipyretics, mannitol, and high-dose barbiturates (Chávez-Bueno & McCracken, 2005).

Depending on the causative organism, the disease may need to be reported to the local health department, and contacts may need to take prophylactic antibiotics, such as rifampin or ciprofloxacin.

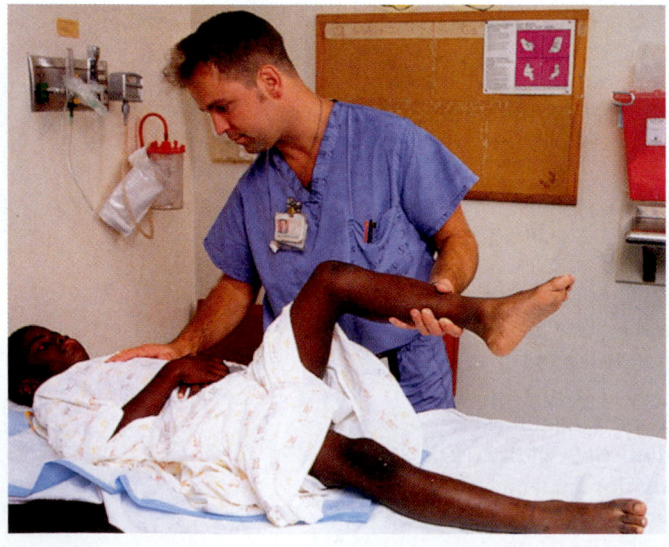

A

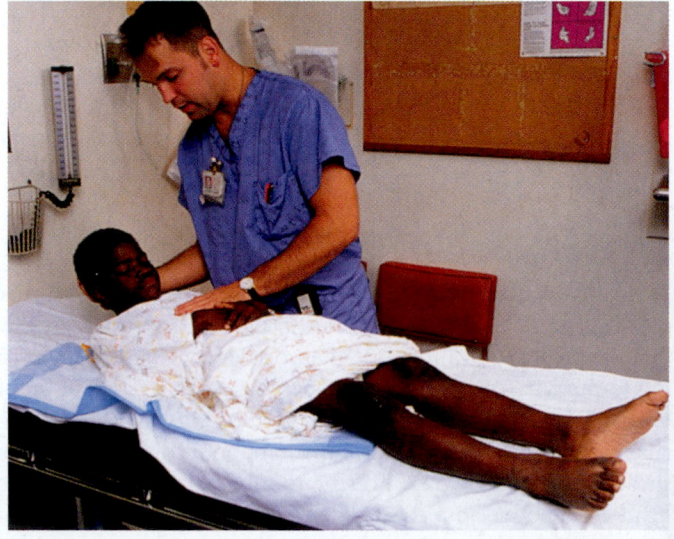

B

Figure 26–9 ➤ A, To test for Kernig's sign, raise the child's leg with the knee flexed. Then extend the child's leg at the knee. If any resistance is noted or pain is felt, the result is a positive Kernig's sign. This is a common finding in meningitis; B, To test Brudzinski sign, flex the child's head while in a supine position. If this action makes the knees or hips flex involuntarily, a positive Brudzinski sign is present. This is a common finding in meningitis.

Infants and children receive nothing by mouth and are started on IV fluids. The IV fluids may initially be restricted to two thirds maintenance as careful monitoring for increased intracranial pressure and for fluid retention associated with SIADH (see Chapter 29 ∞) is initiated. If neither condition is present, fluid restriction is not necessary (Chávez-Bueno & McCracken, 2005). If the child is in shock, however, aggressive fluid resuscitation is performed to maintain an adequate cerebral perfusion pressure.

Some infants and children who have had bacterial meningitis suffer neurologic damage despite early, aggressive management. The most common sequelae involve the cranial nerves, especially the eighth, resulting in hearing loss. In addition, children may develop complications such as seizures, hydrocephalus, subdural effusion, diabetes insipidus, SIADH, developmental delay, learning problems, and behavior problems.

NURSING MANAGEMENT

Nursing Assessment and Diagnosis

Assess the child's physiologic status, including vital signs and level of consciousness. Use the baseline neurologic assessment to help identify changes in the child's condition. Measure head circumference often in infants because of the potential for the obstruction of ventricles causing hydrocephalus. Be alert for signs of a change in the child's condition and response to treatment. Monitor the child's ability to control secretions and to drink sufficient fluids. Monitor intake and output. Assess for any sensory deficits. Identify parents' concerns about this potentially life-threatening condition.

Several nursing diagnoses that may apply to the child with bacterial meningitis are given in the accompanying nursing care plan. Additional nursing diagnoses might include:

- Risk for Aspiration related to altered level of consciousness and poor secretion control
- Risk for Deficient Fluid Volume related to poor oral fluid intake
- Anticipatory Grieving (Parent) related to the child's potentially life-threatening condition
- Caregiver role strain related to a hospitalized child and other family responsibilities

Planning and Implementation

The accompanying Nursing Care Plan summarizes care for the child with bacterial meningitis. Nursing care begins with emergency treatment and continues as the child's condition stabilizes. Monitor respiratory and neurologic status, maintain hydration, administer medications, and prevent complications. Promote the child's comfort with reduced stimulation (dim lights, quiet room) and by placing him or her in a side-lying position. Isolate the child and use standard and droplet precautions until the causative organism is identified and effective treatment is under way.

Monitor the child's response to antibiotic therapy. Observe for signs of gastrointestinal bleeding, which is a potential complication of corticosteroid use. Maintenance and replacement fluids are usually given to children with bacterial meningitis. However, it is important to monitor the serum sodium concentration and urine specific gravity because these children are at risk for SIADH. Fluids are restricted if SIADH is suspected. Sodium chloride, potassium, and sodium acetate or lactate may be administered intravenously to balance sodium excretion.

Respond to parents' concerns about their child's condition, explaining all measures to increase the child's comfort and to treat the illness. Identify ways parents can help meet the child's comfort needs. Parents may also need help figuring out how to meet the needs of other children at home while spending time with the hospitalized child. Ensure that the parents and close family contacts receive prophylaxis, if prescribed.

NURSING CARE PLAN   The Child with Bacterial Meningitis

GOAL	INTERVENTION	RATIONALE	EXPECTED OUTCOME
1. Impaired Spontaneous Ventilation related to level of consciousness and respiratory muscle fatigue			
	NIC Priority Intervention: **Respiratory Monitoring:** *Collection and analysis of patient data to assure airway patency and adequate gas exchange.*		*NOC Suggested Outcome:* **Vital Sign Status:** *Pulse, respiration, and blood pressure are within expected range for the child's age.*
The child's respiratory failure does not progress to respiratory arrest.	• Place the child on a cardiorespiratory monitor with a 20-second alarm.	• The alarm on the monitor alerts staff that the child is having bradycardia or an apneic spell.	The child's respiratory failure is managed with assessment and prompt treatment.
	• Have resuscitation equipment, including oxygen, resuscitation bag with mask, and suction apparatus, at the bedside.	• Equipment should be at the bedside in case of respiratory arrest. Bag-valve-mask ventilation is recommended as the child's respiratory secretions contain bacteria.	
	• Stimulate the child if apneic; if no response, begin manual ventilations and call for emergency resuscitation.	• Stimulation may encourage spontaneous respirations; if not, ventilation is necessary. Calling for emergency resuscitation ensures help in managing the child in a timely manner.	
	• Monitor the heart rate and perform compressions if necessary.	• The apneic child may have bradycardia resulting from cardiac hypoxia.	
2. Ineffective Protection related to infection of cerebrospinal fluid and potential sequelae			
	NIC Priority Intervention: **Neurologic Monitoring:** *Collection and analysis of patient data to prevent or minimize neurologic complications.*		*NOC Suggested Outcome:* **Neurologic Status: Consciousness:** *Extent to which an individual arouses, orients, and attends to the environment.*
The child will suffer minimal CNS injury secondary to infection.	• Administer prescribed antibiotics and corticosteroids as scheduled.	• Antibiotics help eradicate the pathogen and prevent cerebral edema. Corticosteroids diminish inflammatory response and reduce the chance of neurologic sequelae.	The child's condition improves significantly within 48–72 hours (fever decreases and no signs of neurologic sequelae are detected).
	• Note return of fever, nuchal rigidity, or irritability. Monitor vital signs, assess for signs of increased intracranial pressure, measure head circumference once or twice daily. Note changes in responsiveness. Notify the physician immediately if any signs are detected.	• Watching for common sequelae such as subdural effusions or septic arthritis ensures prompt treatment.	
The child will not develop cerebral edema as a result of water retention.	• Monitor for syndrome of inappropriate antidiuretic hormone secretion (SIADH) and watch for signs of increased intracranial pressure (ICP).	• SIADH can be either avoided or quickly managed if recognized early.	Cerebral edema does not develop. If SIADH or increased ICP occurs, the condition is treated promptly so effects are minimal.
	• Perform strict intake and output measurements. Determine urine specific gravity. Check electrolytes and osmolality of both serum and urine. Weigh the child daily. Restrict fluids and give sodium chloride as ordered.	• Low urine output with a high specific gravity is a sign of fluid retention and SIADH. The child is maintained with lower fluids and provided sodium supplements to reduce the possibility for cerebral edema.	

NURSING CARE PLAN   The Child with Bacterial Meningitis (continued)

GOAL	INTERVENTION	RATIONALE	EXPECTED OUTCOME
2. Ineffective Protection related to infection of cerebrospinal fluid and potential sequelae (continued)			
The child will be free of injury resulting from disseminated intravascular coagulation (DIC).	• Be aware of needlesticks that continue to bleed and lesions that continue to ooze. Monitor clotting times.	• Prompt recognition leads to management of the coagulopathy.	The child does not sustain injury from DIC.
	• Administer blood products, vitamin K, or heparin as ordered.	• Prompt recognition allows for early initial treatment of DIC. The child may bleed to death if treatment is delayed.	
The child will be free of injury secondary to shock.	• Monitor vital signs including pulse, respirations, and blood pressure. Note perfusion (capillary refill, central versus proximal pulses). Check level of consciousness. Note urine output.	• Monitoring allows for prompt diagnosis of shock based on clinical signs.	The child recovers from shock quickly with no complications. Prompt management of shock can enhance the child's recovery, since it prevents complications associated with poor perfusion (tissue acidosis and ischemia).
	• Begin fluid resuscitation as ordered.	• Intravenous fluid bolus may improve perfusion.	
	• Administer inotropes if ordered.	• Inotropes enhance perfusion when response to fluid challenge is minimal.	
3. Social Isolation related to decreased level of consciousness and hospitalization			
	NIC Priority Intervention: **Socialization Enhancement:** *Facilitation of the child's ability to interact with others.*		*NOC Suggested Outcome:* **Social Involvement:** *Frequency of an individual's social interactions with persons, groups, or organizations.*
The child's social interaction will be near normal despite isolation.	• Educate parents and other visitors to use proper infection control techniques.	• Family members help fulfill the emotional and social needs of the ill and contagious child.	The child's social and developmental needs are met by family members despite the child's illness and hospitalization.
	• Encourage parents to help with daily activities such as feeding and bathing.	• Parental involvement in the child's care provides the child with a sense of security and emotional well-being. Parents have a sense of control and a feeling that they are doing something to enhance the child's recovery.	
	• Have age-appropriate games and toys in the room. Play with the child. When the child is feeling better, encourage watching television/ videotapes/DVDs or listening to the radio/audiotapes/CDs.	• Providing the child with toys and games as well as sensory stimulation helps the child achieve a sense of well-being.	
The child with any degree of hearing loss will be identified.	• Arrange for hearing assessment prior to discharge.	• Hearing loss is a common complication. Early intervention is needed to promote growth and development.	The child with identified hearing loss is referred to the appropriate specialist or program for intervention.

(continued)

NURSING CARE PLAN The Child with Bacterial Meningitis (continued)

GOAL	INTERVENTION	RATIONALE	EXPECTED OUTCOME
4. Acute Pain related to meningeal irritation			
	NIC Priority Intervention: **Pain Management:** *Alleviation of pain or reduction in pain to a level of comfort acceptable to patient.*		*NOC Suggested Outcome:* **Comfort Level:** *Feelings of physical and psychologic ease.*
The child will be as comfortable as possible.	• Assess pain with age-appropriate pain scale.	• Pain scales provide ability to quantify pain for future comparison.	The child is calm and expresses increased comfort.
	• Minimize tactile stimulation.	• Sensory stimulation increases discomfort.	
	• Allow the child to assume a comfortable position.	• The child determines the most comfortable position. Opisthotonic position, with the head and neck hyperextended, may be the most comfortable.	
	• Keep the lights dim and maintain a quiet environment.	• Dim lights reduce the discomfort from photophobia. Noise can disturb the child.	
	• Provide pain medication as ordered.	• Round the clock pain management promotes comfort and healing.	
5. Risk for Infection (Family and Close Contacts) related to pathogens in the cerebrospinal fluid			
	NIC Priority Intervention: **Infection Control:** *Minimizing the acquisition and transmission of infectious agents.*		*NOC Suggested Outcome:* **Infection Status:** *Presence and extent of infection.*
Caretakers or family members will have no apparent evidence of infection.	• Explain rationale and dose schedule for taking rifampin or ciprofloxacin.	• Rifampin and ciprofloxacin provide prophylaxis for many bacterial pathogens responsible for meningitis.	Family members and other close contacts complete rifampin or ciprofloxacin therapy and avoid becoming infected.

Discharge Planning and Home Care Teaching

Identify and address home care needs well in advance of discharge. Follow-up visits are important to monitor for complications and sequelae. Help parents deal with any physical requirements resulting from the child's illness and any emotional, social, and financial repercussions of the child's condition. Teach parents what to do if the child has a seizure.

Infants and toddlers with neurologic sequelae should be referred to an early intervention program. If the child has had a hearing loss, referral to an otolaryngologist and speech and language specialist should be made. Encourage early identification of other neurologic sequelae, such as learning problems. Children with hearing, learning, or attention disorders need Individualized Education Plans (see Chapter 12 ∞), and parents may need help planning for the child's special educational needs. Refer parents to the appropriate social service agencies for support and assistance.

Adolescents should be encouraged to get the meningococcal vaccine to prevent meningococcal meningitis.

Evaluation

Expected outcomes of nursing care are provided in the accompanying nursing care plan.

Viral (Aseptic) Meningitis

Viral meningitis is an inflammatory response of the meninges characterized by an increased number of blood cells and protein in the cerebrospinal fluid. In the United

States, an enterovirus is often the cause of more than 80% of viral meningitis cases (Prober, 2004).

Generally, the child with aseptic meningitis does not appear as ill as the child with bacterial meningitis. The child may be irritable or lethargic and usually has a fever. Other symptoms include general malaise, headache, photophobia, gastrointestinal distress, upper respiratory symptoms, and a maculopapular rash. The child may also show signs of meningeal irritation such as stiff neck, back pain, and positive Kernig's and Brudzinski signs (see Figure 26–9). The infant may have a tense anterior fontanel. Seizures are rare. Symptoms usually resolve spontaneously within 3 to 10 days.

The child with fever and meningeal signs is hospitalized. Blood, urine, and cerebrospinal fluid analyses are performed. Polymerase chain reaction testing helps detect viral meningitis. Until the diagnosis of aseptic meningitis is confirmed, the child is treated aggressively, as if he or she has bacterial meningitis. Treatment is supportive of symptoms.

Nursing Management

Initial nursing care focuses on providing supportive care as described for the child with bacterial meningitis. Give acetaminophen as ordered to reduce fever, headache, and muscle or joint pain. Keep the room dark and quiet (to decrease stimuli and meningeal irritation), give fluids either intravenously or orally, and promote comfort with proper positioning.

The child and family need information about the disease. Explain medical and nursing procedures in terms that the child and family can understand. Keep parents informed about the child's progress. Once the diagnosis of viral meningitis is made, immediately begin discharge planning and teaching for home care. Explain that recovery may take several weeks but that complete recovery is expected.

Encephalitis

Encephalitis is an acute CNS condition with radiographic or laboratory evidence of brain inflammation (Lewis & Glaser, 2005). Inflammation of the meninges is also common. The incidence is estimated to be 7.3 cases for every 100,000 hospitalizations. Children under 1 year of age have the highest incidence (Lewis & Glaser, 2005).

The encephalitis may occur as a direct or primary infection by an organism that successfully gets past the blood-brain barrier, such as arborviruses, herpes simplex viruses, and rabies. Postinfectious encephalitis occurs days or weeks after an infection, such as with measles or varicella (Lewis & Glaser, 2005). Viruses are believed to cause most cases of encephalitis. Herpes simplex type I is the most common cause after the newborn period, and is associated with a high mortality rate. Those who survive often have significant neurologic sequelae (American Academy of Pediatrics, 2006, p. 365). Other viruses causing encephalitis include enterovirus, Epstein-Barr virus, herpesviruses, arborviruses, varicella, influenza, West Nile virus, and La Crosse encephalitis virus (Lewis & Glaser, 2005). Some bacteria, fungi, and protozoa have been identified as the causative organism in some cases.

Signs and symptoms depend on the causative organism and the location of the infection within the brain. An acute onset of a febrile illness with neurologic signs is the classic manifestation of encephalitis. Initially, the child may have a severe headache and fever, followed by altered mental status or focal neurologic signs. In some cases, the child may have fever, vomiting, and altered mental status or coma as presenting signs. Meningeal irritation signs such as nuchal rigidity, photophobia, and positive Kernig's and Brudzinski signs are common. Other neurologic signs vary. The child may be disoriented or confused, with behavioral or personality changes. Speech disturbances; motor dysfunction such as hemiparesis, ataxia, or weakness; cranial nerve deficits; or alterations in reflex response may be present. Focal or generalized seizures may occur. Progression of signs to coma may occur over hours or days.

Diagnosis is based on history and laboratory findings. Information about recent immunizations, insect bites, or travel to areas where cases of encephalitis are present should be obtained (e.g., West Nile virus or eastern equine encephalitis). Cerebrospinal fluid analysis, blood serologic tests, and nasopharyngeal and stool specimens are evaluated in an attempt to identify pathogens causing the symptoms. Testing for virus-specific immunoglobulin M antibodies with enzyme-linked immunosorbent assay (ELISA) is performed after 5 days of acute illness. The polymerase chain reaction test is used to assay for herpes DNA in the spinal fluid. A CT scan, MRI, and EEG may also be performed. An electroencephalogram (EEG) may help assess seizure activity and help localize the area of the brain affected. Brain biopsy may be performed to diagnose herpes simplex and parasitic infections. Routine blood chemistry and hematology tests are often normal (Lewis & Glaser, 2005).

The child with encephalitis is at risk for seizures, respiratory failure, and increased intracranial pressure and should be cared for in an intensive care unit. Treatment is both pharmacologic and supportive. The child with a suspected bacterial infection should be treated with antibiotics until bacterial pathogens have been ruled out. Acyclovir may be used for herpes viral infections. With postinfectious encephalitis, intravenous immune globulin, corticosteroids, and other immune system modulators are considered (Lewis & Glaser, 2005).

Children with encephalitis have many permanent neurologic sequelae. Although some children recover completely, many more are left with intellectual, motor, visual, or auditory deficits. The cardiovascular system, lungs, or liver may also be affected. Generally, the younger the child, the more serious the illness and the more severe the residual effects.

Nursing Management

Nursing care focuses on monitoring cardiorespiratory function, preventing complications resulting from immobility, reorienting the child, and teaching the parents about the child's condition. This child is usually admitted to the intensive care unit during acute stages.

Monitor the child's cardiorespiratory function. Check the child's airway and ability to handle secretions. Monitor respiratory status by observing color, pulse oximetry readings, and arterial blood gas values. Observe cardiopulmonary status by monitoring heart rate, blood pressure, capillary refill time, and urine output. Provide seizure precautions, and have appropriate equipment for managing seizures at the bedside.

Prevent complications resulting from immobility as described in on page 1039. Maintain skin integrity. Proper positioning with frequent turning is important. When indicated by the physician, perform chest physiotherapy to prevent pneumonia.

The child whose level of consciousness begins to improve may at first be confused and disoriented and may have residual effects of the disease. Orient the child to the hospital environment. Have the family help to reorient the child by bringing favorite stuffed animals or music from home. Engage in therapeutic play (refer to Chapter 13 ∞ for techniques). Give the child age-appropriate toys to encourage a return to normal behavior.

Give the parents information about their child's condition and prognosis. Provide support to the parents and family as they cope with the life-threatening nature of this condition. If the child receives physical, occupational, or speech therapy, explain the treatment regimen to the parents.

DISCHARGE PLANNING AND HOME CARE TEACHING   Encourage parents to take an active role in the child's physical and emotional care in the hospital, and give them written instructions about home care. Encourage the parents to learn specific physical, occupational, and speech therapies so they can work with their child at home between home care visits. Refer parents to home care, social services, family counseling, and support groups. Plan follow-up visits so the child can be evaluated for neurologic sequelae.

Reye's Syndrome

Reye's syndrome is a disorder that includes an acute **encephalopathy** (a cerebral dysfunction caused by a toxic, injury, inflammatory, or anoxic insult that may result in permanent tissue damage) and hepatic dysfunction. In the 1980s, an association was reported between the use of aspirin for influenza or varicella and the subsequent development of Reye's syndrome. The condition has become very rare since most par-

SKILL 7–6
Arterial Blood Gases

SKILL 11–2
Pulse Oximetry

SKILL 11–3
Cardiorespiratory Monitor

ents now give children acetaminophen or ibuprofen rather than aspirin for viral illnesses and flu-like symptoms, and children are immunized against varicella. However, the mortality rate for children who develop the condition is high.

The etiology of Reye's syndrome is unclear. The disorder, an encephalopathy, usually develops after a mild viral illness, such as varicella or influenza, when the child has been given aspirin or aspirin-containing products. The disorder is characterized by cerebral edema, hypoglycemia, and an enlarged, fatty, poorly functioning liver (due to an elevation of short chain fatty acid levels and hyperammonemia).

Reye's syndrome begins with nausea and vomiting, mental status changes, seizures, and progressive unresponsiveness (Padgett, 2006). The condition has five stages that indicate increasing signs of cerebral edema and neurologic dysfunction, as described in Table 26–7.

The diagnosis of Reye's syndrome is based on an abrupt change in the child's level of consciousness and diagnostic laboratory tests that have no other identifiable cause. The child has often progressed to coma or stage III by the time of diagnosis. Cerebrospinal fluid analysis usually reveals white blood cells, while radiographic imaging reveals cerebral edema. Liver enzyme and ammonia levels are elevated, blood glucose levels are below normal, and prothrombin time is prolonged. A liver biopsy is sometimes performed to confirm the diagnosis.

The child with Reye's syndrome should be treated in a pediatric intensive care unit because of the potential for rapid deterioration. The goal of medical management is to provide supportive treatment and to prevent the secondary effects of cerebral edema and metabolic injury. Mechanical ventilation is often needed once the child is comatose. Perform arterial and venous blood pressure monitoring. The child is monitored for signs of increased intracranial pressure, which can be secondary to cerebral edema. Hypoglycemia is treated with intravenous glucose, and electrolytes, blood chemistry, and blood pH are monitored.

Nursing Management

Nursing care focuses on monitoring the child's physical status, providing emotional support, and teaching parents about disease prevention.

Check the child's respiratory and neurologic status frequently, and note any signs of improvement or deterioration. Gradually and repeatedly orient the child who awakens from coma. Refer to the discussion of nursing management of altered states of consciousness at the beginning of this chapter for specific nursing interventions. Monitor laboratory test values for acidosis, an elevation of ammonia levels, or hypoglycemia. Monitor the child's intake and output. Correct imbalances by administering fluids, electrolytes, or medications as ordered. Prevent complications associated with immobility.

Provide emotional support to the parents, who may feel guilty because they did not seek medical attention sooner. Keep them informed about the child's condition,

SKILL 11–7
Arterial Pressure Monitoring

> **NURSING ALERT**
>
> Make sure all parents know to use acetaminophen or ibuprofen when the child has a viral illness such as influenza to prevent the development of Reye's syndrome. Instruct parents to check all over-the-counter medicines for the presence of aspirin compounds prior to giving them to children. Emphasize the importance of obtaining health care whenever a child's condition worsens at the end of a viral illness.

Table 26–7	STAGES OF REYE'S SYNDROME
Stage	**Clinical Manifestations**
I	Vomiting; lethargy; appropriate responses to verbal commands; purposeful responses to pain; brisk pupillary reaction
II	Combativeness; stupor; inappropriate language; confusion; anxiety, fear; purposeful and nonpurposeful responses to pain; sluggish pupillary reaction; conjugate deviation with oculocephalic reflex; hyperactive reflexes; progresses to coma but interrupted by periods of screaming and ranting
III	Coma; decorticate rigidity; conjugate deviation with diminished oculocephalic reflex; sluggish pupillary reaction; decorticate posturing
IV	Coma with brainstem dysfunction; decerebrate rigidity and posturing; inconsistent or absent oculocephalic reflex; loss of corneal reflex; sluggish pupillary reaction
V	Coma with seizures; flaccidity; loss of deep tendon reflexes; respiratory arrest

and prepare them for potential deterioration. Explain treatments to help reduce anxiety. Encourage the parents to participate in the child's care whenever possible.

If the child survives and is discharged, monitoring is needed to observe for sequelae of the illness. Developmental and neurologic deficits may occur and are more severe in children under 2 years of age. Arrange for home nursing visits during the recovery period so that developmental and neurologic status monitoring can be assessed. Be sure the parents know about community resources that can help them deal with the child's recovery.

Guillain-Barré Syndrome (Postinfectious Polyneuritis)

Guillain-Barré syndrome is an acute inflammatory demyelinating polyradiculopathy. This condition may lead to deteriorating motor function and paralysis that progresses in an ascending pattern, as well as paresthesia and areflexia. This disorder affects all ages and genders equally, and occurs in all seasons of the year (Boss, 2006).

Guillain-Barré syndrome is thought to be caused by an immune response to an infectious organism, usually from a gastrointestinal or respiratory viral or bacterial illness about 1 to 3 weeks prior to onset. Associated organisms are *Campylobacter jejuni* and *Mycoplasma pneumoniae*. It has also been associated with immunizations (Boss, 2006). The immune reaction is focused on the peripheral nerve myelin that is attacked by macrophages, resulting in variable demyelination and blocked transmission of nerve impulses to the muscles. The damaged peripheral nerves then begin to atrophy.

Infants have an onset of rapidly progressive severe hypotonia, possible respiratory distress, irritability, and feeding difficulties. Older children have rapidly progressive symmetric weakness and muscle pain with varying degrees of distal paresthesia and numbness in the legs. This ascending weakness spreads to the upper extremities, trunk, chest, neck, face, and head. Deep tendon reflexes may be diminished or absent. The child may develop acute ataxia or an inability to walk. Difficulty swallowing and facial weakness are signs of impending respiratory failure. Respiratory effort may be inadequate for proper ventilation. Cranial nerves may be affected, causing Bell's palsy, for example. A dysfunctional autonomic nervous system may cause such symptoms as a labile blood pressure and cardiac rate, postural hypotension, or profound bradycardia (Sarnat, 2004).

Diagnostic criteria of Guillain-Barré syndrome include progressive motor weakness (minimal weakness of the legs to total paralysis of all extremities), and areflexia of varying degrees. Cerebrospinal fluid analysis reveals twice the limit of normal protein levels, normal glucose level, and fewer than 10 white blood cells per cubic millimeter, a positive indicator of the condition (Sarnat, 2004). Bacterial and viral cultures are usually negative. Electroconduction tests such as electromyography show acute muscle denervation.

Clinical therapy for Guillain-Barré syndrome is intravenous immune globulin (IVIG) for several days when the child cannot ambulate. Guidelines for administration of intravenous immune globulin can be found in Chapter 17 ∞. Responses to intravenous immune globulin are dramatic, often occurring within days. Plasmapheresis, corticosteroids, or immunosuppressive medications are used if there is no response to IVIG. If the child can ambulate, physical therapy and supportive care are provided. The condition is rarely fatal. Use of antibiotics does not change the course of the condition (Sarnat, 2004).

Nursing Management

Nursing care focuses on monitoring respiratory status, meeting nutritional needs, managing autonomic nervous system dysfunction, preventing complications associated with immobility, providing emotional support, and teaching the parents how to care for the child after discharge.

MONITOR CARDIORESPIRATORY STATUS Place the child on a cardiorespiratory monitor to continuously assess the child's cardiorespiratory status, especially in the early phase of illness. Look for such signs as dyspnea, inability to handle secretions, inadequate respiratory effort, and color changes that may indicate the need for endotracheal intubation and mechanical ventilation.

MANAGE AUTONOMIC NERVOUS SYSTEM DYSFUNCTION Monitor the child's vital signs closely for episodes of tachycardia, bradycardia, and hypotension.

NURSING ALERT

The Centers for Disease Control and the Food and Drug Administration have initiated an investigation to determine if there is an association between Menactra, a tetravalent vaccine for meningococcal meningitis, and Guillain-Barré syndrome. While the number of reported cases is low and could have occurred by chance, the timing of the condition 2 to 4 weeks after immunization is of concern. Continued immunization of adolescents is recommended, but parents and adolescents need to be informed about this investigation. Provide parents and adolescents being immunized with information about signs of Guillain-Barré syndrome to be aware of and have them seek medical attention immediately if they occur (Centers for Disease Control, 2005).

RESEARCH

GBS and IVIG

A recent outcome study of some children with Guillain-Barré syndrome (GBS) who were treated with IVIG revealed that approximately 25% of children have residual mild muscle weakness 3 to 10 years after onset of GBS. Approximately 25% of children with good muscle strength had persisting exercise intolerance. The children most likely to have this outcome were those under 9 years who had rapid progression to maximal muscle weakness at the onset of GBS (Vajsar, Fehlings, & Stephens, 2003).

Blood pressure fluctuations and autonomic instability have been linked to asystole (Sarnat, 2004). Observe frequently for decreased responsiveness. Intervene promptly if these or other signs of autonomic nervous system dysfunction are noted.

MEET NUTRITIONAL NEEDS   Assess whether the child is having difficulty swallowing. If the child has no gag reflex, maintain nutritional needs with intravenous supplements or nasogastric tube feedings.

PREVENT COMPLICATIONS   Prevent complications associated with immobility (see the Clinical Tip on page 1039). Ensure good postural alignment, and turn the child every 2 hours. Maintaining skin integrity is also important.

Evaluate the child's muscle tone, strength, and symmetry. When the child's condition begins to improve, recovery of lost strength is the priority. Active exercise is emphasized in physical therapy. Encourage family members to participate in the child's care, especially during the recovery phase. They can help with the activities of daily living and reinforce what the child has learned in physical therapy.

PROVIDE EMOTIONAL SUPPORT   Explain the progression of Guillain-Barré syndrome to the parents and the child during the initial stages. Witnessing a rapid deterioration in their child's physical status can be frightening; therefore, preparation is essential to reduce their anxieties. Be honest when discussing the child's recovery and prognosis.

Have parents bring in the child's favorite toys, dolls, or books to make him or her feel more secure. Playing with or reading to the child can also be comforting.

DISCHARGE PLANNING AND HOME CARE TEACHING   Home care needs should be identified and addressed well in advance of discharge. Support the parents as they prepare for the child's return home, especially when the return to full strength is expected to be slow. Provide referral to home care nurses who can manage all aspects of treatment, rehabilitation, and follow-up. Refer the parents to social workers, who can help with financial arrangements and school considerations.

CARE IN THE COMMUNITY   Help the child to adjust to any residual effects of Guillain-Barré syndrome. Help the child practice exercises learned in physical therapy sessions, and encourage the child to perform activities of daily living, such as brushing the teeth or combing the hair. Refer the child to outpatient rehabilitation programs to promote recovery.

To promote a positive self-image, praise any effort the child makes to be self-sufficient. The child may be frustrated and angry. Allow the child to express these feelings in an appropriate way, either during play or in conversation.

HEADACHES

Children commonly experience headaches. They may be the cause of school absence, decreased extracurricular activity, and poor academic achievement. The majority of children experience a headache by late adolescence. Migraine headaches occur in 3% of children under 7 years of age, and 8–23% of children 11 years and older (Lewis, Ashwal, Hershey et al., 2004).

Headaches have both benign (migraine, inflammatory, and tension) and structural causes.

- Migraines may be triggered by stress; foods containing nitrates, glutamate, caffeine, tyramine, and salt; menses; oral contraceptives; fatigue; and hunger. Another family member often has similar headaches, so there may be a genetic predisposition.
- Tension headaches may be associated with stresses due to school, insecurity, or conflict in the family.
- Medication overuse (rebound) headaches are associated with the frequent use of medications for headaches, more than 2 to 3 times a week. Medications associated with this type of headache include acetaminophen, nonsteroidal anti-inflammatories (NSAIDs), triptans, caffeine, opiates, benzodiazepines, barbiturates, and ergotamines (Reimschisel, 2003).

CLINICAL TIP

An *aura* may give the child warning of an impending migraine headache. Before migraine headaches, children may report seeing spots or a shimmery film that gets larger and affects their vision. In the case of the migraine, the child has time to take medications in an effort to abort the headache. In epilepsy, the child may have time to avoid injury by getting to the floor.

CLINICAL TIP

Examples of foods that are common triggers of migraine headaches include the following: cheese, chocolate, hot dogs, ham, dairy products, citrus fruits, wine, beer, and foods or beverages with monosodium glutamate or caffeine (Millichap & Yee, 2003).

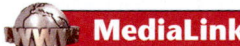

MediaLink

Headache Resources

COMPLEMENTARY THERAPY

Treating Headaches

Mind-body therapies that include biofeedback, self-hypnosis, progressive relaxation, meditation, and cognitive-behavioral therapy have been studied in children and found to be effective in treating the pain associated with headaches. In biofeedback, instruments (α-electroencephalography, muscle electromyography, skin temperature, and temporal pulse feedback) can be used to help the child learn to become aware of physical responses in the body and to learn to control those responses, making them skills the child can use in daily life. Other therapies are often used with biofeedback to enhance the effect (Powers & Andrasik, 2005).

Signs and symptoms of headaches in children and adolescents vary by cause. See Clinical Manifestations of Headaches on the next page.

Diagnosis involves taking a detailed history of the headache characteristics, onset, warning signs, duration, severity, and associated symptoms. The child is assessed for neurologic signs such as altered consciousness, abnormal cranial nerves, papilledema, and motor or sensory deficits, as well as blood pressure and vital signs. Radiologic studies (CT scan or MRI) are used only if a structural problem or pathologic condition is suspected.

Clinical therapy includes relaxation techniques, analgesics, and anti-inflammatory medications. Food elimination diet trials are often used to identify foods that trigger headaches, but they are often unsuccessful. Medications to abort migraines (sumatriptan nasal spray) may be used in adolescents as well as children old enough to identify an aura or warning. Cyproheptadine, beta-blockers, tricyclic antidepressants, and anticonvulsants (valproic acid, topiramate, and gabapentin) may be used prophylactically if headaches significantly interfere with usual activities (Lewis, Scott, & Rendin, 2002).

Nursing Management

Nursing management involves assessing the child for potential neurologic signs associated with headaches and assisting the child and family to identify strategies for relieving the headaches. Encourage the child to keep a calendar or diary of headaches, including the events and stresses occurring at the time. Help the family and child implement the food elimination trial and gradually add foods to identify offending chemical triggers. Make sure the child learns to take the prescribed medications appropriately. Teach the child relaxation techniques (breathing control training, mental imagery, progressive muscle relaxation, and biofeedback) to manage stress and the pain associated with the headaches. Encourage the child to maintain a healthy lifestyle with adequate sleep, healthy eating, regular exercise, and adequate hydration.

See Chapter 23 ∞ for care of the child with a brain tumor.

STRUCTURAL DEFECTS

Microcephaly

Microcephaly indicates a small brain with a head circumference that is more than 3 standard deviations below the mean for age and sex (Johnston & Kinsman, 2004c). It may be caused by chromosomal abnormalities, fetal insult, maternal infection, or destructive insult during infancy, such as infection, metabolic disorder, or anoxia. Children with microcephaly have cognitive impairments. See Chapter 27 ∞ for care of the child with mental retardation.

Hydrocephalus

Hydrocephalus is the body's response to an imbalance between the production and absorption of cerebrospinal fluid (CSF). The condition is often congenital and associated with other CNS malformations. The overall incidence is estimated to be 1 per 2000 births (Ditmyer, 2004). It is commonly associated with myelomeningocele, a spinal fluid-filled meningeal sac that contains a portion of the spinal cord and nerves protruding through a vertebral defect. See page 1066 for care of the child with myelomeningocele. Hydrocephalus can develop as a complication of illness or trauma.

Etiology and Pathophysiology

CSF is produced at a consistent rate of 0.3 mL per minute (Rudy, 2005). When the amount of CSF absorbed is less than the amount produced, the ventricles enlarge. Hydrocephalus may be either communicating or noncommunicating, and congenital and acquired.

- In communicating hydrocephalus, the CSF flows freely between ventricles, normal channels, and pathways, but absorption of the CSF in the subarachnoid space and the arachnoid villi is impaired. Potential causes include postinfectious meningitis, intraventricular hemorrhage, or a congenital malformation in the subarachnoid spaces.

CLINICAL MANIFESTATIONS — HEADACHES

Type of Headache and Cause	Clinical Manifestations	Clinical Therapy
Migraine—vascular, acute recurrent	• Unilateral or bilateral pulsatile throbbing pain lasting for 1 to 72 hours • Moderate or severe intense pain, often in the frontal or temporal region; pain may be aggravated by routine physical activities • Nausea and vomiting • Photophobia and phonophobia • May have visual or motor aura several minutes before headache starts • Preschool-age children may have irritability, restlessness, malaise, head banging, head holding, and sensitivity to light and sound • Relief with sleep	• Ibuprofen, acetaminophen, or naproxen • Medications to abort migraine (supatriptan nasal spray) for adolescents • Relaxation techniques and biofeedback • Food elimination trial to identify food triggers may be attempted • Caffeine and other food trigger avoidance • Noise and light avoidance during acute headache
Tension—muscular contraction, acute recurrent or chronic nonprogressive	• Dull, achy pain in band around head, in neck, and in shoulders that may last for hours or days • Bilateral location • Pressing or tightening pain sensation of mild to moderate intensity • Unlikely to have nausea and vomiting, sensitivity to light or sound, vertigo, or visual disturbances • Pain not aggravated by increased physical activity	• Relaxation techniques • Analgesic and anti-inflammatory medications • Ice pack • Rest
Medication overuse—acute recurrent	• Dull, bilateral, or unilateral pain in frontal area • Occur 5 times a week or 15 times a month • Can vary in character, location, and severity from time to time • Usually increases in frequency and severity over time, paralleling the increase in medication use • Recur with the abortive therapy or when medication wears off	• Withdrawal of all medications for headaches (caffeine, acetaminophen, NSAIDs, and triptans) (Kossoff & Mankad, 2006) • Substitution of medications that do not cause rebound may be used if headaches do not decrease in a month • Clonidine may be used to treat withdrawal symptoms
Inflammatory—sinusitis or dental abscess, acute localized	• Facial pain or tenderness over affected sinus • Dull, constant pressure • Severity of pain varies with head position • Fever	• Analgesic, antipyretic, and anti-inflammatory medications • Antibiotic medications • Cold or heat application
Structural—space-occupying lesion, hemorrhage, increased intracranial pressure, chronic progressive	• Severe pain that is increasing in frequency and severity, often in occipital or frontal location • Pain that awakens child in morning or is present when awakening • Pain increases with coughing, sneezing, or straining • Vomiting that is persistent or preceded by recurrent headache • Abnormal neurologic signs (e.g., double vision, papilledema, strabismus, weakness, ataxia)	• Surgery • Analgesic medications

Data from: Lewis, D., Ashwal, S., Hershey, A., Hirtz, D., Yonker, M., & Silberstein, S. (2004). Practice parameter: Pharmacologic treatment of migraine headache in children and adolescents. *Neurology, 63*(12), 2215–2224; Fisher, P. G. (2005). Help for headaches: A strategy for your busy practice. *Contemporary Pediatrics, 22*(11), 34–40.

- Noncommunicating hydrocephalus is responsible for most cases in children. It results from a blockage in the ventricular system that prevents CSF from entering the subarachnoid space (Figure 26–10 ➤). Enlargement of one or more of the ventricles results. Potential causes include infection, hemorrhage, tumor, surgery, or structural deformity.
- Congenital structural defects causing noncommunicating hydrocephalus include the Chiari II malformation (found in most children with myelomeningocele), aqueduct of Sylvius stenosis (a recessive X-linked cause of hydrocephalus), and the Dandy-Walker syndrome (the fourth ventricle is enlarged because of partial or complete closure of its outlets and a portion of the cerebellum does not develop).

PATHOPHYSIOLOGY ILLUSTRATED

Hydrocephalus

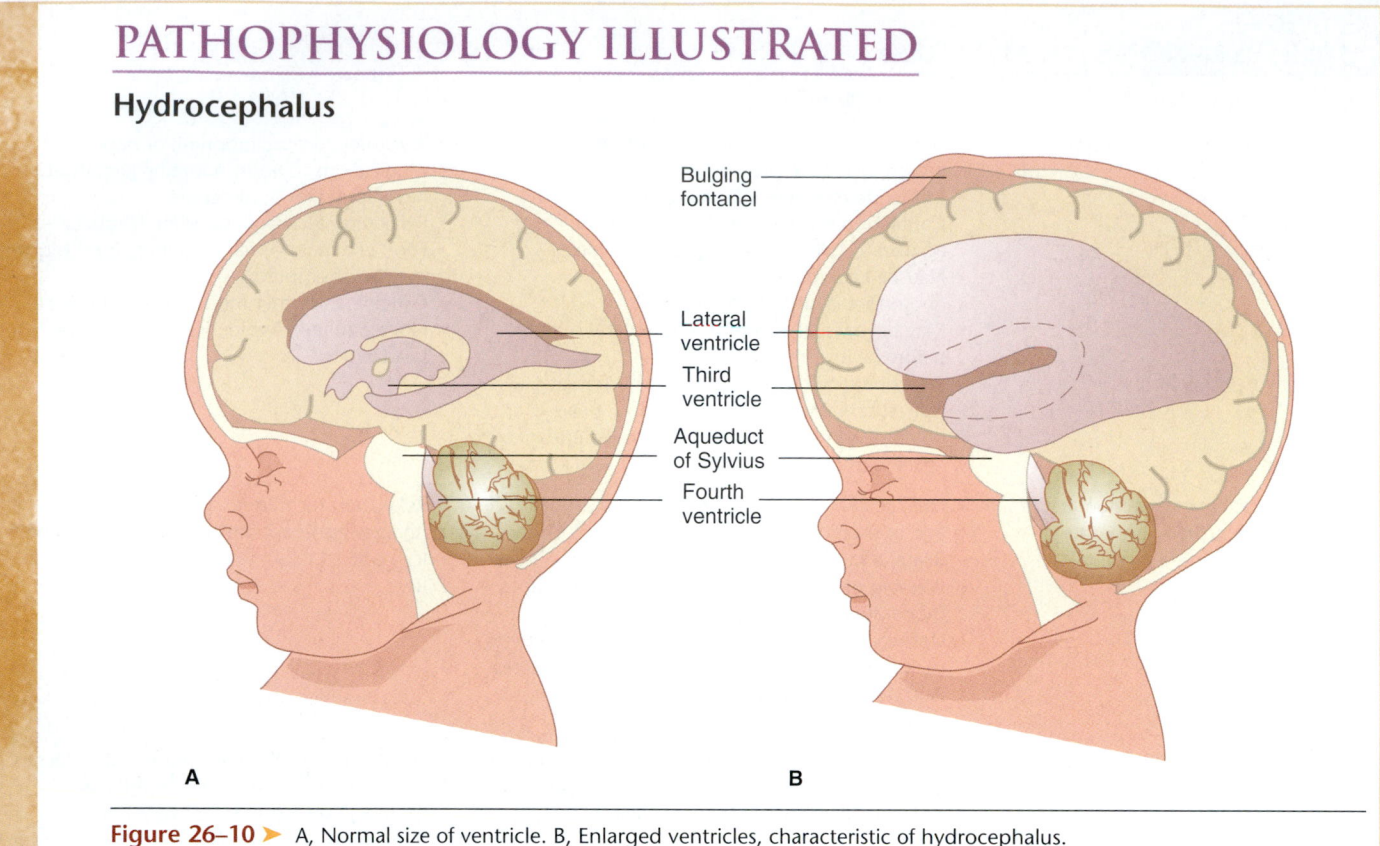

Bulging fontanel

Lateral ventricle

Third ventricle

Aqueduct of Sylvius

Fourth ventricle

A

B

Figure 26–10 ➤ A, Normal size of ventricle. B, Enlarged ventricles, characteristic of hydrocephalus.

> ### ➤ NURSING ALERT
>
> With the Chiari II syndrome there is progressive hydrocephalus along with the myelomeningocele. Symptoms may begin during infancy and consist of stridor, a weak cry, and apnea. An older child may have an abnormal gait, spasticity, and increasing coordination problems. The Chiari II syndrome is associated with an abnormality of the hindbrain that results in kinking of the brainstem and displacement of the pons and medulla into the cervical canal (Johnston & Kinsman, 2004b). Because the structures herniating through the foramen magnum control respiration and the protective reflexes, the child may also have apnea spells, aspiration, and respiratory difficulty. Surgical decompression is needed to treat the condition.

The Chiari syndrome may occur with the Chiari malformation type II in which there is a downward displacement of the cerebellum, brainstem, and fourth ventricle and herniation through the foramen magnum into the cervical spaces. Rapid surgical decompression is needed reduce brainstem compression and to prevent death. Approximately 15% of children with this malformation die by the age of 3 years, and another third have permanent neurologic disability (Stevenson, 2004). A progression of clinical signs again occurs in adolescents and young adults (Lazzaretti & Pearson, 2004).

Clinical Manifestations

The signs and symptoms of hydrocephalus vary with the age of the child, as described in the clinical manifestations table on the next page. The predominant manifestation in infants is a rapidly increasing head circumference (Figure 26–11 ➤). Older children show signs of increased intracranial pressure (see Table 26–4).

■ COLLABORATIVE CARE

Diagnostic Tests

The diagnosis of hydrocephalus may be made prenatally by ultrasound or based on clinical manifestations and neuroimaging studies after birth. If hydrocephalus is detected in the fetus, sonography to detect other anomalies is performed, such as a neural tube defect. In the hospital setting, daily measurements of the infant's head circumference are critical in any infant at risk of developing hydrocephalus. In older children, signs of increased intracranial pressure are noted. CT scanning and MRI diagnose hydrocephalus, and in some cases reveal the anatomic cause. In the infant whose fontanel is still open, ultrasonography or echoencephalography may be used to confirm the diagnosis. Severe congenital hydrocephalus combined with spina bifida is associated with a decreased survival rate of 20–46%, and a chance of normal intelligence in the survivors of 40–52% (Rudy, 2005).

CLINICAL MANIFESTATIONS | HYDROCEPHALUS

Causes	Clinical Manifestations

Congenital structural defect in infancy
Dandy-Walker syndrome
Chiari II malformation
Intraventricular hemorrhage
	Early signs
	  Rapidly increasing head circumference; tense, bulging fontanel, split sutures
	  Bossing (protrusion) of frontal area, face is disproportionate for skull size
	  Difficulty holding head up
	  Macewen's or "cracked-pot" sign with percussion
	  Prominent, distended scalp veins, translucent scalp skin, splitting sutures, bulging anterior fontanel
	  Increased tone or hyperreflexia, Babinski's sign
	  Irritability or lethargy, poor feeding
	  Decline in level of consciousness
	Late signs
	  Apnea
	  Shrill, high-pitched cry
	  Difficulty swallowing or feeding, failure to thrive
	  Vomiting
	  Loss of developmental milestones
	  Sunsetting eyes (sclera visible above iris), 6th cranial nerve palsy
	  Cardiopulmonary depression (severe cases)

Acquired hydrocephalus in older child after closure of sutures Post-infectious Tumor Hemorrhage	No head enlargement Headache upon arising with nausea and vomiting Fussiness, sleepiness, confusion, apathy, or altered level of consciousness Personality change, loss of interest in daily activities Poor judgment or verbal incoherence, worsening school performance, memory loss Ataxia, spasticity, or other alterations in motor development Visual problems (papilledema, blurred vision, double vision) Signs of increased intracranial pressure

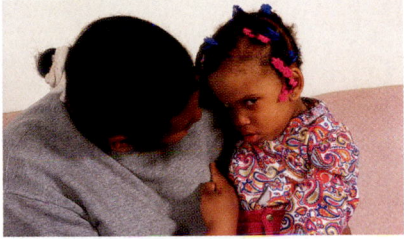

Figure 26–11 ➤ In communicating hydrocephalus, an excessive amount of cerebrospinal fluid accumulates in the subarachnoid space, producing the characteristic head enlargement seen here with the prominent forehead.

Clinical Therapy

Clinical therapy for hydrocephalus involves removing the obstruction (e.g., surgical removal of a tumor) or creating a new CSF pathway to divert excess CSF. A catheter or shunt is placed in the ventricle and passes the CSF to the peritoneal cavity, atrium of the heart, or the pleural spaces. Ventriculoperitoneal shunts (Figure 26–12 ➤) are commonly used, although a ventriculoatrial shunt may be used in older children. Shunt systems consist of four parts: a ventricular catheter, a pumping chamber or reservoir, a one-way pressure valve, and a distal catheter. Initial shunt placement is usually performed early in infancy. Tubing of adequate length is now inserted to accommodate the child's growth and reduce the need for future surgery. Researchers in neuroendoscopy are developing techniques to create a new pathway for CSF to flow between the ventricles and spinal cord in people with obstructive hydrocephalus. The new endoscopy procedure may be used in some future patients to avoid shunt placement (Ditmyer, 2004).

Mechanical complications may include blockage at either the proximal or the distal end of the catheter, kinking of the tubing, or valve breakdown. Infants or children with shunt failure show signs and symptoms of recurrent hydrocephalus and increased intracranial pressure. Shunt failure and ventricular size are confirmed by CT scanning or MRI. Shunt materials and systems continue to be refined in an attempt to reduce mechanical problems.

The most serious complication is shunt infection, which may occur at any time but often occurs within 6 months after placement (Simpkins, 2005). The infection rate is 4% per year, with infants under 6 months of age having the highest rates

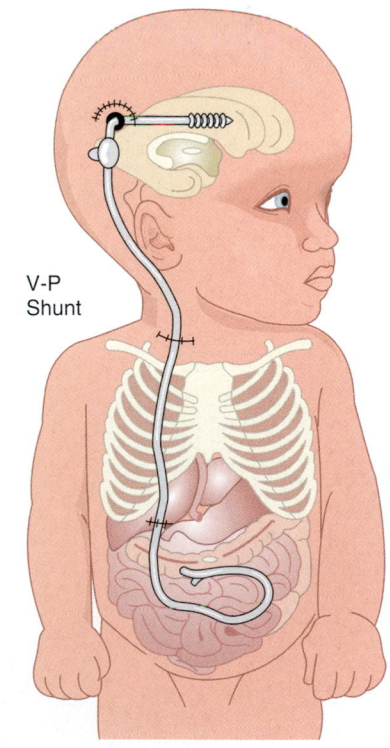

V-P Shunt

Figure 26–12 ➤ A ventriculoperitoneal shunt, commonly used to treat children with hydrocephalus, is usually placed at 3–4 months of age.

(Ditmyer, 2004). Some children who develop shunt infections more than a year after shunt placement have been found to have peritonitis and appendicitis (Simpkins, 2005). The infection may be confirmed by culture of the CSF obtained from the reservoir located in the burr hole (the hole through the skull through which the shunt is placed). The shunt is removed and an external drainage device is placed. Intravenous antibiotics are prescribed until the CSF is sterile. A new shunt is inserted when the CSF cultures are sterile.

Some children, especially those with ventriculoatrial shunts, are placed on the same prophylactic antibiotic treatment regimen used for children with cardiac anomalies to reduce the risk of shunt infections (see the medications table on page 750 in Chapter 21 ∞).

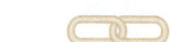

SKILL 6–5
Measuring Head Circumference

■ NURSING MANAGEMENT

Nursing Assessment and Diagnosis

It is important for nurses to become familiar with the clinical manifestations of hydrocephalus to ensure prompt identification and treatment of children with this condition. Measure head circumference of all infants at each well-child visit to detect the condition at an early stage.

Assess the child with a ventriculoperitoneal shunt for signs and symptoms of shunt failure and infection. Important signs of infection include changes in responsiveness and irritability after fever is controlled. Other signs include low grade fever, malaise, headache, and nausea. Measure the infant's head circumference daily when shunt failure is suspected. Report any abnormalities to the physician immediately.

Nursing diagnoses that might be appropriate for the child with hydrocephalus include:

- Risk for Infection related to introduction of infectious organisms during surgery
- Impaired Physical Mobility related to decreased muscle mass to lift the increased weight of head
- Risk for Caregiver Role Strain related to care of a child with a chronic condition or life-threatening illness
- Delayed Growth and Development related to repeated shunt infections and hospitalizations
- Risk for Injury related to potential shunt failure

Planning and Implementation
Hospital-Based Care

Nursing care focuses on providing preoperative and postoperative care and providing emotional support.

Provide preoperative care. Position the child carefully; do not stretch or strain the neck muscles, since they must support the large head. Holding the child may be difficult because of the additional weight of the head. Provide good skin care. Reduce the chances for skin breakdown by placing sheepskin or a lamb's wool blanket under the head. Prevent any other complications associated with immobility (see page 1039).

Attend to the child's special nutritional needs. Because the infant is prone to vomiting, frequent small feedings with frequent burping are beneficial.

After surgery, the child is usually placed in a flat position to prevent rapid CSF drainage. The head of the bed is gradually elevated. Take vital signs every 2 to 4 hours. Maintain aseptic technique when performing incision care. Monitor the child carefully for any signs of shunt malfunction, increased intracranial pressure, or infection.

Support the parents and explain the child's condition and all procedures to be performed. Encourage parents and family to help with the child's care in the hospital when appropriate. Be sympathetic and understanding, and allow parents to express their concerns. If hydrocephalus occurs during early infancy, the parents will be anxious about the impact of the chronic condition and subsequent surgical procedures. If hydrocephalus is secondary to neoplasm, however, the parents' anxieties are compounded by their child's life-threatening illness. Assure parents that most children with shunts lead normal lives; they attend school and interact with others the same way as their peers.

Discharge Planning and Home Care Teaching

Identify and address home care needs well in advance of discharge. Parents must learn how to care for a child with a shunt. Make parents and other family members aware of the signs and symptoms of both shunt failure (signs of increased intracranial pressure) and infection (changes in responsiveness, irritability, malaise, headache, nausea, and low-grade fever). Give them the telephone numbers of the pediatrician and the neurosurgeon; make sure parents understand that they should contact a physician immediately if they suspect a problem. Inform parents that the child may develop a seizure disorder and indicate how to care for the child if a seizure occurs. Refer families to the appropriate home care, social services, and support groups such as the Hydrocephalus Association.

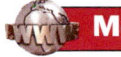 **MediaLink**

Hydrocephalus Support and Resources

Care in the Community

Infants and children need frequent monitoring to ensure proper shunt functioning. Head circumference is measured at each visit to monitor growth. Assess the child for visual problems and cognitive, speech, and motor developmental delays. Refer the child and family to an early intervention program to promote developmental progress. School-age children may need to have an Individualized Education Plan developed (see Chapter 12 ∞). Intellectual functioning outcomes may be associated with the cause of the hydrocephalus. For example, children with uncomplicated congenital causes of hydrocephalus do better than those with brain injury, infection, or intraventricular hemorrhage causes.

Parents should be encouraged to promote an optimal health status by promoting good nutrition and reducing exposure to infections. Parents seeking childcare for their infant should seek a setting with fewer children if possible to decrease exposure to infection. Encourage the use of hand hygiene by all caregivers to reduce the spread of infections. Educate parents about the signs that may indicate a shunt malfunction or infection and to seek medical care immediately, either by calling the physician's office or going to the emergency department. Make sure that parents educate other caregivers and teachers about these signs so that needed care is not delayed. See Families Want to Know: Signs of Shunt Malfunction or Infection.

Teach parents to protect the infant from injury. Do not put infants into a forward-facing car safety seat. These infants have poor head control due to an enlarged head, and this position increases their risk of cervical spine injury and death in a car crash. As the child grows, encourage parents to avoid becoming overprotective and to allow the child to develop normally. Participation in sports with a high potential for head and abdominal impact should be discouraged.

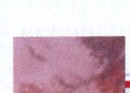 ## FAMILIES WANT TO KNOW

Signs of Shunt Malfunction or Infection

Parents should seek immediate medical attention if the infant or child experiences any of the following signs of shunt malfunction or infection (Simpkins, 2005):

- Headache, progressive or worsening
- Drowsiness or inappropriate sleepiness during the day
- Vomiting
- Personality changes or changes in school performance
- Fever
- Redness or swelling along the shunt tract

Evaluation

Expected outcomes of nursing care include the following:

- The child develops adequate neck muscle control to interact with the environment.
- Shunt infections and malfunctions are identified by the parents and medical attention is sought quickly.
- The child's potential for growth and development is maximized by care and a stimulating environment.

Neural Tube Defects

The neural tube is the tissue that ultimately develops the CNS, including the brain and spinal cord. The incidence of neural tube defects is 0.7 to 1 per 1000 live births in the United States (Padgett, 2006). Types of neural tube defects include the following:

- *Anencephaly.* The brain does not develop above the brainstem.
- *Encephalocele.* A protrusion of meningeal tissue or meningeal-covered brain is observed through a defect in the skull.
- *Spina bifida occulta.* The posterior vertebral arches fail to fuse, most commonly at fifth lumbar or first sacral vertebrae. The spinal cord and meninges lie entirely within the vertebral canal and the condition is usually not visible externally. A tuft of hair, a dermoid cyst, or hemangioma may be found over the site. This is the mildest form of spina bifida.
- *Spina bifida cystica.* A defect in closure of the posterior vertebral arch with protrusion through the bony spine.
- *Meningocele.* A spinal fluid-filled meningeal sac filled with CSF protrudes through a vertebral defect, associated with no abnormalities of the spinal cord. The sac covering the defect may be translucent or membranous. The spinal cord and spinal root are in normal position.
- *Myelomeningocele (spina bifida).* A spinal fluid-filled meningeal sac contains a portion of the meninges; spinal cord or nerve roots protrude through a vertebral defect. Fluid leakage may also occur as the lesion is poorly covered with imperfect tissue.

Myelodysplasia or Spina Bifida

Myelodysplasia (sometimes called myelomeningocele) refers to a malformation of the spinal cord and spinal canal, while spina bifida refers to a defect in one or more vertebrae through which spinal cord contents can protrude. The malformation can occur anywhere along the vertebral column, and it is most common at the lumbar or sacral portion of the spine. This is the most common developmental disorder of the CNS.

Etiology and Pathophysiology

The cause of spina bifida is unknown, although environmental factors such as chemicals (excessive use of alcohol), medications (e.g., valproic acid and carbamazepine used for seizures, isotretinoin for acne), genetic factors, and maternal health conditions (insulin-dependent diabetes mellitus, gestational diabetes, folic acid deficiency, and maternal obesity) have been implicated. The increased incidence of the condition in families indicates a possible genetic influence. Mandatory fortification of all enriched grain products with folate in 1998 has resulted in a 36% reduction in spina bifida among Hispanic births and a 34% reduction among non-Hispanic white births. The rate of reduction was less for non-Hispanic blacks. Similar rates of reduction were found for anencephaly (Williams, Rasmussen, Flores et al., 2005).

Clinical Manifestations

A sac-like protrusion on the infant's back indicates meningocele or myelomeningocele (Figure 26–13 ➤). The clinical manifestations seen depend on the location of the defect: the higher the defect, the greater the neurologic dysfunction as described here:

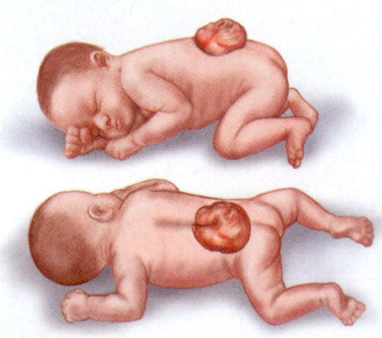

Figure 26–13 ➤ Lumbosacral myelomeningocele is caused by a neural tube defect that results in incomplete closure of the vertebral column. As shown here, the meninges (and sometimes the spinal cord) protrude as a sac-like structure.

- Sensory loss is more pronounced on the back of the legs. Sensory loss around the anus, genitalia, and feet is common.
- Thoracic or lumbar 1-2 level—paralysis of the legs, weakness, and sensory loss in the trunk and lower body region is found.
- Lumbar 3 level—can flex hips and extend the knees; the ankles and toes are paralyzed.
- Lumbar 4-5 level—can flex hips and extend the knees; weak or absent ankle extension, toe flexion, and hip extension.
- Sacral level—mild weakness in ankles and toes; bladder and bowel function may be affected.

Bowel and bladder sphincters may be affected. Renal damage may result from neurologic impairment and urinary retention. Hydrocephalus is usually present in children with myelomeningocele because of the Chiari II malformation that is found in nearly all children with a defect above the sacral level (Johnston & Kinsman, 2004c). The range of potential problems for the child with spina bifida is listed in the clinical manifestations table below.

COLLABORATIVE CARE

Diagnostic Tests

Diagnosis is usually made prenatally, but after birth the lesion is examined and the neurologic status is evaluated. Radiologic imaging by ultrasonography, CT scan, MRI, and flat films of the spinal column can pinpoint the bony defect. Subsequent testing is performed to evaluate bowel and bladder function, neurologic and motor function, and cognitive function.

Clinical Therapy

Surgery to close and repair the lesion usually occurs within 24 to 48 hours of the infant's birth to reduce infection. Depending upon the size of the defect, the excision may

CLINICAL MANIFESTATIONS | MYELODYSPLASIA

Cause	Clinical Manifestations
Interruption of the spinal cord at site of the spinal defect	Loss of motor and sensory function of the abdomen and lower extremities, dependent upon defect level Scoliosis or kyphosis Incontinence of urine or urinary retention Incontinence of feces or constipation Sensory loss around genitalia
Muscle imbalance	Hip abnormalities, hip dysplasia Foot deformities, (e.g., clubfoot)
Chiari II malformation	Hydrocephalus *Infants:* Difficulty swallowing Apnea, respiratory difficulty, inspiratory stridor Weak or poor cry Sustained backward arching of head (opisthotonus) *Older children:* Choking, hoarseness, vocal cord paralysis Disordered breathing during sleep Stiffness or spasticity of arms and hands Loss of feeling or sensation
Brain and spinal cord abnormalities	Learning problems, attention deficit disorder Problems with perceptual motor skills Memory and organization problems Problems with numerical reasoning

be extensive. In some cases, uteromyelomeningocele repairs are performed on the fetus. In cases of spina bifida occulta, surgical intervention is rarely needed.

Braces are used to support joint position and mobility. Assistive devices such as walkers, crutches, and wheelchairs are used to enhance mobility. To minimize the risk for osteoporosis, the diet should ensure adequate calcium and vitamin D, and weight-bearing activities should be encouraged.

Bladder interventions are initated early to prevent kidney damage and to maintain bladder function and urinary continence. Clean intermittent catheterization is performed on a regular schedule to reduce the risk for hydronephrosis and renal damage. Surgical interventions are used if clean intermittent catheterization is not effective in promoting continence. A Mitofanoff procedure that creates a reservoir for urine and a stoma for catheterizing the bladder from the abdominal wall and improves access for catheterization is one surgical option (Zickler & Richardson, 2004). See Figure 26–14 ➤.

Stool softeners and glycerin or bisacodyl suppositories are prescribed for bowel evacuation. Surgery to create a channel between the skin and bowel (Malone antegrade continence enema) is often performed in older children to improve the ease of bowel evacuation management (Zickler & Richardson, 2004).

Prognosis depends on the type of defect, the level of the lesion, and other complicating factors. Children need multiple surgeries and invasive procedures. A team of physicians, nurses, and therapists from the neurosurgery, orthopedic, urology, and physical medicine departments work with the child and family to form a comprehensive care plan.

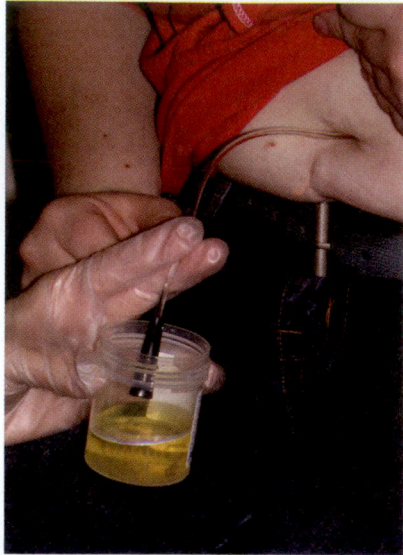

Figure 26–14 ➤ This child has had a Mitranoff procedure to make it easier to perform self-catheterization and maintain modesty. Clean intermittent self-catheterization is performed, and the catheters can be reused until they become brittle. Catheters should be washed with soap and water, rinsed, and stored in a plastic bag.

NURSING MANAGEMENT

Nursing Assessment

Monitor the newborn for integrity of the sac and leakage of cerebrospinal fluid. Assess the extremities for deformities. Frequently assess the vital signs and stay alert for signs of infection. Following surgery, observe the wound healing. Note any signs of infection and cerebrospinal fluid leakage. Measure the head circumference prior to and daily after surgery to assess for potential hydrocephalus. Assess intake and output.

The child with myelodysplasia may be hospitalized for surgery to correct deformities. Assess the child's vital signs, head circumference, responsiveness, and level of pain. Assess neurologic status for any deterioration in function that could be associated with shunt failure or problems with the spinal cord. Assess the range of motion of joints and mobility status. Assess dressing sites for bleeding and draining. Monitor the distal extremities for swelling and circulation. Assess intake and output.

Examples of nursing diagnoses for the child with myelodysplasia include:

- Impaired Physical Mobility related to neuromuscular impairment
- Risk for Latex Allergy Response related to multiple surgical procedures
- Risk for Disproportionate Growth related to caloric intake in excess of needs due to limited mobility
- Impaired Skin Integrity associated with the use of braces and a wheelchair
- Risk for Infection related to urinary retention

Planning and Implementation

Nursing care focuses on providing preoperative and postoperative care, promoting mobility, and providing emotional support.

Cover the sac on the newborn's back with a sterile saline dressing to protect its integrity and monitor for leakage of CSF. Place the infant in a prone position with hips slightly flexed and legs abducted to minimize tension on the sac. Maintain this position using towel rolls placed between the knees. Assess the infant regularly for motor deficits as well as bladder and bowel involvement. Frequently assess the vital signs and stay alert for signs of infection. Feed the infant with the head turned to one side until surgery has been performed. The infant is difficult to handle before surgery, so tactile stimulation such as touching, patting, and cuddling may be comforting.

➤ NURSING ALERT

More than half of the children with myelodysplasia develop a latex allergy during childhood, and the risk for such an allergy increases as the child ages (Liptak, 2002). See Chapter 17 ∞. Anaphylaxis caused by latex exposure in children has been reported. All children with latex allergy need to carry a kit with premeasured adrenaline for emergency treatment of anaphylaxis. Use nonlatex materials when providing care to the child in any setting. The Spina Bifida Association maintains an updated list of products containing latex and potential substitutes (see Table 17–7 ∞ on pages 580–581).

Following surgery, monitor the infant's vital signs carefully. Watch closely for symptoms of infection, especially meningitis. If a ventriculoperitoneal shunt was placed, watch for hydrocephalus, increased intracranial pressure, or infection. Inspect the surgical site for cerebrospinal fluid leakage. The infant should be placed in the prone or side-lying position, or in some cases may be held upright. Splints may be used to maintain extremity alignment.

Support the parents by keeping them informed about their child's status. Allow them to express their frustrations and anger. As soon as parents are able to cope with the child's condition, encourage them to become involved in the child's care in the hospital.

The child with myelodysplasia may be hospitalized for surgery numerous times to correct deformities. Assess the child's vital signs, responsiveness, and level of pain. As the child may have decreased pain sensation in lower extremities, careful assessment is needed. Assess dressing sites for bleeding and drainage. Monitor the distal extremities for swelling and circulation. Use latex precautions with all of these children, whether or not they have latex sensitivity. See Chapter 17 ∞ for information on latex allergy.

Discharge Planning and Home Care Teaching

Identify and address home care needs well in advance of discharge. Make sure family members understand how to care for the child at home. Parents need to learn to perform intermittent catheterization prior to discharge and establish a schedule to perform catheterization about five times daily (Erickson & Ray, 2004). Instruct parents how to position, handle, feed, and perform range of motion exercises. Teach them the signs and symptoms of increased intracranial pressure, hydrocephalus, shunt infection or malfunction, and urinary tract infection. Help them get special devices such as splints, wedges, and rolls, if needed, to prevent complications. Home care nursing should be arranged, if necessary. The home care nurse reinforces the skills learned in the hospital setting and coordinates the numerous healthcare professionals working with the child and family. Refer parents to resource groups such as the Spina Bifida Association of America.

Care in the Community

To reduce complications and promote optimal development, children with myelodysplasia need comprehensive care planned and coordinated by a knowledgeable team of healthcare professionals. This care may be provided in partnership with the primary care physician.

Parents need to catheterize the child at regular intervals during the day, and then at an appropriate age teach the child intermittent self-catheterization (see Chapter 25 ∞). If the child has had a Mitranoff procedure performed, monitor for any signs that the stoma is becoming stenosed. It is important to report stenosis so that dilatation can occur and possibly prevent the need for surgical revision of the stoma (Gray, Blackinton, & White, 2006). When the child begins school, an Individualized Health Plan should be developed to ensure that the child has access to the restroom and assistance as needed for toileting, as well as accommodations for mobility challenges.

Good nutrition planning is important to prevent obesity and to reduce constipation and complications such as fecal impaction. Bowel training is initiated to control bowel evacuation at appropriate times and places. A high-fiber diet helps assure adequate stool. At a convenient time, a glycerin or bisacodyl suppository can be given. Consistency in time of day for bowel evacuation is important.

Promote safety and independent mobility with proper use of braces, walkers, crutches, canes, and in some cases custom-designed wheelchairs and car safety seats (Figure 26–15 ➤). For other safety guidelines, see Families Want to Know: Safety for the Child with Spina Bifida.

Parents are faced with the long-term financial issues of caring for the child who needs regular new adaptive equipment to match growth, as well as other medical supplies. At least 75% of children born with spina bifida generally survive to at least the early adult years (Nehring & Faux, 2006). Parents thus need to learn how to act as the child's case manager, or to work effectively with another person in this role.

CLINICAL TIP
Gentle range of motion exercises should be started as soon as possible to prevent muscle contractures and atrophy. Use caution when performing range of motion because these children have brittle bones that fracture easily.

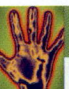
GROWTH & DEVELOPMENT
Self-Care
Treat older children according to their intellectual level, not their motor development. Encourage them to take responsibility for self-care, such as self-catheterization, and recognize their need to control their body functions. Promote interaction with peers in the hospital and participation in activities. If children are hospitalized for an extended time, arrange schooling.

MediaLink
Spina Bifida Resources

CLINICAL TIP
The child who has clean intermittent catheterization performed usually has bacteria in the urine, but this is not treated unless the child becomes symptomatic. Symptoms of a urinary tract infection that should be treated include foul odor or discharge, a change in mood or personality, or fatigue (Gray, Blackinton, & White, 2006).

MediaLink
Health Promotion and Maintenance Overview: Spina Bifida

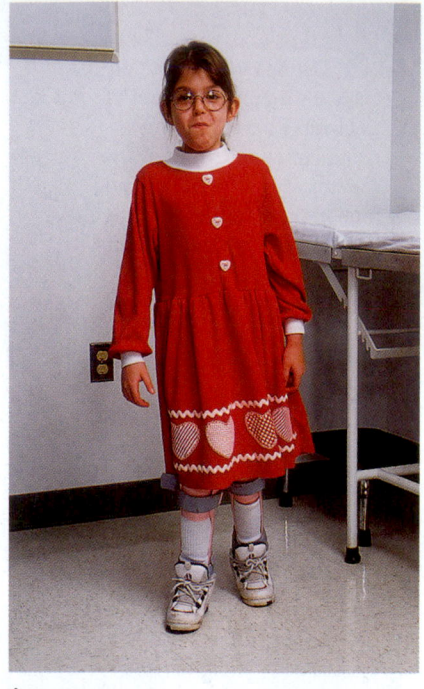
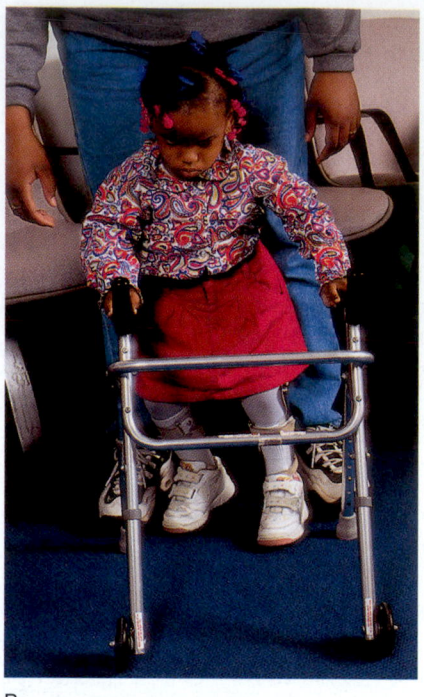
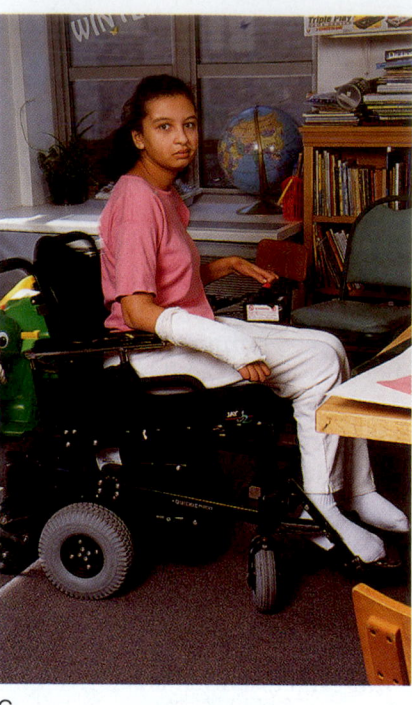

A   B   C

Figure 26–15 ➤ Help determine the best assistive device for the child to gain the most independence for mobilizing and to promote development. The child may change devices in different settings to promote optimal independence. A and B, Braces and walkers may be best for young children to promote an upright posture that encourages a normal interaction with the environment. C, A motorized wheelchair can assist the child with a significant neurologic impairment to achieve independence and mobility.

Craniosynostosis

Craniosynostosis is the premature closing of the cranial sutures during the first 18 to 20 months of life. This condition occurs in up to 1 in 2100 live births, and boys are affected twice as often as girls (Padgett, 2006). Most children have no family history of the condition, although autosomal dominant conditions such as Alpert syndrome and Crouzon syndrome are responsible for some cases (Johnston & Kinsman, 2004a).

Closure of the cranial sutures usually takes place at predetermined times during the child's development. Problems arise if one or more sutures close early. Dysfunctional osteoblasts or osteoclasts are believed to be responsible for the development of craniosynostosis (Johnston & Kinsman, 2004). Bone growth continues in a direction parallel to the prematurely fused suture line, which leads to compensatory overgrowth at normal suture lines and the classic skull deformities associated with craniosynostosis (Figure 26–16A-C ➤).

FAMILIES WANT TO KNOW

Safety for the Child with Spina Bifida

Due to the loss of sensation in the lower extremities, injuries to the skin are not immediately noticed by the child. Several actions routinely taken by the child and family will reduce the risk for injury.

- Each day, check all skin surfaces and pressure points associated with sitting, braces, shoes, and so on, for abrasions, scrapes, reddened areas, and other lesions. Stop using the braces or shoes until the skin heals or redness disappears.
- Keep all skin surfaces clean and dry. Wear socks under braces.

- Use a gel-filled cushion and teach the child to shift his or her position hourly when in the wheelchair to avoid pressure sores.
- Avoid burns to the lower extremities by checking the temperature of bath water and car safety seats in a hot car.
- Take latex precautions as the child is at high risk for latex allergy and avoid latex whenever a nonlatex substitute is available. Be alert for any signs of latex allergy. Inform all healthcare providers about the child's latex allergy.
- Use safe ambulation techniques with walkers, canes, and crutches.

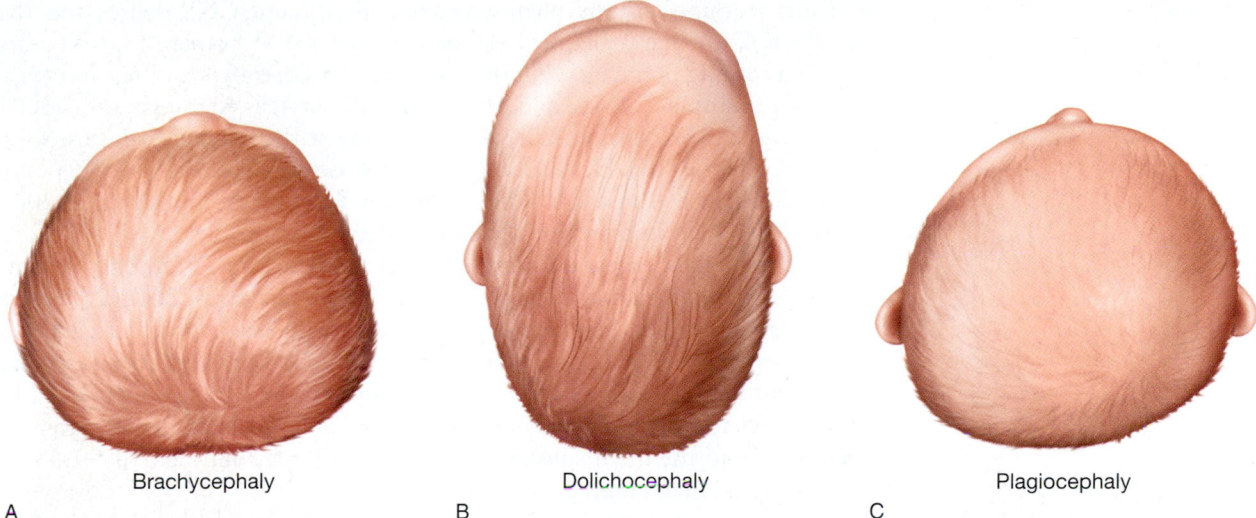

Brachycephaly	Dolichocephaly	Plagiocephaly
A	B	C

Figure 26–16 ➤ In craniosynostosis, the head shape is dependent upon which sutures are involved. A, Brachycephaly or bicoronal synostosis is associated with Crouzon syndrome. The head shape is shortened anterior to posterior and the occiput is flattened. The infant may have hypertelorism and underdeveloped eye orbits with prominent eyes. B, Scaphocephaly or dolichocephaly accounts for more than 50% of cases (Padgett, 2006). Premature closure of the sagittal suture causes a long, narrow skull and flattened parietal bones with a prominent occiput, a broad forehead, and small or absent anterior fontanel. C, Positional plagiocephaly is often asymmetric flattening of the occiput due to preferred position when supine or torticollis.

Diagnosis is made by clinical appearance and measurement of the skull with metal calipers. Palpation of the skull reveals a bony ridge along a suture. Skull radiographs, CT scan, and MRI confirm the diagnosis.

Reconstructive surgery of the skull is performed to promote brain development and vision and to improve cosmetic appearance. Many children need multiple procedures. After surgery, it is important for the incision to remain dry and intact. The nurse should also observe the child for symptoms of increased intracranial pressure (see Table 26–4). Explain to parents that surgery will improve the child's appearance. Assure them that most children with craniosynostosis are healthy, and that their brains develop normally.

Positional Plagiocephaly

Positional *plagiocephaly* (a flattened occiput) and *brachycephaly* (the skull is short in the anteroposterior dimension and wide between the parietal eminences) are seen increasingly in healthy infants because they are put to sleep on their back to prevent Sudden Infant Death Syndrome. See Figure 26–16c. The sutures do not close prematurely, but when the infant's sleep position does not change, the weight of the head flattens the skull. The flattened occiput may be asymmetric when the infant has a positional preference, such as with congenital torticollis. It is speculated that infants who develop these skull shapes do not have enough supervised tummy-time to help correct positional preference (Graham, Kreutzman, Earl et al., 2005).

A helmet device to correct severe cases of positional plagiocephaly or brachycephaly is most effective in infants under 12 months of age and when treatment is initiated at 6 months of age because the skull bones are more malleable. The helmet is worn for 23 hours a day for 3 months. Remolding of the head shape continues after that treatment period because the infant spends more time awake and upright. Younger infants may be successfully treated with positioning and physical therapy for torticollis (Graham, Gomez, Halberg et al., 2005).

NEONATAL ABSTINENCE SYNDROME

Illicit substances that may cause neonatal abstinence syndrome when used by the mother during pregnancy include opiates (heroine, meperidine, methadone), CNS

> ### CLINICAL TIP
>
> Place the infant in a variety of positions for playing, feeding, and carrying to reduce the preference for lying supine in one position and flattening the occiput. Rotate the crib in the room every day so the infant turns the head a different way to look at the door. Rotate the arm used for formula feeding the infant. When the child is awake and alert, place the child in the prone position on the floor to develop neck muscle strength and to interact with nearby objects.

stimulants (cocaine, propoxyphene, amphetamines), and CNS depressants (barbiturates, alcohol, and marijuana). It is estimated that 4.3% of women (15 to 44 years) used illicit drugs during pregnancy, but the rate is much higher (8%) among women ages 15 to 25 years (Substance Abuse and Mental Health Services Administration, 2005). Approximately 45,000 newborns are born annually with prenatal exposure to cocaine (Schiller & Allen, 2005). Heavy or binge alcohol use was reported by 4.1% of pregnant women (Substance Abuse and Mental Health Services Administration, 2005). See Chapter 27 ∞ for information about fetal alcohol syndrome.

Narcotics readily cross the placenta, enter the fetal circulation, and have the same effects on the fetus that they do in the mother. The effect of cocaine on the fetus is decreased placental blood flow that deprives the fetus of essential oxygen and nutrients and an elevated blood pressure and heart rate. The mother's repeated use of narcotics or other substances leads to tolerance and physical dependence in the fetus. If the mother is still actively using drugs at the time of birth, the neonate has signs of abrupt withdrawal from the illicit substance shortly after birth. Between 50–90% of infants born to drug-addicted mothers suffer withdrawal.

Prematurity, intrauterine growth retardation, microcephaly, low birth weight, jitteriness, seizures, hyperexcitability, and poor feeding are common results of prenatal cocaine exposure (Kuehne & Reilly, 2004). These cocaine-exposed newborns may also exhibit hypertonia, tremors, and extensor leg posture, poor sucking, feeding difficulties, less time in quiet sleep, more stressed behaviors such as mouthing and clenched fists, and difficulty regulating their behaviors. The newborn with drug withdrawal from other illicit substances may have irritability and jitteriness. These infants may have excoriated skin, especially on the heels, toes, hands, elbows, nose, or chin, as a result of their continuous movements on the crib sheets. See Clinical Manifestations of Neonatal Abstinence Syndrome below.

The onset of symptoms may be attributed to the type and amount of drug taken by the mother and how soon before birth it was taken. Withdrawal symptoms for opiates usually appear 24 to 48 hours after birth, barbiturate withdrawal symptoms appear between 4 and 14 days after birth, and cocaine or amphetamine withdrawal symptoms appear up to 7 days after birth. Opiates cause the most withdrawal symptoms, but mothers may use multiple substances. Long-term issues for children with cocaine exposure in utero include potential difficulties with language development, attention span, memory, and motor skills (Schiller & Allen, 2005).

Diagnosis is based on the history of maternal substance abuse and physical signs in the infant. EEG abnormalities may be noted. Urine testing provides information on drug use immediately prior to labor, and meconium screening provides information on drug use by the mother for the last half of the pregnancy. The infant's hair may also be tested. If urine is positive, compare the results with medications used during labor and delivery. Chain of custody for specimens may be needed.

Behavioral and neurologic functioning may also be assessed with diagnostic tools such as the Brazelton Neonatal Behavioral Assessment scale. This tool evaluates infants on habituation (ability to respond to and then inhibit response to discrete stimuli when asleep), general arousal level, orientation, quality of movement and tone, autonomic stability, reflexes, and responsiveness when aroused (Campbell, 2003).

Treatment is generally supportive. Infants with cocaine exposure need to have reduced environmental stimuli and swaddling. Medications such as phenobarbitol,

CLINICAL MANIFESTATIONS	NEONATAL ABSTINENCE SYNDROME
System Involved	**Clinical Manifestations**
Central nervous system	Irritability, restlessness, tremors, seizures, high-pitched cry, abnormal sleep patterns, drowsiness, yawning, and hypertonicity
Autonomic nervous system	Sneezing, stuffy nose, sweating, tachycardia, and tachypnea
Gastrointestinal system	Diarrhea, vomiting, and poor feeding

diazepam, methadone, clonidine, and paregoric may be prescribed to alleviate symptoms of drug withdrawal. If the mother is still using illicit drugs, breast-feeding is discouraged since the drugs cross over into milk.

Nursing Management

Prevention and early identification of the infant with neonatal abstinence syndrome is an important nursing role. Providing information for all parents about the risks and effects of various abused substances increases the chance that they will avoid these substances in future pregnancies.

Crying and poor feeding should increase the nurse's suspicion of neonatal abstinence syndrome. Observe the newborn closely for poor sucking, seizures, vomiting and diarrhea, dehydration, and an increased metabolic rate. Many withdrawal symptoms are identical to symptoms of infection, bowel obstruction, electrolyte disorder, hydrocephalus, and intracranial anomaly, so consider the possibility that the infant could have both neonatal abstinence syndrome and another condition.

Provide frequent, small, high-calorie feedings. Formula with 24 calories per ounce may be recommended. Patience is needed when feeding these infants because of poor sucking and swallowing coordination. Teach parents to use a calm approach and soothing voice when feeding. Newborns may initially feed better in the side-lying position while swaddled. Hold the infant with the spine flexed to decrease extensor tone.

Administer prescribed medications, if ordered for drug withdrawal, and monitor the infant's response. Keep in mind, however, that many infants are managed without drugs. Protect the newborn's skin as jitteriness may lead to greater skin surface rubbing against sheets and cause scratches and abrasions.

Assess the strengths, safety, and competence of the mother and other potential caregivers. Determine if the mother is still using illicit drugs and identify other family supports that may help provide the care and safety needed by the newborn. Begin working with the mother and other family members to demonstrate strategies for promoting parent-infant interaction, minimizing stimulation, and promoting feeding. Make plans for careful follow-up by health professionals (social services, physicians, and nurses) so that the infant's safety is assured and the growth and development are monitored and promoted. In some cases, referral to child abuse protective services may be made.

Long-term follow-up care of the child should be planned to ensure regular developmental testing and assessment for catch-up growth, neurobehavioral problems, and fetal alcohol syndrome (as multiple substances could have been used by the mother). The long-term effects of this condition on cognitive function are not known at this time as studies have reported conflicting results (Schiller & Allen, 2005).

Neurofibromatosis

Neurofibromatosis 1, or von Recklinghausen's disease, is an autosomal dominant genetic disorder in which tumors grow along nerves. Skin pigmentation changes and bone deformities also occur. The incidence of the disorder is 1 per 3000–4000 live births. More than 50% of new cases result from a mutation (Hart, 2005). The condition varies in severity, with most individuals having the milder form of the disease. The severe form of the disease can be debilitating when present. The NF1 gene (a tumor suppressor gene) responsible for neurofibromatosis 1 is located on chromosome 17.

The disorder is characterized by multiple light tan colored café-au-lait spots 5 mm or larger seen at birth or by 2 years of age. In darker-skinned children, the spots are darker than surrounding skin. The spots grow to 15 mm or larger in diameter by adulthood. Freckling in the axillary and inguinal areas is common. Lisch nodules, tan or brown benign tumors on the iris of the eye, are a diagnostic sign. Multiple neurofibromas or benign tumors, composed of nervous system tissue and fibrous tissue, grow on or under the skin beginning during puberty. Other findings include plexiform neurofibromas. Skeletal changes include scoliosis as well as thinning or bowing of the tibia, resulting in fractures that fail to heal properly. See Figure 26–17 ▶.

Pain may occur when tumors grow around and compress a nerve or when a tumor grows in the spinal cord. Tumors may develop in the optic nerve (optic glioma) and

> **CLINICAL TIP**
>
> Several techniques are used to calm and soothe the newborn with neonatal abstinence syndrome.
> - Keep the infant in a quiet environment, away from beeping monitors and paging speakers.
> - Keep the lighting subdued and minimize stimulation to promote rest and sleep.
> - Comfort and pacify the infant with swaddling and a pacifier for sucking needs. Rocking along with soothing music may also be calming. Infant massage may also be beneficial in some infants.

Figure 26–17 ➤ Physical signs of neurofibromatosis 1 become more apparent during adolescence. Café-au-lait spots enlarge, axillary freckling appears, and multiple neurofibromas develop. Some children develop plexiform neurofibromas.

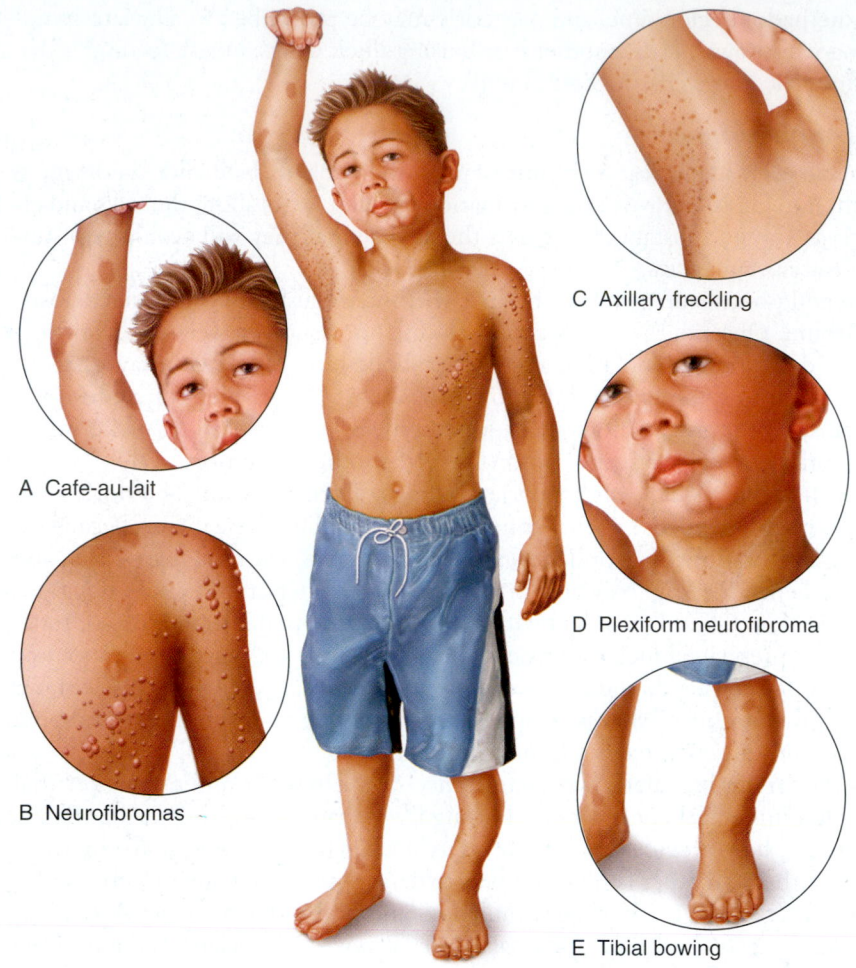

A Cafe-au-lait

B Neurofibromas

C Axillary freckling

D Plexiform neurofibroma

E Tibial bowing

cause various vision deficits or blindness. Precocious puberty may occur with neurofibromatosis 1 when an optic glioma exists and invades the hypothalamus. Delayed puberty with delayed menarche may also occur (Virdis, Street, Bandello et al., 2003). Hypertension may develop in association with renal vascular stenosis or a pheochromocytoma. Affected children may also have learning disabilities, hyperactivity, speech abnormalities, and seizures.

Diagnosis is made in infancy or early childhood by the presence of 6 or more café-au-lait spots, Lisch nodules, small skin tumors, and a positive family history of neurofibromatosis. Radiology imaging (MRI of the brain and radiographs of the spine and other bones) is performed when problems are detected. Ophthalmic examinations should be performed at least annually during childhood to detect optic gliomas, to monitor Lisch nodules, and to detect vision deficits.

Clinical therapy focuses on monitoring the child's growth, development, blood pressure, spine for scoliosis, timing of sexual development, and development of neurofibromas. Genetic counseling is offered. When neurofibromas are disfiguring or cause problems because of their location, surgery may be performed to remove the tumor. Surgical removal of plexiform neurofibromas is more often attempted when tumors are painful, disfiguring, or cause paralysis, or when life-threatening problems develop; however, they may grow back. Most children and adults with mild symptoms can live a normal, productive life.

Nursing Management

The goal of nursing management is to assess the child, identify emerging problems with the disorder, and provide support to the child and family living with the condition.

Nurses assess the child to identify signs of neurofibromatosis, including café-au-lait spots, axillary and inguinal freckling, and small tumors on the body. Vital signs with blood pressure are monitored for hypertension. Vision screening to detect any vision impairment is performed. Monitor growth and development to detect any unusual patterns, identifying signs of early or late pubertal development. Perform scoliosis screening on a frequent basis. Note any evidence of tibial bowing or thinning. School performance should be monitored as learning disabilities and hyperactivity are known problems. Pay attention to any mass that is rapidly enlarging or causing new pain.

Provide psychological support to the child and family. In children with moderate to severe conditions, the tumors will cause cosmetic problems. As tumor development increases during adolescence, problems with self-image and self-esteem are common. The adolescent may have a difficult adjustment to the disorder. Adolescents may fear the response of peers to the tumors and isolate themselves. Identify peers or refer the adolescent to support groups. Assist children and adolescents to learn to live with the disorder. Focus on the child's strengths and encourage continuing development of those strengths.

CEREBRAL PALSY

Cerebral palsy (CP) is a disorder of movement and posture that results from a nonprogressive abnormality of the immature brain occurring in the prenatal, perinatal, or postnatal (up to 2 years) period. CP is the most common chronic disorder of childhood, occurring in an estimated 2 to 3 per 1000 births (Nehring, 2004). Four types of motor dysfunction are seen with cerebral palsy—spastic, dyskinetic, ataxic, and mixed—related to the location of brain insult. Children with severe impairment of mobility and feeding skills have a greater risk of dying during childhood (Liptak & Accardo, 2004).

Etiology and Pathophysiology

Most CP cases are believed to be caused by congenital, hypoxic, ischemic, or infectious intrauterine insults to the CNS (McKearnan, Kieckhefer, Engel et al., 2004). The risk for CP is increased when intrauterine infection (chorioamnionitis) is documented (Van Eerden & Bernstein, 2003). Injury to the immature periventricular white matter in fetuses and premature infants is thought to be the most common cause of cerebral palsy (Johnston, Ferriero, Vannucci et al., 2005). A rate of CP increases with decreasing gestational age; approximately 20% of infants born before 27 weeks' gestational age are diagnosed with CP (Ancel, Livinec, Larroque et al., 2006). Birth asphyxia is believed to account for only 9% of the CP cases. No reduction of incidence of CP was noted since the use of electronic fetal heart rate monitoring was implemented (Van Eerden & Bernstein, 2003). Neonatal sepsis and hyperbilirubinemia place the infant at higher risk. In young children, CNS infection and head trauma are the major sources of acquired brain injury and subsequent motor dysfunction.

Clinical Manifestations

Cerebral palsy is characterized by abnormal muscle tone and lack of coordination with spasticity found in the majority of cases (Table 26–8). Children have a variety of symptoms depending on their ages. See the clinical manifestations table on page 1076 for symptoms by type of central nervous system injury. There is wide variability in symptoms depending on the area of the brain involved and the degree of anoxia. Children with cerebral palsy usually are delayed in meeting developmental milestones. For example, at 6 months of age, they may have persistent back arching, little spontaneous movement, and be unable to sit up. They frequently have other problems, including visual defects such as strabismus, nystagmus, or refractory errors; hearing loss; language delay; speech impediment; or seizures. Feeding may be difficult because of oral motor involvement. Approximately 75% of children with CP have mental retardation or learning disabilities (Liptak & Accardo, 2004).

■ COLLABORATIVE CARE

Diagnostic Tests

Diagnosis is usually based on clinical findings. CP is difficult to diagnose in the early months of life as it must be distinguished from other neurologic conditions and signs

Table 26–8	CLINICAL CHARACTERISTICS OF CEREBRAL PALSY
Clinical Characteristics	**Definitions**
Hypotonia	Floppiness, increased range of motion of joints, diminished reflex response
Hypertonia Rigidity	Tense, tight muscles
Spasticity	Uncoordinated, awkward, stiff movements; scissoring or crossing of the legs; exaggerated reflex reactions
Athetosis	Constant involuntary writhing motions that are more severe distally
Ataxia	Irregularity in muscle coordination or action
Hemiplegia	Involvement of one side of the body, with the upper extremities being more dysfunctional than the lower extremities
Diplegia	Involvement of all extremities, but the lower extremities are more affected than the upper, usually spastic
Quadriplegia	Involvement of all extremities with the arms in flexion and legs in extension

CLINICAL MANIFESTATIONS	CEREBRAL PALSY BY TYPE OF INSULT
Classification and Type of Insult	**Clinical Manifestations**
Spastic Cerebral cortex or pyramidal tract injury 75% of cases	Persistent hypertonia, rigidity Exaggerated deep tendon reflexes Persistent primitive reflexes Leads to contractures and abnormal curvature of the spine
Dyskinetic Extrapyramidal, basal ganglia injury 10–15% of cases	Impairment of voluntary muscle control Bizarre twisting movements Tremors, difficulty with fine and purposeful motor movements Exaggerated posturing Rigid muscle tone when awake and normal or decreased muscle tone when asleep Inconsistent muscle tone that may change hour to hour or day to day
Ataxic Cerebellar (extrapyramidal) injury 5–10% of cases	Abnormalities of voluntary movement involving balance and position of the trunk and limbs Difficulty controlling hand and arm movements during reaching Increased or decreased muscle tone Hypotonia in infancy Muscle instability and wide-based unsteady gait
Mixed Injuries to multiple areas	No dominant motor pattern Unique compensatory movements and posture to maintain control over specific neuromotor deficits Combination of characteristics from other types

may be subtle. Suspicious findings include an infant who is small for age; or has a history of prematurity, low Apgar score (0–3 at 5 minutes), or inflammatory, traumatic, or anoxic event (Van Eerden & Bernstein, 2003). However, the majority of children who develop CP have normal Apgar scores at birth. Ultrasonography can be used to detect fetal and neonatal abnormalities of the brain, such as intraventricular hemorrhage. Neuromotor tests are used to evaluate the presence of normal movement patterns and absence of primitive reflexes and abnormal tone. Once CP is suspected, CT scans, MRI, and positron emission tomography may be performed.

Clinical Therapy

It is not uncommon for children who are delayed in meeting developmental milestones or have neuromuscular abnormalities at 1 year of age to show gradual improvement in function. Half of the infants suspected to be at risk for CP at 1 year of age are unimpaired neurologically by 2 years of age due to physical maturation (Pelligrino, 2002).

Clinical therapy focuses on helping the child develop to his or her maximum level of independence. Referrals are made for physical, occupational, and speech therapy, as well as special education to improve motor function and ability. Braces and splints, serial casting, and positioning devices (prone wedges, standers, and sidelyers) are used to promote range of motion, skeletal alignment, stability, and control of involuntary movements. They are also used to prevent contractures.

Surgical interventions may be required to improve function by balancing muscle power and stabilizing uncontrollable joints. The Achilles' tendon may be lengthened to increase range of motion in the ankle, which allows the heel to touch the floor and thus improves ambulation. The hamstrings may be released to correct knee flexion contractures. Other procedures may be performed to improve hip adduction or correct the foot's natural position. A dorsal rhizotomy may be performed for spastic **diplegia** to cut the afferent fibers that contribute to spasticity; however, some muscle weakness may result from the procedure (Pelligrino, 2002). Physical therapy and occupational therapy promote optimal independent functioning.

Medications are given to control seizures, to control spasms (skeletal muscle relaxants, baclofen, and benzodiazepines), and to minimize gastrointestinal side effects (cimetidine or ranitidine). Baclofen is administered by intrathecal pump to decrease muscle tone and vasospasms when oral administration is ineffective or causes side effects (Pelligrino, 2002). See Figure 26–18 ➤. Botulinum toxin injection into specific muscles is a relatively new therapy used to help control spasticity (Buck, 2003).

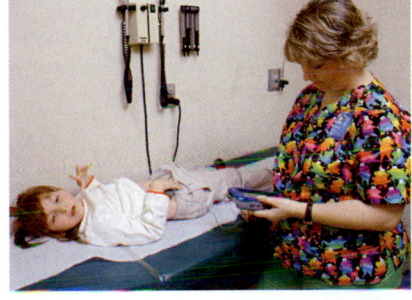

Figure 26–18 ➤ Child having baclofen pump filled.

The prognosis for infants and children with cerebral palsy depends on the level of physical involvement and on the presence of intellectual, visual, or hearing deficits. Early intervention programs can significantly improve performance. Many children with hemiplegia or ataxia show some improvement with maturation and are able to ambulate. Others need assistance with mobility and activities of daily living. They are usually cared for in their homes, although some receive care in long-term care facilities.

NURSING MANAGEMENT

Nursing Assessment and Diagnosis

Be alert for children whose histories indicate an increased risk for CP. Assess all children at each healthcare visit for developmental delays. Note any orthopedic, visual, auditory, or intellectual deficits. Assess for newborn reflexes, which may persist beyond the normal age in a child with cerebral palsy. Identify infants that appear to have an abnormal muscle tone or abnormal posture (arched back, becomes stiff when moving against gravity, neck or extremities have increased or decreased resistance to passive movement). Asymmetric or abnormal crawling by using 2 or 3 extremities indicates a motor problem. Hand dominance before the preschool years is another sign of a motor problem. Record dietary intake as well as height and weight percentiles for children suspected to have or diagnosed with the condition.

Nursing diagnoses for the child with CP vary, depending on the type of cerebral palsy, the particular child's symptoms and age, and the family situation. The accompanying Nursing Care Plan includes several diagnoses that might be appropriate. Additional nursing diagnoses might include:

- Risk for Constipation related to low intake of fiber and fluids and insufficient physical activity

- Impaired Tissue Integrity related to decreased physical mobility and limited self-care ability
- Impaired Verbal Communication related to hearing and/or speech impairment
- Impaired Home Maintenance related to child's developmental disability and inadequate support system
- Chronic Pain related to spasticity and stretching exercises to prevent contractures
- Delayed Growth and development related to lack of muscle strength or limited social interaction

Planning and Implementation

The accompanying Nursing Care Plan summarizes care for the child with CP. Since the condition can range from mild to severe and involve numerous manifestations, interventions need to be adapted to the particular child and family. Nursing care focuses on providing adequate nutrition, maintaining skin integrity, promoting physical mobility, promoting safety, promoting growth and development, teaching parents how to care for the child, and providing emotional support.

Provide Adequate Nutrition

Children with CP require high-calorie diets or supplements to the diet because of feeding difficulties associated with spasticity. Many children have difficulty chewing and swallowing. Give the child small amounts of soft foods at a time. Utensils with large, padded handles may be easier for the child to use.

Maintain Skin Integrity

Take special care to protect the bony prominences from skin breakdown. Monitor the skin under splints and braces for redness. If the skin is red, the braces or splints should be removed and not worn until the redness is gone. (See Families Want to Know: Safety for the Child with Spina Bifida on page 1070.)

Proper body alignment should be maintained at all times. Support the child with pillows, towels, and bolsters whether the child is in bed or in a chair. Support the head and body of a floppy infant. A child with spasticity may have scissored, extended legs, and a child with athetoid movements may be difficult to carry and transport.

Promote Physical Mobility

Range of motion exercises are essential to maintain joint flexibility and to prevent contractures. Consult with the physical therapists who work with the child and help with recommended exercises. Refer parents to the appropriate resources for help getting adaptive devices (Figure 26–19 ➤). Teach parents to position the child to foster flexion rather than extension so that the child can more easily interact with the environment (for example, by bringing objects closer to the face). Encourage parents to bring in the child's *adaptive appliances* (braces, positioning devices) for use during the hospitalization.

Consider the use of therapeutic massage or relaxation training to manage pain associated with spasticity and stretching exercises (McKearnan, Kieckhefer, Engel et al., 2004).

Promote Safety

Safety belts should be used for children in strollers and wheelchairs. Determine if an adaptive car safety seat is needed so the child can be safely transported. A child with chronic seizures should wear a helmet to protect against further injury.

Promote Growth and Development

Remember that many children with CP are physically but not intellectually disabled. Use terminology appropriate for the child's developmental level. Help the child develop a positive self-image to ensure emotional health and social growth. Children with a hearing impairment may need referral to learn American Sign Language or other communication methods. Provide audio and visual activities for the child who is quadriplegic.

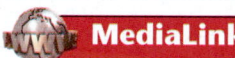

MediaLink

CP Resources

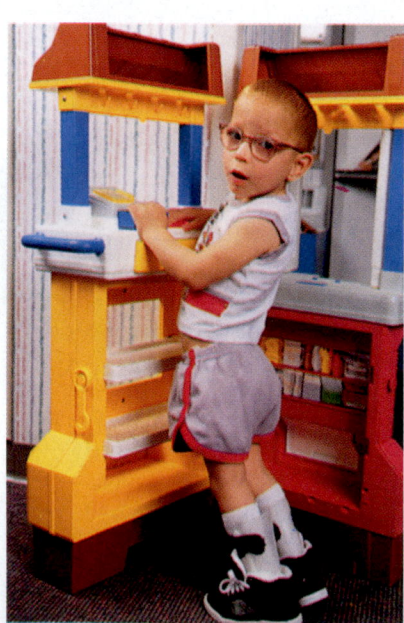

Figure 26–19 ➤ A child with cerebral palsy has abnormal muscle tone and lack of physical coordination. Encourage the parents to find ways for the child to interact with the environment to promote development.

NURSING CARE PLAN   The Child with Cerebral Palsy

GOAL	INTERVENTION	RATIONALE	EXPECTED OUTCOME
1. Impaired Physical Mobility related to decreased muscle strength and control			
	NIC Priority Intervention: **Exercise Therapy, Joint Mobility:** *Use of active and passive body movement to maintain or restore joint flexibility.*		*NOC Suggested Outcome:* **Joint Movement—Active:** *Range of motion of joints with self-initiated movement.*
The child will attain the maximum physical abilities possible.	• Perform development assessment and record age of achievement of milestones (e.g., reaching for objects, sitting).	• Delayed development milestones are common with cerebral palsy. Once the child achieves one milestone, interventions are revised to assist in acquiring the next skill.	The child reaches maximum physical mobility and all developmental milestones.
	• Plan activities to use gross and fine motor skills (e.g., holding pen or eating utensils, toys positioned to encourage reaching and rolling over).	• Many activities of daily living and play activities promote physical development.	
	• Allow time for the child to complete activities.	• The child may perform tasks more slowly than most children.	
	• Perform range of motion exercises every 4 hours for the child unable to move body parts. Position the child to promote tendon stretching (e.g., foot plantar flexion instead of dorsiflexion, legs extended instead of flexed at knees and hips).	• Promotes mobility and increased circulation, and decreases the risk of contractures.	
	• Arrange for and encourage parents to keep appointments with a rehabilitation therapist.	• A regular and frequently reevaluated rehabilitation program assists in promoting development.	
	• Teach the family to maintain appropriate brace wear.	• Adaptive devices are often necessary to maximize physical mobility.	
2. Disturbed Sensory Perception (Visual or Auditory) related to cerebral damage			
	NIC Priority Intervention: **Communication Enhancement: Visual Deficit:** *Assistance with accepting or learning alternative methods for living with diminished vision.*		*NOC Suggested Outcome:* **Sensory Function: Vision:** *Extent to which visual images are sensed, with and without assistive devices.*
The child will receive and benefit from varied forms of sensory and perceptual input.	• Facilitate vision examinations by specialist. Promote the use of glasses and encourage recommended follow-up visits to specialists.	• Glasses often enhance sensory input. Assessment of vision as the child grows may identify needed prescription changes for glasses.	The child receives adequate visual sensory/perceptual input to maximize developmental outcome.
	• Maximize the use of intact senses (e.g., encourage touching of objects, provide auditory stimulation to enhance learning, use computers to promote communication).	• Other senses can compensate for those that are impaired.	

(continued)

NURSING CARE PLAN The Child with Cerebral Palsy (continued)

GOAL	INTERVENTION	RATIONALE	EXPECTED OUTCOME
3. Imbalanced Nutrition: Less Than Body Requirements related to difficulty in chewing and swallowing and high metabolic needs			
	NIC Priority Intervention: **Nutrition Management:** *Assistance with or provision of a balanced dietary intake of foods and fluids.*		*NOC Suggested Outcome:* **Nutritional Status: Nutrient Intake:** *Adequacy of nutrients taken into the body.*
The child will receive nutrients needed for normal growth.	• Monitor height and weight and plot on a growth grid. Perform hydration status assessment.	• Insufficient intake can lead to impaired growth and dehydration.	The child shows normal growth patterns for height, weight, and other physical parameters.
	• Teach the family techniques to promote caloric and nutrient intake: • Position the child upright for feedings. • Place foods far back in the mouth to overcome tongue thrust. • Use soft and blended foods. • Allow extra time for chewing and swallowing. • Obtain adaptive handles for utensils and encourage self-feeding skills.	• Special techniques can facilitate food intake. Adaptive handles may help the child better manage feeding self.	
	• Perform frequent respiratory assessment. Teach the family to avoid aspiration pneumonia. Teach care of gastrostomy and tube feeding technique as appropriate.	• Aspiration pneumonia is a risk for the child with poor swallowing. Special feeding techniques may be needed.	
4. Ineffective Therapeutic Regimen Management: Family related to excessive demands made on family with child's complex care needs			
	NIC Priority Intervention: **Family Mobilization:** *Utilization of family strengths to influence patient's health in a positive direction.*		*NOC Suggested Outcome:* **Family Functioning:** *Ability of the family to meet the needs of its members through developmental transitions.*
The family will adapt to growth and development needs of the child with cerebral palsy.	• Allow chances for parents to verbalize the impact of cerebral palsy on the family. Refer to other parents and support groups.	• The family needs a chance to explore the emotional and social impact of the child's care so they can integrate and grow from the experience.	The child demonstrates appropriate growth and developmental progress. The family successfully supports all of its members.
	• Explore community services for rehabilitation, respite care, childcare, and other needs and refer family as appropriate.	• Diverse services are available and will be needed due to the multiple impacts of cerebral palsy on the child.	
	• During home and office visits, review the child's achievements and praise the family for care provided.	• The child's achievements are positive reinforcement of the family's efforts.	
	• Teach the family skills needed to manage the child's care (e.g., medication administration, muscle stretching, physical rehabilitation, seizure management).	• Complex skills must be learned before they can be performed efficiently.	

NURSING CARE PLAN   The Child with Cerebral Palsy (continued)

GOAL	INTERVENTION	RATIONALE	EXPECTED OUTCOME
4. Ineffective Therapeutic Regimen Management: Family related to excessive demands made on family with child's complex care needs (continued)			
	• Teach case management techniques.	• The child requires care by many specialists. Many parents become case managers to coordinate care.	
	• Involve siblings in the care for the child with cerebral palsy. Review for parents the needs of all children in the family.	• Siblings of the child with cerebral palsy may feel left out because of the care provided. Special efforts contribute to meeting the developmental needs of all family members.	
5. Deficient Diversional Activity (Child) related to poor social skills			
	NIC Priority Intervention: **Recreation Therapy:** *Purposeful use of recreation to promote relaxation and enhancement of social skills.*		*NOC Suggested Outcome:* **Play Participation:** *Use of activities as needed for enjoyment, entertainment, and development by children.*
The child engages in activities that maximize growth and development.	• Refer the family to an early intervention program. Encourage contact with other children. When hospitalized, place the child in a room with other children whenever possible.	• The child needs a variety of activities and contact with other children and adults to maximize development.	The child engages in activities to maximize development.
	• Work with the school to develop an Individualized Education Plan that encourages interaction with peers and a variety of activities that support development.	• The education system is obligated to work with families to provide methods to enhance learning, including social interactions.	
	• Investigate recreational programs for children with disabilities and share information with the parents.	• Recreational programs for children with disabilities may promote social experiences and physical activity.	

Adaptive and assistive technology may be needed to promote mobility and communication. **Assistive technology** is any item, equipment, or product customized for use to promote the functional capabilities and independence of an individual with disabilities. Examples include computers, adaptive utensils, and customized wheelchairs.

Foster Parental Knowledge

Teach parents about the disorder and arrange sessions to teach them about all of the child's special needs. Teach administration, desired effects, and side effects of medications prescribed for seizures. Make sure parents are aware of the need for dental care for children taking anticonvulsants.

Provide Emotional Support

Refer parents to individual and family counseling, if appropriate. Listen to the parents' concerns and encourage them to express their feelings and ask questions. Explain what they can expect from future treatment. Work with other healthcare professionals to help families adjust to this chronic disease.

Care in the Community

Children with CP need continuous support in the community. A case manager such as the parent or nurse is often needed to coordinate care. Parents may need financial assistance to provide for the child's needs and to obtain appliances such as braces, wheelchairs, or adaptive utensils. Children need new adaptive devices, ongoing developmental assessment and care planning, and possibly surgery as they grow. Although the brain lesion does not change, it manifests differently as the child grows. For example, once the child begins to walk, the extensor tone may cause Achilles' cord tightening. Braces may decrease deformities, but surgery may eventually be needed.

Early intervention programs can help parents learn to meet their child's special needs, including physical, occupational, and speech therapy, as well as educational needs. The child often needs an Individualized Education Plan to maximize learning potential (see Chapter 12 ∞). The nurse can be instrumental in helping parents meet the needs of the child with CP in preschools, schools, offices, clinics, and other settings. In addition, the nurse makes referrals as appropriate to support groups, as well as organizations such as the United Cerebral Palsy Association and Shriners Hospitals. Recreational activities may be identified through the National Association of Sports for Cerebral Palsy.

An individualized transition plan developed during adolescence assists the family and adolescent with CP to develop plans for adult living. Vocational training options can be explored. See Chapter 12 ∞. The young adult (18 to 21 years) may be able to move into a group home or live independently, if desired.

Evaluation

Expected outcomes of nursing care for the child with CP are provided on the nursing care plan.

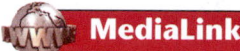

MediaLink

CP Resources and Support

INJURIES OF THE NEUROLOGIC SYSTEM
Traumatic Brain Injury

A traumatic brain injury (TBI) can be defined as any trauma involving the blunt force or penetration to the head that causes a change in level of consciousness or an anatomic abnormality of the brain. Traumatic brain injury is the leading cause of death and disability among children (Blackman, 2005). On an annual basis in children under 15 years, there are 435,000 emergency department visits, 37,000 hospitalizations, and 2685 deaths (Centers for Disease Control, 2006). Children and adolescents with a moderate to severe injury may develop a permanent disability, such as epilepsy, cognitive impairment, learning problems, and behavioral or emotional problems (Adekoya, Thurman, White et al., 2002).

Young children with moderate and severe traumatic brain injury are at risk for long-term cognitive deficits. Most recovery occurs in the first 12 months after injury. Even if the child scores normal on intelligence tests, difficulties with learning skills such as short-term memory, problem solving, sequencing, concrete thinking, and visual-spatial organization are common. No new learning can occur before short-term memory returns (Blackman, 2005).

Etiology and Pathophysiology

Falls are a major cause of unintentional head injuries in young children. Other unintentional injuries leading to hospitalization in children include motor vehicle incidents as passengers, pedestrians, and bicyclists, and being struck by or against an object (Coronado, Johnson, Faul, et al., 2006). Children and adolescents may be injured in rollerblading, skateboarding, and other sports-related incidents. Child abuse, including shaken baby syndrome, accounts for a large number of traumatic brain injuries and deaths in children under 2 years old (Nakagawa & Conway, 2004). See Chapter 6 ∞ for more details on shaken baby syndrome.

Brain injuries can be categorized as either primary or secondary. Primary injuries occur at the time of the insult when the initial cellular damage takes place. These injuries result from either a direct blow to the head (coup injury) or from acceleration-deceleration movement of the brain within the skull (contrecoup injury), as occurred with Antwan in the chapter opening vignette (Figure 26–20 ➤). At the time of

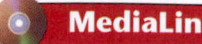

MediaLink

Coup-contracoup Injury Animation

PATHOPHYSIOLOGY ILLUSTRATED

Brain Injury

Subdural vessels are torn

Contrecoup injury results from secondary impact as brain moves forward and then backward within skull

Coup injury results from initial impact

Bruising occurs as brain moves over skull floor

Figure 26–20 ➤ Brain injury can result from a direct blow to the head (coup injury) or the acceleration-deceleration movement of the brain (contrecoup injury). The inertial forces resulting when the head and skull stop moving allow the brain tissue to continue moving within the skull. This results in tearing of nerves, fibers, and blood vessels.

impact, scalp injuries, skull fractures, contusions, and hematomas of brain tissue may occur.

The secondary phase of brain trauma is a biochemical and cellular response to the initial insult. It can be manifested immediately or over hours, days, or weeks. Hypoperfusion of the brain is common in the first 24 hours after serious injury, at the same time the brain has increased metabolic needs. This can lead to ischemia and brain damage. Brain cells are further damaged by the release of amino acids and an inflammatory response that increases the permeability of the blood-brain barrier. Cerebral edema occurs due to cellular swelling, osmolar swelling, and blood-brain barrier injury (Kennedy & Moffatt, 2004). The result is increased intracranial pressure which further compounds brain injury by limiting the blood flow that delivers oxygen and nutrients as well as removes accumulated toxins from cell death.

Clinical Manifestations

The signs and symptoms of brain injuries in children depend on the pathologic features and severity of the injury. The child with a mild brain injury may remain conscious or have brief loss of consciousness (seconds to a few minutes). The child with a moderate brain injury loses consciousness for 5 to 10 minutes. A child with a severe brain injury is usually unconscious for more than 10 minutes and may rapidly show signs of increased intracranial pressure. See the clinical manifestations table on page 1084.

Unconsciousness may result from increased intracranial pressure, edema, hemorrhage, or parenchymal damage to both cerebral cortices or the brainstem. Post-traumatic seizures are common. Children with inflicted TBI are more likely to have retinal hemorrhages, rib fractures, long bone fractures, and skull fractures than children with noninflicted TBI (Keenan, Runyan, Marshall et al., 2004).

Vital signs are important indicators of brain injury. Changes in respiratory effort or periods of apnea can occur secondary to shock, injury to the spinal cord above C4, or damage to or pressure on the medulla. Heart rate and blood pressure are indices of

CLINICAL MANIFESTATIONS	TRAUMATIC BRAIN INJURY BY SEVERITY
Type of Brain Injury	**Clinical Manifestations**
Concussion or mild brain injury	Low-grade headache that won't go away
	Slowness in thinking, acting, speaking, reading
	Memory problems
	Loss of balance, unsteady walking
	Difficulty paying attention or concentrating, change in performance at school
	Feeling tired all the time, change in sleeping pattern
	Change in eating patterns
	Increased sensitivity to lights, sounds, distractions
	Easily irritated
	Lack of motivation or interest in favorite toys
Moderate brain injury	Glasgow Coma Scale score of 9 to 12
	Post-traumatic amnesia for 1 to 24 hours
	Loss of consciousness
Severe brain injury	Glasgow Coma Scale score of 8 or less
	Post-traumatic amnesia greater than 24 hours
	Coma
	Increased intracranial pressure

CLINICAL TIP

Important elements of the history of the head injury include the following:

- If the injury resulted from a fall, what was the distance fallen, what surface did the head strike, where on the head was the primary impact?
- Did the child lose consciousness (for how long), or did the child act confused or dazed after the injury?
- Has the child had a seizure?
- Has the child vomited?

NURSING ALERT

Any infant who arrives in the emergency department with seizures, failure to thrive, vomiting, lethargy, respiratory irregularities, or coma should be evaluated for child abuse (shaken baby syndrome or shaken impact syndrome). The infant has a large head and relatively weak neck muscles. A frustrated adult can shake an infant and cause inertial injuries (acceleration and deceleration) to the head that tear nerve fibers as the brain moves back and forth in the skull. Throwing the infant down onto a solid surface further increases the forces with which the brain hits the back of the skull (Nakagawa & Conway, 2004).

brainstem function. Tachycardia can be a sign of blood loss, shock, hypoxia, anxiety, or pain. **Cushing's triad** is associated with significantly increased intracranial pressure, impending herniation, or compromised blood flow to the brainstem. It is characterized by hypertension, increased systolic pressure with wide pulse pressure, bradycardia, and irregular respirations. Refer to the earlier discussion of altered states of consciousness for more information about increased intracranial pressure.

Reflexes may be hyporesponsive, hyperresponsive, or nonexistent. The child may assume a decorticate, decerebrate, **areflexic** (no response to verbal, sensory, or pain stimulation), or flaccid posture (see Figure 26–4).

■ COLLABORATIVE CARE

Diagnostic Tests

Identifying the severity of a brain injury involves history, observation, examination, and diagnostic testing. Obtain information about how the injury occurred, the child's initial responses and current responses, any loss of consciousness, and the child's memory of the event.

Neurologic evaluation with the pediatric Glasgow Coma Scale is performed frequently to detect changes in the child's condition (see Table 26–3). Cranial nerves are assessed (see Tables 5–20 ∞ and 26–5). Review the discussion of altered states of consciousness at the beginning of this chapter for further details.

Laboratory tests include a complete blood cell count, blood chemistry, toxicology screening, and urinalysis. Radiologic imaging identifies the specific injury. Radiographs detect fractures of the skull and cervical vertebrae. A CT scan detects fractures, intracranial hemorrhage, swelling, and diffuse axonal injury (tearing of nerve fibers throughout the brain). An MRI scan is used during recovery to determine the extent of brain damage. PET scans measure the blood flow in the brain. A fracture indicates a more serious injury. Many children with brain injuries have multiple other injuries. Even though cervical spine injuries are rare, children with a brain injury should have a potential cervical spine injury ruled out by radiologic imaging.

Clinical Therapy

The initial management of a child with a brain injury is based on the child's physiologic status. The airway must be clear and stable, and hypoxia must be prevented. If indicated, the child is intubated, sedated, and chemically paralyzed to protect the airway and prevent aspiration. Hypoxia and hypercapnia have disastrous effects on cerebral function, as they can cause vasodilation and increased intracranial pressure. Mechanical ventilation with supplemental oxygen at the child's normal respiratory rate is often used for the first 24 hours after injury to maintain the oxygenation level. Hyperventilation may be used for a short period in cases of increased intracranial pressure, but prolonged use may cause cerebral ischemia (Adelson, Bratton, Carney et al., 2003).

Shock is treated aggressively with fluid boluses. Maintaining the child's blood pressure within the normal range is essential to keep the brain adequately perfused. This ensures that the brain gets adequate oxygen and nutrients and that the accumulated neurotoxins are removed. Fluid administration is then focused on maintaining the blood pressure. Only after the child is hemodynamically stable will fluids be restricted, if necessary.

Increased intracranial pressure must be controlled. Brain swelling can lead to worsening cerebral ischemia and cerebral edema. If unrelieved, brain contents begin shifting in the cranium that can lead to **herniation** (protrusion of brain contents into the brainstem area). Diuretics such as mannitol or furosemide may be used to decrease intracranial pressure. A continuous infusion of hypertonic saline (3%) is sometimes used for control of increased intracranial pressure (Adelson, Bratton, Carney et al., 2003). Invasive procedures may be necessary to reduce increased intracranial pressure. Burr holes may be made or more extensive surgery may be performed to evacuate a lesion or hematoma. A ventricular catheter may be placed to drain CSF and to monitor pressure. In some cases, the intracranial pressure cannot be controlled and death occurs.

Minimizing pain and stressful stimuli are important steps. Pain and sedation management are used to promote comfort, to help limit unnecessary oxygen consumption by the brain, and to help control intracranial pressure. The environment is kept as quiet as possible. The child's body temperature is kept within normal limits.

If there is no cervical spine injury, the head of the bed is elevated up to 30 degrees. The child's head is kept in the midline to promote venous (jugular) drainage. Hip flexion is avoided. A urinary catheter is inserted to monitor output, and electrolytes should be checked frequently. Nutrition support should be started within 72 hours with total parenteral nutrition or enteral nutrition.

Aggressive support continues until the child regains consciousness and rehabilitation can be initiated. Physical therapists, occupational therapists, and speech therapists are members of the rehabilitation team. The goals of rehabilitation are to promote mobility, regain activities of daily living, perform self-care, and regain language skills (Blackman, 2005). Disabilities that often result from a severe brain injury include: motor and cognitive impairments, feeding disorders, hearing and vision impairments, and communication problems. Reliable predictions of outcome in the child who has suffered a severe brain injury cannot be made until 6 to 12 months postinjury.

NURSING MANAGEMENT
Nursing Assessment and Diagnosis

Assess the child's neurologic status frequently using the guidelines on page 1035 and compare the child's status to baseline findings, noting improvement, stability, or deterioration. Evaluate the child's level of consciousness using the pediatric Glasgow Coma Scale (see Table 26–3). Assess the pupils for size and reactivity, as well as cranial nerves. Monitor vital signs closely. Note decerebrate or decorticate posturing. If a ventricular catheter or bolt is inserted, monitor the actual pressure readings. Changes in these signs may indicate hypoxia, decreased perfusion, shock, or increased intracranial pressure. The cause of any deterioration must be quickly determined and appropriate interventions taken.

Suspect that the child with increased intracranial pressure is in pain, even when unresponsive. Observe for physiologic and behavioral signs of pain.

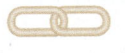

SKILL 6–17
ICP Monitor

LAW & ETHICS

Criteria for Declaring Brain Death

Criteria for declaring brain death involve the following:

- The cause of coma is recognized and sufficient to explain the irreversible stopping of all brain function, and reversible causes of coma have been excluded.
- Clinical evaluation involves testing for the absence of higher brain functioning and brainstem functioning by electroencephalogram or cerebral blood flow testing.
- The age of the child is used to establish the required observation period prior to declaration of brain death. For infants ages 7 days to two months, there must be two examinations separated by at least 48 hours. For infants ages two months to 1 year, there must be two examinations separated by at least 24 hours. For children over 1 year of age, there must be an observation period with two examinations at least 12 hours apart.

Adapted from: Frankel, L. R., & Mathers, L. H. (2004). Withdrawal or withholding of life support, brain death, and organ procurement. In R. E. Behrman, R. M. Kliegman, & H. B. Jepson, *Nelson textbook of pediatrics* (17th ed., pp. 340–342). Philadelphia: Saunders.

CLINICAL TIP

Beliefs that the young age and brain development are protective or brain plasticity allows more recovery after brain injury are changing as research findings emerge. Studies of children with severe TBI are identifying that the immature brain is more vulnerable to diffuse injury. Skills that are not well established are more likely to be disrupted than well-established skills. Functional recovery may be restricted to the younger child's fewer existing skills (Kirkwood, Yeates, & Wilson, 2006).

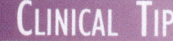
Nursing diagnoses that might be appropriate for the child with a brain injury include:

- Ineffective Cerebral Tissue Perfusion related to hypoventilation, hypovolemia, and/or reduction of arterial blood flow to the brain due to increased intracranial pressure
- Risk for Aspiration related to decreased level of consciousness and loss of protective reflexes
- Risk for Imbalanced Fluid Volume related to therapies for reducing intracranial pressure
- Disturbed Sensory Perception related to central nervous system impairment
- Compromised Family Coping related to life-threatening injury to child

Planning and Implementation
Hospital-Based Care

Nursing care focuses on maintaining cardiopulmonary function, preventing complications, promoting recovery, and providing emotional support. Nursing management is based on prevention of secondary injury and return to an optimal level of function.

Maintain cardiopulmonary function. In the moderately injured child, observe breathing patterns and check color and level of consciousness. Check the pulse oximeter; the oxygen saturation should remain over 95%. Report any sign of decreased oxygenation or signs and symptoms of increased intracranial pressure to the physician immediately (see Table 26–4). Keep suction equipment at the bedside in case aspiration occurs. Avoid suctioning unless essential for airway maintenance because it increases intracranial pressure. Some children need mechanical ventilation to protect the airway and maintain oxygenation.

Reduce physiologic stresses on the body that could increase intracranial pressure. The nurse should minimize unpleasant stimuli when possible, keep the environment quiet, and avoid jarring the bed. Pain management and temperature control are important. Position the child to avoid excessive flexion of the hips and neck that could slow venous circulation. Monitor the effect of nursing procedures on the level of intracranial pressure and determine if the child responds better to clustering procedures than spreading procedures over time. Encourage parents to talk to the child and provide comforting touch.

Administer medications as ordered. Diuretics are often given to remove excess fluid from the body and the brain if the blood pressure is adequate to maintain the cerebral perfusion pressure. Sedatives may be given to decrease the metabolic demands on the brain. Pain medication is provided to promote comfort.

Provide oral care to keep mucous membranes moist and intact, but use care when the gag reflex is absent. Pad and cushion bony prominences, provide skin care, and change the child's position frequently. The eyes should be protected from corneal irritation with ophthalmic ointment and patching. Stool softeners and suppositories should be used as needed to prevent constipation. The side rails of the bed should be padded to protect the child if a seizure occurs.

Promote recovery and prevent physical deformities. Physical, occupational, and speech therapy should begin in the hospital, and often in the intensive care unit. Splinting may be needed to maintain joints in functional positions. Work with these therapists to reinforce exercises and help teach parents the techniques so they can work with the child in the hospital and at home.

After the child survives the critical injury and is moved to a pediatric care unit, begin promoting increased awareness. Using toys, books, music, or games, provide stimulation based on the child's age and ability. Encourage parents to bring in favorite toys, stuffed animals, and tape recordings of the child's favorite music or of family members talking. Assist the family to provide stimulation but to also provide quiet when the child displays agitation.

Provide emotional support to the family in collaboration with the social workers, physicians, psychologists, rehabilitation therapists, and members of the clergy caring for the child and family. All can help the family adjust to having a child with a new disability.

Discharge Planning and Home Care Teaching

Home care needs should be identified and addressed well in advance of discharge. Children with serious brain injuries benefit from inpatient or outpatient rehabilitation to promote optimal achievement of function. A case manager is often needed to coordinate services and resources during rehabilitation. Social services intervention may be needed when brain injury results from child abuse or shaken baby syndrome.

Give parents information about homecare for children with mild or moderate brain injuries and possible behaviors to expect from the child. See the discussion of concussion on the next page. For children with disabilities, determine what adaptations and assistive technology are needed in the home to care for the child, such as a wheelchair, walker, braces, or special bed. Social work and home health agencies can often help the parents make special arrangements.

Care in the Community

Home care nursing may be important for the child with an acquired neurologic dysfunction and prolonged altered consciousness. The home care nurse can take over the case management for the disabled child and make sure the environment is safe. The nurse can teach the family to care for the child's needs, monitor the intake of fluids and foods, as well as position the child and perform range of motion exercises to reduce contractures. Many children with severe brain injuries qualify for Social Security Supplemental Security Income (SSI) benefits or the state program for children with special healthcare needs. Regular follow-up visits are needed to assess the child's recovery and to modify the treatment plan.

Even though the child looks normal within days of a mild or moderate brain injury, parents and teachers need to be aware that brain healing takes up to 6 weeks. Typical behavior during this healing period may include any of the following behaviors: tiring easily, memory loss or forgetfulness, easy distractibility, difficulty concentrating, difficulty following directions, irritability or short temper, and needing help starting and finishing tasks. The child should not be returned to a full school schedule too quickly to prevent fatigue and frustration. Educational assessment should be initiated if recovery takes longer than 6 weeks, and educational accommodations needed are often different from those needed by children with other types of learning disabilities. An Individualized Education Plan is often needed. See Chapter 12 ∞. Children with moderate brain injuries often have problems with attention, problem solving, and speed of information processing. The injury impairs new learning more than the retention of prior learning. Young children are at a special disadvantage because they have not had time to store knowledge and develop learning strategies.

The child or adolescent facing long-term rehabilitation needs support to adjust to the disability and to find the strength to maximize his or her abilities. Identify recreational opportunities for the child with disabilities to promote exercise and self-esteem. The adolescent may need to gain vocational skills and learn to live independently. Refer parents to the Brain Injury Association for further information.

Prevention of brain injury is another important role of the nurse. Encourage parents to obtain, and require children to use, protective helmets for bicycling, skateboarding, inline skating, and other sports. Parents should be encouraged to wear a helmet themselves as role models. Encourage parents to monitor playgrounds for appropriate use of wood chips or cushioning tiles to reduce the severity of injuries associated with falls.

Evaluation

Examples of expected outcomes of nursing care for the child with traumatic brain injury include the following:

- Cerebral perfusion pressure is maintained at an adequate rate to sustain oxygenation of the brain.
- Muscle function is maintained and physical deformities are prevented with range of motion exercises and splinting during the recovery stages of the brain injury.

 MediaLink

Brain Injury Resources and Support

- Parents are supported through the child's acute recovery phase and learn to provide care the child will need at home.
- The child's school performance is monitored and appropriate educational resources are provided to support the child's learning.

Specific Head Injuries
Scalp Injuries

Injuries to the scalp, which can be caused by falls, blunt trauma, or penetration of a foreign body, are usually benign. Although bleeding may be extensive, hypovolemia or shock is uncommon unless the patient is an infant.

Lacerations should be irrigated with copious amounts of sterile normal saline solution and inspected for bony fragments or depressions, CSF leakage with a dural tear, or debris. If the injury is simple, the laceration can be sutured or stapled, and the child discharged from the emergency department. If not, a neurosurgeon should be consulted.

Concussion

A concussion is a mild TBI that usually results from a direct blow to the head, face, or neck that causes an alteration in mental status (e.g., amnesia, dizziness, memory or orientation impairment, unsteady gait), but not necessarily loss of consciousness (Kirkwood, Yeates, & Wilson, 2006). It is secondary to stretching, compression, or shearing of nerve fibers. The injury is metabolic rather than gross structural damage or focal injury. Concussions are categorized by three levels of severity (Table 26–9).

Treatment is supportive. Children are observed in the emergency department for several hours before being sent home with instructions to the parents to watch them closely for decreased responsiveness. Any child who is unconscious for more than 5 minutes or has amnesia of the event may be admitted to the hospital or observed in a short-stay unit to rule out other injury.

Pediatric concussive syndrome, which is believed to be caused by an injury to the brainstem, is seen in children who are less than 3 years old. Toddlers seem stunned at the time of injury, but they do not lose consciousness. Later, however, these children become pale, clammy, and lethargic, and they may vomit. They are usually brought to the hospital for treatment when these symptoms appear. These children may be placed in a short-stay unit for observation and usually recover within 24 hours.

Postconcussive syndrome, which is common in both children and adults, may occur after the initial brain injury. Signs and symptoms can include progressively developing lethargy, disorientation, irritability, and behavior changes within 10 to 30 minutes after the injury. The child may vomit repeatedly, as well as experience pallor and diaphoresis. Symptoms may persist for 1 to 2 hours, and recovery may occur over 2 to 12 hours. Some children have trauma-triggered migraine headaches (Dias, 2004). In adolescents, postconcussive syndrome may involve the development of headaches, dizziness, irritability, and eventually depression that may persist for more than 6 weeks (Theye & Mueller, 2004). Treatment is supportive.

Young athletes suffering a second concussion before complete recovery from the first develop *second impact syndrome*. This syndrome results in acute brain swelling, neu-

CLINICAL TIP

Sports with a high risk for concussion include boxing, field hockey, football, ice hockey, lacrosse, martial arts, soccer, rodeo, wrestling, rugby, baseball, rollerblading, trampolining, and basketball. An estimated 62,800 high school athletes experience a concussion each year, and football accounts for nearly 63% of these cases (Lovell, Collins, Iverson et al., 2003).

Table 26–9	LEVELS OF CONCUSSION SEVERITY
Grade 1	Transient confusion, no loss of consciousness, no post-traumatic amnesia, and duration of mental status abnormalities of less than 15 minutes.
Grade 2	Transient confusion with post-traumatic amnesia, no loss of consciousness, and duration of mental status abnormalities of 15 minutes or longer.
Grade 3	Any loss of consciousness, brief or prolonged.

Adapted from: Quality Standards Subcommittee, American Academy of Neurology. (1997). Practice parameters: The management of concussion in sports. *Neurology, 48,* 581–585.

MediaLink

Assessing Return to Competitive Play Post-Concussion

rologic or cognitive deficits, and sometimes death from the cumulative effect of these concussions. Recommendations should be followed for the management of sports-related concussions to reduce the risk of disability and death. Removal from sports participation ranges from 1 day to the entire season, depending on the severity of the concussion and neurologic symptoms. Testing the child to identify any return of symptoms with a gradual increase in activity may be implemented. Allow the child to return to full game play only when the child is symptom-free (Kirkwood, Yeates, & Wilson, 2006). High school athletes have a slower recovery time from brain injuries than college or adult athletes (Cobb & Battin, 2004). A postconcussive symptom scale is often used to provide uniform information about the actual recovery time from the concussion and to prevent athletes who try to minimize symptoms from returning to play too soon. Individuals with multiple concussions have a longer recovery time (Guskiewicz & McCrea, 2003).

Skull Fractures

A fracture to any of the eight cranial bones is caused by a considerable force to the head. Any area of the skull with swelling or a hematoma should be evaluated for possible fracture. Diagnosis is made by visual inspection, palpation, radiologic study, or CT scan. Treatment should always include neurosurgical consultation.

Management of skull fractures depends on the type and extent of the injury (Table 26–10).

Cerebral Contusion

A cerebral contusion, or the bruising of brain tissue, is secondary to blunt trauma and can occur with either coup or contrecoup injuries (see Figure 26–20). Such injuries are rare in children less than 1 year of age. The temporal or frontal sections of the skull are the most common sites of this injury. Damage to the parenchyma with tears in vessels or tissue, pulping, and subsequent areas of necrosis or infarction may occur.

Table 26–10	**TYPES OF SKULL FRACTURES**
Injury	**Clinical Therapy**
Linear Fracture Results from impact to large area of the skull. Usually no symptoms. May have overlying hematoma or soft-tissue swelling. Most common type of fracture.	If fracture is on temporal bone or crosses sagittal suture line, a CT scan is performed to detect potential epidural hematoma. Consider the possibility of inflicted injury. No treatment is commonly needed.
Depressed Fracture Break in skull itself or an area shattered into many fragments. Pieces of bone may be depressed into brain tissue with hematoma forming on top.	Plain radiographic film or CT scan. Surgery to elevate bone fragments when depression is greater than 5 mm. Tetanus prophylaxis is given as needed. Many are associated with intracranial injury and post-traumatic epilepsy.
Compound Fracture Combination of a full thickness scalp laceration and depressed skull fracture with the bone exposed. Are considered penetrating fractures if the dura is torn.	Visual diagnosis along with radiographic studies. Surgical debridement, a search for foreign bodies, and copious irrigation are performed. Parenteral antibiotics and tetanus prophylaxis are provided as needed.
Basilar Fracture Fracture at the base of the skull that may involve the frontal, ethmoid, sphenoid, temporal, or occipital bones. A dural tear may be present.	Diagnosis is confirmed by signs of blood behind the tympanic membranes, CSF leakage from the nose or ears, periorbital ecchymosis (raccoon eyes), or bruising of the mastoid (Battle sign). CT imaging locates the fracture site. Antibiotics are prescribed. Surgical repair of the site of the CSF leak is performed if the leak persists after 1 to 2 weeks. Transient or permanent cranial nerve injuries occur (e.g., hearing loss).

Data from: Dias, M. S. (2004). Traumatic brain and spinal cord injury. *Pediatric Clinics of North America, 51,* 271–303; Rosman, N. P. (1999). Acute head trauma. In J. A. McMillan, C. D. DeAngelis, R. D. Feigin, & J. B. Warshaw (Eds.), *Oski's pediatrics: Principles and practice* (3rd ed., pp. 603–617). Philadelphia: Lippincott, Williams & Wilkins.

The child may have focal symptoms depending on the area of injury. Altered levels of consciousness range from confusion and disorientation to being obtunded. A CT scan is used for diagnosis.

Treatment involves hospitalization for observation and to rule out other injuries. Surgical treatment is rarely necessary. Sequelae are focal and specific to the area of the brain that was injured. For example, an injury to the left temporal area may affect speech.

Intracranial Hematomas

Intracranial hematomas are space-occupying lesions that expand rapidly or slowly, depending on whether they are arterial or venous in origin. They must be located quickly. Some lesions require evacuation as soon as possible to minimize the secondary effects of the injury. See the clinical manifestations table below for information on cause, symptoms, and clinical therapy.

Penetrating Injuries

Gunshot wounds to the head can damage tissue, bone, and blood vessels. Low-velocity bullets enter but do not exit the skull; instead, they ricochet within the cranial vault, destroying brain tissue and blood vessels. Although the child may be conscious just after the injury, the level of consciousness quickly deteriorates because of the edema surrounding the penetration tract. High-velocity bullets, however, cause immediate, severe damage on impact. See Chapter 6 ∞ for a discussion of violence in childhood.

CT scans evaluate gunshot trauma and pinpoint the location of bullet and bone fragments as well as parenchymal damage. Treatment involves surgical debridement of the tract, evacuation of any hematomas, and removal of accessible bone or bullet particles. Approximately 50% of children with gunshot wounds to the head die. Those who survive may suffer multiple focal deficits and seizures.

CLINICAL MANIFESTATIONS	**INTRACRANIAL HEMATOMAS**	
Type of Hematoma	**Clinical Manifestations**	**Clinical Therapy**
Subdural Hematoma Result of high-velocity impact such as assaults, motor vehicle crashes, child abuse, or fall from considerable height Occurs most frequently in children less than 1 year old Inertial forces cause laceration of a bridging vein or an artery; a venous hematoma forms beneath the dura and presses directly on the brain	Symptoms (may not appear until 48–72 hours after the injury) include: • Loss of consciousness or progressive deterioration in mental status • Nausea or vomiting • Headache • Retinal hemorrhages in both eyes • Fixed and dilated pupil on side of injury • Hemiparesis • Seizures • Fever	• Diagnosis confirmed by CT scan • Treatment involves immediate craniotomy to evacuate the hematoma • Management of increased intracranial pressure; subdural taps may be necessary • Mortality rates range from 42–90%, and morbidity is also high (Dias, 2004) • Damage from the initial inertial injury is compounded by the hematoma
Epidural Hematoma Rare in children, especially those less than 4 years of age Results from blunt trauma (most often falls), motor vehicle crashes, assaults, or baseball to temporal area Temporal and parietal areas are most common sites May be associated with linear skull fracture Rapidly accumulating arterial or venous blood between the skull and the dura	Symptoms include: • Delayed onset, minimal or absent symptoms from initial impact • Rapid deterioration • Sleepiness or lethargy • Persistent and progressive headache • Full fontanel • Paresis of cranial nerves III and VI • Papilledema • Fixed and dilated pupil • Signs of increased intracranial pressure	• Diagnosis confirmed by CT scan • Treatment involves immediate craniotomy to evacuate the hematoma • Prognosis is generally good with mortality below 17% (Dias, 2004) • May be fatal if bleeding is arterial
Intracerebral Hematoma Result of deep contusion or intracerebral laceration (secondary to foreign body, bony penetration, or impalement) Causes diffuse bleeding in parenchyma; there may be a hematoma with associated small areas of bleeding	Symptoms depend upon the size and location of the hematoma, as well as if size is increasing due to uncontrolled bleeding • Altered consciousness • Signs of increased intracranial pressure	• Diagnosis confirmed by CT scan • Surgical treatment not indicated • Neurologic effects depend on size and location of lesion and whether bleeding can be controlled • Hemiplegia or visual loss may result

Impalement injuries frequently occur in children in association with lawn darts or dog bites. All objects must be left in place and removed in the operating room by a neurosurgeon. The child with an impalement injury is at high risk for focal injury and infection. After surgery, children with this type of injury are managed as with other postoperative head injuries, with attention focused on level of consciousness, increased intracranial pressure, and infection control.

Spinal Cord Injury

Children account for about 2–5% of all spinal cord injuries. Half of these injuries occur in the cervical area (Hayes & Arriola, 2005). Motor vehicle crashes are the leading cause of spinal cord injuries, either pedestrian-vehicular, bicycle-vehicular, passenger, or driver-related. Other causes of spinal injuries, especially in toddlers and young children, include falls and child abuse. Recreation or sports-related trauma accounts for more injuries as children grow older. Penetrating injuries such as stab and gunshot wounds are becoming more prevalent.

The mechanism of injury determines the type of lesion that occurs (Figure 26–21 ➤). Hyperflexion injuries (e.g., extreme bending as occurs with whiplash or around a lapbelt)

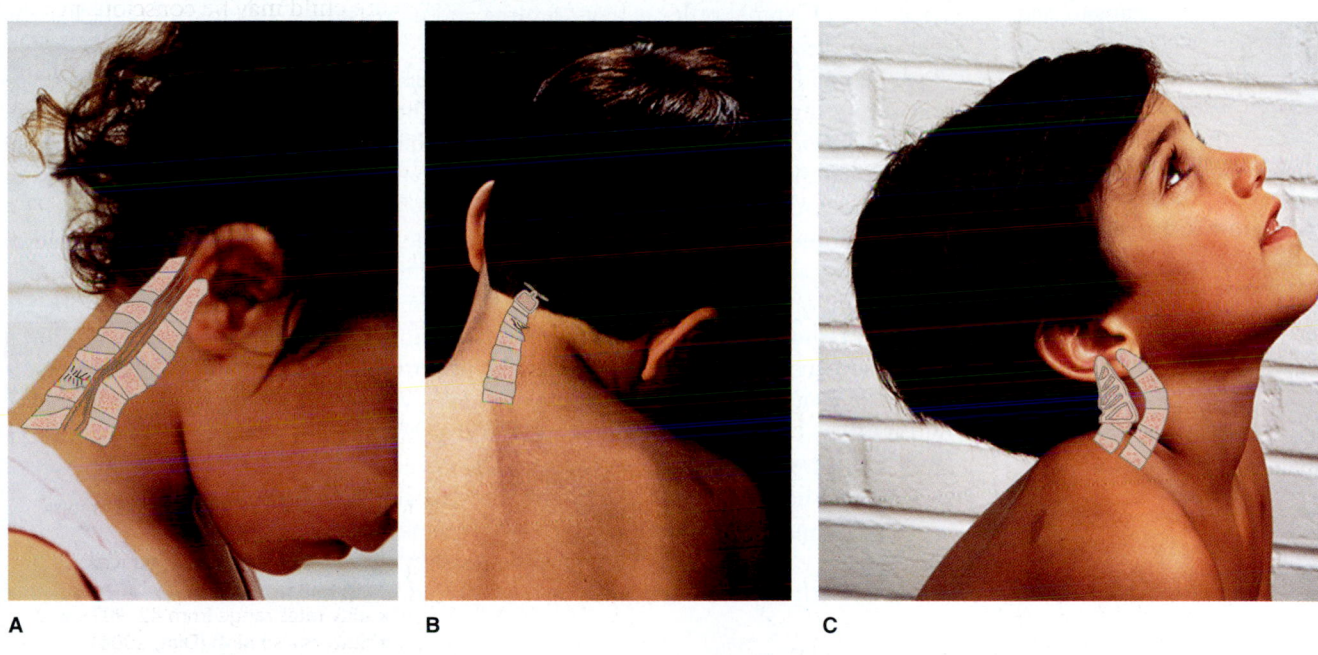

A   B   C

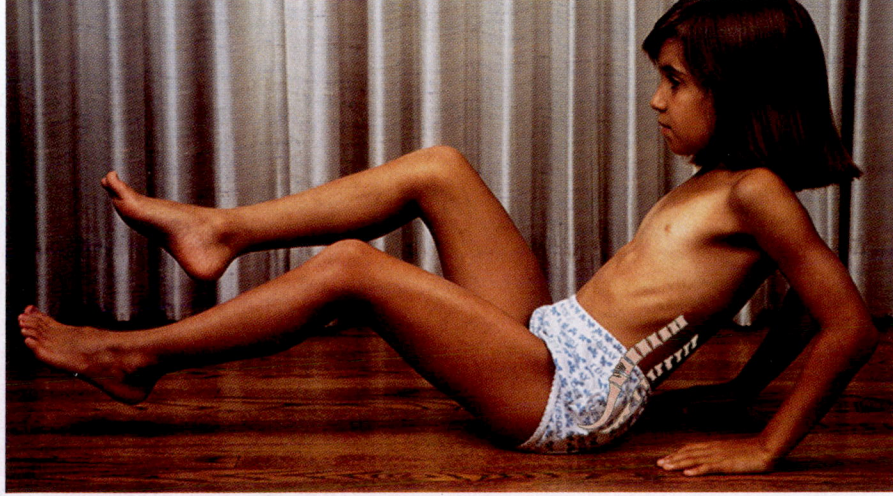

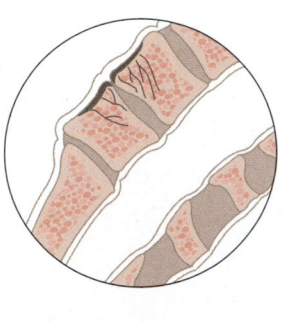

D

Figure 26–21 ➤ Mechanics of injury to the spinal cord. A, Hyperflexion. B, Lateral flexion. C, Extension. D, Compression.

produce tears or avulsions and fractures of vertebral bodies, as well as subluxation and dislocation. Lateral flexion (rotation) may cause joint dislocations or unstable spinal fractures. Extension may result in the so-called hangman's fracture, ligament tears, or avulsion fractures of vertebral bodies, as well as central or posterior spinal cord syndrome. Falling from a height may lead to a compression fracture. Children are prone to specific kinds of spinal cord injuries because of the extreme mobility and flexibility of their spinal column. Table 26–11 describes the spinal cord injuries most common in children.

Spinal cord injuries are classified as complete or incomplete. Complete lesions are irreversible and involve a loss of sensory, motor, and autonomic function below the level of the injury. Incomplete lesions involve varying degrees of sensory, motor, and autonomic function below the level of injury. The higher the level of spinal cord injury, the more severe the neurologic damage. The child is often a victim of multiple trauma and may display signs of hypovolemic shock resulting from other injuries, increased intracranial pressure, or respiratory depression.

At the time of injury, the child is flaccid and areflexic below the lesion. Children can experience spinal shock, in which the child has flaccidity and loss of reflexes, but some return of function occurs within the first 72 hours of injury. As neurologic recovery begins, spinal reflex activity returns and increasing spasticity is seen below the level of the lesion.

The child can also experience neurogenic shock in which there is loss of vasomotor tone and sympathetic innervation of the heart, resulting in hypotension, bradycardia, and peripheral vasodilation (see Chapter 21 ∞). Priapism (prolonged penile erection) may be present. Respiration may be compromised due to paralysis of the diaphragm.

Diagnosis is made by observation, neurologic examination, and radiologic studies (lateral cervical spine and anteroposterior and lateral views of the thoracic and lumbosacral spine). The child's immobilized position is unchanged until radiographs are read by a radiologist and the spine is declared uninjured. In addition, CT scanning, MRI, fluoroscopy, or myelography may be performed. Up to 20–30% of young children who have a spinal cord injury do not have evidence of radiographic abnormality (SCIWORA) because initial films or CT scans show no bony deformity (Dias, 2004). The child is believed to be free of injury; however, profound or progressive paralysis occurs immediately or within 48 hours. An MRI can detect the injury.

Spinal injuries are managed aggressively as the spinal injury extends upward 1 to 2 levels during the immediate hours and days after the injury (Hayes & Arriola, 2005). The child with a spinal cord injury may be placed in skeletal traction or a halo device.

Table 26–11	SPINAL CORD INJURIES IN CHILDREN
Spine Region	**Injury Characteristics**
Cervical region	• Site of 60% of spinal injuries in children through 10 years • Injury above C3 segment causes respiratory arrest and death without ventilator support; many injuries above this level are fatal • Diaphragm function is present when injury is at C5 level • Quadriplegia with some function of upper extremities when injury is at C6–C7 level • Loss of sphincter function, loss of sensation below sternum
Thoracic region	• Site of 20% of injuries, usually between 8 and 14 years • Full control of upper extremities including hands • Poor trunk balance
Thoracolumbar region	• Full control of muscles in abdomen and upper back • Good trunk balance
Lumbar region	• Most injuries occur at the L2 to L4 levels, probably as a result of improperly placed lap belts • Below L3 may have functioning of muscles of upper leg, loss of ankle and foot control

Surgery to reduce and internally fixate the fracture is performed for unstable fractures and dislocations. Decompression of the spinal cord and nerve roots may be performed if the transaction is not complete or if compression by a clot, herniated disk, or other lesion is present and can be relieved.

To decrease neurologic sequelae, methylprednisolone may be administered in high doses to children with motor deficits. Administration must be started within 8 hours of the injury. Gastrointestinal prophylaxis is provided to reduce the risk for an ulcer. Atropine and norepinephrine may be given to manage spinal shock. Pain is managed.

Complications of spinal cord injury include:

- Impaired respiratory function due to a paralyzed diaphragm or diminished vital capacity
- Scoliosis if injury occurs before the skeleton is mature
- Hip instability due to poor acetabular development
- Pathologic fractures of the long bones due to immobilization hypercalcemia
- Pressure sores
- Deep vein thrombosis
- Autonomic dysreflexia

Spasticity, muscle atrophy, increased risk of respiratory problems, weight gain, osteoporosis, and other skeletal problems are long-term issues for many children. An interdisciplinary approach is required to manage the rehabilitation and long-term care needs of the child and family. The goal of rehabilitation is to promote independence in daily activities, as well as mobility, strength, power, and endurance.

Nursing Management

HOSPITAL-BASED CARE   Nursing care focuses on monitoring vital signs, meeting nutritional needs, maintaining skin integrity, promoting independent functioning, encouraging therapeutic play, providing emotional support, and promoting rehabilitation.

Monitor vital signs and be alert for any changes, especially those that may signify increased respiratory difficulty or neurogenic shock (hypotension, bradycardia, and peripheral vasodilation), increased intracranial pressure (see Table 26–4), or autonomic dysreflexia. Monitor intake and output. Monitor bladder and bowel function.

Assess the cranial nerves as they may be affected by swelling around the spinal cord. Note the return of reflexes and change from flaccid tone to spasticity. Identify any changes in level of sensation or motor function.

Ensure adequate nutrition. A child with complete paralysis may require a gastrostomy tube. When the child begins to eat, feed soft foods slowly as the child may have some swallowing difficulties.

Prevent skin breakdown. See Chapter 30 ∞. Observe surgical sites for signs of infection or inflammation. Provide regular traction pin site care according to institutional guidelines.

Promote independent functioning by reinforcing the exercises and skills learned in physical and occupational therapy. Use supports, boots, footboards, splints, and braces as recommended by the therapists to prevent contractures (Figure 26–22 ➤). If hand mobility is limited, explore options for independence. Encourage the child to be as independent as possible in a wheelchair. An important mobility goal is to achieve wheelchair transfer and to perform self-care. Identify adaptive equipment that make these goals possible.

Achieving bowel and bladder control may be difficult, so, intermittent urinary catheterizations may be necessary. Anticipate that constipation will occur and initiate bowel training with a diet high in fiber and the use of stool softeners.

Therapeutic play appropriate for the child's developmental level is an important part of the healing process. Provide as many normal activities for the child as possible, but do not give the child tasks that he or she will have difficulty completing. Child-life teachers or tutors can help the child keep up with schoolwork. Television, videotapes, and music can offer diversion for prolonged hospitalization. Paraplegic children can learn to use their arms and hands to play interactive games.

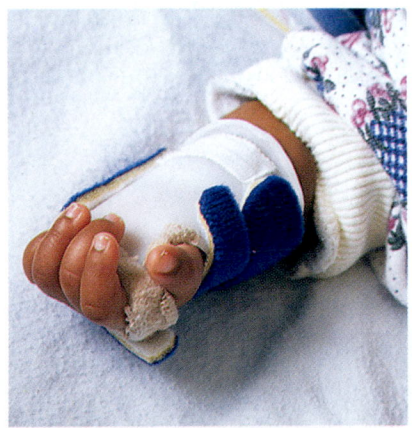

Figure 26–22 ➤ Splints are often used to prevent contractures, thus maintaining optimal functioning of the child's hands or feet.

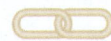

SKILL 13–1
Performing an Indwelling Urinary Catheterization

Devices can also be adapted so that the child can play video games or manipulate the television or radio.

Support the child emotionally. Encourage the child to meet small, short-term goals, including those that involve self-care. Encourage the child to express fears and frustrations.

Be compassionate and understanding. Encourage siblings to visit, answer their questions honestly, and help them to discuss their feelings. Involve the parents and siblings in the child's care as much as possible. When appropriate, encourage the family to help with activities of daily living.

DISCHARGE PLANNING AND HOME CARE TEACHING   Many children are discharged to inpatient rehabilitation facilities. Assist with arrangements for the transfer. Work closely with the child, parents, and other members of the healthcare team concerning placement. Home care needs, reintegration into educational programs, and safety issues should be identified and addressed well in advance of discharge from the rehabilitation facility. Refer families to social services, family counseling, and support groups, if indicated.

Hypoxic-Ischemic Brain Injury (Drowning and Near-Drowning)

Drowning is the process resulting in primary respiratory impairment from submersion/immersion in a liquid medium (Idris, Berg, Bierens et al., 2003). Drowning is the second leading cause of injury-related deaths in children between 1 and 14 years of age (National Center for Injury Prevention and Control, 2004). Children and adolescents under 19 years of age account for 34% (1158) of all drowning deaths in the United States (Burford, Ryan, Stone et al., 2005). Most drownings occur in fresh water such as ponds and residential swimming pools. Boys are more likely to die from drowning than girls.

A child can drown in as little water as it takes to cover the nose and mouth. The events preceding drowning follow a sequential pattern. The child trapped in water panics, struggles, tries to move using swimming motions, and holds his or her breath. Then the child aspirates a small amount of water from the oropharynx, which triggers an involuntary laryngospasm, leading to hypoxia. The child subsequently swallows more water. As the laryngospasm passes, the child breathes water into the lungs. The child may vomit and aspirate stomach contents as well. Aspirated water damages the surfactant in the lungs and impairs the capillary gas exchange in the alveoli. As the arterial oxygen saturation falls, the cardiac output decreases, and hypoxia, hypercarbia, and respiratory acidosis develop (Zuckerbraun & Saladino, 2005). Hypothermia may result because the child's body cools more quickly in water than air, and systemic perfusion decreases as a result. See Chapter 30 ∞ for information on hypothermia. As the child becomes progressively more hypoxic, the cardiac muscle becomes impaired and ultimately the heart stops.

Anoxia is the major insult associated with drowning. Anoxia leads to cerebral edema and increased intracranial pressure. Little can be done to resuscitate the brain, but with aggressive cardiopulmonary resuscitation, more severely brain-injured children are surviving in a permanent vegetative state. When the child is resuscitated, the damaged lungs with inactivated surfactant lead to the development of pulmonary edema, acute respiratory distress syndrome, and pneumonia.

The child who has been immersed exhibits a wide variety of signs and symptoms depending on the length of time underwater, the temperature of the water, the response to the episode, and the initial treatment performed at the scene. Children submerged for short periods (less than 5 to 10 minutes who are resuscitated at the scene) have few symptoms and often fully recover without neurologic impairment. The child who is submerged longer than 25 minutes will likely die or have severe neurologic impairment (Zuckerbraun & Saladino, 2005). Signs and symptoms of the rescued child may be decreased level of consciousness ranging from stupor to total unresponsiveness, apnea or irregular respirations, gastric distention, and seizures.

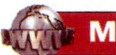

MediaLink

Spinal Cord Injury Resources

GROWTH & DEVELOPMENT

Drowning Age and Location

Between 40–50% of children injured in drowning incidents are under 4 years of age, with peak incidence between ages 1 and 2 years. The majority (78%) of infant drownings are in bathtubs. The most common drowning locations for children 1 to 4 years old are artificial pools (56%). Among children 5 years and older, 63% of drownings occur in natural bodies of fresh water (Zuckerbraun & Saladino, 2005).

Medical intervention begins at the scene of the drowning with immediate ventilation and compressions, when indicated. The sooner CPR is started, the better the child's prognosis. Children still requiring CPR upon arrival at the emergency department are most likely to die or have a significant neurologic impairment (American Academy of Pediatrics, 2003). If the child is severely hypothermic (less than 30°C), active and passive rewarming actions are used during resuscitation. The child is often intubated to prevent aspiration and to provide positive pressure ventilation with supplemental oxygen. An orogastric tube is used to decompress the stomach. Antibiotics are prescribed only if an infection develops unless the water was grossly contaminated.

All surviving drowning victims should be admitted to the hospital for at least 24 hours or observed in a short-stay observation unit for several hours, even when asymptomatic. Many life-threatening complications, including respiratory distress and cerebral edema, may not become evident for at least 12 hours after the incident. Approximately 10% of surviving drowning victims have severe neurologic impairments (Burford, Ryan, Stone et al., 2005).

Nursing Management

Nursing care of the child who survives a drowning incident focuses on monitoring the child's neurologic and cardiopulmonary status and providing emotional support to the family.

Monitor the child's responsiveness, spontaneous respiratory efforts, oxygenation, and pulse. Check the pupils for reactivity. The child should be monitored for signs of complications such as respiratory distress and worsening mental status. Administer prescribed medications and position the child properly. Other nursing interventions, especially for the comatose child, can be found in the earlier discussion of altered states of consciousness.

Provide emotional support to the family. Be nonjudgmental and allow parents to express their feelings. Reassure parents who exhibit guilt reactions that their child is receiving all possible medical treatment. Parents often face an unknown prognosis. See Chapter 14 ∞. Encourage them to seek assistance from social workers, members of the clergy, close friends, and relatives. Arrange for appropriate referrals.

Identify and address home care needs well in advance of discharge. Assist with arrangements for the child with minor deficits. Help the parents decide whether the comatose child will go home or to a long-term care facility.

Drowning can be prevented by education, legislation, and changes in the environment. Infants and toddlers should not be left unattended in a bathtub. Pool owners should erect climb-proof 5-foot fences around all *four* sides of the pool to reduce access to the pool by young children. Local ordinances may require such fences. Pool owners should learn CPR so that immediate resuscitation can begin if a child is found submerged. Adolescents should learn the dangers of mixing alcohol and swimming. Five- and 10-gallon buckets should be kept empty when not in use. Emphasize the importance of closely supervising children when near or in the water, whether at pools, at the beach, or in the bathtub.

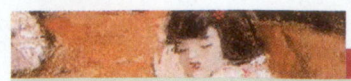

CRITICAL THINKING IN ACTION

Recall Antwan, who experienced a severe traumatic brain injury due to being struck by a car. After 7 days in the intensive care unit, he has been moved to a general care floor. He is still not fully conscious, but quiets when his parents speak to him. He is moving all extremities, but he does not yet follow commands. Antwan will need a rehabilitation program to promote an optimal outcome for his injury and anticipated disabilities.

1. Describe the pathophysiology that could account for Antwan's prolonged diminished responsiveness.

2. Identify age-appropriate sensory stimulation strategies that may help promote Antwan's awareness and improvement in level of consciousness.

3. Describe the neurologic nursing assessment that should be performed on Antwan at regular intervals on the general care unit.

4. Develop a nursing care plan for Antwan, taking into account his diminished responsiveness. Be sure to address nutrition, hydration, and care needs associated with immobility.

 Refer to your Prentice Hall Nursing MediaLink DVD-ROM for answers.

EXPLORE MediaLink 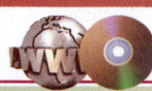 http://www.prenhall.com/ball

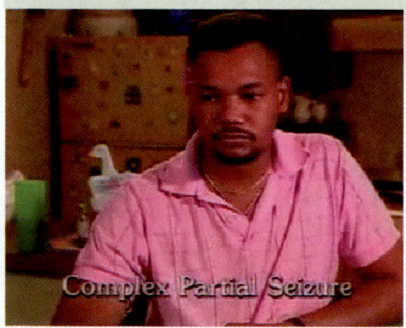

Complex Partial Seizure

Resources for this chapter can be found on the Prentice Hall Nursing MediaLink DVD-ROM accompanying this textbook, and on the Companion Website at http://www.prenhall.com/ball.

DVD-ROM
Audio Glossary
NCLEX-RN® Review
Animations/Videos
  Coup-Contracoup Injury
  Status Epilepticus
  Types of Seizures

COMPANION WEBSITE
Audio Glossary
NCLEX-RN® Review
Care Plan Activity: Care Map
Case Study: Assessing a Child with a Concussion for Return to Competitive Play
MediaLink Application: Reye's Syndrome
WebLinks

REFERENCES

Adekoya, N., Thurman, D. J., White, D. D., & Webb, K. W. (2002). Surveillance for traumatic brain deaths—United States, 1989–1998. *Morbidity and Mortality Weekly Report, 51*(SS-10), 1–14.

Adelson, P. D., Bratton, S. L., Carney, N. A., Chestnut, R. A., duCoudray, H. E. M., Goldstein, B., and others. (2003). Threshhold for treatment of intracranial hypotension: Guidelines for management of severe traumatic brain injury. *Pediatric Critical Care Medicine, 4*(3 Supp), S25–S27.

American Academy of Pediatrics Committee on Infectious Disease. (2006). *Red book: Report of the Committee on Infectious Disease* (27th ed.), Elk Grove Village, IL: Author.

American Academy of Pediatrics Committee on Injury, Violence, and Poison Prevention. (2003). Prevention of drowning in infants, children, and adolescents. *Pediatrics, 112*(2), 440–445.

Ancel, P. Y., Livinec, F., Larroque, B., Marret, S., Arnaud, C., Pierrat, V., et al. (2006). Cerebral palsy among very preterm children in relation to gestational age and neonatal ultrasound abnormalities: The EPAPAGE cohort study. *Pediatrics, 117*(3), 828–835.

Austin, J., Dunn, D., Huster, G., & Rose, D. (1998). Development of scales to measure psychosocial care needs of children with seizures and their parents. *Journal of Neuroscience Nursing, 30*(3), 155–160.

Black, S., Shinefield, H., Baxter, R., Austrian, R., Bracken, L., et al. (2004). Postlicensure surveillance for pneumococcal invasive disease after use of pneumococcal conjugate vaccine in Northern California Kaiser Permanente. *Pediatric Infectious Disease Journal, 23*(6), 485–489.

Blackman, J. A. (2005). Severe brain injury: Helping patient and family on the long road back. *Contemporary Pediatrics, 22*(1), 63–78.

Blair, J., & Selekman, J. (2004). Epilepsy. In P. J. Allen & J. A. Vessey (Eds.), *Primary care of the child with a chronic condition* (4th ed., pp. 469–497). St. Louis: Mosby.

Boss, B. J. (2006). Alterations in neurologic function. In K. L. McCance & S. E. Huether, *Pathophysiology: The biologic basis for disease in adults and children* (5th ed., pp. 547–622). St. Louis: Elsevier Mosby.

Buck, M. L. (2003). Clinical applications for botulinum toxin type A in pediatric patients. *Pediatric Pharmacology, 9*(3), Retrieved April 18, 2003, from http://www.medscape.com/viewarticle/451626

Burford, A. E., Ryan, L. M., Stone, B. J., Hirshon, J. M., & Klein, B. L. (2005). Drowning and near-drowning in children and adolescents. *Pediatric Emergency Care, 21*(9), 610–616.

Campbell, S. (2003). Prenatal cocaine exposure and neonatal/infant outcomes. *Neonatal Network, 22*(1), 19–21.

Centers for Disease Control. (2005). Guillain-Barré syndrome among adolescents who received meningococcal conjugate vaccine. Retrieved April 11, 2006 from http://www.cdc.gov/nip/vacsafe/concerns/gbs/gbs-menactra-facts.pdf

Centers for Disease Control. (2006). What is traumatic brain injury? Retrieved March 3, 2006 from http://www.cdc.gov/ncipc/tbi/TBI.htm

Chávez-Bueno, S., & McCracken, G. H. (2005). Bacterial meningitis in children. *Pediatric Clinics of North America, 52*, 795–810.

Cobb, S., & Battin, B. (2004). Second-impact syndrome. *Journal of School Nursing, 20*(5), 262–267.

Coronado, V. G., Johnson, R. L., Faul, M., & Kegler, S. R. (2006). Incidence rates of hospitalization related to traumatic brain injury—12 states, 2002. *Morbidity and Mortality Weekly Report, 55*(08), 201–204.

Danielpour, M., & Peacock, W. J. (2000). Epilepsy surgery in children. *Clinical Neurosurgery, 47*, 400–421.

Dias, M. S. (2004). Acute traumatic brain and spinal cord injury. *Pediatric Clinics of North America, 51*, 271–303.

Ditmyer, S. (2004). Hydrocephalus. In P. J. Allen & J. A. Vessey (Eds.), *Primary care of the child with a chronic condition* (4th ed., pp. 543–560). St. Louis: Mosby.

Erickson, D. V., & Ray, L. D. (2004). Children with chronic continence problems: The challenges for families. *Journal of Wound and Ostomy Care Nursing, 31*(4), 215–222.

Fadiman, A. (1997). *The spirit catches you and you fall down.* New York: Farrar, Strauss, Giroux.

Fisher, P. G. (2005). Help for headaches: A strategy for your busy practice. *Contemporary Pediatrics, 22*(11), 34–40.

Frankel, L. R., & Mathers, L. H. (2004). Withdrawal or withholding of life support, brain death, and organ procurement. In R. E. Behrman, R. M. Kliegman, & H. B. Jepson, *Nelson textbook of pediatrics* (17th ed., pp. 340–342). Philadelphia: Saunders.

Freeman, J. M. (2003). What every pediatrician should know about the ketogenic diet, *Contemporary Pediatrics, 20*(5), 113–127.

Gill, J. K., & Gieron-Korthals, M. (2002). What pediatricians—and parents—need to know about febrile convulsions. *Contemporary Pediatrics, 19*(5), 139–144.

Goldstein, J. L. (2004). Evaluating new onset seizures in children. *Pediatric Annals, 33*(6), 368–374.

Graham, J. M., Gomez, M., Halberg, A., Earl, D. L., Kreutzman, J. T., Cui, J., & Guo, X. (2005). Management of deformational plagiocephaly: Repositioning versus orthotic therapy. Journal of Pediatrics, 146(2), 258–262.

Graham, J. M., Kreutzman, J., Earl, D., Halberg, A., Samayoa, C., & Guo, X. (2005). Deformational brachycephaly in supine-sleeping infants. *Journal of Pediatrics, 146*(2), 253–257.

Gray, E. H., Blackinton, J., & White, G. M. (2006). Stoma care in the school setting. *Journal of School Nursing, 22*(2), 74–80.

Guskiewicz, K. M., & McCrea, M. (2003). Increased recovery time with multiple sports-related traumatic brain injuries. *Journal of the American Medical Association, 290*, 2549–2563.

Hart, L. (2005). Primary care for patients with neurofibromatosis 1. *The Nurse Practitioner, 30*(6), 38–43.

Hayes, J. S., & Arriola, T. (2005). Pediatric spinal injuries. *Pediatric Nursing, 31*(6), 464–467.

Hightower, S., Carmon, M., & Minick, P. (2002). A qualitative descriptive study of the lived experiences of school-aged children with epilepsy. *Journal of Pediatric Health Care, 16*(3), 131–137.

Idris, A. H., Berg, R., Bierens, J., Bossaert, L., Branche, C., Gabrielli, A., et al. (2003). Recommended guidelines for uniform reporting of data from drowning: The "Utstein style." *Circulation, 108*, 2565–2574.

Johnston, M. V., Ferriero, D. M., Vannucci, S. J., & Hagberg, H. (2005). Models of cerebral palsy: Which ones are best? *Journal of Child Neurology, 20*(12), 984–987.

Johnston, M. V., & Kinsman, S. (2004a). Craniosynostosis. In R. E. Behrman, R. M. Kliegman, & H. B. Jepson, *Nelson textbook of pediatrics* (17th ed., pp. 1992–1993). Philadelphia: Saunders.

Johnston, M. V. & Kinsman, S. (2004b). Hydrocephalus. In R. E. Behrman, R. M. Kliegman, & H. B. Jepson, *Nelson textbook of pediatrics* (17th ed., pp. 1989–1992). Philadelphia: Saunders.

Johnston, M. V., & Kinsman, S. (2004c). Microcephaly. In R. E. Behrman, R. M. Kliegman, & H. B. Jepson, *Nelson textbook of pediatrics* (17th ed., pp. 1988–1989). Philadelphia: Saunders.

Jonas, R., Nguyen, S., Hu, B., Asarnow, R. F., LoPresti, C., Curtiss, S., et al. (2004). Cerebral hemispherectomy: Hospital course, seizure, developmental, language, and motor outcomes. *Neurology, 62*(10), 1712–1721.

Keenan, H. T., Runyan, D. K., Marshall, S. W., Nocera, M. A., & Merten, D. F. (2004). A population-based comparison of clinical and outcome characteristics of young children with serious inflicted and noninflicted traumatic brain injury. *Pediatrics, 114*(3), 633–639.

Kennedy, C. S., & Moffatt, M. (2004). Acute traumatic brain injury in children: Exploring the cutting edge in understanding, therapy, and research. *Clinical Pediatric Emergency Medicine, 5*, 224–238.

Kirkwood, M. W., Yeates, K. O., & Wilson, P. E. (2006). Pediatric sports-related concussion: A review of the clinical management of an oft-neglected population. *Pediatrics, 117*(4), 1359–1371.

Kossoff, E. H., & Mankad, D. N. (2006). Medication-overuse headache in children: Is initial preventive therapy necessary? *Journal of Child Neurology, 21*(1), 45–48.

Kossoff, E. H., Pyzik, P. L., McGrogan, J. R., Vining, E. P. G., & Freeman, J. M. (2002). Efficacy of the ketogenic diet for infantile spasms. *Pediatrics, 109*(5), 780–783.

Kuehne, E. A., & Reilly, M. W. (2004). Prenatal cocaine exposure. In P. Allen, & J. A. Vessey, (Eds.), *Primary care of the child with a chronic condition* (4th ed., pp.708–721). St. Louis: Mosby.

Lazzaretti, C. C., & Pearson, C. (2004). Myelodysplasia. In P. J. Allen & J. A. Vessey (Eds.), *Primary care of the child with a chronic condition* (4th ed., pp. 630–643). St. Louis: Mosby.

Lewis, D., Ashwal, S., Hershey, A., Hirtz, D., Yonker, M., & Silberstein, S. (2004). Practice parameter: Pharmacologic treatment of migraine headache in children and adolescents. *Neurology, 63*(12), 2215–2224.

Lewis, D. W., Scott, D., & Rendin, V. (2002). Treatment of pediatric headache. *Expert Opinion in Pharmacotherapeutics, 3*(10), 1433–1441.

Lewis, P., & Glaser, C. A. (2005). Encephalitis. *Pediatrics in Review, 26*(10), 353–362.

Liptak, G. S. (2002). Neural tube defects. In M. L. Batshaw (Ed.), *Children with disabilities* (5th ed., pp. 467–492). Baltimore: Paul H. Brookes Publishing Co.

Liptak, G. S., & Accardo, P. J. (2004). Health and social outcomes of children with cerebral palsy. *Journal of Pediatrics, 145*(Suppl.), S36–S41.

Lovell, M. R., Collins, M. W., Iverson, G. L., Field, M., Maroon, J. C., et al. (2003). Recovery from mild concussion in high school athletes. *Journal of Neurosurgery, 98*(2), 296–301.

Marin, S. (2005). The impact of epilepsy on the adolescent. *Maternal Child Nursing, 30*(5), 321–326.

McKearnan, K. A., Kieckhefer, G. M., Engel, J. M., Jensen, M. P., & Labyak, S. (2004). Pain in children with cerebral palsy: A review. *Journal of Neuroscience Nursing, 36*(5), 252–259.

McNelis, A., Musick, B., Austin, J., Dunn, D., & Creasy, K. (1998). Psychosocial care needs of children with new-onset seizures. *Journal of Neuroscience Nursing, 30*(3), 161–165.

Millichap, J. G., & Yee, M. M. (2003). The diet factor in pediatric and adolescent migraine. *Pediatric Neurology, 28*(1), 9–15.

Nakagawa, T. A., & Conway, E. E. (2004). Shaken baby syndrome: Recognizing and responding to a lethal danger. *Contemporary Pediatrics, 21*(3), 37–57.

National Center for Injury Prevention and Control. (2004). 10 leading causes of injury deaths, United States 2000–2002, all races, both sexes. Retrieved August 24, 2005, from http://webapp.cdc.gov/cgi-bin/broker.exe

Nehring, W. M. (2004). Cerebral palsy. In P. J. Allen & J. A. Vessey (Eds.), *Primary care of the child with a chronic condition* (4th ed., pp. 327–346). St. Louis, MO: Mosby.

Nehring, W. M., & Faux, S. A. (2006). Transitional and health issues of adults with neural tube defects. *Journal of Nursing Scholarship, 38*(1), 63–70.

Northrup, H., & Volcik, K. A. (2000). Spina bifida and other neural tube defects. *Current Problems in Pediatrics, 30*(10), 317–331.

Padgett, K. (2006). Alterations in neurologic function in children. In K. L. McCance & S. E. Huether, *Pathophysiology: The biologic basis for disease in adults and children* (5th ed., pp. 623–681). St. Louis: Elsevier Mosby.

Pelligrino, L. (2002). Cerebral palsy. In M. L. Batshaw (Ed.), Children with disabilities (5th ed., pp. 443–466). Baltimore: Paul H. Brooks Publishing Co.

Powers, S. W., & Andrasik, F. (2005). Biobehavioral treatment, disability, and psychological effects of pediatric headache. *Pediatric Annals, 34*(6), 461–465.

Prober, C. G. (2004). Central nervous system infections. In R. E. Behrman, R. M. Kliegman, & H. B. Jepson, *Nelson textbook of pediatrics* (17th ed., pp. 2038–2047). Philadelphia: Saunders.

Quality Standards Subcommittee, American Academy of Neurology. (1997). Practice parameters: The management of concussion in sports. *Neurology, 48*, 581–585.

Reimschisel, T. (2003). Breaking the cycle of medication overuse headache. *Contemporary Pediatrics, 20*(10), 101–114.

Rosman, N. P. (1999) Acute head trauma. In J. A. McMillan, C. D. DeAngelis, R. D. Feigin, & J. B. Warshaw (Eds.), *Oski's pediatrics:*

Principles and practice (3rd ed., pp. 603–617). Philadelphia: Lippincott, Williams, & Wilkins.

Rubenstein, J. E., Kossoff, E. H., Pyzik, P. L., Vining, E. P. G., McGrogan, J. R., & Freeman, J. M. (2005). Experience in the use of the ketogenic diet as early therapy. *Journal of Child Neurology, 20*(1), 31–34.

Rudy, C. (2005). Hydrocephalus. *Journal of Pediatric Health Care, 19*(2), 111, 127–128.

Sankar, R. (2004). Initial treatment of epilepsy with antiepileptic drugs. *Neurology, 63*(Suppl 4), S30–S39.

Sarnat, H. B. (2004). Guillain-Barré syndrome. In R. E. Behrman, R. M. Kliegman, & H. B. Jepson, *Nelson textbook of pediatrics* (17th ed., pp. 2080–2081). Philadelphia: Saunders.

Schiller, C., & Allen, P. J., (2005). Follow-up of infants prenatally exposed to cocaine. *Pediatric Nursing, 31*(5), 427–436.

Shinnar, S., & O'Dell, C. (2004). Febrile seizures. *Pediatric Annals, 33*(6), 394–401.

Simpkins, C. J. (2005). Ventriculoperitoneal shunt infections in patients with hydrocephalus. *Pediatric Nursing, 31*(6), 457–462.

Spector, R. E. (2000). *Cultural diversity in health and illness* (5th ed., p. 71). Upper Saddle River, NJ: Prentice Hall Health.

Steinmetz, M. P., Lechner, R. M., & Anderson, J. S. (2003). Atlantooccipital dislocation in children: Presentation, diagnosis, and management. *Neurosurgery Focus, 14*(2). Retrieved March 11, 2003, from http://www.medscape.com/viewarticle/449884_print

Stevenson, K. L. (2004). Chiari type II malformations: Past, present, future.

Neurosurgical Focus, 16(2). Retrieved March 25, 2004, from http://www.medscape,com/viewarticle/470602_print

Substance Abuse and Mental Health Services Administration, Office of Applied Statistics. (2005). Substance use during pregnancy: 2002 and 2003 update. Retrieved April 24, 2006 from http://www.samsha.gov/2k5/pregnancy/pregnancy.pdf

Teasdale, G., & Jennett, B. (1974). Assessment of coma and impaired consciousness. *Lancet, 2*, 81–84; and James, H. E. (1986). Neurologic evaluation and support in the child with acute brain insult. *Pediatric Annals, 15*(1), 16–22.

Theye, F., & Mueller, K. A. (2004). Heads up: Concussions in high school sports. *Clinical Medicine and Research, 2*(3), 165–171.

Vajsar, J., Fehlings, D., & Stephens, D. (2003). Long-term outcome in children with Guillain-Barré syndrome. *Journal of Pediatrics, 142*(3), 305–309.

Van Eerden, P., & Bernstein, P. S. (2003). Summary of the publications, "Neonatal encephalopathy and cerebral palsy: Defining the pathogenesis and pathophysiology" by the ACOG Task Force on Neonatal Encephalopathy and Cerebral Palsy. *Medscape OB/GYN & Women's Health, 8*(2) Retrieved July 10, 2003, from http://www.medscape.com/viewarticle/457882_

Virdis, R., Street, M. E., Bandello, M. A., Tripodi, C., Donadio, A., Villani, A. R., Cagozzi,

L., Garavelli, L., & Bernasconi, S. (2003). Growth and pubertal disorders in neurofibromatosis type 1. *Journal of Pediatric Endocrinology Metabolism, 16*(Supp 2), 289–292.

Weinstein, S. (2002). Epilepsy. In M. L. Batshaw (Ed.), *Children with disabilities* (5th ed., pp. 493–523). Baltimore, MD: Paul H. Brookes Publishing Co.

Wheless, J. W. (2004). Treatment of status epilepticus in children. *Pediatric Annals, 33*(6), 376–383.

Williams, L. J., Rasmussen, S. A., Flores, A., Kirby, R. S., & Edmonds, L. D. (2005). Decline in the prevalence of spina bifida and anencephaly by race/ethnicity: 1995–2002. *Pediatrics, 116*(3), 580–586.

Yassari, R., & Frim, D. (2004). Evaluation and management of the Chiari malformation type 1 for the primary care pediatrician. *Pediatric Clinics of North America, 51*, 477–490.

Youngblut, J. M., Brooten, D., & Kuluz, J. (2005). Parents' reactions at 24–48 hours after a preschool child's head injury. *Pediatric Critical Care Medicine, 6*(5), 550–556.

Zickler, C. F., & Richardson, V. (2004). Achieving continence in children with neurogenic bowel and bladder. *Journal of Pediatric Health Care, 18*(6), 276–283.

Zuckerbraun, N. S., & Saladino, R. A. (2005). Pediatric drowning: Current management strategies for immediate care. *Clinical Pediatric Emergency Medicine, 6*, 49–56.

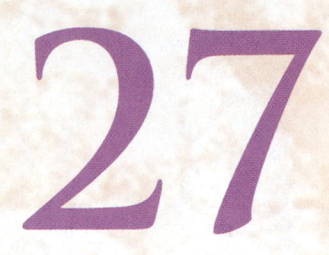

ALTERATIONS in MENTAL HEALTH and COGNITION

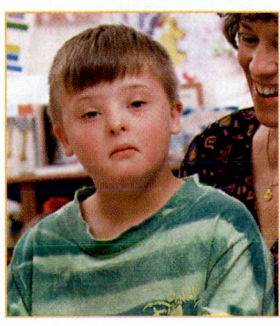

JEREMIAH, a 7-year-old boy with Down syndrome, enjoys attending his special education classroom. Jeremiah is the youngest of four children and was born after an unplanned pregnancy to a mother and father in their forties. Their youngest child at that time was 12 years of age. Although they accepted that they would have another child, Jeremiah's parents learned after an amniocentesis during the pregnancy that their son had Down syndrome. His parents progressed through stages of shock, denial, anger, and sadness. Thanks to a strong support system, they soon learned more about Down syndrome, resolved their grief, and grew to love their infant son. The siblings loved their new brother and seemed to have little trouble accepting the fact that he was different from their original expectations.

During infancy, Jeremiah developed gastroesophageal reflux and frequent otitis media. Since his parents had adequate health care, they were able to seek assistance as needed. When he was almost a year of age, the family enrolled Jeremiah in an early intervention program. He was about 4 months behind in developmental milestone achievement, but through the intervention program he quickly gained fine and gross motor skills. He eventually progressed from the early intervention program to preschool, and recently began attending a special education classroom. The school nurse has worked with the family to review Jeremiah's transport to school, provide information about obtaining and wearing an alert identification bracelet, and monitor his health status in school.

KEY TERMS

adaptive
  functioning **1138**
affect **1136**
agoraphobia **1127**
anhedonia **1121**
behavior
  modification
  1104
cognitive therapy
  1104
coprolalia **1135**
copropraxia **1135**
developmental
  disability **1138**

echolalia **1109**
evidence-based
  practice **1103**
learning disabilities
  1137
mental retardation
  1138
pervasive
  developmental
  disorders (PDDS)
  1108
play therapy **1104**
stereotypy **1109**

MediaLink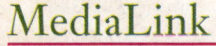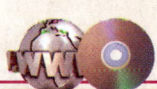

http://www.prenhall.com/ball

See the Prentice Hall Nursing MediaLink DVD-ROM and Companion Website for chapter-specific resources.

LEARNING OUTCOMES

After reading this chapter, you will be able to do the following:

1. Define mental health and describe major mental health disruptions in childhood.

2. Discuss the clinical manifestations of the major mental health disorders of childhood and adolescence.

3. Plan for the nursing management of children and adolescents with mental health disruptions in the hospital and community settings.

4. Describe characteristics of common cognitive disorders of childhood.

5. Plan nursing management for children with cognitive disorders.

6. Establish and evaluate expected outcomes of care for the child with a cognitive disorder.

FOCUS ON
Mental Health and Cognition

PEDIATRIC DIFFERENCES IN BIOPSYCHOLOGICAL INFLUENCES AND FUNCTIONING

Some mental health and cognitive conditions in children originate from a genetic or physiologic cause. Examples include mental retardation and childhood schizophrenia. Often the family and surrounding environments in which children live influence their characteristics and contribute to dysfunctions such as anxiety, depression, and post-traumatic stress disorder. A unique and challenging interplay of genetics and environments influence mental health and cognitive conditions, making diagnosis and treatment challenging.

Children differ from adults both in mental healthcare needs and in the types and progression of mental health disruptions. During childhood, the necessity for bonding and attachment to significant adults forms the cornerstone of the child's healthy mental development. Therefore, young children rely on adults for establishment of mental health. The child's unique genetic makeup couples with these environmental factors, thereby contributing to a state of mental health. Cognitive disorders are also a result of a unique interplay of genetic and environmental causes. The brain develops from the fetal neural tube early in development, with much critical embryology occurring in the fourth to sixth week of gestation (Chamley, Carson, Randall, et al., 2005), at which point many women don't even know they are pregnant. During this time, the brain is not protected by the blood-brain barrier and is at risk for injury from the fetal environment. Environmental conditions such as maternal alcohol ingestion or intake of certain medications can influence the developing fetus's brain.

DIAGNOSTIC PROCEDURES FOR MENTAL HEALTH AND COGNITION

Diagnostic Test	Purpose	Nursing Implications
Magnetic resonance imaging (MRI)	MRI uses a large magnet and radio waves delivered to the body part to be imaged. The energy field produced can be transferred as a visual image to the computer. It is used to image the brain in cases when a structural defect is believed to be causing mental health or cognitive alterations.	• Prepare the child for the procedure, including the size of equipment, sounds, time, and tunnel. • Ensure that the child has no metallic objects or implants and is not connected to metal equipment. • Use sedation for young children, if needed, to ensure that they are still for the procedure; monitor the child with sedation according to guidelines.
Radiograph (x-ray)	Radiographs use irradiation to obtain images and capture them on film for diagnosis and screening. They are not commonly used for mental health or cognitive alterations, but a radiograph fluorescence study may help to diagnose lead in bones (lead poisoning can cause mental retardation).	• Explain the procedure to the child. • Tell the child about the need to hold still for the procedure. Have the child practice holding a breath while being still. • Note that radiopaque materials for tests such as GI studies and IVP administered within 3 days of radiograph may distort images.
Toxicology screening	A variety of blood and urine tests may assist in diagnosing the child who is exposed to toxic substances that are altering mental status and cognition. Examples include alcohol, cocaine, barbiturates, opioids, and environmental contaminants.	• Prepare the child. • Perform the test in a treatment room rather than the child's hospital room or clinic examination room. • Label and transport specimens according to policy.

Data from: Corbett, J. V. (2004). *Laboratory tests and diagnostic procedures with nursing diagnoses* (6th ed.). Upper Saddle River, NJ: Prentice Hall Health.

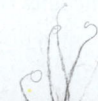

In addition, children with mental health disruptions sometimes display different clinical manifestations for mental illness than adults; therefore, diagnosis is difficult and challenging. For example, a child with a tic syndrome may be mistakenly diagnosed as hyperactive, and the treatment therefore would not be appropriate to the underlying condition. Overall, about one in four or five children and adolescents has a mental health disorder, and 1 in 10 has a disorder that profoundly interferes with daily functioning. However, only 20–30% of these children receive mental health services (Melnyk, Brown, Jones et al., 2003; National Institute for Health Care Management Foundation, 2005).

At birth the brain makes up about 25% of body weight; this percentage decreases to about 2% of weight by adulthood. Most of the brain structure is present at birth, but during the first 5 years of life the brain continues to develop and mature as the young child gains fine and gross motor, social, and language skills. Development and differentiation occurs during childhood spurts with fine motor skills improvement and during adolescent years when perception, motor function, and advanced thinking processes further develop (Chamley, Carson, Randall, et al., 2005). The child remains vulnerable to external forces during periods of brain growth and development. The influence of drugs, poor nutrition, traumatic brain injury, and absence of emotional nurturance are all examples of factors that can interfere with healthly brain and cognitive development.

Examples of diagnostic and laboratory tests used for mental health and cognition are provided in the accompanying table. Use the guidelines below to perform a nursing assessment of the child with a mental health or cognitive alteration.

ASSESSMENT GUIDELINES FOR THE CHILD WITH AN ALTERATION IN MENTAL HEALTH OR COGNITION

Assessment Focus	Assessment Guidelines
History	• Describe prenatal care and problems. Was there any trauma at birth? • Is there a diagnosed mental health disorder in the child or other family members? • Is there a history of any neurological injuries or diseases? • What medications is the child taking?
Growth	• Is growth progressing along the same channel or growth percentile?
Development	• Perform regular developmental screening to identify any variations from expected developmental milestones. Further testing is required if screening suggests any abnormalities. • What is the progression of skills reported by the family? • Are there any unusual capabilities or deficits? • Inquire about progression in school and extracurricular activities.
Social skills	• Describe the relationship between the child and significant adults. Is close attachment evident? Are there signs of attachment disorders such as lack of eye contact, smiles, or response to others in the environment? • Describe the school-age child's daily schedule, including family and peer activities. Does the child have friends and engage in several activities with them on a regular basis? Does the child generally interact well with others? Has the child recently had a change in school performance? • Have the teen describe daily activities and friends. Is there a combination of peer and family influence on personal decision making?
Affect	• Describe facial expression and response to nurse. • Observe body size, position, and posture. • Are interaction behaviors typical for the setting and age of the child? • Does the child display interest in surroundings? • Is the child dressed in an appropriate manner? Does the child establish eye contact?
Appearance	• Is the child's clothing appropriate for age, setting, and developmental level?
Behaviors	• Describe level of consciousness and interaction with surroundings. • Inquire about recent reported changes in behavior (e.g., sleep, eating patterns, communication with others, school performance, friendships, risky activities). • Are problem behaviors identified by the child or parent? • Are there particular events that were associated with problem behaviors?
Life events	• Has the child or family experienced recent stress or trauma? • Has there been any changes in family structure? • Evaluate chronic health conditions in family members.

The purpose of this chapter is to provide the knowledge and tools that can help you to provide appropriate care for children with alterations in mental health or cognition. Much of the care for mental health disruptions is provided by psychiatric-mental health specialists, so the nurse collaborates with these specialists to identify problems, support and carry out therapy, provide education for the family, and refer the family to appropriate resources.

Cognitive conditions are commonly managed by the family and the school personnel. The nurse collaborates with families and school personnel to plan and evaluate care for the child with cognitive conditions such as mental retardation. A thorough knowledge of development is a prerequisite to understanding both mental health disruptions and cognitive conditions since developmental status is often altered in both mental health and cognitive conditions.

Most mental health conditions are treated in community settings, and nurses in these settings play an active role in the treatment and support of the child and family. Nurses may function as case managers, assisting a family to deal with all areas of the child's care. Occasionally a child is hospitalized for treatment of a significant mental health disruption, or is hospitalized for treatment of another health problem and requires continued mental health services.

MENTAL HEALTH ALTERATIONS

Mental health is foundational to a sense of personal well-being, but a variety of conditions cause mental health alterations in children and adolescents. The surgeon general is leading an initiative to examine mental health in the United States and has identified a series of goals and steps toward improving mental health care for children (Department of Health and Human Services, 2004). From the ages of 10 to 21 years, mental health issues are among the top two leading causes of hospitalization in all age groups (see Chapter 1 ∞). This high rate of hospitalization infers that children are not receiving mental health services early, when outpatient care is appropriate and prognosis is best. To confront this childhood mental health crisis, the surgeon general's agenda has established a series of goals:

1. Promote public awareness of children's mental health issues and reduce the stigma associated with mental illness.
2. Continue to develop, disseminate, and implement scientifically proven prevention and treatment services in the field of children's mental health.
3. Improve the assessment of and recognition of mental health needs in children.
4. Eliminate racial/ethnic and socioeconomic disparities in access to mental healthcare services.
5. Improve the infrastructure for children's mental health services, including support for scientifically proven interventions across professions.
6. Increase access to and coordination of quality mental healthcare services.
7. Train frontline providers to recognize and manage mental health issues, and educate mental healthcare providers about scientifically proven prevention and treatment services.
8. Monitor the access to and coordination of quality mental healthcare services. (Department of Health and Human Services, 2004).

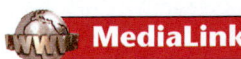

MediaLink

National Mental Health Goals

Nurses are leaders in the field of pediatric mental health care. A recent initiative known as KySS (Keep your children/yourself safe and secure) was launched by nurses in 2001 and was the subject of a summit for health professional collaboration in 2003. The goals of the summit included identification of assessment, implementation, and dissemination strategies for promoting the mental health of children and teens in primary care and alternative care settings, as well as review of evidence-based practice to make recommendations for interventions and needed research areas (Melnyk, Moldenhauer, Tuttle et al., 2003).

Some general clinical manifestations, therapies, and nursing management issues are discussed in the following text. A number of specific conditions, such as developmental and behavioral disorders, attention deficit hyperactivity disorder, mood disorders, anxiety disorders, suicide, tic disorders, and schizophrenia, are described in subsequent sections, along with information about their management.

Clinical Manifestations

The manifestations of mental health alterations in children are varied, but most can be identified through careful developmental and behavioral screening. Children with mental health conditions often do not display usual developmental milestones at the times predicted, may have social interaction problems with family members or other people, or may have demonstrated a change in performance from former developmental achievement. Functional patterns of living such as ability to feed and care for self, regulation of sleep and nutritional intake, and ability to self-regulate during activities may be lacking. Repetitive actions, behavioral instability and outbursts, and withdrawal are other important signs of mental health disruption.

COLLABORATIVE CARE

Many professionals work in the field of mental health and the nurse establishes collaborations with them in caring for children. Teachers may notice changes in behavior and refer a child to the school nurse. The nurse who identifies developmental or behavioral problems may refer the child to a physician, psychiatric mental health nurse practitioner, or psychologist. After diagnosis and the establishment of a treatment plan, the nurse collaborates with others to ensure that the child receives the needed care.

Clinical Therapy

The primary treatment goal in the management of children and adolescents with mental health disorders is to assist the child and family to achieve and maintain an optimal level of functioning through interventions designed to reduce the impact of stressors. Therapeutic interventions and communication are based on the principle that feelings motivate behaviors. Parents and others who are close to the child often fall into the habit of reacting to the child's behaviors rather than trying to find out what feelings may be precipitating the undesirable actions. Although behaviors may be considered in treatment, feelings and life experiences are often explored to provide insight and to lead to behavior change. Medication may be used to enhance and support other therapy, or may be the major therapeutic measure.

TREATMENT MODES   **Evidence-based practice** (EBP) refers to a body of scientific knowledge and its relationship to healthcare services (see further discussion in Chapter 1 ∞). While the research basis for care in all areas of pediatric health is generally scant, there is even less scientific basis to support interventions in mental health services. Nurses must seek to apply evidence-based practice to enhance mental health care when possible, and to participate in research and outcomes measurement so that additional strong evidence can be gathered on the best approaches to care (Burns, 2003; Dulcan, 2005; Hoagwood & Burns, 2005).

Three basic treatment modes based on evidence-based practice are used: individual, family, and group therapy. The choice of treatment mode must take into account the child's age and developmental stage, as well as the family situation and access to care. Most therapists incorporate several intervention strategies simultaneously within these modes. Different strategies are more or less effective and appropriate for children and adolescents in various stages of development. A thorough understanding of developmental needs, expectations, and abilities is therefore essential for mental health professionals. Treatment modes and therapeutic strategies commonly used with children and adolescents are described in the following text.

Individual Therapy   Individual therapy involves only the child and the therapist. Treatment of specific emotional problems or disorders may involve various techniques

such as play therapy, psychodrama, art therapy, and **cognitive therapy** (a technique used to help a person recognize automatic negative thinking). Individual therapy may be short term (four to six sessions) or long term (lasting for several years).

Family Therapy Family therapy involves the exploration of a particular emotional problem and its manifestations among the family members. Family therapy is based on the idea that an individual's emotional symptoms or problems are an expression of emotional symptoms or problems in the family. The focus is on the relationships among the family members, rather than the psychologic conflict within each individual member.

Group Therapy Group therapy involves an ongoing or limited number of sessions in which several individuals participate. The emphasis is on the interpersonal styles of relating to one another in the group. Group therapy is particularly effective with adolescents because of the importance of the peer group at this age. An advantage of group therapy is that stimuli and feedback come from multiple sources (the group members) instead of just one person (the therapist).

THERAPEUTIC STRATEGIES

Play Therapy Play is often called the language or work of the child. From a developmental perspective, children progressively learn to express feelings and needs through action, fantasy, and finally language. The special quality of play buffers children against the pressures and demands of daily life. Play facilitates mastery of developmental stages by strengthening physical and neurologic processes. Play also assists in cognitive learning, setting the stage for problem solving and creativity.

Play therapy is a technique that reveals problems on a fantasy level through the use of toys, dolls, clay, art, and other creative objects. It is often used with preschool and school-age children who are experiencing anxiety, stress, and other specific nonpsychotic mental disorders. Play therapy encourages the child to act out feelings such as anger, hostility, sadness, and fear. It also provides the opportunity for the therapist to help the child understand, on a conscious or unconscious level, personal responses and behavior in a safe, supportive environment.

Art Therapy Children who may be apprehensive about playing can sometimes be encouraged to participate in art therapy, using brief drawing exercises. This technique is appropriate for children of all ages, including adolescents. The drawings can help the therapist gain information about the child, the family, and the interactions between the child and family. However, children's drawings should never be used solely to form a definitive diagnosis.

When used in conjunction with a thorough history and appropriate psychologic testing information, art therapy can guide the child's treatment. These drawing exercises provide an opportunity to help in the healing process. The therapist can assist the child to release feelings of anger, pain, or fear onto paper, where they can be examined objectively. Figures 27–1 to 27–4 ➤ present examples of this technique.

Behavior and Cognitive Therapy **Behavior modification** is a therapeutic technique that uses stimulus and response conditioning to alter inappropriate behaviors. It is used to reinforce desirable behaviors by helping the child to replace maladaptive behaviors with more appropriate ones. This technique is based on the assumption that any learned behavior can be unlearned. Thus, if parents, nurses, teachers, and other adults consistently reinforce desirable behaviors, the child will eventually alter or discontinue undesirable behaviors.

Behavior modification may include (1) removing the child from the home to a more structured environment, such as a hospital, for a brief time, and (2) instructing the parents, teachers, and other appropriate adults to be agents of behavioral change. Several ongoing sessions may be required with the adults involved, using role-play and other techniques. Consistency is the most important principle in the successful use of behavior modification.

Cognitive therapy teaches thinking patterns to change reactions to situations that cause anxiety or other undesirable conditions. Children are taught how their brain and

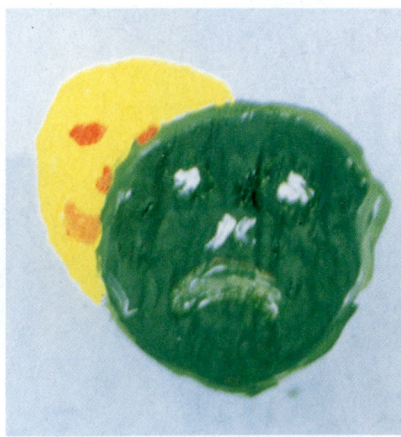

Figure 27–1 ➤ "Me." Drawn by a 14-year-old girl with major depression, anxiety, and school phobia who had experienced multiple losses over several years. Her mother had severe chronic lung problems and diabetes, and the girl had stopped attending school for fear that something would happen to her mother. This drawing represents the girl's obvious feelings of sadness and depression but also indicates a glimmer of hope (represented by the yellow mask coming from behind the dark mask of depression).

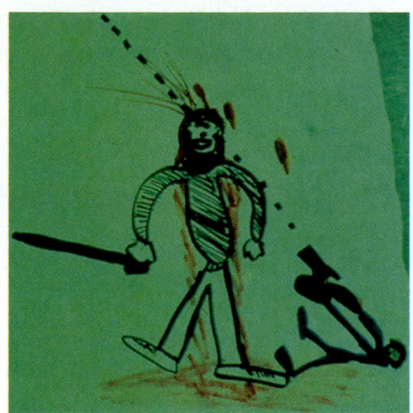

Figure 27–2 ➤ "Self-Portrait." Drawn by a 15-year-old boy who was admitted through the emergency department after a failed suicide attempt by hanging. He had a psychiatric diagnosis of depression and polysubstance abuse (including inhalants and alcohol) and insisted that he was a member of a satanic cult in his hometown. Most of his drawings depicted a preoccupation with violence and suicide. The boy said he always felt a "darkness" like a shadow that followed him around and wanted him dead. His family history was significant for depression and suicide on both his mother's and his father's side. His father also had a lengthy history of polysubstance abuse and alcoholism. The boy was discharged to a long-term residential treatment facility for adolescents.

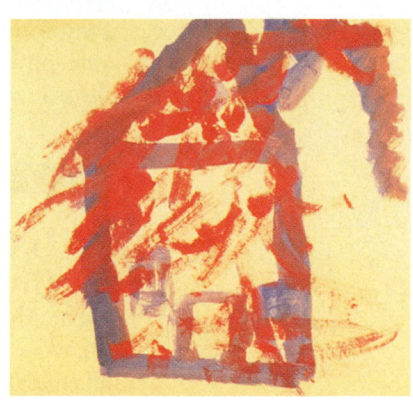

Figure 27–3 ➤ "An Activity." Drawn by an 8-year-old boy who was initially admitted to the medical-surgical floor of a pediatric hospital for dehydration resulting from vomiting and diarrhea. Psychiatric evaluation was ordered for extreme anxiety. These drawings, completed during the initial interview, led to further investigation, which revealed that the child had started a house fire in which his grandmother was killed. The family's home and all their belongings were lost. No one had known that the child had set the fire. Further sessions indicated that he had been setting neighborhood garage fires and watching them burn from a distance.

body are working; this understanding assists them in having control over the experience. Often a combination of cognitive and behavioral approaches is useful in treating children.

Visualization and Guided Imagery   The techniques of visualization and guided imagery begin with specific directions for progressive relaxation according to the child's ability. These forms of therapy use the child's own imagination and positive thinking to reduce stress and anxiety, decrease the experience of pain or discomfort, and promote healing. The techniques are especially useful in the management of anxiety disorders and chronic pain. It is not easy for every child to use his or her imagination in this way, so the technique may not work or be appropriate for every child.

Hypnosis   Hypnosis involves varying degrees of suggestibility and deep relaxation effects. This technique is useful for children and adolescents because they can usually be

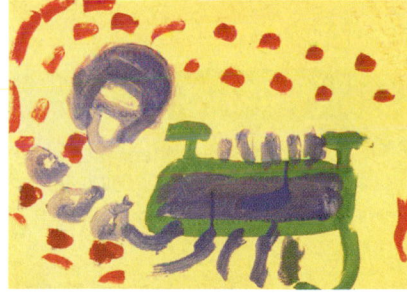

Figure 27–4 ➤ "A Family Activity." By the same boy who drew Figure 27–3. This drawing depicts a recurring incident of physical and emotional abuse by his mother's live-in boyfriend. It shows the family bathtub with feces and blood smeared on the floor and walls. The boy reported that when either he or his 3-year-old brother had a toileting accident the boyfriend would make them go into the bathroom and stand in the bathtub while he smeared the feces on the walls. He would then hit the children and make them clean up the mess. The boy had previously been removed from the mother's custody for neglect. He was transferred from the medical-surgical area to the inpatient children's psychiatric unit, where he received a diagnosis of depression, overanxious disorder, and child abuse (physical and emotional). Charges were filed against the mother's boyfriend and custody of both children was temporarily revoked.

RESEARCH

Art Therapy

The use of drawing as a means for communication with children has been used for many years. Art can be viewed as a window or doorway through which a child's emotions and experiences can be viewed (Driessnack, 2005). This makes it an effective assessment technique with children too young to express certain situations verbally. In addition, it allows them expression of feelings, and thus becomes an intervention. Following a drawing session with a discussion in which the child explains a piece of art is especially helpful.

Art is also versatile and can be accomplished in practically any setting (Driessnack, 2005). One nurse describes the use of drawings with children living in shelters after Hurricane Katrina (Looman, 2006). The author believes that art increased the amount of information a child could communicate and enhanced management of experienced trauma. It was a familiar activity that provided a comfortable space in which children could explore the occurrences and feelings about losing their homes, pets, and/or family and friends.

Nurses who work with children in various settings should consider the use of drawings. Provide a table and drawing materials for children waiting for a healthcare examination, bring art materials to the child in the hospital, and consider the activity with children who have experienced trauma.

hypnotized more easily than adults. Hypnosis is especially helpful in treating physical symptoms with a psychologic component, anxiety, and phobias, as well as managing severe physical symptoms or discomfort (pain or nausea) associated with a physiologic disorder or its treatment (e.g., cancer or juvenile rheumatoid arthritis).

NURSING MANAGEMENT
Nursing Assessment and Diagnosis

Mental health conditions often escalate to a crisis level for families because they are not identified early. In order to avoid serious mental health problems, ongoing assessment of all children for risks is imperative. During all health visits, mental health screening should be integrated into care so that disruptions can be identified. See Chapters 7 to 10 ∞ for specific questions to ask during health promotion and health maintenance visits. When a potential mental health condition exists, the child receives further assessment from a mental health specialist. A resource commonly used is the *Diagnostic and Statistical Manual*, which lists diagnostic criteria for known mental health conditions. The current edition is the DSM-IV-TR (American Psychiatric Association, 2000); its criteria for several conditions are listed throughout this chapter.

Once a mental health problem is identified, the nurse assesses the child for related issues and conditions. Mental health is linked to development so developmental screening tests are administered. Mental health status can influence activity level, physiological parameters, and risk for certain conditions. Therefore, height and weight, review of systems, vital signs, and medication/substance use history are important to perform. Family interactions, stressors, and methods of coping are assessed (see Chapter 2 ∞ for further details on family assessment).

Many nursing diagnoses can be formulated based on particular mental health conditions and child situations. Some examples include:

- Impaired Adjustment related to multiple stressors
- Anxiety related to situational or maturational crises
- Ineffective Coping related to inadequate social support
- Dysfunctional Grieving related to difficulty expressing loss of significant other
- Ineffective Role Performance related to inadequate support system and inadequate linkage with healthcare system

Planning and Implementation
Care in the Hospital

Although most mental health disorders are managed effectively with therapy and/or medication on an outpatient basis, some necessitate admission to an inpatient psychiatric setting. In addition, you may encounter the child with a mental health disorder during hospitalization for a concurrent physiologic problem that requires hospitalization. If a child is hospitalized for a concurrent problem, the child's current level of mental health functioning needs to be assessed in relation to the mental health disorder.

Nursing care includes carrying out the prescribed treatment plan and administering psychotropic medications. The child's medication regimen should be evaluated for administration schedule, dosage, side effects, and effectiveness. Inform the therapist of the child's hospitalization if the child has been hospitalized for a concurrent condition, and consult with the therapist regarding appropriate approaches for the child.

An important nursing intervention is to assure the child's safety. Actions begin in the emergency department if a child is admitted for a mental health crisis. Remove or lock potentially dangerous material in the room such as medications, tubing, and a sharps container. The parent, guardian or health professional should remain with the child at all times. Inform the family member of the need to stay with the child and how to immediately notify the nurse if the adult needs to leave or if the child's condition changes. Part of the initial care is to evaluate risk by asking if the child has tried to hurt him- or herself or been thinking about that. Ask about recent stresses, thoughts of

CULTURE
Definitions of Mental Health

Mental health is defined in different ways by various cultural groups. For most it is a sense of well-being, peace, and productive use of the mind. In many cultures, care of the "spirit" is believed necessary to promote mental health. An identity with one's community and spiritual wholeness is promoted by story telling, singing, and rites of passage. An array of therapies is used to support and restore mental health. Use of certain objects such as bags of herbs may be considered important to preserve mental health. Other therapies may include healers, family and community support, relaxation or meditation, teas and other nutritional products, and exorcism. Find out how individuals and groups define mental health and how they believe health is maintained. Be alert to learn if mental disorders are viewed as a negative stigma or are openly accepted and discussed. Ask about what the family believes will help to enhance the child's mental health and integrate these practices into the plan of care whenever it is safe to do so.

hurting someone else, and why the child thinks he or she has been brought to the emergency room (Meunier-Sham, 2003). If the child is admitted to the psychiatric unit, follow unit policies for ensuring safety for children who are at risk of hurting themselves or others.

Psychiatric hospitalization is a stressful event for all families and both the family and child need supportive care. Continuation of family involvement is critical. See Evidence-Based Practice: Understanding Stress and Mental Healthcare Hospitalization. The nurse frequently is the liaison between the family and the therapist in making follow-up arrangements at the time of discharge. The nurse must be aware of the meaning of mental illness in various cultural groups and the treatments that may be commonly used. These complementary therapies should be integrated within the care plan when considered safe and families must feel that their responses and approaches to the child with a mental disorder are not judged by health professionals.

Care in the Community

The nurse in the community assesses how a child with a mental health disorder is functioning in each part of the microsystem (see Chapter 3 ∞), such as home, childcare, school, and with friends. Risk and protective factors of the child and family are assessed (see Chapter 3). The nurse conducts therapy sessions and performs ongoing evaluation and updates of the child's level of functioning. Changes in the child and family stressors and coping mechanisms are identified, and pharmacologic interventions are evaluated.

Since many children do not receive adequate mental health services, nurses need to be knowledgeable about resources for mental health care and facilitate their use by the child and family. The nurse in the community often acts as a partner to inform other health professionals such as psychiatrists, psychologists, school counselors, teachers, and hospital nurses about the child's mental health status.

EVIDENCE-BASED PRACTICE

Understanding Stress and Mental Healthcare Hospitalization

Problem

Hospitalization for mental health care is always a stressful event. Families frequently do not understand treatment procedures or the child's condition and diagnosis. In addition, treatment may last for several days to months, causing disruption in family roles and routines. Family stresses must be understood so that the nurse can adequately support both the child and the family.

Evidence

A nursing study involved interviews with 38 parents of 29 children who had recently been hospitalized for psychiatric illness. In this qualitative study, themes that emerged during the interviews were analyzed and categorized. Three major categories were identified (Scharer, 2002).

The first was a need for *information*. Parents often did not receive information about admission and unit procedures. Many felt that the physicians and other therapists were hard to reach and did not provide adequate information about the child's condition and treatment. Parents identified a need to have access to hospital records and the child's diagnosis. Such information was viewed as an important link to outpatient facilities where the child was also treated.

The second set of needs was for *instrumental support*. These items included reasonably priced lodging near the hospital, ready access to the hospitalized child, assistance with providing physical care for the hospitalized child, and improved physical environment of the hospital unit and rooms. Some parents voiced a lack of mental health services in their own communities, resulting in lack of care both before and after hospitalization.

The third need was for *emotional support*. Parents often felt isolated and did not know where to turn. They suggested that staff could pro-

vide additional emotional support, and that having a parent to call who had similar experiences would have been helpful.

Implications

The nurse in a psychiatric facility is in a unique position to offer support to the family of the child or adolescent. Information about the unit can be provided by videotape, tour, and written materials. Daily updates on the child's condition and treatment plan are needed. Families must be viewed as partners in the treatment, along with the child and health professionals. Provide an opportunity for parents to ask questions and be sure they understand the diagnosis and treatment.

Consider visiting hours and access to children. If they are limited to certain times, explain the reason to parents. Provide access to a Ronald McDonald House or other low-cost facilities if the parent is from out of town. Provide assistance and instruction with any physical care the child needs. Consider changes that can be made to make the unit more welcoming and pleasant, such as the color of walls, presence of posters and brochures, and general cleanliness.

Facilitate parent-to-parent communication. Ask parents each day about how they feel and what can be done for them. Use empathy and interest to convey support.

Critical Thinking

Why do you think that families find psychiatric facilities frightening or strange? How can you explain the need to remove items with which children could injure themselves or others? What questions will you ask early in the hospitalization to learn about facilities that are present in the home community that can be used for referral upon discharge? How could you locate available treatment options for a family from a community several miles from the hospital? How could support of the family influence the care and condition of their child or adolescent?

Evaluation

Desired outcomes for mental health care depend on the particular condition and the child's situation. Some examples are:

- The child demonstrates the ability to self-restrain compulsive or impulsive behaviors.
- The child successfully adapts to changes in family structure and roles.
- The child verbalizes feelings of productivity and self-worth.
- The family is able to identify and use available social support.
- The child and family demonstrate the ability to draw upon spiritual beliefs for comfort.

DEVELOPMENTAL AND BEHAVIORAL DISORDERS

Autistic Spectrum Disorder

It is estimated that 12–16% of children have a developmental or behavioral disorder. One of the most common sets of disorders is pervasive developmental disorders. **Pervasive developmental disorders (PDDs)** begin in early childhood and are characterized by impaired social interactions and communication, with restricted interests, activities, and behaviors (Centers for Disease Control and Prevention, 2006). The disorders are called "autistic spectrum disorders" and are classified into five types:

- Autistic disorder
- Asperger's syndrome
- Rett's disorder
- Childhood disintegrative disorder
- Pervasive developmental disorder not otherwise specified

About 5.7 children in 1000 have autistic spectrum disorder, with about half of the cases comprised of autistic disorder (commonly called simply autism) (Schieve, Rice, Boyle et al., 2006). This incidence represents a large increase from formerly described levels. Before 1985, about 0.4–0.5 children in 1000 were diagnosed with autistic disorder (Hudson & Dixon, 2003). It is unclear whether there is a true increase in cases or simply improved techniques in making the diagnosis (Jick & Kaye, 2003). The disorder is about four times more common in males than females. Peak age at diagnosis is 6–11 years, but symptoms often begin at 18–24 months of age. Males frequently have mild forms of the disorder and females commonly have associated mental retardation (Jick & Kaye, 2003).

Etiology and Pathophysiology

The cause of autistic disorder is unknown. Genetic transmission is likely since there is high occurrence in twins (Jick & Kaye, 2003). Multiple genes that interact with environmental impact are most likely (Coury & Nash, 2003). Immune responses and neuroanatomy are being investigated as causes. Neurotransmitters such as dopamine, serotonin, and opioids are abnormal in some children and a focus of research. Brain size and therefore head circumference may be enlarged in the young child with the disorder (DiCicco-Bloom, Lord, Zwaigenbaum et al., 2006). Congenital rubella syndrome, fragile X syndrome, phenylketonuria, Down syndrome, and tuberous sclerosis are all associated with a higher than normal incidence (Hudson & Dixon, 2003). Research has indicated that there is no relationship between the measles-mumps-rubella vaccine and reported cases of the disorder (Bechtel, 2003; Wilson, Mills, Ross et al., 2003).

Clinical Manifestations

The essential features typically become apparent by the time a child is 3 years of age. They involve impairments in:

- Social interactions
- Communication
- Adapting to new situations

- Attention span and organizing responses to situations (Volkmar, Wiesner, & Westphal, 2006).

Social interactions are always complex and involve perceptions of the other person as well as social behaviors. The autistic child does not learn the common characteristics of these social interchanges. As a result, the child may be unable to converse normally, may fail to initiate conversations, and may have impaired observations of nonverbal behavior.

Autistic children may manifest disturbances in the rate or sequence of development. A primary finding is impairment in social interactions. Autistic children are unable to relate to people or to respond to social and emotional cues. In addition, they engage in **stereotypy**, or rigid and obsessive behavior. Characteristically these repetitive behaviors in affected children include head banging, twirling in circles, biting themselves, and flapping their hands or arms. Frequently a child's behavior is self-stimulating or self-destructive. Responses to sensory stimuli are frequently abnormal and include an extreme aversion to touch, loud noises, and bright lights. Emotional lability is common (Figure 27–5 ➤).

Communication difficulties or delays in speech and language are common and are often the first symptoms that lead to diagnosis. Absence of babbling and other communication by 1 year, absence of two-word phrases by 2 years, and deterioration of previous language skills are characteristic. Abnormal communication patterns include both verbal and nonverbal communication. Autistic children may eventually learn to talk, in some cases well, but their speech is likely to show certain abnormalities: using "you" in place of "I"; engaging in **echolalia** (a compulsive parroting of what is heard); repeating questions rather than answering them; and having fascination with rhythmic, repetitive songs and verses.

Behaviors of children with autism show several differences from others. They have a great deal of difficulty dealing with new situations, and show agitation and withdrawal when routines are changed. They do not commonly explore objects but have stereotyped behaviors. They may line up objects, play with the same objects over and over, and have certain rituals that must be performed. They often become upset if these normal routines are disrupted. Rituals may involve eating only certain types or colors of foods or eating in specific patterns. Autistic children may manifest disturbances in the rate or sequence of development. They are frequently cognitively impaired but can demonstrate a wide range of intellectual ability and functioning. Cognitive impairment may become manifested early in life by slow developmental progression, particularly in social skills. Some children are impaired in particular areas of development while others are above normal. About 25% have macrocephaly, with reduced head size at birth, followed by excessive growth at 1 to 2 months and 6 to 14 months (Courchesne, Carper, & Akshoomoff, 2003). However, most children have a normal appearance.

The specific clinical manifestation differences among the types of autistic spectrum disorder are listed in the Clinical Manifestations of Autistic Spectrum Disorders table on page 1110.

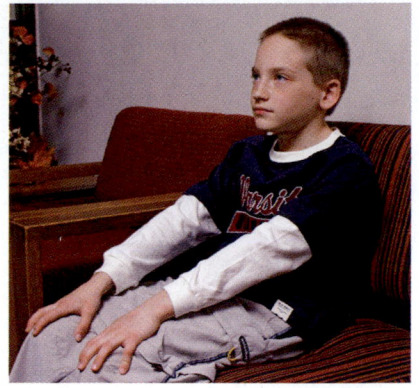

Figure 27–5 ➤ This child with autism sits stiffly in the chair and engages in rhythmic rocking behavior. He has a disengaged appearance and does not readily interact with other children or adults who are in his environment.

■ COLLABORATIVE CARE

Diagnosis is based on the presence of specific criteria, as described in the American Psychiatric Association's *Diagnostic and Statistical Manual of Mental Disorders*, 4th edition (*DSM-IV-TR*). See Table 27–1 for the autistic disorder and the *DSM-IV* for specific criteria for other autistic syndrome disorders. Table 27–2 lists several screening tests that are useful in autistic disorders. Additional testing is done to rule out other causes of the child's behavior. Tests may include neuroimaging (CT scan or MRI), lead screening, DNA analysis, and electroencephalogram. See Chapters 5 and 26 ∞ for further descriptions related to assessment of the neurological system.

Early intervention assists in maximizing the child's potential and establishing helpful support for parents (Giarelli, Souders, Pinto-Martin et al., 2005). Treatment centers on teaching children how to focus and learn, managing behavior to reward

CLINICAL MANIFESTATIONS: AUTISTIC SPECTRUM DISORDERS (PERVASIVE DEVELOPMENTAL DISORDERS)

Disorder	Clinical Manifestations	Clinical Therapy
Autistic disorder	Impaired social, communicative, and behavioral development, usually noted in the first year of life	Early intervention is key to maximal performance. Interventions focus on improving behaviors and communication skills, providing physical and occupational therapy, structuring play interactions with other children, and educating parents about the child's needs.
Asperger's syndrome	Impaired social interactions with normal language development for age; pitch, tone, and other speech characteristics may be abnormal. Verbal skills involving spelling and vocabulary are high, with concept formation, language flexibility, and comprehension low.	Social interactions are the focus of therapy.
Rett's disorder	Early development appears normal and symptoms emerge at 6–18 months. Ataxia, handwringing, intermittent hyperventilation, dementia, and growth retardation show progressive increase. Appears only in females as an X-linked dominant disorder; mutations occur in the gene MeCP2, affecting methyl-CpG-binding protein 2, which is important in brain development.	Early intervention in areas of abnormal behaviors.
Childhood disintegrative disorder	First 2–5 years of development appear normal, followed by deterioration in many areas of functioning. Regression in toileting and other skills may occur. Behaviors finally stabilize at some point without further deterioration.	Focus on areas of developmental function that show abnormality. Individualized Education Plans are needed in school to deal with communication, play, physical therapy, and teaching management skills to parents.
Pervasive developmental disorder not otherwise specified	Severe social impairment without meeting *DSM* criteria for other types of autistic spectrum disorder.	Behavioral therapy focuses on building social skills.

appropriate behaviors, encouraging positive or adaptive coping skills, and facilitating effective communication (Butter, Wynn, & Mulick, 2003). Children are taught how to focus and learn. The goals of treatment are to reduce rigidity or stereotypy (repetitive, obsessive, machinelike movements) and other maladaptive behaviors. Often the child must be physically restrained from aggressive or self-destructive behaviors. Some parents choose to use complementary therapies such as vitamin supplements and dimethylglycine. Foods such as sugar, aspartame, milk products, and wheat are sometimes eliminated from the diet. A variety of complementary practices have been adopted by families, but there is a limited evidence base for these approaches (Levy & Hyman, 2003).

Medications are used with some children to treat associated behavioral disorders but are not effective in treatment of autistic syndrome itself. Medications used for associated conditions may include stimulants, selective serotonin reuptake inhibitors (SSRIs), and mood stabilizers (Lindsay & Aman, 2003). The overall prognosis for autistic children to become functioning members of society is guarded. The extent to which adequate adjustment is achieved varies greatly. However, successful adjustment is more likely for children with higher IQs, adequate speech, and access to specialized programs.

NURSING MANAGEMENT

Nursing Assessment and Diagnosis

The nurse may encounter the child with autism when parents seek care for a suspected hearing impairment, speech difficulty, or developmental delay. Early and frequent developmental screening of all children can help in referral for thorough assessment and identification of cases. Parents may report abnormal interaction such as lack of eye contact, disinterest in cuddling, minimal facial responsiveness, and failure to talk. Be

COMPLEMENTARY THERAPY

Autism Treatments

Some parents who have a child with autism choose to use CAM in an attempt to help the child. A popular treatment approach includes dietary therapy with vitamin A, vitamin C, vitamin B6, magnesium, omega-3 fatty acids, and use of gluten-free or casein-free diets. Drug therapy tried by parents includes secretin, a pancreatic gastrointestinal peptide, and Pepcid or other antacids. Some parents believe that detoxification by limiting certain dietary intake or using Epsom salt baths can be helpful (Levy & Hyman, 2003). Nurses can help parents to evaluate studies on complementary care and encourage them to initiate only one treatment at a time to measure any effectiveness seen. Ask about therapies being used and discuss safeguards to avoid any undesired side effects.

Table 27–2	SCREENING TESTS FOR AUTISM

Test	Source
Clinical Practice Guidelines—Early Intervention Program of the New York State Department of Health	New York State Department of Health
Checklist for Autism in Toddlers (CHAT) or Modified Checklist for Autism in Toddlers (M-CHAT)	Scambler, D., Rogers, S. J., & Wehner, E. A. (2001). Can the checklist for autism in toddlers differentiate young children with autism from those with developmental delays? *Journal of the American Academy of Child* and *Adolescent Psychiatry, 40,* 1457–1463.
Autism Diagnostic Interview—Revised	Lord, C., Rutter, M., & LeConteur, A. (1994). Autism Diagnostic Interview—Revised: A revised version of a diagnostic interview for caregivers of individuals with possible pervasive developmental disorder. *Journal of Autism and Developmental Disorders, 24,* 659–685.
Detection of Autism by Infant Sociability Interview (DAISI)	Hopson, R. P. (1993). *Autism and the development of mind.* Hillsdale, NJ: Erlbaum.
Screening Tool for Autism in Two-Year-Olds	Stone, W. L., Coonrod, E., & Osley, O. (2000). Brief report: Screening Tool for Autism in Two-Year-Olds (STAT): Development and preliminary data. *Journal of Autistic and Developmental Disorders, 30,* 607–612.
Autism Behavior Checklist	Gillberg, C., Nordin, V., & Ehlers, S. (1996). Early detection of autism: Diagnostic instruments for clinicians. *European Child and Adolescent Psychiatry, 5*(2), 67–74.
Autism Diagnostic Observation Schedule—Generic (ADOS-G)	Lord, C., Risi, S., Lambrecht, L., et al. (2000). The Autism Diagnostic Observation Schedule—generic: A standard measure of social and communication deficits associated with the spectrum of autism. *Journal of Autism and Developmental Disorders, 30,* 205–233.
Childhood Autism Rating Scale (CARS)	Schopler, E., Reichler, R. J. & Renner, B. R. (1988). *The Childhood Autism Rating Scale (CARS).* Los Angeles: Western Psychological Services.

Table 27–1	DSM-IV-TR DIAGNOSTIC CRITERIA FOR AUTISTIC DISORDER

A. A total of six or more items from 1, 2, and 3, with at least two from 1, and one each from 2 and 3:
  1. Qualitative impairment in social interaction, as manifested by at least two of the following:
    a. Marked impairment in the use of multiple nonverbal behaviors such as eye-to-eye gaze, facial expression, body posture, and gestures to regulate social interaction
    b. Failure to develop peer relationships appropriate to developmental level
    c. A lack of spontaneous seeking to share enjoyment, interests, or achievements with other people
    d. Lack of social or emotional reciprocity
  2. Qualitative impairments in communication as manifested by at least one of the following:
    a. Delay in, or total lack of, the development of spoken language (not accompanied by an attempt to compensate through alternative modes of communication such as gesture or mime)
    b. In individuals with adequate speech, marked impairment in the ability to initiate or sustain a conversation with others
    c. Stereotyped and repetitive use of language or idiosyncratic language
    d. Lack of varied, spontaneous make-believe play or social imitative play appropriate to developmental level
  3. Restricted repetitive and stereotyped patterns of behavior, interests, and activities, as manifested by at least one of the following:
    a. Encompassing preoccupation with one or more stereotyped and restricted patterns of interest that is abnormal either in intensity or in focus
    b. Apparently inflexible adherence to specific, nonfunctional routines or rituals
    c. Stereotyped and repetitive motor mannerisms (e.g., hand or finger flapping or twisting, or complex whole-body movements)
    d. Persistent preoccupation with parts of objects
B. Delays or abnormal functioning in at least one of the following areas, with onset prior to age 3 years: (1) social interaction, (2) language as used in social communication, or (3) symbolic or imaginative play.
C. The disturbance is not better accounted for by Rett's syndrome or childhood disintegrative disorder.

Reprinted with permission from the *Diagnostic and Statistical Manual of Mental Disorders,* Fourth Edition, Text Revision. Copyright © 2000 American Psychiatric Association.

alert to parental observations that the baby or young child does not look at them or provide other developmental or behavioral cues (Beauchesne & Kelley, 2004). Initial assessment focuses on language development, response to others, and hearing acuity (see Chapters 5 and 19 ∞).

Carefully evaluate the child for history of developmental milestones and refer for abnormalities. Perform developmental screening that considers several areas of development including motor activity, social skills, and language. Recall that the child may have normal performance in one area such as motor skills and delayed development in another area such as language skills. Likewise, language may be normal for age but social interactions may be quite delayed. Include questioning about adaptive skills such as toilet training and feeding patterns. Inquire about school performance since some areas may be normal while others are delayed. Observe the child in play situations and evaluate the use of creative and exploratory play versus more repetitive patterns. Perform hearing and vision screening if possible to rule out sensory problems.

When a child with a diagnosis of autistic disorder is hospitalized for a concurrent problem, obtain a history from the parents regarding the child's routines, rituals, and likes and dislikes, as well as ways to promote interaction and cooperation. Autistic children may carry a special toy or object that they play with during times of stress. Ask parents about these objects and their use.

Ask about the child's behaviors as well as observing them on admission. Obtain a history of acute and chronic illnesses and injuries. Ask about eating patterns and food restrictions. Inquire about CAM in a nonjudgmental and supportive manner.

Nursing diagnoses must be tailored to fit the individual needs of the child. Examples of diagnoses that may be appropriate for children with autistic syndromes include the following:

- Impaired Verbal Communication related to altered perceptions
- Impaired Social Interaction related to developmental disability
- Disturbed Thought Processes related to mental disorder
- Risk for Injury related to cognitive impairment
- Risk for Caregiver Role Strain related to chronicity and demands of child's condition
- Disabled Family Coping: Compromised related to having a child with prolonged disability

Planning and Implementation

Nursing care focuses on stabilizing environmental stimuli, providing supportive care, enhancing communication, maintaining a safe environment, giving the parents anticipatory guidance, and providing emotional support.

Stabilize Environmental Stimuli

Autistic children interpret and respond to the environment differently from other individuals. Sounds that are not distressing to the average person may be interpreted by autistic children as louder, more frightening, and overwhelming. The child needs to be oriented to new settings such as a classroom or the hospital room and may adjust best to a small classroom or a hospital room with only one other child. Encourage parents to bring the child's favorite objects from home, and try to keep these objects in the same places, because the child does not cope well with changes in the environment.

Provide Supportive Care

Developing a trusting relationship with the autistic child is often difficult. Adjust communication techniques and teaching to the child's developmental level. Ask parents about the child's usual home routines, and maintain these routines as much as possible when the child is out of the home. Because self-care abilities are often limited, the child may need assistance to meet basic needs. School programs and Individualized Education Plans (see Chapter 12 ∞) can help the child to learn self-care skills. When possible, schedule daily care and routine procedures at consistent times to maintain predictability. Encourage parents to remain with the hospitalized child and to participate in daily care planning. Parents are integral parts of the treatment team when the child's learning goals are established in early intervention or school programs. Identify rituals for naptime and bedtime, and maintain them to promote rest and sleep. Integrate patterns that facilitate intake of nutritious foods at mealtimes.

Enhance Communication

Because children with autism have impaired communication, nursing care focuses on utilizing and improving communication with the child. Speech is used when possible; short, direct sentences are usually best (Galinat, Barcalow, & Krivda, 2005). If the child responds well to visual cues, then pictures, computers, and other visual aids may form an important part of interaction. Sign language is used with some children.

Maintain a Safe Environment

Monitor autistic children at all times, including bathtime and bedtime. Close supervision is needed to ensure that the child does not obtain any harmful objects or engage in dangerous behaviors. For the child who engages in head banging or other abusive behaviors, bicycle helmets and hand mitts can be the least restrictive method to provide safety. They enable the child to participate in activities and engage in a social environment to the degree possible.

Provide Anticipatory Guidance

Approximately half of all children with autistic disorder require lifelong supervision and support, especially if the disorder is accompanied by mental retardation. Some children may grow up to lead independent lives, although they will have social limitations with impaired interpersonal relationships. Encourage parents to promote the child's development through behavior modification and specialized educational programs. The overall goal is to provide the child with the guidance, education, and support necessary for optimal functioning.

Care in the Community

Families of autistic children need a great deal of support to cope with the challenges of caring for the autistic child. They experience the challenges of families who have a child with a chronic disorder (see Chapter 12 ∞). Participating in parent support groups and learning how to reframe the condition to view its positive aspects are helpful strategies (Luther, Canham, & Cureton, 2005). Help them to identify resources for childcare, such as special toddler programs and preschools. They may need specialized transportation services for the child or other social supports. The child will need an Individualized Education Plan. The parent or primary caretaker often has difficulty obtaining respite care and may need assistance to find suitable resources. Siblings of the autistic child may need help to explain the disorder to their friends or teachers. The nurse can be instrumental in assisting these siblings to understand and explain autism. Family support programs are available in some states to provide assistance to parents.

Genetic counseling should be offered to the family. Information on immunizations is necessary, because parents may have heard about a potential connection between immunization and the disorder. They should be encouraged to have the child immunized on the recommended schedule. Parents may have questions about where to find information on complementary and alternative therapies.

Local support groups for parents of autistic children are available in most areas. Parents can also be referred to the Autism Society of America for information.

Evaluation

Expected outcomes of nursing care for the child with autism are as follows:

- The child with autism performs self-care to maximum potential.
- The child's symptoms will be successfully managed.
- A safe environment is maintained so that the child remains free from injury.
- The child demonstrates consistent developmental progression.
- The child acquires communication strategies that enable socialization with others.

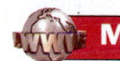

MediaLink

Autism Support and Resources

MediaLink

ADD/ADHD Video

Attention Deficit Disorder and Attention Deficit Hyperactivity Disorder

Attention deficit disorder (ADD) is a variation in central nervous system processing characterized by developmentally inappropriate behaviors involving inattention. When hyperactivity and impulsivity accompany inattention, the disorder is called attention deficit hyperactivity disorder (ADHD). The latter is the more common condition and affects from 4–12% of all school-age children. Boys are affected almost four times more commonly than girls (National Initiative for Children's Healthcare Quality, 2003). It is now known to affect both adolescents and adults. Those with the disorder often continue to manifest at least some of the symptoms as they grow into adulthood. Hyperactivity and impulsivity may improve as the child nears adulthood, with inattentiveness appearing as the most persistent characteristic (McDonnell, Doyle, & Surman, 2003).

Etiology and Pathophysiology

Although a variety of physical and neurologic disorders are associated with ADHD, children with identifiable causes represent a small proportion of this population. Examples of known associations include exposure to high levels of lead in childhood and prenatal exposure to alcohol or tobacco smoke. Other prenatal factors associated with a higher incidence of ADHD include preterm labor, impaired placenta functioning, and impaired oxygenation. Seizures and serious head injury are other potential associations. Genetic factors may be important, as well as family dynamics and environmental characteristics. Although ADHD occurs more commonly within families (25% have a first-degree relative with the disorder), a single gene has not been located and a specific mechanism of genetic transmission is not known. It is believed that a genetic predisposition interacts with the child's environment, so that both factors contribute to the appearance of the condition. Family stress, poverty, and poor nutrition may be contributing factors in some cases. Daily television exposure at ages 1–3 years is associated with attentional problems at 7 years (Christakis, Zimmerman, DiGiuseppe, & McCarty, 2004). There are probably many types of attention deficit, resulting from several different mechanisms that involve interaction of genetic, biological, and environmental risk factors (Gottesman, 2003).

The pathophysiology of ADD/ADHD is unclear but there are some brain characteristics that provide clues. There may be a deficit in the catecholamines dopamine and norepinephrine in some children, lowering the threshold for stimuli input. The disorder is marked by brain maturation delay in the areas of self-regulation. Increased input from stimuli and decreased self-regulation cause the hallmark inability to inhibit stimuli and motor activity. Some children exhibit additional problems such as aggressive behaviors, learning disabilities, and motor disorders.

Clinical Manifestations

Children with ADD and ADHD have problems related to decreased attention span, impulsiveness, and/or increased motor activity (Figure 27–6 ➤). Symptoms can range from mild to severe. The child has difficulty completing tasks, fidgets constantly, is frequently loud, and interrupts others. Sleep disturbances are common. Because of these behaviors, the child often has difficulty developing and maintaining social relationships and may be shunned or teased by other children. This only increases the anxiety of the already compromised child, whose behavior is set on a downward-spiraling course (Brown, Amler, Freeman et al., 2005).

Typically, girls with ADHD show less aggression and impulsiveness than boys, but far more anxiety, mood swings, social withdrawal, rejection, and cognitive and language problems. Girls tend to be older at the time of diagnosis. Children are frequently diagnosed with the disorder soon after beginning school, when demands increase for attentive behavior. See Table 27–3 for DSM-IV-TR diagnostic criteria for attention deficit hyperactivity disorder.

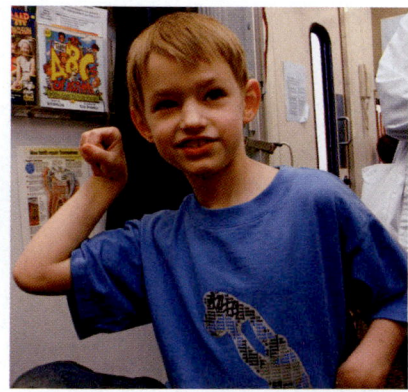

Figure 27–6 ➤ This child with ADHD was challenged by a visit to a healthcare facility for dental care. He found it difficult to remain in the chair for the examination, and once it was over, he rapidly ran from one piece of equipment to another in the facility. He asked what things were for but did not wait for answers. His engaging personality emerged as he posed briefly for a picture. Such behaviors can be exhausting for parents to manage and may create safety hazards in the healthcare setting.

Table 27–3	DSM-IV-TR DIAGNOSTIC CRITERIA FOR ATTENTION DEFICIT HYPERACTIVITY DISORDER

A. Either 1 or 2:
  1. Inattention: Six (or more) of the following symptoms of inattention have persisted for at least 6 months to a degree that is maladaptive and inconsistent with developmental level:
    a. Often fails to give close attention to details or makes careless mistakes in school work, work, and other activities
    b. Often has difficulty sustaining attention in tasks or play activities
    c. Often does not seem to listen when spoken to directly
    d. Often does not follow through on instructions and fails to finish school work, chores, or duties in the workplace (not due to oppositional behavior or failure to understand instructions)
    e. Often has difficulty organizing tasks and activities
    f. Often avoids, dislikes, or is reluctant to engage in tasks that require sustained mental effort (such as school work or homework)
    g. Often loses things necessary for tasks or activities (e.g., toys, school assignments, pencils, books, or tools)
    h. Is often easily distracted by extraneous stimuli
    i. Is often forgetful in daily activities
  2. Hyperactivity-impulsivity: Six (or more) of the following symptoms of hyperactivity-impulsivity have persisted for at least 6 months to a degree that is maladaptive and inconsistent with developmental level:

Hyperactivity
    a. Often fidgets with hands or feet or squirms in seat
    b. Often leaves seat in classroom or in other situations in which remaining seated is expected
    c. Often runs about or climbs excessively in situations in which it is inappropriate (in adolescents or adults, may be limited to subjective feelings of restlessness)
    d. Often has difficulty playing or engaging in leisure activities quietly
    e. Is often "on the go" or acts as if "driven by a motor"
    f. Often talks excessively

Impulsivity
    g. Often blurts out answers before questions have been completed
    h. Often has difficulty awaiting turn
    i. Often interrupts or intrudes on others (e.g., butts into conversations or games)
B. Some hyperactive-impulsive or inattentive symptoms that caused impairment were present before age 7 years.
C. Some impairment from the symptoms is present in two or more settings (e.g., at school [or work] and at home).
D. There must be clear evidence of clinically significant impairment in social, academic, or occupational functioning.
E. The symptoms do not occur exclusively during the course of a pervasive developmental disorder, schizophrenia, or other psychotic disorder and are not better accounted for by another mental disorder (e.g., mood disorder, anxiety disorder, dissociative disorder, or a personality disorder).

Reprinted with permission from the *Diagnostic and Statistical Manual of Mental Disorders,* Fourth Edition, Text Revision. Copyright © 2000 American Psychiatric Association.

■ COLLABORATIVE CARE

Diagnosis begins with a careful history of the child, including family history, birth history, growth and developmental milestones, behaviors such as sleep and eating patterns, progression and patterns in school, social and environmental conditions, and reports from parents and teachers. A physical examination should be performed to rule out neurological diseases and other health problems. The mental health specialist then tests the child and administers questionnaires to the parent and teacher. It is important to identify other conditions that may either mimic as ADD/ADHD or exist in conjunction with the disorders. These might include depression, anxiety, learning disorder, conduct disorder, or oppositional defiant disorder (Adesman, 2003).

Children are usually brought for evaluation when behaviors escalate to the point of interfering with the daily functioning of teachers or parents. When children have learning disabilities or anxiety disorders, the problem is commonly misdiagnosed as

ADHD without further evaluation of the child's symptoms. Obtaining an accurate diagnosis by a pediatric mental health specialist is vital (Brown et al., 2005; Wolraich, Wibbelsman, Brown et al., 2005).

Specific diagnostic criteria (see Table 27–3) must be applied to all children with the potential diagnosis of ADD or ADHD. Behaviors both at home and school or childcare must be evaluated, because abnormal patterns in two settings are needed for diagnosis. The diagnosis of ADD can be difficult due to the absence of hyperactivity behaviors. A variety of tests are available for use by the trained professional in establishing the diagnosis (Table 27–4).

Based on the findings, desired outcomes are established for the child's performance and management of the disorder. Treatment is established to meet the desired behavioral outcomes, and includes a combination of approaches, such as environmental changes, behavior therapy, and pharmacotherapy (Brown et al., 2005). It is expected that treatment will be long term.

Children often benefit from environmental changes. Decreasing stimulation, for example, by turning off television, keeping the environment quiet, and maintaining an orderly and clutter-free desk or study area without distraction, may help the child to stay focused on the task at hand. Another relatively simple change is appropriate classroom placement, preferably in a small class with a teacher who can provide close supervision and a structured daily routine. Consistent limits and expectations should be set for the child. Children living in chaotic homes and communities may function better if the environment can be simplified. When aggressive behaviors occur, therapeutic approaches such as play and group therapy may be useful.

Behavior therapy involves rewarding the child for desired behaviors and applying consequences for undesirable behaviors. Children may be rewarded by praise or earn points toward a movie or other desired outing for staying seated during meals or quietly listening in a classroom. Cues are established so that a child can subtly be reminded when impulsive or hyperactive behaviors are escalating. All adults who are in close contact with the child, such as parents and teachers, must be informed and involved in the established behavioral program.

Children with moderate to severe ADD/ADHD are treated with pharmacotherapy. Methylphenidate (Ritalin, Concerta) is most often prescribed. A skin patch that releases medication over a 9-hour period is now available, facilitating ease of administration (Anderson & Scott, 2006). Usually a favorable response (a decrease in impulsive behaviors and an increase in the ability to sit still and attend to an activity for at least 15 minutes) is seen in the first 10 days of treatment and frequently with the first few doses. Other medications that may be used include dextroamphetamine (Dexedrine or Adderall), the tricyclic antidepressants desipramine and imipramine, and the antidepressant bupropion (Wellbutrin) (Brown et al., 2005; Wolraich et al., 2005). See Medications Used to Treat ADHD.

A variety of other treatments have been attempted for ADHD, and are commonly used by families. Chiropractic manipulation, biofeedback, and dietary interventions

Table 27–4	SCREENING TESTS FOR ADD/ADHD
Test	**Source**
Vanderbilt Parent and Teacher Scales	Wolraich, M. L. (1998). *Journal of Abnormal Child Psychology, 26,* 141; Wolraich, M. L. (2003). *Journal of Pediatric Psychology, 28,* 559.
Connors' Parent and Teacher Rating Scales—Revised—Long Form	Connors, C. K. (1998). *Journal of Abnormal Child Psychology, 26,* 257 and 279.
Swanson, Nolan, and Pelham Questionnaire II Teacher and Parent Rating Scale (SNAP-IV)	Swanson, J. M. (1992). *School-based assessments and interventions for ADD students.* Irvine, CA: KC Publications.
Disruptive Behavior Disorder Scale	Pelham, W. E. (1992). *Journal of the American Academy of Child and Adolescent Psychiatry, 31,* 210.
ADHD Rating Scale	DuPaul, G. J. (1991). *American Academy of Child and Adolescent Psychiatry, 20,* 245.

Adapted from: Liu, Y. H., & Leslie, L. K. (2003). Diagnosing ADHD: Putting AAP guidelines to the test—and into practice. *Contemporary Pediatrics, 20*(12), 51–73.

MEDICATIONS USED TO TREAT *ADHD*

Medication	Action and Indication	Nursing Implications
Methylphenidate	A derivative of piperidine that acts like amphetamine. May work in ADHD treatment by enhancing catecholamine effects in the NS, improving attention span and task performance. Schedule II drug in Schedule of Controlled Substances.	Available in short-acting forms of 5, 10, and 20 mg as Ritalin and Methylin, and in 2.5, 5, and 10 mg forms as Focalin. Also in intermediate-acting forms of 20 mg (Ritalin SR), 10 and 20 mg (Metadate ER and Methylin ER). Available in long-acting forms of 18, 27, 36, and 54 mg (Concerta), 20 mg (Metadate CD), and 20, 30, and 40 mg (Ritalin LA). Transdermal 9-hour patches are now available. The variety of available forms makes it important to read labels carefully and inform families about proper administration of the child's specific type of drug. Periodic growth measurements are needed. Behavior and school performance are monitored.
Amphetamine preparations	Synthetic sympathomimetic amine with stimulant effect on CNS. Increases release of norepinephrine and dopamine by blocking their reuptake. Schedule II drug in Schedule of Controlled Substances.	Available in short-acting forms of 5 mg (Dexedrine), 5 and 10 mg (CextroStat), and 5 and 7.5 mg (Adderall). Intermediate-acting forms include 10, 12.5, 15, 20, and 30 mg Adderall, and 5, 10, and 15 mg Dexedrine Spansules. A long-acting form is 5, 10, 15, 20, 25, or 30 mg Adderall-XR. Read labels and instruct in proper administration. Monitor vital signs and growth measurements periodically.
Atomoxetine	This is the first nonstimulant drug for treatment of ADHD. It inhibits norepinephrine reuptake, decreases hyperactivity and impulsivity of ADHD, and may assist with improving mood and decreasing anxiety.	Available in 10, 18, 25, 40, and 60 mg capsules. Recommended starting dose for children is 0.5 mg/kg/day. Has been shown to have long-lasting effect of 1 day or longer. Side effects are uncommon and transient, with dyspepsia or vomiting, fatigue, decreased appetite, and dizziness most common. Have the child change position slowly if dizziness occurs; caution teen not to drive until effects of drug are clear. Perform periodic growth measurements.

Data adapted from Buck, M. L. (2003); Stein & Baren (2003).

(both elimination diets and supplement use) are examples of common complementary or alternative therapies.

Although ADHD was once thought to be a disorder of childhood that gradually improved with age, it is now believed that symptoms continue into adulthood and that careful management in childhood assists in lessening problems of social functioning later in life.

NURSING MANAGEMENT
Nursing Assessment and Diagnosis
The nurse often encounters the family who is concerned about the child's behavior before a diagnosis has been made. Ask about family and birth history and have the parents describe the child's behaviors. Perform developmental testing and look specifically for attention span and physical activity. Refer the family to their pediatric healthcare home for further assessment, and then to a mental healthcare specialist who is experienced in diagnosing ADHD.

The nurse may encounter the child with ADHD in the hospital when parents bring the child for treatment of an injury (e.g., fracture) or other problem. Explore the parent's report of the child's attention span in detail. Usually within a few minutes in an unstructured setting or waiting area, the child with ADHD becomes restless and searches for distraction. Gather information about the child's activity level and impulsiveness. Be

COMPLEMENTARY THERAPY

ADD and ADHD
There are many claims in the media about what causes ADD and ADHD. Parents may wish to try a variety of approaches in addition to or instead of traditional behavioral therapy and medication. Some common complementary therapies include elimination of dietary components such as highly processed foods, sugar, aspartame, or yeast. Other therapies include use of supplements such as iron, magnesium, zinc, and vitamin B_6. Herbs such as pycnogenol, melatonin, Echinacea, St. John's wort, and gingko biloba are sometimes used, as are visual and auditory training. Parents do not typically tell healthcare providers about the use of herbs; 70–75% have not discussed their use during healthcare visits. Ask parents about alternative therapies used and investigate what is known about them in order to share this information with parents (Cala, Crismon, & Baumgartner, 2003).

alert for information that reveals a serious problem, such as hurting animals or other children. Obtain information about distractibility, attention deficit in activities of daily living, characteristic ways of reacting, and the extent of impulsiveness when the child is receiving medication. Find out how the family manages at home and what treatments are being applied.

Examples of nursing diagnoses that may be appropriate for a child with ADHD include the following:

- Impaired Verbal Communication related to altered perceptions
- Impaired Social Interaction related to chronic episodes of impulsive behavior
- Chronic Low Self-Esteem related to behaviors associated with ADD/ADHD
- Risk for Injury related to high level of impulsiveness and excitability
- Risk for Caregiver Role Strain related to management of the child with unpredictable moods and high energy

Planning and Implementation

Prevention can focus on discouraging regular television exposure for young children from 1–3 years and encouraging daily vigorous physical activity for all children.

Nursing care of the hospitalized child with ADD/ADHD focuses on administering medications, managing the child's environment, implementing behavioral management plans, providing emotional support to the child and family, promoting self-esteem, and ensuring ongoing care. Care in the community includes the same components along with guiding parents to appropriate resources when needed.

Administer Medications

Stimulant and nonstimulant medications increase the child's attention span and decrease distractibility. Be alert for the common side effects of these medications, including anorexia, insomnia, and tachycardia. Administering medication early in the day helps to alleviate insomnia. Anorexia can be managed by giving medication at mealtimes. Careful periodic monitoring of weight, height, and blood pressure is necessary. Instruct families about the abuse potential of stimulant drugs; they should be kept locked and administered only as directed.

Minimize Environmental Distractions

The child may need to be placed in an environment with minimal distractions. When hospitalized, this may mean a room with only one other child. Potentially harmful equipment should be kept out of reach. Television and video game time needs to be monitored and limited. Use shades to darken the room during naps or at bedtime and minimize noise. Teach parents to minimize distractions at home during periods when the child needs to concentrate; for example, when doing school work (Figure 27–7 ➤). Visits to areas such as shopping malls and playgrounds may need to be limited. Plenty of daily exercise and minimal use of television/video games may assist the child in being able to concentrate when needed for school work.

Implement Behavioral Management Plans

Behavior modification programs can help to reduce specific impulsive behaviors. An example is setting up a reward program for the child who has taken medication as ordered or completed a homework assignment. The rewards may be daily as well as weekly or monthly, depending on the child's age. For example, one completed homework assignment might be rewarded with 30 minutes of basketball or a bike ride; assignments completed for a week might be rewarded with participation in an activity of the child's choice on the weekend.

If punishment is necessary, the behavior should be corrected while simultaneously supporting the child as a person. Punishment is generally withdrawal of a privilege, and should follow the offense quickly as the child may not otherwise connect the punishment with the behavior.

Provide Emotional Support

Children with ADD/ADHD offer a special challenge to parents, teachers, and healthcare providers. Parents must cope simultaneously with managing the difficult needs

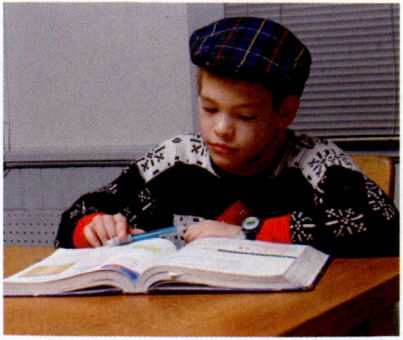

Figure 27–7 ➤ Managing the environment to provide quiet places with minimal distractions is often necessary for the child with ADHD. This boy reads and does homework in a room with few pictures, no music, and only the book with homework on the table. He is also assisted by structure such as a scheduled time for homework, with short breaks to walk around every 10–15 minutes.

and demands of a hard-to-handle child, obtaining appropriate evaluation and treatment, and understanding and accepting the diagnosis, even when the child exhibits different behaviors with different people. Family support is essential. Educate both the parents and the child about the importance of appropriate expectations and consequences of behaviors. Teach skills that will help as the child grows older: making lists of tasks to accomplish; having routines for eating, sleeping, recreation, and school work; minimizing stimuli in the environment when completing work; and asking teachers and friends to identify when behavior is inappropriate. When the child is hospitalized for another condition, the time may provide a brief respite from constant care by the parent. The activity, impulsivity, and general high energy of children with ADHD can fatigue parents. They may wish to spend a few hours each day at home or a nearby residence for families when the child is hospitalized. Ask them how they manage at home and offer ideas for respite care.

Promote Self-Esteem

Help the child to understand the disorder at an appropriate developmental level, and facilitate a trusting relationship with healthcare providers. Assist the child with social skills through the use of role-play, small-group play, and modeling. Promote the child's self-esteem by emphasizing the positive aspects of behavior and treating instances of negative behavior as learning opportunities. Help the child to develop ego strengths (the conscious ability to screen outside stimuli and to control internal demands), which will result in better impulse control and thus increase self-esteem over time. Encourage skills at which the child excels and consider the use of support groups for children in school (Barber, Grubbs, & Cottrell, 2005). Praise the hospitalized child for lying still for a procedure, taking a medication on time, or helping a staff member to carry toys around to other children.

Care in the Community

Most children with ADD/ADHD are only hospitalized when needing care for another condition. Parents need support to understand the diagnosis and to learn how to manage the child. Explain the diagnosis and what is known about attention deficit disorders. Provide written materials, internet sites, and an opportunity to ask questions.

Emphasize the importance of a stable environment, at home as well as at school. At home, the child may have difficulty staying on task. Parents need to consider the child's age and developmental appropriateness of tasks, give clear and simple instructions, and provide frequent reminders to ensure completion. Routines in the evening can promote good sleep patterns.

The nurse can serve as a liaison to teachers and school personnel, or as the case manager for the child. An Individualized Education Plan may be needed (see Chapter 12 ∞), with clear expected outcomes stated for the child's behaviors. Individualized Education Plans or periods of instruction free from the distractions of the entire class may enable the child to improve school performance. Parents may have difficulty understanding the need for these approaches because the child often tests with above-average intelligence. Reinforce the importance of providing a structured environment free from unnecessary external stimuli. Be sure that parents understand behavioral approaches that will help the child, how to administer prescribed medications, and the importance of returning for healthcare visits to monitor for side effects. Medication should be locked safely away at home to keep it away from other children and prevent illegal use of this controlled substance. An Individualized School Health Plan may be needed for medication management. See Families Want to Know: School Suggestions for Children with ADD/ADHD.

Parents may have heard about ADD/ADHD in the media and can have many questions about its cause and management. Providing information about complementary and alternative treatments is a nursing role. The National Institutes of Health sponsors the National Center for Complementary and Alternative Medicine (NCCAM) and is a reliable source for parents and professionals.

As the child grows older, provide explanations about the disorder and information about techniques that will assist in dealing with problems. Emphasize the importance

---

CULTURE

Mental Health and Stigma

Many families who have a child with ADHD or another mental health disorder are embarrassed and feel shame because of the diagnosis, especially in certain cultures such as some Asian groups, and in very structured and highly achieving families. When taking histories from family members, it is best to be sensitive to the stigma some may feel. Ask questions in a private setting and ask about the family's feelings regarding a mental health disorder. Is there someone in their family who they can talk to about the diagnosis? Provide information in a nonjudgmental manner and provide support if appropriate from other families with similar experiences.

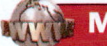 **MediaLink**

National Center for Complementary and Alternative Medicine

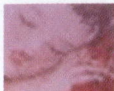

FAMILIES WANT TO KNOW

School Suggestions for Children with ADD/ADHD

Parents can work with teachers to provide for a school environment that fosters attention and learning. Some ideas that may be helpful include:

- Have the child sit near the front of the class.
- Plan a reminder that is apparent to the teacher and student but not to other children when the child needs to concentrate on attention. This might be an object placed on the student's desk or a light hand placed on the shoulder or arm.
- Give instructions verbally and in written form and repeat them more than once.
- Provide opportunities to take notes and make lists of assignments and mark them off when accomplished. Have a planned time to go through the child's backpack daily so notices are seen and homework is completed and in a uniform location.
- Use computers for making lists and taking notes. The child may need to listen in class, record the teacher, and take notes later from the recording.

- If the child has well-developed fine or gross motor skills, integrate motor movement into learning situations whenever possible.
- Provide quiet places with minimal distraction for examinations. Offer additional time.
- Allow time for organizing clothing, desk, and other areas.
- Go over assignments and tests with the child in person to explain areas that are understood and those that need attention.
- Find the child's areas of excellence and allow for performance in these ways. Some children are talented in dance, others in art or extemporaneous speech.
- Never call the child names, make fun of behavior or performance, or call him or her "hyperactive" in front of other children, teachers, or parents.

Adapted from: Call-Schmidt & Maharaj, 2004; Stein & Baren, 2003.

of doing homework or other tasks requiring concentration in a quiet environment without background noise from a television or radio. Encourage children with ADHD to keep assignment notebooks and use checklists to help them accomplish specific tasks.

Evaluation

Expected outcomes of nursing care for the child with ADD or ADHD include the following:

- Parents and child demonstrate understanding of the disorder.
- The family accurately and safely manages medication administration.
- The child demonstrates an increase in attentiveness and decrease in hyperactivity, impulsivity, and sleep disturbance.
- The child displays formation of a positive self-image.
- The child manifests formation of healthy social interactions with peers and family.
- The child achieves educational performance to maximum potential.

MOOD DISORDERS

Depression

Depression is psychological distress that can range from mild to severe. Only in recent years has depression in children been recognized as a clinical condition. Many children referred to child guidance centers and mental health professionals because of behavioral difficulties or poor achievement actually suffer from depression. The incidence of major depression is estimated to be about 0.3% in preschoolers, 2% in prepubertal children, and about 5–10% in adolescents (Dopheide, 2006). Males and females are equally affected until adolescence, when the incidence in girls rapidly increases to a point where they are twice as commonly afflicted. A history of substance abuse and anxiety disorder increases risk, and cultural variations in rates exist (Dopheide, 2006).

Etiology and Pathophysiology

Many theories have been proposed to explain the cause of depression in children and adolescents. Depression may be biologic in origin or a result of learned helplessness,

CULTURE

Depression Rates

Ethnic/racial differences in depression rates exist, with 29% of American Indian youth, 22% of Hispanic youth, 18% of Caucasians, 17% of Asian Americans, and 15% of African American youth displaying signs of depression (Dopheide, 2006).

cognitive distortion, social skills deficit, or family dysfunction. The physiological theory focuses on monoamine neurotransmission. These amines include indolamine, serotonin, norepinephrine, and dopamine; decreased levels are sometimes found in depression. Magnetic resonance imaging has suggested brain changes in individuals who are depressed, suggesting a biological basis (Dopheide, 2006).

Parental depression is a strong predictor of childhood depression. Abuse and neglect, family conflict, parental death, and low socioeconomic status predispose children to depression. Other psychiatric diagnoses are common in children with depression; these include conditions such as ADHD, anxiety disorder, bipolar disease, or substance abuse (Richardson & Katzenellenbogen, 2005).

Clinical Manifestations

Characteristic findings of major depression in children and adolescents include declining school performance; withdrawal from social activities; sleep disturbance (either too much or too little); appetite disturbance (too much or too little); multiple somatic complaints, especially headaches and stomachaches; decreased energy; difficulty concentrating and making decisions; low self-esteem; and feelings of hopelessness. There is much variation among children at different ages in the symptoms displayed, and they often have some but not all of the major criteria.

■ COLLABORATIVE CARE

Careful assessment of the child is the first approach, in order to rule out physical illness that can be linked to depressive symptoms. These may include diabetes, cancer, and some other conditions (Sheikh, Weller, & Weller, 2006). Initial psychiatric assessment is performed by a child psychologist or child psychiatrist. A variety of scales and techniques are used; however, little guidance is available relating to evaluation of children under 6 years of age. Examples of useful tools are the Children's Depression Inventory (CDI), the Revised Children's Manifest Anxiety Scale, the Beck Depressive Inventory, the Preschool Feelings Checklist, the Reynolds Child Depression Scale, the Reynolds Adolescent Depression Scale, and the Center of Epidemiologic Studies Depression Scale for Children (CES-D). The child is assessed for various mental health problems since comorbidities or combination with other disorders is common. Those with a history of bullying and substance abuse are at greater risk (Dopheide, 2006; Jellinek, Patel, & Froehle, 2002).

Treatment may include psychotherapy and psychotropic medication, a combination that is more effective than either approach alone (Treatment for Adolescents with Depression Study Team, 2004). Often a combination of individual, family, and group therapy provides the greatest benefits for young children and adolescents. Involving parents and other family members in the treatment plan is essential. Group therapy is an effective treatment measure for adolescents because of the importance of peer group relationships during the teenage years. Cognitive behavioral therapy may be used with adolescents, and play therapy may be used with younger children (Waslick, Schoenholz, & Pizarro, 2003).

Antidepressant medications, most commonly the selective serotonin reuptake inhibitors (SSRIs); tricyclic antidepressants (TCAs) such as imipramine (Tofranil) and desipramine (Norpramin); and amitriptyline (Elavil) may be prescribed. The only antidepressant approved to treat major depressive disorders in pediatric patients is fluoxetine HCl (Prozac), but others are used by clinicians when the child does not respond to Prozac. Analysis of studies of the TCAs have demonstrated their usefulness in adolescents but not in children (Hazell, O'Connell, Heathcote, & Henry, 2003). See Medications Used to Treat Depression on page 1122.

The SSRIs act to block reuptake of serotonin in the synapse, so that serotonin levels (which influence mood) increase. Although the SSRIs are generally considered safer than some other types of antidepressants, their use in children has been limited, so side effects must be monitored. The major serious side effect of the SSRIs is serotonin syndrome, a condition characterized by agitation, muscle twitching, gastric upset, chills, fever, confusion, and dizziness. Generally the child is started with a low dose, which is

GROWTH & DEVELOPMENT

Symptoms of Depression

Symptoms of depression in children vary according to their developmental levels. *Infants* may fail to eat and grow, while *toddlers* can show regressive behaviors in toileting and other activities. *Preschoolers* have less symbolic and other play activities, and demonstrate self-destructive play themes. They may whine and show irritability, show disinterest, and lack confidence. *School children* may show a decrease in academic performance, increased or decreased activity, somatic complaints, and loss of friends. The older school-age child may talk of running away or show signs of boredom and low self-esteem. The *adolescent* can have a wide array of symptoms such as anxiety, decreased social contact, poor school performance, lack of prior involvement in activities, poor self-care, sleep and eating disturbances, difficulty with parents and teachers, suicidal thoughts, or focus on violence. Sadness and **anhedonia** (inability to experience pleasure) are common at all ages (Dopheide, 2006; Luby, Heffelfinger, Koenig-McNaught et al., 2004; Pruett & Luby, 2004).

MediaLink

Case Study: Depression

NURSING ALERT

Sudden cardiac death has occurred in several children on tricyclic antidepressants (TCA). Because of this risk, serum levels should be monitored and electrocardiograms (ECG) are performed. Specific ECG changes along with a resting heart rate above 100, systolic blood pressure above 130 mmHg, and diastolic blood pressure above 85 mmHg necessitate immediate report to the prescriber.

→ **NURSING ALERT**

Serotonin syndrome, the serious and life-threatening side effect of SSRIs, is caused by overstimulation of serotonin receptors. It is more likely to develop when the child or adolescent is also taking St. John's wort, other antidepressants, alcohol, or diet pills, or abusing drugs such as ecstasy and LSD (Hu, Yang, & Ho, et al., 2005). Be certain to ask questions in a nonjudgmental way about intake of any alternative therapies, other medications, or substance use to identify those most at risk.

NURSING ALERT

There have been reports of increased suicidal ideation and other behavioral changes in children and adolescents taking antidepressant medications. In both the United States and Canada, the medications are now accompanied by clear warnings for use in these age groups. In particular, paroxetine (Paxil) has been implicated in suicidal thoughts and it should not be used in children (Pruett & Luby, 2004). Agencies in both countries have alerted healthcare providers and families of the risks, but leave decisions about medications to the prescribers and families, since the risk of depressive illness in itself carries a risk of harm to the individual. In the United States, the Food and Drug Administration recommends that a patient medication guide be provided to each patient explaining the risks of the drug and precautions to take. Information and instructions are also on the drug label. Nurses must reinforce this important teaching for all families when the child or adolescent receives medication, and emphasize the importance of follow-up visits and prompt reporting of any changes in the child/adolescent behavior.

Data from: U.S. Food and Drug Administration (FDA). FDA Public Health Advisory, October 15, 2004.

increased slowly to minimize the chance of side effects. There have been some reports of children who developed suicidal thoughts and committed suicide while taking SSRIs. Because of these reports and the lack of efficacy evidence, the FDA has cautioned against use of paroxetine in children under 18 years (National Institute of Mental Health, 2004).

■ NURSING MANAGEMENT
Nursing Assessment and Diagnosis

A thorough history and physical examination, including observation of behavior, are obtained at the time of admission. Assess the child for common risk factors for depression (Table 27–5).

Several nursing diagnoses that may be appropriate for the child or adolescent hospitalized with depression are included in the accompanying nursing care plan. Other diagnoses may include the following:

- Imbalanced Nutrition: More than Body Requirements related to eating in response to internal cues other than hunger
- Powerlessness related to sense of helplessness
- Chronic Low Self-Esteem related to negative self-evaluation

MEDICATIONS USED TO TREAT *Depression*

Selective Serotonin Reuptake Inhibitor (SSRI) Drugs Used to Treat Depression

Medication	Pediatric Dose	Adolescent Dose	Selected Side Effects
Fluoxetine (Prozac)	2.5–40 mg every day or 0.5–1 mg/kg/day	10–60 mg every day	Restlessness, headaches, akathesia
Sertraline (Zoloft)	25–125 mg every day or 1.5–3 mg/kg/day	50–200 mg every day	Dry mouth, gastric upset
Paroxetine (Paxil)	5–40 mg every day or 0.25–0.7 mg/kg/day	20–40 mg every day	Dry mouth, weight gain
Fluvoxamine (Luvox)	50–100 mg bid or 1.5–4.5 mg/kg/day	50–300 mg every day	Dry mouth, gastric upset
Citalopram (Celexa)	Little data available	10–40 mg every day	Dry mouth, nausea, sleep disturbance

Note: Data from Shugart, M. A., & Lopez, E. M. (2002). Depression in children and adults. Postgraduate Medicine, 112, 53–61; Walsh, K. H. (2002). Welcome advances in treating youth anxiety disorders, 19(9), 66–82.
Note: Although a variety of SSRIs are used in treatment of children and adolescents, the only approved U.S. FDA medication for major depressive disorder in this age group is Prozac, and the only approved FDA medications for OCD in pediatric age group are Prozac, Zoloft, Luvox, and Anafranil.

Table 27–5	RISK FACTORS FOR CHILD AND ADOLESCENT DEPRESSION		
Child	**Family**		**School and Social Situations**
• Frequent feelings of sadness, sleep problems, loss of interest in activities • Increase in risk taking and impulsivity • Previous suicide attempt • Alcohol or substance abuse • Diagnosed psychotic disorder • Chronic illness and frequent hospitalization	• Parental neglect, abuse, or loss • Dysfunctional family relationships • Family history of depression, suicide, substance abuse, alcoholism, other psychopathology		• Academic pressures and underachievement • Stressful social relationships • Declining participation in social events

Planning and Implementation

Nursing care of the child or adolescent hospitalized for depression includes administering medications and other therapy, and providing supportive care. Monitor vital signs of youth receiving antidepressant medications. Watch for common side effects of the agent(s) used. Carefully monitor for serious side effects of TCAs and SSRIs and be aware that lower doses are used at initiation with doses increasing slowly to the desired level. When dosages are altered, all behavior and ideation changes must be closely monitored. Monitor cardiovascular status, including hypertension and tachycardia; observe motor movement; and record dietary intake. Help parents to evaluate inpatient settings to be certain the care provided will best meet the needs of the child or adolescent. (See Families Want to Know: Selecting Residential and Inpatient Care for the Child with Mental Illness.) Refer to the Nursing Care Plan for specific nursing interventions for the child or adolescent hospitalized with depression.

Discharge Planning and Home Care Teaching

When the child has been hospitalized and is returning home, teach parents to recognize signs and symptoms of worsening depression. Parents should also be taught dosages and side effects of any prescribed medications. Review data in the MedGuide provided by the pharmacy for any medications. Caution parents not to alter dose or discontinue the drug without the guidance and monitoring of the prescriber. Instruct the family to remove guns, ammunition, and other potentially harmful items from the home. Have the family immediately seek emergency care if they are concerned about the child's safety or worsening condition. Refer the family to appropriate healthcare professionals and to support groups for family members dealing with depression.

Care in the Community

Most children with depression are cared for in the community. Maintain regular contact with family members through their healthcare visits to outpatient agencies and by making home visits. Monitor the child's affect, activity, and food intake. School teachers and counselors often are aware of the child's ability to perform in the school setting. Have the family schedule after-school care so young children are not left at home

MediaLink

Depression Support and Resources

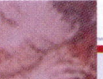

FAMILIES WANT TO KNOW

Selecting Residential and Inpatient Care for the Child with Mental Illness

Families need guidelines to assist them in evaluating inpatient facilities when a child with a mental disorder must be placed in an institution. They can be referred to the National Alliance for the Mentally Ill web site. Nurses can provide questions for the families to ask:

• What is the staff to youth ratio?
• What are the guidelines for chemical and physical restraint?
• Are children isolated alone when behaviors are inappropriate?
• Are children constantly monitored visually when in restraint or when potentially dangerous to self or others?

• Does the child have a full physical and psychological evaluation by a specialist within 24 hours of entry to the facility?
• What professionals review the plan of care and how often?
• To whom can the family speak for regular updates on the child?
• How often can the family visit?
• What services will be covered by insurance?
• What subjective feelings does the family member have when visiting the unit and facility?
• What services will be offered on an ongoing basis upon discharge?

NURSING CARE PLAN The Child or Adolescent Hospitalized With Depression

GOAL	INTERVENTION	RATIONALE	EXPECTED OUTCOME
1. Hopelessness related to long-term stress			
	NIC Priority Intervention: **Hope Instillation:** *Facilitation of the development of a positive outlook.*		NOC Suggested Outcome: **Hope:** *Presence of internal state of optimism that is personally satisfying and life supporting.*
The child or adolescent will discuss feelings of hopelessness.	• Encourage open expression of feelings. Explore hopeless, sad, or lonely feelings. Point out the connection between feelings and behavior. Assess the child or adolescent to identify the precipitating event when feelings of sadness arose.	• Expressing feelings may help to relieve sadness, loneliness, despair, and hopelessness. An accepting and nonjudgmental attitude must be maintained regarding any feelings expressed by the child.	By discharge, the child or adolescent expresses an interest in the future.
	• Encourage the child or adolescent to take part in self-care and unit activities. Use routines to establish feelings of control.	• An active role in self-care and treatment helps the child or adolescent to feel more in control.	
	• Medicate as ordered and document results.	• Antidepressants modify mood to a more hopeful outlook.	
2. Ineffective Individual Coping related to inadequate social support or disturbance in pattern of appraisal of threat			
	NIC Priority Intervention: **Coping Enhancement:** *Assisting a patient to adapt to perceived stressors, changes, or threats which interfere with meeting life demands and roles.*		NOC Suggested Outcome: **Coping:** *Actions to manage stressors that tax an individual's resources.*
The child or adolescent will use effective coping skills.	• Teach positive, effective coping strategies such as guided imagery and relaxation. Assist the child or adolescent to focus on strengths rather than weaknesses.	• Therapeutic techniques can help the child or adolescent to replace negative thoughts and images with more positive and effective beliefs and images. These interventions foster resilience.	The child or adolescent verbalizes and demonstrates ability to cope appropriately for his or her age.
	• Assist the child or adolescent to identify friends, family members, and others who are positive and supportive.	• Helps the child or adolescent to become aware that people can be caring and supportive (thus validating self-esteem).	
3. Impaired Social Interaction related to self-concept disturbance			
	NIC Priority-Intervention: **Socialization Enhancement:** *Facilitation of ability to interact with others.*		NOC Suggests Outcome: **Social Interaction Skills:** *An individual's use of effective interaction behaviors.*
The child or adolescent will participate in and initiate activities and conversation.	• Assist the child or adolescent to identify topics and activities of interest.	• The more the child or adolescent focuses on areas of interest, the less he or she will focus on internal anxiety and depression.	By discharge, the child or adolescent initiates conversation and activities with staff and peers.
	• Encourage interaction with peers and staff.	• Each positive interaction reinforces feelings of success. Each success reinforces the desire for future social interaction.	
	• Facilitate visits from family and friends.	• Reinforces positive and rewarding relationships.	
	• Provide guidance to family regarding interaction that promotes self-esteem.	• The family's existing interaction style is often negative.	

NURSING CARE PLAN The Child or Adolescent Hospitalized With Depression (continued)

GOAL	INTERVENTION	RATIONALE	EXPECTED OUTCOME
4. Imbalanced Nutrition: Less than Body Requirements related to loss of appetite secondary to depression			
	NIC priority Intervention: **Nutrition Management:** *Assistance with or provision of a balanced dietary intake of foods and fluids.*		*NOC Suggested Outcome:* **Nutritional Status:** *Amount of food and fluid taken into the body over a 24-hour period.*
The child or adolescent's daily intake will be adequate to maintain optimal nutritional status.	• Offer nutritious finger foods, sandwiches, and high-calorie liquid supplements frequently throughout the day.	• Convenient easy-to-eat foods encourage the child or adolescent to eat and maintain nutritional status.	The child or adolescent's daily intake will be adequate to maintain optimal nutritional status by discharge.
	• Offer easy-to-carry drinks that are high in vitamins, minerals, and calories.	• These are a convenient method for meeting hydration and electrolyte needs.	
	• Encourage daily vigorous physical activity of at least 30 minutes.	• Physical activity stimulates appetite.	

alone for extended periods. Assist the family in finding support for financial and emotional needs related to managing the child's depression.

Expected outcomes for nursing care of the child with depression are found on the accompanying nursing care plan.

Bipolar Disorder (Manic Depression)

Bipolar disorder is a mental illness in which extreme changes in affect and energy are manifested. Moods most often alter between mania and depression. Children often present with irritability or hyperactivity. About 1% of children and adults suffer from bipolar illness, with a high rate of onset from 15 to 19 years (Lansford, 2005). There is a high rate of attempted suicide as well as other disorders such as ADHD, anxiety, and substance abuse, all of which complicate diagnosis (Kowatch et al., 2005).

When parents or close relatives are affected, the child is more likely to have the disorder. Thus, a genetic etiology is probable. It is believed that genetics and environment interact to create the condition in youth. Brain imaging shows abnormalities of the frontal and prefrontal cortex, the hippocampus, the basal ganglia, and the left amygdala, which is the center for experiencing fear (Schapiro, 2005).

The manic phase of bipolar illness is characterized by hyperactivity and high energy, irritability, explosive outbursts, aggression, and sometimes hallucinations. In the depressive phase, the child is sad, has alterations in sleep and eating patterns, feels worthless, is lacking in energy, and is socially withdrawn, similar to any depressive illness. Mania may be the persistent symptom in children, or rapid cycles of mania and depression can occur throughout the day (Lansford, 2005).

Diagnosis and treatment of bipolar disorder should be performed by mental health specialists. Use of alcohol or illegal drugs should be ruled out as a cause of symptoms, even in children. Since the manic phase is often manifested by hyperactivity, the child may incorrectly be treated with stimulants (see discussion of ADHD earlier in this chapter), thus worsening the disease. While there are criteria for diagnosis of the disorder in adults, the presentation in children differs so diagnosis is difficult. Labile moods and sleep disturbance in children are associated with the condition (Faedda, Baldessarini, Glovinsky, & Austin, 2004; Kowatch et al., 2005). Children rapidly cycle through the depressive and manic phases and the condition may coexist with ADHD (DelBello, Adler, & Strakowski, 2006).

The treatment of bipolar disease involves a variety of drugs used to stabilize mood. Examples include lithium, divalproex, carbamazepine, olanzapine, oxcarbazepine, lamotrigine, quetiapine, and risperidone. Early treatment is key to preventing chronic, serious mental illness (Ferguson-Noyes, 2005; Kowatch et al., 2005). When the condition is under control, treatment for associated conditions such as ADHD or alcohol use can begin.

Nurses are instrumental in identifying children with the disorder, referring to mental health specialists, providing information to families, and monitoring the drugs and psychotherapy for the child. All of the medications used for treatment have side effects that require follow-up and regular monitoring. Assist parents to find resources for health care since medications and other treatments may be costly. Parents and children need information about the disorder since it may recur several times during life. Parents need resources and assistance to deal with the effects of the disorder on the family (Schapiro, 2005).

ANXIETY AND RELATED DISORDERS

A large group of anxiety disorders affects youth as well as adults. Some of the more common types seen in children and adolescents are described in the following text, with detailed nursing management described after the last condition, post-traumatic stress disorder.

Generalized Anxiety Disorder

Anxiety is a subjective feeling of uncertainty and helplessness, usually accompanied by CNS signs, including restlessness, trembling, perspiration, and rapid pulse. Anxiety is second to only substance abuse (see Chapter 6 ∞) in incidence for mental disorders and it is a common mental disorder among children. From 3–12% of children experience generalized anxiety disorder, and 8 to 19 years of age is a common time for its emergence (Hudson, Deveney, & Taylor, 2005). While all children experience anxiety at certain times, those with anxiety disorder are excessively worried about many things and are difficult to reassure. They worry about their health, the safety of the family, their performance in school, and the events in the world. They are not able to distract themselves from the worry. Many youth have accompanying physical complaints, such as headache or stomachache.

Anxiety disorders are strongly linked to familial and genetic factors. They may coexist with other mental health disorders, or children sometimes have more than one type of anxiety (Shear, Jin, Ruscio et al., 2006). Diagnosis is performed by a mental health specialist; treatment is usually cognitive behavior therapy (CBT) and may include medication. CBT can include child or family interventions that focus on relaxation, recognition of feelings, and self-talking. Medications that have been reported to be successful in children include sertraline and fluvoxamine (Hudson, Deveney, & Taylor, 2005).

Separation Anxiety Disorder

Separation anxiety disorder is characterized by an extreme state of uneasiness when in unfamiliar surroundings and often by refusal to visit friends' homes or attend school for at least 2 weeks. It is the most common type of anxiety disorder manifested by children (Cartwright-Hatton, McNicol, & Doublday, 2006). Approximately 75% of children with separation anxiety disorder refuse to attend school (see School Phobia, to follow). This disorder occurs in approximately 4–5% of children and in twice as many girls as boys (Shear et al., 2006; Wren, Bridge, & Birmaher, 2004). The peak age for occurrence is 7 to 9 years. It may be recurrent and become worse periodically.

Children with separation anxiety disorder tend to be perfectionistic, overly compliant, and eager to please. They appear to cling to the parent or caretaker. They may use physical complaints such as headaches, abdominal pain, nausea, and vomiting in an attempt to avoid being away from the parent. Depression frequently accompanies separation anxiety disorder. The resulting avoidant behaviors can interfere with personal growth and development, academic achievement, and social functioning.

Diagnosis is made by a mental health specialist. Treatment includes CBT with both the child and parents. Parents learn about the disorder and how to structure the setting so that the child is expected to attend school. Consistency in expectations is

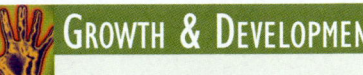

needed since if the child is permitted to stay home some days or has missed school and other activities for longer periods, treatment is more difficult. The child learns what situations cause anxiety and how to handle it. Both parents and the child work out the expectations for behavior for the child with the mental health therapist. School personnel and those from other settings where the child spends time need to be included in the treatment plan. Medication has occasionally been used but only if CBT is not helpful (Jurbergs & Ledley, 2005). The SSRI fluoxetine has been used with a dose of 10–20 mg/day for children and adolescents; the dose may be increased as needed at weekly intervals to a maximum of 60 mg/day (Bindler & Howry, 2005). See the medication table on page 1122.

Panic Disorder

Panic disorder is the presence of recurrent, unexpected panic attacks. These attacks are periods of intense fear and discomfort in the absence of real danger. The risk of panic disorder ranges from 0.4% in adolescent boys, to 0.7% in adolescent girls, and 1.5% in adults. Predictive factors for panic attacks in adolescence include a history of separation anxiety disorder earlier in life, history of parental panic attack, and history of parental chronic illness (Hayward, Wilson, Lagle et al., 2004).

Examples of the physical symptoms experienced are palpitations, sweating, chills, hot flashes, shaking, shortness of breath, choking, chest pain, nausea, and dizziness. The person describes feelings of danger or doom. There may be accompanying agoraphobia in some people. **Agoraphobia** is an anxiety of being in places or situations from which escape may be difficult or embarrassing, or in which help may not be available. The attacks may be continuous or episodic, but generally are chronic in nature.

Diagnosis is made by a mental health specialist. Similar to anxiety, treatment may involve individual and family interventions using CBT, and the use of SSRI medication in some cases.

Obsessive-Compulsive Disorder

Individuals with obsessive-compulsive disorder (OCD) may be mildly or severely affected. From 1–4% of children are affected, and about 80% of adults with OCD were affected in childhood (Lewin, Storch, Adkins et al., 2005). Affected children have recurrent obsessive thoughts, commonly about contamination, harm, sex, or moral concerns. These obsessions are handled through a series of compulsive behaviors that interfere with daily life. Examples of behaviors are excessive handwashing, counting objects, and hoarding substances. These practices may take 1 or more hours each day. Children with OCD differ from adults in several ways. Children have more aggressive obsessions, such as fears of catastrophe, more commonly hoard objects, and are more likely to have religious obsessions. The presence of additional mental health disorders is common (Lewin, Storch, Adkins et al., 2005).

The basal ganglia of the brain are affected and a genetic link is observed. Neurochemical cause may be related to abnormal serotonin metabolism. MRI changes in the globus pallidus and anterior cingulated gyrus of the brain have been noted (Lewin, Storch, Adkins et al., 2005). Poststreptococcal autoimmune disorder may be a cause in some cases.

Diagnosis is made by a mental health specialist. The disorder may have been present for some time before diagnosis as parents tend to overlook or deny the symptoms, and children may hide the behaviors. Treatment may involve CBT, where the feared occurrence is presented and the person learns that no harm will occur. Involvement of the family in treatment is important so that members learn how to handle the child's ritualistic behaviors. Medications, particularly SSRIs, are effective in most children.

Social Phobia or School Phobia

Social phobia (also known as social anxiety disorder) is often manifested by children as school phobia (also called school avoidance or school refusal). It is a persistent, irrational, or excessive fear of negative evaluation or embarrassment in social situations and therefore of attending school. The child may fear being harmed or losing control. Social and school phobia can occur in children as young as 5 years of age, often emerges at 11 or 12 years, but can occur in children up to 16 years (Ginsburg & Grover, 2005).

Children with social phobia may fear asking for directions, ordering food at a restaurant, and speaking in the classroom. Children commonly report that teachers and peers "pick on" them. Somatic complaints are similar to those in children with separation anxiety disorder. Symptoms may be present only on school days and not on weekends or holidays, especially when school phobia is manifested. The social withdrawal that occurs in this disorder further impairs the child since social interactions are needed for normal developmental progression.

Diagnosis is made by a mental health specialist. A variety of instruments are available for assessing social phobia. Treatment includes the family and child, and establishes firm limits for behavioral expectations and consequences. CBT is used, commonly 12- to 16-week group sessions with other youth, and additional sessions involving the family (Ginsburg & Grover, 2005). SSRI medications may sometimes be needed to lessen anxiety in social situations so the child can experience success in these interactions.

Conversion Reaction

Conversion reaction is a disorder in which a disturbance or loss of sensory, motor, or other physical functions suggests neurologic or other somatic disease. The disturbance or loss cannot be explained by any known pathophysiologic mechanism. Instead, psychologic factors are involved. About 3% of the population experiences conversion reactions at some time (American Psychiatric Association, 2000). Adolescence and early adulthood are common times for the onset to occur.

Conversion reactions develop in response to a catastrophic event such as threat, loss, or harm. Clinical manifestations include altered sensations such as blindness or deafness; paralysis or ataxia, including inability to stand or walk and loss of ability to speak (aphonia); involuntary movements, such as pseudoepileptic convulsions; and constant complaints of pain with no physical basis (psychogenic pain). Children under 10 years usually present with gait abnormalities or seizures. The onset of conversion symptoms is usually dramatic and sudden. Symptoms often appear to be neurologic, but on careful examination obvious discrepancies are found. The person is usually calm about the symptoms even though they are serious. Often the child or family members appear indifferent or unconcerned over what healthcare providers consider an overwhelming physical disability.

Children suspected of having a conversion reaction require a complete physical and neurologic evaluation to rule out any possible physiologic basis for the symptoms. Individual and family therapy is usually necessary to identify the source of the psychologic conflict, pain, or need resulting in the conversion symptoms. Pharmacological approaches may also be used (Diseth & Christie, 2005).

Post-Traumatic Stress Disorders

Acute stress disorder can occur after any life-threatening event and is manifested in the first month after exposure to the event. Symptoms include repeatedly reliving the traumatic experience, anxiety, and increased arousal. Similarly, *post-traumatic stress disorder* (PTSD) victims have experienced or witnessed a life-threatening event; however, the symptoms of distress continue for more than 1 month and cause impairment in functioning (Jonker & Hamrin, 2003). Estimates of the incidence of PTSD are hard to obtain. It is assumed that about 40% of youth have an episode of trauma that could lead to PTSD and that 6% have symptoms of the disorder (Caffo & Belaise, 2003).

Etiology and Pathophysiology

Examples of traumatic events that are associated with post-traumatic stress include sexual or other child abuse, rape, car crash, fire, witnessing violence, and having an experience in war (Kaminer, Seedat, & Stein, 2005; Schafer, Barkmann, Riedesser, & Schulte-Markwort, 2006). The events which occurred in the United States on September 11, 2001, are potential causes of post-traumatic stress in children who either had a family member involved, lived near the events, or in some other way were profoundly affected. While the treatment of PTSD is discussed in this section, consult Chapter 6 ∞ for further examples of the types of violence that affect children and methods for reducing youth exposure to violent, traumatic events.

The disorder involves both a traumatic event and the child's reaction to this event. It is believed that brain changes occur in trauma, leading to neurobiological alterations that cause dysfunction of memory. Overreactivity of the amygdala, underreactivity of the prefrontal cortex, and increased dopamine in the medial prefrontal cortex are observed (Brown, 2005). Those with other psychiatric disorders, a family history of psychiatric illness, and severe or lengthy trauma all possess risk factors. Women also are at increased risk.

Clinical Manifestations

The child or adolescent with the disorder has feelings of fear, terror, and helplessness, and may relive the event frequently in thought and nightmares. The child may become emotionally numb in a subconscious attempt to protect the self, but may have a persistently increased state of arousal. The child with PTSD is often irritable and has sleep problems and inattentiveness. There is a state of hypervigilance and exaggerated startle response, such as to touch or loud noises. The person feels detached from others and alone. Even if the child appears to have adapted and functions normally immediately after the traumstic event, several weeks or even months later, the symptoms of PTSD can begin to appear.

The major types of manifestations cluster in three groups: (1) the person repeatedly re-experiences the event, such as in a nightmare or, for young children, in repetitive play about the event; (2) avoidance by purposefully avoiding places or activities that trigger the memory; and (3) arousal such as increased vigilance, and somatic complaints (Brown, 2005).

COLLABORATIVE CARE

The diagnosis is made by a mental health specialist. A history of traumatic events with normal childhood developmental behaviors before the event is characteristic. A variety of instruments are available to screen for symptoms characteristic of the disorder.

Counseling by a mental health specialist is the main therapy for PTSD. CBT is the treatment of choice, with both the child and family members included (Figure 27–8 ➤). A variety of antidepressants and SSRIs can be used for pharmacologic treatment, with the medication tailored to the specific symptoms that are most distressing and which have been resistant to CBT.

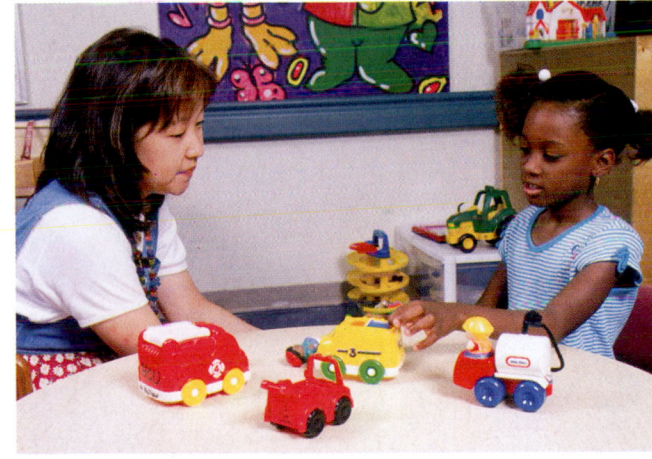

Figure 27–8 ➤ A psychologist uses play therapy to help Cassandra, a young girl who is experiencing PTSD. The child was in a car crash and physically recovered but has experienced nightmares about the event. She also developed a fear of leaving home. The therapist allows Cassandra to play with cars and talk about the event. She uses cognitive-behavior therapy to suggest ways of handling the thoughts and fears. This helps Cassandra to gain control over the event so that it is not so frightening and does not interfere with her functioning in daily life.

NURSING MANAGEMENT

Nursing management for PTSD and other anxiety disorders focuses on partnering with other health professionals and families to relieve the child's anxiety and return him or her to a normal and developmentally appropriate level of functioning.

Nursing Assessment and Diagnosis

Nurses often help to identify PTSD victims and others with anxiety disorders so that care can be obtained. Ask about traumatic events in the past and how the child reacted. Inquire about recent changes in the child's behavior. Include school attendance, complaints of physical illness, sleep patterns, and rituals in behavior. A family history of mental disorders may be useful. See Table 27–6 for an example of a screening tool related to

Table 27–6	SCREENING CHILDREN FOR EFFECTS OF TRAUMATIC EVENTS

Nurses are often effective in screening for events that cause anxiety in children. This a screening tool was initially developed for use after 9/11, but can be used for other traumatic events such as hurricanes, accidents, and violence. If several symptoms are experienced or if the child has impairment in academic or social functioning, a referral should be made to a mental health specialist.

For Children 71 Months of Age and Younger	• *Separation anxiety* • Psychomotor agitation • Regressive behaviors (thumb sucking, bedwetting, fear of darkness) • Persistent and repetitive trauma-related play • Irritability and low frustration tolerance • Disruptive or aggressive behavior • Nightmares, sleep problems
For Children 6 to 11 Years of Age	• Regressive behaviors • Irritability and low frustration tolerance • Disruptive or aggressive behavior • Problems with peers • Nightmares, sleep problems • Extreme withdrawal • Extreme fearfulness • Inability to concentrate • Refusal to attend school • Academic decline • Physical complaints (headaches, stomachaches with a medical basis) • Sadness, feeling hopeless about the future • Emotional numbing or flatness
For Adolescents 12 to 17 Years of Age	• Nightmares, sleep problems • Withdrawal and isolation • Inability to concentrate • School avoidance • Academic decline • Physical complaint without a medical basis • Sadness, feeling hopeless about the future • Suicidal thoughts • Emotional numbing or flatness • Flashbacks • Avoidance of reminders of the traumatic event • First-time or increased use of alcohol or drugs • Problems with peers • Antisocial behavior

From Redlener, I., & Grant, R. (2002). The 9/11 terror attacks: Emotional consequences persist for children. *Contemporary Pediatrics, 19*(9), 49. Used with permission.

9/11. Based on the data gathered, the child's symptoms and the mental health diagnosis, the nurse determines nursing diagnoses. Some examples include:

- Anxiety related to unconscious conflict
- Ineffective Coping related to perceived high degree of threat
- Powerlessness related to chronic mental illness
- Disturbed Sleep Pattern related to anxiety
- Post-Trauma Syndrome related to motor vehicle or other accidents

Planning and Implementation

Nursing care for anxiety disorders focuses on cognitive and behavioral therapies to enhance coping skills. Mental health nurses may conduct group therapy sessions both in inpatient and community settings (Figure 27–9, A&B ➤). Group sessions for children often provide a forum for discussion of fears, an opportunity to enhance skills of working together, and an opportunity to learn coping skills. Being a member of a group

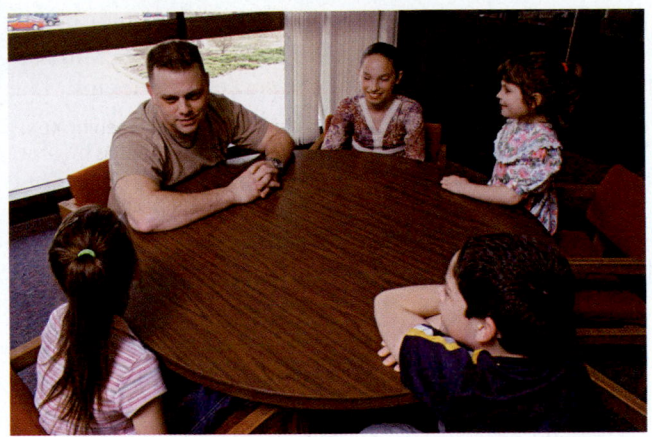
A

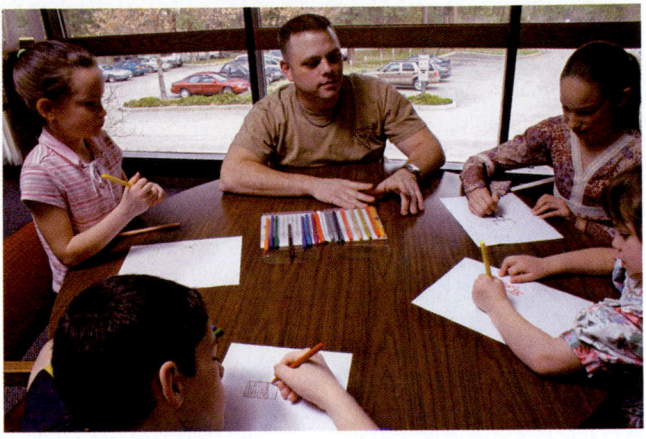
B

Figure 27–9 ➤ A, This nurse conducts a group therapy session for children who have experienced traumatic events and have resulting anxiety disorders. He is clearly engaged, has a positive rapport, and fosters exchanges among the children. B, Playing games and drawing are frequent techniques used in the group, followed by discussion of events and feelings. The children learn from the nurse and each other ways in which they can handle anxiety.

with other children experiencing anxiety or trauma can remove the stigma and allow the child the freedom to explore the behavior and its causes. Several of the techniques described in the chapter beginning, such as drawing pictures and discussing them or telling stories, are techniques used by mental health nurses in child therapy groups.

Children need to learn relaxation techniques. Nurses may teach such techniques or recommend that the child consider participation in yoga or guided imagery classes. Inquire about alternative therapies that the child and family are using or have an interest in beginning, and refer as needed.

Parents or other significant people should be included in the treatment program. Nurses often teach them basic information about the child's diagnosis and therapy. They should be in at least some therapy sessions with the child. Provide resources that they need to get relief from worry about the child, guilt about causing an accident that triggered the child's symptoms, or other feelings related to the diagnosis. (See Families Want to Know: Talking with Children About Traumatic Events.)

Insurance companies may provide limited payment for mental health services. Help the family to see the importance of recommended therapy and assist them to find resources for care, if needed.

School personnel may need to know about the child's treatment. Partner with the families to provide needed information. Some schools have counselors that can

---

COMPLEMENTARY THERAPY

Complementary and Alternative Practice for Mental Health Disorders

- Medications—for example, St. John's wort
- Self-hypnotic relaxation—to reduce pain and anxiety
- Acupuncture—anxiety, depression
- Massage therapy—anxiety, anger, grief
- Reflexology (manual stimulation of specific points on the foot)—anxiety
- Guided imagery—anxiety
- Biofeedback (use of machines to watch muscle or skin responses)—anxiety

---

FAMILIES WANT TO KNOW

Talking with Children About Traumatic Events

Whether a child or adolescent experiences trauma from a car crash, abuse, or environmental event, parents can help to decrease the effects of the stress and prevent the appearance of post-traumatic stress disorder by doing the following:

- Be sure children feel comfortable asking parents, teachers, or others about the events and their feelings.
- Assure children that their feelings are normal and may return over time.
- Be honest and open in responses, without overloading children with more details than they need.
- Be prepared to repeat answers and discuss the same topics many times.

- Get help from counselors who can suggest how to talk with children.
- Use communication methods appropriate at various ages, such as reading books, doing art projects, or drawing.
- Show children that they are loved by spending time and planning activities with them.
- Limit the television and other media time where the child is exposed to violence and traumatic events.
- Restore a sense of normal routines into the child's life.
- Be alert for increasing signs of distress and seek care from a professional if they occur.

be instrumental in carrying out treatment plans at school and acting as a resource in that setting. School personnel may be asked to provide feedback about the child's attendance, performance, and social skills as a measure of the success of therapy. The community or school nurse can relay this information.

Nurses often administer medications to children being treated for anxiety. Be alert for side effects and ensure the family knows how to safely administer the drugs. They should be kept securely locked away. Have the child return for follow-up as needed since some medications may take several weeks to achieve effects, and close monitoring is essential. The child should have a medication alert tag for drugs being taken.

Evaluation

The outcomes of nursing care for the child with anxiety disorder center on return to normal developmental activities, engagement in social relationships, learned coping skills for dealing with stress, and maintenance of safety.

SUICIDE

Suicide is the third leading cause of death in adolescents between 15 and 19 years of age. Over the past 40 years, teenage suicide has nearly tripled, with increases in suicide rates identified in both the United States and Canada (Centers for Disease Control and Prevention, 2004b; Shaw, Fernandes, & Rao, 2005). Suicide accounts for about 12% of deaths in teens, and about 4500 deaths annually in the United States. An analysis of many studies demonstrates that 9.7% of teens report at least one suicide attempt, and 29.9% have suicidal ideation at some time (Evans, Hawton, Rodham et al., 2005).

Boys die as a result of suicide four times more often than girls. This statistic is reversed for suicide attempts, perhaps because boys use lethal methods such as guns, hanging, and jumping more often than girls, who more commonly use drug overdose and wrist cutting (Evans et al., 2005).

It is not unusual for healthcare professionals and parents to label suicide attempts by children and adolescents as accidents. Up to half of childhood suicides may be recorded as accidents; suicide data for children under age 10 years are not maintained. Adults may have difficulty believing that young children, in particular, would have any reason to want to end their lives. For this reason, many children who are brought to the emergency department with indications of a suicide attempt are often classified as unintentional injury victims and released without arrangements for appropriate follow-up care. Accurate identification and treatment are needed for youth at risk of suicide (Pompili, Mancinelli, Girardi et al., 2005).

Many risk factors for suicide exist in children and adolescents (Table 27–7). The most common precursor to adolescent suicide is depression (see previous discussion). Common signs or symptoms of an underlying depression that could lead to suicide include boredom, restlessness, problems with concentration, irritability, lethargy, intentional misbehavior, preoccupation with one's own body or health, discomfort with sexual preference, and excessive dependence on or isolation from others (especially adults or caregivers). The depression may be exacerbated by a recent psychosocial stress such as loss or perceived rejection or ridicule. A previous attempt is also a common risk factor.

The child or adolescent found to be at high risk for suicide may be admitted to a psychiatric unit for care or cared for in a community mental health facility. Treatment may include individual, group, or family therapy. Negotiating a no-suicide contract is one method that may be used with a suicidal youth. In the contract, the child agrees not to attempt suicide during a specified time period. When a suicide attempt is made, the child or adolescent may be hospitalized for 24 hours, kept in a short-term monitoring unit, or sent home under close observation to ensure adequate assessment and monitoring. It is important to provide crisis intervention at the time of the suicide attempt to minimize the opportunity for repeat attempts and begin a therapeutic treatment plan.

Table 27–7	RISK AND PROTECTIVE FACTORS FOR SUICIDE IN CHILDREN AND ADOLESCENTS

Risk Factors	Protective factors
• History of previous attempted suicide • Friend's suicide or attempted suicide • School problems or changes in grades • Pregnancy • Drug use or abuse • Problems with a romantic relationship • Minority sexual practice • Loneliness, withdrawal • Feelings of anxiety • History of chronic family problems • Chronic illness • Physical, emotional, or sexual abuse • History of suicide in a family member • History of depression • Chronic low self-esteem • Change in behavior • Change in weight • Sleep disturbance • Giving away special possessions • Access to firearms and ammunition	• Emotional well-being • Satisfactory school performance • Participation in sports or other group events • Weight satisfaction • Parent/family connectedness • Family issues • School connectedness • Safe school • Safe neighborhood • Caring adult presence at school or elsewhere • Availability of school counseling • School policies on fighting, bullying

NURSING MANAGEMENT

Nursing Assessment and Diagnosis

The major nursing role is in prevention of suicide. All children and adolescents in health promotion visits and emergency rooms should be evaluated for risk. Healthcare providers at health promotion visits should be alert for children with depression (see former discussion), substance abuse, recent stresses, and changes in behavior. Inquire about sleep patterns, feelings of sadness, and use of alcohol and other substances. Gather a family history of mental health disorders, suicide attempts, and stresses. Ask about how often the youth talks with or has meals with the family. Be aware of the risk of self-inflicted accidental strangulation.

Most suicides are committed with firearms, which are usually obtained from the home (Roche, Giner, & Zalsman, 2005). Ask at each healthcare visit if the family has firearms. Encourage them to keep them unloaded, with ammunition and firearms locked in separate locations. Be sure that children and adolescents do not have access to the keys for the locked firearms.

The most important questions to ask of a youth admitted to the emergency room for a suicide attempt are:

- Are you here because you tried to hurt yourself?
- In the past week, have you been having thoughts about hurting yourself?
- Have you ever tried to hurt yourself in the past other than this time?
- Has something very stressful happened to you in the past few weeks (Horowitz, Wang, Koocher et al., 2001)?

Some nursing diagnoses possible for the child at risk of suicide include:

- Risk for Suicide related to hopelessness and substance abuse
- Risk for Self-Directed Violence related to history of suicide attempts, present suicidal ideation, and recent failure in school
- Readiness for Enhanced Family Coping related to recent teen attempted suicide

NURSING ALERT

A tragic cause of accidental suicide in children is that which results from the choking "game." About 25 children annually die in the United States from this practice. When the blood supply to the brain is interrupted and then rushes back, some people report a feeling of euphoria or a "high." Children and adolescents may seek the experience for the feelings it creates and may even become addicted to it. Unfortunately, some children become accidentally strangled and die from the experience. Methods that children use to cut off oxygen include using their hands to apply pressure to the carotids in the neck, or tying belts, cords, towels, and other items to the neck and then around doorways or other solid objects. Some children perform these rituals with others who then rescue them so that they begin breathing; many of the injuries occur when children are alone since there is no one to perform a rescue. Adults can watch for signs such as conjunctival hemorrhage, headaches, bruising in the neck area, periods of disorientation, hoarseness, and finding items tied to doors and other solid objects. Parents can also be alert if the history of a family computer has shown the child's entry to a web site that describes the practice. Nurses in schools and other settings should educate children about the dangers of this strangulation and should provide materials for parents to inform them of the risk (Nativio, 2006).

Planning and Implementation
Care in the Hospital

Many children at risk of suicide or who have just attempted to commit suicide will be admitted to the hospital for a period of monitoring. Therapy is begun and medications can be given under close supervision.

Nursing care centers on taking appropriate precautions to ensure the safety of a child or adolescent at risk of suicide. The child and the environment of the hospital or other setting are monitored for any object that could be used for self-harm. All potentially harmful objects, such as shoestrings, belts, pantyhose, and hair ribbons, are removed. All personal care items (including toothbrush and shampoo) are kept locked at the nursing station and monitored constantly when used by the child.

Children or adolescents who are considered at high risk for suicidal behaviors are attended by a nursing staff member at all times, including while using the bathroom and sleeping. It may be necessary for the child to dress in a plain hospital gown, be kept in a visually monitored seclusion room, or (if seriously impaired and self-abusive) be medicated for restraint for a period of time. Restraints are used only when ordered by the physician and interdisciplinary team caring for the youth. Physical restraint is only a short-term approach to provide immediate safety, if necessary. Chemical (medication) restraint may need to be used to prevent self-injury by the suicidal person. See page 1123 for information to help families evaluate facilities when choosing care for their suicidal child.

Hospitalization continues as long as the child's behavior is self-destructive. Children are referred for intensive individual and family therapy to begin in the hospital and continue after discharge.

Care in the Community

Encourage parents to keep follow-up clinic appointments, to watch for self-destructive behaviors, and to administer any prescribed medications according to the treatment schedule. Arrange home visits and other community resources for families. Fewer than one-half of adolescents who attempt suicide are referred for mental health evaluation and follow-up, so nurses are instrumental in referrals and in encouraging the care that youth need (Fleischman & Barondess, 2004).

Education in all school settings is appropriate to assist children in knowing about resources of help when needed and in identifying peers at risk. Mental health services of all types should be available in and embedded in schools since that is the setting where youth spend much of their time (U.S. Department of Health and Human Services, 2006). Be alert for children and adolescents at risk for suicide in any setting. Assess children and adolescents in schools, outpatient settings, and emergency rooms for the possibility of suicidal behavior. Report threats of suicide and depressive behavior. Recognize that when one suicide has occurred, there may be an increased risk for friends of the victim. Teach students to report to teachers, nurses, or counselors about friends who have threatened suicide or seem depressed or display behaviors different than usual. Nurses often plan with mental health specialists to implement suicide prevention programs in schools and communities (U.S. Department of Health and Human Services, 2006). Provide supportive services to family and friends when suicide occurs. Consult web sites and refer parents as appropriate.

Evaluation

Some desired outcomes related to suicide risk include:

- The family develops coping strategies to support the suicidal member.
- The child or adolescent takes actions to decrease sadness and increase interest in life events.
- The child or adolescent remains safe with no further suicide attempts or ideation.

MediaLink

Suicide Prevention Resources

TIC DISORDERS AND TOURETTE'S SYNDROME

Tics are sudden, rapid, recurrent, nonrhythmic, and brief motor movements or vocalizations. They may involve movement of the head or upper body, blinking of eyes, or a variety of verbal noises. They may be worse during periods of stress or tiredness. About 10–20% of children have mild motor tics at some time which gradually disappear with no intervention. Mid-adolescence is the most common age for tics to appear. When the tics are severe or last over 1 year, they are considered chronic and may require attention from a mental health provider (Schapiro, 2004).

Severe motor tics accompanied by verbal utterances are known as Tourette's syndrome. The syndrome is seen in <1% of children and is often accompanied by other diagnoses such as attention deficit and learning disabilities. Children with Tourette's syndrome may exhibit **coprolalia**, the involuntary utterance of obscenities, profanities, and racial slurs; or **copropraxia**, the involuntary use of obscene gestures (Schapiro, 2004).

There is an underlying genetic cause for tic disorders since about 75% have a family history. Boys are more affected than girls, suggesting an autosomal dominant transfer. The direct pathophysiology of the disorder is unknown, but dopamine, serotonin, and other neurotransmitter and neuropeptide levels are disrupted. Comorbidity commonly involves obsessive compulsive disorder and ADHD.

Careful diagnosis and identification of the disruptive effects of tics are the first steps. Education and reassurance may assist some children with tics. Relaxation and management of stresses in school and other settings may be helpful. The disorders have been treated with haloperidol in adults; pimozide (Orap), a dopamine receptor antagonist, is approved for treatment of childhood tics. Guanfacine and clinidine are sometimes used (Swain & Leckman, 2003).

Nursing care involves supporting parents and encouraging normal developmental progression for the child. Stress should be minimized and relaxation techniques taught. Administer medications and teach families about desired and side effects. If the child's verbal utterances are disruptive in the classroom, partner with families and the school to arrange for home tutors for a while if needed. The nurse can be instrumental in teaching school personnel and other children about the disorder so that they understand the child's behaviors.

TRICHOTILLOMANIA

Trichotillomania, or chronic hair pulling, can affect children and adolescents. Head hair is most commonly pulled, leaving patches of baldness, but eyebrows, eyelashes, and pubic and other body hair may be involved. Incidence is greatest in middle childhood but it can occur earlier or later. Hair pulling may occur in brief periods of stress or over longer periods during sedentary activities.

Trichotillomania is classified as an impulse control disorder. It has similarities to both obsessive-compulsive disorder and to Tourette's syndrome, both described earlier in this chapter (Whitaker, Wolf, & Keuthen, 2003). Behavioral therapy, hypnosis, and SSRI medication therapy are generally used in treatment. Group therapy may be an effective support mechanism that decreases guilt and feelings of isolation regarding the disorder.

People affected by the disorder usually feel shame and guilt. They try to hide the disorder and may not seek help for an extended period. The nurse should be alert for the disorder when head or body hair is missing, someone is wearing a wig, or eyebrows are heavily penciled. An appropriate way to question the child is to say, "Some people pull out their hair. I notice that you have no eyebrows or eyelashes. Is pulling them out something you do?"

Refer the child or adolescent to a healthcare professional. Try to establish a trusting atmosphere that fosters communication about the disorder. Encourage participation in the treatment plan. Ensure follow-up for care so effectiveness of treatment can be measured.

SCHIZOPHRENIA

Schizophrenia, a psychotic disorder that is rare in young children, occurs in 1 in 10,000 children. However, the prevalence of schizophrenia increases after puberty and reaches adult levels by late adolescence (Remschmidt & Theisen, 2005). The disorder most often manifests in youth between 15 and 20 years of age.

The cause of schizophrenia is unknown, but genetic predisposition and neurointegration deficits are suspected causes (Gochman, Greenstein, Sporn et al., 2004; Remschmidt & Theisen, 2005). The brain is altered in the disease, with progressively enlarged ventricles and nervous system arousal. Impaired glucose metabolism is often present. Onset is usually slow with increasing intensity over time. Most often the child demonstrates restlessness, poor appetite, and social withdrawal over a period of several weeks to months. Behavioral problems, slowed development, and minor neurologic symptoms may occur.

The clinical manifestations of schizophrenia are the same in children as in adults. Characteristic behaviors of the schizophrenic individual include social withdrawal, impaired social relationships, flat **affect** (outward appearance of feeling or emotion), regression, loose associations (thought characterized by speech in which ideas shift from one subject to another that is unrelated), poor judgment and problem solving, anxiety, delusions, and hallucinations. Motor abnormalities may include rocking and arm flapping.

During adolescence, acute schizophrenia can occur suddenly while the teenager is making plans to leave home to attend college, marry, or work in another area. Onset of symptoms may be triggered by an important loss (death of a significant other, parent, child, or friend).

Prompt diagnosis can lead to early treatment and more positive outcomes. Clinical therapy for childhood schizophrenia is multifaceted, including individual psychotherapy, family therapy, and various psychotropic medications (antipsychotics such as haloperidol [Haldol], antianxiety agents such as lorazepam [Ativan], antidepressants such as imipramine [Tofranil], and newer antipsychotics such as dozapine, olanzapine, and risperidone) (Remschmidt & Theisen, 2005). Drugs are only moderately effective at controlling hallucinations and delusions, responses vary considerably among individuals, and children may have different responses than adults. Side effects will determine what drugs are used and their duration. Antipsychotic medication is continued for at least 4 to 6 weeks before effectiveness can be determined. Medications often must be continued for several months or years after recovery from an acute schizophrenic episode, although medication-free trials may be attempted in children who have shown an absence of symptoms for 6 to 12 months.

Episodes of acute schizophrenia often require inpatient hospitalization on a psychiatric unit for thorough diagnosis and beginning management. Treatment may include an intensive school-based program in a structured, supervised setting with specially trained professionals. The goal of initial treatment is to reduce or control psychotic episodes and provide a safe, structured environment for the child or adolescent, enabling the child to live each day at an optimal level of functioning. Outpatient care is provided following initial diagnosis and establishment of treatment regimen.

Most children require long-term treatment, including intermittent periods of hospitalization. Children or adolescents whose symptoms are difficult to control and who present a safety risk to themselves or others may require long-term residential treatment. Earlier age at diagnosis and delay in treatment lead to poorer prognosis.

Nursing Management

The nurse may encounter the child or adolescent with schizophrenia during hospitalization for an acute episode, for treatment of another problem, or while working with the individual in the community. Nursing care centers on providing for the child's physical safety and psychologic care, as well as normal growth and development.

Family education and involvement in the treatment plan are essential. The family is taught to monitor the child's symptoms and progression. Educating the child and parents about the risk of recurrence and methods to alleviate side effects of prescribed medications may increase compliance with the treatment plan. The nurse performs assessments of the child for common medication side effects. For example, when excess weight is a potential side effect, frequent growth measurements are made. Neurological assessment and laboratory studies may be needed with some medications.

The family is assisted in establishing educational plans for the child and for integration within the school system. The nurse communicates with school personnel to ensure understanding of the child's condition and ongoing management of the Individualized Education Plan.

COGNITIVE DISORDERS

A wide array of cognitive conditions occur in childhood. Some are mild and not diagnosed until a child has difficulty in school, while others may be associated with physical signs which are visible at birth.

Learning Disabilities

Learning disabilities are a common problem of young children, affecting about 5–10% of school children. They involve neurological conditions in which the brain cannot receive or process information in the normal manner. Often the impairment is only in one or two types of learning, making diagnosis difficult. Common types of learning disorders are listed in the clinical manifestations table below. Children may have difficulty in processing visual information, which may be manifested in reading, writing, and mathematics performance. Others may have more difficulty with oral information, leading to problems in language development and reading (Kelly & Aylward, 2005; National Center for Learning Disabilities, 2004).

The causes of learning disorders are complex. Sometimes they are related to low birth weight or problems during the perinatal period. The disabilities should be diagnosed by a learning specialist such as a psychologist with specialty training. A series of cognitive and developmental tests are most commonly used. Brain scanning with magnetic resonance imaging (MRI) is showing promise for diagnostic clues in the future. There may be a genetic component since their occurrence is more common when other family members are affected. Treatments involve learning how to compensate for the difficulties by using capabilities that are intact. Some children need to have all material written for them, and others need to have verbal presentations. Specific learning goals are established with the assistance of learning specialists. Children with learning disabilities should have Individualized Education Plans (IEP) established with realistic goals for school performance (see Chapter 12 ∞ for further information about IEPs).

Nursing Management

Nurses play a major role in the identification of children with learning disabilities. You may be in contact with families during health promotion visits or other settings when parents relay concerns about the child's performance or difficulty in some aspect of school. Ask about a family history of learning problems and evaluate the child's history for prematurity, low birth weight, head injury, seizure activity, and other chronic health conditions. Assess the child for the following developmental milestones which can indicate learning disability:

- Lack of ability to phrase sentences together by 2½ years
- Inability to use speech that is understandable at least 50% of the time by 3 years
- Inability to ties shoes, button, hop, or cut with scissors by kindergarten
- Inability to sit for a short story by 3–5 years (Kelly & Aylward, 2005)

CLINICAL MANIFESTATIONS	LEARNING DISABILITIES
Disorder	**Clinical Manifestations**
Dyslexia	Difficulty with writing, reading, spelling
Dyscalculia	Mathematics and computation problems
Dysgraphia	Difficulty with writing, spelling, and composition
Dyspraxia	Problems with manual dexterity and coordination

When a child may have a learning disability, refer the family to the school or other testing resource. Partner with the family to plan for the child's learning needs. Help the family to work closely with the child, provide a setting at home to maximize potential for learning, and build healthy self-esteem in the child. Assist the family to work with the school to establish annual goals for the child. A multidisciplinary team commonly works within the school, and includes teachers, therapists, and the family in order to plan for the child's learning needs (Lambros & Leslie, 2005). Most children with learning disabilities can learn to perform well in their areas of strength and compensate for areas of difficulty. Early intervention is key to success and building positive self-image regarding abilities.

Mental Retardation

Mental retardation is defined as significant limitation in intellectual functioning and adaptive behavior. It is manifested in differences in conceptual, social, and practical life skills, and begins before the age of 18 years (American Association of Mental Retardation, 2004). Later events that lead to limitations in function are generally referred to as brain injury. Intellectual functioning is generally characterized by an IQ below 70 to 75 and significant impairments in **adaptive functioning** (the ability of an individual to meet the standards expected for his or her cultural group). The child with mental retardation has adaptive deficits in at least two areas such as communication, self-care, home living, social/interpersonal skills, use of community resources, self-direction, functional academic skills, work, leisure, health, or safety. A low IQ score by itself does not necessarily correlate with impairment in the ability to carry out adaptive skills. The child should be evaluated within the contexts of the individual cultural and community environment. The IQ score and the level of adaptive skills together determine the degree of severity of mental retardation.

Mental retardation is one type of developmental disability. A **developmental disability** is any of a variety of chronic conditions that are characterized by mental and/or physical impairments. Other examples include pervasive developmental disorder, cerebral palsy, and sensory loss. A developmental disability begins by the age of 21 years, and lasts throughout life (Bhasin, Brocksen, Avchen et al., 2006).

Etiology and Pathophysiology

Mental retardation occurs in 12 per 1000 children, a decrease from 15.5 per 1000 one decade ago (Bhasin, Brocksen, Avchen et al., 2006). The causes of mental retardation can be grouped into three general categories: prenatal errors in the development of the CNS, prenatal or postnatal changes in the biologic environment of the person, and external forces leading to CNS damage. In each instance, the precipitating factor causes a change in the form, function, and adaptation of the CNS. Table 27–8 provides examples of common causes of mental retardation for each category.

Three common conditions associated with mental retardation from the prenatal category are Down syndrome, fragile X syndrome, and fetal alcohol syndrome. They will be discussed in greater detail in this section. In the United States, about 1 in 1000 infants, or 5500 infants each year, are born with Down syndrome (Centers for Disease Control and Prevention, 2006). The condition is caused by an extra chromosome; the child has 47 rather than 46 chromosomes (see discussion of genetic transmission in Chapter 3 ∞). The most common chromosome affected is 21, so that the child often

Table 27–8	COMMON CONDITIONS ASSOCIATED WITH MENTAL RETARDATION	
Prenatal Conditions	**Biologic Environment**	**External Forces**
Down syndrome	Inborn errors of metabolism (e.g., phenylketonuria, hypothyroidism)	Traumatic brain injury (e.g., accident)
Fragile X syndrome		Poison ingestion (acute or chronic)
Fetal alcohol syndrome		Hypoxia/anoxic insult
Maternal infection (e.g., rubella, cytomegalovirus)		Infection (e.g., meningitis)
		Environmental deprivation

has trisomy 21, or three copies instead of two of chromosome 21. In addition to mental retardation and physical signs, the child with Down syndrome is at higher risk of developing other conditions such as cardiac defects, hearing loss, strabismus, gastrointestinal problems, orthodontic conditions, thyroid disease, dermatologic conditions, and leukemia (Van Cleve, Cannon, & Cohen, 2006). Jeremiah, who was described in the opening scenario, was born with Down syndrome. He had GI reflux and otitis media frequently as a young child.

Fragile X syndrome is caused by a single recessive gene abnormality on the X chromosome. A permutation to the X chromosome may occur in males or females. When a father or mother passes the faulty X chromosome to a daughter, it may remain as a permutation or may change into a true mutation. The daughter has two X chromosomes and therefore does not manifest this recessive disorder; however, she can give the mutated X chromosome to her son, who becomes affected with fragile X. The mutation of fragile X is on gene FMRP-1, which instructs cells to make a protein necessary for normal brain development. The faulty gene creates a deficiency in the FMR1 protein that leads to brain changes. The condition is often associated with other conditions such as ADHD, anxiety, and autism (Hagerman, 2006).

Fetal alcohol syndrome (FAS) is caused by the effect of ethyl alcohol on the developing fetus. The term *fetal alcohol spectrum disorder (FASD)* describes the wide range of effects from the condition, which can range from FAS to a milder condition called fetal alcohol effects (FAE) (Caley, Shipkey, Winkelman et al., 2006). Alcohol ingestion by the pregnant woman can influence development of many body organs, and its effects can range from mild to severe. In spite of many years of education, alcohol use remains a leading cause of mental retardation, affecting two in 1000 births in the United States, or 8000 to 12,000 infants annually (Troshinksy, 2004).

Chapter 29 ∞ discusses phenylketonuria and hypothyroidism, two common biochemical causes of mental retardation. Other causes involve traumatic brain injury and infections of the CNS (see Chapter 26 ∞).

Clinical Manifestations

Mild mental retardation was originally described as an intelligence quotient (IQ) between 50 and 70, moderate retardation with IQ of 35 to 50, severe retardation with IQ of 20 to 35, and profound retardation with IQ below 20. Although an IQ below 70 is generally considered indicative of retardation, the functional assessment of the child is now considered to be a more accurate identification of children's performance and needs. Children who are mentally retarded manifest delays in all areas of development, including motor movement, language, and adaptive behavior. They usually achieve developmental milestones more slowly than the average child. These developmental delays may be the first indication to parents and care providers of the child's condition.

Mental retardation is sometimes accompanied by sensory impairment, speech problems, motor and orthopedic disabilities, and seizure disorders. Of children with mental retardation, 10–30% manifest one such disorder. Table 27–9 lists several physical characteristics associated with Down syndrome, fragile X syndrome, and fetal alcohol syndrome.

■ COLLABORATIVE CARE

Diagnostic Tests

Mental retardation is diagnosed and initial treatment is planned in a multistep process, and by involving a multidisciplinary team that involves a developmental specialist, physician, geneticist, nurse, teacher, language therapist, and rehabilitation specialists. See Table 27–10 for a description of the *DSM-IV-TR* for mental retardation.

First, a comprehensive history and evaluation of the child's physical characteristics, developmental level, and intellectual and adaptive functioning is carried out. Laboratory tests such as chromosome analysis, blood enzyme levels, lead levels, or cranial imaging provide valuable information in some circumstances. A three-generation family history is performed (Moeschler, Shevell, and the American Academy of Pediatrics, 2006).

MediaLink

Down Syndrome Video

CULTURE

Fetal Alcohol Syndrome

Fetal alcohol syndrome is more common in groups with higher intake of alcohol. The rate in Native American and Alaskan Native communities is 10 times the rate in the population (Troshinksy, 2004). Because some Native American tribes have a high rate of alcoholism, the federal government and some tribes have joined to lower that risk among this ethnic group. On some reservations, such as the Yakama Nation in Washington State, alcoholic beverages are not sold and educational programs are in place.

Table 27–9	CHARACTERISTICS OF THREE COMMON CONDITIONS ASSOCIATED WITH MENTAL RETARDATION

Down Syndrome

(see Figure 27–10 ➤)
Small head (microcephaly)
Flattened forehead
Wide, short neck
Epicanthal eye folds
White spots on eye iris (Brushfield spots)
Congenital cataracts
Flat nose
Small, low-set ears
Protruding tongue
Short broad hands
Simian line on palm
Wide space between first and second toes
Hearing loss
Increased incidence of diabetes, congenital
  heart defect, and leukemia
Hypotonia

Fragile X Syndrome

Long face
Prominent jaw
Large ears
Frequent otitis media
Large testicles
Epicanthal eye folds
Strabismus
High-arched palate
Scoliosis
Pliable joints

Fetal Alcohol Syndrome

(see Figure 27–11 ➤)
Flat midface
Low nasal bridge
Long philtrum with narrow upper lip
Short upturned nose
Poor coordination
Failure to thrive
Skeletal and joint abnormalities
Hearing loss

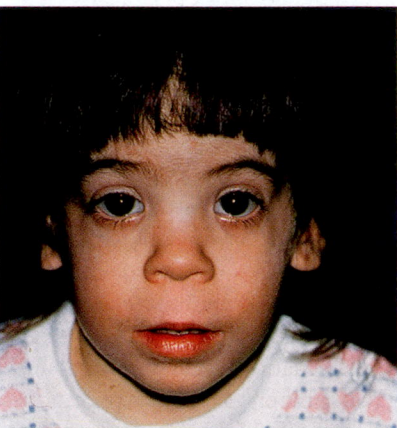

Figure 27–11 ➤ A child with fetal alcohol syndrome.
Courtesy of Dr. Sterling Clarren, Seattle, WA and Vancouver, BC. From Clarren, S. K., & Smith, D. W. (1978). The fetal alcohol syndrome. *New England Journal of Medicine, 298,* 1063–1067.

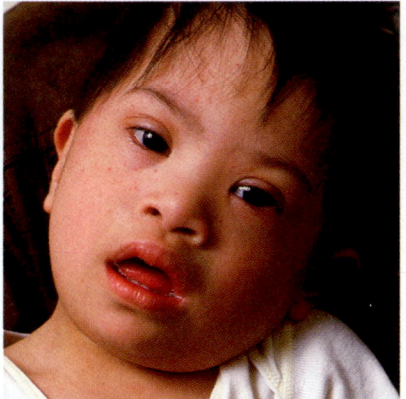

Figure 27–10 ➤ A child with Down syndrome.

LAW & ETHICS

Education for All Handicapped Children Act

The Education for All Handicapped Children Act, P.L. 94–142, provides free appropriate education to all handicapped children between 2 and 21 years of age. Amendments to this act in 1986 (P.L. 99–457) encouraged states to provide early intervention services for infants and toddlers with developmental delay by providing federal funding.

Developmental screening using a test such as the Denver II (see Chapter 7 ∞) can help to identify children who may be at risk. Tests of intellectual and adaptive functioning are performed when mental retardation is suspected. A neurologic examination may indicate asymmetry of movement or strength, irritability or lethargy, or abnormal pitch to an infant's cry. Because mental retardation may be accompanied by physical abnormalities, it is important to observe the child for facial symmetry, distance between the eyes, level of the ears, hair growth, and palmar creases. These abnormalities may be cues to other health problems.

Table 27–10	*DSM-IV-TR* DIAGNOSTIC CRITERIA FOR MENTAL RETARDATION

A. Significantly subaverage intellectual functioning: an IQ of approximately 70 or below on an individually administered IQ test (for infants, a clinical judgment of significantly subaverage intellectual functioning)

B. Concurrent deficits or impairments in present adaptive functioning (i.e., the person's effectiveness in meeting the standards expected for his or her age by his or her cultural group) in at least two of the following areas: communication, self-care, home living, social/interpersonal skills, use of community resources, self-direction, functional academic skills, work, leisure, health, and safety

C. The onset is before age 18 years

Reprinted with permission from the *Diagnostic and Statistical Manual of Mental Disorders,* Fourth Edition, Text Revision. Copyright © 2000 American Psychiatric Association.

Clinical Therapy

Based on the results of the evaluation, a multidisciplinary team plans the support needed to maximize the child's potential for development. Management focuses on early intervention to improve the degree of adaptive functioning. Simultaneous treatment of associated physical, emotional, and behavioral problems is provided. Depending on the child's condition, special education programs and physical or occupational therapy may be necessary (Figure 27–12 ➤).

The child may require supportive care and assistance with ADLs. The plans for intervention change as the child grows and family situations evolve. Some classes and community agencies offer transitional classes when children who are mentally retarded reach adolescence and young adulthood. These services help to teach self-care skills that may enable some youth to live in group homes or other community settings. Families receive help in planning for the child's future as parents look toward retirement. Information is provided on living options, health insurance, work opportunities, and other needs. This can also provide respite services for parents and other family members who have spent much time with the child for many years.

NURSING MANAGEMENT
Nursing Assessment and Diagnosis

Nurses can help to identify children with mental retardation through history taking, observation, and developmental screening during early childhood. The history should provide information about the mental and adaptive functioning of birth parents and other family members, as mental retardation may cluster in some families and conditions such as fragile X syndrome are genetic in origin. The pregnancy and birth history can provide important information relating to alcohol and drug use by the mother during pregnancy. Be alert for a history of difficult pregnancy and problems during delivery.

When genetic conditions in the family predispose family members to mental retardation, careful assessment of the child is needed. Children from deprived environments or those at risk because of environmental factors such as lead poisoning (see Chapter 6 ∞) are more likely to manifest mental retardation.

> **NURSING ALERT**
>
> Prematurity and low birth weight place the child at risk of displaying below-normal cognitive development. The premature and low-birth-weight infant need frequent, thorough neurologic and developmental examinations, particularly in the first 2 years of life. Premature infants are expected to reach developmental milestones at approximately the same age they would reach them if they were born at normal gestational age. For example, an infant born two months prematurely should be evaluated on milestones of an infant two months younger than the infant's current chronological age. The infant gradually catches up and reaches the chronological age milestones by about 2 years of age. Encourage parents to keep health promotion appointments and be sure the child receives developmental screening at each visit.

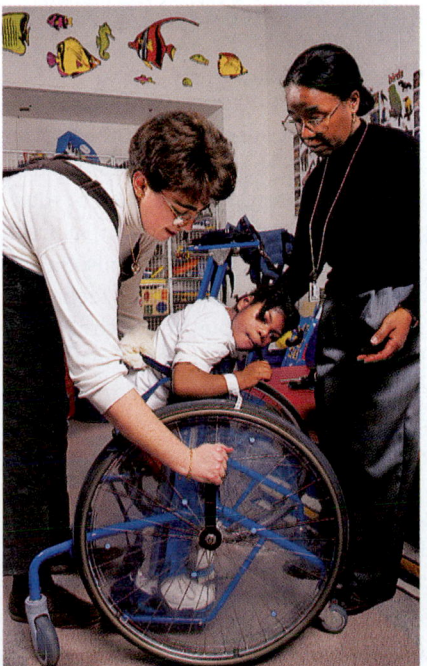

A

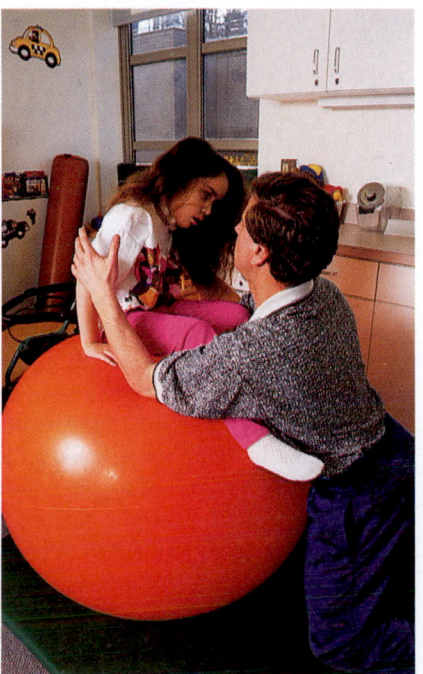

B

Figure 27–12 ➤ Physical therapy is an important component of medical management for many children who are mentally retarded. A, This girl with severe retardation is wheelchair bound, and is being positioned in a mobile prone stander, which enables her to interact in a different manner with her therapists and the environment. B, Physical therapists also provide outpatient care in the community to children with varying degrees of disability.

Many children with mental retardation are not diagnosed with the condition until they reach school age, particularly if the condition is mild or moderate. Early intervention, however, can help to enhance the child's functioning later. During home visits, clinic appointments, in childcare centers, and during hospitalization, be alert for signs of developmental delays, multiple (more than three) physical anomalies associated with a specific condition (see Table 27–9), or neurologic alterations. Developmental assessment should be part of each healthcare visit.

Once the diagnosis of mental retardation has been made, assess the adaptive functioning of the child and family. A functional assessment of the child should be performed, including toileting, dressing, and feeding skills. Assess the child's language, sensory, and psychomotor functioning. Assess the home and community for safety hazards. Observe how the family is managing with the child. Assess the availability of services such as support groups for parents and special education opportunities for children. Evaluate the coping skills of family members.

Several nursing diagnoses may be appropriate for the child with mental retardation, depending on the degree, cause, and outcome of the condition. Diagnoses that relate to impairments in adaptive functioning and family impact include the following:

- Delayed Growth and Development related to neonatal disease or condition
- Imbalanced Nutrition: Less than Body Requirements related to inability to ingest sufficient food
- Self-Care Deficit: Dressing, Toileting, Bathing related to developmental disability
- Impaired Verbal Communication related to developmental disability
- Risk for Injury related to lack of understanding of environmental hazards
- Compromised Family Coping related to the child's developmental variations

Planning and Implementation

Prevention is important for some types of mental retardation. All pregnant women or those who may become pregnant should stop ingestion of alcohol and nonprescription drugs. Encourage regular prenatal visits; this helps to prevent premature births, which have a higher association with mental retardation than birth at term.

Nearly all children with mental retardation are cared for in the community; however, they may have conditions that require periodic hospitalization or frequent healthcare visits. When needed, nursing care focuses on providing emotional support and information to family members, assisting the child with adaptive functioning, and fostering parental management of the child's activities. When possible, the nurse uses preventive teaching to lower the risk of mental retardation.

Provide Emotional Support and Information

Family members need empathy and support both at the time of diagnosis and in the ensuing years. Parents may be in an acute or chronic state of grief over the loss of the perfect child. Encourage them to verbalize their feelings. Introducing them to parents of other mentally retarded children may provide assistance and support as they learn how to manage the child's needs. Discuss the availability of respite care to provide parents with a break from caretaking. Other family members such as grandparents and siblings may also be experiencing grief or guilt and should be given an opportunity to talk about their feelings.

Parents need honest information and answers to their questions about the child's condition. Reinforce information provided by genetic counselors and other healthcare professionals. Parents need to be informed about community resources designed to assist children with mental retardation. Such resources include the Zero to Three Project, special education preschools and schools, county health services, and respite care. Refer parents to Internet sources, and help them to interpret information received and analyze its strengths and limitations. Ask parents if they have questions about Individualized Education Plans (IEP). Refer parents to Internet sources, and help them to interpret information received and analyze its strengths and limitations. Review federal and state laws and services that might be helpful to the family. Examples include:

- Administration on Developmental Disabilities (ADD) is the U.S. organization that ensures that the Developmental Disabilities (DD) Act goals are met. The DD Act implements the Developmental Disabilities and Bill of Rights Act of

2000 and seeks to enhance life through training activities, educating the community, eliminating barriers, and influencing policy (Administration for Children & Families, 2004).

- State Councils on Developmental Disabilities (SCDD) are present in each state to increase integration of children with developmental disabilities.
- Public Law (PL) 94–142 of 1975 mandated that all children, even those with handicaps, be provided with public education and related services.
- Public Law (PL) 99–457 of 1986 expanded the services of PL 94–142 to include children from birth to 5 years who need special education. Its focus is the importance of fostering development and enhancing the capacity of families to meet the needs of children.
- Public Law (PL) 101–336 of 1990 is known as the American Disabilities Act (ADA). It prohibits discrimination and ensures equal opportunity for persons with disabilities in employment, state and local government services, public accommodations, commercial facilities, and transportation.
- Individuals with Disabilities Education Act Amendments (IDEA) of 1997 strengthened the academic expectations and accountability for children with disabilities.

Maintain a Safe Environment

Children with mental retardation require close supervision because they may lack an understanding of common hazards. Ensure safety in the hospital environment. Assist parents to provide safety at home and school and to teach their child necessary skills such as pedestrian safety. Consider both physical and emotional safety. This type of child may be trusting of others and sometimes is at risk for physical or sexual abuse.

Provide Assistance with Adaptive Functioning

Encourage parents' efforts to maximize the child's areas of strength and identify needs related to adaptive behaviors. Refer them to resources to assist in the areas of adaptive functioning in which the child has impairment, such as communication, self-care activities, or social skills. During hospitalization, support parents' efforts to maintain the child's skills in toileting, dressing, and self-care by planning interventions to use the skills being taught at home.

Care in the Community

The child with mental retardation needs ongoing care throughout childhood, and adaptation of interventions as development occurs and the family's needs evolve. Parents often act as case managers for the child's care. Assist parents as necessary to acquire the skills required to coordinate the child's plan of care. Evaluate the child's needs regularly and assist parents with the treatment plan as necessary. Assist with plans for education and for services such as physical or speech therapy. Most children with mental retardation have an Individualized Education Plan designed to meet their specific learning needs. Parents, nurses, and others such as teachers and language therapists are part of the team that establishes this plan. Promote optimal development and socialization. As the child reaches adolescence, education is directed toward a vocation, issues of sexuality, and the goal of independent living, when appropriate.

Specific guidelines for care are available for the child with Down syndrome. These guidelines suggest times for evaluation of hearing, growth, cardiac function, and other areas designed for early identification and treatment of associated disorders (Van Cleve & Cohen, 2006). There are specific growth grids for children with Down syndrome, and specific topics to suggest for anticipatory guidance during healthcare visits.

Evaluation

The expected outcomes of nursing care depend on the child's needs and developmental level. Early in the diagnostic phase, desired outcomes may involve the family's understanding of the diagnosis and the child's special needs. Later outcomes may focus on the child's communication of self-help skills. Outcomes related to cognitive performance and adaptive skills may be developed during childhood.

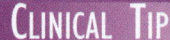

CLINICAL TIP

To determine the impact of the child with mental retardation on the family, ask parents to describe (1) family activities that include the child, (2) strategies that parents and siblings use to deal with community attitudes about the child, and (3) in the case of a child with other disabilities, methods of managing the child's care and planning for future care needs.

MediaLink

Care Plan Activity: Emergency Nursing Care for a Child with a Cognitive Disorder

MediaLink

Mental Retardation Resources and Support

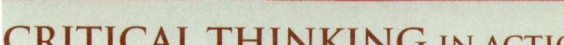

CRITICAL THINKING IN ACTION

Recall the opening scenario. Jeremiah is a 7-year-old child who has Down syndrome. He has been relatively healthy after some GI and ear problems in early childhood. His early intervention programs and now his entrance into school have provided a strong and nurturing environment for learning.

1. How will you decide if the physical growth and psychological development that Jeremiah is demonstrating are what would be expected for a child with his condition? What regular physical assessments are needed, due to some common accompanying health problems seen in children with Down syndrome?

2. Based on his history of frequent otitis media, what assessments will you perform now? See Chapter 19 for ideas.

3. What is the genetic basis for Down syndrome? Why are older parents more at risk for having a child with the syndrome?

4. Plan some physical activities that Jeremiah is likely to enjoy. How will you integrate them into his family and school life?

5. Jeremiah's parents are requesting information about what plans they should make for his care when they start planning for retirement. How can you assist them in locating resources to assist with the future care that Jeremiah will need as he grows into teen years and young adulthood?

 Refer to your Prentice Hall Nursing MediaLink DVD-ROM for answers.

EXPLORE MediaLink

http://www.prenhall.com/ball

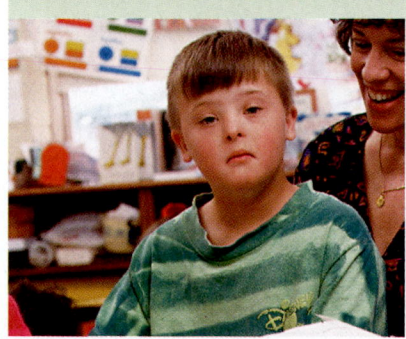

Resources for this chapter can be found on the Prentice Hall Nursing MediaLink DVD-ROM accompanying this textbook, and on the Companion Website at http://www.prenhall.com/ball.

DVD-ROM
Audio Glossary
NCLEX-RN® Review
Animations/Videos
  ADD/ADHD
  Down Syndrome

COMPANION WEBSITE
Audio Glossary
NCLEX-RN® Review
Care Plan Activity: Emergency Nursing Care for a Child
  with a Cognitive Disorder
Case Study: Depression
MediaLink Applications
  Evaluating Mental Health Information on the Internet
  Suicide Rates in Adolescents
WebLinks

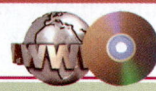

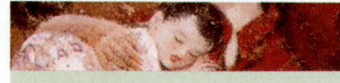

REFERENCES

Adesman, A. (2003). A diagnosis of ADHD? Don't overlook the probability of comorbidity! *Contemporary Pediatrics, 20*(12), 91–106.

Administration for Children and Families. (2004). About ADD. Retrieved July 15, 2005, from http://www.acf.dhhs.gov/programs/add/about/htm

American Association of Mental Retardation. (2004). Definition of mental retardation. Retrieved July 15, 2004, from http://www.aamr.org/Policies/faq_mental_retardation.shtml

American Psychiatric Association. (2000). *Diagnostic and statistical manual of mental disorders* (4th ed., text revision). Washington, DC: American Psychiatric Association.

Anderson, V. R., & Scott, L. J. (2006). Methylphenidate transdermal system: In attention-deficit hyperactivity disorder in children. *Drugs, 66,* 1117–1126.

Barber, S., Grubbs, L., & Cottrell, B. (2005). Self-perception in children with attention deficit/hyperactivity disorder. *Journal of Pediatric Nursing, 20,* 235–245.

Beauchesne, M. A. & Kelley, B. R. (2004). Evidence to support parental concerns as an early indicator of autism in children. *Pediatric Nursing, 30,* 57–67.

Bechtel, B. (2003). New research offers inroads to better understanding of autism. *Infectious Diseases in Children* (September), 14–16.

Bhasin, T. K., Brocksen, S., Avchen, R. N., & Braun, K. V. (2006). Prevalence of four developmental disabilities among children aged 8 years—Metropolitan Atlanta developmental disabilities surveillance program, 1996 and 2000. *Morbidity and Mortality Weekly Report, 55,* SS–1, 1–9.

Binder, R., & Howry, L. (2005). *Pediatric Drug Guide.* Upper Saddle River, NJ: Prentice Hall Health.

Brown, E. J. (2005). Clinical characteristics and efficacious treatment of posttraumatic stress disorder in children and adolescents. *Pediatric Annals, 34,* 139–146.

Brown, R. T., Amler, R. W., Freeman, W. S., Perrin, J. M., Stein, M. T., Feldman, H. M., Pierce, L., Wolraich, M. L. & Committee an Quality Improvement Subcommittee on Attention – Deficit/Hyperactivity Disorder (2005). Treatment of hype activity disorder: Overview of the evidence. *Pediatrics, 115,* e749–e757.

Buck, M. L. (2003). Atomoxetine: A new alternative for the treatment of attention-deficit/hyperactivity disorder. *Pediatric Pharmacology, 9*(2). Retrieved May 7, 2003, from http://www.medscape.com/viewarticle/452714

Burns, B. J. (2003). Children and evidence-based practice. *Psychiatric Clinics of North America, 26,* 955–970.

Butter, E. M., Wynn, J. & Mulick, J. A. (2003). Early intervention critical to autism treatment. *Pediatric Annals, 32,* 677–684.

Caffo, E., & Belaise, C. (2003). Psychological aspects of traumatic injury in children and adolescents. *Child and Adolescent Psychiatric Clinics of North America, 12,* 493–535.

Cala, S., Crismon, M. L., & Baumgartner, J. (2003). A survey of herbal use in children with attention-deficit-hyperactivity disorder or depression. *Pharmacotherapy, 23,* 222–230.

Caley, L. M., Shipkey, N., Winkelman, T., Dunlap, C., & Rivera, S. (2006). Evidence-based review of nursing interventions to prevent secondary disabilities in fetal alcohol spectrum disorder. *Pediatric Nursing, 32,* 155–162.

Call-Schmidt, T., & Maharaj, G. (2004). Using nonpharmacological treatments in conjunction with stimulant medications for children with ADHD. *Journal of Pediatric Health Care, 18,* 255–259.

Cartwright-Hatton, S., McNicol, K., & Doubleday, E. (2006). Anxiety in a neglected population: Prevalence of anxiety disorders in pre-adolescent children. *Clinical Psychology Review, 26,* 817–833.

Centers for Disease Control and Prevention. (2004a). Developmental disabilities. Retrieved July 15, 2004, from http://www.cdc.gov.ncbddd.dd.default.htm

Centers for Disease Control and Prevention. (2004b). Suicide: Fact sheet. Retrieved http//www.cdc.gov/ncipc/factsheets/suifacts.htm

Centers for Disease Control and Prevention. (2006). Improved national prevalence estimates for 18 selected major birth defects—United States, 1999–2001. *Morbidity and Mortality Weekly Report, 54,* 1301–1305.

Chamley, C. A., Carson, P., Randall, D., & Sandwell, M. (2005). *Developmental anatomy and physiology of children.* New York: Elsevier.

Christakis, D. A., Zimmerman, F. J., DiGiuseppe, D. L., & McCarty, C. A. (2004). Early television exposure and subsequent attentional problems in children. *Pediatrics, 113,* 708–713.

Corbett, J. V. (2004). *Laboratory tests and diagnostic procedures with nursing diagnoses* (6th ed.). Upper Saddle River, NJ: Prentice Hall Health.

Courchesne, E., Carper, R., & Akshoomoff, N. (2003). Evidence of brain overgrowth in the first year of life in autism. *Journal of the American Medical Association, 290,* 337–344.

Coury, D. L., & Nash, P. L. (2003). Epidemiology and etiology of autistic spectrum disorders difficult to determine. *Pediatric Annals, 32,* 696–700.

DelBello, M. P., Adler, C. M., & Strakowski, S. M. (2006). The neurophysiology of childhood and adolescent bipolar disorder. *CNS Spectrum, 11,* 298–311.

Department of Health and Human Services. (2004). *Report of the surgeon general's conference on children's mental health: A national action agenda.* Washington, DC: U.S. Department of Health and Human Services.

DiCicco-Bloom, E., Lord, C., Zwaigenbaum, L., Courchesne, E., Dager, S. R., Schmitz, C., Scholtz, R. T., Crawley, J., & Young, L. J. (2006). The developmental neurobiology of autism spectrum disorder. *Journal of Neuroscience, 26,* 6897–6906.

Diseth, T. H., & Christie, H. J. (2005). Trauma-related dissociative (conversion) disorders in children and adolescents—an overview of assessment tools and treatment principles. *Nordic Journal of Psychiatry, 59,* 278–292.

Dopheide, J. A. (2006). Recognizing and treating depression in children and adolescents. *American Journal of Health-Systems Pharmacy, 63,* 233–243.

Driessnack, M. (2005). Children's drawings as facilitators of communication: A meta-analysis. *Journal of Pediatric Nursing, 20,* 415–423.

Dulcan, M. K. (2005). Practitioner perspectives on evidence-based practice. *Child and Adolescent Psychiatric Clinics of North America, 14,* 225–240.

Evans, E., Hawton, K., Rodham, K., & Deeks, J. (2005). The prevalence of suicidal phenomena in adolescents: A systematic review of population-based studies. *Suicide and Life Threatening Behaviors, 35,* 239–250.

Faedda, G. L., Baldessarini, R. J., Glovinsky, I. P., & Austin, N. B. (2004). Pediatric bipolar disorder: Phenomenology and course of illness. *Bipolar Disorders, 6,* 305–313.

Ferguson-Noyes, N. (2005). Bipolar disorder in children. Advance for *Nurse Practitioners, 13*(3), 35–42.

Fleischman, A. R., & Barondess, J. A. (2004). Adolescent suicide: Vigilance and action to reduce the toll. *Contemporary Pediatrics, 21*(12), 27–36.

Galinat, K., Barcalow, K., & Krivda, B. (2005). Caring for children with autism in the school setting. *Journal of School Nursing, 21,* 208–217.

Giarelli, E., Souders, M., Pinto-Martin, J., Bloch, J., & Levy, S. E. (2005). Intervention pilot for parents of children with autistic spectrum disorder. *Pediatric Nursing, 31,* 389–399.

Ginsburg, G. S., & Grover, R. L. (2005). Assessing and treating social phobia in children and adolescents. *Pediatric Annals, 34,* 119–127.

Gochman, P. A., Greenstein, D., Sporn, A., Gogtay, N., Nicolson, R., Keller, A., Lenane, M., Brookner, F., & Rapaport, J. L. (2004). Childhood onset schizophrenia: Familial neurocognitive measures. *Schizophrenia Research, 71,* 43–47.

Gottesman, M. M. (2003). Helping parents make sense of ADHD diagnosis and treatment. *Journal of Pediatric Health Care, 17,* 149–154.

Hagerman, R. J. (2006). Lessons from fragile X regarding neurobiology, autism, and neurodegeneration. *Journal of Developmental and Behavioral Pediatrics, 27,* 63–74.

Hayward, C., Wilson, K. A., Lagle, K., Killen, J. D., & Taylor, B. (2004). Parent-reported predictors of adolescent panic attacks. *Journal of the American Academy of Child and Adolescent Psychiatry, 43,* 613–620.

Hazell, P., O'Connell, D., Heathcote, D., & Henry, D. (2003). Tricyclic drugs for depression in children and adolescents (Cochrane Review). *The Cochrane Library, 2,* Oxford.

Hoagwood, K. E., & Burns, B. J. (2005). Evidence-based practice, part II: Effecting change. *Child and Adolescent Psychiatric Clinics of North America, 14,* xv–xvii.

Horowitz, L. M., Wang, P. S., Koocher, G. P., Burr, B. H., Smith, M. F., Klavon, S., & Cleary, P. D. (2001). Detecting suicide risk in a pediatric emergency department: Development of a brief screening tool. *Pediatrics, 107,* 1133–1137.

Hu, Z. Yang, X., Ho, P. C., Chan, S. Y., Heng, P. W., Chan, E, Duan, W, Koh, H. L., & Zhou, S. (2005). Herb-drug interactions; *A Literature Review Drugs, 65,* 1239–1282.

Hudson, G. T., & Dixon, D. (2003). Autism: Challenges in diagnosis and treatment. *Clinician Reviews, 13,* 45–52.

Hudson, J. L., Deveney, C., & Taylor, L. (2005). Nature, assessment, and treatment of generalized anxiety disorder in children. *Pediatric Annals, 34,* 97–106.

Jellinek, M., Patel, B. P., & Froehle, M. C. (2002). *Bright futures in practice: Mental health. Volume II. Tool kit.* Arlington, VA: National Center for Education in Maternal and Child Health.

Jick, H., & Kaye, J. A. (2003). Epidemiology and possible causes of autism. *Pharmacotherapy, 23,* 1524–1530.

Jonker, B., & Hamrin, V. (2003). Acute stress disorder in children related to violence. *Journal of Child and Adolescent Psychiatric Nursing, 16*(2), 41–51.

Jurbergs, N., & Ledley, D. R. (2005). Separation anxiety disorder. *Pediatric Annals, 34,* 108–115.

Kaminer, D., Seedat, S., & Stein, D. J. (2005). Post-traumatic stress disorder in children. *World Psychiatry, 4,* 121–125.

Kelly, D. P., & Aylward, G. P. (2005). Identifying school performance problems in the pediatric office. *Pediatric Annals, 34,* 288–298.

Kowatch, R., Fristad, M., Birmaher, B., Wagner, K. D., Findling, R. L., Hellander, M., and the Child Psychiatric Workgroup on Bipolar Disorder. (2005). Treatment guidelines for children and adolescents with bipolar disorder. *Journal of American Academy of Child and Adolescent Psychiatry, 44,* 236–239.

Lambros, K. M., & Leslie, L. K. (2005). Management of the child with a learning disorder. *Pediatric Annals, 34,* 275–287.

Lansford, A. H. (2005). The importance of recognizing a child with bipolar disorder. *Contemporary Pediatrics, 22*(2), 69–78.

Levy, S. E., & Hyman, S. L. (2003). Use of complementary and alternative treatment for children with autistic spectrum disorders is increasing. *Pediatric Annals, 32,* 685–691.

Lewin, A. B., Storch, E. A., Adkins, J., Murphy, T. K., & Geffken, G. R. (2005). Current directions in pediatric obsessive-compulsive disorder. *Pediatric Annals, 34,* 128–134.

Lindsay, R. L. & Aman, M. G. (2003). Pharmacologic therapies aid treatment for autism. *Pediatric Annals, 32,* 671–676.

Looman, W. S. (2006). A developmental approach to understanding drawings and narratives from children displaced by Hurricane Katrina. *Journal of Pediatric Health Care, 20,* 158–166.

Luby, J. L., Heffelfinger, A., Koenig-McNaught, A. L., et al. (2004). The Preschool Feelings Checklist: A brief and sensitive screening measure for depression in young children. *Journal of the American Academy of Child and Adolescent Psychiatry, 43*, 708–717.

Liu, Y. H., & Leslie, L. K. (2003). Diagnosing ADHD: Putting AAP guidelines to the test—and into practice. *Contemporary Pediatrics, 20*(12), 51–73.

Luther, E. H., Canham, D. L., & Cureton, V. Y. (2005). Coping and social support for parents of children with autism. *Journal of School Nursing, 21*, 40–47.

McDonnell, J. A., Doyle, R., & Surman, C. (2003). Seeking a link between ADHD medications. *Clinician Reviews, 13*, 110–117.

March, J. S. (2004). Pediatric autoimmune neuropsychiatric disorders associated with streptococcal infection (PANDAS): Implications for clinical practice. *Archives of Pediatrics and Adolescent Medicine, 158*, 927–929.

Melnyk, B. M., Brown, H. E., Jones, D. C., Kreipe, R., & Novak, J. (Eds.). (2003). Improving the mental/psychosocial health of U.S. children and adolescents: Outcomes and implementation strategies from the National KySS Summit. *Journal of Pediatric Health Care, 17*, supplement, S1–S245.

Melnyk, B. M., Moldenhauer, Z., Tuttle, J., Veenema, T. G., Jones, D., & Novak, J. (2003, February). Improving child and adolescent mental health: An evidence-based approach. *Advance for Nurse Practitioners*, 47–52.

Meunier-Sham, J. (2003). Increased volume/length of stay for pediatric mental health patients: One ED's response. *Journal of Emergency Nursing, 29*, 229–239.

Meyer, G. A., & Batshaw, M. L. (2002). Fragile X syndrome. In M. L. Batshaw (Ed.), Children with Disabilities, Baltimore: Paul H. Brookes Publishing Co.

Moeschler, J. B., Shevell, M., and the American Academy of Pediatrics Committee on Genetics. (2006). Clinical genetic evaluation of the child with mental retardation or developmental delays. *Pediatrics, 117*, 2304–2316.

Nash, P. L., & Coury, D. L. (2003). Screening tools assist with diagnosis of autistic spectrum disorders. *Pediatric Annals, 32*, 664–670.

National Center for Learning Disabilities. (2004). Learning disability. Retrieved May 25, 2004, from http://www.ldanatl.org/

National Initiative for Children's Healthcare Quality. (2003). *Improving care for children with ADHD*. Boston: Author.

National Institute for Health Care Management Foundation. (2005). *Children's mental health: An overview and key considerations for health system stakeholders*. Washington, DC: Author.

National Institute of Mental Health. (2004). Antidepressant medications for children: Information for parents and caregivers. Retrieved May 25, 2004, from http://www.nimh.nih.gov/press/StmntAntidepmeds.cfm?Output=PrintM

Nativio, D. G. (2006). Self-inflicted accidental strangulation: The choking game. *American Journal for Nurse Practitioners, 10*(6), 43–48.

Pompili, M., Mancinelli, I., Girardi, P., Ruberto, A., & Tatarelli, R. (2005). Childhood suicide: A major issue in pediatric health care. *Issues in Comprehensive Pediatric Nursing, 28*, 63–68.

Pruett, J. R., & Luby, J. L. (2004). Recent advances in prepubertal mood disorders: Phenomenology and treatment. *Current Opinion in Psychiatry, 17*, 31–36.

Redlener, I. & Grant, R. (2002). The 9/11 terror attacks: Emotional consequences persist for children. *Contemporary Pediatrics, 19*(9), 49.

Remschmidt, J., & Theisen, F. M. (2005). Schizophrenia and related disorders in children and adolescents. *Journal of Neural Transmission, 69*, 121–124.

Richardson, L. P., & Katzenellenbogen, R. (2005). Childhood and adolescent depression: The role of primary care providers in diagnosis and treatment. *Current Problems in Pediatric and Adolescent Health Care, 35*, 6–24.

Roche, A. M., Giner, L., & Zalsman, G. (2005). Suicide in early childhood: A brief review. *International Journal of Adolescent Medical Health, 17*, 221–224.

Schafer, I., Barkmann, C., Riedesser, P., & Schulte-Markwort, M. (2006). Posttraumatic syndromes in children and adolescents after road traffic accidents—a prospective cohort study. *Psychopathology, 39*, 159–164.

Schapiro, N. A. (2004). Tourette's syndrome and obsessive-compulsive disorder. In P. J. Allen & J. A. Vessey, *Primary care of the child with a chronic condition*. St. Louis: Mosby.

Schapiro, N.A. (2005). Bipolar disorders in children and adolescents. *Journal of Pediatric Health Care, 19*, 131–141.

Scharer, K. (2002). What parents of mentally ill children need and want from mental health professionals. *Issues in Mental Health Nursing, 23*, 617–640.

Schieve, L. A., Rice, C., Boyle, C., Visser, S. M., & Blumberg, S. J. (2006). Mental health in the United States: Parental report of diagnosed autism in children age 4–17 years—United States, 2003–2004. *Morbidity and Mortality Weekly Report 55*, 481–487.

Shaw, D., Fernandes, J. R., & Rao, C. (2005). Suicide in children and adolescents: A 10-year retrospective review. *American Journal of Forensic Medicine and Pathology, 26*, 309–315.

Shear, K., Jin, R., Ruscio, A. M., Walters, E. E. & Kessler, R. C. (2006). Prevalence and correlates of estimated *DSM-IV* child and adult separation anxiety disorder in the National Comorbidity Survey Replication. *American Journal of Psychiatry, 163*, 1074–1083.

Sheikh, R. M., Weller, E. B., & Weller, R. A. (2006). Prepubertal depression: Diagnostic and therapeutic dilemmas. *Current Psychiatry Reports, 8*, 121–126.

Shugart, M. A., & Lopez, E. M. (2002). *Depression in children and adults. Postgraduate Medicine, 112*, 53–61; Walsh, K. H. (2002). Welcome advances in treating youth anxiety disorders, 19(9), 66–82.

Stein, M. A., & Barren, M. (2003). Welcome progress in the diagnosis and treatment of ADHD in adolescence. *Contemporary Pediatrics, 20*(8), 83–107.

Suellentrop, K., Morrow, B., Williams, L. & D'Angels, D. (2006). Monitoring progress toward advising material and infant Healthy People 2010 objectives: – 19 states, Pregnancy Risk Assessment Monitoring System (PKAmg) 2000–2003. *Morbidity and Mortality* Weekly Reports, 55 (5509), 1–11.

Swain, J. E., & Leckman, J. F. (2003). Tourette's syndrome in children. *Current Treatment Options in Neurology, 5*, 299–308.

Treatment for Adolescents with Depression Study (TADS) Team. (2004). Fluoxetine, cognitive-behavioral therapy, and their combination for adolescents with depression: Treatment for Adolescents with Depression Study (TADS) randomized controlled trial. *JAMA, 292*, 807–820.

Troshinksy, L. (2004). Fetal alcohol syndrome. Closing the gap. *Newsletter of the Office of Minority Health*. U.S. Department of Health and Human Services, Jan–Feb 2004, 4–5.

U. S. Department of Health and Human Services. (2006). *The current status of mental health in schools: A policy and practice analysis*. Washington, DC: Author.

U. S. Food and Drug Administration (2004). FDA launches a multi-pronged strategy to strengthen safeguards for children treated with antidepressant medications. Retrieved July 10, 2006 from http://www. Fda.gov/bbs/topics/news/2004/NEW01129.html

Van Cleve, S. N., Cannon, S., & Cohen, W. I. (2006). Part II: Clinical practice guidelines for adolescents and young adults with Down syndrome: 12 to 21 years. *Journal of Pediatric Health Care, 20*, 198–205.

Van Cleve, S. N., & Cohen, W. I. (2006). Part I: Clinical practice guidelines for children with Down syndrome from birth to 12 years. *Journal of Pediatric Health Care, 20*, 47–54.

Volkmar, F. R., Wiesner, L. A., & Westphal, A. (2006). Healthcare issues for children on the autism spectrum. *Current Opinions in Psychiatry, 19*, 361–366.

Waslick, B., Schoenholz, D., & Pizarro, R. (2003). Diagnosis and treatment of chronic depression in children and adolescents. *Journal of Psychiatric Practice, 9*, 354–366.

Whitaker, H., Wolf, K. A., & Keuthen, N. (2003). Chronic hair pulling: Recognizing trichotillmania. *Clinician Reviews, 13*(3), 37–44.

Wilens, T. E., et al. (2003). Does stimulant therapy of attention-deficit/hyperactivity disorder beget later substance abuse? A meta-analytic review of the literature. *Pediatrics, 111*, 179–185.

Wilson, K., Mills, E., Ross, C., McGowan, J., & Jadad, A. (2003). Association of autistic spectrum disorder and the measles, mumps, and rubella vaccine: A systematic review of current epidemiological evidence. *Archives of Pediatric and Adolescent Medicine, 157*, 628–634.

Wren, F. J., Bridge, J. A., & Birmaher, B. (2004). Screening for childhood anxiety symptoms in primary care: Integrating child and parent reports. *Journal of the American Academy of Child and Adolescent Psychiatry, 43*, 1364–1371.

Wolraich, M. L., Wibbelsman, C. J., Brown, T. E., Evans, S. W., Gotlieb, E. M., Knight, J. R., Ross, C., Shubiner, H. H., Wender, E. H., & Wilens, T. (2005). Attention-deficit/hyperactivity disorder among adolescents: A review of the diagnosis, treatment, and clinical implications. *Pediatrics, 115*, 1734–1746.

ALTERATIONS IN MUSCULOSKELETAL FUNCTION

28

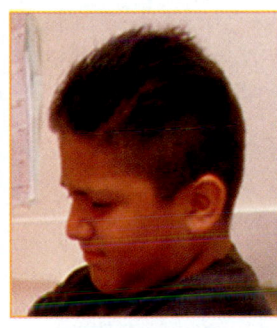

FERNANDO was playing soccer with friends during recess when he twisted his ankle and collapsed in pain. His friends helped him up and into the nurse's office. He is complaining of pain on the right lateral ankle. The nurse inspects the area and finds that it is red and slightly edematous. The foot is warm. Fernando can move his toes, and the pedal pulse is strong. Fernando is more comfortable when the nurse elevates his leg on a chair. She applies an ice bag and takes his vital signs. After a few minutes, Fernando states that his ankle feels better but that it still hurts. The nurse calls his home and his mother comes to take Fernando to the minor emergency center. The nurse calls in a report of the event and Fernando's assessment to the center. Fernando's mother calls later to say that he has a sprain and will need to keep it wrapped and elevated until tomorrow. Fernando is expected back at school in 2 days but will not attend physical education or play outside at recess for about 1 week.

What concerns will Fernando's family have about his injury? What teaching does he need to ensure healing of his ankle? Will any special adaptations be needed in his home and school? Is there any way his injury could have been avoided? The information in this chapter will provide answers to these questions and help to provide effective care for children like Fernando who have musculoskeletal disorders.

KEY TERMS

Blount's disease 1159	osteoblasts 1148
bones 1148	osteoclasts 1148
chondrolysis 1167	osteocytes 1148
compartment	osteopenia 1175
syndrome 1192	osteoporosis 1175
dislocation 1159	osteotomy 1159
dwarfism 1180	periosteum 1148
dysplasia 1159	pseudohypertrophy
equinus 1155	1184
hematopoiesis 1148	rickets 1159
joints 1148	sprain 1151
ligaments 1149	subluxation 1159
muscles 1148	tendons 1149
ossification 1149	varus 1155

MediaLink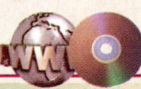

http://www.prenhall.com/ball

See the Prentice Hall Nursing MediaLink DVD-ROM and Companion Website for chapter-specific resources.

LEARNING OUTCOMES

After reading this chapter, you will be able to do the following:

1. Describe pediatric variations in the musculoskeletal system.

2. Plan nursing care for children with structural deformities of the foot, hip, and spine.

3. Recognize signs and symptoms of infectious musculoskeletal disorders and refer for appropriate care.

4. Collaborate with families to plan care for children with musculoskeletal disorders that are chronic or require long-term care.

5. Plan nursing interventions to promote safety and developmental progression in children who require braces, casts, traction, and surgery.

6. Provide nursing care for fractures, including teaching for injury prevention and nursing implementations for the child who has sustained a fracture.

FOCUS ON
The Musculoskeletal System

ANATOMY AND PHYSIOLOGY

The musculoskeletal system is composed of the bones and muscles; of joints, the supporting structures that facilitate movement; and tendons and ligaments that connect parts of the system. Cartilage is the connective tissue precursor to bone, and remains in some structures such as ears and ribs throughout life. Bone formation is a dynamic system at any age, but particularly so in children and adolescents. Children depend on a functioning musculoskeletal system to enable support and movement, which in turn ensures that exposure to various stimuli and normal development can occur.

Bones are composed of osseous or dense connective tissue; they contain an exterior shell or cortex, and an inner, primarily protein, matrix (Figure 28–1 ▸). The cells covering the cortex are called lining cells or compact bone, and protect the bone from penetration by circulating blood cells and other components of circulation; this covering is called the **periosteum**. The inner matrix is comprised of a series of interconnected plates called cancellous, trabecular, or spongy bone. Spaces between these plates are called bone marrow, and this is the area where **hematopoiesis** (production and develop-

ment of blood cells) occurs. In addition to the lining cells found on the bone exterior, other types of cells include **osteoblasts** that synthesize and lay down bone and then attract calcium and phosphates to strengthen the bone; **osteoclasts** that resorb bone in the constant process of bone formation and breakdown; and **osteocytes** that are special osteoblasts that sense and respond to bone pressure and bending in order to direct the process of bone remodeling. The process of bone growth and remodeling is influenced by factors such as pressure (via physical activity), hormones (parathyroid hormone, glucocorticoids, insulin-like growth factor, calcitonin), and external factors (dietary intake of calcium and phosphorus, bisphosphonate drugs, gallium, and so on).

The 206 bones of the human body are comprised of several types. They include:

- *Long bones* such as the fibula, tibia, femur, humerus, and ulna; most childhood growth occurs in these bones
- *Short bones* such as those in the wrist and ankle
- *Flat bones* such as the skull, sternum, and ribs; the ribs retain large components of cartilage even when mature
- *Irregular bones* which have a variety of shapes and sizes, such as vertebrae, pelvis bones, and scapula

Muscles are collections of cells that can contract, causing the accompanying skeleton to move. Muscle fibers require a supply of blood and nerves, and vary from small to quite large in size. Muscle cells develop in response to the stimulation of activity. Types of muscle cells include:

- *Skeletal* (striated) or *voluntary* muscles that involve the biceps, triceps, deltoid, gluteus maximus, and others
- *Smooth* (short-fibered) or *involuntary* muscles such as those in the gastrointestinal tract, lungs, and pupils of the eye
- *Cardiac* (striated, special-function) muscles that ensure the heart's constant contraction and relaxation

Muscles enable parts of the body to flex and extend, abduct and adduct, and carry out other motions (Figure 28–2 ▸). As one muscle flexes, the opposing muscle must extend in order to allow the movement.

Several other structures enable the musculoskeletal system to function. The **joints** are articulations or connections between bones. Fibrous joints provide for little movement (those in the skull are an example), cartilaginous joints allow for slight movement (vertebral joints are a good example), while synovial joints are movable within certain limits (knee,

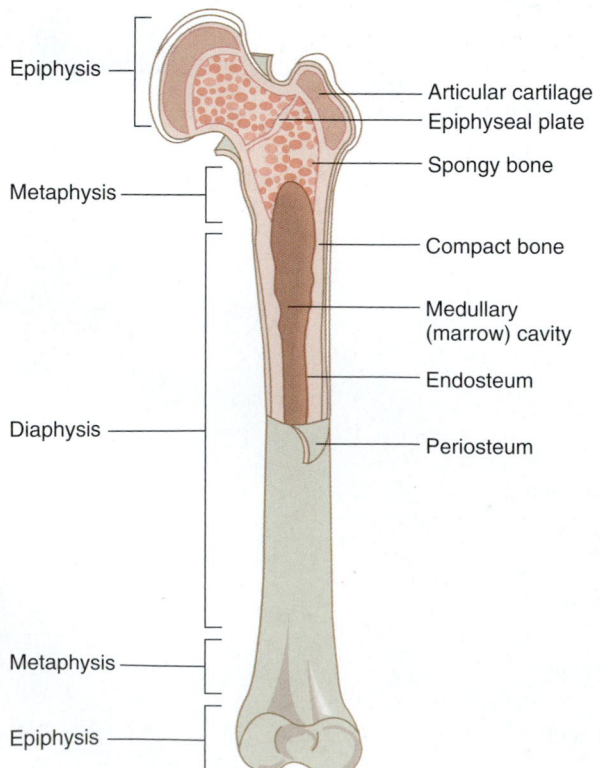

Epiphysis

Metaphysis

Diaphysis

Metaphysis

Epiphysis

Articular cartilage
Epiphyseal plate
Spongy bone
Compact bone
Medullary (marrow) cavity
Endosteum
Periosteum

Figure 28–1 ▸ The composition of long bones.

Varus
An abnormal position of limb that involves bending inward toward the midline of the body

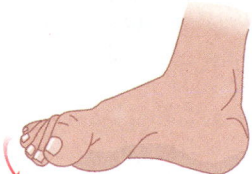

Valgus
An abnormal position of a limb that involves bending outward away from the midline of the body

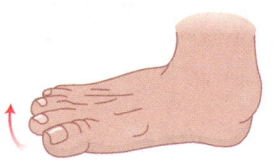

Supination
Lying on the back or placing the hand so that palm faces upward

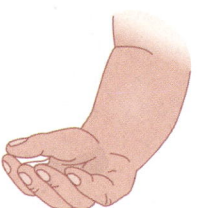

Pronation
Lying on the stomach or placing the hand so the palm faces downward

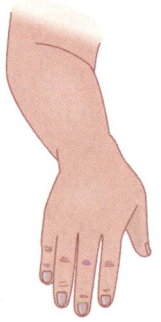

Adduction
Lateral movement of limbs toward the midline of the body

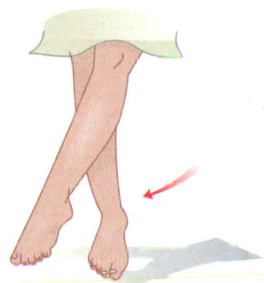

Abduction
Lateral movement of limbs away from the midline of the body

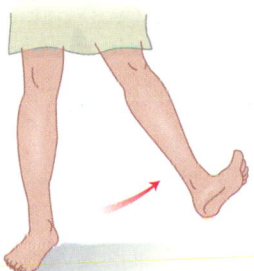

Flexion
A decrease in angle between bones forming a joint

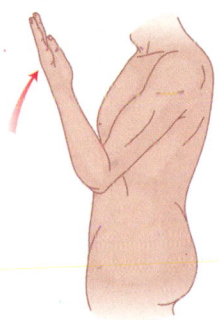

Extension
A movement that brings a limb into a straight position

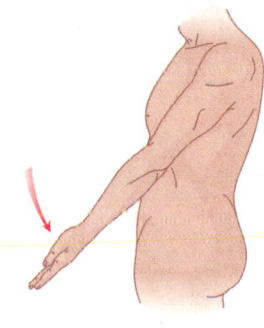

Inversion
Turning inward, usually more than normal

Eversion
Turning outward

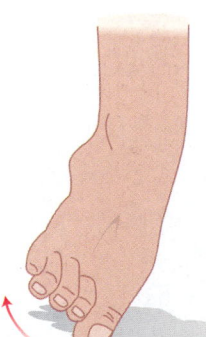

Internal rotation
Rotation of a body part towards the midline of the body

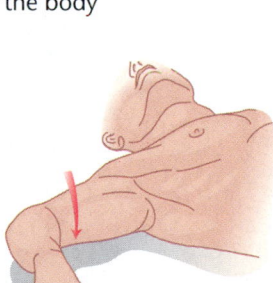

External rotation
Rotation of a body segment away from the midline of the body

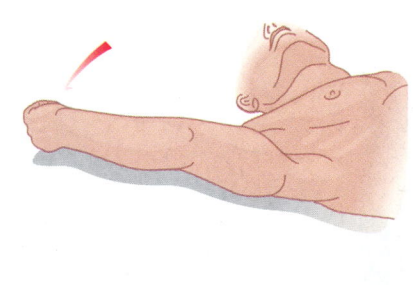

Figure 28–2 ➤ Musculoskeletal positions and joint motions.

hip, elbow, and shoulder are examples). Joints are complex in structure and function, containing the fibrous end of the bone, synovial membrane and fluid, other sacs called bursae, and ligaments. **Ligaments** are tough fibers that bind the ends of bones together. **Tendons** are fibrous bands that connect bone to its accompanying muscles, allowing the bone to move when a muscle contracts or relaxes.

PEDIATRIC DIFFERENCES

Bones

Several differences exist between the bones of children and those of adults. Although primary centers of **ossification** (bone formation) are nearly complete at birth, a fibrous membrane still exists between the cranial bones (fontanels). The posterior fontanel closes between 2 and 3 months of age. The anterior fontanel does not close until approximately 18 months of age, allowing for growth of the brain and skull. Most growth of the skull occurs by 2 years of age, with the skull reaching full size by 16 years (Chamley, Carson, Randall, et al., 2005).

Secondary ossification occurs as the long bones grow. Cartilage cells at the epiphyses (an area enriched with blood cells) are replaced by osteoblasts (immature bone cells), which push the end of the bone away from the shaft and engineer the deposition of calcium within the newly formed bone. Calcium intake during childhood and adolescence is essential to provide adequate bone density that will prevent osteoporosis and fractures in adulthood. See Chapter 4 ∞ for a discussion of inadequate calcium intake during school age and adolescence. Because growth takes place at the epiphyseal plates, injuries to this portion of a long bone are of particular concern in young children. The rapid bone growth of childhood facilitates healing after fractures, but may also lead to "growing pains," as muscles are pulled when bones grow quickly. The ends of the long bones (epiphyses) remain cartilaginous, allowing growth, until approximately age 20 years, when skeletal maturation is complete. At this time, the epi-

physeal plate closes, cartilage at the site is replaced by bone, and only an epiphyseal line remains (Figure 28–3➤).

Children and adolescents may suffer injury to the musculoskeletal system from falls, car crashes, and sports. Fractures are one type of common injury. The long bones of children are porous and less dense than those of adults. For this reason, children's bones can bend, buckle, or break as a result of a simple fall. In addition to the structural differences between the bones of children and adults, there are functional differences in the skeletal system of children. Before birth, the thoracic and sacral regions of the spine are convex curves. As the infant learns to hold up the head, the cervical region becomes concave. When the child learns to stand, the lumbar region also becomes concave. Failure of the spine to assume these final curves results in an abnormal curvature of the spine (kyphosis or lordosis).

Muscles, Tendons, and Ligaments

The muscular system, unlike the skeletal system, is almost completely formed at birth, with any remaining increase achieved in the first year of life. As a child grows, muscles do not increase in number, but rather in length and circumfer-

AS CHILDREN GROW

Musculoskeletal System

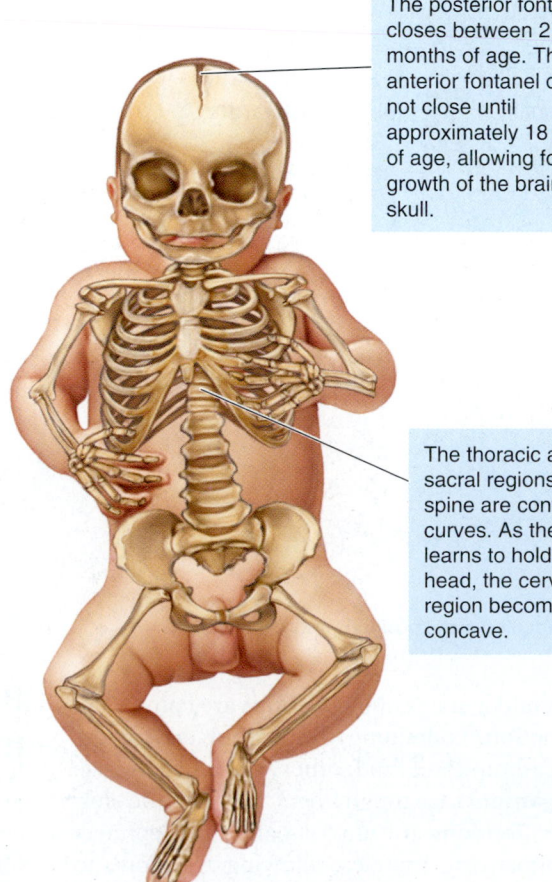

A fibrous membranne still exists between the cranial bones (fontanels). The posterior fontanel closes between 2 and 3 months of age. The anterior fontanel does not close until approximately 18 months of age, allowing for growth of the brain and skull.

The thoracic and sacral regions of the spine are convex curves. As the infant learns to hold up the head, the cervical region becomes concave.

Figure 28–3 ➤ Skeletal and muscle development throughout childhood.

ence. Muscle fibers reach maximum diameter in girls at about 10 years of age, and in boys at 14 years. Muscle strength continues to increase until about 25–30 years of age (Chamley, Carson, Randall, & Sandwell, 2005).

Until puberty, both ligaments and tendons are stronger than bone. When these structural differences are not recognized, a childhood fracture is sometimes mistaken for a sprain. A **sprain** is a tearing of ligaments, the structural sup-

port connecting bones, usually caused when a joint is twisted or otherwise traumatized. Tendons, which connect bones to muscles, grow in length and fibrous tissue as mechanical pressure is placed on them.

Examples of diagnostic and laboratory tests used for the musculoskeletal system are provided in the table on pages 1152–1153. Use the guidelines on page 1153 to perform a nursing assessment of the musculoskeletal system.

AS CHILDREN GROW

Musculoskeletal System

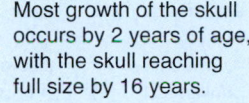
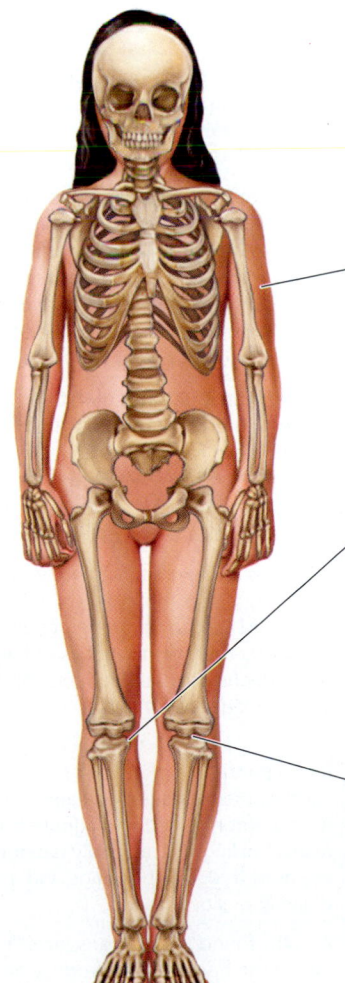

Most growth of the skull occurs by 2 years of age, with the skull reaching full size by 16 years.

The long bones of children are porous and less dense than those of adults, leading to higher rates of fracture.

When the child learns to stand, the lumbar region becomes concave in shape.

As a child grows, muscles do not increase in number, but rather in length and circumference. Muscle fibers reach maximum diameter in girls at about 10 years of age, and in boys at 14 years.

During childhood, cartilage cells at the epiphyses (an area enriched with blood cells) are replaced by osteoblasts (immature bone cells), which push the end of the bone away from the shaft and engineer the deposition of calcium within the newly formed bone.

The rapid bone growth of childhood facilitates healing after fractures, but many also lead to "growing pains" as muscles are pulled when bones grow quickly.

Muscle strength continues to increase until about 25–30 years of age.

The ends of long bones (epiphyses) remain cartilaginous, allowing growth, until approximately age 20 years, when skeletal maturation is complete. At this time the epiphyseal plate closes, cartilage at the site is replaced by bone, and only an epiphyseal line remains.

Until puberty, both ligaments and tendons are stronger than bone. As the child ages and cartilage is replaced by bone, the resulting bone is stronger than ligaments or tendons. Rates of fractures decrease while injuries to ligaments and tendons increase.

Figure 28–3 ➤ Skeletal and muscle development throughout childhood. (continued)

DIAGNOSTIC PROCEDURES/LABORATORY TESTS FOR THE MUSCULOSKELETAL SYSTEM

Diagnostic Procedure	Purpose	Nursing Implications
Arthrogram	A needle is inserted into a joint space, commonly the knee or shoulder, with use of local anesthetic. Samples of joint fluid can be aspirated and then radiopaque dye is injected into the joint cavity. A series of radiographs with the joint in various positions can help in diagnosis of torn cartilage or meniscus.	• Prepare the child and family for the procedure. Local anesthesia is often used, with general anesthesia for very young children. Monitor the child's vital signs before, during, and after the procedure. Support the child when the local anesthetic is inserted.
Bone scan	A phosphate or phosphonate radionuclide is given intravenously and, within several hours, concentrates in the bone. A scintillation camera then scans the body, and can assess for occult fractures, infection, and bone tumors.	• Prepare the child for the test. • If contrast medium is used, obtain history of hypersensitivity to iodine, seafood, or contrast dye from other radiographic procedures. Report to the healthcare provider and staff in the CT scan area. • Start an IV for injection of contrast material. • Sedate young children, if desired, to ensure that they are still; monitor according to sedation guidelines.
Computed tomography (CT)	A narrow beam of radiation examines body sections from different angles, producing a two-dimensional cross-section of the structures. Muscle or bone tumors or other abnormalities may be detected. A contrast media (or dye) can be used to enhance visualization.	• Depending on the body system evaluated, the child may be NPO or require bowel evacuation. • Teach the child about the procedure, including the size of equipment, noises, and length of time. • If contrast medium is used, obtain history of hypersensitivity to iodine, seafood, or contrast dye from other radiographic procedures. Report to the healthcare provider and staff in the CT scan area. • Use sedation for young children, if desired, to ensure that they remain still. Monitor children with sedation according to guidelines.
Dual energy x-ray absorptiometry (DEXA)	Body part to be scanned is placed between two photon energy beams. The bone mineral density and bone mineral concentration can be detected and compared to norms.	• Explain the procedure to the child. • Tell the child about the need to hold still for the procedure. Have the child practice holding a breath while being still.
Electromyelogram	Needle electrodes are inserted into skeletal muscles and muscle activity is measured during rest, voluntary activity, and with electrical stimulation. The test is useful in assisting with diagnosis of muscular dystrophy and to differentiate muscle diseases and lower motor neuron neuropathies such as those caused by hypothyroidism or diabetes.	• Record the child's medications. Inform the child that there may be slight pain when the needle electrodes are inserted. Support the child with age-appropriate relaxation techniques or distraction. Administer analgesics as needed for pain.
Evoked potential	A child who is awake is monitored by electrodes measuring brain and muscle activity. The baseline of electrical activity obtained is then used during later surgery, such as a spinal fusion for scoliosis, in order to monitor innervation to muscle groups and avoid injury to the spinal cord during the surgical procedure.	• Prepare the child for the procedure, including the size of equipment, sounds, and time it will take. Assist the child to relax with quiet music during the test.
Magnetic resonance imaging (MRI)	MRI uses a large magnet and radio waves delivered to the body part to be imaged. The energy field produced can be transferred as a visual image to the computer. Soft-tissue injuries not visible on radiographs, such as ligament and tendon problems, can be diagnosed by MRI.	• Prepare the child for the procedure, including the size of equipment, sounds, time, and tunnel. • Ensure that the child has no metallic objects or implants and is not connected to metal equipment. • Use sedation for young children, if desired, to ensure that they are still for the procedure; monitor the child with sedation according to guidelines.
Radiograph (x-ray)	Radiographs use irradiation to obtain images and capture them on film for diagnostic screening. They are commonly used to diagnose bone fractures and assess healing. Occasionally radiographs of the hand are used to detect bone age and assist in diagnosis of delayed or slow growth.	• Explain the procedure to the child. • Tell the child about the need to hold still for the procedure. Have the child practice holding a breath while being still.
Ultrasound	An ultrasound probe (transducer) is held over the skin above the body part to produce an ultrasound beam to the tissues. The reflected sound waves are then transformed into graphs or pictures of the tissue. It is used to diagnose developmental dysplasia of the hip in infants and used for bone mineral testing in adults.	• Prepare the child for the procedure. • Maintain NPO status if ordered. • Confirm that the child has not received any tests that interfere with results, such as GI series.

DIAGNOSTIC PROCEDURES/LABORATORY TESTS FOR THE MUSCULOSKELETAL SYSTEM (continued)

Laboratory Test	Purpose	Nursing Implications
Alkaline phosphatase (ALP)	Serum ALP provides a clue to the enzyme functioning of liver and bone. While children have levels 1–2 times greater than those in adults, elevations beyond these levels can indicate a variety of conditions such as bone destruction, bone cancer, healing fracture, hyperparathyroidism, vitamin D deficiency, and calcium deficiency. Decreased levels indicate inadequate bone formation and may be seen in conditions such as hypothyroidism, celiac disease, and cystic fibrosis.	• Prepare the child. • Perform the test in a treatment room rather than the child's hospital room or clinic examination room. • Label and transport specimens according to policy.
C-reactive protein (CRP)	C-reactive protein is not normally present in the blood and its presence, like an elevated ESR, often indicates inflammation or infection. It is commonly elevated in juvenile rheumatoid arthritis.	• Prepare the child. • Perform the test in a treatment room rather than the child's hospital room or clinic examination room. • Label and transport specimens according to policy.
Erythrocyte sedimentation rate (ESR or sed rate)	This test, which measures the speed with which RBCs settle in a test tube, is commonly elevated in inflammation, infection, tissue injury, or rheumatologic disorders. The degree of elevation is used to determine the severity of infection, and a decrease in the elevation can indicate improvement in condition. It is commonly elevated in juvenile rheumatoid arthritis. A decreased ESR may be seen in sickle cell anemia.	• Prepare the child. • Perform the test in a treatment room rather than the child's hospital room or clinic examination room. • Label and transport specimens according to policy.
Rheumatoid factor (RF)	This tests for an immunoglobulin present in the blood serum of many individuals with juvenile rheumatoid arthritis.	• Prepare the child. • Perform the test in a treatment room rather than the child's hospital room or clinic examination room. • Label and transport specimens according to policy.

Data from: Corbett, J. V. (2004). *Laboratory tests and diagnostic procedures with nursing diagnoses* (6th ed.). Upper Saddle River, NJ: Prentice Hall Health; Kee, J. L. (2005). *Handbook of laboratory & diagnostic tests with nursing implications* (5th ed.). Upper Saddle River, NJ: Prentice Hall Health.

ASSESSMENT GUIDELINES FOR THE CHILD WITH A MUSCULOSKELETAL SYSTEM ALTERATION

Assessment Focus	Assessment Guidelines
Muscles	• Is muscle mass symmetrical? • Are fine and gross motor movements in line with developmental expectations? • Can you identify any abnormal signs such as asymmetry of movement, tenderness, masses, weakness, hypotonia, hypertonia? • Can the school-age child get up from a lying or sitting position in the usual manner? • Can you describe the child's usual daily physical activity? • Has there been a loss of ability to perform developmental milestones?
Joints	• Are movements smooth and symmetrical? • Are there any signs of tenderness, decreased range of motion, inflammation, crepitus/grinding, or masses? • Do the hips of newborns and infants manifest symmetrical full range of motion? • Were there recent events of trauma such as in sports or a fall?
Bones	• Are there any masses noted? • Are arms and legs the same length? • Is there a recent decrease or change in mobility, such as limping? • Are bones in alignment, or are abnormalities noted such as bowlegs or knock-knees? • Upon spinal screening, is the spine properly aligned (see screening procedure within this chapter)? • In what sports does the child participate? Is recommended protective gear worn?
Tendons and ligaments	• Do all joints move through full range of motion? • Is there any pain upon joint motion or palpation? • Are there feelings of grinding or crepitus as the joint moves? • Has there been a recent sports or other injury? • In what sports does the child participate?

The musculoskeletal system helps the body to protect its vital organs, support weight, control motion, store minerals, and supply red blood cells. Bones provide a rigid framework for the body, muscles provide for active movement, and tendons and ligaments hold the bones and muscles together. Alterations in musculoskeletal functioning thus can have a significant impact on a child's growth and development.

Musculoskeletal disorders may be congenital, such as clubfoot, or acquired, such as osteomyelitis. They may require short- or long-term management, and may be treated on an outpatient basis or require hospitalization. Many musculoskeletal disorders require surgical correction, casting, or braces. This chapter provides a discussion of many of the musculoskeletal disorders of childhood and adolescence. Additional conditions related to this system are fully described in other chapters; for example, bone tumors are presented in Chapter 23 and cerebral palsy in Chapter 26 ∞.

DISORDERS OF THE FEET AND LEGS

Metatarsus Adductus

Metatarsus adductus, the most common congenital foot deformity, is characterized by an inward turning of the forefoot at the tarsometatarsal joints (Figure 28–4►). Often referred to as "intoeing," metatarsus adductus affects male and female infants equally and occurs in approximately 1 in 1000 births, with more common incidence among siblings. This condition is most likely caused by both intrauterine positioning and genetic factors (Gore & Spencer, 2004; Hart, Grottkau, Rebello, & Albright, 2005).

Foot radiographs may be taken and physical assessment of the foot is performed. Treatment depends on the degree of foot flexibility. If the foot can be readily maneuvered past the neutral position, simple exercises may correct the problem (see Families Want to Know: Stretching Exercises for Metatarsus Adductus). Most cases will resolve spontaneously by the time the infant is about 3 months of age. Serial casting is the treatment of choice for curvature angles greater than 15 degrees, or in cases that do not improve. The infant's feet are placed in a position as close to neutral as possible and are held secure with casts. Casts are changed weekly until the desired correction is achieved. Braces and orthopedic shoes may also be used to maintain correction after casting.

Nursing Management

Reassure parents that the child's condition can be corrected. If the child's deformity is mild, teach parents simple stretching exercises that can be performed at each diaper change. If casting is necessary, provide cast care as outlined in Box 28–1 and teach parents how to care for the child in a cast at home. If metatarsus adductus persists into childhood without correction, the challenge is to find shoes that accommodate the unusual shape of the foot.

Clubfoot

Clubfoot, or equinovarus, is a congenital abnormality in which the foot of the newborn is not in the usual position. It occurs in approximately 1 to 3 in 1000 births, affects boys nearly twice as often as girls, and is bilateral in about half of the cases (Gilmore & Thompson, 2003).

Etiology and Pathophysiology

The exact cause of clubfoot is unknown; however, several possible etiologies have been proposed. Some authorities believe abnormal intrauterine positioning causes the de-

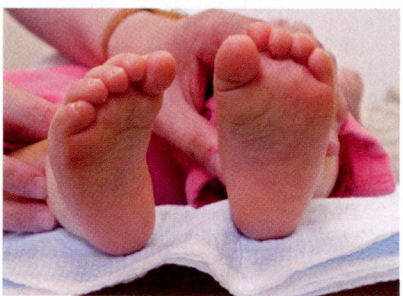

Figure 28–4 ► Metatarsus adductus is characterized by convexity (curvature) of the lateral border of the foot. The child's right foot shows the disorder. Note that the forefoot turns inward and appears out of alignment with the remainder of the foot.

FAMILIES WANT TO KNOW

Stretching Exercises for Metatarsus Adductus

- Hold the infant's foot securely by the heel. Maintain the heel in this position.
- Move the forefoot outward away from the body with the other hand.
- Hold the foot in this position for 5 seconds.
- Repeat five times during each diaper change.

BOX 28–1
NURSING CARE OF THE CHILD IN A CAST

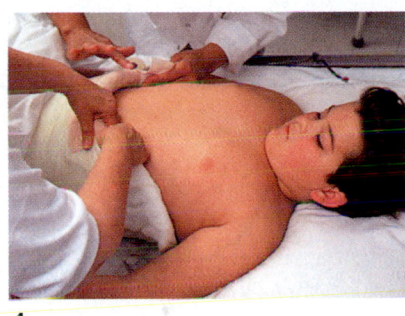

- A plaster cast takes anywhere from 24–48 hours to dry. When handling the cast, be gentle and use the palms of your hands, as fingertips can indent plaster and create pressure areas.
- After the cast is applied, elevate the extremity on a pillow above the level of the heart. Elevation helps to reduce swelling and increases venous return.
- If the cast is applied after surgery, there may be drainage or bleeding through the cast material. Circle the stain and note the date and time on the cast to provide a means of assessing the amount of fluid lost.
- Assess the distal pulses, and check the fingers and toes for color, warmth, capillary refill, and edema. Assess sensation as well as movement. Any deviation from normal may indicate nerve damage or decreased blood supply.
- During the first 24 hours, the casted extremity should be checked every 15–30 minutes for 2 hours, then every 1–2 hours thereafter. The skin should be warm. It should blanch when slight pressure is applied and then return to its normal color within 3 seconds **(1).** For the next 2 days, the casted extremity should be assessed at least every 4 hours.
- Check the edges of the cast for roughness or crumbling. If necessary, pull the inner stockinette over the edge of the cast and tape.
- The rough edges of the cast may also be alleviated by "petaling." This is done by securing adhesive tape to the inside of the cast and pulling it over the edge, covering the jagged or broken pieces of plaster, and securing it to the outer surface of the cast **(2, 3, 4).** Moleskin may be used on the cast as well.

1

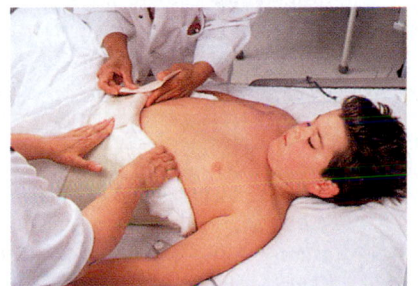

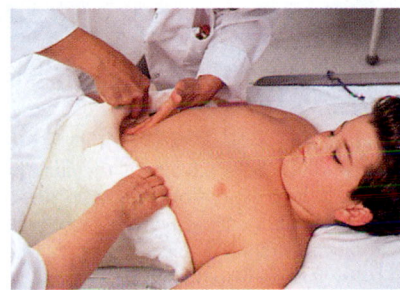

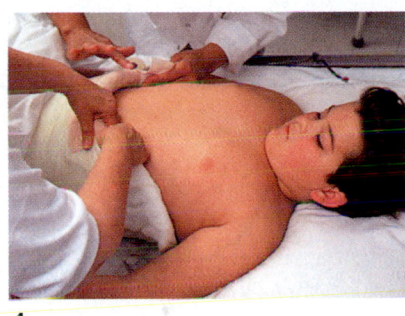

2   3   4

- Keep the cast as clean and dry as possible. Cover the cast with a plastic bag or plastic wrap when the child bathes or showers.
- The skin under the cast may itch; however, do not use powders or lotions near the edges or under the cast as they can cause skin irritation.
- Be sure that children do not put small objects between the casts and their extremities; these actions can cause skin irritation as well as neurovascular compromise.

---

formity. Neuromuscular or vascular problems are suspected as causes by others. Yet other experts believe there is a genetic component, either at the chromosomal level or by the arrest of normal fetal development. A positive family history increases the chance of the deformity, with an occurrence rate 17 times higher in families with affected members than in the general population (Morcuende, 2006).

Clinical Manifestations

A true clubfoot (talipes equinovarus) involves three areas of deformity: the midfoot is directed downward (**equinus**), the hindfoot turns inward (**varus**), and the forefoot curls toward the heel (adduction) and turns upward in partial supination. Most children have a combination of findings, with muscles, tendons, and bones involved. The condition may range from mild to severe involvement, with the latter often associated with additional malformations in the newborn such as meningomyelocele. The foot is small with a shortened Achilles tendon. Muscles in the lower leg are atrophied, but leg lengths are generally normal (Figure 28–5 ➤). Clubhand is a rare occurrence that has similar characteristics to the foot deformity (Figure 28–6 ➤).

■ COLLABORATIVE CARE

Diagnosis is made at birth on the basis of visual inspection, or may be made upon ultrasound at 16–20 weeks' gestation. Radiographs after birth are used to confirm the severity of the condition.

Early treatment is essential to achieve successful correction and reduce the chance of complications. Serial casting is the treatment of choice. Casting should begin as soon as

PATHOPHYSIOLOGY ILLUSTRATED

Bilateral Clubfoot Deformity

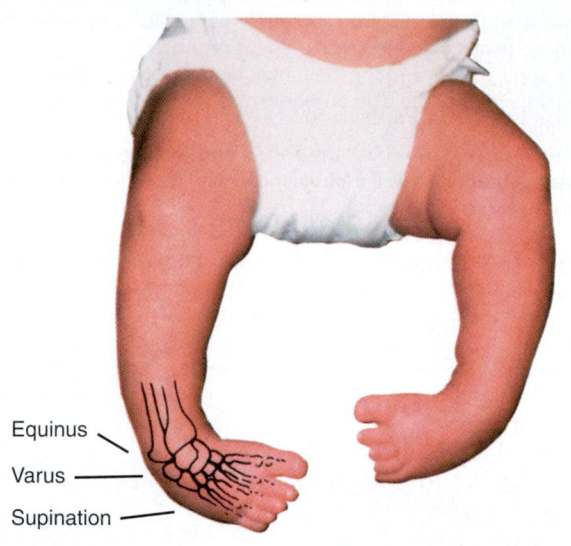

Equinus

Varus

Supination

Figure 28–5 ➤ Parents of a child with clubfoot will have many questions. Can the condition be treated? Will the child be able to walk normally after surgery? Will parents need help caring for the infant? How much will surgery and other care cost? Will any subsequent children have a clubfoot?
Modified from Staheli, L. T. (1992). *Fundamentals of pediatric orthopedics* (p. 5.10). New York: Raven Press.

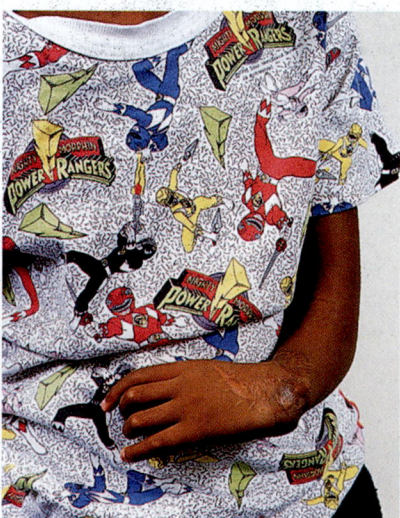

Figure 28–6 ➤ A clubhand deformity is a less common condition than clubfoot.

MediaLink

Care Plan Activity: Postoperative Clubfoot Repair

possible after birth. Timing is critical, because the short bones of the foot, which are primarily cartilaginous at birth, begin to ossify shortly thereafter. The foot is manipulated to achieve maximum correction first of the varus deformity and then of the equinus deformity. A long leg cast is applied to hold the foot in the desired position, which is changed every 1 to 2 weeks. This regimen of manipulation and casting continues for approximately 8 to 12 weeks until maximum correction is achieved. If the deformity has been corrected, the child may begin wearing a splint or reverse last corrective shoes (shaped so that the foot turns outward instead of inward as with usual shoes) to maintain the correction (Gilmore & Thompson, 2003; Morcuende, Dolan, Dietz, & Ponseti, 2004). If the deformity has not been corrected, surgical intervention may be implemented.

The age at which a child undergoes clubfoot surgery varies among surgeons. However, if surgery is needed, it usually occurs when children are between 3 and 12 months of age. The one-stage posteromedial release procedure, which involves realignment of the bones of the foot and release of the constricting soft tissue, is commonly performed. The foot is held in the proper position by one or more stainless steel pins. A cast is then applied with the knee flexed to prevent damage to the pin and to discourage weight bearing (Figure 28–7➤). Casting continues for 6 to 12 weeks. The child may then need to wear a brace or corrective shoes, depending on the severity of the deformity and the surgeon's preference. Alternatively, the Ponseti technique uses a simple Achilles tenotomy following serial manipulation and casting, and is followed by use of a foot-abduction brace (Morcuende, 2006).

NURSING MANAGEMENT
Nursing Assessment and Diagnosis

Nursing assessment, which begins at birth and continues throughout the child's subsequent outpatient casting visits and hospitalization for surgery, includes taking a genetic and birth history, performing a physical examination (including position and appearance of the foot), and assessing the child's motor development and family's coping mechanisms. Because parents will need to bring the child for frequent cast changes, assess access to transportation and other arrangements that are necessary to facilitate these visits.

Nursing diagnoses that may apply to the child with a clubfoot deformity are as follows:

- Impaired Physical Mobility related to prescribed movement restriction of cast
- Risk for Impaired Skin Integrity related to cast
- Risk for Impaired Parenting related to birth of a child with a physical defect
- Health-Seeking Behaviors related to lack of information about deformity, treatment, and home care

Planning and Implementation

Nursing management involves providing emotional support, educating the family about home care of the child in a cast and the importance of keeping appointments at the outpatient facility for cast changes, preparing of the family for the child's hospitalization if surgery is to occur, and providing postsurgical care.

Provide Emotional Support

Clubfoot is a condition that affects both the child and the family. The child's foot deformity is upsetting to parents, and they need emotional support to allay their fears. Helping parents understand the condition and its treatment is essential.

Encourage parents to hold and cuddle the child and to take an active role in the child's care to help promote bonding. Explain that, with treatment, the child will grow and develop normally.

Provide Cast and Brace Care

Routine cast care is outlined in Box 28–1 on page 1155 and is important to ensure skin and neurovascular integrity. Provide support information to the parents during the casting treatment. After serial casting is complete, or following surgery, the child may progress to wearing a brace or special shoe for 6 to 12 months. Braces should fit snugly but should not interfere with neurovascular function. Before the child begins to wear a brace, check the skin for any areas of redness or breakdown. Provide parents with guidelines for brace wear as outlined in the following text. Emphasize that proper skin care is essential. If skin redness develops, arrange to have the fit of the brace evaluated and modified, if necessary.

Provide Postsurgical Care

Routine postoperative care after surgical correction includes neurovascular status checks every 2 hours for the first 24 hours and observing for any swelling around the cast edges. Apply ice bags to the foot, and keep the ankle and foot elevated on a pillow for 24 hours to promote healing and help with venous return. Check for drainage or bleeding. Administer pain medication routinely for 24 to 48 hours. Popliteal or epidural blocks may be placed during surgery and used in the immediate postsurgical period for pain control (Figure 28–8➤). The nurse monitors these blocks for effectiveness and any undesired effects (see Chapter 15 ∞ for detailed instructions on pain management). See the *Clinical Skills Manual* for details on monitoring nerve blocks.

Discharge Planning and Home Care Teaching

Parents should be given written instructions for care of the child with a cast see (Families Want to Know: Care of the Child with a Cast). In addition, assist them in the following ways.

- Demonstrate the use of a sponge bath to protect the cast from water breakdown.
- Discuss several options for clothing that accommodate a cast, for example, one-piece snap suits or sweatpants.

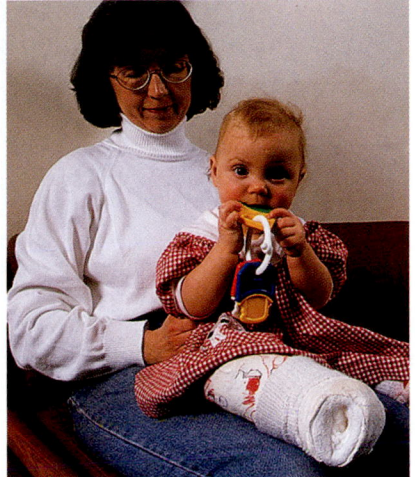

Figure 28–7 ➤ This girl has a long leg cast, which was applied after surgery to correct her clubfoot.

CLINICAL TIP

When an infant is receiving serial casting for clubfoot, recommend that the parent soak the cast off the night before a scheduled cast change. The baby can be placed in a warm bath, during which the cast will start to disintegrate and can be unrolled. This avoids exposure of the baby to the loud sound of the cast cutter, and allows for the infant's leg to be washed and out of the cast overnight. Parents can also be encouraged to bring a bottle to the clinic. If the baby is hungry and feeding, the foot is more easily kept still for the cast application.

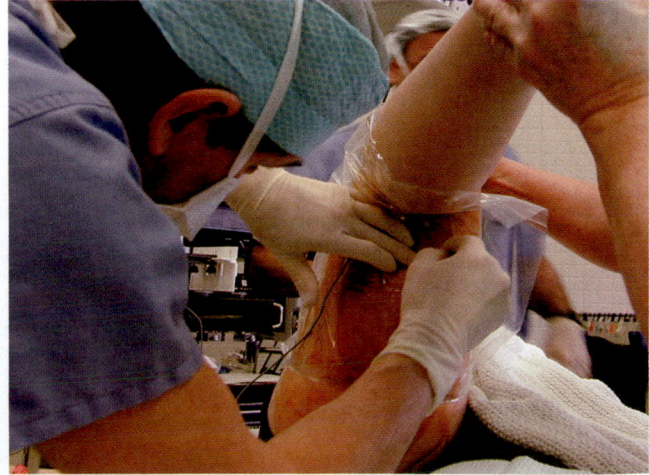

Figure 28–8 ➤ The insertion of a popliteal block during surgery. The site will be wrapped and the tubing connected to an infusion pump. The nurse will monitor the infusion and pain control after surgery.
Courtesy of Shriners Hospital, Spokane, WA.

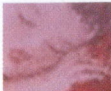

FAMILIES WANT TO KNOW

Care of the Child with a Cast

Skin Care

- Check the skin around the cast edges for irritation, rubbing, or blistering. The skin should be clean and dry.
- Cleanse the skin just under the cast edges and between the toes or fingers with a cotton-tipped applicator and rubbing alcohol. Avoid using lotions, oils, and powders near the cast as they may cause caking.
- Avoid poking sharp objects down inside the cast as this may result in sores.

Cast Care

- Keep the cast dry. Protect plaster with a cast shoe, thick sock, or sling.
- Allow a new, wet cast to air-dry for 24 hours.
- Begin walking on a leg cast only when the physician gives permission.
- Be alert for possible complications
- Verify toes or fingers are pink, not blue or white.

- Keep skin warm; the tips of the toes should blanch when pinched.
- Raise the casted arm or leg above heart level and rest it on pillows to prevent or reduce any swelling.

Notify the Healthcare Provider if Any of the Following Occur

Unusual odor beneath the cast

Tingling

Burning or numbness in the casted arm or leg

Drainage through the cast

Swelling or inability to move the fingers or toes

Slippage of the cast

Cracked, soft, or loose cast

Sudden, unexplained fever

Unusual fussiness or irritability in an infant or child

Blue or white fingers or toes

Pain that is not relieved by any comfort measures (e.g., repositioning or pain medication)

Note: Courtesy of Shriners Hospital for Children, Spokane, WA.

- Discuss potential safety hazards that may result from awkward positioning. Be sure the child is properly situated in a car safety seat for the trip home.
- Suggest that parents make an effort to place toys within the child's reach, because movements of a child in a cast may be slowed.

Once the child progresses to use of special shoes or a brace, provide teaching on brace care for the family. See Families Want to Know: Guidelines for Brace Wear.

Evaluation

Expected outcomes of nursing care include maintenance of skin integrity, recovery without complications after surgery, normal developmental progression of the child, and demonstrated knowledge by parents for care of braces or casts, as needed.

NURSING ALERT

Advise parents that umbrella strollers may not be sturdy enough to support an infant's casted leg. Some infant swings do not provide a foot rest; its absence can contribute to cast slippage or breakdown. Observe the child in the family's car seat to be sure the casted leg is adequately supported. A pillow may need to be placed under the leg for support.

Genu Varum and Genu Valgum

Genu varum (bowlegs) is a deformity in which the knees are widely separated while the ankles are close together and the lower legs are turned inward (varus). In genu valgum (knock-knees), the knees are close together and the lower legs are directed outward

FAMILIES WANT TO KNOW

Guidelines for Brace Wear

- Braces should be as comfortable as possible and the child should have adequate mobility while wearing the brace.
- Begin wearing the brace for periods of 1–2 hours and then progress to 2–4 hours.
- Check the skin at 1 to 2-hour intervals initially, then lengthening to every 4 hours once skin has been clear for several days. If redness is apparent, leave the brace off and allow the skin to clear. If breakdown has occurred, the brace cannot be replaced until healing is complete. (See Chapter 30 ∞ for a discussion of pressure ulcers.)

- Always have the child wear a clean white sock, t-shirt, or other thin white liner beneath the brace. Be sure the liner is wrinkle-free under the brace. Avoid using powders or lotions that can cause skin to break down. Toughen any sensitive areas using alcohol wipes.
- Reapply the brace when the skin returns to its normal color.
- Return to the physician or orthotic specialist if discomfort or red areas persist or if the brace needs adjustment or repair or is outgrown.
- Check the brace daily for rough edges.

(valgus). Chapter 5 ∞ discusses the assessment of bowlegs and knock-knees in children (Figure 28–9➤).

At certain stages of a child's development, the appearance of bowlegs or knock-knees is normal. Until 2 to 3 years, the knees are normally bowed, showing varus alignment, and by 4 to 5 years, some knock-knee or valgus alignment commonly emerges. Persistent genu varum or genu valgum should be evaluated. Two pathologic causes of genu varum are Blount's disease and rickets. **Blount's disease** is characterized by abnormal growth on the medial side of the proximal tibia which causes an increasing varus deformity. It is believed to be due to increasing compression forces across the medial knee and is more common in overweight, Black, and female children (Thompson, 2004b). **Rickets** is a result of inadequate bone mineralization, usually caused by a deficiency of calcium and/or vitamin D (see Chapter 4 ∞ for a description of the association between rickets and diet). Since the bones are decalcified or softened, long bones such as those in the legs may bend into a bowed position. Occasionally rickets is congenital and is caused by an X-linked autosomal dominant or recessive gene with the chromosome location Xp22.31-p21.3. It results in an enzyme deficiency of alkaline phosphatase which in turn leads to excessive inhibitors of bone mineralization. This type of rickets is rare and is called familial hypophosphatemic rickets (FHR).

Measurements, radiographs, arthrography (joint radiographs), MRI, and CT imaging may be used for accurate diagnosis. Braces are often used to correct mild deformities that could worsen as the child grows. Braces for bowlegs are worn at night; those for knock-knees are worn both day and night. Duration of brace wear is determined by the severity of the deformity, which is usually evaluated by radiographs. If the deformity continues to worsen, surgical intervention is necessary. Surgery is common in the treatment of Blount's disease. An **osteotomy** (cutting of the bone) is performed and the tibiofemoral angle surgically corrected. The child is then placed in a cast for approximately 6 to 10 weeks, or until full healing has occurred.

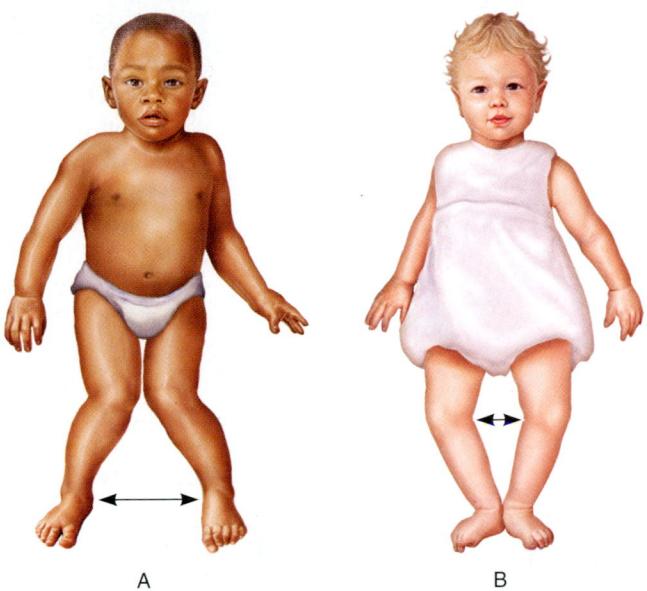

Figure 28–9 ➤ A, Genu valgum or knock-knees. Note that the ankles are far apart when the knees are together. B, Genu varum or bowlegs. The legs are bowed so that the knees are far apart as the child stands.

Nursing Management

Reassure parents that bowlegs and knock-knees are usually a normal part of a child's growth and development. These conditions often resolve in time and require no treatment other than monitoring.

Nursing care focuses on educating the parents and child about the condition and its treatment. Provide the child and family with guidelines for brace wear and maintenance (see page 1158).

DISORDERS OF THE HIP
Developmental Dysplasia of the Hip

Developmental dysplasia of the hip (DDH) refers to a variety of conditions in which the femoral head and the acetabulum are improperly aligned. These conditions include hip instability, **dislocation** (displacement of the bone from its normal articulation with the joint), **subluxation** (in this instance, a partial dislocation), and acetabular **dysplasia** (abnormal cellular or structural development) (Shipman, Helfand, Moyer & Yawn, 2006). In the past, DDH was referred to as congenital dislocated hip (CDH). The disorder's revised name emphasizes that many cases of dislocation, subluxation, and dysplasia occur well after the neonatal period and involve more than a simple dislocation.

Hip instability is present in 1 in 100 newborns, while dislocation occurs in 1.5 to 20 in 1000 births, depending on the studies examined. The condition affects girls four times as often as boys. It can be unilateral or bilateral (Shipman, Helfand, Nygren, & Bougatsos, 2006).

CULTURE

Variations in DDH Rates
Infants who are positioned on cradle boards or traditionally swaddled, as in some Native American cultures, have a high incidence of developmental dysplasia of the hip (DDH). Canadian Indian babies have an incidence of 188 per 1000 births and Navaho Indians in the southwest United States have an incidence of 20 per 1000. However, among cultures in which mothers carry infants on their hips or backs with the infants' legs abducted—as in Korean, Chinese, and some African groups—the incidence of DDH is low (Witt, 2003).

Etiology and Pathophysiology

Although the exact cause of DDH is unknown, genetic factors appear to play a role. DDH is 20 to 50 times more common in first-degree relatives of an infant with the condition than in the general population. If one child of a set of identical twins has DDH, the other twin is affected 30–40% of the time. Some types of DDH are linked to early gestational events at 12 and 18 weeks' gestation, as the lower limbs rotate and surrounding muscles develop. However milder cases may be influenced by mechanical forces in the last month of pregnancy such as breech position or large fetal size, and some cases develop after birth as the hip assumes an extended rather than flexed position (Witt, 2003).

The left hip is involved more often than the right hip as a result of intrauterine positioning of the left side of the fetus against the mother's sacrum. Maternal estrogen may cause laxity of the hip joint and capsule, leading to joint instability, especially in females who respond to these estrogen levels. Cultural factors may also be associated with DDH.

Clinical Manifestations

Common signs and symptoms of DDH include limited abduction of the affected hip, asymmetry of the gluteal and thigh fat folds, and telescoping or pistoning of the thigh (Figure 28–10➤). The older child with untreated DDH walks with a significant limp, which results from telescoping of the femoral head into the pelvis. The longer the disorder goes untreated, the more pronounced the clinical manifestations become, and the worse the prognosis.

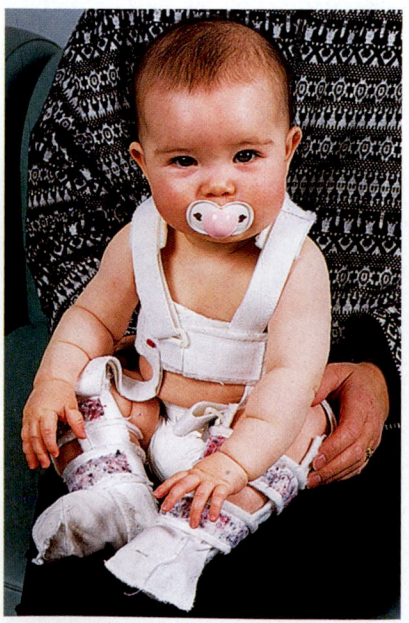

Figure 28–10 ➤ The asymmetry of the gluteal and thigh fat folds is easy to see in this child with developmental dysplasia of the hip.

■ COLLABORATIVE CARE

All infants and young children should be screened for DDH until walking is well established at about 1 year of age (U.S. Preventive Services Task Force, 2006). Physical examination reveals Allis' sign (one knee lower than the other when the knees are flexed) and positive Ortolani–Barlow maneuver in babies under 8 to 12 weeks. Refer to Chapter 5 ∞ for a discussion of the assessment of hip dysplasia in newborns and infants. Radiographs are generally not reliable until approximately 4 months of age, because the pelvis in a newborn is still primarily cartilaginous. Before 4 months, ultrasonography may be useful for diagnosis. After that age, radiographs are used for diagnosis. Radiographs or ultrasound should be considered for the female infant born in the breech position because of the increased risk of DDH in these infants. A family history may also suggest the need for these studies (U.S. Preventive Services Task Force, 2006).

Treatment plans vary according to the child's age. For infants younger than 6 months, the Pavlik harness is the most commonly used method for hip reduction (Figure 28–11➤). The Pavlik harness is a dynamic splint, that is, a splint that allows movement. It ensures hip flexion and abduction and does not allow hip extension or adduction. For infants older than approximately 6 months, skin traction may be used followed by surgery and the application of a spica cast (Figure 28–12➤). In children who are over 18 months of age at the time of diagnosis, surgery and casting are usually necessary and later bracing may also be required.

Early screening, detection, and treatment enable the majority of affected children to attain normal hip function.

Figure 28–11 ➤ The most common treatment for DDH in a child under 3 months of age is a Pavlik harness. A shirt should be worn under the harness to prevent skin irritation (it was omitted for clarity in this photograph).

■ NURSING MANAGEMENT
Nursing Assessment and Diagnosis

Assessment for DDH begins at delivery and continues through all well-child checkups during the first 2 years of life. The specific family history or birth data may indicate a high-risk infant, as does oligohydramnios, large-for-gestational age infant, or breech birth. Instructions for performing the physical examination to assess the infant for DDH are given in Chapter 5 ∞. Further assessments are determined by the treatment provided. Skin assessments are performed on the child in traction or a cast, every few minutes at first and progressing to once or twice daily at home. Respiratory and circulatory assessments are included when the child is immobilized. Ongoing assessment of the child's growth and development are needed. Weigh the casted child once the cast is dry so a baseline casted weight can be used for comparison during the weeks and months while the cast remains in place.

The following nursing diagnoses may apply to the child with DDH:

- Impaired Physical Mobility related to prescribed movement restriction (Pavlik harness, traction, spica cast, brace)
- Risk for Impaired Skin Integrity related to irritation from harness straps or skin traction
- Risk for Altered Urinary Elimination or Constipation related to immobility caused by treatment
- Risk for Imbalanced Nutrition related to decreased appetite
- Risk for Delayed Growth and Development related to limited mobility and potential decreased exposure to stimulation
- Health-Seeking Behavior (Parental) related to lack of information about disease process and treatment

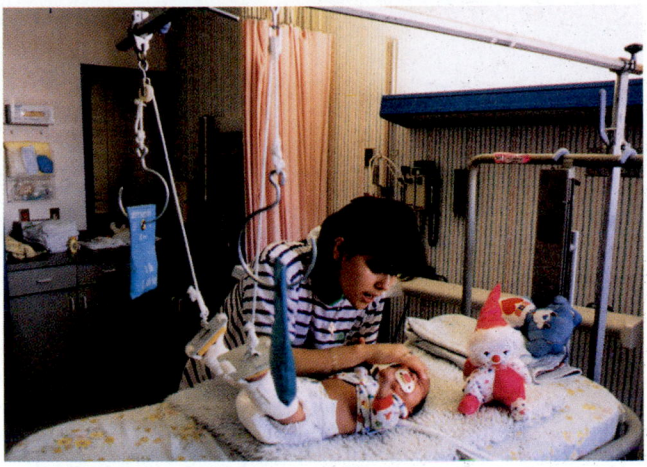

Figure 28–12 ➤ For infants older than 3 months of age, skin traction is commonly used for treatment of DDH.

Planning and Implementation

The infant with DDH is often cared for at home and in outpatient facilities. If surgery is performed, the child is hospitalized for surgery and the immediate postoperative period. Nursing care varies according to the medical treatment and the child's age. Management includes maintaining traction, if ordered; providing cast care; preventing complications resulting from immobility; promoting normal growth and development; and teaching parents how to care for a child in a cast, traction, or a Pavlik harness at home. Because treatment may interfere with the child's normal movement, the treatment plan should take into consideration the child's age and developmental stage.

Maintain Traction

Bryant's traction is the most common form of traction used in the treatment of DDH. (Types of traction are discussed later in the chapter.) Check the traction apparatus frequently to ensure that proper alignment and healing occur. Traction may also be used as a treatment in the home. Give the family careful instruction in how to care for the child in traction. In addition, arrangements should be made for a nurse to make several home visits to set up the traction apparatus and monitor the child's progress after discharge.

Provide Cast Care

The principles of routine cast care presented in Box 28–1 apply to the care of spica casts. Special techniques should be used to help keep the cast clean and dry in children who are not toilet trained. Female and male urinals can be used for older children. Use a plastic lining to protect the cast edges during elimination for older children and use a small disposable diaper to cover the perineum in babies, tucking edges beneath the cast. Be sure to change the diaper frequently to prevent soiling of the cast.

Control Pain

If the child has surgery to correct DDH, pain control in the immediate postoperative period is needed. Assess the child's pain frequently in a method appropriate for age (see Chapter 15 ∞). Administer intravenous and oral pain medications as prescribed. Use

> ### CLINICAL TIP
>
> Inspect the traction apparatus. Ensure the following:
> - Nuts and bolts are tight.
> - Knots are well tied and secured with tape.
> - Weight amounts are correct and weights are hanging free.
> - Ropes are unfrayed.
> - The line of pull is straight.

methods such as holding, rocking, and gentle music to calm the child. An ice bag placed on top of the cast at the operative site may be helpful. Encourage parents to be present and provide care when possible.

If pain is not controlled or if it increases over time, compression at the surgical site may be occurring. Promptly report this to the physician. Pain in the infant may be manifested by a combination of physiological and behavioral changes.

Prevent Complications Resulting from Immobility

Immobilization from traction or a cast can cause alterations in physiologic functioning. Take the following actions to prevent complications:

- Assess breathing patterns and lung sounds frequently for congestion or respiratory compromise.
- Perform skin and neurovascular assessments approximately every 2 hours.
- Use adequate padding and skin wrapping to avoid placing pressure on the popliteal space. Such pressure could lead to nerve damage.
- For the child in a cast, change the child's position every 2 to 3 hours while awake to help avoid areas of pressure and promote increased circulation. The child can be placed either prone or supine or positioned on the floor and supported with pillows.
- Help prevent skin irritation and breakdown in the child with a cast. Use moleskin to provide protection from rough edges. Place tape around the perineal opening of the cast to prevent soiling.
- Increase fluids and fiber in the child's diet, as a change in bowel or bladder status is commonly associated with immobility.
- If permitted by the physician's prescription, release the child from traction for meals and daily care. The time out of traction should not exceed 1 hour per day. Encourage parents to hold and cuddle the child at this time to promote comfort and bonding.

Promote Normal Growth and Development

Engage the child in activities that stimulate the upper extremities and all five senses. Provide stimulating toys such as stacking blocks, brightly colored mobiles, Koosh balls, or musical toys. Position toys within the child's reach and interact with the child as much as possible.

Discharge Planning and Home Care Teaching

Parents must learn how to care for a child in traction or a spica cast at home. The active participation of family members in the daily care of the child while hospitalized gradually increases their confidence in their ability to provide care at home. Home care needs should be identified and addressed well in advance of discharge. Before discharge, be sure the parents have the following information:

- Instructions about general cast care (see pages 1155 and 1158), positioning, bathing, toileting, and age-appropriate diversional activities.
- Importance of performing and reporting changes in neurovascular assessment.
- Instruction regarding the bar between the legs of a hip spica. It is not to be used for holding or lifting the child; it is only for positioning the legs properly. Using the bar to lift can cause the cast to fracture, weaken, or disintegrate.
- Appropriate referrals for periodic assessment by a visiting nurse or home health nurse.
- Family resources to care for the child.

Before discharge, have parents demonstrate how to dress and feed a child in a spica cast. Ensure that safe travel arrangements have been made for the day of discharge. Help parents to obtain an appropriate car safety seat in advance of discharge. Encourage parents to let the child interact with other children at home, and to provide the child in a cast with similar opportunities for play and social activities.

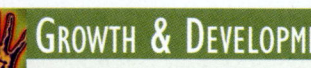

CLINICAL TIP
Neurovascular assessment involves evaluation of temperature, movement, color, capillary refill, and sensation. Even if the child is not old enough to respond to questions about sensation, usually brushing the hands or sheets along the toes elicits a movement from the child and indicates sensation. Report any abnormalities immediately. Keep limbs aligned during traction. For the child in a hip spica, elevate the lower body on pillows immediately after surgery to decrease edema under the cast at the operative site.

GROWTH & DEVELOPMENT

Safe Toys and Casts
Use caution in selecting toys appropriate for the child's developmental age. If the child is in a cast, be sure that toys or parts cannot be swallowed or stuck inside the cast. Place a t-shirt over the cast so that the edges are securely covered and it is difficult for the child to place something under them. Provide toys that are large and soft, use diversion such as play and music to occupy the child's attention, and assess the child frequently.

Care in the Community

Have parents of an infant in a Pavlik harness demonstrate proper application of the harness and care of the infant while in the harness. Teach family members about the daily care (bathing, dressing, and feeding) of the infant. Ideally, the harness is worn 23 hours per day and is removed only for skin checks and bathing. The hips and buttocks should be supported carefully when the infant is out of the harness. Demonstrate how to feed the infant in an upright position to maintain abduction and how to change a diaper without removing the harness. (See Families Want to Know: Guidelines for Pavlik Harness Application.)

Instruct the parents of an infant with a harness or a child in a cast to look for any reddened or irritated areas near the harness or cast edges and to check toes frequently for proper circulation. Frequent repositioning reduces the risk of pressure sores or circulatory compromise. The infant should wear an undershirt and socks under the harness to prevent rubbing of the skin.

Safety precautions are important as the child will not have normal mobility. Parents will need to use a specially designed car seat that accommodates the child with abducted hips (see Families Want to Know: Transporting the Child with Orthopedic Devices). Strollers and cribs should provide sufficient room to protect the legs from injury and to prevent hip adduction.

Evaluation

Expected outcomes for nursing care of the child with developmental dysplasia of the hip include the following

- Skin integrity is maintained.
- The infant shows no complications related to immobility.
- Parents have adequate knowledge of the condition, treatment, and necessary home care.
- A safe environment is maintained for the child.
- The child attains normal mobility by the end of the treatment period.

Legg-Calvé-Perthes Disease

Legg-Calvé-Perthes disease is a self-limiting condition in which there is avascular necrosis of the femoral head. The disease occurs in approximately 1 in 12,000 children and affects boys four times more often than girls. It usually occurs between the ages of 2 and 12 years, with an average age of 7 years at onset. The disease is bilateral in 20% of cases (Thompson, 2004b).

Etiology and Pathophysiology

The necrosis associated with Legg-Calvé-Perthes disease results from an interruption of the blood supply to the femoral epiphysis. How and why this occurs is not completely

FAMILIES WANT TO KNOW

Guidelines for Pavlik Harness Application

1. Position the chest halter at the nipple line and fasten with Velcro.
2. Position the legs and feet in the stirrups, being sure the hips are flexed and abducted. Fasten with Velcro.
3. Connect the chest halter and leg straps in front.
4. Connect the chest halter and leg straps in back.

All the straps are marked at the first fitting with indelible ink so they can be reattached easily after the harness is rinsed and dried.

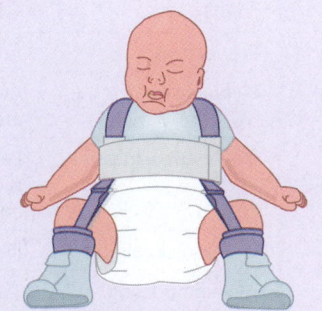
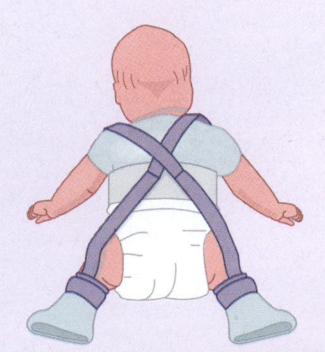

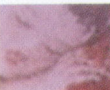

FAMILIES WANT TO KNOW

Transporting the Child with Orthopedic Devices

The American Academy of Pediatrics has established guidelines for transporting children with special healthcare needs.

- Placement in the rear seat is preferable.
- If the front seat must be used, the front passenger airbag should be disconnected. The National Highway and Traffic Safety Administration provides information and assistance (1-888-327-4236).
- Use only car seat transport systems approved for use with children with special needs.
- Install and use seats as instructed.

- When reasonable, a child should be moved from a wheelchair or other special device to the vehicle safety seat.
- Pieces of medical equipment required during transportation (such as monitors or oxygen) or that are being transported with the child (such as wheelchair or walker) should be secured to the floor of the vehicle.
- If the child is transported by school bus, state and federal recommendations for school bus transportation of children with special needs should be followed.
- Keep a cellular phone and emergency equipment in the vehicle.

Note: Adapted from American Academy of Pediatrics (n.d.). Children with Special Health Care Needs. Retrieved on September 12, 2006 from http://www.aap.org/healthtopics/specialneeds.cfm.

CULTURE

Incidence of Legg-Calvé-Perthes Disease

Legg-Calvé-Perthes disease is most common among White, Japanese, and Chinese children. It is less common among Blacks and Native Americans. This suggests a genetic link to the disease, as does the more frequent occurrence in certain families. However, the cause is not known but only theorized (Thompson, 2004b).

understood, but several predisposing factors have been identified. A coagulation system disorder may cause repeated vascular interruptions to the proximal femur. The incidence of this condition is increased in families with a history of the disease, which suggests that genetic factors may play a role. In 17% of the cases, onset of the disease is preceded by a mild traumatic injury, and 10% of children affected have a history of breech birth (Burns, Dunn, Brady et al., 2004). Trauma may cause a subchondral fracture and resultant synovitis, which in turn causes pressure that occludes the blood supply. Children with Legg-Calvé-Perthes disease often have delayed skeletal maturation, increased thyroid levels, and low somatomedin C (insulinlike growth factor). It is more common in those with low birth weight, increased parental age, and exposure to environmental tobacco smoke. Some cultural variations occur.

Clinical Manifestations

Legg-Calvé-Perthes disease progresses through four distinct stages after the original insult (usually unidentified) occurs, over a period of 1 to 4 years. Early symptoms of the disease include a mild pain in the hip or anterior thigh and a limp, which are aggravated by increased activity and relieved by rest. The child favors the affected hip and limits hip movement to avoid discomfort. See Clinical Manifestations of Legg-Calvé-Perthes Disease below.

As the disease progresses, range of motion becomes limited and weakness and muscle wasting develop. The affected thigh is 2 to 3 cm smaller than the unaffected thigh. Prolonged hip irritability may produce muscle spasms and pain increases. Gradually, revascularization begins and pain decreases.

CLINICAL MANIFESTATIONS	LEGG-CALVÉ-PERTHES DISEASE
Stage	**Clinical Manifestations**
Prenecrosis	An insult causes loss of blood supply to the femoral head.
I—Necrosis	Avascular stage (3–6 months); the child is asymptomatic, bone radiographs are normal, and the head of the femur is structurally intact but avascular.
II—Revascularization	Period of 1–4 years characterized by pain and limitation of movement. Bone radiographs show new bone deposition and dead bone resorption. Fracture and deformity of the head of the femur can occur.
III—Bone healing	Reossification takes place; pain decreases.
IV—Remodeling	The disease process is over, pain is absent, and improvement in joint function occurs.

■ COLLABORATIVE CARE

Diagnostic Tests

Because the child's initial symptoms are so mild, parents often do not seek medical attention until symptoms have been present for several months. Diagnosis is made using standard anteroposterior and frog-leg radiographs. As previously noted, radiographs taken early in the course of the disease may be normal or show vague widening of the cartilage space. Bone scans and MRI may show the disease process earlier than radiographs. Laboratory studies of the blood, such as white blood cell count, help to rule out inflammatory synovitis of the hip (Burns et al., 2004).

Clinical Therapy

Medical management and prognosis depend on the degree of femoral involvement and the clinician's decision. Early detection is important. The desired outcome is a pain-free hip that functions properly. To promote healing and prevent deformity, the femoral head must be contained within the hip socket to maintain its sphericity. Observation and examination over time are most commonly used with physical rehabilitation, and occasionally traction or casting. Severe disease may be treated by surgery to release adductor muscles, treat the acetabulum or femur, and restore range of motion (Figure 28–13➤). Prognosis is good if the child is young (under 8 years) and has a mild form of the disorder. Children with untreated disease or those diagnosed late in the disease process may develop osteoarthritis and hip dysfunction later in life. Children may have a short adult height or develop leg length discrepancy (Grzegorzewski, Bowen, Guille, & Glutting, 2003; Kamegaya, Saisu, Ochiai et al., 2004; Herring, Kim, & Browne, 2005).

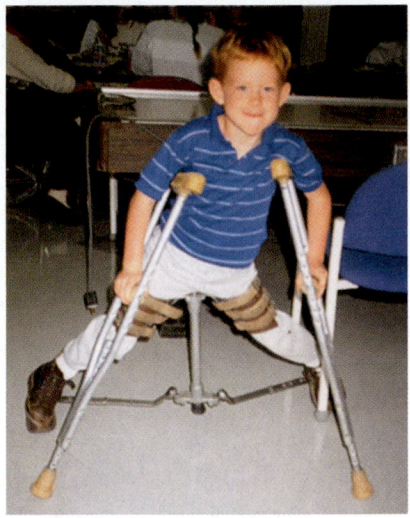

Figure 28–13 ➤ Although the Toronto brace may seem formidable for a child to wear, you can see by this photograph that, as usual, children adapt quite well to it.

■ NURSING MANAGEMENT

Nursing Assessment and Diagnosis

Legg-Calvé-Perthes disease should be suspected in any child, especially a boy age 2 to 12 years, who complains of hip discomfort accompanied by a limp. The school nurse may be the first person to observe the child with symptoms of the disease. The child may complain of pain and have to rest during physical education classes. In this case, immediate referral should be made to the healthcare provider. Question the child who has an apparent limp about pain, and assess the child's range of motion. Ask if the child previously injured the hip.

Nursing diagnoses, which center on altered activities and compliance, may include the following:

- Impaired Physical Mobility related to restriction of treatment
- Risk for Injury related to potential complications resulting from noncompliance with the treatment regimen
- Impaired Adjustment related to duration of treatment
- Deficient Diversional Activity related to forced inactivity
- Potential Disturbed Body Image related to treatment and impaired mobility

Planning and Implementation

Children with Legg-Calvé-Perthes disease often receive all of their treatment at home. Helping the child and family comply with the prescribed treatment plan may be challenging, because children develop the disease at an age when they are usually very active. The child, who may have little pain, often finds immobilization and physical rehabilitation recommendations difficult.

Promote Normal Growth and Development

Parents should be given suggestions to help redirect the child's energy within the limitations in mobility imposed by treatment. A return to school promotes a feeling of normalcy. Coordinate the return to school by facilitating the child's use of an elevator or ramp as needed in that setting. Collaborate with the family to provide instruction for

GROWTH & DEVELOPMENT

Activity and Legg-Calvé-Perthes Treatment

Legg-Calvé-Perthes disease primarily affects boys with an average age of 7 years. These school-age children are industrious and independent. Offer suggestions for activities that redirect energy and promote normal development. These may include horseback riding, which promotes hip abduction; swimming to increase mobility; handcrafts to promote fine motor skills; and computer activities to stimulate cognitive development.

school personnel and other children to foster understanding of the child's condition and treatment. Activities that involve peers also help the child achieve developmental milestones. Help the child adjust to wearing a brace or cast if that is the treatment used.

Care in the Community

Both the child and the family should be aware that treatment generally takes more than 2 years. Emphasize the importance of following the treatment plan to ensure adequate hip containment and proper healing. Teach the family how to care for a child with special devices or following surgery. Follow-up visits should be arranged at regular intervals, and home care visits may be helpful for some families.

Evaluation

Expected outcomes of nursing care are elimination of hip pain and discomfort, normal development during the period of immobilization, and parent and child knowledge of treatment regimen.

Slipped Capital Femoral Epiphysis

Slipped capital femoral epiphysis (SCFE) occurs when the femoral head is displaced from the femoral neck. This condition is seen in 10/100,000 adolescents, commonly during the growth spurt between the ages of 12 and 15 years in boys and 10 and 13 years in girls. Boys are more often affected than girls. Black children are affected more often than other ethnic groups, as are children who are overweight and those with sports injuries or other trauma, a history of radiation therapy, or endocrine disease (Manoff, Banffy, & Winell, 2005).

Etiology and Pathophysiology

The cause of SCFE is unknown. Predisposing factors include obesity, a recent growth spurt, and endocrine disorders such as hypothyroidism and hypogonadism. Slippage of the femoral head occurs at the proximal epiphyseal plate, and the femur displaces from the epiphysis (Figure 28–14▶). Slippage is usually gradual (chronic), but may also result

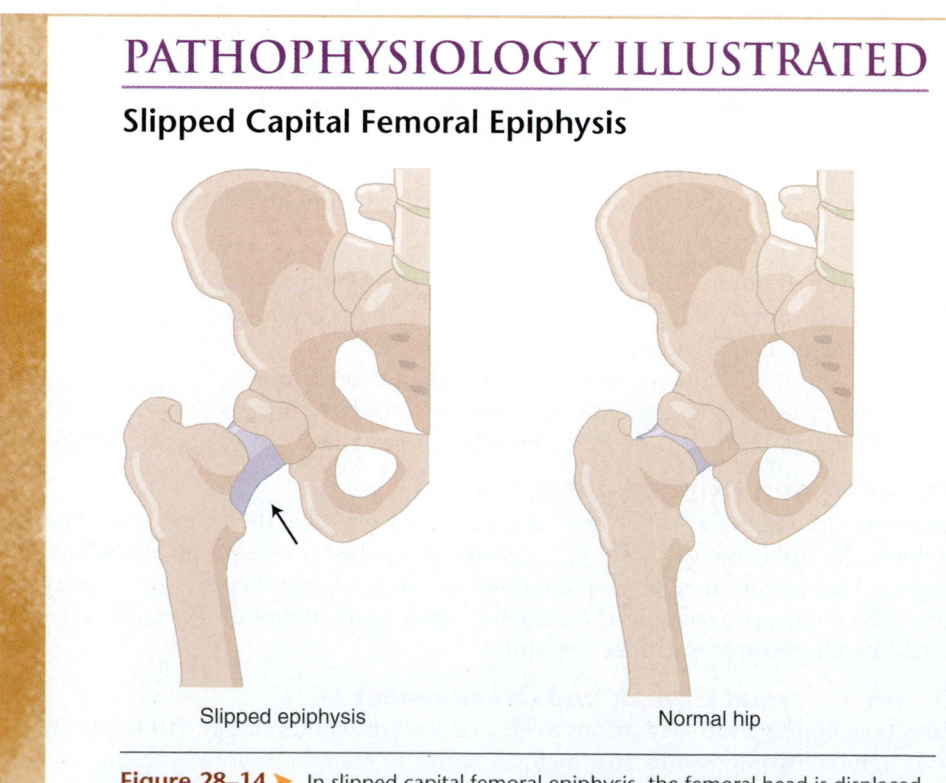

PATHOPHYSIOLOGY ILLUSTRATED

Slipped Capital Femoral Epiphysis

Slipped epiphysis   Normal hip

Figure 28–14 ▶ In slipped capital femoral epiphysis, the femoral head is displaced from the femoral neck at the proximal epiphyseal plate.

from acute trauma. The synovial membrane becomes inflamed, edematous, and painful. If untreated, callous formation occurs, resulting in a deformed hip with limited range of motion (Jingushi & Suenaga, 2004).

Clinical Manifestations

Symptoms include a limp, hip pain, and loss of hip motion. The condition is categorized as acute, chronic, or acute-on-chronic. Acute SCFE has a sudden onset of less than 3 weeks' duration. The child has sudden, severe pain and cannot bear weight. An acute slip may be associated with traumatic injury. Chronic SCFE has a duration of longer than 3 weeks. It presents with persistent hip pain, which is generally aching or mild and can be referred to the thigh, knee, or both. A limp and decreased range of motion may also occur. Acute-on-chronic SCFE is an additional slippage in a child with a chronic condition. The child with a chronic slip sustains a traumatic incident that causes further slippage of the femoral head, causing sudden, severe pain.

COLLABORATIVE CARE

A complete history provides information about risk factors and the development of the condition. Radiographs are used to confirm the diagnosis. A bone scan, ultrasound, CT, and MRI are sometimes performed to verify the extent of injury.

The goal of medical management is to stabilize the femoral head while keeping displacement to a minimum and retaining as much hip function as possible. Surgical treatment is usually necessary; this involves fixation of the epiphysis with screws or pins. If treated early, a single screw into the hip in an outpatient procedure is sufficient for stabilization; in advanced cases, surgery becomes more complicated. More commonly, surgery involves placement of two or three pins placed through the physis into the epiphysis to stabilize the femoral head (Mooney & Podeszwa, 2004). Medical treatment, which is occasionally used, includes a regimen of no weight bearing, bed rest, a spica cast, and Buck or Russell traction (see traction description later in the chapter).

Prognosis is related to the severity of the deformity and the occurrence of complications, such as avascular necrosis of the femoral head or **chondrolysis** (the breaking down and absorption of cartilage).

NURSING MANAGEMENT

Nursing Assessment and Diagnosis

The child usually presents with hip pain or referred pain to the groin, thigh, or knee, and limited mobility. A thorough history is needed to assess for injury as a cause. Assess the child's range of motion, pain, and limp, if apparent. Refer the child for treatment immediately if SCFE is suspected. This condition is considered to be an emergency, and it is essential that the child be treated immediately to keep weight off the affected joint.

Nursing diagnoses that may apply to the child with SCFE are as follows:

- Impaired Physical Mobility related to treatment
- Acute Pain related to hip injury
- Risk for Disturbed Body Image related to treatment
- Risk for Delayed Growth and Development related to mobility restrictions
- Risk for Imbalanced Nutrition: More than Body Requirements related to immobility
- Ineffective Tissue Perfusion: Peripheral related to traction, casting, and other treatments
- Health-Seeking Behaviors (Child and Parent) related to disease process and treatment

Planning and Implementation

SCFE is strongly associated with obesity; therefore, weight control is important for prevention (Manoff, Banffy, & Winell, 2005). Nursing management for the child with a diagnosis of SCFE involves caring for the child in traction or after surgery, administering medications and other pain control interventions, maintaining mobility within the limits imposed by treatment, providing adequate nutrition, educating the child and family about the disorder, providing emotional support, and promoting compliance with the treatment plan.

Encourage Appropriate Nutritional Intake and Physical Activity

A growing adolescent needs adequate amounts of proteins, carbohydrates, and calcium to promote skeletal healing. Provide written instructions about nutritional requirements necessary to promote bone healing and maintain an ideal body weight. If a child is overweight, encourage weight loss by decreasing percent of fat in the diet, as well as controlling caloric intake if it is excessive. This decreases pressure on the femoral epiphysis and can also lead to a more positive self-image. Incorporate upper body exercises into treatment, both to assist in weight control and to build muscle. Physical therapy is useful to facilitate a program of upper body exercise and teach safe ways of increasing the total amount of physical activity.

Provide Emotional Support

Because the onset of SCFE is usually unexpected, the child and family may find themselves facing surgery with little warning. Explain the treatment plan simply and thoroughly. Reassure the child and family that with proper compliance, treatment should be successful.

Discharge Planning and Home Care Teaching

Assist the family to plan for the child's return to school. If attendance is not possible for a period of time due to traction or surgery, arrange for tutors and computer communication with school as needed. Follow-up visits are necessary until the child's epiphyseal plates close. It is not uncommon for SCFE to occur in the other hip. Make sure the child and family are aware of symptoms such as decreased range of motion or pain that could indicate onset of the disorder in the other hip. Tell parents to contact their healthcare provider immediately if these symptoms occur.

Evaluation

Expected outcomes of nursing care for the child with SCFE include maintenance of normal weight and recommended nutritional intake, absence of complications of immobility, successful adaptation to school following treatment, and family recognition the of need for ongoing monitoring for complications.

DISORDERS OF THE SPINE

Scoliosis

Scoliosis is a lateral S- or C-shaped curvature of the spine that is often associated with a rotational deformity of the spine and ribs. Many individuals exhibit some degree of spinal curvature, while curvatures of more than 10 degrees are considered abnormal. Curves are either structural or compensatory, as the spine curves to compensate for a structural deformity along its length. Idiopathic scoliosis occurs most often in girls, especially during the growth spurt between the ages of 10 and 13 years. Early onset of idiopathic scoliosis occurs before 10 years of age and comprises 15% of cases (Thompson, 2004a).

Etiology and Pathophysiology

The cause of scoliosis is complex. Structural scoliosis may be congenital, idiopathic, or acquired (associated with neuromuscular disorders such as muscular dystrophy or myelodysplasia, or secondary to spinal cord injuries).

In idiopathic structural scoliosis (the most common type), the spine for unknown reasons begins to curve laterally, with vertebral rotation. The most common curve is a right thoracic and left lumbar deformity. As the curve progresses, structural changes occur. The ribs on the concave side (inside of the curve) are forced closer together, while the ribs on the convex side separate widely, causing narrowing of the thoracic cage and formation of the rib hump. The lateral curvature affects the vertebral structure. Disk spaces are narrowed on the concave side and spread wider on the convex side, resulting in an asymmetric vertebral canal (Figure 28–15▶).

Scoliosis can also occur in congenital diseases involving the spinal structure and in the musculoskeletal changes seen in conditions such as myelomeningocele, cerebral palsy (see Chapter 26 ∞), or muscular dystrophy. It can also be acquired after injury to the spinal cord. The child in Figure 28–16▶ acquired scoliosis after chemotherapy and radiation to the chest during treatment for cancer.

Clinical Manifestations

The classic signs of scoliosis include truncal asymmetry, uneven shoulders and hips, a one-sided rib hump, and a prominent scapula. However, the child does not complain of pain or discomfort. If diagnosis does not occur before the curvature reaches about 40 degrees, some compensatory problems may develop. Hip and back pain can result, and lung compromise can lead to fatigue or dyspnea with exertion.

■ COLLABORATIVE CARE

Generally, observation and radiographic examination are used to diagnose scoliosis. Additional diagnostic studies include MRI, CT scan, and bone scan, which are used occasionally to assess the degree of curvature.

Early detection is essential to successful treatment. The goal of medical management is to limit or stop progression of the curvature. Adequate treatment and follow-up maximize the child's chances for proper spinal alignment. The treatment regimen chosen depends on the degree and progression of the curvature and the reaction of the child and family to medical management.

Treatment of children with mild scoliosis (curvatures of 10 to 20 degrees) consists of physical rehabilitation to improve posture and muscle tone and to maintain, or possibly increase, flexibility of the spine. Emphasis is placed on bending strength toward the outside of the curve while stretching the inside of the curve. These exercises do not influence the course of condition progression, however, and the child should be evaluated by a physician at 3-month intervals, with radiographic evaluation every 6 months.

Medical management of moderate scoliosis (curvatures of 20 to 40 degrees) includes either regular monitoring of the curve progression or bracing, most commonly with a Boston brace. The goal of wearing a brace is to maintain the existing spinal curvature with no increase. Brace wear begins immediately after diagnosis. To achieve maximum effectiveness, the brace should be worn 23 hours per day. Brace treatment is lengthy and requires a high degree of compliance, which can be difficult for adolescents who view body image or sports involvement as important.

Children with severe scoliosis (curvatures of 40 to 50 degrees or more) require surgery, which involves spinal fusion. The majority of spinal fusions are performed using segmental instrumentation of the spinal cord. Examples of surgical approaches include Luque wires, Coutrel-Dubosset (CD) instrumentation, Texas Scottish Rite Hospital system, and Moss-Miami system (Lonstein, 2006). These treatments stabilize the spine well during surgery, may be accompanied by bone grafting to the spine, and require no long-term therapy or postoperative casting. Following surgery with wires

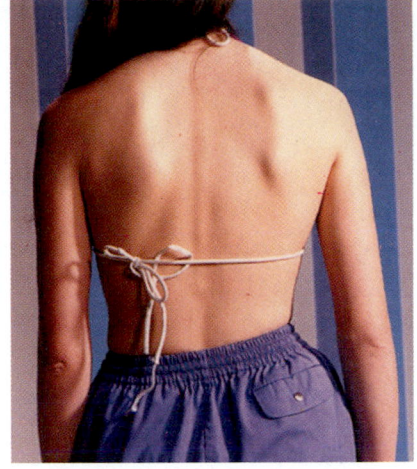

Figure 28–15 ▶ A child may have varying degrees of scoliosis. For mild forms, treatment will focus on strengthening and stretching. Moderate forms will require bracing. Severe forms may necessitate surgery and fusion. Clothes that fit at an angle, such as this teenage girl's shorts, and anatomic asymmetry of the back provide clues for early detection.

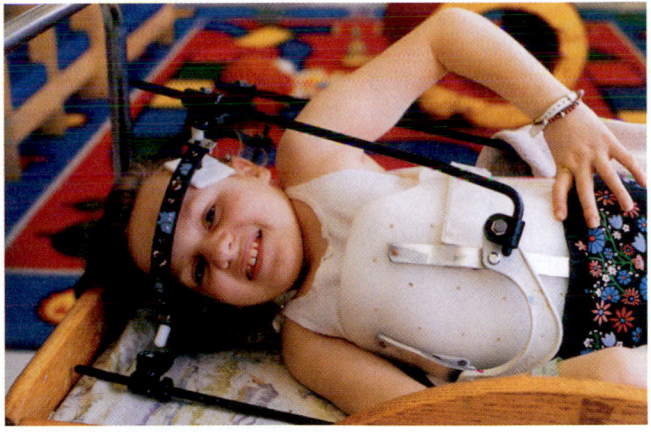

Figure 28–16 ▶ In severe scoliosis, the child may wear a halo brace, shown here, to hold the body in position after surgery.

or instrumentation, the child is on bed rest during a recovery period and then is sometimes fitted with anteroposterior plastic shells (also called thoracolumbar sacral orthotics) that are worn for several months to provide stability for the spine. The wires will remain in the back forever. Occasionally in severe cases, halo traction is used postoperatively to provide support for the unstable spine (see Figure 28–16).

CLINICAL TIP
Scoliosis Screening

From the Front
- Is the head midline?
- Are the shoulders at the same height?
- Is there the same amount of space between the arms and body on each side?

From the Back
- Is the head midline?
- Are the shoulders at the same height?
- Are the scapulae equally prominent and at the same height?
- Is the spine straight?
- Is there the same amount of space between the arms and body on each side?
- Are the hips at the same height?

With the Adolescent Holding Hands Together and Bent Over Slightly
- Are the scapular humps even?

With the Adolescent Holding Hands Together and Bent Over Toward the Floor
- Are the flank humps even?
- Is the spine straight?
- Is there a marked roundness when viewed from the side (evidence of kyphosis)

NURSING MANAGEMENT
Nursing Assessment and Diagnosis

School nurses often screen children for scoliosis, generally in the fifth and seventh grades. This screening is mandated by law in several states. When abnormalities are noted, the child is referred to an orthopedic center for further evaluation. Children should be examined every 6 to 9 months thereafter. If scoliosis is detected, the child's brothers and sisters should be examined and observed closely.

Once scoliosis has been identified, the nurse's focus becomes education and follow-up. Any child with scoliosis should have a comprehensive neurologic, cardiac, and respiratory examination, since the rib cage deformity can influence the functioning of these systems.

The following nursing diagnoses may apply to the child with scoliosis who is not undergoing surgery:

- Risk for Impaired Adjustment to the Exercise Program related to duration and intensity of exercise
- Impaired Physical Mobility related to brace
- Risk for Impaired Skin Integrity related to brace
- Ineffective Breathing Pattern related to rib cage deformity
- Health-Seeking Behaviors (Child and Parent) related to unfamiliarity with disease process
- Disturbed Body Image related to deformity and brace wear

Common nursing diagnoses for the child who is having surgery can be found in the accompanying Nursing Care Plan.

NURSING CARE PLAN The Child Undergoing Surgery For Scoliosis

GOAL	INTERVENTION	RATIONALE	EXPECTED OUTCOME
1. Deficient Knowledge (child and parents) related to lack of information about surgery			
	NIC Priority Intervention: **Teaching, Disease Process and Preoperative:** *Assisting the patient to understand information and mentally prepare for surgery and postoperative recovery.*		*NOC Suggested Outcome:* **Knowledge:** *Extent of understanding conveyed about scoliosis treatment.*
The child and parents will verbalize understanding of the disease, its treatment, and the surgical procedure.	• Teach the child and family about the course of the disease, its signs and symptoms, and treatment. Provide appropriate handouts. Encourage the child and parents to ask questions.	• Understanding and involvement increase motivation and compliance while reducing fear.	The child and family accurately verbalize knowledge about the disease and its treatment. The child and family ask appropriate questions about postoperative care.
	• Begin preoperative teaching at the time of admission. Orient the child to hospital and postoperative procedures. Before surgery, have the child demonstrate log-rolling, range of motion exercises, and the use of an incentive spirometer. Discuss pain management.	• Preoperative teaching and familiarity with hospital procedures reduces the stress related to surgery and postoperative complications.	
2. Ineffective Breathing Pattern related to hypoventilation syndrome			
	NIC Priority Intervention: **Airway Management and Respiratory Monitoring:** *Facilitation of patency of air passages and analysis of patient data.*		*NOC Suggested Outcome:* **Respiratory Status: Ventilation:** *Movement of air in and out of the lungs.*
The child will show no signs of respiratory compromise.	• Monitor respiratory status, especially after the administration of analgesics. Apply pulse oximeter.	• Evaluation of the child's respiratory condition anticipates and avoids complications. Analgesics such as morphine may increase or potentiate respiratory compromise.	The child has no respiratory complications.
	• Administer oxygen if ordered.	• Oxygen increases peripheral oxygen saturation to 95–100%.	
	• Have the child use an incentive spirometer.	• Spirometry increases lung expansion and aeration of the alveoli.	
	• Monitor intake and output.	• Good hydration promotes loose secretions and helps prevent infection.	
	• Reposition the child at least every 2 hours.	• Repositioning ensures inflation of the lung fields.	
3. Risk for Injury related to neurovascular deficit secondary to instrumentation			
	NIC Priority Intervention: **Injury Prevention:** *Instituting special precautions with patient at risk.*		*NOC Suggested Outcome:* **Risk Control:** *Actions to eliminate or reduce modifiable health risks.*

(continued)

GOAL	INTERVENTION	RATIONALE	EXPECTED OUTCOME
3. Risk for Injury related to neurovascular deficit secondary to instrumentation (continued)			
The child's neurovascular system will remain intact as evidenced by circulation, sensation, and motor checks. The child will feel no numbness or tingling.	• Monitor the child's color, circulation, capillary refill, warmth, sensation, and motion in all extremities. Perform neurovascular checks every 2 hours for the first 24 hours and then every 4 hours for the next 48 hours. Record presence of pedal and distal tibial pulses every hour for 48 hours. Report changes and abnormal findings immediately.	• When the spinal column is manipulated during surgery, altered neurovascular status, thrombus formation, and paralysis are possible complications. • Postoperative complications include loss of bowel or bladder control, weakness or paralysis, and impaired vision or sensation.	The child exhibits only temporary alteration (pale skin, faint pulse, and edema occur, but then resolve within the initial postoperative phase). The child returns to the preoperative baseline state by discharge.
	• Have the child wear antiembolism stockings until ambulatory. The stockings may be removed for 1 hour 2–3 times daily.	• Antiembolism stockings prevent blood clots and promote venous return. Thrombus formation is a postoperative risk.	
	• Check for any pain, swelling, or a positive Homans' sign in the legs. Record any evidence of edema.	• Swelling may indicate a tight dressing and tissue damage. A positive Homans' sign and pain may indicate thrombus formation.	
	• Monitor input and output.	• Abnormalities may indicate a fluid shift problem.	
	• Encourage and assist the child with range of motion exercises, both passive and active.	• Activity promotes mobility and reduces risk of thrombus formation.	
4. Pain related to spinal fusion with instrumentation			
	NIC Priority Intervention: **Pain Management:** *Alleviation of pain or a reduction of pain to a level of comfort acceptable to the patient.*		*NOC Suggested Outcome:* **Pain Level:** *Amount of reported or demonstrated pain.*
The child will verbalize an adequate level of comfort or show absence of pain behavior within 1 hour of a specific nursing intervention.	• Assess the level of pain and initiate pain management strategies as soon as possible. Use patient-controlled analgesics if ordered.	• Adequate pain management allows for faster healing and a more cooperative patient. Patient-controlled analgesics may be effective.	The child experiences pain relief early in the postoperative period.
	• Administer pain medication around the clock to help ensure pain relief, especially during the first 48 hours. Monitor epidural blocks and patient-controlled analgesia or other methods used for pain control.	• Medicating around the clock helps to maintain comfort. Monitoring ensures patient safety.	
	• Use nonpharmacologic pain management techniques, such as imagery, relaxation, touch, music, application of heat and cold, and reduced environmental stimulation to supplement medications (see Chapter 15 ∞).	• Alternative treatments also interrupt the pain stimulus and provide relief. Non-pharmacologic methods can be an effective adjunct to pain management.	
	• Document pain assessment, interventions, and the child's reactions.	• Proper documentation guides the selection of the most effective means of pain control.	
	• Reassure the child that some discomfort is expected and that a variety of measures can be tried to reduce discomfort.	• Realistic expectations decrease anxiety and give the child a sense of control.	

GOAL	INTERVENTION	RATIONALE	EXPECTED OUTCOME
5. Impaired Physical Mobility related to movement restrictions and pain			
	NIC Priority Intervention: **Positioning and Ambulation:** *Moving the patient to provide comfort and promote healing, assist with walking.*		*NOC Suggested Outcome:* **Ambulation:** *Ability to walk from place to place.*
The child will maintain proper body alignment and progress with activity as ordered by the physician. If no anteroposterior shell bracing is required the child will have active mobility by the third to fifth postoperative day.	• Resposition the child every 2 hours using the log-roll technique. Support the back, feet, and knees with pillows.	• Proper positioning prevents twisting or turning the spine.	The child is as mobile as appropriate for condition within 3–5 days after surgery.
	• Have the child perform passive and active range of motion exercises every 2 hours for 48 hours and then every 4 hours while awake. Have the child dangle his or her legs at bedside by the second to fourth postoperative day or as ordered by surgeon. Begin ambulation generally by the third to fifth postoperative day. Note any complaints of dizziness, pallor. Proceed slowly.	• Exercises help maintain strength, circulation, and muscle tone. If the spine is stable and the physician has ordered no external support, the child may progress to full ambulation as tolerated. If the spine is not stable, great care must be taken until external supportive devices are used.	
6. Risk for Disturbed Body Image related to treatment			
	NIC Priority Intervention: **Body Image Enhancement:** *Improving conscious and unconscious perceptions toward the body.*		*NOC Suggested Outcome:* **Body Image:** *Positive perception of own appearance and body.*
The child will verbalize feelings about body image and self-esteem in relation to the disease and its treatment. The child will be informed about available support services and use them as needed.	• Encourage independence in daily activities within allowable limits. Use positive reinforcements. Encourage the child to participate in community activities, if possible. Involve the child in scoliosis support groups.	• Involvement in activities demonstrates that a "normal" life is realistic.	The child has a positive self-image and is involved in community activities or support groups.
	• Provide contact with a peer resource person who has undergone treatment for scoliosis.	• Peers are an effective means of support.	
7. Risk for Deficient Knowledge (child and parent) related to lack of information about home care			
	NIC Priority Intervention: **Teaching: Prescribed Treatment:** *Preparing family to understand and perform prescribed treatment.*		*NOC Suggested Outcome:* **Knowledge:** *Extent of understanding conveyed about postoperative treatment and follow-up care.*
The child and family will verbalize reduced anxiety about home care. The child will demonstrate knowledge of self-care and permitted activities.	• Teach cast or brace care as appropriate (see pages 1155–1158). Provide oral and written instructions and a list of activity limitations. Have the child and family demonstrate adequate knowledge.	• Providing education decreases anxiety and increases compliance with treatment plan. Demonstration reinforces the learning process.	The child and family demonstrate home care and implementation of discharge teaching.
	• Arrange for follow-up appointments as ordered by the physician. Encourage the child and family to notify the nurse or physician if they have any questions or concerns.	• Follow-up visits help the nurse and physician evaluate the effectiveness of the treatment plan and patient adjustment to recommended therapy.	

Planning and Implementation

An important aspect of nursing care is patient education. Patient compliance is critical to the success of treatment. Children and their families need to understand the condition and the stages of treatment, particularly adolescents who are undergoing treatment for scoliosis. Children or adolescents facing surgery require education, reassurance, and support. Teach about pain control and the PCA (patient-controlled analgesia) pump. Often the child donates some of his or her own blood prior to surgery, and the family may also donate so is the child's or a family member's blood is transfused in surgery. The adolescent will benefit from learning about deep breathing, positioning, surgical incision, and all other aspects of postoperative care. The accompanying nursing care plan summarizes nursing care for the child undergoing surgery for scoliosis.

Promote Understanding and Acceptance of the Treatment Plan

Provide instructions about exercises that will help to decrease the severity of the spinal curvature. Demonstrate the exercises, and explain their purpose (e.g., to strengthen back muscles). Help the child adjust to wearing a brace. Adolescents, in particular, may be reluctant to wear an external device such as a brace. To promote a sense of control, allow the adolescent to choose when to exercise and when to be out of the brace, within the treatment guidelines. Provide reassurance and encouragement and promote interaction with peers. Suggesting that the adolescent work with a peer support person who is being treated for scoliosis or has had the condition in the past may be beneficial. Provide information about fashionable clothing that can be worn with the brace.

Discharge Planning and Home Care Teaching

Home care needs should be identified and addressed well in advance of discharge after spinal surgery. The child must learn to adapt to a new set of body mechanics. Show the child how to do simple tasks without bending or twisting the torso. Have the child demonstrate the ability to perform activities of daily living before discharge from the hospital. Collaborate with physical therapy/rehabilitation to plan for the youth's needs related to safe and effective movement with the brace.

Activities for the child who has had spinal surgery are commonly limited for a period of time. Restrictions usually should be followed for 6 to 8 months, depending on the type of surgery and the surgeon (See Families Want to Know: Posteperative Activities After Spinal Surgery). Emphasize to both the child and the family the importance of compliance, and give them written discharge instructions. Follow-up visits are important. The child should be examined 4 to 6 weeks after discharge, then every 3 to 4 months for 1 year, and every 1 to 2 years thereafter.

Several organizations provide information and assistance to families of children with scoliosis. Referrals can be made as appropriate.

Evaluation

Expected outcomes of nursing care for the child with scoliosis treated by brace are maintenance of intact skin and compliance with prescribed therapy. Expected outcomes after surgical correction are listed in the accompanying nursing care plan.

Torticollis, Kyphosis, and Lordosis

Torticollis is tilt of the head caused by rotation of the cervical spine. The cause is generally an injury sustained to the sternocleidomastoid muscle at the time of birth or to a cervical spine abnormality. Stretching exercises or surgical lengthening of the sternocleidomastoid muscle are usual treatments. Occasionally the cause of torticollis is visual impairment, leading to constant turning in one direction in order to see with the better eye.

Kyphosis (hunchback) and lordosis (swayback) are two other types of spinal curvature that may occur in children. The type of kyphosis seen in adolescence is most commonly Scheuermann's disease, an abnormality in ossification of anterior vertebral bodies; it differs from the degenerative kyphosis sometimes seen in the elderly. Postural lordosis is a characteristic finding in toddlers, but should disappear by the school-age years.

COMMUNITY CARE

Scoliosis and Airport Screening

Children with metal hardware in their back after scoliosis surgery need to carry an explanation from the physician on airplane flights as they will set off metal detectors in airports. Encourage them to arrive early for flights in order to facilitate transportation screening.

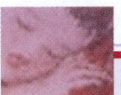

FAMILIES WANT TO KNOW

Postoperative Activities After Spinal Surgery

Recommended	Not Recommended
Lying	Bending or twisting at the waist
Sitting	Lifting more than 10 pounds
Standing	Household chores such as vacuuming, unloading groceries, mowing the lawn, and taking out the garbage
Walking (including normal stair climbing)	Sports such as bicycle riding, horseback riding, skiing, roller blading, skating
Swimming, gentle (not with a cast); diving is not permitted	Physical education classes

Nurses can perform thorough musculoskeletal assessments of children (see Chapter 5 ∞) and refer any children with abnormalities for further evaluation. Clinical therapy depends on the cause and degree of the curvature, and the age of the child at onset. See Clinical Manifestations and Treatment of Kyphosis and Lordosis below.

ADDITIONAL DISORDERS OF THE BONES AND JOINTS

Osteoporosis and Osteopenia

Osteoporosis, a condition in which there is decreased density and mass of bone, promotes the risk of fractures, and is commonly associated with aging. However, children can have **osteoporosis** (also known as metabolic bone disease or a bone mineral density more than 2.5 standard deviations below the norm) related to imbalanced nutrition or other pathological conditions. Osteoporosis is preceded by **osteopenia** or low bone mass, which is between 1 and 2.5 standard deviations below norm (Bowman & Russell, 2006).

Etiology and Pathophysiology

Very-low-birth-weight infants who are premature often have osteopenia of prematurity because much of bone mass is usually acquired in the latter weeks of pregnancy. In addition, they may have other health problems after birth and be unable to ingest enough nutrients to meet metabolic needs for bone growth. Prematures are often less active than other infants, which decreases the amount of mechanical loading on their bones, a factor known to increase bone resorption and decrease bone mass (Eliakim & Nemet, 2005).

CLINICAL MANIFESTATIONS | TREATMENT OF KYPHOSIS AND LORDOSIS

Condition	Clinical Manifestations	Clinical Therapy
Kyphosis Excessive convex curvature of the cervical thoracic spine. (Scheuermann kyphosis is a common type)	*Clinical manifestations:* Visible hunchback or rounded shoulders; shortness of breath or fatigue; pain; abdominal creases and light hamstrings in severe cases. *Diagnostic tests:* Spinal curvature is assessed by having the child bend 90 degrees at the waist and noting roundness at the scapular area from side. Sharp angulation is visible. Diagnosis is confirmed by radiograph.	*Medical therapy:* Exercises are prescribed for mild condition; bracing is commonly used; spinal fusion surgery is performed in severe cases. *Nursing management:* Provide support. Encourage exercises and diligent brace wear. Help the child to deal with the psychologic stress of altered body image.
Lordosis Excessive concave curvature of the lumbar spine with an angle of more than 60 degrees; most common in prepubescent girls and Blacks	*Clinical manifestations:* Presence of sway-back; prominent buttocks; hip flexion contractures; tight hamstrings. *Diagnostic tests:* Spinal curvature is assessed by looking at the standing child from the side. Lumbar lordosis is confirmed by visualizing the spine on standing, lateral radiograph.	*Medical therapy:* Treatment focuses on exercises and postural awareness. Bracing and surgery are rarely prescribed. *Nursing management:* Provide support. Reassure the child and family that the condition is often outgrown as the child matures. Encourage physical conditioning exercises and follow-up examinations on a yearly basis.

A group of children who may show signs of osteoporosis are those who have decreased mechanical loading. Children with spina bifida or cerebral palsy that interferes with ambulation have limited pressure on bones, and bone mass in affected extremities and the spine have lower mass. Some other conditions are associated with lower bone mass, including Turner's syndrome, growth hormone deficiency, osteogenesis imperfecta, juvenile rheumatoid arthritis, and diabetes. Children who are treated for disorders or injuries with casting and bracing are also at high risk of osteoporosis due to immobilization. Children treated for some types of cancer have increased rates of osteoporosis. See Figure 28–17➤ for other effects of immobility on body systems.

Lastly, adolescence is a period when adequate intakes of calcium and vitamin D are needed to maximize bone formation and prevent osteoporosis later in life. Adolescents, particularly females, often do not meet the RDA for these nutrients and are at risk for osteoporosis even though it may not be manifested for years. Other lifestyle patterns of youth that decrease bone formation are smoking, alcohol use, and keeping weight at a very low level. Those with anorexia nervosa are clearly at risk for osteoporosis (Heer, Mika, Grzella et al., 2004).

Clinical Manifestations

Osteoporosis is a silent disease, as is its precursor osteopenia; those who have the disorders are often without signs or symptoms for years. The problem may become apparent when a baby or child has a fracture and radiologic studies make the problem evident.

■ COLLABORATIVE CARE

Bone mineral content and density are measured by single photon absorptiometry (SPA), dual-photon absorptiometry (DPA), and dual-energy x-ray absorptiometry

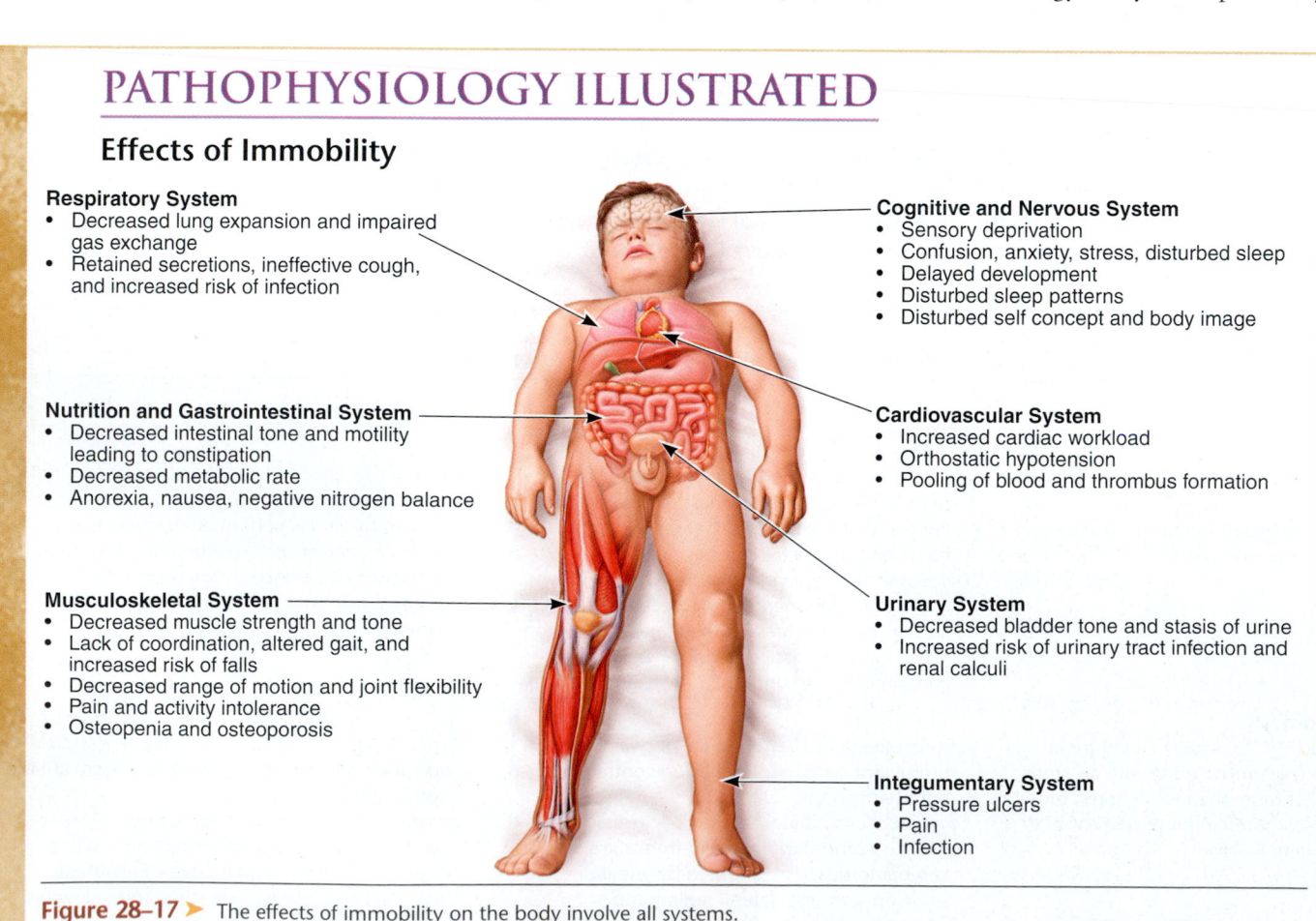

PATHOPHYSIOLOGY ILLUSTRATED

Effects of Immobility

Respiratory System
- Decreased lung expansion and impaired gas exchange
- Retained secretions, ineffective cough, and increased risk of infection

Nutrition and Gastrointestinal System
- Decreased intestinal tone and motility leading to constipation
- Decreased metabolic rate
- Anorexia, nausea, negative nitrogen balance

Musculoskeletal System
- Decreased muscle strength and tone
- Lack of coordination, altered gait, and increased risk of falls
- Decreased range of motion and joint flexibility
- Pain and activity intolerance
- Osteopenia and osteoporosis

Cognitive and Nervous System
- Sensory deprivation
- Confusion, anxiety, stress, disturbed sleep
- Delayed development
- Disturbed sleep patterns
- Disturbed self concept and body image

Cardiovascular System
- Increased cardiac workload
- Orthostatic hypotension
- Pooling of blood and thrombus formation

Urinary System
- Decreased bladder tone and stasis of urine
- Increased risk of urinary tract infection and renal calculi

Integumentary System
- Pressure ulcers
- Pain
- Infection

Figure 28–17 ➤ The effects of immobility on the body involve all systems.

(DEXA). Although uncommonly used, serum studies such as bone-specific alkaline phosphatase, phosphorus, and type-I collagen can be used to measure osteoblastic and osteoclastic activity. Recall that over 90% of the body's calcium is stored in bone, so serum calcium is not reflective of bone density.

Premature newborns at risk for osteopenia of prematurity need collaborative management by neonatologists, neonatal nutritionists, and neonatal nurses. Breast milk is enhanced by adding special fortifiers; premature formula should be used rather than regular baby formula. When babies need enteral or parenteral feedings, calcium to phosphorus ratios are carefully balanced to enhance osteoblastic activity. Extremity range of motion for very-low-birth-weight newborns can decrease bone loss in the period after birth (Litmanovitz, Dolfin, Friedland et al., 2003).

For older children at risk of developing osteoporosis, calcium and vitamin D intake is encouraged and oral supplements may be given. Standing therapy for those who are nonambulatory can provide mechanical weight and enhance bone density (Caulton, Ward, Alsop, Dunn, Adams, & Mughal, 2004). Bisphosphanates, calcitonin, fluoride, and parathyroid hormone may be used to treat children and adolescents with osteoporosis (Unal, Abaci, Bober, & Buyukgebiz, 2006). When a cast or other immobilizing device is removed from a child, a gradually increasing program of exercise in collaboration with physical rehabilitation professionals promotes bone strengthening and lowered risk for fractures or related sequelae.

NURSING MANAGEMENT

Nursing Assessment and Diagnosis

Nurses identify newborns, children, and adolescents at risk of developing low bone mass and density. This is accomplished by identifying diseases putting the child at risk. Ask about exercise and activity patterns, and physical therapy for children who are nonambulatory. Dietary intake is measured periodically for all youth at health promotion visits, and RDAs for calcium, phosphorus, and vitamin D are compared to intake.

Nursing diagnoses that may apply to the child with osteoporosis include the following:

- Imbalanced Nutrition related to inability to consume essential nutrients
- Risk for Injury to Bones related to decreased bone mass and density
- Ineffective Health Maintenance related to inadequate dietary intake

Planning and Implementation

Perform dietary analysis of children at risk (see Chapter 4 ∞ for detailed methods for diet assessment). Refer children at risk to nutritionists and physicians for further education and diagnosis. Suggest referrals to physical rehabilitation to recommend weight bearing exercise. Administer nutritional supplements when prescribed and teach families how to give these medications. Collaborate with families to provide therapy for nonambulatory children that stimulates weight-bearing. Teach parents how to recognize fractures in children who may not have normal sensation and are unable to report them. Swelling, unusual shape of a limb, fussiness of the child, and falls should be promptly reported.

When osteoporosis is due to immobility, many other symptoms occur as well. Be alert for these problems and integrate physical activity in care as much as possible in order to minimize their effects.

Evaluation

Expected outcomes of nursing care for the child with a potential for osteoporosis include adequate intake of recommended amounts of nutrients, absence of fractures, and normal findings on studies of bone mineral content and density.

Osteomyelitis

Osteomyelitis is an infection of the bone, most often one of the long bones of the lower extremity. It may be acute or chronic and may spread into surrounding tissues. Although osteomyelitis may occur at any age, it is most common in children between the ages of 1 and 12 years. Boys are affected two to three times as often as girls, primarily because they have a greater incidence of trauma. Overall incidence is 1 in 5000 youth (Kocher, Lee, & Dolan et al., 2006).

Etiology and Pathophysiology

Osteomyelitis is caused by a microorganism, which is usually bacterial but can be viral or fungal. *Staphylococcus aureus* is the most common causative pathogen, followed by *Escherichia coli*, group B streptococci, *Streptococcus aureus*, *Streptococcus pyogenes*, and *Haemophilus influenzae*. *Kingella kingae* is an increasingly diagnosed pathogen (Frank, Mahoney, & Eppes, 2005). Trauma to the bone or surgical interventions commonly are the initial causes of infection. Osteomyelitis may follow another infection in the body, such as upper respiratory infection.

The infecting organism spreads through the bloodstream or via a penetrating injury to the bone, where it becomes established. Most infections in children begin in the metaphysis (see Figure 28–1), which has a sluggish blood supply. Eventually the infection may penetrate the bone cortex and periosteum. Inflammation and abscess formation can lead to interruption of the blood supply to the underlying bone, involvement of the surrounding soft tissue, and, if the infection is left untreated, to necrosis.

Clinical Manifestations

Symptoms include constant pain, edema, decreased mobility of the infected joint, and fever. Redness over the area may occur. The child may refuse to walk or may limp. Because the onset of acute osteomyelitis is generally rapid, it is sometimes misdiagnosed as a sports injury (Kocher et al., 2006; Kaplan, 2005).

■ COLLABORATIVE CARE

A history suggestive of osteomyelitis includes an upper respiratory infection or blunt trauma followed by pain at the area of a growth plate. Laboratory evaluation shows leukocytosis and an elevated erythrocyte sedimentation rate (ESR) and C-reactive protein (Gutierrez, 2005). The degree of ESR elevation is directly related to the severity of the infection. Radiographs and bone scans may identify the area of involvement. A needle aspiration of the site or a blood culture can confirm the diagnosis and provide a culture of the causative organism.

In children with extensive orthopedic surgery, or in those with immunosuppression, a short course of prophylactic antibiotic may be administered after surgery to prevent infection. Medical management for infection begins with the intravenous administration of a broad spectrum antibiotic, even before culture results are available. Since *S. aureus* is a common cause of infection, the antibiotic should be effective against this organism. Treatment is influenced by the possibility of methicillin-resistant *S. aureus* (MRSA), so beginning antibiotics are usually vancomycin or clindamycin, drugs that are effective against MRSA (see Chapter 18 ∞ for further discussion of MRSA). Once the culture results are obtained, the antibiotic may be altered. Oral antibiotics are given once an adequate response has occurred. However, extended intravenous home therapy may be used. Antibiotic therapy continues for about 3 to 6 weeks. When an adequate response is not obtained within 2 to 3 days, the area may be aspirated again, or surgical drainage may be carried out. Intravenous fluids may be administered to ensure adequate hydration.

Prompt diagnosis and treatment usually result in complete resolution of the infection. The prognosis is related to the initiation of therapy—the earlier treatment begins, the better the outcome. Long-term unfavorable outcomes include disruption of the growth plate, which can interrupt growth and damage the joints from septic arthritis, and recurrent infection.

GROWTH & DEVELOPMENT

Osteomyelitis

Osteomyelitis in a newborn is of great concern, as before 18 months of age the blood vessels cross the growth plates. This creates a higher risk of epiphyseal involvement with resultant limb length discrepancy.

■ NURSING MANAGEMENT

Nursing Assessment and Diagnosis

A thorough history, including information about the onset of symptoms and a history of recent infections or puncture wounds, is essential. Ask about immunization status, especially tetanus. Assess the affected area for signs of redness, edema, pain, and decreased range of motion. Measure vital signs since increased temperature and pulse may provide clues about worsening infection.

Nursing diagnoses that may apply to the child with osteomyelitis are as follows:

- Acute Pain related to biologic injury
- Impaired Physical Mobility related to discomfort
- Risk for Infection (Sepsis) related to spread of infection
- Risk for Imbalanced Nutrition: Less than Body Requirements related to loss of appetite
- Health-Seeking Behaviors (Child and Parent) related to lack of information about disease process

Planning and Implementation

Nursing management focuses on performing cultures and obtaining blood samples, administering antibiotics, protecting the child from the spread of the infection, and encouraging a well-balanced diet with generous amounts of fluid. Standard precautions should be used, with transmission-based precautions for any drainage from the site of infection.

Obtain Cultures and Blood Work

When osteomyelitis is suspected, blood cultures and cultures of any open wound must be performed before the first dose of antibiotic. Obtain continuing blood samples as needed to monitor ESR and C-reactive protein.

Administer Fluids and Medications

Administer intravenous fluids as ordered to maintain the child's hydration status. Antibiotics are administered intravenously at first, then orally. Monitor the intravenous site and provide care for the central line, if used (refer to the *Clinical Skills Manual*). In the early stages of the infection, analgesics are prescribed to relieve the associated pain and joint tenderness.

Protect from the Spread of Infection

Strict aseptic technique and transmission-based precautions should be used during all dressing changes. Children and family members should avoid direct contact with any dressings or drainage. Teach good hygiene practices, including handwashing, to maintain infection control. Take vital signs and evaluate the child frequently for symptoms indicating the spread of infection (e.g., increasing pain, difficulty breathing, increased pulse rate, fever).

Encourage a Well-Balanced Diet

Educate both the child and the parents about healthy dietary choices that promote the healing process. Providing a high-protein diet and extra vitamin C will contribute to this process. Encourage increased fluid intake to provide adequate hydration and circulation.

Discharge Planning and Home Care Teaching

Emphasize the importance of completing the full course of antibiotic therapy, especially for children who have undergone surgical drainage of an abscess or lesion. Some children may be discharged on intravenous antibiotics, in which case the family needs instruction for home administration, as well as referral to a home health agency. Explain that failure to follow the prescribed antibiotic therapy may result in chronic infection. Emphasize the importance of returning for blood analysis to monitor progression of healing.

> **CLINICAL TIP**
>
> When a child has a possible diagnosis of osteomyelitis, ensure that all cultures (blood, wound, etc.) are taken before antibiotic therapy begins. However, the cause of infection is not always identified from culture so ESR and C-reactive protein are followed carefully in these cases to identify if treatment is successful. Some clinicians treat with antibiotics until the ESR is <25 to 30 mm/hour (Givner & Kaplan, 2003).

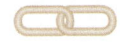

SKILL 9–8
Caring for a Central Venous Catheter Site

COMMUNITY CARE

Schoolwork and the Child Who Is Homebound

If the child is homebound for a period of time during treatment, assist the family in planning for completion of school tasks.

- Contact the school and ask that work be sent home.
- Arrange for a tutor if needed.
- Facilitate computer communication between the child, teacher, and other students.
- Help family members to plan for help at home to monitor the child when they are at work or performing other tasks.
- Refer to financial resources as appropriate for the services the child needs.
- Suggest activities that the child can do at home to foster developmental progression.

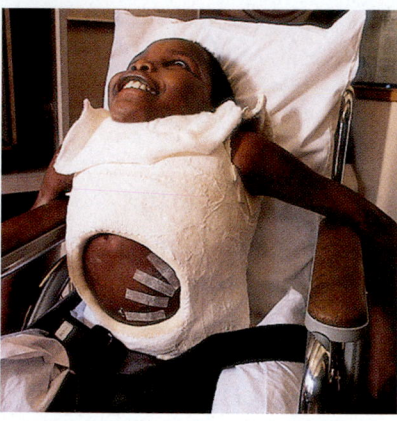

Figure 28–18 ➤ This boy from Kenya had surgery to correct severe kyphosis and scoliosis, caused by tuberculosis of the spine. A Risser cast has been applied to maintain stability of the spine and thoracic cage during healing. Notice the area cut out of the cast to allow for auscultation of the abdomen, as well as to facilitate the child's comfort and adequate intake of food.

Consider the child's age and developmental level to provide suggestions for the family if the child will be immobilized at home. If the child is homebound for the treatment period, assist the family in planning for completion of school tasks.

Evaluation

Expected outcomes of nursing care for the child with osteomyelitis include the following:

- The child shows response to treatment and further absence of signs of infection or sepsis.
- The child completes the prescribed course of antibiotics.
- The family remains free of infection.
- The child ingests adequate intake of fluids and nutrients during the treatment period.
- The child reports absence of pain.
- The child is able to return to normal activities of daily living.

Skeletal Tuberculosis and Septic Arthritis

Skeletal tuberculosis (Figure 28–18➤) and septic arthritis are two infections that, although infrequent, may affect children and adolescents. See Clinical Manifestations and Treatment of Skeletal Tuberculosis and Septic Arthritis on page 1181 for clinical manifestations, diagnostic tests, and medical and nursing management for these infections.

Achondroplasia

Dwarfism is a genetic condition usually resulting in an adult height of 58 inches or less. The most common cause of dwarfism is achondroplasia, which causes short arms and legs. The torso and head are approximately normal size but decreased growth of long bones cause short stature. This is known as disproportionate short stature. Achondroplasia is caused by an abnormal gene of chromosome 4 and occurs in 1 in 26,000 births (March of Dimes, 2004). The gene is coded to produce proteins called fibroblast growth factor receptors. When less receptors are produced, the cells cannot respond normally to signals from growth factors. Achondroplasia may occur as a new genetic mutation with no previous family history or can occur when one or both parents are also dwarfs. There are other less common forms of dwarfism, with about 200 identified types.

Children with achondroplasia have short legs and arms; short fingers with a separation between the middle and ring fingers; and a large, prominent forehead. Hydrocephalus sometimes occurs in children with achondroplasia (see Chapter 26 ∞ for a description of hydrocephalus). Most children with the disorder inherit the gene from one parent. Since only one faulty gene must be present for manifestation of the disorder, it is a dominant characteristic. When a child inherits two copies of the gene from two affected parents, a fatal form of achondroplasia occurs that is characterized by a small thorax, respiratory failure, and death in infancy.

Children with the disorder are diagnosed at birth or shortly after. When there is a family history, genetic testing before or after birth identifies the presence of the faulty gene. Characteristics common in the growth disorder include frequent otitis media, dental malocclusion, bowing of legs, sleep apnea, and marked lordosis can be present during childhood. Low back and leg pain are common as the child grows into adulthood. Perhaps the greatest challenge for families is helping the child to establish a positive self-image in a society that values tall height.

There is currently no treatment for the disorder, although gene therapy and human growth hormone therapy are being explored as possible treatments for the future. Some children and adults with dwarfism have undergone limb lengthening procedures. Other orthopedic intervention may be needed to treat back pain or bone problems. For those children who develop hydrocephalus, insertion of a shunt to divert excess fluid may be needed. Treatment of conditions such as otitis media and malocclusion of teeth is provided.

CLINICAL MANIFESTATIONS   TREATMENT OF SKELETAL TUBERCULOSIS AND SEPTIC ARTHRITIS

Condition	Clinical Manifestations	Diagnostic Tests and Clinical Therapy	Nursing Implications
Skeletal Tuberculosis Rare mycobacterial infection that can be destructive. The spine is the most frequent site of infection (Pott's disease), with joints and other sites sometimes affected.	Depending on the site, pain, limp, severe muscle spasms, kyphosis, muscle atrophy, "doughy" swelling of joints, decreased joint motion, changes in reflexes, low-grade fever.	*Diagnostic tests:* Diagnostic studies include tuberculosis skin test, complete blood count, synovial fluid analysis, and radiographs of affected limb or joint. *Clinical Therapy:* Antibiotic therapy (using a combination of drugs) for 6–9 months is the treatment of choice. The affected site is immobilized. Disease may become resistant to these drugs, and additional drug therapy may be necessary.	Educate the child and family about the disorder and stress the importance of complying with long-term antibiotic therapy. Test all members of the family for tuberculosis. Report the disease to the local health department. Facilitate the immobilization and physical therapy of the child at home.
Septic Arthritis Joint infection of the synovial space most often caused by *Haemophilus influenzae*, *Staphylococcus*, and *Streptococcus*. The most common site of infection is the knee, followed by the hip, ankle, and elbow. Most common in children > 3 years of age.	Fever, pain and local inflammation, joint tenderness, swelling, loss of spontaneous movement. Infant may be irritable, cries when handled, refuses food.	*Diagnostic tests:* CBC with differential ESR, blood cultures. Diagnosis is made based on joint aspiration findings. Results are commonly 100,000 WBCs and 75% neutrophils. Radiographic changes may not be evident until later in the disease process. *Clinical Therapy:* This is a medical emergency requiring prompt treatment to avoid permanent disability. Treatment involves joint aspiration, open drainage, and irrigation, followed by intravenous antibiotic therapy for 3–4 weeks and then oral antibiotics. If the full course of antibiotic treatment is not completed, the child risks recurrent infection and further degeneration of the infected joint.	Educate the child and family about the disorder and emphasize the importance of proper antibiotic therapy. Carefully position the painful joint. Administer antibiotics as ordered. Use transmission-based precautions.

Nursing Management

Nurses play an important role in helping families when a child is diagnosed with achondroplasia. If a parent is a dwarf or there is a positive family history of dwarfism, prenatal genetic counseling should be offered. Explain findings of testing and provide assistance with decision making about pregnancy if needed. Nurses assist parents who have a child with achondroplasia to adjust to the diagnosis, particularly if the parents have had no previous experience with the condition. They may feel guilt and anxiety, so contact with other families who have children with achondroplasia can be a supportive intervention.

Nurses help the child with achondroplasia to develop a positive self-concept during childhood. Many resources are available that provide suggestions about how to foster a positive self-concept, adjust the home to facilitate the dwarf, and assist the child with adjustments in school settings. Partner with school nurses to ensure the child's successful inclusion in all school facilities. While some families decide to explore limb lengthening procedures, most organizations state that focus should be placed on development of a healthy self-image rather than encouraging limb lengthening.

Nurses provide careful assessments of children throughout childhood. Head circumference is especially important in early childhood to identify hydrocephalus if it should occur. Carefully evaluate growth with specialized growth grids for achondroplasia, evaluate dental health at each visit, and perform developmental assessment with special emphasis on gross motor skills. Suggest activities such as swimming and biking that provide activity with little stress on bones. Assist the family by providing resources that assist with planning for car safety seats, methods of adjusting the home, and partnering with the school to provide a supportive atmosphere for the child. Some helpful organizations include Little People of America, Dwarf Athletic Association of America, Human Growth Foundation, The Magic Foundation for Children's Growth and Related Adult Disorders, and March of Dimes. Refer for care for otitis media and provide postoperative care if ear tubes are inserted (see Chapter 19 ∞). Refer to dentists and orthodontists and encourage regular dental care.

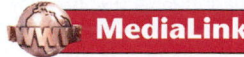

MediaLink

Achondroplasia Resources

Marfan's Syndrome

Marfan's syndrome is another example of a condition inherited in an autosomal dominant manner. About 1 in 5000 children are affected with the syndrome, which manifests with several conditions of connective tissue. The most common problems are cardiac (mitral valve prolapse, aortic regurgitation, abnormal aortic root dimensions), skeletal (pectus excavatum, long arms and digits, scoliosis, elongated head, high arched palate), ocular (lens subluxation), and respiratory (pneumothorax) (Yetman, Huang, Bornemeier, & McCrindle, 2003). The average age for diagnosis is 3 years, and a heart murmur is the usual finding. Careful assessment identifies additional characteristics of the condition along with a positive family history.

No treatment exists for the syndrome, which causes abnormal formation of fibrillin matrix in connective tissue. However, early diagnosis can be successful in treating the cardiac abnormalities with medication or surgery to prevent dissection of the aorta, the major cause of death (de Oliveira, David, Ivanov, et al., 2003). Surgery may be needed to correct scoliosis, pectus excavatum, or pneumothorax. Careful monitoring throughout life is needed to prevent and treat abnormalities associated with the disorder.

Nursing management of Marfan's syndrome begins with identification of infants and children with symptoms of the disorder. Once diagnosed, collaboration with a cardiologist, ophthalmologist, and orthopedist is needed throughout life. The child may require surgery for one or more conditions, can require antibiotics during elective procedures or dental care if the mitral valve is affected, and needs an echocardiogram and other cardiac studies regularly. The nurse may need to explain the disorder to the family and provide referrals for genetic counseling. The child needs support during childhood to learn about the disorder and to manage the medication and monitoring required.

Osteogenesis Imperfecta

Osteogenesis imperfecta (OI), also known as brittle bone disease, is a connective tissue disorder that primarily affects the bones. Children with this condition have fragile bones that are more likely to fracture. The major type of osteogenesis imperfecta occurs in 1 in 30,000 live births and affects boys and girls equally. The underlying disorder is a biochemical defect in the production of collagen. The disease is genetically transmitted, generally in an autosomal dominant inheritance pattern, although some types are transmitted in a recessive pattern. The most common types are caused by mutations on the COLIA1 or COLIA2 genes on chromosomes 17 and 7 (Zeitlin, Fassier, & Glorieux, 2003).

Clinical manifestations include multiple and frequent fractures; blue sclerae; thin, soft skin; increased joint flexibility; enlargement of the anterior fontanel; weak muscles; soft, pliable, brittle bones; and short stature. Most children with OI are short in height and may have decreased range of motion in several joints. Conductive hearing loss can occur by adolescence or young adulthood (Devogelaer & Coppin, 2006).

The disease is classified into four types. In type I disease, the most common form, children have fragile bones, blue sclerae, weakened tooth dentin, and hearing loss that manifests in adolescence. In type II disease, the ribs and skeleton are extensively involved; most children with this form of the disease die in utero or shortly after birth. Type III disease is identified in the newborn period or in infancy when the child sustains numerous fractures and manifests blue sclera. Severe bone fragility and kyphoscoliosis are observed. Most children with type III disease die in childhood as a result of cardiorespiratory failure. Type IV disease is characterized by fractures without other symptoms of the disease. Bowing of the legs and other structural deformities can occur; however, the incidence of fractures decreases beginning in puberty.

Improved knowledge about the genetic transmission of this disease means that some cases of osteogenesis imperfecta can be identified before birth using ultrasound or collagen analysis of chorionic villus cells. In many cases, however, diagnosis of osteogenesis imperfecta is made only when the child has a delay in walking or sustains a fracture. Radiographic evaluation may detect both old and new fractures, and can lead to an erroneous diagnosis of child abuse.

Texts such as dual energy x-ray absorptiometry (DEXA) can be used to measure bone density. Serum alkaline phosphatase may be elevated; other measures of bone metabolism such as serum osteocalcin, procollagen 1 C-terminal peptide, collagen 1 teleopeptide, and urine deoxypyridinoline may be performed occasionally to measure effects of experimental medication. There is no cure for osteogenesis imperfecta. Medical management consists primarily of fracture care and prevention of deformities. The goal is to maximize the child's independence and mobility while minimizing the risk of fractures. Treatment includes physical therapy; casting, bracing, or splinting; surgical stabilization; nutritional management with high vitamin D and calcium; and bisphosphanate medication such as pamidronate. Hematologic stem cell transplant has been used successfully in some children with severe osteogenesis imperfecta and is under further research (Lee & Hui, 2006).

Nursing Management

Nursing care is primarily supportive and focuses on educating the parents and child about the disease and its treatment. The family may have been suspected of child abuse before the disease was diagnosed, and they should be given an explanation about the similar presenting symptoms of these cases. Ask about the child's favorite activities since these will need to be integrated into plans for physical activity and developmental progression. Perform careful growth measures and developmental screening.

To prevent fractures, children with osteogenesis imperfecta must be handled gently. The trunk and extremities should be supported when the child is moved. Such tasks as bathing and diapering may cause fractures and should be performed carefully.

Children usually have several or many fractures during childhood. The period of immobility and casting causes further bone breakdown due to decreased weight bearing, further increasing the chance of fracture. The child should have a well-balanced diet with additional vitamin C, vitamin D, and calcium to encourage healing and bone growth. Calories should be limited to maintain weight at recommended levels since immobility can lead to overweight and the child is generally short for age. Partner with parents if the child is receiving experimental bisphosphanate medication, so that doses are properly administered and serum/urine samples are obtained for monitoring.

When the child needs a fracture stabilized in surgery, or is having rods inserted to strengthen bones, surgical care management is important. Assess the child's vital signs and growth measurements. Obtain accurate weight before surgery and again after with the cast in place. Administer fluids and use pain control techniques such as medication and other comfort measures. Be alert for signs of infection such as osteomyelitis, or respiratory or urinary tract infection. Begin fluids and perform dietary teaching before discharge to promote intake that fosters healing. Follow activity orders precisely to minimize safety hazards for the family. Partner with physical and occupational rehabilitation to plan for the child's return home and to school and to ensure the family can perform range-of-motion exercises and other therapies. Ensure that the family has an approved car safety seat to transport the child.

Emphasize the importance of maintaining normal patterns of growth and development. Toddlers should be helped to explore and interact safely in their environment.

RESEARCH

Pamidronate

Pamidronate is a bone resorption inhibitor that is being used experimentally in children with osteogenesis imperfecta. Low-dose medication is given intravenously every 6 months, and appears to significantly reduce bone fractures and pain. Density of lumbar bones was improved in children receiving the medication. Recently, another bisphosphanate that can be administered orally is showing promise in the treatment of OI (Rauch & Glorieux, 2005; Madenci, Yilmaz, Yilmaz, & Coskun, 2006).

NURSING ALERT

Handle infants with osteogenesis imperfecta gently and use a blanket for additional support when lifting and moving them. Never pull the legs upward when changing a diaper as this can cause a fracture. Instead, gently slip a hand under the hips to raise them, sliding the diaper carefully in, and then bringing it up as the legs are slightly abducted.

MediaLink

OI Resources

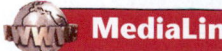

Socialization is essential during the school-age and adolescent years. Encourage exercise, such as swimming, to improve muscle tone and prevent obesity. Independent functioning is promoted by the use of adaptive equipment and motorized wheelchairs. Maintenance of function can depend on proper rehabilitation services. The nurse can arrange and manage such services for the family.

The Osteogenesis Imperfecta Foundation provides information about the disease and can put families in touch with others who have the disease. Parents should receive genetic counseling. For parents who have a child with type II or III OI, the terminal nature of the condition necessitates psychological support, linkage to potential resources, and assistance with managing other tasks of family life (see Chapter 4 ∞ for management of end-of-life care). The siblings and extended family will need support to understand the disease and deal with their feelings and the affected child.

MUSCULAR DYSTROPHIES

The muscular dystrophies are a group of inherited diseases characterized by muscle fiber degeneration and muscle wasting. These disorders can begin early or late in life, and onset can be at birth or gradual. They are all terminal disorders but the progression can vary from a few to many years.

Many kinds of muscular dystrophies affect children and adults. The most common form of childhood muscular dystrophy is Duchenne's muscular dystrophy (pseudohypertrophy), which occurs in 3 in 10,000 live male births (Nereo, Fee, & Hinton, 2003). **Pseudohypertrophy** refers to enlargement of the muscles as a result of their infiltration with fatty tissue. The gene for Duchenne's muscular dystrophy was identified in 1987; it is carried in the Xp21.2 region of the chromosome and is either absent or deleted in affected children. This area codes for a protein called dystrophin which is needed as a muscle membrane stabilizer. A cascade of cellular events occurs, leading to necrosis in the fibers and their replacement by connective tissue. Since this is an X-linked disorder, it is seen only in males. There is similar incidence in various ethnic groups.

Becker muscular dystrophy is also X-linked and affects 1 in 30,000 males (Becker Muscular Dystrophy, no date). Although the gene mutation is similar to Duchenne's, it is milder in form. Other rare muscular dystrophies manifest in infancy, later childhood, or adolescence. There are a variety of genetic mutations ranging from X-linked to autosomal.

Clinical manifestations vary with type of disease. With Duchenne's muscular dystrophy, muscle weakness begins in the lower extremities in early childhood. They compensate for weak lower extremities by using the upper extremity muscles to raise themselves to a standing position (Gower's maneuver) (Figure 28–19▶). The parents may notice the child tripping, toe walking, and displaying enlargement of the calf muscles. By the middle teen years, the child's condition has usually progressed so that walking is not possible. The disease continues to rise, potentially causing conditions such as scoliosis, other musculoskeletal conditions, cardiomyopathy, and respiratory difficulty. Fractures may occur when the child falls. Becker muscular dystrophy is similar but emerges later and more slowly.

The dystrophies of infancy are manifested by generalized weakness and hypotonia. The infant may have difficulty with sucking and swallowing. Ocular problems may be present. Adolescent onset disease is generally milder and slower to progress. Some individuals may live into middle adulthood. See Clinical Manifestations of Muscular Dystrophies of Childhood on page 1186.

Biochemical examinations such as serum enzyme assay, muscle biopsy, and electromyography confirm the diagnosis. Serum creatine kinase (CK) is elevated early in the disease. Dystrophin, the muscle protein that is deficient in muscular dystrophy, can be measured by muscle biopsy. Genetic testing establishes the specific abnormality and type of disease present. Testing of newborns may be offered to families who have one child with the disease since this helps some families to adapt and prepare to the care the child will need (Parsons, Clarke, Hood, Lycett, & Bradley, 2002). Respiratory func-

LAW & ETHICS

Muscular Dystrophy Care

The child with muscular dystrophy has a shortened life span. Parents provide intensive care and require support both physically and emotionally as the child's condition progresses. The child continues to develop in many ways, especially cognitively, as the years pass. Therefore, the needs for explanation and ability to understand the diagnosis change for the child over time. Such a complex chronic disease requires that an interdisciplinary group form a team with collaboration on a regular basis. The child, family, and a variety of health, social, and educational professionals should all be part of the team. The plan of care will include physical, emotional, cognitive, and palliative care; it will evolve and change as the child grows older. Nurses are essential members of the team and may work with families to act as team managers. The key components of the work of the team are:

- Clear communication
- Cooperation
- Cohesiveness
- Commitment
- Collaboration
- Coordination of efforts
- Conflict management
- Consensus decision making
- Caring for the patient (Weidner, 2005)

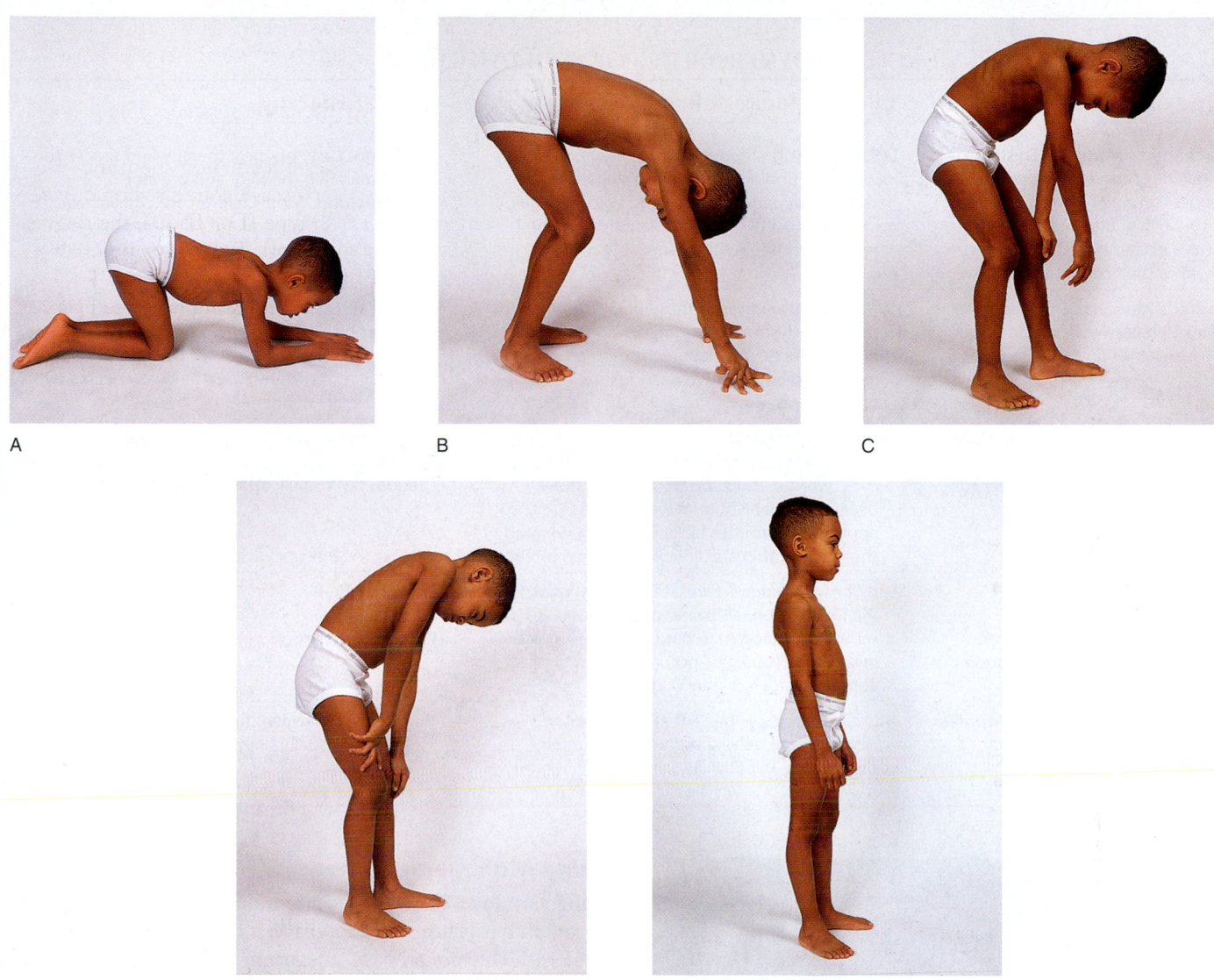

A

B

C

D

E

Figure 28–19 ➤ Since the leg muscles of children with muscular dystrophy are weak, these children must perform the Gower's maneuver to raise themselves to a standing position. A and B, The child first maneuvers to a position supported by arms and legs. C, The child next pushes off the floor and rests one hand on the knee. D and E, The child then pushes himself upright.

tion is measured periodically with pulmonary function tests and overnight pulse oximetry (Beck, Weinberg, Hamnegard et al., 2006). There is no effective treatment for childhood muscular dystrophy. At the present time, research is being directed at several techniques to repair mutations by gene therapy and stem cell therapy (Lee & Hui, 2006). The steroids prednisone and deflazacort may prolong muscle function, preserving walking for a longer period.

Progressive weakness and muscle deformity result in chronic disability (Figure 28–20➤). The goal of medical management is to provide support and prevent complications such as infection or spinal deformities. Respiratory infections are vigorously treated with deep breathing, coughing, nebulizer treatments, and antibiotics. Children and families can benefit from mental health support due to the progressive and terminal nature of the disease. The team approach to managing the child with muscular dystrophy ensures a comprehensive management plan. Team members should include physicians (pediatrician, orthopedic surgeon, neurologist), nurses, physical and occupational therapists, a nutritionist, a psychologist or mental health therapist, and a social worker.

CLINICAL MANIFESTATIONS | MUSCULAR DYSTROPHIES OF CHILDHOOD

Type of Dystrophy	Clinical Manifestations	Clinical Therapy
Duchenne's Muscular Dystrophy X-linked recessive disorder seen in boys (on Xp21 gene); however, 30–50% of affected children have no family history. Onset: within the first 3–4 years of life.	Delayed walking; frequent falls; easily tired when walking, running, or climbing stairs; toe walking, hypertrophied calves; waddling gait; lordosis; positive Gower's maneuver; mental retardation frequently seen.	Supportive care; physical therapy and braces to help maintain mobility and prevent contractures. Most children are wheelchair bound by 12 years of age; death usually occurs during adolescence from respiratory or cardiac failure.
Becker's Muscular Dystrophy X-linked recessive disorder. Onset: usually after 5 years.	Symptoms are similar to those of Duchenne's muscular dystrophy, but milder and delayed; child is mobile until late teens; normal intelligence; congestive heart failure; contractures.	Supportive care, same as for Duchenne's muscular dystrophy. Slow progression (same as for Duchenne's muscular dystrophy); death usually occurs by 30–50 years of age.
Fascioscapulohumeral Muscular Dystrophy Autosomal dominant disorder (on 4q35 chromosome). Onset: later childhood and adolescence.	Face, shoulder girdle, lower limbs affected; unable to raise arms over head; lordosis; cannot close eyes, whistle, smile, or drink from a straw because of inability to move face; characteristic appearance includes facial weakness, winging of the scapula, thin arms, well-developed forearms.	Physical therapy Slow progression; confined to wheelchair as older adult, but usually attains normal life span.
Emery-Dreifuss Muscular Dystrophy X-linked recessive disorder (on Xq28 gene) Onset: childhood.	Early onset of contractures followed by weakness; Achilles tendon, elbow, and spine affected; muscle weakness in upper body follows, with lower body weakness occurring later, cardiac conduction defect may occur.	Physical therapy Surgery Pacemaker insertion
Congenital Muscular Dystrophies Autosomal recessive group of disorders. Onset: present at birth.	Muscle weaknesses present at birth; motor development delay; contractures and joint deformities; hypotonia.	Correction of skeletal deformity (orthosis or surgery). Usually nonprogressive.

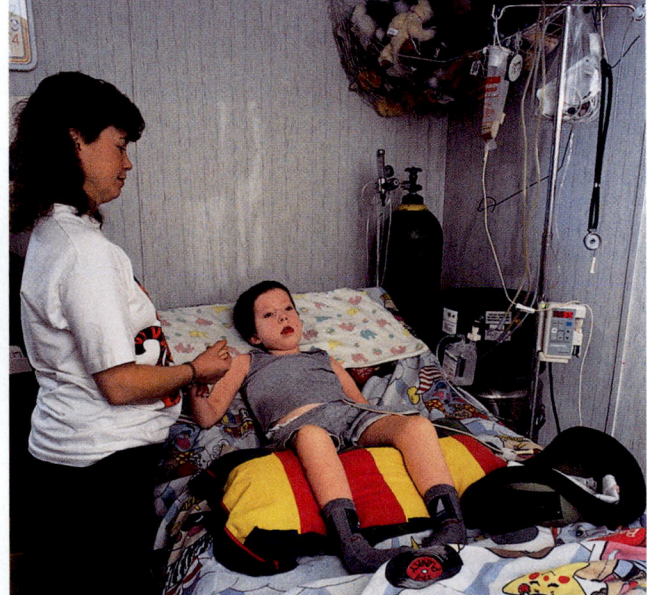

Figure 28–20 ▶ This young boy with muscular dystrophy needs to receive tube feedings and home nursing care. He attends school when possible and is able to use an adapted computer.

Nursing Management

Nursing care focuses on promoting independence and mobility and providing psychosocial support that helps the child and family deal with this progressive, incapacitating disease. Nearly all body systems become involved in the care required, and emotional care is important for the child and family.

Monitor all vital signs as well as cardiac and respiratory functioning. Assess urinary function and frequency of bowel movements. Periodically measure strength and range of motion. Assess mobility via ambulation or assisted device. Perform periodic developmental and nutritional assessments, and provide parents with suggestions for encouraging the child's development. Meet with teachers to evaluate the child's learning needs and functioning in the classroom.

Encourage the child to be independent for as long as possible. Concentrate on what the child can accomplish and do not ask the child to complete tasks that may prove frustrating. Reading books to the child, listening to tapes, and watching television offer the child stimulation during hospitalization. Exercise as tolerated contributes to muscle strength. Physical therapy helps the child ambulate and prevents joint contractures. It is important to provide good back support and posture by keeping the child's body in alignment when confined to a wheelchair.

Maintain the function of body systems by administering oxygen and respiratory therapy as prescribed. Soft foods, gavage, or enteral tube feedings may be needed to promote nutrition. Maintain bowel function with fluids, high-fiber foods, and medications as needed. Monitor and ensure adequate fluid intake and output. Assess for signs of infection. Perform range of motion and provide for physical activity to level of ability. Provide back support and proper posture by keeping the child's body in alignment when in a wheelchair. Splints may be needed to maintain extremities in proper position.

Families may be challenged by the care the child needs. Assist them to find resources to manage this care as well as provide a nurturing environment for other children and family members. Refer the family to financial resources and for respite care as needed. Parents may exhibit feelings of guilt and hopelessness. Encourage parents to express their feelings. Genetic counseling is recommended for the entire family, and it is especially important to identify women who are carriers of one of the X-linked disorders. Siblings may feel neglected because their brother or sister is receiving so much attention. They may also be concerned that they will develop the disease. Encourage the parents to involve siblings in the child's care to reassure them of their importance. Provide ongoing support during hospitalizations, management of home care, and the child's changes in condition. Perform continual assessments of the child's condition, the family management plan, and use of complementary therapies. Refer family members to resource and support groups such as the Muscular Dystrophy Association.

INJURIES TO THE MUSCULOSKELETAL SYSTEM

Musculoskeletal injuries are classified according to the mechanism, the location, and the force of the injury. Athletic participation, car crashes, and other accidents are frequent causes. (see Evidence-Based Practice: Backpack Use and Pain). Strains, sprains, dislocations, and fractures are the most common musculoskeletal injuries in children. Distinguishing among these injuries is often difficult. See Clinical Manifestations of Strains, Sprains, and Dislocations on page 1188. A detailed discussion of fractures follows.

Fractures

A fracture is a break in a bone that occurs when more stress is placed on the bone than the bone can withstand. Fractures, which may occur at any age, occur frequently in children because their bones are less dense and more porous than those of adults.

Etiology and Pathophysiology

Fractures in children may result from direct trauma to a bone (falls, sports injuries, abuse, motor vehicle crashes) or bone diseases (osteogenesis imperfecta) that result in weakening of the bone. Due to their porous nature, the bones of children may bow,

 MediaLink

Muscular Dystrophy Support and Resources

COMPLEMENTARY THERAPY

Muscular Dystrophy

Many families who have a child with muscular dystrophy will use different types of complementary care. The nurse always assesses for such approaches, provides information as needed by the family, makes recommendations for complementary therapies that may be helpful, and cautions against those that could be harmful due to interactions with medications or other problems. Common complementary care used in MD includes dietary enhancement. This enhancement includes certain vitamins, minerals, and omega-3 fatty acids; herbal remedies such as horsetail, oatstraw, and kelp teas; and massage to assist with reduction of muscle spasms (University of Maryland Medical Center, 2004).

Case Study

Fracture Assessment

CLINICAL MANIFESTATIONS | STRAINS, SPRAINS, AND DISLOCATIONS

Condition	Clinical Manifestations	Clinical Therapy
Strain • Stretching or tearing of either a muscle or a tendon, usually from overuse (e.g., back strain resulting from improper or overly heavy lifting, shoulder and elbow tears from baseball).	• Vary according to the type and severity of the strain. Pain can be acute or chronic.	• Rest and support of the injured part until the muscle or tendon heals and normal activity can occur.
Sprain • Stretching or tearing of a ligament, usually caused by a fall, sports injury, or motor vehicle crash (e.g., anterior cruciate ligament [ACL] tear requiring reconstruction).	• Edema, joint immobility, and pain.	• For the first 24–36 hours: **R**est **I**ce **C**ompression **E**levation • After the first 24–36 hours, mobility is gradually increased.
Dislocation • Complete displacement of an articular joint surface, usually associated with a fall, sports injury, or motor vehicle crash. Although almost any joint may be dislocated, most dislocations occur in the shoulder, knee, and hip.	• Pain and tenderness, swelling and obvious deformity, and instability of the joint.	• Varies according to the site and severity of the injury, and consists of: • Shoulder: Open or closed reduction followed by the application of a sling. • Knee: Closed reduction with gentle traction, then immobilization with a splint. • Hip (posterior): Immediate closed reduction or possibly open reduction, traction, or hip spica cast. • Hip (anterior): Immediate closed reduction, extension traction, and hip spica cast.

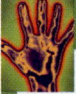

GROWTH & DEVELOPMENT

Stress Fractures

Stress fractures are becoming more common in adolescents who limit their intake of calories and calcium in an attempt to remain lean for sports such as distance running or gymnastics. These fractures may present with chronic pain that changes in intensity. Be alert to this possibility when teenagers' diets and athletic activities place them at risk.

The risk of bone fractures is significantly increased with higher cola consumption and televison viewing time and with lower levels of physical acitivity and lower milk intake (Ma & Jones 2004; Manias, McCabe & Bishop, 2006).

leading to more common greenstick or spiral fractures (Eiff & Hatch, 2003). Trauma may be caused by an acute injury, direct and forceful impact, or overuse such as in chronic and repetitive activities. Children with osteoporosis and osteopenia are more prone to fractures (see description of these conditions earlier in the chapter). Child abuse is a cause of fracture and should be suspected when the type of fracture is uncommon at a given age. For example, femur fractures are most common at 2 to 3 years and in adolescence; a femur fracture in an infant is suggestive of the possibility of abuse (Brown & Fisher, 2004).

Clinical Manifestations

Signs and symptoms of fractures vary depending on the location, type, and nature of the causative injury. Fractures are generally characterized by pain, abnormal positioning, edema, immobility or decreased range of motion, ecchymosis, guarding, and crepitus. Childhood fractures most often involve the clavicle, tibia, ulna, and femur, with distal forearm fractures of the radius or ulna the most common type (Carson, Woolridge, Colletti, & Kilgore, 2006). Fractures to the pelvis are often associated with motor vehicle crashes. Epiphyseal (growth plate) injuries are dangerous in children as they can interfere with future growth at the site. These constitute about 30% of childhood fractures (Eiff & Hatch, 2003). Types of fractures are described using the Salter-Harris classification system (see Figure 28–21 ➤).

■ COLLABORATIVE CARE

Radiographs are useful for determining the exact location and type of fracture. However, in very young children the higher amounts of collagen and cartilage make diagnosis by radiograph challenging. Examination and palpation of the area by a skilled clinician is essential.

PATHOPHYSIOLOGY ILLUSTRATED

Salter-Harris Classification

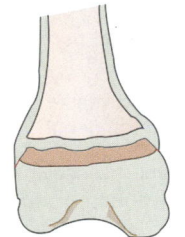 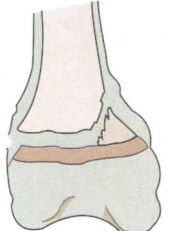 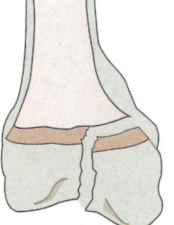 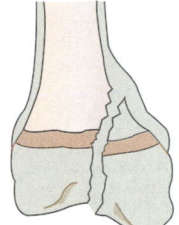 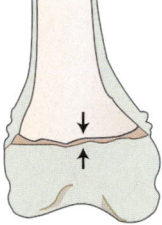

Type I
Common
Growth plate undisturbed
Growth disturbances rare

Type II
Most common
Growth disturbances rare

Type III
Less common
Serious threat to growth
and joint

Type IV
Serious threat to growth

Type V
Rare
Crush injury causes cell death in
 growth plate, resulting in
 arrested growth and limited
 bone length
If growth plate is partially
 destroyed, angular deformities
 may result

Figure 28–21 ➤ The Salter-Harris classification system is based on the angle of the fracture in relation to the epiphysis.

Emergency care focuses on accurate diagnosis, pain management, and establishment of a treatment plan. Medical treatment consists of two basic steps: reduction to realign displaced or fragmented bones, and immobilization so that healing can take place.

A closed reduction aligns the bone by manual manipulation or traction. Conscious sedation or pain management may be used during closed reduction. An open reduction requires surgical alignment of the bone, often using pins, plates, wires, or screws. For open fractures, surgery must also be performed for debridement, to remove dead tissue and clean the wound. Casting is the most common external method of immobilization. Casts may be placed on extremities (short or long leg or arm cast) or the upper body to immobilize the spine, or may be applied from chest to legs to stabilize the pelvis or hips (spica cast). Leg casts may be walking or non-walking casts (Figure 28–22➤). Cast material is either plaster or a synthetic fabric. Other external methods of stabilization include traction and splinting. Pins may be inserted to stabilize the fracture, and can be used with or without casts or traction. A combination of treatments may be needed in the child with multiple fractures following a car crash or other trauma.

Healing of fractures is influenced by factors including age, size of the involved bone, and fracture site. The healing process progresses from cartilaginous callous formation to bone remodeling and bone callus formation (Figure 28–23➤). Fractures heal more quickly in children than in adults. Immobilization is essential for the bone healing process to take place. If a fracture is properly reduced, complications should be minimal (Table 28–1).

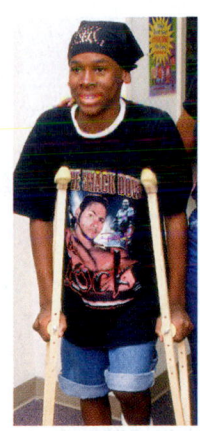

Figure 28–22 ➤ This adolescent had a fracture of the fibula when falling against the metal support on a trampoline. He is using a non-walking cast and crutches. What teaching does he need to ambulate safely with crutches? What questions will be needed to plan safety teaching for his future sporting activities?

NURSING MANAGEMENT
Nursing Assessment and Diagnosis

When dealing with an injured child, be alert to the signs and symptoms of fractures and soft-tissue injuries before moving the child. Try to identify the cause of the injury by asking the child, parents, or other family members what happened. Evaluate pain, swelling, and any abnormal positioning of the injured area. When a child is admitted to the emergency department or hospital, nursing assessment includes the extent of the injury, the degree of pain, and the child's vital signs (respiratory status, pulse, blood pressure).

CLINICAL TIP

When in doubt about the nature of an injury, apply a splint and raise the body part above heart level. Splinting immobilizes the site, prevents further damage, and decreases pain. Be sure to immobilize both the joint above and below the injury. Raising the body part helps to minimize edema and increase comfort.

PATHOPHYSIOLOGY ILLUSTRATED

Process of Bone Healing

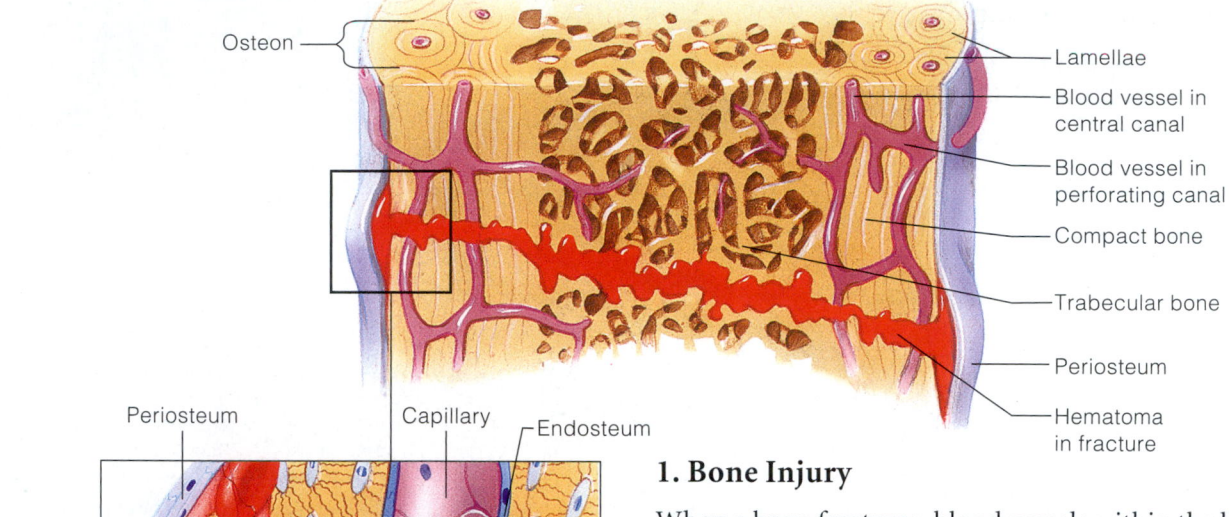

Osteon — Lamellae
Blood vessel in central canal
Blood vessel in perforating canal
Compact bone
Trabecular bone
Periosteum
Hematoma in fracture

1. Bone Injury

When a bone fractures, blood vessels within the bone and surrounding soft tissues tear and begin to bleed, forming a hematoma. Necrotic bone tissue adjacent to the fracture causes an intense inflammatory response characterized by vasodilation, exudate formation, and white cell migration to the fracture site.

Periosteum — Capillary — Endosteum

Fibrin

Bone fragment

Osteocyte

2. Fibrocartilaginous Callus Formation

Clotting factors within the hematoma form a fibrin meshwork. Within 48 hours, fibroblasts and new capillaries growing into the fracture form granulation tissue that gradually replaces the hematoma. Phagocytes begin to remove cell debris.

Osteoblasts, bone-forming cells, proliferate and migrate into the fracture site, forming a fibrocartilaginous callus. The osteoblasts build a web of collagen fibers from both sides of the fracture site that eventually unites to connect bone fragments, thus splinting the bone. Chondroblasts lay down patches of cartilage that provide a base for bone growth.

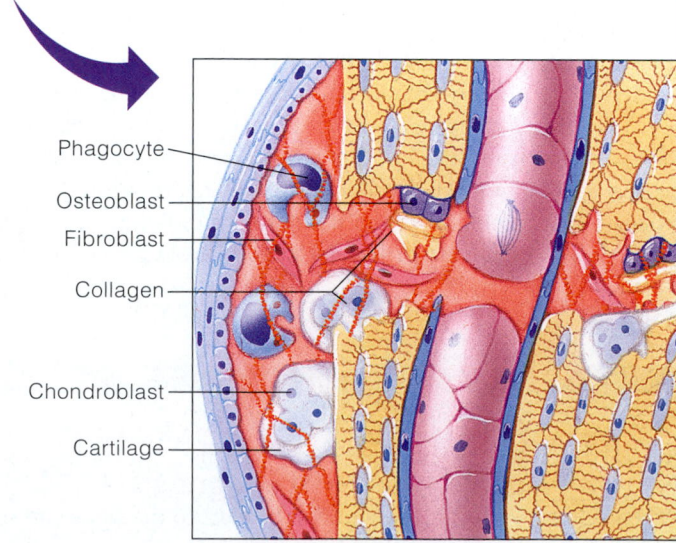

Phagocyte
Osteoblast
Fibroblast
Collagen
Chondroblast
Cartilage

Figure 28–23 ➤ Any injury to the bone brings about a multistep process of bone formation that lasts about 3 months.

PATHOPHYSIOLOGY ILLUSTRATED

Process of Bone Healing (continued)

4. Bone Remodeling

Osteoblasts continue to form new woven bone, which is in turn organized into the lamellar structures of compact bone. Osteoclasts resorb excess callus as it is replaced by mature bone.

As the bone heals and is subjected to the mechanical stress of everyday use, osteoblasts and osteoclasts respond by remodeling the repair site along the lines of force. This ensures that the repaired section of bone eventually resembles the structure of the uninjured part.

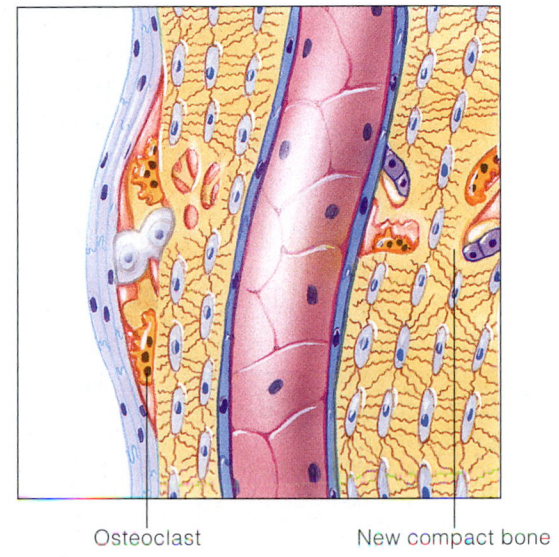

Osteoclast   New compact bone

3. Bony Callus Formation

Osteoblasts continue to proliferate and synthesize collagen fibers and bone matrix, which are gradually mineralized with calcium and mineral salts to form a spongey mass of woven bone. The trabeculae of woven bone bridge the fracture. Osteoclasts migrate to the repair site and begin removing excess bone in the callus. Bony callus formation usually continues for 2 to 3 months.

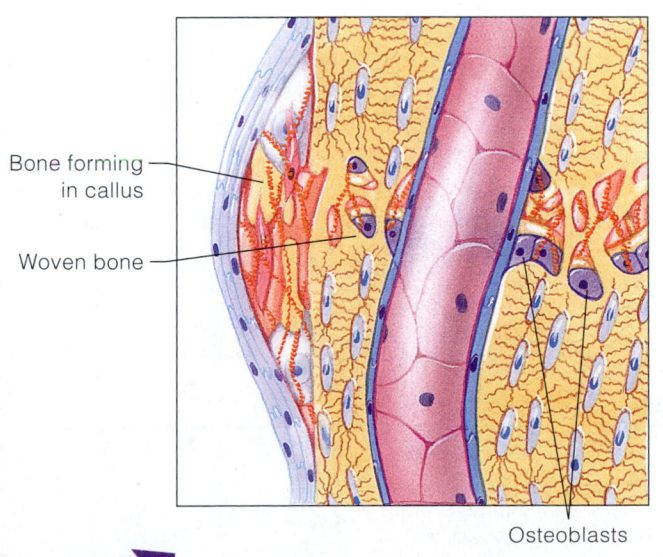

Bone forming in callus

Woven bone

Osteoblasts

Figure 28–23 ➤ (continued)

Table 28-1	COMPLICATIONS OF FRACTURE REDUCTION
Complication	**Clinical Therapy**

Infection
  Acute (may occur with open fractures)
  Chronic (osteomyelitis)
	Debridement, drainage, culture, and treatment with antibiotics

Neurovascular injury resulting from physical nerve damage	Nerve repair
Vascular injury	Vascular repair, amputation, tendon lengthening
Malunion (undesired healed alignment of bone) or delayed union	Corrective osteotomy; prolonged immobilization
Nonunion	Surgical intervention; internal fixation
Leg length discrepancy	Shoe lift

> ### ➤ NURSING ALERT
>
> It is uncommon for children to have repeated fractures. If they occur, make further assessments for their cause. The child may suffer from osteogenesis imperfecta. If attention deficit hyperactivity disorder (ADHD) is present or if the child has a mental health problem, excessive risky behavior may be the cause of fractures. When children are found on radiograph to have several old and healing fractures, or multiple fractures of the same or different bones, they may be victims of physical abuse, particularly if the caretaker's explanation of fracture does not match the clinical picture. An example could be the parent who claims the child fell from a chair, but there is a severe arm fracture and skull fracture. See Chapter 6 for a description of child abuse and Chapter 27 ∞ for a discussion of ADHD.

The following nursing diagnoses may apply to the child with a fracture:

- Acute Pain related to injury
- Risk for Impaired Skin Integrity related to treatment
- Risk for Infection related to open fracture or trauma
- Impaired Physical Mobility related to treatment
- Health-Seeking Behaviors related to lack of information about treatment and expected outcome

Planning and Implementation

Nurses may be in community settings when children experience a fracture, and need to provide emergency care and arrange for transport. Emergency personnel are informed of the assessment data to provide for safe care. In addition, nurses are aware that repeated fractures in the same child can be a sign of other healthcare conditions. Nursing care focuses on care of the child before and after fracture reduction, encouraging mobility as ordered, maintaining skin integrity, preventing infection, and teaching the parents and child how to care for the fracture. If conscious sedation or pain blocks are used, nursing care for these procedures is needed. When caring for a child who has undergone fracture reduction, it is important to be aware of the signs of complications. Notify the physician immediately if these signs occur. The major serious complication is **compartment syndrome**, or a condition of increased pressure in a limited space such as the soft tissue of an extremity, which compromises circulation and nervous innervation (Altizer, 2004). (See Clinical Manifestations of Compartment Syndrome below.)

CLINICAL MANIFESTATIONS | COMPARTMENT SYNDROME

Clinical manifestations begin about 30 minutes after tissue ischemia starts. Major manifestations are:

- Paresthesia (tingling, burning, loss of 2-point discrimination)
- Pain (unrelieved by medication, characterized by crying in the young child)
- Pressure (skin is tense, cast appears tight)
- Pallor* (pale, gray, or white skin tone)
- Paralysis* (weakness or inability to move extremity)
- Pulselessness* (weak or absent pulse)

Check extremities for:
- Color
- Temperature
- Capillary refill
- Peripheral pulses
- Edema
- Sensation
- Motor ability
- Pain

*= late sign
Document results and report changes or abnormal results immediately. (Altizer, 2004; Grottkau, Epps, & Di Scala, 2005).

Maintain Proper Alignment

Immobilization is used to maintain proper alignment of the fracture. Casts and traction are methods used for immobilizing an injured child. Cast care guidelines are included in Box 28–1 on page 1155.

Different types of traction are used, depending on the location and type of fracture (Table 28–2). Nursing care for the child in traction is described in Box 28–2.

Monitor Neurovascular Status

Neurovascular assessment is used for early detection of compartment syndrome, which may occur with a crush injury or when a fracture is reduced. Swelling associated with inflammation reduces blood flow to the affected area, and casting causes further constriction of blood flow. Monitor the child's sensation to touch, temperature, movement, strength of the pulse, and capillary refill time in the extremity distal to the injury. Monitor every 15 minutes after the cast is applied for at least 2 hours and then every 1 to 2 hours, depending on the care facility's policy and the child's condition. Keep the cast elevated above heart level to minimize edema.

Promote Mobility

The amount of mobility the child is allowed is ordered by the physician and restrictions depend on the extent and site of the fracture. Fractures of the hip or pelvis may involve body casts, and providing wheeled carts makes mobility possible. Children with leg fractures can sometimes bear weight on the cast; but if they cannot bear weight, they move around with crutches, walkers, or wheelchairs. See the Clinical Skills Manual for information on crutch walking.

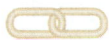

SKILL 14–5
Setting Crutch Height

Discharge Planning and Home Care Teaching

Most fractures can be easily managed at home. Activities are generally limited for approximately 8 weeks. Teach the parents and child cast care, activity restrictions, and how to identify problems that should be reported (see page 1192). Help parents to identify any modifications that may be needed at home and school. The child who has to manage steps at home or school may need special training with crutches or a temporary ramp. Refer parents to home health nurses or home teaching services, if indicated. Provide pertinent teaching to prevent future injuries.

Sports Injuries

Sports injuries are the most common type of injury in youth from 13 to 19 years. Football, cycling, and basketball are the sports most commonly associated with injury (Simon, Bublitz, & Hambidge, 2006). Fernando, who is described in the opening scenario, provides an example of this type of injury. Fractures, which were previously described, are common sports injuries of young athletes. However, a variety of other

---

BOX 28–2
NURSING CARE OF THE CHILD WITH TRACTION OR EXTERNAL FIXATOR

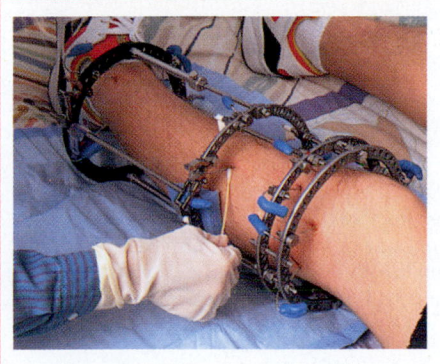

1. Assess the child in traction by first checking the equipment. Make sure that the equipment is in the proper position. Observe both the body appliance and the attached weights and pulleys. Make certain that the child's body is in proper alignment.
2. Assess the skin under the straps and pin insertion sites for any signs of redness, edema, or skin breakdown.
3. Assess the extremity by checking neurovascular status frequently (check warmth, color, distal pulses, capillary refill time, movement, sensation).
4. Provide pin care when ordered using sterile technique. Clean the area surrounding the pin with cotton-tipped applicators saturated with normal saline or half-strength hydrogen peroxide. Clean the area again with sterile water or more saline. Apply an antibacterial ointment, if ordered, using another cotton-tipped applicator.
5. When the traction equipment can be removed, skin care should be performed every 4 hours.
6. Place a sheepskin pad under the child's extremity if orders permit.

| Table 28–2 | **TYPES OF TRACTION** |

Type

Skin Traction
Pull is applied to the skin surface, which puts traction directly on the bones and muscles. Traction is attached to the skin with adhesive materials or straps, or foam boots, belts, or halters.

Dunlop Traction (can be either skeletal or skin)
Used for fracture of the humerus. The arm, which is flexed, is suspended horizontally with straps placed on both the upper and lower portions for pull from both sides.

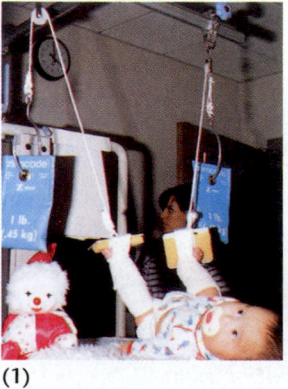 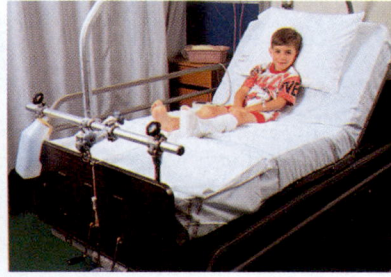

(1) (2)

Bryant Traction (1)
Used specifically for the child under 3 years of age and weighing less than 17.5 kg (35 lb), who has developmental dysplasia of the hip or a fractured femur. This bilateral traction is applied to the child's legs and kept in place by wrapping the legs from foot to thigh with elastic bandages. The hips are flexed at a 90-degree angle, with knees extended. This position is maintained by attaching the traction appliance to weights and pulleys, which are suspended above the crib. The buttocks do not rest on the mattress, but are slightly elevated off the bed.

Buck Traction (2)
Used for knee immobilization; to correct contractures or deformities; or for short-term immobilization of a fracture. It keeps the leg in an extended position, without hip flexion. Traction is applied to the extremity in one direction (straight line) with a single pulley system.

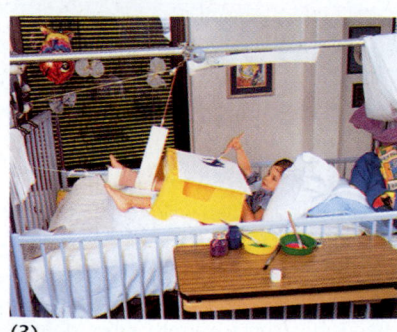

(3)

Russell Traction (3)
Used for fractures of the femur and lower leg. Traction is placed on the lower leg while the knee is suspended in a padded sling. The hips and knees, which are slightly flexed, are immobilized. One force is applied by a double pulley to the foot and another force is applied upward using a sling under the knee and an overhead pulley.

Skeletal Traction
Pull is directly applied to the bone by pins, wires, tongs, or other apparatus that have been surgically placed through the distal end of the bone.

Skeletal Cervical Traction
Used for cervical spine injuries to reduce fractures and dislocations, Crutchfield Gardner-Wells, or Vinke tongs are placed in the skull with burr holes. Weights are attached to the apparatus with a rope and pulley system to the hyperextended head.

Halo Traction
Used to immobilize the head and neck after cervical injury or dislocation. Also used for positioning and immobilization after cervical injury.

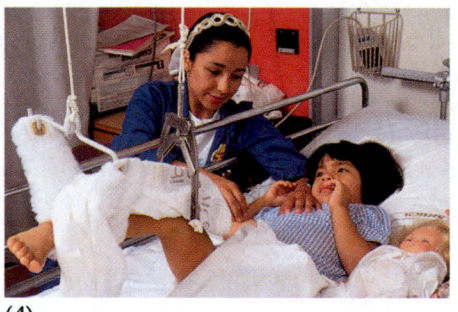

(4)

90-90 Traction (4)
Used for fractures of the femur or tibia. A skeletal pin or wire is surgically placed through the distal part of the femur, while the lower part of the extremity is in a boot cast. Traction ropes and pulleys are applied at the pin site and on the boot cast to maintain the flexion of both the hip and knee at 90 degrees. This traction can also be used for treatment of an upper extremity fracture.

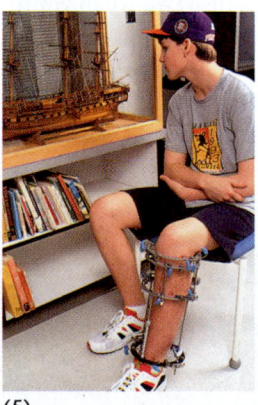

(5)

External Fixators (5)
These devices can be used in the treatment of simple fractures, both open and closed; complex fractures with extensive soft tissue involvement; correction of bony or soft tissue deformities; pseudoarthroses; and limb length discrepancy. They are attached to the extremity by percutaneous transfixing of pins or wires to the bone.

injuries that affect the musculoskeletal system are common in sports. Children and adolescents have characteristics that put them at risk for injury. These include:

- Vulnerability of growth plates to injury, especially distal tibia and fibula.
- Increased joint mobility from lax tendons and ligaments, leading to injury of knee, ankle, and hip.
- Softer bones that lead to fractures and to more common injury to underlying organs.
- Lack of experience in the sport and inadequate training.
- Lack of acceptance of protective gear.
- Impatience with taking the time to heal after injury.

Some common sports injuries are listed in Table 28–3. Treatment for sprains, strains, dislocations and fractures were previously described. Head and neck injuries are discussed in Chapter 26 and dental emergencies in Chapter 19 ∞. A few general approaches to minimize and treat injuries for youth athletes follow.

Athletes can benefit from teaching that enhances performance of their sports and also minimizes the chance of injury. They should receive instruction in correct techniques from a person qualified to coach and supervise children. Encourage youth to gradually increase time and intensity at a sport, rather than immediately playing a new sport for long periods of time. Have parents inquire about the coach's experience and also verify that the coaching staff is prepared in emergency care.

The nurse should be alert for sports injuries during contact with children and adolescents in health promotion visits. Ask about sports participation for all youth, but especially when there are complaints of sore muscles, edema of body parts, and bruises. Perform neurovascular assessment of extremities, including color, temperature, capillary refill time, edema, pulses, sensation, and pain. Phrase questions so that you identify sports such as skate boarding or snow boarding, which may not be performed under supervision or in organized sports programs. Youth may not consider these "sports."

Teach the youth to warm up for 10–15 minutes before participation and to cool down for a corresponding period at the end of an activity. Advise wearing recommended gear for the sport including equipment such as a well-fitted protective helmet, face masks, eye protection, mouth guards, elbow and wrist guards, gloves, knee pads, and shin pads. Parents may need assistance to learn recommended equipment, and to obtain resources for its purchase. Frequent updates are needed as the child grows. Teach the child not to ignore pain.

COMMUNITY CARE

Protective Gear for Sports
When a child has a fracture from sports or other activities, ask details about how the injury occurred. If protective gear is recommended and was not worn, reinforce the need for protection. Suggest financial resources, as necessary.

Table 28–3	COMMON SPORTS INJURIES
Sport	**Types of Injuries**
Baseball	• Hand and finger fractures and sprains • Contusions and sprains of upper or lower extremities; wrists, elbows, knees, and ankles are common sites • Injury to body parts when hit by a ball (i.e., broken teeth, face, head, eye, and chest injuries)
Football	• Head and neck injury such as skull or cervical vertebrae fracture • Pulled muscles or dislocations in shoulders and legs
Gymnastics	• Wrist and elbow fractures and strains • Tendonitis in elbows and ankles/legs
Hockey (ice and inline)	• Dental injury • Leg fractures • Head and neck injuries
Soccer	• Head and neck injury • Strains and fractures of legs
Wrestling	• Fractures and dislocations of upper and lower extremities

Injuries such as muscle strains should be treated promptly. They involve several steps:

- Resting the injury for 24–48 hours; applying ice for 20 minutes four times daily; applying compression with an elastic wrap to provide comfort and decrease edema; elevating the part affected above heart level.
- Gradually increasing motion to the part.
- Adding flexibility and resistance or strengthening exercises.
- Returning gradually to the sport, usually in 2–3 weeks after injury (Harper, 2002).

Partner with the child, family, and other health professionals to plan for activity whenever an injury has occurred. Praise the family and youth for physical activity, which is an important part of a healthy lifestyle. Provide community resources to foster sports participation.

Amputations

Amputation—the complete absence of a body extremity—can be either congenital or acquired. Approximately two-thirds of amputations in children are congenital and one-third are acquired. Congenital amputations can be caused by constrictive amniotic bands, drugs, or irradiation. Acquired amputations are generally associated with trauma or the result of a disease or disorder.

The child with an absent limb should be fitted with a prosthesis as soon as feasible, to foster a positive body image, independence, and self-confidence and to ensure that the child's motor skills develop as normally as possible. The prosthetic device should be reevaluated as the child progresses physically and developmentally. Frequent stump reconstructions are often necessary in children with traumatic amputations, because as children grow, so do their bones, and the skin tends to adhere to the bone. Bone may need to be cut and soft tissue added to keep the stump rounded. Joint fusions or stump lengthenings may also be needed to allow for the effective use of a prosthesis.

Nursing Management

Nursing care focuses on providing emotional support regarding altered body image, managing pain, maintaining skin integrity, and encouraging maximal independent functioning.

Recovering from the loss of a limb is one of the most difficult challenges facing a child. Emphasize what the child can do rather than what he or she cannot do. Good listening skills are important.

The child who has had surgery or a traumatic injury experiences pain. Many of the techniques discussed in Chapter 15 ∞ are useful interventions. After surgery, an epidural may be the treatment of choice. Oral analgesics are used during the period of adaptation to a prosthesis if tenderness is present. Children often regularly experience "phantom" limb pain in the lost extremity (Wilkins, McGrath, Finley, & Katz, 2004).

The child usually begins by wearing the prosthetic device for 1 to 2 hours at a time. Check the skin for any redness or breakdown. If such conditions develop, leave the prosthesis off and allow the skin to clear before reapplying. Have the prosthesis adjusted if necessary, and increase wearing time as tolerated by the child.

Children with amputated limbs quickly learn how to accommodate to the prosthetic device. Make use of physical therapy programs that are specifically designed to help the child perform activities of daily living.

Answer any questions the family has about how to care for the prosthetic device and how to perform skin checks. Encourage parents to allow the child to participate in peer activities that are physically and emotionally challenging. Sporting activities that enable the child to participate using modified equipment are a good way to build self-confidence and motivation. For example, ski centers may offer programs that teach children with physical disabilities how to ski. The Special Olympics is another motivating option for some children. Assess the need for counseling and offer referrals as appropriate.

MediaLink

Special Olympics

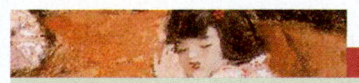

CRITICAL THINKING IN ACTION

Refer back to Fernando in the opening scenario. He is a 12-year-old boy who sustained a sprain during a soccer game at school. Fernando has recently been encouraged to play more sports by his family as he has started to gain weight. He enjoys soccer but is now afraid to play again. Fernando had normal vital signs and neurovascular checks after the injury. He wore an ace wrap for several days and kept his leg elevated with ice for the first day after the injury. The pain gradually decreased and he now has normal range of motion and function of the ankle.

DISCUSSION

1. Describe the benefits of exercise such as soccer for Fernando. How much physical activity should he have every day?

2. Describe all of the assessments you would perform in the immediate period of an injury such as Fernando's. What nursing actions should be taken to prepare him for the transfer to the emergency center by his mother?

3. Describe the soft-tissue injury that occurs in a sprain. What diagnostic tools are useful? Why is rest, elevation, and ice recommended in the initial period?

4. The school nurse plays an important role in preparing for emergencies at school. Outline the items she should keep in the office for treatment of musculoskeletal emergencies.

 Refer to your Prentice Hall Nursing MediaLink DVD-ROM for answers.

EXPLORE MediaLink

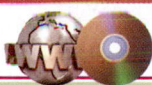 http://www.prenhall.com/ball

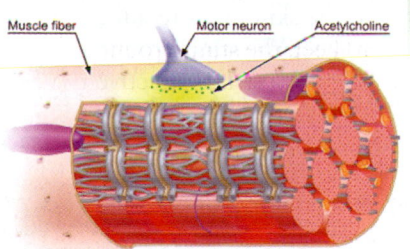

Resources for this chapter can be found on the Prentice Hall Nursing MediaLink DVD-ROM accompanying this textbook, and on the Companion Website at http://www.prenhall.com/ball.

DVD-ROM
Audio Glossary
NCLEX-RN® Review
Animation/Video
   Muscle Physiology

COMPANION WEBSITE
Audio Glossary
NCLEX-RN® Review
Care Plan Activity: Post-operative Clubfoot Repair
Case Study: Fracture Assessment
MediaLink Application: Achondroplasia
WebLinks

REFERENCES

Altizer, L. (2004). Compartment syndrome. *Orthopedic Nursing, 23*, 391–396.

American Academy of Pediatrics (n.d.). Children with Special Health Care Needs. Retrieved on September 12, 2006 from http://www.aap.org/healthtopics/specialneeds.cfm

Beck, J., Weinberg, J., Hamnegard, C. H., Spahija, J., Olofson, J., Grimby, G. Y., & Sindery, C. (2006). Diaphragmatic function in advanced Duchenne muscular dystrophy. Neuromuscular Disorders, 16, 161–167.

Becker Muscular Dytrophy. (n.d.). Becker muscular dystrophy. Retrieved September 12, 2006, from http://www.beckermusculardystrophy.org

Bowman, B. A., & Russell, R. M. (Eds.). (2006). *Present knowledge of nutrition* (9th ed.). Washington, DC: International Life Sciences Institute.

Brown, D., & Fisher, E. (2004). Femur fractures in infants and young children. *American Journal of Public Health, 94*, 558–559.

Burns, C. E., Dunn, A. M., Brady, M. A., Starr, N. B., & Blosser, C. G. (2004). *Pediatric primary care* (3rd ed.). Philadelphia: Saunders.

Carson, S., Woolridge, D. P., Colletti, J. & Kilgore, D. (2006). Pediatric upper extremity injuries, *Pediatric Clinics of North America, 53*, 41–67.

Caulton, J. M., Ward, K. A., Alsop, C. W., Dunn, G., Adams, J. E., & Mughal, M. Z. (2004). A randomized controlled trial of standing programme on bone mineral density in non-ambulant children with cerebral palsy. *Archives of Disease in Childhood, 89*, 131–135.

Chamley, C. A., Carson, P., Randall, D., & Sandwell, M. (2005). *Developmental anatomy and physiology of children*. St. Louis: Elsevier.

Corbett, J. V. (2004). *Laboratory tests and diagnostic procedures with nursing diagnoses* (6th ed.). Upper Saddle River, NJ: Prentice Hall Health.

De Oliveira. N., David, T. E., Ivanov, J., Armstrong, S., Eriksson, M. M., Radowski, H., & Webb, G. (2003). Results of surgery for aortic aneurysm in patients with Marfan syndrome. *Journal of Thoracic and Cardiovascular Surgery, 125*, 789–796.

Devogelaer, J. P., & Coppin, C. (2006). Osteogenesis imperfecta: Current treatment options and future prospects. *Treatments in Endocrinology, 5*, 229–242.

Eiff, M. P., & Hatch, R. L. (2003). Boning up on common pediatric fractures. *Pediatrics, 20*(11), 30–59.

Eliakim, A., & Nemet, D. (2005). Osteopenia of prematurity—The role of exercise in prevention and treatment. *Pediatric Endocrinology Review, 2*, 675–682.

Frank, G., Mahoney, H. M., & Eppes, S. C. (2005). Musculoskeletal infections in children. *Pediatric Clinics of North America, 52*, 1083–1106.

Gilmore, A., & Thompson, G. H. (2003). Common childhood foot deformities. *Consultant for Pediatricians, 2*, 63–71.

Givner, L. B., & Kaplan, S. L. (2003). Bone and joint infections: Pediatrics. Presented at the 40th annual meeting of the Infectious Diseases Society of America. As reported in *Infectious Diseases in Children* (February 2003), p. 82.

Gore, A. L., & Spencer, J. P. (2004). The newborn foot. *American Family Physician, 69*, 865–872.

Grottkau, B. E., Epps, H. R., & Di Scala, C. (2005). Compartment syndrome in children and adolescents. *Journal of Pediatric Surgery, 40*, 678–682.

Grzegorzewski, A., Bowen, J. R., Guille, J. T., & Glutting, J. (2003). Treatment of the collapsed femoral head by containment in Legg-Calve-Perthes disease. *Journal of Pediatric Orthopaedics 23*, 15–19.

Gutierrez, K. (2005). Bone and joint infections in children. *Pediatric Clinics of North America, 52*, 779–794.

Harper, R. S. (2002, December). Back in the game: Preventing and treating athletic injuries in adolescents. *Advance for Nurse Practitioners*, 55–66.

Hart, E. S., Grottkau, B. E., Rebello, G. N., & Albright, M. B. (2005). The newborn foot: Diagnosis and management of common conditions. *Orthopedic Nursing, 24*, 313–321.

Heer, M., Mika, C., Grzella, I., Heussen, N., & Herpetz-Dahlmann, B. (2004). Bone turnover during inpatient nutritional therapy and outpatient follow-up in patients with anorexia nervosa compared with that in healthy control subjects. *American Journal of Clinical Nutrition, 80*, 774–781.

Herring, J. A., Kim, H. T., & Browne, R. (2005). Legg-Calve-Perthes disease. *Journal of Bone and Joint Surgery, 86-A*, 2121–2134.

Jingushi, S., & Suenaga, E. (2004). Slipped capital femoral epiphysis: Etiology and treatment. *Journal of Orthopedic Science, 9*, 214–219.

Kamegaya, M., Saisu, T., Ochiai, N., Hisamitsu, J., & Moriay, H. (2004). A paired study of Perthes' disease comparing conservative and surgical treatment. *Journal of Bone and Joint Surgery, 86*, 1176–1181.

Kaplan, S. L. (2005). Osteomyelitis in children. *Infectious Disease Clinics of North America, 19*, 787–797.

Kee, J. L. (2005). *Handbook of laboratory & diagnostic tests with nursing implications* (5th ed.). Upper Saddle River, NJ: Prentice Hall Health.

Kocher, M. S., Lee, B., Dolan, M., Weinberg, J., & Shulman, S. T. (2006). Pediatric orthopedic infections: Early detection and treatment. *Pediatric Annals, 35*, 112–122.

Lee, E. H., & Hui, J. H. (2006). The potential of stem cells in orthopaedic surgery. *Journal of Bone and Joint Surgery, 88*, 841–851.

Lincoln, T. L., & Suen, P. W. (2003). Common rotational variations in children. *Journal of American Academy of Orthopedic Surgery, 11*, 312–320.

Litmanovitz, I., Dolfin, T., Friedland, O., Arnon, S., Regev, R., Shainkin-Kestenbaum, R., Lis, M., & Eliakim, A. (2003). Early physical activity intervention prevents decrease of bone strength in very low birth weight infants. *Pediatrics, 112*, 15–19.

Lonstein, J. E. (2006). Scoliosis: Surgical versus nonsurgical treatment. *Clinical Orthopaedics and Related Research, 443*, 248–259.

Ma, D. & Jones, G. (2004). Soft drink and milk consumption, physical activity, bone loss, and upper limb fractures in children: A population-based case-control study. *Calcified Tissue International, 75*, 286–291.

Madenci, E., Yilmaz, K., Yilmaz, M., & Coskun, Y. (2006). Aldendronate treatment in osteogenesis imperfecta. *Journal of Clinical Rheumatology, 12*, 53–56.

Manias, K. McCabe, D. & Bishop, N. (2006). Fractures and recurrent fractures in children: varying effects of environment factors as well as bone size and mass. *Bone, 39*, 652–657

Manoff, E. M., Banffy, M. B., & Winell, J. J. (2005). Relationship between body mass index and slipped capital femoral epiphysis. *Journal of Pediatric Orthopedics, 25*, 744–746.

March of Dimes. (2004). Achondroplasia. Retrieved June 1, 2004, from http://www.marchofdimes.com/professionals/681_1204.asp. 3

Mooney, J. F., & Podeszwa, D. A. (2004). The management of slipped capital femoral epiphysis. *Journal of Bone and Joint Surgery, 87*, 1024–1025.

Morcuende, J. A. (2006). Congenital idiopathic clubfoot: Prevention of late deformity and disability by conservative treatment with the Ponseti technique. *Pediatric Annals, 35*, 128–136,

Morcuende, J. A., Dolan, L. A., Dietz, F. R., & Ponseti, I.V. (2004). Radical reduction in the rate of extensive corrective surgery for clubfoot using the Ponseti method. *Pediatrics, 113*, 376–380.

Nereo, N. E., Fee, R. J., & Hinton, V. J. (2003). Parental stress in mothers of boys with Duchenne muscular dystrophy. *Journal of Pediatric Psychology, 28*, 473–484.

Parsons, E. P., Clarke, A. J., Hood, K., Lycett, E., & Bradley, D. M. (2002). Newborn screening for Duchenne muscular dystrophy: A psychosocial study. *Archives of Disease in Childhood, 86*, F91–F95.

Rateau, M. R. (2004). Use of backpacks in children and adolescents. *Orthopaedic Nursing, 23*, 101–105.

Rauch, R., & Glorieux, F. H. (2005). Osteogenesis imperfecta, current and future medical treatment. *American Journal of Genetics, 139*, 31–37.

Sapountzi-Krepia, D., Psychogiou, M., Peterson, D., Zafari, B., Iordanopoulou, E., Michailidou, F., & Christodoulou, A. (2006). The experience of brace treatment in children/adolescents with scoliosis. *Scoliosis, 22*, 8.

Sapountzi-Krepia, D. S., Valavanis, J., Panteleakis, G. P., Zangana, D. T., Vlachojiannis, P. C., & Sapkas, G. S. (2001). Perceptions of body image, happiness and satisfaction in adolescents wearing a Boston brace for scoliosis treatment. *Issues and Innovations in Nursing Practice, 35*, 683–690.

Sheir-Neiss, G. I., Kruse, R. W., Rahman, T., Jacobsen, L. P., & Pelli, J. A. (2003). Association of backpack use and back pain in adolescents. *Spine, 28*, 922–930.

Shipman, S., Helfand, M., Nygren, P., & Bougatsos, C. (2006). Screening for developmental dysplasia of the hip. Evidence synthesis 42. *Agency for Healthcare Research and Quality*, 1–98.

Shipman, S. A., Helfand, M., Moyer, V. A., & Yawn, B. P. (2006). Screening for developmental dysplasia of the hip: A systematic literature review for the U.S. Preventive Services Task Force. *Pediatrics, 117*, e557–e576.

Simon, T. D., Bublitz, C., & Hambidge, S. J. (2006). Emergency department visits among pediatric patients for sports-related injury: Basic epidemiology and impact of race-ethnicity and insurance status. *Pediatric Emergency Care, 22*, 309–315.

Thompson, G. H. (2004a). The spine. In R. E. Behrman, R. M. Kliegman, & H. B. Jenson, *Nelson textbook of pediatrics* (17th ed.). Saunders: Philadelphia.

Thompson, G. H. (2004b). Torsional and angular deformities. In R. E. Behrman, R. M. Kliegman, & H. B. Jenson, *Nelson textbook of pediatrics* (17th ed.). Saunders: Philadelphia. 1161–1169.

Unal, E., Abaci, A., Bober, E., & Buyukgebiz, A. (2006). Efficacy and safety of oral alendronate treatment in children and adolescents with osteoporosis. *Journal of Pediatric Endocrinology and Metabolism, 19*, 523–528.

University of Maryland Medical Center. (2004). Muscular dystrophy. Retreived April 5, 2006, from http://www.umm.edu/altmed/ConsConditions/MuscularDystrophycc.html

U.S. Preventive Services Task Force. (2006). Screening for developmental dyslpasia of the hip: Recommendation statement. *American Family Physician, 73*, 1192–1198.

Van Gent, C., Dols, J. J., de Rover, C. J., Hira Sing, R. A, & de Vet, H. C. (2003). The weight of schoolbags and the occurrence of neck, shoulder, and back pain in young adolescents. *Spine, 28*, 916–921.

Weidner, N. J. (2005). Developing an interdisciplinary palliative care plan for the patient with muscular dystrophy. *Pediatric Annals, 34*, 547–552.

Wilkins, K. L., McGrath, P. J., Finley, G. A., & Katz, J. (2004). Prospective diary study of nonpainful and painful phantom sensations in a preselected sample of child and adolescent amputees reporting phantom limbs. *Clinical Journal of Pain, 20*, 293–301.

Witt, C. (2003). Detecting developmental dysplasia of the hip. *Advances in Neonatal Care, 3*, 65–75.

Yetman, A. T., Huang, P., Bornemeier, R. A., & McCrindle, B. W. (2003). Comparison of outcome of the Marfan syndrome in patients diagnosed at age ≤ 6 years versus those diagnosed at >6 years of age. *American Journal of Cardiology, 91*, 102–103.

Zeitlin, L., Fassier, F., & Glorieux, F. H. (2003). Modern approach to children with osteogenesis imperfecta. *Journal of Pediatric Orthopedics, 12*, 77–87.

ALTERATIONS IN ENDOCRINE AND METABOLIC FUNCTION

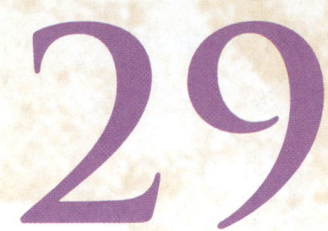

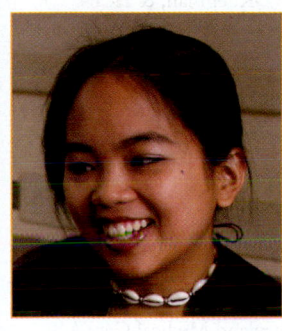

GINA, 16 years old, was diagnosed with type 1 diabetes at the age of 12 years. She has learned about her disease and, with her mother's support, self-manages her condition. She uses frequent blood glucose monitoring and insulin injections to keep her blood sugar within targeted ranges; her control has been confirmed by her HbA1$_c$ blood level. She has also learned to balance her physical activity and food intake by counting carbohydrates so that her insulin requirements do not vary too much each day. In the last few months, she has even been able to work part time in a hair salon while attending high school.

Gina was recently discharged from the hospital for treatment of diabetic ketoacidosis following an episode of influenza with diarrhea and vomiting. She has learned some strategies to manage her diabetes when she is sick. As a result, she has successfully managed minor illnesses and avoided missing too many days of school. However, this last illness was beyond her ability to handle. Gina is anxious to learn if there are ways to avoid future hospitalizations and has recently heard that using an insulin pump might allow her to do a better job managing illnesses. She wants to know the benefits and disadvantages of using an insulin pump compared to her current treatment plan. Would she need to check her blood glucose level as often? What would be the best choice for her after she graduates from high school and begins working full time in a hair salon?

KEY TERMS

acanthosis nigricans **1241**
adrenarche **1202**
bone age **1206**
constitutional growth delay **1205**
dysmenorrhea **1244**
euthyroid **1212**
glucagon **1240**
glycosuria **1225**
goiter **1212**
hormones **1200**
hyperinsulinemia **1240**
inborn errors of metabolism **1205**

insulin deficiency **1225**
insulin resistance **1225**
karyotype **1220**
menarche **1203**
polydipsia **1208**
polyphagia **1225**
polyuria **1208**
pseudohermaphroditism **1219**
puberty **1201**
thelarche **1211**
thyrotoxicosis **1215**
virilization **1219**
water intoxication **1210**

MediaLink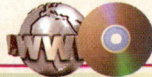

http://www.prenhall.com/ball

See the Prentice Hall Nursing MediaLink DVD-ROM and Companion Website for chapter-specific resources.

LEARNING OUTCOMES

After reading this chapter, you will be able to do the following:

1. Identify the function of important hormones of the endocrine system.
2. Identify signs and symptoms that may indicate a disorder of the endocrine system.
3. Describe differences in pathophysiology between central and nephrogenic diabetes insipidus.
4. Identify three conditions for which short stature is a sign.
5. Develop a nursing care plan for each type of acquired metabolic disorder.
6. Develop a family education plan for the child that needs lifelong cortisol replacement.
7. Distinguish between the nursing care of the child with type 1 and type 2 diabetes.
8. Develop a nursing care plan for the child with an inherited metabolic disorder.

FOCUS ON
The Endocrine System

ANATOMY AND PHYSIOLOGY

The endocrine system controls the cellular activity that regulates growth and body metabolism through the release of hormones. **Hormones** are chemical messengers secreted by various glands that exert controlling effects on the cells of the body. Overlapping with all body systems, the general functions of the endocrine system include the following:

- Differentiation of the reproductive and central nervous systems in the fetus
- Regulation of the pace of growth and development in concert with the central nervous system throughout childhood and adolescence
- Coordination of the male and female reproductive systems, enabling sexual reproduction
- Maintenance of an optimal level of hormones for body functioning
- Maintenance of homeostasis, a healthy internal environment, in the presence of a constantly changing external environment

The endocrine and nervous systems interact to regulate responses within the body and with the external environment.

The hypothalamic-pituitary axis (or system) produces a number of releasing and inhibiting hormones that regulate the function of many endocrine glands, including the thyroid, adrenal, and male and female reproductive glands. The hypothalamus synthesizes many hormones and the pituitary gland works by stimulating or inhibiting the release of these hormones. The pituitary gland also secretes certain hormones. Hormones originating from this axis regulate growth. Other endocrine glands include the parathyroid glands and the islets of Langerhans in the pancreas (Figure 29–1➤). All of these glands secrete hormones into the bloodstream, which carries them to target organs or tissues. Most hormones exert their influence through interaction with receptors in the target cells of specific tissues (Table 29–1).

Hormone secretion regulation occurs through a *negative feedback* mechanism that maintains an optimal internal body environment (Figure 29–2➤). Negative feedback occurs when an endocrine gland or secretory tissue receives a message that the target cells have received an adequate amount of hormone. In response, further secretion is inhibited. Secretion is resumed only when the secretory tissue receives another message indicating that levels of the hormone are low.

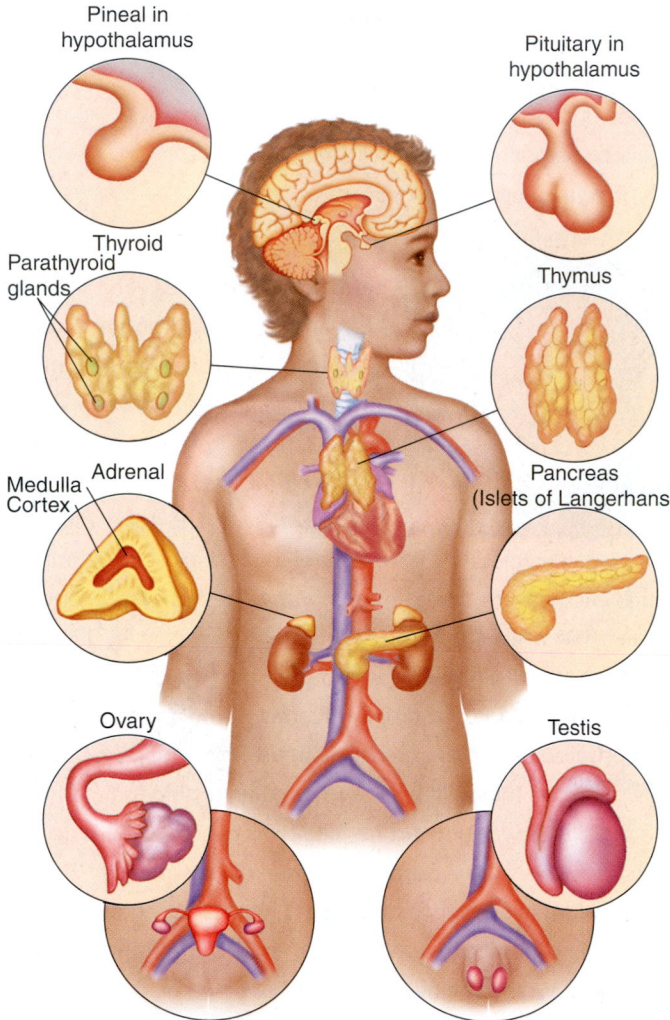

Figure 29–1 ➤ Major organs and glands of the endocrine system.

PEDIATRIC DIFFERENCES

The endocrine system is responsible for sexual differentiation during fetal development. As the embryo develops, the initial reproductive structures are the same (a pair of gonads, two pairs of ducts, and the genital tubercle). Beginning at 7 to 8 weeks of gestation, the male embryo begins secreting testosterone, which causes the gonads to differentiate into testes. The pairs of ducts develop into the vas deferens. The female embryo begins secreting estrogen, causing the gonads to differentiate into ovaries, while the ducts develop into the uterus and the fallopian tubes. The genital tubercle also differentiates and develops the male and female external genitalia.

| Table 29–1 | ENDOCRINE GLANDS AND THEIR FUNCTIONS |

Gland/Hormone	Function
Anterior Pituitary	
Growth hormone (somatotropin)	Regulates metabolic process related to growth
Thyroid-stimulating hormone (TSH)	Stimulates thyroid hormone secretion
Adrenocorticotropic hormone (ACTH) (corticotrophin)	Stimulates secretion of glucocorticoids and androgens
Follicle-stimulating hormone (FSH) (a gonadotropin)	Stimulates secretion of estrogen; stimulates follicle maturation in ovaries. Also critical for sperm production in males.
Luteinizing hormone (LH) and interstitial cell-stimulating hormone (ICSH) (male analogue) (a gonadotropin)	Stimulates secretion of androgens in males and progesterone in females
Prolactin-releasing hormone	Stimulates secretion of prolactin that stimulates the secretion of milk during lactation
Melanocyte-stimulating hormone (MSH)	Stimulates skin pigmentation
Posterior Pituitary	
Antidiuretic hormone (ADH) (vasopressin)	Promotes water reabsorption back into the blood, decreasing urine output
Oxytocin	Stimulates uterine contractions and breast milk letdown reflex
Beta endorphins	May regulate body temperature, food and water intake
Thyroid	
Thyroxine (T_4) and triiodothyronine (T_3)	Regulates metabolic rate of all cells, body heat production; protein, fat, and carbohydrate catabolism in all cells
Thyrocalcitonin	Stimulates bone ossification and development
Parathyroid	
Parathyroid hormone	Regulates serum calcium levels and excretion of phosphorus
Adrenal	
Aldosterone	Increases sodium ion reabsorption, and increases potassium and hydrogen ion excretion in the kidneys
Androgens	Stimulates bone development and secondary sexual characteristics
Cortisol	Stimulates anti-inflammatory reactions, protects from stress
Epinephrine	Activates sympathetic nervous system; stimulates increase in blood pressure and blood glucose levels
Pancreas (Islets of Langerhans)	
Insulin	Facilitates cellular glucose utilization
Glucagon	Increases blood glucose when low by stimulating glycogenolysis
Somatostatin	Inhibits insulin and glucagon secretion; may prevent excess insulin secretion
Ovaries	
Estrogen	Stimulates development of breasts and ova
Progesterone	Stimulates breast glandular development; acts to maintain pregnancy
Testes	
Testosterone	Stimulates production of sperm, development of secondary sexual characteristics, and closure of epiphysis

The endocrine system is also responsible for stimulating growth and development during childhood and adolescence. Growth hormone, produced by the anterior pituitary gland, is secreted in pulses when the child is in stage 4 sleep, stimulates the growth of muscles, and improves bone mineralization (Grimberg & De León, 2005). Multiple hormones in the endocrine system, including the growth hormone, thyroid hormone, adrenal and gonadal androgens, and estrogen, are responsible for skeletal growth and maturation, including the appearance of secondary ossification centers in the bones (Carroll, 2006). Estrogen secretion associated with puberty is a dominant stimulator of increased skeletal maturity that can be detected by examining the child's bone age (Figure 29–3▶) (Lee & Kulin, 2005).

During childhood, the production of sex hormones (estrogen, progesterone, and testosterone) is low. **Puberty** (sexual maturation, lasting an average of 4.5 years) occurs when the gonads begin to secrete increased amounts of the

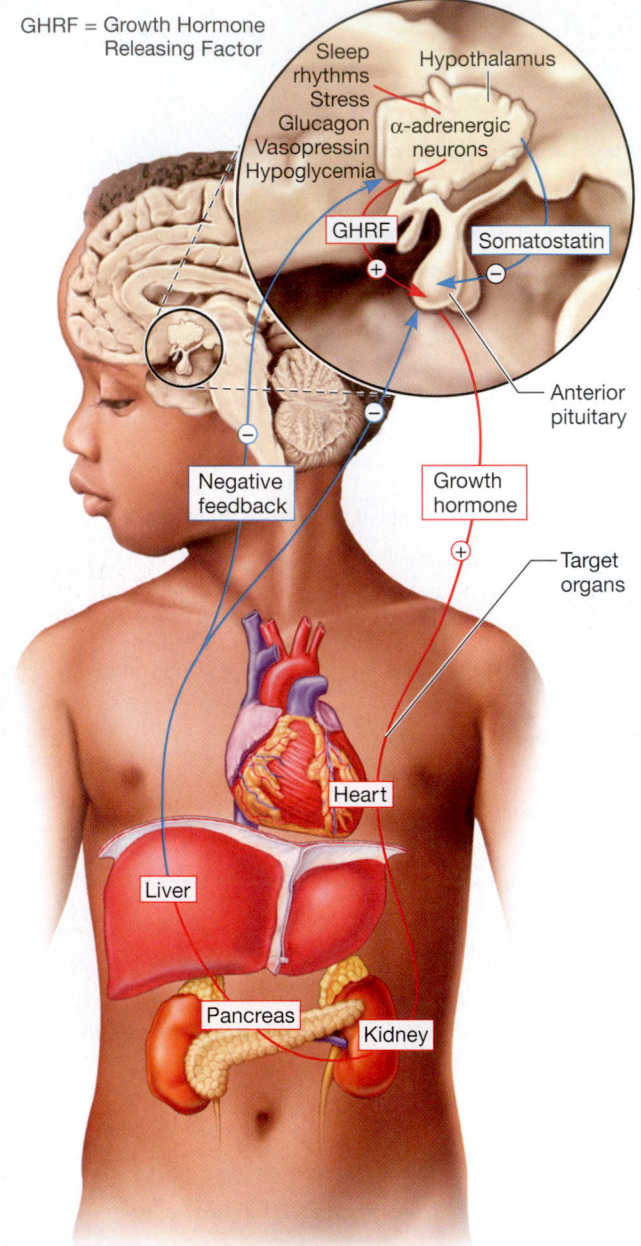

GHRF = Growth Hormone
Releasing Factor

Sleep rhythms
Stress
Glucagon
Vasopressin
Hypoglycemia

Hypothalamus

α-adrenergic neurons

GHRF

Somatostatin

Anterior pituitary

Negative feedback

Growth hormone

Target organs

Heart

Liver

Pancreas

Kidney

Figure 29–2 ➤ Feedback mechanism in hormonal stimulation of the gonads during puberty.

AS CHILDREN GROW

Bone Age

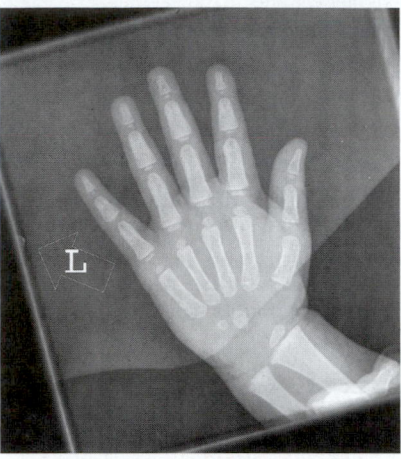

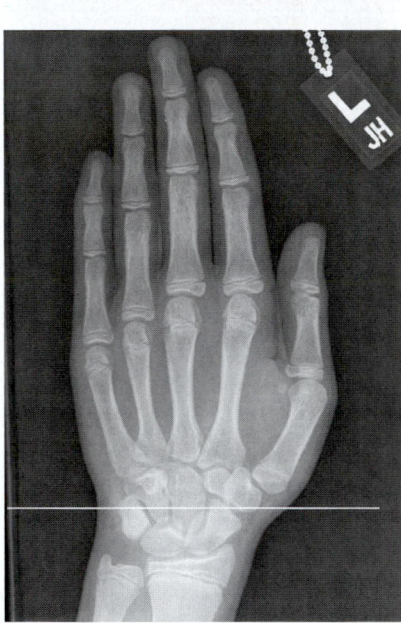

Figure 29–3 ➤ The radiographs of the hand and wrist of a 3-year-old and 13-year-old girl reveal significant differences in skeletal maturation that are closely tied to physiologic maturation. The 3-year-old has many bones in the hand and wrist that have not fully developed. The secretion of estrogen during puberty has resulted in the development and calcification of secondary ossification centers of most of the bones in the hand and wrist of the 13-year-old.
Courtesy, Dorothy Bulas, M.D., Children's National Medical Center.

sex hormones estrogen and androgens. At the average age of 9 years in girls and 11 years in boys, the hypothalamus produces increased amounts of gonadotropin-releasing hormone (GnRH). This hormone stimulates the anterior pituitary gland to secrete luteinizing hormone (LH) and follicle-stimulating hormone (FSH). In boys, LH stimulates testosterone production and FSH stimulates sperm production. In girls, LH and FSH stimulate development and maturation of the ova and ovulation. These hormones in turn stimulate the gonads to secrete more sex hormones, resulting in the development of primary and secondary sex characteristics. They also stimulate the genitalia to grow to adult proportions. At about 6 years of age, the adrenal

glands may begin an increased secretion of adrenal hormones (**adrenarche**) (Lee, 2005). These adrenal hormones lead to the development of increased testicular size, axillary hair and pubic hair, early changes in body growth, and adult body odor. Pubertal development usually follows a specific sequence (accelerated growth, breast development, adrenarche, and menarche) (Pinyerd & Zipf, 2005). See

GROWTH & DEVELOPMENT

Puberty and Weight

Puberty often begins at an earlier age in children of both sexes who have higher weights than average. Delayed puberty is more likely to occur in children who exercise excessively or who have a low body mass index, such as with anorexia nervosa (Pinyerd & Zipf, 2005).

Figures 5–40 , 5–41 , and 5–42 ∞ for the development of secondary sexual characteristics in males and females.

Menarche, the onset of menstruation, occurs in most girls between 11 and 13 years of age, and is a significant sign of sexual maturity. Menstruation is controlled by several hormones (FSH, LH, estrogen, and progesterone), and for 1 to 2 years cycles are anovulatory of variable duration. In contrast, males begin producing sperm once testicular and penile growth has occurred, around 13.5 to 14 years (Pinyerd & Zipf, 2005).

Examples of diagnostic and laboratory tests used to evaluate endocrine conditions are provided in the accompanying table. Use the guidelines on page 1205 to perform a nursing assessment of the endocrine system.

DIAGNOSTIC PROCEDURES AND LABORATORY TESTS USED TO EVALUATE ENDOCRINE SYSTEM FUNCTION

Diagnostic Procedure	Purpose	Nursing Implications
Bone age	Radiographic flat film image of the left hand and wrist is used to assess bone ossification or stage of skeletal maturation.	• Note that no special preparation is needed.
Computed tomography	A narrow beam of radiation examines body sections from different angles, producing a two-dimensional cross-section of a body structure. A contrast media (or dye) can be used to enhance visualization. Used for evaluating the skull and adrenal glands to assess for tumors.	• Assess for any allergy to iodine or seafood, prior allergic reaction to contrast dye. • Tell the child of the need to stay still for the procedure. A small child may need to be sedated. • If dye is used, encourage fluids after the test.
Magnetic resonance imaging (MRI)	A large magnet and radiowaves delivered to the body part to be imaged produce an energy field that is transferred as a visual image to the computer. The brain and abdomen can be imaged for the presence of tumors.	• Tell children about the need to remain still. The small child may need sedation. • Assess the child for iodine or contrast media allergy. • Remove all metal from the body.
Thyroid radioactive iodine uptake (RAI) scan	The radiographic imaging is performed 2 hours, 6 hours, and 24 hours after the child has been given oral or IV radioactive iodine. The scan helps detect hyperthyroidism and hypothyroidism by amount of iodine taken up in the thyroid.	• All sources of iodine in food (enriched breakfast cereal) and medications (vitamins, cough syrup) are avoided for several weeks prior to the test. • Do not allow food or drink for several hours before the initial scan. • Note that allergic problems do not occur, as a very small amount of iodine is used (Corbett, 2004).
Thyroid scan	Radioactive iodine is given by mouth or IV and the scan is performed 30 minutes and 24 hours later. Nodules and tumors may be detected.	• Note that no special preparation is needed. • Do not allow food or drink for several hours before the initial scan.
Laboratory Tests	Purpose	Nursing Implications
ACTH stimulation test	Cortrosyn is given. A series of blood samples are collected to measure the level of ACTH. The test is used to detect adrenal gland reserve and pituitary insufficiency.	• Note that phenytoin and estrogen interfere with the test results. • Check with the laboratory to determine specific blood collection times.
Adrenal (ACTH) suppression test	Dexamethasone is given orally at 11 p.m. to suppress the formation of ACTH. The plasma cortisol level is collected at 8 a.m. the next morning. This test detects a hyperactive adrenal cortex and Cushing's syndrome.	• Have the child fast overnight except for water. • Keep the child at rest in bed when blood is collected. • Do not use a glass collection tube. Place specimen on ice and deliver to the laboratory immediately.

(continued)

DIAGNOSTIC PROCEDURES AND LABORATORY TESTS USED TO EVALUATE ENDOCRINE SYSTEM FUNCTION

Laboratory Test	Purpose	Nursing Implications
Fasting plasma glucose	Measurement of plasma glucose level after fasting for diagnosis of diabetes mellitus.	• Do not allow caloric intake for at least 8 hours, although water is permitted.
Fluid deprivation test	The plasma arginine vasopressin level is tested before and after a 7- to 8-hour period when fluid is prohibited. After completion of the fluid deprivation test, a dose of aqueous vasopressin is administered. The child is given free access to fluids. Differences in urine concentration are evaluated. This test is used to diagnose diabetes insipidus.	• Monitor the child and family closely for any disallowed fluid intake. • Weigh the child, and monitor urine output, specific gravity, osmolality, and serum osmolality every 2 hours or by protocol as the child will become dehydrated. • Notify the physician immediately if 5% weight loss or signs of hypovolemic shock occur.
Hemoglobin A1$_c$	Measurement of glycohemoglobin (red blood cells saturated with glucose) in cases of prolonged hyperglycemia. Helpful in determining control of diabetes.	• No special preparation for the fingerstick sample is needed. • Fasting is not necessary.
Hormone levels	Blood is collected to measure the concentration of a specific hormone (e.g., thyroxine, triiodothyronine, thyroid-stimulating hormone, growth hormone, cortisol, adrenocorticotropin, aldosterone, and parathyroid) in serum or plasma.	• Note that no special preparation is needed. • For a plasma cortisol or serum growth hormone test, take an early morning blood collection when the child is at rest. Have the child fast except for water.
Human chorionic gonadotropin (HCG)	Collection of blood to measure the level of HCG in the serum to detect pregnancy within 1 week of conception.	• Note that no special preparation is needed.
Insulin-like growth factor (IGF-1) and IGFBP-3	Blood is collected to measure the level of these factors. Growth hormone deficiency is excluded if normal.	• Note that no special preparation is needed.
Karyotype	Swab of the buccal mucosa or a blood sample is used to perform a chromosome study to detect errors in chromosome number, shape, and size; provides gender of infant.	• Note that no special preparation is needed.
Newborn metabolic screening	A heelstick is performed on a newborn prior to nursery discharge to collect drops of blood onto a collection card. Screening for up to 29 metabolic conditions is performed.	• Completely fill the circles on the card with blood. • Repeat the screening test at 1 week of age, if desired.
Provocative growth hormone testing	Various medications (e.g., glucagon, artinine, clonidine) are administered. Serial blood samples are collected to see how much the growth hormone level increases. Used to test for growth hormone deficiency.	• Have the child fast overnight, although water is permitted. • Contact the laboratory to identify the timing for collection of blood samples.
Provocative gonadotropin-releasing hormone (GnRH) stimulation	Intravenous or subcutaneous administration of GnRH or its analogue is followed by a series of blood samples to measure the gonadotropins (luteinizing hormone, follicle-stimulating hormone). The test is used to diagnose precocious puberty.	• Check with the laboratory for timing of blood collection.
Thyroid antibodies TPO—thyroid peroxidase TG—thyroglobulin	Collection of a blood specimen to detect the presence of anti-thyroid antibodies. Their presence indicates an autoimmune process.	• Note that no special preparation is needed. • Note if an adolescent is taking oral contraceptives as titer levels may be affected.
24-hour urine	Collection of urine for an entire 24 hours to test the levels of different substances (e. g., cortisol, aldosterone, 17-hydroxycorticosteroid, and catecholamines).	• Have the child void and note the time. Discard this specimen. Have the child collect all urine and place it in the container. Have the child void as close to 24 hours later as possible to obtain the final urine for the specimen. • Refrigerate the specimen or put it on ice. • Check with the laboratory for any needed preservative.

Data from: Corbett, J. V. (2004). *Laboratory tests and diagnostic procedures* (6th ed.). Upper Saddle River, NJ: Prentice Hall; Moshang, T. (2005). *Pediatric endocrinology: The requisites in pediatrics.* St. Louis: Elsevier Mosby.

ASSESSMENT GUIDELINES FOR THE CHILD WITH AN ENDOCRINE CONDITION

Assessment Focus	Assessment Guideline
Growth	• Carefully measure weight, length, or height and plot on a growth curve. • Compare measurements at different ages to assess the growth pattern over time and to assess the growth velocity.
Blood pressure	• Assess blood pressure and compare to expected norms for age. See Table 5–14.
Facial characteristics	• Inspect the face for unusual features such as a protuberant tongue, protuberant eyes, or moon face.
Neck	• Palpate the neck for an enlarged thyroid or goiter.
Muscles	• Assess strength and muscle tone.
Genitalia and secondary sexual characteristics	• Assess external genitalia for signs of ambiguous genitalia, inappropriate size for age. • Determine the child's stage of development for each characteristic (breast and pubic hair for girls, genital and pubic hair for boys) by comparing to the images in Figures 5–40 , 5–41 , and 5–42. • Assess the sexual maturity rating with information in Figure 5–42. Compare the stage of development to the age of the boy or girl to determine early or delayed onset of puberty.
Body odor	• Assess body odor for unusual smell (e.g., sweet, musty, cheesy, sweaty feet).
Skin	• Assess skin color, noting areas of unusual pigmentation.

Endocrine disturbances result in alterations in metabolism, growth and development, and behavior that may have significant implications for children. If not diagnosed and treated early, these conditions can result in delays in growth and development, mental retardation, and, occasionally, death. However, treatment, which usually consists of supplementation of missing hormones, adjustment of hormone levels, or dietary measures, allows most children to live a normal life.

Inborn errors of metabolism—inherited biochemical abnormalities of the urea cycle and amino acid and organic acid metabolism—often have a significant impact on the endocrine system's ability to support growth and development. Some chromosomal abnormalities also result in disturbances in growth and sexual development.

DISORDERS OF PITUITARY FUNCTION

Growth Hormone Deficiency (Hypopituitarism)

Growth hormone deficiency is a disorder caused by decreased activity of the pituitary gland. Because most children with this disorder secrete inadequate amounts of growth hormone, the term *growth hormone deficiency* is often preferred to *hypopituitarism*. The disorder is diagnosed earlier in males than females since males are referred sooner for evaluation of short stature (Grimberg, Kutikov, & Cucchiara, 2005).

The release of growth hormone from the anterior pituitary gland is controlled by the hypothalamus, which secretes releasing and inhibitory factors. Growth hormone stimulates linear growth and bone mineral density, as well as the growth of all body tissues. It also stimulates the synthesis of proteins in the liver, among them the somatomedins or insulin-like growth factors (IGFs), which promote glucose use by the cells and cell proliferation.

Infarction of the pituitary gland (such as that related to sickle cell disease), central nervous system infection, disease, tumors of the pituitary gland or hypothalamus (primarily craniopharyngiomas and gliomas), other brain tumors, cranial irradiation, brain trauma, chemotherapy, and psychosocial deprivation may cause growth hormone deficiency by interfering with the production or release of growth hormone. Dominant or recessive inheritance or a genetic mutation may cause deficiency of growth hormone or abnormalities of hormone receptors (Witchel & Finegold, 2002). Other major causes of short stature include familial short stature, hypothyroidism, Turner's syndrome, **constitutional growth delay** (a late pubertal growth spurt caused by delayed pubertal hormone secretion), chronic renal failure, Cushing's syndrome, inborn error of metabolism, and severe cardiac, pulmonary, or gastrointestinal disease. Psychosocial dwarfism is a syndrome of emotional deprivation that causes suppression of pituitary hormone production, resulting in a transient growth hormone deficiency that is reversed by placing the child in a nurturing environment.

Children with growth hormone deficiency have normal birth weights and lengths. By the age of 1 year, however, they are below the third percentile on the growth chart. They characteristically grow at a rate of less than 5 cm (2 in.) per year. Other characteristic findings in infants include hypoglycemic seizures, hyponatremia, neonatal jaundice, pale optic discs, micropenis, and undescended testicles. Children with growth hormone deficiency tend to be overweight and to have youthful facial features, higher pitched voices, delayed dentition, "ripply" abdominal fat, decreased muscle mass, delayed skeletal maturation, delayed sexual maturation, and hypoglycemia. Slipped capital femoral epiphysis has been associated with growth hormone deficiency (Halac & Zimmerman, 2004a).

Any child whose height is 2 to 3 standard deviations below the mean height for age or whose measurement is falling off the normal growth chart should be evaluated for short stature (Table 29–2). A child whose screening tests reveal low levels of IGF-1 requires further evaluation by a pediatric endocrinologist. A careful history, physical examination, assessment of pubertal development and unusual facies, and radiologic studies are necessary to identify possible causes of short stature. A radiograph of the wrist bones is used to evaluate the stage of bone ossification, and thus the child's **bone age**. Using standardized norms for bone ossification, it can be determined if the child's chronologic age and bone age match. A significantly delayed (less than the child's age) or advanced (greater than the child's age) bone age indicates the possibility of a systemic chronic disease or hormone abnormality. Provocative growth hormone testing, in which various medications (arginine, clonidine, glucagon, insulin, L-dopa) are administered to stimulate release of growth hormone, may be used to confirm growth hormone deficiency.

Treatment depends on the cause of the deficiency. Brain tumors must be treated effectively before growth hormone therapy can be considered. See Chapter 23 ∞. Food and Drug Administration approved uses for growth hormone therapy include growth hormone deficiency, chronic renal insufficiency and pretransplantation, Turner's syndrome, small for gestational age child who has not achieved normal height by age 2 to 3 years, Prader-Willi syndrome, idiopathic short stature unlikely to catch up in height, adults with growth hormone deficiency, and adults with wasting from

Table 29–2	DIAGNOSTIC TESTS FOR SHORT STATURE
Test	**Purpose Related to Short Stature**
IGF-1 and IGFBP-3	Screening test for growth hormone deficiency
MRI of the pituitary gland	To detect pituitary malformation or tumor
Provocative growth hormone testing	Used to test for growth hormone deficiency
Bone age	Identifies potential for additional growth and other possible causes of delayed growth
Karyotype (girls)	Detects Turner's syndrome (see page 1244)
Thyroid function studies	Detects hypothyroidism (see page 1211)
ACTH and cortisol levels	Detects other pituitary hormonal deficiencies
Urine creatinine, pH, specific gravity, urea nitrogen, electrolytes	Detects chronic renal failure (see Chapter 25 ∞)
Complete blood count and erythrocyte sedimentation rate	Screens for inflammatory bowel disease with anemia
Antigliadin antibodies	Screens for celiac disease

Data from: Parks, J. S. (2004). Disorders of the hypothalamus and pituitary gland. In R. E. Behrman, R. M. Kliegman, & H. B. Jenson (Eds.), *Nelson textbook of pediatrics* (17th ed., pp. 1845–1853). Philadelphia, PA: Saunders; Grimberg, A., & DeLéon, D. D. (2005). Disorders in growth. In T. M. Moshang *Pediatric endocrinology: The requisites in pediatrics* (pp. 127–167). St. Louis: Elsevier Mosby.

HIV infection (Lee & Menon, 2005; Wilson, Rose, Cohen et al., 2003). A new drug, Increlex, has recently been approved by the Food and Drug Administration for treatment of children with severe primary deficiency of insulin-like growth factor 1 and who are growth hormone resistant (Food and Drug Administration, 2006).

Most indications for growth hormone replacement require daily or alternate day subcutaneous injections; however, outcomes are improved with more frequent dosing (Lee & Menon, 2005). The child usually experiences increased growth velocity for the first year of treatment, followed by a gradual decrease in growth for subsequent months or years. Growth should progress at least at the normal growth rate for age while maintained on growth hormone treatment. Replacement therapy is continued until either the child achieves an acceptable height or growth velocity drops to less than 2 cm (1 in.) per year. Close monitoring of growth and endocrinology visits every 3 to 4 months are needed. If growth is slower than anticipated, improper preparation and administration of growth hormone and adherence to therapy must be considered (Halac & Zimmerman, 2004a). In some cases, the onset of puberty is delayed with gonadotropin-releasing hormone analogues to provide more time for growth hormone therapy to stimulate growth.

Nursing Management

Nursing care consists of monitoring growth, teaching the child and family about the disorder and its treatment, and providing emotional support. Carefully measure the child's height and weight and plot them on a growth chart.

Teach the parents and child about growth hormone replacement therapy, preparation and administration of subcutaneous injections, rotating injection sites, potential side effects, and actions to take if noticed. Provide the parents with ideas about how to minimize the child's stress associated with daily injections. Give parents educational resources, such as information from the MAGIC Foundation, Human Growth Foundation, and the Short Stature Foundation. Since replacement therapy is expensive (approximately $35,000 per year) and may not be covered by insurance, parents may need financial assistance that is sometimes available from the growth hormone manufacturers.

Children with growth hormone deficiency, especially those due to tumors and trauma from radiation or surgery, may have academic problems because of acquired learning disabilities. Before the child enters school, or returns to school after treatment for a tumor, a comprehensive evaluation should be performed to identify potential problems.

The best results occur when treatment is begun at an early age, before the psychologic effects of short stature become apparent and when attainment of near normal height can be reached. People often treat short children on the basis of their size rather than their age, and such children experience social prejudice about height. Teasing is a common problem. The teenage years may be particularly stressful because of adolescents' characteristic preoccupation with body image.

Encourage parents and teachers to treat the child in an age-appropriate manner. The child should dress in clothing that reflects chronologic age. Emphasize the child's strengths, support independence, and encourage participation in age-appropriate activities to aid in the development of a positive self-image. Suggest that the child take part in sports in which ability does not depend on size (e.g., swimming, gymnastics, wrestling, ice skating, and martial arts). Identifying positive role models, short people who accomplish their goals, also promotes a positive image. Refer the child for counseling, if appropriate.

Growth Hormone Excess (Hyperpituitarism)

Excessive secretion of growth hormone is rare in children, and it is usually caused by a pituitary adenoma. If combined with precocious puberty, a tumor of the hypothalamus may be present. Affected children can grow to 7 or 8 feet in height when oversecretion occurs before closure of the epiphyseal plates. If the disorder occurs after closure of the epiphyseal plates, acromegaly occurs.

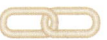

SKILLS 6-2 AND 6-3
Measuring Height and Weight

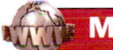

MediaLink

Short Stature Resources

CLINICAL TIP

Encourage the parents to promote optimal nutrition and adequate caloric and iron intake in the child prior to starting and during growth hormone treatment. Lack of adequate nutrition may affect the child's growth response (Zadik, Sinai, Zung et al., 2005).

Because tall stature is valued in our society, assessment of children (particularly boys) with accelerated linear growth is often delayed. Any child whose predicted height exceeds that consistent with parental height should be evaluated for possible growth problems and underlying pathologic conditions.

A complete history is obtained, and physical examination and laboratory testing are performed. Increased levels of IGF-1 establish the diagnosis of growth hormone excess. A bone age radiologic examination is performed to determine if the epiphyseal plates have begun to fuse. Radiologic studies are used to detect a tumor. Thorough evaluation is required to differentiate growth hormone excess from familial tall stature.

Treatment depends on the cause of the excessive growth and may involve surgical removal of a tumor or pituitary gland (hypophysectomy), radiation therapy, or radioactive implants. High doses of sex steroids are given to close the epiphyseal plates. The child may need lifelong pituitary hormone replacement following surgery.

Nursing Management

Tall stature, like short stature, can be stressful for children. Tall children are often treated as if they are older than their chronologic age. Tall adolescents may have problems with self-image, and girls in particular may worry about their appearance.

Nursing care focuses on teaching the parents and child about the disorder and its treatment, providing emotional support, and, if surgery is required, providing preoperative and postoperative teaching and care (see Chapter 13 ∞).

Diabetes Insipidus

Two forms of diabetes insipidus exist: central (neurogenic) antidiuretic hormone (ADH) deficiency and familial nephrogenic diabetes insipidus. Both disorders involve ADH, a hormone secreted by the posterior pituitary gland. In normal circumstances, thirst is the regulator for ADH release (Kache & Ferry, 2005). ADH facilitates concentration of the urine by stimulating reabsorption of water from the distal tubule of the kidney. When ADH is inadequate, the tubules do not resorb water, leading to **polyuria** (passage of a large volume of urine in a given period). Plasma osmolarity, or the concentration of solutes in the blood, is an important factor in ADH secretion.

Diabetes insipidus can occur at any age and results from inadequate production or secretion of ADH or arginine-vasopressin (central or neurogenic diabetes insipidus) or inability of the renal collecting tubules to respond to the ADH. Brain tumors and their treatment are the most common cause of central DI (Kache & Ferry, 2005). Other causes of central diabetes insipidus include brain trauma, central nervous system infection, and neurosurgery. Most cases of nephrogenic diabetes insipidus are genetic, either an X-linked or an autosomal recessive form. Transient nephrogenic diabetes insipidus, however, may be caused by drug toxicity or an adverse drug reaction (Parks, 2004).

Polyuria and **polydipsia** (excessive thirst) are the cardinal signs of diabetes insipidus. Enuresis is common in children. Other signs and symptoms are provided in the clinical manifestations table on the following page. In infants, symptoms may include failure to thrive, poor feeding, and irritability. Their diapers are typically saturated. Although the onset of symptoms is often sudden, the diagnosis is often delayed. Children who can quench their thirst may not complain to parents about symptoms. The child may be obese due to an excessive intake of high-caloric fluids.

In all forms of diabetes insipidus, the urine cannot be concentrated, no matter how dehydrated the child becomes. A dehydration episode usually leads to the diagnosis. The serum sodium concentration and osmolality increase rapidly to pathologic levels. Seizures may occur in response to extreme electrolyte imbalances. Often an unconscious child is admitted to the emergency department with dehydration and hypernatremia.

Initial testing involves serum electrolyte concentrations and a urinalysis including specific gravity and osmolality. Urine osmolality is decreased (less than 300 mOsm/kg), urine specific gravity is decreased (less than 1.005), serum sodium is elevated, and the urine to serum osmolality ratio is less than 1 (Kache & Ferry, 2005). An MRI may be ordered to visualize the pituitary gland to detect a tumor. Diagnosis is confirmed by measuring the plasma arginine vasopressin (AVP) level before

CLINICAL MANIFESTATIONS | DIABETES INSIPIDUS

Cause	Clinical Manifestations	Clinical Therapy
True Diabetes Insipidus ADH deficiency Familial or idiopathic	Polyuria, polydipsia Nocturia, enuresis Thirsty at night, irritable if fluids withheld Constipation, fever, dehydration	Desmopressin acetate
Nephrogenic Diabetes Insipidus Familial, decreased responsiveness of kidneys to ADH	Polyuria, polydipsia Hypernatremia in neonatal period Dehydration, fever, vomiting Mental status changes	Diuretics High fluid intake Salt and protein restricted diet

and during a fluid deprivation test, which is usually conducted in the hospital or in a carefully controlled outpatient setting for up to 8 hours. Fluid intake is prohibited during the procedure. Weight, urine output, specific gravity, and osmolality are measured every 2 hours. The specific gravity remains low (less than 1.005) even after dehydration. A dose of aqueous vasopressin is given after several hours. The response of a decreased urine output and increased urine concentration confirms the diagnosis of central diabetes insipidus. No response to vasopressin is seen in cases of nephrogenic diabetes insipidus. Many children with central diabetes insipidus have deficiencies of other anterior pituitary hormones, so testing for those deficiencies will also be conducted.

Children who can access water and who have an intact thirst mechanism can maintain serum sodium and osmolality status; however, medications decrease polyuria and polydipsia. Fluid management may be the safest and preferred treatment. Infants may be given dilute formula (1/10th strength) to provide needed calories and water (Kache & Ferry, 2005).

Central ADH deficiency is treated by subcutaneous, intranasal, or oral desmopressin acetate (DDAVP). The medication reduces urinary output, enabling the child to live a more normal life with a decrease in thirst, urinary output, and nocturia. The dose of DDAVP, having an effect lasting 8 to 12 hours, must be titered for sufficient coverage of metabolic needs while not high enough to cause water overload. Nephrogenic diabetes insipidus is treated with thiazide diuretics, which promote sodium excretion and stimulate the proximal tubule to reabsorb water. Prostaglandin inhibitors (indomethacin) may also be prescribed to have an additive effect on decreased water excretion. A high fluid intake and a low sodium diet are also ordered (Cheetham & Baylis, 2002). The child's sodium and potassium levels must be carefully monitored to prevent hypernatremia and hypokalemia (see Chapter 16 ∞).

Nursing Management

Nursing care centers on administering medications and teaching parents how to manage the condition and recognize signs of altered fluid status. Educate parents about making fluids available to the child as needed, administering DDAVP, obtaining and recording daily weights, measuring intake and output, and recognizing signs of inadequate fluid intake (see Chapter 16 ∞). The child should consume fluids equal to the amount of output (sometimes as much as 75 mL/kg) (Ferry, 2005). Parents may need to weigh diapers to monitor urine output in infants. Cold fluids are often preferred and help relieve thirst. The child's fluid intake will need to be adjusted to prevent dehydration during an illness. Children often wake to drink fluids at night, but infants will need to have fluids provided. Many infants have coexisting brain damage and need nasogastric or gastrostomy feeding to maintain adequate hydration and nutrition. However, care should be taken to avoid the intake of excessive fluid as the child will not be able to excrete the excess water load with DDAVP treatment. The use of home monitoring for serum sodium levels is being investigated (Green & Landt, 2002).

CLINICAL TIP

During the fluid deprivation test, advise parents that the child will be frustrated and irritable from thirst. No one should drink in front of the child during the testing period. Monitor the child's vital signs, intake, and output carefully. The test is stopped if the child loses 5% of body weight and develops a fever and hypotension (Kache & Ferry, 2005).

NURSING ALERT

When the child with diabetes insipidus has an acute illness, the child's physician should be notified immediately. Dehydration and hypernatremia may develop rapidly, and hypernatremia can cause mental retardation, seizures, and cerebral calcification. Intravenous fluids will be needed to prevent or treat dehydration. See Chapter 16 ∞. Serum sodium and serum osmolality must be carefully monitored.

Syndrome of Inappropriate Antidiuretic Hormone

Syndrome of inappropriate antidiuretic hormone (SIADH) results from an excessive amount of serum ADH. It is seen in children with central nervous system infections, brain tumors, and brain trauma; in children with pulmonary disorders such as pneumonia, asthma, or cystic fibrosis; and in children receiving positive pressure ventilation. Some medications including diuretics and chemotherapy have been associated with SIADH.

Failure of normal feedback mechanisms from the hypothalamus, pituitary gland, and kidney results in excessive secretion of ADH, leading to water reabsorption despite the presence of a low serum osmolality. ADH secretion causes increased permeability of the distal renal tubules and collecting ducts, resulting in water reabsorption, increased intravascular volume, and decreased urine output (Ferry, 2005). Elevated ADH also causes suppression of the renin-angiotensin mechanism and sodium excretion. The outcome is **water intoxication** (an abnormal proportion of water to sodium in the extracellular fluid), hyponatremia, and cellular edema.

Signs include elevated blood pressure, distended jugular veins, crackles in lung fields, weight gain without edema, fluid and electrolyte imbalance, and concentrated urine with decreased urine output. As serum sodium levels continue to fall, lethargy, confusion, headache, and altered level of consciousness, seizures, and coma occur due to cerebral edema.

Laboratory findings include a high urine osmolality (greater than 100 mOsm/kg), elevated specific gravity (greater than 1.025), low serum osmolality (less than 260 mOsm/kg), low serum sodium (less than 125 mM), and decreased BUN (less than 22 mg/dL) (Ferry, 2005).

Treatment includes fluid management, medications, and treatment of the underlying condition when possible. Fluids are restricted to prevent further dilution of the blood. Medications include diuretics, demeclocycline to block action of ADH at the renal collecting tubules, and hypertonic saline IV fluids. Oral urea has recently been evaluated for treatment with promising results (Huang, Feldman, Schwartz et al., 2006). After the acute phase, a daily fluid allowance is calculated to two-thirds maintenance to prevent excess water intake and potential complications such as congestive heart failure or pulmonary edema. See Chapter 16 ∞ for calculation of the maintenance fluid amount for the child.

Nursing Management

Nursing care focuses on preventing injury, monitoring fluid balance, administering medication, and managing nutritional intake. Monitor for level of consciousness, headache, and seizure activity. Implement seizure precautions. Monitor intake and output, serum sodium, urine osmolality, and specific gravity. Educate the parents about the child's fluid restrictions and the hidden sources of water and fluids in foods to help avoid excessive fluid intake. Parents need to understand the importance of weighing the child daily and reporting weight gain that could indicate fluid retention. Lifelong medication may be required depending upon the cause of the disorder. Emphasize the importance of follow-up as the medications have significant side effects (e.g., hypokalemia, renal injury, inhibition of bone growth). Medical alert identification should be worn.

Precocious Puberty

Puberty normally occurs between 8 and 13 years of age in girls and between 9 1/2 and 14 years of age in boys. Precocious puberty is defined as the appearance of any secondary sexual characteristics before 8 years of age in girls (breast development or pubic hair) and 9 years of age in boys (pubic hair) (Pinyerd & Zipf, 2005).

Earlier than expected secretion of the normal hormones responsible for pubertal changes is not usually associated with an endocrine system abnormality (an idiopathic problem). External sources of hormones such as anabolic steroids or estrogen may be identified. Central precocious puberty or true precocious puberty occurs when the hypothalamus is activated to secrete gonadotropin-releasing hormone. In males gonadotropin-dependent precocious puberty is usually the result of a central nervous

CULTURE

Onset of Puberty

Differences exist by race in the onset of puberty and secondary sexual characteristics. African American girls begin puberty between 8 and 9 years of age. Caucasian girls begin puberty by 10 years of age (Herman-Giddens, Slora, Wasserman et al, 1997; Lalwani, Reindollar, & Davis, 2003).

system (CNS) disorder such as an intracranial tumor, and in females it is usually idiopathic (Traggiai & Stanhope, 2003). Other potential causes include brain injury, congenital adrenal hyperplasia, neurofibromatosis, hydrocephalus, and tumors of the ovary, adrenal gland, or testicle.

Isolated signs of premature sexual development such as premature **thelarche** (breast development), premature menarche (vaginal bleeding without other signs of sexual development), and premature adrenarche (development of pubic and axillary sexual hair) before 8 years of age in girls and 9 years in boys often needs no treatment.

Children with central precocious puberty have an advanced bone age (premature skeletal maturation) and may appear unusually tall for their age. Their growth ceases prematurely, however, as the hormones stimulate early closure of the epiphyseal plates, resulting in short stature. Behavior changes may include mood swings and emotional lability.

Serum diagnostic studies include luteinizing hormone (LH), follicle-stimulating hormone (FSH), testosterone, or estradiol. Provocative testing includes gonadotropin-releasing hormone (GnRH) stimulation to confirm the diagnosis. Radiologic imaging of the brain, as well as a bone age, may be performed.

CNS tumors require surgery, radiation, and/or chemotherapy. Treatment may be initiated immediately to slow or stop the progression of sexual development in children below the expected age of puberty. A gonadotropin-releasing hormone analogue (GnRHa) is administered, usually leuprolide acetate (Lupron) injections once a month or nafarelin acetate (Synarel) intranasally twice a day. Treatment often continues until a more normal age for puberty is reached (e.g., 11 years in girls and 12 years in boys). Simple monitoring of growth patterns may be the only intervention for children closer to the lower expected age for puberty to begin.

Nursing Management

Nursing care centers on teaching the child and parents about the condition, administering medication, and providing emotional support. Inform the child in age-appropriate terms that physiologic changes are normal but occurring at an earlier than usual age. Reassure the child that friends will go through the same stages of development eventually. Remember that the child's social, cognitive, and emotional development matches his or her age, even though the physical development is advanced. Determine the family's ability to manage the cost of treatment, which ranges between $6000 and $10,000 a year. Financial assistance may be available through pharmaceutical companies.

Children with precocious puberty often become self-conscious as body changes occur. Parents should be advised to dress the child in a manner appropriate to his or her chronologic age, even though the child may look older. Looser clothing may help hide some of the body changes that are occurring. Provide privacy during examinations. Encourage the child to express his or her feelings about the changes. The child may need to practice role-playing as a coping mechanism to manage teasing by other children. Parents should be advised that they may need to discuss issues of sexuality with the child at an earlier age than normal. Encourage parents to have a discussion with the child's teacher and school nurse to help manage the teasing by other children. Refer the child for counseling, if appropriate.

DISORDERS OF THYROID FUNCTION

Hypothyroidism

Hypothyroidism is a disorder in which levels of active thyroid hormones are decreased. It may be congenital or acquired. Congenital hypothyroidism occurs in approximately 1 in 4000 live births and is twice as common in girls as in boys (Palma Sisto, 2004). In comparison to White infants, it is less prevalent in Black infants but more prevalent in Hispanic infants (Rossi, Caplin, & Alter, 2005). It also occurs more commonly in children with Down syndrome. Acquired hypothyroidism is more common in girls than in boys.

> **CLINICAL TIP**
>
> Hormone levels vary throughout the day, making it difficult to get a measurement of the child's peak hormone level. Provocative testing is used to measure hormone levels when an endocrine condition is suspected. A medication known to stimulate the secretion of the hormone being tested is administered and serial blood samples are collected to measure the child's response.

Etiology and Pathophysiology

Thyroid hormones are important for growth and development and for metabolizing nutrients and energy. When these hormones are not available to stimulate other hormones or specific target cells, growth is delayed and mental retardation develops.

Congenital hypothyroidism is usually caused by a spontaneous gene mutation, an autosomal recessive genetic transmission of an enzyme deficiency, hypoplasia or aplasia of the thyroid gland, failure of the CNS-thyroid feedback mechanism to develop, or iodine deficiency. Mental retardation (cretinism) is irreversible if the disorder is not treated. A small percentage of these cases are caused by hypothalamic-pituitary hypothyroidism and have thyroid-stimulating hormone resistance. Some children have a transient form of congenital hypothyroidism due to transplacental transfer of maternal thyroid-blocking antibodies or antithyroid medications (Eugster, LeMay, Zerin et al., 2004).

Acquired hypothyroidism can be idiopathic or result from autoimmune thyroiditis (Hashimoto's thyroiditis), late-onset thyroid dysfunction, isolated thyroid-stimulating hormone (TSH) deficiency due to pituitary or hypothalamic dysfunction, or exposure to drugs or substances such as lithium that interfere with thyroid hormone synthesis. In the case of Hashimoto's thyroiditis, the thyroid is infiltrated by lymphocytes that cause an autoimmune reaction and an enlarged thyroid. A genetic predisposition to autoimmune thyroiditis and an autosomal dominant inheritance of thyroid antibodies has been identified (Roberts & Ladenson, 2004).

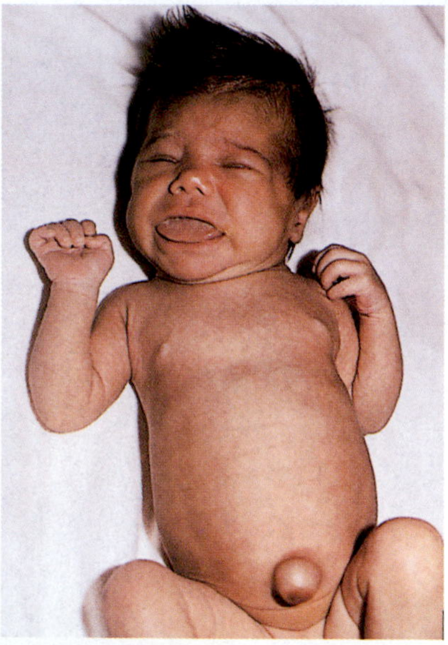

Clinical Manifestations

Infants with congenital hypothyroidism have few clinical signs of the disorder in the first weeks of life. In untreated infants, the characteristic cretinoid features (thickened protuberant tongue, thick lips, dull appearance) appear during the first few months of life (Figure 29–4▶). Other signs include prolonged neonatal jaundice, hypotonia, macroglossia, respiratory distress, bradycardia, decreased pulse pressure, cool extremities, mottling, umbilical hernia, a posterior fontanel larger than 1 cm in diameter, difficulty feeding, lethargy, constipation, and a hoarse cry.

Children with acquired hypothyroidism have many of the same signs as adults: decreased appetite; dry, cool skin; thinning hair or hair loss; depressed deep tendon reflexes; bradycardia; constipation; sensitivity to cold temperatures; abnormal menses; and a **goiter** (a nontender enlarged thyroid gland). Manifestations unique to children include change in past normal growth patterns with a weight increase, decreased height velocity, delayed bone and dental age, muscle hypertrophy with muscle weakness, and delayed or precocious puberty.

Figure 29–4 ▶ Child with congenital hypothyroidism.
Note: From Zitelli, B., & Davis, H. (Eds.). (2002). *Atlas of pediatric physical diagnosis* (4th ed., p. 321). St. Louis, MO: Mosby-Wolfe.

■ COLLABORATIVE CARE

Diagnostic Tests

Congenital hypothyroidism is usually detected during newborn screening of thyroxine (T_4) and TSH levels, which is mandatory in all states. When the T_4 level is low, an elevated TSH level indicates that the disease originated in the thyroid, not the pituitary. The newborn screening test is often performed twice to make sure that the disorder is identified early, once before the newborn leaves the hospital and again at the first healthcare visit at 1 to 2 weeks of age. Rapid feedback from the laboratory reduces the time to diagnosis and the effects of hypothyroidism on the infant's development.

Clinical Therapy

If the T_4 level is below normal and the TSH level is increased, the synthetic thyroid hormone levothyroxine (Synthroid) is prescribed. The recommended starting dose for newborns with congenital hypothyroidism is greater than 10 mcg/kg per day (Rovet, 2005). The dose is increased gradually as the child grows to ensure a **euthyroid** (thyroid hormones in appropriate balance) state. A pediatric endocrinologist monitors treatment. Periodic evaluation of T_4 and TSH serum levels, bone age, and growth parameters is necessary to assess for signs of excess or inadequate thyroid hormone. A trial without medication may be attempted when the child is about 3 years of age if the child has not required increasing doses of levothyroxine to maintain the TSH level. If after 6 weeks the TSH level is elevated, lifelong medication will be needed (Rossi, Caplin, & Alter, 2005).

Antithyroid antibodies are measured in children with a goiter and suspected Hashimoto's thyroiditis, as increased titers of antithyroglobin and antimicrosomal antibodies are often found.

To ensure an adequate growth rate and prevent mental retardation, the hormone must be taken throughout life. Children with congenital hypothyroidism that is diagnosed before 3 months of age have the best prognosis for optimal mental development. Children with acquired hypothyroidism usually have normal growth following a period of catch-up growth. Many adolescents with Hashimoto's thyroiditis have a spontaneous remission.

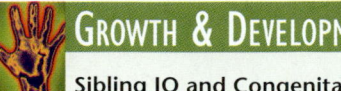

GROWTH & DEVELOPMENT

Sibling IQ and Congenital Hypothyroidism

When comparing the IQ of treated children with congenital hypothyroidism to siblings tested with the same IQ test, the children with congenital hypothyroidism scored significantly lower than their siblings with an average range of 6 to 8 points difference (Rovet, 2005).

NURSING MANAGEMENT

Nursing Assessment and Diagnosis

Routine neonatal screening is performed before discharge from the hospital and is often repeated at the infant's first health visit to evaluate levels of circulating thyroid hormones. Emphasize the importance of these visits and the screening to be performed.

Record the length or height and weight at each follow-up visit and plot on a growth curve. The child is assessed for signs of inadequate growth to determine if the dose of thyroid hormone needs to be adjusted and to monitor compliance with medication. Conduct developmental screening to detect delays in developmental milestones.

Among the nursing diagnoses that might be appropriate for the child with hypothyroidism are:

- Imbalanced Nutrition: Less than Body Requirements related to loss of appetite
- Risk for Delayed Development related to delayed initiation of thyroid replacement therapy
- Risk for Disproportionate Growth related to poor adherence to thyroid hormone therapy
- Constipation related to decreased bowel motility
- Fatigue related to inadequate dose of thyroid medication

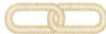

SKILL 7–2
Newborn Screening

Planning and Implementation

Nursing care focuses on teaching the parents and child about the disorder and its treatment and monitoring the child's growth rate. Explain how to administer thyroid hormone, which is only available in tablet form (e.g., tablets can be crushed and mixed in a small amount of formula or applesauce, as long as it can be ensured that the child gets all of the medication). Advise parents that the child may experience temporary sleep disturbances or behavioral changes in response to therapy. Teach the parents how to assess for an increased pulse rate, which could indicate the presence of too much thyroid hormone, and advise them to report problems such as fatigue, which could indicate an improper drug dose that needs to be adjusted.

Caution parents to dress the child appropriately for the season to prevent hypothermia. Modify the child's diet by increasing the amount of fruits and bulk if constipation is a problem.

Reassure the family that the child has the best chance of normal development when the hormone replacement therapy is given as prescribed. Reinforce the importance of follow-up visits to assess growth rate and response to therapy and to regulate drug dosages as the child grows. Periodic assessments of educational achievement are needed. Even with good control, adolescents have persistent visual-spatial deficits, and memory and attention problems. Parents should be informed that in most cases therapy will be lifelong and it is needed to promote the child's mental development. When the cause is genetic, make a referral for genetic counseling.

Evaluation

Expected outcomes of nursing care of the child with hypothyroidism include:

- The child maintains adequate growth of height and weight, following a percentile curve throughout childhood.
- The child's diet contains adequate fruits and bulk to prevent constipation.
- The child's cognitive development is appropriate for age.

Hyperthyroidism

Hyperthyroidism, a disorder of excessive levels of circulating thyroid hormones, is rare in children and adolescents. It is most common in adolescent girls and is almost always due to Graves' disease (Nebesio, Siddiqui, Pescovitz et al., 2002). The disorder may present in the preschool years, but has an increased incidence in adolescence.

Etiology and Pathophysiology

Graves' disease is an autoimmune disorder. Immunoglobulins produced by the B lymphocytes stimulate oversecretion of thyroid hormones, resulting in the clinical symptoms. It has a high familial incidence.

Other less common causes of hyperthyroidism result from thyroiditis and thyroid secreting hormone tumors, including thyroid adenomas and carcinomas, as well as pituitary adenomas. Congenital hyperthyroidism can occur in infants of mothers with Graves' disease because of transplacental transfer of immunoglobulins.

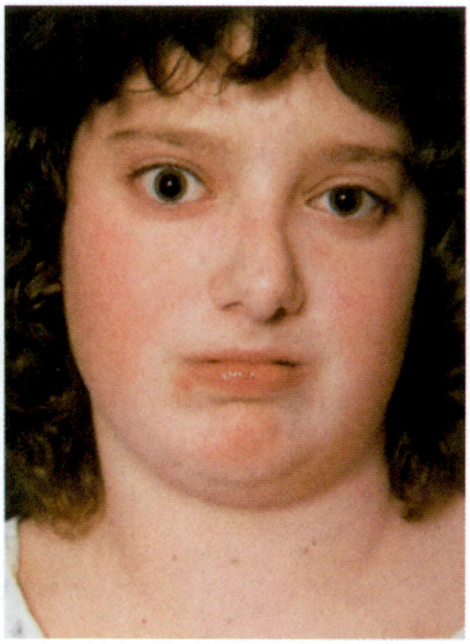

Clinical Manifestations

Signs and symptoms are caused by hyperactivity of the sympathetic nervous system. Characteristic findings include an enlarged, nontender thyroid gland (goiter), prominent eyes (exophthalmos) (Figure 29–5➤), eyelid lag, tachycardia, nervousness, restlessness or irritability, increased appetite with weight loss, emotional lability, heat intolerance, diaphoresis, insomnia, tremor, and muscle weakness. The thyroid gland may be slightly enlarged or grow to three to four times its normal size; feel warm, soft, and fleshy; and have an auditory bruit on auscultation. Onset is subtle, and the condition often goes unrecognized for 1 to 2 years.

Children with Graves' disease usually have difficulty concentrating, behavioral problems, and declining performance in school. They become easily frustrated in the classroom and overheated and fatigued during physical education class. It is difficult for them to relax or sleep. These symptoms usually prompt parents to seek medical treatment for them.

Figure 29–5 ➤ Exophthalmos and an enlarged thyroid in an adolescent with Graves' disease.
Note: From Zitelli, B., & Davis, H. (Eds.). (1997). *Atlas of pediatric physical diagnosis* (3rd ed., p. 271). St. Louis, MO: Mosby-Wolfe.

■ COLLABORATIVE CARE

Diagnostic Tests

Diagnostic studies include laboratory evaluation of serum TSH, T_3 (triiodothyronine) and T_4 levels, and a thyroid scan. T_3 and T_4 levels are markedly elevated while the TSH level is decreased. Serum studies to detect thyroid antibodies (anti-TG and anti-TPO), usually present in Graves' disease and Hashimoto's thyroiditis, are performed. In addition, a thyroid scan is performed to identify nodules or to confirm the high uptake of radioactive iodine associated with Graves' disease.

Clinical Therapy

The goal of clinical therapy is to inhibit excessive secretion of thyroid hormones. Treatment may include antithyroid drug therapy, radiation therapy, or surgery. Drug therapy is most often the initial treatment, but compliance is often a problem because of drug side effects. Methimazole (Tapazole) and propylthiouracil (PTU) are given to inhibit thyroid hormone secretion. PTU therapy can cause temporary side effects, including skin rashes, urticaria, and lymphadenopathy. If rash, fever, or sore throat develops, a healthcare professional should perform hematologic studies. Treatment continues for 18 months to 2 years, or until the thyroid decreases in size and remission occurs (Ginsberg, 2003). Symptoms usually improve within weeks of starting treatment. Beta-adrenergic blocking agents such as propanolol may be given to relieve symptoms of tremors, tachycardia, and restless.

If drug therapy is ineffective, radiation therapy using oral radioactive iodine (131I) is the next treatment choice. Current data do not indicate a relationship between radioactive iodine and cancer or leukemia. It also does not appear to increase the risk of birth defects in future offspring in those treated (Ginsberg, 2003). Thyroidectomy (removal of most of the thyroid) provides an immediate cure and avoids radiation along with possible long-term complications of radioactive iodine (Boger & Perrier, 2004). Manipulation of the parathyroid gland during surgery may result in excess release of parathyroid hormone, leading to hypercalcemia. Severe **thyrotoxicosis** or thyroid "storm" may occur when thyroid hormone is suddenly released into the bloodstream during surgery.

> ### NURSING ALERT
>
> The child who experiences thyrotoxicosis has a fever, diaphoresis, tachycardia, palpitations, muscle weakness, hypertension, and tremors due to sympathetic nervous system hyperactivity. This is a medical emergency, and the condition can progress to shock and, if untreated, death. Treatment includes antithyroid drugs and propranolol. The heart and blood pressure need to be monitored frequently after administration.

NURSING MANAGEMENT

Nursing Assessment and Diagnosis

Assess the child's vital signs, as blood pressure and pulse may be elevated. Keep a record of food intake. Accurate measurement and recording of height and weight are important to establish baselines and identify patterns of growth. Observe the child's behavior, activity, and level of fatigue.

Assess the family's response to the chronic condition, as well as the family's response to the child's disturbing symptoms (e.g., irritability, heat intolerance, and muscle weakness). They also may have concerns with terminology used during discussions about the condition, such as "remission," which may be associated with cancer (Amer, 2005).

Common nursing diagnoses for the child with hyperthyroidism include:

- Ineffective Thermoregulation (Elevated) related to illness and excessive activity of the sympathetic nervous system
- Imbalanced Nutrition: Less than Body Requirements related to high metabolic needs
- Disturbed Body Image related to changes caused by illness (prominent eyes, excessive perspiration, and tremors)
- Fatigue related to hypermetabolic state and sleep deprivation

Planning and Implementation

Nursing care focuses on teaching the child and parents about the disorder and its treatment, promoting rest, providing emotional support, and, if the child needs surgery, providing preoperative and postoperative teaching and care. Promote increased caloric intake by providing five or six moderate meals per day. Encourage the child and family to express their feelings and concerns about the disorder, especially when deciding among the three treatment options or during the period when medication dosage adjustments are frequently needed. Pointing out even slight improvements in the child's condition may increase the child's adherence with therapy.

Children with hyperthyroidism are easily fatigued. Rest periods should be scheduled at school and home and physical activities kept to a minimum until symptoms resolve. Encourage parents to provide a cool environment and allow the child to wear fewer clothes until symptoms subside.

Children who have partial or total removal of the thyroid gland receive antithyroid drugs, such as iodine, for approximately 2 weeks before surgery. Teach the child and parents about drug therapy and instruct parents to watch for side effects of antithyroid drugs, including fever, urticaria, and lymphadenopathy. Provide preoperative teaching (see Chapter 13 ∞), as young children may be fearful about having their throat "cut."

Postoperatively, elevate the head of the bed to 30 degrees and assess the child for bleeding, hoarseness, difficulty breathing, and thyrotoxicosis. A tracheostomy kit, suction supplies, and IV calcium gluconate should be immediately available for emergency treatment of hypocalcemia and respiratory distress.

> ### COMMUNITY CARE
>
> **School and Hormone Therapy**
> Provide information and support to the parents to educate the school nurse and teacher about the child's condition while waiting for the treatment to become effective. Several weeks or months may be needed before the child's hormone levels are stabilized and perceptions of hyperactivity decrease (Amer, 2005). The teacher needs to know that the symptoms are temporary.

Teach the family about the need for lifelong thyroid hormone replacement if radiation or surgery is performed. Encourage the family to adjust food intake to prevent obesity as the child's metabolic rate declines and weight gain may occur. The child should wear a medical alert bracelet. Make sure the child is monitored regularly to ensure that the T_4 level is adequate to sustain growth.

Evaluation

Expected outcomes of nursing care for the child with hyperthyroidism include:

- The child regains lost weight and maintains the previously established growth curve because the T_4 level remains appropriate.
- The child participates in daily activities without experiencing fatigue.

DISORDERS OF THE PARATHYROID

Children usually have four parathyroid glands located posterior to the thyroid gland. Their primary function is to work in conjunction with vitamin D to regulate total body calcium. Ionized calcium influences release of parathyroid hormone, which acts on both bone and the kidney to maintain normal serum levels. The hormone also acts on the kidney to increase vitamin D synthesis, which assists in calcium balance. It is related as well to magnesium and phosphorus balance; low magnesium levels stimulate parathyroid hormone release and the hormone leads to lowered phosphate serum levels.

Hyperparathyroidism

Primary hyperparathyroidism, rare during childhood, is most often the result of a tumor (adenoma) that secretes the hormone without proper regulation (Doyle & DiGeorge, 2004). Secondary hyperparathyroidism is due to disease outside of the parathyroid gland, leading to excessive secretion of parathyroid hormone (Rudock, 2002). This is commonly seen in chronic renal failure when the kidneys are unable to reabsorb calcium, causing low serum calcium levels and stimulating continual secretion of parathyroid hormone to maintain normal serum calcium levels. See Chapter 25 ∞ for further discussion of renal failure.

At any age, symptoms of primary hyperparathyroidism may include bone pain, nephrolithiasis (kidney stones), and pathologic bone fractures. Hypercalcemia may cause symptoms of muscle weakness, peptic ulcer disease, fatigue, volume depletion, and subtle mental disturbance (Viera, 2002). Abdominal pain may be present and may indicate pancreatitis.

There is often a delay between development of symptoms and diagnosis. Elevated serum calcium and parathyroid hormone (PTH) levels are diagnostic (Kollars, Zarroug, van Heerden et al., 2005). Radiographic images may reveal signs of rickets. For primary hyperparathyroidism, surgical parathyroid exploration is performed to remove the adenoma. Surgical cure rate is estimated to be 90% (Viera, 2002). Treatment of secondary hyperparathyroidism focuses on prevention of hypercalcemia utilizing vitamin D replacement and phosphorus binders.

Nursing Management

Nursing care centers on fluid management and electrolyte monitoring. In children who require surgery, assess for respiratory distress and a potential airway obstruction due to edema and a potential hematoma around the tracheal space. Monitor for signs of infection.

Following surgery, educate the child and parents to recognize signs of hypocalcemia and to provide appropriate amounts of calcium supplementation. After diagnosis or after surgical intervention, follow-up is important to monitor serum calcium and phosphorus levels.

Hypoparathyroidism

Primary hypoparathyroidism is rare, but it may result from congenital disorders (parathyroid aplasia, DiGeorge syndrome), surgical removal of the parathyroid glands, disease processes that destroy the parathyroid glands (Wilson's disease, hemochromatosis), or medications (i.e., aluminum, asparagine, doxorubicin, cytosine, arabinoside). The primary result is hypocalcemia and hyperphosphatemia.

Infants may display hyperirritability, muscle rigidity, seizures, vomiting, abdominal distention, apneic episodes, or intermittent cyanosis or twitching. Muscle pain and cramps may progress to numbness, stiffness, and tingling of the hands and feet. A positive Chvostek's sign (spasm of facial muscles after tapping facial nerve) reveals hyperreflexia. Life-threatening tetany and convulsions may occur with severe hypocalcemia (Doyle & DiGeorge, 2004).

Serum calcium and PTH levels are low and serum phosphorus is elevated. Radiographs often demonstrate increased bone density. A 12-lead ECG may demonstrate a prolonged QT interval. In emergencies, intravenous calcium and calcitriol are administered to treat seizures, tetany, life-threatening hypotension, and cardiac arrhythmias. Oral calcitriol and calcium are given for an indefinite time period (Palma Sisto, 2004). Foods with high phosphorus content (dairy products and eggs) are limited.

Nursing Management

Assess and stabilize the airway, breathing, and circulation. In the acute care setting, children should be placed on a cardiorespiratory monitor. Maintain seizure precautions until normal serum calcium levels are attained. Obtain intravenous access and administer calcium supplementation as ordered.

Partner with the family to ensure their understanding of the need for calcium supplementation and reduced intake of phosphorus. Teach the family that periodic monitoring of calcium levels is important. Inform the family that hypoparathyroidism may require lifelong therapy.

DISORDERS OF ADRENAL FUNCTION

Cushing's Disease

Cushing's disease, also called adrenocortical hyperfunction, is characterized by a group of symptoms resulting from excess levels of glucocorticoids (especially cortisol) in the bloodstream. It is rare in children and the true incidence is unknown. During infancy and childhood, most cases of endogenous Cushing's disease are due to a microadenoma pituitary tumor that causes adrenal cortex hyperfunction (Levine & White, 2004). Other causes include hyperplasia of one or both adrenal glands and benign tumors of the adrenal glands. The increased secretion of cortisol alters metabolism.

The initial sign in most children is gradual excessive weight gain followed by growth retardation, hypertension, and mental and behavioral problems. It generally takes up to 2 to 5 years for the child to develop the characteristic "cushingoid" appearance, which includes a moon face (chubby cheeks and a double chin) and fat pads over the shoulders and back (buffalo hump). See the clinical manifestations table below for signs of Cushing's disease.

> **NURSING ALERT**
>
> Dilute intravenous calcium per hospital protocol. Infiltration of IV calcium can cause extravasation and tissue sloughing. Always check the patency of the IV prior to administration. Monitor ECG during administration. Evaluate for hypocalcemia and hypercalcemia after administration.

> **CLINICAL TIP**
>
> The most common reasons for cushingoid features in children are excessive doses of corticosteroids and prolonged use of corticosteroids as treatment for other diseases. Cushingoid features may develop in a shorter time than occurs with Cushing's disease. See Figure 23–10 ∞. Corticosteroids suppress adrenal function when given long term. These children may have Cushing's syndrome.

CLINICAL MANIFESTATIONS	CUSHING'S DISEASE
Cause	**Clinical Manifestations**
Catabolism of protein	Muscle weakness and wasting, capillary weakness and bruising, growth failure with delayed bone age, fatigue
Decreased absorption of calcium from the intestines	Demineralization of bones, osteoporosis
Increased appetite	Weight gain primarily on the trunk, striae on the abdomen, buttocks, thighs
Salt retention	Increased blood volume and hypertension

Diagnosis is based on characteristic physical findings and laboratory values, including increased 24-hour urinary levels of free cortisol, and 17-hydroxycorticosteroid (17-OHCs); and elevated nighttime salivary cortisol level. The child has chronic hyperglycemia and an elevated glycosylated hemoglobin concentration. See Appendix C ∞ for expected laboratory values.

The adrenal suppression test with an 11 p.m. dose of dexamethasone reveals that adrenal cortisol output is not suppressed overnight as would occur in normal children. Computed tomography (CT) and magnetic resonance imaging (MRI) are used to detect the specific location of tumors in the adrenal and pituitary glands.

Surgical removal of the pituitary adenoma is the current treatment of choice when this is the cause of Cushing's disease. Replacement glucocorticoid therapy may be needed for several months after surgery. Irradiation of the pituitary is performed when surgical removal of the adenoma does not substantially reduce cortisol levels. Alternatively, medications may be given for management of hypercortisolism by interrupting adrenal steroid synthesis.

Bilateral removal of the adrenal glands may be necessary in some cases to stop the excessive secretion of cortisol. Lifelong glucocorticoid and mineralcorticoid replacement is required when both adrenal glands are removed. The prognosis for children with malignant adrenal tumors is poor.

Nursing Management

The nurse usually encounters a child with Cushing's disease when the child is hospitalized for diagnostic evaluation or surgery. Nursing assessment includes monitoring the child's vital signs and fluid and nutritional status, and assessing muscle strength and endurance during hospital play activities.

Teach the child and family about the disorder and its treatment, and, for children undergoing surgery, provide preoperative and postoperative teaching and care. Answer any questions the child and family may have and explain all laboratory and diagnostic tests. Explain to parents that the child's cushingoid appearance is reversible with treatment. Refer to Chapter 23 ∞ for general nursing care of the child with cancer. Provide nutritional guidance or refer the child and parents to a nutritionist to promote maintenance of an appropriate weight.

For children who need cortisol replacement therapy because both adrenal glands were surgically removed, administering the drug early in the morning mimics the normal diurnal pattern of cortisol secretion. Cortisol replacement in the postoperative period must be explained carefully to parents. Hydrocortisone (Cortef, Solu-Cortef, cortisone acetate) comes in tablet or injectable form. Parents may need to crush the tablet and mix with a small amount of applesauce, but the entire dose of medication must be taken. The oral preparations of cortisone have a bitter taste and can cause gastric irritation. Giving the dose at mealtimes and using antacids between meals helps reduce these side effects. Teach parents how and when to administer the injectable form—usually when the child is vomiting, has diarrhea, or cannot take the oral medication. Failure to give medication when the child is ill may lead to severe illness and cardiovascular collapse. See Families Want to Know: Hydrocortisone Administration.

> ### → NURSING ALERT
>
> Signs of acute adrenal insufficiency may include increased irritability, headache, confusion, restlessness, nausea and vomiting, diarrhea, abdominal pain, dehydration, fever, loss of appetite, and lethargy. If untreated, the child will go into shock. In newborns, the symptoms include failure to thrive, weakness, vomiting, and dehydration. Hyponatremia and hyperkalemia are key signs.

FAMILIES WANT TO KNOW

Hydrocortisone Administration

Teach the family the following tips regarding hydrocortisone administration:

- Always give the medication on time since the prescribed schedule follows the body's normal cortisol release pattern.
- Never abruptly discontinue the medication.
- If the child has vomiting or diarrhea and is unable to take the medication by mouth, administer the injections to replace oral doses as instructed and notify the physician immediately.

- Higher doses of hydrocortisone are needed when the child is ill.
- Always have injectable hydrocortisone available at home, at school, and everywhere the child travels. An emergency kit should be available at all times to supply cortisol to the child during acute illnesses and stressful situations.

Teach parents to be alert to signs of acute adrenal insufficiency during the withdrawal of corticosteroid therapy, and to inform all healthcare providers of the child's condition and medication. The child should wear a medical alert bracelet at all times.

Congenital Adrenal Hyperplasia

Congenital adrenal hyperplasia, sometimes called adrenogenital syndrome, adrenocortical hyperplasia, or congenital adrenogenital hyperplasia, is an autosomal recessive disorder that causes a deficiency of one of the enzymes necessary for the synthesis of cortisol and aldosterone. It occurs in 1 in 14,000 live births, and males and females are affected equally (Pang, 2003).

Etiology and Pathophysiology

More than 90% of children with congenital adrenal hyperplasia have partial or complete 21-hydroxylase enzyme deficiency that results in inadequate production of aldosterone and cortisol. This form has an autosomal recessive inheritance pattern, and the defective gene CYP21 is located on the short arm of chromosome 6. About 5–8% of children have deficiency of 11β-hydroxylase. Mutations on defective gene CPY11B1 of chromosome 8 result in inadequate cortisol and excess levels of other steroids and testosterone synthesis (Henwood & Katz, 2005). The remaining 2–5% of cases involve deficiencies of other enzymes.

Of the two classic forms of the disorder, 75% are salt-losing, caused by aldosterone deficiency, and 25% are non-salt-losing with **virilization** (the production of masculine secondary sexual characteristics in females). In all forms, increased secretion of ACTH occurs in response to diminished cortisol levels.

During fetal development, the lack of cortisol triggers the pituitary to continue secretion of ACTH. This in turn stimulates overproduction of the adrenal androgens. Virilization of the female external genitalia begins in week 10 of gestation. If untreated after birth, the overproduction of androgens results in accelerated height, early closure of the epiphyseal plates, and premature sexual development with both pubic and axillary hair.

Clinical Manifestations

Congenital adrenal hyperplasia is the most common cause of **pseudohermaphroditism** (ambiguous genitalia) in newborn girls. The female infant is born with an enlarged clitoris and partial or complete labial fusions. The vagina usually has a common opening with the urethra (Figure 29–6 ▶). Severely virilized females may be mistaken for males with cryptorchidism, hypospadias, or micropenis. The uterus, ovaries, and fallopian tubes are normal. The male infant may look normal at birth or may have a slightly enlarged penis and hyperpigmented scrotum. The boy may have tall stature and an adult-sized penis by school age, but the testes are appropriately sized for age. Partial enzyme deficiency produces less obvious symptoms. Precocious puberty, tall stature for age, acne, and excessive muscle development may be noted in both males and females as the child grows. Due to early epiphyseal fusion, adult stature is shorter.

Signs of adrenal insufficiency may be the first indication of the disorder. Recurrent vomiting, dehydration, metabolic acidosis, hypotension, and hypoglycemia are characteristic signs of the salt-wasting form of the disorder. Hypertension with hypokalemic alkalosis is alternately found in children with 11-hydroxylase deficiency.

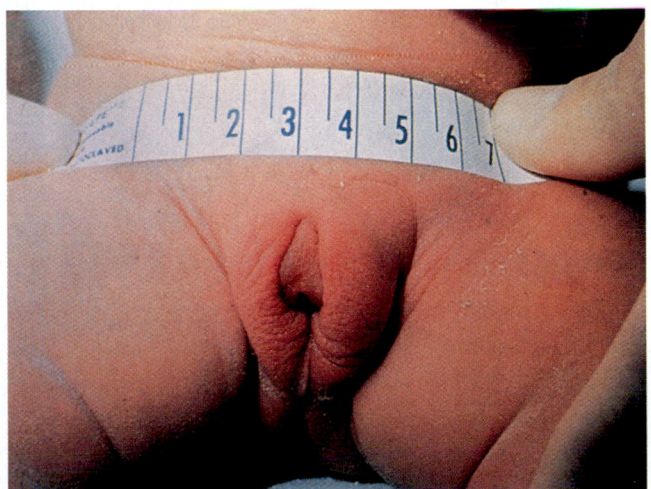

Figure 29–6 ▶ Newborn girl with ambiguous genitalia. Courtesy of Patrick C. Walsh, MD.

◾ COLLABORATIVE CARE

Diagnostic Tests

Diagnosis in infants and children is usually confirmed by laboratory evaluation of serum 17-hydroxyprogesterone (17-OHP) level. Routine newborn screening for congenital adrenal hyperplasia is performed in 44 states (National Newborn Screening and

Genetics Resource Center, 2006). Prenatal diagnosis is available. In instances of ambiguous genitalia, a **karyotype** (a microscopic chromosome study in which the 46 chromosomes of the child are lined up in pairs from largest to smallest to detect errors in chromosome number, shape, and size) determines the infant's gender. Ultrasonography may be used to visualize pelvic structures.

In the salt-wasting form of the disorder, the child may have hyponatremia, hyperkalemia, acidosis, hypoglycemia, a high urine sodium level, and low serum and urinary aldosterone levels. Serum concentrations of testosterone in girls and androstenedione in boys and girls are elevated in affected infants. Measurement of ACTH and 17-OHP levels reveal high readings, while serum cortisol is inappropriately low in comparison to ACTH (Levine & White, 2004). Diagnosis may be delayed in the non-salt-losing form until 3 to 7 years.

Clinical Therapy

The goal of treatment is to suppress adrenal secretion of androgens by replacing deficient hormones. Prenatal steroids may be used when parents have been identified as carriers of congenital adrenal hyperplasia mutations. This may reduce the severe virilization of a female fetus (Henwood & Katz, 2005). Treatment of affected children is accomplished by the lifelong use of oral glucocorticoids (dexamethasone, prednisone, or hydrocortisone). The glucocorticoid replacement reduces secretion of ACTH, which had overstimulated the adrenal cortex. As a result, excessive adrenal androgen production is suppressed. The dose is individualized by monitoring growth parameters, bone age, and hormone levels. If the infant has the salt-wasting form of the disorder, salt is added to the infant's formula and a mineralocorticoid (Florinef) is given to replace the missing hormone. Hormone dosage must be *doubled* or *tripled* during acute illnesses or injury and for surgery. Injectable hydrocortisone is used for severe stress. Adrenalectomy is recommended only in cases when medical therapy is ineffective (Pang, 2003).

Reconstructive surgery of the enlarged clitoris is often performed on girls during the first year of life; however, some centers support waiting until adolescence, allowing the patient to participate in the decision for surgery.

■ NURSING MANAGEMENT

Nursing Assessment and Diagnosis

Assess the infant and child for signs of dehydration, electrolyte imbalance, and hypovolemic shock in the salt-wasting form of the disease. Monitor the airway, breathing, circulation, and responsiveness. Assess vital signs and assess peripheral perfusion (capillary refill, distal pulses, color and temperature of the extremities) frequently to detect early changes in condition.

Assess the parents' emotional response to a child with ambiguous genitalia and a chronic condition. Explore their values and beliefs regarding gender roles and sexuality while awaiting results of the karyotype.

Nursing diagnoses for the child with congenital adrenal hyperplasia might include:

- Impaired Parenting related to a child with undetermined gender identity
- Caregiver Role Strain related to care of a child with a chronic, potentially life-threatening condition
- Risk for Deficient Fluid Volume related to failure of regulatory mechanisms and excess excretion of salt by the kidneys
- Risk for Disproportionate Growth related to accelerated growth and premature closure of epiphyseal plates

Planning and Implementation

Nursing care of the newborn with congenital adrenal hyperplasia focuses on teaching parents about the disorder and its treatment, providing emotional support, and preoperative and postoperative teaching for parents of infants undergoing reconstructive surgery. The administration of glucocorticoids and mineralocorticoids must be carefully controlled

It is often difficult for parents to accept that their infant, whose genitalia look male, is really female. Reassure parents that with medication and surgery the genitalia assume a female appearance and all organs necessary for future childbearing are usually functional. Several surgeries may be performed before 2 years of age and then during adolescence to dilate the vagina. If the parents and surgeon decide to delay surgery until adolescence, psychological support will need to be provided to the parents and child during childhood because of the child's genital appearance. Because of the risk for adrenal insufficiency, the child will most likely be hospitalized for surgery rather than having outpatient surgery.

Nurses can assist parents in educating the child's siblings, grandparents, other family members, and childcare workers about the condition. In the newborn nursery, the infant should be referred to as "your beautiful infant," not "your son" or "your daughter," until gender identity is confirmed.

Inform parents that genetic counseling should be provided for the child during adolescence. Parents considering a future pregnancy should also be informed that prenatal testing may detect congenital adrenal hyperplasia in the fetus. Refer the family for counseling, if indicated.

Care in the Community

The child will need frequent follow-up to monitor growth and appropriate dosage of glucocorticoids. Teach parents about the special problems that develop in the salt-wasting form of the disease during acute illness. Explain the medication regimen and help the family develop an emergency care plan. The child should wear a medical alert bracelet. Teach parents how to administer intramuscular injections of hydrocortisone. (see page 1218). If injectable hydrocortisone is not available, the child needs urgent treatment in an emergency department. The child may become dehydrated quickly and need intravenous fluid and electrolyte replacement in addition to higher doses of hydrocortisone.

An Individualized Health Plan should be developed to inform the school nurse and teachers about the special care needed if the child becomes ill at school. Injectable hydrocortisone should be kept at the school for emergency use.

Evaluation

Expected outcomes of nursing care for congenital adrenal hyperplasia include:

- Parents learn to give glucocorticoids appropriately when the child is ill and prevent episodes of adrenal crisis.
- Families effectively cope with the virilized appearance of the child's genitalia and bond with the child.

Adrenal Insufficiency (Addison's Disease)

Adrenal insufficiency, also known as Addison's disease, is a rare disorder in childhood characterized by a deficiency of glucocorticoids (cortisone) and mineralocorticoids (aldosterone). The majority of cases are caused by an autoimmune process, but it also may be acquired after trauma; with tuberculosis, HIV infection, meningococcemia, or fungal infections that destroy the adrenal glands. The lack of glucocorticoids affects the body's ability to handle stress (Gance-Cleveland, 2003).

Adrenal insufficiency usually develops slowly as the adrenal glands deteriorate. The early signs may not be noticed but include weakness with fatigue; lethargy and emotional lability; anorexia and salt craving; and poor weight gain or weight loss. Skin changes include hyperpigmentation at pressure points, lip borders and gingival margins, nipples, palms and soles, body creases, and scarred areas of the body; and generalized bronzing of the skin or freckling without tan lines, even in winter months. Additional signs include abdominal pain; nausea and vomiting; diarrhea; and symptomatic hypoglycemia. If the child experiences a stressful period (illness, injury, or surgery), acute adrenal insufficiency may occur. Signs of an adrenal crisis include weakness, fever, abdominal pain, hypoglycemia with seizures, hypotension, dehydration, shock, and coma.

Serum cortisol and urinary 17-hydroxycorticoid levels are measured in the early morning. Low levels of serum cortisol are associated with adrenal insufficiency. The ACTH stimulation test is used to detect adrenal gland reserve. Electrolyte values generally reveal low serum sodium, elevated serum potassium, and low fasting blood glucose levels. Computed tomography may be used to visualize the adrenal glands.

Treatment involves replacement of the deficient hormones. Oral hydrocortisone is given in the lowest therapeutic dose to control symptoms and promote normal growth. Fludrocortisone acetate (Florinef) replaces the missing mineralocorticoid in children with aldosterone deficiency. Adrenal crisis is treated by aggressive fluid resuscitation, intravenous glucose, and intravenous hydrocortisone. The precipitating illness or injury is then treated along with adequate doses of glucocorticoid, and maintenance doses of mineralocorticoid. Children will also need increased doses of steroids during periods of increased physiologic stress, such as surgical procedures, illnesses, and injuries. In these cases, the dose of hydrocortisone should be at least tripled and given three times a day for 24 hours or for as long as the stress lasts before resuming the maintenance dose (Henwood & Katz, 2005).

Nursing Management

Nursing management focuses on educating the child and parents about the disorder, providing emotional support, and caring for the child during acute episodes. See the earlier discussion of congenital adrenal hyperplasia for further details.

Pheochromocytoma

Pheochromocytoma is a tumor of the adrenal gland, but it may be extra-adrenal with no anatomic connection. In most cases, these tumors are benign and curable. They can occur in a familial pattern (autosomal dominant trait) with a 3:2 male to female ratio. Most tumors diagnosed in children are identified between the ages of 6 and 14 years. However, most tumors are identified during adult years (Levine & White, 2004). Pheochromocytomas may also be associated with neurofibromatosis. See Chapter 26 ∞.

The tumor causes an excessive release of the catecholamines epinephrine and norepinephrine, leading to hypertension. Clinical manifestations include episodes of hypertension with a systolic reading that may reach 250 mmHg, tachycardia, arrhythmias, palpitations, profuse sweating with cool extremities, flushing, headache, abdominal pain, nausea and vomiting, weight loss, visual disturbances, weakness, polydipsia, and polyuria. The classic triad of signs includes new onset hypertension, new or worsening diabetes mellitus, and hypertensive crisis. Because release of catecholamines (norepinephrine and epinephrine) from the tumor is not continuous, these symptoms occur intermittently. Episodes may occur daily or monthly and generally last minutes to an hour (Failor & Capell, 2003). In some cases, the condition may be silent until a stressor such as surgery causes a hypertensive crisis.

Diagnosis is based on 24-hour urine studies to detect the presence of urinary catecholamines and vanilmandelic acid (VMA) levels (see Appendix C ∞). Radiologic imaging with CT, PET scan, MRI, and ultrasound studies are required to locate the tumor in preparation for surgery. Most are located on the adrenal gland, but they may also be located in the chest, bladder, head, and neck (Failor & Capell, 2003).

The treatment of choice is surgical removal of all identified tumors, which is a cure. However, the procedure is dangerous and may result in pheochromocytoma crisis, manifested by seizures, shock, altered level of consciousness, disseminated intravascular coagulation, rhabdomyolysis (skeletal muscle destruction), and acute renal failure. Alpha- and beta-adrenergic blocking agents to control hypertension, tachycardia, and catecholamine release are given for 10 to 14 days before surgery (Harris & Fawcett, 2002). Plasma catecholamines are used to measure the effectiveness of the preoperative adrenergic blockade. Postoperatively, for several days, a 24-hour urine collection is measured for catecholamines to determine if all tumor sites were removed. With successful removal of all tumor sites, the prognosis is generally good. Follow-up is important to assess for recurrence.

Nursing Management

Nursing care is mainly supportive. Provide preoperative and postoperative teaching and care (see Chapter 13 ∞). Preoperatively, monitor vital signs and observe for signs of complications associated with pheochromocytoma crisis. Administer antihypertensives and watch for any signs of hyperglycemia (see page 1239). Postoperatively, the child may be managed initially in an intensive care unit. Monitor blood pressure, and observe for neurologic signs, respiratory distress, and signs of shock. Lifelong follow-up care with screening for hypertension and increased urinary catecholamine levels is required as symptoms recur if the child has other tumors not yet detected that activate at a later age (Levine & White, 2004).

DISORDERS OF PANCREATIC FUNCTION

Diabetes Mellitus

Diabetes mellitus, the most common metabolic disease in children, is a disorder of hyperglycemia resulting from defects in insulin secretion, insulin action, or both, leading to abnormalities in carbohydrate, protein, and fat metabolism (American Diabetes Association, 2006b). There are two main types of diabetes. Most children have immune-mediated type 1 diabetes, formerly called insulin-dependent diabetes mellitus or juvenile diabetes. However, a disturbingly large number of children are being diagnosed with type 2 diabetes, formerly called noninsulin-dependent diabetes or adult onset diabetes.

Type 1 Diabetes

In the United States, the prevalence of type 1 diabetes among all children ages 19 years and younger is 1.7 per 1000 (Centers for Disease Control and Prevention, 2004). Each year approximately 13,000 children under age 18 years are diagnosed with type 1 diabetes (American Diabetes Association, 2004). Peak incidence occurs in childhood at 5 to 7 years and again at puberty, but it may present at any age (Alemzadeh & Wyatt, 2004). Caucasians experience a higher incidence of type 1 diabetes than other racial groups. Boys and girls are equally affected.

ETIOLOGY AND PATHOPHYSIOLOGY   Type 1 diabetes is a multifactorial disease caused by autoimmune destruction of insulin-producing pancreatic beta cells in genetically predisposed individuals (Sepa, Wahlberg, Vaarala et al., 2005). Type 1 diabetes has familial tendencies but does not show any specific pattern of inheritance. Inheritance of the DR3 and DR4 markers on the human leukocyte antigen (HLA) complex on chromosome 6 increases the likelihood of developing type 1 diabetes. If the child inherits one marker, the child's risk is two to three times higher. If both markers are inherited, the child's risk is 7 to 10 times higher (Alemzadeh & Wyatt, 2004). However, the child inherits a susceptibility to the disease rather than the disease itself. It is believed that an event such as a virus triggers the inflammatory process, resulting in development of islet cell serum antibodies. These antibodies can be detected in the blood years before the development of the clinical symptoms (Weinzimer & Magge, 2005).

Insulin helps transport glucose into the cells so that the body can use it as an energy source. It also prevents the outflow of glucose from the liver to the general circulation. Environmental factors such as enteroviruses or toxins are believed to lead to an autoimmune destruction of the beta cells in the islets of Langerhans (Figure 29–7▶). Antigens are generated that help produce antibodies that indicate

PATHOPHYSIOLOGY ILLUSTRATED

Mechanism of Diabetes Mellitus

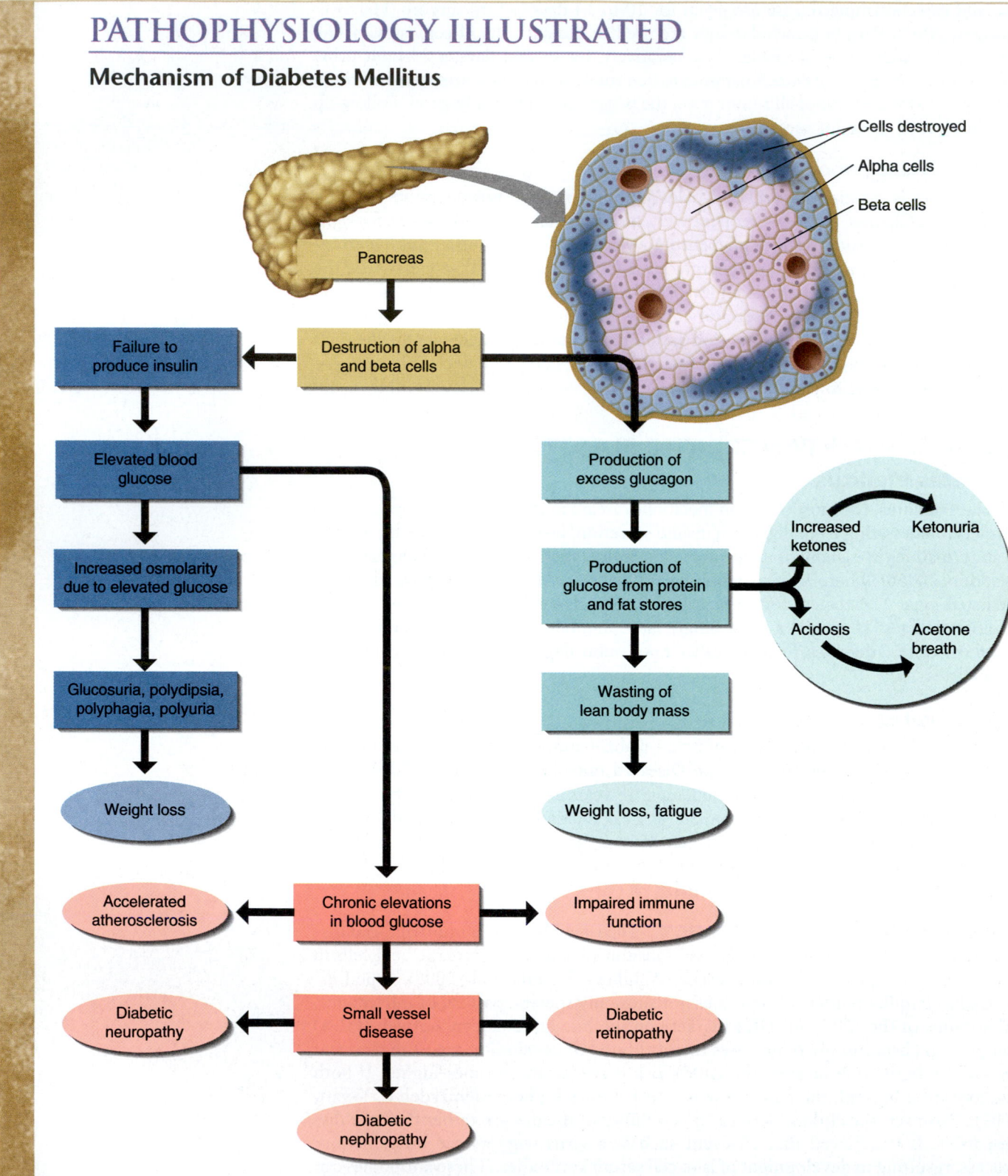

Figure 29–7 ▶ Destruction of the alpha and beta cells in the islets of Langerhans produces multiple metabolic changes. Acute signs and symptoms are followed by short-term and long-term complications if the disease is not well managed.

MediaLink

Physiology of Diabetes

ongoing destruction of the islet cells. As the destruction continues, insulin secretion decreases.

As the secretion of insulin decreases, there is a rise in blood glucose level and a decrease in the glucose level inside the cells. When the renal threshold for glucose (180 mg/dL) is exceeded, **glycosuria** (abnormal amount of glucose in the urine) occurs as a result of osmotic diuresis (Alemzadeh & Wyatt, 2004). Fluids follow the highly osmotic glucose and water is excreted in large volumes (polyuria).

When glucose is unavailable to the cells for metabolism, free fatty acids provide an alternate source of energy. The liver metabolizes fatty acids at an increased rate, producing acetyl coenzyme A (CoA). The by-products of acetyl CoA metabolism (ketone bodies) accumulate in the body, resulting in a state of metabolic acidosis, or ketoacidosis. (Refer to Chapter 16 ∞ for discussion of metabolic acidosis.)

CLINICAL MANIFESTATIONS   The classic signs of type 1 diabetes are polyuria, polydipsia, and **polyphagia** (excessive appetite) with significant weight loss. See Clinical Manifestations of Diabetes by Type below. Other signs include unexplained fatigue or lethargy, headaches, and stomachaches. Enuresis may also occur in a previously toilet-trained child. Adolescent girls may have vaginitis caused by *Candida*, which thrives in the hyperglycemic tissues. Symptoms develop gradually and insidiously but have usually been present less than a month. Approximately 30% of new onset cases of diabetes are ill with diabetic ketoacidosis (DKA), a type of metabolic acidosis (American Diabetes Association, 2005). See page 1237 for more information on DKA. See Box 29–1 for information about cystic fibrosis-related diabetes.

BOX 29–1
CYSTIC FIBROSIS-RELATED DIABETES

Cystic fibrosis-related diabetes (CFRD) has similar features of types 1 and 2 diabetes; however, it is considered a separate condition. In cystic fibrosis, the pancreas does not produce sufficient insulin (as in type 1 diabetes), which is referred to as **insulin deficiency**. Another mechanism of CFRD is **insulin resistance**, in which the body fails to utilize insulin normally, requiring more insulin for metabolism. Insulin deficiency and insulin resistance, combined in the patient with cystic fibrosis, can lead to the development of diabetes more frequently in these patients than in the general population (Cystic Fibrosis Foundation, 2006).

CLINICAL MANIFESTATIONS | DIABETES BY TYPE

Cause	Clinical Manifestations	Clinical Therapy
Type 1—immune-mediated, insulin deficiency due to pancreatic beta-cell destruction	Polyuria, polydipsia Recent weight loss, but may be overweight Ketoacidosis on initial presentation in 30–40% of cases, at continued risk for ketoacidosis Short duration of symptoms Ketosis Initial period of decreased insulin requirement, then need insulin for survival	Blood glucose monitoring Insulin Dietary management, balancing carbohydrate intake to insulin Exercise
Type 2—insulin resistance with relative insulin secretory defect	Obese, little or no weight loss, or may have significant recent weight loss Acanthosis nigricans Long duration of symptoms Polyuria, polydipsia, may be mild or absent Glycosuria without ketonuria in 33% of cases on initial presentation Ketoacidosis on initial presentation in 5–25% of cases Lipid disorders Hypertension Androgen-mediated problems such as acne, hirsutism, menstrual disturbances, polycystic ovary disease Excessive weight gain and fatigue due to insulin resistance	Diet with decreased calories and low-fat foods Decrease sedentary activity time or increase routine physical activity Blood glucose monitoring Oral medication (metformin) to improve insulin sensitivity

COLLABORATIVE CARE

Diagnostic Tests

Diagnosis is based on the presence of classic symptoms and plasma glucose levels as follows (American Diabetes Association, 2005):

- Fasting plasma glucose ≥ 126 mg/dL (7 mmol/L), no caloric intake for at least 8 hours.
- Two-hour plasma glucose ≥ 200 mg/dL (11.1 mmol/L) during an oral glucose tolerance test.
- Plasma glucose concentration ≥ 200 mg/dL (11.1 mmol/L) taken at any time of day regardless of time of last meal.

When an asymptomatic child's screening test reveals an elevated glucose level, confirmation of a second fasting plasma glucose level should be performed. An oral glucose tolerance test is rarely required. Other laboratory tests for known autoantibodies (e.g., glutamic acid decarboxylase (GAD-65), insulin autoantibodies, and islet cell cytoplasmic autoantibodies) can indicate an autoimmune attack against the insulin-producing beta cells of the pancreas, and may be helpful in some cases to distinguish between type 1 and type 2 diabetes. A careful history is necessary to rule out a stress-related illness, corticosteroid use, fracture, acute infection, cystic fibrosis, pancreatitis, or liver disease.

Clinical Therapy

The majority of children (those without diabetic ketoacidosis) can receive initial and ongoing treatment and education in an outpatient program with a diabetes team; however, some children will be hospitalized. Clinical therapy for type 1 diabetes focuses on glycemic control by combining insulin, nutrition management to support growth and maintain blood glucose at near normal levels, an exercise regimen, and psychosocial support.

INSULIN THERAPY Children often need several daily injections of insulin before meals and at bedtime to maintain an optimal blood glucose level. Several forms of insulin are available as identified in the medications table below. Multiple approaches to insulin therapy for children and adolescents are available, and an approach that works for the child and family should be selected.

> ### CLINICAL TIP
> Insulin is usually provided in prepackaged doses of 100 units/mL. Diluted insulin prepared by a pharmacist may be used for infants and toddlers who require a small insulin dosage. Insulin mixtures (e.g., 70% NPH/30% regular, 50% NPH/50% regular, and 75% NPH/25% insulin lispro) are also available. Insulin cartridges, disposable pens, and other devices are available, making insulin easy to carry by adolescents for frequent insulin injections during the day.

MEDICATIONS USED TO TREAT *Diabetes Mellitus and Average Insulin Action Times (Subcutaneous Route)*

Type	Onset	Peak	Duration	Action
Rapid Acting				Insulin is an endogenous hormone, secreted by the beta cells of the pancreas. It lowers the blood glucose level by stimulating glucose passage across cell membranes and uptake into the cells. It also promotes the conversion of glucose to glycogen and inhibits hepatic glucose production from glycogen.
Insulin lispro or Insulin aspart	5–10 min	0.5 to 2 hr	3–4 hr	
Short Acting				
Regular	1/2–1 hr	2–5 hr	6–8 hr	
Intermediate Acting				
NPH or Lente	1–3 hr	5–8 hr	12–18 hr	
Long Acting				
Ultralente	3–4 hr	8–15 hr	22–26 hr	
Very Long Acting				
Glargine or Detemir	1.5–4 hr	None	20–24 hr	

From: Rachmiel, M., Perlman, K., & Daneman, D. (2005). Insulin analogues in children and teens with type 1 diabetes: Advantages and caveats. *Pediatric Clinics of North America, 52,* 1651–1675.

The basal-bolus insulin regimen has been documented to result in stable glycemic control and less hypoglycemia in comparison to other regimens using intermediate and short insulin regimens (American Diabetes Association, 2005). Insulin can be administered by an insulin pump or by multiple daily injections. With basal-bolus therapy, basal insulin is administered once a day using glargine, and then a bolus of rapid-acting insulin is administered with each meal and snack based on the carbohydrate grams consumed. This means that a child may get 6 to 7 injections a day. Stress, infection, and illness may either increase or decrease insulin needs. If basal-bolus therapy for type 1 diabetes is to be effective, the child and family need to do each of the following:

- Monitor the blood glucose four to eight times a day and once a week at midnight and 3 a.m.
- Consistently count carbohydrates consumed
- Anticipate exercise in the daily routine

Continuous subcutaneous insulin infusion (CSII) pump therapy is increasingly used by children and adolescents as the technology makes it possible to more closely match the plasma insulin levels in normal children. CSII pump therapy has been used successfully in children of all ages, including infants and toddlers. Insulin therapy can now be adjusted to the lifestyle of the child or adolescent (Weinzimer, Sikes, Steffen et al., 2005). Advantages and disadvantages of an insulin pump are outlined in Table 29–3. CSII has been found to improve metabolic control in youth with type 1 diabetes (Doyle, Weinzimer, Steffen et al., 2004).

For some children, insulin therapy involves multiple daily injections with combinations of rapid-, short-, intermediate-, or long-acting insulin before meals and at bedtime to maintain blood glucose levels (American Diabetes Association, 2005). One example of multiple daily injection therapy consists of two or three doses of short-acting insulin combined with intermediate-acting insulin (Figure 29–8▶).

The goal of insulin therapy is to maintain a range of blood glucose levels that varies by the child's age. See Table 29–4. Glycemic goals for children younger than 6 years old are generally less tight since they lack the cognitive capacity to recognize and respond to hypoglycemic symptoms (American Diabetes Association, 2004).

CLINICAL TIP

Advantages of rapid-acting insulin in therapy to achieve tight glucose control include:
- Decreased number of nocturnal hypoglycemic episodes
- Matching the insulin to the actual food intake of an infant or toddler; this is very helpful when their food intake is unpredictable
- Flexibility for adolescents concerned about weight gain who do not want to eat a mid-morning snack

Table 29–3	ADVANTAGES AND DISADVANTAGES OF AN INSULIN INFUSION PUMP

Advantages	Disadvantages
• Delivers a continuous infusion of insulin to match the basal rate needed plus an insulin bolus at mealtime to more closely simulate normal pancreatic function • Helps maintain blood glucose control between meals; decreases HbA1$_c$ level • Improves growth in children • Reduces number of injections, reduces number of injection sites, so variation in absorption decreases • New pumps calculate bolus insulin dose to carbohydrates consumed • Allows child to eat with less adherence to a schedule and have more flexible lifestyle • Reduces frequency of severe hypoglycemia and incidence of DKA	• Requires motivated child and supportive parents and healthcare professionals • Requires willingness to live connected to a device (can be disconnected for short periods by removing or clamping the catheter; however, DKA can occur within hours of interruption of insulin flow) • The site must be changed every 2–4 days, at least 1 inch from the last site; involves changing syringe, catheter, and skin setup • Must still monitor blood glucose levels and carbohydrates consumed • Infections can occur at the injection site • Weight gain is common when blood glucose control improves

Data From: Saudek, C. D. (1997). Novel forms of insulin delivery. *Endocrinology and Metabolism Clinics of North America, 26*(3), 599–610; Maniatis, A. K., Klingensmith, G. J., Slover, R. H., Mowry, C. J., & Chase, H. P. (2001). Continuous subcutaneous insulin infusion therapy for children and adolescents: An option for routine diabetes care. *Pediatrics, 107*(2), 351–356; and Miller, M. M. (2003). Insulin pump therapy. *Advance for Nurse Practitioners, 11*(11), 61–66.

Figure 29–8 ➤ Insulin therapy using multiple doses of short-acting insulin combined with intermediate-acting insulin. Blood glucose levels often vary over the 24-hour period in relation to injections and mealtimes.

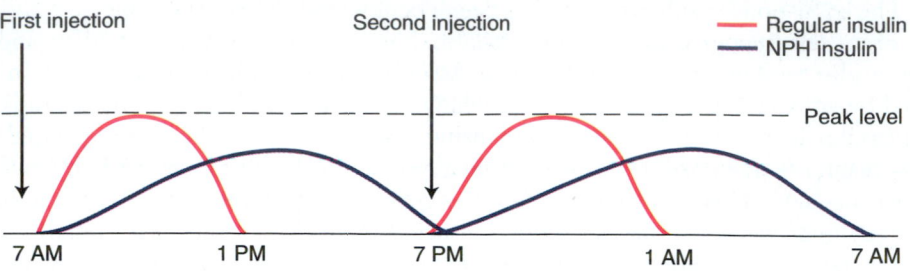

Insulin therapy is evaluated every 3 months with a hemoglobin A1c (HbA1c) level, an objective measurement of glycemic control. It represents the amount of glucose irreversibly attached to the hemoglobin molecule over an extended period (the life span of the red blood cell, approximately 120 days), therefore predicting an index of glucose control over the prior 6 to 8 weeks (Haller, Stalvey, & Silverstein, 2004). The HbA1$_C$ is below 6.2% for individuals without diabetes. See Table 29–4 for the HbA1$_C$ goals for children of different ages. It is also important to determine if the HbA1c matches recorded blood sugars.

EXERCISE PROGRAM   Physical activity is associated with increased insulin sensitivity. Like all children, those with diabetes need 30 to 60 minutes of exercise each day. Regular exercise and fitness improves glucose control, reduces cardiovascular risk factors, contributes to weight loss, and improves overall well-being. Blood lipid levels are also positively affected. However, the child must have an adequate caloric intake to prevent hypoglycemia. Excessive exercise associated with sports requires careful planning and management.

NUTRITION THERAPY   Consideration of the child and family's cultural, lifestyle, and financial issues is important in developing an individualized nutrition plan. Daily caloric requirements are individualized for each child according to his or her needs to support growth and development and for disease management.

Carbohydrate counting provides flexibility in meal planning and is simple for children and adolescents to use. One carbohydrate choice equals 15 grams of carbohydrates. Younger school-age children can consume two to four carbohydrate choices per meal, while older children and adolescents can consume four to six. Additional carbohydrate choices are necessary for more physically active children. Between-meal snacks generally consist of one to two carbohydrate choices, depending on the type of insulin used (Evert, 2004). Generally, one unit of insulin covers 8 grams of carbohydrates, making insulin dosage calculation for meal coverage relatively easy; however, a different ratio of insulin to carbohydrates may be calculated for individual children. If additional carbohydrates are eaten at a meal or snack, the number of insulin units can also be adjusted, providing further flexibility. A high fiber diet is also recommended for improved control of blood glucose.

RESEARCH

Adolescent Diet and Diabetes

The dietary intake of 132 adolescents with diabetes was compared with that of 131 adolescents without diabetes. Both groups had a mean age of 12 years and were comparable by sex, race, ethnicity, and stage of pubertal development. Using a 24-hour recall method, there was no difference in the number of calories consumed by the two groups. The diet of adolescents with diabetes consumed a greater percentage (and more grams) of fat and protein and a smaller percentage of carbohydrates than adolescents without diabetes. Of concern is the greater amount of saturated fat by adolescents with diabetes that may contribute to cardiovascular disease in the future (Helgeson, Viccaro, Becker et al., 2006).

Table 29–4	GOALS FOR BLOOD GLUCOSE AND HEMOGLOBIN A1$_C$ BY AGE OF THE CHILD		
	Blood Glucose Goals		
Age	**Before Meals**	**Bedtime/Overnight**	**Hemoglobin A1$_C$**
Children under 6 years	100 to 180 mg/dL	110 to 200 mg/dL	Greater than 7.5% and less than 8.5%
Children 6 to 12 years	90 to 180 mg/dL	100 to 180 mg/dL	Less than 8%
Adolescents 13 to 19 years	90 to 130 mg/dL	90 to 150 mg/dL	Less than 7.5%

From: American Diabetes Association. (2005). Care of children and adolescents with type 1 diabetes. *Diabetes Care, 28*(1), 193.

Many new developments for diabetes management are being evaluated. Studies of the effectiveness of inhaled insulin for bolus use in addition to injectable basal insulin are being conducted for use by adolescents (Quattrin, Belanger, Bohannon et al., 2004; Rachmiel, Perlman, & Daneman, 2005). Noninvasive or continuous glucose monitoring techniques are in development and will be an important advance when integrated into insulin pumps (Weinzimer, Sikes, Steffen et al., 2005). Pancreatic and islet transplant are not being aggressively pursued until improved immunosuppression therapy regimens are available (Casu, Trucco, & Pietropaolo, 2005).

Complications of type 1 diabetes (retinopathy, heart disease, renal failure, and peripheral vascular disease) result from long-term hyperglycemic effects on the blood vessels. Without careful management, diabetic children may develop renal failure and loss of vision in adulthood. Intensive therapy is expected to reduce the risk for or delay the development of these complications. Risk may be further reduced if the adolescent does not begin smoking and if the blood pressure is controlled.

NURSING MANAGEMENT
Nursing Assessment and Diagnosis

Nursing assessment focuses on a physiologic assessment of the child, but also the environmental, developmental, and psychosocial information that is important to collect to develop a nursing care plan for the family's management of a chronic illness.

Physiologic Assessment

Children are generally admitted to the hospital at the time of diagnosis. Assess the child's physiologic status, focusing on vital signs and level of consciousness. Assess hydration by checking mucous membranes, skin turgor, and urine output. Blood initially is collected hourly to monitor blood gases, glucose, and electrolytes. Once the child is stable, assess dietary and caloric intake and the ability of the child or family to manage care.

Psychosocial Assessment

Parents may feel guilty at the time of diagnosis if they waited to seek care until the child began to experience symptoms of diabetic ketoacidosis. Assess coping mechanisms, family strengths and resources, ability to manage the disease, and educational needs of both the child and parents. Identify family stressors that will cause challenges in long-term diabetes management. Examples of questions to use in assessing the family's strengths and limitations in the child's disease management include:

- Do both parents or the single parent work? What hours?
- Besides the parent(s), who is involved in the child's care?
- What is the child's usual daily schedule? Does the schedule vary on the weekend or any other days of the week?
- Does the child have health insurance? What coverage exists for diabetes education, treatment, and home management?
- Does the child have any cognitive, behavioral, motor, or visual problems coexisting with this condition?
- What other family stressors coexist with the diagnosis?

Developmental Assessment

Assess the child's developmental level, particularly fine motor skills and cognitive level. The child will need to learn how to obtain and read a blood glucose sample or inject insulin. Children can usually perform some of these tasks with supervision by 6 to 8 years of age.

Adolescents perceive type 1 diabetes as a disability and often deny having the disease so they can be like their peers when eating and exercising. Talk with the adolescent and assess problem-solving skills associated with daily condition management, and their ability to manage special circumstances such as illness or changes in exercise. Self-management

MediaLink

Care Plan Activity: An Adolescent with Type 1 Diabetes

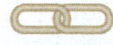
SKILL 8–3
Administering Subcutaneous Injection

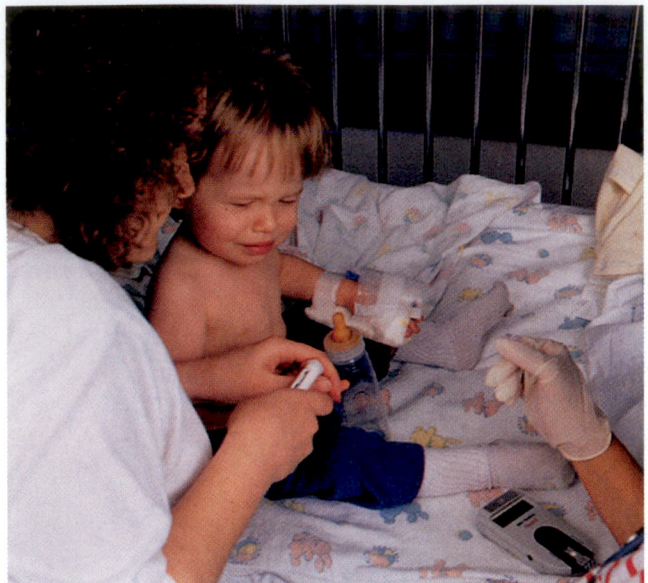

Figure 29–9 ➤ This mother is being taught how to test her child's blood glucose level.

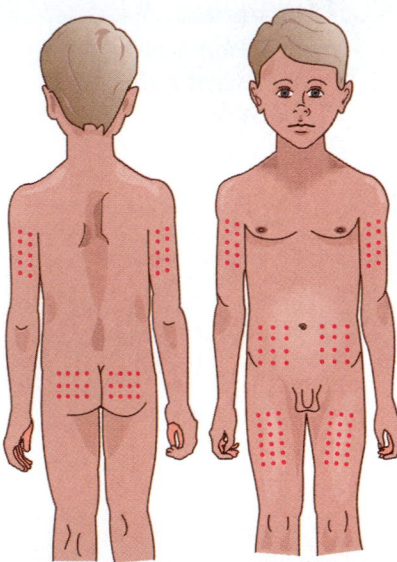

Figure 29–10 ➤ Insulin injection sites. Give all morning insulin in one site (e.g., arms) and all evening insulin in another (e.g., legs) because of different rates of absorption from these sites. Space injections about 1/2 inch (1.25 cm) apart.

GROWTH & DEVELOPMENT

Insulin Requirements
Insulin requirements usually increase as the child grows. Requirements are usually even higher during puberty due to the influences of increased growth hormone and sex hormone secretion (American Diabetes Association, 2005).

is the eventual goal, and the child's responsibilities are gradually increased.

Several diagnoses that may apply to the child newly diagnosed with type 1 diabetes are provided in the accompanying Nursing Care Plans. Additional diagnoses that may be appropriate include the following:

- Risk for Deficient Fluid Volume related to active fluid loss associated with hyperglycemia
- Ineffective Breathing Pattern related to neuromuscular dysfunction associated with metabolic acidosis
- Ineffective Denial related to inability to admit impact of disease on lifestyle

Planning and Implementation

Nursing care focuses on teaching the child and parents about the disease and its management, planning dietary intake, providing emotional support, and planning strategies for daily management in the community. Refer to the accompanying nursing care plans, which summarize nursing care for the child who is hospitalized with newly diagnosed type 1 diabetes, and the child who is receiving care in the community. Some hospitals have developed clinical pathways to streamline and standardize diabetes care.

Provide Education

The nurse is an important member of the management team (physician, nurse, nutritionist, diabetes educator, and social worker) and is usually responsible for educating the child and family. An advance practice nurse or diabetic nurse educator is often responsible for teaching in the clinic setting, since children may be hospitalized only briefly following diagnosis.

The timing and amount of information provided are especially important in the first days following diagnosis. Both the child and parents are very tired, and they are often in a state of shock and disbelief. Information presented during this period needs to be repeated. Use this time to assess learning needs and to answer the family's questions. Provide an overview of diabetes. Initial teaching focuses on the survival skills necessary for home management including the following: insulin administration, blood glucose testing, record keeping, meal planning, and the recognition and treatment of both hypoglycemia and hyperglycemia (Habich, 2006).

Explain the goals of insulin therapy. Teach the child and parents how to draw up and administer insulin and to perform blood glucose tests (Figure 29–9➤). Rotating the injection sites is important to decrease the chances of *lipoatrophy*, loss of subcutaneous tissue, or hypertrophy, in which collagen is replaced by fat cells (Figure 29–10➤). The absorption rate of insulin varies by the site used. Insulin is usually absorbed most rapidly from the abdomen; however, insulin absorption is increased in the extremities with exercise. An understanding of the different types of insulin and their actions is essential.

Once the child and parents demonstrate understanding of this information, teach guidelines for recognizing and managing episodes of hyperglycemia during acute illness and using a sliding scale. A sliding scale indicates specific insulin dosages appropriate for a particular blood glucose level. The family also needs to learn "sick day" care guidelines to prevent diabetic ketoacidosis. (See Families Want to Know: Teaching About Sick Day Guidelines.)

Caution parents to check the blood glucose level of a toddler who is extremely sleepy or irritable, as these can be signs of either hypoglycemia or hyperglycemia.

Manage Food Intake

While no specific meal plan is recommended for children with diabetes, 50–55% of their calories should be carbohydrates, 15–20% of their calories should be protein, and 30% of their calories should be fat (Haller, Atkinson, & Schatz, 2005). The child needs ade-

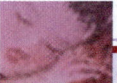

FAMILIES WANT TO KNOW

Teaching About Sick Day Guidelines

When the child with diabetes is sick, parents need to be extra attentive to the child's glycemic control. The following recommendations should be followed (Boland & Grey, 2004):

- Seek medical attention for fever or other signs of infection
- Monitor the blood glucose levels more often than routine (every 1 to 4 hours)
- Test urine ketones when the blood glucose level is greater than 200 mg/dL

- The usual dose of insulin may be increased for high blood glucose levels
- Do not skip doses of insulin
- Maintain a large fluid intake (more than 8 oz hourly) even if the child cannot eat to maintain food and fluid intake; seek medical attention if this is not possible. Fluids should have carbohydrates to maintain the child's usual caloric intake.

---

quate calories to reach or maintain a desirable body weight. The Food Guide Pyramid (see Chapter 4 ∞) may be used to teach the child and family the correct portions and which foods are considered carbohydrates, fats, and proteins. A variety of simple and complex carbohydrates should be eaten. An increased ratio of polyunsaturated fats should be eaten to reduce serum lipid levels.

Eating at consistent intervals is important for glycemic control, whether counting carbohydrates or following a conventional meal plan (three meals a day and three snacks a day). Although the child with diabetes is not restricted from eating any food, the child and parents need to learn about the relationship between foods eaten and insulin needed. Meal plans also need to be adjusted for exercise. Non-nutritive sweeteners such as aspartame and saccharin may be used in moderation. The child and family should learn how to read food labels. The meal plan should be customized, with the assistance of a nutritionist, to the child's age, cultural and family food preferences, and activity level.

Provide Emotional Support

The diagnosis of type 1 diabetes often comes as a shock to the family. If there is a familial history, parents may feel guilty about having caused the disease. The diagnosis of a chronic disease that requires daily management can be difficult to accept. Give parents information about diabetes education programs, put them in touch with other parents of diabetic children, and help them to learn the role they can play in managing the disease. It is important to help the family develop the practices and routines needed to adhere to the regimen of care while they are open to guidance.

Support for the child depends on his or her age and developmental stage. Encourage the child to express feelings about the disease and its management. The adolescent may benefit from contact with other adolescents who have diabetes. See Evidence-Based Practice: Adolescent Diabetes and Quality of Life.

Discharge Planning and Home Care Teaching

Home care needs should be identified and addressed before discharge. Initial survival skills described earlier are taught with the plans for ongoing outpatient education.

Make every effort to incorporate the diabetic regimen (insulin administration, food plan, blood glucose monitoring, and exercise) into the family's present lifestyle. The fewer changes the family has to make, the greater the chance of adherence.

The family and child that is newly diagnosed with diabetes should be made aware of the "honeymoon phase." This is a period during new-onset diabetes when the child has some residual beta-cell function, which reduces exogenous insulin requirements. The child and family may assume this is an indication that the diabetes "is better." However, insulin requirement does eventually return. The duration of this phase varies among individuals.

Make sure the parents inform all healthcare providers that the child has diabetes. Special planning is needed for diagnostic procedures and surgery that require the child to have food withheld for several hours to prevent the child from experiencing hypoglycemia or hyperglycemia.

NURSING CARE PLAN | The Child Hospitalized with Newly Diagnosed Type 1 Diabetes Mellitus

GOAL	INTERVENTION	RATIONALE	EXPECTED OUTCOME
1. Deficient Knowledge (Survival Skills) related to lack of exposure to diabetic management in the newly diagnosed child			
	NIC Priority Intervention: **Individual Teaching:** *Planning, implementation, and evaluating a teaching program designed to address a patient's particular need.*		*NOC Suggested Outcome:* **Knowledge:** *Extent of understanding conveyed about diabetic treatment regimen.*
The child and parents will acquire survival skills for home management.	• Assess the child's developmental level and select an educational approach and self-care activities to match.	• Learning goals for the child must match knowledge and skill expectations appropriate for developmental stage.	The child and parents demonstrate proper technique for blood glucose monitoring, urine testing for ketones, drawing up and injecting insulin doses, and record keeping.
	• Teach blood glucose monitoring, drawing up and injecting insulin, urine testing for ketones, record keeping, survival food guidelines, and when to call the healthcare provider.	• Diabetic management survival skills are needed for initial home management until more extensive education can be completed that permits more independent management.	
	• Use demonstration/return demonstration until the child and family are comfortable with procedures.	• Return demonstration permits evaluation, positive reinforcement, and guidance for modification of techniques.	
The child and parents will recognize signs and symptoms of hypoglycemia and hyperglycemia.	• Teach signs and symptoms of hypoglycemic and hyperglycemic reactions.	• Recognition of and treatment of poor glucose control will prevent progression of symptoms.	The child and family can describe symptoms of hypoglycemia and hyperglycemia.
	• Teach child to test blood glucose when feeling different than usual, and record the reading and symptoms felt.	• Permits child to learn his/her specific symptoms of hyper- and hypoglycemia.	
2. Risk for Injury related to potential episodes of hypoglycemia and diabetic ketoacidosis			
	NIC Priority Intervention: **Risk Identification:** *Analysis of potential risk factors, determination of health risks, and prioritization of risk reduction strategies for an individual or group.*		*NOC Suggested Outcome:* **Risk Control:** *Actions to eliminate or reduce actual, personal, and modifiable health threats.*
The child will experience few episodes of hypoglycemia during hospitalization.	• Assess the child at least every 2 hours for signs of hypoglycemia. If signs are present, check blood glucose to verify and administer the source of quick sugar.	• Hypoglycemia commonly occurs during hospitalization because of change in diet, lack of food intake, or illness.	The child and staff manage episodes of hypoglycemia without a crisis developing.
	• When the child is NPO for a special procedure, verify with physician when food, fluids, and insulin are to be given, or if an intravenous infusion with dextrose is to be given.	• Giving insulin without calorie intake can lead to hypoglycemia. Intravenous dextrose and insulin can be used when the child must be NPO.	
	• Have glucose paste or 50% dextrose solution readily available.	• Dextrose is used for emergency IV treatment of severe hypoglycemia. Glucose paste is used for oral treatment.	

NURSING CARE PLAN The Child Hospitalized with Newly Diagnosed Type 1 Diabetes Mellitus

GOAL	INTERVENTION	RATIONALE	EXPECTED OUTCOME
2. Risk for Injury related to potential episodes of hypoglycemia and diabetic ketoacidosis (continued)			
The child's condition is treated slowly to gradually reverse hyperglycemia and ketoacidosis and to prevent cerebral edema.	• Assess the child's mental status for improvement or deterioration.	• Improvement in mental status may indicate successful treatment. Deterioration may indicate onset of cerebral edema.	The child's hyperglycemia and ketoacidosis resolves without additional complications.
	• Check blood glucose and urine ketones frequently to confirm reduction in blood glucose level and ketosis, to identify the insulin dose for administration.	• Frequent blood glucose and ketone level determination helps assess progress in treating ketoacidosis.	
	• Monitor and control IV fluid intake. Measure output.	• The child with ketoacidosis will be dehydrated. IV fluid intake needs to be carefully controlled to prevent cerebral edema.	
	• Have insulin doses checked by a second nurse.	• Doses are frequently small, and the possibility of error is great.	
The child and parents will demonstrate emergency management of hypoglycemia.	• Identify sources of glucose to give in case of hypoglycemic reaction. Tell the child and parent to carry glucose tablets or paste with them at all times.	• Access to sources of glucose and its rapid administration are important for emergency care.	The child and family can identify several glucose sources for emergencies. The child and family have a source of glucose with them at each visit.
The child and parents will demonstrate management of sick days.	• Teach the child and family to test blood glucose and urine for ketones with acute symptoms and notify the healthcare provider.	• When the child is ill, hyperglycemia needs special management to prevent progression to ketoacidosis.	The child's hyperglycemic episodes do not progress to ketoacidosis.
3. Imbalanced Nutrition: Less than Body Requirements related to glycosuria			
	NIC Priority Intervention: **Nutrition Management:** *Assistance with or provision of a balanced dietary intake of foods and fluids.*		*NOC Suggested Outcome:* **Nutritional Status:** *Extent to which nutrients are available to meet metabolic needs.*
The child will eat a well-balanced diet and maintain normal height and weight proportions.	• Encourage and serve meals and snacks with a consistent number of carbohydrates at the same time each day.	• Keeps blood glucose levels stable during initial disease management stages.	The child regains weight lost and demonstrates normal growth and stable blood glucose levels.
	• Provide a calorie-nonrestricted diet.	• Enables weight lost during onset of diabetes to be regained.	
The child and parents will state understanding of dietary management of type 1 diabetes.	• Make an appointment with a nutritionist who can assess the child's favorite foods and promote their integration into the child's meal plan. Reinforce the dietary information taught.	• The nutritionist can develop dietary recommendations that fit the specific growth needs of the child and include favorite foods, thereby increasing compliance with the meal plan.	The child and parents describe nutritional needs of the child and select the dietary management best suited to the family's and child's eating habits.
	• Provide sample menus and teach the use of carbohydrate counting.	• Assists the family and adolescent with meal planning.	

NURSING CARE PLAN	The Child with Previously Diagnosed Type 1 Diabetes Being Cared for at Home

GOAL	INTERVENTION	RATIONALE	EXPECTED OUTCOME
1. Imbalanced Nutrition: Less than Body Requirements related to chronic illness (type 1 diabetes)			
	NIC Priority Intervention: **Nutrition Management:** *Assistance with or provision of a balanced dietary intake of foods and fluids.*		*NOC Suggested Outcome:* **Nutritional Status: Nutrient Value:** *Adequacy of nutrients taken into body.*
The child will eat a well-balanced diet that maintains weight proportional to height.	• Assess height and weight regularly and plot on growth chart.	• Assesses change in body mass index to identify potential weight problem early.	Diet records indicate meals and snacks have the appropriate distribution of carbohydrates, protein, and fats, and daily caloric intake goals are met.
	• Review the child's 24-hour intake on a weekday and a weekend day to assess adequacy of calories and proportion of carbohydrates, protein, and fats in foods consumed. Obtain information about usual exercise.	• Dietary recall provides information to help guide recommendations for changes in food plans to match growth needs and usual exercise routines.	Food intake is adequate for growth and exercise.
	• Make an appointment with a nutritionist who can assess the child's favorite foods and integrate them into a food plan that controls caloric intake. Encourage the child to keep a food diary.	• Inclusion of the child's favorite foods helps the child adapt to changes in the food plan.	
2. Readiness for Enhanced Family Processes related to management of a chronic disease			
	NIC Priority Intervention: **Family Process Maintenance:** *Minimization of family process disruption effects.*		*NOC Suggested Outcome:* **Family Functioning:** *Ability of family to meet the needs of its members through developmental transitions.*
The child and family will manage the food plan, exercise, blood glucose monitoring, and medications regimen.	• Assess the family's lifestyle and attempt to fit the child's care needs into the family's schedule.	• Fitting the care to the family's lifestyle promotes adherence with regimen.	The child and family make minimal changes in usual lifestyle while managing the type 1 diabetes.
	• Discuss the family's routines for special occasions and vacations. Identify ways to modify the child's management for these occasions.	• It is important for the child to participate in special events with the family and peers as a normal child to promote psychologic development.	
3. Ineffective Coping (Individual) related to inadequate level of confidence in ability to cope			
	NIC Priority Intervention: **Coping Enhancement:** *Assisting a patient to adapt to perceived stressors, changes, or threats which interfere with meeting life demands and roles.*		*NOC Suggested Outcome:* **Coping:** *Actions to manage stressors that tax an individual's resources.*
The child will demonstrate enhanced coping skills.	• Ask how the child has solved problems in the past. Review possible problems the child may encounter. Together evaluate the effectiveness of solutions. Suggest other solutions to consider.	• Children's success in mastering maturational conflicts and daily psychosocial problems will influence their pattern of coping.	The child demonstrates enhanced coping skills and expresses positive attitude toward self. The child displays warmth and affection toward the family.

NURSING CARE PLAN	The Child with Previously Diagnosed Type 1 Diabetes Being Cared for at Home (continued)		
GOAL	**INTERVENTION**	**RATIONALE**	**EXPECTED OUTCOME**
3. Ineffective Coping (Individual) related to inadequate level of confidence in ability to cope (continued)			
The child will develop positive self-esteem.	• Role-plays ways to talk about diabetes with friends and teachers. Encourage the child to express feelings about diabetes to those he or she trusts.	• Sharing information about the condition helps others understand changes in lifestyle needed by the child. Expressing feelings decreases anxiety.	
	• Encourage the child to attend diabetes camp.	• Learning and support networks experienced at camp can promote development of self-esteem.	
	• Encourage the child to continue previous social activities and hobbies.	• Increased social interaction, especially in group sessions, improves self-esteem.	
4. Health-Seeking Behaviors (Child) related to learning self-management of chronic disorder			
	NIC Priority Intervention: **Self-Modification Assistance:** *Reinforcement of self-directed change initiated by the patient to achieve personally important goals.*		*NOC Suggested Outcome:* **Health-Seeking Behavior:** *Actions to promote optimal wellness, recovery, and rehabilitation.*
The child will develop independent ability to manage diabetes care.	• Allow the child to perform as many self-care procedures as possible at each developmental stage.	• Normal growth and development are ensured if the child is encouraged to participate in care from the beginning.	The child is able to perform as many diabetic care techniques as possible for age.
	• Encourage the child to make decisions regarding care. Review decisions and discuss possible alternative solutions. Role-play possible scenarios.	• Trust develops when children sense that their decisions are respected or at least considered by others.	
	• Encourage parents to stay involved even when the adolescent takes primary responsibility for care.	• The child's diabetic control is likely to be better when the parents continue to show interest and supervise care.	
	• Provide 24-hour access to a physician or diabetes nurse educator. Encourage the child to seek help early.	• The child needs to overcome concerns about calling for guidance, and thus maintain better control.	

Provide written materials and refer parents to books and other materials they can use in teaching the child about diabetes. The Juvenile Diabetes Research Foundation and the American Diabetes Association are good sources of information.

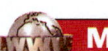 **MediaLink**

Diabetes Resources and Support

Care in the Community

During follow-up visits, ask the child or parents about signs indicating problems of diabetic control. Questions to ask that could help identify problems in diabetic control include:

- Is the child hungry at meals? Between meals?
- How much fluid is the child drinking?
- Has the child been going to the bathroom frequently or had episodes of bedwetting?
- Does the child have dry skin?
- Are there sores on the feet? Do scratches or scrapes take a long time to heal?
- Has the child had any skin infections?

EVIDENCE-BASED PRACTICE

Adolescent Diabetes and Quality of Life

Clinical Question

What factors are associated with how adolescents with diabetes view their quality of life?

Evidence

A descriptive correlational study exploring the quality of life for 69 adolescents with type 1 diabetes versus 75 healthy adolescents revealed that adolescents with diabetes expressed lower life satisfaction and health perception controls. The mean age for both groups was 15 years. The adolescents with diabetes experienced psychological and physiological turmoil while attempting to balance their treatment regimen. Additionally, Caucasian middle adolescents (ages greater than 15 years and less than 17 years) had lower life satisfaction than the younger (greater than 13 years and less than 15 years) and older (greater than 17 years and less than 19 years) adolescents. Differences in level of metabolic control were not associated with worries of life satisfaction among youth with diabetes (Faulkner, 2003). A study involving 115 adolescents with diabetes (ages 11 to 18 years) examined their perception of parental involvement, care, and control in relation to health-related quality of life and metabolic control. Their perceptions were compared to 9345 healthy adolescents and 291 adolescents with physical disabilities. Adolescents with diabetes reported a higher level of parental control than both healthy adolescents and adolescents with disabilities, and this higher level of control was significantly associated with a lower health-related quality of life. Adolescents with diabetes reported a significantly higher health-related quality of life score when they perceived a higher degree of parental care and in-

volvement, and a lower degree of parental control and overprotection. Their HbA1$_C$ level was not significantly related to perceptions of parental care, control, or involvement, potentially because of the challenges of maintaining metabolic control during puberty (Graue, Wentzel-Larsen, Hanestad et al., 2005).

Implications

Developmental tasks of adolescents focus on development of self-concept and self-esteem. This is an important consideration when working with them. Adolescents with type 1 diabetes must also cope with the increasing responsibility for complex self-management, including insulin administration, blood glucose testing, exercise, and nutrition. Self-esteem and self-concept often become linked with the disease as peers react to the differences noted. Life satisfaction, perceived control, and worries associated with having diabetes are important considerations when counseling the teenager and family about diabetic management. Additionally, it is important to know that adolescents value parental involvement and care rather than having it be perceived as a reason for conflict. Parental involvement and supervision is important in helping adolescents transition successfully to self-management of their disease.

Critical Thinking

What are some possible reasons for adolescents in the middle age range to perceive a lower life satisfaction than younger or older adolescents? How will you address quality of life issues with adolescents in different age groups? What questions can be used to explore an adolescent's perceptions of family involvement, care, and control?

- Does the child have changes in mood (depression, unexplained sadness, irritability) or energy level from day to day or throughout the day?
- Have there been any changes in vision?

Record growth measurements and vital signs in the child's chart. Review the child's typical dietary intake and exercise regimens. Assess the child's sexual development using the Tanner staging guidelines (see Chapter 5 ∞). Puberty may be delayed if diabetic control is inadequate. Evaluation for the potential complications of diabetes should be performed annually, including blood for lipid levels, blood pressure, liver and renal function, urine for albumin, an ophthalmologic examination for retinopathy, and a neurologic examination of the extremities for neuropathies.

Education is ongoing, especially for children who develop diabetes at a young age. As they grow and assume more responsibility for their care, remember that they need to learn more about the pathophysiology of the disease and the rationale for its management. New advances in diabetes care needs to be integrated into the ongoing education.

Continually work with the child to help him or her assume responsibility for self-care, and with parents to promote the child's self-care (Figures 29–11▶ and 29–12▶). The child's developmental stage and cognitive level influence his or her readiness to take on responsibility for self-care. Summer camps and other programs for diabetic children are often helpful in providing education and support.

The preschool child's need for autonomy and control can be met by allowing the child to choose snacks or to pick which finger to stick for glucose testing and by helping parents to gather necessary supplies. School-age children can learn to test blood glucose, administer insulin, and keep records. They should be taught how to select foods and portion sizes appropriate for dietary management and how to plan food intake for an exercise program. School-age children need to learn to recognize the signs of hypoglycemia and hyperglycemia, and understand the importance of carrying a rapidly absorbed sugar product.

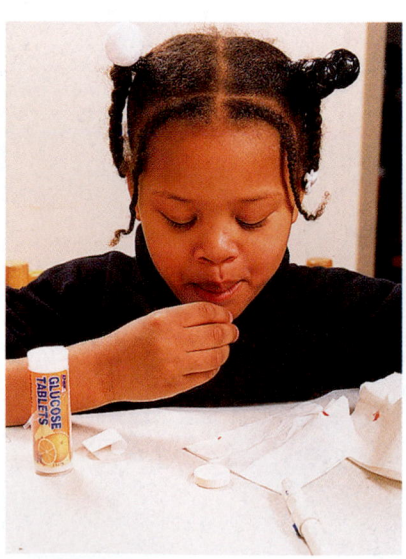

Figure 29–11 ▶ This girl is old enough to understand the need to take glucose tablets or another form of a rapidly absorbed sugar when her blood glucose level is low.

Although adolescents understand explanations about the potential complications of diabetes, they are present-time oriented, and may rebel against the daily regimen of insulin injections, the food plan, and the exercise plan. Successful self-care depends in part on the adolescent's adjustment to the chronic nature of the disease and feelings of being different from peers. Although the adolescent is able to manage self-care, the desire to be like peers may interfere with treatment adherence. Adolescents with high levels of depressive symptoms are at an increased risk for hospitalization (Stewart, Rao, Emslie et al., 2005). Talk with the adolescent to assess his or her mood and to evaluate his or her motivation to manage the meal plan, exercise regimen, blood glucose monitoring, and insulin therapy. Discuss how carbohydrate counting and insulin dose adjustment may provide the flexibility to participate in activities with peers. Collaborate with the adolescent in preparation to assume care, and assist parents in accepting the growing independence from adult supervision. A discussion of the hazards associated with having diabetes and the use of alcohol, drugs, and tobacco should occur.

The child with diabetes should be treated as any other child without a chronic condition, including limit setting and consistent discipline for unacceptable behavior. Children with type 1 diabetes may learn maladaptive behaviors, using their disease to obtain something they want. Teach parents to be alert to signs of maladaption, such as helpless, demanding, or whining behaviors, and any evidence of poor coping. Additional behaviors may include skipping blood glucose testing and losing or damaging equipment. Food may become a battleground for toddlers who are picky eaters, but must eat enough for the insulin dose. Referral for counseling may be appropriate for some families.

The child with type 1 diabetes may develop circulatory and neurologic changes over time. Emphasize the importance of good foot care from an early age; for example, wearing clean cotton socks; changing socks and shoes when they are damp; washing, drying, and powdering feet; and keeping toenails short.

Explain to parents that the child should wear some type of medical alert identification. Help them have an Individual Health Plan developed (see Chapter 12 ∞) to ensure that school administrators and teachers can identify the signs of hypoglycemia or hyperglycemia and provide emergency management.

Evaluation

Expected outcomes of nursing care for children with type 1 diabetes can be found in the Nursing Care Plans on pages 1232–1235.

Diabetic Ketoacidosis

Diabetic ketoacidosis (DKA) is the common and potentially life-threatening condition that occurs primarily in children with type 1 diabetes. Potential causes of DKA include incorrect or missed insulin doses or administration just under the skin, an illness, trauma, or surgery. DKA is found in 20–40% of children with new-onset type 1 diabetes (Haley-Andrews & Mackenzie, 2005).

Insulin deficiency is accompanied by a compensatory increase in hormones (epinephrine, norepinephrine, cortisol, growth hormone, and glucagon) that are released when inadequate glucose is delivered to the cells. The muscle cells break down protein into amino acids that are then converted to glucose by the liver, leading to hyperglycemia. The adipose tissue releases fatty acids that are transformed by the liver into ketone bodies. Their accumulation leads to ketoacidosis. The hyperglycemia causes an osmotic diuresis resulting in dehydration, acidosis, and hyperosmolarity. The rising ketones lead to metabolic acidosis. DKA is associated with severe metabolic, electrolyte, and fluid imbalances. See Chapter 16 ∞.

Characteristic signs of DKA include polyuria, polydipsea, weight loss, abdominal pain, nausea and vomiting, tachycardia, signs of dehydration, flushed ears and cheeks, Kussmaul respirations, acetone breath, altered level of consciousness, and hypotension. Hyperglycemia, glycosuria, and ketonuria are also present. In response to metabolic acidosis, children complain of abdominal or chest pain, nausea, and vomiting. The disorder may progress to electrolyte disturbances, arrhythmias, altered

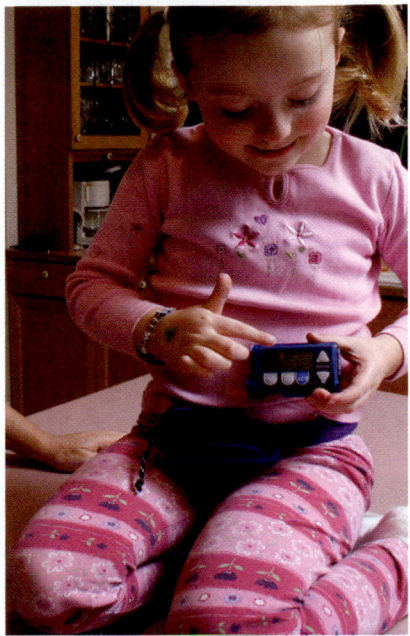

Figure 29–12 ➤ This young girl is learning to check her insulin pump, which she carries in a pouch around her waist.

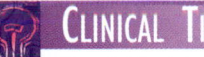

MediaLink

Health Promotion and Maintenance Overview: Diabetes

CLINICAL TIP

The child with diabetes needs an Individual Health Plan (IHP) for management of diabetes while in school or childcare. Information that should be included in the IHP includes: when blood glucose testing should be performed, insulin administration and storage, meals and snacks needed, symptoms and management of hypoglycemia and hyperglycemia. Parents need to ensure that the school or childcare provider has all essential equipment and supplies for the child's management as well as phone numbers for the parents and the child's healthcare provider for diabetes (American Diabetes Association, 2006a).

consciousness, shock, and death if untreated. Cerebral edema is a life-threatening complication associated with treatment that has the following signs and symptoms: headache, irritability, confusion, altered consciousness, vomiting, pupillary changes, irregular respirations, inappropriate slowing of the heart rate, and widening pulse pressure.

DKA is diagnosed by the following criteria: blood glucose level greater than 11 mmol/L (200 mg/dL), a venous pH less than 7.3 and/or bicarbonate less than 15 mmol/L (Dunger, Sperling, Acerini et al., 2004). In addition, the child has glycosuria, ketonuria, and ketones in the blood. Electrolyte disorders also occur (hyperkalemia, hyperchloremia, hyponatremia, hypophosphatemia, hypocalcemia, and hypomagnesemia). The BUN and creatinine are elevated due to dehydration.

The child with DKA is usually hospitalized. Medical management includes isotonic intravenous fluids and electrolytes to treat dehydration and acidosis. Short-acting insulin (0.1 unit/kg per hour) is given by continuous infusion pump to decrease the serum glucose level at a rate not to exceed 100 mg/dL/hr. Faster reduction of hyperglycemia and serum osmolality increases the risk for cerebral edema. Mannitol is kept on standby for treatment of neurologic deterioration. Bicarbonate is not routinely used for treatment of DKA as it places the child at increased risk for hypokalemia, acidosis, and cerebral edema (Glaser, 2005). As insulin is administered, potassium shifts to the cells, resulting in hypokalemia. Potassium supplementation is given only after confirmation of renal function.

Cerebral edema complicates approximately 1% of cases of DKA, and typically occurs 2 to 4 hours after treatment for DKA begins (Dunger, Sperling, Acerini et al., 2004). Cerebral edema is the most common cause of DKA-related deaths (Glaser, 2005). See Chapter 26 ∞ for information about cerebral edema.

NURSING MANAGEMENT   Continuously monitor the child's vital signs, respiratory status, perfusion, and mental status. Assess for changes in neurologic status, respiratory pattern, blood pressure, and heart rate. Attach a cardiac monitor and observe for arrhythmias associated with hypokalemia. Frequently monitor the electrolytes and acid-base status, and the blood glucose levels and urine ketone levels. Monitor intake and output and assess for dehydration.

When the child is severely dehydrated or in shock, intravenous fluids may be given in boluses of 10 to 20 mL/kg rapidly over 5 minutes. See Chapter 21 ∞ for management of hypovolemic shock. Enough fluids are given to reverse the fluid deficit. Replace electrolytes as needed. The insulin infusion must be carefully maintained to control the gradual reduction in hyperglycemia. The child is weaned off of intravenous insulin and transitioned to subcutaneous insulin when clinically stable. Oral feeding is introduced when the child is alert and the glucose level is stabilized.

The prevention of future episodes of DKA is important. As Gina, in the opening scenario, and her parents recognized with this episode of DKA, they need to learn strategies to keep hyperglycemic episodes from progressing to DKA. See the clinical manifestations table on the following page. Sick day care guidelines have been developed for that purpose. For example, the child's urine should be tested for ketones if three or four consecutive blood glucose readings are higher than 200 mg/dL, or if the child is sick. If the child has a high blood glucose and moderate or large amounts of ketones, treatment with extra insulin and fluids can be initiated. This monitoring is especially important when the child has significant stressors such as an illness. It is important for the child and family to know that insulin is needed even when the child is not eating to counter the hormones secreted in response to the stressor. See Families Want to Know: Preventing DKA.

Hypoglycemia

Hypoglycemia can develop within minutes in children with type 1 diabetes mellitus. The symptoms outlined in the clinical manifestations box on the following page may occur when blood glucose levels suddenly drop or fall below 70 mg/dL. Children are at risk of hypoglycemia due to their rapid growth rates, unpredictable eating habits, and physical activity. Severe hypoglycemia episodes may occur at night in children

---

CLINICAL TIP

Insulin binds to IV tubing. Let 50 to 100 mL run through new IV tubing to saturate all the binding sites. This assures that the full dose of insulin reaches the child from the outset.

CLINICAL MANIFESTATIONS | HYPOGLYCEMIA AND HYPERGLYCEMIA

Cause	Clinical Manifestations	Clinical Therapy
Hypoglycemia • Insulin dose too high for food eaten • Insulin injection into muscle • Too much exercise for insulin dose • Too long between meals/snacks • Too few carbohydrates eaten • Illness, stress	*Rapid onset* Irritability, nervousness, tremors, shaky feeling, difficulty concentrating or speaking, behavior change, confusion, repeating something over and over Unconsciousness, seizure, shallow breathing, tachycardia Pallor, sweating Moist mucous membranes, hunger Headache, dizziness, blurred vision, double vision, photophobia Numb lips or mouth	If conscious, give 15 grams of carbohydrate. Wait 15 minutes and recheck blood glucose level. Give another 15 grams of carbohydrate if blood glucose level is 70 mg/dL or less. Recheck the blood glucose level in 15 minutes. If unconscious, give glucagon by injection.
Hyperglycemia • Insulin dose too low for food eaten • Illness or injury, stress • Too many carbohydrates eaten • Meals/snacks too close together • Insulin injected just under skin or injected into hypertrophied areas • Decreased activity	*Gradual onset* Lethargy, sleepiness, slowed responses, or confusion Deep, rapid breathing Flushed skin, dry skin Gradual onset Lethargy, sleepiness, slowed responses, or confusion Deep, rapid breathing Flushed skin, dry skin Dry mucous membranes, thirst, hunger, dehydration Weakness, fatigue Headache, abdominal pain, nausea, vomiting Blurred vision Shock	Additional insulin given at usual injection time. Sliding scale insulin doses for specific blood glucose levels when ill or injured. Extra injections if hyperglycemia and moderate to large ketones. Increased fluids.

who are treated with two to three injections per day. Other common causes include an error in insulin dosage, errors in injection technique, inadequate calories because of missed meals, or exercise without a corresponding increase in caloric intake. Severe hypoglycemia can cause seizures.

Hypoglycemia can be diagnosed on the basis of the sudden onset of signs and symptoms. See the clinical manifestations table above. A blood glucose reading should be taken to confirm the diagnosis, since signs of hyperglycemia and hypoglycemia may be difficult to distinguish. Give glucose immediately but only in the form of a low-fat carbohydrate-containing snack or drink, sugar gel, glucose tablets, or glucose paste. The fat in the frosting, candy bars, and other higher fat snacks prevents the sugar from working quickly. In the hospital, administer an intravenous infusion of dextrose or

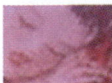

FAMILIES WANT TO KNOW

Preventing DKA

Call the child's healthcare provider if the child has the following signs (Boland & Grey, 2004):

- Vomiting more than two times or for longer than 4 hours
- More than five diarrheal stools
- Sick and cannot eat
- Altered mental status

- Temperature over 102°F (38.9°C)
- Blood glucose greater than 400 mg/dL on two separate readings, or greater than 200 mg/dL and moderate to large ketones
- Large ketones are present, acetone breath
- Evidence of a bacterial infection or urinary tract infection
- Trouble breathing

glucagons to prevent progression of symptoms. If the child becomes unconscious, sugar gel or glucose paste can be squeezed onto the gums or a glucagon injection can be given.

NURSING MANAGEMENT   Teach parents and children about the signs of hypoglycemia and the appropriate action to take. (See Families Want to Know: Treating Hypoglycemic Episodes.) Parents should be encouraged to check the child's blood glucose level when any signs of hypo- or hyperglycemia are noticed to help them learn which signs in their child are associated with hypoglycemia. Teach parents to give an intramuscular or subcutaneous dose of **glucagon** (a hormone produced by the pancreas that helps release stored glucose from the liver) for severe cases of hypoglycemia. Reinforce the importance of balancing dietary intake, insulin, and exercise every day. Since the effects of glucose, dextrose, and glucagon are temporary, additional snacks or a meal is provided once the child is alert. Monitor the child continually for several hours after treatment.

Type 2 Diabetes

Type 2 diabetes is a disease associated with obesity and insulin resistance (an impairment in insulin receptors on cell membranes, leading to inability to transfer sufficient amounts of glucose into cells). While it is sometimes connected to an insulin secretory defect in the pancreas (caused by a decrease in the beta-cell weight and number) and insulin deficiency (Gungor & Arslanian, 2004), it is more commonly associated with decreased insulin receptors at the cellular level. Significant risk factors for type 2 diabetes include obesity, low levels of physical activity, a diet high in fat, minority race (African American, Hispanic, Native American/Alaskan Native, or Asian/Pacific Islander), and family history of diabetes (Alemzadeh & Wyatt, 2004; Berry, Urban, & Grey, 2006b). Several genes on chromosomes 1q, 12q, 20q, and 7q are associated with the predisposition for development of type 2 diabetes (Vivian, 2006). Most children are diagnosed between the ages of 8 and 19 years (Berry, Urban, & Grey, 2006b).

The increasing number of children being diagnosed with type 2 diabetes has caused significant concern in the healthcare community. Up to 45% of children with a new diagnosis of diabetes have type 2 (Fagot-Campagna, Pettitt, Engelgau et al., 2000).

ETIOLOGY AND PATHOPHYSIOLOGY   Type 2 diabetes is a complex metabolic disorder with the central abnormality being insulin resistance. With the increased body weight, the visceral fat produces a cytokine hormone (tumor necrosis factor) that desensitizes the insulin receptor within cells to insulin. The pancreatic cells produce more insulin in an attempt to facilitate glucose transfer into the cells and to overcome the insulin resistance. This results in **hyperinsulinemia** (elevated insulin levels in the blood). The child maintains a balance between hyperinsulinemia and insulin resistance and a normal glycemic state. As insulin resistance worsens, the islet of Langerhans beta cells fail in their ability to hypersecrete insulin. This leads to impaired glucose tolerance and develops into overt diabetes. The onset of puberty and increased secretion of

FAMILIES WANT TO KNOW

Treating Hypoglycemic Episodes

- If the child shows signs of hypoglycemia (pallor, sweating, tremors, dizziness, numb lips or mouth, confusion, irritability, altered mental status), test the blood glucose level.
- Assist the child to do the test as skills needed to get an accurate reading deteriorate with altered mental status.
- If the blood glucose reading is 70 mg/dL or less, give glucose rapidly. Use one of the following to give 15 gm of rapid-acting glucose to raise the blood sugar level:
  - 1/2 cup fruit juice
  - 1/2 cup of regular cola or soda
- 1 small box raisins
- 3 to 4 glucose tablets
- Wait 15 minutes and recheck the blood glucose level. Repeat the rapid-acting glucose if it is still 70/mg/dL or less. Recheck the blood glucose level in another 15 minutes.
- Once blood sugar has returned to at least 80 mg/dL, give a more substantial snack such as cheese and crackers if the next meal will be more than 30 minutes later or an activity or exercise is planned.
- If the child is unconscious, administer IM or SQ glucagon.

the growth hormone is believed to be a contributing factor in the development of insulin resistance (Vivian, 2006).

CLINICAL MANIFESTATIONS   Signs and symptoms of type 2 diabetes upon initial presentation are usually different from type 1. See the clinical manifestations table on page 1225. Onset is more insidious, and a history of polydipsia and polyuria is uncommon (Alemzadeh & Wyatt, 2004). **Acanthosis nigricans**, hyperpigmentation and thickening of the skin with velvety irregularities in the skin folds of the neck, axillae, elbows, knees, groin, and abdomen, is a common finding associated with chronic hyperinsulinemia (Figure 29–13➤). The child is usually obese, with a high waist circumference. The child may present in diabetic ketoacidosis.

COLLABORATIVE CARE

Diagnostic Tests

Blood glucose levels of 200 mg/dL or greater without fasting, or a fasting glucose of 126 mg/dL or greater, are diagnostic of diabetes. Hemoglobin $A1_C$ provides an accurate indicator of the average serum glucose level for the past 120 days (life of a red blood cell). Urine is tested and ketones are found in about 50% of children. Islet cell autoantibodies, fasting insulin levels, glutamic acid decarboxylase autoantibody test (GAD-65), and C-peptid level are used to differentiate between type 1 and type 2 diabetes. The child with type 2 diabetes has normal or elevated fasting insulin and C-peptid levels while these levels are normally low in the child with type 1 diabetes. Islet cell and GAD-65 autoantibodies will not be present in the child with type 2 diabetes (Berry, Urban, & Grey, 2006a). A fasting lipid profile is obtained since dyslipidemia (primarily low HDL-C and elevated triglycerides) is usually present. High blood pressure for age, gender, and height percentile is also seen.

Clinical Therapy

The multiple goals for managing the child with type 2 diabetes include the following: normalizing the blood glucose and $HbA1_C$ levels, decreasing weight, increasing exercise, normalizing lipid profile and blood pressure, and preventing complications. Nutrition education and weight loss is the major therapy. The child needs to have gradual sustained weight loss, metabolic control of blood glucose levels, exercise, and emotional support.

If the child or adolescent presents with severe hyperglycemia or diabetic ketoacidosis, insulin will be required to gain initial glycemic control. Once metabolic control is achieved, oral medication (metformin) is initiated as the child is weaned off of insulin. Metformin is used when diet and exercise efforts are inadequate to control hyperglycemia. Metformin improves the sensitivity of target cells to insulin, slows the gastrointestinal absorption of glucose, and reduces the hepatic and renal glucose production. It can be used when there is normal liver and kidney function and no ketosis. The dosage may be gradually increased to improve metabolic control. If additional medication is needed, sulfonylurea or meglitinides may be used; however, they are not approved for use in children in the United States due to liver toxicity (Alemzadeh & Wyatt, 2004). Insulin may only be needed for periods of increased stress, but the adolescent may ultimately need insulin for glycemic control if weight and exercise goals are not met.

NURSING MANAGEMENT

Nursing Assessment and Diagnosis

Because the child with type 2 diabetes often does not have an acute onset, assess any child with a BMI greater than the 85th percentile for age and gender for signs of insulin resistance (acanthosis nigricans, hypertension, and dyslipidemia). Family history

> **NURSING ALERT**
>
> Several cases of children and adolescents with previously undiagnosed type 2 diabetes have been reported to have a hyperglycemic hyperosmolar state (HHS) that was confused with diabetic ketoacidosis and had a very high mortality rate. These children had life-threatening dehydration. Diagnostic criteria for HHS are blood glucose of greater than 600 mg/dL, serum carbon dioxide concentration of greater than 15 mmol/L, and serum osmolality greater than 320 mOsm/kg. Small amounts of ketones are present in the urine and sometimes in blood. The child's level of consciousness is significantly impaired with stupor or coma (Morales & Rosenbloom, 2004).

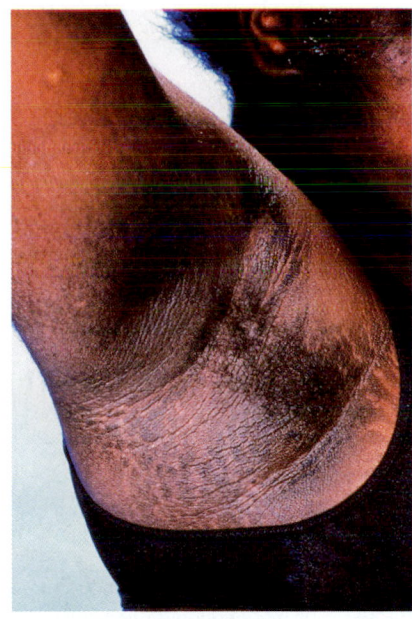

Figure 29–13 ➤ Acanthosis nigricans.
Courtesy of Audrey Austin, M.D., Children's National Medical Center, Washington, D.C.

CLINICAL TIP

Both the American Diabetes Association and the American Academy of Pediatrics recommend diabetes screening for children over 10 years of age when the child has a body mass index (BMI) greater than the 85th percentile for age and gender and at least two additional risk factors (Vivian, 2006):

- Family history of type 2 diabetes in a first- or second-degree relative
- Member of a high risk racial or ethnic group, such as Native American, African American, Hispanic, Asian American, or Pacific Islander
- Signs of insulin resistance or associated condition such as acanthosis nigricans, hypertension, dyslipidemia, or polycystic ovary syndrome

CLINICAL TIP

The American Diabetic Association considers a fasting glucose level of 100–125 mg/dL (5.6–6.9 mmol/l) to be an *impaired fasting glucose*, and a 2-hour postload glucose level of 140–199 mg/dL to be an *impaired glucose tolerance*. Individuals with impaired fasting glucose and/or impaired glucose tolerance are now referred to as having "pre-diabetes," indicating that they have a relatively high risk for development of diabetes (American Diabetes Association, 2006b).

CLINICAL TIP

Early intervention is needed to reduce the incidence of type 2 diabetes in an at-risk child, as well as potential complications, such as hypertension. Identify children at risk by carefully analyzing the family history, height, weight, and blood pressure measurements. Plot the growth measurements on the growth chart to identify the child who is overweight or at risk for overweight. Compare the blood pressure reading to the table of values for age, sex, and height to identify the risk for hypertension. Plan further interventions based upon the findings (Bindler & Bruya, 2006).

of diabetes in an overweight child is a reason to begin screening for the condition. Once the child has been diagnosed, monitor the child's blood glucose levels and blood pressure. Assess the child's diet and activity patterns to determine appropriate changes for disease management. Also consider evaluating the siblings for diabetes.

Nursing diagnoses that may apply to the child with type 2 diabetes include:

- Imbalanced Nutrition, More than Body Requirements related to high fat food intake and inadequate exercise
- Activity Intolerance related to sedentary lifestyle and disease state (insulin resistance)
- Fatigue related to disease state (insulin resistance)
- Ineffective Therapeutic Regimen Management (Family and Individual) related to family conflict over changing eating patterns
- Situational Low Self-Esteem related to situational crisis associated with diagnosis of new-onset chronic illness

Planning and Implementation

The child with type 2 diabetes may be hospitalized at the time of diagnosis because of ketoacidosis. However, the nurse in an inpatient setting is more likely to encounter this child when hospitalized for another condition or during healthcare visits in clinics or schools. Nursing care focuses on managing the child's blood glucose levels and hypertension during the hospitalization, assessing growth and dietary intake, evaluating goals for weight loss and exercise programs, and reviewing the child's knowledge about diabetes and strategies for management at home.

Care in the Community

Since the child is usually diagnosed and managed on an outpatient basis, nursing care focuses on teaching the child and parents about the disease and its management, managing dietary intake, providing emotional support, and planning strategies for daily management in the community.

Educate the child and family about the disease and lifestyle changes required for effective management of the condition. Focus on the need to increase activity with routine exercise of at least 30 to 60 minutes daily and by decreasing sedentary activity time, such as computer and television viewing time to no more than 2 hours daily. Customize the activity strategy for each child with motivation to develop a regular routine.

Work with the family to substitute alternatives to high-calorie and high-fat foods with a meal plan sensitive to the family's resources and ethnic preferences. Suggestions include limiting fast food and using fruits and vegetables as snacks rather than foods high in fat and sugar. Assess the child's height, weight, and BMI on each visit, and plot on the appropriate growth curve for age and gender on each visit. A gradual sustained weight loss or decrease in BMI is the goal. If the child is experiencing a growth height spurt, maintenance of weight rather than weight loss is the goal. Encourage the entire family to make dietary changes, especially since other family members are also at risk for the condition. The nutritional patterns in the family are a key part of treatment.

Teach the child and family to perform home blood glucose testing to monitor glycemic control. This will let the child and family know that efforts to manage the disease are successful. Take $HbA1_C$ levels at each visit to determine the average blood glucose level for the past 3 months. A $HbA1_C$ level of 7% or less is the goal. When dietary control and exercise are not successful in reducing blood glucose levels, teach the child and family about the prescribed oral medication.

Give the child and family chances to talk about the impact of the disease on their lives. Identify resources for information about strategies that have worked for other families. Identify local support groups and peer groups for the family and child.

Make sure the child gets annual evaluations for potential complications of diabetes. The tests to be performed include blood for lipid levels and lipoproteins, blood pressure, liver and renal function, urine for albumin, an eye exam for retinopathy, and a neurologic exam of the extremities for neuropathies. The child with type 2 diabetes has the same risk for developing long-term vascular complications as the child with type 1 diabetes when hyperglycemia is poorly controlled.

Evaluation

Examples of expected outcomes of nursing care include:

- The child decreases sedentary activity time to under 2 hours a day.
- The child's daily intake of fruits and vegetables increases to 5 to 8 daily and total fat intake decreases to less than 30% of total calories.
- The child's body mass index slowly and consistently decreases.

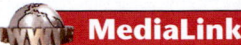

MediaLink

Type 2 Diabetes Resources

DISORDERS OF GONADAL FUNCTION

Gynecomastia

Gynecomastia is the presence of unilateral or bilateral enlarged breast tissue that occurs in about 65% of boys during puberty, usually at 13 to 14 years (Pinyerd & Zipf, 2005). It is sometimes confused with subcutaneous fat pads in obese boys. Gynecomastia occurs when the ratio of estrogen to testosterone is greater than the usual male ratio. It is also associated with Klinefelter's syndrome and drugs that increase the circulating concentration of prolactin such as marijuana, tricyclic antidepressants, and calcium channel blockers. The condition usually disappears in 1 to 2 years, and the amount of breast tissue varies among boys.

Nursing care focuses on reassuring the boy and his parents that gynecomastia is common and transient. Because of the body image concerns common during adolescence, embarrassment is a frequent problem. Recommend clothing styles and other methods to camouflage the enlarged breasts.

Amenorrhea

Amenorrhea, or lack of menstruation, may be primary or secondary. Criteria for primary amenorrhea include absence of menarche by age 14.5 years in association with no growth or development of secondary sexual characteristics or absence of menses by age 16 when secondary sexual characteristics and growth are present.

Secondary amenorrhea is the cessation of menstrual periods 6 months or 3 cycles after menstruation has begun; it is characterized by an absence of spontaneous bleeding for at least 120 days. Pregnancy is the most common cause of secondary amenorrhea in adolescents. It is common for adolescents to have irregular menstrual cycles and duration of the menstrual period for 1 to 2 years after menarche. A large number of cycles are anovulatory for the first 2 years after menarche.

Primary amenorrhea is most often caused by structural defects of the reproductive system; chromosomal abnormalities (such as Turner's syndrome); or hypothalamic or pituitary tumors, thyroid dysfunction, or polycystic ovary syndrome. No underlying pathologic condition is found in some adolescents. Primary or secondary amenorrhea may be found in competitive athletes and in youth with anorexia nervosa (see Chapter 4 ∞).

A thorough history (including sexual activity), physical examination, and laboratory evaluation are required to determine the cause of amenorrhea. The history focuses on asking questions about recent excessive weight loss or gain; excessive physical activity or sports training; chronic illness; use of illegal drugs, birth control pills, or phenothiazines; emotional problems; and age of the mother at menarche. The physical examination focuses on evaluating the adolescent's stage of sexual development and assessing for hirsutism (see Chapter 5 ∞). A vaginal exam is performed to determine vaginal patency and if the vaginal mucosa is estrogenized. A pregnancy test is performed. Bone age and hormone levels are evaluated (estrogen, LH, FSH, and prolactin).

Treatment of amenorrhea depends on the specific cause. The most common approach is to prescribe birth control pills containing both estrogen and progesterone. Athletic teenagers are encouraged to eat a well-balanced, high-calorie diet. Calcium

---

GROWTH & DEVELOPMENT

Female Athletics and Inadequate Nutrition

Girls competing in sports such as gymnastics, ballet, and long-distance running need to maintain a low weight and an ideal body type. The inadequate nutrition and strenuous activity may cause the hypothalamus to inhibit gonadotropin-releasing hormone and to increase corticotropin secretion. Low serum estradiol levels result (Sanfilippo, 2004). Amenorrhea or oligomenorrhea and bone demineralization often result. This, in turn, may increase the girl's risk of fractures and osteoporosis in young adulthood. See Chapter 28 ∞.

supplements may be ordered. Estrogen with progesterone in low doses may be prescribed for athletes to reduce the risk for osteoporosis. Nursing management centers on patient education and emotional support. The goal is to maintain normal growth and development.

Dysmenorrhea

Dysmenorrhea (menstrual pain or cramping) is a common complaint of adolescent girls. Primary dysmenorrhea occurs in the absence of pathologic disorders. Dysmenorrhea accounts for more hours of missed school by females than any other cause. The prevalence increases from 38–39% at age 12 years or Tanner stage III, to 66–72% at age 17 years or Tanner stage V. Approximately 15% of adolescent females are incapacitated by dysmenorrhea for 1 to 3 days a month (Slap, 2003).

Primary dysmenorrhea is usually caused by an increased secretion of prostaglandins that are produced during the ovulatory cycle. Prostaglandin causes smooth muscle contraction in the uterus, leading to ischemia and pain. In secondary dysmenorrhea, a pathologic condition, such as endometriosis or pelvic inflammatory disease, has been identified.

Dysmenorrhea usually occurs prior to the beginning of the menstrual period and ends on the second day of the period. The cramping pain in the lower abdomen and pelvic region ranges from mild to severe and varies with the individual. Pain may also radiate to the back or thighs. Other symptoms may include nausea, headache, backache, vomiting, diarrhea, fatigue, and urinary frequency.

A gynecological examination may be conducted to rule out any structural abnormalities for primary and secondary dysmenorrhea. Uterine, rectovaginal, and adnexal tenderness is found in 76% of adolescents with endometriosis (Slap, 2003). Vaginal and cervical cultures are taken when a sexually transmitted infection is possible. See Chapter 25 ∞.

The treatment of choice is nonsteroidal anti-inflammatory drugs (NSAIDs) such as ibuprofen and naproxen sodium. These drugs inhibit prostaglandin synthesis, which leads to a reduction in uterine activity and pain. Oral contraceptives may be prescribed to prevent ovulation and to decrease prostaglandin production. An increase in protein, magnesium, calcium, and vitamin B_6 may help relieve symptoms.

Nursing Management

Nursing care centers on providing patient education and emotional support. For females with chronic dysmenorrhea, instruct the adolescent to keep a calendar and begin taking NSAIDs 1 day before the onset of the menstrual period. The medications should be taken with food to minimize side effects.

DISORDERS RELATED TO SEX CHROMOSOME ABNORMALITIES

Turner's Syndrome

Turner's syndrome is the most common sex chromosome abnormality in females. Affected girls have a missing, partial absence of, or abnormal X chromosome. It occurs in approximately 1 in 2000 to 5000 live female births (Halac & Zimmerman, 2004a). The cause of the chromosomal error is unknown. Approximately 99% of fetuses with the disorder are spontaneously aborted. In the absence of one X chromosome, the oocytes in the ovaries disappear and are nearly all gone by age 2 years. Other specific clinical manifestations are related to specific missing genes.

Characteristic clinical findings in the newborn include lymphedema of the hands and feet, a webbed neck, and a low hairline. During childhood, short stature becomes apparent (less than 5th percentile). During adolescence, there is a lack of breast development, pubertal delay, and amenorrhea. Other characteristic signs include cubitus valgus (increased angle at the elbow); scoliosis; broad chest with widely spaced nipples; hyperconvex fingernails; and dark and pigmented nevi (Figure 29–14▶). Few girls have all of these features.

COMPLEMENTARY THERAPY

Dysmenorrhea

Guided imagery, hypnosis, meditation, chiropractic massage, and reflexology are non-pharmacologic methods that may be useful in the relief of dysmenorrhea. Application of a heating pad may also be helpful. Intake of vitamin B6 with B complex vitamins, vitamin E, calcium, and magnesium may help relieve symptoms of dysmenorrhea (Shuler, Huebscher, Miller et al., 2004).

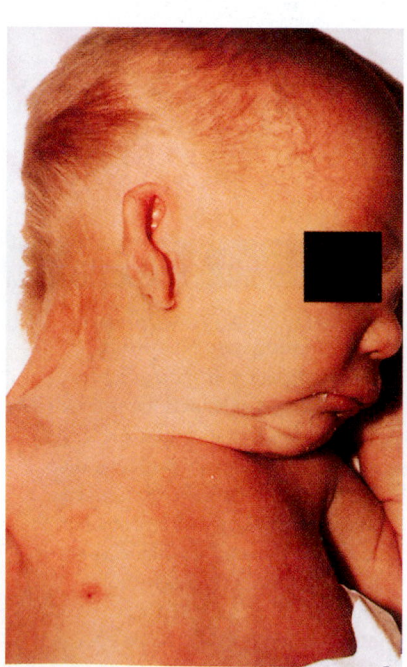

Figure 29–14 ▶ What characteristic physical manifestations of Turner syndrome can you identify in this girl? Note: From Zitelli, B. J., & Davis, H. W. (Eds.). (1997). *Atlas of Pediatric physical diagnosis*, (3rd ed., p. 14, Fig. 1–19a). St. Louis: Mosby.

Growth usually proceeds at a normal rate for the first 2 to 3 years of life and then slows. Breast tissue, which begins to bud at about 10 to 12 years, fails to develop fully. Only in rare instances does a girl with Turner's syndrome menstruate spontaneously or become able to conceive. Without treatment, final height is approximately 20 cm (7.8 in.) lower than the expected mean adult female height (Misra & Lee, 2005).

Among the conditions that may be associated with Turner's syndrome are congenital heart disease; coarctation of aorta; hypertension; kidney malformations; congenital lymphedema; hypothyroidism or Hashimoto's thyroiditis; hearing loss; ptosis, myopia, or amblyopia (lazy eye); inflammatory bowel disease; idiopathic hypertension; and scoliosis.

The condition is diagnosed definitively by a karyotype, which reveals the classic 45,X chromosome pattern or 46,XX pattern with one misshapen X chromosome. Turner's syndrome may be detected during prenatal testing with chorionic villus sampling or amniocentesis. Increased levels of alpha-fetoprotein, estradiol, and human chorionic gonadotropin, maternal progesterone, and inhibin A may be detected (Karnis & Reindollar, 2003).

Because of the incidence of certain disorders associated with Turner's syndrome, additional diagnostic testing should be performed at the time of diagnosis: echocardiogram to detect cardiac anomalies, renal ultrasound to detect kidney malformations, and hearing evaluations (Parker, Wyatt, Blethen et al., 2003).

Treatment involves careful monitoring of the child's growth. A growth chart made especially for girls with Turner's syndrome is available from the Turner Syndrome Society. Growth hormone therapy may be prescribed to promote growth during childhood and therapy can be begun at age 2 years (Halac & Zimmerman, 2004a). Low-dose estrogen therapy is usually begun after 12 years of age with a gradual dosage increase to mimic natural puberty (Tyler & Edman, 2004). This treatment produces pubertal changes such as breast development and pubic hair. Progesterone is added to the estrogen therapy to initiate cyclic menstrual periods.

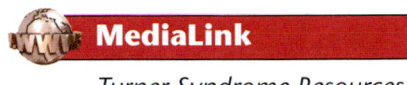

Turner Syndrome Resources

Nursing Management

Nursing assessment is focused on monitoring growth rates and observing for signs of cardiac, renal, gastrointestinal, vision, hearing, musculoskeletal, or thyroid dysfunction. Carefully measure the child's height and plot on the growth curve. Teach the family the correct administration of growth hormone and potential side effects.

The lack of growth and sexual development associated with Turner's syndrome presents problems not only for physical growth but also for psychosocial development. The girl's perception of her body and how she differs from peers affects self-image, self-consciousness, and self-esteem. In the United States, cultural values place importance on attaining normal to tall stature. Short children tend to be treated according to their size rather than their age. Emphasis is also placed on sexual maturity. Encourage parents to treat the child by her chronological age rather than size. The nurse can be instrumental in helping the child adapt to the condition and gain self-esteem. Be an active listener and reinforce abilities and skills that the girl exhibits. Encourage parents to provide support. The Turner Syndrome Society can provide additional information about the disorder for parents and adolescents.

Even though their intelligence is generally normal, these children have a higher incidence of learning problems because of memory, attention-deficit disorder, and visual-spatial deficits that affect performance on mathematical and manual dexterity tasks (Tyler & Edman, 2004).

Klinefelter's Syndrome

Klinefelter's syndrome is a common genetic condition that occurs in boys who have an extra X chromosome (usually 47,XXY). It occurs in approximately 1 in 600 male live births (Misra & Lee, 2005). It is the single most common cause of hypogonadism (decreased secretory activity of the gonad), androgen deficiency, and infertility in males.

Most infants appear normal at birth. The condition is usually diagnosed during the school-age years when the boy's behavior becomes a problem in the classroom. Boys with Klinefelter's syndrome may have delayed language development and auditory processing problems that are frustrating to the child. Intelligence quotient (IQ) scores may be similar to those of siblings, but academic difficulty is common because of memory, data retrieval skills, and verbal processing problems (Misra & Lee, 2005). Boys with Klinefelter's syndrome are tall and thin, with overly long arms and legs. The arm span is greater than height by 2 cm or more. The onset of puberty may be delayed with an abnormal progression. Testicular size is decreased at all ages. Less facial and body hair may develop. Gynecomastia is a characteristic finding. Associated conditions that occur with Klinefelter's syndrome include cardiac anomalies, pulmonary disease, dental abnormalities, and scoliosis.

Chromosomal analysis revealing one or more extra X chromosomes confirms the diagnosis. The goal of treatment is to stimulate masculinization and the development of secondary sex characteristics when adolescence is delayed. Testosterone replacement is begun when the boy is 11 or 12 years of age. A testosterone preparation is given by intramuscular injection every 3 to 4 weeks to maintain serum testosterone levels within the normal range. The dose is increased gradually until an adult dose is reached between 15 and 17 years of age; however, this does not improve fertility. Hormone treatment helps improve psychologic well-being and social functioning (Misra & Lee, 2005). It also helps to promote normal body proportions and prevent gynecomastia.

Nursing Management

Nursing care consists of educating the parents and child about the syndrome, evaluating the child's and family's coping mechanisms, assisting with school problems, and reinforcing the child's strengths. Encourage parents to channel their son's energy into areas that will provide opportunities for success and productive experiences. Emphasize the importance of rewarding the boy's successes in school, sports, or hobbies. Make genetic counseling available to adolescents, if indicated, because sexual functioning and fertility may be impaired.

INBORN ERRORS OF METABOLISM

Inborn errors of metabolism are inherited biochemical abnormalities of the urea cycle, amino acid, and organic acid metabolism. Therefore, protein, carbohydrate, fat, electrolyte, blood, and respiratory metabolism can be affected. Individually they are rare disorders; however, as a group they are a significant health problem in infancy.

The biochemical defect usually causes an abnormal chemical by-product to accumulate in the blood, urine, or tissues or results in a decreased amount of normal enzymes. Most disorders are associated with protein intolerance, and symptoms develop shortly after formula or breast milk feedings are begun.

Clinical manifestations usually occur within days or weeks of birth. Signs and symptoms may include lethargy and poor feeding, persistent vomiting, abnormal muscle tone and seizures, apnea and tachycardia, and an unusual urine or body odor (musty, sweet odor of maple syrup or burnt sugar, or cheesy or sweaty feet).

Newborn screening has been demonstrated to save lives and to prevent serious disability. The March of Dimes recommends that newborn screening tests for 29 disorders that have effective treatment be made available to all newborns (March of Dimes, 2006). In most states, newborn screening programs lead to the detection of several conditions before symptoms develop.

In some cases, disorders associated with inborn errors of metabolism are not detected until signs and symptoms are present. Initial laboratory tests include measurement of serum glucose, electrolytes, blood gases, and serum ammonia. Test results make it possible to classify the disorder by the presence of hypoglycemia, metabolic acidosis, hyperammonemia, or liver dysfunction. Further diagnostic laboratory tests are then performed on newborns with positive results.

Treatment, when available, focuses on replacing or reducing the amount of the substance causing the biochemical abnormality.

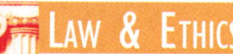

LAW & ETHICS

Neonatal Screening

As of May 2006, neonatal screening for congenital hypothyroidism, sickle cell disease, sickle C disease, sickle beta thalassemia, galactosemia, and phenylketonuria is mandated by state law in all 50 states. The majority of states also offer the newborn screening for the other disorders (National Newborn Screening and Genetics Resource Center, 2006). Many states obtain parental consent or allow parents to choose not to have their newborn screened.

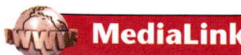

MediaLink

March of Dimes

Four of the more common inborn errors of metabolism—phenylketonuria, galactosemia, fatty acid oxidation defects, and maple syrup urine disease—are presented here. Congenital hypothyroidism and congenital adrenal hyperplasia, which are also considered inborn errors of metabolism, were discussed earlier in this chapter.

Phenylketonuria

Phenylketonuria (PKU) is an autosomal recessive inherited disorder of amino acid metabolism that affects the body's use of protein. It is caused by a mutation of the phenylalanine hydroxylase gene. The incidence is greater than 1 in 25,000 live births per year in the U. S. population (March of Dimes, 2006).

Children with PKU have a deficiency of the liver enzyme phenylalanine hydroxylase that normally breaks down the essential amino acid phenylalanine into tyrosine. As a result, phenylalanine accumulates in the blood, causing a musty or mousey body and urine odor, irritability, vomiting, hyperactivity, hypertonia, hyperreflexive deep tendon reflexes, seizures, and an eczema-like rash (Rezvani, 2004). Persistence of elevated phenylalanine leads to disruption of cellular processes of myelination and protein synthesis, and results in a seizure disorder and untreatable mental retardation.

Infants appear normal at birth except for lighter skin complexion than their non-affected siblings. If diagnosis is delayed, a mousey or musty body odor is noted and mental retardation may be severe. Microcephaly, prominent maxilla and widely spaced teeth, enamel hypoplasia, and growth retardation are other common findings in untreated children (Rezvani, 2004).

Screening for PKU is required by state law in all 50 states. For best results, the newborn should have begun formula or breast milk feeding before specimen collection. Early hospital discharge places newborns at risk for false negative screening tests if screened within 24 hours of birth. Screening needs to occur no sooner than 48 hours after birth, or the test should be repeated at 1 to 2 weeks of age, even when the initial screening test is negative. If the test shows elevated levels of plasma phenylalanine, a repeat quantitative test is performed. If the second test is positive, the family is referred to an outpatient treatment center. Serum phenylalanine should be measured periodically throughout life. Levels greater than 15 mg/dL are considered dangerous.

PKU is treated using special formulas (e.g., Lofenalac, Minafen, and Albumaid XP) and a diet low in phenylalanine to keep plasma phenylalanine levels between 2 and 6 mg/dL. The diet must also meet the child's needs for optimal growth. Breastfeeding is possible if phenylalanine levels are monitored. High-protein foods (meats and dairy products) and aspartame are avoided because they contain large amounts of phenylalanine. Elemental medical foods (modified protein hydrosylates in which the phenylalanine has been removed) are used instead. The low-phenylalanine diet should be maintained throughout life. If dietary control is lost before 6 years of age, there is a significant impact on IQ. The low phenylalanine diet is especially important for adolescent females and women prior to conception and during pregnancy to prevent congenital anomalies (low birth weight, microcephaly, mental retardation, and congenital heart defects) in the fetus (Rouse & Azen, 2004).

Nursing Management

Nursing care is mainly supportive and focuses on teaching parents about the disorder and its management. The low-phenylalanine diet is a rigid, strict diet that excludes many foods. Educate the family about sources of phenylalanine, and refer the family to a nutritionist to establish an appropriate meal plan. Parents and children need a great deal of support to promote compliance. The formula and elemental medical food costs are relatively high. The formula is usually reimbursed by insurance, but negotiations with health plans may help parents obtain some support for medical foods. The current recommendation is for all patients to remain on the phenylalanine restricted diet for life (Rezvani, 2004).

Like children with diabetes mellitus, children with PKU may rebel against the dietary limitations in an effort to be like their peers. Reinforcement of the need for

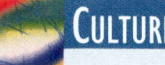

CULTURE

PKU

PKU is rare in African American, Latin American, Ashkenazi Jewish, and Japanese populations (Read & Charbonneau, 2004). It is more commonly found in isolated communities with numerous intermarriages between families over several generations.

dietary control is important during this time. Educate the child's teacher and school nurse about the child's special meal plan in an effort to encourage compliance while the child is at school.

Refer parents of an affected child who are considering a future pregnancy and adolescents with the disorder for genetic counseling.

Galactosemia

Galactosemia, a disorder of carbohydrate metabolism, has an autosomal recessive inheritance pattern. It occurs in greater than 1 in 50,000 live births (March of Dimes, 2006).

Galactosemia results from a deficiency of the liver enzyme galactose 1-phosphate uridyltransferase (GALT), one of three enzymes needed to convert galactose to glucose. The lack of enzyme leads to an accumulation of galactose metabolites in the eyes, liver, kidney, and brain, rapidly damaging the organs and causing life-threatening problems. Children become susceptible to gram-negative sepsis.

Early signs include poor sucking, failure to gain weight due to vomiting followed by diarrhea, hypoglycemia, and an enlarged liver. Later signs include mental retardation, jaundice, ascites, sepsis, lethargy, seizures, hypotonia, cataracts, and coma. Babies may die within 1 month of birth without treatment, usually due to sepsis. When diagnosis is not made at birth, damage to the liver (cirrhosis) and brain (mental retardation) become progressively more severe and irreversible.

Routine newborn screening for galactosemia is performed in almost all U. S. newborn screening programs (Larsson & Therrell, 2002). Infants who are not screened at birth are identified once they become symptomatic. The diagnosis is based upon history, physical examination, and laboratory tests (galactose, AST, and ALT are abnormally high). Urine specimens are checked for reducing substances (the Clinitest is positive and the Clinistix is negative) in several specimens while the infant is receiving human milk or formula with lactose.

Treatment involves placing infants on a lactose- or galactose-free formula (e.g., Nutramigen, a meat-based or soybean formula), which remains the child's milk substitute for life. Improvement in the infant's condition is generally seen within 24 hours. A galactose-free diet (no milk or cheese products, including foods with dry milk products) is prescribed when the infant is ready for solids. In spite of compliance with the diet, complications (learning disabilities, speech defects, ovarian failure, and neurologic syndromes) develop in many children.

Nursing Management

Nursing management focuses on educating the parents and child about the disorder and required diet, assessing coping abilities, and providing emotional support. Refer the family to a nutritionist for diet counseling. Families must learn to screen foods for added milk solids and to avoid medications, such as antibiotics, that have lactose fillers. Calcium supplementation may be needed. Advise parents that several galactose-free cheeses are sold commercially. Because the disorder is inherited, refer the family for genetic counseling.

Defects in Fatty Acid Oxidation

Mitochondrial oxidation of fatty acids is an energy-producing pathway that becomes essential during periods of starvation, when the body fuel converts from carbohydrate to fat. Gene defects can occur in nearly every stage in the fatty acid oxidation pathway, resulting in many subclasses of fatty acid oxidation defects. All of these defects are autosomal recessive traits that occur in both males and females. Most patients have a northwestern European ancestry (Venditti & Stanley, 2004).

Screening has revealed that fatty acid oxidation disorders are among the most common inborn errors of metabolism. Some of these defects include medium-chain acyl-CoA dehydrogenase (MCAD) deficiency (most common), long-chain acyl-CoA dehydrogenase (LCHAD) deficiency, and plasma carnitine deficiency. If undiagnosed, these disorders can lead to serious complications affecting the heart, liver, eyes, and muscular system, and can even cause death.

SKILL 7–7
Applying a Urine Collection Bag (Infant)

The most common presentation is an acute onset life-threatening coma and hypoglycemia induced by a period of fasting. Other manifestations often include cardiomyopathy, hepatomegaly, and muscle weakness. Infants and children can be asymptomatic except for times during fasting or stress.

Diagnosis can occur during routine newborn screening when laboratories use mass spectrometry. Most cases are identified during an acute presentation of symptoms when laboratory evaluation may include blood gases, electrolytes, hepatic profile, plasma lactate, plasma amino acids, urine organic acids, acylcarnitine profile, quantitative carnitine levels, and urine for ketones. Hypoglycemia is usually present and ketone levels are unusually low. Liver function tests demonstrate elevated transaminases, urea, and ammonia. Plasma and tissue concentrations of total carnitine are reduced. Skin biopsies are often obtained for fibroblast analysis. Physical examination may reveal hepatomegaly due to fatty infiltration.

Treatment of acute illnesses with 10% dextrose is needed to suppress lipolysis. Chronic therapy is to avoid fasting, ensuring that no more than 10 hours pass before food is eaten. Carnitine supplementation may be required in some disorders as it is useful in preventing low blood sugar and assists in removing metabolic waste from cells.

Nursing Management

Nursing management involves educating parents about the importance of frequent feedings and avoidance of fasting. These children should not go longer than 8 to 12 hours without food. Infants should be fed around the clock every 2 to 4 hours. If the infant or child is unable to sustain oral intake during an acute illness, he or she must be referred to the hospital for intravenous dextrose supplementation. Even simple infections such as an ear infection or influenza can become life-threatening for these children. Several snack foods and meals of low-fat and high-carbohydrate foods (i.e., cereal, pasta) are recommended throughout the day. Genetic counseling should be offered to the family. If one child in the family is diagnosed with the disorder, their siblings should also be tested, even if they are asymptomatic.

Maple Syrup Urine Disease

Maple syrup urine disease (MSUD), a disorder of amino acid metabolism, has an autosomal recessive inheritance pattern. It is rare (found in less than 1 in 100,000 live births) but has a higher incidence among some Pennsylvania Mennonites.

In MSUD, three essential amino acids (leucine, isoleucine, and valine) cannot be metabolized because of absent or defective enzyme branched-chain alpha-ketoacid dehydrogenase. This results in alpha ketoacidosis. All three amino acids are essential to form normal structures such as the hair, skin, and muscle. Leucine has the potential to build up in the brain and cause cerebral edema, progressive neurologic impairment, and death.

Within 3 to 7 days of life, the newborn develops symptoms of poor appetite, lethargy, vomiting, variable muscle tone, irritability, seizures, high-pitched cry, and a sweet odor of maple syrup in the body fluids. The symptoms may quickly progress to coma and death if not treated (Larsson & Therrell, 2002).

Most but not all states require newborn screening for this condition. Diagnosis is made with laboratory tests of the urine for positive ketones and blood tests for elevated leucine, isoleucine, alloisoleucine (a stereoisomer of isoleucine not normally found in the blood), and valine.

Treatment during the acute stage involves removal of the branch-chained amino acids and their metabolites from the tissues and body fluids. Some critically ill infants may require dialysis to remove these compounds as renal clearance is poor. Lifelong treatment with specially designed medical formulas and foods rich in amino acids, calories, vitamins, minerals, and other nutrients is required. These special medical foods have the three amino acids removed. The child needs special low-protein foods that are adequate for growth with enough calories to support twice the child's basal metabolic rate. Daily urine testing is required to determine if ketones are being excreted, an indication that the body is in a catabolic state. A liver transplant has been performed in a few affected children who were subsequently able to tolerate a normal diet (Rezvani & Rosenblatt, 2004). The long-term prognosis of affected children is guarded as severe ketoacidosis, cerebral edema, and death may occur during stressful situations such as infection and surgery.

Nursing Management

Nursing care includes educating the family about the disorder and special dietary requirements. The parents need to learn how to mix the child's special formula with natural protein source, amino acid supplements, and water. The child needs formula even when ill; parents should have a sick day plan to prevent ketoacidosis. The child should be permitted moderate exercise only to prevent increases in leucine levels. Help families identify sources of information or support groups who can share recipes and tips for managing the child's condition.

When the child starts childcare or school, it is important for teachers and other care providers to know foods the child should avoid and a list of snacks that can be used for special occasions. The child should have formula and other supplements available to ensure a steady intake of calories during the day. An Individual Health Plan should be developed with the school nurse so that teachers and other school personnel are informed.

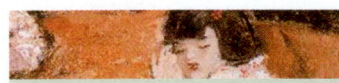

MediaLink

Inborn Errors of Metabolism Resources

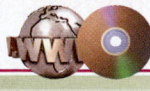

CRITICAL THINKING IN ACTION

Recall 16-year-old Gina in the opening scenario who has had type 1 diabetes since 12 years of age. She has just experienced hospitalization for diabetic ketoacidosis following an acute illness. She has been self-managing her diabetes with blood glucose testing, carbohydrate counting, and basal-bolus insulin injections five times a day. However, she does not get much exercise. Learning to manage this disease as a teenager has been difficult, because she wants to eat the same foods and participate in the same activities as her friends.

DISCUSSION

1. What strategies might help a newly diagnosed adolescent assume increasing responsibilities for self-management of diabetes?

2. What pathophysiologic changes occur with an illness or injury that lead to the need for careful monitoring and additional insulin?

3. Gina is interested in discussing use of an insulin pump. What are some advantages and disadvantages of using an insulin pump? How would Gina's diabetes management change?

4. Gina does not routinely exercise. What information should be discussed with Gina about the importance and benefits of exercise in her current and future health?

 Refer to your Prentice Hall Nursing MediaLink DVD-ROM for answers.

EXPLORE MediaLink http://www.prenhall.com/ball

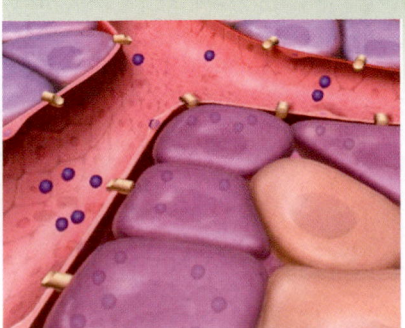

Resources for this chapter can be found on the Prentice Hall Nursing MediaLink DVD-ROM accompanying this textbook, and on the Companion Website at http://www.prenhall.com/ball.

DVD-ROM

Audio Glossary
NCLEX-RN® Review
Animations/Videos
  Hypothalamic-Pituitary Axis
  Physiology of Diabetes
  Responding to Hypoglycemia

COMPANION WEBSITE

Audio Glossary
NCLEX-RN® Review
Care Plan Activity: Adolescent with Type 1 Diabetes
Case Study: Child with Type 1 Diabetes Returning to School
MediaLink Application: Turner's Syndrome
WebLinks

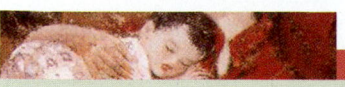

REFERENCES

Alemzadeh, R., & Wyatt, D. T. (2004). Diabetes mellitus in children. In R. E. Berhman, R. M. Kliegman, & H. B. Jenson (Eds.), *Nelson textbook of pediatrics* (17th ed., pp. 1947–1972). Philadelphia: W.B. Saunders Company.

Amer, K. S. (2005). Advances in assessment, diagnosis, and treatment of hyperthyroidism in children. *Journal of Pediatric Nursing, 20*(2), 119–126.

American Diabetes Association. (2004). Diabetes statistics for youth. Retrieved February 1, 2005, from http://www.diabetes.org/utils/printthispage.jsp?PageID-STATISTICS_233184

American Diabetes Association. (2005). Care of children and adolescents with type 1 diabetes. *Diabetes Care, 28*(1), 186–212.

American Diabetes Association. (2006a). Diabetes care in the school and day care setting. *Diabetes Care, 29*(Suppl. 1), S49–S55.

American Diabetes Association (2006b). Diagnosis and classification of diabetes mellitus. *Diabetes Care, 29*(Supp. 1), S43–S48.

Berry, D., Urban, A., & Grey, M. (2006a). Management of type 2 diabetes in youth (Part 2). *Journal of Pediatric Health Care, 20*(2), 88–97.

Berry, D., Urban, A., & Grey, M. (2006b). Understanding the development and prevention of type 2 diabetes in youth (Part 1). *Journal of Pediatric Health Care, 20*(1), 3–10.

Bindler, R. M., & Bruya, M. A. (2006). Evidence for identifying children at risk for being overweight, cardiovascular disease, and type 2 diabetes in primary care. *Journal of Pediatric Health Care, 20*(2), 82–87.

Boger, M. S., & Perrier, N. D. (2004). Advantages and disadvantages of surgical therapy and optional extent of thyroidectomy for the treatment of hyperthyroidism. *Surgical Clinics of North America, 84*, 849–874.

Boland, E. A., & Grey, M. (2004). Diabetes mellitus (Types 1 and 2). In P. J. Allen & J. A. Vessey (Eds.), *Primary care of the child with a chronic condition* (4th ed., pp. 426–444). St. Louis, MO: Mosby.

Brosnan, C. A., Upchurch, S., & Schreiner, B. (2001). Type 2 diabetes in children and adolescents: An emerging disease. *Journal of Pediatric Health Care, 15*(4), 187–193.

Carroll, K. L. (2006). Alterations of musculoskeletal function in children. In K. L. McCance & S. E. Huether, *Pathophysiology: The biologic basis for disease in adults and children* (5th ed., pp. 1547–1571). St. Louis: Elsevier Mosby.

Casu, A., Trucco, M., & Pietropaolo, M. (2005). A look at the future: Prediction, prevention, and cure including islet transplantation and stem cell therapy. *Pediatric Clinics of North America, 52*, 1779–1804.

Centers for Disease Control and Prevention. (2004). Diabetes projects. Retrieved December 10, 2004, from http://www.cdc.gov/diabetes/projects/cda2.htm

Cheetham, T., & Baylis, P. H. (2002). Diabetes insipidus in children. *Pediatric Drugs, 4*(12), 785–796.

Corbett, J. V. (2004). *Laboratory tests and diagnostic procedures* (6th ed.). Upper Saddle River, NJ: Prentice Hall Health.

Cystic Fibrosis Foundation. (2006). Nutrition: Cystic fibrosis: Changes through life. Retrieved May 29, 2006, from http://www.cff.org/UploadedFiles/living_with_cf/Files/Nutrition

Doyle, D. A., & DiGeorge, A. M. (2004). Disorders of the parathyroid. In R. E. Berhman, R. M. Kliegman, & H. B. Jenson (Eds.), *Nelson textbook of pediatrics* (17th ed., pp. 1890–1898). Philadelphia: W.B. Saunders Company.

Doyle, E. A., Weinzimer, S. A., Steffen, A. T., Ahern, J. H., Vincent, M., & Tamborlane, W. V. (2004). A randomized prospective trial comparing the efficacy of continuous subcutaneous insulin infusion with multiple daily injections using insulin glargine. *Diabetes Care, 27*(7), 1554–1558.

Dunger, D. B., Sperling, M. A., Acerini, C. L., Bohn, D. J., Daneman, D., Danne, T. P. A., et al. (2004). European Society for Paediatric Endocrinology/Lawson Wilkins Pediatric Endocrine Society consensus statement on diabetic ketoacidosis in children and adolescents. *Pediatrics, 113*(2), e133–e140.

Eugster, E. A., LeMay, D., Zerin, J. M., & Pescovitz, O. H. (2004). Definitive diagnosis in children with congenital hypothyroidism. *Journal of Pediatrics, 144*, 643–647.

Evert, A. B. (2004). Tools and techniques for working with young people with diabetes. *Diabetes Spectrum, 17*(1), 8–14.

Fagot-Campagna, A., Pettitt, D. J., Engelgau, M. M., Burrows, N. R., Geiss, L. S., et al. (2000). Type 2 diabetes among North American children and adolescents: An epidemiologic review and public health perspective. *Journal of Pediatrics, 136*(5), 664–672.

Failor, R. A., & Capell, P. T. (2003). Hyperaldosteronism and pheochromocytoma: New tricks and tests. *Primary Care: Clinics in Office Practice, 30*(4), 801–820viii.

Faulkner, M. S. (2003). Quality of life for adolescents with type 1 diabetes: Parental and youth perspectives. *Pediatric Nursing, 29*(5), 362–368.

Ferry, R. J. (2005). Salt wasting and the syndrome of inappropriate antidiuretic hormone. In T. M. Moshange, *Pediatric endocrinology: The requisites for pediatrics* (pp. 269–274). St. Louis: Elsevier Mosby.

Food and Drug Administration. (2006). Mecasermin injection (marketed as Increlex). Retrieved May 19, 2006, from http://www.fda.gov/cder/drug/InfoSheets/patient/MecaserminPIS.pdf

Gance-Cleveland, B. (2003). Adaptation to Addison's disease in a child: A case study. *Journal of Pediatric Health Care, 17*(6), 301–310.

Ginsberg, J. (2003). Diagnosis and management of Graves' disease. *Canadian Medical Association Journal, 168*(5), 575–585.

Glaser, N. (2005). Pediatric diabetic ketoacidosis and hyperglycemic hyperosmolar state. *Pediatric Clinics of North America, 52*, 1611–1635.

Graue, M., Wentzel-Larsen, T., Hanestad, B. R., & Sovik, O. (2005). Health-related quality of life and metabolic control in adolescents with diabetes: The role of parental care, control, and involvement. *Journal of Pediatric Nursing, 20*(5), 373.

Green, R. P., & Landt, M. (2002). Home sodium monitoring in patients with diabetes insipidus. *Journal of Pediatrics, 141*, 618–624.

Grimberg, A., & De León, D. D. (2005). Disorders of growth. In T. M. Moshange, *Pediatric endocrinology: The requisites for pediatrics* (pp. 127–167). St. Louis: Elsevier Mosby.

Grimberg, A., Kutikov, J. K., & Cucchiara, A. J. (2005). Sex differences in patients referred for evaluation of poor growth. *Journal of Pediatrics, 146*(2), 212–216.

Gungor, N., & Arslanian, S. (2004). Progressive beta cell failure in type 2 diabetes mellitus of youth. *Journal of Pediatrics, 144*(5), 656–659.

Habich, M. (2006). Establishing a standard for pediatric inpatient diabetes education. *Pediatric Nursing, 32*(2), 113–115.

Halac, I., & Zimmerman, D. (2004a). Coordinating care for children with Turner syndrome. *Pediatric Annals, 33*(3), 189–196.

Halac, I., & Zimmerman, D. (2004b). Managing growth hormone treatment in pediatric patients. *Pediatric Annals, 33*(3), 183–190.

Haley-Andrews, S., & Mackenzie, J. E. (2005). Pediatric diabetic ketoacidosis: Clinical presentations and nursing considerations. *Pediatric Emergency Care, 21*(9), 624–628.

Haller, M. J., Atkinson, M. A., & Schatz, D. (2005). Type 1 diabetes mellitus: Etiology, presentation, and management. *Pediatric Clinics of North America, 52*, 1553–1578.

Haller, M. J., Stalvey, M. S., & Silverstein, J. H. (2004). Predictors of control of diabetes: Monitoring may be the key. *Journal of Pediatrics, 144*(5), 660–661.

Harris, G. D., & Fawcett, G. F. (2002). Hypertensive endocrine disorders. *Clinics in Family Practice, 4*(3), 585–600.

Helgeson, V. S., Viccaro, L., Becker, D., Escobar, O., & Siminerio, L. (2006). Diet of adolescents with and without diabetes. *Diabetes Care, 29*(5), 982–987.

Henwood, M. J., & Katz, L. E. L. (2005). Disorders of the adrenal gland. In T. M. Moshange, *Pediatric endocrinology: The requisites for pediatrics* (pp. 193–213). St. Louis: Elsevier Mosby.

Herman-Giddens, M. E., Slora, E. J., Wasserman, R. C., Bourdony, C. J., Bhapkar, M. V., Koch, G. G., et al. (1997). Secondary sexual characteristics and menses in young girls seen in office practice: A study from the pediatric research in office settings network. *Pediatrics, 99*(4), 505–512.

Huang, E. A., Feldman, B. J., Schwartz, I. D., Geller, D. H., Rosenthal, S. M., & Gitelman, S. E. (2006). Oral urea for the treatment of chronic syndrome of inappropriate antidiuresis in children. *Journal of Pediatrics, 148*, 128–131.

Kache, S., & Ferry, R. J. (2005). Diabetes insipidus. In T. M. Moshange, *Pediatric endocrinology: The requisites for pediatrics* (pp. 257–267). St. Louis: Elsevier Mosby.

Karnis, M. F., & Reindollar, R. H. (2003). Turner syndrome in adolescence. *Obstetrics and Gynecology Clinics of North America, 30*, 303–320.

Kollars, J., Zarroug, A. E., van Heerden, J., Lteif, A., Stavlo, P., et al. (2005). Primary hyperthyroidism in pediatric patients. *Pediatrics, 115*(4), 974–980.

Lalwani, S., Reindollar, R. H., & Davis, A. J. (2003). Normal onset of puberty: Have the definitions changed? *Obstetrics and Gynecology Clinics, 30*(2), 279–286.

Larsson, A., & Therrell, B. L. (2002). Newborn screening: The role of the obstetrician. *Clinical Obstetrics and Gynecology, 45*(3), 697–732.

Lee, J. M., & Menon, R. K. (2005). Growth hormone for short children without growth deficiency: Issues and practices. *Contemporary Pediatrics, 22*(10), 46–53.

Lee, P. A. (2005). Early pubertal development. In T. M. Moshange, *Pediatric endocrinology: The requisites for pediatrics* (pp. 73–86). St. Louis: Elsevier Mosby.

Lee, P. A., & Kulin, H. E. (2005). Normal pubertal development. In T. M. Moshange, *Pediatric endocrinology: The requisites for pediatrics* (pp. 63–71). St. Louis: Elsevier Mosby.

Levine, L. S., & White, P. C. (2004). Disorders of the adrenal glands. In R. E. Behrman, R. M. Kliegman, & H. B. Jenson (Eds.), *Nelson textbook of pediatrics* (17th ed., pp. 1898–1921). Philadelphia: W.B. Saunders Company.

Maniatis, A. K., Klingensmith, G. J., Slover, R. H., Mowry, C. J., & Chase, H. P. (2001). Continuous subcutaneous insulin infusion therapy for children and adolescents: An option for routine diabetes care. *Pediatrics, 107*(2), 351–356.

March of Dimes. (2006). Quick reference: Recommended newborn screening tests: 29 disorders. Retrieved May 22, 2006, from http://www.marchofdimes.com/printableArticles/14332_15455.asp

Miller, M. M. (2003). Insulin pump therapy. *Advance for Nurse Practitioners, 11*(11), 61–66.

Misra, M., & Lee, M. M. (2005). Delayed puberty. In T. M. Moshange, *Pediatric endocrinology: The requisites for pediatrics* (pp. 87–101). St. Louis: Elsevier Mosby.

Morales, A. E., & Rosenbloom, A. L. (2004). Death caused by hyperglycemic hyperosmolar state at the onset of type 2 diabetes. *Journal of Pediatrics, 144*, 270–273.

National Newborn Screening and Genetics Resource Center. (2006). National newborn screening status report. Retrieved May 22, 2006 from http://genes-r-us.uthscsa.edu/nbsdisorders.pdf

Nebesio, T. D., Siddiqui, A. R., Pescovitz, O. H., & Eugster, E. A. (2002). Time course to hypothyroidism after fixed-dose radioblation therapy of Graves' disease in children. *Journal of Pediatrics, 141*(1), 99–103.

Palma Sisto, P. A. (2004). Endocrine disorders in the neonate. *Pediatric Clinics of North America, 51*(4), 1141–1168.

Pang, S. (2003). Newborn screening for congenital adrenal hyperplasia. *Pediatric Annals, 32*(8), 516–523.

Parker, K. L., Wyatt, D. T., Blethen, S. L., Baptista, J., & Price, L. (2003). Screening girls with Turner syndrome: The National Cooperative Growth Study experience. *Journal of Pediatrics, 143*, 133–135.

Parks, J. S. (2004). Disorders of the hypothalamus and pituitary gland. In R. E. Behrman, R. M. Kliegman, & H. B. Jenson (Eds.), *Nelson textbook of pediatrics* (17th ed., pp. 1845–1853). Philadelphia, PA: Saunders.

Pinyerd, B., & Zipf, W. B. (2005). Puberty—Timing is everything. *Journal of Pediatric Nursing, 20*(2), 75–82.

Quattrin, T., Belanger, A., Bohannon, N. J. V., & Schwartz, S. L. (2004). Efficacy and safety of inhaled insulin (Exubera) compared with subcutaneous insulin therapy in patients with type 1 diabetes. *Diabetes Care, 27*(11), 2622–2627.

Rachmiel, M., Perlman, K., & Daneman, D. (2005). Insulin analogues in children and teens with type 1 diabetes: Advantages and caveats. *Pediatric Clinics of North America, 52*, 1651–1675.

Read, C.Y., & Charbonneau, R. M. (2004). Phenylketonuria. In P. J. Allen & J. A. Vessey (Eds.), *Primary care of the child with a chronic condition* (4th ed., pp. 667–681). St. Louis, MO: Mosby.

Rezvani, I. (2004). Defects in metabolism of amino acids. In R. E. Behrman, R. M. Kliegman, & H. B. Jenson (Eds.), *Nelson textbook of pediatrics* (17th ed., pp. 398–402). Philadelphia: W.B. Saunders Company.

Rezvani, I., & Rosenblatt, D. S. (2004). Valine, leucine, isoleucine and related organic acidemias. In R. E. Behrman, R. M. Kliegman, & H. B. Jenson (Eds.), *Nelson textbook of pediatrics* (17th ed., pp. 409–421). Philadelphia: W.B. Saunders Company.

Roberts, C. G. P., & Ladenson, P.W. (2004). Hypothyroidism. *Lancet, 363*(9411), 793–803.

Rossi, W. C., Caplin, N., & Alter, C. A. (2005). Thyroid disorders in children. In T. M. Moshange, *Pediatric endocrinology: The requisites for pediatrics* (pp. 171–190). St. Louis: Elsevier Mosby.

Rouse, B., & Azen, C. (2004). Effect of high maternal blood phenylalanine on offspring congenital anomalies and developmental outcome at ages 4 and 6 years: The importance of strict dietary control preconception and throughout pregnancy. *Journal of Pediatrics, 144*, 235–239.

Rovet, J. F. (2005). Children with congenital hypothyroidism and their siblings: Do they really differ? *Pediatrics, 115*(1), e52–e57.

Rudock, A. S. (2002). Secondary hyperparathyroidism—current concepts and controversies. *Clinics in Family Practice, 4*(3), 639–642.

Sanfilippo, J. S. (2004). Gynecologic problems of childhood. In R. E. Behrman, R. M. Kliegman, & H. B. Jenson (Eds.), *Nelson textbook of pediatrics* (17th ed., pp. 1827–1844). Philadelphia: W.B. Saunders Company.

Saudek, C. D. (1997). Novel forms of insulin delivery. *Endocrinology and Metabolism Clinics of North America, 26*(3), 599–610.

Sepa, A., Wahlberg, J., Vaarala, O., Frodi, A., & Ludvigsson, J. (2005). Psychological stress may induce diabetes-related autoimmunity in infancy. *Diabetes Care, 28*(2), 290–295.

Shuler, P., Huebscher, Miller, H., & Rauckharst, L. (2004). Genitourinary concerns. In R. Huebscher & P. Shuler. *Natural alternative and complementary health care practices* (pp. 567–657). St. Louis: Mosby.

Slap, G. B. (2003). Menstrual disorders in adolescence. *Best Practice and Research Clinical Obstetrics & Gynecology, 17*(1), 75–92.

Stewart, S. M., Rao, U., Emslie, G. J., Klein, D., & White, P. C. (2005). Depressive symptoms predict hospitalization for adolescents with type 1 diabetes mellitus. *Pediatrics, 115*(5), 1315–1319.

Traggiai, C., & Stanhope, R. (2003). Disorders of pubertal development. *Best Practice and Research Clinical Obstetrics and Gynecology, 17*(1), 41–56.

Tyler, C., & Edman, J. C. (2004). Down syndrome, Turner syndrome, and Klinefelter syndrome: Primary care throughout the life span. *Primary Care Clinics for Office Practitioners, 31*, 627–648.

Venditti, C. P., & Stanley, C. A. (2004). Defects in metabolism of lipids. In R. E. Behrman, R. M. Kliegman, & H. B. Jenson (Eds.), *Nelson textbook of pediatrics* (17th ed., pp. 433–438). Philadelphia: W.B. Saunders Company.

Viera, A. J. (2002). Hyperparathyroidism. *Clinics in Family Practice, 4*(3), 627–638.

Vivian, E. M. (2006). Type 2 diabetes in children and adolescents—The next epidemic? *Current Medical Residents Opinion, 22*(2), 297–306.

Weinzimer, S. A., & Magge, S. (2005). Type 1 diabetes mellitus in children. In T. M. Moshange, *Pediatric endocrinology: The requisites for pediatrics* (pp. 3–18). St. Louis: Elsevier Mosby.

Weinzimer, S. A., Sikes, K. A., Steffen, A. T., & Tamborlane, W. V. (2005). Insulin pump treatment of childhood type 1 diabetes. *Pediatric Clinics of North America, 52*, 1677–1688.

Wilson, T. A., Rose, S. R., Cohen, P., Rogol, A. D., Backeljauw, P., et al. (2003). Update of guidelines for the use of growth hormone in children: the Lawson Wilkins Pediatric Endocrinology Society Drug and Therapeutics Committee. *Journal of Pediatrics, 143*(4), 415–421.

Witchel, S. F., & Finegold, D. N. (2002). Endocrinology. In B. J. Zitelli & H. W. Davis, *Atlas of pediatric physical diagnosis* (4th ed., pp. 315–336.). St. Louis: Mosby.

Zadik, Z., Sinai, T., Zung, A., & Reifen, R. (2005). Effect of nutrition on growth in short stature before and during growth-hormone therapy. *Pediatrics, 116*(1), 68–72.

ALTERATIONS IN SKIN INTEGRITY

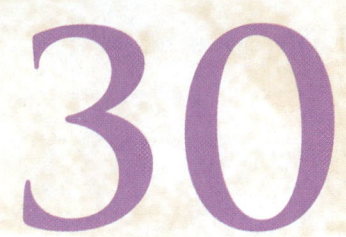

30

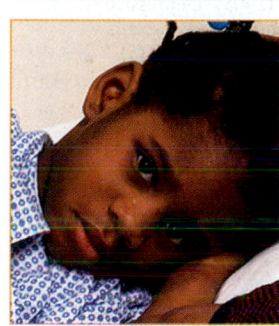

Shanelle, 6 years old, was admitted to the hospital with a deep partial-thickness burn after dropping a bowl of soup on her leg. By her second day of hospitalization, it was determined that Shanelle's burn was not full thickness and would need no skin grafting. Because parents often have a difficult time doing dressing changes due to the amount of pain it causes the child, Shanelle was discharged with twice weekly dressing changes scheduled in the hospital's burn clinic.

Shanelle has come into the clinic for her first debridement and a dressing change since being discharged 3 days ago. Shanelle's mother gave her the pain medication prescribed prior to leaving home for the clinic visit, but Shanelle is still anxious about how much the dressing change is going to hurt. Her mother is encouraged to stay with her during the dressing change and provide support. When the dressing and the exudate are removed, granulation tissue is seen and no odor indicating infection is present. Topical medication and the burn dressing are applied.

After the dressing change, some time is spent talking with Shanelle's mother. She reports that Shanelle has been eating the recommended high-protein, high-calorie diet to promote wound healing. She is concerned about how much trouble Shanelle has extending her leg and walking. She knows the movement hurts when it stretches the burned skin, but she wonders if Shanelle is moving her leg enough. She also wants to know what else she can do to help Shanelle cope with the burn injury.

MediaLink

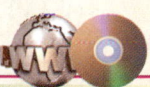

http://www.prenhall.com/ball

See the Prentice Hall Nursing MediaLink DVD-ROM and Companion Website for chapter-specific resources.

LEARNING OUTCOMES

After reading this chapter, you will able to do the following:

1. Describe important differences in the anatomy and physiology of the child's skin.
2. Identify the characteristics of different skin lesions caused by irritants, drug reactions, mites, infection, and injury.
3. Describe the stages of wound healing.
4. Identify the skin conditions that have a hereditary cause or hereditary predisposition.
5. Develop nursing care plans for a child with alterations in skin integrity, including dermatitis, infectious disorders, and infestations.
6. Develop an education plan for adolescents with acne to promote self-care.
7. Describe the process to measure the extent of burns and burn severity in children.
8. Develop a nursing care plan for the child with a full-thickness burn injury.
9. Identify preventive strategies to reduce the risk of injury from bites and stings.

FOCUS ON
The Integument System

ANATOMY AND PHYSIOLOGY

The skin is the largest organ in the body and performs several essential functions. The skin protects underlying tissues from invasion by microorganisms and from trauma. The nerves in the skin enable the perception of touch, pain, pressure, heat, and cold. The skin also assists the body to regulate its temperature. Dilation of blood vessels and the secretion of sweat by the eccrine sweat glands, functioning under the control of the central nervous system, enable the body to release excess heat. The sweat glands, secreting a solution of water, electrolytes, and urea, also help to rid the body of toxins. The skin supplements the body's intake of vitamin D by synthesizing this vitamin from ultraviolet light.

The skin has three distinct layers: the epidermis, the dermis, and the subcutaneous fatty layer that separates the skin from the underlying tissue (Figure 30–1➤). The **epidermis** is the thin, rapidly growing, outermost layer of skin. Skin is continually shed by the **stratum corneum**, the superficial layer of

the epidermis. The thickness of the epidermis varies by location on the body (e.g., 0.3 mm on the eyelids and 1.5 mm on the soles of the feet) (Nicol, Huether, & Weber, 2006). The epidermis contains the melanocytes that synthesize and secrete melanin when the skin is exposed to ultraviolet light. The Langerhans cells within the epidermis initiate the skin's immune response when exposed to environmental antigens.

The **dermis**, the middle layer of the skin, is mostly composed of connective tissue, which allows the skin to stretch and contract with movement. Nerves, muscles, hair follicles, sebaceous and sweat glands, lymph channels, and blood vessels are all contained within the dermis. Mast cells located within the dermis play a role in the skin's hypersensitivity reactions.

The third skin layer, the subcutaneous layer, connects the dermis to the muscle below. This layer of fat cells helps insulate the body from cold temperatures. The sebaceous glands appear all over the body except on the palms of the hands and soles of the feet, and are connected with hair follicles in most

Figure 30–1 ➤ Layers of the skin with accessory structures.

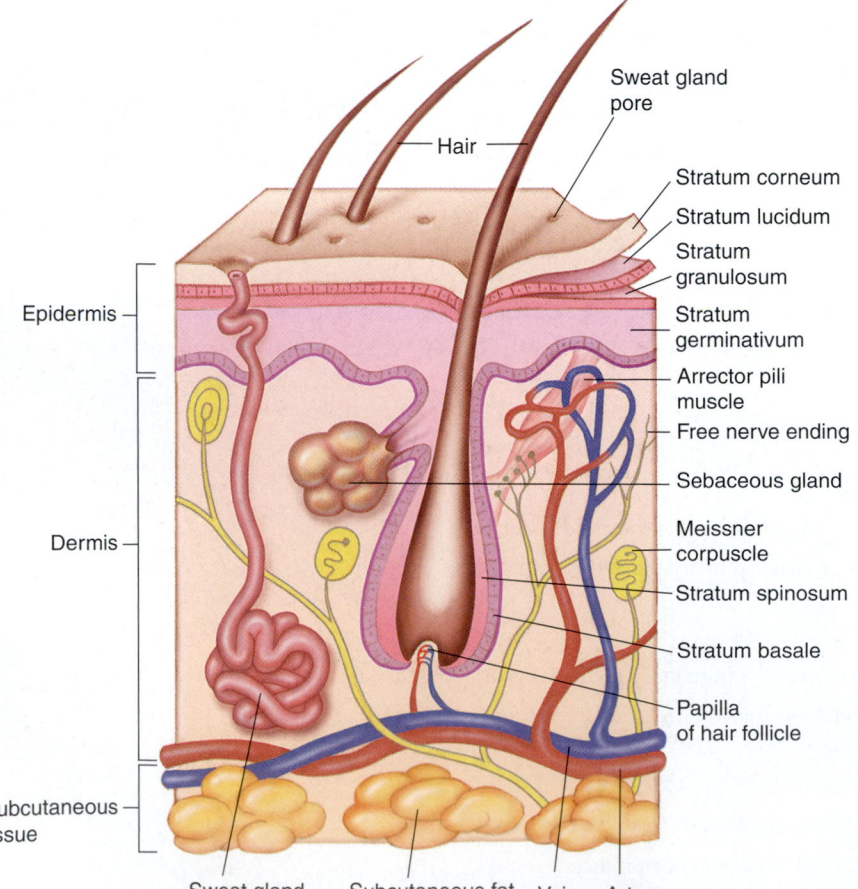

cases. Sebum, a lipid substance produced and secreted into the hair follicle or directly onto the skin, lubricates the skin and hair, prevents excessive evaporation from the skin, and inhibits the growth of bacteria (Chamley, 2005).

Eccrine sweat glands, located in the dermis, open onto the skin's surface. All eccrine sweat glands are present, structurally mature, and functional at birth in a term infant. They secrete an odorless, watery fluid containing sodium, chloride, urea, and other body wastes in response to changes in body temperature. As body temperature increases, the glands increase their production of sweat; its evaporation cools the body.

Fewer apocrine sweat glands are primarily located in the axillary and genital areas, and they become functional at puberty. The apocrine sweat gland secretions contain more lipids and proteins. Decomposition of the fluid secreted by these glands leads to body odor.

PEDIATRIC DIFFERENCES

The newborn's skin is covered by vernix caseosa in utero, a greasy substance containing shed cells that cover and protect the fetal skin from amniotic fluid and urine (Chamley, 2005).

It has many important properties: anti-infective, anti-oxidant, moisturizer, and wound healing agents (Stokowski, 2006).

The newborn's skin is the largest organ of the body, accounting for about 4% of the body weight (Chamley, 2005). The infant's skin is thin, about 1 mm thick at birth, with little underlying subcutaneous fat. The skin grows to 2 mm thick by adulthood. With thinner skin and less subcutaneous fat, the infant loses heat more rapidly, has greater difficulty regulating body temperature, and becomes more easily chilled than an older child or an adult. The thinner skin also leads to increased absorption of harmful chemical substances and topical medications. The infant's skin contains more water than an adult's and has loosely attached cells. As the infant grows, the skin toughens and becomes less hydrated, making it less susceptible to bacteria (Figure 30–2➤).

Melanin, a peptide present in the skin and synthesized by an enzyme in melanocytes, influences skin color. The amount of melanin present at birth is low, accounting for the lighter skin in newborns of all races. Newborns and young infants are therefore more susceptible to the harmful effects of the sun (Chamley, 2005).

AS CHILDREN GROW

Integumentary System Changes

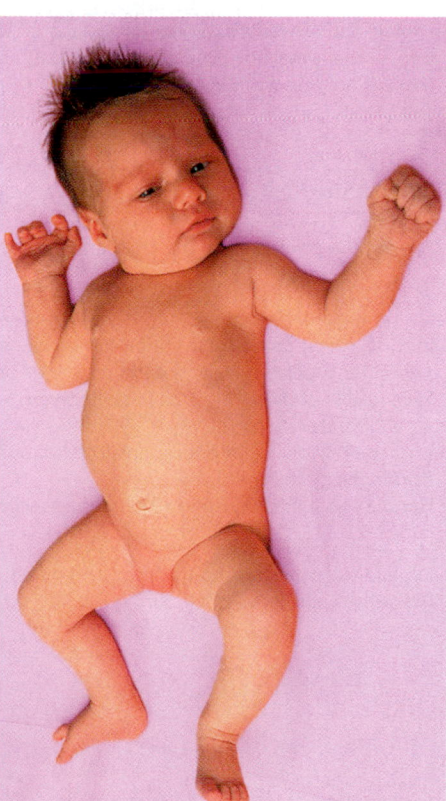

Newborns
Skin is very thin
Epidermis is loosely bound to the dermis, friction can cause separation of the layers with blistering
Eccrine sweat glands function, produce sweat in response to heat and emotional stimuli
Apocrine sweat glands are small and nonfunctional
Less melanin is present at birth so skin is lighter colored

Adolescents
Skin thickens
Epidermis and dermis are tightly bound, increasing resistance to infection and irritation
Eccrine sweat glands achieve full function, after puberty males sweat more than females
Apocrine sweat glands mature during puberty
Melanin is at adult levels, determining skin color and serving as a shield against ultraviolet radiation

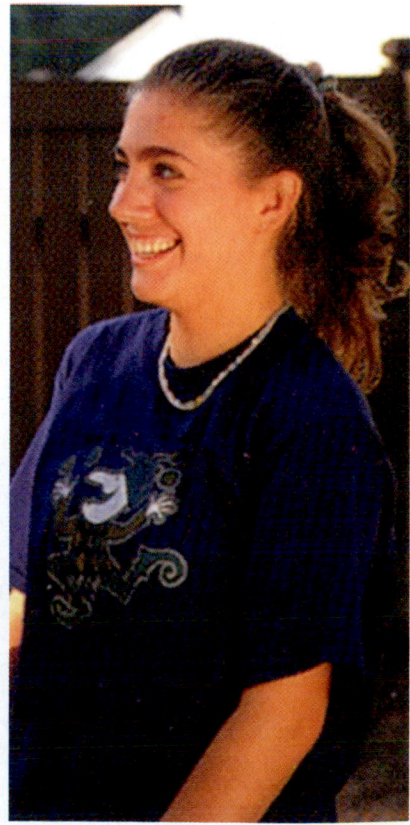

Figure 30–2 ➤ The structures of the skin mature during childhood, reaching adult function at puberty.

Sebaceous glands function at birth, although somewhat immaturely. Apocrine glands, located mainly in the axillary and genital areas, do not function until puberty.

Examples of diagnostic and laboratory tests used to evaluate skin conditions are provided in the accompanying table. Use the guidelines on the next page to perform a nursing assessment of the integument system.

DIAGNOSTIC PROCEDURES AND LABORATORY TESTS USED TO EVALUATE THE INTEGUMENT

Diagnostic Procedure	Purpose	Nursing Implications
Computed tomography	The CT scan produces a narrow radiograph beam that examines a body structure from different angles, producing a two-dimensional cross-section of the structures. CT of a hemangioma evaluates the size of the lesion and pressure on vital organs and other tissues. CT may also be used to identify injury to anatomic structures following a dog bite.	• Inquire about allergy to iodine, seafood, or contrast dye used for other radiographic procedures. Antihistamines and/or steroids may be ordered prior to the procedure if an allergic reaction is suspected. Assess for an allergic reaction during the procedure. • Prepare the child for the test by describing size of equipment, noises and other sensations that will be experienced, and how the child can help during the procedure. • When sedation is required to help keep an infant or small child still, monitor the child according to agency guidelines.
Radiograph	Radiographs use irradiation to obtain images and capture them on film for diagnostic and screening purposes. They can be used to assess damage to the skull, soft tissue, and vital organs following dog bites.	• Explain the procedure to parents and the child. Inform them that more than one radiograph may be taken from different angles to detect problems. Explain that modern equipment decreases radiation exposure. • Tell the child about the need to hold still for the test. Have the child practice holding still and holding a breath in preparation for the test.
Ultrasound	A noninvasive procedure by placing an ultrasound transducer over the area of the body, producing an ultrasound beam to the tissues. The reflected sound waves are transformed into scan graphs. Ultrasound is used to visualize the size of a hemangioma and compression on other structures.	• Administer sedation as prescribed. • Explain the procedure to parents and the child. Inform them that the procedure is painless, and there is no radiation exposure. • Tell the child to remain still during the procedure.

Laboratory Tests	Purpose	Nursing Implications
Complete blood count	The CBC assesses WBC and differential, providing evidence of infection and whether it is of bacterial or viral origin.	• Explain the procedure to the child and parents.
Cultures	Cultures are taken to isolate microorganisms causing body tissue or body fluid infection. Common cultures taken include: • Wound • Blood A Gram stain may be performed on a smear taken from the wound culture to detect gram + or gram−organisms.	• In most cases, do not give antibiotics or sulfonamides until after specimen collection, as they may cause false results. If these drugs have been given, list them on a laboratory slip. • Immediately deliver all specimens to the laboratory, or refrigerate the specimen. • Handle the specimen using strict aseptic technique.
Skin scraping	A thin layer of skin is scraped from a wound. The scraping may be examined under the microscope to see moving mites, nits, and feces associated with scabies. The scraping may be placed in potassium hydroxide (KOH) solution, heated, and examined under the microscope. Rows and chains of spores reveal a fungal infection.	• Explain the procedure to the child and parents. • Assist the child to hold still during the skin scraping.
Wood's lamp	Shining the ultraviolet light of the Wood's lamp on skin or hair helps identify fungus that fluoresces bright yellow-green.	• Explain the test to the child and parents. • Tell the child that there will be no pain.

Data from: Corbett, J. V. (2004). Laboratory tests and diagnostic procedures (6th ed.). Upper Saddle River, NJ: Prentice Hall.

ASSESSMENT GUIDELINES FOR THE CHILD WITH A SKIN CONDITION

Assessment Focus	Assessment Guidelines
Skin characteristics	• Inspect the skin for color, elevations, and imperfections. • Palpate the skin for texture, moisture, temperature, turgor, and edema.
Hair	• Inspect the scalp hair for color, distribution, and cleanliness. Inspect for nits (lice eggs) that adhere to the hair. • Inspect for areas of hair loss or broken hairs.
Lesions	• Describe skin lesions according to the characteristics listed in Figure 5–7 ∞ and Table 30–3. Note erythema, signs of scratching (excoriation), or secondary infection. • Identify the location or distribution of lesions on the body (e.g., generalized, diaper area, flexor surfaces). • Palpate lesions for induration and temperature. • Measure the size of lesions (length, width, and height when appropriate).
Pain	• Assess level of pain when present.
Temperature	• Assess the body temperature.
Family history	• Identify family members with allergies.

SKIN LESIONS

Skin lesions vary in size, shape, color, and texture characteristics. The two major types of skin lesions are primary lesions and secondary lesions. Primary lesions arise from previously healthy skin and include macules, patches, papules, nodules, tumors, vesicles, pustules, bullae, and wheals (see Figure 5–7 ∞). Secondary lesions result from changes in primary lesions. They include crusts, scales, **lichenification** (thickening of the skin with increased visibility of normal skin furrows), scars, keloids, excoriation, fissures, erosion, and ulcers (Table 30–1). It is important for the nurse to be able to identify and describe the primary and secondary skin lesions and understand their underlying cause and treatment. See the Complementary Therapy table on the next page.

Table 30–1	COMMON SECONDARY SKIN LESIONS AND ASSOCIATED CONDITIONS

Lesion Name	Description	Example
Crust	Dried residue of serum, pus, or blood	Impetigo
Scale	Thin flake of exfoliated epidermis	Dandruff, psoriasis
Lichenification	Thickening of skin with increased visibility of normal skin furrows	Eczema (atopic dermatitis)
Scar	Replacement of destroyed tissue with fibrous tissue	Healed surgical incision
Keloid	Overdevelopment or hypertrophy of scar that extends beyond wound edges and above skin line due to excess collagen	Healed skin area following traumatic injury
Excoriation	Abrasion or scratch mark	Scratched insect bite
Fissure	Linear crack in skin	Tinea pedis (athlete's foot)
Erosion	Loss of superficial epidermis; moist but does not bleed	Ruptured chickenpox vesicle
Ulcer	Deeper loss of skin surface; bleeding or scarring may ensue	Chancre
Comedone	A plug of sebaceous and keratin material in a hair follicle	Acne
Burrow	A narrow, raised irregular channel caused by a parasite	Scabies
Telangiectasia	Dilated, superficial blood vessels	Birthmark

COMPLEMENTARY THERAPY

Condition	Complementary Therapy	Use
Poison ivy	Aloe, calendula, oatmeal (topical)	Relief from itching
Atopic dermatitis	Evening primrose oil (oral)	Decreases excoriations and lichenification Decreases need for antihistamines for itching
Accelerated wound healing, burns, abrasions	Aloe vera gel (topical)	Antimicrobial effects, bacteriostatic, bacteriocidal
Skin inflammation	Chamomile (topical)	Wound drying, antimicrobial properties
Acne	5% tea tree oil (topical)	Antibiotic, decreases open and closed comedomes

From Gardner, P., Coles, D., & Kemper, K. J. (2001). The skinny on herbal remedies for dermatologic disorders. *Contemporary Pediatrics, 18*(7), 103–114.

MediaLink

Integument Repair Animation

WOUND HEALING

Wound healing occurs in three overlapping phases: inflammation, reconstruction, and maturation, so the wound fills in, seals, and finally shrinks (Trask, Rote, & Huether, 2006). See Figure 30–3 ▶.

Inflammation, the initial response at the injury site, lasts approximately 3 to 5 days. This phase prepares the injury site for the repair process. The blood coagulates as platelets, red blood cells, and fibrin gather to form a clot. This seals the wound and unites wound edges, preventing bacterial invasion. Vasodilation, which occurs shortly after injury, allows leukocytes to travel to the injury site, where they ingest bacteria and debris.

Reconstruction or **epithelialization** (the process by which epithelial cells grow into the wound from surrounding healthy tissue), the second phase, may last from 5 days to 2 weeks, depending on the extent of the injury. Capillary budding to reestablish the blood flow and natural **debridement** (enzyme action by macrophages and neutrophils to clean the lesion and dissolve the clot or scab) occur. The wound contracts. Fibroblasts multiply, producing collagen and granulation tissue to fill the wound to skin level. A fine layer of epithelial cells forms over the site.

Maturation or remodeling, the third phase, involves continued collagen production for scar production. Although the scar gradually strengthens and devascularizes, it will never be as strong as healthy skin. Maturation can take months to years, depending on the extent of the injury. Formation of a **keloid**, a scar that extends beyond the original boundaries of the wound, is caused by an imbalance between collagen synthesis and collagen breakdown. The cause is unknown, but there is a familial tendency. A **hypertrophic scar** is one that is raised but stays within the original boundaries of the wound.

DERMATITIS

Many skin inflammations occur in early childhood. Most are easily treated and do not have long-term consequences. Dermatitis is a condition in which the skin changes in response to external stimuli. The four most common types of dermatitis in infants, children, and adolescents are contact dermatitis, diaper dermatitis, seborrheic dermatitis, and eczema (atopic dermatitis). It is important to understand that these skin disorders bring emotional problems for the family and child. Be sympathetic and remember that the family and child can see the skin condition and need to be reassured that the child is not infectious.

PATHOPHYSIOLOGY ILLUSTRATED

Phases of Wound Healing

Inflammation (3–5 days)
Clot formation that seals the wound with fibrin and trapped cells and platelets
Increased blood flow to area carrying exudate with phagocytes and lymphocytes to the site
Increased capillary permeability, causing swelling
Dilute toxic products released by dying cells. Phagocytosis

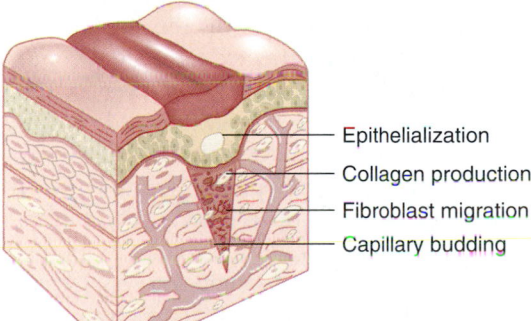

Inflammation

- Swelling/inflammation
- Clotting and wound sealing
- Neutrophils and monocytes (phagocytosis)
- Increased capillary permeability

Figure 30–3 ➤ Wound healing occurs in three phases: Inflammation, reconstruction, and scar maturation.
Note: From Trask, B. C., Rote, N. S., & Huether, S. E. (2006). Innate immunity: Inflammation. In K. L. McCance & S. E. Huether, *Pathophysiology: The biologic basis for disease in adults and children* (5th ed., pp. 175–209). St. Louis: Elsevier Mosby.

Reconstruction (4 days to 2 weeks)
Debridement or cleanup of the site, fibrinolytic enzymes dissolve the fibrin clots
Regeneration of destroyed cells if injury is minor
Collagen production for scar formation occurs when tissue is too injured to regenerate
Epithelialization with granulation tissue that includes capillary budding and becomes scar tissue
Wound contraction, inward movement of the wound edge

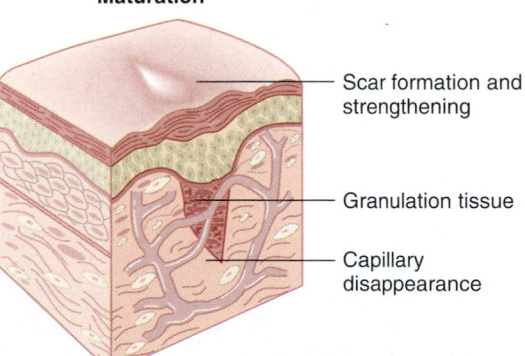

Reconstruction

- Epithelialization
- Collagen production
- Fibroblast migration
- Capillary budding

Maturation (Months to 2 Years)
Remodeling of the site as scar tissue forms
Scar formation and strengthening
Capillary disappearance from scar tissue

Maturation

- Scar formation and strengthening
- Granulation tissue
- Capillary disappearance

Contact Dermatitis

Contact dermatitis is an inflammation of the skin that occurs in response to direct contact with an allergen or irritant. It is a common problem for children of all age groups.

When an external irritant causes contact dermatitis, an inflammatory response occurs, but there is no immune response. Common irritants include soaps, detergents, fabric softeners, bleaches, lotions, urine, and stool. Sweating and friction enhance the absorption of the allergen or irritant. Photodermatitis can result when the child has contact with a chemical found in such plants and vegetables as citrus fruits, celery, parsley, and ragweed that sensitizes the skin to radioviolet light. Following sun exposure, the child develops erythema and blistering at the site of the exposure that then becomes hyperpigmented. The hyperpigmentation fades over 2 to 3 months (Khachemoune, Khechmoune, & Blanc, 2006).

Allergic contact dermatitis is a delayed hypersensitivity reaction. An antigen is absorbed from the skin's surface during the initial sensitization phase, and an immune memory is created. Generally, repeated exposures or a long-term exposure are required to cause the immune response and the dermatitis. Common allergens include poison ivy, poison oak, lanolin, neomycin and bacitracin, rubber, chemicals in shoe leather, nickel, formaldehyde, fragrances, and latex. Children may have both irritant and allergic reactions to latex, found in many types of hospital equipment and supplies, as well as in products in the home and community (see Chapter 17 ∞).

The allergic contact dermatitis is characterized by erythema, edema, pruritis, vesicles, or bullae that rupture, ooze, and crust. The rash is usually limited to the area of contact. Symptoms of allergic contact dermatitis develop several hours after exposure and after the immunologic response has been activated. Symptoms can last up to 3 to 4 weeks without treatment. In contrast, irritant contact dermatitis is a discrete area of redness that corresponds to the exposure location. The rash usually develops within a few hours of contact, peaks within 24 hours, and quickly resolves with removal of the irritant.

The distribution of the lesions provides clues about the source and identity of the allergen. See Table 30–2. Patch testing may be used to identify the allergen. Treatment involves removing the offending agent (e.g., clothes, plant, soap). Calamine lotion can be applied to the affected skin. Cool compresses with aluminum acetate (Burow's solution) promote drying. Wet dressings and colloidal oatmeal soaks relieve itching. Antihistamines may be given for a sedative effect when the child is too irritable to sleep. Acute allergic contact dermatitis is managed with medium potency topical corticosteroids when less than 10% of the body surface area is affected; however, they should not be applied to open lesions. The topical corticosteroids are applied to the affected area twice a day for 2 to 3 weeks. Stopping the treatment too soon can cause rebound dermatitis. Reactions to poison ivy covering more than 10% of the body surface area require treatment with oral corticosteroids for 7 to 14 days and a tapered dose for 7 to 10 additional days.

Nursing Management

Patient education for home care management focuses on care of the skin and prevention of future exposures. Teach parents how to apply topical corticosteroids and to keep using the ointment for 2 to 3 weeks even when the skin shows signs of healing. When oatmeal soaks are used, caution parents that the tub will be slippery, and to pat the child dry to leave the oatmeal film in place. Wet dressings may be soothing and help loosen crusts. Burow's or Domeboro solution applied to blistered or oozing lesions for 20 minutes daily helps dry lesions (Allen, 2004). Familiarize parents with the symptoms of infection in the affected area (i.e., increased redness, oozing, fever) and tell them when to return for follow-up care. See Families Want to Know: Exposure to Poison Ivy or Poison Oak.

Table 30–2	DISTRIBUTION OF LESIONS BY TYPE OF ALLERGEN	
Distribution of Lesion	**Allergen**
Face, eyelids	Cosmetics, skin care products, nail cosmetics
Ear lobes, neck	Nickel, fragrances
Lips, mouth	Oral hygiene products, gum, lipstick
Trunk	Snaps on pants, moisturizers, cleansers
Dorsal aspects of toes and feet	Rubber or leather chemical in shoes

Adapted from: Timm-Knudson, V. L., Johnson, J. S., Ortiz, K. J., & Yiannias, J. A. (2006). Allergic contact dermatitis to preservatives. *Dermatologic Nursing, 18*(2), 130–136; and Weston, W. L., & Bruckner, A. (2000). Allergic contact dermatitis. *Pediatric Clinics of North America, 47*(4), 897–907.

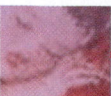

FAMILIES WANT TO KNOW

Exposure to Poison Ivy or Poison Oak

- React quickly after contact. Wash off sap with Zanfel® (a product that removes poison ivy sap) soap and water and scrub under the nails within 10 minutes if possible.
- Do not rub fingers exposed to poison ivy against broken skin or in eyes.
- Avoid hugging a pet exposed to poison ivy until after it has been bathed.
- Launder clothing worn during exposure, and wash hands after handling exposed clothing.

- Wear vinyl gloves to handle plants (cloth and rubber gloves allow sap to penetrate).
- Search the yard and remove all plants. Do not burn plants removed. A person with a sensitivity may inhale the smoke and develop airway inflammation.
- For children with sensitivity to poison ivy, an over-the-counter barrier cream such as IvyBlock® can help prevent skin penetration of plant oil.

Teach parents to avoid exposure to allergens or irritants. Advise parents to wash all clothes before the first wearing and to rinse clothes an extra time to remove all the soap. Mild soap should be used to clean the skin. Place a barrier between the irritant (e.g., metal, shoe leather) and the skin. If a nickel allergy exists, avoid use of nickel jewelry and belt buckles.

Diaper Dermatitis

Diaper dermatitis, a common cause of irritant contact dermatitis, occurs in approximately one-third of young children, usually in a mild form. It is most common in infants from 4 to 12 months of age. Diaper dermatitis is a primary reaction to urine, feces, moisture, or friction. Urine and feces interact with the skin to cause dermatitis. The urine increases the wetness and pH of the skin, increasing abrasion and its permeability to irritants and microbes. Fecal organisms provide more irritants.

Candida albicans, a secondary infection, is a common complication of diaper dermatitis or antibiotic therapy for another condition. It is frequently the underlying cause of severe diaper rash. Diaper candidiasis often occurs simultaneously with oral candidiasis (see later discussion).

The rash is characterized by glazed red plaques over skin in contact with the diaper area. Usually the perineum, genitals, and buttocks are affected, and the skin folds are spared. In severe cases, the infant develops a rash that is fiery red, raised, and confluent. Pustules with tenderness can also be present (Figure 30–4▶). When a secondary infection with *Candida albicans* occurs, the rash has bright red scaly plaques with sharp margins in the skin folds. Small papules and pustules may be seen, along with satellite lesions.

Mild diaper dermatitis is treated with a barrier or protective sealant such as zinc oxide, Desitin, or Balmex. Treatment for moderate or severe diaper dermatitis involves application of low or moderate potency (0.25% or 1%) hydrocortisone cream with each diaper change for 5 to 7 days and good basic hygiene. The cream must be applied before any protective sealant is used. Diaper candidiasis is treated with alternating applications of 1% hydrocortisone cream and antifungal creams (clotrimazole or nystatin) applied to the affected areas at diaper change. An oral antifungal agent may be given to clear the candidiasis from the intestines. Fluorinated topical corticosteroids should not be used because of the higher rate of absorption through damaged skin.

Nursing Management

Severe diaper dermatitis can be a major source of stress for parents who must deal with a child in constant discomfort. Instruct parents to change the diaper as soon as the infant is wet, or at least every 2 hours during the day and once during the night.

Encourage parents to use superabsorbent disposable diapers, which tend to reduce the frequency and severity of diaper dermatitis. When wet, these diapers form a gel that keeps the skin drier than cloth diapers. However, parents should avoid waiting until the diaper is saturated to change it. Tell parents to avoid using tight diapers and waterproof pants. A & D ointment, zinc oxide, Desitin, and Balmex can be

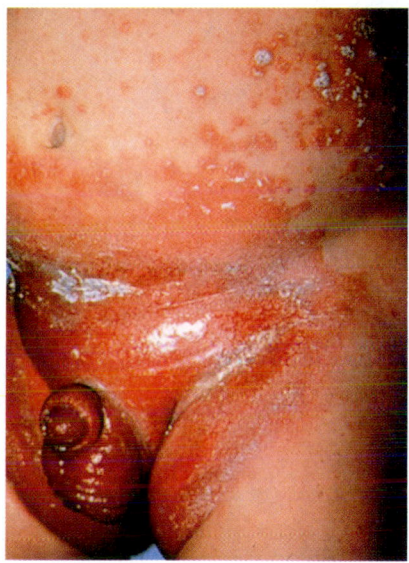

Figure 30–4 ▶ Diaper dermatitis. Note the skin fold that is free of inflammation. Courtesy of the Centers for Disease Control, Atlanta, GA.

used to protect the skin from urine and stool. Mineral oil on a cloth may be helpful in removing pastes from the skin once or twice a day so that fresh medications may be applied.

Advise parents to wash the perianal area with warm water and a mild soap (such as Dove or Tone) or a cleanser not needing water (Aquanil HC lotion or Cetaphil) only after a bowel movement. Soaps remove lipids and make the skin more permeable to irritants (Borkowski, 2004). Advise parents to use soft paper towels with water or baby wipes without alcohol at other times. Talcum powder is abrasive and offers no protection (Atherton, 2004). Exposing the diaper area to air helps aid healing; for example, parents could allow the child to go without a diaper while lying on an absorbent pad or cloth. Watch for signs of infection since the skin is damaged and can allow infectious organisms to grow. If this occurs, additional treatment will be needed.

Seborrheic Dermatitis

Seborrheic dermatitis is a recurrent inflammatory skin condition thought to be caused by an overgrowth of *Pityrosporum* yeast, commonly found in areas of sebaceous gland activity. The condition is influenced by hormones and associated with an oily complexion. The rash is found over the areas of the body where the sebaceous glands are most plentiful: scalp (cradle cap), forehead, and postauricular and periorbital areas. It may also occur on the skin of the eyelids, inguinal area, or nasolabial folds. The condition is frequently seen in infants up to 3 months of age and adolescents.

Common symptoms are pruritus and a mildly erythematous, adherent, waxy scaling of the scalp (or "dandruff"). Yellow-red patches with greasy scaling may be present, typically on the scalp and nasolabial folds on the face, behind the ears, on the upper chest, and sometimes on the **intertriginous** (skin folds of the neck, axillae, antecubital fossa) areas (Figure 30–5 ➤). The rash itches less than atopic dermatitis.

Treatment for seborrheic dermatitis consists of daily shampooing with a medicated shampoo (e.g., Selsun or Head and Shoulders). An emollient is left on the scalp for about 20 minutes to soften the crusts. The scales are removed by brushing with the fingertips, a baby hairbrush, or soft toothbrush. The hair is then rinsed thoroughly. Lesions on the body can be treated with shampoos containing selenium sulfide or salicylic acid. Use baby shampoo to wash lesions on the eyelids and eyelashes. Treatments are continued for several days after the lesions disappear. Topical corticosteroids are used to treat seborrhea that is not on the scalp; however, avoid using topical corticosteroids around the eyes.

Nursing Management

Teach new parents to wash the infant's hair regularly with each bath. Reassure parents that gentle cleansing will not harm the infant's "soft spot." Demonstrate bathing to show them the proper technique, if necessary. Follow-up is seldom necessary, as the condition resolves with treatment. Advise adolescents that emotional distress may trigger future flare-ups and to initiate treatment promptly when symptoms begin.

Atopic Dermatitis (Eczema)

Atopic dermatitis, also called eczema, is a chronic, superficial inflammatory skin disorder characterized by intense pruritus. The condition affects infants, children, and adolescents. It is common, and is believed to affect up to 20% of young schoolchildren (Dohil & Eichenfield, 2005). Up to 65% of children who develop the condition do so during the first year of life, and in 90% by 5 years of age (Schachner, Lamerson, Sheehan et al., 2005). Some children have recurrent symptoms that continue into adulthood.

Etiology and Pathophysiology

The etiology of atopic dermatitis is unknown, but an immune disorder of the skin is influenced by a genetic predisposition, and external environmental triggers may be involved. Children have T-cell activation and excessive production of immunoglobulin E (IgE). See Chapter 17 ∞ for a discussion of IgE. The disorder tends to occur in children with hereditary allergic tendencies **(atopy)**. If one parent has allergies (e.g., hay fever, asthma, or contact dermatitis), the child has a 60% greater chance of having

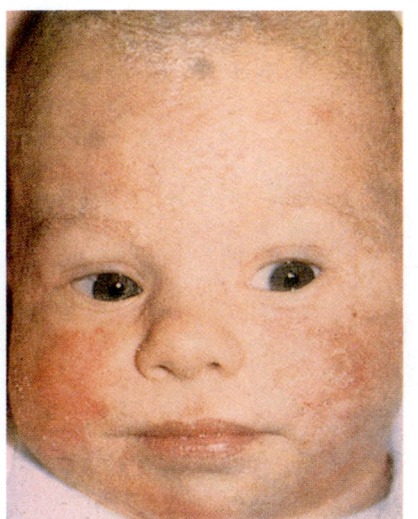

Figure 30–5 ➤ Seborrheic dermatitis.

allergies. This increases to 80% if both parents have allergies (Cheigh, 2003). Food allergens are an important cause of atopic dermatitis in young infants. Several factors exacerbate the condition: triggers (house mites, animal dander, pollens), food allergies, irritants (soaps, detergents, chemicals, solvents, abrasive clothing), hormonal changes, and emotional stress. The immune abnormalities predispose children to viral and *Staphylococcus aureus* skin infections (Tharp, 2005). Atopic dermatitis differs from contact dermatitis in that it is a chronic immune disorder with genetic, environmental, metabolic, and infectious triggers (Dohil & Eichenfield, 2005).

Children with eczema have **xerosis**, generally dry skin that is more likely to crack and fissure. The barrier function of the skin is impaired, leading to increased water loss from the epidermis and decreased elasticity. When the skin is chronically dry, irritants have a greater chance to penetrate, and the child is more susceptible to infection.

Clinical Manifestations

Acute atopic dermatitis is characterized by pruritus and erythematous patches with vesicles, exudate, and crusts (Figure 30–6➤). Subacute atopic dermatitis is characterized by scaling with erythema and excoriation. Some patches may weep. There are often postinflammatory pigment changes. Symptoms of chronic atopic dermatitis are pruritus, dryness, scaling, and lichenification. Inflammation usually occurs on the face, upper arms, back, upper thighs, and back of the hands and feet. Skin folds such as the antecubital and popliteal areas are often affected. The itching interferes with sleep and causes irritability. The child moves so much due to itching discomfort that a perception of hyperactivity may occur. Exacerbations of atopic dermatitis are related to factors such as allergies, dry skin, high and low ambient temperatures, perspiring, scratching, anxiety, stress, and skin irritants (e.g., detergents, wool, other rough fabrics). Erythema and warmth may indicate a secondary bacterial infection.

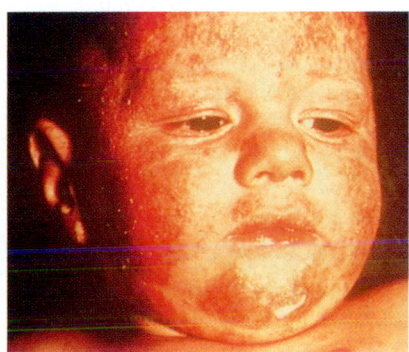

Figure 30–6 ➤ Chronic eczema.

See the clinical manifestations table below for the characteristics of the three forms of atopic dermatitis: infantile (ages 2 months to 2 years), childhood (ages 2 years to puberty), and adolescent. Children typically have numerous relapses, but atopic dermatitis may resolve in some when they begin to have respiratory symptoms. Other children continue to have atopic dermatitis into adulthood (Tharp, 2005).

CLINICAL MANIFESTATIONS | ECZEMA

Type	Clinical Manifestations	Outcome
Infantile (2 months to 2 years)	Exudative, crusty, papulovesicular, and erythematous lesions on cheeks, scalp, forehead, neck, trunk, and extensor surfaces of extremities Diaper area spared because skin is damp and the diaper protects the area from scratching Intensely pruritic, child wiggles to rub and scratch areas out of reach Lichenification after the child can scratch at about 2 months of age	50% of cases resolve by age 2 to 3 years
Childhood (2 years to puberty)	Erythematous, dry, scaly or weeping, well-circumscribed, papular, more thickened and lichenified lesions on flexor surfaces of extremities, neck, and retroauricular folds Once toilet trained, buttocks are affected	Subacute and chronic 75% of cases have no recurrence after adolescence
Adolescent (puberty and onward)	Much the same as childhood eczema but generalized form is less acute Localized areas affected may include eyelids, where earlobe touches the face, fingertips, toes, nipple, and the vulvar area	May recur as it is more often a chronic inflammation

COMPLEMENTARY THERAPY

Chinese Medical Herbs for Atopic Dermatitis

One or more of the components of Zemaphyte, a mixture of plant extracts based on Chinese herbal therapy, has been found effective in treatment of 37 children with atopic dermatitis (Latchman, Xu, Poulter et al., 2002). The mixture contains 10 primary herbs that are ground, placed in teabags, and boiled for 90 minutes. The herbs include the following: Ledebouriella seseloides, Potentilla chinensis, Clematis armandii, Rehmannia glutinosa, Paeonia lactoflora, Lophatherum gracile, Dictamnus dasycarpus, Tribulus terrestris, Glycyrrhiza uralensis, and Schizonepeta tenuifolia.

Children should not eat food 1 hour prior to drinking the warm mixture. If the liquid is too unpleasant tasting to drink, it can be freeze-dried into granules to put into a capsule. Significant improvements in skin lesion severity were noted in children who completed a year of treatment without significant adverse effects.

■ COLLABORATIVE CARE

Diagnostic Tests

Atopic dermatitis is distinguished from other forms of dermatitis by its age-specific patterns, chronic and relapsing nature, pruritus, xerosis, and family history. No laboratory tests are diagnostic; however, the child may have an elevated immunoglobulin E level, as well as positive skin tests to a variety of food and inhalant allergens (Nicol, Huether, & Weber, 2006).

Clinical Therapy

As there is no cure for atopic dermatitis, the goals of treatment are to hydrate and lubricate the skin, reduce pruritus, minimize inflammatory changes, and try to determine what triggers flares. The cardinal principle of topical therapy for oozing or weeping is "wet on wet." If lesions are weeping, wet compresses (cotton cloths) soaked in aluminum acetate solution are sometimes used. The skin is lubricated by applying occlusive topical ointment after bathing to trap moisture and prevent drying. Moisturizing ointments and creams (e.g., Eucerin cream, Aquaphor ointment, Vanicream, Cetaphil cream, SBR-Lipocream, and white petrolatum) should be applied three to four times a day or whenever the skin feels dry.

Topical corticosteroids reduce inflammation. Ointments are preferred over creams because of their occlusive effect, which ensures a stronger barrier and absorption into the skin. Hydrocortisone 1–2.5% or triamcinolone 0.1% is usually the drug of choice; however, many different preparations and strengths exist. Corticosteroids are used two times daily for 2 weeks and must be applied before the skin moisturizer is used. Newer corticosteroid ointments such as fluticasone propionate and mometasone furoate are effective for once-daily use (Dohil & Eichenfield, 2005). Lower potency ointments are used for thinner skin areas, such as the face, diaper area, and skin folds. A more potent ointment is used for flares, with tapering to lower potency as the dermatitis improves. When the dermatitis resolves, topical corticosteroids are tapered in freqency of application and potency, and then discontinued. Topical steroids are not used on healthy skin to reduce the risk for steroid side effects. Oral corticosteroids may be used for an acute exacerbation; however, there is often a rebound effect (i.e., after the medication is discontinued, the rash returns). Complementary therapy may also be beneficial. See Medications Used to Treat Atopic Dermatitis on page 1265.

Topical antibiotics are used to treat excoriated, open lesions and those that appear infected. Oral antibiotics are often given to reduce the *Staphylococcus aureus* population, as these organisms can trigger an immune cascade that increases pruritus. Oral and topical antibiotics are often used in 7-to 10-day intervals rather than continuously to reduce the risk of drug-resistant organisms getting established (Shwayder, 2003). Superinfections with herpes simplex may be treated with acyclovir.

Immunomodulator ointments (Tacrolimus and Pimecrolimus) are increasingly used as a second-line treatment for some children, but they may be too expensive for some families. The medication has been approved by the FDA for children over 2 years of age for short-term or intermittent treatment who are not responsive to conventional therapy. Recent warnings of increased risk for lymphoma and skin cancer associated with duration of use may be of concern to parents (Food and Drug Administration, 2005a). However, advocates of these immunomodulator ointments have identified the significant potential side effects to topical corticosteroids such as skin atrophy, hypopigmentation, and suppression of the hypothalamic-pituitary axis when used long term, indicating that all treatments have risks (Tharp, 2005).

Antihistamine agents such as dyphenhydramine (Benadryl) or hydroxyzine (Vistaril and Atarax) have a limited effect on itching, but the sedative effect may help promote sleep. Methods to reduce pruritus include environmental controls, such as humidification in the winter and air conditioning in the summer. A humidifier counteracts dryness of the surrounding air, minimizing loss of skin moisture. Air conditioning limits unnecessary sweating that can exacerbate inflamed areas.

MEDICATIONS USED TO TREAT *Atopic Dermatitis*

Medications	Action	Adverse Effects

Emollients
  Eucerin cream
  Aquaphor ointment
  Vanicream
  Cetaphil cream
  SBR-Lipocream
  White petrolatum
	Helps lubricate the skin when applied immediately after bathing.	Fragrances and preservatives in products may cause irritation.
		Fragrance-free or bland emollients should be used.

Oral antihistamines	Control of itching and sedating effect when given at night.	Sleepiness and interference with school if given during the day.

Antibiotics
  Topical
  Oral
	Treat cutaneous skin superinfections.	Hypersensitivity reaction.

Corticosteroids
  Topical
  Oral
	Anti-inflammatory.	Skin atrophy, suppression of the hypothalamic-pituitary-adrenal axis (see Chapter 29 ∞). Can induce glaucoma or cataract formation if used around eyes.

Immunomodulators
  Tacrolimus ointment
  Pimecrolimus (Elidel,
  SDZ ASM 981)
	Inhibiting T-lymphocyte activation. Inhibit release of cytokines and inflammatory mediators from anti-IgE-activated skin mast cells and basophils.
	Often used on face rather than topical corticosteroids.
		Topical application may cause a sensation of burning, redness, and itching for the first few days of therapy. These symptoms generally decrease after a few days of treatment. Tacrolimus helps promote skin healing and breaks the cycle of itching and scratching (Schachner, Lamerson, Sheehan et al., 2005).
		Sunscreens should be used because of potential increased risk for skin cancer with sun exposure. Approved for children over 2 years of age.

Breast milk is hypoallergenic, and exclusive breast-feeding for the first 3 months of life may be associated with a lower incidence of atopic dermatitis in infants with a positive family history. Introduction of solid foods at a later age, after 4 months, can result in decreased atopic dermatitis during the first 4 years of life. In some children, avoidance of highly allergenic foods such as eggs, wheat, milk, and peanuts from the diets of infants and lactating mothers may improve the skin condition (Cheigh, 2003). When regular therapy does not result in improvements in skin condition, an allergy specialist may help identify food and other environmental allergens that trigger the atopic dermatitis. See Chapter 17 ∞.

NURSING MANAGEMENT

Nursing Assessment and Diagnosis

Take a thorough history, including any family history of allergy, environmental or dietary factors, and past exacerbations. Note distribution and type of lesions. What makes the skin condition worsen or flare (e.g., a food, wool clothing, soap)? What is the impact of the skin lesions on the child's comfort level?

How does the family describe living with a child who has atopic dermatitis? What impact is the skin disorder having on the child and family? Do the child, siblings, or other family members have disturbed sleep because of the child's scratching? Is the child's self-esteem disturbed? What other stresses have the child's skin disorder placed on the family's quality of life? How is the child's appearance impacting the family's social relationships? What are the family's concerns with medication use?

RESEARCH

Probiotic Use

A recent study evaluated the benefit of an 8-week trial of twice daily oral probiotic (Lactobacillus fermentum) compared with a placebo in 53 children ages 6 to 18 months. Children had moderate or severe atopic dermatitis at the beginning of the study. Children continued their usual treatment with topical steroids as needed. After 16 weeks, 92% of the children in the probiotic group had a less severe atopic dermatitis than the children (63%) receiving the placebo. Supplementation with a probiotic may be beneficial in young children with moderate to severe atopic dermatitis (Weston, Halbert, Richmond et al., 2005).

MediaLink

Care Plan Activity: Atopic Dermatitis

Common nursing diagnoses that may be appropriate for the child with atopic dermatitis include:

- Impaired Tissue Integrity related to chemical irritants and mechanical factors (abrasive clothing)
- Disturbed Sleep Pattern related to prolonged physical discomfort (itching)
- Risk for Infection related to breaks in skin barrier
- Chronic Low Self-Esteem related to chronic illness and peer reaction to visible skin lesions
- Ineffective Therapeutic Regimen Management (families) related to excessive demands made on the family to keep the condition under control

Planning and Implementation

Nursing management focuses on education and emotional support. Atopic dermatitis can be controlled, but there is no cure. Advise parents that the lesions are not contagious and will not usually result in scarring. Help parents and adolescents deal with the frustration of the acute flares of the condition by reinforcing that remissions do occur even with consistent home care.

Teach parents or adolescents to avoid using harsh or perfumed soaps or bubble bath. Bathing with tepid water once or twice a day with a mild soap (e.g., Dove or Tone) is recommended. Washing clean skin with soap and hot water dries it out and may increase itching. Pat the skin dry or air-dry. Moisturizers should be applied within 3 minutes of exiting the bath to help promote absorption and retention of moisture. If the child bathes only once a day, moisturizer should still be used twice a day. Wet wraps over severely affected skin may be used for a couple of days to replace moisture; however, the use of wet wraps for several days increases the risk for infection (Barham & Yosipovitch, 2005).

Teach parents and adolescents how to apply topical ointments or creams. A thin layer over the entire area should be applied twice a day. The medication should be rubbed in gently and completely. Treatment should continue until the skin clears. Instruct parents to place clean cotton gloves or socks over the infant or young child's hands and to keep the child's fingernails cut short to decrease scratching and reduce the chance of secondary infection.

Atopic dermatitis produces visible changes that can affect a child's self-confidence and self-esteem. Identify activities that the child can participate in to improve self-esteem. Even though humidity and sweating can make atopic dermatitis worse, have the child shower after a sporting event or strenuous activity to clean the skin. Needed medications and lubricants can then be applied. Encourage the child to wear loose cotton clothing. Wool clothing and clothing washed in harsh laundry detergents should be avoided because it can increase skin irritation and pruritus.

When atopic dermatitis is difficult to manage, it is more stressful and can have a more profound effect on the child's and family's quality of life. The use of immunomodulators in children with moderate or severe atopic dermatitis significantly improves the quality of life in children and adults as measured by daily activities, feelings, relationships, and sleep (Schachner, Lamerson, Sheehan et al., 2005; Whalley, Huels, McKenna et al., 2002).

A daily massage using emollients may reduce redness, scaling, lichenification, excoriation, and pruritis. This may improve the child's disposition and comfort.

Food allergies are commonly identified as a trigger for atopic dermatitis. Educate parents that increased itching within hours of eating a food may be associated with an atopic dermatitis flare. Teach parents how to control the skin inflammation that results, as previously described. Once a specific food allergy has been identified, refer the parents to a nutritionist for counseling about alternative food options that will fulfill daily nutritional requirements. Tell parents that food allergies can change, so foods connected with atopic dermatitis can sometimes be safely eaten later in life. Different food sensitivities may also develop. Refer the family to the Food Allergy Network.

CLINICAL TIP

Wet wraps may be used for a few days during acute flares of atopic dermatitis to enhance the penetration of medications and to add moisture to the skin. Lower potency corticosteroid ointments should be used to reduce the amount of systemic absorption. Before wet wraps are applied, the child is bathed in lukewarm water with a soap-free cleanser, the prescribed topical corticosteroid ointment is applied to the affected areas, and an emollient is applied to all the skin. A warm wet layer (e.g., a form-fitting T-shirt) is then applied over the treated skin and covered with a dry layer, such as pajamas. The wet layer should be moistened about every 2 hours during the night (Barham & Yosipovitch, 2005).

NURSING ALERT

Avoid the use of fluorinated corticosteroids on the face, genitalia, and skin folds where absorption of the medication is increased due to thinness of skin in these areas. Occlusive dressings, such as may occur with a tight-fitting diaper, further increase potential absorption. The absorption of large amounts of steroids through the skin can lead to adrenal suppression. The lowest concentration of topical corticosteroids should also be used in these areas. Posterior cataracts and glaucoma are a potential adverse effect of topical corticosteroid use around the eyes. Other adverse effects may include skin atrophy due to decreased collagen synthesis and striae after 3 to 4 weeks of therapy.

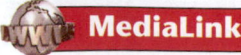

MediaLink

Food Allergy Network

Evaluation

Expected outcomes of nursing care include the following:

- Control of the child's atopic dermatitis is maintained and no infection occurs.
- Parents identify triggers of the child's atopic dermatitis and avoid or eliminate them.
- The child's and family's sleep is minimally disturbed by itching.

DRUG REACTIONS

Adverse reactions to over-the-counter or prescription medications are relatively common. Children with drug allergies usually have reactions after ingestion (e.g., aspirin, antibiotics, sedatives), injection (e.g., penicillin), or direct skin contact with medications. Drug sensitivities may result from variations in an individual's ability to tolerate a particular drug or drug concentration, or from allergic responses. (See Chapter 17 ∞ for a description of allergic reactions.)

Sensitivity reactions to a drug not previously administered may take up to 7 days to develop. If the child has been sensitized to a drug, the reaction is almost immediate. The most common reactions in children are erythematous macules and papules or urticaria, which may be pruritic. Drugs most likely to cause sensitivity reactions such as maculopapular eruptions, urticaria, and pruritis include the following: sulfonamides, anticonvulsants, antibiotics (penicillins, cephalosporins, erythromycin, vancomycin), and NSAIDs (Boguniewicz, 2004). Some drug reactions such as Stevens-Johnson syndrome and toxic epidermal necrolysis, as described in the clinical manifestations table on the next page, can be life threatening. Be alert to the possibility of serious drug reactions that may become a medical emergency.

The treatment of choice for most drug sensitivity reactions is discontinuation of the causative drug. In some cases, a drug may be continued with careful monitoring when a sensitivity reaction occurs because it is the best treatment choice. Supportive measures should be taken to decrease the intensity of the reaction. An antihistamine may be used to block the release of histamine, which causes the rash. Topical corticosteroids, cool compresses, and baths may also be prescribed for pruritus. For some severe drug reactions, the child must be hospitalized and treated on a burn unit.

Nursing Management

Teach parents to be alert for the signs of drug sensitivity reactions. Obtain a careful history of the child's past reactions to medications before starting new therapies. If a reaction occurs, discontinue the medication until the physician is notified.

ACNE

Acne, a chronic inflammatory disorder of the pilosebaceous hair follicles on the face and trunk, is the most common skin disorder in adolescents. It is triggered by the increased androgen production of puberty and the overproduction of sebum. The prevalence in adolescents ages 12 to 16 years is estimated to approach 50–85% (Rudy, 2003). Acne is found in all ethnic groups and is present equally in males and females. Acne may also occur in neonates in response to maternal androgen hormones. This form of acne usually develops between 2 and 4 weeks of age and resolves by 4 to 6 months of age.

Etiology and Pathophysiology

Acne is caused by the interaction of several factors: increased sebum production, abnormal follicular shedding of skin cells that are more adherent than normal, and an overgrowth of the *Propionibacterium acnes (P. acnes)* bacteria in the hair follicle. The extra sebum caused by androgen secretion mixes with the shed skin cells and causes them to clump together. The keratin and sebum that usually flow to the skin surface are obstructed in the follicular canal, causing comedones (whiteheads and blackheads). The

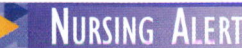

NURSING ALERT

Children with a true drug allergy (having a past serious systemic reaction) should never be treated with that drug again. Prominently mark the child's records so that all allergies are easily identified. The child should wear a medical alert bracelet.

MediaLink

Acne Animation

CLINICAL MANIFESTATIONS · DRUG REACTIONS

Type of Reaction	Clinical Manifestations	Clinical Therapy
Allergic drug reaction Most commonly caused by sulfonamides, tetracyclines, NSAIDs, oral contraceptives, barbiturates, and phenolphthalein	Erythematous macules and papules. Pruritis. Urticaria, may move among body parts. A fixed drug reaction may commonly involve the face, genitals, sacrum. Recurrent localized target lesions may be seen with repeated exposure; healing with hyperpigmentation of the center may be seen (Cohen, 2002).	Remove offending drug Topical antipruritics Oral antihistamines Lubricate skin when scaly Systemic corticosteroids if no response to other treatment
Erythema multiforme Hypersensitivity or toxic reaction to a drug (sulfonamides, anticonvulsants, and NSAIDs) or infectious agent (*Mycoplasma pneumoniae*, herpes simplex)	Widespread pruritic macules and plaques. Target lesions with a central dusky zone surrounded by rings of alternating edema and inflammation. May progress to blisters and bullous lesions.	Remove offending drug and treat infection with alternate medication Supportive care Oral antihistamines Topical antipruritics Analgesics Cool compresses or baths Topical corticosteroids are sometimes prescribed
Stevens-Johnson syndrome (SJS) and Toxic epidermal necrolysis (TEN) Potential life-threatening hypersensitivity reaction or autoimmune response to NSAIDs, sulfa, antibiotics, and anticonvulsants or reaction to an infectious agent Believed to be a form of the same disease and the most severe form of erythema multiforme	Prodrome of an upper respiratory infection for 1 to 7 days with cough, coryza, sore throat, fever, malaise, headache, muscle aches, and joint pain in some cases. Skin lesions are blistering and crusting on the mucous membranes and redness in the eyes. Bullae and erosions may spread to cover up to 10–30% of the skin surface in SJS, 10%–30% of the skin surface in overlapping SJS and TEN, and to more than 30% of the skin surface in TEN. Full-thickness epidermis peels off in sheets easily with light pressure (Nikolsky's sign). Corneal blistering can lead to blindness. Respiratory and gastrointestinal tracts may have mucosal sloughing. Causes hypopigmentation in children with dark skin, but hyperpigmentation in children with white skin. Hyperpigmentation fades over time. Signs of sepsis.	May be cared for in a burn center, see page 1286. Debridement of blisters and necrotic epidermis Gentle cleaning with saline or Burow's solution (aluminum acetate) compresses Pain management Sterile nonadherent dressings Wounds may be covered with biosynthetic dressing, human allografts to reduce infection and pain IV immune globulin has been used successfully in a few cases (Metry, Jung, & Levy, 2003) Intensive nutritional support Ophthalmic consultation and eye care Corticosteroid use is controversial; may increase the child's risk for sepsis and gastrointestinal tract hemorrhage

Note: Data from: Nicol, N. H., Huether, S. E., & Weber, R. (2006). Structure, function, and disorders of the integument. In K. L. McCance & S. E. Huether, *Pathophysiology: The biologic basis for disease in adults and children* (5th ed, pp. 1589–1590). St. Louis: Elsevier Mosby; Schmidt, C. E. (2003). A 12-month-old girl with maculopapular lesions and lower extremity edema. *Journal of Emergency Nursing, 29*(3), 204–207; Cohen, B. A. (2002). Plaques: Oval, itchy, and red: What's your diagnosis? *Contemporary Pediatrics, 19*(4), 36–41; Sheridan, R. L., Schulz, J. T., Ryan, C. M., Schnitzer, J. J., Lawlor, D., et al. (2002). Long-term consequences of toxic epidermal necrolysis in children. *Pediatrics, 109*(1), 74–78; Metry, D. W., Jung, P., & Levy, M. L. (2003). Use of intravenous immunoglobulin in children with Stevens-Johnson Syndrome and toxic epidermal necrolysis: Seven cases and review of the literature. *Pediatrics, 112*(6), 1430–1436.

sebum behind the comedone is an ideal environment for the anaerobic *P. acneces,* and this bacterium metabolizes the sebum, dilating the pores and causing an inflammatory reaction. When the inflammatory reaction is close to the surface, a papule or pustule develops. If the inflammatory reaction is deeper, a larger papule or nodule develops. Extensive rupture and inflammation leads to cysts that can result in scars. Although acne follows familial trends, data have not yet defined a pattern of inheritance. Medications associated with the appearance of acne lesions include androgens, corticosteroids (topical, oral, intravenous), immunosuppressants (e.g., cyclosporin), phenytoin, lithium, and isoniazid (Rudy, 2003; Silverberg, Silverberg, & Silverberg, 2005). Other factors that can trigger acne include friction of the skin from hairbands, helmets, and hats, as well as oil-based cosmetics. Females may have an exacerbation of acne with changes in the hormone levels associated with the menstrual cycle.

Clinical Manifestations

Noninflammatory acne involves a follicular plug (comedone) that precedes inflammatory acne lesions. There are three main types of acne: comedomal (characterized by open and closed comedones), papulopustular (characterized by papules and pustules) (Figure 30–7 ➤), and cystic (characterized by nodules and cysts). Closed comedones are flesh-colored papules with tiny follicular openings called whiteheads. Open comedones are found when the follicular plug has enlarged and dilated the follicular opening, called blackheads. Lesions occur most often on the face, upper chest, shoulders, and back. Scars form when the surrounding dermis is damaged. Types of scars may include the following: ice pick (small, deep, punched out pits), atrophic macules, hypertrophic scars or keloids, or broad sloping depressions (Woodard, 2002).

■ COLLABORATIVE CARE

Diagnostic Tests

Diagnosis is based upon the examination of the skin. A child under 8 years of age who develops acne should be evaluated for signs of precocious puberty (Silverberg, Silverberg, & Silverberg, 2005). See Chapter 29 ∞ .

Clinical Therapy

The goal of treatment is to suppress lesions until the condition is outgrown, thus preventing infection and scarring, and minimizing psychologic distress. The severity of skin lesions is graded, and treatment is customized to the severity level. See treatment protocols for acne below.

Benzoyl peroxide, a topical keratolytic, is an antimicrobial and breaks down comedones. Benzoyl peroxide comes in many preparations and strengths. Other topical keratolytics include azelaic acid 20%, salicylic acid, and sulfur. Topical antibiotics help reduce the colonization of bacteria and reduce inflammation.

Topical retinoids (tretinoin, adapalene, tazarotene) slow desquamation and decrease the adherence of shed cells within the follicles leading to reduced follicular plugging. Newer topic retinoids approved by the FDA for acne treatment include dapsone gel and nicotinamide. Dryness and scaling of the skin are typical after several days of treatment. It may seem as if the condition is worsening in the first 1 to 3 weeks of treatment, but with continued treatment, the skin adapts (Rudy, 2003). Adolescents with dry or more sensitive skin should use creams while those with more oily skin should use gels.

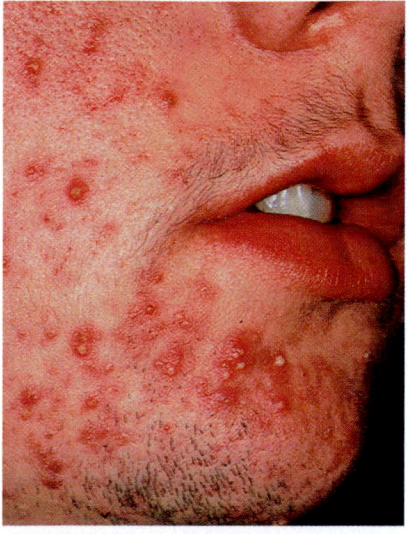

Figure 30–7 ➤ Pustular acne can have a significant effect on an adolescent's self-esteem.
Note: From Habif, T. P. (1990). *Clinical dermatology: A color guide to diagnosis and therapy* (2nd ed., p. 113). St. Louis, MO: Mosby-Year Book.

CULTURE

Acne Lesions and Skin Color
Inflammatory acne in adolescents with darker skin color is associated with a hyperpigmented macule. Extra pigment gets deposited in the areas of inflammation and this color change can last for 4 months or longer. If inflammation is controlled with acne therapy, the hyperpigmented areas may fade over time; however, keloid scars that can develop will not recede (Rudy, 2003).

MEDICATIONS USED TO TREAT *Acne*

Severity and Appearance	Treatment
Grade I (mild) Comedonal acne (comedones only)	Tretinoin (Retin-A) 0.025% cream daily (to comedones only), in the evening, salicylic acid, adapalene, tazarotene
Grade II (moderate) Papulopustular acne (red papules, pustules)	2.5% benzoyl peroxide gel, Tretinoin (Retin-A) in evening, topical antibiotics (clindamycin, erythromycin, tetracycline) twice a day, azaleic acid cream twice a day
Grade III (severe) Cystic acne (red papules, many pustules, cysts)	Tretinoin (Retin-A) and benzoyl peroxide twice a day, oral antibiotics (tetracycline, minocycline, or doxycycline)
Grade IV Pustulocystic nodular (severe, resistant to other treatment)	Isotretinoin (Accutane)

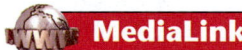
Oral antibiotics are used for moderate or severe acne. Generally, 3 months are needed for medication to be effective. After a positive response to oral antibiotics and topical acne medications, the antibiotic dose is tapered to the lowest dose that maintains acne control when used in combination with topical medications. Increasing numbers of cases of bacterial resistance to antibiotics have been noted. A recurrence or flare-up of acne after it has been controlled may indicate that the bacteria have developed resistance to the antibiotic. The antibiotic may need to be replaced to find one that is effective.

Isotretinoin (Accutane) is reserved for the most serious cases that are not responsive to other therapies. Isotretinoin acts on the skin by reducing sebaceous gland size and thus decreasing sebum secretion. The drug blocks follicular keratinization and has antiacne properties. Because of its teratogenicity and potential adverse reactions, the Food and Drug Administration established the iPLEDGE program, which requires that prescribers, pharmacies, and individuals taking isotretinoin agree to accept specific responsibilities designed to minimize pregnancy exposures. Patients must be counseled, have monthly pregnancy tests, and be monitored for liver function, cholesterol, and triglycerides (Food and Drug Administration, 2005b).

Oral contraceptives have been approved by the FDA for treatment of acne (Keri, 2006). Spiralatone is sometimes prescribed due to its action in decreasing sebum production; when prescribed with oral contraceptives, its action is enhanced (Woodard, 2002).

NURSING MANAGEMENT

Nursing Assessment and Diagnosis

Physical assessment should include documentation regarding distribution, type, and severity of acne lesions. Assess the adolescent's and parents' knowledge about the cause and treatment of acne. Also explore the amount of emotional distress the acne is causing the adolescent.

Common nursing diagnoses are presented in the accompanying Nursing Care Plan: The Adolescent with Acne.

Planning and Implementation

Nursing care for the adolescent with acne is summarized in the accompanying nursing care plan. Nursing management focuses on educating the child and parents about acne and its treatment. Advise adolescents to wash their hands before touching affected areas and to avoid picking or squeezing the lesions. Remind them that the inflammation occurs with the rupture of lesions below the skin surface, which picking and squeezing may cause. In addition, advise them to avoid using any cleansing products that have a greasy base, to shampoo hair regularly (to treat seborrhea that can accompany acne), to expect flare-ups despite treatment, and to eat a well-balanced diet. See Families Want to Know: Caring for Acne.

Topical medications should be spread in a thin film over the skin, according to directions. Emphasize that treatment is often long term, and there may be an increased flare a few weeks after starting topical medications. This is not a sign that the regimen is failing. Significant improvement may not be seen until at least 6 to 12 weeks after the start of treatment.

Correct misconceptions about dietary causes. Although no food has been found to cause acne or an increase in severity of lesions, good nutrition is important. Teach parents and children that increased sweating, as well as heat and humidity, may exacerbate acne. Emotional stress may increase adrenal androgen production, resulting in increased sebum production and acne flares.

Caution patients using tretinoin that this medication is **phototoxic** (a rapid nonimmunologic reaction of the skin when exposed to sunlight), resulting in sunburn with even minimal exposure. A noncomedonic sunscreen should be used. Teach correct procedures

NURSING CARE PLAN   The Adolescent with Acne

GOAL	INTERVENTION	RATIONALE	EXPECTED OUTCOME
1. Effective, Individual Therapeutic Regimen Management related to hygiene and skin care			
	NIC Priority Intervention **Health Education:** *Developing and providing instruction and learning experiences to facilitate voluntary adaptation of behavior conducive to health in individuals, families, groups, or communities.*		*NOC Suggested Outcome* **Symptom Control Behavior:** *Personal actions to minimize perceived adverse changes in physical and emotional functioning.*

The adolescent will verbalize proper hygiene, nutrition, and treatment of acne.	• Teach good skin care:
	  • Wash skin with mild soap and water twice a day.
	  • Do not use astringents or abrasive cleansers.
	  • Avoid vigorous scrubbing.
	  • Apply topical retinoid 20 minutes after washing and drying the face.
	• Wash hands frequently and especially after eating greasy foods.
		• Good hygiene and appropriate skin care reduce surface oils and bacteria, which intensify inflammatory reactions.	The adolescent exhibits good hygiene habits.

	• Praise good habits.	• Positive reinforcement encourages continued effort.	
	• Advise the adolescent to wash hair with antiseborrheic shampoo, avoid oil-based cosmetics or lotions.	• Treats seborrhea, which frequently accompanies acne. Oil-based preparations can obstruct sebaceous glands, exacerbating acne.	
	• Encourage a balanced diet, adequate fluids, exercise, and adequate rest.	• Adequate nutrients, water, and exercise promote healthy skin.	
	• Encourage the adolescent to keep a diary of health and diet habits.	• A record may help identify associations with flare-ups that can be avoided in the future.	
The adolescent will verbalize understanding of the treatment regimen.	• Educate the adolescent about medications (action, side effects, dosage, method of application).	• Proper application of medication enhances healing of lesions.	The adolescent implements the treatment regimen as outlined, resulting in a noticeable reduction in lesions.
	• Encourage application of tretinoin at night. Encourage use of noncomedonic sunscreens of at least SPF 30.	• Helps reduce sensitivity to sun and avoid sunburn.	
	• Educate the adolescent about time needed for response and importance of daily compliance.	• May take up to 3 months for significant improvement to occur. The adolescent needs a reason to continue with the care plan.	
2. Disturbed Body Image related to biophysical factors (visible facial lesions)			
	NIC Priority Intervention **Self-Esteem Enhancement:** *Assisting a patient to increase his personal judgment of self-worth.*		*NOC Suggested Outcome* **Self-Esteem:** *Personal judgment of self-worth.*
The adolescent will demonstrate increased self-confidence and self-esteem.	• Establish a rapport with the adolescent.	• A trusting relationship promotes verbalization of concerns and fears.	The adolescent freely discusses concerns and fears.

NURSING CARE PLAN The Adolescent with Acne (continued)

GOAL	INTERVENTION	RATIONALE	EXPECTED OUTCOME
2. Disturbed Body Image related to biophysical factors (visible facial lesions) (continued)			
	• Provide education about the condition and therapy modalities.	• Providing information better enables the adolescent to take control of the condition.	The adolescent demonstrates active involvement in own care.
	• Encourage the adolescent to be responsible for treatment and follow-up, and give positive reinforcement.	• Responsibility reinforces sense of self-esteem.	The adolescent shows increased confidence, as demonstrated by involvement in extracurricular activities.
	• Encourage the adolescent to become involved with school activities and peers.	• Involvement in activities helps enhance self-esteem and allows the adolescent to explore new experiences and friendships.	

for taking other prescribed drugs, such as tetracycline and isotretinoin (Accutane), and discuss possible side effects. Emphasize the importance of return visits to the adolescent's healthcare provider to monitor medication side effects.

Psychologic support is an important aspect of care. Because adolescents are preoccupied with their body image and peer relationships, they often find having acne embarrassing. Depression, anxiety, and social withdrawal have been noted in some adolescents. Encourage them to express their feelings and refer for counseling, if necessary.

Evaluation

Expected outcomes of nursing care can be found in Nursing Care Plan: The Adolescent with Acne.

INFECTIOUS DISORDERS

Bacterial Infections

Bacterial infections commonly occur in children due to minor skin injuries. The most common superficial infections include impetigo and folliculitis. Cellulitis is a more serious and deeper bacterial skin infection.

Impetigo

Impetigo is a highly contagious, superficial (epidermal) infection caused by streptococci, staphylococci, or both. The most common sites are the face and around the

FAMILIES WANT TO KNOW

Caring for Acne

- Wash the hands frequently and avoid touching the face to reduce the transfer of oils (e.g., from greasy foods) and bacteria to the face. Avoid picking and squeezing pimples.
- Use gentle cleansers to wash the face twice a day. Do not use abrasive sponges or cloths. Wait 20 minutes until the skin is thoroughly dry before applying topical medications.
- Avoid the use of astringents and aftershaves that contain alcohol and may further dry the skin.
- Avoid hats or gear that can cause friction and occlusion of the skin.
- Limit the use of pomades or petrolatum-based hair products. Keep hair spray and other hair products away from the face.
- Use noncomedonic (for acne-prone skin) moisturizers.
- Use oil-free or water-based makeup. Avoid waterproof makeup.
- Use noncomedonic sunscreen or protective clothing even on cloudy days.
- Continue daily therapies, even when acne has improved significantly, so acne does not return.

mouth, the hands, the neck, and the extremities. It is the most common bacterial skin condition in children.

Minor skin abrasions, lacerations, insect bites, burns, and dermatitis provide the portal for the infectious agent commonly present in the environment. *Staphylococcus aureus, Group A beta hemolytic streptococcus,* or both together are usually responsible. Staphylococcus aureus colonizes on the skin and mucous membranes, particularly in the nose and throat. This infection occurs more commonly in children who are in close physical contact with others, such as in childcare settings, or who have poor hygiene. The child may develop multiple lesions through self-inoculation.

Impetigo lesions begin as a vesicle or pustule surrounded by edema and redness, usually at a site that has been injured. This progresses to an exudative and crusting stage. The initially serous vesicular fluid becomes cloudy, and the vesicle ruptures, leaving a honey-colored crust covering an ulcerated base. Common sites include the intertriginous areas, and moist skin folds such as in the neck, axillae, or diaper area. The rash may spread to the face and extremities by self-inoculation. In bullous impetigo, vesicles develop on intact skin. The vesicles, stimulated by a toxin, enlarge into bullae with straw-colored fluid (Figure 30–8▶). The bullae rupture easily, leaving a red weeping surface on which a thin honey-colored crust forms. When the crust is removed a moist, erythematous lesion with a collar of skin around the erosion is seen.

Impetigo may be diagnosed by physical appearance; however, a Gram stain and bacterial culture may sometimes be required.

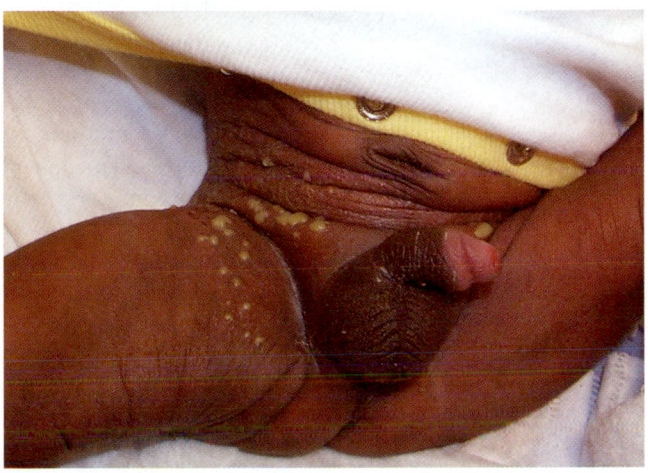

Figure 30–8 ▶ Bullous impetigo.
Courtesy of Dr. William H. Sorey, University of Mississippi Medical Center.

Local treatment involves removal of the crusts and application of a topical antibiotic. Crusts are soaked in warm water and gently scrubbed off with an antiseptic soap. A topical bactericidal ointment (such as bacitracin, or mupirocin) is applied for 5 to 7 days. If there is no response to topical antibiotics, a skin culture and systemic antibiotic (e.g., dicloxacillin or erythromycin) may be needed. Bullous impetigo is treated with systemic antibiotics. Methicillin-resistant *Staphylococcus aureus* is becoming more common and identifying the antibiotic to which it is sensitive is important. In children with bullous impetigo, an oral antibiotic may be used. The infection is communicable for 48 hours after antibiotic ointment treatment is begun.

If the child has a history of recurrent impetigo, determine if a person in contact with the child is a nasal carrier of *Staphylococcus aureus.* The carrier can be effectively treated with topical mupirocin ointment applied to the nares two times daily for 5 days (McLeod, 2004).

NURSING MANAGEMENT   Advise parents that they must continue oral or topical medications for the full number of days prescribed. If the child's lesions do not start to improve within 24 hours with the care previously described, the healthcare provider should be contacted. A culture may be needed.

Tell the parents to observe all close contacts and family members for lesions. Caution them that an infected child should not share towels or toiletries with others and that all linens and clothing used by the child should be washed separately with detergent in hot water. Fingernails should be kept short and clean to prevent spreading infection by scratching. Inform the child's childcare center about the infection, so staff can sanitize toys and surfaces. The child can return to the childcare center after 24 hours of treatment. Athletes should not return to practice or compete until the treatment is determined to be effective. In some cases, a physician's note may be required, such as for wrestlers who have close skin contact with other athletes.

Increased cases of skin infected with methicillin-resistant *Staphylococcus aureus* have been reported among athletes in high school, particularly when skin-to-skin contact or trauma occurs or when items are shared. Educate parents, adolescents, coaches, and teachers about the importance of a regular schedule for cleaning equipment, having athletes shower with soap and water after all practice sessions, and discouraging the sharing of protective equipment, towels, and clothing. Wounds should be covered to reduce exposure of other athletes to infection (Centers for Disease Control, 2003a). Skin infections that worsen rather than heal with regular topical antibiotics should be seen by a healthcare provider.

Folliculitis

Folliculitis is a superficial inflammation of the pilosebaceous hair follicle caused by infection, trauma, or irritation. The causative organism is usually *Staphylococcus aureus*, but it may also be caused by *Pityrosporum*. The condition is common in children and teenagers because of increased sweat production. Folliculitis may be associated with *Pseudomonas aeruginosa* exposure in a poorly chlorinated pool or hot tub.

Symptoms include pain or pruritus, localized swelling, and the formation of tiny dome-shaped, yellowish pustules and red papules at follicular openings with surrounding erythema. Individual lesions may become deeper and form an abscess (furuncle). Lesions are usually seen in clusters on the face, scalp, trunk, and extremities. Ruptured lesions heal with hyperpigmentation and no scarring. Some children have fever, aching, and flu-like symptoms. If associated with *Pseudomonas* exposure in a pool or hot tub, lesions may develop on areas covered by bathing suits.

Treatment of inflamed follicles consists of washing the affected area with a topical antibacterial cleanser and water, followed by application of hot compresses for 20 minutes, four times a day. A benzoyl peroxide gel or wash or another drying agent will also help clear the infection. Complications are rare. If lesions do not resolve within a week, the child may need systemic antibiotics (e.g., cephalexin or dicloxacillin) and, if the infection is deep, incision and drainage.

NURSING MANAGEMENT   Nursing management focuses on educating the parents and child about prevention. Advise children to shower daily and shortly after exercise, to cleanse with an antibacterial soap, and to wear loose cotton clothing. Talk with parents about the importance of maintaining the correct pH level and chlorine concentration in swimming pools and hot tubs. Bathing suits of affected children should be laundered and well dried before the next use.

Cellulitis

Cellulitis is an acute inflammation of the dermis and underlying connective tissue characterized by red or lilac, tender, warm, edematous skin that may have an ill-defined, nonelevated border. The condition usually occurs on the face and extremities as a result of trauma or a compromised skin barrier.

ETIOLOGY AND PATHOPHYSIOLOGY   Children with cellulitis often have a history of trauma, impetigo, folliculitis, or recent otitis media. Common causative organisms are *Staphylococcus aureus, Streptococcus pneumoniae, Haemophilus influenzae,* and beta-hemolytic and group A *streptococcus*. The condition may also result from a nearby abscess or sinusitis. Onset is usually rapid.

CLINICAL MANIFESTATIONS   Children with cellulitis have a rapid onset and they appear ill. Classic signs and symptoms include erythema, edema of the face or infected limb, warmth, and tenderness around the infected site (Figure 30–9►). Other symptoms include fever, chills, malaise, and enlargement and tenderness of regional lymph nodes. Lymphangitis may be present. In some cases, a rapidly progressive lesion may result in septicemia.

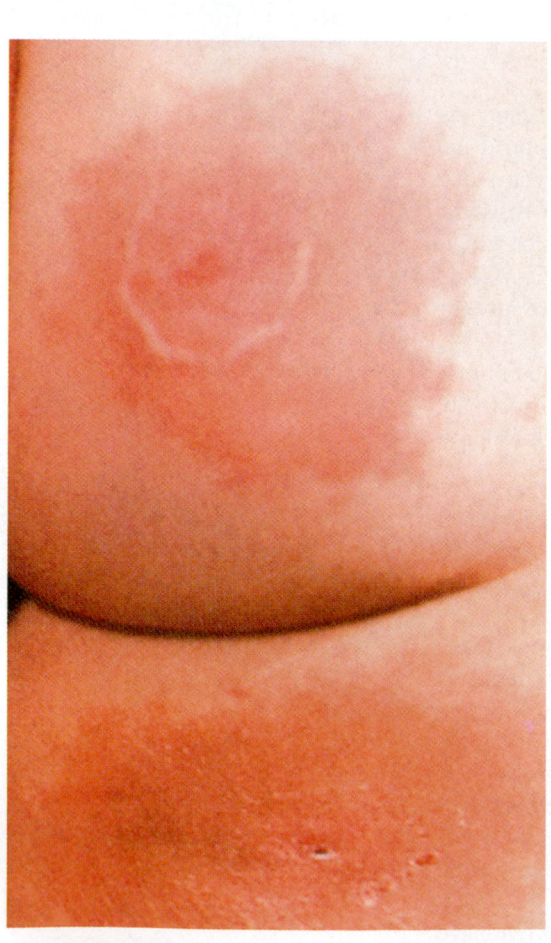

Figure 30–9 ► Characteristic appearance of cellulitis. Note: From Ben-Amitai, D., & Ashkenazi, S. (1993). Common bacterial skin infections in children. *Pediatric Annals, 22*(4), 226. Photograph courtesy of Dr. Aryeh Metzker.

COLLABORATIVE CARE

Diagnostic Tests

Blood studies may show an increase in white blood cells. Cultures are taken by needle aspiration, if possible, to identify the causative organisms. Blood cultures are taken if the child has a toxic (very ill) appearance.

Clinical Therapy

If the face is involved, antibiotic therapy is administered to avoid serious complications. (Periorbital cellulitis is discussed in Chapter 19 ∞.) Children with severe cases or a large affected surface area are treated with systemic antibiotics and analgesics in the hospital to prevent sepsis. Children with cellulitis on the trunk, limbs, or perianal area may be treated on an outpatient basis with oral antibiotics. Recovery begins within 48 hours, but therapy should continue for at least 10 days. Untreated cellulitis or cellulitis that does not respond to treatment can lead to osteomyelitis, arthritis, or serious systemic infection.

SKILL 7–14
Obtaining a Sample for Wound Culture

NURSING MANAGEMENT

Nursing Assessment and Diagnosis

Assessment centers on recognition of infection, documentation of location and related symptoms, and monitoring of vital signs.

Among the nursing diagnoses that may be appropriate for the child with cellulitis are:

- Impaired Skin Integrity related to mechanical factors (injury, the inflammatory process, and presence of infection)
- Acute Pain related to injury agents (swelling and inflammation of the skin)
- Interrupted Family Processes related to home care needs of the child with acute illness

Planning and Implementation

Because of the risk of sepsis, cellulitis is managed carefully. Administer prescribed oral or IV antibiotics as scheduled. Supportive care includes warm compresses to the affected area four times daily, elevation of the affected limb, and bed rest. Outpatient follow-up is crucial to ensure response to therapy.

Advise parents about possible complications, such as abscess formation. Instruct parents of children treated at home to contact their healthcare provider if the child has any of the following signs:

- Spread of the infected area in the 24- to 48-hour period after the start of treatment
- Temperature over 38.3°C (101°F)
- Increased lethargy

Reinforce to parents the importance of compliance with the treatment regimen and the seriousness of the possible complications.

Evaluation

Expected outcomes of nursing care include pain control, adherence with administration of antibiotics, and resolution of the infection without progression to systemic infection.

Viral Infectious Disorders

Molluscum Contagiosum

Molluscum contagiosum is a skin infection caused by a poxvirus. It is transmitted by direct contact, by contact with contaminated objects, or by sexual contact. The incubation period is weeks to months (Smolinski & Yan, 2005). The infection most commonly occurs in children between 1 and 5 years, and it is more common in children with atopic dermatitis. Patients who are immunosuppressed have a higher incidence of the infection and a much greater number of lesions (Smolinksi & Yan, 2005).

The individual lesions are pearl-like, flesh-colored smooth papules about 1 to 5 mm in size with a central depression. A plug of cheesy material can be expressed when the lesion is punctured. Lesions may appear anywhere on the body, but tend to be seen more commonly on the face, trunk, and extremities. In adolescents, lesions are more common on the inner thighs, genital, and pubic areas. The palms and soles are not involved. Children may have few to hundreds of lesions. The lesions often disappear spontaneously in 6 to 18 months, but the condition can continue for several years.

In mild cases, no intervention is needed (Smolinski & Yan, 2005). Clinical therapy may involve the daily application of tretinoin to irritate the skin and stimulate the immune system to respond to the viral condition. Curettage preceeded by topical anesthesia or **cryotherapy** (freezing each lesion with liquid nitrogen) may be performed by dermatologists. All lesions should be treated to prevent self-inoculation. Scarring may result from clinical therapy. Secondary infections are treated with topical or oral antibiotics.

NURSING MANAGEMENT   Nursing education focuses on reducing disease transmission. Infected children should avoid public swimming pools, hot tubs, and other joint bathing situations as the virus is more easily transmitted when the skin is wet. Towels and sponges should not be shared.

The skin should be washed daily with gentle fragrance-free cleansers, followed by application of a hypoallergenic moisturizer or emollient to the entire skin surface. If tretinoin is selected as a therapy, educate the parents how to apply the lotion. Teach parents to recognize potential secondary infections.

When intervention such as curettage or cryotherapy is performed, inform the child about what will happen, and then provide distraction during the procedure to reduce anxiety. Assure that the child has adequate topical anesthetic to minimize any pain from the intervention.

Warts (Papillomavirus)

Several types of human papillomavirus infect epithelial cells and cause warts. Various types of warts are found in children: common warts that appear on any skin surface and plantar warts found on the feet. The human papillomavirus is commonly transmitted by direct skin-to-skin contact or mucous membrane contact. The virus also survives on various surfaces, and transmission can occur with contact, such as plantar warts from locker room floors. The incubation period may be 2 to 6 months; however, a latency period may exist in some cases. Children with immune compromise are more susceptible and often have numerous warts.

Common warts appear as skin-colored, rough, scaly papules and nodules on exposed skin surfaces. Individual and multiple warts may be seen, or large plaques may form if autoinoculation occurs. Warts usually cause no pain or itching unless in skin surface areas or creases that become irritated. Plantar warts appear as papules and plaques on the bottom of feet that grow inward and cause pain. Small black dots result from thrombosed vessels on the surface of the warts caused by weight bearing.

No intervention may be recommended as warts often resolve spontaneously over a couple of years and clinical therapy may be traumatic for children. Application of duct tape that is changed every 1 to 3 days over a couple of months is often effective and painless (Smolinski & Yan, 2005). The tape is thought to work by stimulating the immune system through irritation (Focht, Spicer, & Fairchok, 2002). Clinical therapy may be provided when warts have a negative social stigma. Therapy usually involves some form of destruction, such as cryotherapy, application of caustic substances or peeling agents, electrocautery, and laser therapy. Treatment is not always successful and may result in scarring. Immunologic medications (oral and topical) are being investigated for use in treating warts.

NURSING MANAGEMENT   Educate the parents and child about the application of peeling agents and caustic substances when prescribed for home use. If the reaction to the substance is painful, encourage the parents to reduce the frequency of the treatment until the pain subsides and then to resume the original treatment schedule. Successful treatment may take several months, and the parents and child may need encouragement to continue the therapy and remain optimistic.

Other viral skin conditions are described in Chapter 18 ∞ .

Fungal Infections
Oral Candidiasis (Thrush)

Oral candidiasis (moniliasis or thrush) is a fungal infection that occurs as an acute condition in newborns (usually acquired during birth from the vaginal canal of an infected mother). It is also a chronic condition in young children who have an immune disorder, regularly use a corticosteroid inhaler, or are receiving antibiotics that have disturbed the normal flora, allowing the fungus to grow.

Oral thrush is characterized by white patches that look like coagulated milk on the oral mucosa and may bleed when removed (Figure 30–10➤). Milk residue can be removed from the oral mucosa with gentle swabbing. With candidiasis, however, attempts at gentle removal are unsuccessful. The infant may refuse to nurse or feed because of discomfort and pain. The infant may also have diaper dermatitis superinfection with candidiasis. Fever is usually not present.

Treatment involves oral nystatin suspension or clotrimazole, which is applied to the mouth and tongue after feedings. Fluconazole or itraconazole may be used for immunocompromised patients with oropharyngeal candidiasis. If infection is severe, occurs in the esophagus, or invades other body systems, oral fluconazole or intravenous amphotericin B may be prescribed for a minimum of 21 days.

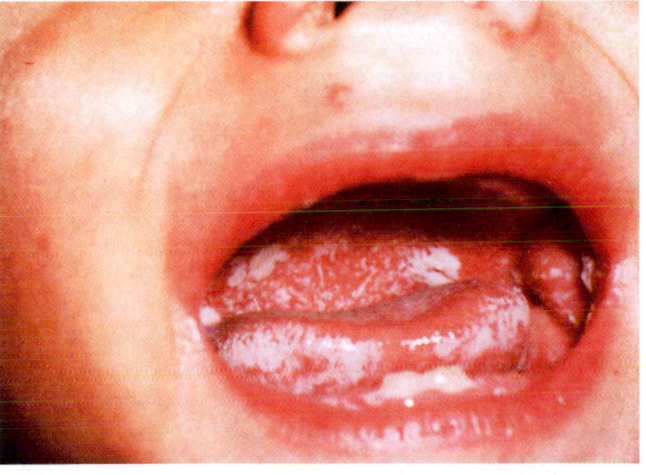

Figure 30–10 ➤ Thrush, an acute pseudomembranous form of oral candidiasis, is a common fungal infection in infants and children.
Note: From Zitelli, B. J., & Davis, H. W. (Eds.). (1997). *Atlas of pediatric physical diagnosis,* (3rd ed., p. 104, Fig. 4–50a). St. Louis: Mosby.

NURSING MANAGEMENT   Educate parents to give the oral medication to infants. Parents should use a swab to apply the suspension to the buccal mucosa and tongue surfaces, allowing the infant to swallow the remaining suspension. Older children should be told to swish the solution around in the mouth before swallowing it.

To prevent a reinfection, educate parents about sterilizing bottle nipples and pacifiers. Breast-feeding mothers should be treated as the breasts may have become infected from contact with lesions in the infant's mouth. A commercial antiseptic spray may be used on toys that cannot be autoclaved, but follow directions carefully so the child does not ingest any harmful residue. Teach parents and older children with asthma to rinse the mouth well with water after using a corticosteroid inhaler to prevent candidiasis. If a spacer is used, it should also be rinsed with water after use.

Dermatophytoses (Ringworm)

Dermatophytoses are fungal infections that affect the skin, hair, or nails. Children of all ages may be affected. Dermatophytoses may be spread from person to person, from animal to person, or by contact with an inanimate object (e.g., clothing or linens) belonging to an infected individual. The most common infections are tinea capitis, tinea corporis, tinea cruris, and tinea pedis. See the clinical manifestations table on the next page for common organisms, signs and symptoms, and clinical therapy.

Diagnosis may be confirmed through microscopic examination of the hair and scalp scrapings using a potassium hydroxide (KOH) wet mount to reveal rows and chains of spores within the hair shaft. A fungal culture can also be taken from a scalp lesion by rubbing a cotton-tipped applicator across the scalp and placing it in a throat culture tube. A Wood's lamp is also useful in identifying some forms of tinea that fluoresce

CULTURE

Tinea Capitis
While tinea capitis can occur in any racial or ethnic group, it is most prevalent in African American children. This is believed to be due to immunological factors, genetic factors, or hair care practices. For this reason, any African American child with scaling in the scalp should be screened for tinea capitis (Elewski & Krowchuk, 2001).

CLINICAL MANIFESTATIONS TINEA INFECTIONS

Site, Incidence, and Common Dermatophyte	Clinical Manifestations	Clinical Therapy
Tinea capitis (scalp) *Trichophyton tonsurans* *Trichophyton violaceum* *Trichophyton soudanense* *Trichophyton verricosum* *Microsporum canis* Usually prepubertal children between 1 and 10 years 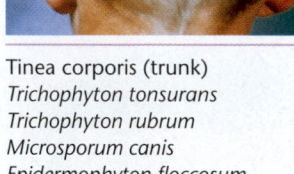	Circumscribed hair loss Broken hairs; black, dotted stubbed appearance where weakened hair has broken off Diffuse fine scaling, may appear as seborrhea with yellow greasy scales Many scaly pustular bald areas with indistinct margins Mild itching **Kerion**—large purulent tender boggy mass on scalp with drainage Papules, pustules, and crusting on scalp Suboccipital or posterior cervical nodes	Griseofulvin orally for 6 to 8 weeks, or 2 weeks after symptoms disappear OR Terbutafine orally for 2 to 4 weeks Selenium sulfide shampoo two to three times weekly, leave on for 10 minutes before rinsing to help eliminate scalp spores Alternate antifungal agents used when children do not tolerate or respond to griseofulvin include fluconazole, itraconazole, and terbinafine (not approved by FDA for children less than 12 years of age)
Tinea corporis (trunk) *Trichophyton tonsurans* *Trichophyton rubrum* *Microsporum canis* *Epidermophyton floccosum* Children and adolescents 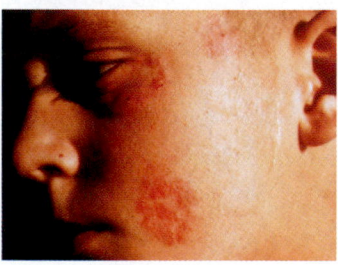	Pink, scaly circular patch with an expanding border, may be scaly or erythematous throughout Slightly raised borders with a clearing center Usually acquired from contact with infected humans, cats, dogs, or horses (Monroe, 2005)	Topical cream (e.g., clotrimazole, miconazole, ketoconazole, naftifine, or terbinafine) twice a day for 4 weeks. Avoid combination with a topical steroid preparation as this may lead to a persistent or recurrent infection Wash body with selenium sulfide shampoo An oral antifungal agent may be needed for extensive lesions, hair follicle involvement, or no response to topical therapy
Tinea cruris ("jock itch") *Epidermophyton floccosum* *Trichophyton rubrum* Rare before adolescence	Annular lesions Scaly, erythematous eruption symmetric bilaterally, may spread to abdomen, buttocks, and upper thighs, usually spare penis and scrotum May have elevated lesions, papules, or vesicles Tinea pedis may have been spread by hand to groin area	Topical antifungal agent such as imidazole for 2 weeks or butenafine, naftifine, or terbinafine for 1 week Wash body with selenium sulfide shampoo Decrease moisture and occlusion to area
Tinea pedis ("athlete's foot") *Trichophyton rubrum* *Trichophyton mentagrophytes* *Epidermophyton floccosum* Children and adolescents	Vesicles or erosions on instep or between toes (fissures, red scaly) Peeling maceration and fissures in lateral toe web spaces (indicate secondary bacterial involvement) Dry scaly patches or plaques with mild erythema on plantar and lateral surfaces of foot Itching	Broad spectrum topical antifungal agent that has antibacterial properties (e.g., econazole or ciclopirox) Keep feet dry with absorbent talc Allow to air dry Use 100% cotton socks, change twice daily

Photographs of tinea capitis and tinea corporis courtesy of the Centers for Disease Control and Prevention, Atlanta, GA.

under ultraviolet light; for example, tinea caused by a *Microsporum* infection flouresces a brilliant green under the Wood's lamp (American Academy of Pediatrics, 2006, p. 655). *Trichophyton tonsurans*, the most common cause of tinea capitis, does not fluoresce. An oral antifungal agent (e.g., griseofulvin, terbinafine) is usually prescribed for tinea capitis. Resistance is developing to griseofulvin, so high doses for 8 to 12 weeks are needed. Terbinofine is often effective with a 2- to 4-week course of medication; however, the FDA has not yet approved its use for tinea capitis (Fleece, Gaughan, & Aronoff, 2004).

NURSING MANAGEMENT All members of the family and household pets should be assessed for fungal lesions. Since person-to-person transmission is common, personal contact with hair and sharing hair accessories, brushes, and hats should be avoided. In some cases, there may be an asymptomatic carrier in the family, in which case everyone should be treated. Teach parents and older children or teenagers that fungi are found in soil and animals and are transmitted through direct contact.

Advise parents to give oral griseofulvin with fatty foods such as whole milk or peanut butter to enhance absorption. The medications must be used for the entire prescribed period, even if the lesions are gone, to prevent recurrence of the infection. For children with *tinea cruris*, encourage loose-fitting undergarments to promote dryness. With *tinea pedis*, feet should be kept clean and dry and nails clipped short. Encourage the use of 100% cotton socks that keep moisture away from the skin. Encourage children to wear shower shoes in public showers and locker rooms.

Parents of children with tinea capitis should be told that hair regrowth is slow and may take 6 to 12 months. In some cases hair loss is permanent, which can be particularly stressful for older children or adolescents. Provide emotional support.

INFESTATIONS
Pediculosis Capitis (Lice)

Pediculosis capitis is a lice infestation of the hair and scalp. Infestation occurs among children of all socioeconomic levels. Parents or teachers may be the first to notice lice, or healthcare providers may spot them during routine examination (see Chapter 5 ∞). Outbreaks occur periodically among preschool and school-age children, particularly those in day care and elementary school. Head lice are much less common in African American children (Leung, Fong, & Pinto-Rojas, 2005).

Head lice live and reproduce only on humans and are transmitted by direct hair-to-hair contact or indirect contact such as sharing of hair accessories, brushes, hats, towels, and bedding. Lice do not fly or jump, but they can crawl quickly. The female louse lays her eggs (nits) on the hair shaft, close to the scalp for food, moisture, and warmth (see Figure 5–8 ∞). The incubation period for eggs to hatch is 8 to 10 days. Lice feed on human blood several times a day.

Clinical manifestations include intense pruritus and complaints of "dandruff" that sticks to the hair (actually the nits) and "bugs" in the hair. Nits look like silvery white, yellow, or darker 1-mm teardrops adhering to one side of the hair shaft. Secondary effects of scratching include inflammation, pustules, and bacterial infection. Nits are found most commonly behind the ears and at the base of the head. Lice are wingless insects about the size of a sesame seed (2 to 3 mm long). They move quickly away from light and are not often seen. Occipital and posterior cervical lymph nodes are frequently palpable.

Treatment involves a pediculicide shampoo, such as pyrethrum with an enzymatic lice egg remover, or an ovicidal rinse, such as 1% permethrin (Nix). Permethrin cream rinse is applied to washed and towel-dried hair. The preparation is applied, left in place for 10 minutes, and then rinsed. The hair is towel dried, and the nits are removed with a fine-toothed comb. A second treatment is needed in 7 to 10 days as the neurotoxin is not effective on nits. Permethrin resistance has been reported, but a 5% concentration is effective. Lindane shampoo was removed from the U.S. market in 2003 because of lice resistance and toxicity (Leung, Fong, & Pinto-Rojas, 2005). See the medications adminstration table on the next page for products used to treat lice. Of home remedies (vinegar, isopropyl alcohol, olive oil, mayonnaise, melted butter, and petroleum jelly), only petroleum jelly caused significant louse mortality and allowed only 6% of eggs to hatch. None of the other home remedy products were an effective means of louse control (Takano-Lee, Edman, Mullens et al., 2004).

Nursing Management

Carefully assess children who have been exposed to head lice using a bright light and magnifying glass (see Chapter 5 ∞). To avoid potential reinfestation of other children, change gloves frequently when assessing several children in a classroom setting.

MEDICATIONS USED TO TREAT *Head Lice*

Name of Medication/Preparation	Nursing Considerations
Insecticide Free Lice R Gone Lice Away Enzyme Shampoo LiceFreee!	Apply all products to dry hair.
Hair Clean 1-2-3	Cover with shower cap overnight.
Oil, petrolatum jelly, mayonnaise	Used as a rinse to loosen nits.
Distilled white vinegar used as a rinse	Used as a rinse to loosen nits.
Formic acid used as a rinse	
Cetaphil cleanser	Apply lotion to a wet scalp and dry it with a hair dryer to shrink wrap and suffocate lice (Pearlman, 2004).

First-Line Pesticide Treatment
Permethrin 1% Crème Rinse—Nix
Pyrethrin shampoo (0.17–0.33%) or
  Piperonyl butoxide (2–4%)—Rid, A-200,
  R&C, Triple X, Pronto, Tegrin-LT, InnoGel Plus
	Should be applied to dry hair and scalp. Massage into the hair one section at a time. Wet hair dilutes the product and may contribute to treatment failure.

Second-Line Pesticide Treatment Malathion 0.5—Ovide lotion Lindane 1% or "lindano"—Kwell, limited effectiveness due to resistance	Apply to dry scalp and hair until soaked and allowed to dry naturally. Leave on for 8 to 12 hours. Do not expose the child to electric heat sources as the malathion treatment contains flammable alcohol.
Non-FDA Approved Trimethoprim/sulfamethoxazole Ivermectin—antiparasitic	Drug in bloodstream is ingested by louse, destroys bacterial flora in louse intestine. Does not treat the nits.

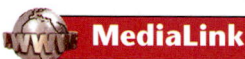

MediaLink

Head Lice Education

Infestation with lice can be upsetting for both the child and family. Emphasize to the family that anyone can get lice. Thorough interventions and education are essential for effective treatment. All contacts of the child should be examined for infestation and should be treated as necessary. Tell parents that children infested with lice should return to childcare or school the day after the first pediculicide treatment. Teach the child not to share clothing, headwear, or combs.

Explain to parents that the shampoo and rinses prescribed are pesticides and must be used for the time specified and as directed. Hair conditioners should not be used prior to applying a pediculicide as it may reduce the ovicide activity. An extra bottle of shampoo may be needed if the child has extra long hair. Keep these products out of the eyes and mouth of the child during their use as they will irritate mucous membranes.

To remove nits, use a small-toothed comb, tweezers, and a basin filled with water or isopropyl alcohol to dip and clean the comb and tweezers. Comb 1-inch sections from the scalp outward and pin these out of the way when done. Nits adhere to the hair shaft and must be manually pulled down the shaft with the comb, tweezers, or fingernails. All nits should be removed. Have blunt-nosed scissors available to cut a hair shaft below the level of the nit when the nit cannot be removed. Put the child under a bright light and use distractions such as a video to keep the child occupied during the procedure. An alternate therapy for boys is to cut off the hair in a close buzz cut. A shorter haircut for girls may also help with nit removal.

Although lice can survive for only about 3 days away from a human host, shed nits may hatch 8 to 10 days later. For this reason, the child's bedding and clothing should be changed daily, laundered in hot water with detergent, and dried in a hot dryer for 20 minutes. Nonessential bedding and clothing can be stored in a tightly sealed bag for 2 to 3 weeks and then washed. Hair accessories, brushes, and combs should be discarded or soaked in hot soapy water (54.4°C [130°F]) for 10 minutes. Vacuum furniture and carpets and treat them with a hot iron when possible. Use of an insecticide in the home to kill the lice on carpets, furniture, and other items with which young children and pets come into contact is not recommended. Seal toys and other personal items that cannot be washed or dry cleaned in a plastic bag for 2 weeks.

Scabies

Scabies is a highly contagious infestation caused by the mite *Sarcoptes scabiei*. It is spread by skin-to-skin contact and through sexual contact. Children of all ages and both sexes can be affected.

The female mite burrows into the outer layer of the epidermis (stratum corneum) to lay her eggs, leaving a trail of debris and feces. The larvae hatch in approximately 2 to 4 days and proceed toward the surface of the skin. The larvae emerge and dig new burrows. The mite matures and mates, repeating the cycle every 14 to 17 days. Hypersensitivity to the ova and mite feces causes irritation and intense pruritus approximately 2 to 6 weeks after infestation (Johnston & Sladden, 2005). Nodules, which can persist for weeks after effective treatment, develop as a granulomatous response to the dead mite antigens and feces. Because the mite usually takes at least 45 minutes to burrow into the skin, transient contact is unlikely to cause infestation.

Symptoms include a rash with various types of lesions (papules, vesicles, pustules, and nodules), severe pruritus that worsens at night, and restlessness. Lesions are usually located in the palms of the hands, webs of the fingers, in the intergluteal folds, or around the axillae, wrists, elbows, inner thighs, and waist (Figure 30–11➤). In children under 2 years, insteps of the feet, as well as the head, neck, and face, can be affected. The burrow lesions may appear as a threadlike, grayish line on the skin surface 1 to 10 cm in length, which may end in a pinpoint vesicle. Burrows are often more easily seen on the hands and feet. The lesion may have been obliterated by the child's scratching and secondary infection. The lesions may look like widespread atopic dermatitis.

Diagnosis is confirmed by examination under the microscope of scrapings from a burrow, which reveals actively moving mites, fecal pellets, eggs, or nits. Treatment involves application of a scabicide, such as 5% permethrin lotion, over the entire body with special attention to the hands, fingers, feet, toes, and under the nails. The scabicide should be applied to the face, neck, ears, and scalp, but avoid getting the medication in the eyes (Sladden & Johnston, 2005).

Application of 5% permethrin lotion or malathion (Ovide) is preceded by a warm soap and water bath. The skin must be cool and dry before the lotion is applied to reduce excessive absorption of the scabicide. The lotion is left in place for 8 to 12 hours (overnight) before it is washed off. A second treatment is used 1 week later. Topical and oral invermectin is a new antiparasitic product with FDA approval for children weighing more than 15 kg. All close contacts, members of the household, and childcare contacts should be treated at the same time, even if they have no symptoms. Treatment failure is usually due to inadequate treatment or reinfestation by an untreated contact (Johnston & Sladden, 2005).

Itching may persist for 6 weeks after treatment. An oral antihistamine (e.g., Benadryl, Atarax) may be prescribed to help relieve itching. Antibiotics may be needed when a secondary infection occurs.

Nursing Management

Educate parents about the proper application of the scabicide. Make sure parents understand the importance of keeping the medication on the skin for the full 8 to 12 hours. The child should have scabicide reapplied to the hands if hands are washed or if the child sucks the fingers or thumb. Mitts or socks over the hands of young children may reduce the chance of ingesting the scabicide by placing the fingers in the mouth.

Advise parents that scabies is transmitted by close contact and is very contagious. All clothing, bedding, and pillowcases used by the child should be changed daily, washed with hot water, and ironed before reuse. Nonwashable toys and other items should be sealed in plastic bags for 5 to 7 days.

Family members who are not infected should avoid touching the affected child until after treatment is completed. If they do, they should wash their hands well. Inform the parents about signs of secondary infections and that itching and nodules may

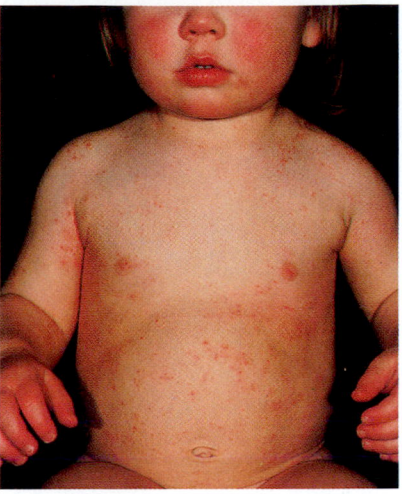

Figure 30–11 ➤ Diffuse scabies in an infant. The lesions are most numerous around the axillae, chest, and abdomen. *Note:* From Habif, T. P. (1990). *Clinical dermatology: A color guide to diagnosis and therapy* (2nd ed., p. 298). St. Louis, MO: Mosby-Year Book.

CLINICAL TIP

Make sure the scabicide lotion is applied to every skin surface below the neck, even between fingers and toes, the genitalia, and under freshly cleaned fingernails. Apply scabicide to the scalp, ears, face, and forehead of children up to 2 years of age (Johnston & Sladden, 2005). If the hands are washed or the infant sucks his or her fingers during the treatment period of 12 hours, the lotion should be reapplied.

persist for weeks after effective treatment. Encourage the use of emollients as the treatment dries the skin.

Scabies, like pediculosis, can be embarrassing or upsetting for the child and family. Educate the child and parents about the condition, its spread, and treatment measures to prevent recurrence.

INFANTILE HEMANGIOMAS

Vascular tumors or hemangiomas occur in 1–3% of all neonates; however, by the age of 1 year, approximately 10% of infants are affected. An increased incidence has been noted in girls and preterm infants weighing less than 1500 grams. The head and neck are common sites (Miller & Frieden, 2005). The risk for a hemangioma is greater in children of women who had chorionic villus sampling during pregnancy (Cohen, 2005).

Hemangiomas may initially arise from embolized placental tissue or a mutation that arrests vascular differentiation. This may be one reason for the rapid growth of hemangiomas in the first few months of life (Miller & Frieden, 2005). Vascular tumors are neoplasms of endothelial cells and increased numbers of small blood vessels that undergo rapid growth and proliferation during the first 6 to 10 months of life that may lead to ulceration. This phase is followed by a slow **involution** (process of decreasing in size) that is completed in 95% of children by adolescence (Cohen, 2004). Hemangiomas may be superficial (located in the epidermis), deep (located in the dermis or subcutaneous tissue), or mixed superficial and deep. A large facial hemangioma may be associated with PHACE syndrome (*P*osterior fossa malformation, large facial *H*emangioma, *A*rterial anomalies, *C*ardiac defects, and *E*ye abnormalities) (Morel, Hogeling, & Eichenfield, 2005). When multiple hemangiomas are found, some may be in major organs, such as the liver. Complications caused by the rapid growth and pressure against or obstruction of vital structures may occur (Miller & Frieden, 2005).

- Airway compromise, stridor, and eating difficulty may occur when the hemangioma is in the lower face or beard area.
- Amblyopia, strabismus, and astigmatism when the hemangioma is near the eye.
- Renal abnormalities, imperforate anus, tethered cord, and bony anomalies of the sacrum when the hemangioma is in the lumbosacral area.

Infantile hemangiomas begin as barely visible telangiectasia or red macules that begin to grow rapidly and become bright red and compressible. Superficial hemangiomas are bright red vascular cutaneous plaques that resemble strawberries. Deep hemangiomas appear as bluish tumors covered with normal-appearing epidermis. Mixed hemangiomas have features of both superficial and deep tumors. The lesions, appearing any place on the body, are minimally compressible and have no bruit or thrill. As the hemangioma involutes, signs of tissue atrophy, wrinkles, telangiectasias, and hypopigmentation may be noted.

Initial diagnosis is by physical examination and monitoring the growth of the vascular tumor. When a vital organ could become obstructed, ultrasound, computed tomography, or magnetic resonance imaging may be performed.

Some hemangiomas are monitored and receive no treatment. Hemangiomas in problem areas may be treated by high doses of systemic corticosteroids during the proliferation phase to slow the growth (Cohen, 2004). Injections of corticosteroids into small localized hemangiomas are sometimes performed. Pulsed dye laser treatment at 2- to 3-week intervals is used for superficial hemangiomas during the proliferative phase. The hemangioma will darken for 1 to 2 weeks, the darkness will fade to red, and eventual lightening of the treated skin surface occurs.

Nursing Management

Assess the distribution of the hemangioma and consider the potential for complications as it goes through a rapid growth stage. Monitor the child for signs of any complications, such as ulceration or stridor that could be associated with compression on the

---

CLINICAL TIP

A port-wine stain is a capillary malformation. When the port-wine stain is on one side of the face in the distribution of the trigeminal nerve, it may indicate the presence of Sturge-Weber syndrome, an intracranial vascular anomaly. Children with Sturge-Weber syndrome are at high risk for glaucoma and may develop seizures, mental retardation, and hemiplegia during the first few years of life (Cohen, 2004). Regular ophthalmic examinations should be scheduled (Morel, Hogeling, & Eichenfield, 2005).

airway. Assess the parents' response to the infant's appearance and how they are managing interactions with friends and family about the infant's changing appearance. Take photos of the infant at each visit so that parents have a record of improvements once therapy is initiated.

Teach the parents about the type of vascular lesion and potential treatment options. When corticosteroids are prescribed, teach the parents about administration, the need to take full course as prescribed, and potential side effects. Inform parents about the possible ulceration of a rapidly growing hemangioma, what signs to expect, and how to protect the skin until the infant is seen by the physican.

Talk with parents about comments received about the infant's appearance and provide some possible responses that parents can make. To promote attachment, help the parents see the infant's positive characteristics, such as responsiveness and smiling. Show photos of other children with similar lesions who have completed therapy to show that improvements in appearance are gradual, but possible.

Teach parents to protect the skin surface from trauma after pulsed dye laser treatments and to keep the infant's nails short to prevent scratching. Cleanse the area treated with water and pat it dry. Inform parents to avoid sun exposure for several weeks after the treatments, and to use sunscreen in the future.

INJURIES TO THE SKIN

Pressure Ulcers

An increasing number of children with disabilities are cared for in hospital, community, and home care settings. Many are at risk for skin breakdown and pressure ulcers. Children at greatest risk are those with limited mobility or high activity, sensory deficits, the inability to change positions, or incontinence (Table 30–3). The incidence of pressure ulcers at any stage in children within a pediatric intensive care unit has been reported to be as high as 27% (Curley, Quigley, & Lin, 2003).

Soft tissues may be compressed between a bony prominence and another surface. Tissue ischemia occurs when high pressure is maintained over a short period of time or low pressure is maintained over a prolonged time. The cells are deprived of oxygen and nutrients, and metabolic waste products accumulate, injuring the soft tissue. Without appropriate intervention, the injury progresses rapidly and a pressure ulcer forms (Figure 30–12▶).

The earliest sign of skin damage is an area of redness that does not go away within 30 minutes of removing the pressure or skin irritant. Children with dark skin may have persistent red, blue, or purple discoloration. As the injury progresses, the skin looks rubbed or raw like an abrasion or blister. Damage then extends through the epidermis and dermis, forming an ulcer. The ulcer then deepens to underlying muscles, bone, or connective tissue unless treated. Secondary infection may occur.

Initial treatment for early stages of skin damage involves removing pressure from the affected site until the skin has healed. Children who use leg braces for alignment and mobility are often put in wheelchairs. Children who use wheelchairs are often put

Table 30–3	SITES AND POTENTIAL CAUSES OF PRESSURE ULCERS	
Sites	**Potential Causes**
Occipital region of scalp, ear	Inability to lift head
Sacrum and buttocks	Confinement to bed or wheelchair
Legs and feet	Leg braces, casts
Spine and neck	Scoliosis brace
Knees and elbows	Rubbing against bedsheet
Sternum, iliac crest	Ventilated in prone position

PATHOPHYSIOLOGY ILLUSTRATED

The Four Stages of Ulcer Formation

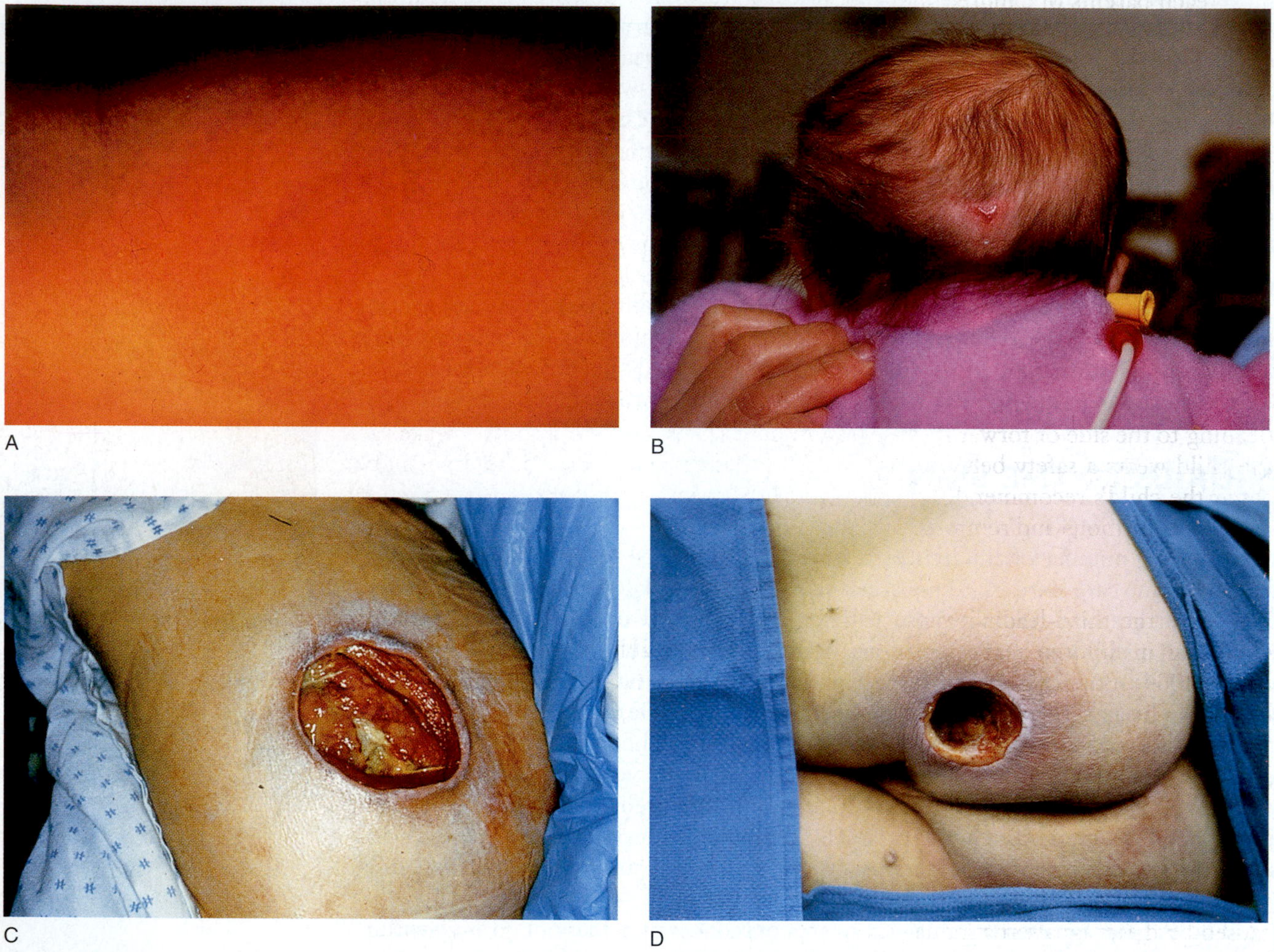

Figure 30–12 ➤ A, Stage 1, nonblanchable erythema of intact skin. B, Stage 2, blister or abrasion, partial-thickness loss with damage through epidermis, dermis, or both. C, Stage 3, full thickness loss with exposure of subcutaneous tissue. D, Stage 4, full-thickness loss that extends to muscle, bone, or supporting tissues.
Courtesy of Sandra Quigley, Children's Hospital, Boston, MA.

GROWTH & DEVELOPMENT

Pressure Sites
The site of greatest pressure in infants and young children is the occiput. Older children have increased pressure on the sacral and occipital areas.

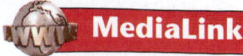
MediaLink

Braden Q Scale

on bed rest on a pressure-reducing surface. Frequent repositioning is needed. A transparent film may be applied to affected red skin to minimize friction. Pressure ulcers are treated with dressings, such as hydrocolloids, gels or hydrogels, and calcium alginates.

Nursing Management

Carefully inspect the dependent skin surfaces of all infants and children confined to bed at least three times in each 24-hour period. The Braden Q scale can be used for children under 5 years, and the Braden scale can be used for older children in the critical care setting. Evaluate the risk for skin damage based on factors that can contribute to skin breakdown. Identify the size (diameter and depth) and character of the skin lesion. Note any signs of infection, the appearance of wound edges, type of tissue at the wound base, and drainage.

Follow guidelines for pressure ulcer prevention in children with chronic conditions and in the critical care unit, such as increased ambulation, frequent position changes, pressure-reducing surfaces, and moisture barriers. If the child is incontinent, change the diaper frequently to keep the skin clean and dry. Provide wound care and dressing changes according to agency guidelines. These guidelines may include saline irrigation, debridement, and a dressing appropriate for the wound condition. Avoid using tape to hold dressings in place unless a protective skin barrier is used.

Teach parents of children with braces to inspect the skin under the braces every day for irritation (redness or blisters). Help the child to use a mirror with a long handle to inspect skin on the bottom and sides of the feet, behind the knees, and on the lower legs. Check all edges of the braces for roughness or breakage that can pinch or scrape the skin. If any skin irritation is seen and redness does not go away within 30 minutes, do not put the brace back on until the skin heals. Inform the child's physician so that treatment can be started immediately. To prevent braces from rubbing on bare skin, have the child wear cotton socks under the braces and make sure the shoes are large enough to accommodate the brace, socks, and the foot (Figure 30–13➤). Advise parents to return to a prosthetist regularly for brace refitting as the child grows.

Children who use a wheelchair are at risk for skin breakdown on the buttocks and lower back from the pressure of sitting for hours. A wheelchair gel or foam cushion can distribute and shift the child's weight when sitting in the chair. Teach the child to change position frequently by doing wheelchair push-ups or by shifting the weight (leaning to the side or forward) for several minutes every 10 to 15 minutes. Make sure the child wears a safety belt when sitting in the wheelchair. Teach school personnel about the child's recommended protocol so they can provide opportunities in school to change positions and reinforce the routine.

Burns

Burns are the third-leading cause of injury deaths (after motor vehicle crashes and drowning) in children between 1 and 14 years of age (Forum on Child and Family Statistics, 2004). Boys between the ages of 1 and 4 years are twice as likely as girls to be burned. The national average age of pediatric burn patients is 32 months. Nearly 100,000 children less than 15 years of age are treated in U.S. emergency departments annually for burns (Perry, 2003).

There are four main types of burns: thermal, chemical, electrical, and radioactive. Thermal burns, the most common in children, result from flames, scalds (such as hot water or grease), or contact with hot objects (such as a wood stove or curling iron). Chemical burns occur when children touch or ingest caustic agents. Electrical burns are caused by direct or alternating current in electrical wires, appliances, or high-voltage wires. Radiation burns result from exposure to radioactive substances or sunlight. About 10–25% of all burns in children are due to child abuse, and most occur in children under 3 years of age (Horner, 2005). See Chapter 6 ∞ for a description of child abuse.

Etiology and Pathophysiology

Children at different developmental stages are at risk for different types of burns.

- Infants are most often injured by thermal burns (scalding liquids, house fires).
- Toddlers are at risk for thermal burns (pulling hot liquids or grease onto themselves) (Figure 30–14➤), electrical burns (biting electrical cords) (Figure 30–15➤), contact burns, and chemical burns (ingesting cleaning agents and other substances) associated with exploring the environment.
- Preschool-age children are most often injured by scalding or contact with hot appliances (curling irons, ovens).
- School-age children are at risk for thermal burns (playing with matches, fireworks), electrical burns (climbing high-voltage towers, climbing trees, and contact with electrical wires), and chemical burns

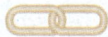

SKILL 14–1
Wound Irrigation

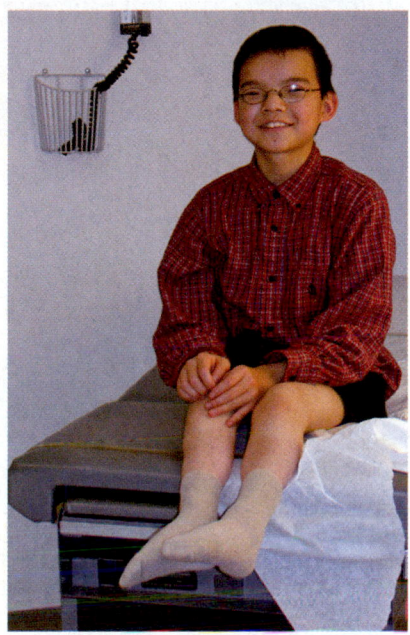

Figure 30–13 ➤ Sam has meningomyelocele. He wears socks under his braces to help prevent them from rubbing directly against his skin. He uses crutches and a wheelchair for mobility. What other measures should Sam and his parents take to prevent skin breakdown?

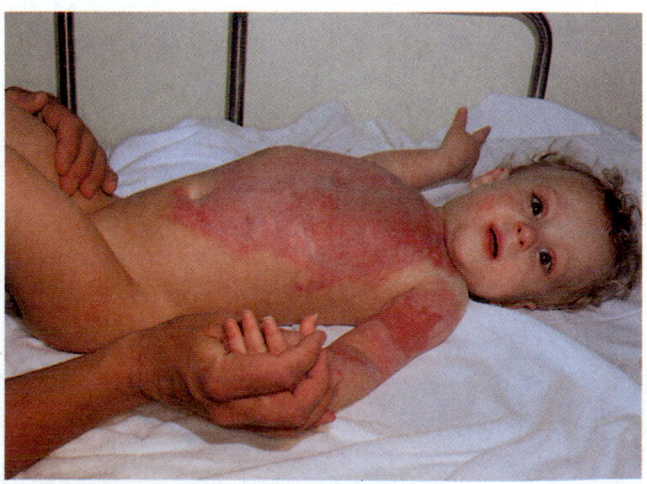

Figure 30–14 ➤ Thermal (scald) burns are the most common burn injury in infancy.

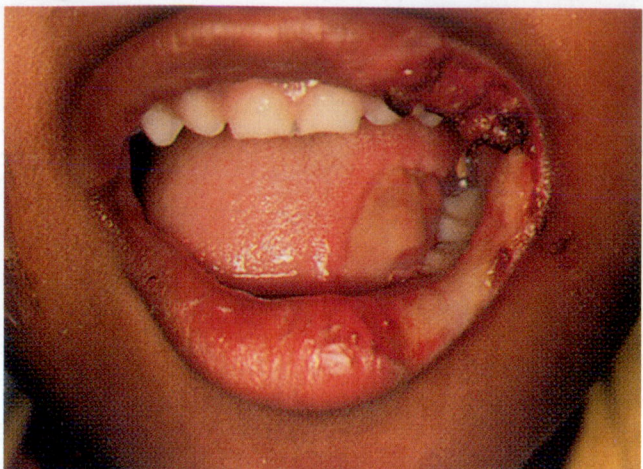

Figure 30–15 ➤ Electrical burn caused by biting on an electrical cord. The burn is caused when the current arcs through the lips, often causing a full-thickness injury through the mucosa, muscle, nerves, and blood vessels. The labial artery may be injured and cause significant bleeding once the eschar falls off after 2 to 3 weeks. Courtesy Dr. Lezley McIveen, Department of Dentistry, Children's National Medical Center, Washington, DC.

(combustion experiments) associated with their curiosity and interest in experimentation.

- Adolescents also experience thermal, chemical, and electrical burns.

Immediately after the burn, intense vasoconstriction occurs in response to substances released by the injured cells. Ischemia due to vasoconstriction may increase the depth of the burn injury. Then vasoactive hormones are released that increase capillary permeability. This permits fluid and plasma to shift into the interstitial spaces causing edema and decreased volume circulating in the blood vessels. Capillary integrity is not restored for 18 to 36 hours after the burn injury. The child loses increased water and heat through the injured epidermis. The child's metabolic rate and need for calories increase in the attempt to maintain body temperature.

Clinical Manifestations

Burns are classified by, and have specific clinical manifestations associated with, burn depth (Figure 30–16➤). Burn depth may be defined as partial thickness or full thickness. Partial-thickness burns, in which the injured tissue can regenerate and heal, may be either first or second degree. Full-thickness burns, in which the injured tissue cannot regenerate, are also known as third-degree burns. The depth of the burn depends upon the temperature and duration of the heat application, and on the ability of tissues to dissipate the transferred energy. Signs of infection include purulent drainage, swelling, erythema, discoloration of wound margins, and pain in the uninjured skin around the wound (Sheridan, 2005a).

■ COLLABORATIVE CARE

Diagnostic Tests

Burn severity is determined by the depth of the burn injury, percentage of body surface area (BSA) affected, and involvement of specific body parts. A Lund and Browder chart with BSA distributions for various body parts at different ages is used to calculate the area affected by the burn injury (Figure 30–17➤). The palm of a child's hand (without fingers and thumb) is 1% of his or her body surface area and can be used to make a quick estimate of the burn size (Merz, Schrand, Mertens et al., 2003).

Once the affected BSA is calculated, the burn can be classified as minor, moderate, or major (Table 30–4). Children with moderate and major burns require hospitalization, and those with major burns will usually be transferred to a burn center.

The involvement of specific body parts or specific burn distributions increases the burn severity, regardless of the percentage of BSA affected. Burns to the face, hands, feet, or perineal area are treated as major injuries because of the potential for cosmetic and functional impairment. **Circumferential** burns (injury completely surrounding the thorax or an extremity), anterior chest burns, and smoke inhalation are also classified as major burns.

Clinical Therapy

INITIAL TREATMENT The first step is to ensure that the child has an airway, is breathing, and has a pulse. Then stop the burning process by removing jewelry and clothing. Moist soaks or ice (if a small surface area is affected) are used to stop the burning process and to relieve pain. A tetanus vaccine booster is given if more than 5 years have passed since the last vaccine, or when the child has not completed the full vaccine series.

TREATMENT OF MAJOR BURNS The goals of treatment include: decrease burn fluid losses, prevent infection, control pain, promote nutrition, and salvage all viable tissue. Fluid replacement is necessary to maintain the cardiovascular and renal systems

PATHOPHYSIOLOGY ILLUSTRATED

Classification of Burns by Depth

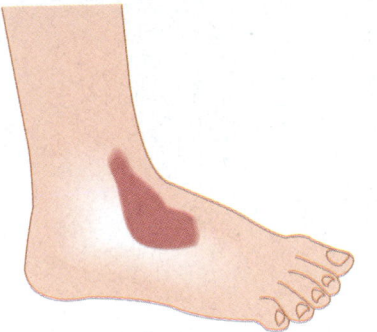

Superficial Partial Thickness (First Degree)
Damages only outer layer of skin; burn is painful and red; heals in a few days (e.g., sunburn)

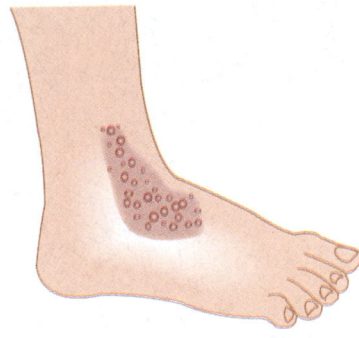

Partial Thickness (Second Degree)
Involves epidermis and upper layers of dermis; may have sparing of sweat gland and sebaceous glands; heals in 10–14 days

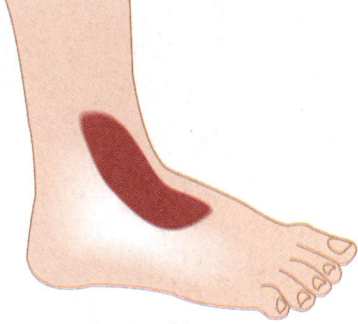

Full Thickness (Third Degree)
Involves all of epidermis and demis; may also involve underlying tissue; nerve ending usually destroyed; requires skin grafting

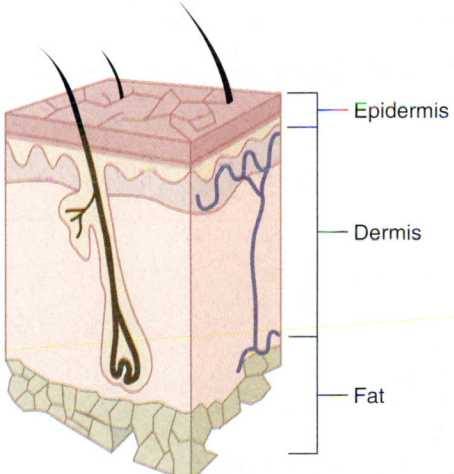

Erythema, blanches on pressure, no bullae, peeling after a few days due to premature cell death

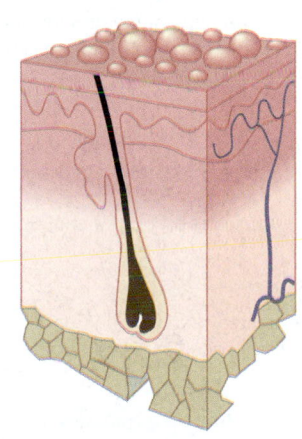

Blisters or bullae, erythema, blanches on pressure, pain and sensitivity to cold air, minimal scar formation

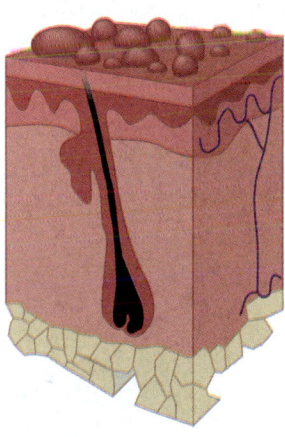

Skin may appear brown, black, deep cherry red, white to gray, waxy or translucent, usually no pain, injured area may appear sunken

Figure 30–16 ▶ Burn characteristics by depth of injury.

and to prevent hypovolemic shock in cases of major burn injury. Fluid shifts from the vasculature to the interstitial spaces (third spacing) soon after the burn and can result in hypovolemic shock. Fluid replacement for the first 24 hours after the injury is based on a fluid volume formula calculated from the child's body weight, affected BSA, and normal maintenance needs. The Parkland and Galveston formulas are two examples used for this calculation. Lactated Ringer's or normal saline solution is the preferred fluid. The administered fluid volume is reduced after 24 to 48 hours once the capillary integrity is restored. Efforts are focused on maintaining the child's temperature because heat is lost rapidly through burned skin.

Fever is a normal, expected outcome of any significant burn injury, but it is not always a sign of infection. Treatment may include analgesics, ice packs, cooling blankets, or cool hydrotherapy sessions. Infection is a frequent complication, and wounds are cultured to identify specific organisms for antibiotic therapy rather than routinely giving prophylactic antibiotic treatment (Sheridan, 2005b).

CLINICAL TIP

The Parkland formula is 4 mL/kg weight /% body surface area burned. This fluid volume is added to the child's maintenance fluid needs for 24 hours. Half of the total volume calculated for the 24-hour period is infused over the first 8 hours, starting at the time of the burn rather than arrival time in the emergency department. The remainder is distributed evenly over the next 16 hours. Children with an inhalation injury need additional fluids (Merz, Schrand, Mertens et al., 2003).

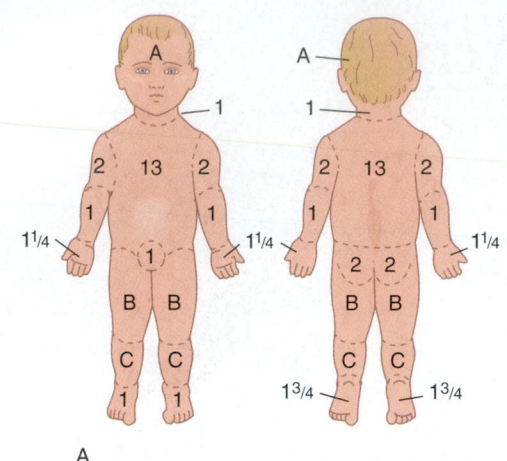

Relative Percentages of Areas Affected by Growth

Area	Age in years					
	0	1	5	10	11	Adult
A = 1/2 of head	9 1/2	8 1/2	6 1/2	5 1/2	4 1/2	3 1/2
B = 1/2 of one thigh	2 3/4	3 1/4	4	4 1/2	4 1/2	4 3/4
C = 1/2 of one lower leg	2 1/2	2 1/2	2 3/4	3	3 1/4	3 1/2

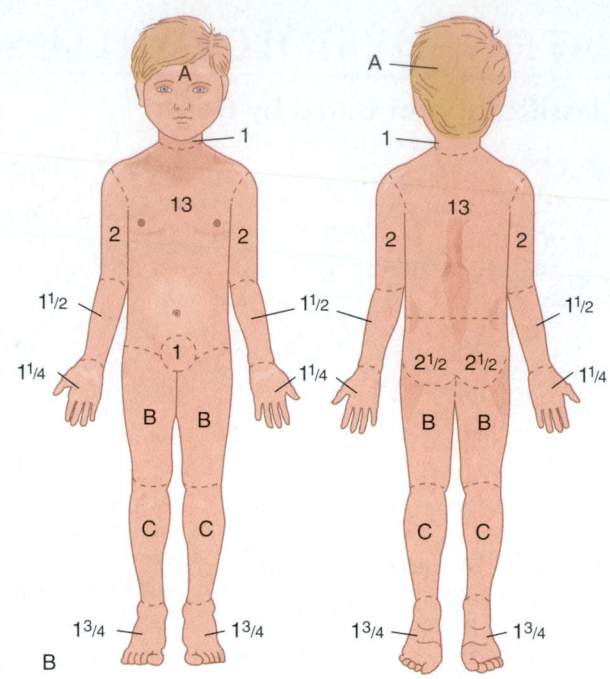

Figure 30–17 ➤ Lund and Browder chart for determining percentage of body surface areas in pediatric burn injuries, A, Infant; B, Child of 5 years. *Note:* From Artz, C. P., & Moncrief, J. A. (1969). *The treatment of burns* (2nd ed.). Philadelphia: Saunders. Adapted.

Table 30–4	CLASSIFICATION OF BURN SEVERITY

Minor

Can be treated as an outpatient	Partial thickness < 10% BSA
	Full thickness < 2% BSA

Moderate

Can be treated in a burn unit or general hospital	Partial thickness of 10–20% BSA
	Full thickness 3–10% BSA

Major

Should be treated in a specialized burn center	Partial thickness of > 20% BSA
	Full thickness of > 10% BSA
	Burns involving face, eyes, ears, hands, feet, and perineum that may result in cosmetic or functional impairment
	Burns complicated by inhalation injury, major trauma, and preexisting chronic conditions

From Perry, C. M. (2003). Thermal injuries. In P. A. Maloney-Harmon & S. J. Czerwinski (Eds.), *Nursing care of the pediatric trauma patient* (p. 279). St. Louis: Saunders.

Continuous enteral feedings are often begun within 6 hours of a major burn injury to support the child's nutritional requirements for increased calories and additional protein. These nutrients are needed for the significantly increased metabolic rate and to support healing and the body's stress response to injury. Vitamins A and C, and supplemental zinc, are also helpful for wound healing (Merz, Schrand, Mertens et al., 2003).

Aggressive pain management with intravenous opioids is needed around the clock and for all procedures. The burns cause a significant emotional overlay that increases the perception of pain. See Chapter 15 ∞. Cimetidine or other H₂ blockers may be ordered to prevent a burn stress ulcer.

Special consideration is needed when burns involve certain areas of the body:

- Deep partial-thickness and full-thickness burns develop **eschar** (the tough leathery scab that forms over severely burned areas) with no elasticity. When the burn is circumferential, blood flow can become restricted due to edema and cause tissue hypoxia. Assess for an increase in cyanosis, deep-tissue pain, and capillary refill time, and a decreased pulse distal to a circumferential burn. If you detect these signs, notify the physician immediately. An **escharotomy** (incision into the constricting tissue) may be necessary to restore peripheral circulation.

- Facial burns usually cause significant edema. Care must be taken to ensure airway patency. An ophthalmologist should be consulted for burns to the eye to assess damage and prescribe treatment. If the lips are burned, an infant may be unable to suck.
- Burns of the hands require careful management to maintain function. Special splinting and physical therapy are usually necessary.
- Perineal burns are at higher risk for infection because of frequent contamination with urine and stool. Frequent dressing changes are required. A urinary catheter is usually inserted but is removed once hydration status is stable to minimize the risk of urinary tract infection.

WOUND MANAGEMENT   Burn wound care has several goals: (1) to remove necrotic tissue and speed wound debridement, (2) to maintain moist wound conditions and adequate circulation, (3) to conserve body heat and fluids, (4) to protect the wound from infection, and (5) to control scarring and prevent scar contracture. Several treatment regimens are used to achieve these goals.

When the child has an extensive burn, the entire body is bathed to initiate debridement (removal of dead tissue to speed the healing process). Sedation and anesthesiology support may be ordered for pain management during debridement. Intact blisters provide a natural, pain-free, sterile dressing; however, some healthcare providers believe the fluid provides a medium for bacterial infection. Some burn centers keep blisters intact and others break them open. In either case, the tissues should be carefully cut away when the blisters are broken to prepare the wound for grafting.

Various options are used for wound management after debridement. Traditional burn care for a partial-thickness injury involves the use of antibacterial agents, such as silver sufadiazine (Silvadene), mafenide acetate (Sulfamylon), aqueous silver nitrate, or bacitracin after initial cleansing. Dressings are added to cover the burned area and changed once or twice daily. Newer silver-based antimicrobial dressings have been developed that provide a sustained release delivery of silver, and the dressing also functions to absorb exudate from the wound (Figure 30–18▶). Dressings can be left in place for several days (Duffy, McLaughlin, & Eichelberger, 2006). When the dressing is removed, a layer of eschar may also be debrided. These dressing changes are often painful, so pharmacologic and nonpharmacologic pain management is needed. See Chapter 15 ∞.

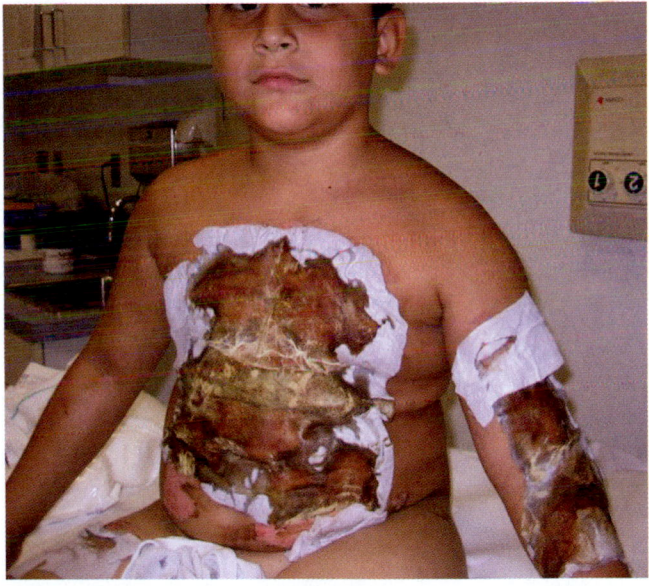

Figure 30–18 ▶   Child with a scald burn treated with an Aquacel AG® dressing, one of the newer silver-embedded dressings. Note the absorbed exudate that is visible through the burn dressing. Courtesy of Martin Eichelberger, MD, and Lisa Ring, RN, PNP, Children's National Medical Center.

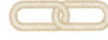

SKILLS 10–2 THROUGH 10–4
Pain Management Techniques

Hydrotherapy (whirlpool) baths may be given to cleanse extensive wounds before debridement, to increase vasodilation and circulation, and to speed healing. The water loosens exudate, topical medications, and dead tissue. As a rule, tap water is used for debridement. Gentle washing is necessary to protect new epithelial cells. Granulation tissue forms as a result of daily debridement. Alternatively, the dressings that adhere to the skin may be soaked to help loosen them. Superficial second-degree burns reepithelialize within 3 weeks.

Skin grafting is necessary with any deep second- or third-degree burn. Often a temporary skin substitute or allograft (cadaver skin from a skin bank) is used to cover a second-degree burn until healing occurs. An allograft also covers and improves the condition of a deep second- and third-degree burn until **autografting** (use of healthy skin taken from a nonburned area of the child's body) can be performed. The graft is placed after the wound is debrided in the operating room to reveal healthy, bleeding tissue. This

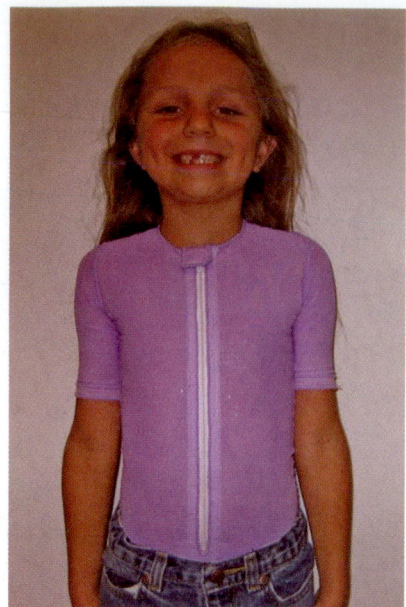

A

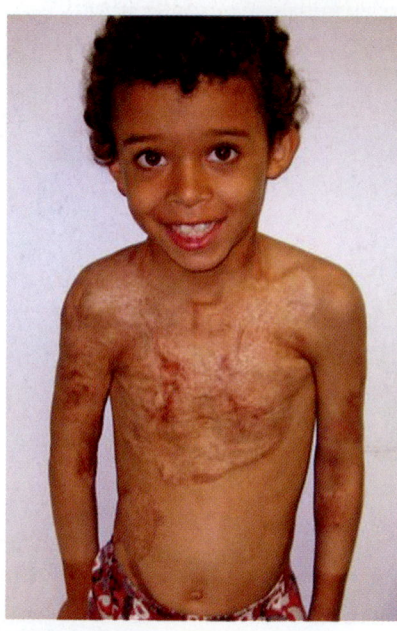

B

Figure 30–19 ➤ A, Pressure garment used to reduce hypertrophic scarring from a burn on the chest. B, Hypertrophic scar on the chest. Courtesy of Martin Eichelberger, MD, and Lisa Ring, RN, PNP, Children's National Medical Center.

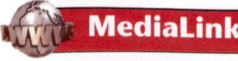

SKILL 13–1
Performing an Indwelling Urinary Catheterization

MediaLink

Burn Resources and Support

forms a protective barrier over the wound surface to decrease infection risk and to protect against fluid loss. An autograft is permanent. The donor site (where the autograft was harvested) is a new wound, causing pain and requiring close monitoring for signs of infection.

Various temporary skin substitutes, such as Integra or Biobrane, may be applied to debrided skin to form a protective barrier over the wound surface. This covering is effective in decreasing infection risk and pain, protecting against fluid loss, and promoting revascularization (Merz, Schrand, Merten et al., 2003).

During the rehabilitation stage, pressure garments (e.g., Jobst®) are used to reduce development of hypertrophic scarring and contractures (Figure 30–19A➤). Such garments are worn 23 hours a day for 6 to 8 months to shorten the time of scar maturation and to reduce the thickness of the scars (Figure 30–19B➤) (Perry, 2003). Cosmetic surgery may be needed to improve the child's appearance.

■ NURSING MANAGEMENT
Nursing Assessment and Diagnosis

Nursing assessment first focuses on the potential for life-threatening injuries that need immediate care. After the child's condition has been stabilized, the history, physical assessment, and psychosocial assessment are performed.

Emergency Assessment

Emergency assessment is based on the ABCs of basic life support (airway, breathing, and circulation). Assessment of the airway is necessary, especially when there are signs of smoke inhalation or burns to the face and neck. It is important to identify other potential injuries when the mechanism of injury includes a fall or explosion. Identify signs of respiratory distress and any potential bleeding source. A weak, thready pulse; tachycardia; and pallor are important signs of early shock that may provide clues to an internal injury.

History

Obtain information about the type of burn (e.g., thermal, electrical, chemical) and a complete history. If a burn injury was preventable, parents may be emotionally stressed by feelings of guilt. Take care to avoid sounding accusatory when questioning parents about the injury. Be alert for the potential of child abuse when the history does not match the burn injury. Signs of child abuse include glove and stocking burns, burns that spare flexor surfaces such as on the perineum, contact burns from cigarettes or irons, and zebra burn lines from contact with a hot grate (Figure 30–20➤). Photographs are often taken to document these burn injuries. Child neglect can be a factor in the burn of an inadequately supervised child. When taking a burn history, carefully document the type of injury, time of injury, people present at the time of the injury, first aid administered, and history of other unusual injuries or emergency department visits.

Physical Assessment

Assess the extent of burn injury (depth and body surface area affected). Frequently monitor the vital signs, control pain, and weigh the child daily. Monitor the child's circulatory and respiratory status to identify signs of hypovolemia in the first 24 hours or fluid overload as capillary integrity is restored. Perform a head-to-toe assessment at the beginning of every shift followed by system-specific assessments, depending on clinical findings and changes in the child's status. Monitor electrolytes as well as intake and output carefully. A urinary catheter may be inserted to enable close monitoring of urine output. Be alert to signs of infection such as purulent drainage, odor, and edematous, red, or discolored wound margins.

Psychosocial Assessment

Assess the child's concerns over appearance and the stress of hospitalization. Determine if the child has memories or nightmares about the burn and arrange psychologic support as needed. Talk with parents to identify their level of stress and feelings of guilt. Identify any family stressors that may need to be addressed during the child's care.

Common nursing diagnoses for the child with a major burn injury are included in the accompanying Nursing Care Plan: The Child with a Major Burn Injury. Additional nursing diagnoses for the child with a major burn might include:

- Impaired Physical Mobility related to movement prescriptions (limb immobilization) and pain
- Disturbed Body Image related to burn injury
- Anxiety related to situational crisis and threat of death or disfigurement

Planning and Implementation

Nursing care focuses on performing burn care, preventing complications, and providing emotional support. Care of the burned child involves various treatments designed to promote healing and prevent complications. These include dressing changes, hydrotherapy, antibiotic therapy, pain management, physical therapy, play therapy, psychological support, and possibly skin grafting.

Begin pain and sedation management as soon as possible for the initial debridement to reduce the stress on the child. Fluids should be administered at the rate prescribed for resuscitation for the first 24 hours. Soak charred clothing off with sterile saline and clip any hair within 2 inches of the burn to keep it out of the burn site. Cleanse the burn with mild soap and water and remove any foreign matter. If a chemical is the burning agent, remove the clothing and wash with lots of water. Elevate burned extremities.

Wound Care

The burned area is debrided and cleaned, often with an chemical enzyme. Then an antibacterial/antimicrobial medication or dressing is applied. Medications are often covered with dressings. At each dressing change, the wound needs to be assessed for appearance, exudate, odor, appearance of surrounding tissue, and presence of granulation tissue.

A semipermeable wound membrane may be applied to clean superficial partial-thickness burns. These membranes protect the burned tissue from trauma, prevent fluid loss, create a moist environment for healing, and provide a physical barrier to bacteria. Monitor the burn under the transparent membrane carefully for infection which could potentially cause sepsis or a deepening burn wound (Sheridan, 2005a). When the burn heals, the wound membrane loosens, permitting it to be trimmed.

Allografts or autografts may be placed in the operating room after debridement to prepare the burned tissue for the graft. Following the grafting procedure, wet dressings with antibiotic solution are used for several days, followed by other dry dressings with antibiotics. Splints may be required to promote healing when the skin over a joint is burned. The child may be on bed rest for several days following an autograft to protect the graft until it has a vascular supply. Donor sites are treated as separate wounds.

Nutrition Support

Enteral feeding may be needed initially by the child with extensive burns until the child is able to eat. Once the child is able to eat, provide a diet high in protein and calories. Identify food items that the child likes, and encourage the family to bring food in that the child may prefer to eat. Provide small frequent feedings to increase the number of calories consumed each day.

Prevent Complications

Severe complications of burns include infections, pneumonia, and renal failure, as well as possible irreversible loss of function of the burned area. The healthcare team's goal is to prevent complications. Parents need to be involved in their child's care and to learn how to change dressings, assess for infection and dehydration, and perform range-of-motion exercises to aid in the child's recovery.

Provide Emotional Support

Burned children have received a profound insult to their body and their self-image. Fear and anxiety about disfigurement and scarring are common, especially among adolescents. The shock and pain of the injury cause increased stress, as do the unfamiliar surroundings and presence of healthcare providers. Psychologic support is

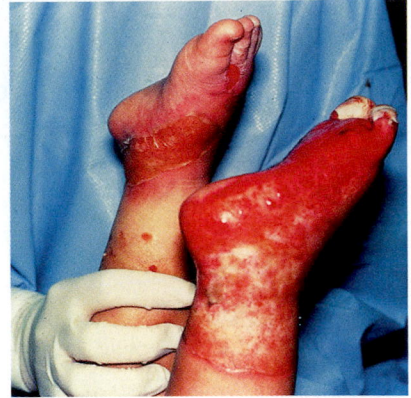

A

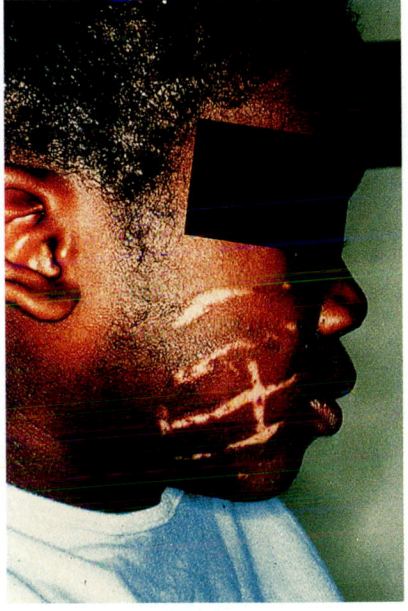

B

Figure 30–20 ▶ Burn injuries associated with child abuse. A, Burns of the hands or feet that are distributed like gloves or stockings indicate dipping in hot water. B, Zebra burns from a grate. Courtesy of American Academy of Pediatrics, Elk Grove Village, IL, and the Kempe Children's Center, Denver, CO.

NURSING CARE PLAN The Child with a Major Burn Injury

GOAL	INTERVENTION	RATIONALE	EXPECTED OUTCOME
1. Acute Pain related to physical injury agents			
	NIC Priority Intervention **Pain Management:** *Alleviation of pain or a reduction in pain to a level of comfort that is acceptable to the patient.*		*NOC Suggested Outcome* **Comfort Level:** *Feelings of physical and psychologic ease.*
The child will verbalize adequate relief from pain and will be able to perform activities of daily living (ADLs).	• Assess the level of pain frequently using pain scales (see Chapter 15 ∞).	• Pain scale provides objective measurement. Pain is always present, but changes in location and intensity may indicate complications.	The child verbalizes adequate relief from pain and is able to perform ADLs.
	• Cover burns as much as possible.	• Temperature changes or movement of air causes pain.	
	• Change the child's position frequently. Perform range-of-motion exercises.	• Reduces joint stiffness and prevents contractures.	
	• Encourage verbalization about pain.	• Provides outlet for emotions and helps the child cope.	
	• Provide diversional activities.	• Helps lessen focus on pain.	
	• Promote uninterrupted sleep with use of medications.	• Sleep deprivation can increase pain perception.	
	• Use analgesics before all dressing changes and burn care.	• Helps to reduce pain and decreases anxiety for subsequent dressing changes.	
2. Risk for Infection related to trauma and destruction of skin barrier			
	NIC Priority Intervention **Infection Protection:** *Prevention and early detection of infection in a patient at risk.*		*NOC Suggested Outcome* **Risk Control:** *Actions to eliminate or reduce actual, personal, and modifiable health threats.*
The child will be free of infection during the healing process.	• Take vital signs frequently.	• A fever may be an early sign of infection, but it is also a common response to the burn injury.	The child either stays free of secondary infection, or has infection diagnosed and treated early.
	• Use standard precautions (gown, gloves, mask) when wounds of a major burn are exposed. Limit visitors (no one with an upper respiratory infection or other communicable disease).	• Reduces risk of wound contamination.	
	• Clip hair around burns.	• Hair harbors bacteria.	
	• Keep burn dressings clean and dry.	• Helps reduce the number of bacteria introduced to the burned site.	
	• Do not place the IV in any burned area.	• Reduces risk of wound contamination.	
	• Administer oral or IV antibiotics for diagnosed infections as prescribed.	• Antibiotics administered as prescribed help to clear the infection quickly.	

NURSING CARE PLAN   The Child with a Major Burn Injury (continued)

GOAL	INTERVENTION	RATIONALE	EXPECTED OUTCOME
**3. Risk for Deficient Fluid Volume** related to loss of fluids through wounds and to subsequent excess fluid intake			
	NIC Priority Intervention **Fluid Management:** *Promotion of fluid balance and prevention of complications resulting from abnormal or undesired fluid levels.*		*NOC Suggested Outcome* **Fluid Balance:** *Balance of water in the intracellular and extracellular compartments of the body.*
The child will maintain adequate urine output.	• Monitor vital signs, central venous pressure, capillary refill time, pulses.	• The child is initially at risk for hypovolemic shock and needs fluid resuscitation (see Chapter 21 ∞).	The child maintains normal urine output and burn site edema is not excessive.
	• Administer IV and oral fluids as ordered.	• Careful calculation of fluid needs and ensuring proper intake helps keep the child properly hydrated and reduces the risk for renal damage.	
	• Estimate insensible fluid losses.	• Losses are increased during the first 72 hours after burn injury; may need replacement. Plasma is lost through burn site because of capillary damage.	
	• Monitor intake and output.	• The child is at risk for fluid overload during hydration, and for edema in the tissues at the burn site.	
	• Weigh child daily.	• Significant weight loss or gain can help determine fluid imbalances.	
	• Insert urinary catheter.	• Helps maintain accurate output measurement during critical care stage.	
	• Monitor for hyponatremia and hypercalcemia (see Chapter 16 ∞).	• Sodium is lost with burn fluid and potassium is lost from damaged cells, causing electrolyte imbalances.	
**4. Ineffective Peripheral Tissue Perfusion** related to mechanical reduction of venous and/or arterial blood flow (edema) of circumferential burns			
	NIC Priority Intervention **Circulatory Care:** *Promotion of arterial and venous circulation.*		*NOC Suggested Outcomes* **Tissue Perfusion (Peripheral):** *Extent to which blood flows through the small vessels of the extremities and maintains tissue function.*
The child will maintain adequate perfusion in burned extremities.	• Elevate extremities. Check distal pulse hourly. Notify the physician of decreased or absent pulses.	• Elevation helps to reduce dependent edema by promoting venous return. Dependent edema can constrict peripheral circulation.	The child has no episodes of poor perfusion in the burned extremity.
	• Assess extent of eschar for potential for constriction of circulation.	• Eschar that is circumferential can constrict peripheral circulation in edematous extremity.	
**5. Ineffective Breathing Pattern** related to respiratory muscle fatigue due to smoke inhalation and airway edema			
	NIC Priority Intervention **Respiratory Monitoring:** *Collection and analysis of patient data to ensure airway patency and adequate gas exchange.*		*NOC Suggested Outcomes* **Vital Signs Status:** *Temperature, pulse, respiration, and blood pressure within expected range for the individual.*

(continued)

NURSING CARE PLAN The Child with a Major Burn Injury (continued)

GOAL	INTERVENTION	RATIONALE	EXPECTED OUTCOME
5. Ineffective Breathing Pattern related to respiratory muscle fatigue due to smoke inhalation and airway edema (continued)			
The child will maintain or demonstrate improvement in breathing pattern.	• Closely monitor quality of respirations, breath sounds, mucous secretions, pulse oximetry.	• Excess fluid replacement can cause pulmonary edema; toxins from burning products can cause airway inflammation.	The child has regular and unlabored breathing pattern.
	• Provide thorough pulmonary care.	• Pulmonary care assists in removal of secretions to prevent infection.	
	• Elevate head of bed. Keep intubation tube at bedside.	• Dyspnea, nasal flaring, and air hunger (respiratory distress) may develop. Emergency airway management may be needed.	
	• Administer corticosteroids, as prescribed.	• Reduces airway edema.	
6. Impaired Physical Mobility related to joint stiffness due to burns			
	NIC Priority Intervention **Exercise Therapy, Joint Mobility:** *Use of active or passive body movement to maintain or restore joint flexibility.*		*NOC Suggested Outcome* **Joint Movement (Active):** *Range of motion of joints with self-initiated movement.*
The child will maintain maximum range of motion.	• Arrange physical and occupational therapy twice daily for stretching and range-of-motion exercises. Splint as ordered. Encourage independent activities of daily living.	• Positioning in alignment and range-of-motion exercises prevent contractures. Self-care should be encouraged when appropriate.	The child maintains maximum range of motion without contractures.
7. Imbalanced Nutrition: Less than Body requirements related to high metabolic needs			
	NIC Priority Intervention **Nutrition Management:** *Assistance with or provision of balanced dietary intake of foods and fluids.*		*NOC Suggested Outcome* **Nutritional Status:** *Extent to which nutrients are available to meet metabolic needs.*
The child will maintain weight and demonstrate adequate serum albumin and hydration.	• Provide an opportunity to choose meals. Offer a variety of high-calorie and high-protein foods. Provide snacks.	• Encourages intake. General malaise and anorexia lead to poor healing.	The child maintains weight, adequate hydration, and normal serum albumin.
	• Encourage the child to have meals with other children.	• Socialization improves intake.	
	• Provide a multivitamin supplement.	• Vitamin C aids zinc absorption; zinc aids in healing.	
	• Substitute milk and juices for water. • Provide nasogastric feedings as needed.	• A child with a burn greater than 10% of BSA cannot usually meet nutrition requirements without assistance.	
	• Weigh the child daily.	• Provides objective evaluation.	
8. Anxiety (Child) related to threat to or change in health status			
	NIC Priority Intervention **Anxiety Reduction:** *Minimizing apprehension, dread, foreboding, or uneasiness related to an unidentified source of anticipated danger.*		*NOC Suggested Outcome* **Coping:** *Actions to manage stressors that tax an individual's resources.*

NURSING CARE PLAN The Child with a Major Burn Injury (continued)

GOAL	INTERVENTION	RATIONALE	EXPECTED OUTCOME
8. Anxiety (Child) related to threat to or change in health status (continued)			
The child will verbalize reduced anxiety.	• Provide continuity of care providers.	• Helps to build a trusting relationship.	The child expresses and shows signs of reduced anxiety.
	• Encourage parents to stay with the child; calls from home; pictures from classmates.	• Familiar surroundings, people, and items encourage relaxation.	
	• Group tasks and activities.	• Reduces overstimulation and encourages rest.	
9. Anxiety (Parent) related to situational crisis			
	NIC Priority Intervention **Coping Enhancement:** *Assisting a patient to adapt to perceived stressors, changes, or threats that interfere with meeting life demands and roles.*		*NOC Suggested Outcome* **Anxiety Control:** *Ability to eliminate or reduce feelings of apprehension and tension from an unidentified source.*
Parents will verbalize decreased anxiety.	• Provide educational materials about healing, grafting, dressing changes, and course of action.	• Knowledge reduces anxiety.	Parents state decreased anxiety and describe plans and solve problems related to care of the child at home.
	• Be flexible when teaching parents about wound care.	• Adults learn in many different ways.	
	• Refer to social services or parent support group.	• Allows for venting of fears and guilt feelings, and provides exchange of ideas on dealing with hospitalization and long-term care.	

therefore essential to the child's recovery. Social workers, chaplains, art therapists, child life specialists, and play therapists are all trained to help the child and family deal with the stressors of recovery. Make appropriate referrals to ensure that the child and family receive necessary services.

An attitude of genuine interest and concern by the nurse is essential. Orient the child to his or her surroundings frequently and give ample preparation for procedures, when possible. Continuity of care providers is important in developing a trusting relationship with the child and family. Encourage the child and parents to voice concerns, and show understanding and support.

Play therapy is encouraged for children, even if they can only observe initially. Play therapy serves several purposes for the child with a major burn:

- It provides an outlet for frustration, independence, and creativity.
- It promotes activities that challenge range of motion.
- It normalizes the child's daily routine.
- It encourages the child, who sees the progress other children make day by day.

Families are at risk for emotional stress. Warn them to expect edema and changes in the child's body with the injury response. Parents often feel guilty and responsible for the child's injury. Help parents focus on recovery rather than past actions. Fear usually results from lack of knowledge about the severity of the burn and the child's status, especially in the early stages of burn care and admission to the hospital ICU. Include the family in the child's care whenever possible. The family needs information and frequent updates. This promotes trust between the family and the healthcare team.

Severe morbidity is likely with major burns. Significant scarring may occur regardless of autografting. Contractures and loss of function are also possible. Inadequate fluid replacement may lead to irreversible renal damage or cardiac damage, necessitating close follow-up unrelated to the actual burn injury. Children with extensive burns require comprehensive follow-up, sometimes involving repeated hospitalizations for surgery to release burn contractures, perform new grafting, or perform cosmetic surgery for scar revision.

Discharge Planning and Home Care Teaching

Identify and address home care needs well in advance of discharge. Thorough assessment is necessary to identify the family's needs related to the child's discharge home or to a rehabilitation facility. Discharge planning may include instructing parents in nutrition and diet needs, safety in the home, protection of the burned area, signs of infection and actions to take, use of pressure garments, and range of motion exercises to prevent contractures.

Provide support and encouragement to parents as they learn how to care for the child with burns. Many parents find it difficult to perform dressing change procedures they know will inflict pain to their child. Many burn centers now perform burn dressing changes in a burn clinic until the parent is proficient in dressing changes, or dressings are used that reduce the frequency of burn dressing changes needed. When parents provide dressing changes, provide pain medication and guidelines for how soon to give the medication before the dressing change. Specific guidelines for dressing changes should be outlined so that parents and healthcare team members have the same focus. Parents should first observe care being performed and then provide repeat demonstrations until competent.

Care in the Community

Care of the child with a burn requires long-term therapy and rehabilitation. Nurses in clinic and home care settings continue the care provided during hospitalization. Long-term care commonly occurs in the home, with frequent visits to healthcare professionals. Children with extensive burns or with burns in locations where scarring may limit function must often wear a pressure (Jobst®) garment, and sometimes a face mask if the face was burned (see Figure 30–19A). The garment is used 23 hours a day, and is removed only for bathing and laundry of the garment. Garments are worn for 6 months until the scar is mature (Macintyre & Baird, 2006). The pressure garment may present a threat to the child's body image, but it is an important way to decrease scarring. Scarring may also be managed through drug injections or surgery (i.e., revision, grafting, or Z-plasty). Help families understand the need for the special garments and masks and how to clean and care for them.

Continued physical therapy and occupational therapy are often needed to increase strength and dexterity in performing self-care skills and to prevent contractures. Emphasis is placed on returning to normal activities of daily living as soon as possible, such as returning to school. Some children have home tutors or computer connections to school for a time to ensure opportunities for learning while decreasing their risk of exposure to infection.

School reentry is often a traumatic experience, especially for older children and adolescents, because of the fear of rejection, decreased self-esteem, and impaired body image. The child's primary nurse, social worker, and child life specialist may visit the school of a child with a burn injury before the child returns to school—bringing photographs of the child, pressure garments, or other items—to inform classmates and allow them to explore their feelings about the child's burn injury. Several communities offer support groups for families and children with burn injuries. Referral to these groups may be beneficial.

A major role of nurses in the community is prevention. Provide burn prevention information to parents at each health promotion visit. Become involved with a Safe Kids coalition or local firefighters to help educate families and caregivers about ways to prevent scald burns and house fires.

CLINICAL TIP

Moisturizing creams can be used after healing to relieve residual drying. The healed skin is very sensitive to sunburn, so cover the area or use a sunscreen. Sunscreen also helps prevent hyperpigmentation after burn healing.

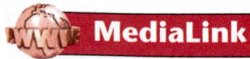
MediaLink

Burn Prevention

Management of Minor Burns

Many children with minor burns are cared for at home after an initial visit to the emergency department or urgent care clinic. Discuss home remedies for minor burn care. (See Families Want to Know: Caring for Minor Burns.) For superficial burns covering a small area, use moist soaks to stop the burning process and to relieve pain. Any open blisters are debrided, and a thin layer of an antibiotic medication (e.g., silver sulfadiazine) is spread over the burn. Do not place this medication close to the eyes or mouth. Bacitracin is often used for burns on the face. The burn is then covered with one or two layers of gauze. Burn dressings should be changed twice daily. This involves cleaning the burn and reapplying antibiotic cream.

Tell parents to increase the child's fluid intake to compensate for loss of fluid through damaged skin. A high-calorie, high-protein diet is necessary to meet the increased nutritional requirements of healing. Acetaminophen (Tylenol) with codeine is often given, especially before dressing changes. Infection is a common complication. Educate the parents to observe for signs of infection (inflammation extending under the dressing, bad odor, excessive exudates, and fever), and notify the physician immediately if noticed. The child should be seen within 48 hours of treatment to monitor progress. Reinforce to parents the importance of follow-up appointments.

Sunburn

Sunburn is a burn injury to the outer layer of skin caused by excess sun exposure, or sun exposure after taking phototoxic drugs (acne medication, some antibiotics, birth control pills) (American Academy of Dermatology, 2006). Young children have less melanin to protect their skin against harmful ultraviolet rays. A childhood sun exposure history that includes intense repeated sunburns and chronic sun exposure for the purpose of tanning is strongly associated with the development of skin cancer (Maguire-Eisen, Rothman, & Demierre, 2005). Melanoma is the most common cancer in individuals less than 30 years of age, and the rate of melanoma is increasing rapidly in children and adolescents (Centers for Disease Control, 2002; Oliveria, Saraiya, Geller et al., 2006). Avoiding sunburn during childhood is believed to be more important than protecting skin during adulthood.

Erythema and skin tenderness usually develop between 30 minutes and 4 hours after exposure to sunlight. Increased vasodilation and vascular permeability result in the extravasation of fluid to the tissues and white blood cell migration to the damaged skin. The erythema peaks at 24 hours. Prolonged exposure can result in edema, vesiculation, bullae, or ulceration. Systemic complaints include malaise, insomnia (because of skin tenderness), fatigue, headaches, and chilling (because of rapid heat loss).

Treatment is generally supportive. Pain can be relieved by cool compresses followed by application of a low-potency topical corticosteroid (on unblistered skin). Children with severe sunburn may need nonsteroidal anti-inflammatory drugs (NSAIDs) for pain relief and to reduce inflammation. See Chapter 15 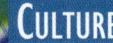 for information on NSAIDs.

Nursing Management

Educate parents and children about preventing sunburn. (See Families Want to Know: Preventing Sunburn.) Advise them that repeated sunburns may lead to permanent skin damage, skin cancer, cataracts, and premature aging of the skin. Recommend to parents that children use sunscreens, use a sunblock such as zinc oxide, wear protective

---

CULTURE

Litargirio Use

When taking a history about methods used to treat minor burns in children, inquire about the use of "litargirio." This is a traditional remedy used for burn and wound healing, and as a deodorant and foot fungicide in the Dominican Republic. The powder is sold in small packets at specialty stores that cater to Spanish-speaking populations. It contains up to 79% lead and can cause lead toxicity in children (FDA, 2003).

NURSING ALERT

Behaviors and skin characteristics that increase the risk for pediatric melanoma include light-colored eyes, freckling, fair skin, blond or red hair, family history of melanoma, blistering sunburns before 12 years of age, frequent sun exposure without the use of sunscreen, melanocytic nevi, and immunosuppression (Strouse, Fears, Tucker et al., 2005).

COMMUNITY CARE

UV Rays

Harmful exposure to ultraviolet (UV) rays is more intense in the summer, at higher altitudes, and closer to the equator. The UV index is published in most newspapers to report the ultraviolet intensity expected for the day in any given community. Encourage parents to monitor the UV index and use it as a guide for the use of sunscreen and protective covering when children play outside.

FAMILIES WANT TO KNOW

Caring for Minor Burns

- Place burn under cool, running water to stop the burning process and to help reduce pain.
- Do not use ice as it can cause more damage to the injured skin.
- Remove all clothing and jewelry from the burned area.
- Apply a topical antibiotic such as Bacitracin to the burned area on the face.

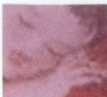

FAMILIES WANT TO KNOW

Preventing Sunburn

- Keep children out of direct sunlight as much as possible, especially the midday sun. Avoid scheduling outdoor activities during the hours of maximum exposure (10 a.m. to 2 p.m.).
- When outdoors, minimize exposed skin by wearing hats and long-sleeved, closely woven cotton clothing and pants; wear T-shirts while swimming. Special sun protection clothing is now available from some manufacturers.
- Be aware that water, concrete, and sand reflect sunlight and increase exposure up to 90% by reflecting up to 85% of the ultraviolet rays.
- Use sunscreen (at least 15 SPF) consistently for all sun exposure. For optimal protection, apply as thickly as directed to all exposed areas 30 to 45 minutes before sun exposure. Remember to apply it behind the knees and on the ears, eye areas, and neck. Reapply every 2 hours as needed, or sooner if swimming, toweling off, or perspiring heavily.

- Use a waterproof sunscreen when swimming; this provides protection in water for approximately 60 to 80 minutes. Then reapply. Avoid getting waterproof sunscreen in the eyes because it causes severe pain and a chemical burn. Call the Poison Control Center immediately for guidance.
- Protect newborns from sun exposure. Avoid using sunscreens in infants less than 6 months of age because they may absorb the chemicals through their skin.
- Remember that a child can be burned even on a cloudy day. Up to 80% of ultraviolet rays can penetrate the cloud cover.
- If the child is taking any medications, check with your healthcare practitioner before exposure (some medications cause hypersensitivity to sunlight).
- Adolescents should avoid indoor tanning facilities and artificial tanning devices as the rays used are as damaging to the skin as the sun.

clothing and hats, and limit the amount of time they spend in the sun. Children should also wear sunglasses with 99% ultraviolet blockage. See Evidence-Based Practice: Education to Prevent Sunburn.

Hypothermia

Hypothermia is a condition in which the core body temperature falls below 35°C (95°F). This occurs when the heat produced by the body is less than the heat lost. Hypothermia is a life-threatening emergency that can occur in any season and any geographic location. Infants and young children are at risk because of immature temperature regulatory mechanisms, thinner skin, limited subcutaneous fat, and high skin surface area to body mass ratio. Adolescents are at risk due to risk-taking behaviors such as drug and alcohol use and engaging in remote outdoor activities without proper equipment or clothing.

Hypothermia is associated with near-drowning episodes because body heat is lost more quickly in water, as compared with air. As the core body temperature falls, the body tries to conserve the core temperature at the expense of the extremities. Increased muscle tone and an increased metabolic rate occur. Shivering is the body's attempt to rewarm the blood before it returns to the body's core. Other causes of hypothermia include exposure to a cold environment, ingestion of alcohol or barbiturates, trauma or a brain disorder that interferes with temperature regulation, and overwhelming sepsis.

Symptoms of mild hypothermia (32° to 35°C [90° to 95°F]) include fatigue, slurred speech, poor coordination and clumsiness, confusion and poor judgment, inappropriate behavior, shivering, tachycardia, and tachypnea. Symptoms of moderate hypothermia (28° to 32°C [82° to 90°F]) include depressed mental status, no shivering, depressed respirations, slow pulse or irregular heartbeat, low blood pressure, pale or cyanotic color, hallucinations, and coma. Profound hypothermia (body temperature below 28°C [82°F]) results in absence of respirations and pulse, ventricular fibrillation, dilated and unresponsive pupils, and coma.

Clinical therapy focuses on resuscitation, if necessary, and gradual core body rewarming. The child who has been immersed in cold water for a long time (up to 30 to 45 minutes) should receive CPR and active rewarming until the body temperature returns to normal because the hypothermia may have preserved vital organs. Warmed IV fluids are needed to expand blood volume and promote cardiac output. Assess body temperature with a rectal probe inserted about 15 cm. Provide active rewarming with warmed IV fluids, warm humidified oxygen, and warm packs to the trunk of the body and in core circulation areas (axilla, groin, and posterior neck). The goal is to rewarm

EVIDENCE-BASED PRACTICE

Education to Prevent Sunburn

Problem/Clinical Question

Excessive exposure to ultraviolet (UV) radiation during childhood and adolescence is associated with the development of skin cancer during adulthood. Which prevention strategies successfully promote reduced sun exposure in children and adolescents to help reverse the dramatic increase in skin cancer attributed to UV radiation exposure?

Evidence

The parents of 77 children seen in a medical clinic in Florida were surveyed about attitudes and practices related to sun protection for their children. Less than 50% of parents reported regular use of sun protection for their children despite some knowledge of sun protection measures and consequences of sun exposure. Their children were outside 1 to 4 hours a day. Sunscreen was the most common sun protection measure used, but half of the parents felt it was okay to stay outside longer when sunscreen was used. This practice potentially increased the overall sun exposure for these children (Johnson, Davy, Boyett et al., 2001). When these same parents were asked about sun protection counseling received by the child's physician, those who received enthusiastic counseling perceived that sun protection was important for their children. Of the 21 parents who received enthusiastic sun protection counseling, more than 40% of them reported increased sun protection habits, and they were more likely to teach their child safe sun habits. (Davy, Boyett, Weathers et al., 2002). A national telephone survey of 651 parents of children ages 5 to 12 years was conducted to assess the parent's skin cancer knowledge, sun protection behavior, and perceived

risk of skin cancer, as well as the child's sun protection behavior, and the parent's and child's vigilance in sunscreen use. Results indicated that children were more likely to get sunburns when parents also got sunburns. When both parents and children were vigilant in using sunscreen, children were less likely to get sunburns. (O'Riordan, Geller, Brooks et al., 2003). A 1- to 2-hour sun exposure education program for children between 5 and 15 years was developed by the Environmental Protection Agency and evaluated in 85 schools across the country. When compared to children in schools that did not receive the education, study children were more likely to report a change in attitude about the healthier look with a suntan, and intentions to play in the shade more frequently. There were no changes in plans to wear sunscreen, sunglasses, or protective clothing (Geller, Rutsch, Kenausis, et al., 2003).

Implications

Successful strategies to reduce exposure to UV radiation have not yet been identified. Information about sun protection behaviors indicates a need for education and behavior change by parents and children. Parents are also important role models for their children in sun protection behavior. Regularly wearing a hat, sunglasses, covering skin, and staying in the shade should also be encouraged. Since an effective education strategy has not been identified, an alternate strategy, such as policy changes to reduce sun exposure in childcare and school settings, may be more effective.

Critical Thinking

Develop guidelines that a childcare center could use for the reduction of UV radiation exposure by enrolled infants and children.

---

the core body temperature by 1° to 2°C (2° to 4°F) per hour (Centers for Disease Control and Prevention, 2006). Active rewarming is also used for moderate hypothermia. For mild hypothermia (temperature above 35°C [95°F]), passive rewarming with blankets and external heat lamps may be all that are necessary.

Nursing Management

Monitor vital signs and urine output during active rewarming and assess for cold-related injuries. See the following section on frostbite.

Prevention is a primary nursing goal. Educate parents to layer children's clothing in cold climates, recognize signs of hypothermia, decrease time of exposure to cold, and know how to treat mild hypothermia. Teach school-age children and adolescents who go on camping and hunting trips how to recognize and manage hypothermia in themselves and others. Teach preventive techniques such as to avoid riding snow mobiles or walking on ice that is not known to be deep enough to support the weight.

If a child becomes hypothermic during an outing such as a camping trip, a warm person should get into a sleeping bag (or under the blankets) next to the child. This action will warm the child and prevent further heat loss. First aid for hypothermia includes moving the child to a dry area, removing any wet clothing, and protecting the child from further environmental exposure. Wrap the child in dry blankets or dress in warm, dry clothing, and encourage the child to drink a warm, high-calorie liquid, if able.

Frostbite

Frostbite is a cold injury that results from overexposure of the skin cells to temperatures low enough to cause crystal formation. Frostbite develops in tissues exposed to temperatures below freezing for more than an hour when environmental protection is inadequate. Areas of the body at high risk for frostbite include the hands, feet, cheeks, nose, and ears. Ice crystallizes in the tissues, resulting in dehydration of the cells and ischemic damage.

NURSING ALERT

Frostbite can also occur if a chemical ice pack (found in many first aid kits) is left in contact with the skin for too long a period of time. Avoid using these chemical packs in children if possible. When a chemical ice pack is used, cover it with a few layers of clothing or towel and monitor the skin under the pack frequently. Remove the chemical ice pack if the skin starts to looks white or has decreased sensation. Remove the ice pack periodically to allow the skin to rewarm.

With cold exposure, the skin loses sensation and vascular constriction occurs. As ice crystals develop in the extracellular fluid, water moves out of the cells. As the cold injury progresses, cells are progressively damaged due to ischemia and vascular stasis. This environment sets the stage for gangrene (Nield & Nanda, 2005).

Clinical manifestations depend on the severity and depth of the cellular damage after rewarming (Nicol, Huether, & Weber, 2006).

- *Superficial skin affected.* Numb, central white area surrounded by redness and edema, no blistering.
- *Full-thickness skin affected.* Erythema, vesicle formation with clear or pink fluid, surrounded by edema and redness.
- *Full-thickness and subcutaneous skin affected.* Local edema, grayish-blue color, hemorrhagic vesicles, tissue necrosis.
- *Deeper cold injury.* Deep cyanosis, no vesicles or local edema, necrosis of subcutaneous tissue or lower, possibly involving the muscles or tendons.

The skin at first appears pale and is numb. Rapid rewarming causes a flush and the sensation of tingling, burning, or prickling in the affected area. The erythema and mild swelling develop into bullae. The extent of injury usually is not initially apparent.

If frostbite is suspected, get the child to a warmer environment, loosen all constricting clothing, and remove any wet clothes. Because the frostbitten area is numb, extreme caution is needed to protect it from any trauma. Obtain health care as soon as possible. Rewarming is done slowly to decrease the chance of cellular damage. Immerse the affected part for 10 to 15 minutes in water warmed to between 38 and 40°C (100.4 and 104°F). Analgesics are needed because thawing causes significant pain. Gently clean the affected skin with saline. Cover the exposed skin loosely with sterile dressings and elevate the affected extremity. As the extent of the cold injury is gradually revealed, the ruptured vesicles and eschar are debrided. Wound care may be similar to that provided to a child with burns. Whirlpool and physical therapy treatment are important to improve circulation and maintain function. Amputation may be needed when circulation is not restored.

Nursing Management

As with hypothermia, the goal of management is prevention. Teach parents to layer the children's clothing for warmth and to pack extra blankets and clothing if cold temperatures are expected during outdoor activities. Hats covering the ears should be worn. Teach adolescents how to avoid frostbite during hunting and other cold weather expeditions. Wet clothing should be changed quickly.

Early care is instrumental in minimizing permanent injury. Severe frostbite requires hospitalization, fluid management, dressing changes, and careful attention to diet. Provide emotional support to the child and family while they wait to learn the full extent of the injury and disability.

Bites

Animal Bites

Approximately 150,000 dog bites occur among children under 14 years of age and require treatment in the emergency department, with injury rates highest among children between 5 and 9 years of age (Centers for Disease Control, 2003b). Dog bites are among the most frequent injuries to children requiring emergency department care. More than half of dog bite victims are children under 14 years of age (Melnick, 2005). Children, especially those between 5 and 9 years, followed by those less than 5 years are at greater risk, and more boys are bitten than girls (Melnick, 2005). Most dogs involved are known by the child, and most happen in the home or a familiar place. Bites are often associated with the child's inappropriate behavior, such as teasing, rough play, or interfering with feeding or the care of puppies. Other animals that may bite include cats, birds, turtles, and wild animals such as bats, squirrels, and raccoons. See Families Want to Know: Preventing Animal Bites.

Dog bites tend to be crushing, rather than clean, sharp lacerations. Cat bites tend to be puncture wounds. Assessment includes noting the location and number of puncture wounds, abrasions, lacerations, and crushing injuries, redness or swelling at entry

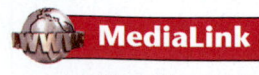

MediaLink

Dog Bite Statistics

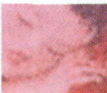

FAMILIES WANT TO KNOW

Preventing Animal Bites

- Never leave a young child alone with an animal.
- Do not buy or adopt a pet unless you are confident of your child's ability to respect it.
- Spay or neuter the pet to reduce aggression.
- Teach children the following rules:
  - Avoid all unfamiliar animals and report them to a parent.
  - Avoid contact with all wild animals.
  - Do not touch an animal when it is eating, sleeping, or nursing puppies.
  - Do not try to separate fighting dogs.
- Never overexcite an animal, even in play. Do not roughhouse or play games that stimulate aggressive behavior.
- Never tease or throw objects at an animal.
- Never put your face close to an animal. Seek permission before hugging or petting an animal.
- If approached by a dog, stay calm, stand still, talk softly, and back away slowly until the dog loses interest; don't run.
- If attacked, stand still like a tree. If knocked down, curl into a ball and protect the face and neck.
- If an animal (wild or unknown) is sick or acting strangely, notify the health department.

sites, redness extending out from the site (possible cellulitis), and any drainage related to the bite. Check for nerve, muscle, tendon, or vascular damage. Carefully document findings. Head and neck bites require radiographic examination to rule out any associated injury, such as trauma to the airway or breathing structures or a depressed skull fracture.

To decrease infection, initial treatment involves wound irrigation, removal of devitalized tissue, and a clean dressing. Sedation and pain management may be needed for some children. Small wounds may be closed with adhesive strips rather than suturing because of the potential for infection. Severe bites sometimes require surgical closure or reconstruction. Wounds over joints should be immobilized and elevated. Cat bites often result in puncture wounds, 50% of which become infected (American Academy of Pediatrics, 2006, p. 191). Puncture wounds should not be irrigated or sutured. Cat bites can result in septic arthritis and osteomyelitis if a bone or joint is punctured. Antibiotics and early treatment can greatly decrease these complications.

Dog bites should be reported and the dog should be observed for 10 days for signs of rabies. Cat bites are also dangerous as fewer cats are immunized against rabies. Bites by wild animals in areas with endemic rabies require rabies prophylaxis. Human rabies immune globulin (HRIG) or human diploid cell rabies (HDCV) vaccine should be given to all children bitten by wild animals in which rabies cannot be excluded, as well as to children bitten by domestic animals (cats and dogs) suspected or proven to be rabid. See Chapter 18 ∞ for information about rabies and rabies prophylaxis.

Human Bites

Human bites are more common than most people realize. They may occur among toddlers and young children, and adolescents also receive human bites in association with an altercation (Merchant, Fuerch, Becker et al., 2005). Because the mouth harbors many bacteria, infection is fairly common. Assess the risk for hepatitis B and HIV infection. Antibiotics may be prescribed to prevent systemic complications. Initial treatment includes irrigating with sterile saline and debridement. Instruct parents about how to care for the wound. Follow-up is important to watch for infection.

NURSING MANAGEMENT   If a child is bitten by an animal, take a complete and accurate history that includes the following information: extent of the injury, circumstances surrounding the attack, present location of the animal, and attempts to assess the animal's health.

Wound care is important. To decrease infection in nonpuncture wounds, high-pressure wound irrigation with large quantities of sterile saline or lactated Ringer's solution is performed rather than scrubbing. One method of high pressure irrigation involves the use of an 18-gauge needle attached to a 60cc syringe filled with saline. Apply a clean dressing and elevate the affected body part to reduce bleeding. Check the child's immunization record to determine whether a tetanus booster is necessary. Debridement of puncture wounds may be performed in the operating room.

As children with bites are often cared for at home, teach the parents about the normal healing process, proper wound care, and the signs and symptoms of infection that indicate a need to return for care. Give the parents information about the symptoms of and potential for post-traumatic stress syndrome following a dog bite (Peters, Sottiaux, Appelboom et al., 2004). Encourage parents to inform the child's healthcare provider if symptoms occur.

Educate parents about preventing animal and human bites and the importance of teaching children appropriate behavior around other children and animals. Parents and children need to understand that any dog may bite at any time. See Families Want to Know: Preventing Animal Bites. When human bites occur in a childcare or school setting, inform parents about the bite so they can discuss potential risks and follow-up with a healthcare provider.

Insect Bites and Stings

Insect bites and stings occur frequently in children and usually are not a cause for concern. Exceptions include bites or stings by insects that carry parasites or communicable diseases (ticks, mosquitoes), those of venomous insects (spiders), and those that produce an allergic reaction. Up to 3% of the population is sensitized to bee stings and have a generalized response to stings (Steen, Carbonaro, & Schwartz, 2004). (For a discussion of communicable diseases carried by ticks and mosquitos, e.g., Lyme disease and Rocky Mountain spotted fever, see Chapter 18 ∞.)

See the clinical manifestations table on the next page for signs of insect bites and stings and their treatment.

NURSING MANAGEMENT The goal of nursing care is prevention. Become familiar with the harmful insects in your area, so you can identify them and recognize their effects. Children should be taught to avoid spiders and other biting or stinging insects. Many commercial repellents are available. Most products contain DEET (diethyltoluamide), picaridin, or oil of lemon eucalyptus and are effective against many insects including mosquitoes, fleas, ticks, and chiggers. However, DEET does not repel stinging insects. The repellent should be reapplied if washed off by sweating or getting wet. Wash DEET off the skin with soap and water once the child is back indoors. Caution parents to avoid overuse of products containing DEET, especially with infants and small children. Do not apply to a young child's hands, as they may rub it into the eyes and mouth. Cases of toxic encephalopathy have been reported following repeated use on children's bedding and clothing (American Academy of Pediatrics, 2006, p. 198). It is believed that a combination of DEET with sunscreens may decrease the sunscreen's effectiveness, so limit the sun exposure for these children.

Warn parents against using heavily perfumed shampoos, powders, soaps, or lotions, or dressing children in bright clothing when outdoors, as these may attract insects. Avoid eating sweet foods and beverages outdoors as these will attract bees and wasps. Pour beverages into a cup or use a straw rather than drinking directly from a can to prevent stings to the mouth and lips by unseen bees.

Household pets may be a source of fleas or ticks. Use preventive treatments against fleas and ticks if pets are allowed prolonged contact with children.

When a known allergy to *Hymenoptera* (bees or wasps) has occurred, the child should wear a medical alert identification and carry an emergency kit with epinephrine (EpiPen). Teach parents and school personnel how to administer the EpiPen, and then to call 9-1-1 for emergency care and transport as the epinephrine's effectiveness lasts only about 20 minutes. Desensitization injections may be given.

Snake Bites

Venomous snakes are found in most areas of the country. During warm months, snakes are active and likely to bite if disturbed. Fortunately, many bites are dry, delivering no venom. Fatalities are rare. Rattlesnake, copperhead, and cottonmouth venom is composed of enzymes and toxins that cause hemolysis and tissue necrosis (Singletary, Rochman, Bodmer et al., 2005). Coral snake venom causes neuromuscular paralysis.

CLINICAL MANIFESTATIONS | INSECT BITES AND STINGS

Type	Clinical Manifestation	Clinical Therapy
Mosquitoes and Fleas Local inflammation results from injected foreign protein or chemicals.	Local reactions: • Discrete, red papules and edema at the bite site with itching, burning, pain, and hives; minimal discomfort • Pruritic wheals and bullae tend to develop with repeat exposure Systemic reactions: • Wheezing, urticaria • Laryngeal edema • Shock	• Cold compresses or ice applied to the site • Antihistamine medication • Systemic reactions need emergency medical treatment
Bee or Wasp Sting Hymenoptera Venoms contain enzymes that affect vascular tone and permeability.	Local reactions: • Mild, local pain • Erythema and edema Systemic reactions: • Generalized urticaria, flushing, angioedema, pruritis • Wheezing • Anaphylaxis is rare	• Remove stinger as soon as possible • Use ice or cold compresses and elevate extremity • Massage a dash of meat tenderizer (papain powder) and a drop of water into the skin for 5 minutes to relieve the pain • Antihistamine medication • Treat systemic reactions with glucocorticoids and antihistamines or epinephrine • Desensitization for severe reactions
Fire Ants Venom is hemolytic and neurotoxic, causing a histaminelike response.	Local reactions: • A black center at the point of the bite, or trail of lesions across skin • Initial wheal becomes a vesicle in a few hours; in 24 hours, the fluid is cloudy, and the vesicle has a red halo • Pruritis, erythema, edema, induration • Systemic and anaphylactic reactions can occur	• Ice or cold compresses • Antihistamine medication • Elevate extremity Systemic reactions—same as bees and wasps
Black Widow Spider Venom is neurotoxic.	• Stinging sensation at time of bite • Localized edema and erythema, two fang marks, petechiae branching from site • Systemic reaction in 1–3 hours, symptoms peak in 3–12 hours, diminish in 72 hours • Muscle rigidity of torso and abdomen, priapism, muscle cramps near the bite • Malaise, sweating, nausea, vomiting, dizziness, restlessness, insomnia • Hypertension and arrhythmias • Oliguria	• Ice • Diazepam for muscle spasms • Opioids for pain management • Antihistamine medication • Hydrocortisone may decrease the inflammatory response • Antivenom IV is used in severe reactions after negative skin test for hypersensitivity to horse serum
Brown Recluse Spider Venom contains proteolytic enzymes and sphingomyelinase D, a cytotoxic factor.	• Itching, pain, and erythema at bite site in first 6 to 12 hours, evolves to purple bull's eye lesion that signals beginning of necrosis; reddish blisters; a white ring is surrounded by an irregular erythematous ring (Zeglin, 2005) • Severe progressive reactions may occur in 12–72 hours, including fever, chills, restlessness, malaise, joint pain, and nausea and vomiting	• Ice or cold compresses • Cleanse the wound and provide good wound care • Analgesics • Oral anti-inflammatory agent • Antibiotics for secondary infection • Excision and skin grafting in cases of severe necrosis

Puncture marks, white wheal, and burning sensation appear at the site of the bite. Pain, erythema, bruising, and edema rapidly develop and extend from the site for up to 24 hours. The swelling may progress without treatment to involve the entire extremity. The extremity has tense skin, tenderness, paresthesia, and pain with movement and may look similar to an extremity with compartment syndrome. Systemic signs include dizziness, tachycardia, nausea, vomiting, diarrhea, diaphoresis, and chills. Children may receive a higher concentration of venom for body mass than adults and may have a more severe response to the bite. Such a severe response may include

CLINICAL TIP

Tourniquets and excision of the bite is no longer recommended. Attempts to catch the snake may result in a second victim. However, attempt to identify the type of snake that caused the bite.

hypotension, altered consciousness, and bleeding from mulitple sites (disseminated intravascular coagulation), pulmonary edema, and renal failure.

Clinical therapy involves immobilization of the extremity and a cold compress to slow the spread of the venom. Laboratory studies include complete blood count, platelet count, coagulation studies, electrolytes, and renal function. The Poison Control Center is contacted to obtain treatment guidelines. Specific antivenom is usually administered within 4 to 6 hours. CroFab®, a newer antivenom used for cottonmouth, copperhead, and rattlesnake bites, is available, but limited data on its use in children exists (Schmidt, 2005). Because antivenom contains a hyperimmune horse serum product, anaphylaxis or delayed serum sickness may develop. The use of antivenom is usually determined after consultation with the Poison Control Center. A skin test may be performed first to detect hypersensitivity. Analgesics are needed, but avoid the use of NSAIDs in victims with coagulopathy (Singletary, Rochman, Bodmer et al., 2005). Antihistamines are often given in anticipation of a hypersensitivity reaction. A tetanus booster is given if vaccination status is unknown, the tetanus series is incomplete, or it has been 10 or more years since the last vaccination. Antibiotics are not administered unless an infection develops.

NURSING MANAGEMENT Nursing care involves assessing the child for initial and progressive signs of the venom's effect. Monitor the child's vital signs and the distal extremity's neurovascular status. First aid involves immobilizing the extremity, keeping it in a dependent position to slow the spread of venom, and using cold compresses. Rings or constricting items should be quickly removed from the injured extremity. Clean the wound with germicidal soap and water. Keep the child quiet and calm to slow the circulation. Help the child identify the snake from pictures of snakes common to the area; however, keep in mind that other venomous snakes may be kept as exotic pets.

The antivenom is diluted in saline and slowly administered intravenously as ordered. Help locate additional antivenom if the hospital does not have an adequate supply. Monitor the child for progressive signs of venom effect, and for antivenom hypersensitivity. Provide skin care for the swollen and tense skin to prevent abrasions and to prevent additional injury. Monitor the site for necrosis and secondary infection. Provide emotional support to the child and family.

As children with bites are often cared for at home, teach the parents about the normal healing process, proper wound care, and the signs and symptoms of infection. Teach children and their family to avoid future snakebites. When in areas where snakes may live, the child should wear protective clothing such as leather boots, avoid reaching into areas where snakes may hide, and avoid any actions that may provoke a snake.

Contusions

Contusions are soft-tissue injuries that have a variety of causes. Often it is difficult to assess whether an injury has caused underlying tissue damage. An injury does not have to break the skin to result in internal damage. Radiographic examination may be necessary to rule out broken bones or further tissue damage. Signs and symptoms that indicate a need for treatment include swelling that does not subside within 72 hours, intense pain, inability to move the injured part, and infection.

Elevate the injured extremity and apply ice as soon as possible after injury. This can reduce inflammation and swelling in the area.

Foreign Bodies

Many skin injuries result from penetration of foreign particles. Common substances include gravel from abrasions, bee stingers, and splinters. Treatment of superficial foreign bodies involves irrigating the wound to try to forcibly dislodge the debris. A deeply embedded foreign body is best removed under medical supervision to avoid permanent injury or scarring.

Lacerations

Lacerations are caused by cuts or tears to the skin. In many cases, the cut is minor and can be managed at home with gentle cleansing, antibiotic ointment, and a bandage. More extensive lacerations and those on the face or over joints often need closing to promote healing and reduce scarring. Laceration repair is performed after wound cleansing and appropriate local analgesia to control pain. Sutures or dermal adhesive may be used. Sutures are usually removed about 7 days later.

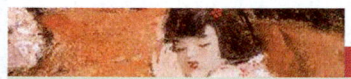

CRITICAL THINKING IN ACTION

Recall Shanelle, 6 years old, who was admitted to and discharged from the hospital with a deep partial-thickness burn after dropping a bowl of soup on her leg. She is making her first visit to the burn clinic for a burn dressing change 3 days after discharge. Shanelle will return to the burn clinic for dressing changes twice a week until the burn is healed.

Shanelle was given pain medication before leaving home in anticipation of the discomfort of the burn dressing change, but she is still anxious about the dressing change and fears that it will still hurt. Shanelle's mother has had no difficulty identifying high-calorie foods for her to eat, but she it not sure if Shanelle is getting enough extra protein to promote the wound healing. Shanelle also avoids walking because it hurts when she straightens her leg. Her mother found a wheelchair for Shanelle when she arrived at the hos-

pital this morning because Shanelle is too heavy to carry as far as the burn clinic.

1. What signs of infection must you watch for?

2. What are some complementary therapies for pain management that can be used during the burn dressing changes?

3. What suggestions can you make to encourage Shanelle to extend and use her leg, despite the pain movement causes?

4. What are some foods or strategies that Shanelle's mother can use for home food preparation at each meal to provide the high-protein and high-calorie diet needed for healing?

 Refer to your Prentice Hall Nursing MediaLink DVD-ROM for answers.

EXPLORE MediaLink 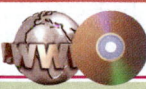 http://www.prenhall.com.ball

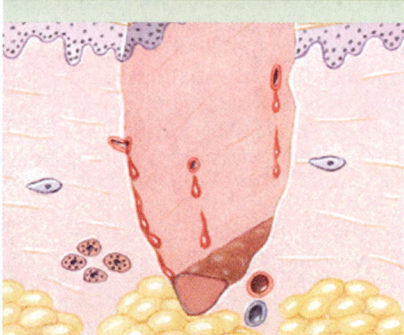

Resources for this chapter can be found on the Prentice Hall Nursing MediaLink DVD-ROM accompanying this textbook, and on the Companion Website at http://www.prenhall.com/ball.

DVD-ROM
Audio Glossary
NCLEX RN®Review
Animations/Videos
   Acne
   Integument Repair

COMPANION WEBSITE
Audio Glossary
NCLEX-RN® Review
Care Plan Activity: Atopic Dermatitis
Case Study: Atopic Dermatitis
MediaLink Applications
   Adolescents and Acne
   Head Lice
   Reduce Potential for Burns in Young Children
WebLinks

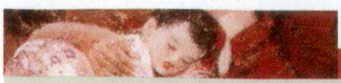

REFERENCES

Allen, P. L. J. (2004). Leaves of three, let them be: If it were only that easy! *Pediatric Nursing, 30*(2), 129–135.

American Academy of Dermatology. (2006). The sun and your skin. Retreived June 24, 2006, from http://www.aad.org/public/Publications/pamphlets/SunandSkin.htm.

American Academy of Pediatrics Committee on Infectious Disease. (2006). *Red book, Report of the committee on infectious disease* (27th ed.). Elk Grove Village, IL: Author.

Atherton, D. J. (2004). A review of the pathophysiology, prevention and treatment of irritant diaper dermatitis. *Current Medical Resident Opinion, 20*(5), 645–649.

Barham, K. L., & Yosipovitch, G. (2005). It's a wrap: The use of wet pajamas in wet-wrap dressings for atopic dermatitis. *Dermatology Nursing, 17*(5), 365–367.

Boguniewicz, M. (2004). Adverse reactions to drugs, In R. E. Behrman, R. M. Kliegman, & H. B. Jenson, *Nelson textbook of pediatrics* (17th ed., pp. 783–786). Philadelphia: Saunders.

Borkowski, S. (2004). Diaper rash care and management. *Pediatric Nursing, 30*(6), 467–470.

Centers for Disease Control and Prevention. (2002). Guidelines for school programs to prevent cancer. *Morbidity and Mortality Weekly Report, 51*(RR-4), 1–18.

Centers for Disease Control and Prevention. (2003a). Methicillin-resistant *Staphylococcus aureus* infections among competitive sports participants—Colorado, Indiana, Pennsylvania, and Los Angeles County, 2000–2003. *Morbidity and Mortality Weekly Report, 52*(33), 793–795.

Centers for Disease Control and Prevention. (2003b). Nonfatal dogbites–Related injuries treated in hospital emergency departments–United States, 2001. *Morbidity and Mortality Weekly Report, 52*(26), 605–610.

Centers for Disease Control and Prevention. (2006). Hypothermia-related deaths—United States, 1999–2002 and 2005. *Morbidity and Mortality Weekly Report, 55*(10), 282–284.

Chamley, C. A. (2005). Development of the integumentary system. In C. A. Chamley, P. Carson, D. Randall, & M. Sandwell, *Developmental anatomy and physiology of children: A practical approach* (pp 37–58), Edinburgh: Elsevier Church Livington.

Cheigh, N. H. (2003). Managing a common disorder in children: Atopic dermatitis. *Journal of Pediatric Health Care, 17*(2), 84–88.

Cohen, B. A. (2002). Plaques: Oval, itchy, and red: What's your diagnosis? *Contemporary Pediatrics, 19*(4), 36–41.

Cohen, B.A. (2004). Another baby and another cutaneous lesion—and more on efficient recognition and management. *Contemporary Pediatrics, 21*(10), 39–57.

Cohen, S. G. (2005). Hemangiomas in infancy and childhood. *Advance for Nurse Practitioners, 13*(11), 41–44.

Corbett, J. V. (2004). Laboratory tests and diagnostic procedures (6th ed.). Upper Saddle River, NJ: Prentice Hall

Curley, M. A. Q., Quigley, S. M., & Lin, M. (2003). Pressure ulcers in pediatric intensive care: Incidence and associated factors. *Pediatric Critical Care Medicine, 4*(3), 284–290.

Davy, L., Boyett, T., Weathers, L., Campbell, R. J., & Roetzheim, R. B. (2002). Sun protection counseling by pediatricians. *Ambulatory Pediatrics, 2*(3), 207–211.

Dohil, M. A., & Eichenfield, L. F. (2005). A treatment approach for atopic dermatitis. *Pediatric Annals, 34*(3), 201–210.

Duffy, B. J., McLaughlin, P. M., & Eichelberger, M. R. (2006). Assessment, triage, and early management of burns in children. *Pediatric Emergency Medicine, 7,* 82–93.

Elewski, B. E., & Krowchuk, D. P. (2001, September). Update on tinea capitis: Reaching consensus. *Contemporary Pediatrics, 18,* S11–S14.

Fleece, D., Gaughan, J. P., & Aronoff, S. C. (2004). Griseofulvin versus terbinafine in the treatment of tinea capitis: A meta-analysis of randomized clinical trials. *Pediatrics, 114*(5), 1312–1315.

Focht, D. R., Spicer, C., & Fairchok, M. P. (2002). The efficacy of duct tape vs. cryotherapy in the treatment of verruca vulgaris (the common wart). *Archives of Pediatric and Adolescent Medicine, 156,* 971–974.

Food and Drug Administration. (2003). FDA issues health advisory regarding labeling changes for lindane products, Retrieved 3/31/2003 from http://www.fda.gov/bbs/topics/ANSWERS/2003/ANS01205.html

Food and Drug Administration. (2005a). FDA public health advisory: Elidel (pimecrolimus) and Protopic (tacrolimus) ointment. Retrieved April 3, 2005, from www.fda.gov/cder/drug/advisory/elidel_protopic.htm

Food and Drug Administration. (2005b). FDA public health advisory: Strengthened risk management program for isotretinoin. Retrieved August 23, 2005, from http://www.fda.gov/cder/drug/advisory/isotretinoin2005.htm

Forum on Child and Family Statistics. (2004). America's Children 2004. Retrieved February 9, 2005, from http://childstats.gov/ac2004/tables/health7b.asp

Gardner, P., Coles, D., & Kemper, K. J. (2001). The skinny on herbal remedies for dermatologic disorders. *Contemporary Pediatrics, 18*(7), 103–114.

Geller, A., Rutsch, L., Kenausis, K., & Zhang, Z. (2003). Evaluation of the SunWise school program. *Journal of School Nursing, 19*(2), 93–99.

Grant, E. J. (2004). Burn prevention. *Critical Care Nursing Clinics of North America, 16,* 127–138.

Horner, G. (2005). Physical abuse: Recognition and reporting. *Journal of Pediatric Health Care, 19*(1), 4–11.

Johnson, K., Davy, L., Boyett, T., Weathers, L., & Roetzheim, R. G. (2001). Sun protection practices for children: Knowledge, attitudes, and parent behaviors. *Archives of Pediatric and Adolescent Medicine, 155*(8), 891–896.

Johnston, G., & Sladden, M. (2005, Sept. 17). Scabies: Diagnosis and treatment. *British Medical Journal, 331,* 619–622.

Keri, J. E. (2006). Acne: Improving skin and self-esteem. *Pediatric Annals, 35*(3), 174–179.

Khachemoune, A., Khechmoune, K., & Blanc, D. (2006). Assessing phytophotodermatitis: Boy with erythema and blisters on both hands. *Dermatologic Nursing, 18*(2), 153–154.

Latchman, Y. E., Xu, X. J., Poulter, L.W., Ruston, M. H. A., & Brostoff, J. (2002). Chinese medical herbs in the treatment of atopic dermatitis. *ACI International, 14*(1), 4–9.

Leung, A. K. C., Fong, J. H. S., & Pinto-Rojas, A. (2005). Pediculosis capitus. *Journal of Pediatric Health Care, 19*(6), 369–378.

Macintyre, L., & Baird, M. (2006). Pressure garments for use in the treatment of hypertrophic scars—a review of the problems associated with their use. *Burns, 32,* 10–15.

Maguire-Eisen, M., Rothman, K., & Demierre, M. F. (2005). The ABCs of sun protection in children. *Dermatology Nursing, 17*(6), 419–433.

McLeod, R. P. (2004). Lumps, bumps, and things that go itch in your office! *Journal of School Nursing, 20*(6), 361–362.

Melnick, A. (2005). Dog bites man *is* new—how pediatricians can spread the word to parents and patients. *Contempoary Pediatrics, 22* (12), 55–64

Merchant, R. C., Fuerch, J., Becker, B. M., & Mayer, K. H. (2005). Comparison of the epidemiology of human bites evaluated at three U.S. pediatric emergency departments. *Pediatric Emergency Care, 21*(12), 833–838.

Merz, J., Schrand, C., Mertens, D., Foote, C., Porter, K., & Regnold, L. (2003). Wound care of the pediatric burn patient. *AACN Clinical Issues, 14*(4), 429–441.

Metry, D. W., Jung, P., & Levy, M. L. (2003). Use of intravenous immunoglobulin in children with Stevens-Johnson Syndome and toxic epidermal necrolysis: Seven cases and review of the literature. *Pediatrics, 112*(6), 1430–1436.

Miller, T., & Frieden, I. J. (2005). Hemangiomas: New insights and classification. *Pediatric Annals, 34*(3), 179–187.

Monroe, J. R. (2005). All that is round is not fungal. *Clinician Reviews, 15*(2), 46–53.

Morel, K. D., Hogeling, M., & Eichenfield, L. F. (2005). More than skin deep: Cutaneous signs of systemic disease. *Contemporary Pediatrics, 22*(2), 48–56.

Nicol, N. H., Huether, S. E., & Weber, R. (2006). Structure, function, and disorders of the integument. In K. L. McCance & S. E. Huether, *Pathophysiology: The biologic basis for disease in adults and children*, (5th ed, pp. 1573–1607). St. Louis: Elsevier Mosby.

Nield, L. S., & Nanda, S. (2005). Cold injuries: A guide to preventing and treating hypothermia and frostbite. *Consultant for Pediatricians, 4*(9), 427–434.

Oliveria, S. A., Saraiya, M., Geller, A. C., Heneghan, M. K., & Jorgensen, C. (2006). Sun exposure and risk of melanoma. *Archives of Disease in Childhood, 91,* 131–138.

O'Riordan, D. L., Geller, A. C., Brooks, D. R., Zhang, Z., & Miller, D. R. (2003). Sunburn reduction through parental role modeling and sunscreen vigilance. *Journal of Pediatrics, 142*, 67–72.

Pearlman, D. L. (2004). A simple treatment for head lice: Dry-on, suffocation based pediculicide. *Pediatrics, 114*, 275–279.

Perry, C. M. (2003). Thermal injuries. In P. A. Maloney-Harmon & S. J. Czerwinski (Eds.), *Nursing care of the pediatric trauma patient* (pp. 277–294). St. Louis: Saunders.

Peters, V., Sottiaux, M., Appelboom, J., & Kahn, A. (2004). Posttraumatic stress disorder after dog bites in children. *Journal of Pediatrics, 144*, 121–122.

Richards, C. A. (2006, April). Treatment tips for common dermatologic problems in ethnic patients. *Infectious Diseases in Children*, 66–67.

Rudy, S. J. (2003). Overview of the evaluation and management of acne vulgaris. *Pediatric Nursing, 29*(4), 287–293.

Schachner, L., Field, T., Hernandez-Ruif, M., Duarte, A. M., & Krasnegor., J. (1998). Atopic dermatitis symptoms decreased in children following massage therapy. *Pediatric Dermatology, 15*(5), 390–395.

Schachner, L. A., Lamerson, C., Sheehan, M. P., Boguniewicz, M., Mosser, J., et al. (2005). Tacrolimus ointment 0.03% is safe and effective for the treatment of mild to moderate atopic dermatitis in pediatric patients: Results from a randomized, double-blind, vehicle-controlled study. *Pediatrics, 116*(3), e334–e342.

Schmidt, C. E. (2003). A 12-month-old girl with maculopapular lesions and lower extremity edema. *Journal of Emergency Nursing, 29*(3), 204–207.

Schmidt, J. M. (2005). Antivenom therapy for snakebites in children: Is there evidence? *Current Opinion in Pediatrics, 17*, 234–238.

Sheridan, R. L. (2005a). Outpatient burn care in the emergency department. *Pediatric Emergency Care, 21*(7), 449–456.

Sheridan, R. L. (2005b). Sepsis in pediatric burn patients. *Pediatric Critical Care Medicine, 6*(3, suppl), S112–S119.

Sheridan, R. L., Schulz, J. T., Ryan, C. M., Schnitzer, J. J., Lawlor, D., et al. (2002). Long-term consequences of toxic epidermal necrolysis in children. *Pediatrics, 109*(1), 74–78.

Shwayder, T. (2003). Five common skin problems—and a string of pearls for managing them. *Contemporary Pediatrics, 20*(7), 34–54.

Silverberg, N. B., Silverberg, J. I., & Silverberg, A. I. (2005). Eradicating acne vulgaris of puberty: What makes for optimal therapy? *Contemporary Pediatrics, 22*(10 supp), 12–22.

Singletary, E. M., Rochman, A. S., Bodmer, J. C. A., & Holstege, C. P. (2005). Envenomations. *Medical Clinics of North America, 89*, 1195–1224.

Sladden, M. J., & Johnston, G. A. (2005). More common skin infections in children. *British Medical Journal, 330*, 1194–1198.

Smolinski, K. N., & Yan, A. C. (2005). How and when to treat molluscum contagiosum and warts in children. *Pediatric Annals, 34*(3), 211–221.

Steen, C. J., Carbonaro, P. A., & Schwartz, R. A. (2004). Arthropods in dermatology. *Journal of American Academy of Dermatology, 50*, 819–842.

Stowkowski, L. A. (2006). Neonatal skin: Back to nature? Medscape Pediatrics. Retrieved January 3, 2006, from http://www.medscape.com/viewarticle/519767?src=mp

Strouse, J. J., Fears, T. R., Tucker, M. A., & Wayne, A. S. (2005). Pediatric melanoma: Risk factor and survival analysis of the surveillance, epidemiology, and end results database. *Journal of Clinical Oncology, 23*, 4735–4741.

Takano-Lee, M., Edman, J. D., Mullens, B. A., & Clark, J. M. (2004). Home remedies to control head lice: Assessment of home remedies to control the human head louse, *Pediculus humanus capitis* (Anoplura: Pediculidae). *Journal of Pediatric Nursing, 19*(6), 393–398.

Tharp, M. D. (2005). A multifaceted approach to the treatment of atopic dermatitis. *Medscape Dermatology, 6*(1). Retrieved July 5, 2005, from http://www.medscape.com/viewarticle/506964

Timm-Knudson, V. L., Johnson, J. S., Ortiz, K. J., & Yiannias, J. A. (2006). Allergic contact dermatitis to preservatives. *Dermatologic Nursing, 18*(2), 130–136.

Trask, B. C., Rote, N. S., & Huether, S. E. (2006). Innate immunity: Inflammation. In K. L. McCance & S. E. Huether, *Pathophysiology: The biologic basis for disease in adults and children* (5th ed, pp. 175–209). St. Louis: Elsevier Mosby.

Weston, S., Halbert, A., Richmond, P., & Prescott, S. L. (2005). Effects of probiotics on atopic dermatitis: A randomized controlled trial. *Archives of Disease in Childhood, 90*, 892–897.

Weston, W. L., & Bruckner, A. (2000). Allergic contact dermatitis. *Pediatric Clinics of North America, 47*(4), 897–907.

Whalley, D., Huels, J., McKenna, S. P., & van Assche, D. (2002). The benefit of pimecrolumus on parents' quality of life in the treatment of pediatric atopic dermatitis. *Pediatrics, 110*(6), 1133–1136.

Woodard, I. (2002). Adolescent acne: A stepwise approach to management. *Topics in Advanced Practice Nursing eJournal, 2*(2). Retrieved September 24, 2003, from http://www.medscape.com/viewarticle/430534

Zeglin, D. (2005). Brown recluse spider bites. *American Journal of Nursing, 105*(2), 64–68.

Appendix A

Physical Growth Charts

Figure A–1 ➤

Classification of newborns based on maturity and intrauterine growth.

Sources: Adapted from Lubchenco, L. O., Hansman, C., & Boyd, E. (1966). Intrauterine growth in length and head circumference as estimated from live births at gestational ages from 26 to 42 weeks. *Pediatrics, 37,* 403–408; Battaglia, F. C., & Lubchenco, L. O. (1967). A practical classification of newborn infants by weight and gestational age. *Journal of Pediatrics, 71,* 159.

CLASSIFICATION OF NEWBORNS— BASED ON MATURITY AND INTRAUTERINE GROWTH

Symbols: X-1st Exam O-2nd Exam

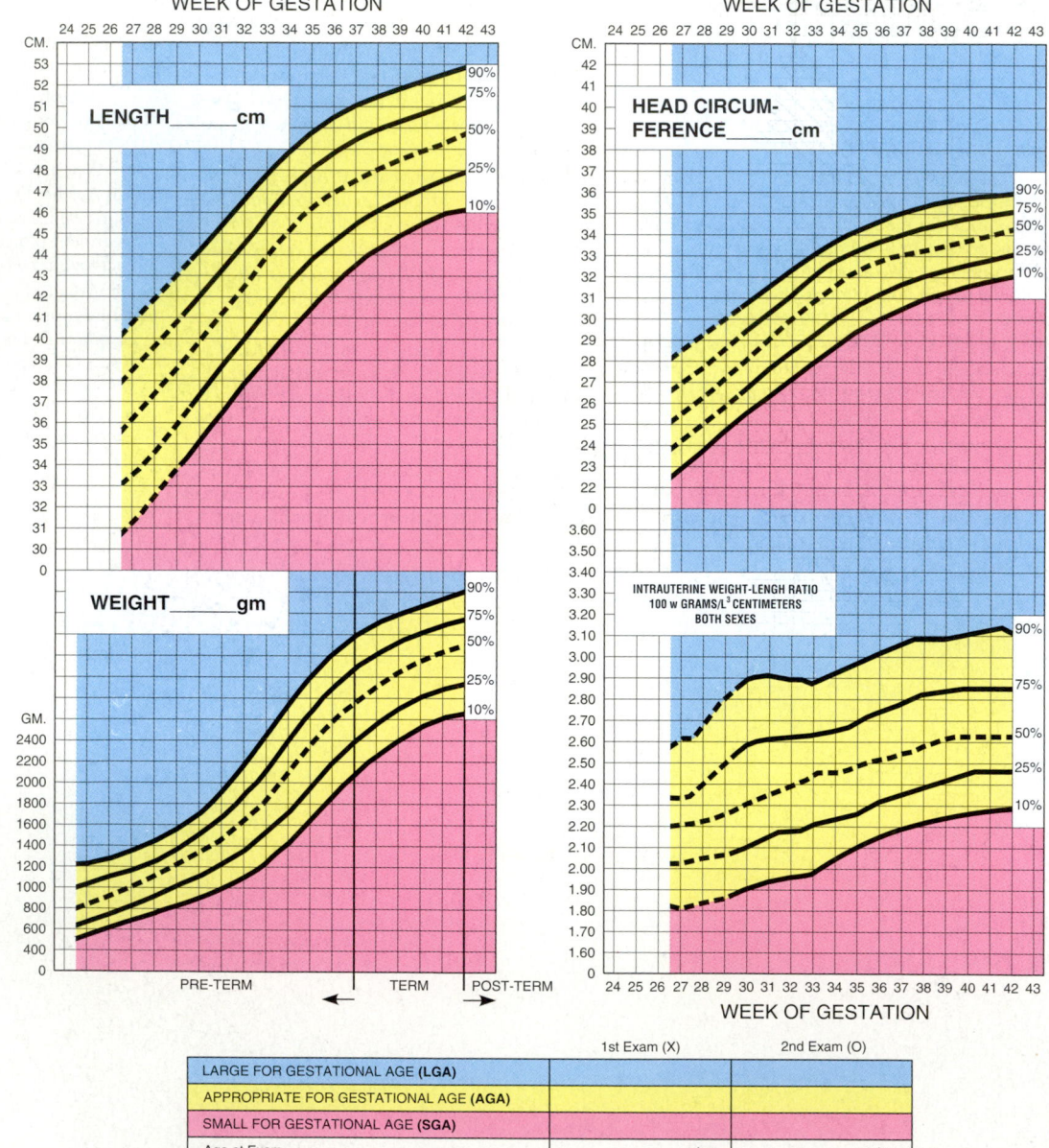

	1st Exam (X)	2nd Exam (O)
LARGE FOR GESTATIONAL AGE (**LGA**)		
APPROPRIATE FOR GESTATIONAL AGE (**AGA**)		
SMALL FOR GESTATIONAL AGE (**SGA**)		
Age at Exam	hrs	hrs
Signature of Examiner	M.D.	M.D.

Birth to 36 months: Boys
Length-for-age and Weight-for-age percentiles

NAME _____

RECORD # _____

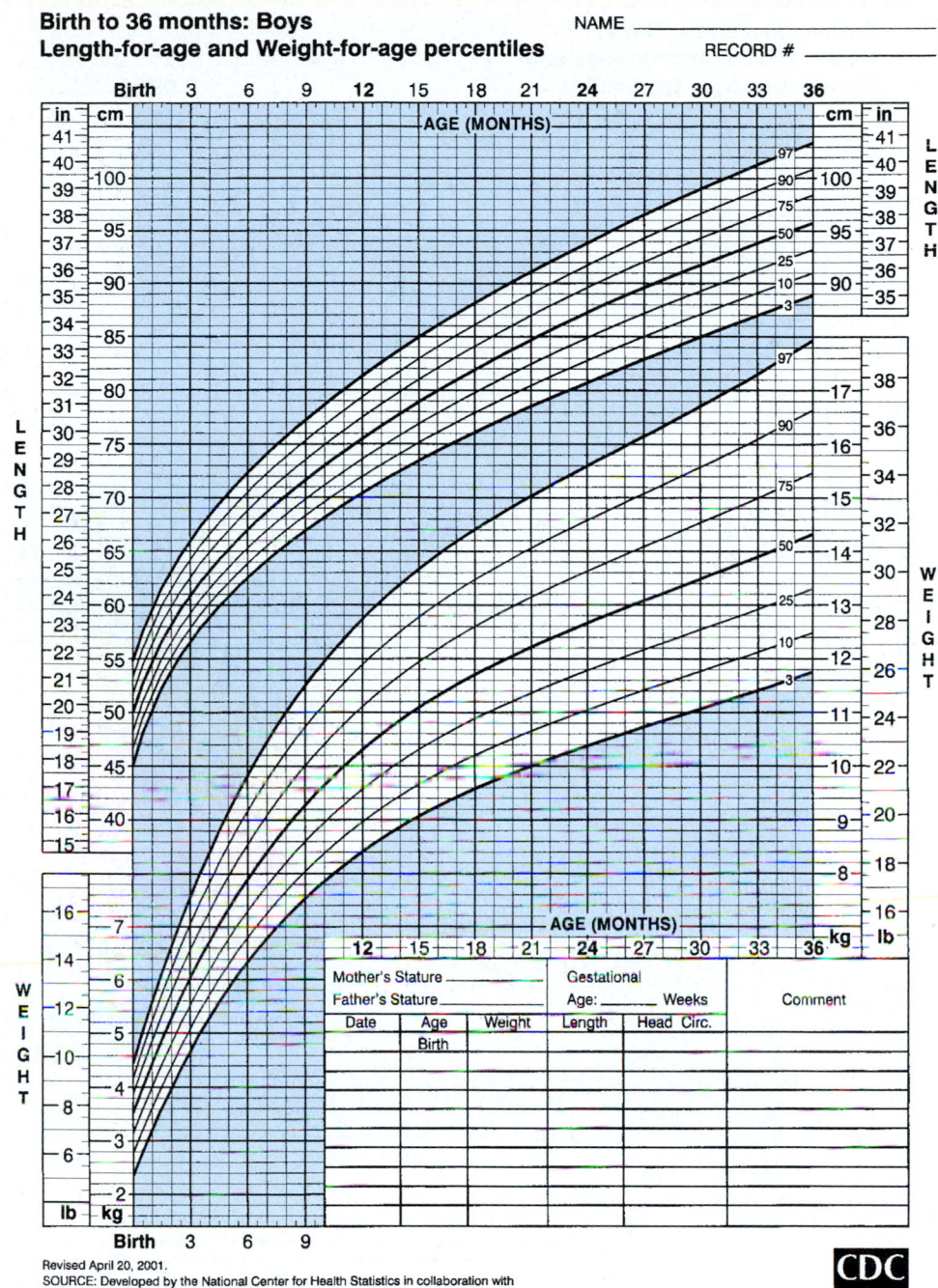

Revised April 20, 2001.
SOURCE: Developed by the National Center for Health Statistics in collaboration with
   the National Center for Chronic Disease Prevention and Health Promotion (2000).
   http://www.cdc.gov/growthcharts

Figure A–2 ➤ Physical growth percentiles for length and weight—boys: birth to 36 months. From CDC, 2001. *www.cdc.gov/growthcharts*

Figure A–3 ➤ Physical growth percentiles for head circumference, weight for length—boys: birth to 36 months.

From CDC, 2001. *www.cdc.gov/growthcharts*

Birth to 36 months: Boys
Head circumference-for-age and
Weight-for-length percentiles

NAME _____

RECORD # _____

SOURCE: Developed by the National Center for Health Statistics in collaboration with
the National Center for Chronic Disease Prevention and Health Promotion (2000).
http://www.cdc.gov/growthcharts

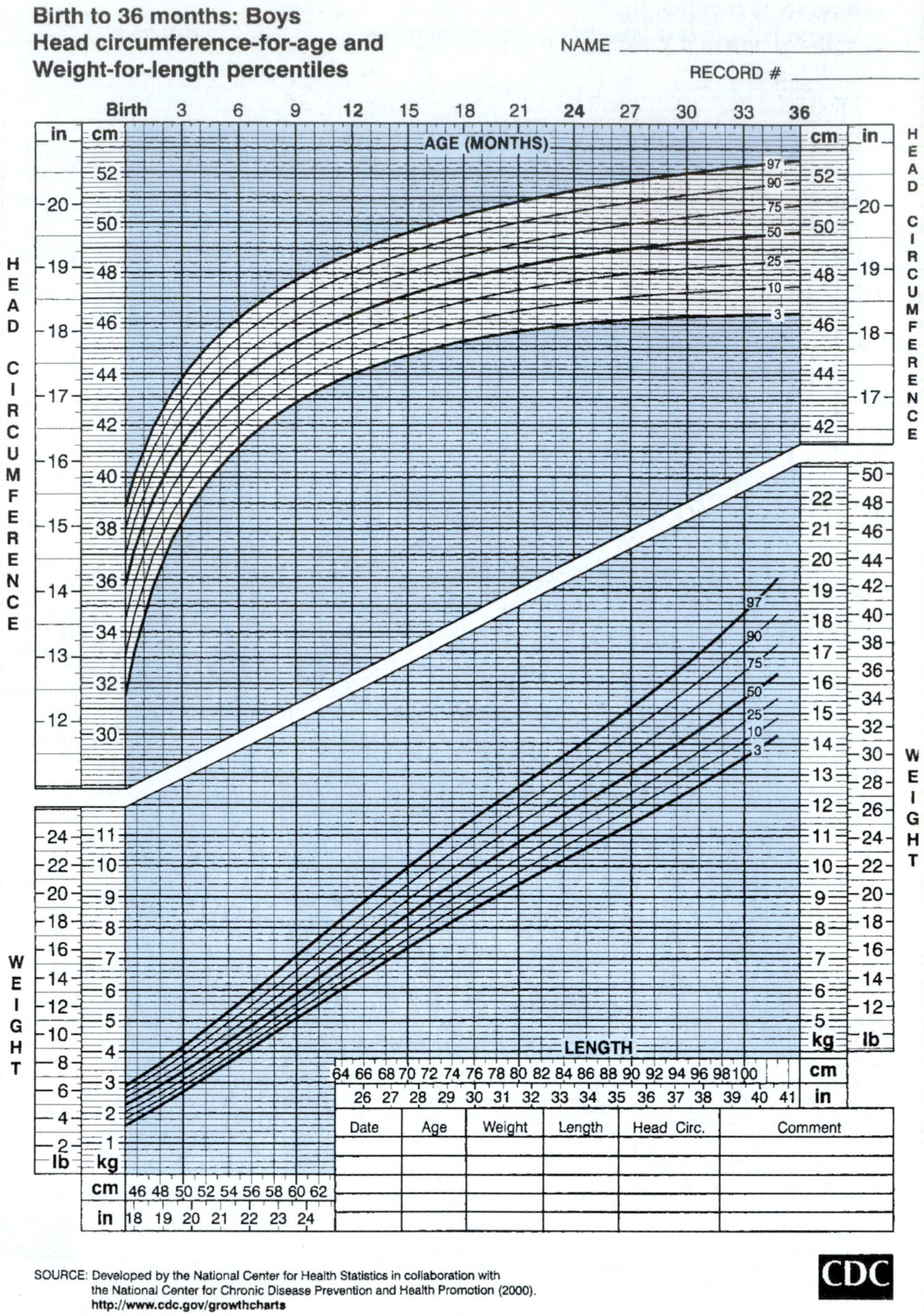

Birth to 36 months: Girls
Length-for-age and Weight-for-age percentiles

NAME _____

RECORD # _____

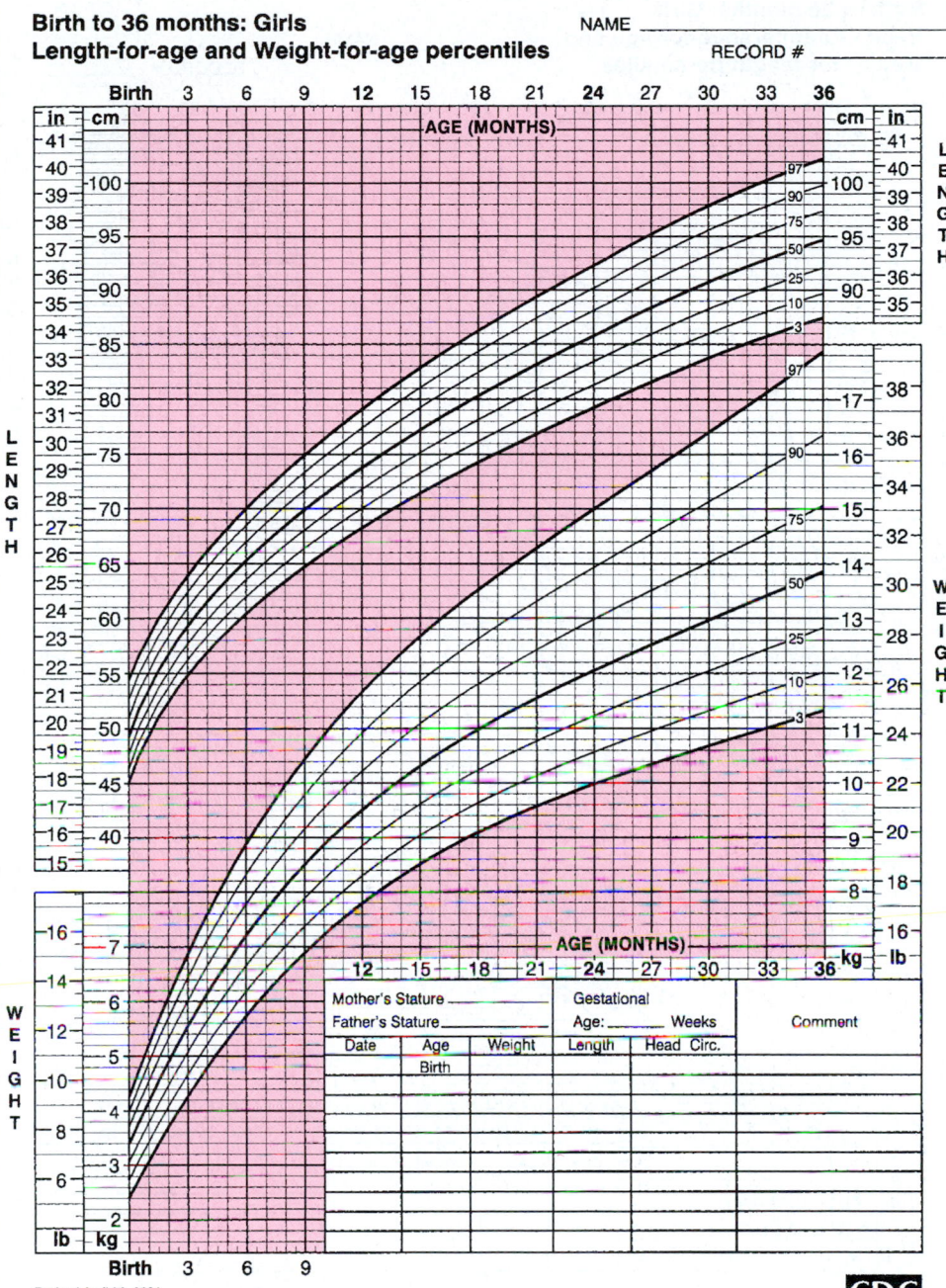

Revised April 20, 2001.
SOURCE: Developed by the National Center for Health Statistics in collaboration with
the National Center for Chronic Disease Prevention and Health Promotion (2000).
http://www.cdc.gov/growthcharts

Figure A–4 ➤ Physical growth percentiles for length and weight—girls: birth to 36 months.
From CDC, 2001. *www.cdc.gov/growthcharts*

Figure A–5 ➤ Physical growth percentiles for head circumference, weight for length—girls: birth to 36 months.

From CDC, 2001. *www.cdc.gov/growthcharts*

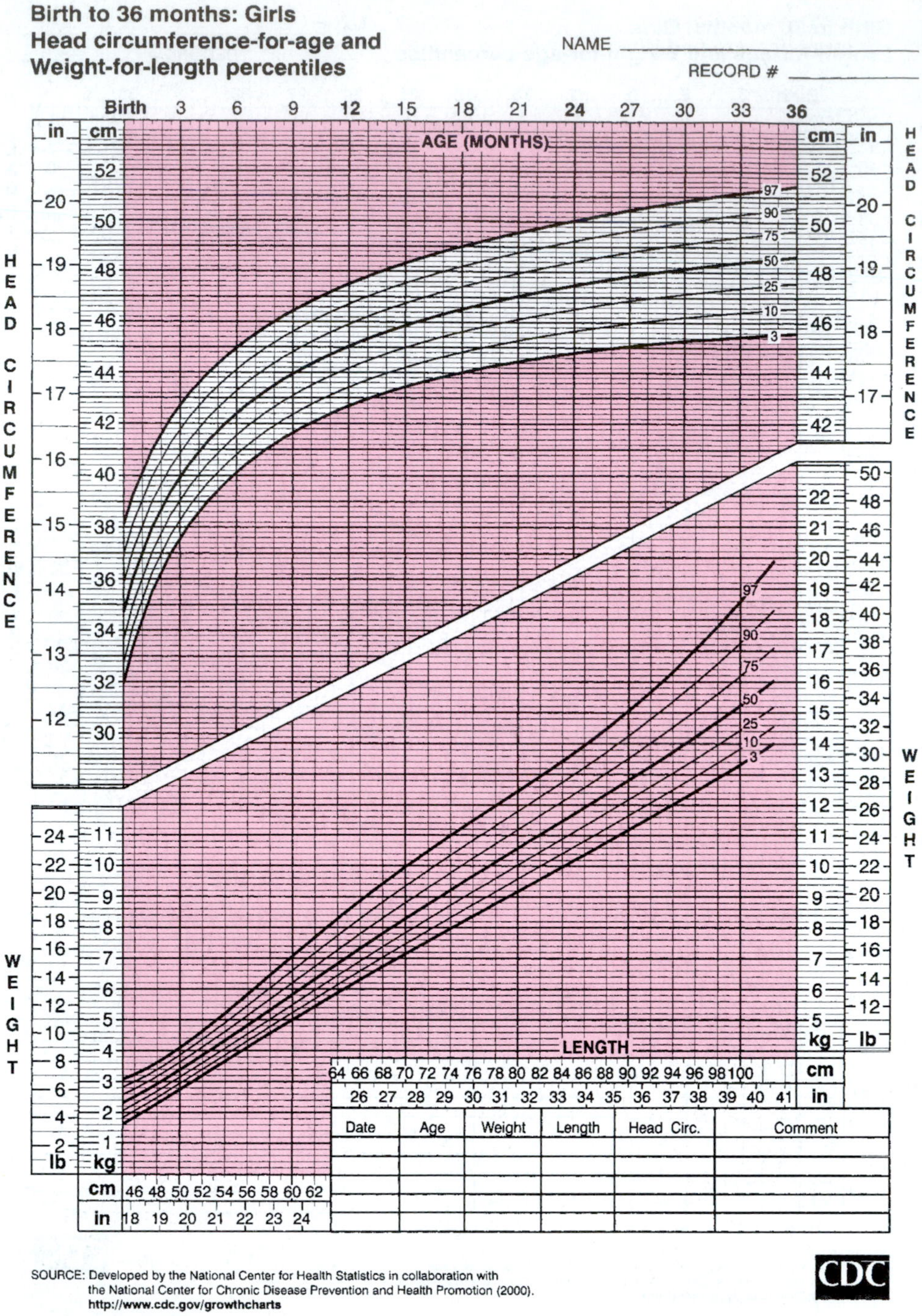

**Birth to 36 months: Girls
Head circumference-for-age and
Weight-for-length percentiles**

NAME _____

RECORD # _____

Date	Age	Weight	Length	Head Circ.	Comment

2 to 20 years: Boys
Stature-for-age and Weight-for-age percentiles

NAME _____

RECORD # _____

Figure A–6 ➤ Physical growth percentiles for stature and weight according to age—boys: 2 to 20 years.
From CDC, 2001. *www.cdc.gov/growthcharts*

Mother's Stature _____   Father's Stature _____

Date	Age	Weight	Stature	BMI*

*To Calculate BMI: Weight (kg) ÷ Stature (cm) ÷ Stature (cm) x 10,000
or Weight (lb) ÷ Stature (in) ÷ Stature (in) x 703

AGE (YEARS)

STATURE

WEIGHT

Revised and corrected November 21, 2000.
SOURCE: Developed by the National Center for Health Statistics in collaboration with
the National Center for Chronic Disease Prevention and Health Promotion (2000).
http://www.cdc.gov/growthcharts

CDC

Figure A–7 ➤ Physical growth percentiles for body mass index according to age—boys: 2 to 20 years.

From CDC, 2001. *www.cdc.gov/growthcharts*

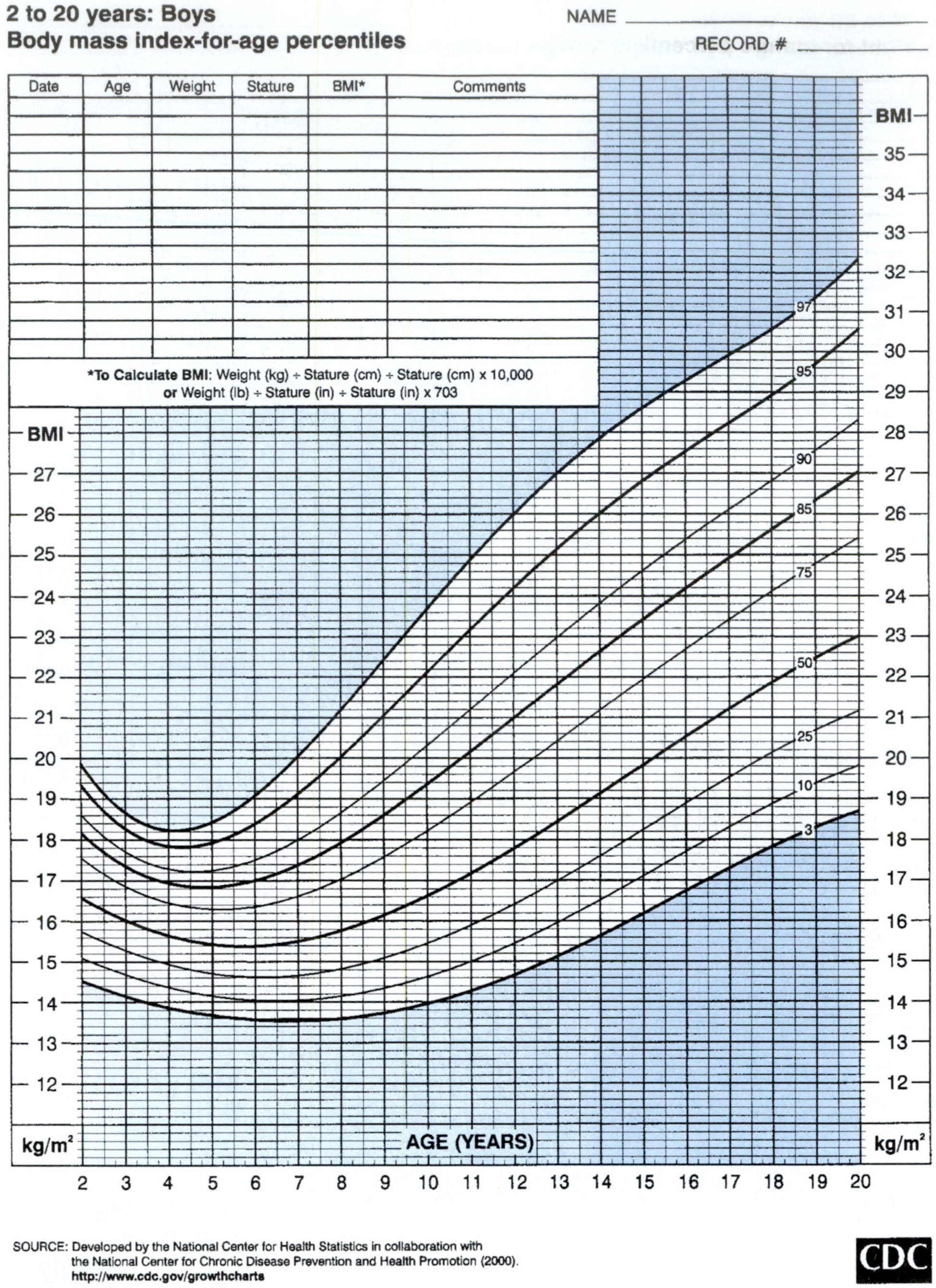

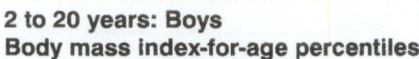

2 to 20 years: Boys
Body mass index-for-age percentiles

Date	Age	Weight	Stature	BMI*	Comments

*To Calculate BMI: Weight (kg) ÷ Stature (cm) ÷ Stature (cm) x 10,000
or Weight (lb) ÷ Stature (in) ÷ Stature (in) x 703

AGE (YEARS)

Weight-for-stature percentiles: Boys

NAME _____

RECORD # _____

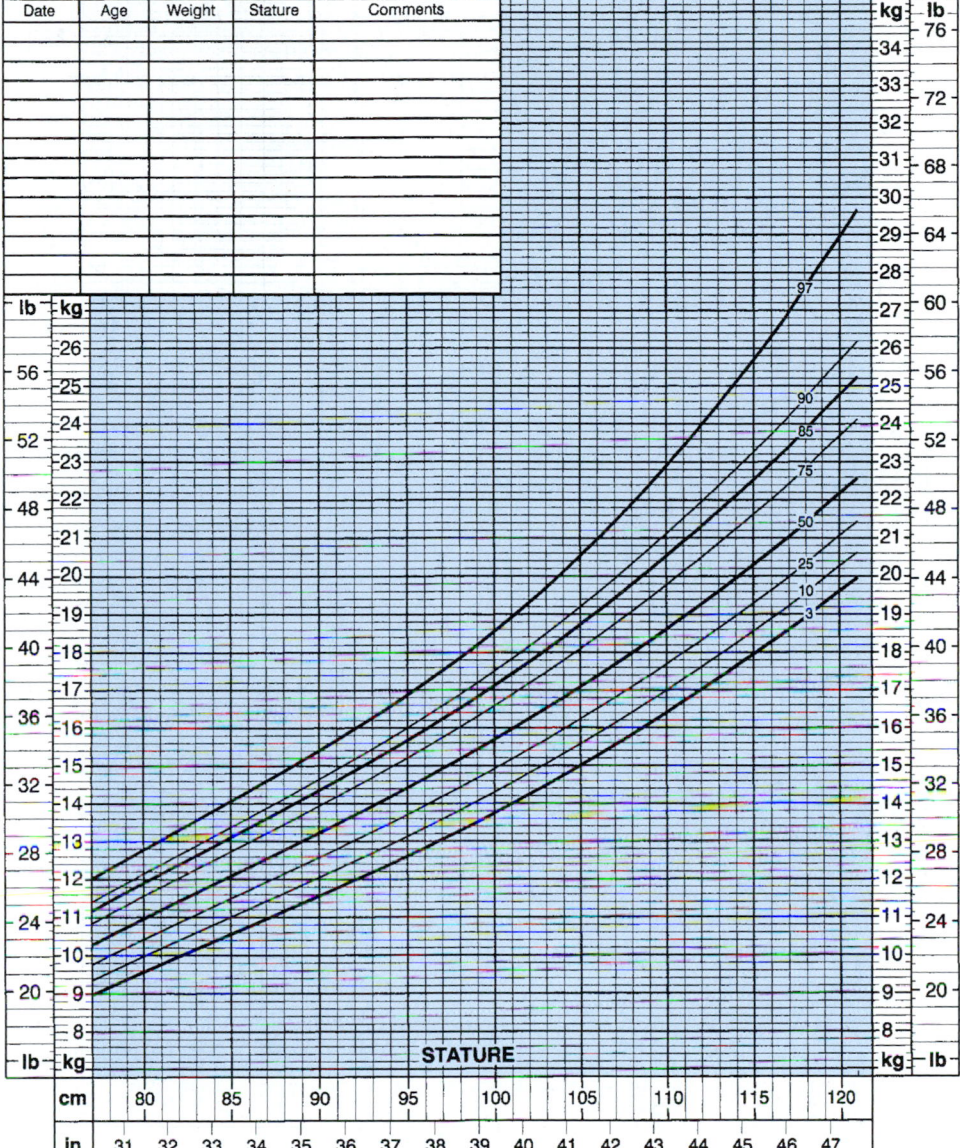

Date	Age	Weight	Stature	Comments

STATURE

SOURCE: Developed by the National Center for Health Statistics in collaboration with
the National Center for Chronic Disease Prevention and Health Promotion (2000).
http://www.cdc.gov/growthcharts

Figure A–8 ➤ **Physical growth percentiles for weight for stature—boys: 2 to 20 years.**
From CDC, 2001. *www.cdc.gov/growthcharts*

Figure A–9 ➤ Physical growth percentiles for stature and weight according to age—girls: 2 to 20 years.

From CDC, 2001. *www.cdc.gov/growthcharts*

2 to 20 years: Girls
Stature-for-age and Weight-for-age percentiles

NAME _____

RECORD # _____

Revised and corrected November 21, 2000.
SOURCE: Developed by the National Center for Health Statistics in collaboration with
the National Center for Chronic Disease Prevention and Health Promotion (2000).
http://www.cdc.gov/growthcharts

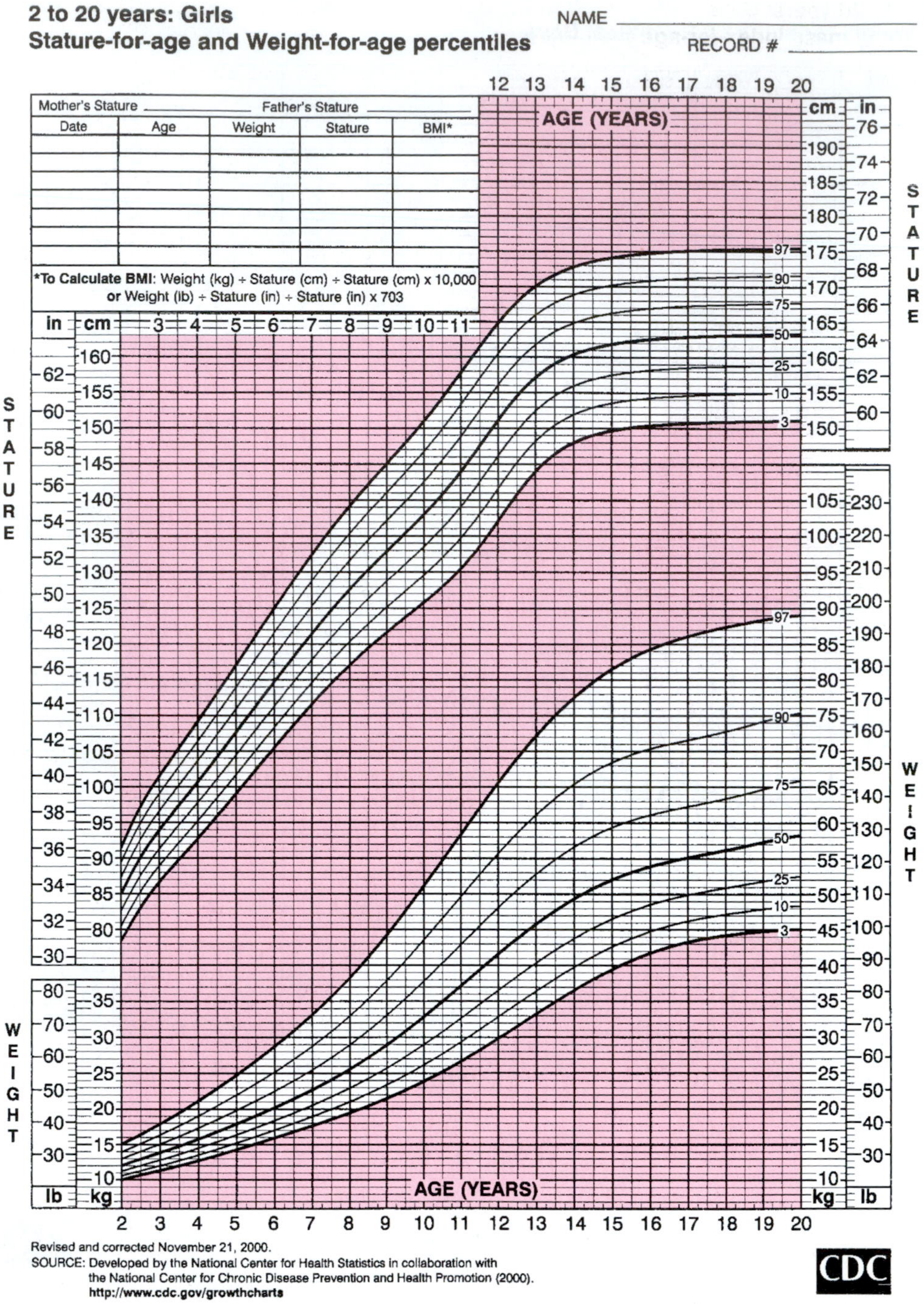

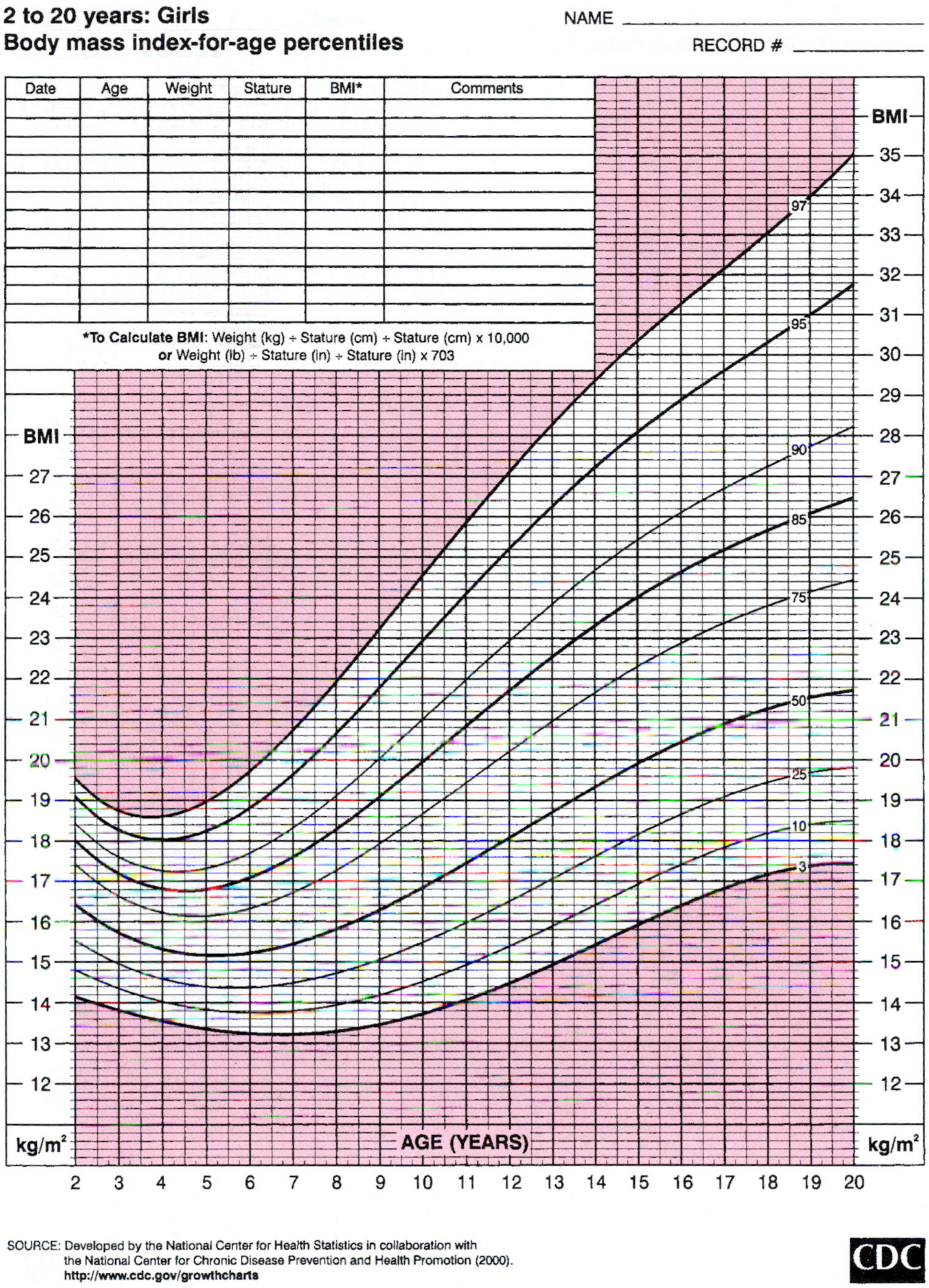

2 to 20 years: Girls
Body mass index-for-age percentiles

NAME _____

RECORD # _____

Date	Age	Weight	Stature	BMI*	Comments

*To Calculate BMI: Weight (kg) ÷ Stature (cm) ÷ Stature (cm) x 10,000
or Weight (lb) ÷ Stature (in) ÷ Stature (in) x 703

BMI

97
95
90
85
75
50
25
10
3

BMI

35
34
33
32
31
30
29
28
27
26
25
24
23
22
21
20
19
18
17
16
15
14
13
12

kg/m²   AGE (YEARS)   kg/m²

2 3 4 5 6 7 8 9 10 11 12 13 14 15 16 17 18 19 20

SOURCE: Developed by the National Center for Health Statistics in collaboration with
the National Center for Chronic Disease Prevention and Health Promotion (2000).
http://www.cdc.gov/growthcharts

Figure A–10 ➤ Physical growth percentiles for body mass index according to age—girls: 2 to 20 years.
From CDC, 2001. *www.cdc.gov/ growthcharts*

Figure A–11 ➤ Physical growth percentiles for weight for stature—girls: 2 to 20 years.

From CDC, 2001. *www.cdc.gov/growthcharts*

Weight-for-stature percentiles: Girls

NAME _____

RECORD # _____

Date	Age	Weight	Stature	Comments

Percentile curves labeled: 97, 90, 85, 75, 50, 25, 10, 3

STATURE

cm: 80, 85, 90, 95, 100, 105, 110, 115, 120

in: 31, 32, 33, 34, 35, 36, 37, 38, 39, 40, 41, 42, 43, 44, 45, 46, 47

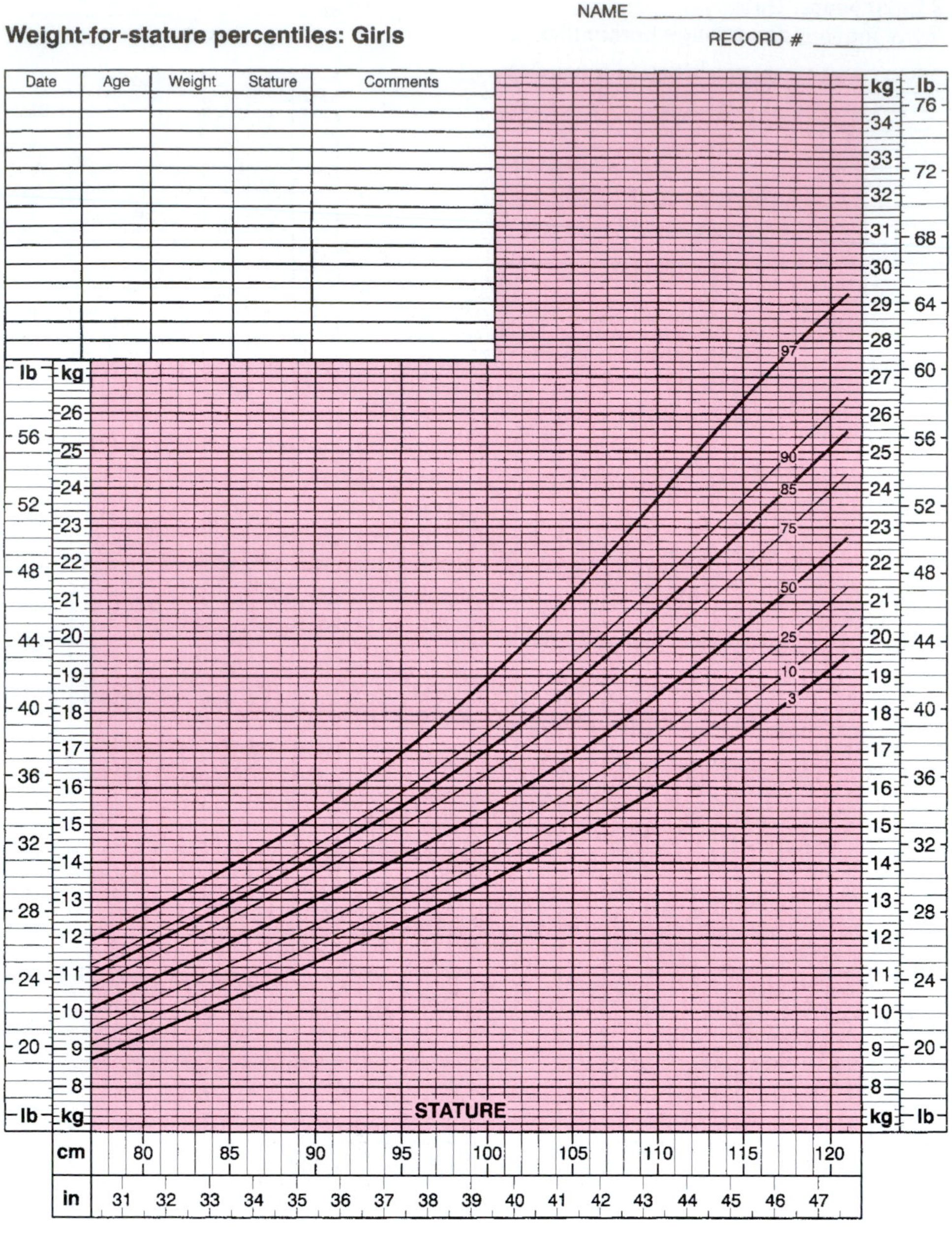

SOURCE: Developed by the National Center for Health Statistics in collaboration with
the National Center for Chronic Disease Prevention and Health Promotion (2000).
http://www.cdc.gov/growthcharts

Appendix B
Dietary Reference Intakes

Table B–1	DIETARY REFERENCE INTAKES									
	Age	Vitamin A (mcg/d)	Vitamin D (mcg/d)	Vitamin E (mg/d α-tocopherol)	Vitamin K (mcg/d)	Vitamin C (mg/d)	Thiamin (mg/d)	Riboflavin (mg/d)	Niacin (mg/d)	Vitamin B₆ (mg/d)
Infants	0–6 months	400*	5*	4*	2.0*	40*	0.2*	0.3*	−0.2*	0.1*
	7–12 months	500*	5*	5*	2.5*	50*	0.3*	0.4*	−0.4*	0.3*
Children	1–3 years	300	5*	6	30*	15	0.5	0.5	6	0.5
	4–8 years	400	5*	7	55*	25	0.6	0.6	8	0.6
Males	9–13 years	600	5*	11	60*	45	0.9	0.9	12	1.0
	14–18 years	900	5*	15	75*	75	1.2	1.3	16	1.3
Females	9–13 years	600	5*	11	60*	45	0.9	0.9	12	1.0
	14–18 years	700	5*	15	75*	65	1.0	1.0	14	1.2

*Values are Adequate Intakes (AIs) rather than Recommended Dietary Allowances (RDAs). All other values on the chart are RDAs. See Chapter 4 for a discussion of nutrient requirements.

Note: All data from Otten, J.J., Hellwig, J.P., & Meyers, L.D. (eds.) (2006). *Dietary reference intakes: The essential guide to nutrient requirements.* Washington, DC: National Academies Press.

Table B–2	DIETARY REFERENCE INTAKE FOR WATER (L/D)			
	Age	From Food	From Beverages	Total
Infants	0–6 months	0	0.7	0.7*
	7–12 months	0.2	0.6	0.8*
Children	1–3 years	0.4	0.9	1.3*
	4–8 years	0.5	1.2	1.7*
Males	9–13 years	0.6	1.8	2.4*
	14–18 years	0.7	2.6	3.3*
Females	9–13 years	0.5	1.6	2.1*
	14–18 years	0.5	1.8	2.3*

*Values are Adequate Intakes.

Folate (mcg/d)	Vitamin B$_{12}$ (mcg/d)	Calcium (mg/d)	Phosphorus (mg/d)	Magnesium (mg/d)	Iron (mg/d)	Zinc (mg/d)	Iodine (mcg/d)	Selenium (mcg/d)	Potassium (g/d)	Sodium (g/d)
65*	0.4*	210*	100*	30*	0.27*	2.0*	110*	15*	0.4*	0.12*
80*	0.5*	270*	275*	75*	11	3	130*	20*	0.7*	0.37*
150	0.9	500*	460	80	7	3	90	20	3*	1*
200	1.2	800*	500	130	10	5	90	30	3.8*	1.2*
300	1.8	1300*	1250	240	8	8	120	40	4.5*	1.5*
400	2.4	1300*	1250	240	11	11	150	55	4.5*	1.5*
300	1.8	1300*	1250	410	8	8	120	40	4*	1.5*
400	2.4	1300*	1250	360	15	9	150	55	4.7*	1.5*

Table B–3 | RECOMMENDED DIETARY ALLOWANCES

	Age	Protein	Carbohydrate	Polyunsaturated Fatty Acids n-6	Polyunsaturated Fatty Acids n-3	Total Fat	Fiber
Infants	0–6 months	9.1 g/d or 1.52 g/kg/d*	60 g/d*	4.4 g/d	0.5 g/d	31 g/d	NE
	7–12 months	1.5 g/kd/g	95 g/d*	4.6 g/d	0.5 g/d	30 g/d	NE
Children	1–3 years	1.1 g/kg/d or 13 g/d	130 g/d	7 g/d (linoleic)	0.7 g/d (α-linolenic)	NE	19 g/d
	4–8 years	0.95 g/kg/d or 19 g/d	130 g/d	10 g/d (linoleic)	0.9 g/d (α-linolenic)	NE	25 g/d
Males	9–13 years	0.95 g/kg/d or 34g/d	130 g/d	12 g/d (linoleic)	1.2 g/d (α-linolenic)	NE	31 g/d
	14–18 years	0.85 g/kg/d or 52 g/d	130 g/d	16 g/d (linoleic)	1.6 g/d (α-linolenic)	NE	38 g/d
Females	9–13 years	0.95 g/kg/d or 34 g/d	130 g/d	10 g/d (linoleic)	1.0 g/d (α-linolenic)	NE	26 g/d
	14–18 years	0.85 g/kg/d or 46 g/d	130 g/d	11 g/d (linoleic)	1.1 g/d (α-linolenic)	NE	26 g/d

*Values are Adequate Intakes (AIs) rather than Recommended Dietary Allowances (RDAs). All other values on charts are RDAs. NE = not established

All data from Otten, J.J., Hellwig, J.P., & Meyers, L.D. (eds.) (2006). *Dietary reference intakes: The essential guide to nutrient requirements.* Washington, DC: National Academies Press.

Appendix C
Selected Pediatric Laboratory Values

All laboratory value ranges listed are approximate. Consult your local laboratory for guidelines as to normal values for the specific testing procedures used.

NORMAL VALUE RANGES: BLOOD

Albumin (S)[1]

1 mo–1 year: 2.8–4.8 g/dL
1–18 years: 3.2–4.7

Alkaline Phosphatase (S)[1]

Age	Males Units/L	Females Units/L
1–30 days	75–316	48–406
1–3 years	104–345	108–317
4–6 years	93–309	96–297
7–9 years	86–315	69–325
10–12 years	42–362	51–332
13–15 years	74–390	50–162
16–18 years	52–171	47–119

Blood Chemistry

Chloride (S, P)[1]:

< 1 year: 96–111 mmol/L
1–17 years: 102–112 mmol/L

Glucose (S, P)[1]:

54–117 mg/dL (3.00–6.49 mmol/L)

Magnesium (P, S)[1]:

1.6–2.5 mg/dL (0.7–1 mmol/L)

Osmolality (S)[1]:

280–300 mOsm/kg

Potassium (S, P)[1]:

3.3–4.7 mmol/L

Sodium (P, S)[1]:

132–141 mmol/L

Urea Nitrogen (S, P)[1]:

1–13 years   4–17 mg/dL (1.1–4.6 mmol/L)
14–19 years   7–21 mg/dL (1.9–5.7 mmol/L)

Blood Gases

Carbon Dioxide, Partial Pressure (Pco$_2$)(B)[1]:

Infant: 27–41 mmHg (3.6–5.5 kPa)
Children: 32–48 mmHg (4.3–6.4 kPa)

Oxygen, Partial Pressure (Po$_2$) (B)[1]:

> 1 day   83–108 mmHg (11–14.4 pKa)

Bicarbonate, Actual (P)[2]:

Calculated from pH and Paco2
Newborns: 17.2–23.6 mmol/L
Children: 18–25 mmol/L

PH (B)[1]:

0–6 months   7.18–7.50
6–12 months   7.27–7.49

Base Excess (B)[1]:

Infant: −7 to −1 mmol/L
Child: −4 to +2 mmol/L
Thereafter: −3 to +3 mmol/L

Oxygen Saturation (B)[1]:

Newborns: 85–90%
Thereafter: 95–99%

KEY for Type of Specimen: S = serum; B = whole blood; P = plasma

Cholesterol (S)[3]

Total Cholesterol:

Borderline > 170 mg/dL
Elevated > 200 mg/dL

High-Density Lipoprotein:

< 35 mg/dL

Low-Density Lipoprotein:

Borderline > 110 mg/dL
Elevated > 130 mg/dL

Triglycerides:

<150 mg/dL

C-Reactive Protein (CRP) (P, S)[1]

0.068–8.2 mg/L

Hemoglobin Alc (B)[1]

Normal: 4–7%
Stable diabetic patients: 8–10%

Hemoglobin Electrophoresis (B)[2]

A_1 hemoglobin: 96–98.5% of total hemoglobin
A_2 hemoglobin: 1.5–4% of total hemoglobin

Hematology Values (B)

Values for children 2 to 12 years

Red Blood Cell (RBC)[1]:

$3.89–4.96 \times 10^{12}$/L

Hemoglobin (HGB)[1]:

10.2–13.4 g/dL

Hematocrit (HCT)[1]:

31.7–39.3%

Mean Corpuscular Volume (MCV)[1]:

72.7–86.5 micrometer^3

Mean Corpuscular Hemoglobin (MCH)[1]:

24.1–29.4 picograms

Mean Corpuscular Hemoglobin Concentration (MCHC)[1]:

32.4–35.3%

Reticulocyte Count[1]:

0.8–2.2%

Sedimentation Rate (Micro)[2]:

<2 years: 1–5 mm/hr
>2 years: 1–8 mm/hr

White Blood Cell (WBC)[1]:

$5.4–11 \times 10^9$/L

Differential[1]:

Neutrophils	34.3–72.9%
Eosinophils	2.4–4.8%
Basophils	1%
Lymphocyte	13.5–52.8%
Atypical lymphocytes	2.6–5.6%
Monocytes	3.5–13.4%

Iron-Related Values

Ferritin (P, S)[1]:

1–6 months:	47–449 ng/mL
Thereafter:	47–110 ng/mL

Iron (S, P)[1]:

5–11 am: 20–105 mcg/dL (3.6–18.8 micromol/L)

Iron-Binding Capacity (S, P)[1]:

1–5 years:	268–441 mcg/dL (48–79 micromol/L)
6–9 years:	240–508 mcg/dL (43–91 micromol/L)
10–19 years:	290–575 mcg/dL (52–103 micromol/L)

Lead (B)[1]

0–15 years   <5 mcg/dL

Thyroid Hormones

Thyroid-Stimulating Hormone (TSH) (P, S)[1]

Age	Males	Females
1–30 days	0.52–16 mUnit/L	0.72–13.1 mUnit/L
1 mo–5 yr	0.55–7.1 mUnit/L	0.46–8.1 mUnit/L
6–18 yrs	0.37–6 mUnit/L	0.36–5.8 mUnit/L

Thyroxine (T4) (S, P)[1]

Age	Males	Females
1–30 days	5.9–21.5 mg/dL	6.3–21.5 mg/dL
1–6 years	6.1–13.1 mg/dL	7.1–14.1 mg/dL
7–12 years	6.7–13.4 mg/dL	6.1–12.1 mg/dL
13–15 years	4.8–11.5 mg/dL	5.8–11.2 mg/dL
16–18 years	5.9–11.5 mg/dL	5.2–13.2 mg/dL

Thyroxine, "Free" (Free T4)(S, P)[1]

1–12 months:	0.76–2 ng/dL
1–5 years:	0.9–1.72 ng/dL
6–18 years:	0.81–1.68 ng/dL

Throxine-Binding Globulin (TBG) (P)[1]

0–6 years:	16.2–33.8 mg/L
7–12 years:	15–29.2 mg/L
13–18 years:	13.4–28.7 mg/L

Triiodothyronine (T3) (S)[1]:
0–11 years: 90–260 ng/dL
12–18 years: 100–210 ng/dL

NORMAL VALUE RANGES: URINE

Addis Count[2]

Red cells (12-hr specimen): <1 million
White cells (12-hr specimen): <2 million
Casts (12-hr specimen): <10,000
Protein (12-hr specimen): <55 mg

Catecholamines (Norepinephrine, Epinephrine)[1]

Values in mmol/mol creatinine

Age	Norepinephrine	Epinephrine
<1 year	0.017–0.207	0–0.232
1–4 years	0.017–0.194	0–0.051
4–10 years	0.018–0.072	0.003–0.057
10–18 years	0.003–0.07	0.001–0.027

Chloride[2]

Infants: 1.7–8.5 mmol/24 hr
Children: 17–34 mmol/24 hr
Adults: 140–240 mmol/24 hr

Creatine[2]

18–58 mg/L   1.37–4.42 mmol/L

Creatinine[1]

3–8 years: 0.11–0.68 g/24 hr
9–12 years: 0.17–1.41 g/24 hr
13–17 years: 0.29–1.87 g/24 hr
Adults: 0.63–2.50 g/24 hr

Osmolality[2]

Infants: 50–600 mosm/L
Older children: 50–1400 mosm/L

Phosphorus, Tubular Reabsorption[2]

78–97%

Potassium[2]

26–123 mmol/L

Specific Gravity

1.01–1.03

NORMAL VALUE RANGES: SWEAT
Electrolytes[1]

Normal: <40 mmol/L for both sodium and chloride
Patients with cystic fibrosis: >60 mmol/L for both sodium
   and chloride

NORMAL VALUE RANGES: CEREBROSPINAL FLUID

Protein[1]

< 1 month: 15–153 mg/dL
< 3 months: 15–93 mg/dL
>3 months: 15–45 mg/dL

Glucose[1]

All ages: 60–80% of blood glucose

Adapted from:
[1] Soldin, S. J., Brugnara, C., & Wong, E. C. (2003). *Pediatric reference ranges* (4th ed.). Washington, DC: AACC Press.
[2] Hay, W. W., Hayward, A. R., Levin, M. J., Sondheimer, J. M., & Associate Authors. (2003). *Current pediatric diagnosis and treatment* (16th ed.). New York: Lange Medical Books/McGraw Hill.
[3] Kavey, R. W., Daniels, S. R., Lauer, R. M., Atkins, D. L., Hayman, L. L., & Taubert, K. (2003). American Heart Association guidelines for primary prevention of atherosclerotic cardiovascular disease beginning in childhood. *Journal of Pediatrics, 142*, 368–372.

Temperature and Weight Conversion

°C	°F
35	95
35.2	95.4
35.4	95.7
35.6	96.1
35.8	96.4
36	96.8
36.2	97.2
36.4	97.5
36.6	97.9
36.8	98.2
37	98.6
37.2	99
37.4	99.3
37.6	99.7
37.8	100
38	100.4
38.2	100.8
38.4	101.1
38.6	101.5
38.8	101.8
39	102.2
39.2	102.6
39.4	102.9
39.6	103.3
39.8	103.6
40	104
40.2	104.4
40.4	104.7
40.6	105.1
40.8	105.4
41	105.8

Temperature Conversion Formula

$°F = (°C × 9/5) − 32$ or $(°C × 1.8) + 32$

$°C = (°F − 32) × 5/9$ or $(°F − 32) × 0.55$

Weight Conversion Formula

$lb/2.2 = kilograms$

$kg × 2.2 = pounds$

Example:

40 lb = 40/2.2 = 18.2 kg

20 kg = 20 × 2.2 = 44 lb

Index

Page numbers followed by italic *f* indicate figures and those followed by italic *t* or *b* indicate tables or boxes.

Pearson Education, Inc.

YOU SHOULD CAREFULLY READ THE TERMS AND CONDITIONS BEFORE USING THIS DVD-ROM PACKAGE. USING THIS DVD-ROM PACKAGE INDICATES YOUR ACCEPTANCE OF THESE TERMS AND CONDITIONS.

Pearson Education, Inc. provides this program and licenses its use. You assume responsibility for the selection of the program to achieve your intended results, and for the installation, use, and results obtained from the program. This license extends only to use of the program in the United States or countries in which the program is marketed by authorized distributors.

LICENSE GRANT

You hereby accept a nonexclusive, nontransferable, permanent license to install and use the program ON A SINGLE COMPUTER at any given time. You may copy the program solely for backup or archival purposes in support of your use of the program on the single computer. You may not modify, translate, disassemble, decompile, or reverse engineer the program, in whole or in part.

TERM

The License is effective until terminated. Pearson Education, Inc. reserves the right to terminate this License automatically if any provision of the License is violated. You may terminate the License at any time. To terminate this License, you must return the program, including documentation, along with a written warranty stating that all copies in your possession have been returned or destroyed.

LIMITED WARRANTY

THE PROGRAM IS PROVIDED "AS IS" WITHOUT WARRANTY OF ANY KIND, EITHER EXPRESSED OR IMPLIED, INCLUDING, BUT NOT LIMITED TO, THE IMPLIED WARRANTIES OR MERCHANTABILITY AND FITNESS FOR A PARTICULAR PURPOSE. THE ENTIRE RISK AS TO THE QUALITY AND PERFORMANCE OF THE PROGRAM IS WITH YOU. SHOULD THE PROGRAM PROVE DEFECTIVE, YOU (AND NOT PRENTICE-HALL, INC. OR ANY AUTHORIZED DEALER) ASSUME THE ENTIRE COST OF ALL NECESSARY SERVICING, REPAIR, OR CORRECTION. NO ORAL OR WRITTEN INFORMATION OR ADVICE GIVEN BY PRENTICE-HALL, INC., ITS DEALERS, DISTRIBUTORS, OR AGENTS SHALL CREATE A WARRANTY OR INCREASE THE SCOPE OF THIS WARRANTY.

SOME STATES DO NOT ALLOW THE EXCLUSION OF IMPLIED WARRANTIES, SO THE ABOVE EXCLUSION MAY NOT APPLY TO YOU. THIS WARRANTY GIVES YOU SPECIFIC LEGAL RIGHTS AND YOU MAY ALSO HAVE OTHER LEGAL RIGHTS THAT VARY FROM STATE TO STATE.

Pearson Education, Inc. does not warrant that the functions contained in the program will meet your requirements or that the operation of the program will be uninterrupted or error-free.

However, Pearson Education, Inc. warrants the DVD-ROM on which the program is furnished to be free from defects in material and workmanship under normal use for a period of ninety (90) days from the date of delivery to you as evidenced by a copy of your receipt.

The program should not be relied on as the sole basis to solve a problem whose incorrect solution could result in injury to person or property. If the program is employed in such a manner, it is at the user's own risk and Pearson Education, Inc. explicitly disclaims all liability for such misuse.

LIMITATION OF REMEDIES

Pearson Education, Inc.'s entire liability and your exclusive remedy shall be:

1. the replacement of any DVD-ROM not meeting Pearson Education, Inc.'s "LIMITED WARRANTY" and that is returned to Pearson Education, or
2. if Pearson Education is unable to deliver a replacement DVD-ROM that is free of defects in materials or workmanship, you may terminate this agreement by returning the program.

IN NO EVENT WILL PRENTICE-HALL, INC. BE LIABLE TO YOU FOR ANY DAMAGES, INCLUDING ANY LOST PROFITS, LOST SAVINGS, OR OTHER INCIDENTAL OR CONSEQUENTIAL DAMAGES ARISING OUT OF THE USE OR INABILITY TO USE SUCH PROGRAM EVEN IF PRENTICE-HALL, INC. OR AN AUTHORIZED DISTRIBUTOR HAS BEEN ADVISED OF THE POSSIBILITY OF SUCH DAMAGES, OR FOR ANY CLAIM BY ANY OTHER PARTY.

SOME STATES DO NOT ALLOW FOR THE LIMITATION OR EXCLUSION OF LIABILITY FOR INCIDENTAL OR CONSEQUENTIAL DAMAGES, SO THE ABOVE LIMITATION OR EXCLUSION MAY NOT APPLY TO YOU.

GENERAL

You may not sublicense, assign, or transfer the license of the program. Any attempt to sublicense, assign or transfer any of the rights, duties, or obligations hereunder is void.

This Agreement will be governed by the laws of the State of New York.

Should you have any questions concerning this Agreement, you may contact Pearson Education, Inc. by writing to:

Director of New Media
Higher Education Division
Pearson Education, Inc.
One Lake Street
Upper Saddle River, NJ 07458

Should you have any questions concerning technical support, you may contact:

Product Support Department: Monday–Friday 8:00 A.M. –8:00 P.M. and Sunday 5:00 P.M.-12:00 A.M. (All times listed are Eastern). 1-800-677-6337

You can also get support by filling out the web form located at http://247.prenhall.com

YOU ACKNOWLEDGE THAT YOU HAVE READ THIS AGREEMENT, UNDERSTAND IT, AND AGREE TO BE BOUND BY ITS TERMS AND CONDITIONS. YOU FURTHER AGREE THAT IT IS THE COMPLETE AND EXCLUSIVE STATEMENT OF THE AGREEMENT BETWEEN US THAT SUPERSEDES ANY PROPOSAL OR PRIOR AGREEMENT, ORAL OR WRITTEN, AND ANY OTHER COMMUNICATIONS BETWEEN US RELATING TO THE SUBJECT MATTER OF THIS AGREEMENT.